Brief Contents

THE PARAMEDIC

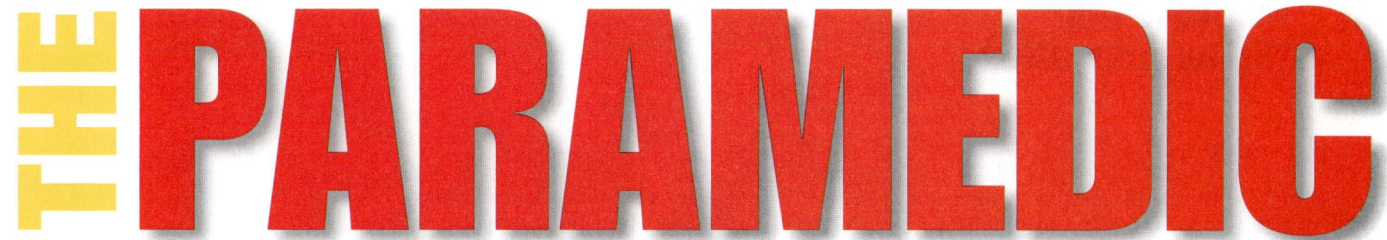

THE PARAMEDIC

Will Chapleau, EMT-P, RN, TNS

Manager, ATLS Program
American College of Surgeons
Chicago, Illinois

Angel Clark Burba, MS, EMT-P, NCEE

Associate Professor
EMS Program Director
Howard Community College
Columbia, Maryland

and

Volunteer Paramedic, Boonsboro Volunteer Rescue Service
Boonsboro, Maryland

Peter T. Pons, MD

Emergency Physician
Denver, Colorado

David Page, MS, NREMT-P

Faculty, Emergency Health Services Department
Inver Hills Community College
Inver Grove Heights, Minnesota

and

Field Paramedic
Allina Medical Transportation
St. Paul, Minnesota

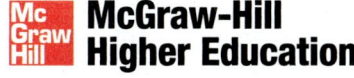 **McGraw-Hill
Higher Education**

Boston   Burr Ridge, IL   Dubuque, IA   New York   San Francisco   St. Louis
Bangkok   Bogotá   Caracas   Kuala Lumpur   Lisbon   London   Madrid   Mexico City
Milan   Montreal   New Delhi   Santiago   Seoul   Singapore   Sydney   Taipei   Toronto

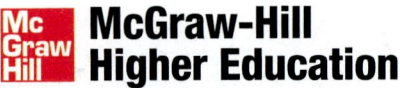

ISBN 978–0–07–352071–1
MHID 0–07–352071–3

Vice President/Editor in Chief: *Elizabeth Haefele*
Vice President/Director of Marketing: *John E. Biernat*
Sponsoring Editor: *Linda Schreiber*
Consulting Editor: *Claire Merrick*
Outside Developmental Services: *Laura Horowitz*
Editorial Coordinator: *Michelle L. Zeal*
Marketing Manager: *Kelly Curran*
Lead Media Producer: *Damian Moshak*
Director, Editing/Design/Production: *Jess Ann Kosic*
Lead Project Manager: *Mary E. Powers*
Senior Production Supervisor: *Sherry L. Kane*
Cover/Interior Designer: *Laurie B. Janssen*
Senior Photo Research Coordinator: *John C. Leland*
Photo Research: *Mary Reeg*
Compositor: *Aptara*
Typeface: *10/12 Melior*
Printer: *R. R. Donnelley Willard, OH*
(USE) Cover Image: © *Richard Gaul/GettyImages*, © *Daniel Templeton/Alamy, Industrial Sidestreets/Photodisc*

The credits section for this book begins on page C-1 and is considered an extension of the copyright page.

Library of Congress Cataloging-in-Publication Data

The paramedic / Will Chapleau ... [et al.]. – 1st ed.
    p. cm.
Includes index.
ISBN 978–0–07–352071–1 — ISBN 0–07–352071–3 (alk. paper)
  1. Medical emergencies. 2. Emergency medical technicians. I. Chapleau, Will.
  [DNLM: 1. Emergency Medical Technicians. 2. Emergency Medical Services. WX
215 P222 2007]
  RC86.7.P362 2008
  616.02'5–dc22
                                        2006053069

www.mhhe.com

Dedication

We'd like to dedicate this book to providers everywhere. Whether we've worked with you in the field, you were a student in our classrooms, or you're reading our book now, we have been, and are, honored by the experiences we've shared and the trust you've placed in us.

We'd also like to dedicate this book to our families. Like all EMS providers, our families have sacrificed in support of a noble career that they knew we were dedicated to. Their support to us during the process of developing this text and support materials was invaluable in giving us the confidence to put in the long hours required to produce quality materials, secure in the knowledge that they loved and supported us. So to

> Will's wife, Kathy, and his children, Abby (and her husband, Alfie, and son, Rocco), Paul, and Alex
>
> Angel's husband, Brian, and her mother, who she says never let her quit anything
>
> Peter's wife, Kathy
>
> David's wife, Elizabeth, and their children, Alexander, Andrew, and Michael

we offer our appreciation and thanks for loving us and supporting us in this task in the service of our profession.

Brief Contents

Contents

chapter 11

The Normal Physical Examination   195

chapter 12

Airway Management, Ventilation, and Oxygenation   214

chapter **13**

Shock Overview   259

chapter **14**

Patient Assessment   274

chapter **15**

Pharmacology   295

chapter 16

chapter 17

part 3

Trauma   352

chapter 18

chapter 19

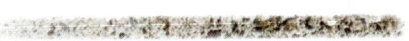

Medical Issues   563

chapter **28**

chapter 29

Cardiology   590

Section I: Physiology and ECG Interpretation   590

chapter 32

Allergies and Anaphylaxis   789

chapter 33

Infectious and Communicable Diseases   806

chapter 34

Gastroenterology   839

chapter 35

chapter 36

chapter 37

chapter **38**

Environmental Conditions   928

chapter **39**

Eyes, Ears, Nose, and Throat   958

chapter **40**

Behavioral and Psychiatric Disorders   974

chapter 41

Obstetrics and Gynecology   995

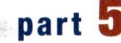 **part 5**

Special Populations   1026

chapter 42

Neonatology   1027

chapter 43

Pediatric Patients   1048

chapter **44**

chapter **45**

chapter **54**

Special Events and Mass Gatherings   1298

chapter **55**

Responding to WMD Events   1308

Foreword

Ever since the first EMT book was written, there have been two philosophies chosen by the authors for the reader: One type is to provide for the minimal required information and to meet only the minimum standards required by the profession. At the other end of the spectrum is the philosophy that it is written to be all-inclusive. This will give the student reader (and ultimately patient care provider) the strongest possible knowledge foundation.

If you or your family were to become sick or injured in the middle of the night, in the blowing snow or in the cold rain, would you want the EMT taking care of you to be the very best possible *or* simply one who has taken the course to "get by"?

This book is not a "get by" book. This book is not written by "get by" authors. This book is not edited by "get by" editors. Just open this book and look at the four editors—four better people in the United States to write such a book could not have been chosen.

If you buy such a book, you want to know that it is on the cutting edge of medical science, just as this book was written, and with these contributors and editors you know that it is. You also want to know that, if another edition is required, the second edition will also be on the cutting edge. Again, no one would expect less from these editors.

Take a look at the chapter elements. They are all there (as you would expect by these authors), but in addition they are organized in such a manner that they provide an easy format for learning. Students want to know that they're learning in the most efficient way available, not in an awkward, inefficient way.

Science has frequently been ignored in prehospital books. It is "logical" that it should be there; therefore, no question is made of the literature to find out if it truly is correct. This book looks at the evidence: need to know vs. nice to know. This has been an argument since the first textbook was written. These authors have not tried to get by with only the need-to-know information; they have put together the nice-to-know information that separates the good EMT from the superb EMT. Although the nice-to-know information may never be "required," the nice-to-know information promotes understanding. It is understanding that makes a superb paramedic.

You can't learn without appropriate visuals. On the other hand, a "picture book" of "prehospital gory pictures" does nothing except to sell books. The authors have done an outstanding job of not including gore, but having put in only the information that is important in providing education that can allow students to offer the best patient care possible.

So, who is to be served by this textbook? The patient—and this book is designed exactly to do that. The authors know what it takes to educate an outstanding paramedic. They have provided information to do so in a very easy format to use with a bottom line as the patient. If you want to take care of the sickest patients around, you need the very best textbook to provide you this information. And that textbook is sitting here in front of you.

Norman E. McSwain, Jr., MD, FACS, NREMT-P
Professor of Surgery
Tulane University
New Orleans, Louisiana

Preface

The Paramedic comes to you through the concerted efforts of the authors, contributors, and publisher to produce a text that reflects the depth and breadth of modern Advanced Life Support in the field of emergency medical services, which continues to define itself in response to the needs of its patients.

From the beginning, the team of authors and contributors set out not just to cover the material dictated by national standard curricula but also to provide the depth of science and history that explains the anatomy and function of patients when they are well and how their bodies respond when they become sick or injured.

As you review the table of contents, you'll see that we've added chapters you may have not seen in prehospital texts before. We believed it was important to break the book up into body systems and topic areas. This allows for time to be spent on each body system and operational topic area, giving us the chance to expand on the information previously available in typical prehospital texts and to be able to show the connections to other systems and operational topics.

Chapter Elements

Several chapter elements are used throughout the text to highlight objectives, important concepts, and helpful tips.

Evidence

Reading through the chapters you'll notice an important difference from texts you may have used in the past. This text is fully referenced. In the age of evidence-based medicine, we felt it important that our text be referenced to the science that supports the knowledge and standards of practice within the field. Throughout the text, when we make a statement of fact, you'll find the science to support the statement in the notes at the end of each chapter.

Need to Know

Each chapter begins with Need to Know objectives. These are things every paramedic should know, and the supporting content is clearly described in the chapter.

Sick/Not Yet Sick

These tables are designed to give the reader a sense of how the patients change from well to sick or injured.

Do/Ask

When applicable, you'll find Do/Ask tables at the beginning of the chapter. These guide readers through actions and questions appropriate to the patients the chapter describes.

Anatomy, Physiology, and Pathophysiology

An essential element of becoming a good EMS clinician is an understanding of the human body and its response to illness or injury. In addition to a general overview of anatomy in the first section of the book, each clinical chapter includes relevant anatomy, physiology, and pathophysiology content.

Nice to Know

Whereas the Need to Know objectives cover the absolutes, the history of EMS and the experiences of our authors and contributors bring Nice to Know pieces of information that enhance the material being studied and the paramedic's role in patient interactions.

Working in the Gray Zone

All of us working in medicine know that we don't work in a world of black and white, but a world of gray. Working in the Gray Zone will take the reader into these gray areas and help make sense of situations that don't lend themselves to memorized algorithmic responses.

Connections

As educators, we all feel strongly about how things tie together—that is, how one body system is tied to another and how an action on one system can affect other systems. This book reflects those intersections. Throughout the text, we have placed Connections boxes to direct the reader to related information in other chapters.

DOT Objectives

Although most EMS texts cover the Department of Transportation curriculum objectives, in *The Paramedic* we wanted to make more direct correlations. Throughout the text, the DOT objectives are listed at the points in the text where they are covered. Students looking for those relationships and educators looking for those connections will find the DOT numbers at the end of the appropriate paragraphs.

EMS Core Content

As the nation's EMS education system moves from the 1998 DOT curriculum toward educational standards and core content, it is important for *The Paramedic* to include as many of these as possible. The core content was used to develop the objectives for each chapter. A detailed list of objectives can be found in the instructor materials and the workbook that accompany this book.

Art and Photos

We thought a great deal about art. We set out in our early discussion to create a scholarly text. High-end texts often have little art and photos, whereas lower-level texts that may have less content tend to have a great deal of visual support. In *The Paramedic*, the photos, drawings, and other visual aids throughout the text were carefully selected to enhance the material in the chapter. Our

objective was not just to break up the text for appearance sake but to elucidate through artwork the key points being made in each of the chapters.

Accountability

There are lots of options for educators and students looking for textbooks. We felt strongly that our book needed to be accountable to the educators who select the text for their programs and the students who purchase our book. We took that thought to work with us every day as we wrote and edited *The Paramedic,* and we will continue to follow that sense of commitment as we work to ensure that our text and ancillaries are accountable to the science of our practice and the needs of the faculty and students we serve, as well as the patients they will treat in the field.

W. C.
A. B.
P. P.
D. P.

Contributors

Maija Anderson, RN, DNP *(chapter 43)*
Nursing Education Editor
Emergency Nurses Association
Des Plaines, Illinois

Catherine A. Parvensky Barwell, RN, EMT-P, MEd *(chapter 46)*
President, Integrated Learning
  Technology, Inc.
West Chester, Pennsylvania
and
EMT Instructor Trainer
Good Fellowship Ambulance & EMS Training
  Institute

Vikhyat S. Bebarta, MD *(chapter 35)*
Director of Medical Toxicology
Department of Emergency Medicine
Wilford Hall Medical Center
San Antonio, Texas

Carl J. Bonnett, MD *(chapter 21)*
Department of Emergency Medicine
Denver Health Medical Center
Denver, Colorado

Kevin Boone, BSN, EMT-P *(chapter 47)*
Paramedic Captain
San Francisco Fire Department
San Francisco, California

Joseph A. Browning, MD *(chapter 29(II))*
Minneapolis Heart Institute
Abbott Northwestern Hospital
Minneapolis, Minnesota

Angel Clark Burba, MS, EMT-P, NCEE *(chapters 1, 5, 15)*
Associate Professor
EMS Program Director
Howard Community College
Columbia, Maryland
and
Paramedic, Boonsboro Volunteer Rescue Service
Boonsboro, Maryland

Christopher Buresh, MD, FAAP *(chapter 18)*
Chief Resident, Emergency Medicine
Department of Emergency Medicine
University of Iowa Hospitals and Clinics
Iowa City, Iowa

Michael Casner, MD, *(chapter 33)*
Assistant EMS Medical Director
San Francisco Fire Department
and
Assistant Clinical Professor of Medicine
San Francisco General Hospital
University of California, San Francisco

Will Chapleau, EMT-P, RN, TNS *(chapter 1, 9, 27)*
Manager, ATLS Program
American College of Surgeons
Chicago, Illinois

Christopher B. Colwell, MD, FACEP *(chapter 34)*
Medical Director
Denver Paramedic Division and Denver Fire Department
and
Associate Professor, Department of Surgery, Division of
  Emergency Medicine
University of Colorado Health Sciences Center
and
Associate Director, Department of Emergency Medicine
Denver Health Medical Center

Megan Corry, MA, NREMT-P *(chapter 30)*
Paramedic Program Director
City College of San Francisco
San Francisco, California

Jeffrey A. Coto, RN, MS, CCNS, CCRN *(chapter 42)*
Clinical Director, Pediatric Emergency Services
& Pediatric Level I Trauma Center
University of Chicago Hospitals
Comer Children's Hospital
Chicago, Illinois

Amanda J. Cotter, MS, NREMT-P *(chapters 16, 37)*
Clinical/Internship Coordinator
Department of Emergency Medical Technology
Greenville Technical College
Greenville, South Carolina

Steven Cotter, MBA, NREMT-P *(chapter 51)*
Director
Laurens County Emergency Medical Services
Laurens, South Carolina

Catherine B. Custalow, MD, PhD *(chapter 7)*
Assistant Professor
Department of Emergency Medicine
University of Virginia Health System
Charlottesville, Virginia

Kerry Dixon, RN, CPM, LM, MSN-CNMc *(chapter 41)*
Frontier School of Midwifery & Family Nursing
St. Paul, Minnesota

Daryl Doering, BA, NREMT-P *(chapters 35, 53)*
Emergency Health Services Department Faculty,
Inver Hills Community College
Inver Grove Heights, Minnesota
and
Field Paramedic
Allina Medical Transportation
St. Paul, Minnesota

William Dunn, BA, NREMT-P *(chapter 23)*
Training Supervisor
Eagle County Health Service District
Vail, Colorado
and
Paramedic
Denver Health Medical Center, Paramedic Division
Denver, Colorado

Kim M. Feldhaus, MD *(chapter 45)*
Departments of Emergency Medicine
Boulder Community Hospital
Boulder, Colorado
and
Denver Health Medical Center
Denver, Colorado

Patrick L. Finley, PhD *(chapter 2)*
Associate Professor
Health Sciences Division
Howard Community College
Columbia, Maryland

Ray Fowler, MD, FACEP *(chapter 12)*
University of Texas Southwestern Medical Center
Emergency Medical Section
Dallas, Texas

Ryan C. Fringer, MD *(chapter 19)*
William Beaumont Hospital
Department of Emergency Medicine
Royal Oak, Michigan

Daniel R. Gerard, MS, RN, MICP *(chapter 49)*
EMS Education Coordinator
City of Alameda Fire Department
Alameda, California

Denise H. Graham, RN, BSN, CLNC *(chapter 17)*
Chief Executive Officer
MidAtlantic Legal Consultants
Comus, Maryland

Michael Guttenberg, DO, FACEP *(chapter 24)*
Director, Emergency Medicine
St. Joseph's Medical Center
Yonkers, New York

Jason S. Haukoos, MD, MS *(chapter 13)*
Assistant Professor
Department of Emergency Medicine
Denver Health Medical Center
Department of Preventive Medicine and Biometrics
University of Colorado Health Sciences Center
Denver, Colorado

Kennon Heard, MD *(chapter 35)*
Medical Toxicology Fellowship Director
Rocky Mountain Poison and Drug Center
Denver, Colorado

Timothy D. Henry, MD *(chapter 29(II))*
Minneapolis Heart Institute
Abbott Northwestern Hospital
Minneapolis, Minnesota

Jeffrey D. Ho, MD, FACEP *(chapters 9, 17, 52)*
Assistant Professor of Emergency Medicine
University of Minnesota Medical School
and
Faculty Emergency Physician
Hennepin County Medical Center
Minneapolis, Minnesota
and
Medical Director
City of Edina Public Safety
Associate Medical Director
Hennepin County EMS
Hennepin County, Minnesota
and
Deputy Sheriff
Meeker County Sherrif's Office
Meeker County, Minnesota

Arthur Hsieh, MA, NREMT-P *(chapter 11, 14)*
Chief Operating Officer
San Francisco Paramedic Association
San Francisco, California

Joseph Jensen, RN, EMT-P *(chapter 25, 26)*
Regions Hospital EMS
St. Paul, Minnesota

John Jerome, BS, EMT-P *(chapter 50)*
Battalion Chief, EMS Training Branch
Howard County Fire Rescue
Columbia, Maryland

I. Kevin Johnson, AS, BS, NREMT-P *(chapter 29(I))*
Emergency Health Services Department Faculty
Inver Hills Community College
Inver Grove Heights, Minnesota
and
Paramedic
Allina Medical Transportation
St. Paul, Minnesota

Nicholas C. Johnson, MD *(chapter 20)*
Emergency Medicine Staff Physician
Abbott Northwestern Hospital
Minneapolis, Minnesota

Christopher Kahn, MD *(chapter 54)*
Fellow, Emergency Medical Services and Disaster
Medical Services
Department of Emergency Medicine
University of California, Irvine

Ralph Katieb, NREMT-P *(chapter 48)*
Ridgeview Medical Center Ambulance
Watertown, Minnesota

John L. Kendall, MD *(chapter 23)*
Department of Emergency Medicine
Denver Health Medical Center
Denver, Colorado

Tara Khan, DO *(chapter 24)*
New York Methodist Hospital
Brooklyn, New York

Andrew L. Knaut, MD, PhD, FACEP *(chapter 39)*
Department of Emergency Medicine
Porter Hospitals
Denver, Colorado

Kristi Koenig, MD, FACEP *(chapter 54)*
Professor of Clinical Emergency Medicine
Director of Public Health Preparedness
Department of Emergency Medicine
University of California, Irvine

Gordon Kokx, BA, NREMT-P *(chapter 3)*
Associate Professor, EMS Program Director
College of Southern Idaho
Twin Falls, Idaho

Mark D. Lindquist, MD *(chapters 9, 17, 36, 52)*
St. Mary's Regional Health Center and St. Mary's EMS
Detroit Lakes, Minnesota
and
Medical Director, Becker County Sheriff, Detroit Lakes
Police and Fire Department
EMS Medical Director, State of Minnesota

Jeffrey T. Lindsey, PhD, CFO, EMT-P *(chapter 22)*
Estero Fire Rescue
Estero, Florida

Keith Lurie, MD *(chapter 29(I))*
Professor of Emergency Medicine and Internal
Medicine
University of Minnesota and Hennepin County Medical
Center
and
Chief Medical Officer
Advanced Circulatory Systems, Inc.
Minneapolis, Minnesota

Vincent J. Markovchick, MD, FAAEM, FACEP
(chapter 5)
Director, Emergency Medical Services
Denver Health Medical Center
and
Professor of Surgery
Division of Emergency Medicine
University of Colorado
Denver, Colorado

Kevin McVaney, MD *(chapter 12)*
Department of Emergency Medicine
Denver Health Medical Center
Denver, Colorado
and
Medical Director
Denver Health Paramedic School

Paul Murphy, MA, MSHA, Paramedic *(chapter 31)*
Healthcare Consultant
Denver, Colorado

Marc C. Newell, MD *(chapter 29(II))*
Minneapolis Heart Institute
Abbott Northwestern Hospital
Minneapolis, Minnesota

Mike Nugent, BA, EMT-P *(chapter 55)*
Chief Paramedic
Denver Health Paramedic Division
Denver, Colorado

Kristen A. Olson, Esquire *(chapter 4)*
Judicial Law Clerk
Court of Common Pleas
York, Pennsylvania

David I. Page, MS, NREMT-P *(chapters 10, 40, 48)*
Faculty, Emergency Health Services Department
Inver Hills Community College
Inver Grove Heights, Minnesota
and
Field Paramedic
Allina Medical Transportation
St. Paul, Minnesota

Lana Parsons, MS, MA, ANP-C *(chapter 26)*
Burn Trauma Coordinator
Johns Hopkins Burn Center
Johns Hopkins Bayside Medical Center
Baltimore, Maryland

Jim Radcliffe, BS, NREMT-P *(chapter 27)*
EMS Coordinator
R. Adams Cowley Shock Trauma Center
University of Maryland Medical Center
Baltimore, Maryland

Lee Ridge, EMT-P, FP-C *(chapter 18)*
Program Assistant
Director Emergency Medicine Simulation Center
University of Iowa Hospitals & Clinics
Iowa City, Iowa

Austin G. Rinker, Jr., MS, NREMT-P *(chapters 25, 32)*
Paramedic
Community Rescue Service, Inc.
Hagerstown, Maryland
and
Program Coordinator
Paramedic Emergency Services Program
Hagerstown Community College
Hagerstown, Maryland

Paul Satterlee, MD *(chapter 27)*
North Memorial Medical Center
Robbinsdale, Minnesota
and
Century College EMS Program
White Bear Lake, Minnesota

Robert S. Schwartz, MD, FAHA, FACC *(chapter 29(II))*
Medical Director
Minneapolis Heart Institute
Abbott Northwestern Hospital
Minneapolis, Minnesota

Kevin G. Seaman, MD, FACEP *(chapter 28)*
Clinical Assistant Professor
University of Maryland, Baltimore County
Baltimore, Maryland
and
Medical Director Howard County Fire Rescue
Columbia, Maryland

Lee Shockley, MD *(chapter 38)*
Denver Health Medical Center
Denver, Colorado

Robert Swor *(chapter 19)*
Director of EMS Programs
William Beaumont Hospital
Department of Emergency Medicine
Royal Oak, Michigan

Matthew M. Thielman, MD *(chapter 29(II))*
Minneapolis Heart Institute
Abbott Northwestern Hospital
Minneapolis, Minnesota

David Tierney, MD *(chapter 29(II))*
Minneapolis Heart Institute
Abbott Northwestern Hospital
Minneapolis, Minnesota

Melissa Tschohl, MD *(chapter 22)*
Regions Hospital
St. Paul, Minnesota

Patricia Turner *(chapter 8)*
Professor
Howard Community College
Columbia, Maryland

Barbara Unger, BS, RN, FAACVPR *(chapter 29(II))*
Minneapolis Heart Institute
Abbott Northwestern Hospital
Minneapolis, Minnesota

Robert Vroman, BS, NREMT-P *(chapter 6)*
EMS Instructor
HealthONE EMS
Englewood, Colorado

Robert K. Waddell II, EMT-P, BS, BA *(chapter 43)*
National Chair
Emergency Pediatric Care (EPC) Program
National Association of Emergency Medical Technicians
  Cheyenne, Wyoming

Roy Karl Werner, MD, MS *(chapter 18)*
Infinity Healthcare
SwedishAmerican Hospital
Department of Emergency Medicine
Rockford, Illinois

Jean B. Will, EdD, MSN, RN, CEN, EMT-P *(chapter 44)*
Director, Disaster Medicine and Management Program
Philadelphia University
Philadelphia, Pennsylvania

Matthew Willems NREMT-P *(endpapers)*
Inver Hills Community College
St. Paul, Minnesota

Stephen R. Wirth, Esquire *(chapter 4)*
Page, Wolfberg & Wirth, LLC
Mechanicsburg, Pennsylvania

Douglas M. Wolfberg, Esquire *(chapter 4)*
Page, Wolfberg & Wirth, LLC
Mechanicsburg, Pennsylvania

Stephen J. Wolf, MD *(chapter 21)*
Denver Health Medical Center
Department of Emergency Medicine
Denver, Colorado

Acknowledgments

We've been blessed to spend our careers in a profession that we truly love, in the service of providers who are dedicated to the care of the sick and injured. Our collective experiences in diverse environments all over the world have enriched us and influenced our work, and this textbook is a testament to that collective experience.

We are thankful to all of the contributors, who put so much of themselves into their submissions, and the reviewers, whose comments were helpful in ensuring the utility of this work.

This book was made possible by Claire Merrick, who brought us together. Claire's willingness to support and encourage a new standard for paramedic textbooks, to secure the needed resources from a publisher new to the EMS market, and to stick with us over the long haul was the engine that made this project accomplish its goals. We hope this book earns a place on Claire's bookshelf, already filled with decades of the landmark EMS textbooks she has published.

Kelly Trakalo was the developmental editor who built our foundation and jump started the process. Her talent and passion for this project gave us the fuel for a great beginning. She was matched by our "knight in shining armor," Laura Horowitz, who picked us up midstream without missing a beat and brought this book to a successful conclusion.

Art Hsieh and Kevin Boone were key members of our editorial team, in addition to being the authors of the worktext. With unrelenting humor, they were instrumental in steering the project, creating the chapter objectives, spending countless hours on photo shoots, video editing, and researching clinical standards. With the help of Nancy Peterson, the supplement materials they have created complement this text perfectly and will surely set a new standard for the industry. We are both proud and grateful to have had such a great editorial team and such great support from McGraw-Hill.

We are most grateful to Barbara Aehlert for loaning us so many images from her fine book *Emergency Medical Responders;* David Shier, Jackie Butler, and Ricki Lewis for images from Hole's *Human Anatomy & Physiology;* Michael McKinley and Valerie Dean O'Loughlin for illustrations from *Human Anatomy;* and Bruce Shade and Keith Wesley for illustrations from *Fast & Easy ECGs,* all published by McGraw-Hill. Michael Johnson and his staff were a pleasure to work with as they assisted us with an online system for test item review and cataloging of DOT objectives that was as helpful as it was innovative.

Thanks to Mary Powers and Mary Reeg, who spent countless hours steering us through the production process that resulted in this wonderful book.

Finally, and most importantly, we thank you, the faculty and students who have trusted us to provide you with the best materials possible to play a role in making you the best that EMS has to offer to our patients.

Reviewers

Linda M. Abrahamson, BA, RN, EMTP
Silver Cross Hospital/Joliet Junior College
Joliet, Illinois

David K. Anderson, BS, EMT-P
NW Regional Training Center
Vancouver, Washington

Romney C. Andersen
Assistant Chief
Walter Reed National Military Medical Center
Bethesda, Maryland

Katherine Bakes, MD
UCHSC/Denver Health Medical Center
Denver, Colorado

Augie Bamonti III, BA, EMT-P
AFB Consulting, Inc.
Chicago Heights, Illinois

Christopher Callahan, MD
Attending Physician in Emergency Medicine
St. Francis Regional Medical Center
Shakopee, Minnesota
and
Supplemental Consultant in Emergency Medicine
Mayo Clinic
Rochester, Minnesota

Chris Caulkins, MPH, FF-EMT-P
Program Director
Century College
White Bear Lake, Minnesota
and
Firefighter-Paramedic
Woodbury Public Safety Department
Woodbury, Minnesota

Gregory M. Cole, BS, NREMT-P, CCEMT-P, FP-C
Emergency Technology Department
Jones County Junior College
Ellisville, Mississippi

Jon S. Cooper, NREMT-P, MICRB
Baltimore City Fire AND EMS Academy
EMS Training Division
Baltimore, Maryland

Steven Cotter, MBA, NREMT-P
Director
Laurens County Emergency Medical Services
Laurens, South Carolina

Larry Davis
Independent Consultant
Corpus Christi, Texas

Mike DeLoach, BS, NREMT-P
Program Director
South Plains College EMS Programs
Lubbock, Texas

Pamela Drexel
Executive Director
Brain Trauma Foundation
New York, New York

Marti Driscoll
Assistant Professor, Clinical Coordinator
Daytona Beach Community College
Daytona Beach, Florida

Hunter Elliott
The Center for Emergency Health Services
Williamsburg, Virginia

Richard Ellis, NREMT-P, BSOE
United States Air Force
Robins AFB, Georgia

Craig Felty, RN, BSN, CEN, EMT-P
Advocate South Suburban Hospital
Hazel Crest, Illinois

William E. Gandy, JD, LP
TechPro Services, Incorporated
EMS Academy
Abilene, Texas

Adiel Garcia, NREMT-P, RDMS, BAT
EMS Program Director
University of Texas at Brownsville
Brownsville, Texas

Dan Garner
Education Affiliates
Medix School, Atlanta EMS Department
Smyrna, Georgia

Peter Glusker, MD-PhD, FAAN, FACP
Adjunct Clinical Assistant Professor
Stanford Department of Neurosciences
Palo Alto, California

Robin Goede, FF/NREMT-Paramedic, AAS, BA
St. Louis Community College
St. Louis, Missouri

John Gosford, BS, EMT-P
EMS Coordinator, Associate Professor
Lake City Community College
Lake City, Florida

Tim Hardy, AAS, FF/EMT-LP
Department of Emergency Medical Services
Blinn College
Bryan, Texas

Anthony S. Harbour, MED, NREMT-P
Director
Southern Virginia EMS
Richmond, Virginia

Bernard Heilicser DO, MS, FACEP, FACOEP
South Cook County EMS System
Harvey, Illinois

David J. Hendricks, MD
Associate Director of Emergency Medicine
Griffin Hospital
Derby, Connecticut

Lindi Holt, NREMT-P, PhD
Clarian Health/Methodist Hospital
Indianapolis, Indiana

Sandy L. Hunter, PhD, NREMT-P
Emergency Medical Care Program
Eastern Kentucky University
Richmond, Kentucky

Andy Jagoda
Emergency Medicine Department
Mount Sinai School of Medicine
New York, New York

Koren Kaye, MD
Regions Hospital EMS
St. Paul, Minnesota

Gordon A. Kokx, BA, NREMT-P
Associate Professor, EMS Program Director
College of Southern Idaho
Twin Falls, Idaho

Al Landry, EMT-P
National EMS Academy
Lafayette, Louisiana

Jeffrey T. Lindsey, PhD, EMT-P
Estero Fire Rescue
Estero, Florida

Michael McGowan, NREMT-P, Flight Paramedic, Airmedic One Flight
Program Director
Florida Medical Training Institute
Melbourne, Florida

Louis N. Molino, Sr., CET
Training Program Manager
Fire & Safety Specialists, Inc.
College Station, Texas

Liz Mrak, NREMT-P
National EMS Academy
Lafayette, Louisiana

Stephen J. Nardozzi, BA, EMT-P
Westchester Community College
Valhalla, New York

Nikhil Natarajan
Adjunct Professor, SUNY Ulster
Nursing and Public Safety Department
Stone Ridge, New York

Hemant Nayah, MD, MPH, FACEP
Education Director
Griffin Hospital
Derby, Connecticut

Chris Nolette, NREMT-P, LP
Emergency Medical Services Department
Riverside Community College
Riverside, California

Deputy Chief Kevin J. O'Hara, MS, EMT-P
Nassau County EMS Academy
East Meadow, New York
William Seifarth, MS, NREMT-P
Associate Director
Education, Licensure & Certification Department
Maryland Institute for EMS Systems
Baltimore, Maryland

Jerry Overton
Executive Director
Richmond Ambulance Authority
Richmond, Virginia

Terry Arend Provo
Director of Clinical Trials
Advanced Circulatory Systems, Inc.
Eden Prairie, Minnesota

Jim Radcliffe
EMS Coordinator
R. Adams Cowley Shock Trauma Center
University of Maryland Medical Center
Baltimore, Maryland

Christoph Redelsteiner, MS, MSW, EMT-P
Chief of EMS
Vienna Red Cross EMS
and
Director, Emergency Health Services Management Program
Danube University
Vienna, Austria

Jennifer D. Reese, NREMT-P
Paramedic Coordinator
Center for Emergency Health Services
Williamsburg, Virginia

Christopher M. Rockefeller, NREMT-P
Instructor, Adjunct Faculty
Center for Emergency Health Services
Williamsburg, Virginia

Joseph R. Ross, NREMT-P
Lieutenant, Paramedic EMS Educator
EMS Training Group
Howard County Fire and Rescue Training Academy
Clarksville, Maryland

Christopher T. Ryther, MS, NREMT-P
Paramedics Department
American River College
Sacramento, California

Paul Satterlee, MD
North Memorial Medical Center
Robbinsdale, Minnesota
and
Century College EMS Program
White Bear Lake, Minnesota

Patrick Sennett, EMT-P
Advocate Good Samaritan Hospital, Emergency Medical
   Services System
Downers Grove, Illinois

James Shiplet, AAS, LP, EMSC
EMS Education Coordinator
Collin County Community College
McKinney, Texas

Kelly B. Simkins, NREMT-P
Program Manager, Emergency Services
Laramie County Community College
Cheyenne, Wyoming

Kenneth J. Sternig, MS-EHS, BSN, EMTP
Emergency Medical Services Education
Milwaukee County EMS Education Center
Milwaukee, Wisconsin

Kimberly Stotts, RN
South Cook County EMS
Harvey, Illinois

Susan Tarr
University of Wisconsin, River Falls
River Falls, Wisconsin

John E. Tartt, MPH, EMT-P
School of Emergency Medical Science
Carolinas College of Health Sciences
Charlotte, North Carolina

Stephen J. Teale
Emergency Services Department
Wisconsin Technical College System
Madison, Wisconsin

Annmary E. Thomas, MEd, NREMT-P
Drexel University
Philadelphia, Pennsylvania

Mitch Trahan
National EMS Academy
Lafayette, Louisiana

Meghan Treitz
Arapahoe Community College
Littleton, Colorado

Ross Utter, MHS, PA-C
Griffin Hospital
Derby, Connecticut

Robert K. (Bob) Waddell II
Cheyenne, Wyoming

Nathan C. Walk, MD
St. Louis, Missouri

Jimmy Walker, EMT-P
S.C. Midlands EMS
Gaston, South Carolina

Thomas Wyatt, MD
Mercy Hospital Emergency Department
Coon Rapids, Minnesota

Instructor Manual Acknowledgments

Much hard work and craftsmanship has been dedicated to the Instructor Productivity Center that accompanies this textbook. A team of talented educators contributed their best lesson plans, images, and creativity to bring together the most comprehensive paramedic teaching resource ever assembled for an EMS textbook. We graciously acknowledge the invaluable assistance of the following individuals:

Development Team

Kenna Dick, NREMT-P
Edina Police Department
Edina, Minnesota

Catherine Eaton, BA, NREMT-P
North Ambulance
Minneapolis, Minnesota

Darcy Ebert, NREMT-P
Allina Medical Transportation
Buffalo, Minnesota

Timothy Howey, BA, NREMT-P
Stevens County Ambulance
Morris, Minnesota

David Page MS, NREMT-P
Inver Hills Community College
St. Paul, Minnesota

Nancy Peterson
Developmental Editor
Catonsville, Maryland

Lesson Plan Contributors

Matthew Bogan, BS, NREMT-P
Allina Medical Transportation
St. Paul, Minnesota

Lisa Breitinger, RN, BSN, Flight Nurse EMT-B
Paramedic Program Director
Tacoma Fire Department
Tacoma, Washington

Toryono Green
Northwest Emergency Medical Education
Puyallup, Washington

Mark Dascalos, BA, EMT-P
Allina Medical Transportation
St. Paul, Minnesota

Robin Goede, FF/NREMT–Paramedic, AAS, BA
St. Louis Community College
St. Louis, Missouri

William E. Gandy, JD, LP
TechPro Services, Incorporated
EMS Academy
Abilene, Texas

Adam Longman, BA, NREMT-P
Allina Medical Transportation
St. Paul, Minnesota

Christopher Matek, NREMT-P
EMS Training Coordinator
Image Trend Inc.
Lakeville, Minnesota
and
Paramedic/Instructor
ALF Ambulance
Apple Valley, Minnesota

Nicole Petroff, BA, NREMT-P
Allina Medical Transportation
St. Paul, Minnesota

Christopher M. Rockefeller, NREMT-P
Faculty Instructor
The Center for Emergency Health Sciences
Williamsburg, Virginia

For the Student

As you begin using this text, you will notice an overall approach to writing and recurring themes of deliberate design. First, the text is patient-centered as it embraces the concept that the patient comes first, the writing style is focused on the patient at the center and builds into what will become your approach to the assessment and treatment of your own patients.

Textbook Features

You'll read about the textbook features in the preface and the user's guide, but there are a few that we would like to point out to you:

- We sincerely hope that, as a paramedic graduate, you appreciate the importance of research to support and improve your practice. One of the most exciting features of this text is that it is fully referenced. For the first time in the history of EMS publishing, you will not have to wonder "where did these authors come up with that information?" The note citations in the chapters link you to the *Notes* section at the end of each chapter, where you'll find the research on which the comments were based. This is also a good list of resources for additional reading.
- At the beginning of each chapter, you will see *Do/ Ask and Sick/Not Yet Sick* boxes. These boxes identify the assessment actions and interview questions that you will be able to apply pertaining to the chapter material.
- At the beginning of the chapters are *Need to Know* boxes that emphasize the content that you must know, and throughout the chapters are *Nice to Know* boxes that give information that will enhance your knowledge base and critical-thinking skills.
- To be a "critical thinker," the paramedic needs to recognize interdependencies. Throughout our text, you will find *Connections* boxes that tie the content being discussed at that point of the chapter to material in other chapters.
- Thousands of images showing skills, traumatic conditions, and illnesses in detail never published before are waiting for you in the *Online Learning Center* and *student worktext.*
- The text is oriented to the street. Information is provided because it is relevant to the work of the paramedic, not for its own sake. *Street Secrets* are

provided throughout the text to guide you through applying what you have learned.
- We felt strongly that, besides strong support in the area of anatomy, the paramedic student needs to know how the body functions normally and how it functions when it is sick or injured. For this reason, this text has more pathophysiology than you'll find in any other prehospital text.

Supplements

In addition to the textbook, there are several supplements that will help round out your education and give you experiences to practice and test yourself. These include the student workbook, *The Paramedic Companion: A Case-Based Worktext,* with its accompanying student DVD, and the Online Learning Center www. mhhe.com/chapleau1e.

Drug Reference

Listing drugs and dosages in texts can be problematic. Protocols and changes in drugs and the way they are used can make texts less relevant to students and teachers if they are not up to date. For this reason, we are proud to offer the *Clinician's Pocket Drug Reference.* Packaged with the text, this reference provides key content and the latest information about the drugs that paramedics may have in their drug boxes, as well as the drugs commonly prescribed to patients. Links are also provided to make sure that you and the faculty have the latest drug information available.

Online Learning Center

The Online Learning Center, which can be accessed at www.mhhe.com/chapleau1e offers you an array of creative resources, testing tools, and multimedia learning experiences. The content includes the following:

- Step-by-Steps in a video format that show skills being performed correctly; text "bubbles" and arrows point to key aspects of skill performance
- PDF versions of approximately 100 Skill Sheets
- Audio Glossary with pronunciations of key terms
- Chapter-by-chapter quiz bank, including questions keyed to photographs and video clips, such as "Show Me" video clips that show real people experiencing

real medical emergencies and Patient Perspective video clips of interviews/vignettes with victims and survivors

- Anatomy and physiology animations
- Drug administration animation
- Games and exercises, such as drug flashcards, ECG exercises, and puzzles

Worktext

The Paramedic Companion: A Case-Based Worktext is a nontraditional workbook that can be used throughout the paramedic curriculum and is tightly integrated with the main textbook. *The Paramedic Companion* goes beyond the simple "review and test" approach of most workbooks. Instead, it supports your exploration of the art and science of prehospital medicine by providing a rich palette of learning tools, images, and video to better explain concepts and techniques. *The Paramedic Companion* speaks clearly and directly to you, the paramedic student. The material in each chapter revolves around "Need to Know" content, based on the DOT objectives, that the authors of both the textbook and the worktext felt was absolutely necessary for you to master before moving on to the next section or chapter. All features in the worktext were designed to ensure that you can successfully master these key content areas. These include the following:

- Are You Ready? opening vignettes with related questions to help you dive into the chapter content
- Active Learning exercises and activities
- You Are There, reality-based cases that address core content and progress to give you a realistic learning experience and help you integrate what you have been learning
- Test Yourself quizzes, which are chapter-based
- Need to Know objectives
- Need to Do skill sections keyed to Skill Sheets and Step-by-Steps
- Connections that tie the worktext to the textbook and to other related resources
- Secrets, hints, and tips from seasoned paramedics
- Drug Boxes that summarize key information about relevant drugs

- I Spy exercises that quiz you after you study a photograph of a patient encounter or emergency scene
- Answers to all questions, provided at the end of each chapter for your convenience

Problem-Based Learning Cases (PBLs) are also included in the worktext to support major content areas. Problem-based learning employs an open-ended, Socratic approach to student learning. By exercising critical-thinking skills, you are encouraged to answer the questions through research and analysis.

In addition, multimedia tools on the accompanying DVD will create an educational space that is rich with information. This robust DVD provides a tremendous learning advantage. Its content includes the following:

- Step-by-Steps that show skills being performed correctly; text "bubbles" and arrows point to key aspects of skill performance
- National Registry Skill Practice clips showing "Do's and Don'ts"
- PDF versions of approximately 100 Skill Sheets
- Audio Glossary with pronunciations of key terms
- Chapter-by-chapter quiz bank, including questions keyed to photographs and video clips
- Anatomy and physiology animations
- Drug administration animations
- Games and exercises, such as drug flashcards, ECG exercises, and puzzles
- I Spy exercises with detailed photographs and accompanying questions

From the beginning of this project, we set out to make this book a complete guide through your paramedic training experience. We felt strongly that the book should reflect our actual practice and that we should not distract you with elements that were not part of the job. We wanted to go to great depths to give you the breadth of knowledge needed to determine the needs of your patients and to treat them appropriately based on those needs.

We hope you enjoy this book and that it guides you through your paramedic training.

User's Guide

This User's Guide will show you how to use the features of *The Paramedic* to enhance your paramedic training.

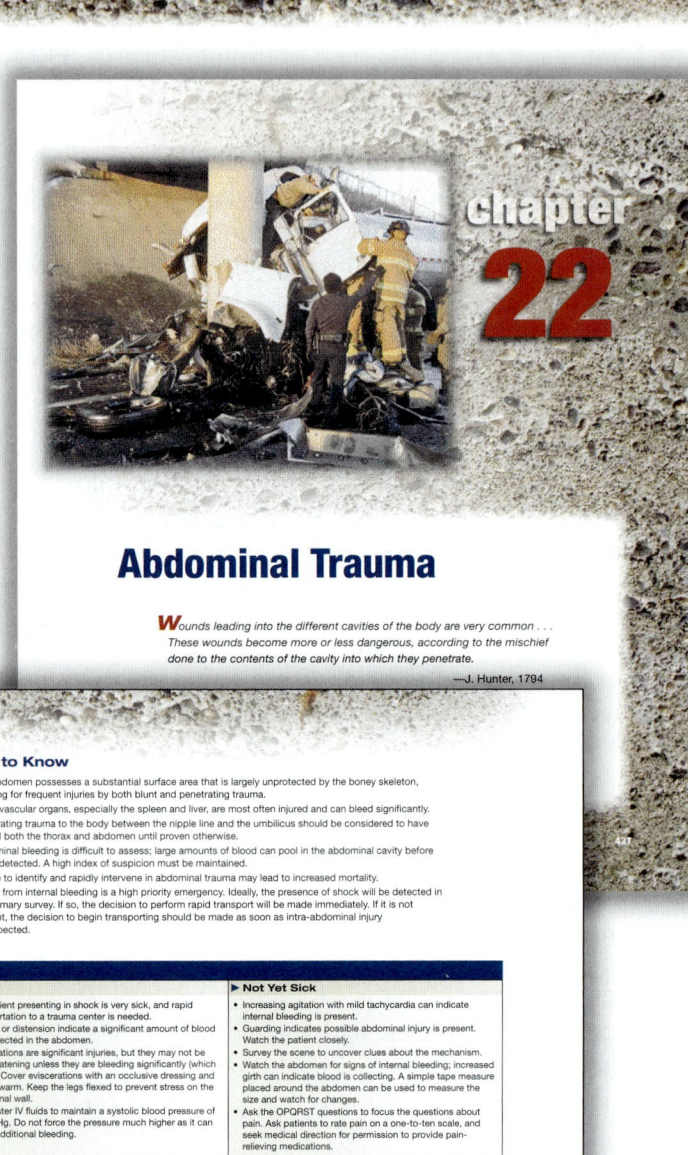

Need to Know The primary objectives for the chapter are stated in the Need to Know list. You can read this list before you read the chapter and again when you have finished it as a review of the material. Expecting a test in class? Have a clinical shift in a particular area of the hospital? This quick summary can help you zero in on the most important elements of the chapter.

Sick/Not Yet Sick In the field, you will often need to make rapid decisions about the severity of your patients. Building on the Sick/Not Yet Sick continuum described in Chapter 10 and used throughout the text, this box will help you identify key signs and symptoms that differentiate critical ("sick") patients from more stable ("not-yet-sick") patients. We use the term "not-yet-sick" because we know how rapidly a patient's condition can change. In these boxes, we have also identified key elements that signal a change in patient condition.

Street Secrets From the real-world experience of the 73 contributors to this text, Street Secrets share words of wisdom—and warning—that only experienced paramedics know.

Connections You will find that, in paramedicine, many procedures, medications, and physiology concepts are applied to multiple conditions. This feature helps you make a connection to material that is explained in a different chapter. Making these connections will help you link important concepts together and improve your understanding and retention of the material.

DOT Objectives The content in the textbook is linked to the Department of Transportation Objectives—National Standard Curriculum which represent the critical information paramedics need to know. Your instructors and some certification exams use these objectives as guides to create lessons and test questions. This reference will show you exactly where you have met the DOT standards.

Skill Sheets Cross-references to the 94 Skill Sheets and 45 Step-by-Steps (found at the Online Learning Center and in the Student Worktext and/or DVD) are included throughout the text. The Skill Sheets will help you in labs as you practice skills. The Step-by-Step demonstrations are detailed visual "maps" that will guide you in learning the practical elements of being a paramedic.

Illustrations Figures have been carefully chosen and created to enhance your understanding of important concepts.

Notes This is the first evidence-based paramedic textbook to be published. Although much research is needed in EMS, we have included state-of-the-art information whenever possible. More than 150 peer-reviewed medical journals are cited, as well as dozens of medical textbooks and websites.

Glossary An extensive glossary can be found at the end of the book. All key terms are bolded in the text.

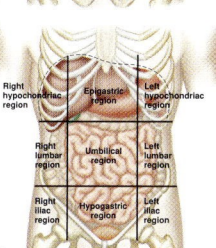
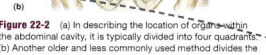

Photographs   A picture paints a thousand words. From the field to the hospital, vibrant photographs support the text and clarify concepts. Look for hundreds of photos in the textbook and thousands more images used to create our Step-by-Step skill demonstrations and online media-based questions.

Working in the Gray Zone   EMS is often not black and white. Controversial and complicated procedures and topics are described in special boxes to help you gain an understanding of the complexity of the field.

Nice to Know   These boxes present that extra information that will help you rise above the standard. You may decide to come back to these after you have mastered the basics, or dive into the additional material during your paramedic education program.

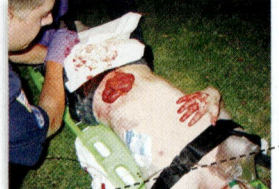

Ancillaries

Additional Learning Resources

This powerful learning tool also includes the following:

www.mhhe.com/chapleau1e

Online Learning Center

- Chapter-based review questions
- Audio Glossary
- A&P animations
- Drug administration animation
- A&P games and exercises
- ECG exercises
- Drug flashcards
- Skill sheets
- Step-by-Step skills in Shockwave format
- National Registry Practical Examination Evaluation forms

The Paramedic Companion: A Case-Based Worktext

This nontraditional workbook goes beyond the simple "review and test" approach of most workbooks. Instead, *The Paramedic Companion* supports your exploration of the art and science of prehospital medicine by providing a rich palette of learning tools, images, and even video to better explain concepts and techniques. Key features include the following:

- Progressive Case Scenarios with questions and answers
- Active Learning activities
- Multiple-choice quizzes
- Need to Know narrative explanations
- Step-by-Step illustrated skills
- Street Secrets
- Full-color illustrations
- Problem-Based Learning Cases

"Tell me and I will forget,
   Show me, and I might remember,
      Involve me and I will understand."

Confucious

Paramedic instructors will be stunned by the resources that support this text. In the preceding Preface and For the Student sections, we have described the elements of the text that will guide students through their experience with this book and in your classroom. We believe this full-featured text will serve as the foundation for building strong cognitive knowledge and beginning the critical-thinking process. Your students will have the tools to prepare for a classroom and lab experience with unprecedented interactivity and rich media. The ancillaries we have developed offer a full range of features to accommodate various teaching and learning styles. The materials speak to the structure needed for the left brain to organize new information and are visually appealing to the right brain. If you are a traditional lecturer, you will find it easy to use the lesson plans and slides. If you are a nontraditional instructor, you will find alternative slides and active learning exercises to complement each lesson. We are confident that the depth and variety of these tools will support you in producing the best prepared graduates.

Guiding Principles for Instructor Materials

The materials we have designed for this text incorporate cutting edge concepts in teaching and learning. As with the rest of this text, these concepts are supported by strong research and evidence for "best practices." These concepts include the following:

- **Patient-focused lessons:** As much as possible, the lessons include vignettes, scenarios, and street secrets that are focused on real people. You should be able easily to see that learning is centered on assessing and treating people, not just their illness or injury.
- **Responsive lecture format:** Optional critical-thinking questions, active learning exercises, and audience participation questions are embedded in the lecture.
- **Multiple-choice questions:** To prepare the student for better test performance, each chapter includes multiple-choice items that are presented in-line with the lecture, or they can be administered as a pre- or postlecture quiz.
- **Scenario-based learning and guided lecture process:** This style of lecture can be used by asking the student to put into practice what they have learned in the assigned chapter reading. Each lesson begins with a practical, real-life case and ends with a detailed scenario. You can encourage students to report what they already know about the subject of the lecture and clarify errors or focus on additional depth of new information. The scenarios at the conclusion of the lessons can be as simple as a quick review of the lecture, or they can be used as a tool for problem-based learning and lab simulation.
- **"Show me" concepts:** Throughout the Instructor Manual, we have elected to "show" as much as possible, using rich photographs and detailed illustrations. The photos take up most, if not all, of the slide space. These slides will impact your students and are enriched with simple animations to improve understanding and minimize student fatigue. Never before has a paramedic textbook package used this many images. Word slides have been kept to a minimum and detailed notes help you use the image-based slides more effectively.
- **Instructor notes:** For the first time in an EMS slide set, the notes for each slide are contained in the Notes section of PowerPoint, making them immediately available during lecture. This convenient, state-of-the-art method allows you to view the notes while the students view the slide and does not require additional printing. Extra tips, references, and full text explanations will help you prepare and deliver a lecture without having to carry an extra manual.
- **Anatomy and physiology:** McGraw-Hill Higher Education publishes some of the world's best anatomy and physiology textbooks. We have packed the slide set, DVD, and Online Learning Center full of detailed A&P images, illustrations, and even video animations. Add these to your PowerPoint slides, show them by themselves, or simply assign the students to view them online. Our hope is that concepts, such as sodium-channels and action potentials of cardiac cells, will become much more fun for you to explain and your students to learn.

- **Step-by-Step Skill PowerPoint slides:** You will notice that detailed explanations of step-by-step procedures for skills have been printed in the worktext. We have organized the book and worktext in the same manner as you teach it in class, focusing the book on cognitive learning and keeping the hands-on practical (psychomotor) domain for the more active learning worktext. In addition to organizing the material in the same way that it is taught in class, this allows the student to take a smaller book to practical skills labs and allows you to have separate PowerPoint slides that focus on each of the skills you demonstrate. Forty-five Step-by-Step PowerPoint presentations are included. These include stunning close-ups of each skill and never-before-seen realism for each skill. You can use them "as is" or customize the order of the steps or particular technique that is unique to your program or region.

- **The future:** Although we have included references to the current 1998 National Standard Curriculum in our entire array of instructor tools, we are also prepared for the new standards. The editors and chapter contributors used the Core Content and Practice Analysis Tasks to guide the objectives and content for the chapter. Instructors can search the lesson files (PowerPoint or Word documents) for key DOT objectives by number or key word using the standard search function in the Windows start menu. Each item in the test bank relates back to the current curriculum as well.

- **Instructor-developed material:** The instructor material for this book was developed by a cadre of experienced instructors with over 100 years of combined teaching experience. Teaching tips, tricks, and key lesson objectives were incorporated from each of the Instructor Manual contributors. The slides were built by the instructor development team with you, the students, and the patients in mind.

Student Supplements

Please familiarize yourself with the supplements offered to students (detailed in For the Student), which include the following:

- *Clinician's Pocket Drug Reference,* which is packaged with each text
- Online Learning Center, which can be accessed at www.mhhe.com/chapleau1e, offers the student an array of creative resources, testing tools, and multimedia learning experiences; you have full access to this resource
- *The Paramedic Companion: A Case-Based Worktext,* a nontraditional workbook that can be used throughout the paramedic curriculum and is tightly integrated with the main textbook; *The Paramedic Companion* goes beyond the simple "review and test" approach of most workbooks and instead supports students' exploration of the art and science of prehospital medicine by providing a rich palette of learning tools, images, and video to better explain concepts and techniques

- Student DVD, which includes multimedia tools that create an educational space that is rich with information

Instructor Supplements

For the instructor, we have developed a stunning array of tools that we believe will give you what you need to build the course you want, rather than building your course around available resources.

The Instructor Productivity Center, provided on DVD, contains the following content:

- Lesson plans for each chapter
  - Creative PowerPoint presentation, which include case studies, lecture notes, animations, photographs, video clips, handouts, games, and exercises
  - Word document with Need to Know objectives (including Practice Analysis Tasks, National EMS Core Content, Paramedic National Standard Curriculum Objectives, and Unit Terminal Objectives); Need to Know Bullets; Teacher Toolbox; Skills information; and extra Case Scenarios
- Computerized test generator with 1,100 questions
- Image collection
- Step-by-Steps in a Shockwave video and PowerPoint format that show skills being performed correctly; text "bubbles" and arrows point to key aspects of skill performance
- National Registry Skill Practice clips showing "Do's and Don'ts"
- PDF and Word versions of approximately 100 Skill Sheets
- Anatomy and physiology animations
- Drug administration animation
- I Spy exercises with photographs and accompanying questions

Instructors can also access the **Online Learning Center** at www.mhhe.com/chapleau1e for the following:

- Chapter-by-chapter student quiz bank, including questions keyed to photographs and video clips, such as "Show Me" video clips that show real people experiencing real medical emergencies and Patient Perspective video clips of interviews/vignettes with victims and survivors

- Audio Glossary with pronunciations of key terms
- Games and exercises, such as drug flashcards, ECG and A&P exercises, and puzzles

While this gives you some sense of what we've brought to publication in support of our text and the educators who choose to use it; it is just the beginning of a commitment to continue to find ways to provide resources to our readers and educators. Use our publications secure in the knowledge that this is a dynamic process and we will continue to enhance existing resources and build new ones based on the feedback from you, the instructors who have placed your trust in us. We are grateful for that trust and will continue to work to show that we are worthy of that trust.

About the Authors

Will Chapleau, EMT-P, RN, TNS is the manager of the Advanced Trauma Life Support program for the American College of Surgeons. He has been a paramedic for over 30 years, a trauma nurse specialist 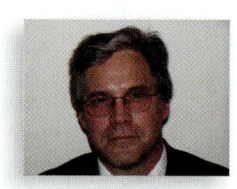 for 18 years and an EMS educator for over 20 years. He has worked in the field as a paramedic/firefighter with over 13 years of fire service experience, including 6 years as chief of Chicago Heights Fire Department. His nursing experience includes trauma, emergency services and intensive care service. He has also coordinated college and hospital basic and advanced primary and secondary educational programs. He serves on the board of directors of the National Association of EMTs and has been the chairman of the PreHospital Trauma Life Support Division since 1996. He also serves on the board of directors of the National Association of EMS Educators and the Society of Trauma Nurses; and he has served as the administrative division chair of The National Association of EMS Physicians. He has published several texts and numerous articles on EMS and Emergency Services and has lectured all over the world.

Angel Clark Burba, MS, EMT-P, NCEE is currently serving on the board of directors and is president elect for the National Association of EMS Educators. She is the assistant professor and program director for the EMS Program at Howard Community College in Columbia, Maryland. She has been an EMS 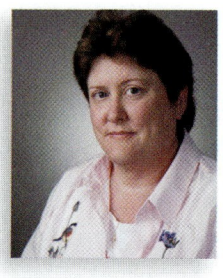 provider for over 28 years and an EMS educator for over 25. Besides teaching and conference presentations, she has contributed to many EMS publications, journals, and textbooks. She is the instructional designer of the NAEMSE Foundations of Education EMS Instructor Course and co-chaired the task force that wrote the 2002 DOT NHTSA Guidelines for Educating the EMS Instructor.

Peter T. Pons, MD, is an emergency physician who has been actively involved with prehospital care and disaster preparedness for over 25 years. He has been on the medical staff of Denver Health Medical Center (formerly Denver General 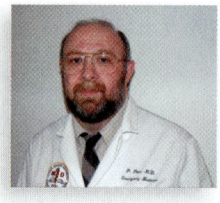 Hospital) and is a professor in the Division of Emergency Medicine in the Department of Surgery at the University of Colorado Health Sciences Center. Dr. Pons served as the medical director for several EMS systems, including two fire-department-based and one third-service-based.

David Page, MS, NREMT-P, a native of Mexico, is a full-time faculty member at Inver Hills Community College in St. Paul, Minnesota. He started his EMS career in 1985 as a junior member of the Bethesda Chevy-Chase Rescue Squad outside of Washington, D.C., and has been 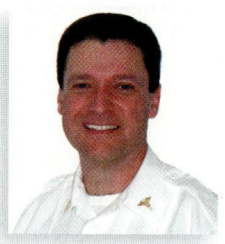 teaching paramedics since 1989. He has worked in Boston, Massachusetts; Fort Worth, Texas; and Denver, Colorado. Since 1989, he has served as a field paramedic for Allina Medical Transportation, a hospital-based emergency ambulance service in the Minneapolis–St. Paul area. He loves to teach and to learn. He holds a master's degree in experiential education from Minnesota State University and a bachelor's degree in human services from Macalester College. He is a frequent speaker at national conferences focusing on clinical competency, research, web-based education, and crisis intervention. He is fluent in French, Spanish, and English.

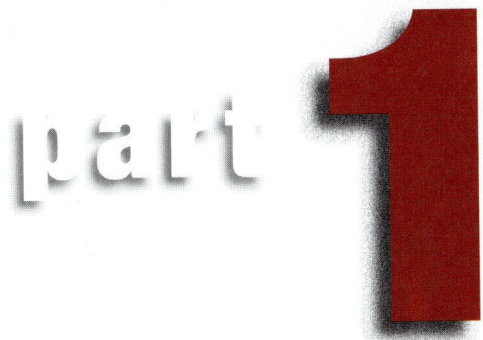

part **1**

Foundations

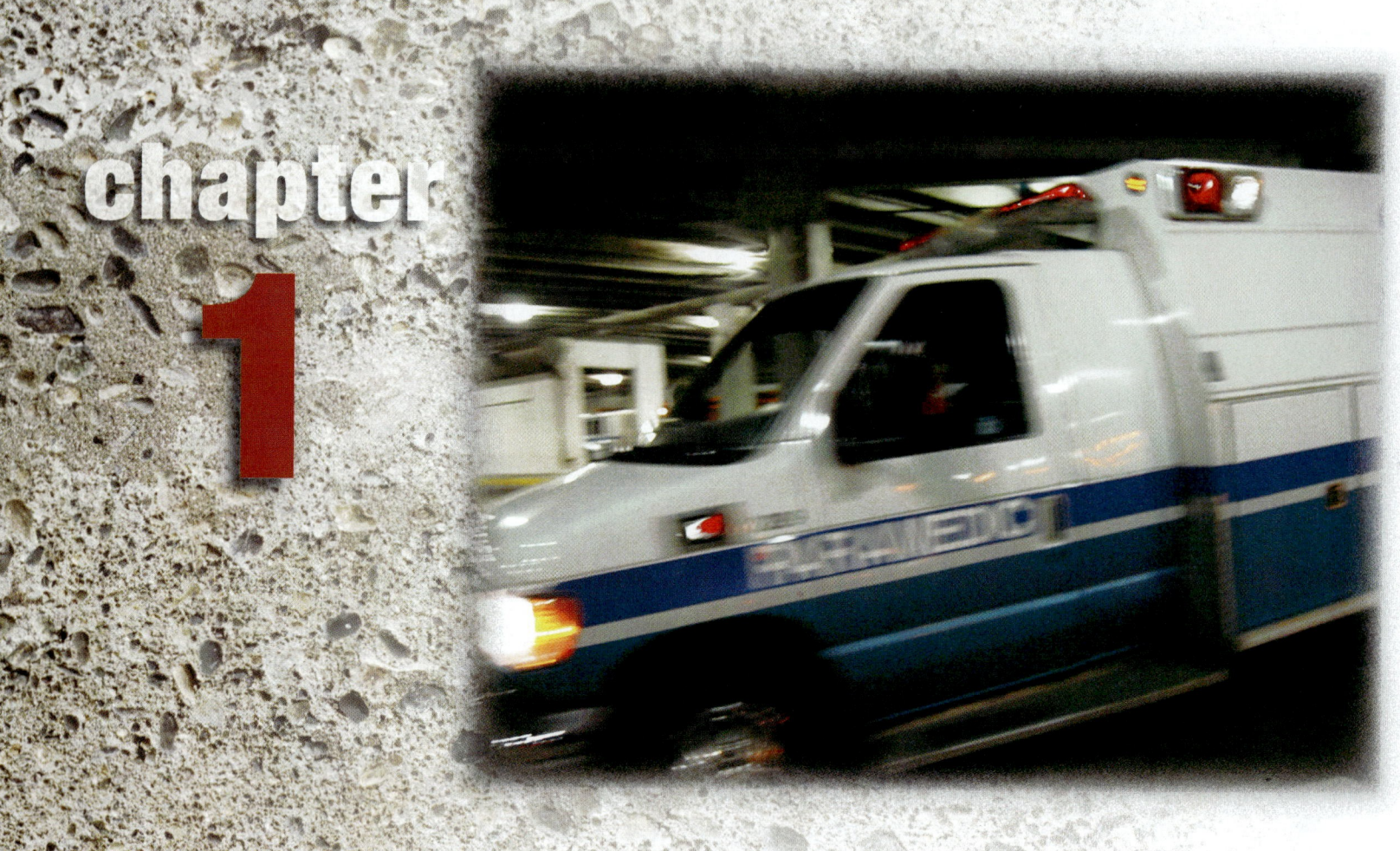

The EMS Profession

"*I*n nothing do men more nearly approach the gods than in doing good to their fellow men."

—Cicero

Need to Know

▶ The attributes and behaviors required of an EMS professional
▶ The importance of recognizing that EMS is a single component of the entire health care system and that all must work as a team to better serve the patient
▶ The levels of provider that make up the EMS profession
▶ The historical milestones that have shaped and defined the EMS profession
▶ The role you play in shaping the future of EMS

Introduction

The word *crisis* is a strong word that carries images of catastrophe and people in need. While many want a pathway through life that avoids confronting crisis, those who choose the emergency medical service (EMS) profession are drawn to it. Paramedics willingly accept being the healthcare providers called upon when situations are at their worst. When it comes to serving the patient, EMS is a part of a larger team composed of many medical and public safety professionals who are all held to high standards in order to ensure the public good. Learning to work as a team is an essential skill for a paramedic to master. The work of a paramedic is rewarding, but it can be frustrating and stressful at times. DOT 1-1.1

As you begin your journey to become a paramedic, it is important to understand what the emergency medical services profession is all about. Certainly the work as a paramedic calls for a swift response to a crisis, but a majority of your time is spent dealing with routine situations that often seem like a crisis to the patient but may not in fact be a threat to life. Customer service occurs with every patient interaction. Regardless of the severity of the situation, in every encounter there will be an opportunity to provide a high level of customer service.

This chapter is an introduction to the EMS profession. It will reflect on how the current EMS system grew from its beginnings and look ahead to the future. The regulatory processes of EMS will be discussed, along with key federal, state, local, and private organizations that influence how paramedics are taught, credentialed, and monitored. This chapter will explore how the profession moved from disorganized pockets of emergency services provided on the battlefield to the well coordinated system of interrelated services that make up the modern EMS system.

Working within a Structured System as Part of a Team

EMS is provided by a diverse population of emergency responders. **Responder** is a generic term used to describe a person with any level of credential in the

EMS profession. Not only do trained prehospital care providers have to work together, but EMS providers also have to be prepared to work within an emergency response structure that includes interaction with police, fire, rescue, other public safety agencies, and even military personnel or tribal authorities. EMS providers are called upon to provide medical support and assistance to other members of the team as well as to patients and bystanders. Whether or not you receive a salary for your services, all members of the EMS team are expected to perform their duties in a professional manner.

EMS providers are often cross trained in other areas of health care [paramedic nurse or emergency medical technician (EMT) respiratory technician] or other areas of public safety [emergency medical responder (EMR), fire fighter, or state trooper]. A provider may have another career altogether, and EMS may be a part-time job or a volunteer pastime.

EMS personnel are part of a health care profession that also has multiple layers. The primary role of the paramedic is providing emergency care to patients outside of the hospital setting.[1] This can take place in many locations, in medical settings as well as homes and in public places. Clinics and doctors' offices see patients who may need to be transferred to other facilities. Outpatient facilities provide care ranging from physical therapy to radiation therapy, dialysis, outpatient surgery, and many other services. They may need EMS to transfer a patient between home and their facility. Long- and short-term residential facilities and programs often have patients with no ability to transport themselves between facilities. EMS is also often called to move patients from one hospital to another that offers specialized care or one that is closer to the patient's family or better able to serve the patient's unique needs. DOT 1-1.21, 1-1.22, 1-1.32

The profession of EMS cannot be pigeonholed into a single type of service delivery model or have a single description of duties and responsibilities. Box 1-1 is taken directly from the 1995 National Standard Curricula for Paramedic. This is a description of the paramedic profession. Box 1-2, which is from the objectives of the same curricula, describes some of the attributes and behaviors required of a paramedic.

BOX 1-1 Description of the Profession of Paramedic

Paramedics have fulfilled prescribed requirements by a credentialing agency to practice the art and science of out-of-hospital medicine in conjunction with medical direction. Through performance of assessments and providing medical care, their goal is to prevent and reduce mortality and morbidity due to illness and injury. Paramedics primarily provide care to emergency patients in an out-of-hospital setting.

Paramedics possess the knowledge, skills, and attitudes consistent with the expectations of the public and the profession. Paramedics recognize that they are an essential component of the continuum of care and serve as linkages among health resources.

Paramedics strive to maintain high quality, reasonable cost healthcare by delivering patients directly to appropriate facilities. As an advocate for patients,

paramedics seek to be proactive in affecting long term healthcare by working in conjunction with other provider agencies, networks, and organizations. The emerging roles and responsibilities of the paramedic include public education, health promotion, and participation in injury and illness prevention programs. As the scope of service continues to expand, the paramedic will function as a facilitator of access to care, as well as an initial treatment provider.

Paramedics are responsible and accountable to medical direction, the public, and their peers. Paramedics recognize the importance of research and actively participate in the design, development, evaluation and publication of research. Paramedics seek to take part in life-long professional development and peer evaluation, and assume an active role in professional and community organizations.[19]

BOX 1-2 Professional Behaviors Expected of Paramedics

Integrity
Empathy
Self-motivation
Appropriate appearance and personal hygiene
Self-confidence
Good written and verbal communication skills

Effective time management
Teamwork and diplomacy
Respect
Patient advocacy
Careful delivery of services

The aspects of professionalism required to be a paramedic carry over into your personal life as well. Once you are a paramedic you are recognized as such whether you are on duty or not, and your actions are judged by others. DOT 1-1.5, 1-1.15, 1-1.16

CONNECTIONS Chapter 3: Professional Ethics will discuss professionalism in more detail.

Wherever you enter into the system in caring for a patient, you will be interacting with other health care professionals as well as EMS peers. Nurses, allied health technicians, physicians, and specialists will give you patient reports, and you in turn will give reports back to them. Because of this, you must be able to speak professionally and communicate well with all team members you encounter. To be effective in EMS you must develop relationships based on professional confidence and trust. You must appreciate and

respect the roles that each member of the health care team plays in patient management. The better you are at working within this structure, the better the benefit to your patients. Medical terminology, including anatomical terms and pharmacology, is used by the EMS community to effectively pass information from one provider to the next. Your knowledge and proper use of these terms, including how to spell them, is essential to good communication.

CONNECTIONS Chapter 6: Medical Terminology will give you an overview of terminology you will need as a paramedic.

EMS providers are getting more involved in research initiatives. Data collected from many services across the country are being used to develop protocols that directly impact patient care. Improvements in the quality of the medical services being delivered often arise through research. Quality improvement

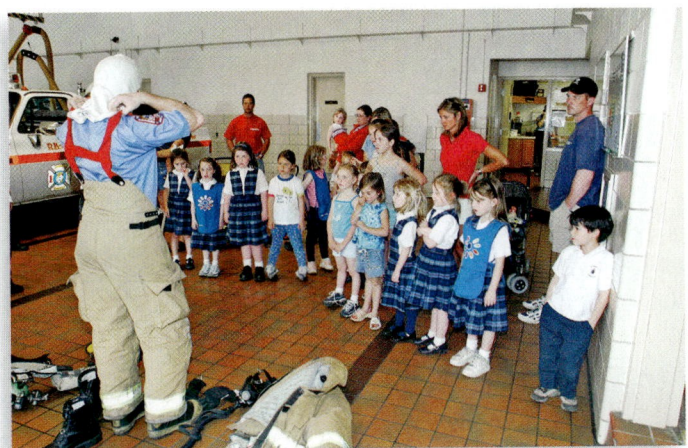

Figure 1-1   Emergency medical responders should educate the public about accessing the EMS system and preventing injuries.

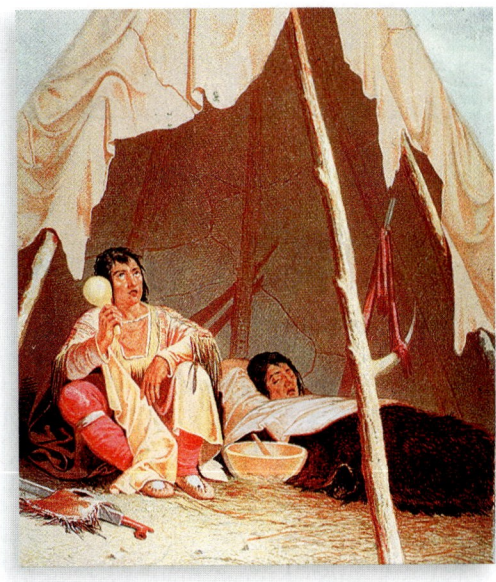

Figure 1-2   Healers, shaman, and medicine men and women provided medical care to the sick and injured for centuries.

activities benefit all aspects of EMS, not just patient care. They provide systems with the ability to identify the best practices in all aspects of performance. DOT 1-1.29, 1-1.34, 1-1.35

EMS professionals are finding themselves increasingly involved in public health initiatives. You have a large role in the surveillance of the health of your communities, and you can be of assistance in educating and caring for the populations you serve. Paramedics may assess blood pressures at community health fairs, give presentations on home safety to school children, or help the elderly in their community make their homes safer places to live by helping prevent trips and falls (Figure 1-1). DOT 1-1.17, 1-1.19, 1-1.33

Street Secrets

Encourage the public to visit you in the station to learn about the services you provide. Many people do not know the difference between the various levels of EMS providers and may not appreciate the work paramedics do. Inviting the public to an open house is a way of helping them learn about our work. It also helps establish relationships that can help later when EMS needs an advocate. DOT 1-1.20

Major Milestones in the Development of the EMS System

In searching for the origins of EMS, we find them in our own beginnings as a society. Even in the absence of a coordinated response to an emergency, altruistic citizens would rush to the aid of the sick and injured, try to alleviate their suffering, and transport them to someone able to help. DOT 1-1.2, 1-1.3

In our earliest times, the healer went to the patient. History is filled with many cultural accounts of healers, shaman, and medicine men and women coming to the aid of the sick and injured (Figure 1-2). As time went by, the art of healing began to mix with the science of medicine. As humanity industrialized, the medical professional became stationary and patients started coming to the healer. When hospitals began to arise, the era of the traveling medical professional stopped in all but the most remote parts of the world. The interest in medical care outside of the hospital seems to have renewed with the advent of large military conquests and the need to transport the wounded to physicians. Box 1-3 lists some of the milestones that had an impact upon the development of our EMS system.[2] DOT 1-1.11, 1-1.13

Over two hundred years ago, Napoleon's Chief Surgeon, Dr. Dominique-Jean Larrey, wrote the earliest recorded specifications for ambulances.[2] Like many advancements in emergency medical care, it was inspired by warfare. In the United States, the development of the ambulance, and the first ambulance system, occurred during the Civil War. This work was strongly influenced by a disastrous evacuation attempt of wounded soldiers following the Battle of Bull Run on July 21, 1861, in Manassas, Virginia. As a response to the disaster at Bull Run, the Rucker ambulance was developed. Designed by Brigadier General Daniel H. Rucker, it could carry patients either seated or on stretchers. It also had the capability of carrying water and supplies used in caring for the wounded (Figure 1-3).

Around this same time, battlefield physician, Jonathan Letterman, M.D., devised a plan of ambulance

BOX 1-3 Major Milestones of National Impact

1966	NAS-NRC Report (the "White Paper")
1966	National Highway Safety Act
1968	9-1-1 designated the national emergency telephone number
1969	DOT NHTSA leads in the development of EMS curricula
1970	National Registry of EMTs founded
1971	White House EMS Demonstration Projects
1972	Robert Wood Johnson Foundation Projects
1973	EMSS Act (PL 93-154)
1975	American Medical Association recognizes paramedicine as an allied health profession
1975	National Association of EMTs formed
1976	EMSS Act (PL 94-573, extension of PL 93-154)
1979	EMSS Act (PL-96-142, extension of PL 94-573)
1981	Prevention Health Service Block Grant (PL 97-35)
1984	DOT NHTSA NSC revised
1993	National EMS Education and Practice Blueprint
1994	NREMT Practice Analysis
1994–1995	DOT NHTSA NSC revised
1995	National Association of EMS Educators formed
1996	Agenda for the Future
2000	Education Agenda for the Future
2005	National Core Content
2005	National Scope of Practice
2006	Institute of Medicine Report "Future of EMS Core Series: EMS at the Crossroads"
In progress	National EMS Education Standards

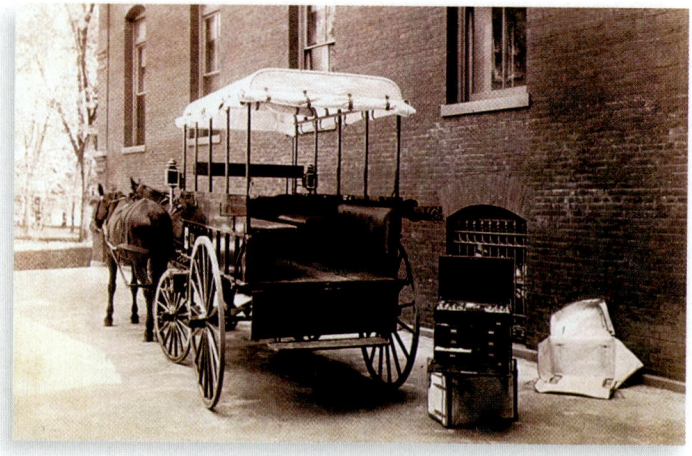

Figure 1-3 The Rucker ambulance, used during the American Civil War, ushered in the development of patient transport systems in the United States.

operations that was fairly comprehensive. It not only detailed how to deploy ambulances and where to transport patients, but also described the duties and qualifications for the "stewards" who staffed the vehicles. Prior to Letterman's plan, the few litter-bearers present on the battlefield were generally soldiers considered "unfit" for duty. Letterman did not want unfit soldiers; he wanted trained professionals who cared about the patient. He made the position of ambulance steward a desirable one, one where a soldier had to be fit for duty, meet certain qualifications, and perform well under supervision.

In 1865 as the Civil War came to a close, Cincinnati General Hospital started the first ambulance service in America. Soon after, services at Grady Hospital in Atlanta and Charity Hospital in New Orleans started. Grady ambulance service is still in operation today and holds the distinction of being the nation's longest continuously running ambulance service (Figure 1-4).

The military continued to improve its ability to care for injured soldiers with each successive conflict. With each major conflict, the military noted decreased death rates among battle casualties. In World War I the death rate was 8%. In World War II the rate was cut nearly in half to 4.5%. In the Korean Conflict the rates dropped to 2.5%, and in the Vietnam War the fatality rate from battlefield wounds was less than 2%.[3] But the same was not true for civilians. Soldiers injured in battle in a foreign country had a better chance of receiving state-of-the-art care than civilians injured at home.

Physicians returning from military duty began applying the lessons learned on the battlefield in their own communities. Ideas like organized trauma systems and trained nonphysician response personnel were gaining attention. At this point, ambulances were provided in a variety of service models including hospital based, volunteer rescue companies, and funeral homes.

The 1940s and 1950s

In 1949, John. E. Gordon demonstrated through scientific inquiry how the prevention of accidents could be brought into the mainstream of scientific medicine.[4] He

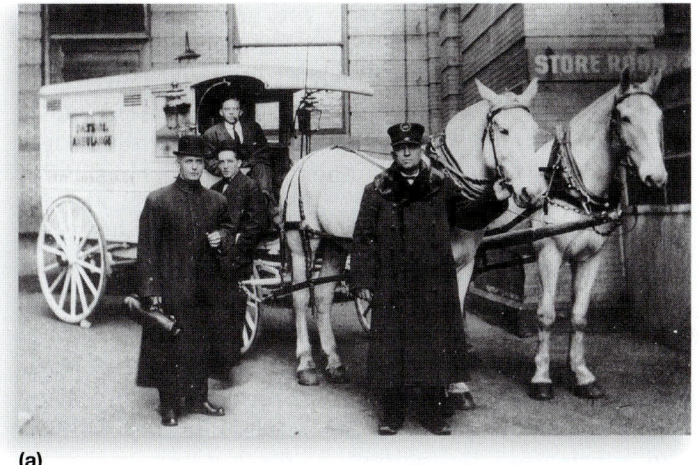
(a)

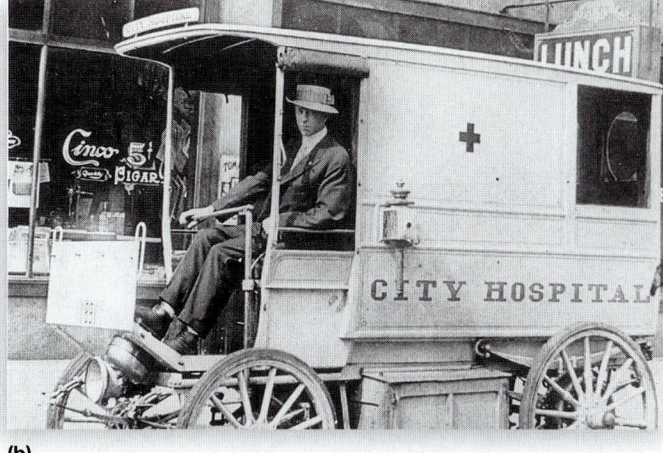
(b)

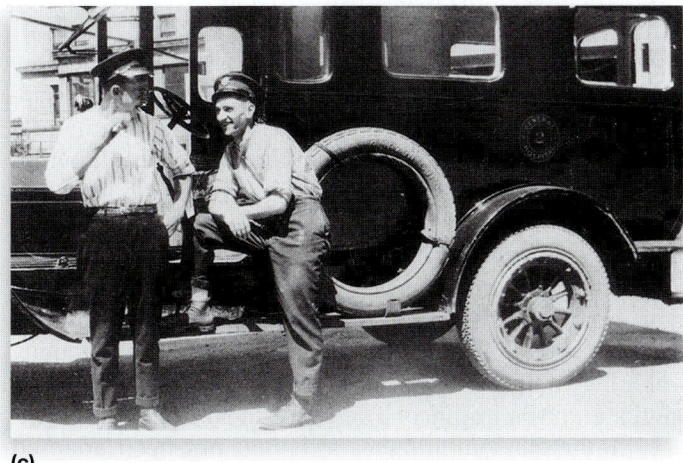
(c)

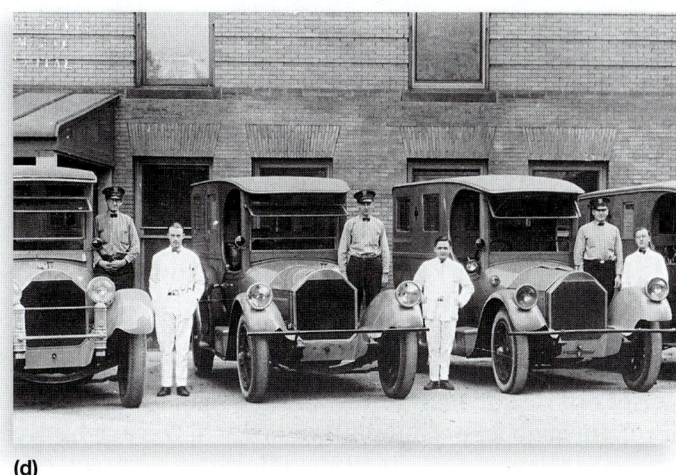
(d)

Figure 1-4   Early ambulances: (a) 1894, (b) 1912, (c) 1919, and (d) 1920s fleet. *Source:* Hennepin County Medical Center EMS.

proposed that accidents be viewed in epidemiologic terms. Epidemiology is the branch of medical science that deals with the incidence, distribution, and control of disease in the population. A principle of epidemiology is to compare disease to a three-legged stool: one leg is the host with the disease, one the disease-causing agent, and the other the environment where the host and disease live (Figure 1-5). If any leg of a three-legged stool is removed, the stool cannot stand, and the same is true for disease: remove one "leg" and the disease cannot survive. Gordon, along with a few other researchers at the time, felt that this approach would lead to creative thinking in how to stop the disease of "accidents" from spreading. Thinking along these lines was novel at the time but would eventually prove invaluable in the development of EMS systems.

CONNECTIONS   Chapter 33: Infectious and Communicable Diseases will discuss epidemiology principles in more detail.

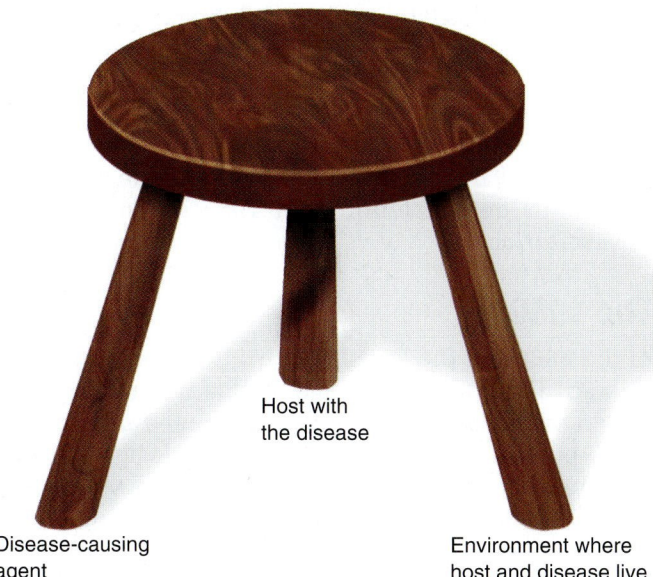

Host with the disease

Disease-causing agent

Environment where host and disease live

Figure 1-5   Disease can be compared to a three-legged stool. If one leg is removed, the disease, like the stool, cannot stand (survive).

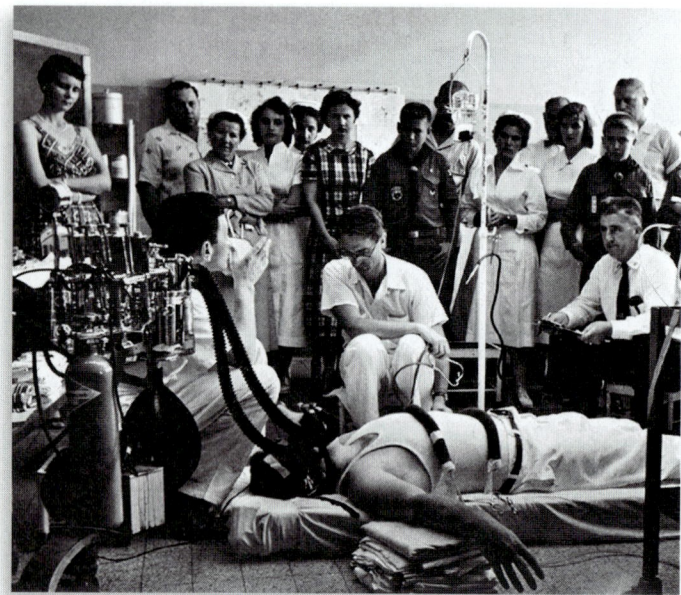

Figure 1-6 In the mid-1950s, Dr. Peter Safar taught volunteers to perform mouth-to-mouth ventilation and kept chemically paralyzed volunteers alive.

The 1950s marked the birth of the "breath of life" (mouth-to-mouth respiration) as a technique being taught to rescuers. Dr. Peter Safar, often referred to as the "Father of Resuscitation," was troubled by the variety of rescue techniques being used and sought to find, through experimentation, which were actually effective (Figure 1-6). In 1956 in Baltimore, Maryland, he gathered healthy volunteer medical residents to participate in the experiments. The volunteers were given the potent drug curare to paralyze them and stop their breathing. They were ventilated by the mouth-to-mouth method by male firefighters, Boy Scouts, and nonmedical women from the hospital auxiliary. All these individuals were trained by Dr. Safar to perform mouth-to-mouth. Dr. Safar demonstrated that nonbreathing patients could be successfully ventilated by his newly trained rescuers. He published his results and techniques in 1957 in *The ABCs of Resuscitation.*

The 1960s

In the 1960s, at the Royal Victoria Hospital in Belfast, Ireland, Dr. Frank Pantridge staffed a converted van with a driver, a nurse, a physician, a medical student, and a portable defibrillator (which he designed). This was the first recorded effort to build an EMS service with medical professionals of varying training levels. It would serve as a model for similar system development activities in other countries, including the United States.

During his presidential campaign in 1960, John F. Kennedy declared that "traffic accidents constitute

one of the greatest, perhaps the greatest, of the nation's public health problems."[5] After his election, the Department of Labor was tasked with assisting in the development of federal legislation to establish safety standards for motor vehicles. The Bureau of Budget and the Department of Commerce were working under similar direction.

Throughout the early part of the 1960s, the Division of Emergency Health Services (DEHS) in the United States Department of Health, Education, and Welfare (DHEW) was the only federal office that assumed significant responsibilities in improving EMS. They operated with minimal funding and limited authority. They focused most of their attention on disaster preparedness and information dissemination. For that time in history, this office was the closest thing to a federal lead agency for EMS.

In 1965 the President's Commission on Highway Safety published their final report "Health, Medical Care and Transportation of the Injured."[6] The recommendations called for a national accident response program with the purpose of working toward the reduction of death and injuries from accidents. This report noted that 50% of the ambulance services in the U.S. were being provided by approximately 12,000 morticians. The reason cited was that their vehicles could accommodate the stretchers. There were no assembly line emergency vehicles being produced, and there were no vehicle design standards in place. The report also noted that military helicopter ambulances still had not been adapted to peacetime needs, ambulance medical equipment and supplies were inadequate, ambulance attendants lacked training, and there was a need for discrete medical radio channels.

The Highway Safety Act of 1966

During his State of the Union Address in 1966, President Lyndon Johnson promised to send to Congress a Traffic Safety Act. This was the first time a President advocated for a direct federal role in highway safety. With passage of the Highway Safety Act in 1966, the National Highway Traffic Safety Agency and the National Traffic Safety Agency were combined to form the Highway Safety Bureau within the Federal Highway Administration of the Department of Transportation (Figure 1-7). In discussing this watershed event, Dr. David Boyd (one of the early leaders in EMS politics) states:[2]

> In the history of medical and social science there are few, if any, instances of a complex and novel idea that has made its way so quickly from the mimeograph papers of professional meetings and journals of learned societies to the statute books of the nation. There are probably none where the process has occurred with such unanimity and essential support in the space of nine months, at the initiative of the President, by the

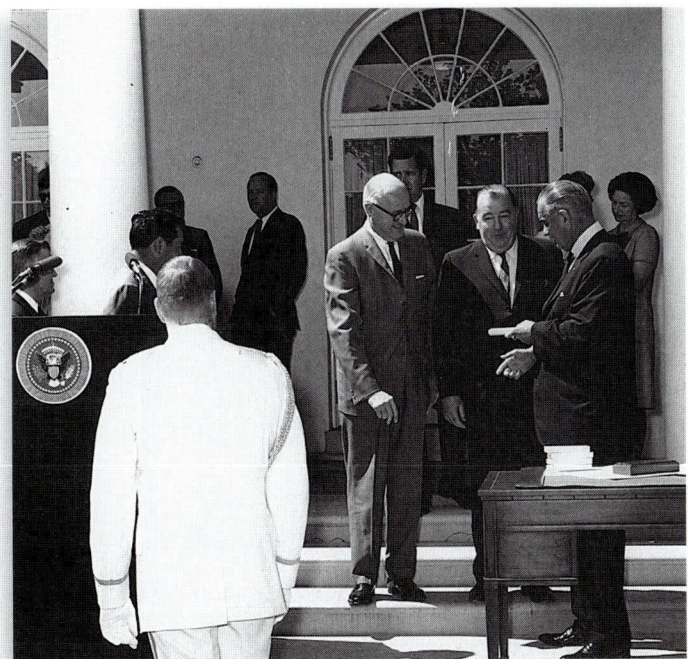

Figure 1-7   President Lyndon B. Johnson after signing the 1966 Highway Safety Act to form the Highway Safety Bureau within the Federal Highway Administration within the Department of Transportation.

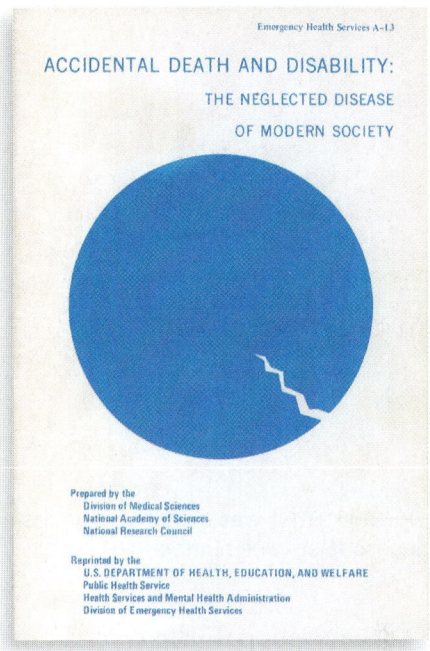

Figure 1-8   *Accidental Death and Disability,* also called "The White Paper," is one of the most important documents that shaped the modern EMS system.

unanimous vote of the Congress, and with the wholly honorable acquiescence of the industries involved. Rarely have Americans witnessed a more dramatic instance of responsive and responsible government in action or a more dramatic transfer of power.

The White Paper

Any document which provides a vision for change that has a national or international scope is often called a **"white paper."** This usually occurs retrospectively when the importance of such a work is recognized for the historical contribution it made.

In 1966, the National Academy of Sciences–National Research Council (NAS–NRC) published a report entitled "Accidental Death and Disability, The Neglected Disease of Modern Society" (Figure 1-8).[7] For the first time **trauma** was officially recognized and classified as a disease process. Once the majority of the medical scientists began thinking of accidents as a form of disease, proven clinical and public health models of management could be applied to help "cure" the disease. This represented a huge step forward in the progress of treating injuries as well as illness.

The report was the result of four years of work by subcommittees focusing on trauma, shock, and anesthesia. The committee members reviewed and studied ambulance services, communication systems, and hospital emergency departments. They also looked at all available research on each topic. Some of the many accomplishments of these task force members included a revision of the American National Red Cross first aid textbook, formal statements on cardiopulmonary resuscitation, and a call for disaster survey studies.

Virtually overnight "Accidental Death and Disability" became known as "The White Paper." Much of what has come to pass in EMS was envisioned by this document. It became the blueprint for EMS systems design and development.

In 1966 the American Trauma Society was established. In 1967 Dr. Eugene Nagle was training firefighters as "paramedics" in Miami, Florida. Between 1968 and 1970, paramedic training programs were started in Seattle, Washington; Columbus, Ohio; and Los Angeles, California. Many of the first instructors in these programs were doctors and nurses. There were no standardized curricula specific to EMS, and there were no formal job descriptions or provider levels established.

Dr. Pantridge published a report in the British medical journal *Lancet* in August of 1967 that his ambulance system in Ireland had resuscitated 5 of 300 patients.[8] Virtually overnight, pioneering physicians like Nagel (Miami, Florida), Cobb (Seattle, Washington), Lewis and Criley (Los Angeles, California), Lambrew (Nassau County, New York), Grace and Nolte (New York), and Warren (Columbus, Ohio) modeled programs based upon Pantridge's.

In 1968 the American Telephone and Telegraph Company (AT&T) designated 9-1-1 as the national emergency phone number (Figure 1-9).

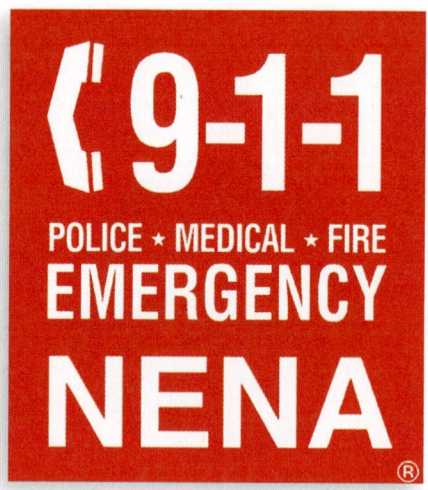

Figure 1-9   In 1968, 9-1-1 was designated as the national emergency access telephone number.

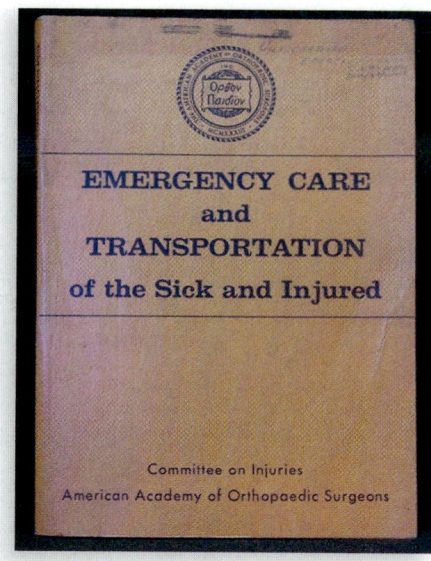

Figure 1-10   In 1969, the American Academy of Orthopedic Surgeons (AAOS) created the first EMT-Ambulance training course and wrote the accompanying textbook. It is now affectionately called the "Orange Book" because of its bright orange cover. This was the only textbook specifically written for training EMS providers for many years.

In 1969, the National Highway Transportation Safety Administration of the Department of Transportation (NHTSA DOT) led a team to develop the first standardized curricula for training EMS providers. The National Standard Curricula (NSC) for training the Emergency Medical Technician—Ambulance (or EMT-A) was the result. Curricula for Paramedics, Intermediates, First Responders, and Emergency Medical Dispatchers followed. A curriculum was also developed for the training of EMS Instructors.

The Committee on Trauma of the American College of Surgeons and the Committee on Injuries of the American College of Orthopedic Surgeons hosted the first national conference on EMS in May 1969. They published "Recommendations for an Approach to an Urgent National Problem."[9] This paper called for immediate attention and control of both the transportation of the injured and the communications systems used to dispatch them. In 1969 the American Academy of Orthopedic Surgeons (AAOS) created the first EMT-Ambulance training course and wrote the accompanying textbook, affectionately called the "Orange Book" because of its bright orange-colored cover (Figure 1-10). This was the only textbook written specifically for training EMS providers for many years. Also in 1969, the Commission on Emergency Medical Services, a subcommittee of the American Medical Association (AMA), published the "Guide for Program Planning: Emergency Medical Service Technician." This document laid an additional foundation for system planning and development.

The 1970s

In 1970 the **National Registry of Emergency Medical Technicians (NREMT),** or "the Registry" as it is often called, began service to the EMS profession. This non-profit group provides a nationally recognized method of credentialing all levels of EMT by developing testing instruments. The mission of the NREMT is "to serve as the national EMS certification organization by providing a valid, uniform process to assess the knowledge and skills required for competent practice required by (EMS) professionals throughout their careers and by maintaining a registry of certification status."[10] Although membership in the NREMT is voluntary, in many states NREMT certification is a requirement to practice as an EMS provider. The Registry is one of the leaders in supporting research into best practices in educational evaluation processes. Boxes 1-4 and 1-5 describe some of the excellent work contributed by the NREMT.

In 1972, a television show called *Emergency!* hit the airwaves and forever changed what the public knew about EMS. The show originally aired between 1972 and 1977. It showed the life of a two-man cross trained paramedic crew from the Los Angeles County fire department. They responded to emergencies in a non-transporting heavy duty utility truck, and scenes were shown both in and out of the hospital and at the fire station. This show introduced the country to paramedics and influenced the career choices of many men and women who grew up in the 1970s (Figure 1-11).

The buildup of emergency service continued in the early 1970s with Dr. David Boyd organizing a statewide trauma system for Illinois that became a national model. At the same time Dr. R. Adams Cowley in Baltimore was developing one of the first trauma centers in the

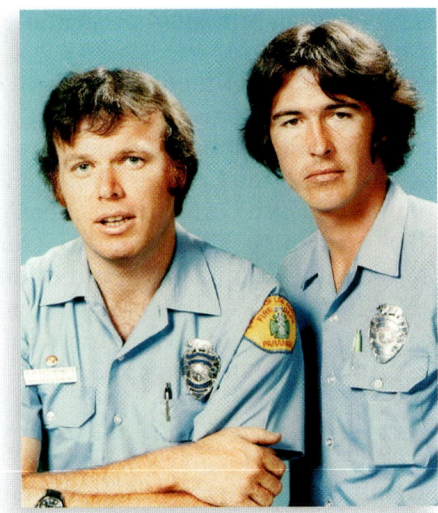

Figure 1-11 Johnny and Roy, the paramedics in the 1972 television show *Emergency!* introduced the nation to paramedics and emergency medical services (EMS).

BOX 1-5   The Practice Analysis

Since 1994, the National Registry of Emergency Medical Technicians (NREMT) has conducted the National EMS Practice Analysis. They began this process with the intent of using the information gathered about the actual practice of prehospital care to develop the blueprint for their certification tests. Conducted every five years, the data from this survey have proven invaluable in helping the NREMT design their exams. The survey has also helped in the redesign of EMS to reflect actual clinical practice. Several of the documents described in the Agenda for the Future, such as the National Scope of Practice and the EMS Education Standards, relied heavily on the Practice Analysis for their development.

world and was working closely with state authorities to set up their own statewide EMS regulatory body called the Maryland Institute for Emergency Medical Services System, or MIEMSS. Controversy still exists over which state's system was developed first, but both should be very proud of their accomplishments and pioneering efforts.[11]

In September of 1972, the Committee on EMS from the NAS-NRC circulated a paper that stated that EMS was still "one of the weakest links in the delivery of health care in the nation."[12] At the time there were 61 federal agencies with an identified role or resources available for EMS support, but none was

BOX 1-4   The LEADS Project

An important research project funded by the NREMT is the LEADS project. In 1998, NREMT brought together a group of people that included state EMS directors, state training coordinators, system managers, emergency physicians, educators, researchers, and the NREMT staff to begin the **Longitudinal Emergency Medical Technician Attributes and Demographics Study,** or LEADS. Conducted annually, this study seeks to define and describe the components of the EMS profession. It includes profiles of the people in EMS and examines their working conditions. This important ongoing survey contributes to the body of knowledge about this profession and allows designers of systems, educational programs, and many other EMS activities to make educated decisions backed by research.

designed as the "lead agency." The report urged the development of a coordinating body, which it called a National Emergency Medical Services Council, to be placed in the Executive Office of the President. The report also urged the development of a national Center for Disaster Emergency Medical Services be established. Unfortunately these recommendations were not implemented.

On January 20, 1973, President Nixon, in his State of the Union Message, directed the DHEW to develop new ways of organizing EMS.[13] He specifically mentioned that "by improving communication, transportation, and the training of emergency personnel, we can save many thousands of lives that would otherwise be lost to accidents and sudden illnesses" (Figure 1-12). He cited Congress's accomplishments the previous year

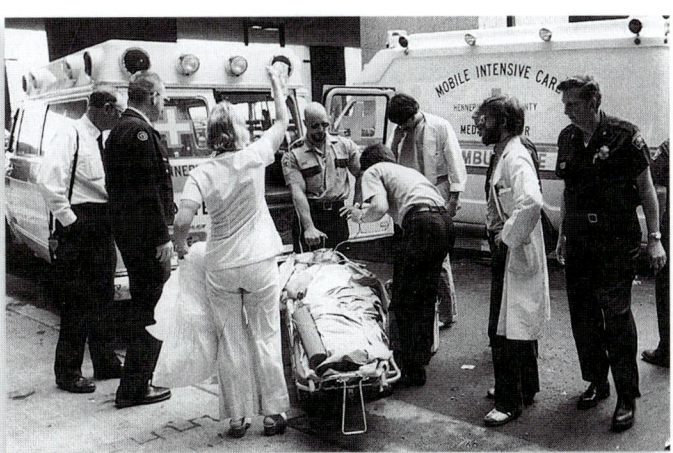

Figure 1-12 Even in the early days of the profession, the positive impact of EMS upon the community was being felt.

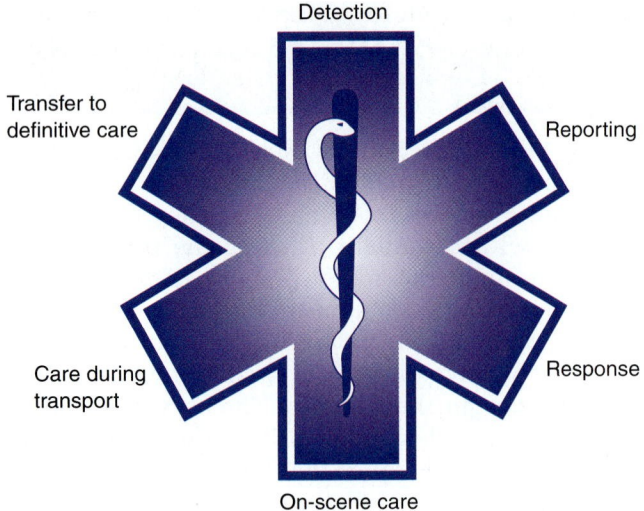

Detection

Transfer to definitive care

Reporting

Care during transport

Response

On-scene care

Figure 1-13 The Star of Life was designated as the symbol for EMS in 1977.

in developing occupational health and safety programs and added his desire to expand this to include air traffic safety, boating safety, and highway safety. The response by DHEW was to fund the development of five EMS systems in the United States. The purpose was to establish systems that other states could model as they designed their own systems.

Star of Life: The EMS Symbol

In 1973 Dr. Leo Schwartz, then the Chief of the EMS branch of the National Highway Traffic Safety Administration (NHTSA), designed the **Star of Life** to identify EMS vehicles and personnel (Figure 1-13). This six-sided star was registered as the symbol for EMS in February of 1977. Each of the bars of the star represents one element of EMS: Detection, Reporting, Response, On-scene care, Care during transport, and Transfer to definitive care. The staff encircled by a snake in the center of the star represents both medicine and

healing. It comes from the symbol of the American Medical Association (AMA).

The AMA symbol came from the "Staff of Asklepios." Greek mythology tells us that Asklepios was the son of the god Apollo, and he learned the art of healing from Cheron the Centaur. Asklepios' knowledge intimidated Zeus (the king of the Greek gods). He was afraid that Asklepios' skill would render all men immortal. Zeus slew Asklepios with a thunderbolt but later raised him from the dead and made him a god.

The use of the star of life is monitored by NHTSA, and its use is allowed on all things specific to EMS.

The EMSS Act of 1973

The biggest national push for EMS came in 1973 with the passage of PL 93-154: The **EMS Systems Act.** Under the Department of Health Education and Welfare, the act provided for funding for planning, implementation, and coordinating EMS systems. President Ford signed the act in 1974.

This act established 303 EMS regions across the nation. The intent was to provide "wall-to-wall" coverage by EMS for handling multiple injured trauma patients with major central nervous system injuries. Approximately one-third of the regions were split over state lines, and mutual aid agreements had to be worked out. A lead agency was designated within each region as well. This agency was tasked with planning and designing an EMS system that addressed all 15 of the components found in the EMSS Act (Box 1-6).

Major provisions of the EMSS Act were

- To establish a lead agency for EMS in the federal government
- Make grants and contract awards for EMS system development
- Promulgate DHEW EMS systems requirements (the 15 components)

BOX 1-6 The 15 Components of an EMS System Described in the EMSS Act of 1973 (PL 93-154)

1. Manpower
2. Training
3. Communications
4. Transportation
5. Facilities
6. Critical care units
7. Use of public safety agencies
8. Consumer participation
9. Accessibility of care
10. Transfer of patients
11. Standardized medical record keeping
12. Consumer information and education
13. Independent review and evaluation
14. Disaster linkage
15. Mutual aid agreements

- Provide extensive technical assistance to support EMS system design and development (called the Technical Assistance Program, or TAP)
- Provide leadership to the Interagency Committee (IAC) on EMS (The IAC EMS group would later become the Federal Interagency Committee on EMS, or FICEMS.)

The EMSS Act of 1973 was amended two times, in 1976 and in 1979. All grants from the DHEW required a systematic approach be utilized in all projects. Because the monies awarded were closely tied to this rule, much of the vision of developing EMS from a systems approach was accomplished.

The Technical Assistance Program (TAP) established state and regional lead agencies, promoted physician leadership in EMS, implemented clinically sound patient-oriented care delivery systems, facilitated the development of national professional system and care standards (including medical control), and helped obtain professional, political, and public support for the regional EMS systems.

Work by the TAP in the area of patient-oriented care focused on the following seven areas: major accident trauma, burn injuries, spinal cord injuries, acute coronary syndromes/heart attacks, poisonings, high-risk infants and mothers, and behavioral and psychiatric emergencies.

Work by the TAP in the area of medical control focused on the role of an EMS provider as a physician extender. In all of the EMS system models supported by federal initiatives, quality medical control was established as the responsibility of physicians. All services provided by EMS needed to be rendered under appropriate medical supervision and meet the regional systems and national standards for patient care. This included the treatment of all three categories of patients:

- Critical
- Emergent
- Nonemergent

Care rendered in the out-of-hospital setting must have the same accountability measures in place as the care given in the traditional hospital setting.[2] Medical oversight (control) can occur directly and indirectly. Control through protocols and standing orders is an example of off-line oversight. On-line medical oversight occurs with real time consultation from a physician (or approved designee) via telephone, two-way radio, satellite, or other device to permit two-way interaction. Today, the cellular telephone has come into use in EMS communication. DOT 1-1.23, 1-1.24, 1-1.27

The development of medical direction and medical directors was further enhanced by the efforts of the **National Association of EMS Physicians (NAEMSP),** the **American College of Surgeons Committee on Trauma (ACS COT),** and the **American College of Emergency Medical Physicians (ACEP).** These physician groups have been instrumental in the training of physicians on directing EMS services and the science that defines Paramedic practice. DOT 1-1.28

CONNECTIONS Medical control and direction will be discussed in more detail in Chapter 4: Legal Issues.

The final element of note to discuss about the EMSS Act was the establishment of the Interagency Committee on Emergency Medical Services (IAC EMS). This committee was composed of 23 federal members and five public members. Four working groups were established within IAC EMS to focus on training, transportation, communications, and financing and administration.

When funding for the EMSS Act ended after the 1979 extension, this group mostly dissolved, and efforts to coordinate EMS on a federal level became disorganized. What did survive of this original group was called the **Federal Interagency Committee on EMS,** or **FICEMS.** Many of the federal agencies continued to support EMS via grants and technical assistance. Most notable among these were the efforts in the late 1980s through the mid-1990s to continue with curricula revisions and the development of the Agenda for the Future, which ushered in the next wave of development in EMS.

In 1974 the Government Services Administration (GSA), the agency charged with buying ambulances for the federal government, developed the KKK-A-1822 ambulance specifications. This set the first *minimum* specification criteria for ambulances. It provided specifications for electrical systems, oxygen securing brackets, internal and external lighting, and ambulance body types. DOT 1-1.25, 1-1.26

CONNECTIONS See Chapter 49: Ambulance Operations for more detail on ambulance specifications.

The update of this document includes specifications on infant transporters, ambient temperature ranges, static load for ambulance bodies, grab rail specifications, cot retention and securing devices, and carbon monoxide levels. It is important to note that compliance with the KKK specifications is not a law; these are a set of ambulance specifications used by federal agencies that purchase ambulances. The current version of these specifications is designated as KKK-A-1822E.

In 1975 the American Medical Association (AMA) recognized EMS and the EMT-Paramedic as an allied health occupation.

In 1975 the **National Association of EMTs (NAEMT)** was formed. The Association represents EMTs on a national level by participating in policy development and concensus building. NAEMT has over 20,000 members and serves all provider levels (emergency medical responder through paramedic), both volunteer and career providers. NAEMT's mission statement is "to represent and serve Emergency Medical Services personnel through advocacy, educational programs and research."[14]

The 1980s

In 1988 the American College of Emergency Physicians (ACEP) built by consensus the first list of recommendations of equipment and supplies to carry on various types of transportation vehicles such as ambulances, vans, and helicopters. In 2000 ACEP issued a joint recommendation with the American College of Surgeons Committee on Trauma (ACS COT) to improve and expand upon its original 1988 recommendations. The ACEP/ACS COT recommendations are important because they identify the equipment required for basic life support and advanced life support ambulances. They do not specify the minimum number of bandages or number of doses of medication to carry. Instead, they state "equipment requirements will vary, depending on the certification levels of the providers, population densities, geographic and economic conditions of the region, and other factors."[15] This document takes into account that each community may have different requirements, based on a variety of factors, to adequately stock each vehicle.

The Twenty-First Century

On June 14, 2006, the Institute of Medicine (IOM) of the National Academies (National Academy of Sciences) released a report, Future of Emergency Care Series: Emergency Medical Services at the Crossroads.[16] This report strongly recommended that Congress establish a lead agency for emergency and trauma care within two years of the publication of the report and recommended that the agency be housed in the Department of Health and Human Services.

Evidence-Based Medicine Practices

As the twentieth century came to an end and the twenty-first century was ushered in, EMS again found itself at a crossroads. The practice of medicine was moving toward a more evidence-based approach called **evidenced-based medicine,** or **EBM.** The art of medicine has traditionally been defined as a combination of medical knowledge (including scientific evidence), intuition, and judgment in the care of patients.[17] The advent of an evidence-based approach placed renewed emphasis on the science component of medical practice. This is not meant to replace the artistic element of medicine but is instead a refocusing on the importance research should play in the decision-making process. DOT 1-1.18

EBM has a variety of approaches, but the following four steps are common to most approaches:

- **Step one:** Formulate the patient management question to be answered.
- **Step two:** Search the medical literature for applicable research data.
- **Step three:** Appraise the evidence gathered with regard to its validity and relevance.
- **Step four:** Integrate the information into clinical practices, taking into account the unique needs of every patient. DOT 1-1.36

Step one of the EBM process begins with a question about what treatments should be provided to patients. An example: What breast cancer treatment will provide the greatest chance of survival five years from the time of diagnosis? (For purposes of illustrating the concept of EMB, we will use an overly simplified example. This question alone has many factors to consider including: In what stage was the cancer detected? What is the age, race, sex, weight, etc. of the patient, and how does that matter in survival? As you can see, a "simple" question can have many dimensions.)

Step two requires a search to find all available research on the topic. This step can take months to complete on some topic areas. It may also lead to the realization that more research into that area needs to occur.

Step three sorts out the research and decides if it is of good quality. Research studies on breast cancer may be grouped in many different ways: by patient type, by stage of cancer process, by treatment options available to the patient, by cost of treatment options, etc. It can also be sorted by the type of study that was conducted and whether the final study was published. If the study was published, what is the reputation of the journal?

In step three, each piece of evidence must be reviewed critically for validity and relevance. Validity asks if the research methods used to gather the data resulted in unbiased and "truthful" information. DOT 1-1.37 Was the study well constructed? Did the researcher stand to gain from a favorable or unfavorable outcome so that their data may be biased? How many subjects (patients) were included in the study, and does this number represent a true sample of the actual population?

Relevance of the data is determined as well. This asks if the data presented are connected in a meaningful way to answer the question you are asking. An example would be if one study found that all patients who had breast cancer also got a minimum of four hours of sleep every night. While this may be interesting information, it may not be very relevant since most people get at least four hours of sleep every night. If another study found that all patients diagnosed with stage four breast cancer (the worst type) survived the following five years with a particular therapy regimen, this would be very relevant to the original question and worthy of further consideration.

Step four of the EMB approach is to take all of the research that was determined to be valid and reliable and develop a treatment plan. The answer for the original question about breast cancer may include drug therapy, radiation, surgery, and lifestyle modification, among other treatments. From this, a practice guideline may be recommended.

While using EBM principles seems like an elegant way to practice medicine, it is difficult to bring this approach into prehospital care. There is surprisingly little actual research on EMS practice (compared to other areas of medicine), so there is not a lot of information to draw upon to design treatment guidelines. Even a seemingly easy question appropriate for EMS, like "What type of immobilization device is appropriate for a majority of patients in low speed motor vehicle collisions with minimal injuries?" has limited research available to make a national policy decision or practice guideline. DOT 1-1.25

For years, EMS has drawn from practice guidelines from the emergency department and taken them into the out-of-hospital environment. This may or may not be appropriate or effective, for a variety of reasons that are not within the scope of this discussion to even begin to explore. Questions such as, "What do our patients need from us?" and "What improves patient outcomes?" are currently being asked of EMS, and these serve as a good starting point for our research efforts. Research that is cited throughout this text is beginning to show that there are definite interventions that improve patient outcomes while other interventions should not be done or should wait until the patient is in the hospital setting.

A variety of initiatives have begun in an attempt to look at what EMS personnel are currently doing, whether or not it is effective, and what else should be done to provide the highest level of care for patients. These initiatives are looking at every aspect of EMS. Training, staffing, protocols, and system designs are all currently under the microscope. Some national initiatives have focused on reviewing where the EMS system currently is and where it should go in the future. The Agenda for the Future has provided the vision for the future direction of EMS. This document speaks to all aspects of EMS, including the role of research in directing our clinical decision-making process.

BOX 1-7   The SEERP Project

With a grant from NHTSA, the National Association of EMS Educators conducted the State of EMS Education Research Project or SEERP. The purpose of this survey was to determine more about EMS educators. It asked who they are, who they work for, what their resources are, what their education levels are, whether they are paid or volunteer, how many hours they work, and what their experience levels are. For the first time, a snapshot was taken of what EMS education is, what resources are available to the educators, how they are providing education, and how they prepare for it. This information, along with the analysis of patients' needs and clinical practice, will help build better EMS education systems.

CONNECTIONS   See Boxes 1-4 and 1-5 (page 11) about the LEADS project and Practice Analysis and Box 1-7: The SEERP Project, above, to get more information on some exciting projects.

The Future Direction of EMS

In 1993 the DOT NHTSA began a formal, national, multidisciplinary consensus process to develop the *National EMS Education and Practice Blueprint.* This was the first attempt to determine the total number of the various EMS provider levels across the nation. The purpose of the *Blueprint,* which was published in 1994, was to gain consensus for the establishment of nationally recognized levels of EMS providers and to develop a nationally recognized scope of practice for EMS paramedicine, a framework for future curriculum development projects, and a standardized pathway for states to deal with legal recognition and reciprocity.

This was a consensus process, which involved all levels of stakeholder in EMS. It set the stage for future EMS consensus activities. Although over 50 distinct provider levels were identified, four distinct and fairly consistently structured provider levels were noted: First Responder, EMT-Basic, EMT-Intermediate, and EMT-Paramedic. These four closely matched the four levels the DOT NHTSA national standard curricula supported.

In 1994 and 1995 the DOT NHTSA contracted with private agencies for the purpose of revising the DOT NSC. This was the second time the curricula was undergoing revision. The first revision cycle occurred in 1984 and was conducted by the National Council of State EMS Training Coordinators (NCSEMSTC) under contract from the DOT NHTSA.

In 1995 the National Association of EMS Educators (NAEMSE) was founded. This group, which has over 4,600 members, is a professional organization made up of EMS educators, instructors, program directors, clinical coordinators, field training coaches, and any other person interested in educating any level of EMS provider. NAEMSE, under DOT NHTSA contract, led a task force that revised the DOT NHTSA EMS Instructor NSC. This document was released in 2002. NAEMSE is also taking the lead, under another DOT NHTSA contract, in the development of the National EMS Education Standards (which will be discussed later in this chapter). The mission of the NAEMSE is: "to inspire excellence in EMS education and lifelong learning."[18]

The Agenda for the Future

In 1996, the National Highway Traffic Safety Administration published the EMS **Agenda for the Future,** or "the Agenda" as it is also known. This was a federally funded position paper completed by the National Association of EMS Physicians (NAEMSP) in conjunction with the National Association of State EMS Directors (NASEMSD).[19] The Agenda was crafted by a task force brought together by NHTSA and made up of leadership from the EMS community including government officials, educators, providers, administrators, physicians, medical directors, and interested citizens from the community. These stakeholders were charged to develop a strategic plan to take EMS into the new millennium. This document was intended to be used by government and private organizations at local, state and national levels to guide planning, policy making, and decision making. DOT 1-1.12

In the final analysis, the Agenda built upon the original elements of an EMS system and also integrated new advances in technology and patient care. The original 15 *components* from the EMSS Act of 1973 were reshuffled and realigned, and became 14 *attributes* (See Box 1-8 for a list of the attributes). The vision of the Agenda is for the EMS systems of the past (which should contain all 15 components) to focus on achieving the 14 attributes as they move toward the future. In addition, accreditation of EMS services, standardization of scope of practice, national quality standards, and national certification and licensure are being implemented in an effort to

Nice to Know

In 2006, the National Association of State EMS Directors (NASEMSD) and the National Association of State EMS Training Coordinators (NASEMSTC) merged into a single organization called the **National Association of State EMS Officials (NASEMSO).**

BOX 1-8   The 14 Attributes from the Agenda for the Future

Integration of Health Services
EMS Research
Legislation and Regulation
System Finance
Human Resources
Medical Direction
Education Systems
Public Education
Prevention
Public Access
Communication Systems
Clinical Care
Information Systems
Evaluation

move the profession from pockets of excellent systems to a national system of excellent quality. DOT 1-1.14

In December, 1996, NHTSA convened an EMS Education Conference with representatives of more than 30 EMS stakeholders to identify the next logical Agenda implementation steps for the EMS community. The following recommendations emerged from this process:

- The *National EMS Education and Practice Blueprint* (the *Blueprint*) from 1993 is a valuable component of the EMS education system. It should be revised by a multidisciplinary panel, led by NHTSA, to more explicitly identify core educational content for each provider level.

- *National EMS Education Standards* are necessary, but need not include specific declarative material or lesson plans. NHTSA should support and facilitate the development of National EMS Education Standards.

- The *Blueprint* and *National EMS Education Standards* should be revised periodically (with major revision recommended every five to seven years and minor updates every two to three years).

In January of 1998, NHTSA gathered together stakeholders for a Blueprint Modeling Group (which was eventually called the "Blue Ribbon Panel") to determine the process for revising the blueprint and implementing the recommendations from the 1996 Education Conference. It was ultimately decided that the Blueprint represented a part of a much broader EMS education system that needed development. The Blue Ribbon Panel was renamed the EMS Education Task Force. This Task Force defined the elements of the education system and described the interrelationships necessary to achieve the vision of the Agenda.

In 2000 this group produced a document entitled **The EMS Education Agenda for the Future: A Systems Approach.** The document proposed an improved structured system to train the next generation of EMS professionals. The proposed system would enhance consistency in education quality in an effort to improve the competence of entry level providers. The proposed educational system had five elements: National Core Content, National EMS Scope of Practice, National EMS Education Standards, National EMS Certification, and National EMS Education Program Accreditation. The National EMS Core Content and the Scope of Practice have been completed, and as this text was under development, educators have gathered to create the Education Standards.

The National Core Content (published in 2005) is a comprehensive listing of the skills and knowledge essential to a practicing prehospital care provider. This document was created by the National Association of EMS Physicians (NAEMSP) and ACEP. It is based on the Emergency Medicine Model and was developed through a comprehensive survey of Emergency Department physicians. The Core Content was used to guide depth and importance in the development of this text.

The National Scope of Practice (published in 2005) divides prehospital care into its discrete levels of delivery. This defines the four levels of prehospital care delivery as Emergency Medical Responder, Emergency Medical Technician, Advanced Emergency Medical Technician and Paramedic. This document was created by EMS professionals brought together by NHTSA and further determines what knowledge base and skills are appropriate for each level.

The National EMS Education Standards takes the place of the DOT National Standard Curricula. This document sets minimal terminal learning objectives for each level of practice. The task force was concerned about consistency in adhering to standards of education that were advocated in the recommendations for *National EMS Education Program Accreditation.* Accreditation is provided through nonprofit independent agencies whose direction is represented by leaders from every facet of EMS. This process helps to ensure program quality to protect students and the patients they will ultimately treat. Finally, *National EMS Certification* was recommended as it provides for national adherence to standards of practice for evaluating competence levels of entry level providers.

Current Levels of Prehospital Care (From the National Scope of Practice)

Currently, prehospital care is provided in levels of care according to the amount of training the responders have received and the types of skills they perform. The following four levels of prehospital care providers were identified: Emergency Medical Responder (EMR), Emergency Medical Technician (EMT), Advanced Emergency Medical Technician (AEMT), and Paramedic. DOT 1-1.4

These levels represent two categories of care: basic life support (BLS) and advanced life support (ALS). Care given at the basic life support level is mostly supportive of the airway, breathing, and circulation with primarily non-invasive techniques. Solid BLS level care is the foundation upon which ALS level care is built.

ALS level care includes all aspects of BLS level care and includes more invasive techniques like fluid therapy, medication administration with nonprescribed medications, and other skills like performance of cardiac monitoring and intubation. As the scope of practice is currently written, the EMR and EMT levels of provider are BLS, and the AEMT and paramedic are ALS.

Emergency Medical Responder

Emergency Medical Responders used to be called First Responder until the Scope of Practice document changed it in 2005. The training these professionals receive is designed to ensure that the people arriving first on the scene will have the skills necessary to be a bridge between the immediate event and the arrival of personnel with more equipment and supplies. EMRs are often police and firefighters, but they also include industrial, school, recreational facility, security, and office personnel. In recent years, many private citizens have received this training to be better able to assist responders by working with the patient prior to their arrival and providing any assistance necessary once they arrive. An EMR training program is typically 40 hours. Topics covered include calming and reassuring the patient, controlling bleeding, providing CPR, and maybe even using automatic external defibrillators (AEDs). Generally, EMRs do not work on patient transport teams; however, in some areas EMRs may work with an EMT or Paramedic on a transport team.

Emergency Medical Technician

An **Emergency Medical Technician** or **EMT** provides basic life support and may also transport patients (Figure 1-14). This training includes the use of oxygen, glucose, and activated charcoal and assisting patients in administering their own medications. EMTs are trained to use AEDs, and some are trained in the use of advanced airway techniques. Emergency child birth, bleeding and bandaging, splinting, and a variety of medical emergencies are covered during EMT training. Emergency vehicle operations, incident command, and orientation training in the areas of rescue, hazmat, and technical rescue are included in the curriculum. An EMT training program has a minimum of 120 hours, but many programs are longer.

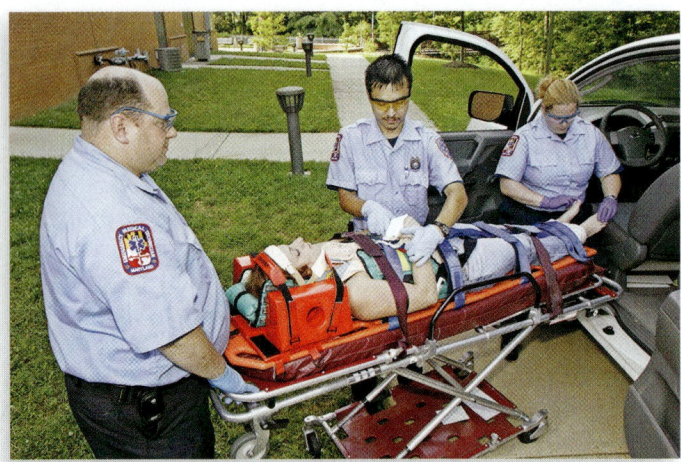

Figure 1-14 The BLS level EMT is considered the entry-level provider for many EMS systems.

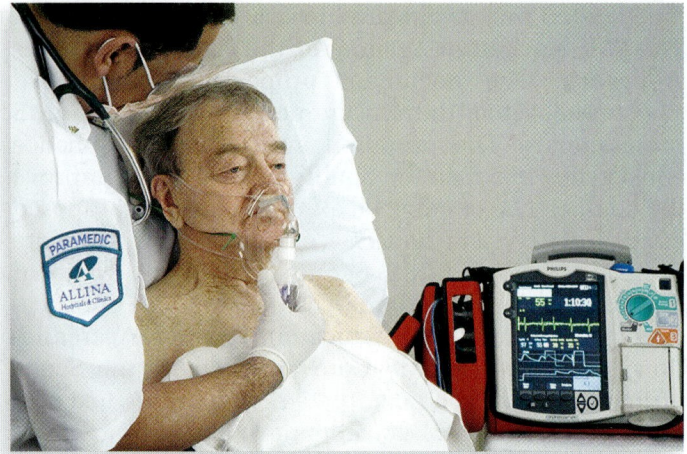

Figure 1-15 Paramedics perform basic and advanced-level EMS care.

Advanced EMT

AEMTs are trained to do a limited number of advanced skills. While the training and scope of practice of the AEMT will vary from state to state, advanced life support skills including advanced airway, intravenous fluids, limited medications, the recognition of noncirculating heart rhythms, and defibrillation are among those commonly found within this group. This level of provider closely resembles the previous EMT-Intermediate levels. The number of hours of a training program varies significantly.

Paramedic

Currently the **paramedic** level is the highest training level for the EMS profession. The DOT curriculum does not recommend a minimum number of hours for a paramedic program, but many are longer than 2,000 hours. During the course of a paramedic's training, didactic and practical skill training is supported by numerous clinical experiences in a variety of environments both in the field and in the hospital. Paramedics' skills include IV insertion and administration of medications, ECG monitoring and defibrillating, and advanced airway management (Figure 1-15).

Licensure, Certification, Reciprocity, Recertification, and Continuing Education

Prehospital care providers are certified or licensed according to individual state law once they complete a state approved training program and pass all state sanctioned licensure or certification evaluations. These evaluations are typically both a written and practical

(skills-based) examination. Once licensed or certified, prehospital care providers must complete regular continuing education to maintain their eligibility to provide patient care. For example, the certified NREMT paramedic is on a two year recertification cycle. To recertify, he or she must provide documentation verifying the appropriate continuing education has occurred before recertification is granted. DOT 1-1.6,1-1.7, 1-1.10

State rules and regulations describe the number of hours to be completed, and whether refresher or re-licensure/certification exams or evaluations are required. These rules may also provide for specific content elements to be covered or may include the need to take additional certification courses like the American Heart Association's Advanced Cardiac Life Support (ACLS) course. As discussed earlier in the chapter, both initial certification and recertification processes are available on a national level through the NREMT as well as through individual states. DOT 1-1.8

Licensure and certification are the two legal processes in place to provide permission for an individual to provide paramedic level care or to verify the competency of a person to provide care. The actual definition of each term varies from state to state. Each jurisdiction that grants permission to function as a paramedic will have specific terminology, and you bear the responsibility to understand what this means and how it impacts you as a professional. Different counties, cities, or ambulance services may have additional certification requirements that go above and beyond the state or national guidelines. DOT 1-1.7

Generally, **licensure** allows a recognized competent authority to grant permission to an individual to engage in a business or occupation that would be otherwise unlawful.[20] (The actual example cited in the dictionary is a reference to the granting of a license to practice medicine.) **Certification** is described in the same dictionary as "the state of being certified." It focuses the attention on the idea that certification is a process that indicates proficiency has been attained, but it does not actually establish the permission to practice prehospital care as an EMS provider. In other words, a certification process says you are competent to do the job, but it does not give you permission to do the job. Licensure gives you permission to do the job.

Reciprocity is a legally recognized method that allows an EMS provider to transfer his or her license or certification from one jurisdiction to another. Because of the myriad provider levels across the country, it is difficult for people to move from one place to another and take EMS credentials with them. It may even be hard to move from one county or region to another within the same state. As more states buy into and support the standardization brought about through the work of the EMS Agenda for the Future, it will become easier for a paramedic to obtain reciprocity. Until that happens, make sure you contact the state EMS agency wherever you plan to move and begin the process of obtaining reciprocity as soon as possible. Sometimes it is as simple as providing your card or certificate for verification, and other times proof of the education program curricula, proof from your original jurisdiction of your status, and a series of interviews and tests will be required to obtain reciprocity. DOT 1-1.7

Street Secrets

Make sure you keep copies of all syllabi, transcripts, schedules, etc. from any EMS training program you attend, as well as maintain current contact information for the facility that provided the training. It will make the process of gaining reciprocity much easier if this information is readily available.

Recertification is a process of verifying that the competencies required for each level of provider have been maintained over time. Many skills, such as needle thoracostomy (chest decompression), are taught to paramedic students, but the frequency of performing this skill on an actual patient is rare in many EMS systems.

Even if a paramedic never performs a skill like needle thoracostomy, it is nonetheless a skill that is established as a minimal competency, so it must be maintained. Recertification is the mechanism for verifying continued competency. A recertification process may include knowledge testing as well as psychomotor skills testing. EMS services may also utilize a process which tracks skills as they are performed on actual patients. A recertification process may include an opportunity for the paramedic to attend workshops or alternative training opportunities to verify continued competency of any skill not tracked on

patients. It is up to each individual paramedic to monitor this process and ensure that all records are up-to-date and accurate. Paramedics who do not monitor this process may find inaccurate or incomplete records when the time comes for recertification, which can pose many problems including suspension, loss of patient care privileges, or even loss of employment.

Continuing education is different from recertification. While recertification ensures competency is maintained in certain areas, continuing education provides for a means to gain new knowledge. The knowledge and skills from the initial training program establish the *entry level* of the paramedic. These are the minimum elements required to provide paramedic level care. Completion of licensure or certification testing establishes you are ready to begin the real education process, where you will apply it all to real patient care challenges. Passing the paramedic program and obtaining licensure or certification is step one in a journey of a lifetime of learning. Continuing education provides opportunities to expand upon the foundation established in the initial training program. DOT 1-1.9

Summary

EMS is dynamic and evolving. Although the roots are in wartime, the focus of the profession is on providing quality patient care to try to preserve life. The attributes and behaviors expected of this field hold the paramedic to a very high standard. EMS is a small, but critical, piece of the total spectrum of patient care. Compared to other parts of medicine, EMS is relatively young, with most of the major innovations in ambulances, patient stretchers, and gear designed specifically for field use coming in the final quarter of the last century. The future for EMS is bright. The role you play in shaping the future can be as important as you choose it to be, as long as you stay focused on quality customer service and perform as a professional.

Notes

1. Emergency Medical Technician Paramedic: National Standard Curriculum (EMT-P), United States Department of Transportation. www.nhtsa.dot.gov/people/injury/EMS/EMT-P/index.htm (accessed October 11, 2006).
2. David R. Boyd, Richard F. Edlich, and Sylvia Micik, *Systems Approach to Emergency Medical Care* (New York: Appleton-Century-Crofts, 1983).
3. L. D. Heaton, Army Medical Services Activities in Viet Nam. *Military Medicine* 131(19):646.
4. J. E. Gordon, The Epidemiology of Accidents. *American Journal of Public Health* 39(1949):504–515.
5. J. F. Kennedy, quotation from campaign speech. Published in "Report of the Secretary's Advisory Committee on Traffic Safety," U.S. Department of HEW, USGPO, February 28, 1968, 11.

6. *Highway Safety Program Standard Emergency Medical Services Report No. 1700,* House of Representatives, 89th Cong., 2d sess., 1966, 17.

7. *Accidental Death and Disability: The Neglected Disease of Modern Society* (Washington, DC: NAS-NRC, 1966).

8. J. F. Pantridge, J. S. Geddes, "A Mobile-Intensive Care Unit in the Management of Myocardial Infarction." *Lancet,* 2(1967):271.

9. "Emergency Medical Services: Recommendations for an Approach to an Urgent National Problem." Proceedings of the Airlie Conference on Emergency Medical Services, Airlie House, Warrenton, VA, May 5–6, 1969. American College of Surgeons and the American Academy of Orthopedic Surgeons, 1969.

10. NREMT Mission Statement. http://nremt.org/about/mission_statement.asp (accessed April 10, 2006).

11. Jon Franklin and Alan Doelp, *Shock-Trauma* (New York: St. Martin's Press, 1980).

12. *National Research Council Committee Calls for Expanded Emergency Medical Services System.* Washington, DC: National Academy of Sciences-National Research Council, 1972.

13. President's State of the Union Message, Richard M. Nixon, House of Representatives, 92nd Congress, Washington, DC, January 20, 1972.

14. National Association of EMTs. http://www.naemt.org/aboutNAEMT/(accessed April 10, 2006).

15. American College of Emergency Physicians, American College of Surgeons. *Equipment for Ambulances* (Chicago, IL: American College of Surgeons, 2000).

16. Institute of Medicine of the National Academies. *Future of Emergency Care Series: Emergency Medical Services at the Crossroads* (Washington, DC: The National Academies Press, 2006), p. 5.

17. D. L. Kasper, E. Braunwald, A. S. Fauci, S. L. Hauser, D. L. Longo, J. L. Jameson, and K. J. Isselbacher, eds., *Harrison's Principles of Internal Medicine,* 16th ed., McGraw-Hill's AccessMedicine (accessed October 11, 2006).

18. The National Association of EMS Educators. http://naemse.org/ (accessed April 10, 2006).

19. The National Highway Traffic Administration. http://www.nhtsa.dot.gov/people/injury/ems/EdAgenda/final/emstoc.html (accessed April 11, 2006).

20. *Webster's Medical Desk Dictionary* (Springfield, MA: Merriam-Webster, Inc., 1986).

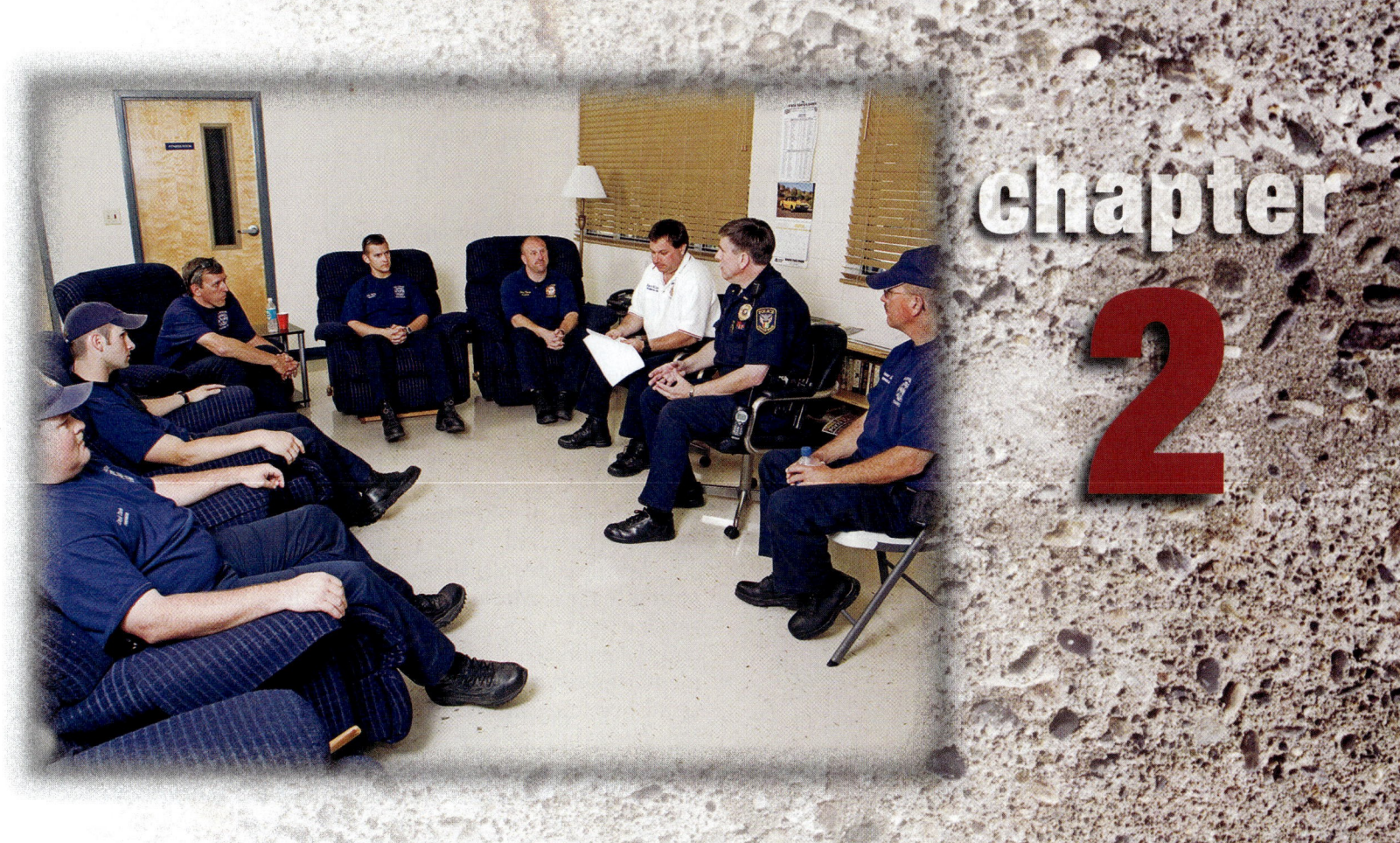

The Well-Being of the Paramedic

"**A** wise man ought to recognize that health is his most valuable possession."

—Hippocrates

Need to Know

▶ Individual responsibilities of a paramedic in promoting, modeling, and maintaining wellness
▶ Behavior choices that prevent wellness and ways to avoid those behaviors
▶ Behaviors that promote wellness and ways to build them into your lifestyle
▶ Appropriate management strategies to deal with the stress inherent in the EMS profession

Introduction

Paramedics provide extensive prehospital and emergency care and may work for fire departments, private ambulance services, police departments, or hospitals.[1] Paramedics often work between 45 and 60 hours a week. Because emergency services function 24 hours a day, paramedics sometimes have irregular working hours and are often on call for extended periods of time.[2]

The duties of the paramedic range from covering unique or critical life-threatening emergencies to covering the nonemergency or routine. The working environment is demanding and often unpredictable. The paramedic may have to lift, carry, walk, stand, crawl, kneel, or bend to perform these duties. Heavy lifting is often required. Physical fitness is critical to maintaining a long and healthy career in EMS. Paramedics work in all types of weather and under various conditions. Additionally, there is risk of noise-induced hearing loss from sirens, potential exposure to infectious diseases, and possible violence from drug impaired, mentally altered, or unstable patients.

The work of a paramedic is not only physically strenuous but also intellectually and emotionally demanding. It often involves high levels of stress, dealing with life-and-death situations, many of which have poor outcomes, and suffering patients. EMS providers must be able to remain calm, focused, and capable of critical decision-making even under difficult and highly stressful situations.[2,3]

The maintenance of well-being allows for both excellent job performance and the ability to meet the demands of the profession. It also leads to increased health and vitality in your personal life as well.

Being healthy is much more than just not being sick or injured. Optimal health or "wellness" involves maintaining *quality* in your life. To achieve this requires balance in all aspects of life including the physical, intellectual, emotional, environmental, social, spiritual, and occupational areas. Attaining a "high level" of wellness, as outlined in this chapter, can improve both your lifespan and your quality of life.[4] DOT 1-2.1, 1-2.2

Disease, Injury, and Death

Although being healthy involves much more than just not being sick or injured, this discussion of wellness will start by focusing on the absence of wellness: disease, injury, and death.

Morbidity and Mortality

The pie graph in Figure 2-1 shows the current average life expectancy in the United States. Notice that while the average lifespan is approximately 78 years in length, typically 12 of those years are affected by disease or accidents.[5] Often the disease- and injury-affected years come in the last 12 years of life, but not always. One of the goals of achieving and maintaining wellness is to increase the quality of each year of life.

Two measures of health and wellness are morbidity and mortality rates. **Morbidity rates** show how many people get sick from various diseases or are injured in accidents, and the collected statistics are published by the government. Understanding morbidity numbers helps to understand possible causes of diseases and injuries as well as the effects they have on a person's ability to function.

Mortality is a component of morbidity—it is the number of individuals who die from the illness or injury being studied. Research into mortality tries to identify the cause of fatal diseases and accidents. Although morbidity and mortality are important to all components of medical science, public health is the branch devoted to examining both morbidity and mortality in terms of demographic factors such as age group, gender, ethnicity, geographic location, and socioeconomic status.

CONNECTIONS Chapter 1: The EMS Profession discussed the historical roots of EMS and identified that EMS has roots in public health. The Department of Health, Education, and Welfare in particular was one of the first federal agencies that assumed a leadership role in developing EMS in the U.S. EMS continues to play a pivotal role in public health as advocates for, and participants in, prevention programs and public education.

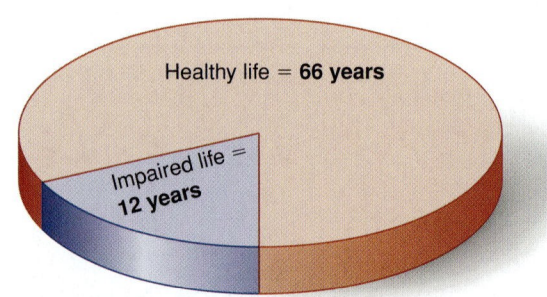

Life expectancy in the U.S. = **78 years**

Figure 2-1 Life expectancy in the United States.

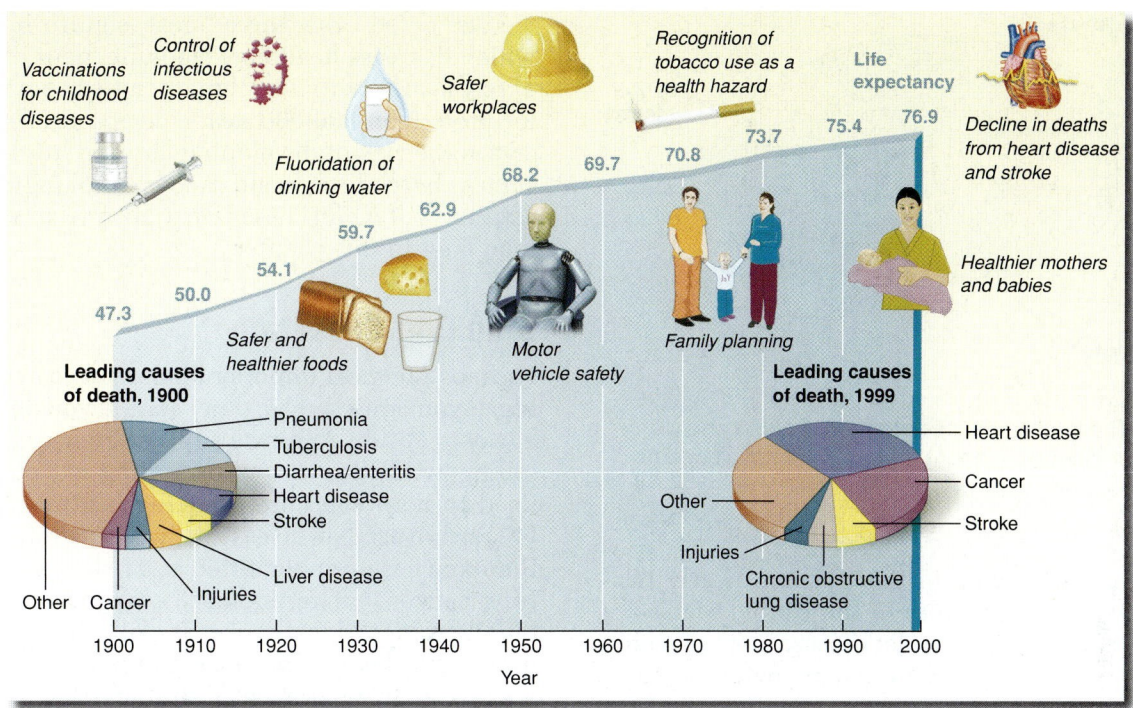

Figure 2-2   Causes of death in the United States in the 1900s. Notice how improvements in the environment, medical technology, and lifestyle lead to a decrease in the death rate and an increase in life expectancy.

Analysis of morbidity and mortality rates helps determine what behavioral and environmental factors affect health and safety. Examining these rates allows a better understanding of what can be done to reduce risks of injury, disease, and death. It also helps identify what can be done to impact personal wellness.

During the early 1900s, the average lifespan in the United States was 47 years of age. At that time, the leading causes of death included tuberculosis, cholera, and influenza.[5] These diseases are termed **infectious** because they are caused by various pathogens or disease-causing agents such as viruses, bacteria, and fungi. Infectious diseases tend to be acute in nature, which means they progress rapidly, causing sickness and even death.

> A **pathogen** is any substance (protein, bacteria, virus, etc.) that is capable of causing a disease.

As stated previously in this chapter, the average life expectancy today is nearly 78 years. The two biggest killers in this country are cardiovascular disease and cancer. Other major causes of death include cerebrovascular disease (strokes) and chronic obstructive pulmonary diseases (COPD) such as emphysema and chronic bronchitis. All of these diseases collectively are known as **chronic lifestyle diseases** because they take many years to develop and are almost always directly related to lifestyle habits and choices.[5]

Various factors resulted in a change of the primary cause of death in the United States from infectious disease to diseases of lifestyle behaviors. Improvements such as the development of vaccines, clean water supplies, sanitation, and food refrigeration and preservation have brought about a dramatic reduction in morbidity and mortality from infectious disease. Many of these factors are not present in other countries, especially underdeveloped, or "third world" nations. This helps to explain why the leading cause of death in such countries remains infectious diseases.

Examine Figure 2-2. It illustrates the changes that have taken place in our country over the last 100 years related to improved health status.[6] The two pie charts in the figure compare the causes of death in 1900 and 1999. Notice how the death rate declines steadily as improvements in the environment, medical technology, and lifestyle have occurred.

Behavior Choices with a Negative Impact on Wellness

As you can see from Figure 2-2, when you examine the current causes of sickness, injury, and death you find that many causes are directly related to behavioral choices. Individuals who focus on making healthy choices are said to lead a wellness-oriented lifestyle.

Research has shown that 83% of the deaths in the U.S. that occur before the age of 65 are preventable.[7]

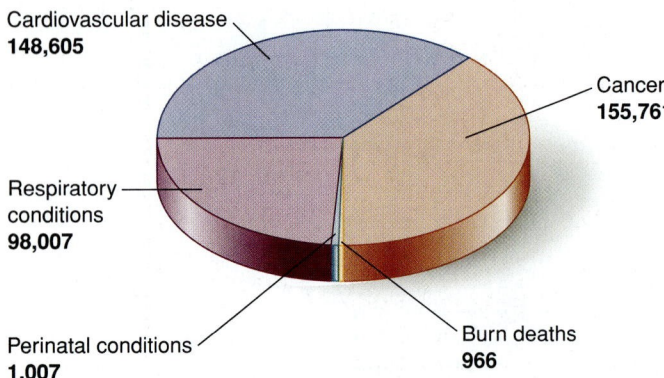

Cardiovascular disease
148,605

Cancer
155,761

Respiratory conditions
98,007

Perinatal conditions
1,007

Burn deaths
966

Figure 2-3 The leading causes of death. Cancer and cardiovascular disease account for two-thirds of all deaths in America.

As previously mentioned in this chapter, nearly two-thirds of all deaths each year in the United States are due to cancer and cardiovascular disease, both of which are caused primarily by individual behavior choices.[5] The graph in Figure 2-3 shows the leading causes of death across all age groups. More than 50% of disease is related to lifestyle behaviors, 20% is related to environmental factors, 10% is impacted by the level and type of healthcare you receive, and 16% is related to hereditary/genetic factors.[6] From a practical standpoint, you have the potential to control more than 80% of your risk of developing disease.[8]

Take another look at the figures, and think about the choices that lead to these diseases. Once you have determined which behaviors you should adopt as well as which ones to minimize or eliminate, you will better understand how to achieve wellness and a better quality of life. DOT- 1-2.3

Reducing the Threat of Disease and Injury

Reducing your risk of disease involves controlling or eliminating those behaviors that cause disease as well as engaging in behaviors that promote well-being. The best way to reduce the potential threat of disease and injury is through prevention. There are many measures you can take to help reduce your risks.

Adopting good diet and exercise practices is a big step in improving your well-being and reducing risks. Regular medical screenings for various diseases are big steps towards disease prevention. Responsible use of alcohol and avoiding drug abuse will help to reduce your potential for addictions, as well as any accidents caused while under the influence. Following safety procedures and practices will help to reduce exposure to motor vehicle accidents, toxins, and disease-causing agents.

As noted, the three most significant behaviors which decrease health are smoking, poor diet, and lack of physical activity. Combined, these behaviors account for more than 800,000 deaths every year. All three increase the risk of developing chronic lifestyle diseases such as heart disease and cancer. Smoking and physical activity will be discussed next; nutrition will be examined later in this chapter.

Smoking Cessation

Perhaps the most important behavior to avoid is smoking. If you don't smoke, don't start. If you do smoke, find a way to quit by joining a support group, taking a class, talking with your doctor, or finding any other way you need to help you quit. Smoking is a major risk factor for cardiovascular disease as well as stroke and COPD. Smoking has been identified as a risk factor not only for lung cancer, but for stomach, esophageal, pancreatic, bladder, and cervical cancer as well. Table 2-1 shows the number of deaths that occur in the U.S. each year that are caused by or connected to smoking.[9]

Cigarette smoking is the single most preventable cause of premature death in the United States. Each year, more than 400,000 Americans die from cigarette smoking. In fact, one in every five deaths is smoking related. Every year, smoking kills more than 276,000 men and 142,000 women.[9] Between 1960 and 1990, the number of lung cancer deaths among women increased by more than 400%, far surpassing deaths from breast cancer by over 20,000 each year.[10,11] Men who smoke increase their risk of death from lung cancer by more than 22 times that of a nonsmoker. Their risk of dying from emphysema or bronchitis is 10 times higher than their nonsmoking counterparts.[12]

Smokeless tobacco users are also at risk for cancer. The two main types of smokeless tobacco used in the United States are chewing tobacco (which is chopped up loose leaf, solid blocks called "plugs," or twisted leaves), and snuff (which is finely ground). Snuff can be inhaled into the nose, but most users of both forms place it into their mouths between their gums and cheeks. So far, 28 carcinogens (cancer causing agents) have been found in smokeless tobacco, and users are at high risk for developing oral cancer.[13] Three percent of adults are smokeless tobacco users and nearly 90% of those users are men.[14] An estimated 7% of high school students and 3% of middle school students use smokeless tobacco.[15,16]

Secondhand smoke is a major health concern. **Secondhand smoke** is the smoke that enters the air from the burning end of a cigarette, cigar, or pipe that has not been inhaled into the lungs. Because it is unfiltered when compared to the smoke inhaled by the smoker, it has twice the tar and nicotine as well as three times the benzopyrene, which is a known carcinogen. Secondhand

TABLE 2-1   **Causes of Death in the United States in 2004**

This data includes all deaths which were attributed to or directly caused by smoking or the use of tobacco products.

Disease	Men	Women	Overall
Cancers			
Lung	81,179	35,741	116,920
Lung from environmentally transmitted smoke (second-hand smoke)	1,055	1,945	3,000
Other	21,659	9,743	31,402
Total	**103,893**	**47,429**	**151,322**
Cardiovascular diseases			
Hypertension	3,233	2,151	5,450
Heart disease	88,644	45,591	134,235
Stroke	14,978	8,303	23,281
Other	11,682	5,172	16,854
Total	**118,603**	**61,117**	**179,820**
Respiratory diseases			
Pneumonia	11,292	7,881	19,173
Bronchitis/emphysema	9,234	5,541	14,865
Chronic airway obstruction	30,385	18,579	48,982
Other	787	668	1,455
Total	**51,788**	**32,689**	**84,475**
Diseases among infants	1,006	705	1,711
Burn deaths	863	499	1,362
All causes	**276,153**	**142,537**	**418,690**

Source: http://www.cdc.gov/tobacco/research_data/health_consequences/mortali.htm. Extracted April 2006.

smoke also has almost three times the carbon monoxide and three times the ammonia of the inhaled smoke. About 85% of the smoke in a room where someone is smoking comes from secondhand smoke. The Environmental Protection Agency estimates that an average of 3,000 lung cancer deaths per year are due to secondhand smoke.[17] More than 35,000 coronary heart disease deaths occur annually among adult nonsmokers as a result of exposure to secondhand smoke.[18]

Smoking cessation reduces the risk of heart attack and death from heart disease by 50% or more. Quitting smoking also helps reduce the impact of atherosclerosis (fatty plaque buildup in arteries), blood clots, peripheral arteriosclerosis (fatty buildup in peripheral arteries), and the rates of chronic obstructive pulmonary disease. Within one year of quitting smoking, the risk is reduced by 50%. After 15 years of not smoking, the risks of heart disease and stroke are similar to that for people who have never smoked.[19] DOT 1-2.16

Eliminating smoking from one's life usually involves determination and personal commitment. The decision to quit is a healthy one. The U.S. Department of Health and Human Services has provided several guidelines for quitting smoking.[20] If you plan to quit, set a quit date. Change the environment in which you live and work to eliminate any smoking reminders and temptations. Examples include getting rid of all cigarettes and ashtrays, and not letting people smoke in your home, car, or place of work. Avoid social situations where you might be tempted to smoke. Try to distract yourself from urges to smoke. Use substitute behaviors like exercising, reading, or socializing. Calculate the dollar amount that would be spent on smoking in one year, and instead use the money saved to plan a celebration or vacation on the one year anniversary of quitting.

Studies have shown that you have a better chance of quitting successfully if you have help. You can get support in many ways including from family and friends, health counselors, health care providers, and individual, group, or telephone counselors. Learn to manage your stress. Often high or sudden stress triggers smoking behavior.

Often medications can be used to help you stop smoking. Several are available including the nicotine patch, nicotine gum, nicotine inhaler, and nicotine nasal spray. Note that all of these products contain nicotine. If you do use medication, make sure to ask your healthcare provider for advice, and carefully read the information on the package.

Be prepared if you relapse. A relapse does not mean you have failed, merely that you have stumbled briefly. Most relapses occur within the first three months after quitting. Do not be discouraged if it happens to you. Refocus on your objective and move forward. Remember, most people try several times before finally quitting.

Cardiovascular Disease and Stroke Prevention

Arteriosclerosis occurs when an artery becomes blocked so that it can no longer supply muscles or organs with the oxygen that is needed for metabolism. Arteriosclerosis reduces blood flow to various areas of the body, especially the legs. When arteriosclerosis occurs, pain often occurs. If the blockage is in the heart, the pain is called angina.

CONNECTIONS Chapter 28: Pulmonary explores cardiac and vascular diseases in detail. Chapter 8: Physiology Overview also describes the body when it is in and out of a state of balance. While the focus of this chapter is wellness, if you want additional information on the pathophysiology of cardiovascular disease, please refer to those chapters.

The most common cause of blockage in the heart or brain is a build-up of fatty deposits, called **plaque,** within the lining of the blood vessels. This condition is also called "hardening of the arteries." This reduces the arteries' diameters and decreases the amount of blood that can freely flow through them. The fatty build-up places increased strain on the heart which must work harder to force blood through the narrower vessels. The build-up also reduces the elasticity of the blood vessels which further increases the amount of force necessary to pump blood through them. Narrower blood vessels also mean an increased risk of additional blockage from blood clots or gas bubbles which may be in the cardio-vascular system.

The three most significant risk factors for heart disease and stroke are smoking and other tobacco use, unhealthy diet, and lack of physical activity. These behaviors can lead to serious physical problems including high blood fats (hyperlipidemia) or cholesterol, high blood pressure (hypertension), and high blood sugar (diabetes). These conditions may lead to atherosclerosis.

Prevention of heart disease and stroke involves controlling risky behaviors that lead to the development of hyperlipidemia, hypertension, and diabetes. Regular checkups can help to catch early signs of these diseases. DOT 2-2.8 If you are on medication to help control high blood pressure, high cholesterol, or angina, it is vital that the regimen be followed as prescribed by the doctor. Figure 2-4 has additional information on strategies to reduce the risk of cardiovascular disease and stroke.[6]

Do More

- Eat a diet rich in fruits, vegetables, whole grains, and low-fat or fat-free dairy products. Eat 5–9 servings of fruits and vegetables each day.

- Eat several servings of high-fiber foods each day.

- Eat 2 or more servings of fish per week; try a few servings of nuts and soy foods each week.

- Choose unsaturated fats rather than saturated and trans fats.

- Be physically active; do both aerobic exercise and strength training on a regular basis.

- Achieve and maintain a healthy weight.

- Develop effective strategies for handling stress and anger. Nurture old friendships and family ties, and make new friends; pay attention to your spiritual side.

- Obtain recommended screening tests and follow your physician's recommendations.

Do Less

- Don't use tobacco in any form: cigarettes, spit tobacco, cigars, pipes, bidis, or clove cigarettes.

- Avoid exposure to environmental tobacco smoke.

- Limit consumption of fats, especially trans fats and saturated fats.

- Limit consumption of cholesterol, added sugars, and refined carbohydrates.

- Avoid excessive alcohol consumption—no more than one drink per day for women and two drinks per day for men.

- Limit consumption of salt to no more then 2400 mg of sodium per day.

- Avoid excess stress, anger, and hostility.

Figure 2-4 Choices and behaviors to do more, and less, to better your chances of avoiding cancer and living in good health.

Cancer Prevention

While heart disease is the leading cause of disease across all age groups, the leading cause of death for those under the age of 85 is cancer. Almost 50% of men and over 33% of women in the United States will develop cancer during their lifetimes.[21]

Cancer occurs when cells grow in an abnormal and uncontrolled fashion. Most forms of cancer occur as tumors; however, some do not. A tumor is a mass of tissue that has no physiological purpose. Not all tumors are the product of cancers.[6] Cancer cells can travel from one location in the body to another, where they can start to grow, developing additional tumors. This process of cancer cell migration is termed metastasis. Cancer does not have to metastasize to be fatal.

Preventing cancer means avoiding or reducing those risk factors that may predispose you to developing cancer. Figure 2-4 describes the things to do and avoid to reduce your risk of cancer.[6] Risk factors for cancer include tobacco use (smoking and chewing), non-nutritious diet, infectious diseases, chemical exposure, and radiation exposure. These five risk factors account for approximately 75 percent of all cancers. As with cardiovascular disease, tobacco use, poor diet, and lack of physical activity are more likely to put you at

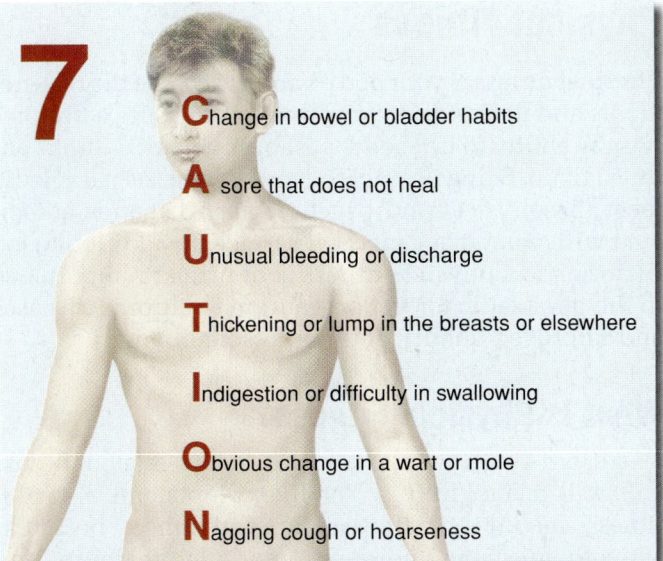

7
Change in bowel or bladder habits

A sore that does not heal

Unusual bleeding or discharge

Thickening or lump in the breasts or elsewhere

Indigestion or difficulty in swallowing

Obvious change in a wart or mole

Nagging cough or hoarseness

Figure 2-5   Look for these CAUTIONs. If any of them show up, consult with your doctor immediately for additional evaluation and screening for cancer. Early detection is one of the best ways to beat the disease.

risk for developing cancer. Approximately one-third of all cancer deaths are related to lack of physical activity and unhealthy diet.[21] The sooner a cancer is found and treatment begins, the better the chance of living. Identifying cancer as soon as possible is vital. Figure 2-5 provides the CAUTION method for recognizing signs of potential cancer.[6] DOT 1-2.8

Wellness

The World Health Organization (WHO) defines **health** as a state of being that involves "more than freedom from illness, disease, and debilitating conditions."[22] They also included in their description the need for a positive component of health identified here as "quality of life." Wellness therefore requires both health and a positive quality of life.

Wellness is a concept that has been widely used and promoted by medical, health, nutrition, and fitness professionals as well as the general public. Various definitions of wellness have been developed over the last 50 years. These early definitions were often inadequate or too complicated to be useful in understanding what strategies were needed to attain wellness. Recent research has provided the following functional definition of **wellness:**

> Wellness is a multidimensional state of being describing the existence of positive health in an individual as exemplified by quality of life and a sense of well-being.[23]

The Dimensions of Wellness

Wellness is seen as encompassing the physical, intellectual, and emotional dimensions of the individual. Other components are the social, environmental, and spiritual dimensions of wellness.

The physical dimension of wellness involves regular exercise, eating nutritiously, and getting adequate recuperative sleep. Safe sexual practices as well as avoiding alcohol and drug use/abuse are aspects of this component. Physical well-being involves regular self-tests, checkups, rehabilitation, proper medication use, and taking the time to rest and heal when sick.

The intellectual dimension of wellness involves the ability to think critically and make healthy choices. A person with a high level of intellectual wellness can reason and think straight, even under stress. Intellectual wellness involves the perception of life as it really is and that you can respond to life's changes in appropriate ways. Emotionally healthy people strive to maintain psychological balance and understand when to express their emotions appropriately and comfortably. Emotional well-being requires acknowledging one's feelings without being overwhelmed or controlled by them.

The social dimension of wellness involves having satisfying relationships and interacting well with others. It includes an appreciation for diversity. The idea of being well socially also involves having a social support network of friends, family, and others who can be called upon during times of need. This group should be concerned about your welfare and steer you towards making healthy choices. Social health should also involve a feeling of connectedness to the community.

The environmental component of wellness refers to the ways your environment impacts you. It includes protecting yourself from hazards that are present in the air, water, and soil. The environmental component is a critical component for the EMS professional. Scene safety is one of the primary responsibilities of every member of the EMS team. In addition to ensuring scene safety upon arrival, providers should be on alert for changes to scene safety throughout the entire call. DOT 1-2.10

CONNECTIONS   Chapter 9: Safety and Scene Size Up will discuss all aspects of safety including scene, individual, team, bystander, patient, and vehicle operations. Personal protective equipment and supplies will also be discussed.

Spiritual wellness is an awareness and practice of that which provides your life with meaning and purpose. Spiritual health fosters a sense of connection with others, nature, and the universe. It may come from religion, philosophy, ethics, morals, environmental sensitivity, or any other source that has a deep level of personal importance for you. Spiritual health also includes maintaining faith and hope, even after setbacks occur.

Some wellness professionals also include a seventh dimension or component of wellness related to one's job. Occupational well-being involves finding meaning and satisfaction with your school, work, and leisure pursuits. The occupational component of wellness also includes being able to work with others to accomplish the objectives required for your job.

High-Level Wellness

As previously discussed in this chapter, having a high level of wellness is more than just being free of illness. It is a matter of integrating and balancing the many dimensions of wellness. The more balanced your dimensions are, the higher the level of wellness you possess (Figure 2-6). The less balanced your dimensions, the more you are susceptible to disease and experience sickness.

Wellness is never static—it is always changing. Throughout your life, you move up and down the wellness continuum. At times you have a high level of wellness, and then illness strikes. The healthier your lifestyles and the more positive your behaviors, the greater your potential for attaining and sustaining a state of wellness. To that end, it is important for you as a paramedic to actively improve, maintain, and promote your own wellness. DOT 1-2.3

As a paramedic, you also have the responsibility of encouraging wellness in the public through education and by example. As individuals approach you for information about healthy living, you will be provided the opportunity to encourage wellness through education. It is important to maintain a list of wellness and community resources that, when the opportunity arises during patient interaction, you can pass on to the willing listener.

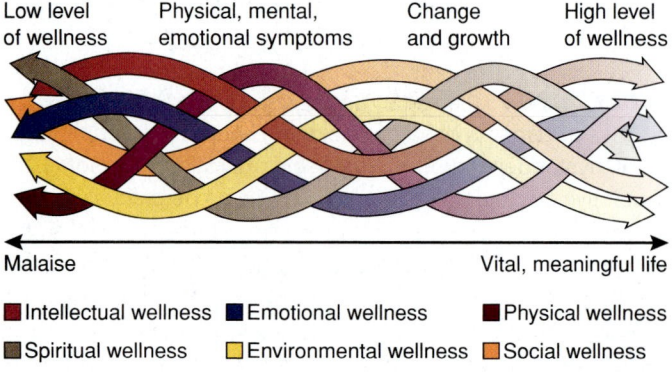

| Low level of wellness | Physical, mental, emotional symptoms | Change and growth | High level of wellness |

Malaise   Vital, meaningful life

■ Intellectual wellness ■ Emotional wellness ■ Physical wellness
■ Spiritual wellness □ Environmental wellness ■ Social wellness

Figure 2-6 The key to high-level wellness is in balancing all of the dimensions.

Physical Fitness

Physical fitness is your body's ability to meet the requirements and demands of your work and leisure activities. It is the ability to lift, bend, climb, and work without undue fatigue. Being physically fit will help the paramedic meet the physical and psychological demands associated with emergency medical service. In addition to job performance, physical fitness is of primary importance to the paramedic for the prevention of chronic diseases and improved quality of their personal lives.

What Is Physical Fitness?

There are two types of fitness: health-related fitness and skill-related fitness. The five components of health fitness include cardiovascular endurance, muscular strength, muscular endurance, muscular flexibility, and body composition. Skill-related fitness includes many components involved with athletic performance including agility, speed, power, stamina, balance, and coordination. Of prime importance for the paramedic is the development of health-related fitness. With that in mind, each of the components of health-related fitness and how you can develop them will be discussed. DOT 1-2.6

Cardiovascular endurance is the ability of the heart, lungs, and blood vessels to supply the muscles of the body with oxygen and fuel during prolonged exercise. Cardiovascular endurance is sometimes referred to as cardio-respiratory or aerobic endurance. Exercising aerobically over time strengthens your cardiovascular system. This occurs because the capacity of the cardiovascular system to use oxygen and other fuels improves. Basically, your system becomes more efficient. You can develop your cardio-respiratory endurance by participating in activities such as walking, jogging, swimming, cycling, aerobic dance, and many others.

Muscular strength is defined as the amount of force produced by a muscle during a single maximal contraction. In practical terms, it would be the amount of weight you could lift one time. Good muscular strength is necessary for the paramedic since virtually every emergency call involves some type of lifting.[3] Greater muscle mass also increases your metabolic rate, making it important to overall body composition. Muscular strength can be improved and maintained through various resistance training methods including free weights, weight machines, and resistance tubing.

Muscular endurance is the ability to contract your muscles repeatedly under sub-maximal resistance. It allows you to perform repeated movements without undue fatigue. It is important for good posture and injury prevention. Both everyday life and most leisure and fitness activities are enhanced by good muscle endurance. Muscular endurance is developed by stressing muscles with a greater load (weight) than they are used to.

Muscular flexibility involves the capacity to move your joints through their full range of motion. Proper muscular flexibility helps improve posture and reduce lower back problems. It is necessary for bending and lifting. You can improve and maintain your flexibility through stretching exercises, either as part of your regular exercise program or through classes such as yoga.

Body composition is defined as the ratio of your fat weight to your total body weight. It is usually expressed as the percentage of body fat. For you to have a healthy body composition, you should have a relatively low amount of body fat. Excessive body fat has been identified as a great threat to our health and well-being. It has been demonstrated to increase the risk leading to, accelerating, and exacerbating (worsening) many chronic diseases including heart disease, high blood pressure, and diabetes. The concepts of body weight, overweight, and obesity will be discussed later in this chapter.

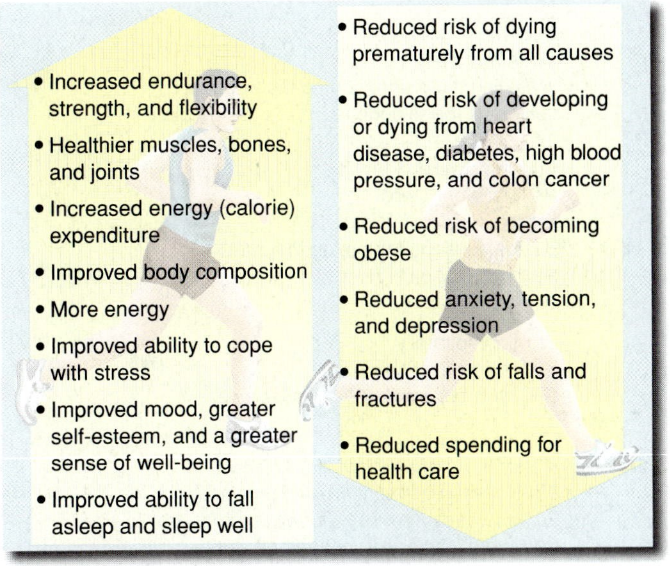

Benefits of Regular Physical Activity

The benefits of physical activity are far-reaching. On average, physically active people outlive those who are inactive.[24] Research has established the benefits of physical activity as well as the risks of inactivity.[25] Evidence has demonstrated that physical inactivity is a major risk factor for a variety of diseases including cardiovascular and metabolic diseases. A direct connection has been established between physical activity and lower death rates from heart attack, stroke, high blood pressure, diabetes, and some cancers. Physical activity has been shown to reduce stress as well as the effects of psychological conditions such as anxiety and depression. Further, exercise has been shown to improve motor performance in the elderly and reduce the effects of Alzheimer's disease.

For the paramedic, the benefits of exercise include increased energy levels and reduced stress levels for better job performance. Physical activity improves cardiovascular endurance and reduces the risk of heart and various other diseases. It also increases muscular strength, muscular endurance, and muscular flexibility which help to protect against injury, decrease back pain, and improve posture. Unless you perform regular strength exercises, you will lose up to one-half pound of muscle every year of life after the age of 25. Muscle is a very active tissue with high energy requirements, even when you are asleep; your muscles are responsible for over 25% of your calorie use. An increase in muscle tissue causes a corresponding increase in the number of calories your body will burn, even at rest.[6] Exercise can provide opportunities for social interaction as well as enjoyment for its own sake.[26] Figure 2-7 summarizes many of the benefits the paramedic can achieve with exercise.[4]

- Increased endurance, strength, and flexibility
- Healthier muscles, bones, and joints
- Increased energy (calorie) expenditure
- Improved body composition
- More energy
- Improved ability to cope with stress
- Improved mood, greater self-esteem, and a greater sense of well-being
- Improved ability to fall asleep and sleep well

- Reduced risk of dying prematurely from all causes
- Reduced risk of developing or dying from heart disease, diabetes, high blood pressure, and colon cancer
- Reduced risk of becoming obese
- Reduced anxiety, tension, and depression
- Reduced risk of falls and fractures
- Reduced spending for health care

Figure 2-7   Some of the benefits of exercise.

Beginning and Maintaining an Exercise Program

When seeking to incorporate physical activity into your life, several questions will probably come to mind. How much activity is enough? How can you fit exercise into a shift schedule? What sort of activity is appropriate?

Exercise and physical activity should fit into your life. Make choices based upon personal interests, personality, and lifestyle. The two most important considerations when establishing an exercise program are interest and convenience.[25] It should be something you want to do, an activity you enjoy or believe you would enjoy. Think about your preference for individual activities such as running versus group or class activities such as aerobic dance. Trying to exercise when you don't enjoy what you're doing tends to lead to a loss of interest and motivation.

Street Secrets

One way to get in some exercise is to work out with your fellow crewmembers. Play team sports such as basketball, volleyball, or softball while waiting for calls. Some EMS services provide exercise equipment or weight rooms for employees or have special arrangements with local gyms for on-duty crews. At a minimum, you should stretch for several minutes prior to the start of your shift and every few hours, particularly if you are not running a lot of calls. Use the back bumper of the ambulance to stretch against and practice taking the cot in and out of the ambulance a few times, performing deep knee bends while lifting it in and out.

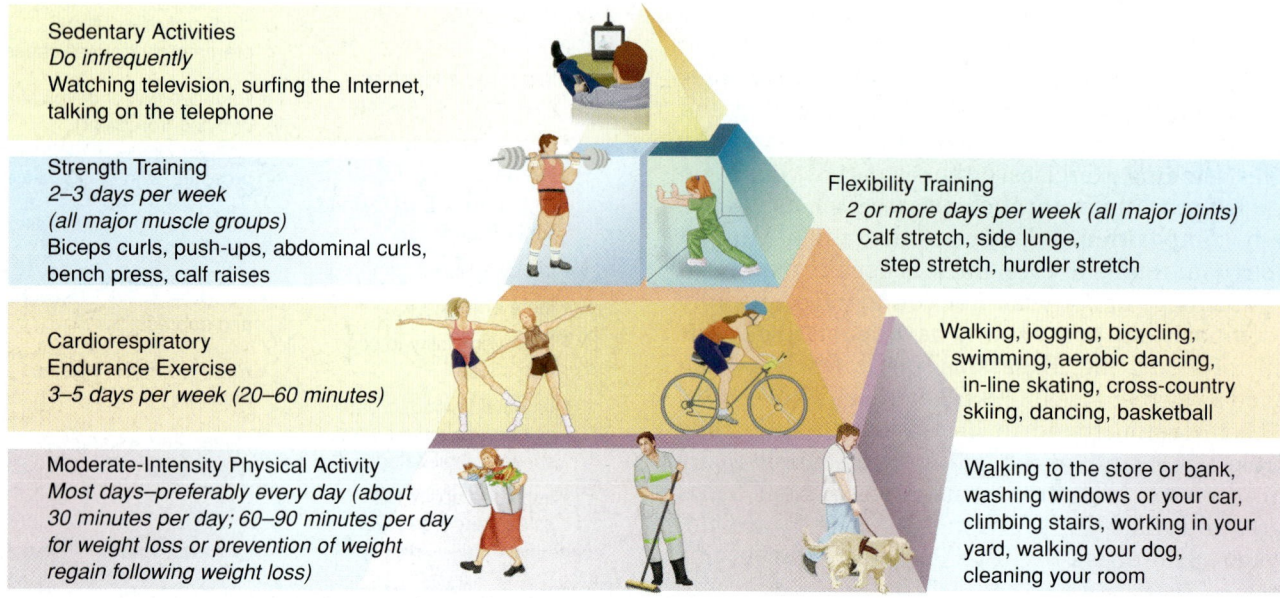

Sedentary Activities
Do infrequently
Watching television, surfing the Internet,
talking on the telephone

Strength Training
2–3 days per week
(all major muscle groups)
Biceps curls, push-ups, abdominal curls,
bench press, calf raises

Flexibility Training
2 or more days per week (all major joints)
Calf stretch, side lunge,
step stretch, hurdler stretch

Cardiorespiratory
Endurance Exercise
3–5 days per week (20–60 minutes)

Walking, jogging, bicycling,
swimming, aerobic dancing,
in-line skating, cross-country
skiing, dancing, basketball

Moderate-Intensity Physical Activity
Most days–preferably every day (about
30 minutes per day; 60–90 minutes per day
for weight loss or prevention of weight
regain following weight loss)

Walking to the store or bank,
washing windows or your car,
climbing stairs, working in your
yard, walking your dog,
cleaning your room

Figure 2-8 An activity pyramid can be helpful in seeing how much of each type of exercise to build into your exercise program.

You should find a time that is relatively convenient to your schedule. Nothing kills an exercise program faster than procrastination. To be successful, your exercise time should be a regular part of your daily schedule. Try to keep the same time for exercise each day if possible. Determine where physical activity fits into your schedule and stick to that time. Further considerations include the accessibility to facilities or equipment. For example, if you like to swim, you would obviously need a pool. Other considerations will include expense and other personal obligations that may require your time.

The U.S. government developed an activity pyramid to help in planning an exercise program. Review the pyramid in Figure 2-8 to see how you can incorporate the different aspects of physical fitness into your exercise program.[6]

Nutrition

Eating right is essential for growth, development, and improving and maintaining wellness. It is also important for reducing the risk of death or disability from chronic diseases. It has been estimated that dietary changes could reduce cancer deaths in the United States by as much as 35%.[27]

Dietary factors are an important consideration in preventable illnesses and premature deaths in the United States. Dietary factors are associated with four of the ten leading causes of death including cardiovascular disease, some types of cancer, stroke, and type 2 diabetes. These health conditions are estimated to cost society over $200 billion each year in medical expenses and lost productivity.[28] DOT 1-2.4

Components of a Healthy Diet

Food can be divided into different components based on how the body uses it. The body requires proteins, fats, carbohydrates, fiber, vitamins, minerals, and water. Carbohydrates and fats supply energy. Proteins help build muscles, hormones, enzymes, antibodies, and cell membranes as well as supplying energy when needed. Vitamins and minerals are essential in many chemical reactions and body functions. Fiber is important to the digestive process. All of the components of nutrition are found in the food you eat provided the diet is balanced.

Many dietary components are involved in the relationship between nutrition and health.[28] Consumption of too much saturated fat and too few vegetables, fruits, and grain products is of great concern. Only 3% of all individuals meet four of the five recommendations for the intake of grains, fruits, vegetables, milk products, and meat and bean food groups. Only one-fourth of U.S. adults eat the recommended numbers and types of servings of fruits and vegetables each day.[27]

Fat should supply no more than 25–30% of average total daily calories. This means no more than 65 grams of fat in a 2000-calorie-per-day diet. Complex carbohydrates should provide 55–65% of total daily calories. Simple carbohydrates should make up no more than 10–15% of the total calories. The recommended amount of protein is 10–15% of total daily calories.

Aim for fitness.

1. Aim for a healthy weight.
2. Be physically active each day.

Following these two guidelines will help keep you and your family healthy and fit. Healthy eating and regular physical activity enable people of all ages to work productively, enjoy life, and feel their best. They also help children grow, develop, and do well in school.

Build a healthy base.

3. Let the Pyramid guide your food choices.
4. Choose a variety of grains daily, especially whole grains.
5. Choose a variety of fruits and vegetables daily.
6. Keep food safe to eat.

Following these four guidelines builds a base for healthy eating. Let the Food Guide Pyramid guide you so that you get the nutrients your body needs each day. Make grains, fruits, and vegetables the foundation of your meals. This forms a base for good nutrition and good health and may reduce your risk of certain chronic diseases. Be flexible and adventurous—try new choices from these three groups in place of some less nutritious or higher calorie foods you usually eat. Whatever you eat, always take steps to keep your food safe to eat.

Choose sensibly.

7. Choose a diet that is low in saturated fat and cholesterol and moderate in total fat.
8. Choose beverages and foods to moderate your intake of sugars.
9. Choose and prepare foods with less salt.
10. If you drink alcoholic beverages, do so in moderation.

These four guidelines help you make sensible choices that promote health and reduce the risk of certain chronic diseases. You can enjoy all foods as part of a healthy diet as long as you don't overdo it on fat (especially saturated fat), sugars, salt, and alcohol. Read labels to identify foods that are higher in saturated fats, sugars and salt (sodium).

Figure 2-9 Follow an ABC approach to incorporate the 10 strategies for improving nutrition and wellness.

Street Secrets

The common practice in EMS is to drink a lot of coffee or other caffeinated beverages during long shifts. However, drinking caffeinated fluids actually dehydrates your body. If you are feeling thirsty, you are already dehydrated. Make sure you drink at least eight to twelve glasses of water every 24 hours. If you are working in a stressful, hot, or humid environment, you will need more.

Guidelines for Healthy Nutrition

Eating is essential to survival, is vital for health, and provides pleasurable experiences. Many people make poor or inappropriate choices which may mean a less than perfect diet. How do you make better choices for optimal nutrition?

The U.S. Department of Health and Human Services and the U.S. Department of Agriculture have established guidelines to provide direction in choosing a healthy diet.[29] "Dietary Guidelines for Americans" provides advice for people two years and older about positive dietary practices that promote health and reduce risk for major chronic diseases. The Dietary Guidelines are based upon three principles: 1) aim for fitness, 2) build a healthy base, and 3) make sensible choices. The Guidelines list ten simple strategies for improving nutrition and wellness. These are presented in Figure 2-9.

The Food Guide Pyramid

The **Food Guide Pyramid** is an outline of what to eat each day and is based on the principles of moderation, variety, and balance.[30] It is based on a recommended number of servings from the six food groups.

1. Breads, cereal, rice, and pasta should provide six to eleven servings.
2. Vegetables should provide three to five servings.
3. Fruit should provide two to four servings.
4. Milk, yogurt, and cheese should provide two to three servings.

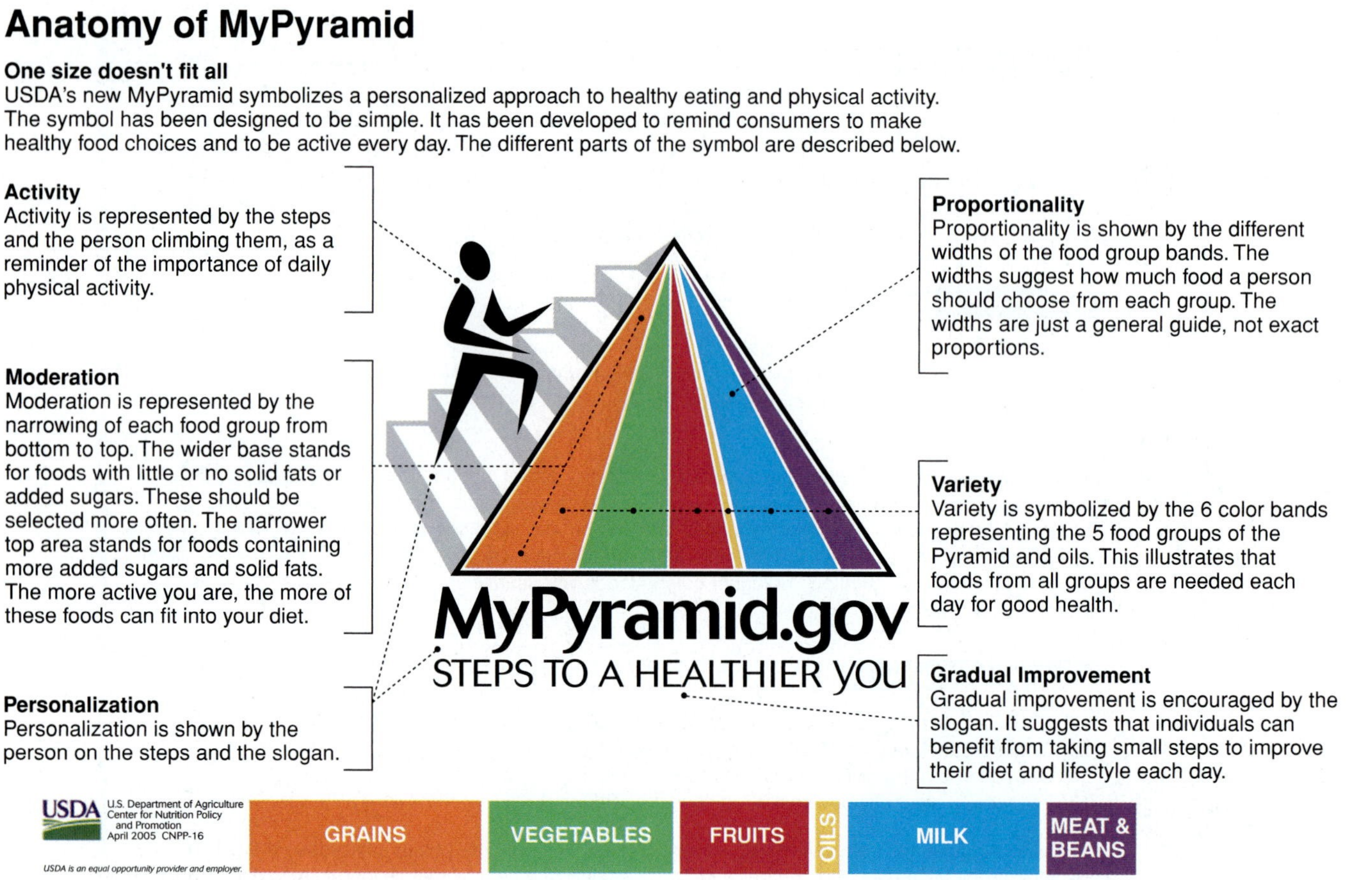

Anatomy of MyPyramid

One size doesn't fit all
USDA's new MyPyramid symbolizes a personalized approach to healthy eating and physical activity. The symbol has been designed to be simple. It has been developed to remind consumers to make healthy food choices and to be active every day. The different parts of the symbol are described below.

Activity
Activity is represented by the steps and the person climbing them, as a reminder of the importance of daily physical activity.

Moderation
Moderation is represented by the narrowing of each food group from bottom to top. The wider base stands for foods with little or no solid fats or added sugars. These should be selected more often. The narrower top area stands for foods containing more added sugars and solid fats. The more active you are, the more of these foods can fit into your diet.

Personalization
Personalization is shown by the person on the steps and the slogan.

Proportionality
Proportionality is shown by the different widths of the food group bands. The widths suggest how much food a person should choose from each group. The widths are just a general guide, not exact proportions.

Variety
Variety is symbolized by the 6 color bands representing the 5 food groups of the Pyramid and oils. This illustrates that foods from all groups are needed each day for good health.

Gradual Improvement
Gradual improvement is encouraged by the slogan. It suggests that individuals can benefit from taking small steps to improve their diet and lifestyle each day.

MyPyramid.gov
STEPS TO A HEALTHIER YOU

USDA
U.S. Department of Agriculture
Center for Nutrition Policy and Promotion
April 2005 CNPP-16
USDA is an equal opportunity provider and employer.

GRAINS VEGETABLES FRUITS OILS MILK MEAT & BEANS

Figure 2-10 The Food Guide Pyramid can help you make nutritious eating choices.

5. Meat, poultry, fish, dry beans, eggs, and nuts should provide two to three servings.
6. Fats, oils, and sweets should not replace foods from other groups; the total amounts consumed should be determined by overall needs.

Fruits and vegetables provide essential vitamins, minerals, and fiber associated with good health. Low fat diets rich in fiber-containing grain products, fruits, and vegetables may reduce the risk of heart disease and some types of cancer. Milk products provide protein, vitamins, and minerals and are the best source of calcium. Fats, oils, and sweets should be used sparingly since they provide calories and little else. Water is also essential to keeping hydrated, converting food into energy, carrying nutrients throughout the body, and removing waste.

The pyramid can be used to create food plans that meet all known nutritional needs. Figure 2-10 is the Food Guide Pyramid.[30] The United States Department of Agriculture provides the public with detailed information on using the Food Guide Pyramid for personal nutrition as well as tools for creating a healthy diet. These can be found at http://www.mypyramid.gov/. Go to this website; plug in your age, sex, and activity level; and you will receive your own "Pyramid Plan" with detailed information on the appropriate dietary needs, including

the number and size of portions, for you. There are also meal tracking worksheets and other tools to aid you in creating a healthy, well-balanced diet.

The American Diabetes Association has a free resource available through their website at https://www.diabetes.org/home.jsp. This resource applies to everyone, not just diabetics. Diabetes PHD (Personal Health Decisions) is a powerful new risk assessment tool used to explore the effects of a wide variety of health care interventions, including weight loss, smoking cessation, and taking certain medications.

Food Labels and Healthy Eating

Food labels are required for most packaged foods. In the "Nutrition Facts" panel on the label, manufacturers are required to provide information on certain nutrients (Figure 2-11).[31] Reading food labels helps you make better choices about what foods to use in your diet. All food labels list nutrient content by weight as well as amounts of fat, saturated fat, cholesterol, protein, dietary fiber, and sodium in each serving. Unpackaged foods such as meat, poultry, fruits, and vegetables do not have labels.[31]

The order in which information appears on the label is indicative of the importance of the particular dietary recommendation. The serving size provides

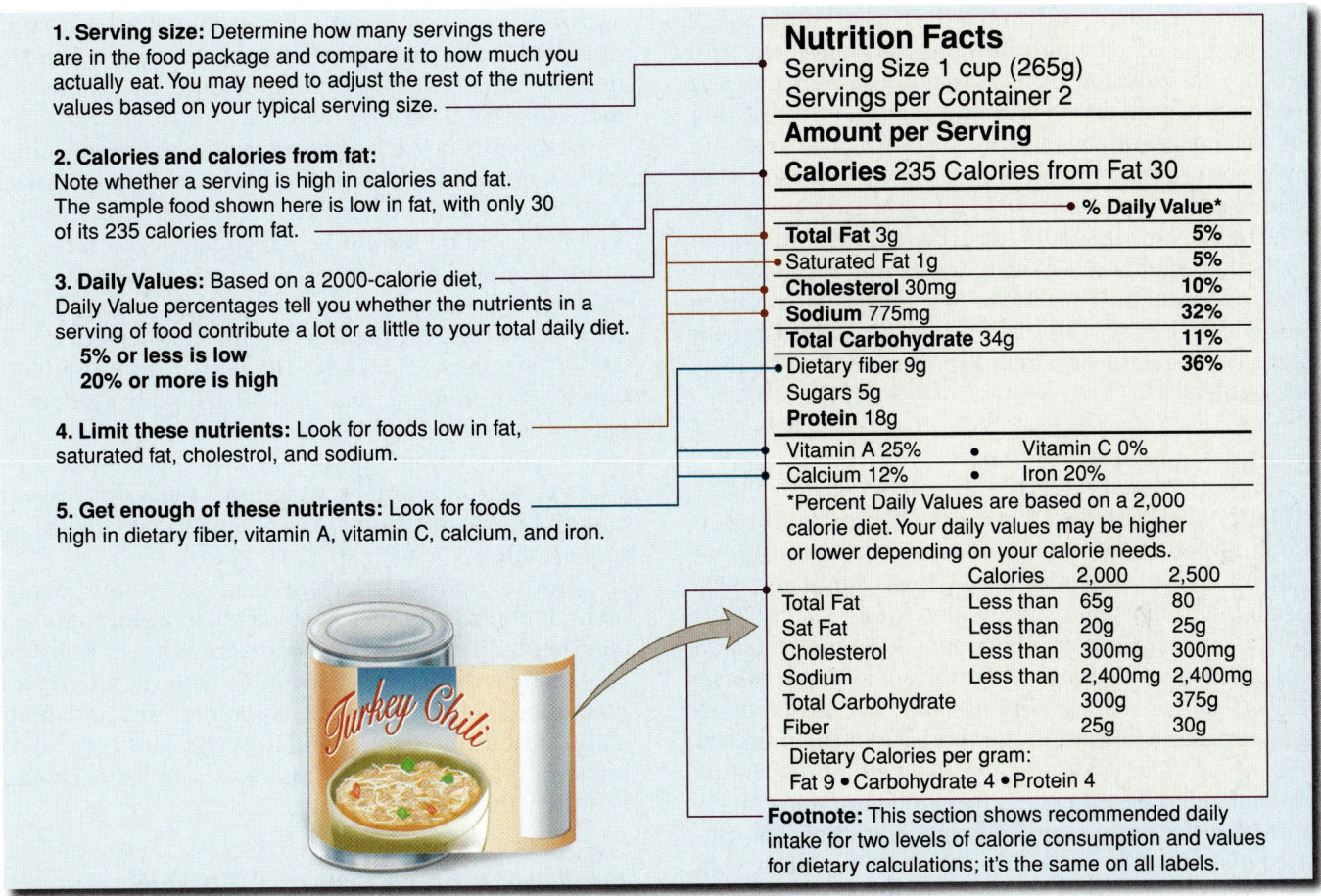

1. **Serving size:** Determine how many servings there are in the food package and compare it to how much you actually eat. You may need to adjust the rest of the nutrient values based on your typical serving size.

2. **Calories and calories from fat:** Note whether a serving is high in calories and fat. The sample food shown here is low in fat, with only 30 of its 235 calories from fat.

3. **Daily Values:** Based on a 2000-calorie diet, Daily Value percentages tell you whether the nutrients in a serving of food contribute a lot or a little to your total daily diet.
   5% or less is low
   20% or more is high

4. **Limit these nutrients:** Look for foods low in fat, saturated fat, cholestrol, and sodium.

5. **Get enough of these nutrients:** Look for foods high in dietary fiber, vitamin A, vitamin C, calcium, and iron.

Nutrition Facts
Serving Size 1 cup (265g)
Servings per Container 2

Amount per Serving

Calories 235 Calories from Fat 30

% Daily Value*

Total Fat 3g	5%
Saturated Fat 1g	5%
Cholesterol 30mg	10%
Sodium 775mg	32%
Total Carbohydrate 34g	11%
Dietary fiber 9g	36%
Sugars 5g	
Protein 18g	

Vitamin A 25%	•	Vitamin C 0%
Calcium 12%	•	Iron 20%

*Percent Daily Values are based on a 2,000 calorie diet. Your daily values may be higher or lower depending on your calorie needs.

		Calories	2,000	2,500
Total Fat	Less than		65g	80
Sat Fat	Less than		20g	25g
Cholesterol	Less than		300mg	300mg
Sodium	Less than		2,400mg	2,400mg
Total Carbohydrate			300g	375g
Fiber			25g	30g

Dietary Calories per gram:
Fat 9 • Carbohydrate 4 • Protein 4

Footnote: This section shows recommended daily intake for two levels of calorie consumption and values for dietary calculations; it's the same on all labels.

Figure 2-11   Learn to read the label. Lots of valuable information is available here.

the basis for the nutritional information found on the label. The Daily Value (DV) is the amount of a particular nutrient you should be getting each day. The percent Daily Value (% DV) provides consumers an easy way to determine how much of that particular nutrient is found in the food. The ingredient list is another part of the food label that is important for consumers to use. The U.S. Department of Agriculture requires a list on all foods that have more than one ingredient. Each of the ingredients is listed in descending order from largest to smallest amount of that ingredient found in the food.

Eating on the Go

The paramedic often works long and irregular hours. The opportunity to eat food that is prepared in a healthy manner may be limited during work hours. As a paramedic, you will have to be especially careful to manage your nutrition away from home.

Be careful about quick and easy sources of food including fast food restaurants, vending machines, and convenience stores. Develop good strategies for meeting your nutritional needs on the go. Plan your meals ahead

of time. Pack your lunch. Pack healthy snacks that are low in calories, fat, and sugar.

Here are some guidelines for packing meals and snacks.[32] Make sure to use a freezer gel pack in an insulated cooler to ensure that food will stay at 40 degrees Fahrenheit or below. Any food kept above that temperature should be eaten within two hours. Fill resealable bags with raw vegetables such as bell peppers, carrot sticks, cauliflower, broccoli, and snow peas. Apple slices with a sprinkle of lemon juice, bananas, a small bunch (a small handful) of seedless grapes, and small boxes of raisins are also good choices. Take along the single-portion sizes of boxed or canned foods. Low-sodium vegetable juice, individual packages of fat-free milk, and low-sodium instant soups are all recommended. You can always fill a thermos with canned or homemade soup. Small boxes of ready-to-eat cereal, dried fruits, whole-grain crackers, and vacuum-packed tuna are great for packed meals. Stock your home pantry with single servings of nutritious non-perishable foods so you can "grab and run" if you are in a hurry instead of stopping for fast food along the way.

The U.S. Department of Agriculture provides recommendations for times you are unable to prepare your meals at home and must purchase your food.[33] Watch portion sizes when purchasing food at the grocery store or ordering from a restaurant. When at the grocery store, plan ahead and buy enough nutrient-rich foods for meals and snacks for the entire week to avoid impulse buying when you are hungry. Get a sandwich on whole-grain bread instead of white bread. Drink only low-fat/fat-free milk, water, or other drinks that do not have added sugars. In a restaurant, opt for steamed, grilled, or broiled dishes instead of those that are fried or sautéed. When working a long shift, pack fresh fruit and cut-up vegetables to avoid impulsive, less healthy snack choices.

Weight Control

The National Health and Nutritional Examination Survey conducted from 1999 to 2002 found that approximately 65% of all U.S. adults were overweight and 30% were obese.[4] This same survey also found that 16% of children and adolescents between the ages of 6 and 19 years old were also overweight. High fat, high calorie diets and physical inactivity are the two most important factors contributing to the increase in the numbers of overweight and obese people in this country. Being overweight or obese is a major risk factor for certain chronic diseases and conditions such as diabetes, cardiovascular disease, unhealthy cholesterol levels, impaired heart function, hypertension, cancer, and other disorders.[34] Obesity may also lead to depression, low self-esteem, and eating disorders.

The words over-fat, overweight, and obese are often used interchangeably. However, they are not the same. Overweight refers to an excess of body weight that includes all tissues such as fat, bone, and muscle. Over-fat refers to an excess of body fat. Obesity refers specifically to an extreme excess of body fat. It is possible to be overweight without being obese, as with a football player who has a substantial amount of muscle mass. It is possible to be over-fat without being overweight, as in the case of a very sedentary person who is within the desirable weight range but who nevertheless has an excess amount of body fat. However, many overweight people are also obese, and vice versa.[35]

Energy in the form of calories comes from food and is used for fueling body reactions (metabolism), for digestion, and for fueling physical activity. One pound of fat equals 2,700 to 3,500 calories, depending on several factors including fitness, weight, and gender. A calorie is a measure of the amount of energy stored in your body, typically in the form of fat. Maintaining, gaining, or losing weight is based on the simple concept of energy balance or imbalance.

Because fat contains more calories than either carbohydrates or protein (9 calories per gram for fat as compared with 4 calories per gram for carbohydrates

and protein), it is usually the focus of weight control diets. Reducing fat in your diet will also reduce the total number of calories. Fat intake should be limited to no more than 30% of total calories.

Alcoholic beverages provide no nutritional value, in other words "empty calories," and contain 7 calories per gram. If you do consume alcohol, one way of controlling your weight would be to reduce or eliminate your alcohol intake.

Weight control is based on controlling calorie balance as well as on making healthy choices every day. Avoid fad diets, especially those that do not advocate variety, moderation, and balance in the food groups eaten. Be wary of weight control or weight loss diets that exclude whole components or types of food such as severe carbohydrate restrictions. Such diets may not contain all the nutrients you need and may be difficult to maintain.

Limiting portion sizes is crucial to weight management; it may also be an easier way to monitor intake than calorie-counting. Protein or carbohydrates consumed in excess will be stored by the body as fat. Keeping your diet high in complex carbohydrates and moderate in protein is recommended for weight control. Eating small, frequent meals four to six times each day is healthier than skipping meals. DOT 1-2.5

The Rhythms of Life and Shift Work

You were meant to sleep at night and work during the day. The responsibilities of a paramedic's job may require that you sleep during the day and work at night, or worse, alternate shifts so that sometimes you are sleeping at night and other times during the day. In general, following these types of patterns is problematic. Shift-work is a significant source of stress for the paramedic.

Emergency services are provided to the public 24 hours a day, 7 days a week. Because of this, paramedics are often required to work 8-, 10-, 12-, or 24-hour shifts. There are some EMS services that use 48- to 96-hour shifts. Also, if your service provides emergency response in addition to routine response, you may be required to extend your work shift into the next one or come in at a time other than your usual shift to assist in the event of a disaster or multiple casualty incident. Shift-work has been shown to be associated with hypertension, cardiovascular disease, obesity, increased triglycerides, impaired glucose tolerance, increased sleep disorders, increased risk of accidents, greater use of health care services, interference of social life and social problems, and increased psychological problems.[36]

For years, the transportation sector has recognized how important sleep and rest are and how much the lack of sleep and fatigue affects safety. For this reason, tough federal laws are in place outlining how many hours a truck driver can drive before a mandatory rest or sleep cycle must occur. In recent years, a number of states have considered legislation to limit the use of mandatory overtime for health care workers, but to date, no state has enacted any law preventing it.

In April, 2004, the Centers for Disease Control (CDC) Office of Workplace Safety and Health published a document on overtime and extended work shifts. The intent was to pull together any recent research on the effects of overtime and long work shifts on illness, injury, and health. The researchers found 52 studies published between 1995 and 2002 from 15 countries. Only five studies came from the United States. The studies looked at various aspects of the issues of overtime and shift work in a variety of professions. The researchers defined overtime as working more than 40 hours per week and an extended work shift as any that was longer than 8 hours.

It is difficult to draw significant conclusions from these studies because they examined so many different variables, but some trends seemed to emerge from the information. Here are some of the findings:[37]

- Sixteen of 22 studies addressing general health effects believed overtime was associated with a perception of poorer general health, increased injury rates, more illness, or increased mortality
- In two studies overtime was associated with unhealthy weight gain
- In four studies of workers of 12-hour shifts, after nine hours workers experienced decreased alertness, increased fatigue, lower cognitive function, difficulty keeping focused while performing a task, and increased injuries (No studies like this were done on workers on shifts longer than 12 hours.)
- Two studies examining physician performance found deterioration of cognitive performance after 12 hours into very long shifts
- Two studies comparing 12-hour day and night shifts found the night shift workers reported more fatigue, smoking, and alcohol use
- Two studies in Japan found a twofold increase in the number of heart attacks in workers who reported working 61 or more hours per week or who had taken less than two days off per month
- One study reported upper extremity fatigue in workers who worked four 12-hour night shifts per week

A person tends to function best when maintaining a normal 40-hour work week, working during the day and sleeping at night. This cycle is termed a circadian rhythm.[37] Your circadian rhythm is also referred to as your biological clock. The timing of your own biological clock occurs in three ways. The first way is by the schedule of your meals. The second is through your social interactions and scheduled activities. The third

TABLE 2-2   Epworth Sleepiness Scale

Situation	Chance of dozing
Sitting and reading	_____
Watching TV	_____
Sitting inactive in a public place (like a movie theatre)	_____
As a car passenger riding for an hour without a break	_____
Lying down to rest in the afternoon	_____
Sitting and talking with someone	_____
Sitting quietly after lunch (without alcohol)	_____
In a car, while stopped for a few minutes at a traffic light	_____

Score each block as follows:

0 = Would never doze

1 = Slight chance of dozing

2 = Moderate chance of dozing

3 = High chance of dozing

Results: A score of 10 is definite cause for concern as it indicates significant daytime sleepiness.

Source: From the Nebraska Rural Health and Safety Coalition. Funded by a grant from the W.K. Kellogg Foundation. Nebraska Rural Health and Safety Coalition, University of Nebraska.

and most dominant force influencing your biological clock is the sun. DOT 1-2.7

Not everyone, however, suffers ill-effects from the stress of shift-work. Some people tolerate this type of schedule better than others. However, even if you find the night shift tolerable, you should change the shift periodically so that you're not doing a night shift all the time.

Most adults need seven to eight hours of sleep per night.[38] The Epworth Sleepiness Scale is useful in determining if the amount of sleep is enough. Table 2-2 has the scale. People who are well-rested feel alert and do not have the urge to nap. Sleepiness may indicate sleep deprivation is present. People who are sleep deprived are more likely to have accidents in the early to mid-afternoon and in the very early morning hours. These are the times when everyone is the least alert. Fill out the scale for yourself. If you score higher than 10, it is a warning to you to try and get more sleep.

Stress

As reported by the National Institute for Occupational Safety and Health database at www.cdc.gov, on January 13, 2001, a 43-year-old fire fighter wearing turnout gear and self-contained breathing apparatus (SCBA) was working a fire. He vented the second story roof, entered the structure, and exited out the first floor on a normal rotation 15 minutes later. He reported to the ambulance and said he was feeling light-headed. He collapsed and died despite CPR and ACLS care. The coroner ruled the cause of death as hypertension, heart disease, and smoke inhalation after the autopsy revealed an enlarged heart and evidence of acute pulmonary edema. On December 13, 2002, a 29-year-old male EMT student was found dead in the bathroom. He had just finished taking the state EMT written exam. A heart attack was ruled as his cause of death. There was no evidence of drugs, alcohol, or stimulants in his body. On January 27, 2004, a 35-year-old male fire fighter paramedic collapsed after jogging one mile as part of the conditioning portion of an EMS training program. His cause of death was ruled atherosclerotic heart disease.

Everyone experiences stress. It is a constant force in everyone's life, and even when it isn't perceived, it is there. Excessive levels of stress and inability to deal with it in a healthy fashion have been shown to be a leading risk factor for many chronic diseases including heart disease, hypertension, ulcers, arthritis, diabetes, cancer, alcoholism, depression, and suicide. The cost of stress in the United States has been estimated at between $20 and $100 billion per year.[39]

What Is Stress?

While stress occurs in all aspects of life, job stress in particular is of concern for the EMS profession. The National Institute for Occupational Safety and Health defines **job stress** as "harmful physical and emotional responses that occur when requirements of the job do not match the capabilities, resources or needs of the worker."[40] Job stress can lead to poor health and even injuries. The Bureau of Labor and Statistics reports that workers who must take time off from work because of stress, anxiety, and other related causes are typically off work for 20 days.

Your body seeks to maintain a physiological and psychological balance. This balance is termed **homeostasis.** Your body makes constant adjustments to maintain homeostasis, and stress impacts this process by tending to keep the body away from homeostasis through constant stimulation.

Anything that results in chemical or emotional stimulation, and thus imbalance, is termed stress. The circumstance that causes stress is called a **stressor,** and the physiologic reaction to the stressor is the **stress response.** In general, stressors are identified as either positive or negative.

Eustress is stress which results in positive consequences, so it is sometimes called "good stress." **Distress** results in negative consequences. Whether it is eustress or distress, your body reacts in a similar fashion to both

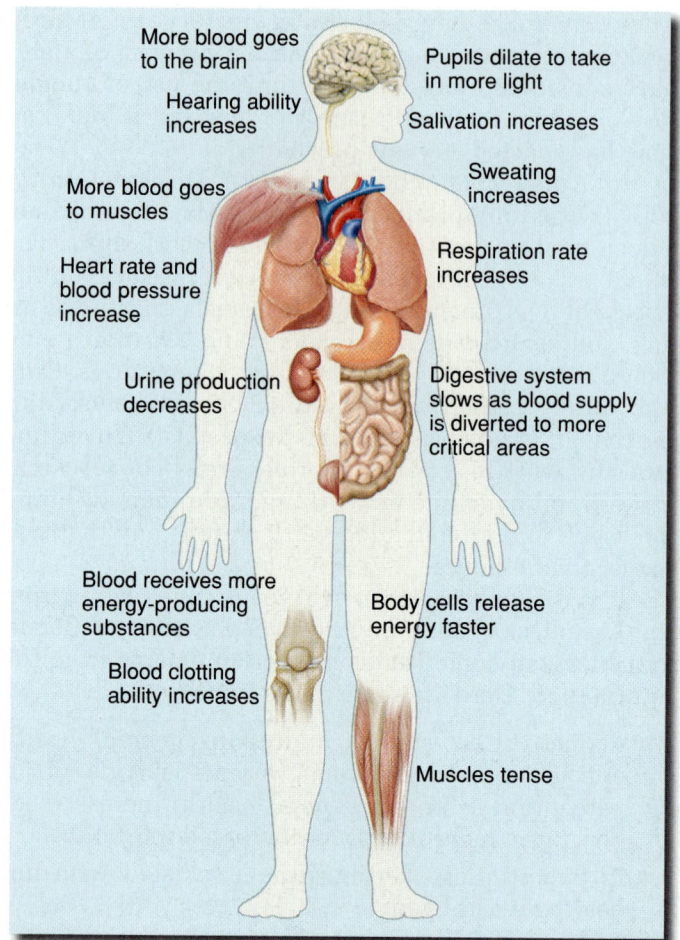

More blood goes to the brain

Hearing ability increases

More blood goes to muscles

Heart rate and blood pressure increase

Urine production decreases

Blood receives more energy-producing substances

Blood clotting ability increases

Pupils dilate to take in more light

Salivation increases

Sweating increases

Respiration rate increases

Digestive system slows as blood supply is diverted to more critical areas

Body cells release energy faster

Muscles tense

Figure 2-12   The body's response to triggering of the fight or flight response. This is the alarm phase of the GAS response.

forms of stressors. Another name for the stress response is the **fight-or-flight response.** The fight-or-flight response is the result of a set of physiological and psychological reactions to a stressful situation. These responses are illustrated in Figure 2-12. DOT 1-2.20

CONNECTIONS Chapter 8: Physiology Overview will discuss the fight-or-flight response in detail, including the connection it has to the autonomic nervous system and the impact it has upon body processes such as blood pressure and cardiac function.

Stress is a risk factor for many diseases and conditions. When stress is constant, your body is continuously subjected to the physiological and psychological reactions of the stress response. This can lead to many health problems. Chronic high blood pressure; atherosclerosis; cardiovascular disease; emotional problems; decreased immunity leading to colds, infections, asthma and allergies; cancer; and flare-ups of other chronic diseases can result from stress. Other health concerns related to excessive stress include headaches and migraines, insomnia and fatigue, injuries, complications during pregnancy, and psychological problems.[6]

The General Adaptation Syndrome

Early research on stress and the response to it was conducted by a scientist named Hans Selye. He called his theory of stress and its relationship to disease the **general adaptation syndrome** *or* **GAS.** The general adaptation syndrome involves three stages. The initial stage, *alarm,* occurs when the person is presented with a stressor. The alarm stage is the triggering of the fight-or-flight reaction. During the alarm stage, the heart rate and blood pressure increase and mental acuity increases. The person may feel anxious and may even sweat. The next stage, *resistance,* occurs when a person develops a new level of homeostasis to deal with the sustained level of added stress. Some people never stop living on the edge because they continue to add stimulation to their body. Caffeine, smoking, and adrenalin-producing activities all continue to stress the body. Like a drug, over time this changes the person so they begin to "need" to have that same level of stress to function. Eventually the effect of all stressors wears off (if they don't kill you first), and this is when the *exhaustion* stage sets in. The exhaustion stage, as described by Selye, results in the depletion of resources which not only leaves the body vulnerable to disease, but also weakens its ability to respond to the next stressor that comes along. It is now believed that, over time, the stress response itself is a cause of disease (Box 2-1). DOT 1-2.17, 1-2.19

Signs of Stress

Early warning signs of job stress include: headache, sleep disturbances, difficulty concentrating, short temper, upset stomach, job dissatisfaction, and low morale.[40]

The **National Institute for Occupational Safety and Health (NIOSH)** identifies both worker characteristics and working conditions that contribute to stress. The

experts do not yet agree which element is more important, but they do agree that both play a role as the two primary causes of job stress. The following six job conditions are identified by the NIOSH as the leading causes of stress:[41]

- The design of tasks (a heavy workload, infrequent breaks, shift work and long working hours, and situations that provide little sense of control)
- Management style (lack of participation by workers in decision-making, poor communication in organizations, and lack of family-friendly policies)
- Interpersonal relationships (a poor social environment with a lack of support or help from coworkers and supervisors)
- Work roles (conflicting or uncertain job expectations, too much responsibility, or doing too many tasks)
- Career concerns (job insecurity; lack of opportunity for growth, advancement, or promotion; rapid changes for which the workers are unprepared)
- Environmental conditions (unpleasant or dangerous physical conditions such as crowding, noise, air pollution, or ergonomic problems) DOT 1-2.18, 1-2.20

Ninety-nine percent of your body's response to stress is related to your perception of the stressor. Except for certain disease-causing agents and toxins, the way you see the stressor accounts for the intensity of your stress response to a particular stress situation.

Any major life change, whether positive or negative, can be a source of stress. The presence of multiple stressors has been associated with various health problems. Everyday hassles and problems often accumulate and cause stress-related troubles. Money and time issues can contribute to the stress. Changes in interpersonal relationships and establishing new relationships are sources of stress. Prejudice and discrimination are forms of stress created by the community and society. Even though EMS is more stressful than many other careers, many paramedics do not believe they are affected by a high level of stress. This is called *unrealistic optimism.* Unrealistic optimism can lead to an inability to assess problems (because of a lack of awareness of them) and inability to cope effectively with them.

Identifying Sources of Stress Found in the EMS Profession

A review of the six causes of stress listed previously reveals that many of the characteristics are inherent in the EMS profession. One of the most prominent stressors in the EMS profession is the responsibility for the life and safety of others.[41]

Low pay; conflicts with management or coworkers; lack of respect from other health care professionals; old, outdated, and poorly maintained equipment and

---

BOX 2-1 The General Adaptive Syndrome

The GAS has three phases:

1. Alarm
2. Resistance
3. Exhaustion

If an intervention occurs to stop any stage, the entire GAS response can be stopped—reducing the stress level. For the best results, the intervention should happen before stage three occurs.

vehicles; and lack of sleep have all been identified as stressors for the emergency services worker.

The environment in which the paramedic must work is filled with stress. Sirens, cries for help, moans of pain, angry or threatening voices, blaring sirens, and roaring engines are examples of noise stressors in the emergency environment. Weather conditions can add aggravation to the stress of the environment. Emergency driving, traffic, and crowds can be frustrating. Dealing with hazardous materials, waiting on scene for additional assistance, or intoxicated and abusive patients or bystanders can add tension to the emergency services workers' environment. DOT 1-2.22

When the stress experienced by paramedics becomes overwhelming, they may experience "burnout." If you reflect back on the GAS model discussed earlier, burnout is a typical presentation of phase three, exhaustion. Burnout affects the mental and physical health of paramedics as well as their ability to perform the duties of their job.[43] It usually occurs as a result of overwork—too many shifts, too many hours on shift, and not enough time to rest and recuperate. The effects of burnout have been documented.[41] They can include high job turnover, increased absenteeism, and low morale as well as physical exhaustion, insomnia, increased substance abuse, and marital and family problems. Burnout leads to a decrease in the quality of care provided to patients.

Managing Your Stress

The goal of stress management is to reduce the physiological and emotional impact of stress. This can be achieved through the use of strategies which will help control your stress in three ways. One, reduce the physiological effects of stress on your body, or "quiet the internal" environment. Second, "quiet" the external environment to help manage those stressors. Third, learn to adjust perceptions and emotional responses to stress-causing events. The NIOSH report on job stress noted that jobs that were viewed as "challenging" by employees did not result in distress or eustress to the workers. Challenges at work served to energize and motivate the employees and resulted in them reporting feeling relaxed instead of stressed.[40] DOT 1-2.23

Learning relaxation techniques helps to reduce the impact stress has on your body and your mind. Perhaps the simplest and easiest method for relaxing is through deep breathing. Begin by taking slow and deep breathes. Focus on breathing, imagining that you are pushing the air you inhale down to the bottom of the lungs. This simple technique will help to reduce the stressor's effects and help you to function better.

Learning additional relaxation methods and maintaining healthy lifestyle behaviors will help decrease the impact of the stress response. Additionally, learning other relaxation techniques such as biofeedback, progressive relaxation, Tai Chi, meditation, and visual imagery are highly recommended. These methods help cushion the consequences of high levels of stress. Beginning or continuing a hobby or recreational pursuit will also provide a means of relaxation and stress release.

Healthy nutrition habits, especially limiting the intake of caffeine, fat, and sugar, is vital to your ability to deal with stress. Physical activity is essential to controlling both short- and long-term impacts of stress. We know that regular exercise will reduce your stress response. Other healthy practices such as getting enough sleep help to quiet the internal environment.

Learn effective time management. Develop a time management plan. Make short- and long-term goals and decide your priorities. Most importantly, establish a schedule. Keep a calendar for your extended schedule and a daily to do list. Make sure you schedule exercise as well as recreation. Don't forget to schedule quiet time as well. Every waking moment of the day does not have to be scheduled. Rest and recuperation is just as important as work. Avoid overextending your schedule by trying to take on too many tasks. Learn to say "no" without feeling guilty.

Your perception of stressors can help improve how you deal with stress. Paramedics face many negative stressors. It is vital that you keep a positive attitude and maintain your sense of humor. Learn to "let things go" that you have no control over. Be realistic in your expectations of performance for yourself and your co-workers. Develop your critical thinking and problem solving skills. The better prepared you are to perform your job the better you will feel about it and the less stress it will cause.

Seek help when you feel overwhelmed. Find a mentor and share your concerns with that person. A mentor is someone you trust and respect and is someone who has your best interests in mind. A mentor will guide you in the right direction. A mentor will not always tell you what you want to hear but will tell you what you need to hear. Select somebody you want to be like, who has strong values and a good moral character. This relationship should go both directions, with both of you growing and developing from the experience. The person you choose does not have to be a member of the health care team, but if they are you can benefit from their experience in EMS. DOT 1-2.26

Learning to Live with Death and Dying

Death occurs when the body is no longer able to function. Traditionally, death was defined as occurring when the heart stopped beating and respiration ceased. Resuscitation techniques have proven that not to be true in all cases. Presently, death is believed to occur when the brain ceases to function. Even though death may be defined in clinical terms, it affects your social, emotional, and spiritual well-being.

As a paramedic, some of the most severe causes of stress will be the line-of-duty death of a coworker, a child, or sometimes even the death of any adult. In this profession, death is something you may come face-to-face with on a regular basis. It is important to be aware of how both the patients and their family members could respond to impending death or death. Even if a patient has a terminal disease, the patient may be experiencing fear and anxiety. It is possible the dying patient will express emotions of anger, guilt, depression, and hostility. These strong emotions may be directed at you or your team. When dealing with patients, remain calm. Be honest about the seriousness of their conditions. Speak with hope, avoiding negative statements that may exacerbate their emotional states. Do not make false reassurances or claims that "everything is going to be alright." Instead, reassure them that you are giving them the best care you can, and allow them to talk and vent their feelings. One of the most important things you can say in these situations is "I'm sorry." DOT 1-2.27

If the situation allows, you may give patients some time alone with their loved ones so they can say good-bye in private. Stay close by to provide support to the family. In most states, any death that occurs outside of the hospital setting is required to have law enforcement presence to ensure that no crime has been committed. Even if the death is expected, as when the patient has a terminal illness and is under hospice care, law enforcement should be called to the scene to take a formal report and record the time of death. In these situations, it may be appropriate to remain at the scene

and render emotional support to the family members and friends. They may need direction to call the funeral home or call other family members to the scene. In the immediate minutes following a death, the loved ones will not be able to make good decisions or stay focused. They are overwhelmed with thoughts of what just happened, their past, and their future. Compassion displayed by the EMS team can help them gather their thoughts and focus their attention.

When dealing with grieving family members, always be sincere and supportive. Realize that the family, like the patient, may also be angry, hostile, depressed, or resentful. Also, you should be aware of the grieving process the family members may be going through. Figure 2-13 illustrates the stages of the grieving process. It is important to recognize that personal and cultural customs will impact how an individual expresses emotions during the grieving process. DOT 1-2.28

CONNECTIONS Chapter 48: Patients from Diverse Cultures will discuss the implications of culture on all aspects of caring for patients, including dealing with patients and families in the grief process. It is important to remember that different cultures view death in different ways. Some celebrate it, and others are grief stricken. Some do not show emotions, and others may seem to exaggerate their responses. Try not to feel embarrassed, surprised, or alarmed when dealing with their emotional responses.

Especially difficult for the paramedic will be the care of a critically ill or dying child. The death of a child is tragic for both the child's family and the EMS team. Allow a parent or relative to remain with the child, if

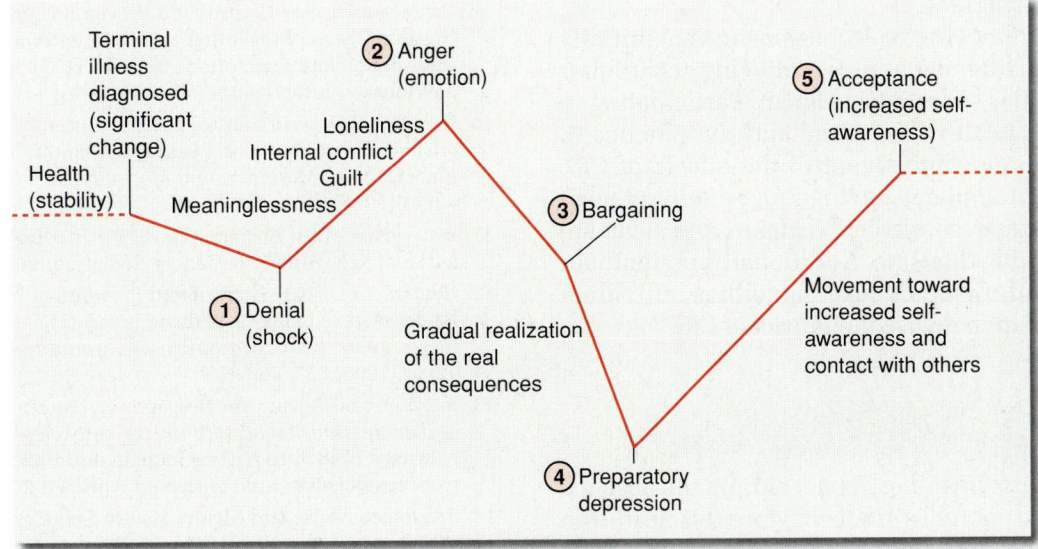

Figure 2-13 The stages of death and dying. Remember, not all patients exhibit all of these behaviors or go through the process in this order. This is the most common path people take when grieving.

possible. Never refer to the child as "the deceased" or "the body." Use the patient's name whenever possible. Inform the family of what happened in clear, jargon-free language, answer questions tactfully and honestly, and provide as much information as possible without jeopardizing an investigation. It is important to use the words "dead" and "death" instead of "passed on," "crossed over," or any of the other phrases commonly used instead of "death." DOT 1-2.29

Physical contact can be very comforting, but take your cues from the people on the scene. If they move towards you like they need to be hugged, hug them. Do not be afraid to offer comfort, such as a shoulder on which to cry. Ask the parents if they would like to have someone contacted to assist them such as a relative, clergy member, neighbor, coworker, or grief specialist.[43] The death of a child may lead to critical incidence stress for the paramedic.

Critical Incident Stress

Events that elicit strong emotional reactions for the paramedic are termed critical incidents. The great stress that these events can bring forth can create lasting effects for the paramedic and is termed **critical incident stress (CIS)**. CIS is also known as traumatic stress, combat fatigue, and rapid onset burnout. Such events are uncommon.

Short term responses to CIS can include various psychological and physical symptoms.[43] These can include hand tremors, chin and lip shakes, headaches, and stomach distress. Jumpiness, over alertness, over protectiveness, and social withdrawal are also symptoms. CIS can lead to weakened thought processes, reduced judgment, and loss of job skills. If not treated, the experience of CIS can lead to **Post-Traumatic Stress Disorder (PTSD)** which in turn may lead to substance abuse, alcoholism, depression, and suicide.

Critical Incident Stress Management can initially involve many of the same stress-relieving techniques practiced in regular stress management. Participating in regular exercise, healthy nutrition, and the practice of relaxation techniques helps control the effects of CIS. Making and keeping plans, having fun, remaining positive, and avoiding drugs, alcohol, caffeine, and sugar are all important during this time. Additionally, preincident education and follow-up counseling (either individual or family) may help to defuse the impact of CIS.[44] DOT 1-2.24

Summary

Wellness is a choice. Wellness is not simply the absence of disease; it also includes life behaviors that lead to a good quality of life. Wellness encompasses many aspects of a life, including physical, emotional, intellectual, social, environmental and spiritual dimensions, and job satisfaction. High-level wellness occurs when a person

has attained wellness in nearly all of these areas and is able to maintain and sustain that balance. This occurs only when poor behavior choices are removed and replaced by healthy choices. Healthy choices include eliminating the use of tobacco and drugs, using alcohol in moderation (or eliminating it completely), minimizing or avoiding stimulants such as caffeine, maintaining the proper body weight, eating a nutritious diet, exercising regularly, managing stress, and getting enough recuperative sleep and relaxation. Stress causes cardiovascular disease, stroke, and many other diseases. The paramedic is exposed to stress on a regular basis. In order to perform at optimal levels, managing stress is critically important. It is the best choice to make if you want a long and healthy career in EMS.

Notes

1. U.S. Department of Transportation National Highway Traffic Safety Administration. *EMT-Paramedic National Standard Curriculum* (Washington, DC: Government Printing Office, 1998).
2. Emergency Medical Technicians and Paramedics, http://www.bls.gov/oco/pdf/ocos101.pdf (accessed April 11, 2006).
3. DOT NHTSA EMT-Paramedic National Standard Curricula. *Job Description for the Paramedic* (1997).
4. T. D. Fahey, P. M. Insel, and W. T. Roth, *Fit & Well: Core Concepts and Labs in Physical Fitness and Wellness Brief Edition,* 6th ed. (New York: McGraw-Hill 2004).
5. Centers for Disease Control, National Center for Health Statistics. "Deaths: Preliminary Data for 2003." *National Vital Statistics Reports* 53 (February 28, 2005): 15.
6. P. M. Insel and W. T. Roth, *Core Concepts in Health,* 10th ed. (New York: McGraw-Hill, 2005).
7. W. W. K. Hoeger, and S. A. Hoeger, *Principles and Labs for Fitness and Wellness* (Belmont, CA: Thomson Wadsworth, 2005).
8. T. A. Murphy and D. Murphy, *The Wellness for Life Workbook* (San Diego: Fitness Publications, 1987).
9. Center for Disease Control and Prevention, National Center for Chronic Disease Prevention and Health Promotion. Tobacco Information and Preventions Source (TIPS). http://www.cdc.gov/tobacco/hlthcon.htm (accessed April 11, 2006).
10. Centers for Disease Control and Prevention. "Smoking-attributable mortality and years of potential life lost—United States, 1990." *Morbidity and Mortality Weekly Report* 42(33)(1993):645-8.
11. American Cancer Society, *Cancer Facts & Figures—1996* (Atlanta, GA: American Cancer Society, 1996).
12. Centers for Disease Control and Prevention. "Mortality trends for selected smoking-related and breast cancer—United States, 1950–1990." *Morbidity and Mortality Weekly Report* 42(44)(1993):857, 863–6.
13. International Agency for Research on Cancer (IARC). *Summaries and evaluations tobacco products, smokeless (Group 1).* February 1998. http://www.inchem.org/documents/iarc/suppl7/tobaccosmokeless.html (accessed April 11, 2006).
14. Substance Abuse and Mental Health Services Administration. *Results from the 2004 National Survey on Drug Use and Health. Detailed Tables.* Rockville, MD: Substance Abuse and Mental Health Services Administration, Office of Applied Studies; 2005. http://oas.samhsa.gov/nhsda/2k3tabs/Sect2peTabs1to56.htm#tab2.39b (accessed April 11, 2006).

15. Centers for Disease Control & Prevention. Youth Risk Behavior Surveillance—United States, 2003. *CDC Surveillance Summaries 2004* 53(SS–2):1–96.

16. Centers for Disease Control & Prevention. Tobacco use, access, and exposure to tobacco in media among middle and high school students—United States, 2004. *Morbidity and Mortality Weekly Report* 54(12)(2005):297–301.

17. U.S. Environmental Protection Agency. *Respiratory Health Effects of Passive Smoking: Lung Cancer and Other Disorders* (Washington, DC: U.S. Environmental Protection Agency, Office of Health and Environmental Assessment, Office of Research and Development, 1992).

18. Centers for Disease Control & Prevention. "Annual smoking-attributable mortality, years of potential life lost, and economic costs—United States, 1995–1999." *Morbidity and Mortality Weekly Report* 51(14)(2002):300–303.

19. American Heart Association. (2005). Smoking Cessation. http://www.americanheart.org/presenter.jhtml?identifier=4731 (accessed April 11, 2006).

20. Agency for Health Research and Quality. (2000). You Can Quit Smoking Consumer Guide. http://www.ahrq.gov/consumer/tobacco/quits.htm (accessed April 11, 2006).

21. American Cancer Society. (2005). Detailed Guide: Cancer. http://www.cancer.org/docroot/CRI/CRI_2_3x.asp?dt=72 (accessed April 11, 2006).

22. World Health Organization (2003). WHO Definition of Health. http://www.who.int/about/definition/en/ (accessed April 11, 2006).

23. President's Council of Physical Fitness and Sports, *Toward a Uniform Definition of Wellness: A Commentary* 3 (December 2001): 15.

24. Centers for Disease Control and Prevention. (2001). Healthy People 2010, Chapter 22. http://www.healthypeople.gov/Document/HTML/Volume2/22Physical.htm (accessed April 11, 2006).

25. J. M. Johnson & S. D. Ballin, "Surgeon General's Report on Physical Activity and Health Is Hailed as a Historic Step Toward a Healthier Nation." *Circulation* 94 (1996):2045.

26. V. Pierson, Starting an Exercise Program. http://primusweb.com/fitnesspartner/library/activity/startexercise.htm (accessed July 24, 2006).

27. HealthierUS.gov (2005). Nutrition. Eat a Nutritious Diet. http://www.healthierus.gov/nutrition.html (accessed April 11, 2006).

28. Food and Drug Administration & National Institutes of Health. (2001). http://www.healthypeople.gov/Document/pdf/Volume2/19Nutrition.pdf (accessed April 11, 2006).

29. U.S. Department of Health and Human Services & U.S. Department of Agriculture. (2005). Aim . . . Build . . . Choose . . . for Good Health. http://www.health.gov/dietaryguidelines/dga2000/document/default.htm (accessed April 11, 2006).

30. U.S. Department of Health and Human Services & U.S. Department of Agriculture. (2005). Anatomy of My Pyramid. http://www.mypyramid.gov/downloads/MyPyramid_Anatomy.pdf (accessed April 11, 2006).

31. U.S. Department of Health and Human Services & U.S. Department of Agriculture. (2005). Working Together... Dietary Guidelines, Food Guidance System, Food Label. http://www.health.gov/dietaryguidelines/dga2005/toolkit/together.htm (accessed April 11, 2006).

32. R. Webb, "Healthy meals on-the-go." *Diabetes Forecast* 56, 9 (September 2003): 39–42.

33. U.S. Department of Health and Human Services & U.S. Department of Agriculture. (2005). Don't Give In When You Eat Out And Are On The Go. http://www.health.gov/dietaryguidelines/dga2005/document/media/OnTheGo.pdf (accessed April 11, 2006).

34. K. M. Flegal, M. D. Carroll, R. J. Kuczmarski, and C. L. Johnson, "Overweight and obesity in the United States: Prevalence and trends, 1960–1994." *International Journal of Obesity* 22(1998):39–47.

35. *Clinical Guidelines on the Identification, Evaluation, and Treatment of Overweight and Obesity in Adults.* (Bethesda, MD: National Institutes of Health: National Heart, Lung, and Blood Institute. June 1998.)

36. DHHS CDC NIOSH, "Overtime and Extended Work Shifts: Recent Findings on Illness, Injuries, and Health Behaviors." April 2004. Publication number 2004-143.

37. D. Argenti, "Mastering your circadian rhythm: sleep is vital to maintaining health and fitness on the night shift." *American Fitness*, v20 i1(Jan.–Feb. 2002):29(5).

38. Sleep Deprivation: Causes and Consequences. National Ag Safety Database. http://www.cdc.gov/nasd/docs/d000707-d000800/d000705/d000705.html (accessed April 11, 2006).

39. United States Fire Administration, *EMS Safety: Techniques and Applications* (2005). (Emmitsburg, MD: U. S. Fire Administration.)

40. Stress at Work. DHHS (NIOSH) Publication number 99-101. Publication date: January 5, 2002. Page 6.

41. A. A. Mikolaj, "Emergency Services Stress." In *Stress Management for the Emergency Care Provider* (Upper Saddle River, NJ: Prentice-Hall, 2005).

42. F. J. McMahan, *Paramedics and Burnout: Coping and Prevention Suggestions.* http://www.giftfromwithin.org/pdf/burnout.pdf

43. For First Responders: Dealing with the Sudden Death of a Child. http://www.compassionatefriends.org/Brochures/first_responders.htm (accessed April 11, 2006).

44. M. Nordberg, *Rescuing the Rescuer: Critical Incident Stress Management.* http://www.advancedrt.com/articles/rtarticles/RTCISD.html (accessed April 11, 2006).

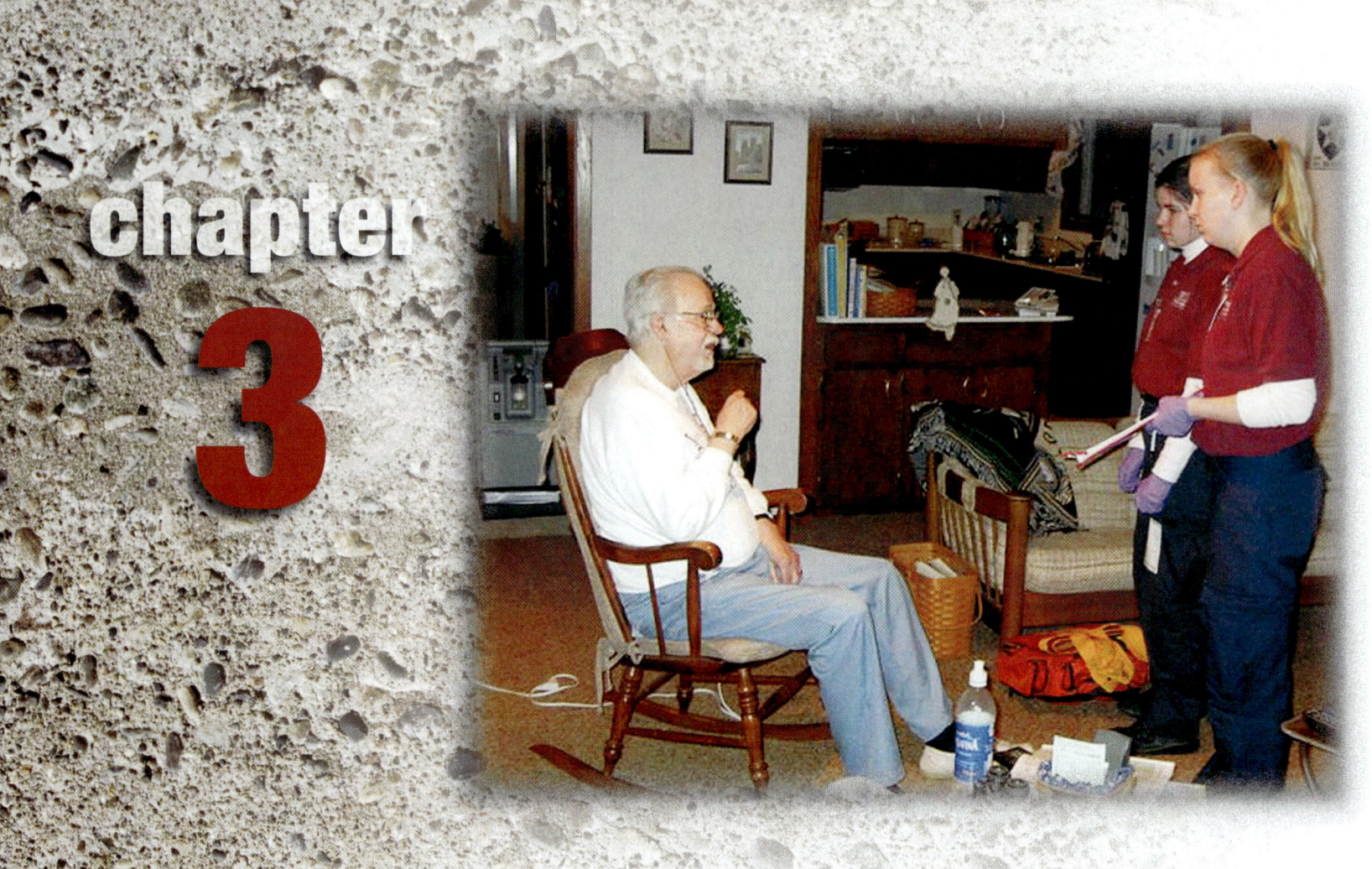

Professional Ethics

"No one cares how much you know until they know how much you care."

—John Maxwell

Need to know

▶ The ethical characteristics appropriate for EMS professionals to practice in their personal and professional lives.

▶ The principles described in the EMT Code of Ethics.

▶ All laws, rules, regulations, policies, procedures, protocols, and standing orders of the paramedic's organization so care can be rendered in an ethical manner.

▶ How to rehearse ethical dilemma situations with coworkers and begin to develop problem solving abilities for those times when they arise.

▶ Problem solving tools to aid in working through ethical dilemmas. This will help the paramedic develop a systematic and consistent approach.

▶ Do	▶ Ask
• Familiarize yourself with the EMT code of ethics	• Ask EMS officials about system ethics policies
• Familiarize yourself with ethical principles ensuring patients rights	• Ask supervisors and system officials about policies regarding DNRs, advance directives, and durable power of attorney
• Familiarize yourself with state law and system policy regarding care without consent	• Ask supervisors about documentation in care situations involving ethical dilemmas
• Endeavor to honor the patient's wishes unless the patient is unable or not lawfully able to make decisions	• Ask the patient for permission to care for him or her unless otherwise directed by law and policy

Introduction

Most of us have met individuals in healthcare who are very intelligent and have excellent psychomotor skills, and yet they are not always professional in their actions. As you read in Chapter 1, a paramedic must be professional at all times. This includes professional behavior in all the domains we operate within: cognitive (thinking abilities), psychomotor (ability to perform technical skills), and affective (behaviors, feelings, and emotions). Inextricably tied to being a professional is demonstrating correct affective behaviors like being ethical, hence the idea of **professional ethics.** The concept of professional ethics is one that encompasses the practice of all paramedics, whether on or off duty. How you react in difficult situations, how you make difficult decisions regarding resuscitation and patient consent or refusal, as well as living right in your personal life is always a reflection on the profession.

In this age, the line between what was traditionally defined as right and wrong is overshadowed by moral and ethical relativist thinking that believes that there is no absolute right or wrong or that what is right or wrong should be left to the judgment of each individual. Regardless of what personal view is held, every paramedic must have a clear understanding of the proper behavior expected of a healthcare professional. Books detailing the manner in which a profession emerges and develops from a particular field have one uniform concept—that to become a profession, the group of individuals making up that profession must agree to rules, regulations, and codes of conduct that distinguish them in their profession. Without this type of self-awareness and standard setting, many argue that a profession truly does not exist. If you reflect on the path the EMS profession has taken in the past several decades, you can see this unfold in the choices many of our leaders have made.

As in the past, many of the ethical challenges we face today will impact the rules and laws we live by in the future. This chapter will discuss the concepts and issues surrounding professional ethics and lay the foundation for the principles in place to be used by EMS professionals. Box 3-1 lists the terminology used in the study of ethics. You will see these terms used throughout this chapter. This chapter will discuss some tools and skills that may be helpful as you confront the inevitable ethical dilemmas found within the paramedic practice of medicine.

An Overview of Ethics

Defining Ethics

The word *ethics* comes to us from the Greek word for "character" and relates directly to personal standards based on what is right and wrong.[1] For paramedics, **ethics** are the set of principles and standards that determine what is right and wrong conduct within the profession. Paramedics enter homes and environments (often without invitation), invade personal space, ask questions about private and embarrassing issues, undress and touch patients all over their bodies, put patients

BOX 3-1 Terminology Used in the Study of Ethics and Morals

Advocacy: Active support, especially the act of pleading or arguing for patients who cannot plead or argue for themselves.

Autonomy: Self dependent; having the right to choose a course of treatment based on personal beliefs independent of the influence of others.

Beneficence: Kind, charitable, benefiting; acting in the best interest of the patient.

Bioethics: The study of the ethical and moral implications of new biological discoveries and biomedical advances, as in the fields of genetic engineering and drug research.

Ethics: Personal or professional standards relating to character and what is right or wrong.

Futility: Having no practical result; in healthcare it may mean all efforts are failing or the intervention will not result in a positive outcome.

Justice: Quality of being fair, especially in regards to allocating proper healthcare resources to patients.

Morals: Social standards, specifically how humans act (either good or bad), in a society.

Nonmalfeasance: Without misconduct or wrongdoing.

Teamwork: Cooperative effort by the members of a group or team to achieve a common goal.

Veracity: Telling the truth and being honest.

Virtue: Moral excellence and righteousness; goodness.

---

into positions where they are totally dependant for information, and perform painful and invasive procedures. It is vital to earn and maintain the public's trust in order to do the work required of a paramedic. To do so, paramedics must live as upstanding citizens with good and decent character, often putting the interest of others before their own to assume the role of patient advocate. DOT 1-5.1, 1-5.3

As the definition of ethics relates to both personal and professional standards, **morals** relate to societal standards, specifically how humans act, either good or bad, as they live and function within a society. Recent news reports have shown several cases of EMS providers engaging in poor ethical and moral behaviors such as embezzlement, sexual misconduct, selling drugs, and operating an emergency vehicle under the influence of alcohol.[2] It is easy to agree that such behavior is unprofessional and lacking in ethics and character. Actions such as these are reprehensible and do significant damage to our profession. The small fraction of offenders cast a negative mark on all, and you must continually evaluate your own behavior to prevent further incidents. DOT 1-5.2

Some situations arise where appropriate ethical choices may not be clear.

- An ambulance crew transports a homeless person to a hospital for evaluation, but the crew refuses to uncover the patient and look for injuries because they know that in doing so the odor from the patient will fill the back of the ambulance.
- An EMS provider causes an intoxicated person undue pain and handles the patient roughly in order to let the patient know that driving while intoxicated is unacceptable behavior.

In both of these situations, the lines between ethical and unethical behaviors may be blurred. Each illustrates that although patient care is being performed, the attitude or actions of the provider may not reflect the highest ethical standards. In the absence of clearly articulated standards, such as those found within the EMT Code of Ethics, these lines can blur even further.

Occasionally veteran EMS personnel have told students or new paramedics, "What you learn in class is one thing, but this is the way it's *really* done in the field." That statement implies that what is taught in class is not applicable in the "real world." Unfortunately, those uttering such phrases are often the individuals most likely to compromise their standards and integrity when ethical dilemmas arise. We will not mature as a profession until the ethics discussed in class are practiced in the field. As paramedics, we are called to live our lives in a decent ethical and moral fashion. By doing so, we are worthy of the trust our patients place in us, and we fulfill a required component of our profession.

The EMT Code of Ethics

In order to establish a standard of professional behavior in practice, every profession needs an ethical code by which it can be measured. In emergency healthcare there are ethical codes for physicians, nurses, and EMTs. Dr. Charles Gillespie wrote the *EMT Code of Ethics*. This code, found in Box 3-2, was formally adopted by the National Association of EMTs in 1978.[3] For many years, it was traditional for graduating EMT professionals to swear an oath to uphold the Code of Ethics (Box 3-3). Although this is still practiced in some services, today

BOX 3-2 EMT Code of Ethics

Professional status as an Emergency Medical Technician and Emergency Medical Technician-Paramedic is maintained and enriched by the willingness of the individual practitioner to accept and fulfill obligations to society, other medical professionals, and the profession of Emergency Medical Technician. As an Emergency Medical Technician-Paramedic, I solemnly pledge myself to the following code of professional ethics:

A fundamental responsibility of the Emergency Medical Technician is to conserve life, to alleviate suffering, to promote health, to do no harm, and to encourage the quality, and equal availability of emergency medical care.

The Emergency Medical Technician provides services based on human need, with respect for human dignity, unrestricted by consideration of nationality, race, creed, color, or status.

The Emergency Medical Technician does not use professional knowledge and skills in any enterprise detrimental to the public well-being.

The Emergency Medical Technician respects and holds in confidence all information of a confidential nature obtained in the course of professional work unless required by law to divulge such information.

The Emergency Medical Technician, as a citizen, understands and upholds the law and performs the duties of citizenship; as a professional, the Emergency Medical Technician has the never-ending responsibility to work with concerned citizens and other health care professionals in promoting a high standard of emergency medical care to all people.

The Emergency Medical Technician shall maintain professional competence and demonstrate concern for the competence of other members of the Emergency Medical Services health care team.

An Emergency Medical Technician assumes responsibility in defining and upholding standards of professional practice and education.

The Emergency Medical Technician assumes responsibility for individual professional actions and judgment, both in dependent and independent emergency functions, and knows and upholds the laws which affect the practice of the Emergency Medical Technician.

An Emergency Medical Technician has the responsibility to be aware of and participate in matters of legislation affecting the Emergency Medical Service System.

The Emergency Medical Technician, or groups of Emergency Medical Technicians, who advertise professional service, do so in conformity with the dignity of the profession.

The Emergency Medical Technician has an obligation to protect the public by not delegating to a person less qualified, any service which requires the professional competence of an Emergency Medical Technician.

The Emergency Medical Technician will work harmoniously with and sustain confidence in Emergency Medical Technician associates, the nurses, the physicians, and other members of the Emergency Medical Services health care team.

The Emergency Medical Technician refuses to participate in unethical procedures, and assumes the responsibility to expose incompetence or unethical conduct of others to the appropriate authority in a proper and professional manner.

Source: www.naemt.org
Written by: Charles Gillespie M.D.
Adopted by The National Association of Emergency Medical Technicians, 1978.

BOX 3-3 EMT Oath for Paramedics

Be it pledged as an Emergency Medical Technician, I will honor the physical and judicial laws of God and man. I will follow that regimen which, according to my ability and judgment, I consider for the benefit of patients and abstain from whatever is deleterious and mischievous, nor shall I suggest any such counsel. Into whatever homes I enter, I will go into them for the benefit of only the sick and injured, never revealing what I see or hear in the lives of men unless required by law.

I shall also share my medical knowledge with those who may benefit from what I have learned. I will serve unselfishly and continuously in order to help make a better world for all mankind.

While I continue to keep this oath unviolated, may it be granted to me to enjoy life, and the practice of the art, respected by all men, in all times. Should I trespass or violate this oath, may the reverse be my lot.

So help me God.

Source: www.naemt.org
Written by: Charles B. Gillespie, M.D.
Adopted by the National Association of Emergency Medical Technicians, 1978

the custom of taking an oath upon entering a profession has all but disappeared from most areas of allied health and medicine, and many textbooks do not even reference such codes.

The EMT Code of Ethics is a powerfully written document that contains the very essence of what our professional nature as EMS providers should be. As you read the Code of Ethics, think of the many principles that describe our appropriate professional attitude. We must remember that although cognitive knowledge and psychomotor skills are important, professional conduct is often our greatest gift of service to our patients. In our pursuit to become excellent providers, we should commit the principles of the Code of Ethics to memory and review them on a regular basis to remind us both of our profound responsibilities and also the type of individuals we are expected to be as paramedics.

Answering Ethical Dilemmas

Ethical situations and dilemmas commonly arise in EMS, and paramedics must have the necessary skills to deal with them effectively. Such situations must be dealt with quickly in order to allow for appropriate patient care to continue. Experience is a wonderful tool to help you make ethical decisions. As you encounter ethical dilemmas and questions, you will develop wisdom and answers that can be carried forward to help in handling future situations. Box 3-4 lists key factors to remember when answering ethical questions.[4] The rules described in this box can help bridge the gap as you gain experience in dealing with ethical dilemmas.

It is very difficult when faced with an ethical question not to be influenced by emotion. Family members, bystanders, and even your own personal beliefs and experiences influence your emotions and subsequently

your ability to make objective decisions. Recognizing this, you should make every effort to use objective reason as you deal with ethical questions.

If patients are competent, they have every right to decide what is appropriate, even if you do not agree with their choices. This can be difficult for you to resolve, yet the law is very clear. It states in no uncertain terms that a competent adult has the right of self-determination, even if the decision made is not the best decision medically. DOT 1-5.4

Street Secrets

While ethical situations may sometimes be unclear, one principle of behavior is very clear: Never do anything that is obviously morally wrong.

K.V. Iserson and his associates developed a rapid approach to solving ethical dilemmas in the emergency setting that can also be used in the out-of-hospital environment.[5] By using the following three tests found in Box 3-5, your ethical decisions can be made with greater speed and certainty. DOT 1-5.3

First, the *Impartiality Test* asks "Would I accept the proposed treatment if I were in the patient's situation?" To answer this question, you must put yourself in the patient's place. Ask if you would want the treatment you are suggesting. This question will help remind you to provide the patient information about the risks and benefits of treatment so the patient can make an informed decision. Next, the *Universalizability Test* asks: "Would I want this action performed in relevantly similar circumstances?" Is the treatment universally accepted, and would I want to receive it if I were in a similar situation? Finally, the *Interpersonal Justifiability Test* asks, "Can I justify or defend my actions to others?" If you proceed, will you be able to defend that your choice to proceed was an appropriate one? It may mean explaining your choices and treatments to the patient, family members, medical director, EMS supervisor, receiving facility staff, or others who may question your actions.

By using these three tests, paramedics can resolve many difficult ethical questions. It is also crucial to remember that medical control exists to help paramedics. It is always wise to involve the consulting physician or medical director to get their opinion on difficult matters involving ethical conflicts. Since morals are based on what is right and wrong behavior from a societal perspective, another good rule of thumb is to never do anything obviously morally wrong. In doing so, many of the ethical dilemmas one will face will, by default, have an obvious answer.

BOX 3-4 Rules of Thumb for Answering Ethical Questions

1. Emotions should not be a factor in making decisions.
2. The questions should be answered with reason and logic.
3. Answers must not be based on what other people think is right or wrong.
4. Individuals must answer the questions for themselves.

BOX 3-5 · A Three-Step Process to Solving Ethical Dilemmas in the Emergency Setting

Step One: Perform the *Impartiality Test*

- Ask yourself: **"Would I accept the proposed treatment if I were in the patient's situation?"**
- If NO, do not proceed with the proposed treatment.
- If YES, go to Step Two.

Step Two: Perform the *Universalizability Test*

- Ask yourself: **"Would I want this action performed in relevantly similar circumstances?"**

- If NO, do not proceed with the proposed treatment.
- If YES, go to Step Three.

Step Three: Perform the *Interpersonal Justifiability Test*

- Ask yourself: **"Can I justify or defend my actions to others?"**
- If NO, do not proceed with the proposed treatment.
- If YES, continue with treatment.

Street Secrets

Work with your administrators and medical director when you are in doubt about an ethical issue. These individuals may offer a level of objectivity that those of you dealing directly with the situation may lack.

Ethical Tests in Healthcare

The Fundamental Question to Ask: What Is in the Patient's Best Interest?

All ethical tests in healthcare should begin with the premise of a single question: What is in the patient's best interest? One of the primary responsibilities of the paramedic is to serve as an advocate for patients. This means you speak on their behalf when they cannot. Serving as an advocate must occur whether you believe the patient warrants your protection or not. Patients do not have to earn your advocacy; it is a required component of your professional duties and responsibilities.[4]

Although this may seem simple enough, it can become complicated. In order to determine what is best for the patient, often you must first determine the patient's wishes. When it comes to resuscitation, for example, some patients want everything possible to be done for them, while others want no resuscitation efforts at all and may wish that efforts stop immediately when they become pulseless (Figure 3-1). It is important to remember that what *you* would want and what *the patient* actually wants may be two entirely different things.

In the absence of clearly specified instructions to the contrary you "err on the side of treatment" since your job is to provide patient care. This means that if

you seem to have a choice to make between providing and withholding treatment, the logical choice to make is to provide treatment until such time that information is found to change that decision. This is based upon the first standard for patient care.[6] It comes to EMS from physicians and is the Latin phrase "Primum non nocere." This is translated to mean "first do no harm." This doctrine is the premise by which all treatment regimens are judged.

Primum non nocere: First do no harm.

Determining what a patient wants can be achieved in various ways. If the patient is conscious and competent, simply asking the patient's wishes is easy. Prewritten statements directing care decisions such as advance directives, do not resuscitate orders, and living wills provide information when the patient is incompetent or unconscious. Lastly, family input may be utilized as a guide although it cannot supersede legal documents. DOT 1-5.4

"Incompetent" means that the patient is not capable of making decisions that would represent the patient's best interest. Testing this ability is not simple and can involve lengthy legal proceedings. Generally, patients under the influence of mind-altering substances such as drugs or alcohol should not be considered competent to make appropriate medical decisions.

The role of "good faith" becomes important in the course of making ethical decisions. **Good faith** can be defined as: "Acting honestly and without deception."[7] A more specific definition for EMS would be to put the concept in the form of the question: "Is the paramedic acting in an appropriate way, just as another paramedic would act, in the patient's best interest?" Remember

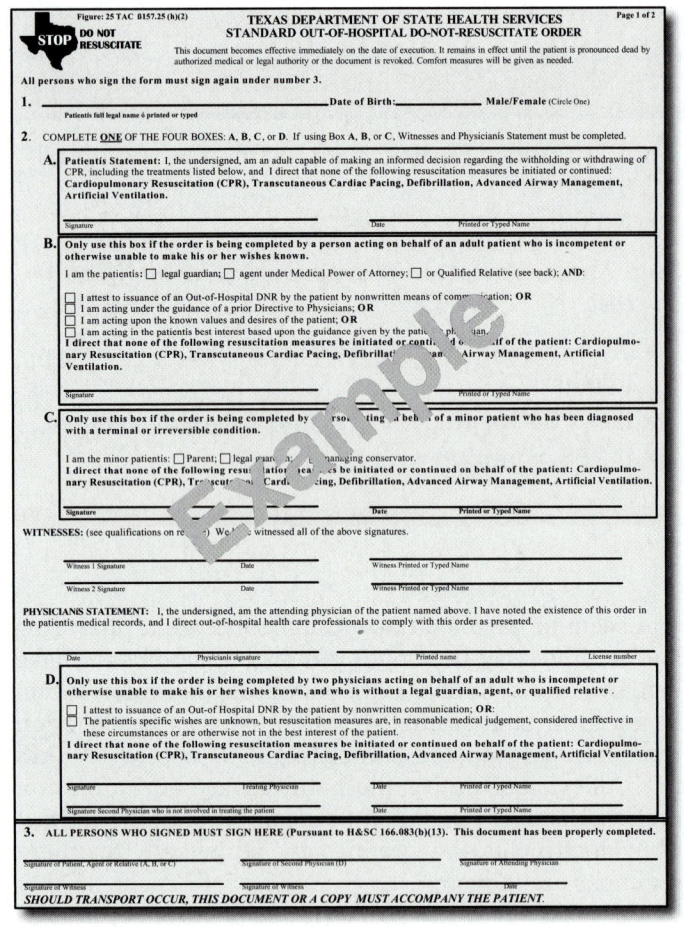

Figure 3-1   Advance directives such as Do Not Resuscitate (DNR) Orders, Do Not Attempt Resuscitation (DNAR) Orders, Living Wills, and others help guide questions regarding resuscitation.

that sometimes this does not mean aggressive treatment but instead honoring a patient's wishes to have treatment withheld.

Global Concepts of Ethics

Many of the world's moral and ethical foundations are rooted in religious culture. It is fascinating to note that nearly all of the world's major religions have some similarity in their common views of acceptable ethical behavior. In a global perspective, ethics can be largely summed up using the Golden Rule from the Judeo/Christian ethic, which states: "Do unto others as you would have them do unto you." The premise of this concept is that you would want to be treated in an ethical fashion so you should treat others with good ethics.

The three mainstays of ethical healthcare are:

1. Provide benefit to the patient
2. Avoid harm to the patient
3. Recognize patient autonomy

Autonomy means that the individual is considered distinct and self-governing.

By providing a benefit to the patient, avoiding further harm, and recognizing patient autonomy, you will have fulfilled the ethical obligation you have to every patient. DOT 1-5.8

Resolving Ethical Dilemmas

Occasionally the global concepts discussed conflict with one another. As a paramedic you must be able to find a solution that allows you to meet your patient's needs and continue to be that patient's advocate. Consider the following case study.

Case 1

You are working as a paramedic in a busy high performance EMS system, have given morphine to a patient with chest pain, and have delivered him to a very busy Emergency Department (ED). As you enter the ED, you are notified by dispatch that you have another emergency call pending. There is not an RN available to take your patient, but an ED tech who is an EMT-B

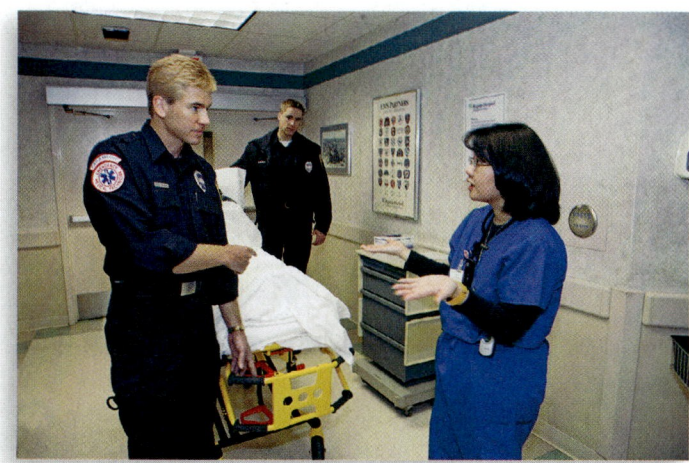

Figure 3-2 Is it okay to leave your patient with a lower level care provider?

hears your predicament and says, "Just leave the patient with me. I take care of patients like this all the time" (Figure 3-2).

Questions: What are the ethical and legal implications of leaving the patient with the EMT-B? What would you do?

Answers: Leaving a patient with an individual of lesser training after initiating care constitutes abandonment. The principles of virtue, teamwork, beneficence, justice, nonmalfeasance, veracity, and advocacy would all have been violated in this situation (see Box 3-1 for definitions). The proper thing to do would be to advise dispatch of the situation and wait until a healthcare professional of equal or higher training from the hospital can assume patient care.

Resolving Dilemmas in the Healthcare Community

Situations can be present in the healthcare community or within the public sector. Within the healthcare community, three main adjuncts help us to resolve ethical dilemmas:[4]

1. Follow established standards of care.
2. Use research and treatment protocols to help guide decision making.
3. Perform prospective and retrospective reviews of decisions.

Established standards of care are solid tools to help determine if a treatment or procedure is ethical. They provide a reference as to what the accepted course of treatment should be. When a paramedic steps outside the established standards, ethical danger usually lurks nearby.

Research and treatment protocols are also a benefit when attempting to resolve an ethical dilemma. Treatment protocols provide specific guidelines for patient care that are recognized and approved by the appropriate authority of the EMS system. They also must meet regional or state guidelines. Research can be helpful in determining future treatments and protocols. As EMS moves from anecdotal treatments to a more evidence-based practice, research will play a greater role in developing policies and procedures. It should be noted, however, that just because a research study on a treatment is published in medical literature, it does not make it ethically or legally acceptable to perform the treatment until it is approved by the medical director and medical control authority.

Street Secrets

Stay current on research. It will help you stay informed of new innovations and anticipate changes that will come to your system. The more informed you are, the more opportunities you will have to help influence and drive changes that will be made in your profession.

Prospective and retrospective reviews of decisions can also be very helpful in the healthcare setting when working through ethical dilemmas. Reviewing potential ethical situations either before (a prospective approach) actual situations or after (a retrospective approach) they occur can prove valuable tools to use when faced with similar situations in the future. Challenge coworkers and partners to provide input regarding their behavior choices. Seek input from experienced professionals you trust and respect. Work with your administrators and medical director to learn how to apply the rules and regulations that are in place governing policies and procedures. These exercises are similar to disaster plan exercises; they test the processes and policies and help every member of the team learn to understand how the organization believes issues should be handled.

Resolving Dilemmas in the Public Community

Within the public community, ethical dilemmas are traditionally addressed in two ways: through the creation of laws that protect patient rights (see Box 3-6 for an example of one state's Patients' Bill of Rights) and by the use of advance directives (see Figure 3-1).

CONNECTIONS See Chapter 4: Legal Issues for more information on the laws pertaining to patient rights.

BOX 3-6 Patients' Bill of Rights

As a patient in a hospital in New York State, you have the right, consistent with law, to:

1. Understand and use these rights. If for any reason you do not understand or you need help, the hospital MUST provide assistance, including an interpreter.

2. Receive treatment without discrimination as to race, color, religion, sex, national origin, disability, sexual orientation or source of payment.

3. Receive considerate and respectful care in a clean and safe environment free of unnecessary restraints.

4. Receive emergency care if you need it.

5. Be informed of the name and position of the doctor who will be in charge of your care in the hospital.

6. Know the names, positions and functions of any hospital staff involved in your care and refuse their treatment, examination or observation.

7. A no smoking room.

8. Receive complete information about your diagnosis, treatment and prognosis.

9. Receive all the information that you need to give informed consent for any proposed procedure or treatment. This information shall include the possible risks and benefits of the procedure or treatment.

10. Receive all the information you need to give informed consent for an order not to resuscitate. You also have the right to designate an individual to give this consent for you if you are too ill to do so. If you would like additional information, please ask for a copy of the pamphlet "Do Not Resuscitate Orders—A Guide for Patients and Families."

11. Refuse treatment and be told what effect this may have on your health.

12. Refuse to take part in research. In deciding whether or not to participate, you have the right to a full explanation.

13. Privacy while in the hospital and confidentiality of all information and records regarding your care.

14. Participate in all decisions about your treatment and discharge from the hospital. The hospital must provide you with a written discharge plan and written description of how you can appeal your discharge.

15. Review your medical record without charge. Obtain a copy of your medical record for which the hospital can charge a reasonable fee. You cannot be denied a copy solely because you cannot afford to pay.

16. Receive an itemized bill and explanation of all charges.

17. Complain without fear of reprisals about the care and services you are receiving and to have the hospital respond to you and if you request it, a written response. If you are not satisfied with the hospital's response, you can complain to the New York State Health Department. The hospital must provide you with the State Health Department telephone number.

18. Authorize those family members and other adults who will be given priority to visit consistent with your ability to receive visitors.

19. Make known your wishes in regard to anatomical gifts. You may document your wishes in your health care proxy or on a donor card, available from the hospital.

Public Health Law(PHL)2803 (1)(g)Patient's Rights, 10NYCRR, 405.7,405.7(a)(1),405.7(c)

Laws provide patients with rights such as the right to receive emergency care regardless of their race, color, religion, sex, national origin, disability, sexual orientation, or ability to pay. By having such laws, no one can be refused lifesaving care.

A significant way patients can help minimize ethical dilemmas is through the adoption of an advance directive such as a living will. These documents make a patient's wishes regarding medical treatment known in the event they are unable to speak for themselves. As their name implies, advance directives are written in advance of their need, so family members are not left to guess what should be done for the patient. They are witnessed and signed by nonfamily members as well as the patient.

Very public battles have ensued within families whose members each claimed they knew what the patient would have wanted although an advance directive was not available. The 2005 case of Terri Schiavo in Florida dealt with a brain-damaged woman who was being kept alive in a nursing home by a feeding tube. Medical authorities differed on how severe her condition was, and family members were divided in their desires for patient care. Her husband claimed she always said she would not want to be kept alive in a persistent vegetative state. Her parents disagreed, challenged his claims, and wished to have her supported in the condition she was in. After a very public seven-year battle that went all the way to Congress, the president, and the Supreme Court, Ms. Schiavo's feeding tube was removed and she eventually died.[8] The presence of an advance directive would have removed the guesswork in this situation and ensured the patient's wishes were honored. DOT 1-5.6

As a paramedic, you can promote the use of advance directives in your community and set an example by completing your own. Discuss your wishes with your family members, so they will be informed and able to act upon your wishes. Keep copies of the document in a location that is known to family members. DOT 1-5.7

Ethical Issues in Contemporary Practice

Allocation of Resources

The allocation of resources in EMS is most often determined by need—when there is an emergency, someone responds to lend assistance. This system works well as long as there are enough resources to provide equal care to all people (a concept known as *true parity*). Problems arise however, when there are not enough resources to meet the public's need. These types of situations may be caused by such things as multiple casualty incidents and disasters, economic barriers (not enough funding to provide adequate service), or staffing shortages.

During a mass casualty incident, a system of sorting, called **triage**, is used to save the greatest number of lives. Typically the critical (but salvageable) patients are transported first, followed by potentially unstable patients, and then the stable patients. Patients with catastrophic injuries may not be treated if their injuries are so resource intensive that treating them will result in delayed care of many other individuals. These patients are considered unsalvageable and are often moved to a secure, private, and, if possible, quiet, location where they die out of the view of the media, salvageable patients, bystanders, and rescuers. In these situations, mature senior healthcare professionals often are the best equipped emotionally to work with the patients in these predeath holding areas. DOT 1-5.5

CONNECTIONS See Chapter 50: Medical Incident Command for more information on triage and handling disaster situations.

Another concept of resource allocation is based upon need. It would not be ethical to place an ambulance in a jurisdiction where very few people live at the expense of an area where the majority of the population resides. This is one of the factors EMS planners try to determine when deciding station locations. Lastly, a concept exists for resource allocation based on the premise that patients, through their payment of taxes, have earned the right to have care provided. An example of this might be an area with political support that decides to provide the highest degree of care with the most expensive equipment and training. DOT 1-5.5

Decisions Surrounding Resuscitation

When considering resuscitation there are many potential ethical dilemmas that a paramedic may encounter. The focal point is determining what the patient really wants. If there is a valid advance directive present, the patient's wishes are usually clear. Many times, however, things are not so easily determined. Many factors come into play in a situation where someone is to be resuscitated. Family dynamics, survivor's guilt, economic gain, and even criminal activity can affect the decision either to proceed or to cease resuscitation efforts. As stated before, it is always best, when in doubt, to begin resuscitation efforts.

A unique situation that bears mentioning is the resuscitation call where care has been initiated and an advance directive is later found. If the document is valid and approved for use in your state, most agencies will mandate or allow you to cease resuscitative efforts. Given this situation, it is imperative to know your local protocols and involve medical control in the decision process. If protocol requires resuscitative efforts continue while a family member searches for a misplaced advance directive, explain this with compassion, diplomacy, and professionalism.

Confidentiality

Confidentiality is a fundamental legal right of every patient. Paramedics who violate this right may be sued or may face legal charges or disciplinary action. It could lead to loss of wages or employment and profound embarrassment to you, your agency, and the profession. In 1996 the United States Congress passed the **Health Insurance Portability and Accountability Act (HIPAA).** HIPAA details strict patient privacy guidelines for both personal and medical information. Violators may be fined up to $250,000 and/or imprisoned for up to 10 years for the malicious distribution of protected patient information.[9] Remember what is written in the EMT Code: "The Emergency Medical Technician respects and holds in confidence all information of a confidential nature obtained in the course of professional work unless required by law to divulge such information."

CONNECTIONS HIPAA laws will be discussed in more detail in Chapter 4: Legal Issues and 17: Documentation and Communication.

As strict as the policies and laws are surrounding confidentiality, there may be occasional situations which arise that will require divulging information to fulfill other laws. Examples include when there is a risk to public health, such as in cases of infectious disease like tuberculosis, or with the mandatory reporting of suspected child and elder abuse or neglect and domestic violence. In the latter situation, the patient may be at risk for further harm if the suspected abuse is not reported. Another example is when a healthcare provider is subpoenaed under court order to provide information in a case. It is crucial to be aware of rules, laws, regulations, policies, and procedures and consult with an attorney when appropriate. DOT 1-5.6

Consent

You should not treat a competent patient without first obtaining consent. As with confidentiality, consent to medical procedures is a fundamental right of everyone. DOT 1-5.4

All competent patients have the right to make decisions regarding the amount and type of healthcare they wish to receive.

Consent is also described as the "fundamental element of the patient-physician relationship."[4] As it is with physicians, so it is with paramedics and all healthcare professionals. EMS must always value and respect the patient's autonomy. Before performing any treatment, explain the procedure, risks, benefits, and alternatives so the patient can make an informed decision whether or not to allow the procedure. This process results in what is called actual and informed consent. Exceptions to this may occur if the patient is deemed incompetent, is unconscious, or is a minor who is less than the age of consent established for that particular state. When the patient is incapable of providing actual consent, the patient may be treated under the doctrine of implied consent. *Implied consent* states that a reasonable person in a similar situation would likely want treatment and provide consent. DOT 1-5.8

CONNECTIONS Chapter 4: Legal Issues contains more information on the various types of consent, along with definitions and descriptions of each type.

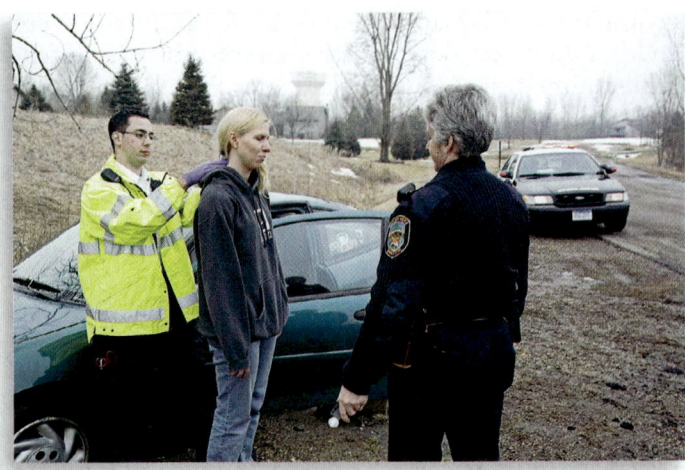

Figure 3-3   Is this patient competent to refuse treatment?

Case 2

You are on scene at an automobile crash of one car (Figure 3-3). There is one patient, an unrestrained 25-year-old female, who states there is no need for you to be there, and she denies calling 9-1-1 from her cell phone. She admits to having "one beer" an hour ago. You believe the mechanism of injury is significant and convince her to let you assess for injuries. She answers questions, acts appropriately, and has stable vital signs. Upon assessing her neck, you note deformity, and she winces from neck pain. She reports "tingling" in her extremities but seems to have no other injuries. You explain to her the potential significance of her injury, and she absolutely refuses to be treated and transported. You decide her risk to herself is too great, forcefully restrain her by immobilizing her to a rigid long backboard, and transport her to the local emergency department for care of a suspected spinal injury. She protests the entire time.

Question: What are the ethical and legal implications of your actions? DOT 1-5.10

Answer: The patient always has a right to refuse care as long as she is competent—even when she is injured. The challenge in this scenario is to determine competence before any additional actions are taken. Law enforcement can be of great assistance in a situation such as this. If the patient is determined to be intoxicated by law enforcement, she can be put into protective custody and then treated. If the patient is not intoxicated, she is capable of making treatment decisions, and you have no right to forcefully immobilize and transport her against her will. To do so is unethical. It violates the ethical principles of virtue, beneficence, justice, autonomy, morals, nonmalfeasance, and advocacy. Legally, your actions may constitute battery (unlawful touching of another), false imprisonment, or perhaps even kidnapping.

Key issues in determining implied consent are twofold. First, does the patient understand the medical issues at hand? Risks as well as benefits of treatment should be explained in language and terms the patient can understand. Patients should be questioned to test their understanding of what they have been told, and clarifications to the conversation should be made until you believe they understand what has been said. Second, can the patient make an informed decision that is in his or her best interest? Just because patients can understand the medical issues at hand does not necessarily mean they can make an informed decision, and vise-versa. If there is disease, injury, or intoxicating substances impairing their judgment, it is best to consider them incapable of competent decision-making abilities.

Applying Ethical Principles to Patient Care Situations

When considering the application of ethical principles to patient care situations, remember the obligation to provide care in all circumstances, including futile ones that seem destined to have a poor outcome, like death. Also consider the need to remain a patient advocate, the need for professional accountability, and your role as a physician extender. As mentioned previously in this chapter, the best time to think about possible ethical issues is *before* they happen. Although it is impossible to plan for every ethical dilemma that may present itself, it is a good idea to practice ahead of time how to handle various situations.

Care in Futile Situations

Futility of medical care is defined as the point in the medical care process when all interventions are failing or will not result in a positive outcome. Many times, in eagerness to save all patients, paramedics are reluctant to admit the situation has reached the stage of futility. In the early years of the profession, paramedics were required to begin resuscitation on every patient in cardiac arrest and continue resuscitation efforts until arrival at the hospital where a physician would pronounce the patient dead. Recently, that process has changed. Now when paramedics determine the situation is futile, they often either have a protocol or standing order to guide them in ceasing resuscitative efforts in the field. Such regulations may require direct physician consultation via phone or radio prior to stopping resuscitation. That being said, it is also important that paramedics are aware of special situations where, although the situation may appear futile, the patient may still have a chance of survival (such as patients suffering from hypothermia or cold water drowning or who have been struck by lightning) and resuscitation attempts may be appropriate.

The American Heart Association states,"It is inappropriate, futile, and ethically unacceptable to routinely continue prehospital resuscitative efforts and require ambulance transport and ongoing CPR for all patients. Likewise it is inappropriate for clinicians to routinely apply rules for stopping resuscitative efforts without thinking about the particular clinical situation."[10]

Certainly, to make such difficult decisions, it is always best for paramedics to involve their medical control physician to make a collaborative decision. In the rare occasion a medical control physician is unavailable, it is crucial to have standing orders in place that clearly delineate the appropriate actions to be taken.

Obligation to Provide Care

Paramedics are obligated to be kind and charitable, perform in a beneficial manner, and act in the best interest of every patient. It can be very challenging to maintain composure when patients are exhibiting threatening or hostile behavior. Regardless of patient actions, healthcare professionals must always exhibit beneficence toward the patient. This does not mean you must allow yourself to be assaulted or battered while performing patient care. Scene safety is an ongoing necessity, and you must protect yourself, your partner(s), bystanders, and your patient from harm.

Another important facet to consider is that of a patient's ability to pay for services. By federal law, you are not allowed to deny emergency care to any patient based upon his or her ability to pay. This type of "economic triage" is absolutely illegal, immoral, and unethical, regardless of your type of service.

Occasionally, you will transport patients who belong to insurance programs or special medical groups such as Health Maintenance Organizations (HMOs) that require them to be treated in a specific healthcare setting. Never let this interfere with providing appropriate emergency care. Always transport patients to the closest appropriate emergency facility, regardless of their insurance or healthcare plan. If the emergency situation permits and your protocols allow, you may be authorized to transport these patients to facilities that they request. Complying with these requests is appropriate in the right situations and demonstrates a high level of patient satisfaction.

You may encounter hospitals that advise transport of uninsured patients to publicly funded hospitals or other facilities. You must immediately report this unethical and illegal behavior, which is called "patient dumping," to the proper authorities in your area.

A special situation involves your actions when you are not on duty. Every state in America has a form of the Good Samaritan Law which protects EMS providers who are not officially on duty (in either a paid, unpaid, or volunteer capacity) who provide medical assistance.

Often, these laws include provisions requiring the paramedics perform their actions in good faith and within their scope of medical practice. Although most states do not consider it a legal obligation for an off-duty paramedic to provide medical assistance, many states consider it an ethical obligation. It is important to be aware of pertinent legal and ethical stipulations in your system.

CONNECTIONS Good Samaritan Laws and the Duty to Act are discussed in more detail in Chapter 4: Legal Issues.

Patient Advocacy

As an ethical responsibility to your patients, you must always practice patient advocacy. By promoting and protecting your patients' rights, you will be helping them get the care and attention they are entitled to and deserve.

Paramedic Accountability

Since paramedics are given great responsibility, they are also held to high ethical standards. Paramedics are ethically accountable to the public, their patients, medical director, and EMS system. Paramedics are required to follow protocols, standing orders, and online and offline medical direction. You must always strive to give the best care possible to your patients. Accomplishing this will include being aware of the environment for clues and dangers, doing a thorough history and assessment, and developing a comprehensive prehospital emergency care plan. By always doing what is in the best interest of your patient, you will fulfill your duty to be accountable to every patient you encounter. DOT 1-5.9

In a similar fashion, by being accountable to both your medical director and medical control physicians, you will instill in them a sense of confidence, so they will trust your abilities and allow you to practice to your full potential. For example, if you have a good reputation as a paramedic, the medical control physicians will be more likely to trust your judgment and allow you to exercise that judgment. If the medical director questions your decisions or patient care choices, you must be ready to provide a rationale in a professional, nondefensive manner.

Since you are also accountable to your EMS system, you must always function in a professional manner and be a good reflection of the profession. Another ethical requirement is for you to report any unethical behavior by your colleagues to the proper authority. This is usually a very difficult task but one that must be done. Any time you fail to speak up about unethical behavior, you are, in a sense, approving of it.

Finally, you are accountable to your protocols and standing orders. It is your responsibility to know the details of these documents, so that you can follow them at a second's notice in any situation. By doing so, your patients, medical director, medical control physicians, and the EMS system will be better served.

Role as Physician Extender

As a paramedic, you are literally an extension of the physician under whose supervision you work; because of this, you are the eyes, ears, nose, and touch of the physician in the prehospital environment. Vital to this role is your ability to communicate what you find to the physician in order to provide the best and most efficient care. The relationship between the physician and paramedic is most often one of excellence and trust. There are a few situations, however, that could pose potential legal and ethical violations.

It is possible you may receive an order from a physician that goes against your standard of care. This often occurs when physicians are new to your system or are just learning your protocols, but it can happen at other times as well. Whether you are the designated team leader for this patient encounter, you are ethically and morally a party to any care given or withheld, even that which is ordered by a physician during consultation. If something is not consistent with the standard of care, you have an obligation to discuss that with the person giving the order, so the person understands it is out of the normal routine.

Case 3

You have a patient in a medical clinic who is in ventricular tachycardia. A physician on the scene is giving a dose of 1 gram of Lidocaine by IV bolus to the patient. You know that your protocols sometimes vary from hospital dosages, but you also recognize that this is way too much by any standard of care. You ask the physician if 1 gram is the dose he wishes to give, and he insists that it is (Figure 3-4).

Question: What are the ethical implications of this call if you let the physician give this dose? DOT 1-5.11

Answer: If you administered the ordered dose yourself, you would commit a legal and ethical violation. This is inconsistent with the standard of care and is potentially a fatal action. The principles you would have violated would be virtue, teamwork, beneficence, justice, veracity, and advocacy. Those same violations apply to allowing the physician to proceed. One course of action would be to contact online medical direction and discuss this with the online physician. Another would be to report this to your supervisor. Although this is a very difficult situation, you should attempt to reasonably intervene so that this physician does not proceed.

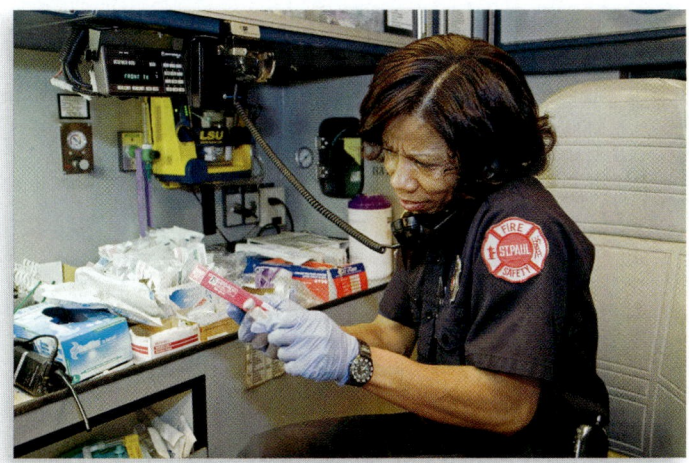

Figure 3-4 What would you do if you were given an order to administer an excessive dose of medication?

Common Areas of Ethical Concern

Nearly every patient you encounter can present you with a potential ethical situation. A few of the unique ethical situations that are common and are especially important to be aware of in your practice are abandonment, competence, and resuscitation.[11] An additional unique (and seldom mentioned) situation is that of patients with vague complaints.

Abandonment

Since **abandonment** involves initiating patient care and then leaving the patient (or leaving the patient with a lesser trained individual), the ethical implications are immense. In an ethics investigation, the obvious question will be: "Why was the patient abandoned?" In today's age of rapid-paced, high performance EMS systems and overcrowded emergency departments, situations can present themselves to leave patients before the proper individual has taken over the care you have initiated.

Competence

Determining patient competence can be a major challenge in the out-of-hospital environment and can be another source of ethical compromise. In an ethics investigation, the question asked will be "Was the patient competent to make a decision regarding his or her healthcare?" As discussed previously in this chapter, all adult patients have a legal right to determine what happens to their bodies but only if they are of sound mind and are competent to do so. As healthcare costs, insurance rates, and malpractice litigations are increasing at record levels, the question of who gets care and to what level becomes increasingly important.

Resuscitation

Resuscitation is a common area of ethical concern to EMS providers. With the existence of advance directives such as Do Not Attempt Resuscitation Orders and living wills, paramedics must be guided by what the legal documents direct. Most difficulties arise when a patient has expressed wishes to someone but has not written a legal document stating such wishes. You must have a clear understanding of the laws in your area that govern these situations. Typically, if there is doubt whether or not to resuscitate, you should attempt resuscitation.

Patients with Vague Complaints

Many patients you will be called to assist are not experiencing emergencies by the standards you apply for emergency situations. People call EMS for all kinds of situations, some of which are vague or nonspecific in nature. Many times patients are emotionally upset or lonely. These types of calls can try your patience.

It is important to keep in mind that it is not up to you to judge a patient's place in life, and the mere fact the patient called for an ambulance should signal a problem. Granted, they may not have life-threatening medical emergencies, but these patients may need some type of referral to social services or a program that can help them with their problems. Remember that being ethical is keeping in mind the global picture. For individuals who do not routinely experience emergencies, what seems like a minor situation to you can overwhelm their coping mechanisms and result in a call to 9-1-1 for assistance.

Summary

Ethical challenges are as common in the field of paramedicine as they are in life. Understanding ethics and how it applies to various patient care situations is paramount for appropriate professional behavior. As a paramedic, strong ethics are vital in both personal and professional life. When ethical dilemmas arise, it is important to have an understanding of the appropriate tools to use to resolve these situations. A firm knowledge of your protocols and standing orders is critical.

Key issues critical to solving ethical dilemmas on a system level involve the allocation of resources and decisions surrounding resuscitation, confidentiality, and consent. The ability to apply the ethical principles you have learned will allow you to practice at the highest ethical level and be a compliment to your profession.

Notes

1. Online Etymology Dictionary. http://www.etymonline.com/index.php?term=ethics (accessed July 25, 2002).

2. M. Zavadsky, *Let's add a new "E" in EMS . . .* (June 2005). http://www.emsnetwork.org/artman/publish/article_15890.shtml (accessed June 16, 2005).

3. C. Gillespe, MD, *EMT Code of Ethics.* http://www.naemt.org/aboutEMSAndCareers/emt_code_of_ethics.htm (accessed July 24, 2006).

4. U.S. Department of Transportation National Highway Traffic Safety Administration: *EMT-Paramedic National Standard Curriculum* (Washington, DC, 1998).

5. K. Iserson et al., *Ethics in Emergency Medicine*, 2nd ed. (Tucson, AZ: Galen Press, 1995).

6. *Hippocratic Oath (Modern Version),* Public Domain, 1993.

7. 'Lectric Law Library. http://www.lectlaw.com/def/g011.htm (accessed June 22, 2005).

8. R. Phillips et al., *'May God give grace to our family' Terri Schiavo dies amid legal, ethical battle* (April 11, 2005). http://www.cnn.com/2005/US/03/31/schiavo/ (accessed June 19, 2005).

9. U.S. Department of Health and Human Services, *Summary of the HIPAA Privacy Rule* (May 2003). http://www.hhs.gov/ocr/privacysummary.pdf (accessed June 18, 2005).

10. American Heart Association, *ACLS Provider Manual* (Dallas, TX, 2000).

11. G. L. Larkin and R. L. Fowler, "Essential ethics for EMS: cardinal virtues and core principles." *Emerg Med Clin North Am.* 20(4) (November 2002). http://www.ncbi.nlm.nih.gov/entrez/query.fcgi?cmd=Retrieve&db=pubmed&dopt=Abstract&list_uids=12476886&query_hl=1 (accessed June 20, 2005).

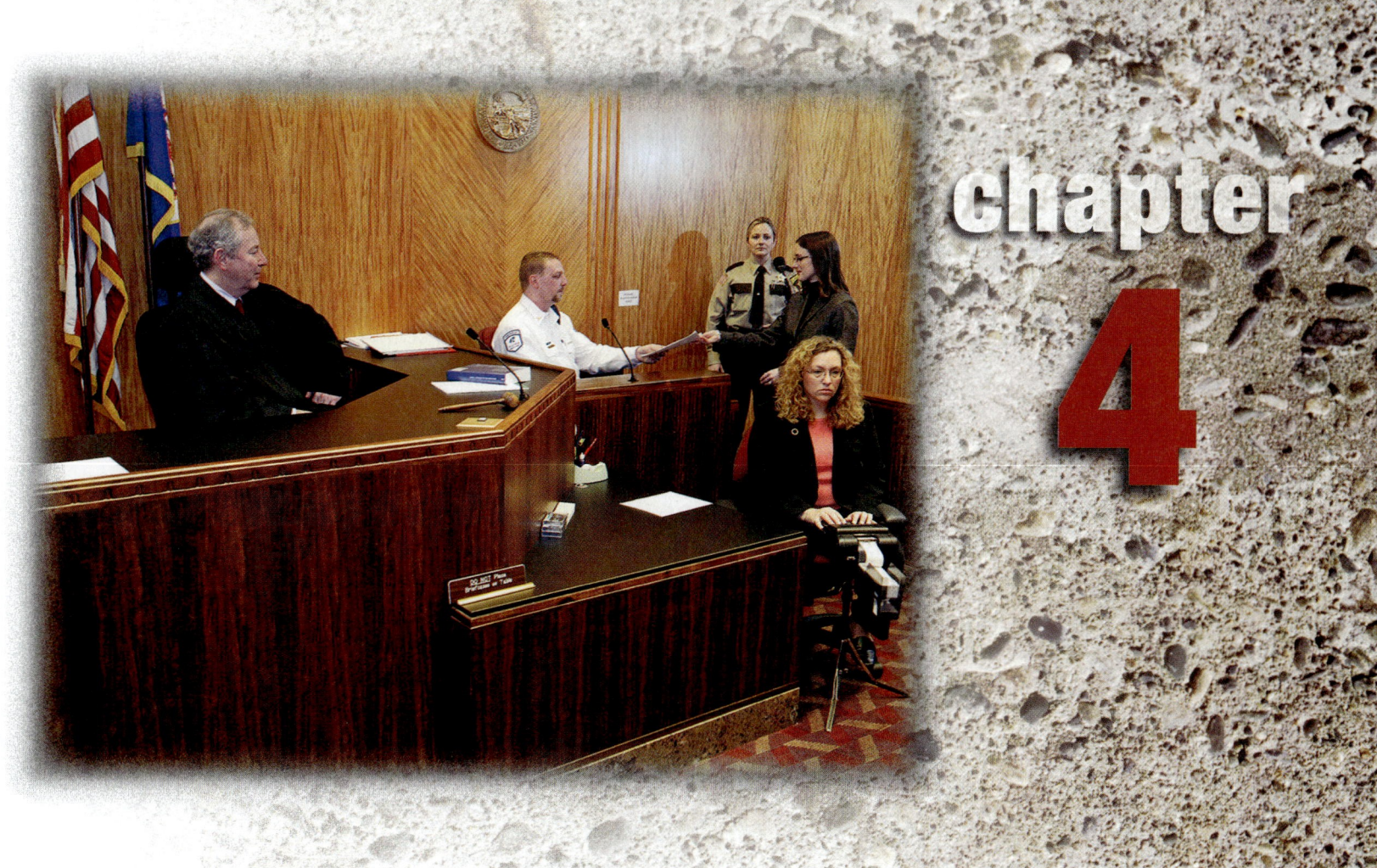

chapter 4

Legal Issues

> **"L**aw has been called a bottomless pit, not so much because of its depth, as that its windings are so obscure nobody can see the end."
>
> —George P. Morris

Need to Know

▶ Consent is legally required prior to providing EMS care, and every reasonable attempt should be made to attain it before you treat patients.

▶ Always "err on the side of treatment," meaning the job of an EMS provider is to perform patient care services, so when there is doubt if the patient needs service, continue to provide care as you look for other information or obtain medical direction.

▶ A professional appearance and actions, coupled with a high regard for patient satisfaction, are your best legal defenses.

▶ Know what circumstances require additional reporting to social service, public service, or law enforcement agencies.

▶ Understand the elements of malpractice/negligence and how to avoid it.

Do/Ask	
▶ **Do**	▶ **Ask**
• Keep patients informed of what is going on and what procedures you will perform on them or actions you are taking on their behalf. • Ensure you understand all of the laws, rules, and regulations that apply in the performance of your duties. • Ensure appropriate documentation is done on every patient care experience and in all situations likely to raise legal questions.	• Obtain consent before treating every patient that is conscious and capable.

Introduction

Paramedics and other EMS providers are subject to many types of laws, rules, and regulations in the performance of their duties, which originate at many levels. Most of the legal requirements for EMS exist at the state and local government levels; however, there are some federal laws that also apply. Laws pertinent to EMS span the spectrum of law and can be categorized under the headings of administrative, civil, and criminal.

In general, states typically establish the laws and regulations dealing with provider certification or licensing, scope of practice, disciplinary enforcement, and related issues.[1] In addition, many states establish the rules and regulations that oversee the licensing and operation of ambulance vehicles.[2] Regulation of advance directives (also known as Do Not Resuscitate (DNR)) is done by the states as well.[3] DOT 1-4.7h

Local government agencies, such as cities, counties, ambulance districts, local EMS agencies, or other entities may establish ordinances, rules, regulations, or protocols that govern issues such as response times, clinical practice, patient destination, and other issues.[4] The federal government establishes laws and regulations relating to reimbursement for ambulance services (Medicare), as well as requirements dealing with patient privacy and confidentiality, and the security of electronic information (HIPAA—the Health Insurance Portability and Accountability Act).[5,6] Federal law also addresses patient destination and hospital diversion issues (EMTALA—the Emergency Medical Treatment and Active Labor Act).[7] DOT 1-4.2, 1-4.7f

Street Secrets

It is in your best interest to know the pertinent laws and regulations that govern your practice of paramedicine. You should always maintain the stance that nobody is ever going to care more about issues that pertain to you than you. Ignorance of the law is never a good defensive strategy.

There are also several categories of law that relate to the delivery of EMS and the providers of field care. Administrative laws and regulations are typically overseen and enforced by government agencies, such as a state EMS office, which is usually part of a state health department or similar agency. These administrative agencies can impose disciplinary sanctions such as revocation or suspension of a provider's certification.[8]

Civil law is the area of the law that concerns itself with issues such as professional malpractice and other types of **tort** actions, which will be explained in more detail later in this chapter. Civil law is typically enforced through the court system, most often at the state level, and involves private litigants, including a plaintiff (typically an injured party seeking redress of a perceived injury) and a defendant (the party against whom liability is claimed). A common area of civil law encountered by EMS providers is tort law. A "tort" is merely the legal word for a "wrong" under the law, and torts can be either unintentional or intentional, as discussed later in this chapter.

Criminal law has increasingly been applied in EMS, often involving issues related to vehicle operations, drug diversion, and other activities.[9] Criminal laws are enforced by the government—including the local, state, or federal government. Penalties such as fines and imprisonment can be imposed from criminal proceedings. DOT 1-4.3

Nice to Know

Loss of licensure, certification, or the privilege to work or volunteer as an EMS provider can occur during any type of legal action, civil or criminal.

Chapter 3: Professional Ethics discusses the ethical considerations of EMS law. Ethics and morals are firmly rooted in legal principles, and legal principles help guide and shape ethics and morals as well. Legal responsibilities are typically placed upon the EMS professional externally. In other words, they are written regulations that are agreed upon (typically through voting or consensus building) by the government or other leadership body that guides the practice of a profession. They establish the framework the professional operates within. Ethics and morals represent the behavioral choices and decisions each individual makes in fulfilling his or her legal obligations. They can be strongly influenced by the culture of each professional, but they are also impacted by personal and internal forces such as innate personality, prior choices, family influences, and upbringing. **See Skill Sheet 64: Documentation and Skill Sheet 65: Physical Restraints (also see Step-by-Step 65: Physical Restraints).** DOT 1-4.1

State Laws and Regulations

A paramedic student first becomes exposed to the legal requirements imposed by state regulatory agencies when the student initially seeks to become an EMT. In all states, the educational programs and process of certifying, first as a basic EMT and then as a paramedic, are defined and overseen by the state agency granted that authority and responsibility. The regulatory agency sets the minimum educational requirements and often administers the tests utilized to certify EMTs at all levels.

As was mentioned earlier in this chapter, the state agency also has the authority and responsibility to ensure that an EMT is performing appropriately and can impose sanctions such as suspension or revocation of

Nice to Know

Many states utilize the NREMT examination process. For those states, the NREMT has been granted permission to conduct testing of their citizens, and the state has agreed that they will accept the results of the testing process either in lieu of (to replace) or in addition to their own testing process. Although the NREMT process is recognized as a valid process, it is within the scope of authority of each individual state to accept or not accept the certification granted through the NREMT testing process.

EMT certification. In such instances, administrative agencies must afford an affected provider with **due process** regarding disciplinary action involving the provider's certification. Typically, due process involves, at a minimum, notice of the charges and proposed disciplinary action and an opportunity to be heard regarding those charges, prior to any disciplinary action being taken. DOT 1-4.4

All states also require that a physician oversee the quality of the medical care that is provided by EMTs and ambulance services.[10]

CONNECTIONS Chapter 1: The EMS Profession describes the political processes that EMS went through in the 1900s to become a profession. Other professional groups within medicine, particularly physicians, were instrumental in providing leadership and direction for EMS. These groups continue to partner with EMS as it continues to grow and develop as a profession.

The Standard of Care and the Scope of Practice

As discussed in Chapter 1, the profession of EMS experienced a tremendous burst of growth and development over the last four decades of the twentieth century. During the early years in the 1960s and 1970s, the depth and breadth of the scope of practice for EMS was largely unknown, and the individuals and agencies providing the oversight and development were understandably cautious in how fast they allowed the profession to grow.

The capabilities and thirst for knowledge of the early pioneers in EMS led to an increasing expansion of the skill sets and knowledge base. Additionally, advances in the portability and ease of use of many medical devices and procedures allowed more and more tools such as cardiac monitoring, 12 lead ECG, blood gas analysis, and glucose monitoring to come into the prehospital setting.

At a federal level, there has always been guidance on the curricula, which has then provided some foundation for the actual scope (or size) of the out-of-hospital competencies and expectations for the profession. Collectively this has always been known as the **scope of practice.** Also, because this has represented the national focus, it can be argued that this then represents the accepted **standard of care.** The standard of care as defined legally explains the behaviors expected of similarly trained, competent individuals within a profession. It is often the basis of legal decisions when EMS issues are brought into the legal setting.

Until the development of the *Scope of Practice* in 2005, there has never been an actual document that outlined the scope on a national level. The development of this document was conducted over months, and it could be argued that it has actually taken the lifetime of the profession to accomplish. It was formed via a consensus process that included input and comment from all aspects of the EMS community and their stakeholders.

Adherence to the actual *Scope of Practice* on a state level is voluntary. The federal government has yet to exercise any authority to compel (or mandate) states to adhere to the *Scope* as defined. Many states align very closely to the *Scope of Practice,* and others have developed solid EMS systems that are not closely aligned to it. Some states may resist changing to the new *Scope,* and that resistance can have very legitimate reasons as well as sentimental or even illogical ones. The way a state defines its EMS provider levels and the scope of practice it allows these providers to operate under represents its individual scope of practice. DOT 1-4.8

Medical Direction and Oversight

An integral part of the delivery of EMS is physician oversight of the delivery of patient care. Physician direction and oversight of the system typically is divided into several categories based upon when that oversight occurs. The categories for physician direction are usually defined as prospective, concurrent, or retrospective, and medical control is exercised both on-line and off-line. DOT 1-4.9

Street Secrets

Many paramedics are afraid to speak on the radio. There are a variety of reasons for this, but many of them seem to stem from lack of confidence in communicating or fear of appearing to have inadequate knowledge. You should practice performing medical consultations until you gain proficiency, and with that will come the confidence. Seek medical direction whenever you are unsure how to proceed and any time your protocols require it.

Prospective medical control includes the development of clinical practice standards such as training curricula, protocols, and other such clinical standards. These standards establish, in advance, the parameters for EMS clinical practice and set forth the expectations that EMS providers must satisfy in the delivery of patient care. In some EMS systems, physician medical directors are also required to prospectively approve paramedics for work in the field, typically upon the completion of a required course of training or preceptorship. In some states, a paramedic can be removed from clinical practice when a medical director believes the paramedic is not functioning according to prescribed standards.[11]

Concurrent medical direction or control occurs when a paramedic consults with a physician or other advanced health care professional via telephone, radio, or other electronic means, permitting the physician and paramedic to collaboratively decide on the best course of action in the delivery of patient care. Technological advancements have and will continue to impact the delivery of concurrent medical direction, with the ability to transmit real-time video and clinical information in digital form improving the accuracy and timeliness of clinical decision-making at the patient's bedside (Figure 4-1).

Retrospective medical direction or control is typically exercised through quality improvement mechanisms such as chart reviews, case reviews, and other methods after patient care has been completed. Retrospective medical control allows paramedics and their medical directors to evaluate the effectiveness of care rendered and discover opportunities for improvement in skills, protocols, or other aspects of patient care delivery.

The legal relationship between a paramedic and physician varies from state to state. As indicated above, some states grant local medical directors authority to approve or disapprove individual paramedics for clinical practice. Other states concentrate this authority at the county or regional level, and still others reserve this

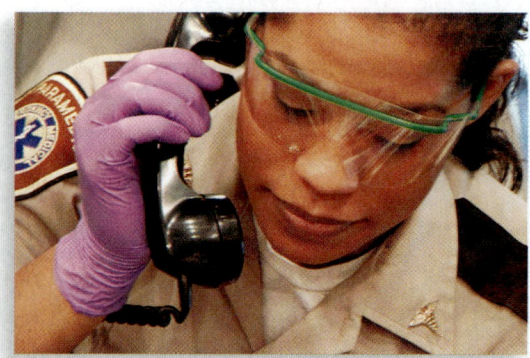

Figure 4-1 Telephones, radios, and other communication techniques enable paramedics to consult directly with other medical professionals from the emergency healthcare team.

authority for the state level.[11] In some states, physicians have advisory roles regarding clinical practice but are given less or no operational control over the functioning of the EMS system. In other states, physicians play a key role in the administration and oversight of the entire system.[11]

Subject to individual state laws that grant physicians the authority to approve or oversee paramedic practice, paramedics are typically individually certified or licensed by the state. This means that paramedics have their own, discrete scope of practice and are subject to specific state laws and regulations that govern their practice and the care they deliver. The concept of derivative authority to practice—i.e., the notion of a paramedic practicing "under" a physician's license—is, for the most part, outdated and inaccurate. Paramedics are independently licensed or certified professionals, subject to the physician direction or oversight granted to medical directors under the law. DOT 1-4.4, 1-4.7r

Patient Decision-Making and Self-Determination

An important legal concept that has evolved over the past several decades is the concept of patient self-determination. The principle of **patient self-determination** or **patient autonomy** states that patients are to be the primary decision-makers with regard to the medical care they receive. However, some patients are unable to make informed decisions about their condition or their treatment, and, in some cases, the law impacts medical decision-making. The principles of consent, refusal of care, and advance directives are three areas of the law where principles of patient self-determination come most sharply into view.

CONNECTIONS Chapter 3: Professional Ethics discusses consent from the ethical perspective and asks you to consider what is in the best interests of your patients. It asks you always to remember that you are there to serve as an advocate for patients who may be unable to make good decisions on their own behalf. Consider reading Chapter 3 if you are unclear on the connections between ethics and the law as this can help you understand the concepts discussed here.

Consent

The concept of **consent** for health care is informed permission given by a competent patient, or the patient's legally responsible decision-maker, for care or transportation by EMS providers. DOT 1-4.7g

The cornerstone of consent is that the patient or responsible decision maker is fully informed of the

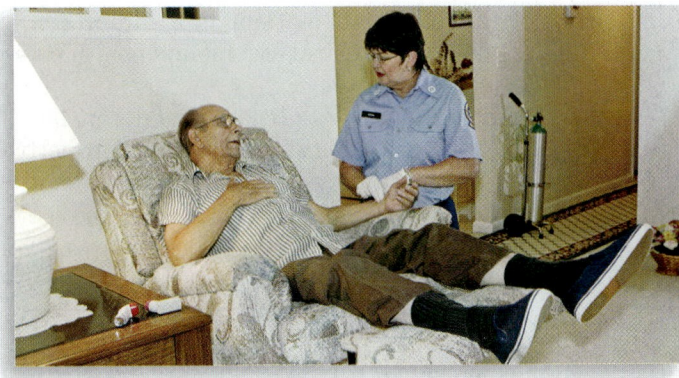

Figure 4-2   Paramedic informing the patient of her planned actions and obtaining informed consent to treat.

patient's condition, the risks of nontreatment, and the benefits of treatment.

For consent to be valid, it must be informed.

That is, the patient must be given sufficient information, in language the patient can understand, to make an *informed* decision as to whether or not to accept a particular course of treatment (Figure 4-2). The information about the patient's condition, benefit of treatment, and potential risks from refusing treatment must be provided in simple terms that are free of the medical jargon that healthcare providers use on a routine basis to communicate among themselves.[12]

The patient or responsible decision-maker must also be competent to grant consent for care (or to refuse it). A person must be legally competent—meaning old enough to grant consent (typically 18 years of age)—and mentally competent—meaning that the person is able to understand the information given to make an informed decision regarding healthcare.

Consent can be expressed or implied. **Expressed consent** is given directly by patients or their responsible decision-maker either verbally or through some physical action that the patient desires treatment. Nonverbal, physical expressions of consent may include, for example, a nod of the head or rolling up a sleeve to allow the paramedic to initiate IV access. If the patient's legally responsible decision-maker is not present at the scene (for instance, a minor's parents are at work), the legally responsible decision-maker can give consent by telephone, so long as that person is properly informed of the patient's condition and the risks/benefits discussed above. In a true emergency, when informed consent is not available, treatment can be rendered under the doctrine of implied consent.[13] DOT 1-4.17

Implied consent means that an emergency health care provider may presume that a patient who is ill or injured and for any reason is unable to give consent (unconscious, incapacitated, patient is a minor, etc.) would consent to the delivery of emergency health care necessitated by the condition.

A competent patient who gives consent can later withdraw that consent, so long as the patient is properly informed of the risks of that course of action. DOT 1-4.16

Working in the Gray Zone

It is difficult to handle situations when patients refuse to provide consent and you honestly believe they should grant it. Remember that ultimately a capable patient has the right to refuse care—even if it is an unreasonable course of action in your eyes. Continue to treat the patient in the areas they have given consent. You may persuade them to accept more care once they see you are genuinely concerned. Demonstrating disapproval for their decision may make the situation worse, or cause undesirable behaviors on their part to escalate.

Consent of Minors

When treating a minor (who, in most states, is defined as a person under 18 years of age), paramedics must be mindful of the fact that minors are not given the authority to be able to consent for medical treatment or to make a decision to refuse care. Therefore, it follows that any consent or refusal form signed by a minor on the minor's own behalf is quite likely invalid and unenforceable. DOT 1-4.7o

Nevertheless, some states permit minors to make their own medical decisions in certain circumstances.[14] State law varies widely on this subject, so be sure to consult with authorities in your system to determine under what circumstances a minor may make a healthcare decision in your state. Some of the situations in which minors are most often permitted to make medical decisions under state laws include minors who are pregnant, minors in need of psychiatric or mental health care, minors seeking treatment for drug and alcohol addiction, or minors in need of emergency healthcare.

A term often used in healthcare—sometimes erroneously—is the term "emancipated minor." An **emancipated minor** is typically a self-supporting minor, and this status is often dependent upon the minor receiving an actual court order of emancipation. DOT 1-4.7j

Wherever the law grants the ability of a patient to make a medical decision, that decision-making authority can typically be exercised by a legal representative on behalf of the patient. In the case of a minor, this can include a parent or legal guardian. In the case of a minor whose parents are divorced, either parent is

typically empowered to make medical decisions on behalf of the minor, unless the parent's rights have been completely severed with regard to the minor.[15] A **legal guardian** is typically someone with court-appointed authority or other authority recognized under the law to make decisions for a minor.

Working in the Gray Zone

Use all the tools at your disposal, including medical direction, when you are unsure of legal issues that arise. Sharing the decision-making process with supervisors and other members of the healthcare team helps you make better decisions—particularly when you are in a stressful situation.

In some cases, government agencies with temporary custody of a minor are empowered to make healthcare decisions for the minor on an emergency basis. For instance, child welfare agencies may grant consent for emergency healthcare for a minor in their custody under the principle of *parens patriae,* which, literally translated, means "parent of the country."[16]

The principle of *in loco parentis* empowers school officials to "stand in place of the parent" for purposes of controlling the conduct and behavior of children in school. It gives teachers the authority to make healthcare decisions for a child in the absence of the parents in cases that involve a medical emergency in which delay in care might endanger the child's well-being.[17]

Legal Representatives

Adults who have reached the age of majority (typically 18 in most states) can also have legal representatives for healthcare decision-making purposes. A competent adult can appoint a legal representative in a document called a **power of attorney** (also referred to as a **health care power of attorney** or **medical durable power of attorney**).[18] The person appointed to act as the patient's legal representative is typically called the *agent.* The agent is, subject to state law, permitted to exercise the powers granted in the power of attorney document. Adults can also have court-appointed legal guardians who are authorized to make medical decisions on their behalf. In most cases, the agent is granted this decision-making authority when the patient has become incapacitated and is unable to make decisions for himself or herself.[19]

Some states have laws that grant other family members the ability to make healthcare decisions on behalf of an incompetent or incapacitated patient. For instance, some state laws grant authority to a spouse, son/daughter, sibling, or other relative to make emergency healthcare decisions on behalf of an incapacitated person in need of health care.[19]

Refusal of Care

Closely related to the notion of patient consent is the concept of **refusal of care.** The basic rule is

> A competent patient (or legally responsible decision maker) who is properly informed of the risks of nontreatment and the benefits of treatment is permitted to refuse medical care and/or transportation, even if that care would save the person's life.

In any refusal situation, it is important to determine if the patient is both legally and mentally competent to make an informed refusal decision and that the patient understands the risks of refusal. Any patient refusal of care should be carefully documented.

CONNECTIONS See Chapter 17: Documentation and Communication for more detailed coverage of documentation of refusal of care. **Skill Sheet 64: Documentation has more information.**

A competent patient who is fully informed of the risks may make a decision to refuse medical care or transportation even if that decision is likely a bad decision from a medical perspective. Whenever possible, obtain physician consultation in a refusal of care situation (some protocols require it). Have the patient or responsible decision-maker speak directly to the medical control physician if possible, as consultation with a physician may sometimes change the patient's decision to refuse care (Figure 4-3). DOT 1-4.18, 1-4.19, 1-4.28

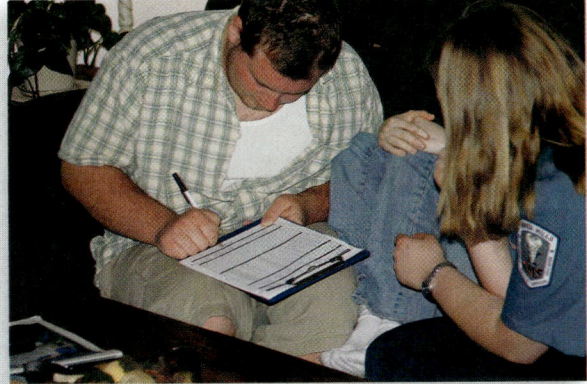

Figure 4-3 Competent patients have the legal right to refuse care and treatment, even when they have a life-threatening problem. Documenting patient refusal is very important. A signature on the patient care form is one way to document the refusal.

When documenting a refusal of care and the patient refuses to sign the form, see if a family member or someone who knows the patient personally is willing to sign the form. Often, handwritten signatures are unreadable. In addition to the signature, print the person's name and relationship to the patient, and obtain contact information for that person.

Abandonment

Abandonment involves initiating patient care and then leaving the patient before turning the patient over to another medical professional capable of continuing to render the appropriate level of care to the patient. An obvious example of this is leaving the scene without treating or transporting the patient when a physician evaluation is warranted. A less obvious example is when a paramedic leaves the patient in the care of a lesser trained individual, such as an EMT, when the patient really needs ALS-level care. DOT 1-4.7

Sometimes it is appropriate for an EMT to take over caring for a patient. It may represent good medical decision-making and good use of scarce medical resources. However, whenever a paramedic transitions care to an EMT or Advanced EMT, the paramedic should consult with the individual assuming care to insure the individual understands the situation and feels capable of continuing to care for the patient. If there is any hesitation by the EMT or AEMT crew to care for the patient, the paramedic should continue care and address the issue at a later time. DOT 1-4.20

Advance Directives/DNROs

Most, if not all, states have laws pertaining to advance directives for health care.[20] An **advance directive** is a document in which a competent person gives instructions to be followed with respect to healthcare in the event the person later becomes incapacitated and is unable to make or communicate those decisions to others. An advance directive typically does not become effective unless it is documented in writing and until the patient becomes terminally ill or enters a permanent vegetative or nonresponsive state. State law varies on the ability of paramedics and other EMS providers to honor advance directives for health care. DOT 1-4.7b, 1-4.25

A majority of states have also adopted specific EMS or out-of-hospital **Do Not Resuscitate Order (DNRO or DNR) programs.**[21] Although these programs vary from state to state, they share common characteristics. For instance, most state EMS DNR programs feature an approved means of identifying patients with valid DNR orders. These identification methods often include a DNR bracelet, necklace, form, or card.

Though this also varies by state, if a person is subject to a verified and valid out-of-hospital DNR order, DNR typically means that the paramedic shall withhold cardiac compressions, intubation, artificial ventilation, resuscitative drugs, defibrillation, and other invasive resuscitative measures. In addition, some states allow a patient to specify individually which of these interventions they do not want performed and which they will allow. In all cases, however, paramedics should still administer other appropriate care to a DNR patient as indicated, such as supplemental oxygen, pain control, basic airway management, and other basic steps for a patient's physical comfort.

"Do not resuscitate" does **not** mean "do not treat" or "do not transport."

Nice to Know

Palliative care is the term applied to care measures meant to provide comfort to the patient. Often when lifesaving therapy is not allowed, palliative measures are appropriate. It allows for humane and compassionate treatment when lifesaving measures are not allowed.

Patient Destination and Hospital Diversion Issues

One area of increasing regulation and controversy in EMS involves the choice of hospital destination. There is, in many states, what can best be described as tension between the principles of patient autonomy (the right of patients to make their own healthcare decisions) and the protocols and regulations of EMS oversight agencies, which often restrict or attempt to restrict the exercise of those rights by patients. This most often occurs in an effort to take a patient to the most appropriate hospital given the patient's problem, which may not be the patient's hospital of choice. Often, the situation arises where the ambulance service needs to take the patient to a nearby hospital in order to get the ambulance back into service, but the patient would prefer a different hospital.

While the principle of patient self-determination firmly holds that legally and mentally competent patients are free to make decisions about their health care—including whether or not to receive health care

and from which providers to receive it—some EMS systems have specific protocols in place addressing the issue of patient destination. For instance, most states have trauma patient destination protocols that require transport (under certain circumstances) to a trauma center instead of a facility without emergent trauma capabilities.[22] In other cases, patients who meet other specialty care criteria, such as critically burned, cardiac, stroke, or pediatric patients, are also directed by protocols to specialty centers rather than community hospitals, even if those hospitals are closer.[22]

These types of protocols can place the paramedic in a difficult position—choosing between the requirements of a protocol and the clearly expressed wishes of a competent patient.

Generally, providers should follow applicable system protocols, and any variation from those protocols should be handled only in consultation with medical control authorities.

Diversion Issues

In some cases, hospitals may issue diversionary orders to incoming ambulances, directing them to transport the patient to an alternate destination. Typically this is because of inadequate resources in the hospital's emergency department due to excess patient demand. Some EMS systems refer to this concept using terminology such as "ER diversion," "hospital bypass," or "hospital re-route" (Figure 4-4). DOT 1-4.21, 1-4.22

Regardless of what this issue is called, Federal law imposes significant constraints on this practice. Specifically, the Emergency Medical Treatment and Active Labor Act (EMTALA) permits a hospital to issue a diversionary order only when it lacks the staff or

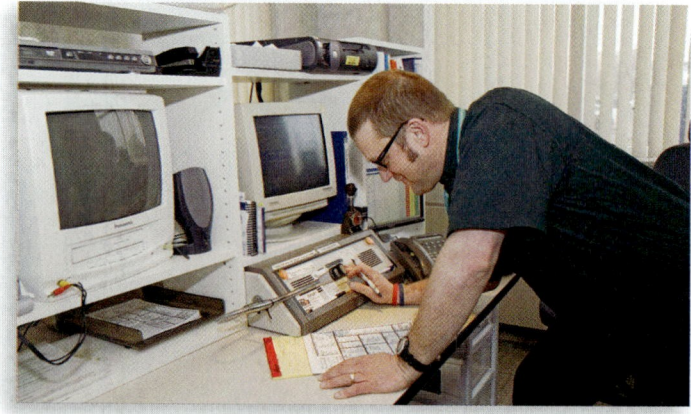

Figure 4-4 Medical Resource Communication Center diverting an incoming ambulance. In some systems, a computer system can assist in determining the latest hospital bed status for receiving facilities.

resources to handle an additional emergency patient.[23] In addition, regardless of the issuance of a diversionary order, a hospital *must* accept a patient who comes on to the hospital's property. It must also perform a medical screening examination on that patient without undue delay. If the medical screening examination reveals the presence of an emergency medical condition, the hospital must provide stabilizing treatment to that patient, without regard to the patient's ability to pay. In addition, EMTALA, in most cases, prohibits the transfer of a patient to another facility until the patient is stabilized, which is why the law is often referred to as the "patient anti-dumping law."

EMTALA requires that:

- Hospitals must allow patients on the premises admission into the emergency department.
- Appropriate medical professionals must perform medical screening of the patient for life-threatening conditions without undue delay.
- If a life-threatening condition is detected, the hospital must provide treatment (stabilization) regardless of the patient's ability to pay.
- The patient cannot be transferred until the patient is stabilized (unless transferring the patient is required to stabilize him or her).

EMTALA regulations also make it clear that ambulances owned and operated by the hospital are considered "hospital property" for purposes of determining when a hospital's EMTALA duties apply. In most cases, a patient must be transported back to the hospital that owns the ambulance in order for the hospital to be able to perform the required medical screening examination on its patient, unless one of the law's exceptions applies. In some cases, such as where a physician gives a medical direction order to transport the patient to a different facility, and where that physician is not affiliated with the hospital that owns and operates the ambulance, the patient may be transported to a different destination. In addition, the hospital-owned ambulance may transport the patient to a different hospital when the ambulance is functioning as part of an organized EMS system and protocols regarding patient destination are in place.

Privacy and Confidentiality

Federal law establishes privacy protection applicable to almost every type of healthcare provider in the United States, including ambulance and EMS providers. This Federal law is known as **HIPAA**—the **Health Insurance Portability and Accountability Act.**[24] HIPAA requires that all individually identifiable health information—commonly referred to as **PHI or Protected Health Information**—be safeguarded and used only for purposes specifically permitted by the regulations. DOT 1-4.15

For instance, HIPAA permits PHI to be used for purposes of treatment, payment, and healthcare operations. This means that providers involved in the care of the patient can freely share appropriate information for treatment purposes. Providers can also use a patient's PHI to submit claims and invoices for their services. Providers may also use a patient's PHI—provided they use only the minimum amount of PHI necessary—for operational purposes such as quality improvement and other management functions.

HIPAA greatly restricts the types of disclosures of PHI that a healthcare provider may make to law enforcement officers. For instance, certain limited information can be shared with law enforcement upon their request to identify or locate a suspect or a fugitive. The HIPAA Privacy Rule provides very detailed information about the situations in which a release of PHI to law enforcement is permitted. HIPAA also restricts the disclosure of PHI to the media and to others.

Every entity that is subject to HIPAA is required to have a privacy officer in place and to provide training to all of its workforce members regarding the organization's privacy practices. Healthcare providers are also required, in most circumstances, to give patients a "notice of privacy practices" describing the organization's privacy policies and informing patients of their healthcare privacy rights.

Although Federal law establishes a "floor," or baseline, of privacy protection, state laws also address issues of privacy and confidentiality. Under HIPAA, conflicting state laws are preempted, that is, superseded, by HIPAA, meaning that HIPAA, and not the state law, controls patient privacy issues. However, if a state law is more stringent in protecting patient privacy than HIPAA, the state law then applies. In many states, laws that deal with the confidentiality of HIV or AIDS-related information may be more stringent than HIPAA. In addition, state laws pertaining to issues such as mental health or substance abuse may also be more stringent than HIPAA, and thus still applicable.

Working in the Gray Zone

HIPAA laws are constantly evolving, and therefore it is difficult to discuss the law in great detail. Make sure you stay connected with local, regional, and state legal resources to ensure you have the most current information.

Negligence

Unfortunately, paramedics will occasionally be involved in claims of medical negligence. One of the most common types of legal actions in which paramedics (and other EMS and healthcare providers of all types) find themselves is a negligence case. Simply defined,

> **Negligence** is the failure to act as a reasonably prudent and careful person would under similar circumstances. DOT 1-4.7p

In the healthcare context, negligence is referred to as **malpractice** (Figure 4-5). Negligence/malpractice actions fall under the heading of unintentional torts. An **unintentional tort** is one that the defendant did not mean to commit; it is simply a case where a bad outcome may occur due to the failure to exercise reasonable care.

Regardless of the level of training, certification, or licensure held by the health care provider, there are four elements that a plaintiff must prove in order to impose malpractice liability upon a healthcare provider in a negligence case.[25]

Elements of Negligence/Malpractice

1. Duty to Act exists (the EMS provider is obligated to assess and treat the patient)
2. Breach of Duty by omission (not doing something you should have) or commission (doing something improperly)
3. Damages (Injury or harm occurs to the patient)
4. Proximate Causation (a link exists between the duty to act and the injury) DOT 1-4.10

Duty

The first element that must be established in a malpractice case is the concept of **duty.** This means that the plaintiff must establish that the defendant had a legal

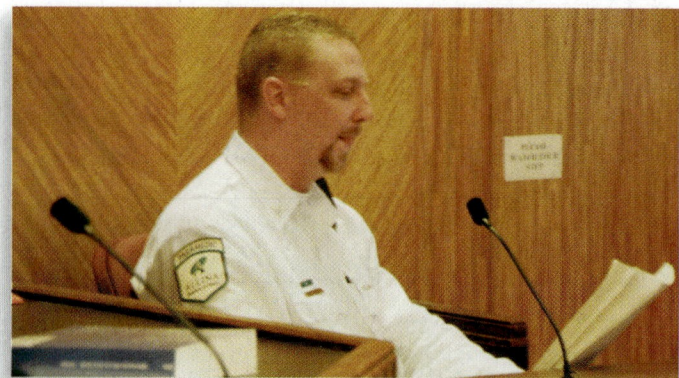

Figure 4-5 Legal proceedings are occurring with greater frequency. Your best defense is to strictly adhere to good patient care practices and to be knowledgeable of the rules and regulations that govern your practice.

duty—a legal relationship—to the plaintiff. Ordinarily, a paramedic who is dispatched to assist a person in need has formed a legal relationship with that person that gives rise to a legal duty under the law of negligence. In contrast, a healthcare provider who just happens upon the scene of an accident as a passerby and who was not summoned to the scene as part of his or her job duties typically does not have a legal duty to act in such a circumstance. Of course, whether or not the provider feels compelled to act out of a sense of *moral* duty is an entirely different question, and that is ordinarily up to the individual provider. DOT 1-4.7i

> **CONNECTIONS** Chapter 3: Professional Ethics explores duty to act from the ethical perspective in more detail.

The existence of a legal duty typically means that the paramedic must act with due regard for the patient and provide the applicable standard of care with respect to that patient. The standard of care will be discussed in more detail in the next section.

Breach of Duty

The second element that a plaintiff must prove in a malpractice case against a paramedic, or any other health care provider for that matter, is a **breach of duty.** This means that the paramedic must be found to have violated a legal duty owed to the plaintiff. Exactly what duty is owed to a patient and how it is breached or violated depends entirely upon the circumstances.

A breach of duty exists where the provider fails to provide the standard of care for the need of that patient. The standard of care is, generally speaking, what a similar, reasonably prudent paramedic would do under similar circumstances. Therefore, the standard of care is measured objectively, rather than subjectively, in a malpractice case. DOT 1-4.7e, 1-4.8

Evidence of the standard of care can come from many sources. If there is an existing applicable law or regulation, violation of such a requirement by the paramedic can constitute *negligence per se,* which basically means that the plaintiff can establish negligence without needing to prove what would be reasonable and prudent under similar circumstances.[26] Other sources of the standard of care can be protocols or applicable policies or procedures. Documents such as the National Standard Curriculum or EMS textbooks such as this one can also be used to establish evidence of the standard of care. In most cases, evidence of the standard of care, and its violation by a paramedic or other healthcare provider, is established in court through the testimony of one or more expert witnesses.

In short, whenever a paramedic fails to exercise the degree of care that would be exercised by a reasonably prudent paramedic under similar circumstances, a breach of duty can be found.

> ## Working in the Gray Zone
>
> Duty to act has two elements: omission and commission. Breach of duty can occur from doing something wrong or *from not doing something right* when it is the right time or circumstance to do it.

Damages (Harm or Injury)

The third element that must be established in a negligence case is damages. **Damages**—in a malpractice case—typically refer to harm or other losses sustained by the injured party (the plaintiff) as a result of the negligence of the defendant. The remedy for damages in a malpractice case is money—financial compensation to the injured party. There are many components to the damages that can be awarded in a malpractice case including medical expenses, pain and suffering, funeral expenses, wage loss, and others.

Causation

Finally, the fourth element that a plaintiff must prove to bring a successful malpractice case against a paramedic is the element of causation. Simply put, **causation** means that the negligence of the defendant likely caused or created the harm sustained by the plaintiff. Although under the law, the concept of causation has many aspects and is a good deal more complicated, the basic idea is one of foreseeability—whether or not the harm that befell the plaintiff is reasonably foreseeable by the defendant. To be a legal cause of a plaintiff's harm, a defendant's negligent conduct must ordinarily be a substantial factor in causing that harm. DOT 1-4.7q

There can be more than one legal cause of a plaintiff's harm, and one defendant's negligence does not excuse the negligence of another defendant. For instance, a patient who is initially injured in a vehicle accident by another driver who runs a stop sign and then who is the victim of medical malpractice by the responding paramedics, would have viable negligence cases against both the negligent driver and the paramedics.

Intentional Torts

Negligence actions fall under an area of the law known as "unintentional torts." Paramedics and other EMS providers can also be subject to intentional torts. In contrast to an unintentional tort, an intentional tort is one in which the defendant meant to cause the harmful action. DOT 1-4.7u

Some of the most common types of intentional torts as applied to EMS providers include assault, battery, false imprisonment, and defamation.[27]

Assault is placing a patient in a position where he fears for his safety or perceives you mean to cause him some sort of injury or harm. Threatening a patient that you will twist her sprained arm unless she calms down and obeys your directions is an example of assault. **Battery** is the touching of or contact with another person without that person's consent. Taken to the extreme end of the spectrum, any patient care rendered without actual consent could potentially be considered battery. DOT 1-4.7c, 1-4.7d, 1-4.23

False imprisonment is the confinement of a person against his or her will or without the person's consent. Acts such as securing a patient to a stretcher or a backboard, immobilizing a patient, or placing a person in an ambulance can, without proper consent (whether express or implied), constitute false imprisonment. DOT 1-4.7k

Defamation is saying or publicizing something untrue about a person that tends to injure that person's character or blacken the person's reputation. For instance, disclosing false information about a patient—such as telling another person that "Mr. Smith has HIV"—can constitute the tort of defamation when that information is untrue. (It can also constitute invasion of privacy or a HIPAA violation even if it is true.)

> Defamation can be in verbal form (which is called "slander") or in written form, in which case it is called "libel." DOT 1-4.7n, 1-4.7s

Defenses and Immunity Laws

While paramedics and other EMS providers can be sued for malpractice or other types of malfeasance, most states have laws that assist providers in defending themselves when faced with these types of lawsuits.[28] For instance, many state EMS laws contain **immunity** provisions (often called Good Samaritan laws) that protect paramedics for acts of ordinary negligence or for acts or omissions done in good faith.[29] **Good Samaritan laws** may also offer protection in some cases, although these laws ordinarily exist for the benefit of individuals who rendered aid to an injured person but otherwise had no legal duty to do so (Figure 4-6).[30] In some states, there are also specific legal protections for volunteers.[31] Paramedics who work for public agencies may also enjoy a form of local government immunity when acting within the course and scope of their official duties. DOT 1-4.7l, 1-4.14

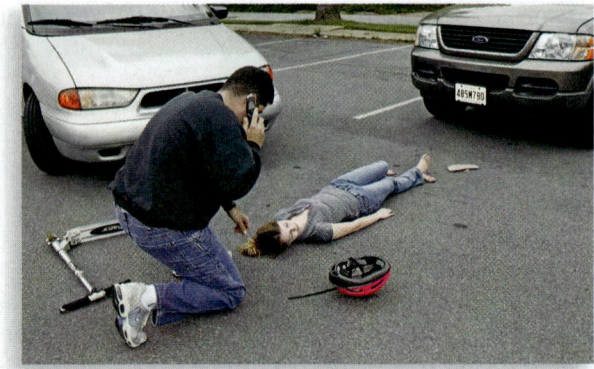

Figure 4-6   Good Samaritan calling 9-1-1 at the scene of a pedestrian struck by a car.

Nice to Know

Good Samaritan, or "Good Sam" Laws as they are also called, arose in California in the mid-1900s following an increasing number of lawsuits against doctors when they stopped to render aid to patients in motor vehicle crashes. Every state in the U.S. has some type of Good Sam law, but when and how that applies to certified and licensed healthcare providers (including the EMS professional) varies.

The common thread in most immunity statutes is that most offer protection only when the paramedic acts in good faith and only for acts of ordinary negligence. Most immunity laws do not offer any protection for intentional or reckless acts or acts of gross negligence. The difference between ordinary and gross negligence can be subjective, however, and is most often decided by a judge relatively early in a court case. Therefore, paramedics and other EMS providers should not think of immunity statutes as a hammock on which they can rest but as a safety net on which they can rely if necessary.

Though relatively few cases against paramedics go all the way to trial, an individual paramedic is entitled to offer a vigorous defense in a malpractice case. Most often, this defense involves attacking the elements of breach of duty or causation in court (i.e., whether or not the standard of care was violated or whether or not any breach of a standard of care was the legal cause of the plaintiff's harm). Most EMS organizations carry malpractice insurance (called **"professional liability" insurance**), and under those policies the insurer (provided it is given prompt notice of the claim) is obligated to provide a defense for the organization's paramedics in malpractice cases. As part of that defense, the insurer must typically hire a lawyer to represent the interests of the paramedic. Some paramedics or EMS organizations still retain their own personal lawyer to oversee these types of cases in conjunction with the lawyer hired by the insurer. DOT 1-4.7n, 2-1.13

Working in the Gray Zone

You should consult with your personal legal adviser whether or not it is in your best interest to carry your own liability insurance coverage in addition to the coverage offered by your employer or EMS agency.

Criminal Law

Although it is rare, paramedics are becoming involved in an increasing number of criminal cases. One common type of criminal case involving EMS providers is related to the emergency operation of the ambulance (Figure 4-7). Ambulance crashes are a common source of litigation, often resulting in criminal charges.[32] Where an emergency vehicle operator's conduct crosses the line from mere negligence to reckless or intentional is often difficult to determine, however, law enforcement agencies with increasing frequency are charging ambulance or other emergency vehicle operators with vehicle code or other criminal law violations. Driver training, prudent use of lights and sirens, and a continuing commitment to drive with due regard for the safety of others are the best ways to avoid both civil and criminal liability in the operation of emergency vehicles. DOT 1-2.12, 1-2.14

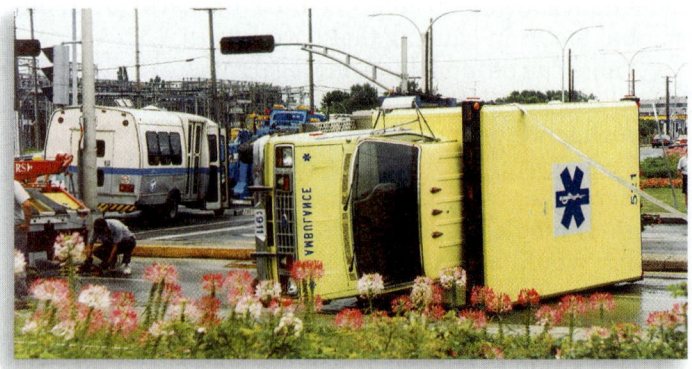

Figure 4-7   Just like any other member of society, EMS personnel are held accountable for traffic accidents they cause.

Another area of criminal liability in EMS has involved drug diversion or drug-related illegal behaviors.[33] Paramedics use many medications and solutions in the course of their duties, and most of those constitute controlled substances (that require a prescription) under state and federal law. Drug abuse or addiction among healthcare providers is well known and in many cases leads to theft of supplies in order to feed the addiction. In other cases, paramedics have diverted drugs in order to sell them. Special care should be taken to ensure the security and accountability of controlled substances in the EMS environment. Drugs should be locked and stored in accordance with applicable laws, regulations, or policies and inventoried at regular intervals.

Working in the Gray Zone

Giving patients drugs to use later so they do not have to contact the EMS service is also considered a diversion. An example would be a paramedic leaving behind some naloxone on the scene for heroin users to use the next time they overdose. Another example might be giving a patient an epinephrine autoinjector to replace the personally prescribed pen just used. Although these actions may seem altruistic, they are misguided and should not occur. It can be very difficult to balance doing the right thing legally with treating patients to personal perceived levels of compassion. If you have a strong interest in this area, get involved with groups that influence political and cultural changes so you can help protect all the citizens you serve.

Reporting Requirements

Some situations paramedics encounter require that they be reported to public health or public safety agencies. Paramedics may be required to make the report personally to the agency or patient care facility, or they may be required to make the report through their chain of command within their organization. Requirements will vary from state to state and agency to agency. Reports may be made verbally or in writing, and this requirement will vary as well. Some situations that typically require additional reporting requirements include:

- Criminal activity: drug possession, manufacture or distribution of drugs, weapons possession, theft of property, illegal possession of property, etc. (Reporting requirements vary significantly. Consult with your agency's legal department for the reporting requirements.)
- Perceived threats to homeland security or perceived terrorist activities
- Animal attacks and bites or animals in situations of misuse or abuse
- Violent actions against others: domestic abuse, elder abuse, and child abuse or neglect, sexual assault, etc.
- Discriminatory or harassing behaviors
- Suspicion of communicable, infectious, or sexually transmitted diseases DOT 1-4.6

Use of Restraints

Occasionally EMS providers face situations where patients require the use of restraints in order to assess, treat, or transport them. Patients who are in need of care, and are also incompetent to make good patient care decisions, may pose a physical threat to the EMS care providers. This can occur with the use of mind-altering substances such as drugs or alcohol, but it can also occur due to illness or injuries. Metabolic disturbance, psychological illness and disease, head trauma, blood loss, and other life-threatening problems can render a patient incompetent to make rational decisions. The human brain, once deprived of oxygen or glucose from any cause, may be incapable of rational thoughts, decisions, or behaviors. Unfortunately, hypoxia or hypoglycemia does not lead to an improvement in personality and decision-making. Usually the opposite is true, and the patient becomes argumentative, irrational, and perhaps even combative.

Public safety law enforcement professionals are specifically trained to handle patients who are uncooperative or out of control and not acting in the best interest of themselves or the public. Sometimes they are not present, however, when a patient or situation escalates out of control, so paramedics should know how to de-escalate the situation and regain control of the scene. Chapter 10: Therapeutic Communications and History Taking discusses tips and techniques to use to provide therapeutic communications.

The use of restraints is governed by law, and, as with many laws and regulations in EMS, there is variability from state to state. Any regulation on the use of restraints should include language for the reasonable use of enough force to ensure personal safety for the EMS providers and other public safety personnel. No law allows public safety personnel to then become the aggressor and continue to harm the individual further. DOT 1-4.24

Several resources, including textbooks and continuing education courses, address personal safety while performing EMS care. Chapter 9: Safety and Scene Size-Up discusses some of these concepts as well.

Summary

Laws govern EMS providers as they do all other professions. Paramedics have a duty to be aware of the laws that pertain to them. Knowledgeable paramedics are better prepared to deal with circumstances as they arise on the job.

The laws pertaining to EMS providers establish the guidelines that mold and shape the profession. Certain laws that EMS providers should be aware of are those that provide for control and guidance such as medical direction and oversight. They also provide necessary protections for both the providers of care as well as the people receiving care. Laws originate at the Federal level, such as Medicare or HIPAA; state level, such as Pennsylvania's EMS Act; or at a local level as when counties or townships enact special rules that are only meant to be enforced within those communities.

It is important to know the people that direct EMS and that provide immediate oversight for the providers. There are different types of medical direction (prospective, concurrent, and retrospective) that govern medical treatments and decision-making processes.

EMS providers should be aware of torts that can be brought against paramedics, such as false imprisonment and battery or in situations where providers do not follow the directions of those persons they are attempting to care for. More importantly, it is becoming common for criminal charges to be filed against EMS providers for such things as ambulance accidents and drug diversion. It should be noted that while "Good Samaritan" laws do provide immunity to EMS providers, in many situations they do not and cannot serve to protect against every possible infraction on the part of providers. Any person who plans to work as an EMS provider or paramedic should make themselves aware of laws that govern the profession since those laws exist for the protection of providers and patients alike.

Notes

Notes on References:

P.S. = Pennsylvania Statutes Annotated
Pa. C.S.A. = Pennsylvania Consolidated Statutes Annotated
Rest. 2d Torts = Second Restatement of the Law of Torts
U.S.C.A. = United States Code Annotated

1. Pennsylvania: 35 P.S. §6931 (Emergency medical services personnel)
   Minnesota: MN ST §144E.001 (Emergency medical services regulatory board, general provisions)
   Virginia: Va. Code Ann. §32.1-111.5 (Certification and recertification of emergency medical services personnel)
   Ohio: OH ST §4765.01 (Emergency medical services)
2. Pennsylvania: 35 P.S. §6932 (Minimum standards for ambulance service)
   Alabama: Ala.Code 1975 §22-18-3 (Rules and regulations as to training, licensing, etc., of ambulance drivers and emergency medical technicians foundation and operation, licensing, etc. of vehicles.)
   California: West's Ann.Cal.Vehicle Code §2512 (Regulations governing ambulance service; ambulance driver's handbook)
   Maine: ME ST T. 32 §86 (Ambulance services and nontransporting medical services); ME ST T. 32 §87 (Ambulances)
   Missouri: V.A.M.S. 190.105 (Ambulance license required, exceptions)
3. Pennsylvania: 20 Pa. C.S.A. §54A01-A13 ("Do-Not-Resuscitate" Act)
   Maryland: MD Code, Health—General, §5-602 (Advanced directive)
   West Virginia: WV ST §16-30C-1 ("Do Not Resuscitate Act")
   North Carolina: N.C.G.S.A. §90-21.17 (Portable do not resuscitate order)
   New Jersey: N.J.S.A. 26:2H-53 (New Jersey Advance Directives for Health Care Act)
4. 35 P.S. §§6921-6938 (Pennsylvania EMS Act of 1985)
5. §4531(b)(2) of the Balanced Budget Act (BBA) of 1997 added a new section 1834(1) to the Social Security Act (SSA); sec 1834 [42 U.S.C. 1395m] (Special Payment Rules For Particular Items And Services)
6. Pub. L. 104-191 (Public Law 104-191, 104th Congress, enacted August 21, 1996)
7. 42 U.S.C.A. §1395dd (Examination and treatment for emergency medical conditions and women in labor)
8. 35 P.S. §6931(j.1) (Suspension, revocation, or refusal of department certification or recognition)
9. "Paramedic charged with stealing drugs" http://www.newschannel5.com/content/news/18967.asp (May 2, 2006).
   "Paramedic drug case heads to trial" http://www.timesherald.com/site/news.cfm?newsid=16393225&BRD=1672&PAG=461&dept_id=33380&rfi=6 (March 29, 2006).
   "Paramedic ordered to seek drug treatment for stealing painkillers" http://www.wkyc.com/news/news_article.aspx?storyid=47137 (February 2, 2006).
10. 35 P.S. §§6921-6938 (Pennsylvania EMS Act of 1985)
11. Jonathan Busko, MD, "Medical Control" http://www.emedicine.com/emerg/topic716.htm (April 12, 2006).
12. Pennsylvania: 40 P.S. §130.504 (Informed Consent)
    California: V.T.C.A., Civil Practice & Remedies Code §74-105 (Manner of Disclosure)
    Oregon: O.R.S. §677.097 (Obtaining informed consent of patient)
    District of Columbia: DC ST §7-1231.07 (Consent to mental health services and mental health supports.)
13. 35 P.S. §6933 (Limitation for liability for failure to obtain consent)
14. Pennsylvania: P.S. §2511(b) (Rights of Minors)
    New Jersey: N.J.S.A. 9:17A-1 (Consent by minor to performance of medical or surgical care and procedure by hospital or licensed physician)
    Maine: ME ST T. 22, Subt. 2, Pt. 3, Chapter 260 (Consent of Minors for Health Services)
15. 42 Pa. C.S.A. §6357 (Rights And Duties Of Legal Custodian)
16. 23 Pa. C.S.A. §5424 (Temporary Emergency Jurisdiction)
17. D.O.F., D.J.F. and M.F. v. Lewisburg Area School District Board of School Directors 868 A.2d 28 (Pa.Cmwlth., 2004.) While the school district does stand "*in loco parentis,*" this status does not invest schools with all authority of parents over children. Instead, it provides for such control as is necessary to prevent infractions of discipline and interference with the educational process. *Axtell v. LaPenna, 323 F.Supp. 1077, 1080 (W.D.Pa.1971).*
    Guerrieri v. Tyson 24 A.2d 468 (147 Pa.Super. 239, 1942) These teachers stood *in loco parentis* to the child, but there is

nothing in that relationship which will justify defendants' acts. Under the delegated parental authority implied from the relationship of teacher and pupil, a teacher may inflict reasonable corporal punishment on a pupil to enforce discipline *(Harris et al. v. Galilley, Appellant, 125 Pa.Super. 505, 189 A. 779),* but there is no implied delegation of authority to exercise her lay judgment, as a parent may, in the matter of the treatment of injury or disease suffered by a pupil. Treatment of the minor plaintiff's hand was not necessary in this case; defendants were not acting in an emergency. The defendants were not school nurses and neither of them had any medical training or experience. Whether treatment of the infected finger was necessary was a question for the boy's parents to decide.

18. 20 Pa. C.S.A. §5604 (Durable Powers Of Attorney)
19. 20 Pa. C.S.A. §5604(b) (Durable Powers Of Attorney)
20. 20 Pa. C.S.A. §54A01-A13 ("Do-Not-Resuscitate" Act)
21. Pennsylvania: 20 Pa.C.S.A. §54A04 (Advance directive for health care)
    New Jersey: N.J.S.A. 26:2H-56 (Executing an advance directive)
    Oklahoma: OK ST T. 63 §3131.5, Chapter 61A (Oklahoma Do-Not-Resuscitate Act)
22. Pennsylvania: *Trauma Patient destination Protocol Statewide Air Medical Transport Protocol*
    http://www.dsf.health.state.pa.us/health/lib/health/ems/airtraumatriage.pdf
    New York: *Emergency Patient Destinations and Hospital Diversion*
    http://www.nyhealth.gov/nysdoh/ems/policy/06-01.htm
    Virginia: Appendix H: *Ambulance Destination Policy*
    http:www.tidewaterems.org/protocols/2003%20Protocols/Appendix%20H%20Ambulance%20Pt%20Destination%20Policy.pdf
    California, Santa Clara County: EMS Agency, Prehospital Care Manual, Policy 602; Effective Date March 1, 2006
    www.sccgov.org/SCC/docs%2FEmergency%20Medical%20Services%20(DEP)%2Fattachments%2F2.10.06%20602%20Prehospital%20Patient%20Destination%20Feb%202006%20Revision.pdf
23. 42 USC §1395dd (Emergency Medical Treatment and Active Labor Act)
24. Pub. L. 104-191 (Public Law 104-191, 104th Congress, enacted August 21, 1996)
25. Rest. 2d Torts §281 (Statement Of The Elements Of A Cause Of Action For Negligence)
26. Restatement (Third) of Torts (proposed final draft) §14, Comment *a*
27. *Lemann v. Essen Lane Daiquiris, Inc.* (923 So.2d 627) (2006) According to plaintiffs' averments, if a person refuses to go to the hospital, the paramedics may be held liable for respecting his rights and not taking him. In order to avoid this liability, the paramedics would be forced to violate the person's statutorily granted refusal rights and transport him against his will, thus, leaving themselves vulnerable to suit for the tort of false imprisonment or battery. The EMS defendants label this dilemma as a "no-win situation." Indeed, allowing EMS personnel to be subject to possible litigation for making one of two choices would represent a choice between Scylla and Charybdis, particularly in this matter where Parker was alert, oriented, in no distress, and denied unconsciousness.
    Easton v. Sutter Coast Hosp. (80 Cal.App.4th 485, 95 Cal. Rptr.2d 316) (2000) Plaintiffs have failed to allege facts

establishing that the conduct of which they complain was not lawfully privileged—that is, Winchester's removal to the hospital by the paramedics at the direction of the deputies. Having failed to allege that her removal to the hospital (where their complaint alleges she was intubated and treated for three days) was unprivileged; they have failed to plead a cause of action for false imprisonment.
Naeem v. Bensalem Tp. (Not Reported in F.Supp.2d, 2005 WL 696763 E.D.Pa.) (2005) In this action, Plaintiff has sued Defendants Bensalem Township, Bensalem Township Police Department, Officer Jack Gohl, Officer Clark, Officer Reilly, Officer Maren, Officer Domanico, and Paramedic Daniel MacIntosh for an alleged police assault occurring on or about May 5, 2002. Plaintiff asserts two § 1983 civil rights claims. Plaintiff's First Cause of Action pursuant to § 1983 is for the alleged assault. The Second Cause of Action is for a purported "cover up" of the assault. Plaintiff also asserts state law claims of assault and battery, intentional infliction of emotional distress, and conspiracy against all Defendants.

28. 42 Pa. C.S.A. §8331 (Medical Good Samaritan Civil Immunity)
29. 42 Pa. C.S.A. §8331.2 (Good Samaritan civil immunity for use of automated external defibrillator); §8331 (Medical Good Samaritan Civil Immunity)
30. Rest. 2d Torts §314.323 (Duty To Act For Protection Of Others)
31. Pennsylvania: 42 Pa.C.S.A. §8332 (Nonmedical good Samaritan civil immunity)
    Alabama: Ala.Code 1975 §6-5-336 (Volunteers) "The Volunteer Service Act."
    Texas: V.T.C.A., Civil Practice & Remedies Code §84.004 (Volunteer Liability)
    Florida: West's F.S.A. §768.1355 (Florida Volunteer Protection Act)
32. *Kik v. Sbraccia* (708 N.W.2d 766) Parents of deceased infant and infant's estate brought action against ambulance driver and township that owned and operated ambulance, alleging wrongful death and loss of consortium based on infant's death following premature birth that occurred when ambulance carrying mother crashed and caused mother to go into premature labor.
    LeBlanc v. Acadian Ambulance Service, Inc. (746 So.2d 665) Motorist brought action against ambulance company to recover damages for injuries sustained when motorist was struck by ambulance.
    Bell v. Community Ambulance Service Agency for Northern Des Moines County (579 N.W.2d 330) Motorist brought action against ambulance driver, ambulance service and townships which utilized service for injuries sustained in collision with ambulance.
33. "Officials Look Into Charges On Missing E.M.S. Drugs"
    http://query.nytimes.com/gst/fullpage.html?sec=health&res=9906EED81639F930A35752C1A963958260 (November 3, 1995).
    "Fire station plagued by pattern of missing drugs; A paramedic admits stealing vials of a powerful painkiller, but police don't know who stole the morphine."
    http://www.sptimes.com/2005/07/01/Northpinellas/Fire_station_plagued_.shtml (July 1, 2005).
    "Ft. Lauderdale Paramedics Disciplined in Drug-Theft Scandal"
    http://info.jems.com/jems/news03/news12e.html.

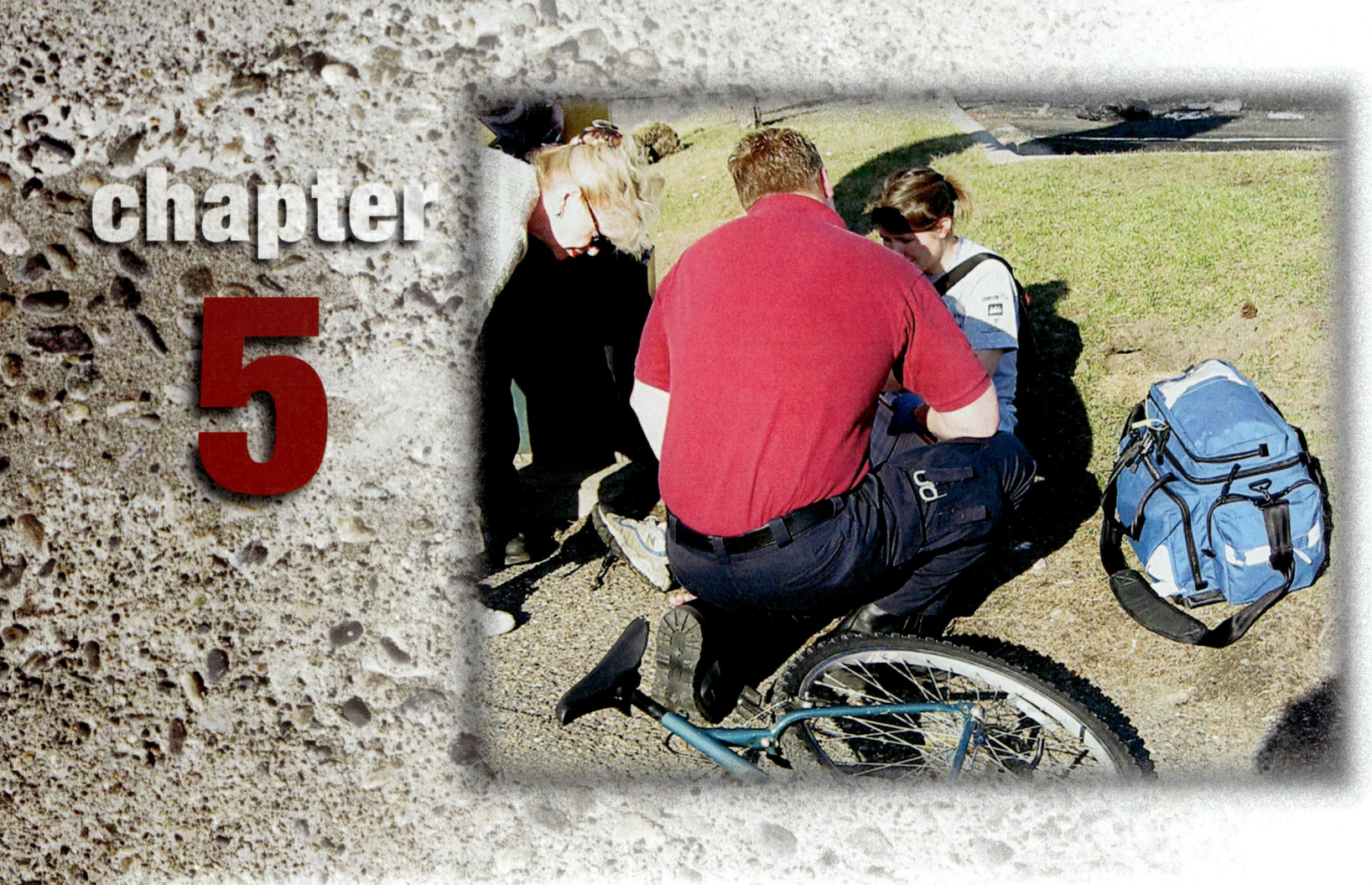

Clinical Decision-Making

"**I**t is extremely difficult for a physician who puts too much trust in what he reads to form a proper decision from what he sees."

—Andrew Boorde (1490?–1549), English Physician and Author

Need to Know

► Paramedics do not diagnose disease in the same manner as physicians. Paramedics assess signs and symptoms and formulate treatment plans based upon their findings without the benefit of the diagnostic studies available in the hospital. The approach paramedics utilize is called "assessment-based management."

► Paramedics need to understand the subtle differences in patient presentation between a patient who is "not sick," "sick," and "not yet sick."

► There is a difference in how problems are solved by both novice and expert paramedics. Novices can learn from the strategies experts use and build upon their own skills, but experience is the only real way to become an expert.

► Knowing when enough information is gathered to form an assessment of the problem needs to be balanced with the need, and timing of when, to manage the patient—particularly when the problem is life-threatening.

► Critical thinking skills can be developed, and there are some methods commonly used by physicians that may be useful in EMS.

► Biased thought processes result in difficulties in problem solving. Being aware of possible biases and consciously filtering for them can minimize the impact they have on critical thinking.

Introduction

A paramedic is called upon to make clinical decisions with every patient interaction. This chapter will focus on the initial approach to patient encounters and how to safely navigate the sometimes turbulent waters of clinical decision-making.

Unfortunately EMS has limited research regarding how clinical decisions are made by paramedics in the field. In fact, medicine in general has more evidence gathered on how doctors *should* make clinical decisions than on how they actually *do* make decisions. There are many empirical studies based upon analyzing experience of nonmedical problem-solving behavior that we can draw upon to make some assumptions about how we expect paramedics to make decisions.[1]

Research has described the problem-solving behaviors of individuals who are considered novice compared to those who are experienced. Once again however, not much of this research has targeted the paramedic profession. If we draw upon the general research on how novice and expert physicians problem solve, we may be able to apply some of these observations to paramedics. Of course there is a risk in doing this, as physicians and paramedics are products of vastly different amounts of education, but the assumption is, since paramedics are "physician extenders," there may be some common ground in the problem-solving process. **This chapter uses Skill Sheets 32: Primary Survey (and Step-by-Step 32: Primary Survey) and 88: NREMT Oral Station.**

What Is Critical Thinking?

Researchers who study the mind and how people think and learn use very specific terminology for the processes being discussed in this chapter. For the purposes of this chapter, and throughout this textbook, the words **critical thinking** will have the following meaning: having the ability to *think about the processes used to solve problems* as well as having the ability to solve problems. According to Bloom's Taxonomy of Learning, this ability, which he called metacognition, represents the highest level of thinking a person is capable of reaching.[2]

The approach to problem solving and critical thinking described in this chapter is something that, if used, should minimize the chances of the paramedic overlooking a problem and not recognizing a potential life-threatening situation.

Elements of the EMS Critical Thinking Process

During a call, the EMS critical thinking process starts with the information provided by the dispatcher (Figure 5-1). It continues with information gathered on the scene from the patient, family, and bystanders. It includes objective clues such as mechanism of injury, patient position, and environmental conditions. It also includes objective findings from the vital signs and physical examination and subjective findings from the history and interview. All of this must be gathered together, analyzed, and filtered in a logical and focused manner.

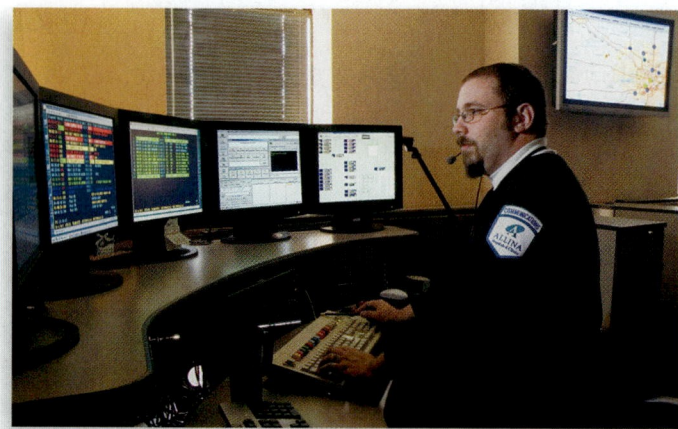

Figure 5-1   Dispatchers give paramedics initial information about patients.

Objective findings are those that are measurable or observable by the paramedic. **Subjective findings** are those that the patient (or someone else) tells you.

Vomiting can be either subjective or objective. If the patient says "I vomited two times," that is subjective information. If the patient vomits while you are present, it is objective information. "Nausea" is subjective because it is not something you see; it is a feeling or sensation from the patient's perspective. Subjective and objective clues are equally important in making an assessment.

After information is gathered, an appropriate management plan must be developed and then implemented. This management plan will be based upon system protocols and the paramedic's ability to apply judgment and exercise appropriate independent decision-making. DOT 7-1.1

The out-of-hospital environment is very different from the more controlled hospital environment. The paramedic has unique pressures that affect the ability to provide care, including adverse weather conditions, poor lighting, uneven terrain, and even a possible shortage of equipment, supplies, or team members. These sorts of situations will not likely occur in the in-hospital setting. Critical thinking and problem solving often must occur during stressful situations, so paramedics must be able to think and work effectively under pressure.

The following are a few of the factors that must be taken into account when approaching and evaluating a patient and making medical decisions:

- The spectrum of prehospital care ranges from obvious critical life threats, to the potential, and sometimes not so easy to recognize, life threats, to non-life-threatening situations. The majority of patients encountered will most likely have non-life-threatening presentations, even in services that focus on providing responses to 9-1-1 emergency calls.

- Standing orders, protocols, and guidelines are important tools to use in managing patients. However, all of these have limitations, and not all patient situations will "fit" these tools. Therefore, the paramedic must be capable of exercising independent thinking and sound judgment.

How the EMS Decision-Making Process Differs from the Physician Process

The decision-making process for both the physician and the EMS provider involves gathering, evaluating, and synthesizing information. There are, however, substantial differences between the purposes of the two processes, the most notable of which is the need for the physician to make an actual diagnosis of the problem. The act of diagnosis has three purposes: to summarize information, to guide treatment, and to aid in research.[3]

Fortunately for the paramedic, managing patients effectively in the out-of-hospital setting will not depend upon diagnosing their problem. Instead, it centers upon the ability to gather pertinent information; recognize the severity of the signs and symptoms; prevent or correct abnormalities that impact the airway, breathing, and circulation; and provide safe, expeditious transportation to the most appropriate facility capable of caring for the patient.[4] The Paramedic National Standard Curricula calls this type of clinical decision-making process an assessment-based approach.

Why Doesn't a Diagnosis Matter in the Prehospital Setting?

Many diseases have similar presentations of symptoms and signs making a definitive diagnosis difficult, even in the best of circumstances. Take, for example, patients who present with abdominal pain, nausea, and vomiting. The list of diseases and processes that contain similar signs and symptoms (or *differential diagnosis*) of these three problems is vast. The patient could have any number of vascular problems such as a dissecting aortic aneurysm or a heart attack. The issue could be an obstetrical or gynecological problem such as an ectopic pregnancy or a sexually transmitted disease. The problem could be the result of disease in any organ in the abdominal cavity. The patient could have a bacterial or viral infection, toxicologic problem, poisoning, etc. The list seems endless. Even in the hospital, it is not always possible to formally diagnose every patient's complaint.

Sick, Not Sick, and Not Yet Sick

Caring for this patient is not dependent on determining the underlying cause of a problem; it is in recognizing whether or not the problem poses a threat to the patient's life or health. Chapter 11: The Normal Physical Examination, will discuss the difference between normal and abnormal patient presentations. Chapter 11 focuses on a recurrent thread that is found throughout this textbook, the concept of a patient being either "sick," "not sick," or "not yet sick."

The idea of "sick" should be easy to understand: sick patients have abnormal vital signs, evidence of shock, or a clinical presentation suggesting that their lives are at risk if they do not see a physician immediately. In some cases, they are so sick that resuscitation efforts must begin before they can be taken to the physician. A person with a heart attack, stroke, or multi-system trauma is an example of a sick patient.

Some patients are obviously not sick. They call for an ambulance for a variety of reasons, and in some cases a routine or nonemergent transport is all that is required. These patients will still receive an assessment, but they may or may not receive any treatment in the prehospital setting. They still need to be monitored throughout the transport and receive compassionate and professional patient care.

The patients who are in between "sick" and "not sick" can be the most difficult for both experienced and novice paramedics to handle. These patients do not appear sick at the moment, or sick enough to warrant aggressive resuscitation measures, but if they are not watched carefully and handled correctly, they can become very sick and may even die. These patients are referred to as "not yet sick." They are the difficult patients to assess as well as treat. These are the groups of patients who benefit most from a paramedic's experience and ability to perform a thorough

Working in the Gray Zone

Medical books contain thousands of descriptions of diseases. Unfortunately, patients do not read these books before they get sick. You get what you get, and their presentation often does not match what the textbook says. Sorting through the signs and symptoms will not be so important if the patient is lying there and not breathing. Appropriate interventional treatments must always be balanced with gathering information and performing an assessment. What makes patient care difficult, especially for the novice provider, is knowing where the balance between assessment and treatment lies. The old adage "experience is the best teacher" is true for the practice of paramedicine.

assessment and anticipate the potential for the patients to have serious problems. The following are examples of patients who could be in the "not yet sick" group:

- A 22-year-old with stable vital signs who has a broken ankle from a fall off a step ladder. The patient says she slipped but does not remember falling, and she has a mild headache.
- A 25-year-old with flushed itchy skin with no history of allergies who was stung by a bee. The vital signs are stable, and the patient is not having any trouble breathing.
- A 64-year-old with "mild" chest pain and stable vital signs who says, "I think I am going to die."

Differences between Novices and Experts in Problem Solving

Much of the art in paramedicine is in developing the ability to evaluate patients and determine if their problems are significant enough to jeopardize their lives. This is not an easy skill to master. The expert is the individual who has enough knowledge, gained through experience, to be able to function at a consistently high level in the areas of critical thinking and decision-making. A large part of becoming an expert is acquiring a vast amount of knowledge in a particular field.[5] Estimates indicate that it takes 10 years or 10,000 hours of study focused in a particular field to become an expert.[6]

Experienced physicians rely heavily on their experience and are capable of performing rapid evaluations and prompt treatments.[1] Paramedics who draw from their own experience improve performance as well. Physicians must possess skill in the decision-making process, so that they can integrate the findings of diagnostic tests into the appropriate treatment plan. Although paramedics may not be performing a host of "tests," they perform a targeted physical examination, gather information through the patient history, and compare what they know about abnormal findings with normal findings in order to develop a treatment plan.

Novice physicians have been known to use a shotgun approach to decision-making.[7] These individuals hope to hit the target (an accurate diagnosis) by shooting with a wide variety of tests and procedures. These novices often do not even know what their actual target is, but by covering all the possibilities, something likely hits the mark. Anybody who has watched a new paramedic struggle with decisions during a cardiac arrest likely has seen this same behavior.

By contrast, experts have specific targets in mind and efficiently adjust their strategies to reach their goals. In the case of physicians, they perform a patient history and physical assessment, and then they pick a few tests to confirm their suspicion. Expert paramedics take the signs and symptoms presented and begin by ruling out the most likely life-threatening problems, then work their way down to less life-threatening problems.

Emergency physicians cannot make a definitive diagnosis in every patient situation. This is true regardless of whether the doctor is a novice or an expert. Research is being conducted to determine how many patients are being misdiagnosed or are not fully diagnosed before being sent home. One multi-center study of emergency departments published in the *Annals of Emergency Medicine* in 2006 concluded "the majority of ED patients with severely elevated blood pressure do not receive the evaluation, medical regimen modification, and discharge instructions advised by current guidelines."[8] Paramedics who miss or misinterpret assessment findings place their patients at risk as well.

Paramedic Clinical Reasoning

Physician clinical reasoning has two aspects:

1. Using cognitive (thinking) shortcuts as a way of organizing complex or unstructured information collected in the clinical evaluation
2. Using diagnostic hypothesis to consolidate the information and determine the best course of treatment.[1]

Cognitive shortcuts useful to paramedics, such as pattern matching, will be defined and described in the following sections. Since paramedics do not need to diagnose, the second piece can be altered to fit the paramedic's needs, and the process will be approached from the assessment perspective previously discussed.

Working in the Gray Zone

A good paramedic knows what to do to treat a patient. An excellent paramedic not only knows what to do, but also has the wisdom to know when and how far to go to treat the patient. For example, giving 2 mg of naloxone will most likely (but not always) wake up a heroin addict, resulting in a very uncooperative patient. Giving small amounts of naloxone a little at a time until breathing resumes (your true goal) keeps the patient alive and sleeping peacefully without precipitating acute narcotic withdrawal.

Street Secrets

Once your assessment is complete, always assume the most serious potential problem is present, never the most likely or most benign. Rule out and treat the life-threatening conditions first, then manage any other problems that are encountered as your time with the patient permits.

The overriding question that must be answered in all patient encounters is, "What is the most serious possible cause of this patient's presenting signs and symptoms?" The reason why it is important to combine the assessment elements before making a decision on treatment is that there are certain conditions in which a "normal" vital sign, when combined with a specific chief complaint, is indicative of a life-threatening situation. Here are three examples of situations when findings are "normal" but the patient is still very "sick":

- **Example 1:** A patient with reactive airway disease (asthma) has been short of breath for many hours. The patient has bilateral wheezing and a respiratory rate of less than 16. The normal adult respiratory rate is 12–20; however, asthmatics with bronchospasm and increased work in breathing generally should be breathing more than 20 times per minute. The respiratory rate in this patient may indicate the patient is tiring, is becoming hypoxic, and is starting to retain carbon dioxide. All of this could result in increased somnolence (sleepiness), respiratory depression, and respiratory arrest (Figure 5-2).
- **Example 2:** A patient with normal vital signs who is life-threatened is a patient who presents in hypovolemic shock or acute pericardial tamponade. Such patients are initially tachycardic, which is a normal compensatory response. If their normal status is hypertensive, as they become "hypotensive" and their condition worsens, their blood pressure reading may be in the "normal" range. When their blood pressure finally falls below normal readings, they are truly in critical condition. These are patients who are in danger of cardiac arrest and who must have aggressive therapeutic interventions. In this

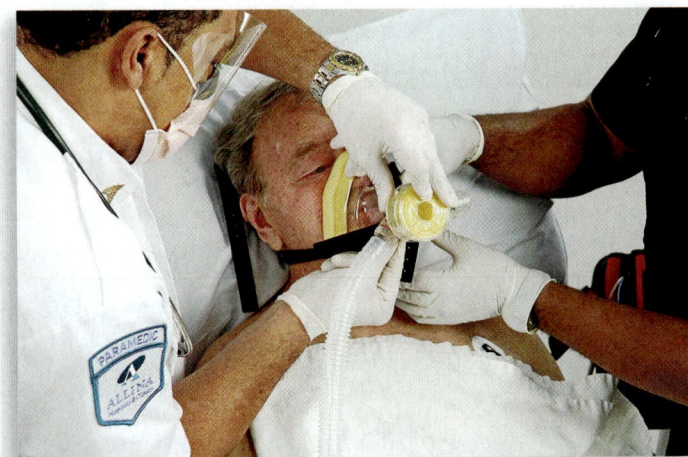

Figure 5-2 Making a decision between intubation and use of continuous positive airway pressure (CPAP) can be difficult; you may be able to avoid more invasive procedures with early interventions.

case, it is important to recognize that the "normal" blood pressure reading actually represented the beginning of the development of shock.

■ ***Example 3:*** A well-conditioned athlete who presents with a major mechanism of injury to the abdomen and has a resting pulse of 72 and a normal blood pressure. For this individual, this is tachycardia and is a manifestation of early-compensated hypovolemic shock. Athletes of this caliber usually have resting heart rates of 40–50 beats per minute.[9]

Any of these patients could be assessed at a time when they are transitioning between a not sick appearance and a sick appearance. If the paramedic maintains a high index of suspicion for the development of problems, is aware of when "normal" is not really normal, and monitors the patient closely, the outcome for the patient can be a positive one. If the paramedic encounters the patient at the beginning of the problem and is very attentive and manages the patient appropriately, the patient may never transition from the not yet sick state into the sick state.

Street Secrets

Always remember that there is a huge uncontrollable aspect of patient care called "fate." Everyone has a time to die, and despite your best efforts, some patients will. Sometimes, even when you do not perform at your best, the patient will survive. That too is fate in action.

Strategies for Critical Thinking

Medical and educational research has identified some elements and procedures that enhance the decision-making process. Here is a brief discussion of pattern recognition and heuristics. Both strategies apply to the paramedic critical thinking process. **Review Skill Sheet 88: NREMT Oral Station before continuing on with this section. As you read the sheet, think about the various steps and procedures described within each category of the sheet. This information can help you organize your approach to the patient.**

Pattern Recognition

Experts can recall patterns and processes that are helpful from previous problem-solving activities to use in handling new problems. A study of world-class chess players calculated they had a memory of an average of 50,000 chessboard patterns.[10] What makes this valuable is that each possible pattern is associated with several moves. If an individual can rapidly recognize patterns, it is possible to move quickly through a problem.[3] EMS can use this technique during assessment-based management. **Review Skill Sheet 32: Primary Survey**

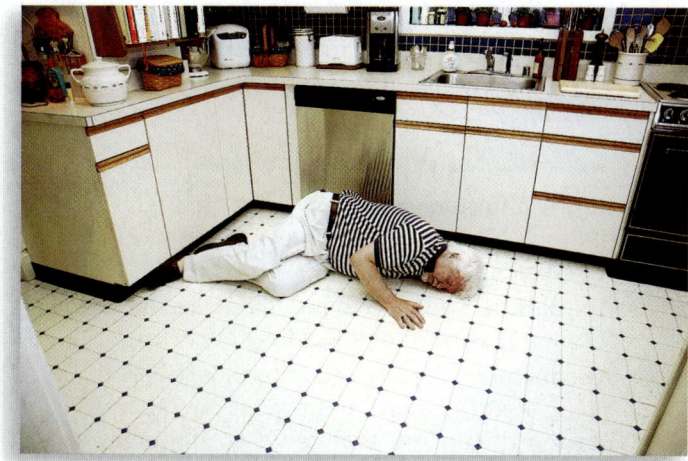

Figure: 5-3 A scene size-up will provide clues for pattern matching. Always look around the scene for any visible clues that can help you piece together the story of what happened.

(and Step-by-Step 32: Primary Survey) as you read through the following scenario.

Here is an example. Look at Figure 5-3. You are in the home of Mr. Jones. He is lying on his left side in the middle of the kitchen floor. There is no blood on the floor, and his wife says she assisted him to the floor when he collapsed while standing. The floor is dry, and there are no rugs near his feet. He is not moving or breathing, and his skin looks gray. DOT 7-1.14

You know you must position the patient flat on his back in order to assess and treat him. Before making this move, you quickly scan the environment for any signs of trauma. With the history from his wife and not finding any evidence of trauma, you know you can likely rule out cervical injury at this time. Because of this you do not need to put on a cervical collar or order cervical immobilization.

Several patterns were assessed in the first few moments with this patient. Focusing on only the scene size-up, there was an assessment for environmental clues for trauma, and the position of the patient in relationship to the environment was noted. Because the floor lacked blood, the position of the patient suggested he collapsed while standing (ground level fall), and there is a lack of any other clues to suggest trauma (step ladder, slippery floor, weapon, heavy object, etc.), you move quickly through the trauma recognition pattern. With the information gathered in this assessment, trauma was ruled out (at this time) because there was no pattern or evidence indicating it, so the assessment moved on to the next appropriate step.

Other Heuristics

Heuristics (pronounced HUE-wrist-icks) is the term for any strategy or technique that helps direct attention and focus while thinking. Heuristics are used in learning,

> ### BOX 5-1 Three Types of Heuristic Problem-Solving Behavior for EMS
>
> - **Representativeness:** you have enough information to believe a particular disease is represented.
> - **Availability:** you make judgments based on the frequency of similar situations occurring.
> - **Anchoring:** you begin with the most likely cause as the anchor and then the signs and symptoms needed to confirm that cause are the ones you assess for first.

discovering, and problem solving. The word comes from the Greek word "eureka" which loosely translated means "I found it!" The term was introduced in the fourth century AD by Pappus of Alexandria,[11] and the study of heuristics has persisted throughout the ages to modern times. Heuristic processes have been studied extensively in virtually every profession, including medicine.

Any problem-solving behavior can produce incorrect or inexact results at times. Success is most likely when heuristic techniques are used to solve problems in commonly occurring situations.[11] This points out the need to have a strong foundation in the basic knowledge, principles, and processes of a profession before any problem-solving methods should be used. Bias is a problem sometimes encountered when using heuristic approaches. Some elements of bias will be discussed in context but will also be presented later in this chapter.

There are many forms of heuristic problem-solving behavior. Medical professionals rely on three basic types of heuristics when problem solving: representativeness heuristic, availability heuristic, and anchoring heuristic.[3] Box 5-1 lists these types.

Representativeness Heuristic

The **representativeness heuristic** means that the situation provides enough information for the paramedic to believe that the current signs and symptoms represent a particular disease. The technique of pattern recognition just discussed employs a representativeness approach, so think of that as the example.

A problem with representativeness occurs when a paramedic does not change to another pattern when it is obvious a match does not exist or when an excessive amount of time is spent without patient treatment occurring. For the example with Mr. Jones, if the paramedic had insisted on ruling out trauma completely, there may

have been a delay in the care Mr. Jones needed while trauma-focused activities occurred. In treating Mr. Jones, time should not have been spent in that phase of his care, cutting off all of his clothes and palpating his body from head to toe looking for injuries. That behavior may be appropriate later if time permitted. What the paramedic in the example did should be enough to rule out trauma at this point in the call. Switching focus from trauma to beginning the ABC assessment was appropriate.

Availability Heuristic

The **availability heuristic** involves making judgments based upon the frequency of similar situations occurring. A simple example of this is when a flu epidemic occurs. If every patient that the EMS service transports has the same signs and symptoms and the hospital diagnosis is consistently the same, then the chances are good that the next patient you encounter with those same signs and symptoms has the flu.

An immediate problem that comes to mind with this approach is something called "tunnel vision." When **tunnel vision** occurs, the field of focus is too narrow and possibilities that should be considered for the cause of the problem may not be considered. The next patient with those same signs and symptoms may not have the flu. Again, if the signs and symptoms that are presented are managed appropriately then there is no problem from the prehospital perspective. If, however, signs or symptoms are ignored by the paramedic because they do not match the expected cause of the problem, the patient may be mismanaged.

Think back to Mr. Jones. Let us say that, as the call continued, the paramedic next had Mr. Jones lying on his back and was assessing his ABCs. The paramedic was convinced Mr. Jones had a heart attack and was in cardiac arrest, and so far the evidence seemed to be favoring that assessment. An EMT crewmember was giving Mr. Jones two breaths with a bag-mask ventilation device and the chest did not rise. The paramedic told the EMT to reposition the head and try again. The paramedic checked for a pulse at the neck. Because there was no pulse, he ordered the third crewmember, an EMT ambulance driver, to begin CPR.

The paramedic continues to treat the patient for a cardiac arrest but does not notice that the chest was not rising with bag valve mask (BVM) ventilations. The EMT does not speak up, and Mr. Jones continues to have a blocked airway. The paramedic does not figure this out until he takes over BVM ventilation in order to perform intubation. The paramedic had tunnel vision by attributing the problem to a sudden death cardiac arrest instead of a foreign body airway obstruction-induced sudden death.

An experienced paramedic will use the availability heuristic differently than a novice paramedic when the patient falls into the "not yet sick" category. For example, an experienced paramedic has seen 20 elderly patients in the last few years with an acute onset of painless difficulty breathing. Every one of those patients was diagnosed in the ED with a heart attack. That same paramedic may quickly move from thinking the problem is respiratory to cardiac if a patient with a similar age and problem presents again. The novice paramedic faced with a similar situation may focus more on a respiratory cause and exhaust that line of reasoning before moving toward a cardiac consideration.

Hopefully, each of these patients received a thorough assessment and appropriate management of the presenting signs and symptoms, but that may not be the case. Unless the novice paramedic is routinely performing cardiac monitoring for patients with respiratory complaints, these two patients may not receive the same care. The novice paramedic may not obtain an ECG or look for signs of a cardiac problem until very late in the care process. As you will discover later when you learn about cardiac emergencies, the passage of time makes a big difference in the outcome of serious cardiac emergencies.

Working in the Gray Zone

As the technology available in the prehospital environment is increasing, the use of tools such as the cardiac monitor, pulse oximeter, and end-tidal CO_2 detector are becoming more common. These devices are minimally invasive and are good tools to assess for possible cardiovascular or respiratory problems. They are becoming a standard of care for most cardiac and respiratory emergencies as well as serious trauma situations.

Anchoring Heuristic

The **anchoring heuristic** is a problem-solving strategy that begins with the most likely cause as the anchor, and then assessment begins for the signs and symptoms needed to confirm that cause. Think back to the flu epidemic example used earlier in this chapter. If a paramedic uses an anchoring heuristic, the initial approach begins with the assumption that flu is the cause. The paramedic would then perform a targeted history and physical exam to verify that the patient has the flu.

This can be a powerful tool, but it is used incorrectly when the paramedic does not perform a thorough enough assessment or gather enough history to justify the conclusions reached. For example, the most likely cause of fever, chills, and body aches in the middle of a flu

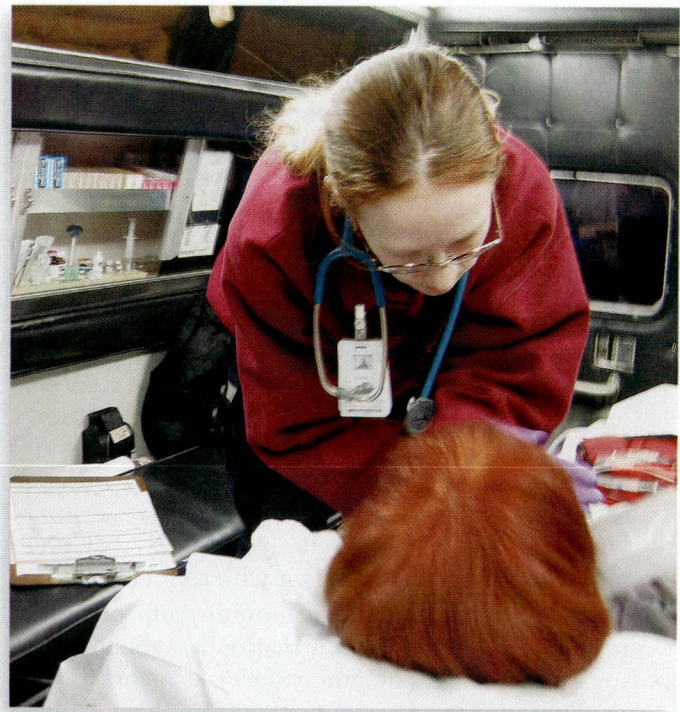

Figure 5-4 A thorough physical exam can help you differentiate between a patient who is in serious distress versus one who is not yet showing signs of being sick.

epidemic is the flu. But there are a host of other diseases with the same signs and symptoms.

Important negative findings (called **pertinent negatives**) are often as important as positive findings in establishing and refining the actual cause of the problem. There are certain medical conditions that must be considered with the presentation of certain signs and symptoms. Meningitis for example is one of those diseases that falls into the group of illnesses that present with "fever, chills, and body aches." Meningitis is often accompanied by headache and a stiff neck. Certain forms of meningitis are highly contagious and also have high mortality. If the paramedic treating a patient during the flu epidemic does not ask about or examine for (rule out) the presence of a stiff neck or headache, the life and health of the patient, crew, and bystanders could be in jeopardy if meningitis is the real disease (Figure 5-4).

Street Secrets

Experienced paramedics value pertinent negatives as much as positive findings. With some diseases, such as infectious diseases, they are critical to safety. In some cases, pertinent negative findings are more important than other signs and symptoms.

Each of these heuristic approaches—representativeness, availability, and anchoring—can help paramedics focus and fine tune their problem-solving abilities. The list below presents some additional suggestions that can help you improve your critical thinking abilities:[3]

DOT 7-1.4, 7-1.5

- *Tolerate uncertainty, avoid premature closure, and consider alternatives:* Any decision-making process will not be perfect, neither will the presentation of every patient fit into neat packages. Know when to stop gathering information and begin treatment, but also know when more information is needed. Making a snap judgment as to the patient's problem prior to fully assessing the patient is not appropriate, neither is delaying patient care until each potential cause is fully explored. Avoid tunnel vision by being open to the possibility that there may be other things going on with the patient.

- *Separate distracting information from pertinent information:* A lot of information is available during every patient encounter. There is an art to sorting out the "need to know" from the "nice to know" and the "don't need to know" information. Using heuristics can help with the filtering process.

- *Be alert for fresh evidence, particularly evidence that demands a revision or deletion of the assessment conclusion:* Until a person is dead, that person is in a dynamic state. The person can improve or deteriorate rapidly. Your treatment strategies must be flexible as well.

- *Value negative evidence as much as positive evidence:* Ruling out and searching for pertinent negatives are critical to the appropriate assessment and treatment process. Missed pertinent negative findings can result in disastrous consequences.

- *Be prepared to commit yourself when you have gathered enough evidence:* Know when it is appropriate to switch to treatment, and know when you do not have enough information to begin a course of treatment.

Roadblocks to Effective Critical Thinking

Decision-making and critical thinking may be affected by a number of factors. Bias and fallacies can lead a paramedic off track. **Fallacies** are nothing more than something that is not true. A fallacy can occur from deliberate or accidental misinformation. If a fallacy is not recognized, it can skew the critical thinking process. Paramedics should be on guard against fallacies by constantly questioning the information they receive and examining it for untruthfulness.

Bias

Bias, in regard to the critical thinking process, is a tendency or prejudice. As a tendency, bias will steer you toward one line of thinking or reasoning rather than another. As a prejudice, bias often stops you from going down one thought pathway or another.

We all have biases. Our experiences in life, interactions with others, ethics, morals, and values all bring bias into our lives. A memorable negative or positive outcome can impact future decisions. A person's point of view can introduce bias: a treatment that saves nine out of ten lives may be preferred over one that sacrifices one life to save nine others—even though the outcome is identical. Chapter 3: Professional Ethics discusses bias with regard to ethical and moral behavior and, although that is one consideration, it is not the entire focus of this discussion on bias. Paramedics should be constantly on guard for bias and consider its impact in the decision making process. The following is a list of the more commonly studied biases found in the cognitive (thinking) process.[12] DOT 7-1.3

Hindsight: The tendency to see past events as being predictive of future outcomes. Example: The paramedic "knows" the patient is going to have a seizure because every time she responds to that address it is for a seizure. This bias may result in tunnel vision.

Focalism: The tendency to place too much importance on one aspect of an event that causes an error in accurately predicting a future outcome. Example: The paramedic is focused on the appearance of a mangled fractured upper extremity in the driver of an automobile collision. The paramedic does not notice that the windshield has a "spiderweb" appearance and that the patient is not responding to questions appropriately. The paramedic allows the broken arm to distract him from noting there could be another, more serious traumatic brain injury. This is an example of tunnel vision.

Fundamental attribution error: The tendency for a paramedic to overemphasize personality-based explanations for behaviors in others while underemphasizing the role of the situation on the same behavior. Example: A paramedic thinks the patient is overly dramatic in complaining about the pain while starting an IV. The paramedic assumes this is due to the patient's ethnic background because she knows this particular group tends to be dramatic when injured. However, the paramedic fails to notice that the IV slipped out of the vein and that the fluid is flowing into the subcutaneous tissue of the arm (infiltrating), causing bruising, tissue damage, and edema (swelling) at the IV site. In addition to falling victim to tunnel vision, this is also unprofessional.

Confirmation bias: The tendency to search for and interpret information in a way that confirms your preconceptions. Example: The paramedic knows that most calls received between the hours of 2 and 4 a.m. are from people driving home from a night of partying. When the team is called for a motor vehicle crash at 3 a.m. and the patient is "acting bizarre" and "smelling of alcohol," she is treated for the trauma and the doctor in the ED is told she is intoxicated. Later it is revealed the patient was on her way to start her early morning work shift, she had a diabetic emergency, and there were no drugs or alcohol in her blood.

Self-serving bias: The tendency to claim more responsibility for successes than failures. It may also manifest itself as a tendency for people to evaluate information in a way that is beneficial to their interests. Example: The patient has chicken pox and is in the stage of the disease where he has itchy, crusty patches. As you treat him, you suggest he soak in the bathtub adding oatmeal and baking soda to the water. The patient sees you on the street two weeks later and happily tells you your treatment "cured" him. You thank him, and you both part ways. This innocent-appearing example is self-serving. The paramedic walked away with undue credit for the natural progression of a disease running its course. This is not very professional behavior.

Controlling Bias in the Decision-Making Process

Although there has been much research into bias and fallacies in the medical profession, it has not had much effect upon clinical practice.[3] Two possible reasons seem to point out why. One of the most notable is that clinicians will concede that others may make a mistake but state they are unlikely to do so. Based upon the previous discussion, you can see the fallacy in this thinking: it is self-serving.

Another reason cited was that although there are some recognized patterns of heuristics to follow, expert clinicians do not follow a fixed pattern in patient examinations.[7] Instead, experts allow the situation that is unfolding to guide them as they direct their assessment and treatment plan.

Patient presentations are diverse, and their problems evolve over time. Paramedics must be flexible to be effective. The information presented within this chapter is meant to offer assistance in the development of critical thinking skills. It cannot present an algorithm or flow chart to follow. As you continue through this textbook and each body system is explored, some tips, pearls, and bits of wisdom will be shared which are specific to the disease of that system.

Every novice paramedic needs to practice the skill of critical thinking in order to learn it. It is also important to observe expert paramedics in action, modeling the behavior that makes sense to them and learning from any mistakes they observe in their own behavior or the behavior of others.

Street Secrets

Be observant for experts in all aspects of medicine as well as the EMS profession. There are expert EMRs, EMTs, and AEMTs who will serve as good role models. As you "move up the ladder" in EMS, remember where you came from and never forget that professionalism is a common thread throughout EMS.

A paramedic must always guard against making social judgments about any patient. For example, a patient who appears to be psychotic or intoxicated may actually be hypotensive, hypoxic, or hypoglycemic. It is difficult to avoid making judgments on patients who abuse or frequently call for an emergency transport when none is needed. For example, the alcoholic patient who calls 9-1-1 may have a life-threatening cause of altered mental status. Each and every call should be approached with the same question: "What is the most serious possible cause of this patient's presenting signs and symptoms?" It is imperative to avoid making social judgments about patients. DOT 7-1.2

Critical Thinking Skills in Action

An important decision is the most appropriate destination for the patient. When a paramedic has a choice of patient care destinations (i.e., trauma centers, burn centers, psychiatric hospitals, cardiac care, or stroke specialty units), it is important to determine the appropriate destination early in the patient encounter. DOT 7-1.6, 7-1.7, 7-1.11

Patients with multiple trauma or penetrating injury should go to a high-level trauma center. Other patients that should be considered for trauma centers are those who will likely need emergent operative intervention, for example, an elderly male who has acute onset of flank pain and syncope or near syncope. This must be considered to be a ruptured abdominal aortic aneurysm until proven otherwise, and he is best managed in a setting where an operating room is immediately available.

Patients who appear to have had a stroke or cerebral vascular accident should be considered for transport to a stroke center. Also, patients who have the clinical

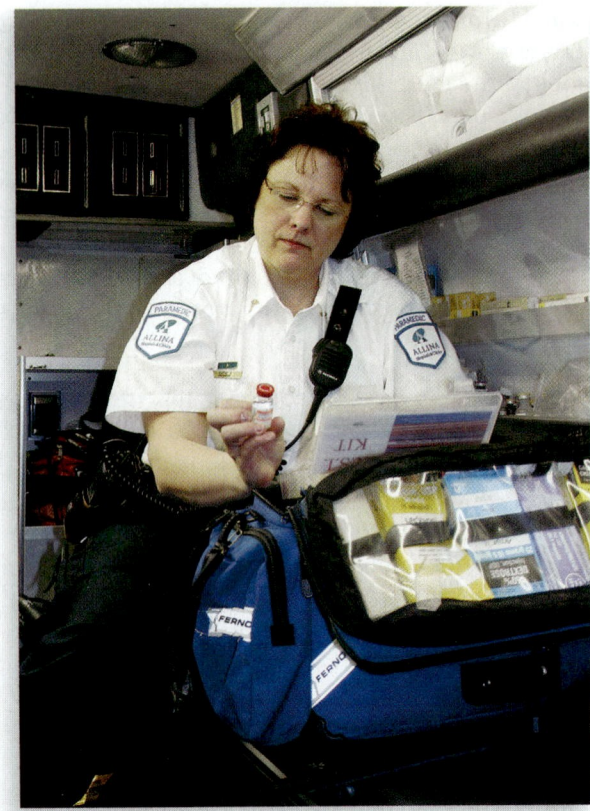

Figure 5-5 Thorough equipment checks—including checking the expiration date of medications—are part of being prepared to respond to any emergency

signs and symptoms of an acute myocardial infarction should be taken to a facility that specializes in cardiac care. By initially taking the patient to the appropriate destination, unnecessary delays will be avoided.

Failure to take the necessary equipment to the patient and failure to mobilize adequate personnel to support the management of the care of the patient are common pitfalls. Always take an ECG monitor-defibrillator, airway kit with oxygen, and IV kit with cardiac drugs to every patient that dispatch information indicates as "sick" or "not yet sick" (Figure 5-5). Chest pain and trouble breathing are two problems that should always receive this type of response. The paramedic should be on high alert for the possible development of life-threatening complications, even if the patient appears "not sick" in your initial impression. DOT 7-1.9, 7-1.10

Another pitfall that may be encountered is performing assessments out of sequence, so a life threatening problem, when it arises, cannot be handled. An example of this can easily happen when treating a patient with chest pain. If the paramedic suspects a heart attack, the paramedic may connect the patient to a cardiac monitor and obtain a 12-lead ECG before taking measures to maintain the basic ABCs. DOT-1.15

Although further cardiac assessment is appropriate, if the patient suddenly deteriorates into ventricular tachycardia with hypotension, an IV is not established, and oxygen is not given to the patient, this is a problem. To remain focused and on task, the paramedic should always ask, "What is life-threatening about this situation?" Thinking about this will remind you to get ready for a change to happen. Often an IV needs to be in place to anticipate resuscitation efforts. For that reason, placing an IV is likely a higher priority than obtaining a 12-lead ECG tracing.

It is important for the paramedic always to continuously reassess every patient. Reassessment may reveal problems that were not noted before, switching the patient between the "not sick," "not yet sick," and "sick" categories. At times this may alert the paramedic to revise the impression of the patient and to formulate a different destination or field treatment plan.[9] DOT 7-1.16

At the end of each call, it is helpful to reflect on the decisions made, what may have been done differently, and what can be done better in the future. Seek input from the emergency department personnel who treated your patients. At an appropriate time, ask questions of the emergency physician, nurses, and other staff members and be open to constructive suggestions on how to improve performance.

Everyone who provides medical care, from the emergency medical responder to the subspecialty physician, makes mistakes and could do things better. The most important thing that you can do as a medical professional is to recognize and learn from your mistakes, to critically evaluate your care of each patient, and to ask yourself if there is anything you could have done better. Keeping an open mind and critically critiquing your care of every patient enhances the clinical experience. As discussed in Chapter 1: The EMS Profession and Chapter 2: The Well-Being of the Paramedic, there is no better way to minimize job-related stress than to do the job well. Continuously learning with every opportunity will help you gain more experience and more confidence.

Summary

Paramedics do not diagnose diseases in the same manner that physicians do. Paramedics assess signs and symptoms and formulate treatment plans based upon their findings. The approach paramedics utilize is called "assessment-based management."

Paramedics need to understand the subtle differences in patient presentation between a patient who is "not sick," "sick," and "not yet sick." Sometimes the patients at each end of the spectrum are easier to identify than those in the middle. Maintaining a high level of alertness with every patient contact is one way of catching changes in the patient's condition as it occurs.

Knowing when enough information is gathered to form an assessment of the problem needs to be balanced with the need to manage the patient. This is particularly true when managing life-threatening and potentially life-threatening problems.

There is a difference in how problems are solved by both novice and expert paramedics. Novices can learn from the strategies experts use to build their own skills, but experience is the only real way to become an expert. Critical thinking skills can be developed, and there are some heuristic tools commonly used by physicians that may be useful in EMS. Bias thought processes result in difficulties in problem solving. Being aware of possible biases and consciously filtering for them can minimize the impact they have on critical thinking.

A compulsive, organized approach to every patient encountered is the rule. If you obtain a chief complaint, a focused history around this complaint, and a complete set of accurately taken vital signs and critically interpret them in light of the patient's presenting complaint, an accurate assessment of the underlying problem may be formulated. Appropriate resuscitative measures should be undertaken, and an appropriate disposition should be made on all patients.

Notes

1. D. L. Kasper, E. Braunwald, A. S. Fauci, S. L. Hauser, D. L. Longo, J. L. Jameson, and K. J. Isselbacher, eds., *Harrison's Principles of Internal Medicine,* 16th ed., McGraw-Hill's AccessMedicine (accessed October 18, 2006).

2. D. Cason (ed.), *Foundations of Education: An EMS Approach* (St. Louis, MO: National Association of EMS Educators, Mosby, Inc., 2006), p. 78.

3. Michael H. Ebert, Peter T. Loosen, and Barry Nurcombe, *Current Diagnosis and Treatment in Psychiatry* (McGraw-Hill's AccessMedicine (accessed October 18, 2006).

4. Emergency Medical Technician Paramedic: National Standard Curriculum (EMT-P), United States Department of Transportation. www.nhtsa.dot.gov/people/injury/EMS/EMT-P/index.htm (accessed October 18, 2006).

5. P. A. Alexander, "Domain knowledge: Evolving themes and emerging concerns," *Educational Psychologist* 27 (1992): 33–51.

6. H. A. Simon, "The information processing view of mind," *American Psychologist* 50 (1995): 507–508.

7. D. L. Kasper, E. Braunwald, A. S. Fauci, S. L. Hauser, D. L. Longo, J. L. Jameson, and K. J. Isselbacher, eds., *Harrison's Principles of Internal Medicine,* 16th ed., McGraw-Hill's AccessMedicine (accessed October 18, 2006).

8. D. J. Karras, L. K. Kruus, J. J. Cienki, M. M. Wald, W. K. Chiang, P. Shayne, J. W. Ufberg, R. A. Harrigan, D. A. Wald, and K. L. Heilpern, "Evaluation and treatment of patients with severely elevated blood pressure in academic emergency departments: a multicenter study. Temple University School of Medicine, Philadelphia, PA 19140, USA" *Annals of Emergency Medicine* 47(3) (March 2006):230–6.

9. D. Bobes and V. J. Markovchick, "Decision Making and Critical Interpretation of Vital Signs," *Prehospital Emergency Care Secrets,* 1st ed. (Philadelphia: Hanley & Belfus, 1998), 105–108.

10. Anita Woolfolk, *Educational Psychology,* 9th ed. (Upper Saddle River, NJ: Pearson Education, 2004), p. 293.

11. K. N. Anderson, L. E. Anderson, W. D. Glanze eds., *Mosby's Medical Nursing and Allied Health Dictionary,* 4th ed., Mosby YearBook Inc. St. Louis, 1994, p. 737.

12. K. N. Anderson, L. E. Anderson, W. D. Glanze eds., *Mosby's Medical Nursing and Allied Health Dictionary,* 4th ed., Mosby YearBook Inc. St. Louis, 1994, p. 184.

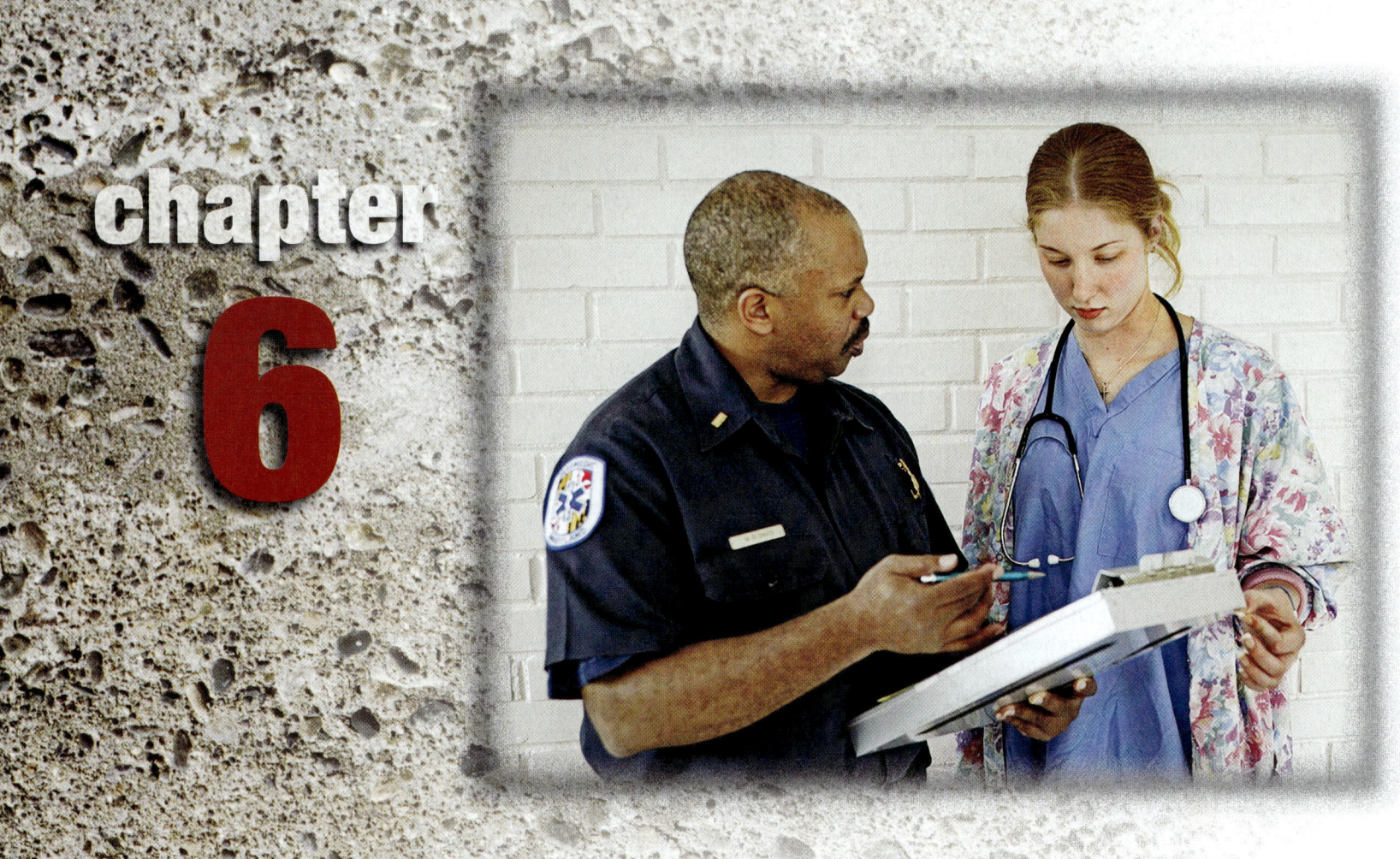

Medical Terminology

*"**W**hat's in a name? That which we call a rose by any other word would smell as sweet."*

—From *Romeo and Juliet* (II, ii, 1–2)

Sir William Shakespeare

Need to Know

▶ Medical terminology is the language of medicine, and using it properly is essential professional behavior.

▶ Medical terms are easier to understand and comprehend if you know the meaning of the root or main part of the word as well as the prefix (the beginning of the word) and suffix (the end of the word), which both serve to modify the root.

▶ Memorizing is a good way to begin learning medical terminology, but using it often is the best way to learn it.

Introduction

As a medical professional, you will elicit information from a patient by obtaining a history and performing a physical exam as the patient tells you the "story" of the illness or injury. This story is then formulated into a hypothesis and diagnosis of the most likely cause of the current complaint, so you can provide the most effective treatment for the patient's condition. Much of your training and education will focus on these elements of your role in medicine. However, you must also be able to pass along the information you gain to other healthcare providers to avoid disruption of the continuum of care, as well as the loss of valuable information. DOT 3-5.1, 3-6.1

Use of Medical Terminology

Every profession has its own language and method of communication that is unique to that group. The medical profession is no different, and the language of medicine is medical terminology.[1] Paramedics typically speak common language with the patient but need to switch to medical terminology to communicate with other members of the healthcare team. Appropriate use of medical terminology is essential. It allows quick and efficient communication in a commonly accepted

Working in the Gray Zone

Unfortunately medical terminology, and particularly the use of abbreviations, has not been standardized in EMS. Some states have provided lists of recommended abbreviations and terms to use, and many ambulance services have adopted lists that are approved for use within their service. If your service does not have an approved list, consult with your EMS lead agency (local, regional, state, or tribal) for more direction. Hospitals and accreditation agencies such as the Joint Commission on Accreditation of Healthcare Organizations (JCAHO) may also be of assistance. DOT 3-5.9

format, so that all those involved in the patient's care will be informed of conditions, findings, and procedures. DOT 3-5.4, 3-6.2

When to Use Medical Terminology

In order to be an effective method of communication, medical terminology must be used appropriately. The use of medical terms with patients and family members, however, will often lead to ineffective communication and confusion. This can easily lead to a misdiagnosis or mistreatment of the patient. As a general rule, you should use lay terms when communicating with patients, family members, and bystanders. Medical terminology should be used only when communicating with other medical professionals.

Take, for example, a respiratory emergency. Asking patients about "dyspnea" may not provide the information you need, but asking about their "breathing trouble" will provide better information. In some instances, you may have to use terms from the local culture when communicating with a patient. For example, if you understand the culture you are dealing with, asking the patient about "smothering spells" in a nonjudgmental fashion may provide the in-depth history you are looking for.[2] Your knowledge of locally used terms will be of great benefit in aiding effective communication. DOT 3-5.5, 3-5.6, 3-5.7, 3-6.2

Street Secrets

Patients often admire EMS providers and look at you with awe and respect. Avoid using a lot of terminology and jargon to "show them how smart you are." But also, do not speak down to your patients. Use good communication skills, along with appropriate words and phrases, and continually test their understanding of what you are saying to avoid miscommunication.

CONNECTIONS Chapter 10: Therapeutic Communications and History Taking will discuss more strategies on effective ways to communicate.

Spelling and Word Selection

Appropriate use of medical terminology in documentation is crucial to proper written communication. Correct spelling is of the utmost importance. Not only will misspelled words cause your competence and knowledge to be questioned, but also utilizing an inappropriate word or spelling can relay an entirely different meaning. DOT 3-5.8, 3-5.9, 3-5.10, 3-6.6, 3-6.9, 3-6.10

CONNECTIONS The JCAHO provides a listing of medical terms, symbols, and abbreviations that are found to cause documentation confusion and errors.[3] This list, called the "Do Not Use" list, is updated on an annual basis and is included in Chapter 17: Documentation. It is a good resource and should be used by EMS.

If you are unsure of the medical term for difficulty swallowing, it is better to write "the patient experienced difficulty swallowing" rather than trying to guess and write something inaccurate like "the patient experienced dysphasia." The latter comment states the patient had difficulty speaking rather than swallowing.

The paramedic must be diligent in spelling accuracy. *Cholecystectomy* is preferred over "removal of the gallbladder"; however, "removal of the gallbladder" would be better than *colesistectomy* (a misspelling). Similarly, it is better to write "placed a needle in the chest" rather than misspelling *thoracentesis* as *thorocenteses*. Many medical terms are difficult to spell because they begin with a silent letter or have a silent letter within them. Many terms with different meanings have very similar spellings. If you are unsure of the spelling or meaning of a word, always look it up before using it in your documentation. Box 6-1 gives a list of terms that are often confused.

Origins of Medical Terms

Learning medical terminology seems like learning a foreign language. In some aspects, this is true, as most medical terms are based in Greek or Latin.[4] Medical terms are also broken into two categories: descriptive terms and eponyms.

- **Descriptive terms** describe the shape, color, function, or some other characteristic of what has been named.
- **Eponyms** are terms that are named after those who first discovered or described something or who first diagnosed a disease.[5]

The difficulty with eponyms is that they give no indication as to what is being discussed [and are not commonly used] outside of the particular field of medicine

BOX 6-1 Commonly Confused Terms

Abduct	Adduct
Aphasia	Aphagia
Athero	Arthro
Dysphasia	Dysphagia
Humeral	Humoral
Humerus	Humorous
Ilium	Ileum
Intra-	Inter-
Malleolus	Malleus
Mucus	Mucous
Pera-	Peri-
Perineal	Peroneal
Principle	Principal

to which they are connected. For example, Wilson's block is the most common form of a right bundle branch block, and Wirsung's duct is the pancreatic duct, but neither name provides any clue as to the meaning. A cardiologist or endocrinologist may know these eponyms, but other medical professionals may not. Some diseases, structures, or processes are known entirely by the name derived from the eponym, such as Cushing's syndrome (rather than pituitary basophilism) or Korsakoff's syndrome (rather than dysmnesic psychosis). Because of the confusion they cause, there is a move away from the use of eponyms. To find an extensive list of medical eponyms along with biographical information about the founder of the term visit http://www.whonamedit.com/.

Constructing Medical Terms

The key to learning and understanding medical terminology is recognizing that all words are made up of several parts. Imagine a child playing with toy building bricks; by combining the various shapes and sizes, an infinite number of objects can be created. The same concept applies in the construction of medical terms. Rather than memorizing the meaning of thousands of medical terms, it is far better to learn the various parts that are combined to create these terms and derive the appropriate word you need. All medical terms are composed of a *root word,* which may have a *prefix* and/or a *suffix* attached to further define the term (Figure 6-1).

When defining a medical term, begin with the back of the word (the suffix), then move to the front of the

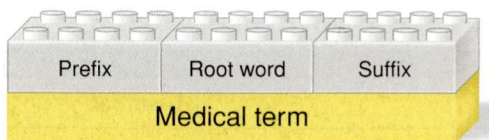

Prefix | Root word | Suffix

Medical term

Figure 6-1 Building a medical term is easy once you understand the basic rules.

word (the prefix), and finish with the middle of the word (the root).[6] For example, *cardiomyopathy* would be defined as "an abnormal condition or illness *(pathy)* of the heart *(cardio)* muscle *(myo)*," and *hypoxemia* would be an "abnormal blood condition *(emia)* with low *(hypo)* oxygen *(ox)*."

Root Words

The foundation of any medical term is the root word. This is the portion that gives the central meaning of the word and describes the "what" portion of the term. Many word roots are nouns. Root words determine what body system, part, disease, etc. is being discussed and forms the base to which prefixes and suffixes are attached. It is important to note that some words may have more than one root. An example is *cardiovascular,* which means the heart and blood vessels.

Prefixes

Prefixes are attached to the front of a root word to *modify* or *qualify* its meaning; they *do not change* the meaning of the root word. Prefixes tell the what, where, when, and how of the term by giving additional information.

A prefix does not change the meaning of the root word, but it does change the meaning of the whole medical term.

To determine if a word part is a prefix or a root word, simply remove the part in question. For example the root "*pnea*" pertains to breath, or respirations. The prefix "*tachy*" means fast. Combined, they form the term tachypnea, or fast respirations. When removing "*tachy*" from the word, the portion left still refers to respirations. This indicates that "*tachy*" is a prefix.

If you take away a prefix from a term, you only remove the *what, when, where,* or *how* of the term. If you remove the root word, you remove the *what,* the basic meaning of the word.

Suffixes

Suffixes are attached to the end of a root word (or combining form) to give further definition and meaning to the medical term. The other role of a suffix is to change the part of speech of the word. The addition of a suffix can change the root word from a noun, which describes a person, place, thing, or quality, to an adjective, which is a word that describes a noun or a verb that describes action or movement.

Most root words need a suffix attached to them as they cannot stand alone as a complete word.

Combining Forms

Many times root words cannot be pronounced in medical terms in their original form. To facilitate the pronunciation of these terms, a vowel is added to the root word. This combination of a root word and a vowel is called the *combining form.* Most commonly the letter "*o*" is used to create the combining form of a root word. For example, an "*o*" is added to *frontonasal* (relating to the frontal and nasal bones) making it easier to say than *frontnasal.* You may occasionally see another vowel used like "*a*" or "*i*" as in venisection. For general rules regarding the use of combining forms, see Box 6-2. When learning medical terminology you will often see forward slashes "/" placed between word parts to separate them into their various components. These are to assist you in identifying prefixes, root words, combining vowels, and suffixes. However, they are not used when writing the word in your medical reports.

BOX 6-2 **Rules for Combining Forms**

1. When the suffix begins with a consonant, the combining form of the root word is used.
2. When the suffix begins with a vowel, the root word is used, not the combining form.
3. The combining form is always used between two root words in a compound word, even when the second root word begins with a vowel.
4. A combining vowel is not used between a prefix and a root word.

TABLE 6-1 Plural Endings

Singular Ending	Example	Pluralizing Rule	Example
Words ending in any consonant or vowel except *s, x, y, or z*	Joint, Muscle	Add *–s* to the end of the word	Joints, Muscles
Words ending in *s, x, or z,* **but not those ending in ax or ix**	Viru**s**, Refle**x**	Add *–es* to the end of the word	Virus**es**, Reflex**es**
Words ending in *ax or ix*	Pneumothor**ax**, Append**ix**	Remove the *–x* and add *–ces* to the end of the word	Pneumothora**ces**, Append**ices**
Words ending in *y* where the *y* is preceded by a consonant	Thyroidecto**my**	Remove the *–y* and add *–ies* to the end of the word	Thyroidectom**ies**
Words ending in *y* where the *y* is preceded by a vowel	Bo**y**	Retain the *–y* and add an *–s* to the end of the word	Boy**s**
Words ending in *a*	Lamin**a**	Add an *–e* to the end of the word	Lamina**e**
Words ending in *en*	Foram**en**	Remove the *–en* and add *–ina* to the end of the word	Foram**ina**
Words ending in *ma*	Fibro**ma**	Add *–ta* to the end of the word	Fibroma**ta**
Words ending in *nx*	Phary**nx**, Phala**nx**	Remove the *–x* and add *–ges* to the word	Phary**nges**, Phalan**ges**
Words ending in *on*	Enterozo**on**, Gangli**on**	Remove the *–on* and add an *–a*	Enterozo**a**, Gangli**a**
Words ending in *sis*	Neuro**sis**	Remove the *–sis* and add an *–ses*	Neuro**ses**
Words ending in *um*	Pericardi**um**, Dat**um**	Remove the *–um* and add an *–a*	Pericardi**a**, Dat**a**
Words ending in *us*	Fung**us**, Staphylococc**us**	Remove the *–us* and add an *–i*	Fung**i**, Staphylococc**i**

Plural Words

Many spelling errors occur when writing plural medical terms. Plural words in the English language are often formed by adding an *–s* or *–es* to the end of the word. As mentioned before in this chapter, most medical terms are derived from Greek and Latin words. As a result, pluralizing these words will follow the rules of those languages. See Table 6-1 for rules regarding forming these words.

Abbreviations

Abbreviations are commonly used in medicine to shorten longer medical terms and descriptions. As with medical terms, abbreviations are generally derived from the original Greek or Latin term they represent. As a result, simply looking at an abbreviation may not indicate what it represents, and rote memorization is often required. The end of this chapter contains a list of common abbreviations used in medicine; however, your EMS service will most likely have a list of abbreviations approved for use in your patient care reports. In the event such a list does not exist, only use abbreviations that are commonly accepted in order to avoid confusion, and when in doubt, write out the term. Always avoid abbreviations that you create; these will have no meaning to those

reading your report and will result in an ineffective transfer of information. DOT 3-6.3, 3-6.10, 3-6.12

Street Secrets

Be consistent in the abbreviations used. Patient care reports are *legal documents* and as such may be entered into court records during a trial or lawsuit. If you are inconsistent in any area of your documentation, including using unauthorized abbreviations, it may be difficult to reconstruct the meaning later on, which can be a disadvantage in court. DOT 3-5.11, 3-6.14

The Next Step

As mentioned earlier in the chapter, the key to learning medical terminology is memorization. The remaining pages contain lists of prefixes, root words, suffixes, and self-assessment exercises. During your paramedic education and career, you should refer to these lists, and use correct medical terminology as often as possible. Like any language, the more you use it, the easier it will be to use. Remember, this chapter is only an introduction to medical terminology. There are several self-study references available to further your knowledge of the language of medicine.

Prefixes

Prefix	Meaning	Prefix	Meaning
a-	without or lack of	in-	not, unable. Appears as *im-* when preceding the letters *b, p,* or *m.*
ab-, abs-	away from		
acr-	pertaining to an extremity		
ad-	toward	infra-	below, beneath
ambi-	both, both sides	inter-	between
an-	without or lack of	intra-	within
ana-	up, toward, apart	iso-	equal, same
ante-, antero-	before, in front of	latero-	lateral, to one side
anti-	against, opposite	macr-, macro-	large, long
apo-	derived, separate	mal-	bad, inadequate
aut-, auto-	self	medi-, medio-	middle, median
bi-	two	meg-, mega-, megalo-	enlarged
brachy-	short	mega-	one million
brady-	slow	mes-, mesio-, meso-	middle, median
cata-	down	meta-	change, beyond, after
circum-	around, about	micr-, micro-	small, (also one millionth)
co-, col-, com-, con-, cor-	together, with, in association	mid-	middle, median
contra-	against, opposite	mon-, mono-	one, single
de-	away from	multi-	many
dextr-, dextro-	right, toward the right, on the right side	neo-	new, recent
		nulli-	none
di-	twice, double; also separation or taking apart	odyn-, odyno-	pain
		olig-, oligo-	few, little, minimal
dia-	through, across, completely	oophor-, oophoro-	pertaining to the ovary
dif-, dir-, dis-	separation or taking apart	pachy-	thick
diplo-	double	pan-, pant-, panto-	all
dors-, dorso-	the back or the back side	para-	abnormal or departure from normal; closely related to or beside
dys-	difficulty, painful, bad		
ec-, ect-, ecto-	outer, on the outside		
em-	in, or within. Only used when preceding the letters *b, p,* or *m.*	per-	through, thoroughly, intensely
		peri-	around
		pluri-	several
en-	in, or within. Appears as em- when preceding the letters b, p, or m	poly-	many, multiple
		post-	behind, after
end-, endo-	within, inner	pre-	before, anterior
epi-	on, upon, over	pro-	before, forward, precursor of
eu-	good, normal	pseudo-	false
ex-, exo-	external, outside	quad-, quadra-, quadri-	four
extra-	without, outside of	re-	again, back
hemi-	half	retro-	backwards, behind
hetero-	different	semi-	partial, half
homo-	same	sinistro-	left, towards the left, on the left side
hyper-	over, excessive, above normal		
hypo-	under, deficient, below normal	sub-	beneath, under, less than normal, inferior
im-	not, unable. Only used when preceding the letters *b, p,* or *m.*		
		super-	in excess, above, superior

(continued)

Prefixes (*continued*)

Prefix	Meaning	Prefix	Meaning
supra-	positioned above the part referenced by the word it is joined to	*tri-*	three
		ultra-	beyond, excess
sy-, syl-, sym-, syn-, sys-	together	*un-*	not
tachy-	rapid, fast	*uni-*	one
trans-	across, through, beyond		

Colorful Prefixes

Prefix	Meaning	Prefix	Meaning
alb-	white	*melan-, melano-*	black
chlor-, chloro-	green	*purpur-, purpuro-*	purple
cyan-, cyano-	blue	*rose-, roseo-*	rose, pink
eosin-, eosino-	rosy	*rube-*	*red*
erythr-, erythro-	red	*xanth-, xantho-*	yellow
leuk-, leuko-	white		

Root Words and Combining Forms

Root Word/ Combining Vowel	Meaning	Root Word/ Combining Vowel	Meaning
abdomin/o	abdomen	*capn/o*	carbon dioxide
acu/o	needle, sharp	*carcin/o*	cancer
aden/o	gland	*cardi/o*	heart
adip/o	fat	*carp/o*	wrist
adren/o	adrenal glands	*cephal/o*	head
aer/o	air, gas	*cerebell/o*	cerebellum
alge, algesi, algio, algo	pain	*cerebr/o*	cerebrum
algesia	sensitive to pain	*cervic/o*	neck, cervix
alveoli/o	air sac, alveolus	*chol(e), cholo*	bile
andr/o	male	*cholecyst/o*	gall bladder
angi/o	vessel	*chondri/o, chondr/o*	cartilage
arteri/o	arteries	*col/o*	colon
arthr/o	joint	*cost/o*	rib
ather/o	plaque, fatty substance	*crani/o*	head or cranium
atri/o	atrium	*cutane/o*	skin
axill/o	armpit	*cyst/o, cysti*	bladder
bacill/i	bacteria	*cyt/o*	cell
bacteri/o	bacteria	*derm/o, derma, dermat/o*	skin
blast/o	the process of budding by cells or tissue	*duoden/o*	duodenum
		emesis	backward flow
blephar/o	eyelid	*encephal/o*	brain
brachi/o	arm	*enter/o*	intestines
bronch/o, bronchi	bronchus	*epiglott/o*	epiglottis
bucc/o	cheek	*esophag/o*	esophagus
calc/o, calci/o	calcium	*esthesi/o*	sensation, perception

Root Words and Combining Forms (*continued*)

Root Word/ Combining Vowel	Meaning	Root Word/ Combining Vowel	Meaning
fasci/o	fascia	*osseo, ossi*	bone
fibr/o	fiber, fibrous	*ost(e), osteo*	bones
galact/o	pertaining to milk	*ot/o*	ear
gastr/o	stomach	*path/o*	disease
gen/o	precursor, producing	*ped/o, pedi*	child or foot
gloss/o	tongue	*peritone/o*	peritoneum
glyc/o	sugar	*phag/o*	eating, devouring, swallowing
gnath/o	jaw	*pharyng/o*	pharynx
gyn/o, gyne, gyneco	women	*phleb/o*	veins
hem/o, hema, hemat/o	blood	*phon/o*	sound, speech
hepa, hepat/o hepatic/o	liver	*pleur/o*	pleura
histi/o, histo	tissue	*phren/o, phreni, phrenico*	diaphragm
hydr/o	water, hydrogen	*pneum/o, pneum/a, pneumat/o, pneumon/o*	air, gas, the lungs, or breathing
hyster/o	uterus		
iatr/o	physician, treatment	*proct/o*	the anus or rectum
idio	unknown	*psych/o, psyche*	mind
immun/o	immune	*pulmon/o*	lung
kerat/o	cornea	*py/o*	pus
kyph/o	hump, bent	*pyel/o*	renal pelvis
lact/o, lacti	milk	*rect/o*	rectum
lapar/o	pertaining to the loins (less properly, but more commonly, the abdomen in general)	*ren/o, reni*	kidney
		rhabdomy/o	striated muscle
		rhin/o	nose
		salping/o	a tube
laryng/o	larynx	*sarc/o*	flesh
lingu/o	pertaining to the tongue	*schiz/o*	split, division
lip/o	fat, lipid	*scler/o*	hardness
lith/o	a stone, calculus, or calcification	*somat/o, somatic/o*	body
		spir/o	breath, breathe
lymph/o	lymph or the lymphatic system	*splen/o*	spleen
mast/o	pertaining to the breast	*spondyl/o*	vertebra
mediastin/o	mediastinum	*staphyl/o*	a grouping, a bunch, grapelike clusters
mening/o	meninges		
muc/o	mucus	*sten/o*	narrowness, constriction
my/o	pertaining to muscle	*stern/o*	sternum
myel/o	bone marrow or the spinal cord and medulla oblongata	*terato*	fetus with deficient, misplaced, or grossly misshapen body parts
myring/o	tympanic membrane	*therm/o*	heat
myx/o-	mucus	*thorac/o, thoracico*	the chest or thorax
nat/o	birth	*thromb/o*	blood clot
necr/o	death, necrosis	*thym/o*	thymus gland
nephr/o	kidney	*thyr/o*	thyroid gland
neur/o, neuri	nerve, the nervous system	*trache/o*	trachea
ocul/o	eye	*ur/o*	urine, urinary tract
opthalm/o	eye	*vascul/o*	blood vessel
orchi/o, orchid/o	testes	*ven/o, veni*	vein
orth/o	straight, right, in proper order	*vertebr/o*	vertebra

Suffixes

Suffix	Meaning	Suffix	Meaning
-a	converts a root word to a noun	-ic	pertaining to
-ac	pertaining to	-ical	pertaining to
-ad	toward, in the direction of	-ion	process
-al	pertaining to	-ism	condition, disease
-algia	pain	-itis	inflammation
-an	pertaining to	-ium	changes the root word to a noun
-ar	pertaining to	-ive	nature of, quality of
-ary	pertaining to	-ize	to take away
-ase	an enzyme	-lepsy	condition of
-asthenia	weakness	-leptic	having seizures
-ate	use, action	-logist	one who practices
-blast	immature, forming	-logy	the study of
-cele	hernia, protrusion	-lysis	the destruction of
-centesis	puncture, usually to withdraw fluid	-lytic	destroying
-cidal	destroying, killing	-malacia	softening
-cide	destroying, killing	-mania	obsession, abnormal love for
-cise	cut	-megaly	enlargement of
-cle	small	-meter	measuring device
-coccus	round	-metry	measurement
-crine	secreting	-oid	like or resembling
-crit	separate	-ole	small
-cyte	cell	-oma	tumor
-cytosis	condition of the cells	-opia	vision
-dynia	pain	-opsia	vision
-eal	pertaining to	-ose	pertaining to or like
-ectasis	expansion, dilation	-osis	condition
-ectomy	surgical removal	-ostomy	surgical opening
-ectopia	displacement	-otomy	incision into, cutting into
-edema	swelling	-ous	pertaining to
-ema	condition	-paresis	weakness, slight paralysis
-emesis	vomiting	-parous	producing, bearing
-emia	condition of the blood	-pathy	disease
-emic	relating to the blood	-penia	few, deficiency
-er	someone who	-pexy	surgical fixation
-esthesia	sensation	-phasia	speech, speaking
-gen	producing	-phobia	fear, usually abnormal
-genesis	production of	-phoria	feeling
-genic	producing	-phrenia	of the mind
-gnosis	knowledge of	-phylaxis	protection
-gram	a recording	-physis	growing
-graph	a recording instrument	-plasia	formation
-graphy	the process of recording	-plasm	formation
-ia	condition	-plasty	surgical repair
-iac	pertaining to	-plegia	paralysis
-iasis	pathological condition	-pnea	breath
-iatric	pertaining to medicine or to a physician	-poiesis	formation
		-poietic	forming

Suffixes (*continued*)

Suffix	Meaning	Suffix	Meaning
-ptosis	drooping, falling	-stasis	stopping, constant
-rrhage	excessive flow	-static	maintaining a constant state
-rrhagia	heavy discharge	-stenosis	narrowing
-rrhaphy	surgical suturing	-therapy	treatment
-rrhea	flowing	-tic	pertaining to
-rhexis	rupture	-trophy	nutrition
-sclerosis	hardening	-tropic	turning toward, having an affinity for
-scope	instrument for viewing or observing	-um	converts a root word into a noun
-scopy	viewing or observation		
-sis	condition	-uria	condition of the urine
-spasm	contraction	-version	turning backward
-stalsis	contraction, constriction	-y	condition

Directions, Locations, and Movement

Term	Meaning	Term	Meaning
abduction	to move away from	hypogastric	immediately below the umbilicus
adduction	to move toward		
anterior	at the front of the body or surface	inferior	below or directed downward
		inversion	turning inward
apex	the tip or top	lateral	situated to the side
base	the bottom or lower part	medial	at or near the middle
caudal	toward the feet or tail	posterior	at the back of the body
cephalic	toward the head	pronation	turning the palm downward
circumduction	movement in a circular motion	prone	lying face down
deep	away from the surface	protraction	moving a body part forward
distal	away from the center of the body or point of origin	proximal	near the center of the body or point of origin
dorsal	at the back of the body or surface	retraction	moving a body part backward
		rotation	movement of a body part around a point
dorsiflexion	bending a body part backward		
		superficial	near the surface
epigastric	immediately above the stomach	superior	above another structure
		supination	turning the palm upward
eversion	turning outward	supine	lying face up
extension	straightening a limb	ventral	at or toward the front of the body
flexion	bending a limb		

Common Medical Abbreviations

Those commonly in use but listed on the JCAHO "Do Not Use" list are so marked. DOT 3-6.3

Abbreviation	Meaning	Abbreviation	Meaning
+ or ⊕	plus (positive)	A&P	auscultation and percussion
− or ⊖	minus (negative)	ARD	acute respiratory disease
@	At (considered for future listing on the Do Not Use list)	ARDS	adult respiratory distress syndrome
~	approximately	a.s.	left ear
↑ or ⇡	increase, upper	ASA	Asprin (considered for future listing on the Do Not Use list)
↓ or ⇣	decrease, lower		
=	equal	ASCVD	arteriosclerotic cardiovascular disease
≠	unequal		
♀	female	ASD	atrial setpal defect
♂	male	ASHD	arteriosclerotic heart disease
>	greater than (considered for future listing on the Do Not Use list)	a.u.	each ear
		AV	atrioventricular
		BBS	bilateral breath sounds
<	less than (considered for future listing on the Do Not Use list)	b.i.d.	twice a day
		BGL	blood glucose level
→	leading to	B-K	below the knee
Δ	change	BKA	below the knee amputation
ā	before	BM	bowel movement, bag-mask
AAO	awake, alert, and oriented	BP	blood pressure
AB	abortion	bpm	beats per minute
ABC	airway, breathing, and circulation	BS	breath sounds
abd	abdomen	BSA	body surface area
AAA	abdominal aortic aneurysm	BVM	bag valve mask
ABG	arterial blood gas	c̄	with
a.c.	before meals	CC	chief complaint
AC	antecubital	cc	Cubic centimeter (considered for future listing on the Do Not Use list—write "ml" instead)
ACE-I	angiotensin converting enzyme inhibitor		
ACLS	advanced cardiac life support		
a.d.	right ear	c/o	complains of
ADD	attention deficit disorder	C-section	caesarean section
ADH	anti-diuretic hormone (DO NOT USE per the JCAHO Do not use list)	C-spine	cervical spine
		C(1-7)	cervical vertebra (1-7)
		CA	cancer
ADL	activities of daily living	CABG	coronary artery bypass graft
AF	atrial fibrillation	CAD	coronary artery disease
A-Fib	atrial fibrillation	cath	catheter
A-flutter	atrial flutter	CBC	complete blood count
A-K	above the knee	CBG	capillary blood glucose
AKA	above the knee amputation or alcoholic ketoacidosis	CHD	coronary heart disease
		CHF	congestive heart failure
ALS	advanced life support	CHI	closed head injury
a.m.	morning	cm	centimeter
AMA	against medical advice	CMS	circulation, motor, sensation
AMI	acute myocardial infarction	CNS	central nervous system
AP or A/P	anteriorposterior	CO	cardiac output, carbon monoxide

Common Medical Abbreviations (*continued*)

Abbreviation	Meaning	Abbreviation	Meaning
COPD	chronic obstructive pulmonary disease	GERD	gastroesophageal reflux disease
CP	chest pain or cerebral palsy	GI	gastrointestinal
CPAP	continuous positive airway pressure	GSW	gunshot wound
		GU	genitourinary
CPK	creatine phosphokinase	gyn, GYN	gynecology
CPR	cardiopulmonary resuscitation	g	gram
CRF	chronic renal failure	gtt(s)	drop(s)
CSF	cerebrospinal fluid	HA	headache
CSID	cervical spine immobilization device	HBV	hepatitis B virus
		h.s.	bedtime; hour of sleep
CTA	clear to auscultation	HCT, Hct	hematocrit
CVA	cerebrovascular accident, costovertebral angle	HD	hemodialysis
		HEENT	head, eyes, ears, nose, and throat
CVD	cerebrovascular disease		
CXR	chest x-ray	H&P	history and physical
dc	discontinue	HPI	history of present illness
Dig	Digoxin (considered for future listing on the Do Not Use list)	HR	heart rate
		HTN	hypertension
DIP	distal interphalangeal	Hx	history
DM	diabetes mellitus	IBD	inflammatory bowel disease
DOA	dead on arrival	IBS	irritable bowel syndrome
DOB	date of birth	ICS	intercostal space
DOE	dyspnea on exertion	ICP	intracranial pressure
DOS	dead on scene	ID	intradermal
DNR	do not resuscitate	IDDM	insulin-dependant diabetes mellitus
DT	delirium tremens		
DTR	deep tendon reflex	IM	intramuscular
DVT	deep vein thrombosis	inj	injection
Dx or dx	diagnosis	I&O, I/O	intake and output
ECG or EKG	electrocardiogram	IO	intraosseus
EDC	estimated date of confinement	IPPD	intermittent positive pressure breathing
EENT	eyes, ears, nose, and throat		
EMS	emergency medical services	IV	intravenous
EMT	emergency medical technician	IVCD	intraventricular conduction delay
EOM	extraocular movement		
EOMI	extraocular movements intact	JVD	jugular venous distension
epi	Epinephrine (considered for future listing on the Do Not Use list)	KVO	keep vein open
		l	liter
		L or Ⓛ	left
ETA	estimated time of arrival	LAC or lac	laceration
ETOH	Alcohol (considered for future listing on the Do Not Use list)	LR	lactated ringers
		LBBB	left bundle branch block
ETT	endotracheal tube	LLL	left lower lobe
FB	foreign body	LLQ	left lower quadrant
FBAO	foreign body airway obstruction	LMP	last menstrual period
		LOC	level of consciousness
Fx	fracture	loc	loss of consciousness

Common Medical Abbreviations (*continued*)

Abbreviation	Meaning	Abbreviation	Meaning
lpm	liters per minute	OTC	over the counter
LSB	long spine board	p	after
LUL	left upper lobe	PAC	premature atrial contraction
LUQ	left upper quadrant	PE	physical exam, pulmonary embolus
LVH	left ventricular hypertrophy		
MAL	mid axillary line	PEEP	positive end expiratory pressure
MAOI	monoamine oxidase inhibitor	PCN	Penicillin (considered for future listing on the Do Not Use list)
mcg	microgram		
MCI	mass casualty incident	PERRL	pupils equal round and reactive to light
MCL	midclavicular line		
MDI	metered dose inhaler	PERRLA	pupils equal round and reactive to light and accommodation
meds	medications		
mEq	milliequivalent	PID	pelvic inflammatory disease
mg	milligram	PIP	proximal interphalangeal joint
MI	myocardial infarction	p.m.	evening
MIP	middle interphalangeal	PMH	past medical history
ml	milliliter	PMP	previous menstrual period
mm	millimeter	PMS	premenstrual syndrome
mmHg	millimeters of mercury	pn	pain
MS	multiple sclerosis	PND	paroxysmal nocturnal dyspnea
MVC	motor vehicle collision	p.o.	by mouth
MVP	mitral valve prolapse	PRN, p.r.n.	as needed
$NaHCO_3$	sodium bicarbonate (considered for future listing on the Do Not Use list)	pt	patient
		PTA	prior to arrival
		PVC	premature ventricular contraction
NC	nasal cannula	pwd	pink, warm, and dry
NG	nasogastric	q	Every (DO NOT USE per the JCAHO Do not use list)
NPA	nasopharyngeal airway		
NS	normal saline	q.d.	every day (DO NOT USE per the JCAHO Do not use list)
N&V or N+V	nausea and vomiting		
N&V&D or N+V+D	nausea and vomiting and diarrhea	q.h.	every hour (DO NOT USE per the JCAHO Do not use list)
NIDDM	noninsulin-dependant diabetes mellitus	q.i.d.	four times a day
		RBBB	right bundle branch block
NKA	no known allergies	RBC	red blood cell count
NKDA	no known drug allergies	resp	respirations
NPO	nothing by mouth	RLL	right lower lobe
NRB	nonrebreather mask	RLQ	right lower quadrant
NRM	nonrebreather mask	RML	right middle lobe
NSAID	nonsteroidal anti-inflammatory drug	R/O	rule out
		ROM	range of motion
NSR	normal sinus rhythm	RUL	right upper lobe
NTG	nitroglycerin (considered for future listing on the Do Not Use list)	RUQ	right upper quadrant
		s̄	without
OB	obstetric	SA	sinoatrial, sexual assault
OCD	obsessive compulsive disorder	SAH	subarachnoid hemorrhage
OD	overdose	s.c., SC, subq	subcutaneously
OPA	oropharyngeal airway	SIDS	sudden infant death syndrome

Common Medical Abbreviations (*continued*)

Abbreviation	Meaning	Abbreviation	Meaning
SL	sublingual	Tx	treatment
S&S, S+S	signs and symptoms	UA, U/A	upon arrival
SV	stroke volume	unc	unconscious
Sx	symptoms	unk	unknown
t.i.d.	three times a day	URI	upper respiratory infection
TB	tuberculosis	UTI	urinary tract infection
TIA	transient ischemic attack	V-fib	ventricular fibrillation
TKO	to keep open	V-tach	ventricular tachycardia
TMJ	temporomandibular joint	y/o	years old

Summary

Understanding medical terminology is a critical component in making use of the language of the paramedic profession. Knowing the rules used to build medical terms will help in determining the meaning of words even when exposed to them for the first time.

Notes

1. J. Rice, *Medical Terminology with Human Anatomy,* 2nd ed. (East Norwalk, CT: Appleton & Lange, 1991).
2. N. Thierer and L. Breitbard, *Medical Terminology; Language for Healthcare,* 2nd ed. (New York, NY: McGraw-Hill, 2006).
3. Official "Do Not Use" List. http://www.jointcommission.org/PatientSafety/DoNotUseList (accessed April 11, 2006).
4. *Stedman's Medical Dictionary,* 26th ed. (Baltimore, MD: Williams and Wilkins, 1995).
5. Webster's Medical Desk Dictionary (Springfield, MA: Merriam-Webster, Inc., 1986), p. 10a.
6. *Tabers Cyclopedic Medical Dictionary,* 20th ed. (Philadelphia, PA: F. A. Davis Company, 2005).

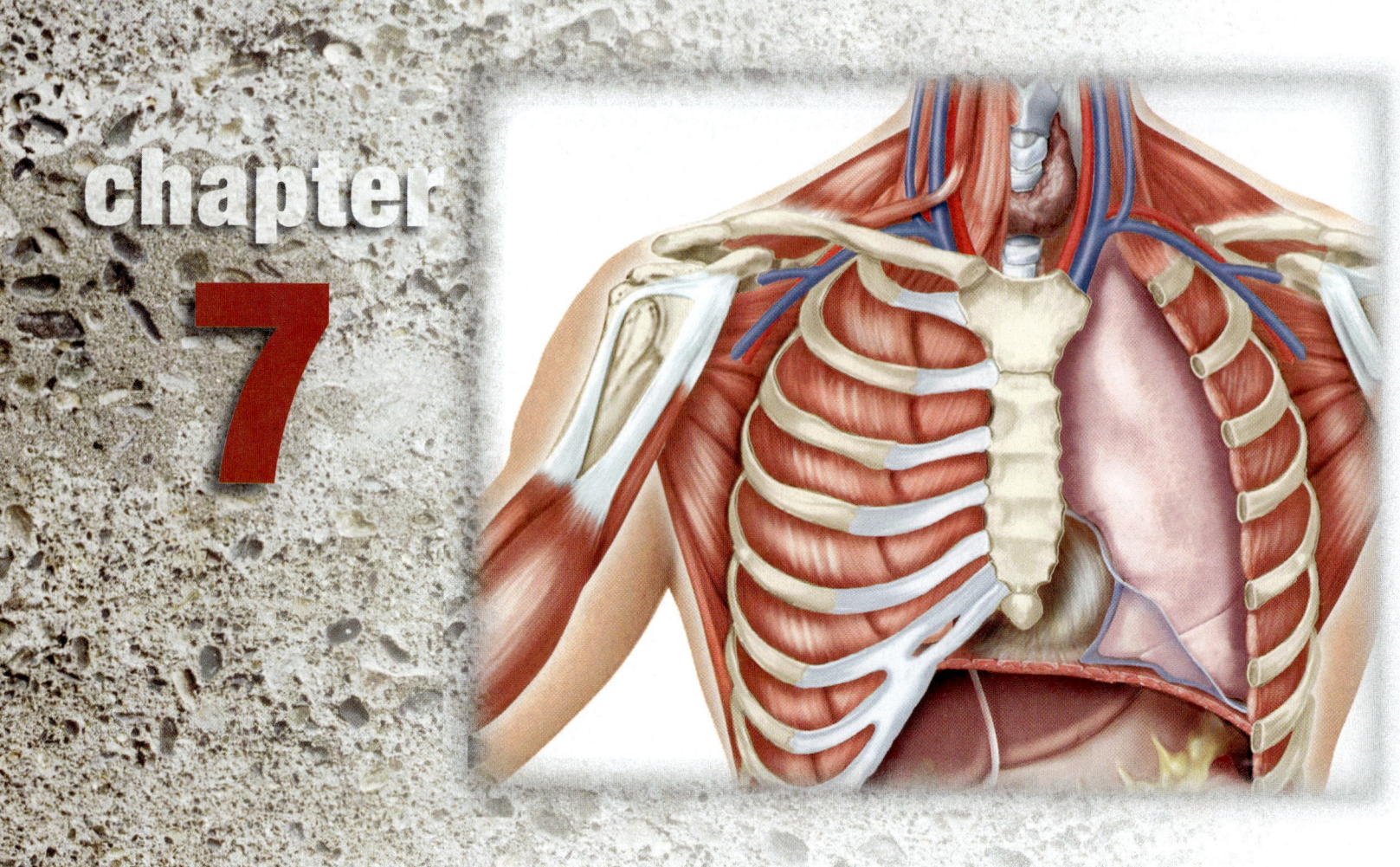

Anatomy Overview

"**H**uman ingenuity may make various inventions but it never will devise any inventions more beautiful, nor more simple, nor more to the purpose than nature does; because in her inventions, nothing is lacking and nothing is superfluous."

—Leonardo Da Vinci, 1452–1519

Need to Know

▶ Understand and appreciate the anatomy that is pertinent to the tasks performed by paramedics. This will enable you to better perform assessments and treatments and will help you critically consider how anatomy impacts the performance of these duties.

▶ Learn how to pronounce the names of anatomical structures, so you can communicate more effectively with other members of the health care team.

▶ Understand the interworking relationships organs have with each other and which organs are grouped together to form systems.

▶ Understand how the structure of the body (bones, muscles, joints, connective tissues, etc.) affects movement.

Introduction

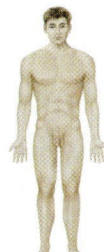

Anatomy is the branch of study that deals with the structure and organization of living things. It comes from the Greek term, *anatome,* in which *ana* means *up* and *tome* means *cutting,* hence, the cutting up of the body, as in dissection.

The goal of this anatomic overview is to familiarize you with the basic details of body structure, so you will have a foundation to understand the more detailed physiology, pathology, and therapeutics that will be specifically presented later in this textbook. This chapter is organized in the same way that a paramedic will approach a secondary survey: from head to toe. Future chapters will explore the detailed aspects of anatomy as it relates to each of the topic-specific chapters.

Anatomical Terminology

It is essential for healthcare providers to learn anatomic terminology to keep communication consistent and accurate among team members—dispatchers, EMS personnel, hospital personnel, etc. Anatomical terms are described below. All of the terms apply to the **anatomical position,** which is when the subject is standing erect (upright) with the eyes facing forward, the arms hanging down at the sides, and the palms of the hands facing forward (Figure 7-1).

For consistency, it is an agreed-upon convention to describe locations on the body in reference to an individual in the anatomical position. This is true even if the patient is lying down or sitting. Additionally, you should report the actual position the patient is in when met by EMS. Many patient care reports include an outline drawing of a person in the anatomical position, making it possible for the treating paramedic to draw in locations of injuries to increase accuracy in reporting (Figure 7-2).

The body is then described by locating body parts relative to each other:

■ **Anterior** or **ventral** is toward the front of the body.

■ **Posterior** or **dorsal** is toward the back of the body.

■ **Frontal** refers to any structure that is toward the anterior surface of the body.

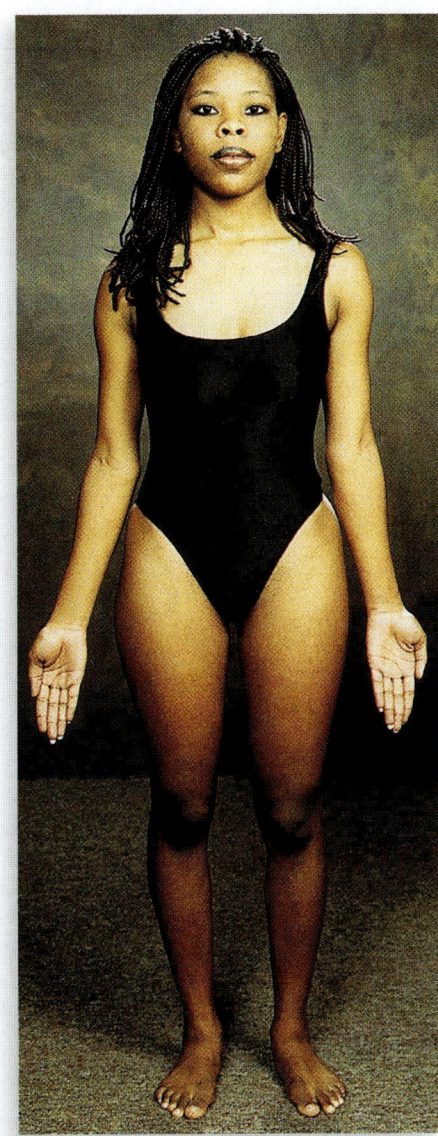

Figure 7-1 The anatomical position is the common point of reference used to describe the locations of problems found on the body.

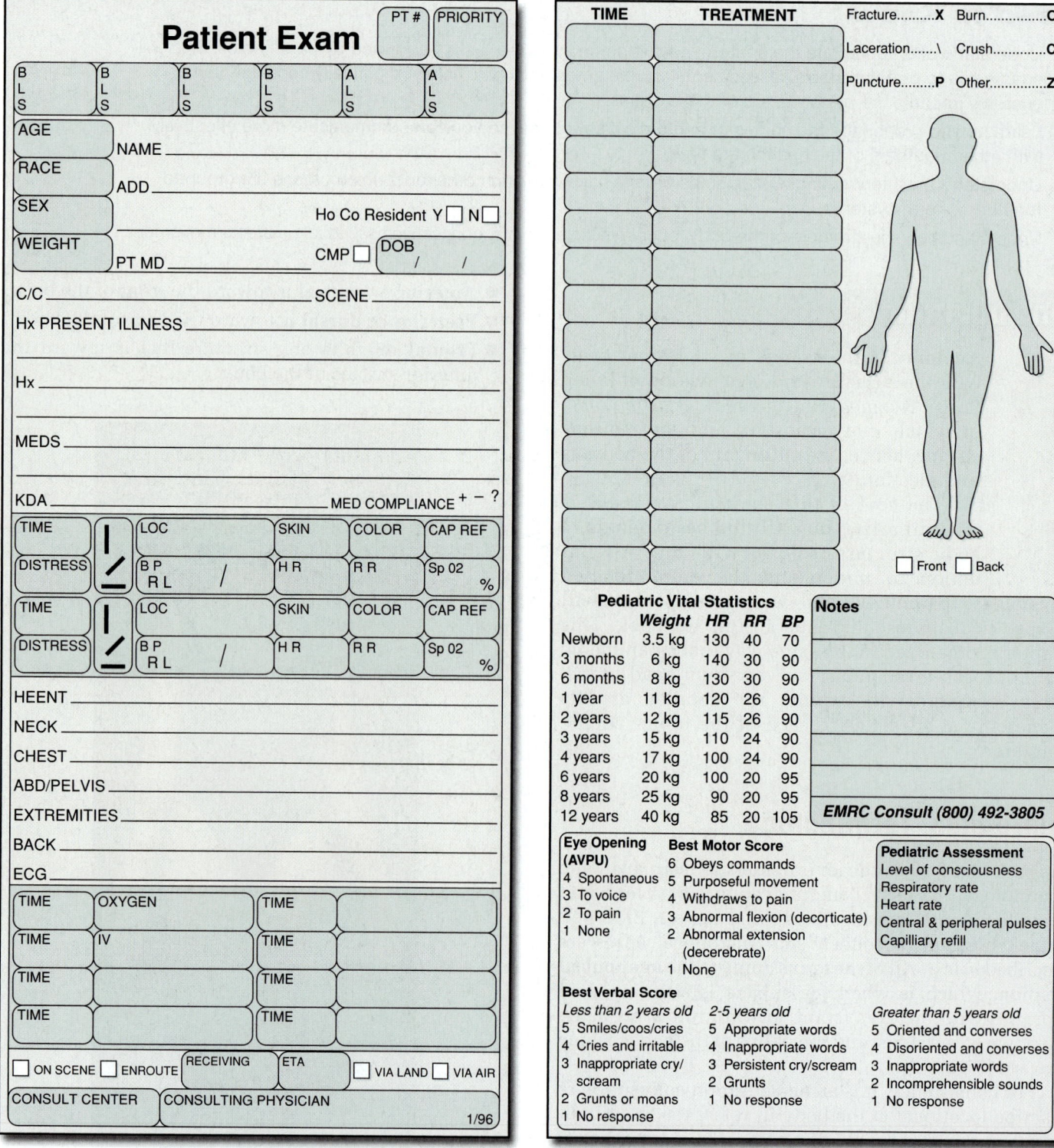

Figure 7-2 Many patient care reports have a drawing to assist the paramedic in identifying the location of injuries.

For example, a cut on the calf would be posterior, and a cut on the knee would be anterior.

The body is also described by using imaginary lines, called **planes,** sliced through it (see Figure 7-3):

- The **midsagittal plane** passes through the midline of the body and divides it into equal left and right halves.
- A **sagittal plane** is any dividing line that runs parallel to the midsaggital plane.

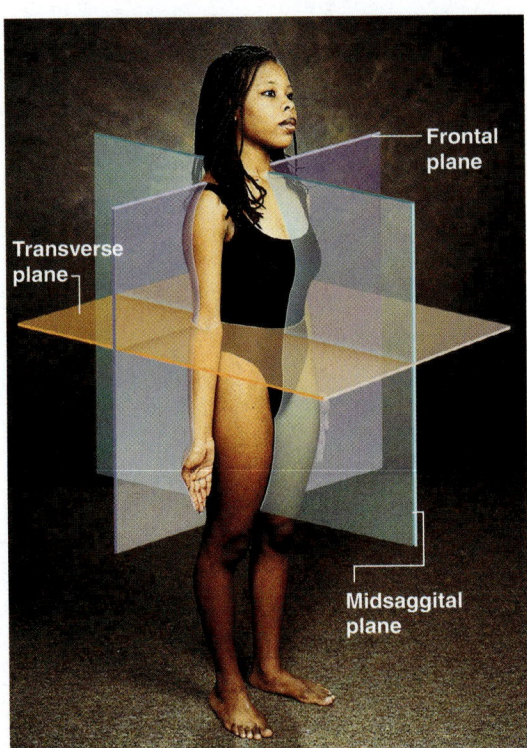

Figure 7-3 Planes help divide the body into specific areas. Because the planes are individually named, communication between members of the health care team is more accurate.

- **Medial** means toward the midline.
- **Lateral** means away from the midline.

For example, the heart is medial compared to the kidney, but the kidney is medial compared to the axilla (arm pit).

- **Transverse planes** section the body crosswise into top and bottom pieces, and these planes run at 90-degree angles to saggital planes (see Figure 7-3).

The horizontal line that runs through the umbilicus (belly button) to help divide the abdomen into four quadrants is an example of a transverse plane.

There are additional terms used to describe direction (Figure 7-4). Some of the more commonly used terms include the following:

- **Craniad** or **cephalad** means toward the head.
- **Caudad** is toward the tail.
- **Superior** means toward the top.
- **Inferior** means toward the feet.
- **Superficial** is toward the exterior.
- **Deep** is toward the interior.
- **Proximal** is nearer to the trunk of the body when compared to another point.
- **Distal** is farther from the trunk when compared to another point.

A bruise on the elbow is proximal to a bruise on the hand. If you compare that same bruise to the axilla (armpit), it would be described as distal. If you were basing that same bruise on the anatomical position, you would describe it as distal because it is on an extremity and away from the midsaggital line.

You should report the position the patient is found in and include it in your written patient care document. This will help the receiving medical team visualize the scene and aid in police reconstruction efforts if they are conducting an investigation. It can also help clarify or provide context for injury patterns or explain marks, bruises, injuries, or other physical findings to people who are later assessing the patient. Use the following terms to describe the patient position:

- **Supine** means lying horizontal with the face upward.
- **Prone** is lying horizontal with the face downward.
- **Lateral recumbent** is lying on the side (record which side, left or right).
- **Trendelenburg position** was established for the operating room. The patient is lying supine with the head of the table angled downward at about a 45-degree angle, and the arms are hanging loosely off the bed. EMS uses a modified version of this when they elevate the feet above the head to treat for shock.

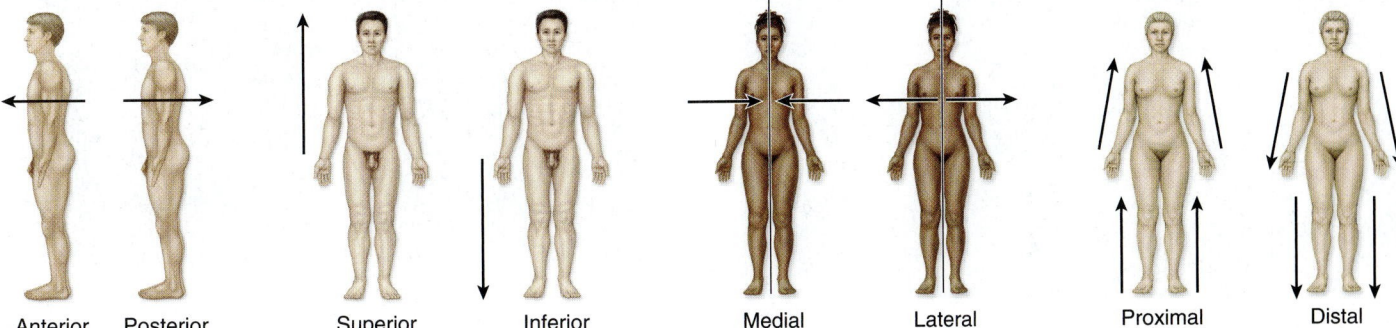

Anterior   Posterior   Superior   Inferior   Medial   Lateral   Proximal   Distal

Figure 7-4 Common medical terms that describe the relationship of various parts of the body.

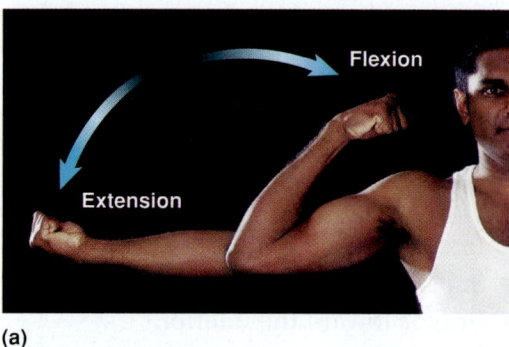

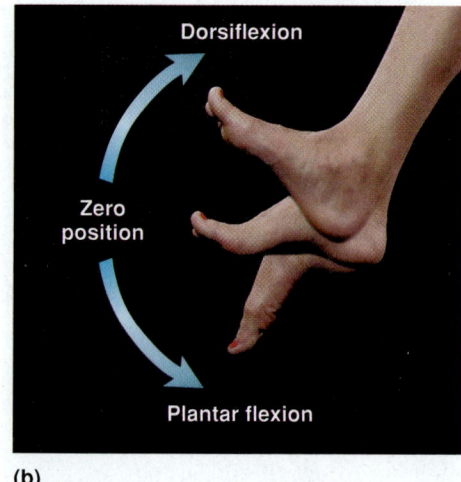

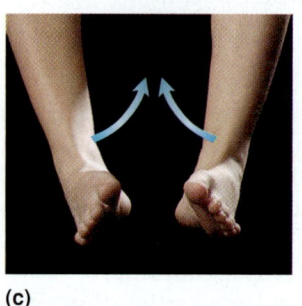

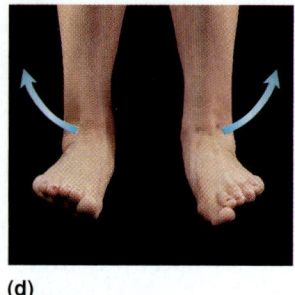

Figure 7-5   A joint of the body illustrating joint motions. (a and b) Flexion and extension. (c) Inversion. (d) Eversion.

■ **Reverse Trendelenburg** (which is mostly a jargon term for EMS) places the patient supine and then elevates the head of the bed up to 45 degrees. The body should be flat to the bed. Many medical people confuse reverse Trendelenburg and Fowler's position, but in true Trendelenburg the patient is lying flat on the surface and the surface changes positions.

■ **Fowler's position** has the patient sitting (bent at the hip) from a supine position. The patient may be positioned anywhere from a few degrees up to 90 degrees. Some people refer to "semi-Fowlers" position as a Fowlers position that is 45 degrees or less.

Finally, joint movements are described as follows (Figures 7-5, 7-6, 7-7, and 7-8):

■ **Abduction** is a movement away from the body.
■ **Adduction** is a movement toward the body.
■ **Flexion** is the act of bending.

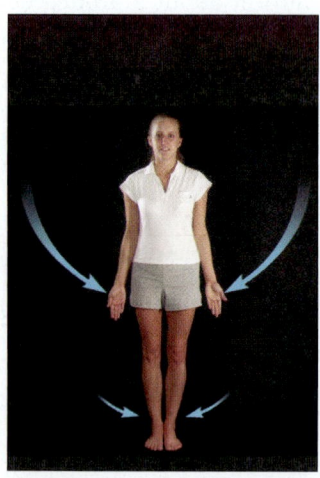

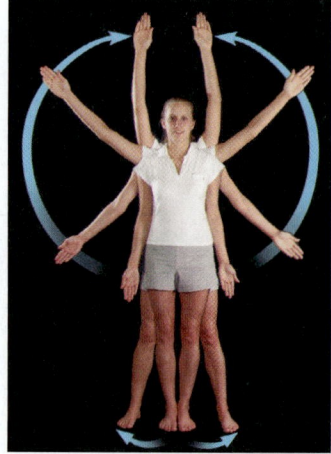

Figure 7-6   Adduction brings a joint into the body and abduction moves it away.

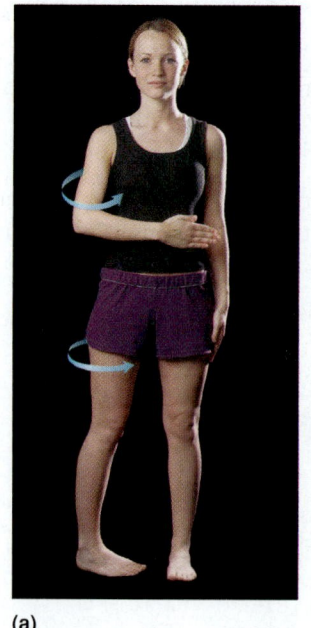

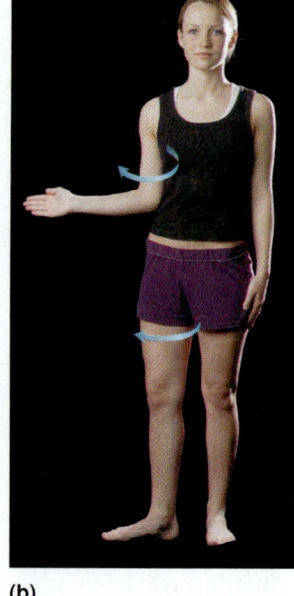

Figure 7-7   (a) Internal rotation is closer to the center, or midline, of the body while (b) external rotation is away from the body.

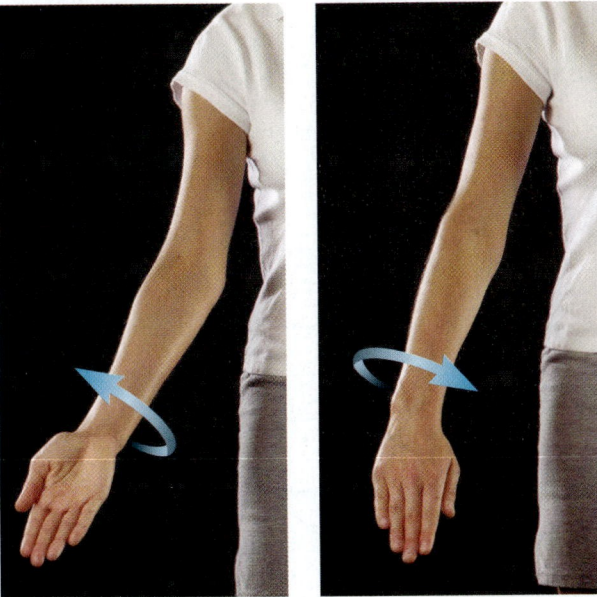

Figure 7-8 Supination and pronation are rotational movements that turn the body part away from the midline (supination) or toward the midline (pronation).

- **Extension** is the act of straightening.
- **Pronation** is the act of rotating the arm so that the palm of the hand is facing downward.
- **Supination** is the act of rotating the arm so that the palm of the hand is facing up (think of holding a soup bowl on the palm).

Anatomy of the Head and Neck

The Skull and Brain

The bony skull surrounds the brain, eyes, and hearing apparatus of the ears to protect them from injury. The frontal, occipital, parietal, temporal, sphenoid, and ethmoid bones are the major bones that make up the skull. Arteries, veins, and the 12 cranial nerves pass through foramina (openings) at the base of the skull. As the spinal cord exits through the largest opening (foraman magnum) in the base of the skull, nerve fibers and tracts cross over from one side to the other so that the nerves arising from the right side of the brain innervate the left side of the body and vice versa. The eyes are protected by the bony orbits of the face. (See Figures 7-9, 7-10, 7-11, and 7-12).

The brain is divided into multiple parts, each with a different function (Figure 7-13). There are two **cerebral hemispheres** divided into **frontal, parietal, temporal,** and **occipital lobes,** and they are joined together by the corpus collosum (Figure 7-14). The **cerebrum** has many functions, including sensory and motor control as well as higher mental functions. The **cerebellum,** located inferior to the cerebrum, coordinates fine motor control, posture, and balance. The **brainstem** is made up of the midbrain, pons, and medulla oblongata (Figure 7-15). The **midbrain** connects the brainstem with both the cerebrum and the cerebellum and controls eye movements and motor coordination. The **pons** helps coordinate the function

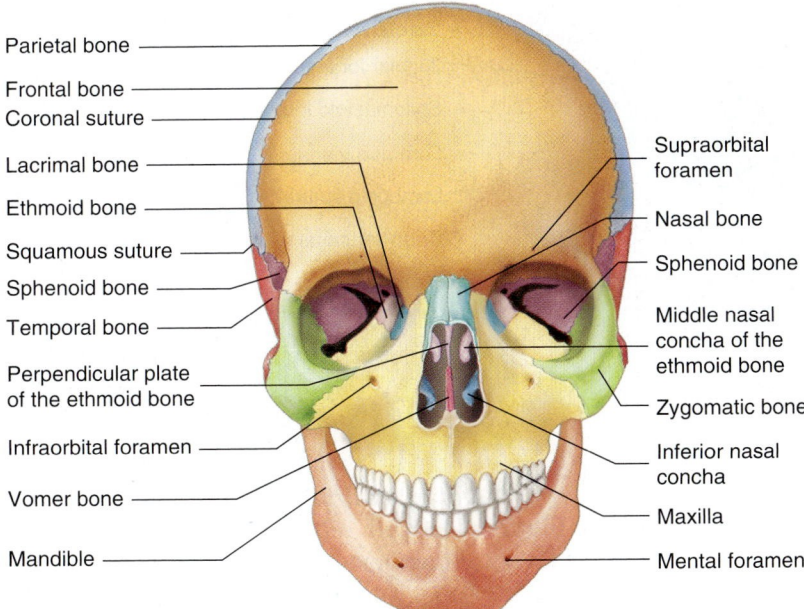

Figure 7-9 The anterior view of the skull.

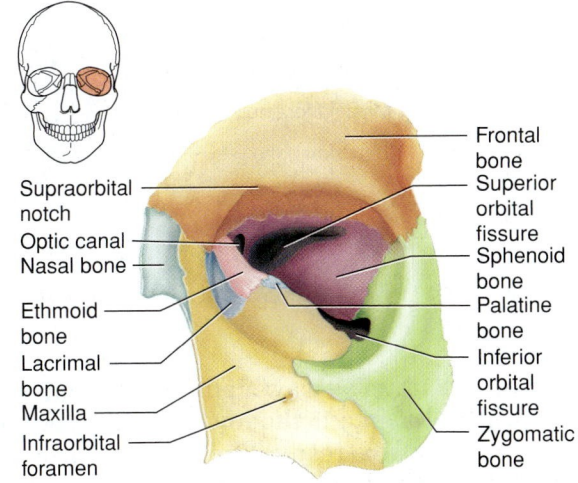

Figure 7-10 The cranial and facial bones help protect the eye.

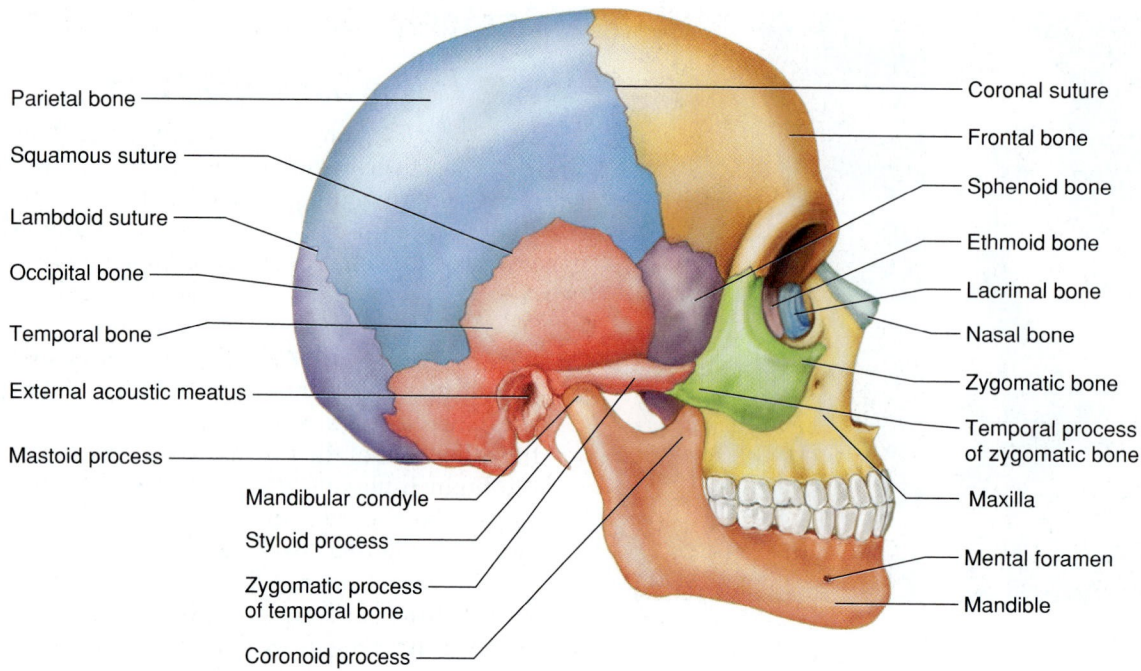

Figure 7-11   The lateral view of the skull.

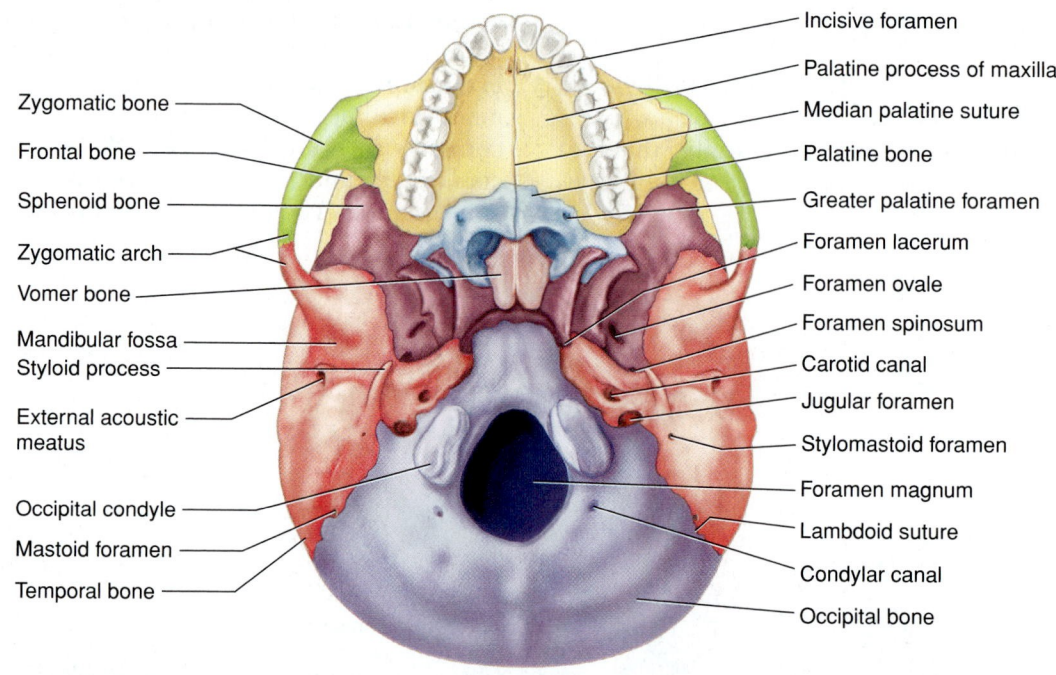

Figure 7-12   The inferior view of the skull.

of the cerebellum by way of pontocerebellar tracts. The **medulla oblongata** is the lowest portion of the brainstem and controls respiration and cardiac activity. At the base of the brain, the medulla oblongata travels through the foramen magnum and attaches the brain to the spinal cord. Twelve pairs of cranial nerves arise directly from the brain and provide innervation to the face (see Figure 7-16 and Table 7-1).

Three layers of **meninges** surround the brain and spinal cord (Figure 7-17). The **pia mater** adheres closely to the brain and spinal cord. The **arachnoid membrane** is the second layer of the meninges and has a spiderweb-like

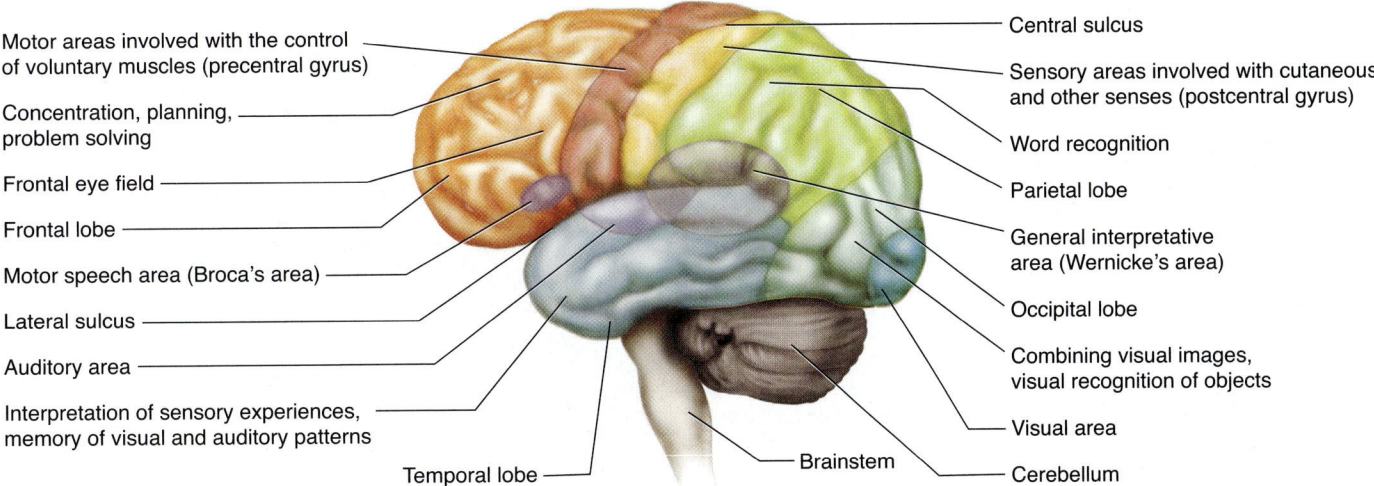

Motor areas involved with the control of voluntary muscles (precentral gyrus)

Concentration, planning, problem solving

Frontal eye field

Frontal lobe

Motor speech area (Broca's area)

Lateral sulcus

Auditory area

Interpretation of sensory experiences, memory of visual and auditory patterns

Temporal lobe

Brainstem

Central sulcus

Sensory areas involved with cutaneous and other senses (postcentral gyrus)

Word recognition

Parietal lobe

General interpretative area (Wernicke's area)

Occipital lobe

Combining visual images, visual recognition of objects

Visual area

Cerebellum

Figure 7-13 A map of the brain identifying which parts are responsible for the various senses, thought processes, and memory.

appearance. The **subarachnoid space** lies between these two layers and contains the cerebrospinal fluid. The outer layer of the meninges is thick and fibrous and is called the **dura mater.** The space between the arachnoid membrane and the dura mater is called the subdural space. Outside of the dura mater is the **epidural space,** which is located between the inside of the skull and the dura mater. The third and fourth ventricles are connected by the **cerebral aqueduct** and contain cerebrospinal fluid.

The **pituitary gland** is found at the base of the brain and is suspended by a stalk (Figure 7-18). The **sella turcica** is a protective bone that surrounds it. It is an endocrine organ. The posterior pituitary secretes **oxytocin** and **antidiuretic hormone (ADH).** The anterior pituitary secretes **thyroid stimulating hormone (TSH), adrenocorticotropin hormone (ACTH), follicle stimulating hormone (FSH), luteinizing hormone (LH),** and **prolactin.**

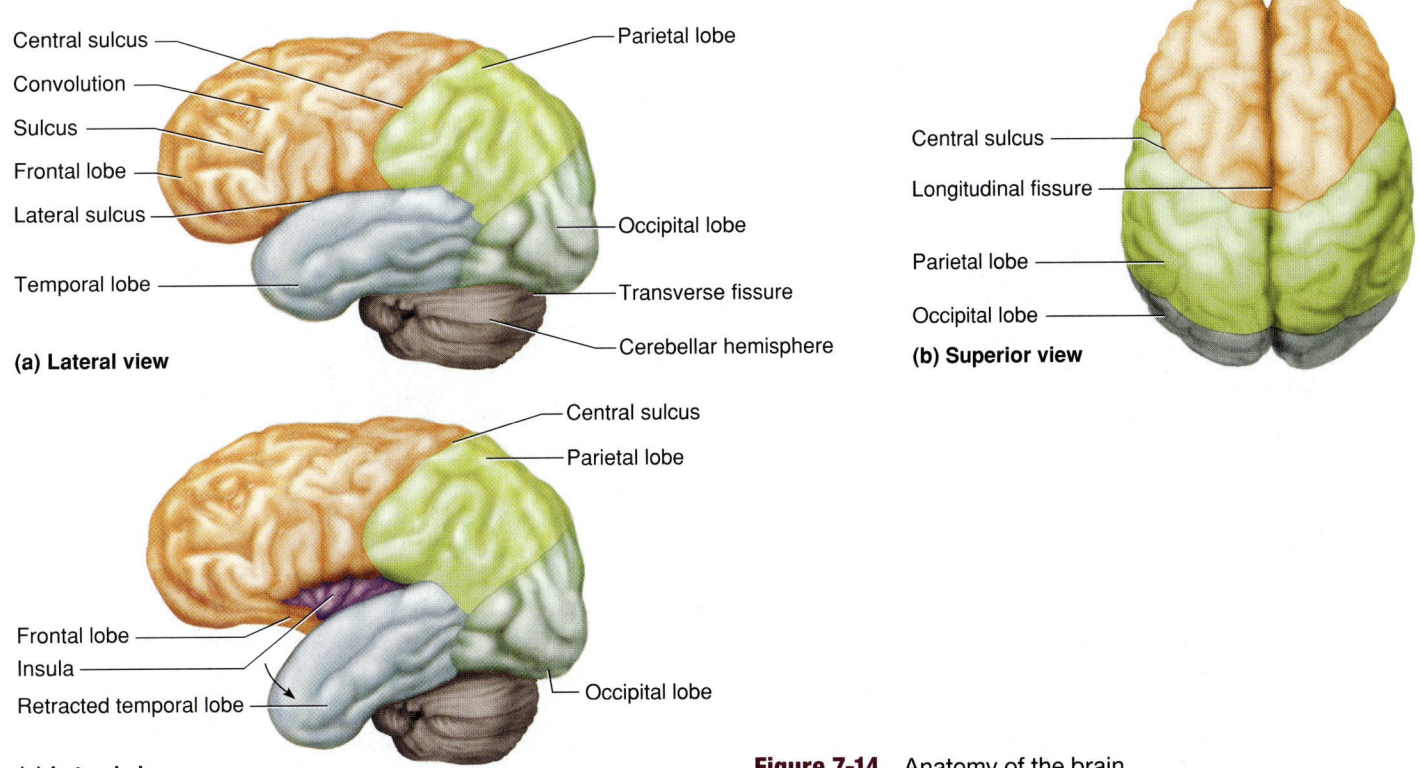

Central sulcus

Convolution

Sulcus

Frontal lobe

Lateral sulcus

Temporal lobe

Parietal lobe

Occipital lobe

Transverse fissure

Cerebellar hemisphere

(a) Lateral view

Central sulcus

Longitudinal fissure

Parietal lobe

Occipital lobe

(b) Superior view

Central sulcus

Parietal lobe

Frontal lobe

Insula

Retracted temporal lobe

Occipital lobe

(c) Lateral view

Figure 7-14 Anatomy of the brain.

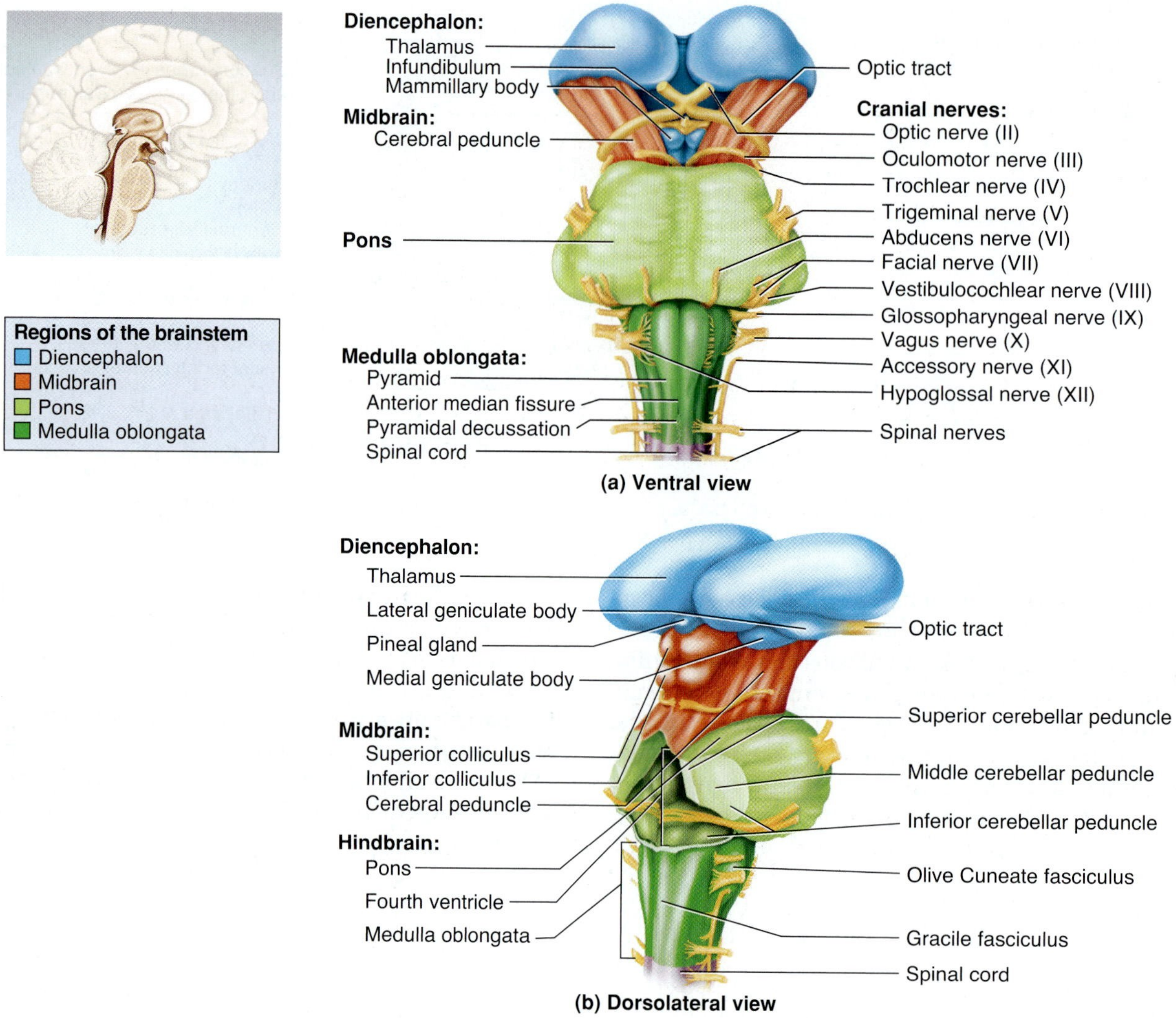

Regions of the brainstem
- Diencephalon
- Midbrain
- Pons
- Medulla oblongata

Diencephalon:
Thalamus
Infundibulum
Mammillary body

Optic tract

Midbrain:
Cerebral peduncle

Pons

Cranial nerves:
Optic nerve (II)
Oculomotor nerve (III)
Trochlear nerve (IV)
Trigeminal nerve (V)
Abducens nerve (VI)
Facial nerve (VII)
Vestibulocochlear nerve (VIII)
Glossopharyngeal nerve (IX)
Vagus nerve (X)
Accessory nerve (XI)
Hypoglossal nerve (XII)

Medulla oblongata:
Pyramid
Anterior median fissure
Pyramidal decussation
Spinal cord

Spinal nerves

(a) Ventral view

Diencephalon:
Thalamus
Lateral geniculate body
Pineal gland
Medial geniculate body

Optic tract

Midbrain:
Superior colliculus
Inferior colliculus
Cerebral peduncle

Superior cerebellar peduncle

Middle cerebellar peduncle

Inferior cerebellar peduncle

Hindbrain:
Pons
Fourth ventricle
Medulla oblongata

Olive Cuneate fasciculus

Gracile fasciculus

Spinal cord

(b) Dorsolateral view

Figure 7-15 The midbrain, pons, and medulla oblongata comprise the brainstem.

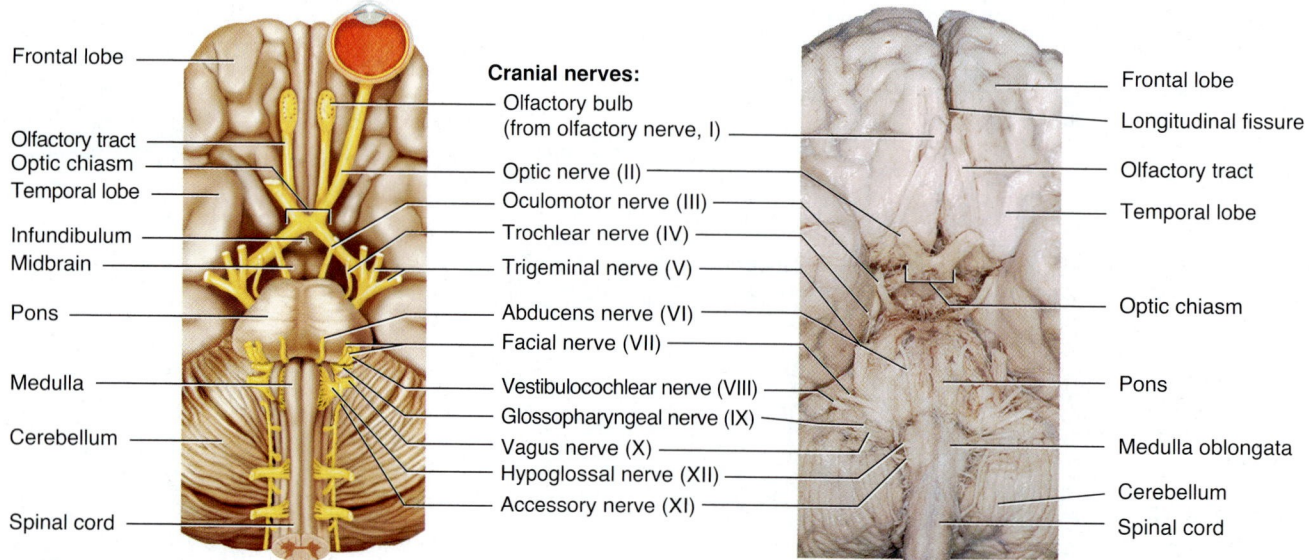

Frontal lobe

Olfactory tract
Optic chiasm
Temporal lobe

Infundibulum
Midbrain

Pons

Medulla

Cerebellum

Spinal cord

Cranial nerves:
Olfactory bulb
(from olfactory nerve, I)
Optic nerve (II)
Oculomotor nerve (III)
Trochlear nerve (IV)
Trigeminal nerve (V)
Abducens nerve (VI)
Facial nerve (VII)
Vestibulocochlear nerve (VIII)
Glossopharyngeal nerve (IX)
Vagus nerve (X)
Hypoglossal nerve (XII)
Accessory nerve (XI)

Frontal lobe

Longitudinal fissure

Olfactory tract

Temporal lobe

Optic chiasm

Pons

Medulla oblongata

Cerebellum

Spinal cord

Figure 7-16 The cranial nerves arise directly from the brain and control many of the senses.

TABLE 7-1   Cranial Nerves

Number	Name	Function
I	Olfactory	Sense of smell
II	Optic	Sight
III	Oculomotor	Controls four of the six eye muscles, controls eyelid (upper), constricts pupil
IV	Trochlear	Controls one of the six eye muscles
V	Trigeminal	Sensation of face, control of muscles for chewing
VI	Abducens	Controls one of the six eye muscles
VII	Facial	Controls muscles of facial expression, taste sensation, tear, and salivary gland
VIII	Vestibulocochlear (Auditory)	Hearing and balance
IX	Glossopharyngeal	Taste and sensation to back of tongue
X	Vagus	Sensory and motor function of palate, pharynx, and larynx
XI	Accessory	Motor to neck and back muscles (trapezius and sternocleidomastoid)
XII	Hypoglossal	Motor function of tongue muscles

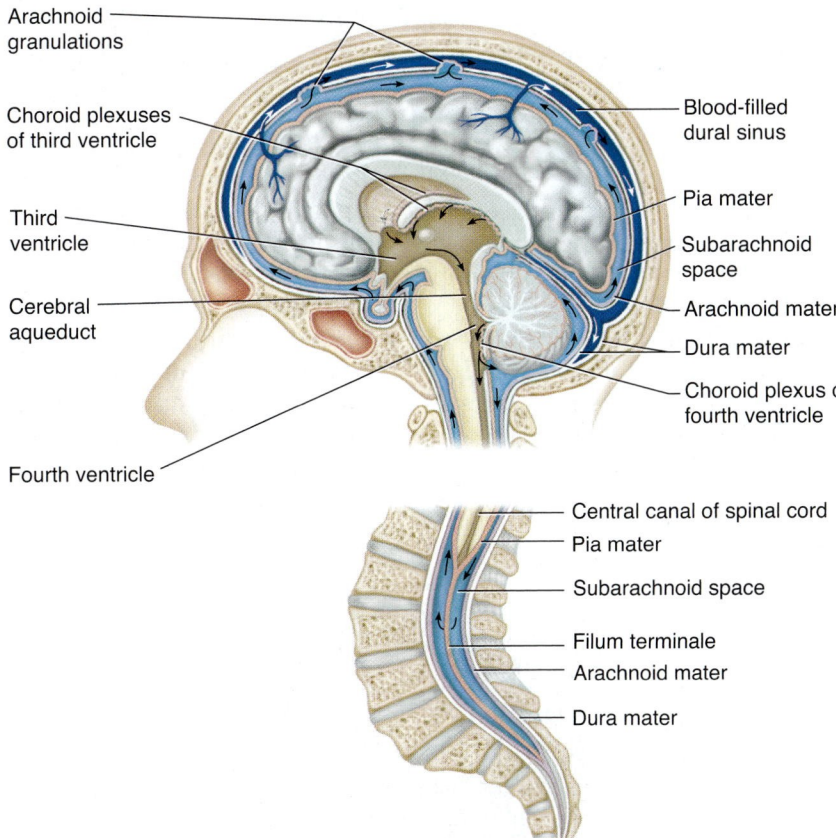

Figure 7-17   Meninges cover and protect the brain and spinal cord.

The Eyes, Ears, and Nose

The Eyes

The outermost portion of the eye is the **cornea.** Behind the cornea is the fluid-filled anterior chamber. The colored part of the eye is the **iris** with its central opening, called the pupil, which is the anterior limit of the posterior chamber. Moving posteriorly, the **lens,** which focuses images and light onto the **retina,** is next. Beyond the lens is the **vitreous humor** through which images, focused by the lens, travel to the sensory retina located at the posterior aspect of the vitreous chamber. The **optic nerve** then transmits impulses to the brain where they are interpreted as images (Figure 7-19).

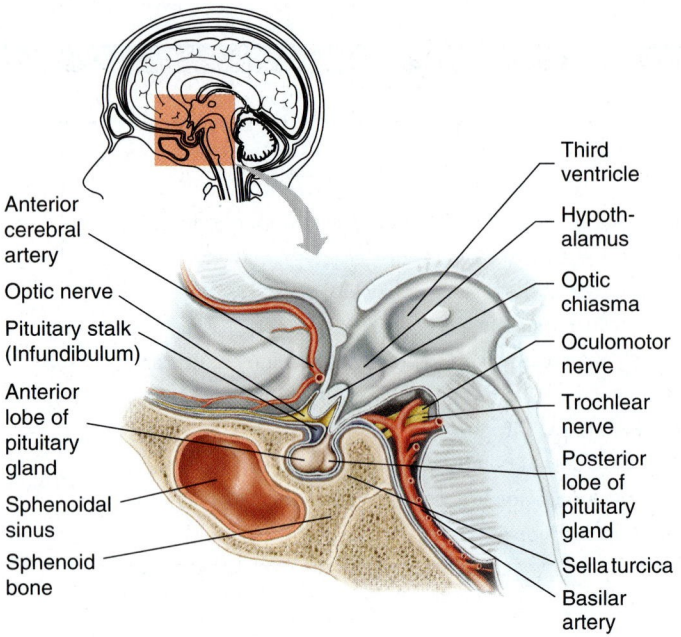

Figure 7-18 The pituitary gland is found at the base of the brain.

The Ears

There are three main divisions to the ear. The external ear consists of the **auricle** (commonly thought of as the ears on the outside of the head) and the ear canal leading into the middle ear. The **middle ear** is a cavity in the temporal bone. The **eustachian tube** balances pressures in the middle ear. Secretions from the eustachian tube, **lacrimal duct,** and the **sinuses** all empty into the **nasopharynx.** The **internal ear** is a series of cavities between the middle ear and the internal acoustic meatus (Figure 7-20).

The Nose

The nose is the outermost region or cover to the uppermost portion of the airway. The two **nares** open into the external nose and are divided by the **nasal septum.** Within the nares are three curved shelves of bone called the **inferior, middle,** and **superior concha.** These chambers lead into the nasal cavity. The **nasal cavities** are divided into three regions. The **nasal vestibule,** a small space just beyond the nares, is lined by skin and filtering hair follicles. The **respiratory region** is the largest of the three. It has a rich vascular supply lined by epithelium, mostly mucous-producing cells. The **olfactory region** at the apex of the nasal cavities contains the olfactory receptors. Besides giving us the sense of smell through the olfactory receptors, the nose humidifies and filters inspired air.

CONNECTIONS More on eyes, ears, nose, and throat can be found in Chapter 39.

The Airway and Neck

The airway begins in the mouth and the nose (Figure 7-21). The purpose of the upper airway is to warm and humidify air that is inspired as it moves to the lungs. Air enters the nose by way of the nares and then passes posteriorly into the nasopharynx. Hairs in the nose filter the air. The nasal bones, nasal cartilage, and a portion of the maxilla form the nose. A cartilaginous **septum** divides the nose into right and left nares. The mucosa of the nose is very vascular and susceptible to bleeding. Turbinates are shelf-like structures inside the nose that cause turbulent flow of the air as it enters the nose. Their purpose is to precipitate, or filter out, particulate matter.

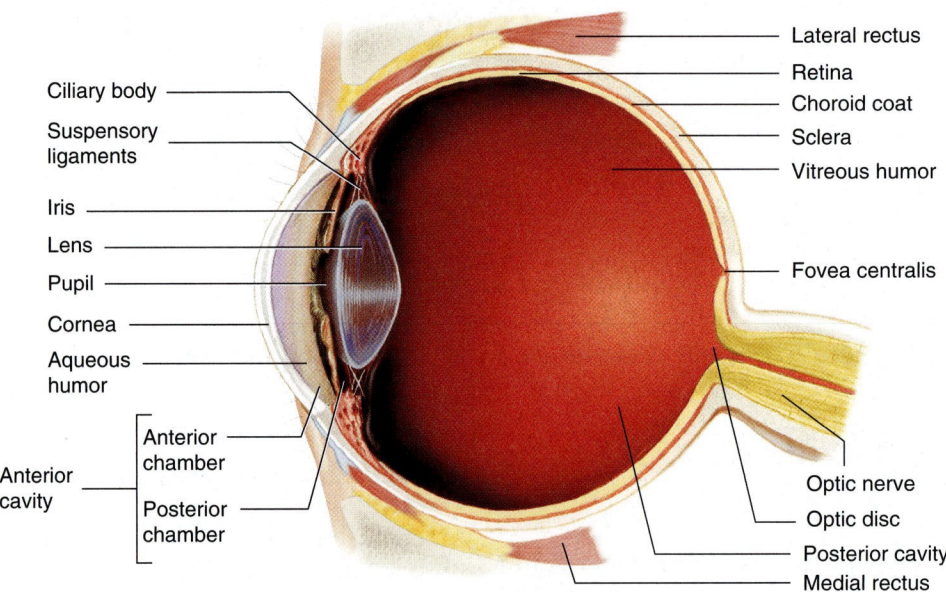

Figure 7-19 The optic nerve connects the eye directly to the brain.

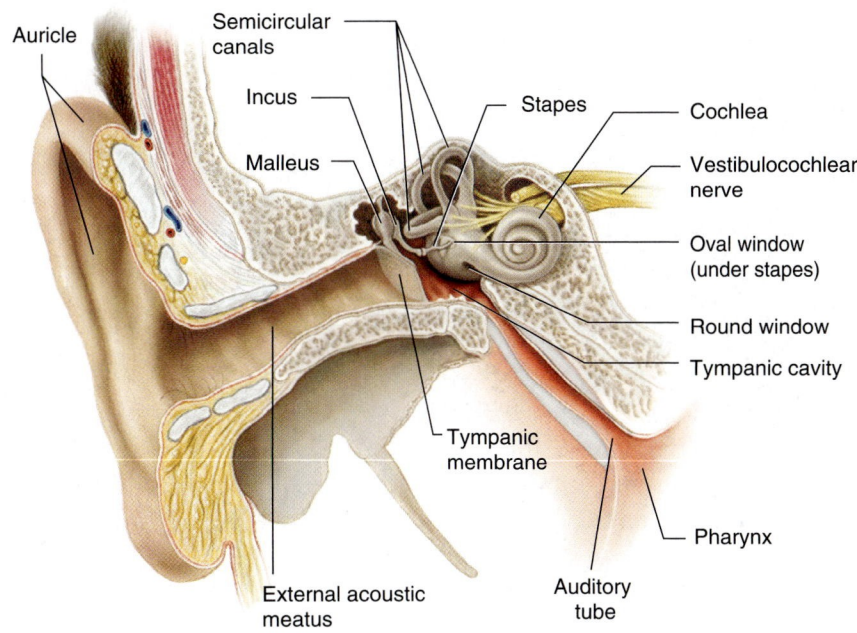

Figure 7-20   Anatomy of the ear and hearing apparatus.

The **oropharynx** is the space bounded by the palate to just above the tip of the epiglottis below, where the hypopharynx begins. This area includes the teeth, the tongue, and posterior pharynx.

The **gastrointestinal system** breaks down complex nutrients into a form that the body can use for energy. Digestion begins in the oral cavity where the tongue, lips, cheeks, and gums contain food, so that the teeth

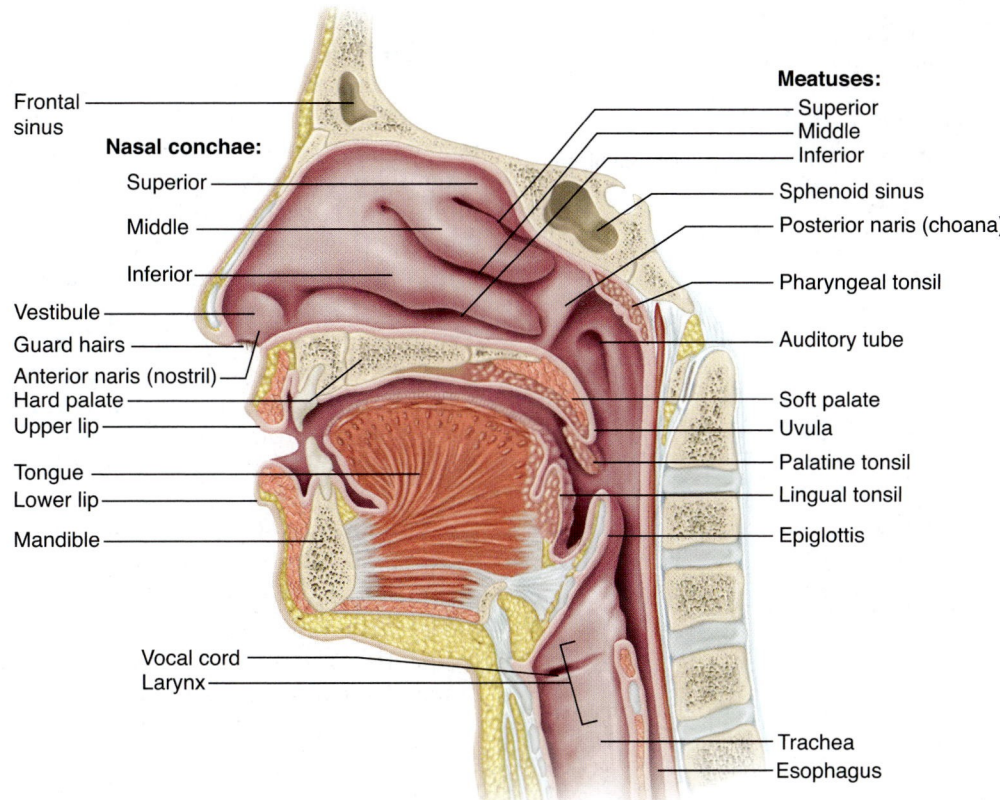

Figure 7-21   The upper airway. The vocal cords, found within the glottic opening in the thyroid cartilage, separate the upper airway from the lower one.

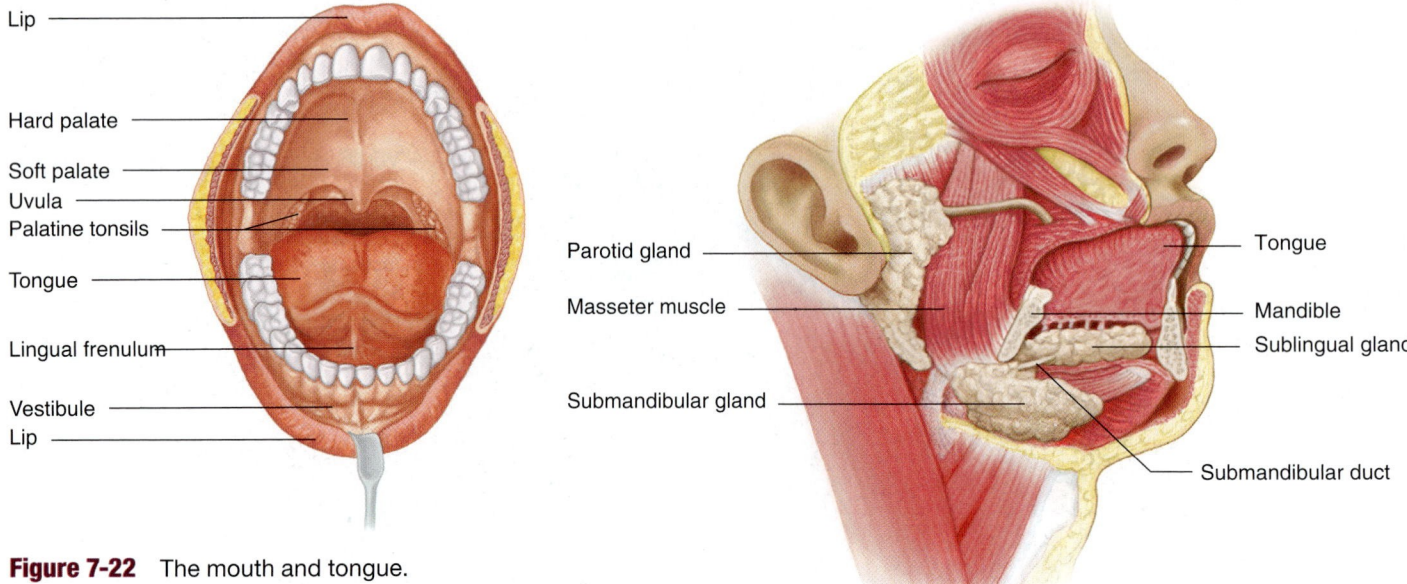

Lip

Hard palate

Soft palate
Uvula
Palatine tonsils

Tongue

Lingual frenulum

Vestibule
Lip

Parotid gland

Masseter muscle

Submandibular gland

Tongue

Mandible
Sublingual gland

Submandibular duct

Figure 7-22   The mouth and tongue.

Figure 7-23   Enzyme secretions from the salivary glands lubricate and digest food.

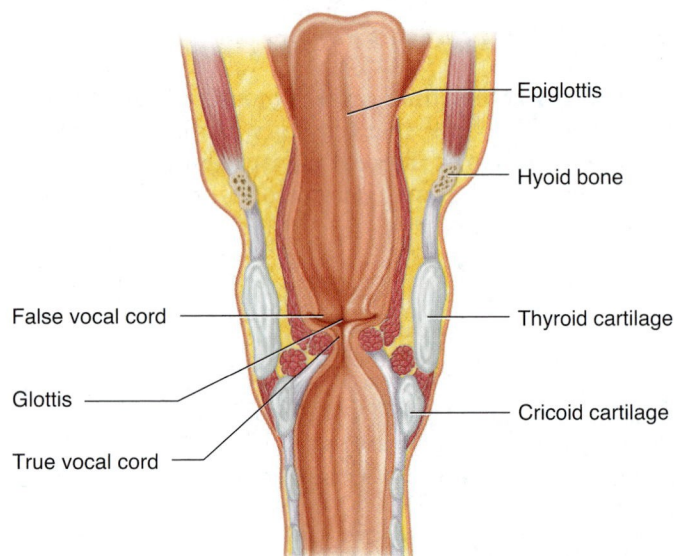

Epiglottis

Hyoid bone

False vocal cord

Thyroid cartilage

Glottis

Cricoid cartilage

True vocal cord

(a) View from behind

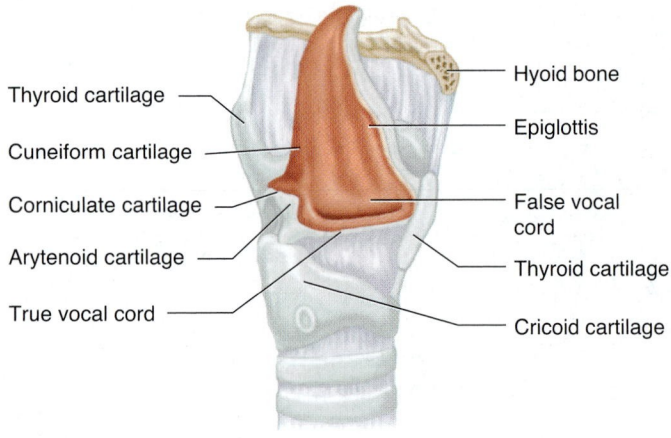

Thyroid cartilage

Cuneiform cartilage

Corniculate cartilage

Arytenoid cartilage

True vocal cord

Hyoid bone

Epiglottis

False vocal
cord

Thyroid cartilage

Cricoid cartilage

(b) Lateral view

Figure 7-24   Structures of the larynx and glottic opening.

can chew it into smaller sized pieces that can be swallowed. The tongue is mainly muscular and aids in speech, taste, chewing, and swallowing (Figure 7-22). Three types of **salivary glands** (parotid, submandibular, and sublingual) lubricate the food and release digestive secretions into the oral cavity (Figure 7-23).

The **hypopharynx** is just inferior to the oropharynx. It is home to the **epiglottis,** which serves to protect the airway from aspirated food during swallowing. The **laryngopharynx** is the lowest part of the upper airway. It contains the **larynx,** the **vocal cords,** the **arytenoid folds,** and the **trachea** (Figure 7-24). **Glottis** is a term for the space between the arytenoid folds and vocal cords. The vocal cords serve as the dividing point between the upper and lower airway (Figure 7-25). The **esophagus** lies just posterior to the larynx and trachea. Cartilaginous structures, including the **thyroid cartilage,** the **cricoid cartilage,** and the **arytenoid cartilage,** protect the esophagus from injury. The **hyoid bone** also protects the esophagus (Figure 7-26). From this point, air passes through the trachea into the lower airway.

The **thyroid gland** is another endocrine organ lying in the anterior neck, with most of its structure located just inferior to the larynx. The gland is divided into two lobes, with a narrow band of tissue called the **isthmus** connecting them (Figure 7-27). The thyroid gland secretes **thyroxine** and **triiodothyronine,** and these secretions regulate the body's metabolism. The **parathyroid glands** are four small endocrine glands posterior to the thyroid gland (Figure 7-28). They regulate the level of calcium in the body. Paramedics must be careful not to damage the thyroid and parathyroid glands when performing procedures such as cricothyrotomy.

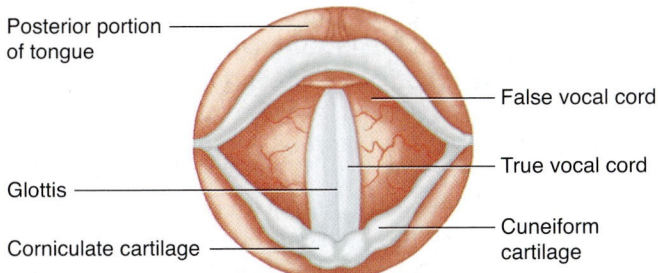

Posterior portion of tongue

False vocal cord

True vocal cord

Glottis

Cuneiform cartilage

Corniculate cartilage

(a) Vocal cords in closed position

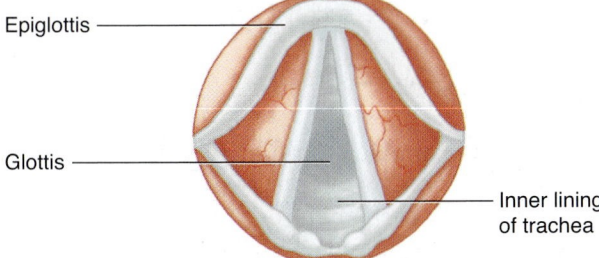

Epiglottis

Glottis

Inner lining of trachea

(b) Vocal cords in open position

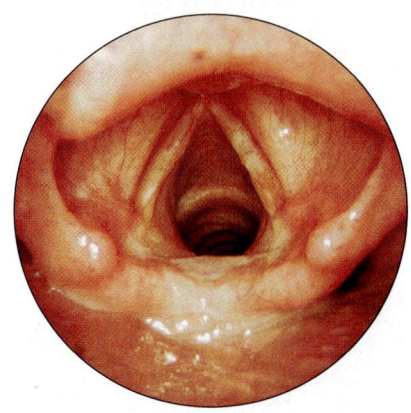

(c) Vocal cords open

Figure 7-25 The vocal cords divide the upper and lower airway.

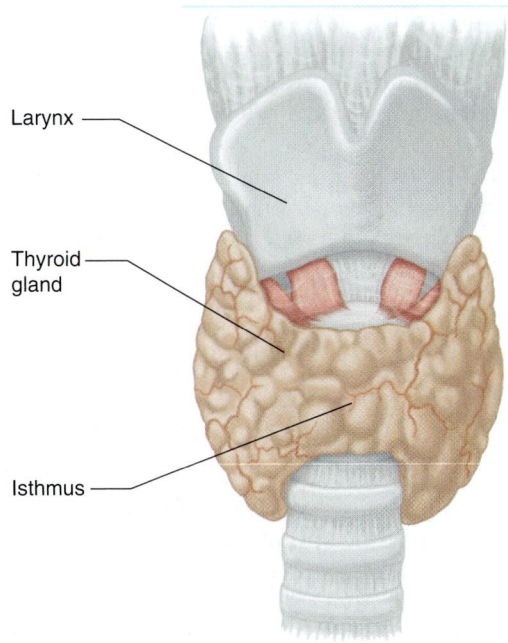

Larynx

Thyroid gland

Isthmus

Figure 7-27 The thyroid gland lies anterior to the thyroid cartilage. It has a rich blood supply and bleeds freely when injured.

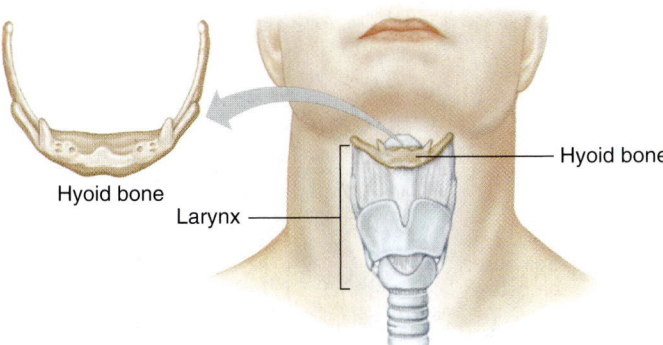

Hyoid bone

Hyoid bone

Larynx

Figure 7-26 The hyoid bone, which is found at the top of the thyroid cartilage, is the only bone in the body that does not articulate (attach) directly to another bone. It is easily broken with direct trauma.

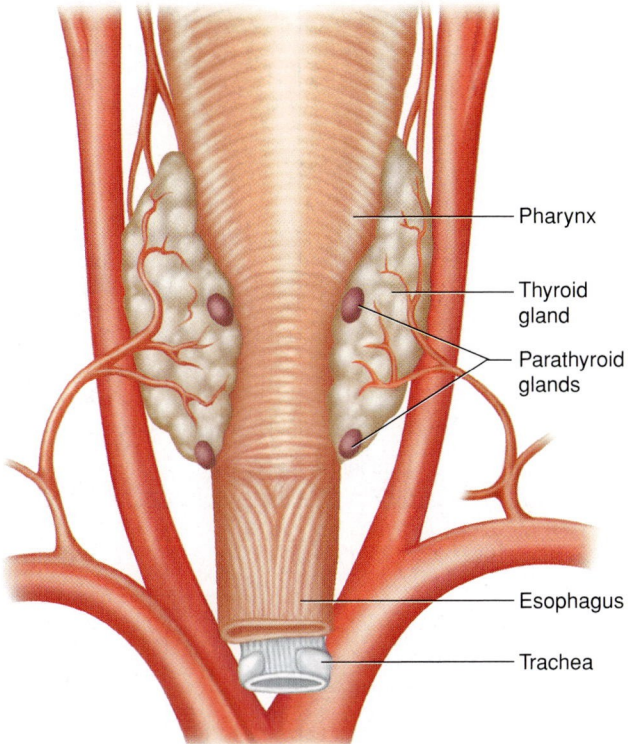

Pharynx

Thyroid gland

Parathyroid glands

Esophagus

Trachea

Posterior view

Figure 7-28 The parathyroid glands are found on the posterior surface of the thyroid.

Muscles in the back of the neck provide for extension of the head and neck and help to maintain posture. Other muscles, including the **trapezius** and **sternocleidomastoid muscles,** help to turn the head from side to side.

CONNECTIONS More on the head, face and neck can be found in Chapter 12: Airway Management, Ventilation, and Oxygenation; Chapter 20: Head, Face, and Neck Trauma; and Chapter 30: Neurology.

Anatomy of the Back and Spinal Cord

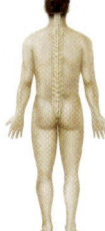

Vertebrae

Thirty-three **vertebral bones** surround and protect the **spinal cord** (Figure 7-29). This includes seven cervical, twelve thoracic, five lumbar, five sacral, and four coccygeal vertebrae, which are usually fused together. At approximately the level of the second lumbar vertebra, the spinal cord as a single entity splits into many nerve rootlets. Because of its resemblance to a horse's tail, it is named the **cauda equina.** All along the length of the spinal cord, at each vertebral level, the 31 pairs of spinal nerve roots exit by way of the **intervertebral foramina** to innervate the various organs and structures of the body (Figure 7-30).

Several landmarks can help you identify vertebral levels. The spine and the inferior edge of the scapula are at the level of the third and the seventh thoracic vertebrae, respectively. The **iliac crest** is at the level of the fourth lumbar vertebra, and the posterior superior iliac spine is at the level of the second sacral vertebra.

Nerves

Spinal reflexes are in place to rapidly protect the body from harm. If a peripheral nerve senses pain, such as touching something sharp, inward-going **afferent nerves** transmit a signal to the spinal cord. Through a reflex arc, the signal to draw away from the threat is returned by outward-going **efferent nerves** toward the appropriate muscles (Figure 7-31).

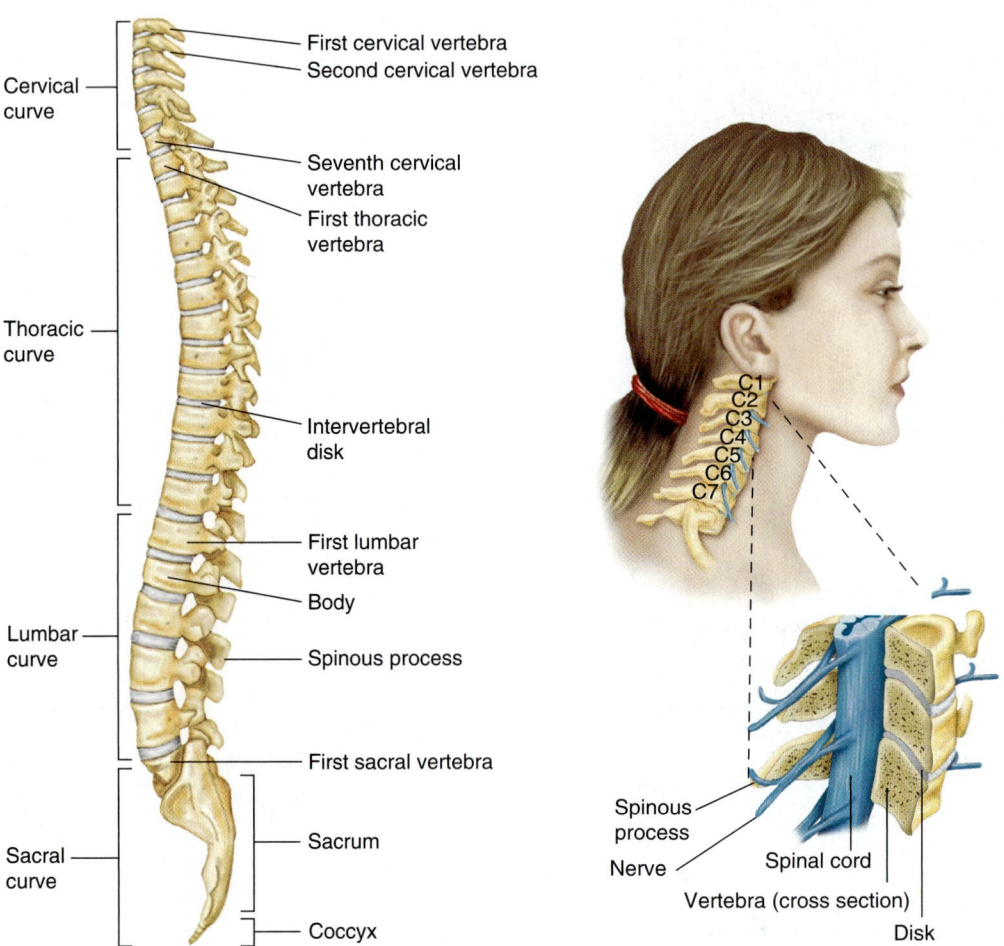

Figure 7-29 The spinal cord passes through the vertebra, and nerves branch off the cord, passing between the spinous processes of the vertebra.

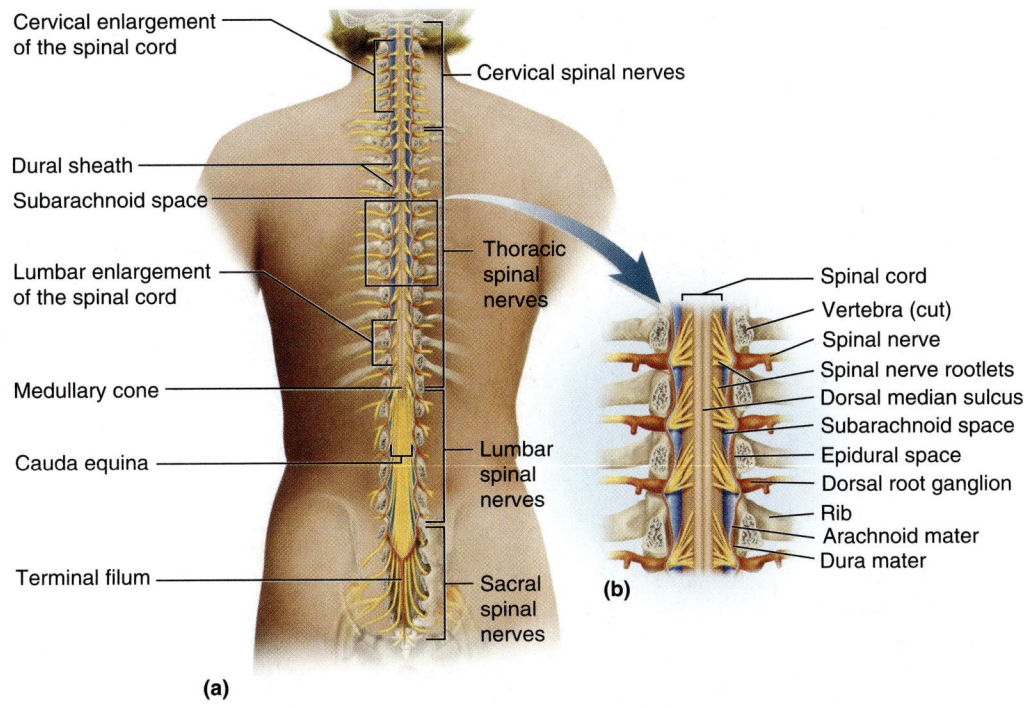

Figure 7-30   Spinal nerves branch off of the spinal cord.

Back Muscles

Muscles in the back provide for extension and help to maintain posture. Superficial muscles of the back articulate with (articulate means to attach directly to or come together to form a joint) and allow for movement of the upper limbs. These include the **trapezius**, the **latissimus dorsi**, the **levator scapulae**, the **rhomboideus major**, the **rhomboideus minor**, and the **serratus anterior** (Figure 7-32). The **semispinalis capitis** and **cervicis** pull the head back posteriorly. The erector spinae muscles maintain erect posture and extend from the sacrum and iliac crest to the back of the head.

CONNECTIONS   More on the spine can be found in Chapter 23: Spinal Trauma.

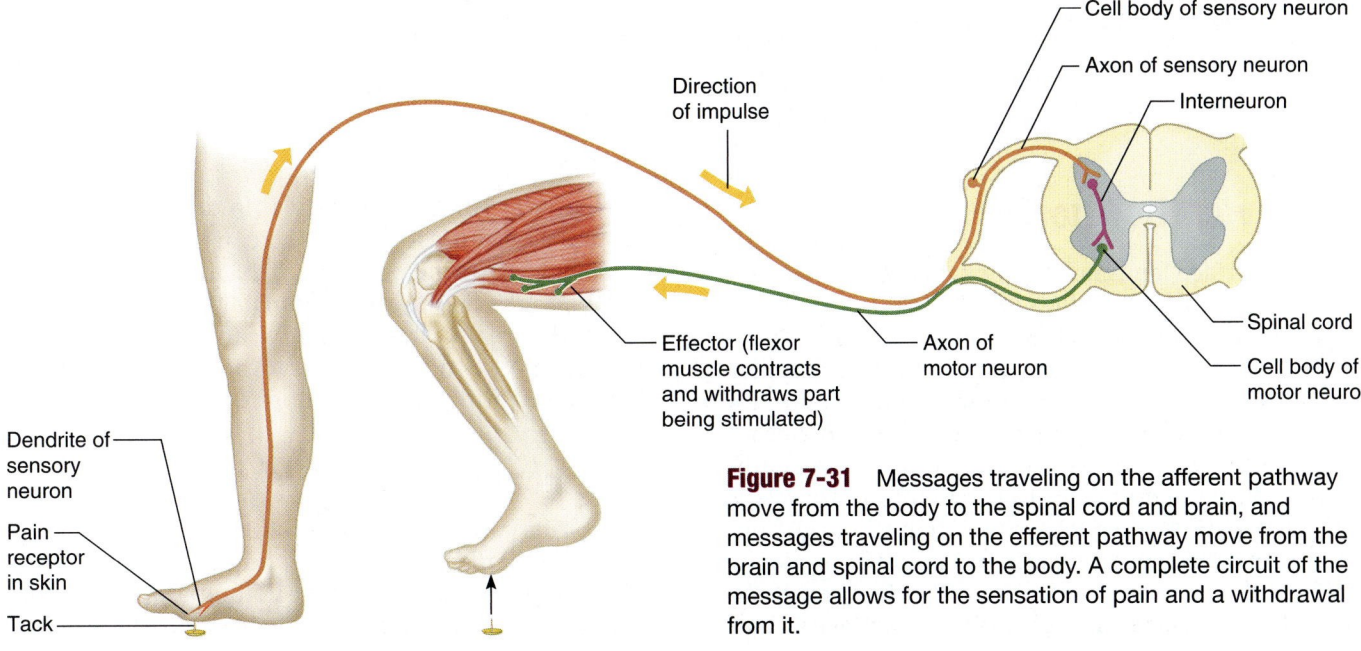

Figure 7-31   Messages traveling on the afferent pathway move from the body to the spinal cord and brain, and messages traveling on the efferent pathway move from the brain and spinal cord to the body. A complete circuit of the message allows for the sensation of pain and a withdrawal from it.

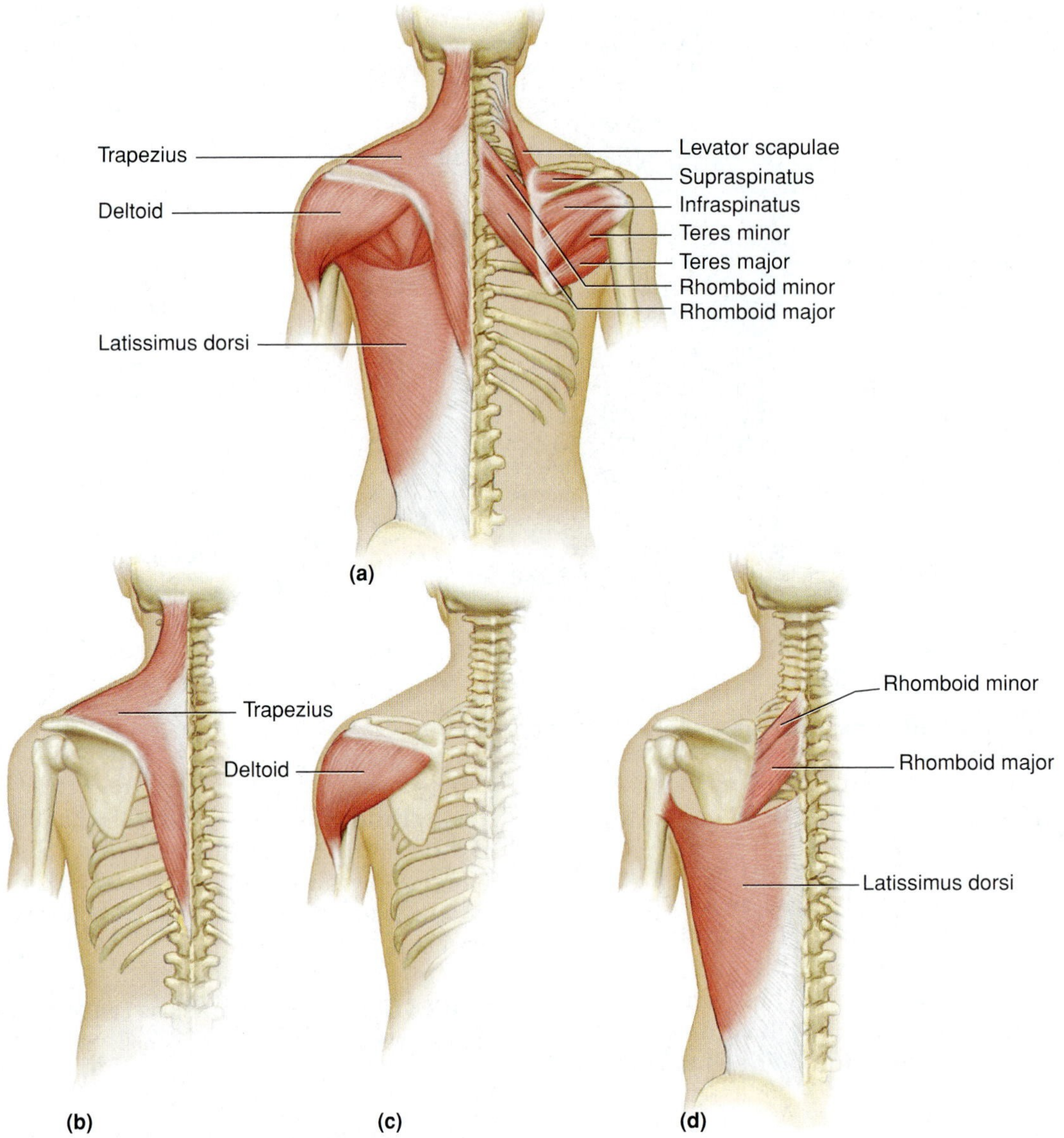

Trapezius

Deltoid

Latissimus dorsi

Levator scapulae
Supraspinatus
Infraspinatus
Teres minor
Teres major
Rhomboid minor
Rhomboid major

(a)

Trapezius

Deltoid

Rhomboid minor

Rhomboid major

Latissimus dorsi

(b)   **(c)**   **(d)**

Figure 7-32   Muscles of the back.

Anatomy of the Thorax

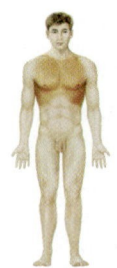

Surface landmarks delineate useful divisions of the **thorax** (Figure 7-33). The mid-axillary line is a vertical line drawn from the middle of the axilla downward. The mid-clavicular line is a vertical line drawn from the middle of the clavicle downward. The mid-sternal line is a vertical line drawn from the center of the manubrium to the xiphoid process. It separates the right chest (hemithorax) from the left chest. The costal margin is the lower border of the ribs and their cartilages. The costochondral junction is between the ribs and their cartilages. The mid-scapular line is a vertical line drawn through the scapula. The suprasternal notch can be palpated at the upper border of the sternum. The nipple in the male usually marks the fourth intercostal space. All of these landmarks are important to know, and they are valuable reference points when you perform an assessment and physical examination on a patient.

The Ribcage

Twelve ribs can be found and palpated on the body (see Figure 7-34 and Plate A at the end of the chapter). Posteriorly, they articulate with the vertebrae and anteriorly, with the costal cartilages. The costal cartilages of ribs

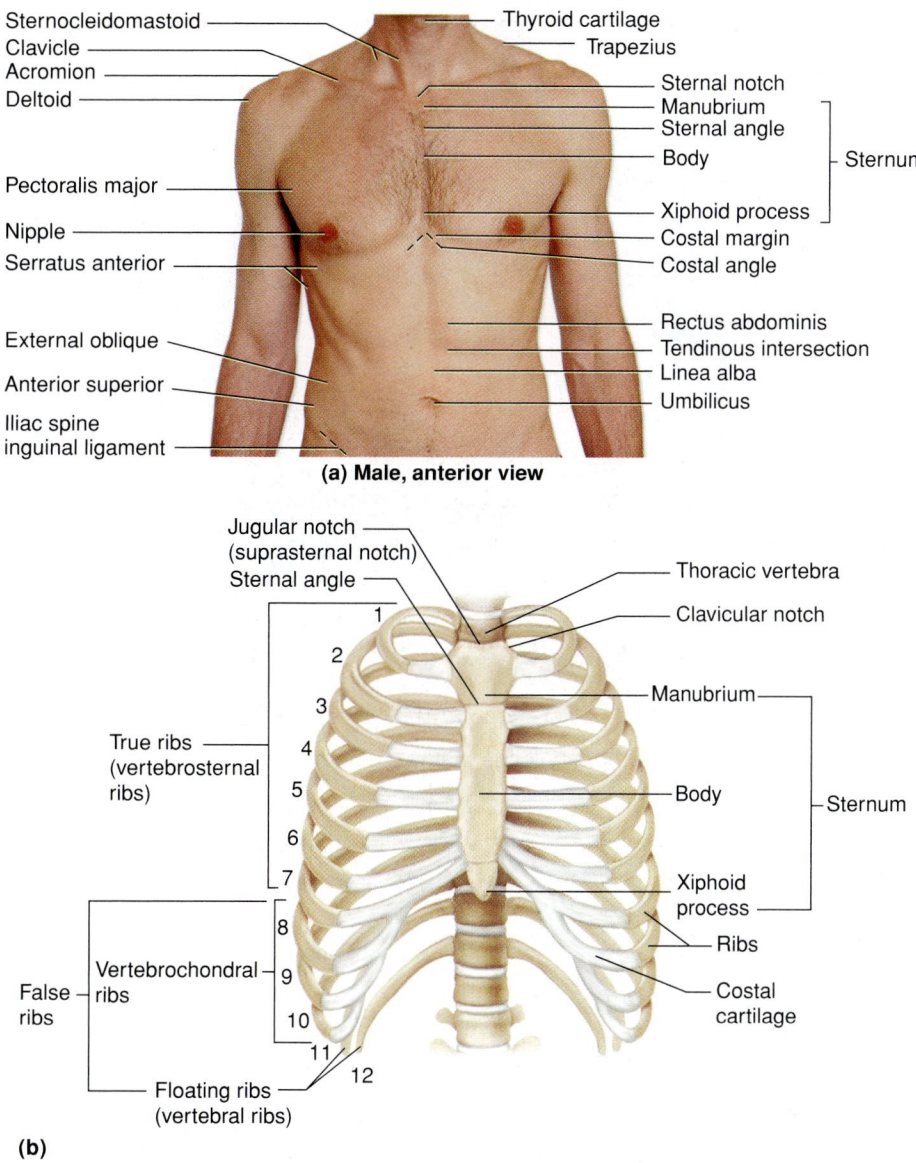

(a) Male, anterior view

(b)

Figure 7-33   Surface landmarks on the thorax help identify anatomic structures.

one through seven articulate with the sternum. The cartilages of ribs eight through ten share a common structure, and together they join into the seventh rib. The eleventh and twelfth ribs have cartilage anteriorly but are free-floating without any attachment to the sternum. An intercostal bundle made up of a nerve, artery and vein is found running along the underside of each rib (Figure 7-35). The ribs protect many vital organs including the heart, lungs, and some upper abdominal organs such as the liver, spleen, and kidneys. Movement of the ribs and diaphragm is important for respiration. The phrenic nerve innervates the diaphragm and, therefore, is involved with respiration. It passes through the thorax on its way to the diaphragm (Figure 7-36).

The Heart

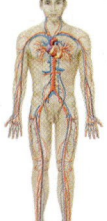

The heart is located in the center of the chest and slightly to the left of the center (midline) (see Figure 7-37 and Plate B at the end of the chapter). The heart is surrounded by a protective sac called the **pericardium** which is divided into two layers. There is a small amount of pericardial fluid between these two layers, providing lubrication when the heart contracts. There are three layers of heart muscle: the **epicardium,** the **myocardium** (forming the bulk of the heart muscle), and the **endocardium,** which is in contact with the blood (Figure 7-38).

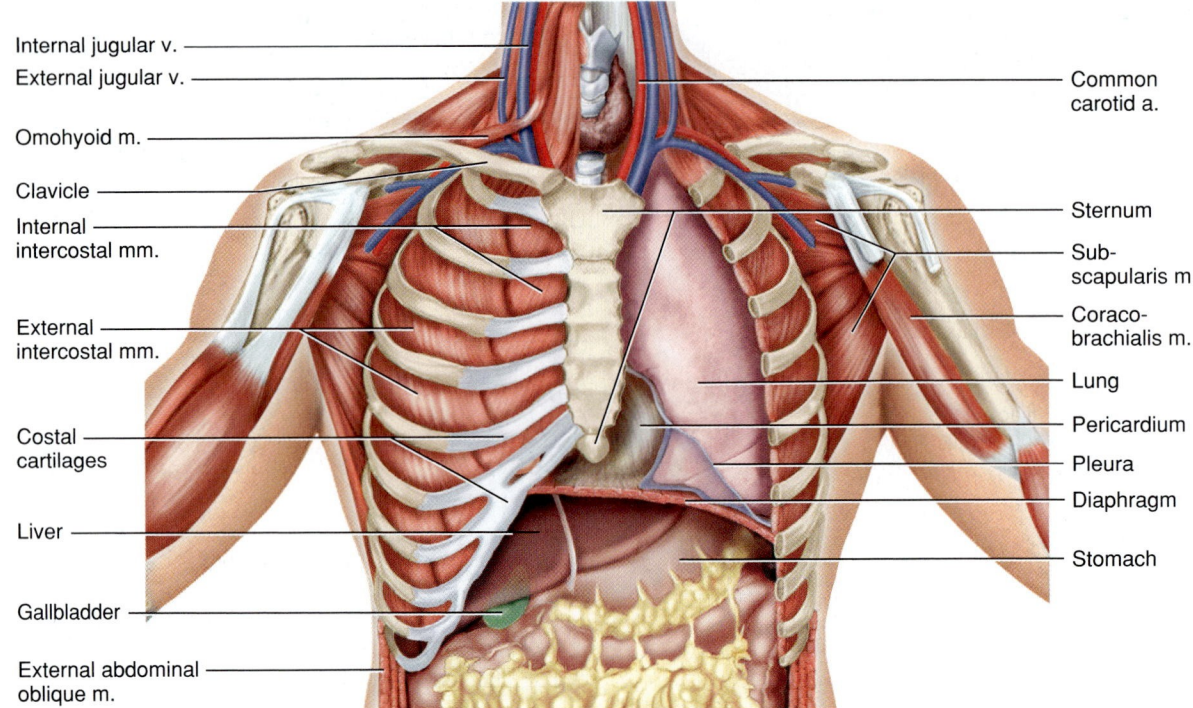

Internal jugular v.
External jugular v.
Omohyoid m.
Clavicle
Internal intercostal mm.
External intercostal mm.
Costal cartilages
Liver
Gallbladder
External abdominal oblique m.

Common carotid a.
Sternum
Sub-scapularis m.
Coraco-brachialis m.
Lung
Pericardium
Pleura
Diaphragm
Stomach

Figure 7-34   Twelve pairs of ribs make up the thoracic cage that protects the heart, lungs, and great vessels.

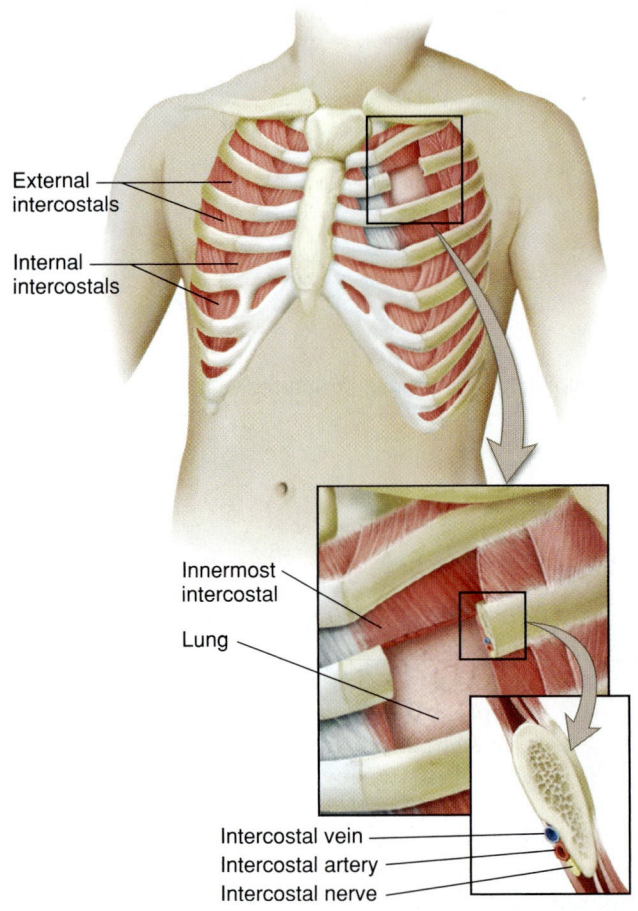

External intercostals
Internal intercostals
Innermost intercostal
Lung
Intercostal vein
Intercostal artery
Intercostal nerve

Figure 7-35   Nerves, arteries, and veins line the posterior surface of each rib.

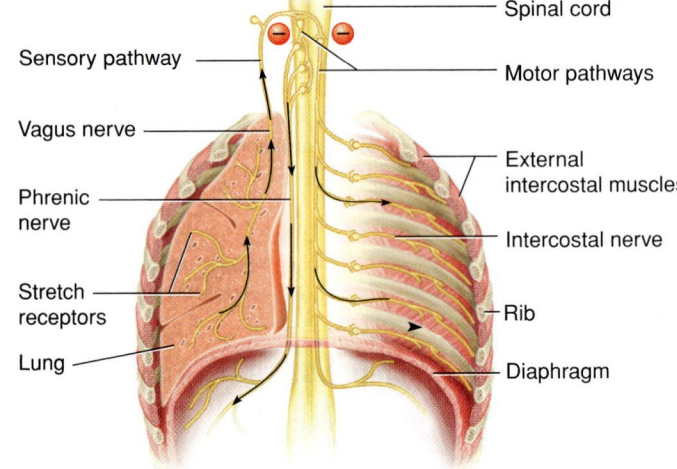

Spinal cord
Sensory pathway
Motor pathways
Vagus nerve
Phrenic nerve
External intercostal muscles
Intercostal nerve
Stretch receptors
Rib
Lung
Diaphragm

Figure 7-36   The phrenic nerve leaves the spinal cord from near the fourth cervical vertebra and travels to innervate the diaphragm and other structures.

The heart has four chambers. Two of these are called **atria** and are superior to the remaining two chambers, which are called **ventricles** (Figure 7-39). There are four valves in the heart, two lying between the atria and ventricles on both sides of the heart and two lying between the ventricles and the major vessels on both sides of the heart. The atrioventricular valve leaflets are attached to the ventricular papillary muscles by way of specialized fibers called the **chordae tendinae** (Figure 7-40). These fibers prevent the leaflets from prolapsing into the atria when the ventricles contract.

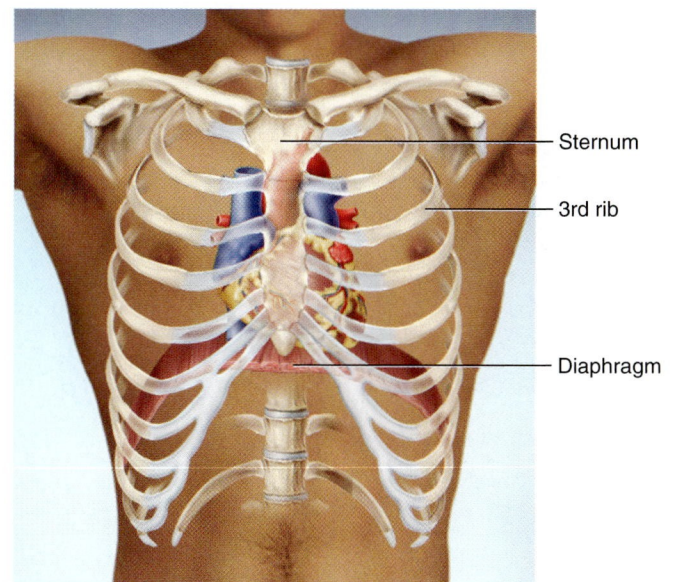

Figure 7-37   The heart is located slightly left of the midline in the chest.

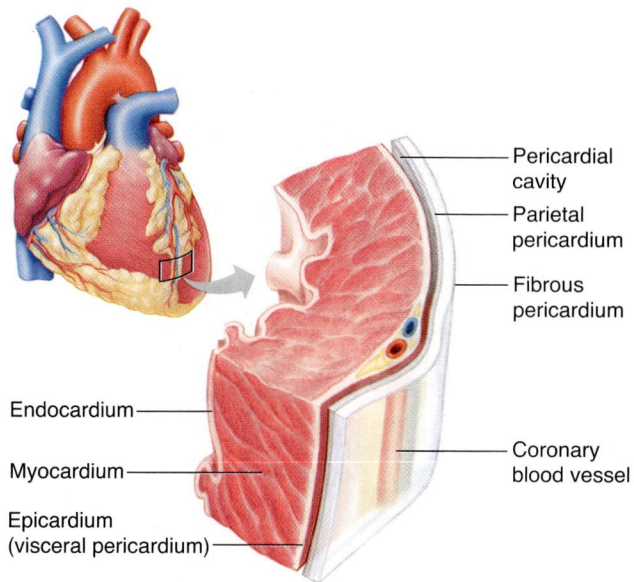

Figure 7-38   The layers of the heart and pericardium.

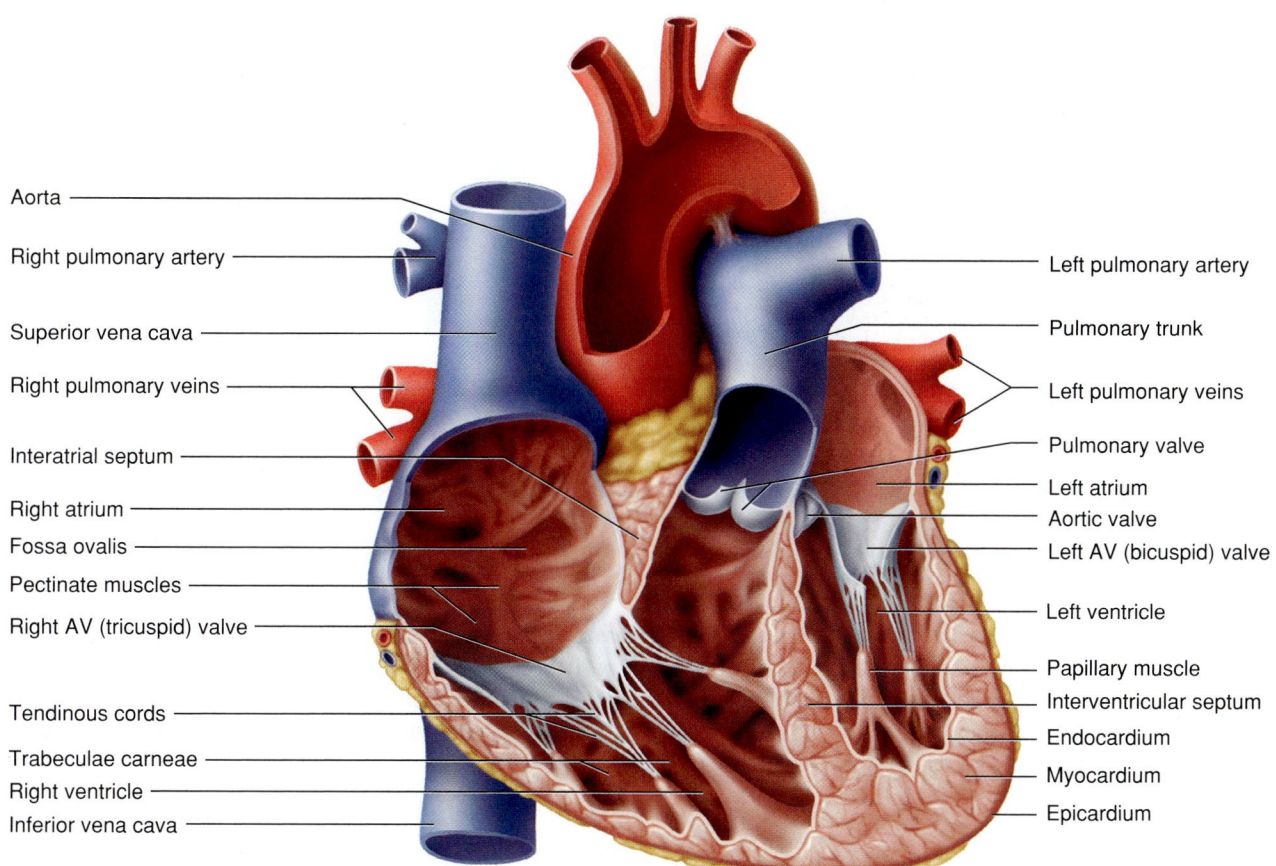

Figure 7-39   A view of the interior of the heart showing both atria, both ventricles, and the location of the four valves.

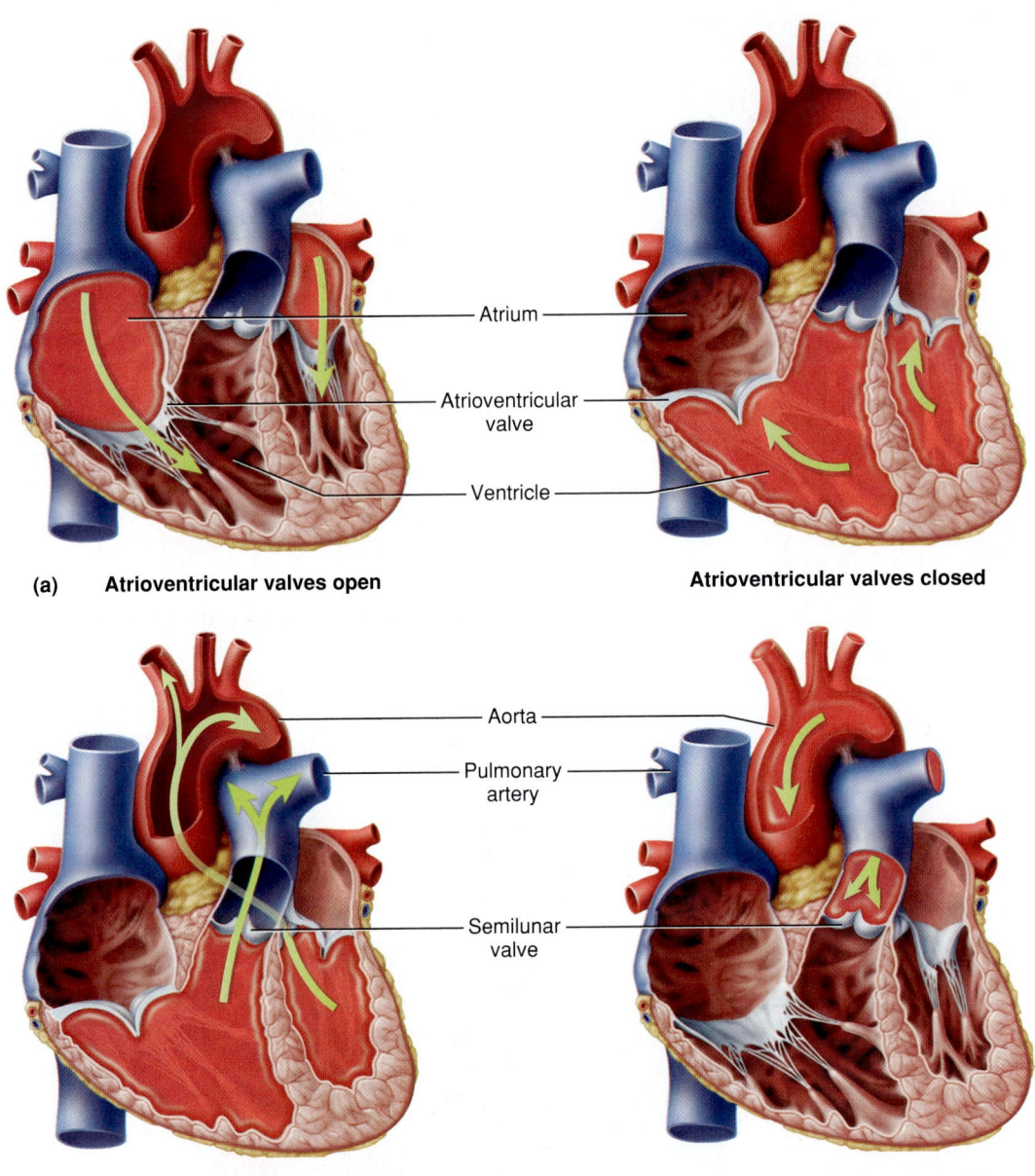

Atrium

Atrioventricular valve

Ventricle

(a) **Atrioventricular valves open**

Atrioventricular valves closed

Aorta

Pulmonary artery

Semilunar valve

(b) **Semilunar valves open**

Semilunar valves closed

Figure 7-40 **Operation of the Heart Valves.** (a) The atrioventricular valves. When atrial pressure is greater than ventricular pressure, the valve opens and blood flows through (green arrows). When ventricular pressure rises above atrial pressure, the blood in the ventricle pushes the valve cusps closed. (b) The semilunar valves. When the pressure in the ventricle is greater than the pressure in the artery, the valve is forced open and blood is ejected. When ventricular pressure is lower than arterial pressure, arterial blood holds the valve closed.

The heart sounds heard with a stethoscope result from the opening and closing of the valves. The valves serve to prevent the backward flow of blood as the chambers of the heart contract.

Following the blood on its passage through the heart illustrates the function of the various chambers, valves, and vessels. Deoxygenated blood from the peripheral and coronary veins enters the right atrium by way of the **superior vena cava** and the **inferior vena cava.** Blood then passes into the right ventricle via the right atrioventricular valve, which is named the **tricuspid**

valve because of its three leaflets. The blood from the right ventricle passes into the **pulmonary arteries** by way of the **pulmonic valve.** These are the only arteries that carry deoxygenated blood (Figure 7-41).

The Great Vessels

The blood is oxygenated by the lungs and returns to the heart by way of the pulmonary veins, passing into the left atrium. These are the only veins in the body that carry oxygenated blood. Blood from the left atrium

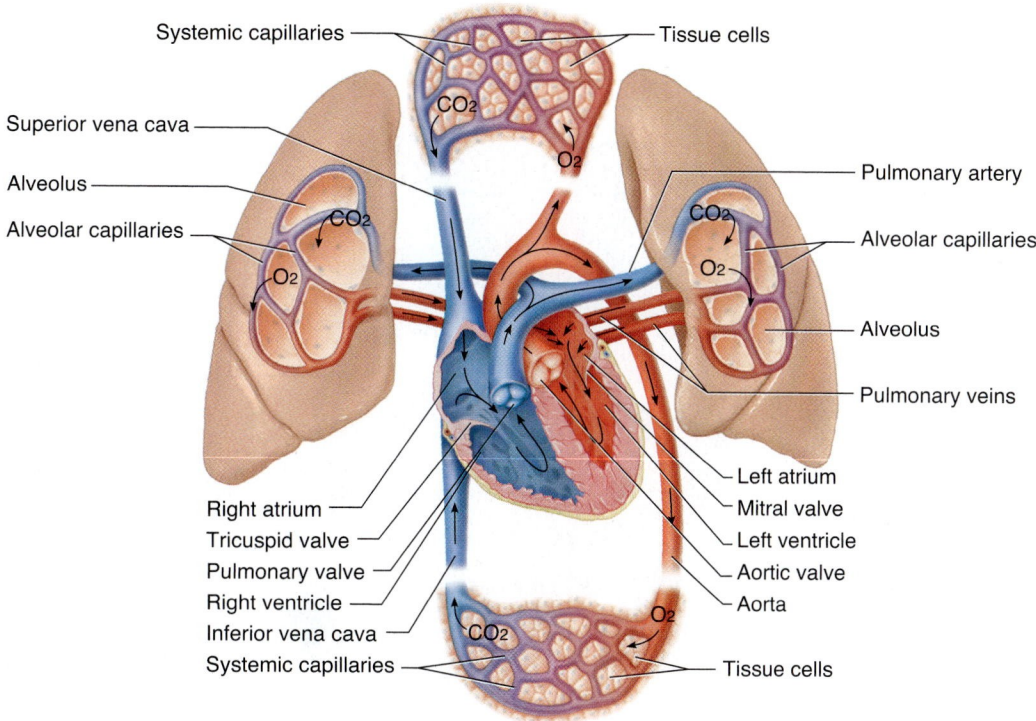

Figure 7-41 Blood moving through the heart and lungs.

passes into the left ventricle by way of the left **atrioventricular bicuspid valve.** The bicuspid valve is called the **mitral valve** because of its resemblance to the bishop's hat, which is called a miter. Blood then is pumped by the left ventricle, through the **aortic valve,** and into the **aorta** for distribution throughout the body.

Blood vessels are made up of three layers surrounding a **lumen,** which is the opening of the vessels. The **tunica intima** is the innermost layer; it is smooth and allows the free flow of blood. **Tunica media** is the middle muscular layer; it controls the size of the lumen. The **tunica adventitia** is the outermost fibrous layer; it defines the maximum lumen size when the muscles relax (Figure 7-42).

The coronary arteries branch off of the aorta just beyond the aortic valve (Figure 7-43). The heart receives its perfusion (oxygen supply) during the relaxation phase (diastole) of the cardiac cycle, when the ventricles are relaxing following the contraction needed for emptying. The left coronary artery divides into two branches, the left anterior descending artery and the circumflex artery. The right coronary artery divides into the posterior descending artery and the marginal artery. Coronary veins remove the deoxygenated blood and converge to form the coronary sinus, which in turn empties into the right atrium.

The cardiac musculature is specially modified so that the heart is able to contract spontaneously without an external stimulus. This property, called **automaticity,**

then permits the heart to generate its own electrical impulse. The **sinoatrial node (SAN)** normally sets the heart rate and functions as a pacemaker. The conduction wave travels next to the **atrioventricular node (AVN)** located in the inferior portion of the interatrial septum. From the AVN, the impulse travels through the bundle of His and down the interventricular septum and divides into the right and left bundle branches which distribute the impulse to the rest of the heart muscle (Figure 7-44).

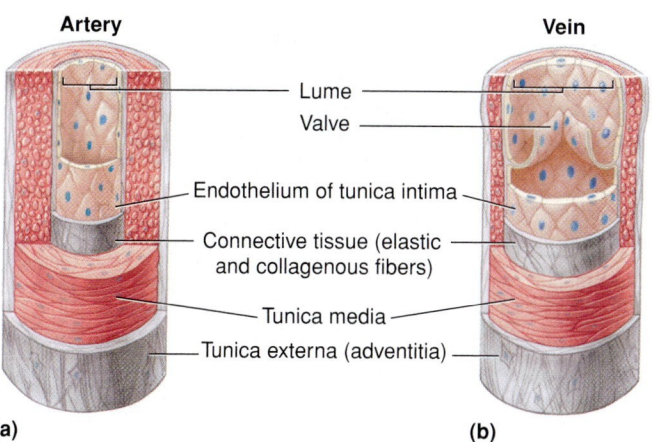

Figure 7-42 The tunica, or layers, that make up the blood vessels.

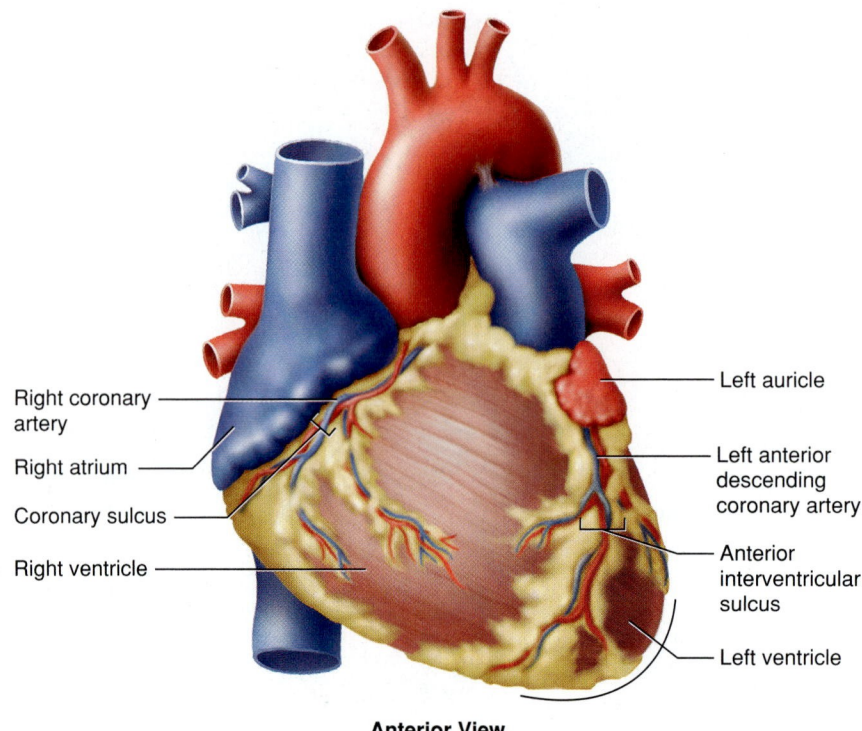

Anterior View

Figure 7-43   The coronary arteries provide oxygenated blood to the muscle cells of the heart.

The heart rate is further regulated by the **autonomic nervous system (ANS),** which is made up of the sympathetic and the parasympathetic nervous system divisions. The **sympathetic system** prepares the body for stressful situations (fight or flight), and the **parasympathetic nervous system** controls vegetative functions (feed and breed). These two systems have opposing functions, but under normal conditions, they balance each other out.

CONNECTIONS More on the chest can be found in Chapter 21: Thoracic Trauma. More on the heart can be found in Chapter 29: Cardiology.

Airways and Lungs

The respiratory system provides oxygen to the body, while removing carbon dioxide and other waste products. The upper airway was discussed previously in this chapter. The lower airway begins with the C-shaped rings of cartilage that form and support the trachea and keep it from collapsing (see Plate C at the end of the chapter). Cilia and mucous-producing cells are found within specialized respiratory epithelium. **Cilia** are hair-like structures that move particulate matter out of the trachea and into the mouth where it can be removed by swallowing or coughing. The trachea divides at the carina into the right and left mainstem **bronchi,** which then divide into secondary bronchi (Figure 7-45). Further subdivisions form **respiratory bronchioles, alveolar ducts,** and **alveolar sacs.** Oxygen and carbon dioxide are exchanged within the alveoli (Figures 7-46 and 7-47). The alveoli remain

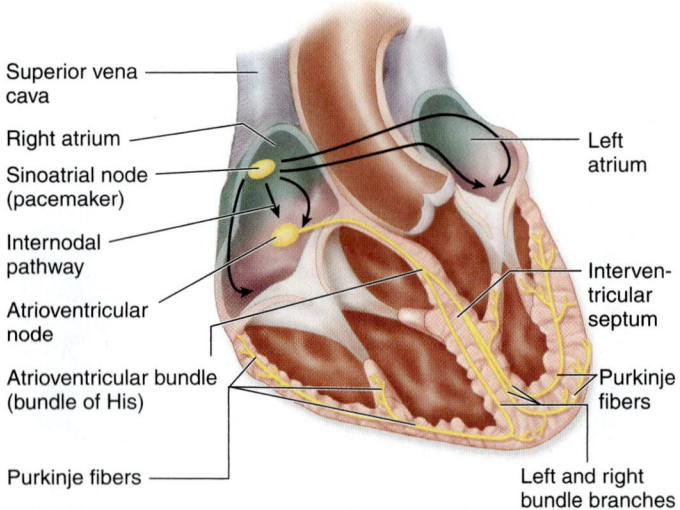

Figure 7-44   The electrical conduction of the heart.

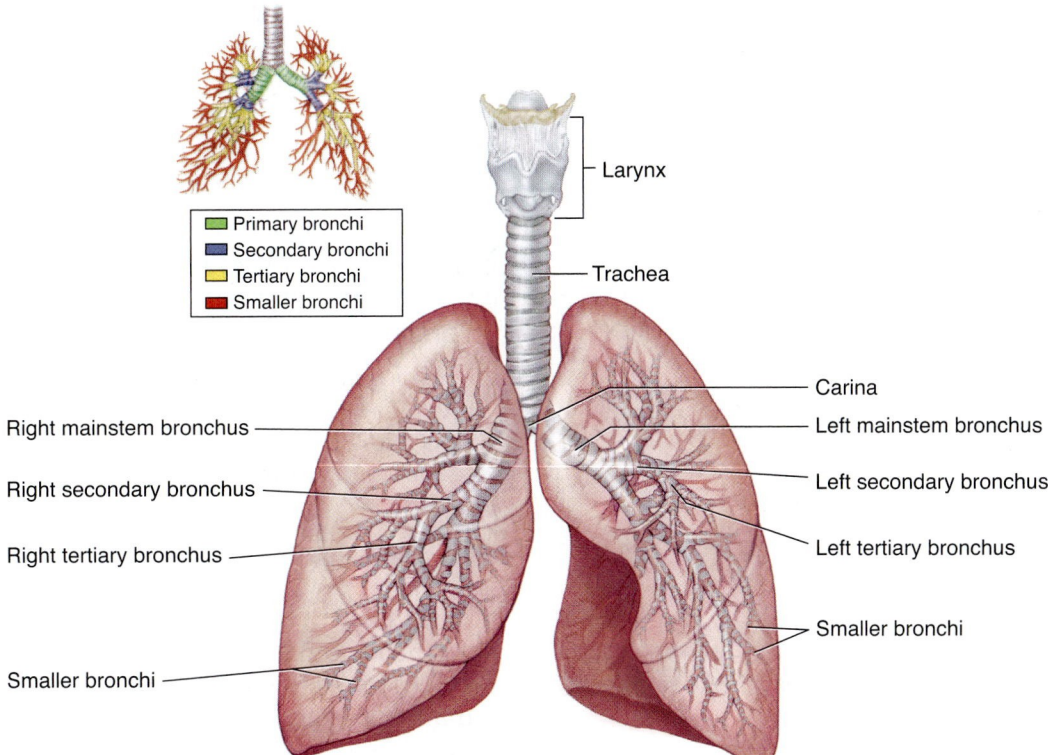

Figure 7-45   Anatomy of the respiratory tract. The carina is the point where the trachea bifurcates (splits into two) and the left and right mainstem bronchi begin.

open because of a substance called surfactant that decreases the surface tension of the alveoli.

The **parenchyma** of the lung is made up of primary pulmonary lobules. The right lung has three lobes that are called the upper, middle, and lower lobes. The left lung has only two lobes, which are the upper and lower lobes (see Figure 7-48 and Plate B at the end of the chapter). Connective tissues called **pleura** cover the lungs. The visceral pleura covers the lungs and is insensate. The parietal pleura lines the thoracic cavity and contains nerve fibers. Normally, the visceral pleura and parietal pleura closely adhere to one another. However, air, fluid, or blood can get between the two pleura and separate them, especially after

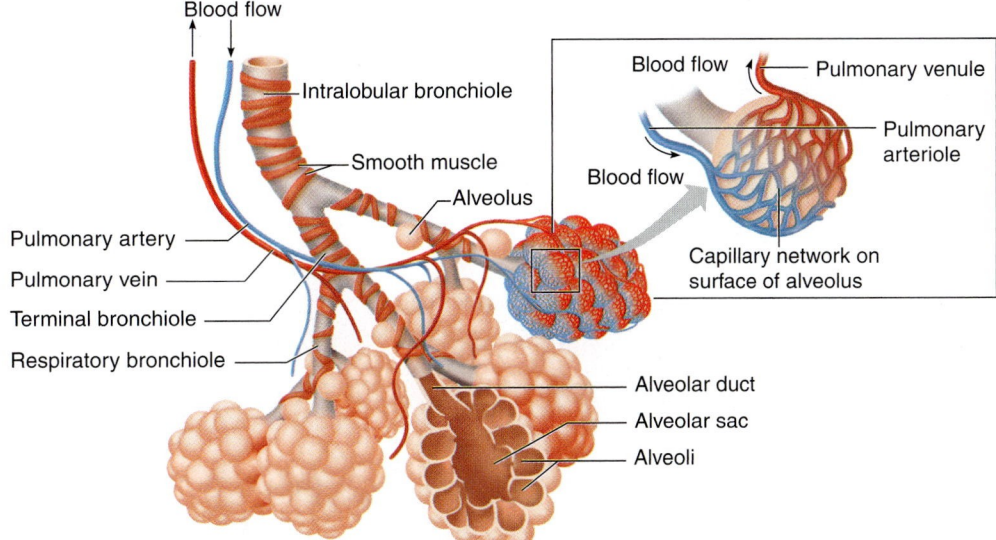

Figure 7-46   The alveoli and terminal bronchioles located proximal to the alveoli are the site of gas exchange within the capillary beds of the lungs.

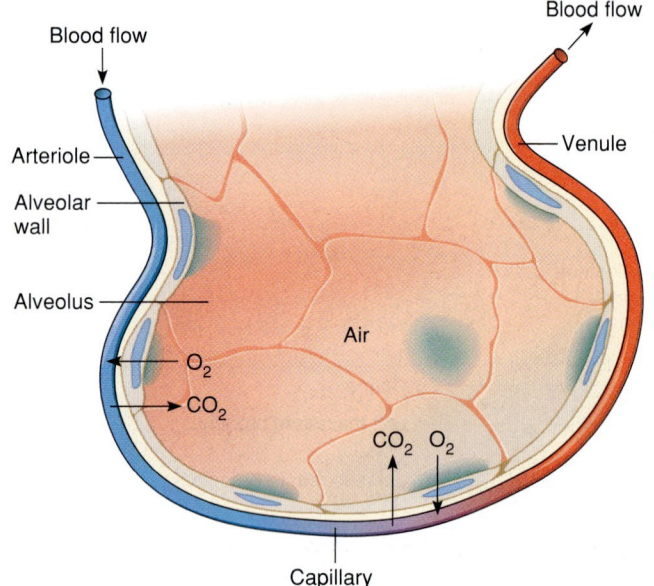

Figure 7-47   Oxygen and carbon dioxide freely diffuse between the alveoli and the hemoglobin of the red blood cell. The alveoli and blood cells are brought into close contact because of the capillary network that covers over the outer surface of the alveoli.

traumatic injury to the chest. This potential space is called the pleural space and normally contains a small amount of pleural fluid that lubricates the lung during the movement associated with breathing (Figure 7-49).

Nice to Know

Parenchyma

The parenchyma is the functional tissue that forms an organ. It is different from the supporting structures that hold an organ in place. In the case of the lung, it is the tissue where gas exchange takes place.

Blood supplies the lungs by two separate systems. First, as mentioned previously in this chapter, the pulmonary artery transports deoxygenated blood from the heart into the lungs for oxygenation. The oxygenated

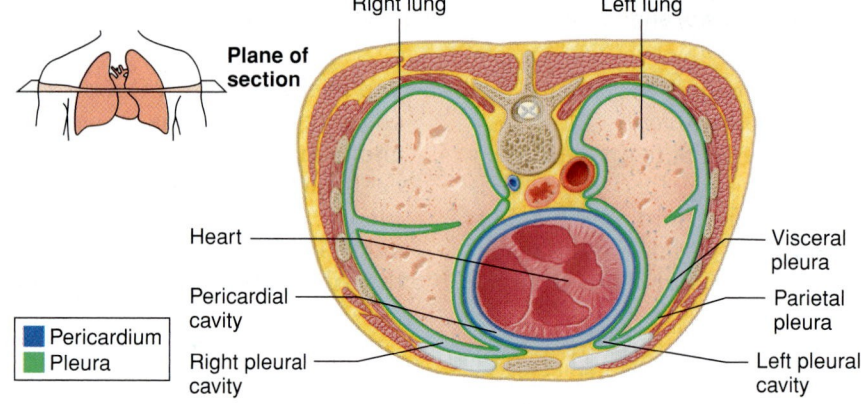

Figure 7-48   The potential spaces between the pleural membranes are shown here as actual spaces.

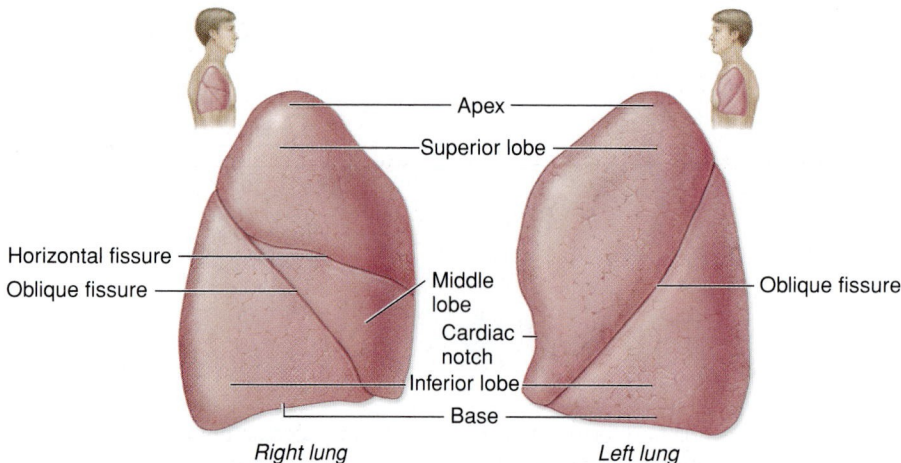

Figure 7-49   The left lung has two lobes while the right has three.

blood then passes back to the heart by way of the pulmonary veins for subsequent distribution to the rest of the body. Secondly, the lungs themselves receive blood from the bronchial arteries which are branches of the aorta. Blood is returned by veins called the **azygos** and **hemiazygos** into the superior vena cava and back to the heart.

In addition to the major organs of the pulmonary and circulatory systems, the thorax also contains the initial portion of the gastrointestinal tract, the esophagus, and the vagus nerve which helps to control the heart rate (Figure 7-50).

CONNECTIONS More on the lungs can be found in Chapter 28: Pulmonary. More on the airways can be found in Chapter 12: Airway Management, Ventilation, and Oxygenation.

The Abdomen

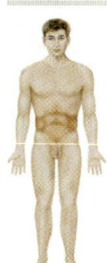

The abdomen is generally divided into four quadrants. A midsaggital line spanning from the xiphoid process to the symphysis pubis separates the right from the left. This line is halved by a horizontal line through the umbilicus to separate the upper from the lower quadrants. The lateral aspect of the abdomen is often called the flank. The point where the twelfth rib attaches to its corresponding vertebra can be found on the back and is called the **costovertebral angle (CVA).** The right upper quadrant (RUQ) contains the liver, gallbladder, head of the pancreas, part of the duodenum, right kidney, and part of the colon. The left upper quadrant (LUQ) contains the spleen, the tail of the pancreas, the stomach, the left kidney, and part of the colon. The right lower quadrant (RLQ) contains the appendix, the ascending colon, the small intestine, and, in the female, the right ovary and the right fallopian tube. The left lower quadrant (LLQ) contains the small intestine, descending colon, left ovary, and left fallopian tube (Figure 7-51).

Digestive Tract

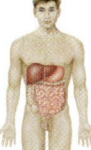

The **esophagus** transports food from the mouth to the stomach by way of voluntary and involuntary muscles during the process of swallowing. The **gastroesophageal junction** is the gateway to the stomach and may, at times, allow regurgitation of stomach acid into the esophagus. The **stomach** is located mostly in the left upper quadrant and continues digestion started by saliva by secreting hydrochloric acid, which further breaks down the food (see Plate B at the end of the chapter).

Partially digested food (called **chyme** once it is ejected from the stomach) next enters into the small intestine. **Peristalsis** is the rhythmic movement of the muscles of the digestive system that continues to propel the chyme through the intestinal tract for processing. The **duodenum** is the most proximal part of the small intestine, followed by the **jejunum,** and then the **ileum.** The common bile duct is a conduit for digestive secretions from the liver and pancreas, and the duct empties into the duodenum. The **liver** is located in the right upper quadrant of the abdomen and secretes bile to emulsify and break down fats. It also detoxifies many substances.

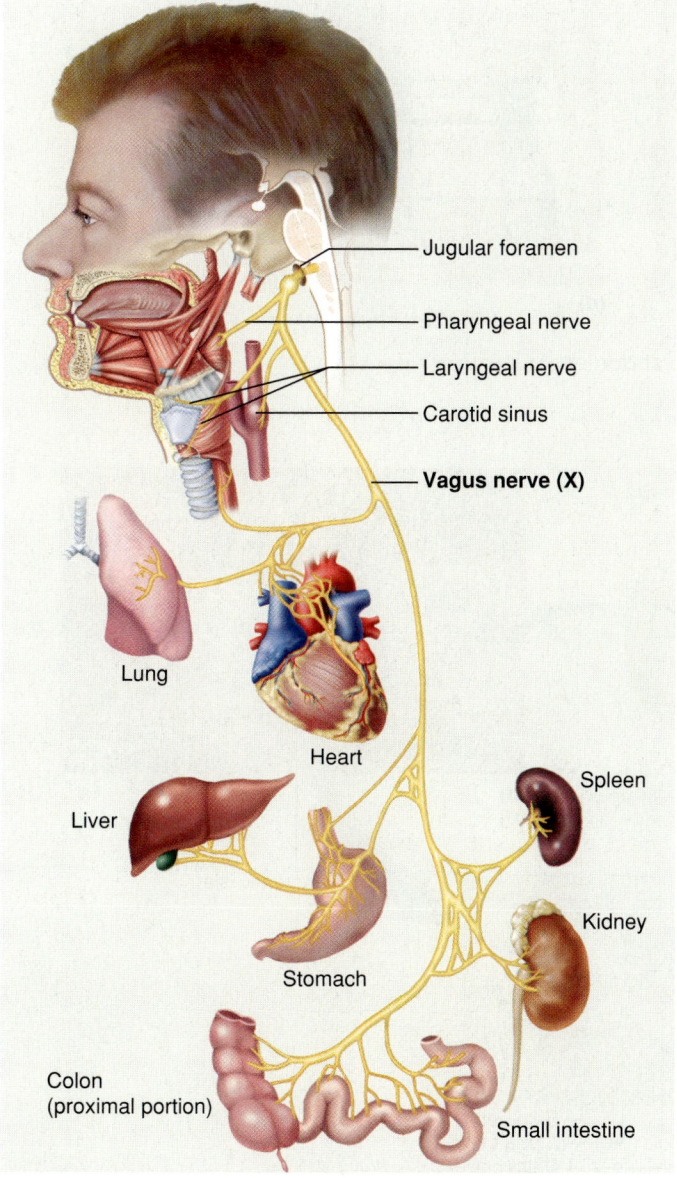

Jugular foramen

Pharyngeal nerve

Laryngeal nerve

Carotid sinus

Vagus nerve (X)

Lung

Heart

Spleen

Liver

Kidney

Stomach

Colon (proximal portion)

Small intestine

Figure 7-50 Cranial nerve X, the vagus nerve, slows the heart rate down and exhibits parasympathetic nervous system control in the heart.

Quadrants

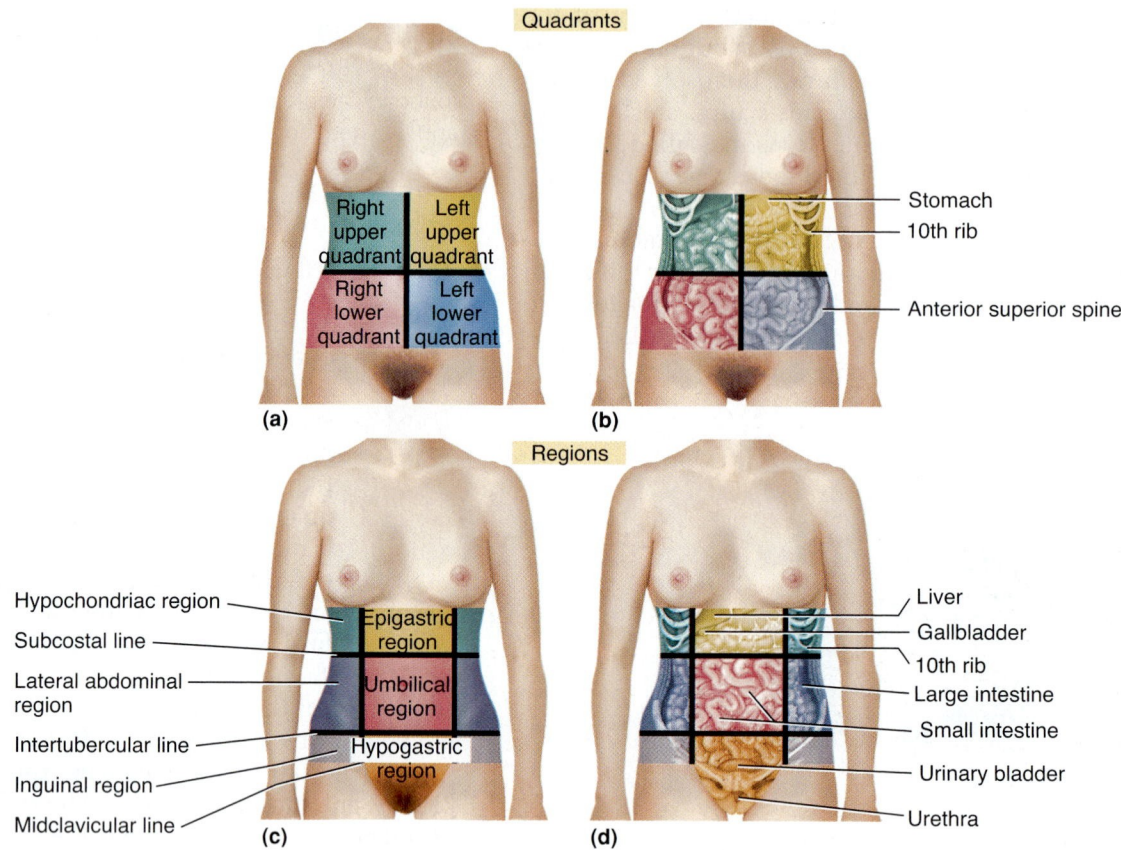

(a)

(b)

Stomach
10th rib

Anterior superior spine

Regions

Hypochondriac region
Subcostal line
Lateral abdominal region
Intertubercular line
Inguinal region
Midclavicular line

Epigastric region
Umbilical region
Hypogastric region

(c)

(d)

Liver
Gallbladder
10th rib
Large intestine
Small intestine
Urinary bladder
Urethra

Figure 7-51   The regions and quadrants of the abdomen.

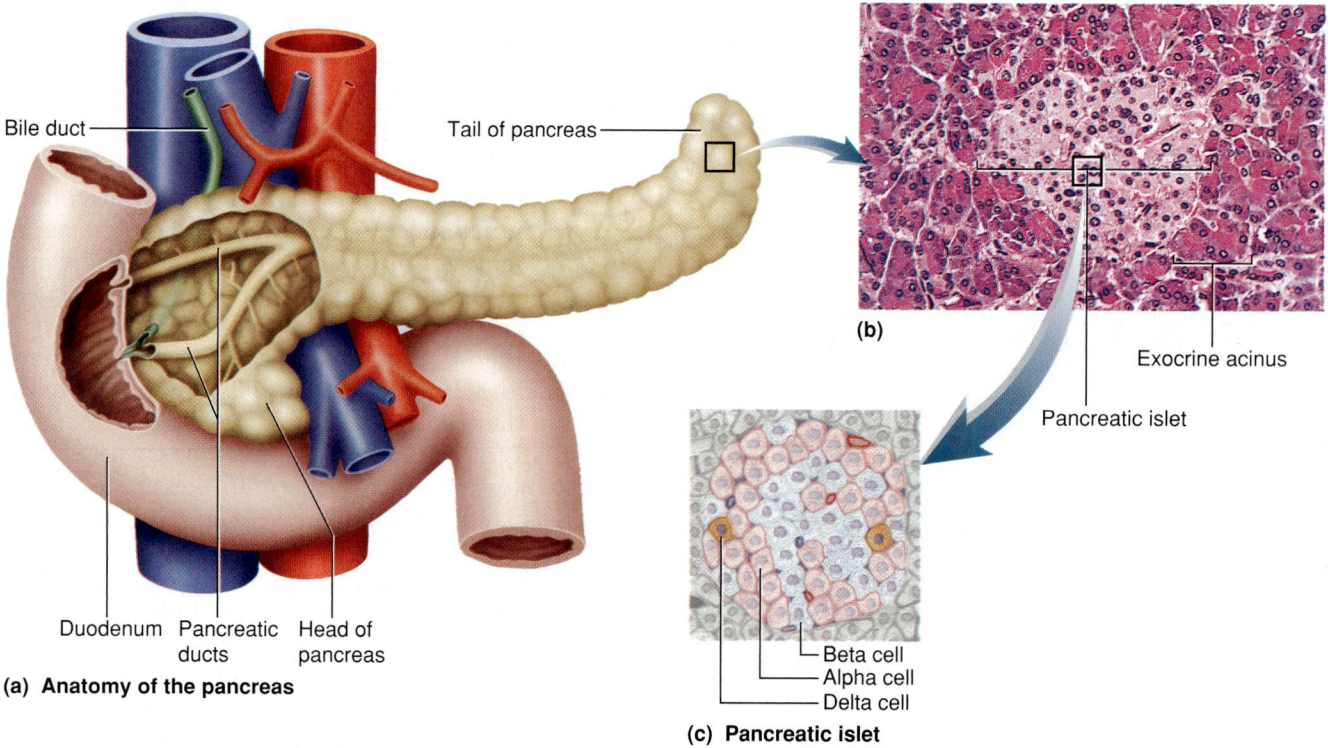

Bile duct

Tail of pancreas

(b)

Exocrine acinus

Pancreatic islet

Duodenum   Pancreatic   Head of
ducts   pancreas

(a) Anatomy of the pancreas

Beta cell
Alpha cell
Delta cell

(c) Pancreatic islet

Figure 7-52   The pancreas secretes glucagon, insulin, and somatostatin.

The **pancreas** is located in both of the upper quadrants (primarily in the LUQ) and has both endocrine and exocrine functions (see Plate C at the end of the chapter). Its exocrine function is to secrete digestive enzymes while its endocrine function is to release hormones from the Islets of Langerhans. There are three distinct types of cells. The alpha cells secrete glucagon, the beta cells secrete insulin, and the delta cells secrete somatostatin (Figure 7-52).

The food then passes from the small intestine into the large intestine by way of the ileocecal valve. The **appendix** is a rudimentary structure located in the cecum, which is the most proximal portion of the large intestine. The colon is divided into four parts: ascending, transverse, descending, and sigmoid. The most distal portion is the rectum, which is located in the pelvis. Having traversed the entire digestive tract, the stool is evacuated from the body by way of the anus. The anus has a muscular sphincter to aid in retaining the stool.

Abdominal Muscles

Layers of abdominal wall muscles protect the abdominal organs and also provide for movement in the region between the lowest ribs and the pelvis. The **rectus abdominis muscle** runs vertically and functions as the main flexor. The **transversus abdominis, external oblique,** and **internal oblique muscles** assist in rotation, flexion, and lateral movements of the trunk (see Plate A at the end of the chapter).

Abdominal Circulation

Branches of the aorta supply blood to the abdominal organs (see Plate C at the end of the chapter). The first branch is the **celiac trunk** which supplies arterial blood to the stomach, part of the duodenum, liver, gallbladder, pancreas, and spleen. Arterial blood flows to the kidneys by way of the **renal arteries.** The superior mesenteric artery supplies the remaining portions of the duodenum and the proximal colon up to two-thirds of the way along the transverse colon. The inferior mesenteric artery supplies the remainder of the colon (Figure 7-53).

The **portal venous system** is a specialized group of veins that receives blood from the gastrointestinal organs so that it can be taken directly to the liver for processing.

CONNECTIONS More on the abdomen can be found in Chapter 22: Abdominal Trauma and Chapter 34: Gastroenterology.

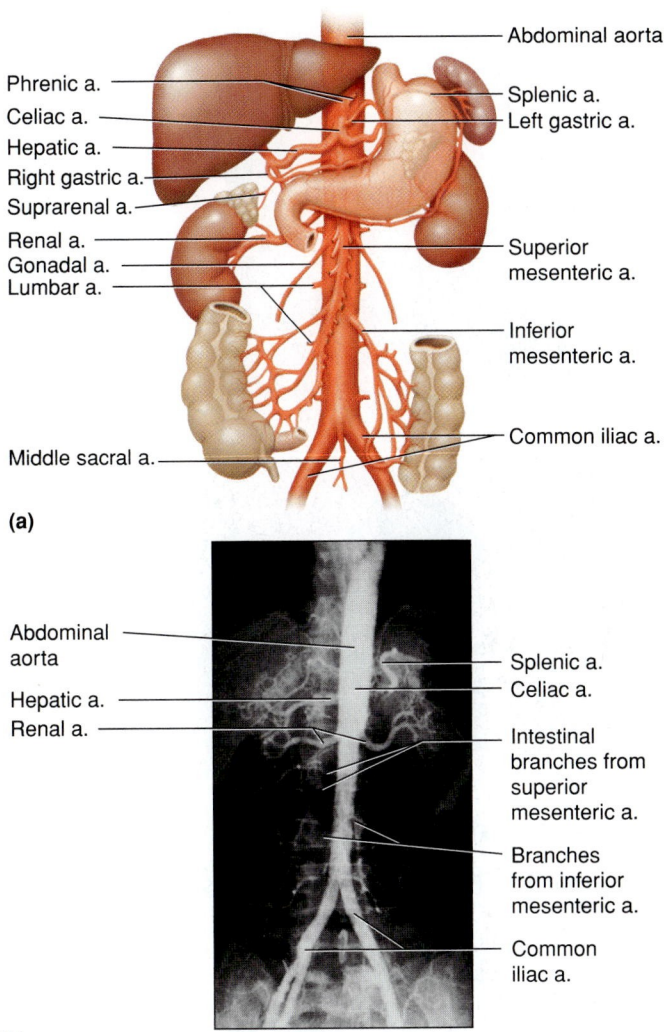

(a)

(b)

Figure 7-53 The abdominal aorta.

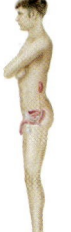

Pelvis and Genitourinary System

The **genitourinary system** consists of the kidneys, ureters, bladder, and urethra. It is important in the elimination of waste products. The kidneys also play a major role in the regulation of water, electrolytes, blood pressure, and many other essential body functions.

Kidneys

The **kidneys** are a pair of organs situated on the posterior and upper abdominal wall (see Plate C at the end of the chapter). The **adrenal glands** are **endocrine organs** located at the superior pole of the kidneys, and they are divided into two parts. The adrenal medulla (sympathetic component of the autonomic nervous system) secretes both epinephrine and norepinephrine, commonly known as catecholamines. The adrenal cortex secretes three steroid hormones which are the

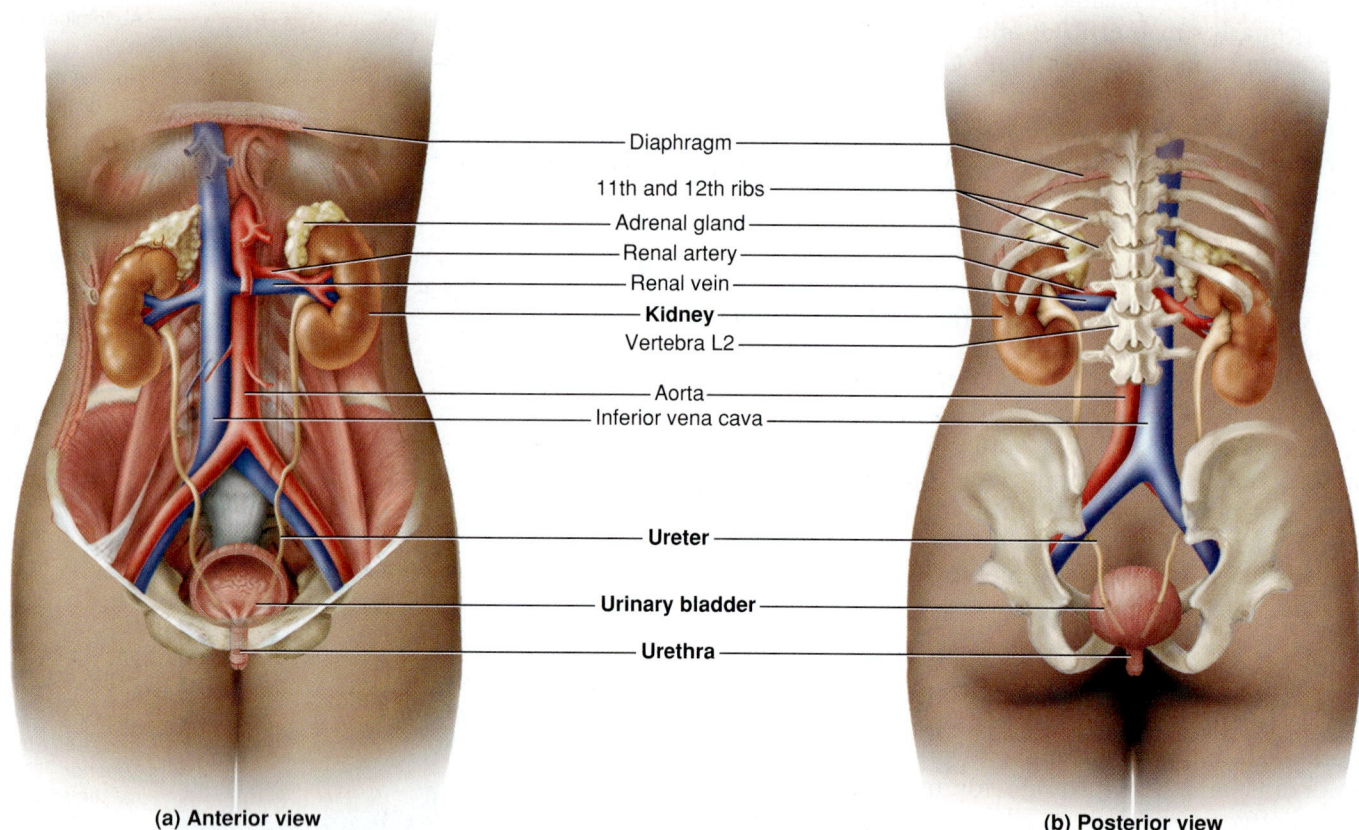

Diaphragm
11th and 12th ribs
Adrenal gland
Renal artery
Renal vein
Kidney
Vertebra L2
Aorta
Inferior vena cava

Ureter

Urinary bladder

Urethra

(a) Anterior view   **(b) Posterior view**

Figure 7-54   The organs and structures of the urinary system.

glucocorticoids, the mineralocorticoids, and the androgenic hormones (Figure 7-54).

From the kidneys, blood returns to the inferior vena cava by way of the renal veins. After filtration in the kidney, urine empties into the ureters and finally into the bladder for excretion by the urethra.

CONNECTIONS More on the genitourinary system can be found in Chapter 36: Urology.

Bladder

The **bladder** is a muscular organ that can distend to hold great volumes of urine. In the female, the **urethra** is located just anterior to the vaginal opening and is only 2–3 cm in length. In the male, the urethra is much longer and goes through the prostate and the length of the penis before becoming the urethral opening.

Reproductive Organs

Female Reproductive Organs

In the female, the reproductive organs are contained entirely in the pelvis (see Plate C at the end of the chapter). The **gonads** are endocrine organs that regulate reproduction. In the female, the gonads are called **ovaries** and are located in the pelvis next to the **fallopian tubes** and **uterus.** The development of the ovum takes place under the influence of estrogen and progesterone, which are secreted by the ovaries. The secretion of these hormones is under the control of luteinizing hormone (LH) and follicle stimulating hormone (FSH). The ovaries release eggs by a process known as **ovulation.** Once the egg has been released from the ovary, it travels down one of the paired fallopian tubes which empty into the uterus (Figure 7-55).

If a sperm cell from the male combines with the female's ovum, they become a conceptus, which is also called an **embryo.** This process is called **fertilization** and ordinarily takes place in the fallopian tube. The embryo usually implants in the uterus. The fundus is the superior portion of the uterus which can stretch from 5 cm to the size of a newborn baby. The lining of the uterus is called the **endometrium,** and it develops and thickens during each menstrual cycle in order to be receptive to the implantation of an embryo. If fertilization is not successful, the lining subsequently sloughs off and a menstrual period occurs as it sheds.

The **cervix** is the lower portion of the uterus that opens into the **vagina,** and it is this structure that can dilate to as much as 10 cm to allow passage of a baby

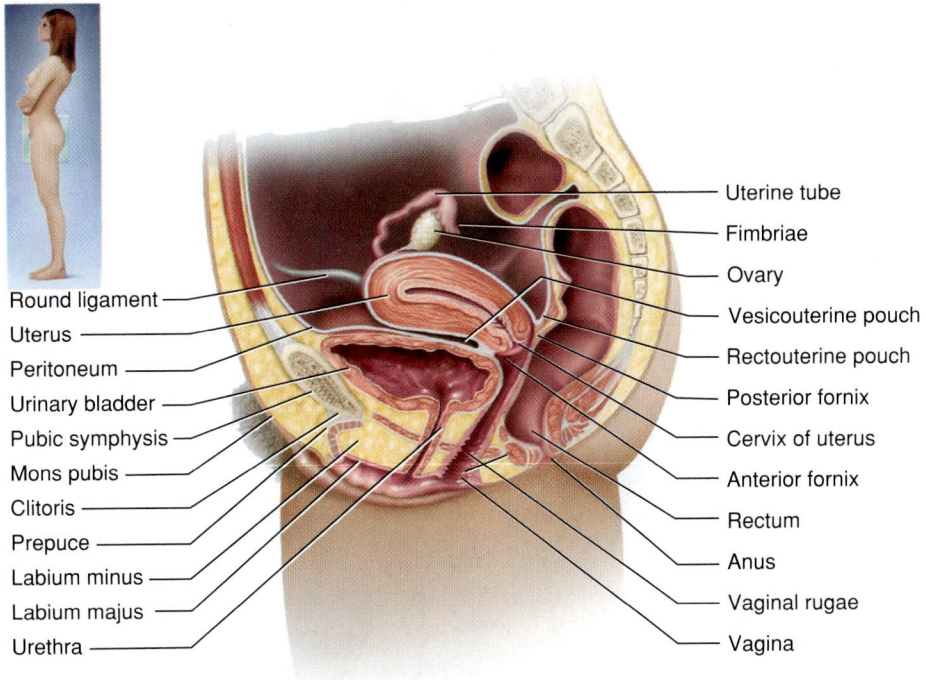

Figure 7-55   Female reproductive organs and structures.

during labor and delivery. The vagina is a structure connecting the cervix to the perineum. Between the vaginal opening and the anus is an area called the **perineum.** The urethra in the female is located just anterior to the vaginal opening. The labia minora and majora protect the urethra and vagina from injury.

Once a pregnancy has been established, the **placenta** is formed very early. It is an organ that serves as the interface between the mother and the fetus. Oxygen and carbon dioxide are exchanged here. It carries important nutrients for the fetus and removes waste products. The placenta is connected to the fetus by the **umbilical cord.** The umbilical cord has two arteries and one vein. The vein carries oxygenated blood to the fetus, and the arteries return deoxygenated blood to the placenta and the mother. The **amniotic sac** is a protective fluid-filled sac which surrounds the fetus as it develops (Figure 7-56).

CONNECTIONS More on the female reproductive system can be found in Chapter 41: Obstetrics and Gynecology.

Male Reproductive Organs

In the male reproductive system, the gonads—called **testes**—are located entirely within the scrotum (see Plate B at the end of the chapter). The **scrotum** is a pouch formed by the dartos muscle and skin in which the testes lie surrounded by the tunica vaginalis. The testes release sperm, but they also make and secrete

testosterone. The penis consists of two corpora cavernosa which separate and attach to the ischiopubic ramus. The ischiocavernosus muscles cover the corpora cavernosa as they diverge, and they function to restrict venous blood egress during erection. The urethra is surrounded by tissue called the corpus spongiosum which becomes the glans penis distally. The spermatic cord suspends the testes and contains the vas deferens, the veins, and artery of the testes. The urethra in the male passes through the prostate gland. Secretions from the prostate and seminal vesicle combine with sperm from the testicle by way of the **vas deferens.** Semen is emptied by way of the penile urethra during ejaculation.

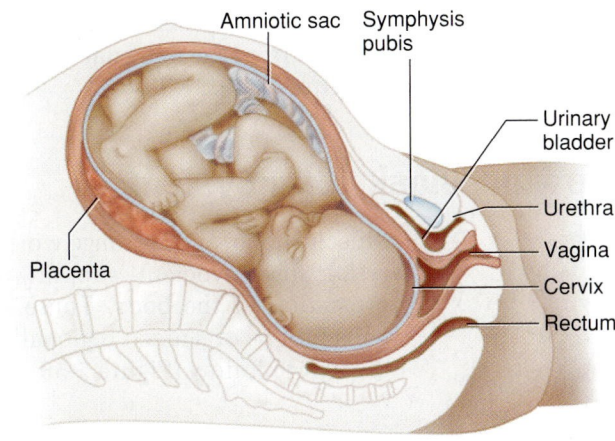

Figure 7-56   A fetus developing inside a uterus.

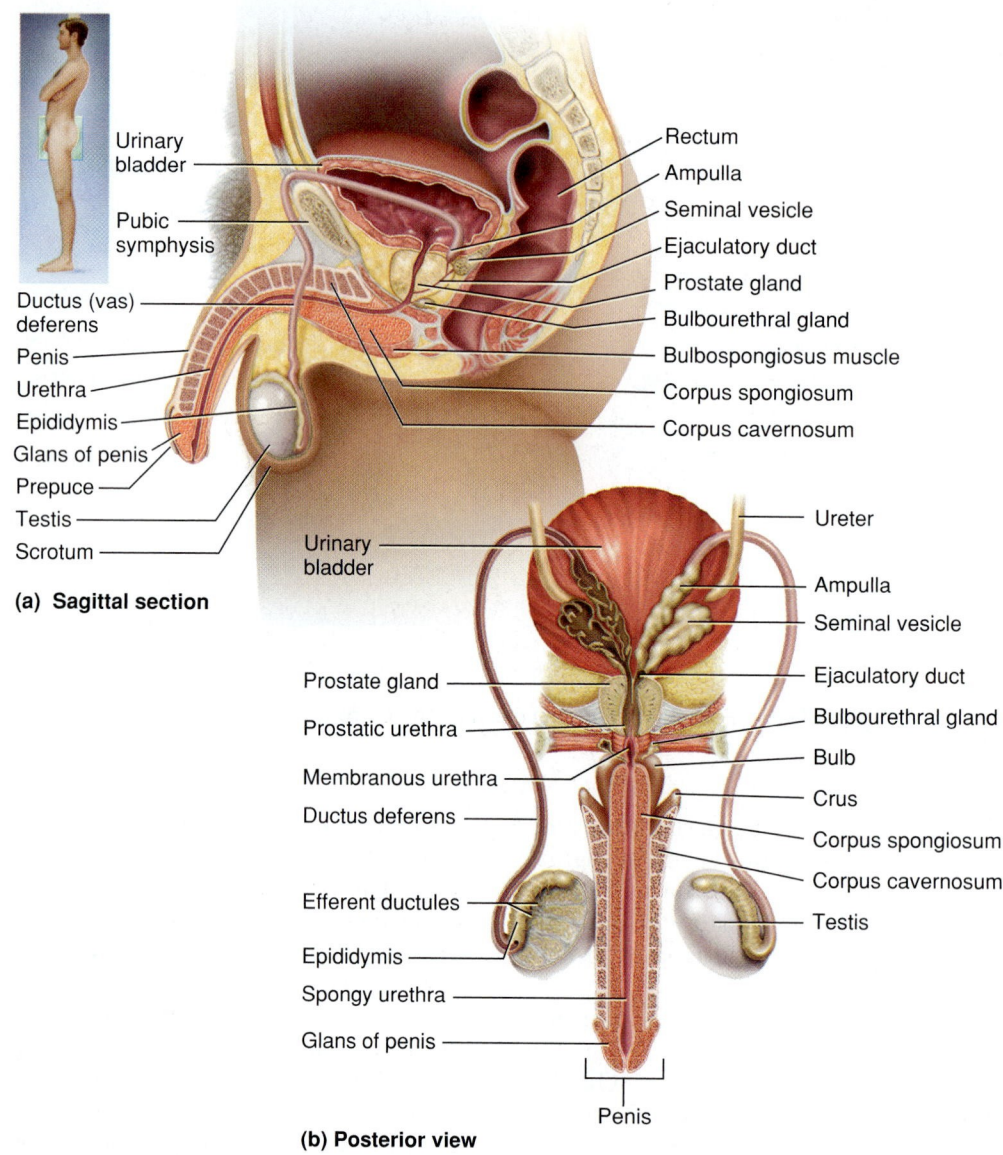

Urinary bladder
Pubic symphysis
Ductus (vas) deferens
Penis
Urethra
Epididymis
Glans of penis
Prepuce
Testis
Scrotum

Rectum
Ampulla
Seminal vesicle
Ejaculatory duct
Prostate gland
Bulbourethral gland
Bulbospongiosus muscle
Corpus spongiosum
Corpus cavernosum

(a) Sagittal section

Urinary bladder
Prostate gland
Prostatic urethra
Membranous urethra
Ductus deferens
Efferent ductules
Epididymis
Spongy urethra
Glans of penis

Ureter
Ampulla
Seminal vesicle
Ejaculatory duct
Bulbourethral gland
Bulb
Crus
Corpus spongiosum
Corpus cavernosum
Testis

Penis

(b) Posterior view

Figure 7-57   The male reproductive organs and structures.

The pudendal nerve stimulates muscles in this area and supplies sensation to the skin of the external genitalia, perineum, and anus (Figure 7-57).

The Musculoskeletal System

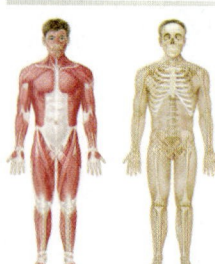

Muscle, bone, and cartilage work together for movement, support, and protection of the body. These systems will be organized regionally in the text to follow (Figure 7-58).

The Upper Limbs

Bones and Joints of the Upper Limbs

The **clavicles** articulate medially with the **sternum** to form the sternoclavicular joints and articulate laterally with the **scapula** to form the acromio-clavicular (AC) joints. The AC joints connect the trunk with the upper limbs. The supraspinatous, infraspinatous, subscapularis, and teres minor muscles form the **rotator cuffs.** These muscles span from the scapula to the humerus and provide stability of the shoulders at the glenohumeral joints. The **humerus** articulates with the **radius** and the **ulna** at the elbow joint which in turn articulates with the **carpal bones** at the wrist. The carpal bones articulate with the metacarpal bones to

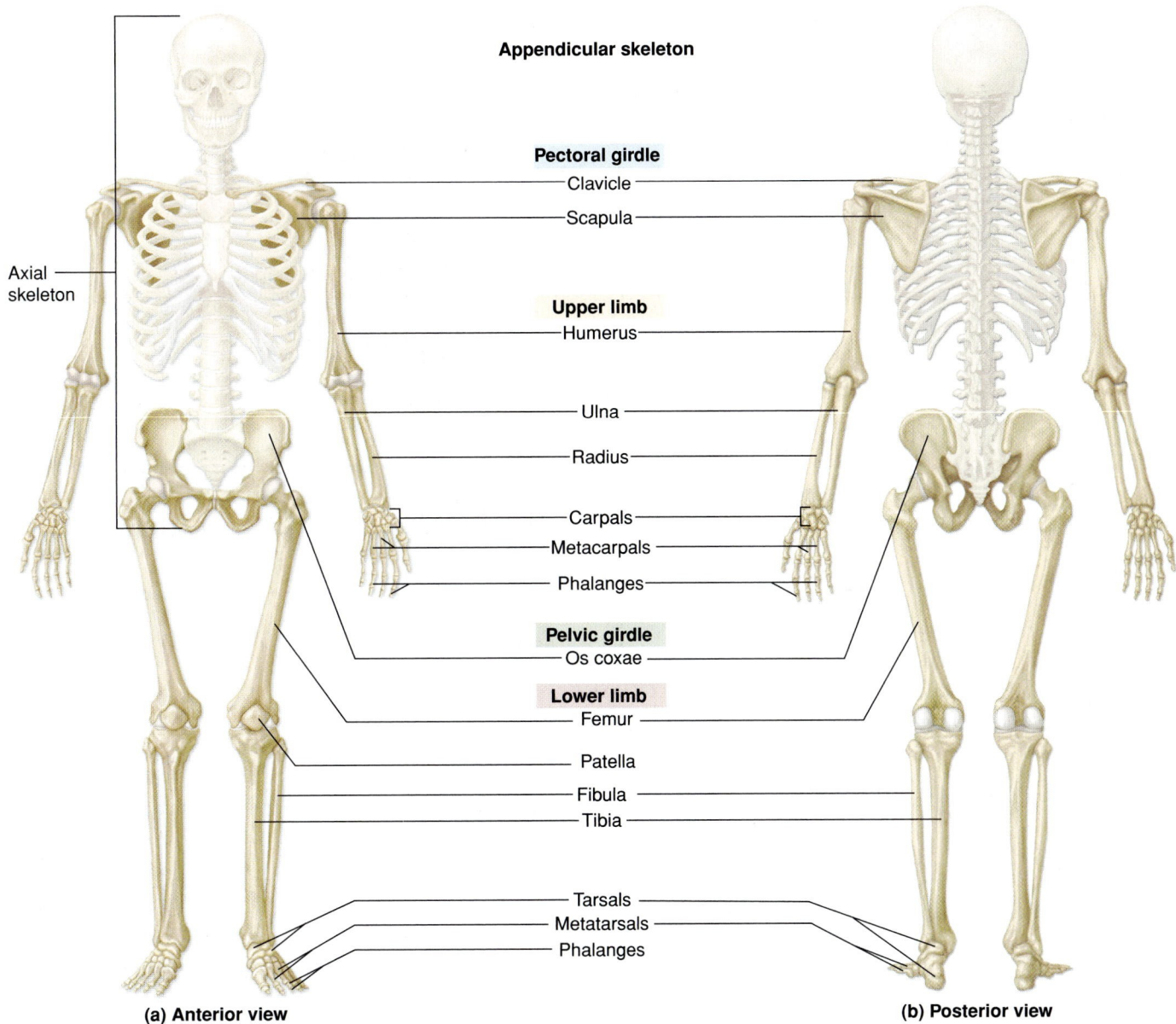

Appendicular skeleton

Pectoral girdle
Clavicle
Scapula

Axial
skeleton

Upper limb
Humerus

Ulna

Radius

Carpals
Metacarpals
Phalanges

Pelvic girdle
Os coxae

Lower limb
Femur

Patella
Fibula
Tibia

Tarsals
Metatarsals
Phalanges

(a) Anterior view   **(b) Posterior view**

Figure 7-58 The bones of the skeletal system.

form the carpometacarpal joints. The metacarpals articulate with the **phalanges** to form the metacarpophalangeal joints. Finally, the phalanges articulate with each other to form the interphalangeal joints (Figure 7-59).

Muscles and Nerves of the Upper Limbs

There are five main nerves in the arms that arise from a complicated network of nerve roots to supply the arms and hands. These nerves are named the musculocutaneous, axillary, radial, median, and ulnar nerves. The muscles of the upper arms and forearms

are divided into anterior and posterior compartments by fascia. The muscles of the anterior compartments are innervated by the musculocutaneous nerve and cause flexion of the elbows. The muscles of the posterior compartment are innervated by the radial nerve and cause extension at the elbows. The muscles of the anterior compartment of the forearm are innervated by the ulnar and median nerves and cause flexion at the wrists and the fingers. The muscles of the posterior compartment of the forearm are innervated by the radial nerve and cause extension at the wrists and fingers. The forearms can be rotated on their longitudinal axis to cause pronation and supination. The hands

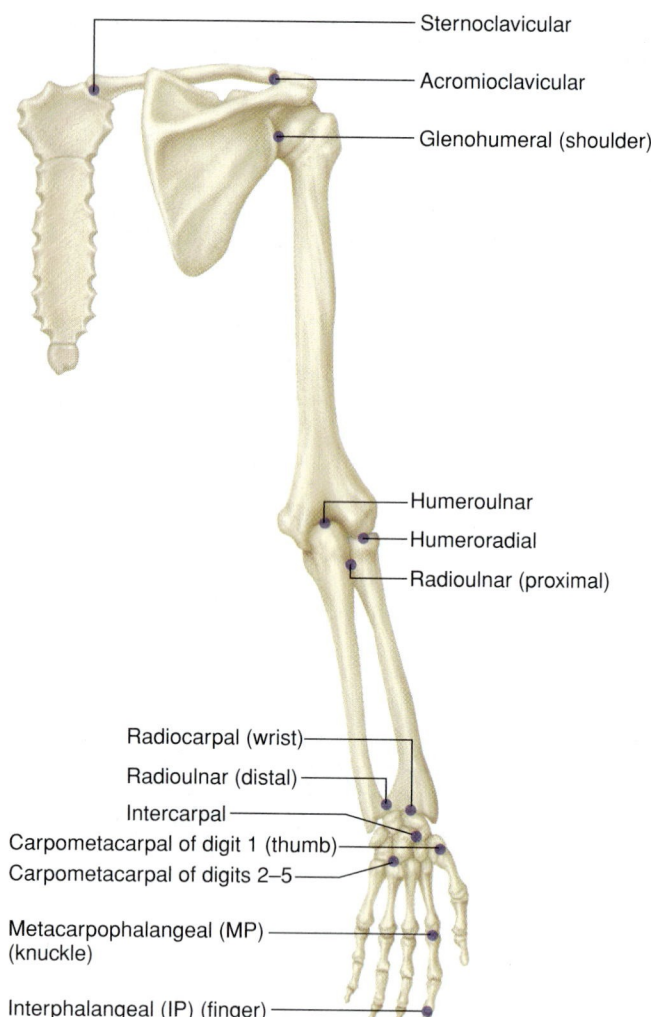

Figure 7-59   Joints of the upper extremities.

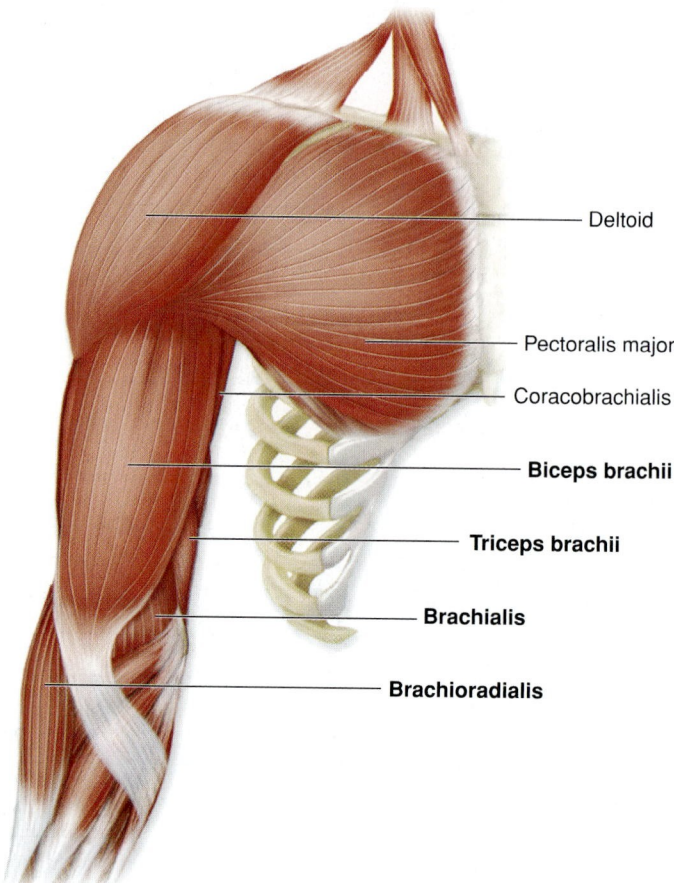

Figure 7-60   Muscles of the upper extremity.

have many small muscles, and this, along with the mobility of the thumbs, brings about the dexterity of the hands (Figure 7-60).

Blood Supply to the Upper Limbs

The **subclavian arteries** are found under the clavicle (see Plate B at the end of the chapter). At the first rib, they are renamed the **axillary arteries.** They are named the **brachial arteries** in the anterior compartments of the upper arms. At the elbows, the arteries divide into the radial and ulnar arteries which can both be palpated on the ventral surfaces of the wrists. The radial artery travels down the anterior compartment of the forearm. The ulnar artery travels down the anterior compartment of the forearm but also supplies a branch to the posterior compartment. Both the radial and ulnar arteries supply bloodflow to the hands. They are joined

together in the hands via the palmer arches. Deep veins follow the corresponding arteries. There are two major superficial veins in the arms. The basilic vein will be found on the medial aspect of the arm while the cephalic vein can be found on the lateral aspect of the arm. There are communicating vessels between the two. These vessels are commonly used for intravenous access and blood draws (Figure 7-61).

The Lower Limbs
Bones and Joints of the Lower Limbs

The ischium, ilium, and pubis bones fuse together to form two sides of the **pelvis.** This structure articulates with the sacrum at the sacroiliac joints. These joints form the connection of the trunk with the legs. The hip joint is a ball-and-socket joint formed by the acetabulum of the pelvis and the head of the femur. The knee joint is formed by the articulation of the femur with the **tibia** and **fibula.** The knee joint is

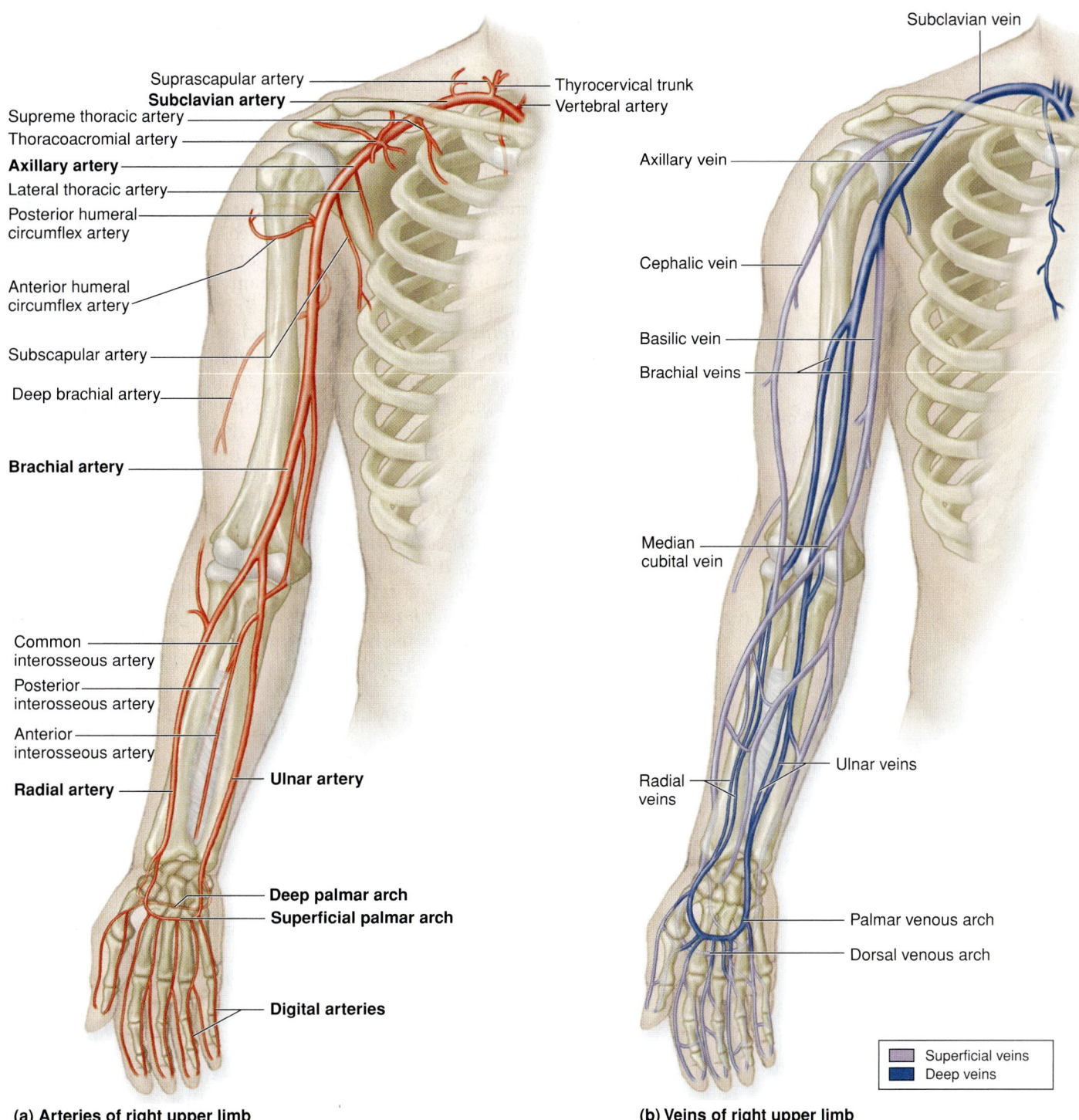

Suprascapular artery
Subclavian artery
Supreme thoracic artery
Thoracoacromial artery
Axillary artery
Lateral thoracic artery
Posterior humeral circumflex artery

Anterior humeral circumflex artery

Subscapular artery

Deep brachial artery

Brachial artery

Common interosseous artery
Posterior interosseous artery
Anterior interosseous artery
Radial artery

Thyrocervical trunk
Vertebral artery

Ulnar artery

Deep palmar arch
Superficial palmar arch

Digital arteries

(a) Arteries of right upper limb

Subclavian vein

Axillary vein

Cephalic vein

Basilic vein
Brachial veins

Median cubital vein

Radial veins
Ulnar veins

Palmar venous arch
Dorsal venous arch

| | Superficial veins |
| | Deep veins |

(b) Veins of right upper limb

Figure 7-61   The vascular system for the upper extremity. Note how the vessels pass near the joint and lie close to the bones.

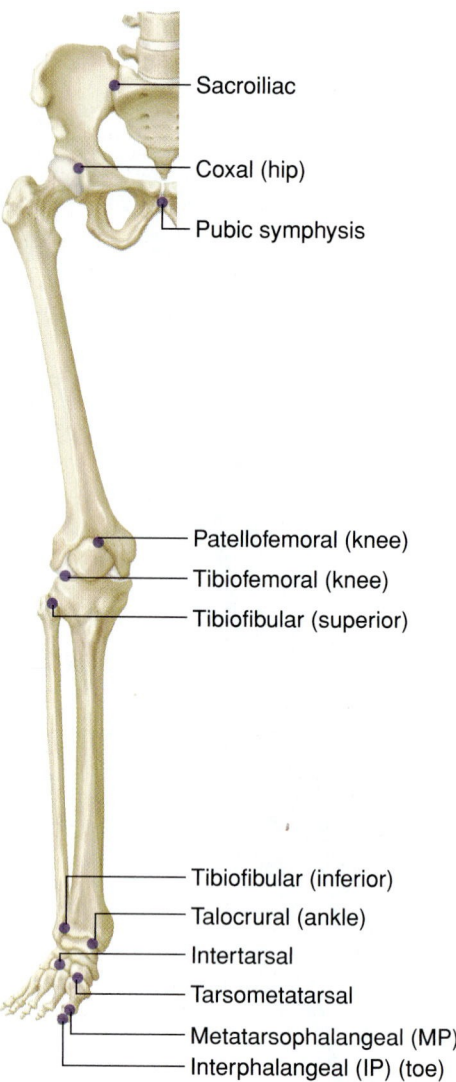

- Sacroiliac
- Coxal (hip)
- Pubic symphysis
- Patellofemoral (knee)
- Tibiofemoral (knee)
- Tibiofibular (superior)
- Tibiofibular (inferior)
- Talocrural (ankle)
- Intertarsal
- Tarsometatarsal
- Metatarsophalangeal (MP)
- Interphalangeal (IP) (toe)

Figure 7-62   Joints of the lower extremity.

stabilized by the medial and lateral menisci and by the medial and lateral collateral ligaments. The ankles are hinge joints connecting the tibias and fibulas with the talus bones of the feet. The talus bones articulate with the tarsal bones to form the talotarsal joints. The tarsal bones articulate with the metatarsal bones forming the tarsometatarsal joints. The metatarsal bones articulate with the phalanges to form the metatarsophalangeal joints. Finally, phalanges articulate with one another to form the interphalangeal joints (Figure 7-62).

Muscles and Nerves of the Lower Limbs

The muscles of the anterior compartments of the thigh (the **quadriceps**) are innervated by the musculocutaneous nerve and cause extension of the knee. The muscles of the adductor compartments of the thigh are innervated by the obturator nerve and cause adduction of the thigh. The muscles of the posterior compartments of the thigh (the **hamstrings**) are innervated by the sciatic nerve and cause extension of the hips and flexion of the knees. There are four compartments in the lower legs, which are named the anterior, lateral, deep posterior, and superficial posterior compartments. The branches of the sciatic nerves innervate the muscles of the lower legs. The muscles of the lower legs can cause flexion of the ankles, extension of the ankles (also called dorsiflexion), and support for the arches of the feet. They can also cause inversion and eversion of the feet (Figure 7-63).

Blood Supply to the Lower Limbs

At the level of the inguinal ligaments, the external iliac arteries divide into the **femoral** and the **deep femoral arteries.** An important relationship exists with the neurovascular structures in this region. A mnemonic (NAVEL) is useful to remember the order of the structures in the groin.

Proceeding from lateral to medial, NAVEL stands for:

N Nerve
A Artery
V Vein
E Empty Space
L Lymphatics

Behind the knees, the femoral arteries become the **popliteal arteries.** Below the popliteal spaces, the arteries divide to form the anterior and posterior tibial arteries to supply the anterior and posterior compartments, respectively. When the anterior and posterior tibial arteries cross the ankles, they become the **dorsalis pedis arteries** and the **posterior tibial arteries,** respectively. These pulses are easily palpated at the ankles. The main superficial veins in the leg are the great saphenous and the small saphenous veins (Figure 7-64).

CONNECTIONS More on the limbs can be found in Chapter 24: Skeletal Trauma and Chapter 25: Soft Tissue and Muscle Trauma.

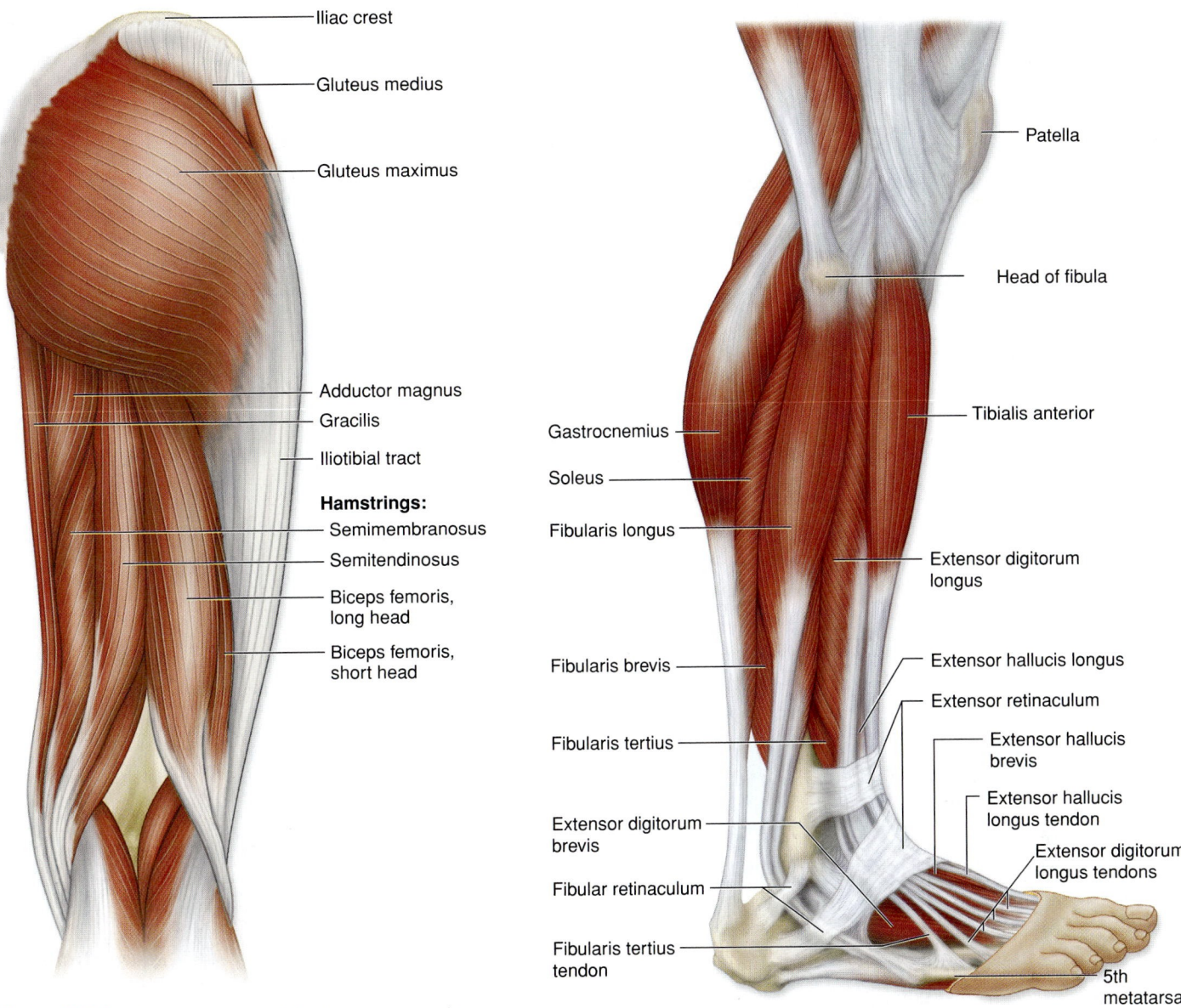

Iliac crest

Gluteus medius

Gluteus maximus

Adductor magnus

Gracilis

Iliotibial tract

Hamstrings:

Semimembranosus

Semitendinosus

Biceps femoris, long head

Biceps femoris, short head

Patella

Head of fibula

Tibialis anterior

Gastrocnemius

Soleus

Fibularis longus

Extensor digitorum longus

Fibularis brevis

Extensor hallucis longus

Extensor retinaculum

Fibularis tertius

Extensor hallucis brevis

Extensor hallucis longus tendon

Extensor digitorum brevis

Extensor digitorum longus tendons

Fibular retinaculum

Fibularis tertius tendon

5th metatarsal

Figure 7-63 Major muscles of the lower extremity.

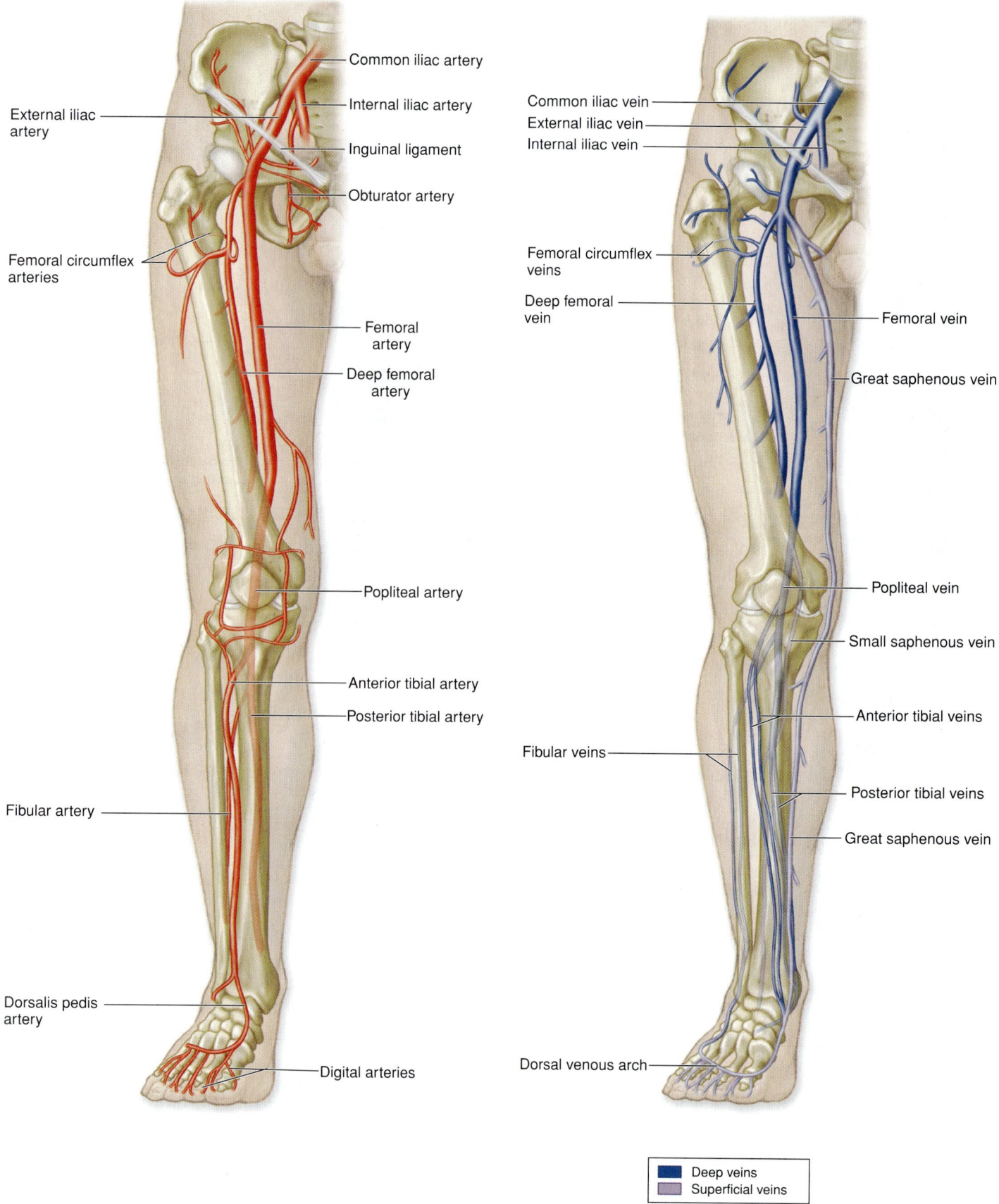

Common iliac artery

Internal iliac artery

External iliac artery

Inguinal ligament

Obturator artery

Femoral circumflex arteries

Femoral artery

Deep femoral artery

Popliteal artery

Anterior tibial artery

Posterior tibial artery

Fibular artery

Dorsalis pedis artery

Digital arteries

Common iliac vein

External iliac vein

Internal iliac vein

Femoral circumflex veins

Deep femoral vein

Femoral vein

Great saphenous vein

Popliteal vein

Small saphenous vein

Anterior tibial veins

Fibular veins

Posterior tibial veins

Great saphenous vein

Dorsal venous arch

Deep veins
Superficial veins

Figure 7-64 Vessels of the lower extremity. The femoral artery is a large vessel. It is difficult to control bleeding when this artery is damaged.

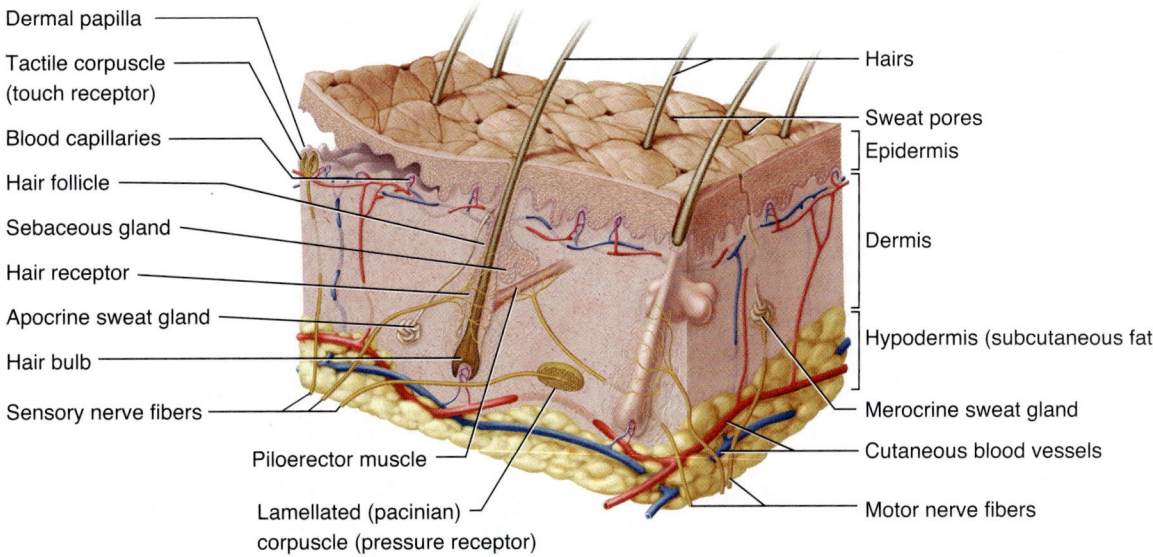

Dermal papilla

Tactile corpuscle (touch receptor)

Blood capillaries

Hair follicle

Sebaceous gland

Hair receptor

Apocrine sweat gland

Hair bulb

Sensory nerve fibers

Piloerector muscle

Lamellated (pacinian) corpuscle (pressure receptor)

Hairs

Sweat pores

Epidermis

Dermis

Hypodermis (subcutaneous fat)

Merocrine sweat gland

Cutaneous blood vessels

Motor nerve fibers

Figure 7-65 The layers of the skin.

Integumentary System

Skin covers the body and is made up of three layers. The **epidermis** is the outermost layer of the skin. It is a layer composed of dead and dying cells that are being pushed outward by the new cells underneath. The **dermis** is located below the epidermis. It produces and houses glands, blood vessels, and nerves associated with the skin. **Sebaceous glands** secrete sebum (a fatty substance) into the hair follicles, and this keeps the skin pliable and waterproof. Also found in this layer are sudoriferous glands that secrete sweat. The subcutaneous layer of the skin is the **hypodermis** and is composed of adipose tissue (fat) and connective tissue (Figure 7-65).

CONNECTIONS More on the skin can be found in Chapter 25: Soft Tissue and Muscle Trauma and Chapter 26: Burn Trauma.

Summary

This brief review of anatomy is provided to familiarize paramedics with the structure of the human body. The goal is to provide enough detail to understand the physiology, pathology, and therapeutics discussed elsewhere in this book. If further detail is desired, there are many textbooks devoted entirely to the discipline of anatomy, and the reader is encouraged to delve more deeply into the intricacies of the human body.

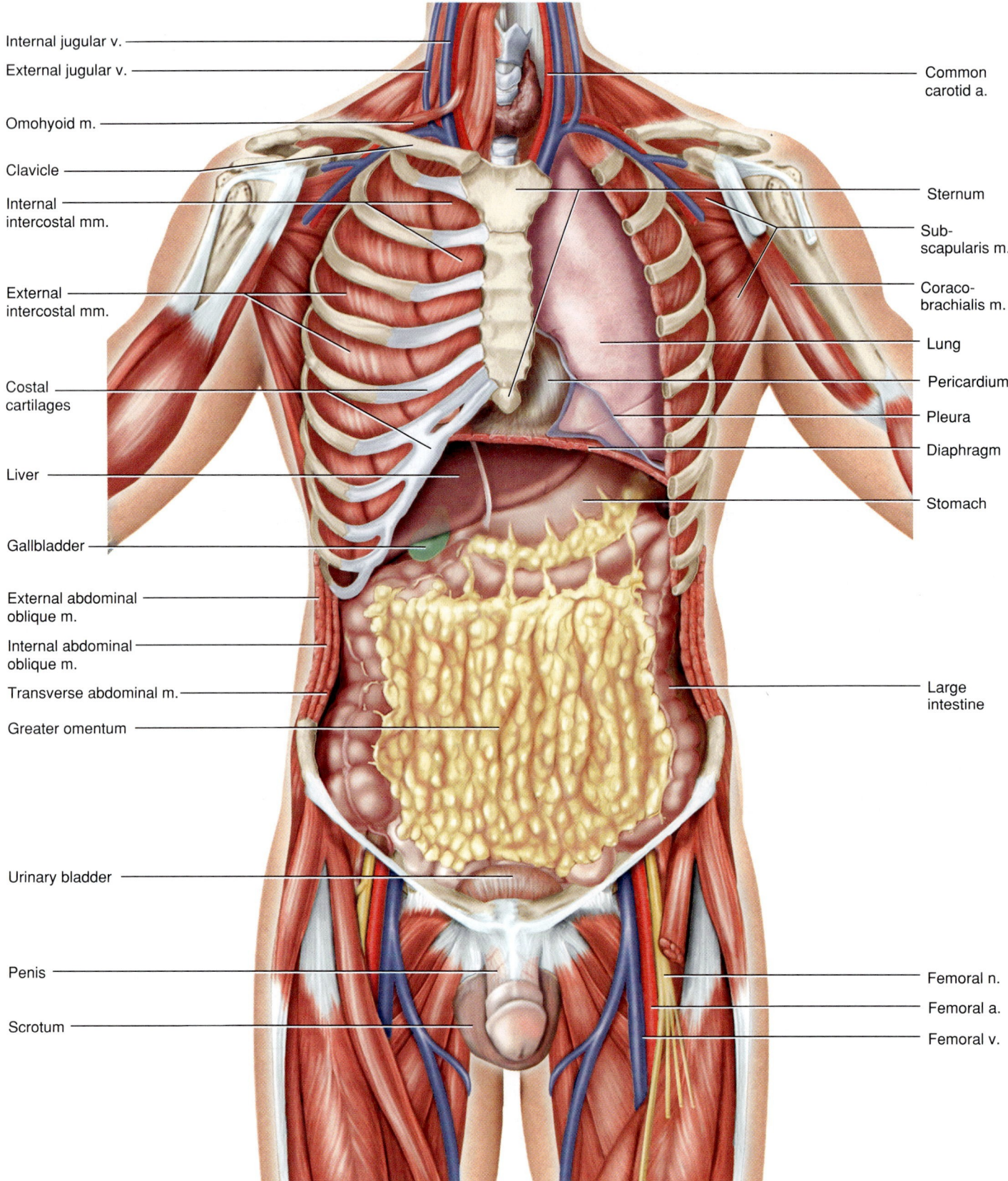

Internal jugular v.

External jugular v.

Omohyoid m.

Clavicle

Internal
intercostal mm.

External
intercostal mm.

Costal
cartilages

Liver

Gallbladder

External abdominal
oblique m.

Internal abdominal
oblique m.

Transverse abdominal m.

Greater omentum

Urinary bladder

Penis

Scrotum

Common
carotid a.

Sternum

Sub-
scapularis m.

Coraco-
brachialis m.

Lung

Pericardium

Pleura

Diaphragm

Stomach

Large
intestine

Femoral n.

Femoral a.

Femoral v.

Plate A   Anatomy at the level of the rib cage and greater omentum (male). The ventral body wall is removed, and the ribs, intercostal muscles, and pleura are removed from the anatomical left (a. = artery; v. = vein; m. = muscle; mm. = muscles; n. = nerve).

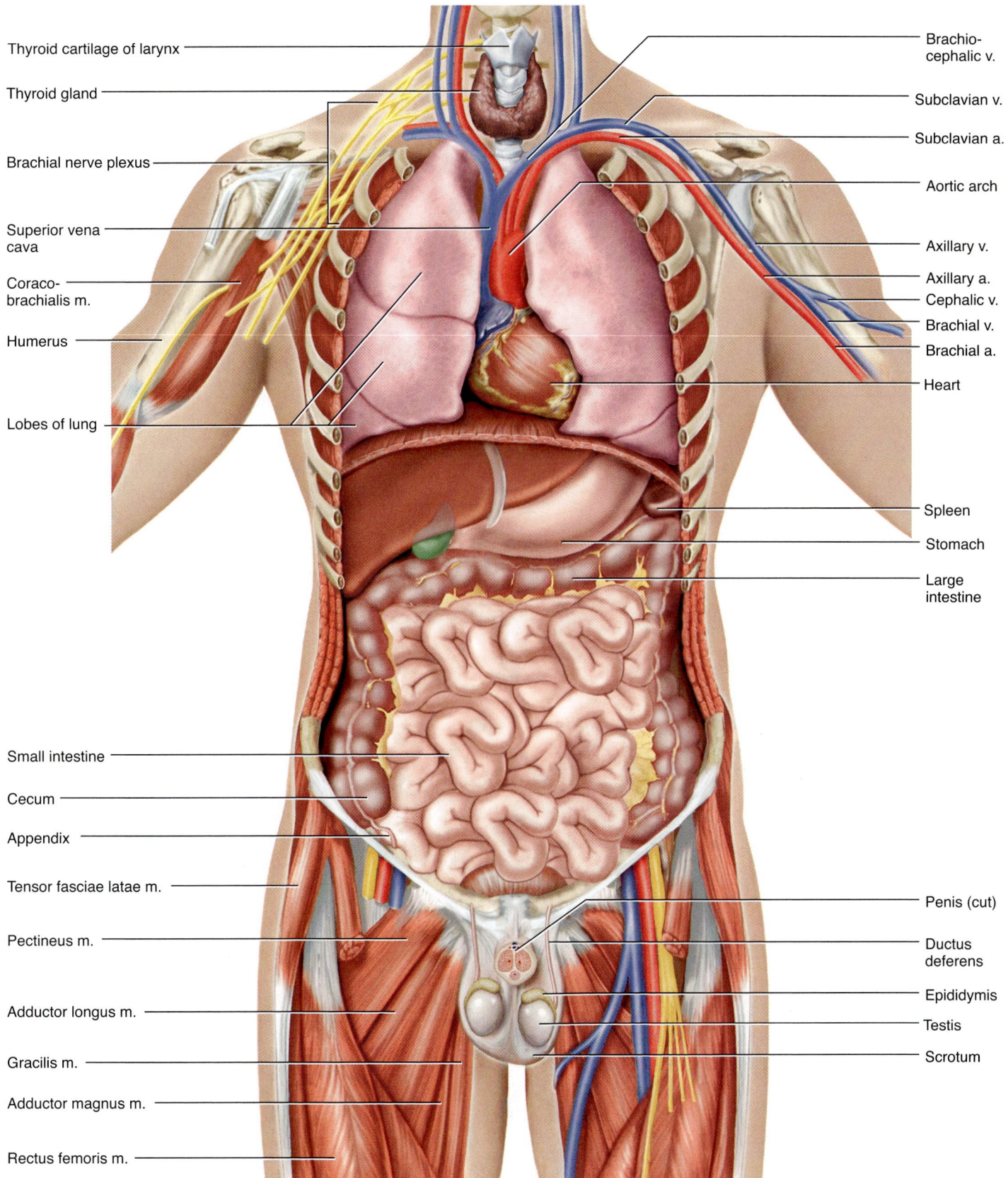

Thyroid cartilage of larynx

Thyroid gland

Brachial nerve plexus

Superior vena cava

Coraco-brachialis m.

Humerus

Lobes of lung

Small intestine

Cecum

Appendix

Tensor fasciae latae m.

Pectineus m.

Adductor longus m.

Gracilis m.

Adductor magnus m.

Rectus femoris m.

Brachio-cephalic v.

Subclavian v.

Subclavian a.

Aortic arch

Axillary v.

Axillary a.
Cephalic v.
Brachial v.
Brachial a.

Heart

Spleen

Stomach

Large intestine

Penis (cut)

Ductus deferens

Epididymis

Testis

Scrotum

Plate B   Anatomy at the level of the lungs and intestines (male). The sternum, ribs, and greater omentum are removed (a. = artery; v. = vein; m. = muscle).

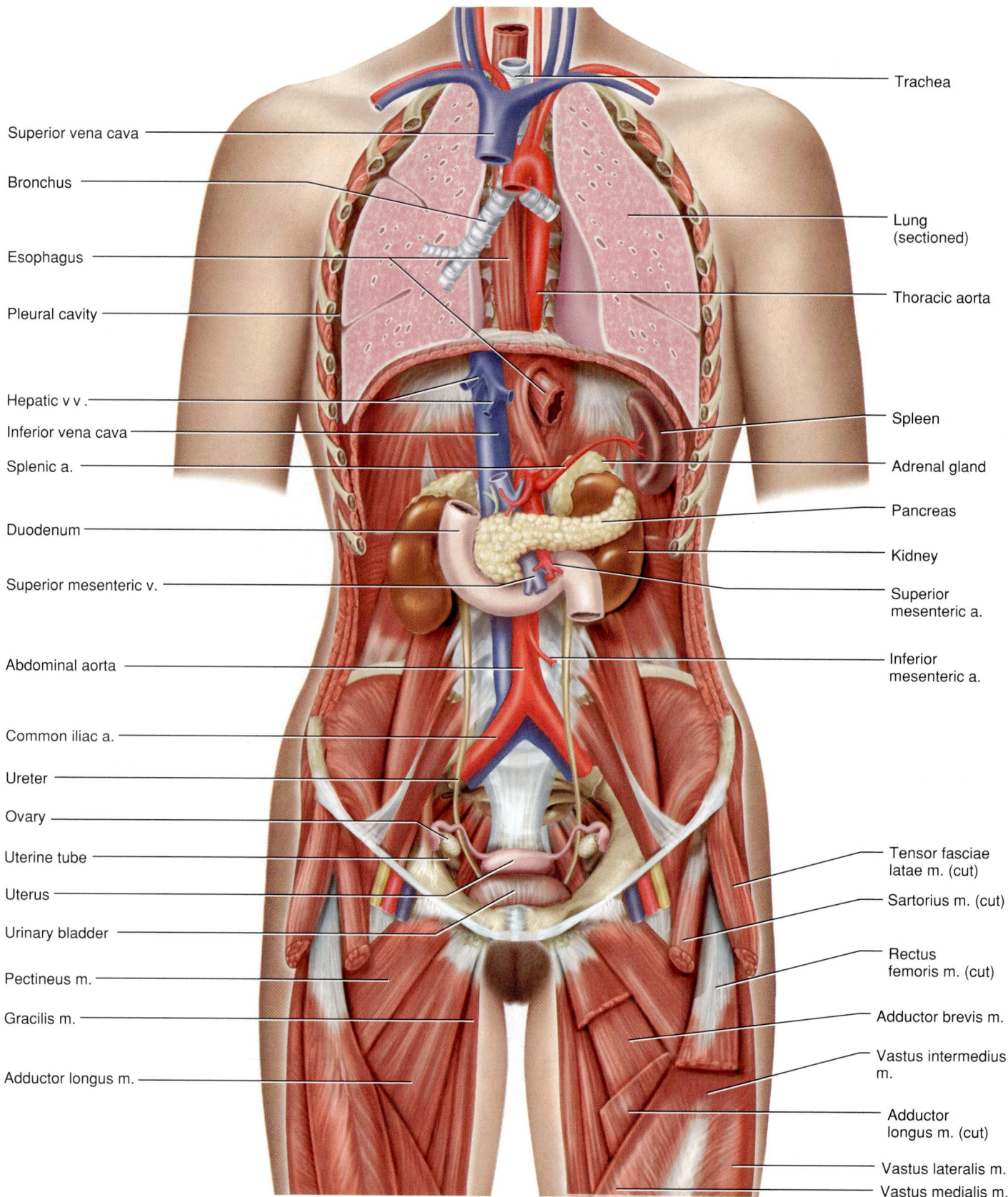

Trachea

Superior vena cava

Bronchus

Esophagus

Pleural cavity

Lung (sectioned)

Thoracic aorta

Hepatic v v .

Inferior vena cava

Splenic a.

Duodenum

Superior mesenteric v.

Abdominal aorta

Common iliac a.

Ureter

Ovary

Uterine tube

Uterus

Urinary bladder

Pectineus m.

Gracilis m.

Adductor longus m.

Spleen

Adrenal gland

Pancreas

Kidney

Superior mesenteric a.

Inferior mesenteric a.

Tensor fasciae latae m. (cut)

Sartorius m. (cut)

Rectus femoris m. (cut)

Adductor brevis m.

Vastus intermedius m.

Adductor longus m. (cut)

Vastus lateralis m.

Vastus medialis m.

Plate C Anatomy at the level of the retroperitoneal viscera (female). The heart is removed, the lungs are frontally sectioned, and the viscera of the peritoneal itself are removed (a. = artery; v. = vein; vv. = veins; m. = muscle).

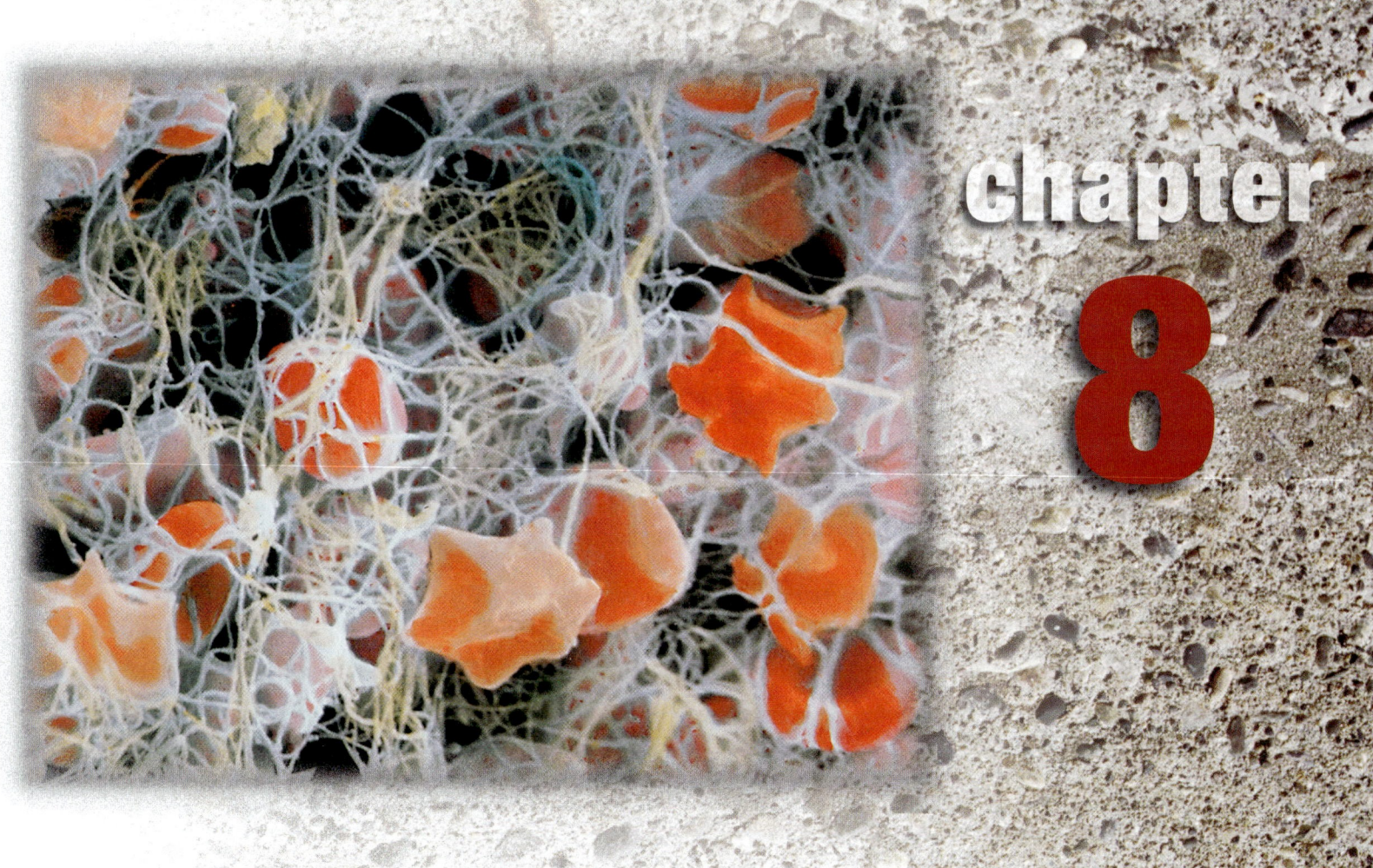

Physiology Overview

"*Every bodily action is coordinated by conference calls between millions of neurons in the brain. Imagine a multinational corporation with 35 billion employees who stay in constant touch with each other and are capable of making trillions of decisions every millisecond.*"

—Geoffrey Simmons from: *What Darwin Didn't Know,* 2004

Need to Know

▶ A basic foundation of anatomy and physiology is essential for understanding the signs and symptoms of the various diseases and traumatic conditions presented by patients.

▶ Understanding basic principles of physiology will allow you to focus the history and physical examination toward elements pertinent to the situation presented.

▶ Understanding how various body systems are interrelated will help you think through medical problems. As you recall these relationships, you will be reminded of related assessments you may need to perform in order to obtain a complete picture of the patient's ailment.

▶ Aerobic metabolism is normal. Anaerobic metabolism is not, and it leads to the production of lactic acid and the buildup of wastes in the blood that result in acidosis, organ impairment, organ failure, and eventually death, if untreated.

▶ An intact and functioning heart and circulatory system and adequate blood volume with the appropriate amount of oxygen and nutrients are required for homeostasis.

▶ The sympathetic, parasympathetic, and endocrine systems exert control over the heart and blood vessels.

▶ Although patients do not read the "signs and symptoms manual" when they become sick, they often exhibit patterns that can be predicted or anticipated by the paramedic who has a good understanding of pathophysiology.

▶ Sometimes signs or symptoms can be subtle. Narrowing pulse pressure, which is a decreasing difference between the systolic and diastolic blood pressure reading, may go unnoticed if only one blood pressure reading is obtained. The key is continuous monitoring.

▶ Sick	▶ Not Yet Sick
• Many vital signs that are abnormal (based on the patient's age, sex, weight, and preexisting medical conditions) should prompt you to consider that the patient is in need of aggressive attention. • Patients should be closely monitored with multiple sets of vital signs obtained, so the paramedic can observe the patient for trends. This can make the difference in noticing a patient deteriorating into early shock versus waiting to find an irreparable drop in blood pressure signaling perhaps an irreversible shock state has begun.	• Often a single vital sign that is abnormal should trigger an aggressive search for other more subtle changes taking place. • Ask the patient about habits (such as smoking, drinking, etc.) that will impact upon disease processes.

Introduction

Physiology is the branch of the biological sciences that studies the functions of a living organism and its component parts, including all chemical and physical processes.[1] The physiological processes of multicellular organisms can be examined at several levels of complexity—molecular, cellular, tissue, organ, organ system, and, finally, the entire organism. A true understanding of human physiology requires both the examination of basic individual processes, such as the generation of a heart beat, and an integrated view of processes, such as how the heart rate changes to help an organism adapt to states of anxiety, hypothermia, or hypoxia. Understanding physiology creates a better understanding of how you will help the human body overcome illness and injury. For example, the blood clot shown in the opening photo is your best friend when you are trying to stop a patient from bleeding to death. It is also your worst enemy when it has blocked the passage of oxygen to heart or lung tissue. Understanding how the body forms and destroys blood clots is essential to understanding why you administer thrombolytics to heart attack victims and apply hemostatic dressings to spurting arteries.

Regulation and Maintenance

Tissue cells cannot function properly unless they receive adequate nutrients and oxygen; are able to eliminate wastes and carbon dioxide; live in an environment that provides stable pH, temperature, fluid and electrolyte balance; and aquire a mechanism for appropriate stimulation.

Nutrients are used by cells to synthesize more complex molecules, such as proteins, complex carbohydrates, lipids, and nucleic acids such as DNA and RNA.

Some of these molecules are structural; lipids, for example, are components of all cell membranes, and protein filaments stabilize the position of organelles within the cell. Other complex molecules act as enzymes (complex proteins made by cells that catalyze [promote] a chemical reaction). Still others such as antibodies, signaling molecules, antigens, receptors, and ion channels, are involved in motility (movement) and contraction or are involved in the regulation of DNA expression, cell division, and metabolism.

Metabolism is a term that includes all of the chemical reactions that take place in an organism. Some of the reactions taking place in cells are **catabolic;** these reactions release the energy contained in the chemical bonds of complex molecules. Other reactions are **anabolic;** these reactions consume energy and are used to synthesize large biomolecules. At any given time, a cell is accomplishing both catabolic and anabolic reactions. Although individual, specialized cells have a range of metabolic rates (for example, neurons and liver cells have a very active metabolism while bone cells have a slow metabolism), all cells are continually synthesizing (making) and degrading molecules. These metabolic reactions require enzymes and may also require nutrients, energy, and oxygen.

Reactions that require an oxygen environment are called **aerobic,** and reactions that occur without the use of or need for oxygen are called **anaerobic.** Metabolic reactions typically release waste products, such as carbon dioxide (CO_2), acids, urea, creatinine, and heat, that need to be removed from the extracellular environment. If these wastes remain in close proximity to the cell, they can damage or kill the cell.

A very important function of nutrients is to serve as energy sources. Cells require energy to grow, synthesize proteins, transport molecules and ions through membranes, move, divide, and change shape. Cells extract energy from nutrient molecules in a process called cellular respiration. The extracted energy is then transferred to the chemical bonds of adenosine triphosphate (ATP) and related molecules. ATP acts as a "carrier molecule" for energy. Excess energy can also be stored as glycogen (a glucose polymer) or as lipid (fat) for conversion to ATP when additional energy is needed.

Most energy-transferring reactions in cells are called oxidation-reduction reactions, in which one molecule loses electrons and becomes "oxidized" and another molecule accepts electrons and becomes "reduced." The reactions of cellular respiration take place in three steps: glycolysis, the Krebs (citric acid) Cycle, and electron transport.

Glycolysis

In **glycolysis,** glucose is reduced in 10 consecutive catabolic (energy releasing) reactions. Glucose is the primary carbohydrate used for ATP generation in most cells.

Amino acids (derived from proteins), glycerol, and fatty acids (derived from triglycerides) can also be used for ATP generation by acting as substrates in glycolysis or the Kreb's Cycle. As a result of this pathway, pyruvic acid is generated, and the energy released is used to generate two ATP molecules and two molecules of the energy carrier molecule $NADH + H^+$.

The reaction of glycolysis is anaerobic; it takes place in the cytosol of the cell and does not require oxygen in order to occur. The pyruvic acid generated in glycolysis may be converted to lactic acid in a subsequent reaction that also does not require oxygen, and this process occurs in muscle cells of the body.

This form of metabolism (anaerobic) is not very efficient as it uses a lot of raw product and yields little gain; one molecule of glucose yields two ATP molecules and two molecules of pyruvate. Alternatively, the pyruvic acid can be taken into the mitochondria of the cell, and in the presence of oxygen (O_2) be further oxidized in reactions of aerobic metabolism. Mitochondria are specialized organelles (internal cell structures) rich in fats, proteins, and enzymes that produce energy for the cell through cellular respiration. These reactions generate CO_2 and H_2O and approximately 30 to 32 ATP per glucose molecule.

The aerobic metabolism of glucose, therefore, has a higher energy yield than the anaerobic reactions.

Hypoxia

Hypoxia is defined as a lack of adequate O_2 in cells, resulting in an impairment of tissue function (see Box 8-1). Hypoxia can result from many causes:

- A lack of O_2 in the environment (high altitude)
- An inability to take O_2 into the body (in lung or airway disease or a reduced rate of ventilation)[1]
- Reduced O_2 carrying capacity of the blood (hemorrhage, carbon monoxide poisoning, anemia)
- Poor blood circulation (heart disease, thrombosis)
- An inability of cells to utilize O_2 (cyanide poisoning)
- Any state in which O_2 consumption exceeds O_2 delivery

The exact consequences of hypoxia will depend on how much oxygen a particular cell requires. Neurons, for example, continuously require substantial oxygen to meet their metabolic needs. Therefore brain cells deprived of oxygen beyond four to six minutes begin to die.[2] Hepatocytes (liver cells) and skeletal muscle cells can survive for longer periods of time in low oxygen states, even up to several hours.

Without sufficient O_2 for aerobic metabolism, hypoxic cells are forced to generate ATP by anaerobic methods which may cause a state of energy deficiency,

BOX 8-1 What Is the Difference Between Hypoxia and Hypoxemia?

The amount of oxygen available to the tissues is a function of the arterial oxygen content (amount of oxygen in blood) and blood flow. Tissue hypoxia occurs in states of low cardiac output, low hemoglobin concentration, or low saturation of oxygen. **Hypoxia** is literally defined as a low oxygen state. It does not describe where, within the body, it is taking place, meaning it does not specify the blood as the site. The term hypoxia is also used to describe the condition of insufficient oxygen delivery to body tissues. Using the term in this manner creates confusion between hypoxia and hypoxemia.

Hypoxemia is an abnormally low arterial oxygen tension within the blood. In most situations when cardiac output (defined as stroke volume × heart rate) is within a normal range, hypoxia is most commonly caused by hypoxemia.

The terms hypoxia and hypoxemia are often used interchangeably; however, one state can occur without the other. For example, patients with chronic lung disease (such as COPD) may have a low oxygen level within the blood (hypoxemia), but because they have polycythemia (a higher than normal amount of red blood cells), they may have no tissue hypoxia. An alternative example can occur in a patient with anemia (a lower than normal number of functional red blood cells) who may have tissue hypoxia despite having a normal oxygen saturation level. Hypoxemia is arbitrarily defined in many medical references as a PaO_2 less than 60 mm Hg.

Systemic effects from chronic hypoxemia include the following:

- Increased RBC production.
- Pulmonary and cerebral hypertension; stress failure of pulmonary capillaries.
- Localized vasodilation in hypoxic tissues (except for lungs) causing cerebral edema.

a decrease in cellular pH **(acidosis),** and an increase in intracellular phosphate. The acidosis can adversely affect a wide array of cellular processes, including enzyme function, DNA and RNA structure and replication, protein synthesis, and membrane transport.

Acidosis alone can lead to cell, tissue, or organ death.

Street Secrets

When you find an increased respiratory rate, consider metabolic acidosis as a possible cause. This can help direct your attention as you assess and treat the patient.

Free Radicals

Hypoxia can also lead to the accumulation of dangerous chemicals called **free radicals.** These free radicals are partially reduced, meaning they contain an unpaired electron in their outer orbits. Because of this, they are unstable and highly reactive, and they quickly interact with other molecules in the cell, especially membrane phospholipids, cellular proteins, and nucleic acids, in an effort to "steal" another electron to complete their pairs. Free radicals have a life span of a fraction of a second.[3] When a free radical takes an electron, the af-

fected phospholipid, protein, or nucleic acid becomes damaged. This damage can lead to, among other things, loss of membrane integrity, alterations in calcium (Ca^{+2}) homeostasis, cancer, or premature cell death. Although cells contain natural antioxidant substances that utilize a number of strategies to prevent free radical accumulation, hypoxic cells may generate too many free radicals for the antioxidants to be effective.

CONNECTIONS Chapter 2: The Well-Being of the Paramedic focuses on healthy dietary choices and discusses foods that are rich in antioxidants and help rid the body of free radicals.

Homeostasis

Individual cells of the body may fail to function properly if the chemical, physical, or electrical property of the environment outside the cell (extracellular) is disrupted. Most of the processes that occur in the body function to maintain relative internal stability even when external conditions are fluctuating. For example, when you get dehydrated, you become thirsty; when you are overheated, you sweat; and when you are oxygen deficient, you may hyperventilate.

This property of organisms that drives them to remain in a healthy well-balanced state, called **homeostasis,** is the central, unifying theme of physiology. Disease often results when homeostasis is not maintained. Unresolved

Nice to Know

The term *physiology* is credited to French physician and philosopher, Jean Fernel (1497?–1559) who used the term to describe the study of the body's function. He is quoted as saying "Anatomy is to physiology as geography is to history; it describes the theatre of events."

dehydration can lead to decreased blood pressure and electrolyte imbalance; hyperthermia can lead to central nervous dysfunction; and hypoxia can result in acidosis, cellular edema, and toxemia. Any of these conditions may cause death.

Physiologic control mechanisms continuously monitor and make adjustments to variables, such as fluid volume, core body temperature, and blood oxygen, to maintain them within acceptable ranges. The acceptable value for any variable is called its **setpoint.**[4] Setpoints are each determined genetically but may be heavily influenced by external conditions as individuals adjust to changes. There are many examples of variables maintained in this way. Table 8-1 shows some of the normal variables and their normal ranges.

The control of a variable can be accomplished locally by cells. In these simple cases, the cells detect a change in a variable internally, or in the extracellular environment, and execute a corrective action. A common example of this is vascular autoregulation.[5] When the cells of a tissue are metabolically active, the O_2 levels and pH (described later in this chapter) fall, and the CO_2 levels and temperature rise. Cells that line the blood vessels respond by releasing paracrine factors that act locally to relax the muscles of the blood vessel wall. (**Paracrine regulation** refers to factors released by one cell that act on an adjacent cell in the same tissue.) The blood vessel then dilates, improving the blood flow to and from the area. For example, when the hormone somatostatin is secreted by pancreatic islet α cells

TABLE 8-1 Examples of Set Points Maintained By Control Mechanisms

Variable	Normal Range
Plasma pH	7.35–7.45
Plasma potassium (K^+)	3.8–5.5 mEq/L
Plasma glucose (fasting)	70–100 mg/dl
Temperature (adult)	96.8–99.5°F
Respiratory rate (adult)	12–20/minute

(alpha cells), it inhibits insulin secretion from nearby β cells (beta cells).[3]

Reflex pathways, called control mechanisms, utilize structures outside of the affected organs to accomplish regulation. Each control mechanism has three essential elements: receptors, a control center, and effectors. **A receptor** is activated when a variable moves outside of its desirable range. A **control (integration) center** assesses information registered by the receptor, compares it to its normal set point, and initiates a corrective change. One or more **effectors** are then triggered. Effectors are the structures of the body that actually accomplish the desired effect.[6]

A receptor is a specific site on or inside a cell, a whole cell, or a group of cells together that receive messages. These messages can be chemical, electrical, or both (electrochemical). An example of a control center is seen in the regulation of levels of the thyroid hormone. A small reduction in thyroid hormone triggers a rapid increase of thyrotropin-releasing hormone (TRH) and thyroid-stimulating hormone (TSH) secretion. This results in stimulation of the thyroid gland and increased thyroid hormone production. When thyroid hormone levels return to normal, a negative feedback loop suppresses TRH and TSH, and homeostasis of thyroid hormone levels is attained.[3] The effector in the above example is the thyroid gland in the neck, and the control center is located in the anterior pituitary gland in the brain.

Electrical and chemical messages are passed from receptors to control (integration) centers along **afferent pathways** and from control centers to effectors along **efferent pathways.** Control centers are typically located in the central nervous system or in endocrine glands. Afferent and efferent pathways are typically signaled by nerves or hormones.

Examples of afferent pathways in the body are the arterial receptors found primarily in the arch of the aorta and in the carotid sinuses. These receptors respond to both the force of blood coursing through the vessels (called the pulsatile force) and mean arterial pressure. The pressures from these two factors result in transmission of a signal to make adjustments in blood pressure.[7]

Efferent pathways are in operation when a patient responds to a blood volume loss with an increased heart rate and contraction force. Signals from the brain travel down the sympathetic nervous system to the heart to increase both the rate and force of contractions in an attempt to preserve cardiac output and the blood pressure (Figure 8-1).[8]

In most control systems, the output (or result) of the effector is a reversal of the original change, which serves to restore the variable to its normal acceptable range. However, because of the manner in which this works, either by shutting down or reacting to a change in progress, it is called a negative feedback mechanism

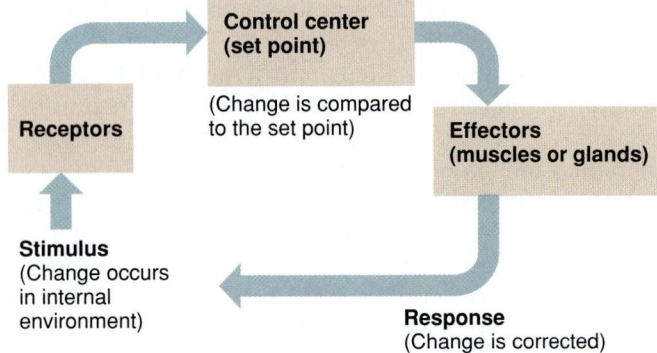

Figure 8-1   During homeostasis, physiologic control systems keep regulated variables within a desired range.

Integration and Control

Most control (integration) centers are located either in endocrine organs or in the central nervous system. The endocrine system is composed of glands that manufacture and secrete hormones into the blood. Figure 8-3 shows the endocrine system and its major glands.

Hormones are chemicals produced by living cells that circulate in the blood to signal organs and tissues to release other chemicals or affect processes and systems. Hormones can be divided into five major classes (see Table 8-2):

1. Amino acid derivatives such as dopamine, catecholamines, and thyroid hormone.
2. Small neuropeptides such as gonadotropin-releasing hormone (GnRH), thyrotropin-releasing hormone (TRH), somatostatin, and vasopressin.
3. Large proteins such as insulin or luteinizing hormone (LH) produced by endocrine glands.
4. Steroid hormones such as cortisol and estrogen that are synthesized from cholesterol-based precursors.
5. Vitamin derivatives such as vitamin A and D[3].

Hormones bind to specific target cell receptors and stimulate a range of responses depending on the nature of the hormone, the receptor, and the target cell. The functions of hormones include control of growth; development and reproduction; regulation of nutrient

(Figure 8-2a). These **negative feedback mechanisms** are designed to minimize deviation from the normal set point and maintain homeostasis.

There are examples of mechanisms in which the effectors act to move the stimulus farther away from its set point, and these regulatory mechanisms are called positive feedback mechanisms (Figure 8-2b). These **positive feedback mechanisms** do not accomplish homeostasis, meaning they do not readjust back to the set point. They actually magnify the deviation from the set point. There is not as much known about positive feedback mechanisms, and the manner in which they function is poorly understood.[3]

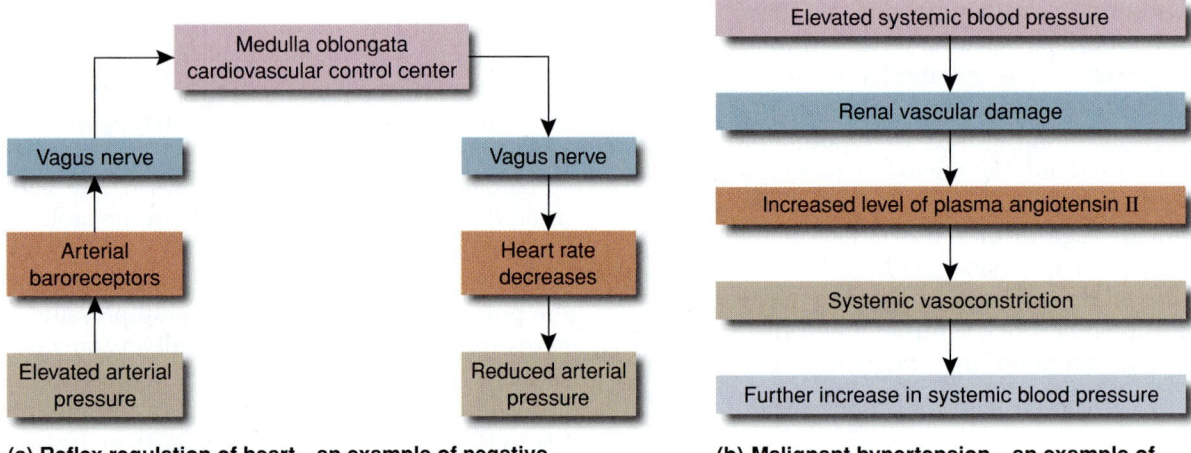

(a) Reflex regulation of heart—an example of negative feedback

(b) Malignant hypertension—an example of positive feedback

Figure 8-2   Examples of negative and positive feedback. (a) Negative feedback: The stimulus—elevated arterial pressure—activates baroreceptors located in arteries. The vagus nerve acts as an afferent pathway and sends impulses to the medulla oblongata, which contains the cardiovascular control center. The vagus nerve acts as an efferent pathway, sending impulses to the heart (effector). The heart rate is decreased. When heart rate decreases, arterial pressure decreases. (b) Malignant hypertension is an example of a positive feedback mechanism. Hypertension can lead to organ damage. Highly susceptible organs include the brain, kidney, and structures of the cardiovascular system. As shown here, high blood pressure leads to damage of blood vessels in the kidney. Reduced blood flow in the kidney leads to hypoxia. This condition initiates a series of reactions that leads to an increase in the plasma levels of a vasoconstricting chemical called angiotensin II. The induced systemic vasoconstriction causes a further increase in systemic blood pressure.

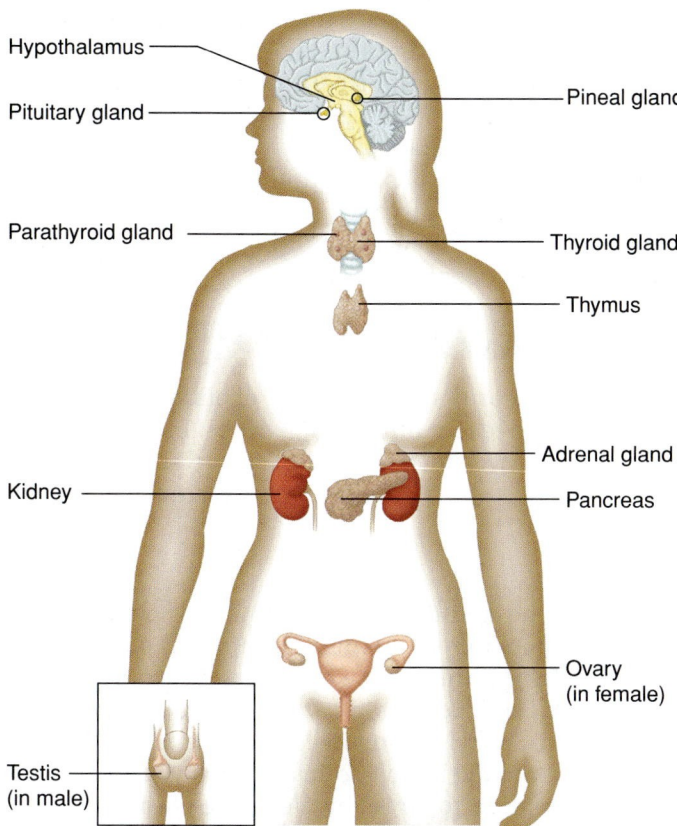

Figure 8-3 The location of the major endocrine organs of the endocrine system.

TABLE 8-2 The Five Major Classes of Hormones

Hormone Type	Examples
Amino acid derivatives	dopamine catecholamines (Epinephrine, norepinephrine, isoproterenol) thyroid hormone
Small neuropeptides	gonadotropin-releasing hormone (GnRH) thyrotropin-releasing hormone (TRH) somatostatin vasopressin (antidiuretic hormone or ADH)
Large proteins produced by endocrine glands	insulin luteinizing hormone (LH)
Steroid hormones synthesized from cholesterol-based precursors	cortisol and estrogen
Vitamin derivatives	Vitamin A Vitamin D

and electrolyte concentration; control of water balance, body temperature, and metabolism; and the coordination of adaptive responses to external stimuli (for example, stress). Table 8-3 lists some of the targets and effects of selected endocrine gland hormones.

TABLE 8-3 Selected Hormones, Targets, and Effects

Hormone	Source	Target Organ: Effect
Oxytocin	Hypothalamus	Breast: triggers lactation Uterus: initiates labor and triggers uterine contractions
Prolactin	Anterior pituitary	Breast: stimulates milk production
Antidiuretic (ADH) hormone	Hypothalamus	Kidney: water reabsorption
Growth hormone	Anterior pituitary	Many tissues: growth and metabolism, mobilizes fats, spares glucose
Thyroid hormone	Thyroid gland	Many tissues: growth, metabolism, and development
Parathyroid hormone	Parathyroid glands	Bone, kidney, intestine: increases plasma Ca^{+2} levels
Glucagon	Pancreas	Liver, many tissues: stimulates glucose production and elevated blood glucose, stimulates fat breakdown
Insulin	Pancreas	Many tissues: stimulates glucose uptake by cells, inhibits glycogen breakdown, stimulates the conversion of glucose to fat
Aldosterone	Adrenal cortex	Kidney: promotes Na^+ retention and K^+ elimination
Cortisol	Adrenal cortex	Many tissues: stimulates glucose production and elevated blood glucose, stimulates fat breakdown, suppresses inflammation and immune responses
Norepinephrine, epinephrine	Adrenal medulla	Cardiac muscle, smooth muscle, glands: elevates heart rate and force of contraction, increases metabolic rate, induces constriction of arteries and increases arterial pressure
Testosterone	Testes	Many tissues, sperm production, secondary sex characteristics, maturation of reproductive organs
Progesterone	Ovaries	Many tissues: breast development, cyclical changes in the uterine lining, fetal development

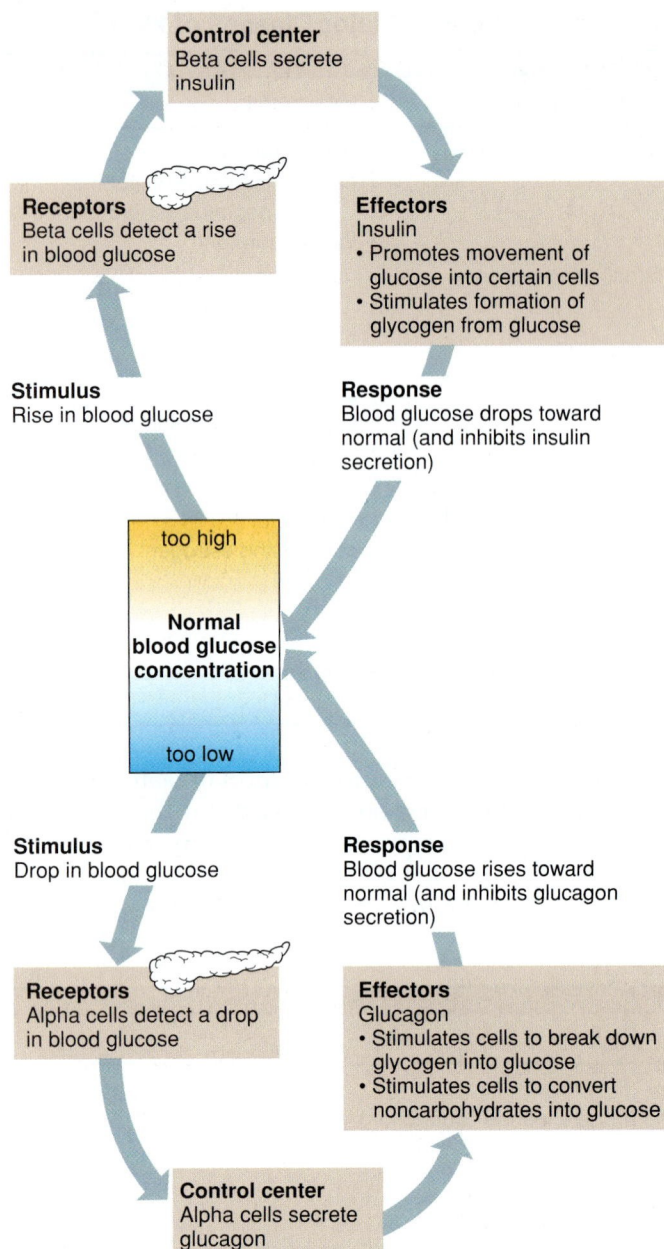

Control center
Beta cells secrete insulin

Receptors
Beta cells detect a rise in blood glucose

Effectors
Insulin
• Promotes movement of glucose into certain cells
• Stimulates formation of glycogen from glucose

Stimulus
Rise in blood glucose

Response
Blood glucose drops toward normal (and inhibits insulin secretion)

too high

Normal blood glucose concentration

too low

Stimulus
Drop in blood glucose

Response
Blood glucose rises toward normal (and inhibits glucagon secretion)

Receptors
Alpha cells detect a drop in blood glucose

Effectors
Glucagon
• Stimulates cells to break down glycogen into glucose
• Stimulates cells to convert noncarbohydrates into glucose

Control center
Alpha cells secrete glucagon

Figure 8-4 Insulin and glucagon regulate blood glucose levels. The pancreas is the control center for the variable blood glucose level. Homeostasis of blood glucose is noted with nonfasting levels between 80 and 120 mg/dL.

The endocrine system is involved in homeostatic regulation in two ways: (1) serving as a control center and (2) producing hormones. An endocrine gland itself can serve as a control center for a variable, as in the case of control of plasma glucose by the pancreatic hormones insulin and glucagon (Figure 8-4).

When plasma glucose rises after eating, the beta cells of the pancreas release the hormone insulin; insulin reduces plasma glucose by stimulating cells of the body to take up and use glucose for fuel, to convert glucose to glycogen or fatty acids, and to activate protein and triglyceride synthesis. This results in a lowering of blood glucose levels back to the normal range. When plasma glucose falls, alpha cells of the pancreas release the antagonistic hormone glucagon; glucagon elevates plasma glucose by converting glycogen, amino acids, and lactic acid to glucose. Another example of endocrine glands that serve as control centers are the parathyroid glands and thyroid gland that regulate plasma Ca^{+2} concentrations.

Street Secrets

Antagonism results when two chemicals work in opposition to each other. The drugs morphine and naloxone are classic examples of this. Naloxone binds to the same receptor sites as morphine and blocks its effects.

Endocrine glands can also be activated by other control centers to release their hormones. For example, stress can trigger the release of adrenocorticotropic hormone (ACTH) from the anterior pituitary gland (Figure 8-5). ACTH acts on its target cells in the adrenal cortex, stimulating them to release cortisol. Cortisol mediates adaptation to stress by elevating plasma glucose levels and by enhancing the effects of the catecholamines epinephrine and norepinephrine.

Nervous System Control

The **central nervous system (CNS)** is composed of the brain and spinal cord (see Figure 8-6 for details). The CNS contains many important control centers including those that regulate water balance, skeletal muscle tone, digestion, heart rate, blood pressure, and ventilation. Receptors communicate messages to the CNS using afferent neurons, and messages are delivered to effectors (muscles and glands) by efferent neurons. The efferent division of the nervous system is divided into two parts: somatic and autonomic. The **somatic branch** is used to activate skeletal muscles. The **autonomic branch** is used to activate cardiac muscle, smooth muscle, and glands.

The autonomic branch is subdivided into two branches: a **sympathetic** branch and a **parasympathetic** branch.

Although these two branches generally innervate the same structures, they have vastly different effects (see Figure 8-7).

The goal of the parasympathetic nervous system (PNS) is to help the body conserve energy resources and maintain a state of "rest and digest." As a result, parasympathetic nervous system activity is associated with reduced heart rate, reduced mean arterial blood pressure, and bronchoconstriction (which increases airway

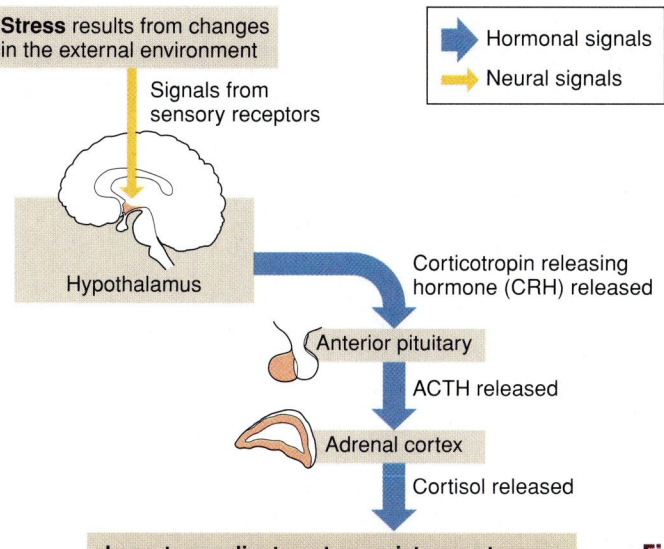

Stress results from changes in the external environment

Signals from sensory receptors

Hypothalamus

Corticotropin releasing hormone (CRH) released

Anterior pituitary

ACTH released

Adrenal cortex

Cortisol released

Hormonal signals
Neural signals

Long-term adjustment or resistance stage

• Increase in blood concentration of amino acids.
• Increased release of fatty acids.
• Increased glucose formed from noncarbohydrates—amino acids (from proteins) and glycerol (from fats).

Figure 8-5   A long-term stress response is seen when ACTH is released from the anterior pituitary. This leads to retention of water and sodium which increases blood pressure and volume. Proteins and fats are either converted to glucose or broken down and used for energy and the blood sugar levels rise. Unfortunately long term stress suppresses the immune system.

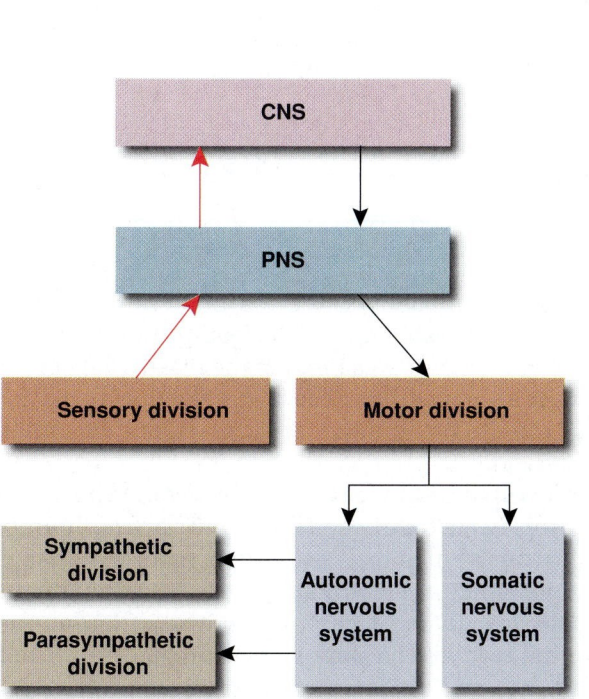

Figure 8-6   The central nervous system is made up of the brain and spinal cord. The CNS branches off to form the peripheral nervous system which has two divisions: sensory and motor. The motor division branches into the autonomic and somatic branches and the autonomic branches one more time into the sympathetic and parasympathetic divisions.

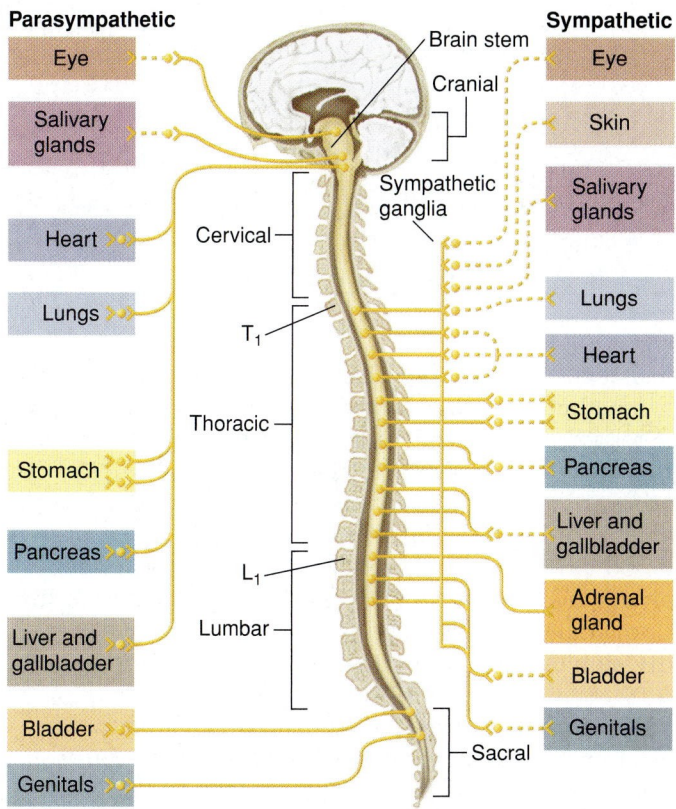

Figure 8-7   The brain and spinal cord showing where specific nerves leave the CNS and travel to target organs and tissues. Note that in this illustration, the parasympathetic nerves are on the left and the sympathetic are on the right.

TABLE 8-4 Effects of Autonomic Stimulation on Various Visceral Effectors

Effector Location	Response to Sympathetic Stimulation	Response to Parasympathetic Stimulation
Integumentary system		
Apocrine glands	Increased secretion	No action
Eccrine glands	Increased secretion (cholinergic effect)	No action
Special senses		
Iris of eye	Dilation	Constriction
Tear gland	Slightly increased secretion	Greatly increased secretion
Endocrine system		
Adrenal cortex	Increased secretion	No action
Adrenal medulla	Increased secretion	No action
Digestive system		
Muscle of gallbladder wall	Relaxation	Contraction
Muscle of intestinal wall	Decreased peristaltic action	Increased peristaltic action
Muscle of internal anal sphincter	Contraction	Relaxation
Pancreatic glands	Reduced secretion	Greatly increased secretion
Salivary glands	Reduced secretion	Greatly increased secretion
Respiratory system		
Muscles in walls of bronchioles	Dilation	Constriction
Cardiovascular system		
Blood vessels supplying muscles	Constriction (alpha adrenergic) Dilation (beta adrenergic)	No action
Blood vessels supplying skin	Constriction	No action
Blood vessels supplying heart (coronary arteries)	Dilation (beta adrenergic) Constriction (alpha adrenergic)	No action
Muscles in wall of heart	Increased contraction rate	Decreased contraction rate
Urinary system		
Muscle of bladder wall	Relaxation	Contraction
Muscle of internal urethral sphincter	Contraction	Relaxation
Reproductive systems		
Blood vessels to penis and clitoris	No action	Dilation leading to erection of penis and clitoris
Muscles associated with internal reproductive organs	Male ejaculation, female orgasm	

resistance and reduces air flow during ventilation). The sympathetic nervous system (SNS), on the other hand, is responsible for the "flight or fight" response, a state in which energy reserves are mobilized to deal with crisis. Sympathetic nervous system activity is associated with increased heart rate, increased mean arterial blood pressure, and bronchodilation (which reduces airway resistance and increases air flow during ventilation). Table 8-4 summarizes the effects seen when each division of the autonomic nervous system is triggered.

CONNECTIONS Chapter 15: Pharmacology has additional detail on the sympathetic and parasympathetic nervous system and describes many of the receptors found in each branch.

Figure 8-8 provides classification of some of the **ligands** that interact with hormone receptors. The term *ligand* is used to describe a group of cells, ions, or molecules that connect to a central atom in a complex of cells or tissues. Some of the ligands and the receptors they react with are presented in the figure. This provides you with a perspective of the complex inter-relationships that exist in the human body; it is not meant to be memorized.

In comparison to the endocrine system where efferent signaling is accomplished by slower-acting hormones, the nervous system uses nerve cells (neurons) that propagate quick-acting electrical signals (action potentials) in its pathway. In most cases, however, when an action potential reaches the end of a neuron, neutrotransmitter molecules are released from the neurotransmitter. Figure 8-9 shows two relationships: the hypothalamic-pituitary-target gland and the endocrine glands of the parathyroid and pancreatic islet cells.

Neurotransmitter is the name given to chemicals, such as epinephrine or acetylcholine, that serve to move (or transmit) a nerve impulse across a synapse. These

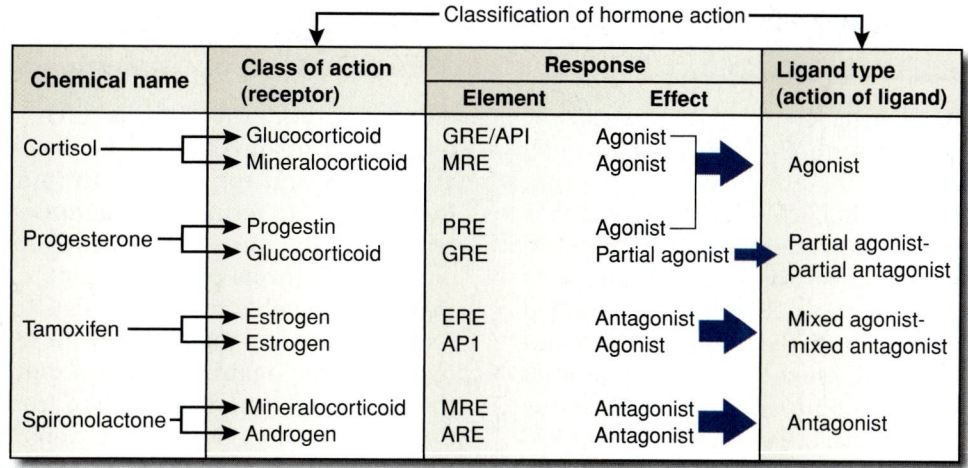

Figure 8-8 Shown are examples of different types of **ligands** with classification of the type of ligand and the receptors through which they interact. (GRE, glucocorticoid response element; AP1, activating protein 1; MRE, mineralocorticoid response element; PRE, progesterone response element; ERE, estrogen response element; ARE, androgen response element.)

neurotransmitter molecules diffuse across a small synaptic gap (space) at the end of the nerve to the target tissue (skeletal muscle, smooth muscle, gland, or another nerve cell) and bind to specific receptors on the target tissue membrane. Once bound, they exhibit a specific effect: Carry a message forward, block other messages from binding, and speed up the message transmission, among other effects. See Box 8-2 for additional information.

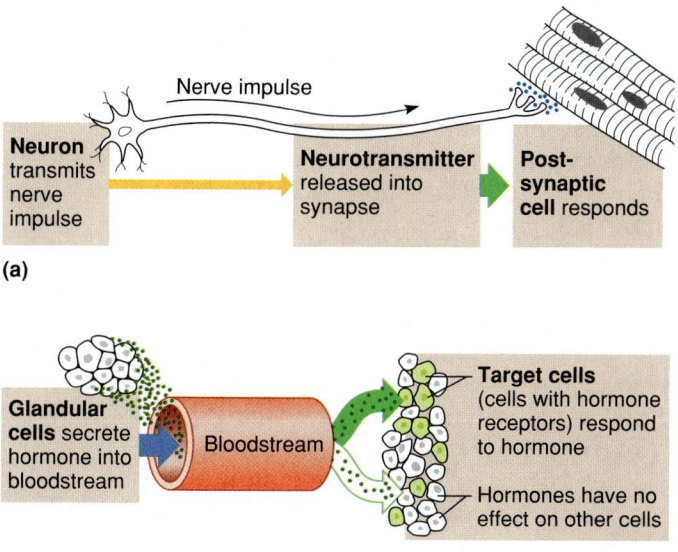

Figure 8-9 Chemical communication. (a) Neurons release neurotransmitters into synapses, affecting postsynaptic cells. (b) Glands release hormones into the bloodstream. Blood carries hormone molecules throughout the body, but only target cells respond.

Synapses

Synapses exist between afferent (sensory) neurons and CNS neurons, between neurons in the CNS, and between efferent neurons and their effectors (Figure 8-10). There are a staggering number of neurotransmitters that have been discovered, and they are classified in a number of ways.[8,3] One useful classification system groups neurotransmitters into categories based on their molecular structure: acetylcholine, amino acids, amines (derived from amino acids), polypeptides, purines, gasses, and lipids. A neurotransmitter may have several types of receptors that it can bind to (Table 8-5).

The existence of abundant types of neurotransmitters, the varied receptors available for individual neurotransmitters, and different types of target cells bearing these receptors enables neurotransmitters to induce a range of physiologic responses. For example, when norepinephrine (NE) binds to alpha$_1$ receptors present on vascular smooth muscle in the skin or GI tract, the result is vasoconstriction. NE also binds to beta$_2$ receptors present on vascular smooth muscle in skeletal muscles, inducing vasodilation.

Neurotransmitter molecules are inactivated, or removed, from synapses rapidly. Inactivation mechanisms usually rely on specific enzymes that degrade the neurotransmitter. Other neurotransmitters are taken back into the cell neuron that secreted it, or by another cell, or they diffuse away from the synapse.[3]

Many body systems contribute to the homeostatic maintenance of the extracellular environment, most importantly the cardiovascular, respiratory, digestive, and urinary systems. The cardiovascular system is essential for delivering O_2, nutrients, and hormones to the cells

BOX 8-2   What Is an Action Potential?

All body cells are electrically polarized (positively or negatively charged) with the inside of the cell more negatively charged than the outside of the cell. The difference in the electrical charge (voltage) is called the **resting membrane potential.** Electrochemical signals will cause the cell to change its resting membrane potential. This change, called the **action potential,** allows the signal to transmit from one cell to the next. Once the action potential threshold level is overcome, the cell membrane changes, and ions (electrically charged particles) can pass through the cell, changing the cell's charge. The cell then moves through three phases or states: **depolarization, repolarization,** and **polarization,** which is also called the resting or ready state. During depolarization, the ion balance changes as ions move into and out of the cell. Depolarization eventually peaks, and repolarization immediately begins. Repolarization returns the membrane to the original ready state by moving (pumping) ions back to their original positions on either side of the membrane. Because the cell's membrane has the ability to reset itself back to the ready state, the process can occur over and over again. The action potential represents the period of time from when the cell reaches the threshold energy level and depolarization begins until repolarization has reestablished the ready state. This process occurs in phases, and not every cell has an identical number of phases or identical timing intervals within each phase.[3]

of the body and for removing CO_2, wastes and the heat generated by cell metabolism. The respiratory system is responsible for taking O_2 into the body and eliminating CO_2. The digestive system is used for the intake and assimilation of nutrients. The urinary system is important for eliminating wastes, regulating ion and water balance, and controlling pH.

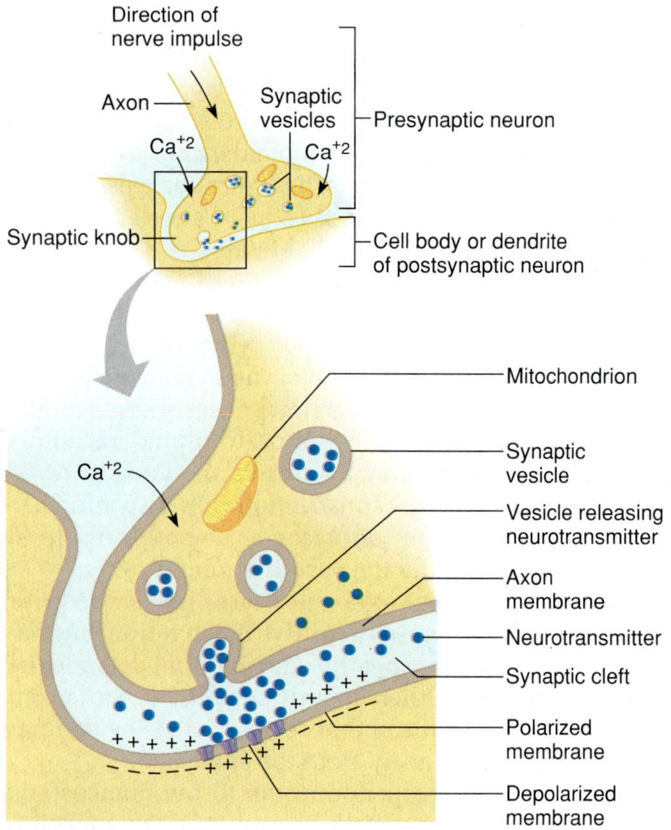

The Cardiovascular System

The cardiovascular system is responsible for circulating blood throughout the body. The heart is a muscular pump whose function is to collect blood from veins and eject blood into arteries. The heart is an organ made primarily of cardiac muscle. Cardiac muscle has several vital properties (see Table 8-6): **contractility** (the ability of muscle cells to shorten), **extensibility** (the ability to lengthen, within limits, without damage), **rhythmicity** and **automaticity** (the ability to regularly generate an electrical impulse to trigger contraction in the absence of an external stimulus), **conductivity** (the ability to spread the impulse), and **irritability** (the ability to respond to external stimuli).

The heart has an inherent contraction rate between 60–100 beats per minute (bpm) in the normal adult. Sinus bradycardia exists when the sinus rate is < 60 beats per minute, and sinus tachycardia is > 100 beats per minute. The normal value of the intrinsic heart rate (in beats per minute) can be calculated by the following formula: $118.1 - (0.57 \times age)$.[3,5]

A **cardiac cycle** is the time period extending from one heart beat to the next heart beat, and includes both **systole** (contraction) and **diastole** (relaxation) of the atria and the ventricles (Figure 8-11).[5] Blood, like other substances in nature, flows from areas of high pressure to areas of lower pressure. Compressing a fluid elevates its pressure. Pressure in the atria or ventricles of the heart is low when the heart muscle is in diastole and the chamber is enlarged (volume is high). Conversely, pressure in the atria or ventricle of the heart is elevated

Figure 8-10 Synapses serve as a bridge between one structure (like a nerve) and another (like a nerve or organ). Electrical messages are carried across the synaptic bridge to the other side.

TABLE 8-5   **Neurotransmitters**

Name	Type of Molecule	Receptors	Targets	Effect
Acetylcholine	Derived from choline and acetyl CoA	Nicotinic	Skeletal muscle cells, CNS	Excitatory at skeletal muscle; elsewhere, excitatory or inhibitory
		Muscarinic	CNS, ANS (parasympathetic targets and some sympathetic targets)	E.G., stimulates skeletal muscle contraction; reduces the heart rate, constricts the pupil, facilitates glutamate release in the CNS
Catecholamines			CNS	
Norepinephrine	Derived from amino acids (phenylalanine and tyrosine)	α and β adrenergic	CNS (brain) and ANS (a few sympathetic targets)	Excitatory or inhibitory; e.g., stimulates ventilation, increases heart rate and contraction force, generally induces vasoconstriction, except in heart, skeletal muscle, and skin
Dopamine			CNS (brain) and ANS (a few sympathetic targets)	Excitatory or inhibitory; e.g., involved in preventing muscle rigidity; induces euphoria; regulates prolactin release; involved in the regulation of renal function, blood pressure, and sodium homeostasis
Serotonin (5HT)	Derived from the amino acid tryptophan	5HT (many subtypes exist)	Many targets, including CNS (brain, spinal cord), GI tract, and platelets	Excitatory or inhibitory; e.g., involved in sleep, mood, appetite, nausea, and vomiting
GABA (γ amino butyric acid)	Derived from the amino acid glutamate	GABA-A and GABA-B	CNS and the retina	Generally inhibitory
Glutamate	Amino acid	AMPA, NMDA, Kainate, mGlu	CNS (brain and spinal cord)	Generally excitatory
Endorphin, enkephalin, dynorphin	Peptides	Mu, delta, kappa, sigma, epsilon	CNS (brain and spinal cord)	Generally inhibitory; e.g., analgesia

TABLE 8-6   **Cardiac Properties**

Property	Effect Seen
Automaticity	Ability to generate a spontaneous depolarization enabling the SA or AV node to pace the heart's electrical conduction system
Contractility	The ability of muscle cells to shorten (contract). **Inotropy:** affecting muscular contractility
Extensibility	The ability for cardiac muscle cells to stretch and lengthen without damage
Irritability	The property that permits the heart to react to electrical (nerve) stimuli
Rhythmicity	Ability to regularly generate an action potential in the conduction system. **Chronotropy:** affecting the heart rate
Conductivity	Ability of a nerve impulse to move through the electrical conduction pathway. **Dromotropy:** affecting the conductivity

when the heart muscle is in systole and the chamber is reduced in size (volume is small). The chambers fill with blood during periods of diastole and eject blood during periods of systole.

Stroke Volume

The arteries of the body receive blood from the ventricles and deliver it to the cells of the body. The right ventricle delivers deoxygenated blood to the pulmonary arteries in the lung, and the left ventricle delivers oxygenated blood to the arteries of systemic circulation. **Stroke volume** (in mL/min) is the amount of blood ejected by a ventricle each time it contracts. Stroke volume averages 70 mL per heart beat. Stroke volume has three major influences: (1) the length of the muscle cell at the start of contraction (also called preload), (2) the contractility of the muscle, and (3) the pressure the muscle must overcome when expelling the blood from the chamber (called the afterload).[3] Preload and afterload will be described in detail later in this chapter. Problems with the size or shape of the ventricle and dysfunction of the valves can also affect stroke volume.[5]

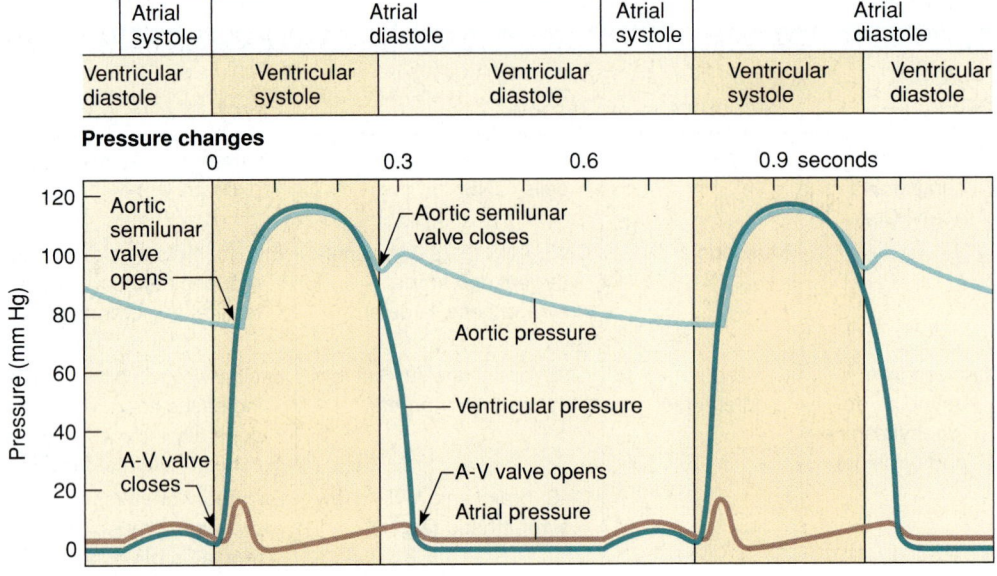

	Atrial systole	Atrial diastole		Atrial systole	Atrial diastole	
Ventricular diastole	Ventricular systole	Ventricular diastole		Ventricular systole	Ventricular diastole	

Figure 8-11 The relationship between cardiac pressure and stroke volume. Note that as pressure rises, stroke volume is declining.

Cardiac Output

Cardiac output, the volume of blood ejected by one ventricle per minute, is a measure of the heart's pumping effectiveness. Cardiac output is calculated by multiplying stroke volume (mL/beat) times the heart rate (beats/min).

The equation for cardiac output is $CO = SV \times HR$.

Example Calculate the CO for a normal adult with a heart rate of 72 bpm

$$\text{Cardiac Output (CO)} = \text{Stroke Volume (mL/beat)} \times \text{Heart Rate (bpm)}$$
$$CO = 70 \text{ mL/beat} \times 72 \text{ bpm}$$
$$CO = 5040 \text{ mL/min} \approx 5 \text{ L/min}$$

Cardiac output is directly proportional to heart rate in healthy, normal individuals. The average cardiac output, at rest, is approximately 5 liters/minute.

The average blood volume for an individual is estimated with the following equation: Blood volume = 65 mL/kg × body weight in kg.[5] For example, an adult weighing 85 kg would have approximately 5.5 L of blood (65 mL/kg × 85 kg = 5525 mL). The average adult blood volume is 5 liters; this means that each ventricle ejects the body's entire blood volume every minute under resting conditions. In persons with normal cardiac function, the cardiac output rises by more than 500 mL/min for each 100 mL increase in O_2 consumption per minute.[3] In individuals who are not actively exercising (sedentary), the cardiac output during maximal exercise increases approximately four times to an average of 20–22 L/min. In highly trained athletes, the CO may rise eight times to 30–40 L/min.[9]

This difference between resting cardiac output and maximum cardiac output is called the **cardiac reserve.** It is important to remember that the right ventricle and the left ventricle eject the same volume of blood each minute. If right ventricular output exceeded left ventricular output, blood would pool in the lungs; if left ventricular output exceeded right ventricular output, blood would pool in systemic circulation.

Changes in cardiac output can be accomplished by changing stroke volume, heart rate, or both. **Stroke volume,** the volume of blood ejected from a ventricle per beat, is defined by the equation: Stroke Volume, SV (mL/beat) = End Diastolic Volume (EDV) − End Systolic Volume (ESV) or SV = EDV − ESV. **End diastolic volume** is the volume of blood in the ventricle after it has finished filling (at rest, it averages 135 mL). The **end systolic volume** is the volume of blood remaining in the ventricle after systole (at rest, it averages 65 mL). Therefore, a sample average stroke volume for a person with an EDV of 135 and an ESV of 65 would be 70 mL/min (135 − 65 = 70).

The end diastolic volume is also called the **preload.**

CONNECTIONS See Chapter 7: Anatomy Overview, Figure 7-40, to see a diagram of the heart.

As mentioned previously, the stroke volume is influenced by the following factors: the EDV (preload), the strength of cardiac contraction, and arterial pressure (afterload). Since EDV is the volume of blood that the ventricle receives during the cardiac cycle, it follows that EDV increases whenever the veins deliver large volumes of blood to the ventricles. The volume of blood delivered to the heart during the cardiac cycle, called the **venous return,** is influenced by several factors: total blood volume, venous constriction or venous compression of large veins, skeletal muscle activity, and pressure changes in the heart, abdomen, and thorax during ventilation.

An increased total blood volume leads to an increased blood volume in veins and increased venous pressure. Constriction or compression of veins elevates pressure. Contracting skeletal muscles act externally on veins, especially in the extremities, squeezing them and elevating pressure. Because blood moves from areas of high pressure to areas of lower pressure, in each case, venous return is increased.

While inhaling, the size of the thorax increases and thoracic pressure decreases; at the same time, abdominal pressure increases as the contracting diaphragm flattens and moves towards the abdomen. A pressure gradient develops because of abdominal vein compression and thoracic vein expansion, triggering the movement of blood from the abdomen into the thorax and the heart. Another factor that increases EDV is increased time for ventricular filling (increased length of ventricular diastole).

Once the EDV has accumulated in a ventricle, it must move forward into an elastic artery of either the pulmonary circulation or the aorta. The amount of blood that leaves the ventricle (stroke volume) is dependant on the pressure gradient between the ventricle and the artery (afterload). Stroke volume, then, will be increased whenever ventricular pressure is elevated or arterial pressure is reduced.

The pressure within all the arteries and vessels of the circulatory system contributes to the pressure creating the afterload. The single most powerful determinant of the pressure created is the diameter of the lumen of the vessel the blood must flow through.[9] As blood vessels contract and the lumen diameter becomes smaller, pressure increases. Minimal amounts of pressure are contributed by the length of the vessel and the viscosity (thickness) of the blood. The pressure within the vasculature is called the systemic vascular resistance, or SVR.

Often the SVR and afterload are described as the same thing.[5]

Although the EMS provider does not have the clinical tools to measure systemic vascular resistance, a discussion of the components is included in order to clarify its

BOX 8-3 What Is Mean Arterial Pressure?

Systolic blood pressure (SBP) is measured at the peak of the systolic contraction of the ventricles. The lowest pressure is recorded at the midpoint in the diastolic relaxation phase during ventricular filling. This pressure is the diastolic arterial blood pressure (DBP). Pulse pressure is the difference between the SBP and the DBP. This measurement is obtained by weighting the averages to account for normal pressure changes occurring on a continual basis. This average over time is called the mean arterial pressure, or MAP. It can be estimated by using the following formula:

$$MAP = \frac{(SBP) + 2(DBP)}{3}$$

physiology. SVR can be calculated with the following equation:

$$SVR = 80 \times \frac{MAP - CVP}{CO}$$

MAP is **mean arterial pressure** and is measured in mm/Hg (see Box 8-3 for a discussion of MAP). CVP is **central venous pressure.** It is measured in the hospital setting by catheters inserted into the internal jugular or other suitable vein. It is generally not a prehospital procedure. CO is measured as liters per minute. The systolic blood pressure reading may be used as an approximation of left ventricle afterload pressure if the patient does not have any chronic changes in the size or shape of the heart.[5]

Frank Starling's Law of the Heart

Factors that elevate ventricular pressure include increasing the length (stretch) of cardiac muscle fibers prior to contraction and increasing the contractility.[9] The force of contraction generated by a cardiac muscle fiber is directly related to its resting length; when ventricles fill with increasing volumes of blood, the force of contraction increases proportionately. This relationship, called **Starling's Law of the Heart,** enables the heart to adapt to increasing venous return. (It is possible to overstretch cardiac muscle fibers; when that happens, there is a reduction in contractile force and possible cardiac failure.)

Starling's Law describes the relationship between CO and left ventricular end-diastolic volume and states that when the heart rate is constant, cardiac output is directly proportional to preload, until excessive end-diastolic volumes are reached. At that point, cardiac output does not appreciably change or may even decrease.[9] **Contractility** refers to changes in contractile force independent of muscle fiber length; factors that increase contractility are said to have a positive inotropic (contractile) effect and include the sympathetic nervous system and drugs (such as digitalis). Factors that reduce contractility are said to have a negative inotropic effect and include β adrenergic blockers and calcium channel blockers.

Nice to Know

Inotropic refers to muscle contractility. Positive inotropic effects promote muscle contractility, and negative effects suppress contractility.

The Impact of Heart Rate on Cardiac Output

Changes in heart rate also affect cardiac output. According to the equation, elevated heart rates lead to increased cardiac output while reduced heart rates lead to reduced cardiac output. However, at very high heart rates (usually > 170 bpm), the shorter duration of diastole limits the time available for ventricular filling. In these circumstances, the stroke volume falls (due to decreased length of diastole) so much so that the cardiac output decreases, despite an increase in heart rate.

Factors that elevate heart rate are said to have a positive chronotropic effect. These factors include an increase in sympathetic nervous system activity, a decrease in parasympathetic nervous system activity, and several drugs (such as isoproterenol). Conversely, negative chronotropic factors include decreased sympathetic nervous system activity, increased parasympathetic activity (increased vagal tone), and several drugs (such as digitalis).

Heart Rate and Venous Return

There is also a relationship between heart rate and venous return. When venous return increases, the pressure in the right atrium and vena cava increases, and the heart rate increases. This response, called the **right atrial reflex,** or **Bainbridge reflex,** allows the heart to eject a volume of blood that is equal to the volume it receives. This reflex is most active when the initial heart rate is low (it would be ineffective to increase the heart rate so much that it couldn't fill). Figure 8-12 summarizes the factors that affect cardiac output.

Blood ejected from the right ventricle enters the elastic arteries of the pulmonary circulation while blood ejected from the left ventricle enters the elastic arteries of the systemic circulation. The elastic arteries that receive blood from the heart expand when they receive a stroke volume (during ventricular systole); the pressure recorded in an artery at this time is called systolic arterial pressure (P_s). These arteries then recoil back on that blood during ventricular diastole and drive the blood into smaller, muscular arteries; the pressure recorded in the artery at the end of this period is called diastolic arterial pressure (P_d).

When arterial pressure is measured using a sphygmomanometer (BP cuff), it is recorded as P_s/P_d (see Figure 8-13). That is, for a blood pressure recorded as 110/68, the systolic arterial pressure is 110 mmHg, and the diastolic pressure is 68 mmHg.

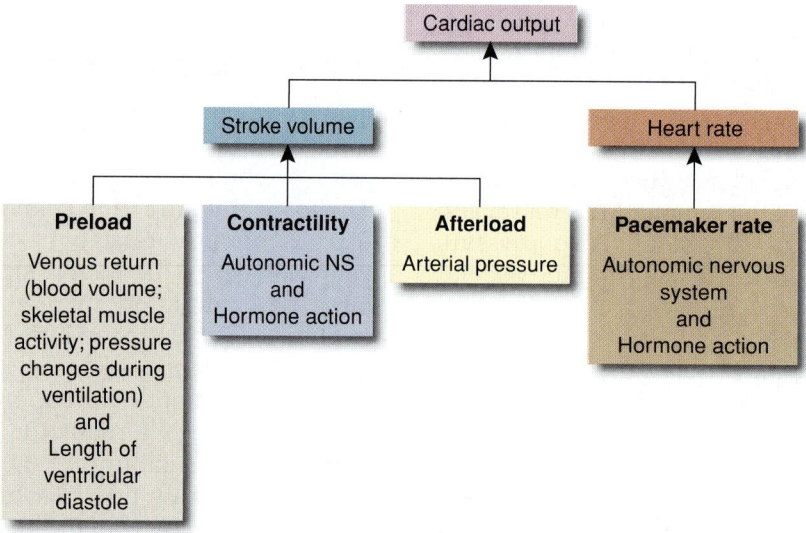

Figure 8-12   Factors that affect cardiac output

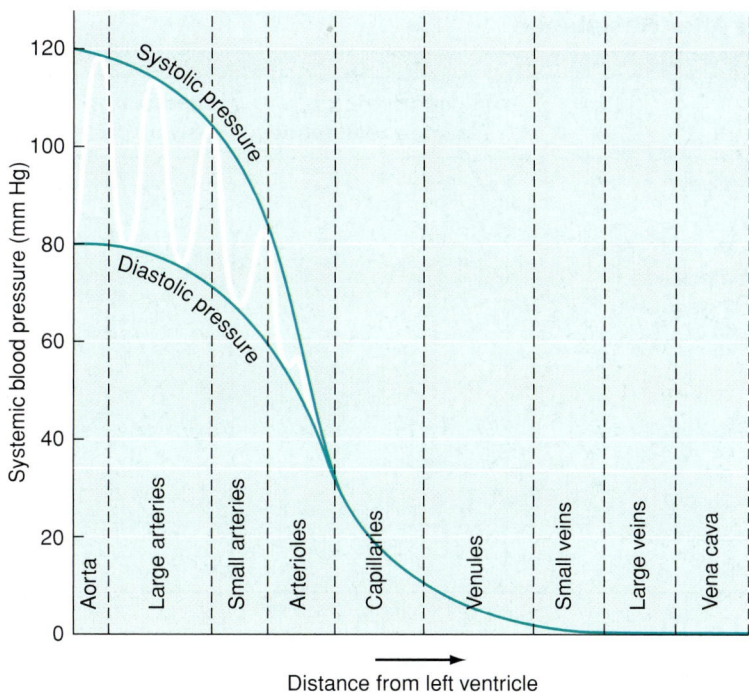

Figure 8-13 Pressures found within the systemic circulatory vessels of the body. Note the variability of pressure seen within the aorta. The pressure drops from the time blood exits the left side of the heart and it hits the lowest point just prior to entering the right side of the heart. Once blood reaches the capillary beds it is approximately 20 mm/Hg.

The difference between the systolic arterial pressure (P_s) and the diastolic arterial pressure (P_d) is called the pulse pressure.[3]

The change in pressure that occurs in arteries during the cardiac cycle can be felt as a pulse, or pressure wave. The strength of the pressure wave decreases as it travels through arteries to capillaries and cannot be felt in veins. Because blood pressure is highest in elastic arteries, blood moves into muscular arteries and arterioles and then the capillaries, venules, veins, and ultimately returns to the atria of the heart.

The average pressure in elastic arteries, that drives blood flow, is called mean arterial pressure (MAP) (see Box 8-3). Mean arterial pressure can be calculated as follows:

Mean arterial pressure (MAP) = [(SBP) + 2(DBP)] ÷ 3

or

$$MAP = \frac{(SBP) + 2(DBP)}{3}$$

Mean arterial pressure is important because it reflects the average pressure driving blood flow into smaller vessels during the cardiac cycle.[5] Note that mean arterial pressure is not an average of systolic and diastolic pressure; mean arterial pressure is actually closer to diastolic pressure because the ventricles spend more time in diastole than they do in systole during the cardiac cycle. For a cardiac cycle lasting 0.8 seconds, ventricular systole lasts for 0.3 seconds, and ventricular diastole lasts for 0.55 seconds. (Remember, these overlap somewhat as cells transition from one state to the next.)

Frictional Resistance to Blood Flow

While a blood pressure gradient is the driving force for blood flow, blood flow is opposed by frictional resistance. Blood encounters resistance when it flows against the walls of a blood vessel or when formed elements of the blood contact each other. Pulmonary vascular resistance (PVR) is the sum of all resistance in pulmonary circulation (averages (155–255 (dyne · sec)/cm), and systemic vascular resistance (SVR) is the sum of all resistance in systemic circulation (averages 900–1200 dyn · sec/cm).[5] Note that PVR is about one-fifth of systemic vascular resistance. Therefore, blood flow is directly proportional to the pressure gradient and inversely proportional to resistance:

$$Blood\ flow = \frac{Mean\ arterial\ pressure - Venous\ pressure}{Resistance}$$

Resistance, opposition to blood flow, is described by this equation:

$$Resistance = \frac{Vessel\ length \times Blood\ viscosity}{[Vessel\ radius]^4}$$

TABLE 8-7   **Chemicals that Alter Resistance**

Name	Source	Vasoconstrictor/ Elevates resistance	Vasodilator/ Lowers resistance	Other effects
Angiotensin II	Renin pathway	✓		Stimulates the secretion of aldosterone
Antidiuretic hormone (ADH)*	Hypothalamus (secreted from the posterior pituitary gland)	✓		Water retention and increased blood volume
Atrial natriuretic peptide	Atrial cardiac muscle		✓	Na+ elimination and decreased blood volume
Epinephrine/ Norepinephrine (NE)	Adrenal medulla	✓ (generally)		Increased heart rate and contractility
Nitric oxide	Endothelial cells		✓	
Endothelin	Endothelial cells	✓		
Histamine	Tissue cells		✓	

*at very high concentrations

The only variable in this equation that normally fluctuates is the radius of the blood vessel.[9] Most of the resistance encountered in the circulation of blood is in arterioles. When arterioles constrict, resistance increases and flow decreases. Factors that increase arteriolar resistance include the increased activity of the sympathetic nervous system and hormones, such as angiotensin II. Table 8-7 lists some of the important chemical factors that affect vessel diameter.

Remember that blood must flow from ventricles into elastic arteries and then from elastic arteries into the smaller vessels of circulation. Thus, it is important that MAP be low enough to accommodate ventricular ejection but high enough to facilitate blood flow to capillary beds. **Hypertension,** or elevated pressure, in arteries is dangerous because it can damage arterial walls and because it increases the workload on the ventricles. **Hypotension,** or reduced arterial pressure, is dangerous because it can lead to inadequate tissue perfusion.[10]

If you substitute "cardiac output" for blood flow and assume that venous pressure is 0 mmHg, a rearrangement of the above equations provides the following relationship:

Mean arterial pressure = Cardiac output × Resistance

Therefore, any factor that increases cardiac output or resistance, increases MAP; conversely, any factor that lowers cardiac output or resistance lowers MAP.

Both neural and endocrine regulatory mechanisms exist for controlling MAP. The baroreceptor (pressure sensing) reflex utilizes control centers in the medulla oblongata; the cardiac center controls heart rate, and the vasomotor center controls vascular resistance. The vasomotor center normally activates a tonic (contracted) state of vascular constriction, a state called vasomotor tone.[9]

The Vasomotor Center

When mean arterial pressure falls, baroreceptors found in the aortic arch and in the carotid sinus are activated.[9] Afferent nerves in cranial nerves IX (glosspharyngeal) and X (vagus) activate these control centers. The cardiac center sends a message through the sympathetic cardiac thoracic nerves to activate the sinoatrial (SA) node to increase the heart rate and increase cardiac contractility (to increase stroke volume). Both of these processes elevate cardiac output and, as a result, mean arterial pressure.

The vasomotor center responds to a decrease in mean arterial pressure by activating vasoconstriction, resulting in increased resistance and increased mean arterial pressure. Conversely, an increased pressure in the aortic arch and carotid sinus leads to activation of parasympathetic vagal outflow to the SA node and a reduction in heart rate. The vasomotor center decreases sympathetic outflow to blood vessels, which results in vasodilation and decreased resistance (Figure 8-14).

Chemoreceptors

Along with the baroreceptors present in the aortic arch and the carotid sinus, chemoreceptors are present to adjust MAP relative to plasma O_2 and pH. When plasma O_2 falls or pH falls, mean arterial pressure rises; conversely, if plasma O_2 rises or pH rises, mean arterial pressure falls. This allows mean arterial pressure to be adjusted relative to changes in metabolic rate. Elevated metabolic rate is characterized by reduced O_2, elevated

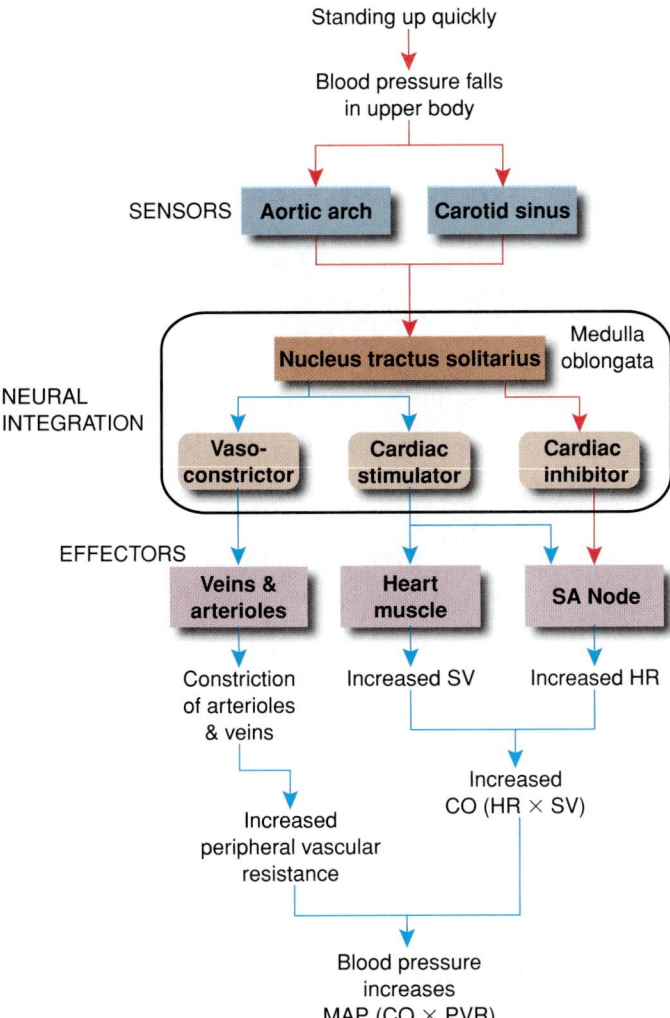

Figure 8-14 The baroreceptor reflex, which is triggered every time a person stands up, quickly adjusts the blood pressure back into the normal range. This is just one of the many baroreceptor control mechanisms.

CO_2, and reduced pH; reduction in metabolic rate is characterized by elevated O_2, reduced CO_2, and elevated pH.

Blood flows from elastic arteries into muscular arteries and arterioles that dilate and constrict to distribute blood to organs and tissues. Tissues receive blood according to their metabolic needs. During exercise, blood flow is directed to skeletal muscle, cardiac muscle, and the skin (for thermoregulation); while at rest, blood flow is directed to the digestive viscera and kidneys. The arterioles that supply these organs respond to local factors, increasing their diameter (thereby increasing blood flow) in response to reduced tissue O_2, reduced pH, elevated CO_2, elevated temperature, and elevated potassium (K^+).

Blood that flows from arterioles into capillary beds has a reduced velocity; this facilitates the diffusion of small nutrients and O_2 into intracellular fluid and the diffusion of CO_2 and waste products into the blood. Larger solutes such as proteins can pass through capillary walls by a process called transcytosis.[9] Bulk flow refers to the movement of water and dissolved solutes through capillary walls because of osmotic and hydrostatic pressure.

Additional Pressures within the Body

Hydrostatic pressure (fluid pressure) exists in both the capillary and in the interstitial fluid; fluid will move from an area of high hydrostatic pressure to an area of lower hydrostatic pressure. The presence of solutes (particles) in blood plasma and in interstitial fluid creates an additional pressure called **osmotic pressure**. Proteins are normally more concentrated in blood plasma than in interstitial fluid, so fluid is drawn into the capillary (blood osmotic pressure is greater than interstitial fluid osmotic pressure). **Net filtration pressure** indicates how much pressure is acting on fluid to move it through the wall of a capillary (see Figure 8-15):

Net filtration pressure =
  {Capillary hydrostatic pressure
  + Interstitial fluid osmotic pressure}
  − {Blood osmotic pressure
  + Interstitial fluid hydrostatic pressure}

Typically, fluid and dissolved solutes leave the capillary and enter the interstitial fluid at the arteriolar end of a capillary, and a smaller amount of fluid is reabsorbed into the capillary at its venous end. The fluid that is not reabsorbed back into the capillary must be absorbed by the lymphatic system, or tissue swelling (edema) will result. Edema can impair tissue function and compress blood vessels; this is particularly dangerous when edema occurs in the lungs or in the brain. Systemic edema involves a shift of fluid from the blood into the interstitial spaces, which results in reduced blood volume and reduced mean arterial pressure; this is a potentially lethal condition.

The cardiovascular system exists to perfuse tissues. Shock, a generalized failure to deliver oxygenated blood to tissues, can result from a variety of causes including the following:

- Heart failure leading to reduced cardiac output (called cardiogenic shock).
- Reduction in blood volume which leads to reduced stroke volume and cardiac output (called hypovolemic shock).
- Bacterial toxins which induce vasodilation and reduced resistance (called septic shock).
- Failure of the vasomotor center to maintain vasomotor tone (neurogenic or vascular shock).

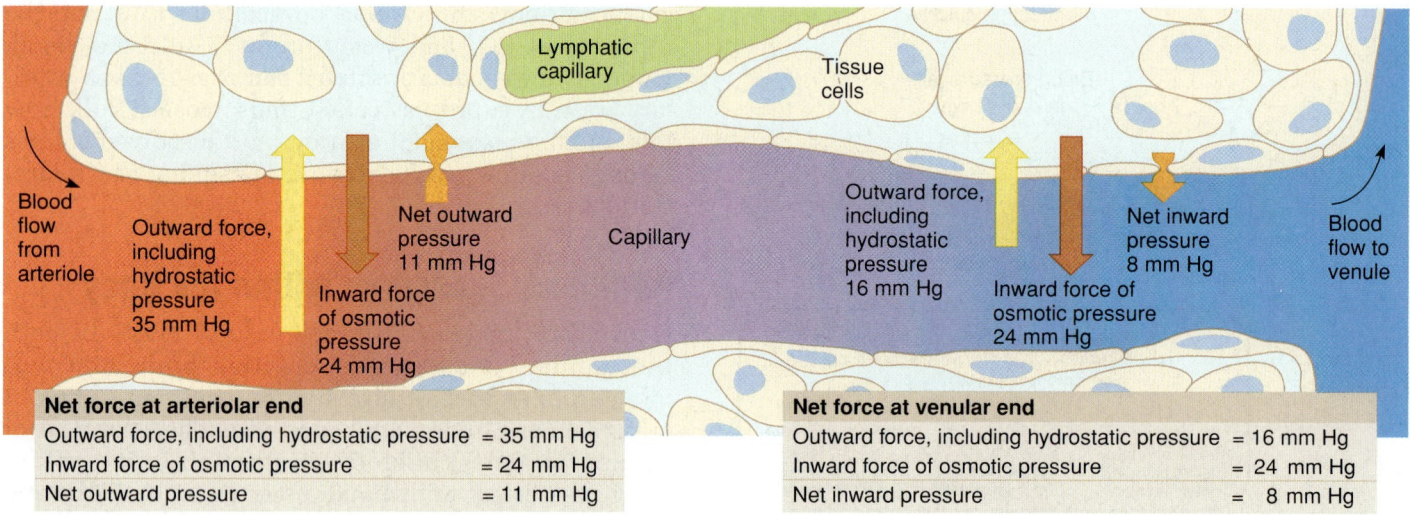

Figure 8-15 Capillary net filtration pressure (NFP). As blood enters the proximal end of the capillary bed, NFP is high enough to force fluids out of the capillary. Oxygen is pushed out also, and it can travel to neighboring cells. At the distal end of the capillary bed, NFP is low, and some fluids move back in bringing CO_2 and wastes along for removal from the body.

- Massive immune reactions that lead to systemic vasodilation and increased capillary permeability (called anaphylactic shock).

For most types of shock, low blood pressure and reduced urine formation clinically characterize this disorder. Cells may sustain irreversible damage from a lack of O_2 and a buildup of waste products.

CONNECTIONS See Chapter 13: Shock Overview and Chapter 19: Trauma and Hemorrhagic Shock for more information on shock.

The Respiratory System

The respiratory system functions to bring O_2 into the blood and remove CO_2 from the blood. The organs of the respiratory system largely function as conduits for air to flow into alveoli (during inspiration) and out of alveoli (during expiration). Air, like blood, flows from areas of high pressure to areas of low pressure and is impeded by resistance. Thus in order to inhale, atmospheric pressure must be higher than intra-alveolar pressure, and in order to exhale, intra-alveolar pressure, must be higher than atmospheric pressure.

The phrenic and intercostal nerves are used to reduce intra-alveolar pressure and accomplish inhalation. The diaphragm is stimulated to contract by the phrenic nerve, which causes it to pull lower toward the abdomen. Then the external intercostal muscles are stimulated to contract by the intercostal nerve, which in turn raises and opens the rib cage. The end result of both of these processes is that the size of the thorax increases, and the intrathoracic pressure decreases.

As the lungs expand, intra-alveolar pressure falls. As this process is occurring, air is being pulled in, because of the drop in pressure, to fill the lungs. At the peak of this process, the contracted muscles transition from their contraction phase to relaxation, and they begin to relax and shorten. The muscle fibers return back to their normal size, and the chest cavity size decreases. As the thorax gets smaller, the intra-alveolar pressure rises. As the pressure continues to rise, it elevates to just slightly above atmospheric pressure. Air now passively flows out from the alveoli and tracheobronchial tree, and exhalation occurs (Figure 8-16).

Ventilation and Respiration

Ventilation is the mechanical process of air flowing into and out of the structures of the respiratory system.[5] This process is often misnamed respiration, which over time has become a common substitute term. However, **respiration** is actually the exchange of the gasses oxygen and carbon dioxide that occurs in the lung and tissues. In the lung, respiration occurs between the alveoli and pulmonary capillary membrane. Within the capillary beds, oxygen and carbon dioxide diffuse between the cells of the tissues and the red blood cells within the capillary beds.

The actual definitions and the working definitions of respiration and ventilation are further confused when terms such as **"respiratory rate"** are used. This term would be correct if it were called the ventilation rate instead of the respiratory rate since what is actually counted is the number of cycles of inhalation and exhalation that occur in one minute. Conventional use of terminology has lead to the use of the "respiratory rate"

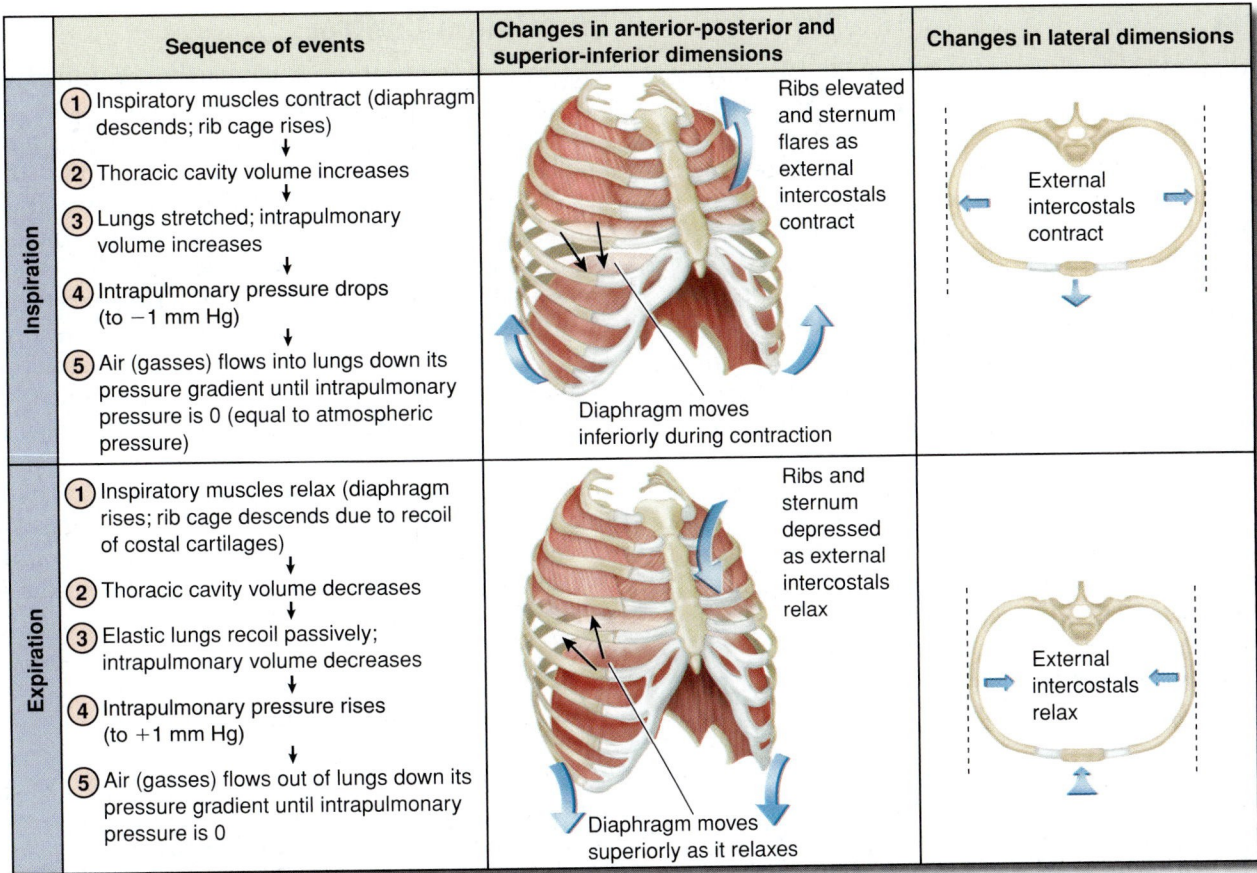

	Sequence of events	Changes in anterior-posterior and superior-inferior dimensions	Changes in lateral dimensions
Inspiration	① Inspiratory muscles contract (diaphragm descends; rib cage rises) ↓ ② Thoracic cavity volume increases ↓ ③ Lungs stretched; intrapulmonary volume increases ↓ ④ Intrapulmonary pressure drops (to −1 mm Hg) ↓ ⑤ Air (gasses) flows into lungs down its pressure gradient until intrapulmonary pressure is 0 (equal to atmospheric pressure)	Ribs elevated and sternum flares as external intercostals contract Diaphragm moves inferiorly during contraction	External intercostals contract
Expiration	① Inspiratory muscles relax (diaphragm rises; rib cage descends due to recoil of costal cartilages) ↓ ② Thoracic cavity volume decreases ↓ ③ Elastic lungs recoil passively; intrapulmonary volume decreases ↓ ④ Intrapulmonary pressure rises (to +1 mm Hg) ↓ ⑤ Air (gasses) flows out of lungs down its pressure gradient until intrapulmonary pressure is 0	Ribs and sternum depressed as external intercostals relax Diaphragm moves superiorly as it relaxes	External intercostals relax

Figure 8-16   Pressure changes in the thorax during ventilation.

instead of ventilation rate to describe this process. The term **ventilation rate** is often applied to mean the number of ventilation breaths given when performing bag mask ventilation or when the patient is connected to a ventilator or other device forcing air into the patient. **Minute ventilation** is calculated as the amount (volume) of air moved in and out of the lungs multiplied by the minute respiratory rate.[11]

Respiration

Oxygen diffuses from the inhaled air in alveoli, which has a high pO_2, into the blood of pulmonary capillaries, which has a lower pO_2.[7] (See Table 8-8 for information on pO_2 and other related terms.) The oxygen binds to hemoglobin and is carried by arterial blood to tissue cells. A small amount of the plasma O_2 dissolves in water (1.5%), and the majority (98.5%) enters the erythrocytes and combines with hemoglobin. Each hemoglobin molecule can carry up to four O_2 molecules.[11] When this oxygenated blood flows into tissue capillaries, the O_2 diffuses from the capillary blood into the interstitial fluid. Under normal resting conditions, about 25% of the O_2 carried by the blood is released to tissue cells. Additional O_2 can be released when tissues

are metabolically active; hemoglobin loses affinity for O_2 and releases additional O_2 whenever tissue pO_2 falls, tissue pH falls, tissue pCO_2 rises, or tissue temperature rises.

TABLE 8-8   Respiration Terminology

Value	Definition
FiO_2	The percent concentration of oxygen in inspired air, ventilator, or a blood oxygenator
pO_2	Partial pressure of O_2 in a mixture of gasses or in solution; measured in mm Hg
SaO_2	The percentage of available hemoglobin binding sites in arterial blood occupied by oxygen
PaO_2	Partial pressure of O_2 dissolved in the plasma of arterial blood
$PaCO_2$	Partial pressure of CO_2 dissolved in the plasma of arterial blood
pCO_2	Partial pressure of CO_2 in a mixture of gasses or in solution; measured in mm Hg
$SaCO_2$	The percentage of available hemoglobin binding sites in arterial blood occupied by CO_2

Hypoxia

The amount of O_2 carried by the blood depends on the amount of O_2 present in the alveoli. This requires an adequate supply of O_2 in the environment and requires effective ventilation. Hypoxia, which was described earlier in this chapter, is present with a lower than expected oxygen level which results in less oxygen reaching the target cells and tissues of the body. Any disease that increases airway resistance or impairs the ability of air passageways to change size (and alveolar pressure) will decrease O_2 diffusion into the plasma. Blood O_2 also depends on the presence of erythrocytes (red blood cells) and the presence of an adequate amount of functional hemoglobin. Compensation for hypoxemia includes an increased rate of ventilation (if plasma pO_2 falls below 60 mmHg), increased vasomotor tone (sensitivity of carotid and aortic chemoreceptors increases), and increased erythropoiesis (red blood cell production). The kidney synthesizes and secretes the hormone erythropoietin when blood pO_2 falls. Erythropoietin travels in the blood and binds to pro-erythroblasts, stimulating their development into red blood cells.

Working in the Gray Zone

Although the body can compensate for gradual chronic hypoxia by increasing the number of red blood cells, this compensating mechanism will not be seen acutely when you encounter a traumatically injured patient. These patients will need emergent attention to control further blood loss, and treatment for shock will include providing an increased concentration of oxygen in the air they are breathing in order to maximize the amount of oxygen carried by their decreased amount of red blood cells.

Carbonic Acid

Carbon dioxide (CO_2), a waste product produced by tissue cells, diffuses into tissue capillaries and is carried in venous blood to the alveoli. The CO_2 is carried in three ways: a small amount (about 7%) dissolves in the plasma, approximately 23% binds to hemoglobin, and most of the CO_2 reacts with water to form H_2CO_3 (carbonic acid).[11] The carbonic acid yields HCO_3^- (bicarbonate). When these various forms of CO_2 reach the lungs, the CO_2 will diffuse out of the capillary into the alveoli and be eliminated from the body during exhalation.

$$HCO_3^- + H^+ = CO_2 + H_2O$$

Ventilation Control

The rate of ventilation is primarily controlled by the respiratory centers of the medulla oblongata.[5] These centers are most sensitive to changes in plasma pCO_2 and the pH of cerebrospinal fluid. Elevated pCO_2 causes systemic acidosis, and reduced pCO_2 causes alkalosis. These are serious alterations in pH that can be lethal if uncorrected. When pCO_2 rises, the respiratory center activates an increased rate of ventilation **(hyperventilation)** to allow the body to exhale CO_2. Conversely, when pCO_2 falls, the respiratory center activates a decreased rate of ventilation **(hypoventilation)** to allow the body to retain CO_2. Hypoventilation, to retain CO_2, also means that O_2 intake is reduced. This is generally not a problem since hemoglobin normally releases only 25% of the O_2 that it is carrying to tissues.[9] The extra O_2 acts as a reserve that can be critically important under conditions of hypoventilation (think about swimming under water without taking a breath).

The Urinary System

Blood flowing through tissues picks up waste products that must be eliminated from the body. The kidneys are responsible for eliminating waste products, including urea, uric acid, and creatinine. They are also responsible for eliminating excess ions, excess water, neurotransmitters and other drugs, and excess acid (H^+). The kidneys must manufacture at least 500 mL of urine daily to eliminate the accumulated wastes, but the average daily urine volume is closer to 720–1200 mL (30–50 mL/hr).[2]

The kidneys utilize mechanisms of filtration and secretion to manufacture urine. Blood pressure is the driving force for filtration, and when blood pressure falls, urine output falls.[3] During filtration, plasma components smaller than the larger proteins move from renal capillaries into epithelial renal tubules (nephrons). These particles form a substance called filtrate.[12]

Water Conservation

The kidneys require pressure to filter the blood, and there are many mechanisms in place to ensure that renal pressure is maintained. Perhaps the most important of these mechanisms, systemically, is the **renin-angiotensin mechanism.** When renal pressure falls, or when the renal filtrate is dilute or slow moving, renin is released from kidney cells into the blood. Renin is an enzyme that acts on angiotensinogen (an inactive plasma protein), forming angiotensin I. Angiotensin I is acted on by angiotensin converting enzymes (ACE) to form angiotensin II. Angiotensin II is a potent vascoconstrictor that elevates systemic pressure by elevating resistance with vasoconstriction. Angiotensin II also acts on the adrenal cortex and stimulates the release of aldosterone. Aldosterone acts on renal tubules to increase retention of Na^+ and H_2O, and it also triggers the secretion of K^+ into the urine. The retention of Na^+ and H_2O elevates the blood volume, end diastolic volume, stroke volume, and mean arterial pressure. The SNS can also trigger renin release from the kidney when systemic pressure falls; this is independent of the use of renin to elevate renal filtration pressure.[9,11,5]

Kidneys are stimulated to restore H_2O to the body by **antidiuretic hormone** (ADH), which is also called vasopressin. ADH is a small peptide that enables the body to conserve H_2O. ADH is manufactured by the hypothalamus and is stored and secreted by the posterior pituitary gland. ADH is released from the posterior pituitary gland when the blood plasma becomes too concentrated with solute (particles) or when blood pressure falls. It stimulates the cells of kidney tubules to manufacture membrane water channels from proteins. These channels are called aquaporins.[3] These channels provide a mechanism for water that was filtered out to return to the bloodstream. In the absence of ADH, individuals eliminate large amounts of water.

Water Excretion

Atrial natriuretic peptide (ANP) is a peptide hormone produced by atrial myocardial cells that acts as an antagonist to aldosterone and ADH.[8] ANP is released when atrial pressure increases, as it might if the blood volume were too high (it is released during hypervolumetric conditions or during congestive heart failure). This hormone appears to decrease aldosterone secretion by the adrenal cortex, increase the rate of renal filtrate formation, decrease Na^+ retention, and decrease renin release. As a result, ANP causes a reduction in blood volume, a reduction in cardiac

Working in the Gray Zone

Because ADH release is triggered by blood osmolarity it is unlikely that an acute blood loss will trigger its release. An acute blood loss will cause a loss of all components of the blood: plasma, red and white cells, and all the wastes and nutrients it was carrying. A concentration and accumulation of wastes will increase osmolar pressure and will trigger ADH release. With an acute blood loss, the blood pressure is preserved through vasoconstriction and increased work by the heart (increased rate and contraction force).

output, and a reduction in mean arterial pressure. The kidneys also play a vital role in the regulation of plasma pH by secreting H^+ into the urine and adding $NaHCO_3$ to the blood.

The Acid/Base Balance

The amount, or concentration, of hydrogen ions in the body is the basis for the measurement of **pH.** The normal values for blood, interstitial fluid, intracellular fluid, and many other fluids of the body are well-known, and Figure 8-17 lists the pH of several body fluids. Normal pH values differ among the various body fluids. The pH is measured on a standard scale (values < 7 are labeled acidic; 7 is neutral; and values > 7 are labeled basic or alkaline). The pH of blood plasma normally ranges from 7.35–7.45, which is slightly alkaline compared to neutral (7.0).

The maintenance of normal pH values is important because alterations in pH can affect protein structure and, therefore, function. Enzymes, membrane channels, and structural proteins are sensitive to the pH of their local environments. The cells of the body generate acids from internal metabolism (for example lactic acid

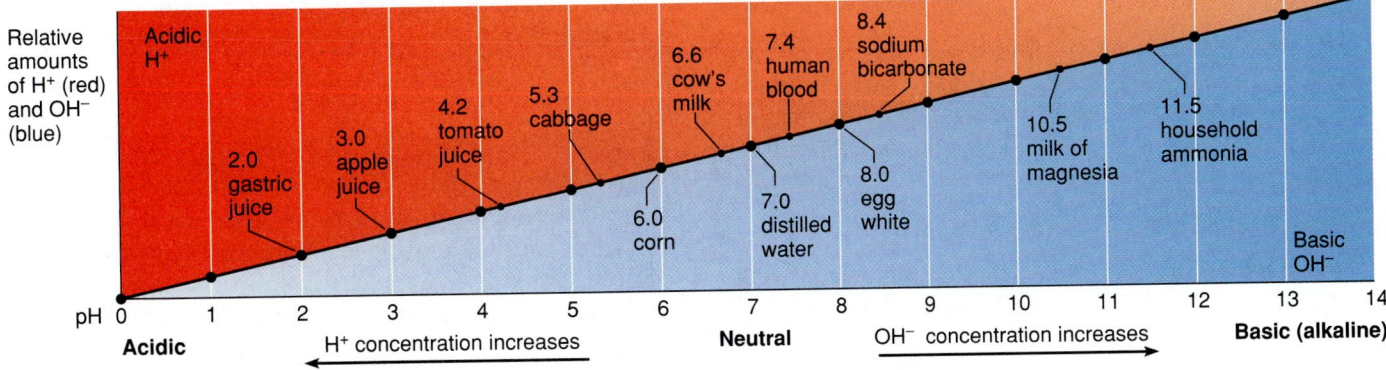

Figure 8-17 This pH scale shows the pH of blood and other body fluids along with many other common liquids.

produced by anaerobic metabolism). Foods can also be a source of acids (such as fatty acids and amino acids).

One of the primary sources of acid for body regulation is CO_2 since CO_2 can react with water to form H_2CO_3 (carbonic acid). CO_2 is produced by the body's metabolism at approximately the same rate as oxygen consumption. At rest, this value is about 3 mL/kg per minute, but it may increase dramatically with heavy exercise.[13]

Street Secrets

pH can affect medication effectiveness. Many medications are either weak acids or weak bases. The membrane of a cell is altered by changes in pH, resulting in changes to the permeability (ease of passage) of substances into and out of the cell. These changes in pH may affect the ability of some drugs to cross into the cells. All of the catecholamine drugs (including epinephrine) are especially susceptible to the pH of the blood. This means that patients in an acidotic state caused by cardiac arrest may not be responsive to epinephrine until a more normal pH level is restored.

Acidosis and Alkalosis

Acidosis is a condition in which plasma pH falls below 7.35; it can lead to, among other things, central nervous system depression, lethargy, coma, and death. **Alkalosis** is a condition in which the plasma pH rises above 7.45; it can lead to hyperexcitability, numbness and tingling, muscle tetany (spasms brought on by mineral imbalance), muscle paralysis, and death.

pH Buffers

The body maintains pH using buffers, by controlling the ventilation rate and acidifying the urine.[7] **Buffers** are substances that act to prevent fluctuations in pH. The primary buffer system operating in blood plasma is the plasma proteins; amino acids can bind to H^+ to prevent acidosis or donate H^+ to prevent alkalosis. A good example of a protein buffer is the hemoglobin found in red blood cells.

Another buffer system found in plasma is the $NaHCO_3$ (sodium bicarbonate) and H_2CO_3 (carbonic acid) buffer pair. These compounds work as a team to prevent fluctuations in either the acidic or alkaline direction. Sodium bicarbonate buffers excess acids as follows:

$$NaHCO_3 + H^+ \rightarrow Na^+ + H_2CO_3$$

The products are Na^+ and carbonic acid, a very weak acid. Carbonic acid buffers excess base as follows:

$$H_2CO_3 + OH^- \rightarrow H_2O + HCO_3^-$$

The OH^- (base) binds to H^+ in the H_2CO_3 molecule forming water and bicarbonate ion.

Even though most buffering is accomplished by plasma proteins, the $NaHCO_3/H_2CO_3$ buffer system is a clinically important buffer system because the amount of each substance fluctuates relative to ventilation rate and renal function. The amount of H_2CO_3 is dependant on the ventilation rate since it is formed from CO_2 and H_2O. Therefore, hyperventilation decreases pCO_2, decreases H_2CO_3, and leads to alkalosis (less base is being buffered); this is called respiratory alkalosis. Healthy kidneys will respond by eliminating $NaHCO_3$ in the urine.

CONNECTIONS The kidneys' corrective measures for acid or base imbalances take hours or days to occur. These will not be seen in the acute emergency situation. Chapter 13: Shock Overview will discuss the acid base balance in more detail.

Normally, the reaction between CO_2 and water occurs slowly, but carbonic anhydrase reversibly accelerates this reaction several thousand times.[13] CO_2 rapidly diffuses across the luminal membrane (in the blood tubule) into the epithelial cell where it reacts with water to form H_2CO_3, a reaction catalyzed by cytoplasmic carbonic anhydrase.

Respiratory and Metabolic Considerations

Hypoventilation increases pCO_2, increases H_2CO_3, and leads to respiratory acidosis (where more acid builds up). When respiratory acidosis occurs, healthy kidneys will respond (or compensate) by eliminating H^+ in the urine and adding $NaHCO_3$ to plasma.

Any other cause of alkalosis or acidosis is called metabolic. For metabolic conditions, both the kidneys and the lungs can attempt compensation. During metabolic acidosis, the kidneys will eliminate H^+ and add $NaHCO_3$ to the blood, and hyperventilation will occur. During metabolic alkalosis, the kidneys will not eliminate H^+, and hypoventilation will occur. Box 8-4 gives you a guide to use to distinguish between metabolic and respiratory causes of alkalosis and acidosis.

Summary

A basic foundation of anatomy and physiology is essential for understanding the signs and symptoms of the various diseases and traumatic conditions presented by patients. Understanding basic principles of physiology will allow you to focus the history and physical examinations toward elements pertinent to the situation presented. Table 8-9 provides a summary of the formulas covered in this chapter.

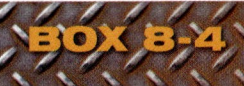

BOX 8-4 Distinguishing Between Metabolic and Respiratory Causes of Acidosis and Alkalosis

Acidosis

	Respiratory	Metabolic
Problem	Elevated pCO_2	Not related to pCO_2
Some causes	Hypoventilation (trauma to respiratory centers, excess sedatives) Poor diffusion of gasses (COPD, pulmonary edema, infection) Respiratory muscle weakness (muscular dystrophy)	Diabetic acidosis, lactic acidosis, $NaHCO_3$ loss (severe diarrhea), high fat intake, ingested substances (aspirin, methanol, bleach)
Compensation	Kidney reabsorbs $NaHCO_3$ and excretes H^+	Hyperventilation, kidney reabsorbs $NaHCO_3$ and excretes H^+

Alkalosis

	Respiratory	Metabolic
Problem	Reduced pCO_2	Not related to pCO_2
Some causes	Hyperventilation (excessive artificial ventilation, anxiety, fever, pain, intentional overbreathing, encephalitis, adaptation to high altitudes, chronic hypoxia)	Vomiting, increased ingestion of alkalai, GI suction
Compensation	Kidney eliminates $NaHCO_3$ and reabsorbs H^+	Hypoventilation, kidney eliminates $NaHCO_3$ and reabsorbs H^+

Note: Remember the following reference ranges:
plasma $NaHCO_3$:   22–28 mEq/L
plasma pCO_2:   33–44 mmHg
plasma pH   7.35–7.45

TABLE 8-9 Summary of Formulas

Stroke volume = End diastolic volume − End systolic volume	$SV = EDV - ESV$
Cardiac output	$CO = SV \times HR$
Blood pressure	$BP = SVR \times CO$ or $BP = SVR \times SV \times HR$
Blood volume	$BV = 65$ mL/kg $\times$ body weight in kg
Preload = End diastolic volume	EDV = Amount in ventricle at the end of the diastolic phase (filling) of the cardiac cycle
Systemic vascular resistance = Afterload	$SVR = 80 \times \dfrac{MAP - CVP}{CO}$
Mean arterial pressure	$MAP = \dfrac{(SBP) + 2(DBP)}{3}$
Blood flow	$\text{Blood flow} = \dfrac{\text{Mean arterial pressure} - \text{Venous pressure}}{\text{Resistance}}$
Net filtration pressure	Net filtration pressure = {Capillary hydrostatic pressure + Interstitial fluid osmotic pressure} − {Blood osmotic pressure + Interstitial fluid hydrostatic pressure}
Carbonic acid equation	$HCO_3^- + H^+ = CO_2 + H_2O$
Sodium bicarbonate buffering equation	$NaHCO_3 + H^+ \rightarrow Na^+ + H_2CO_3$
Carbonate acid buffering equation	$H_2CO_3 + OH^- \rightarrow H_2O + HCO_3^-$

Notes

1. Dee Unglaub Silverthorn, *Human Physiology, An Integrated Approach,* 3rd ed. (San Francisco: Pearson Education, 2003), p. 2.

2. C. K. Stone and R. L. Humphries, *Current Emergency Diagnosis and Treatment* McGraw-Hill's AccessMedicine (accessed October 26, 2006).

3. D. L. Kasper, E. Braunwald, A. S. Fauci, S. L. Hauser, D. L. Longo, J. L. Jamesonm, and K. J. Isselbacher, eds., *Harrison's Principles of Internal Medicine,* 16th ed. McGraw-Hill's AccessMedicine (accessed October 26, 2006).

4. J. P. Pooler and D. C. Eaton, *Vander's Renal Physiology,* 6th ed. McGraw-Hill's AccessMedicine (accessed October 26, 2006).

5. G. E. Morgan, M. S. Mikhail, and M. J. Murray, *Clinical Anesthesiology,* 4th ed. McGraw-Hill's AccessMedicine (accessed October 26, 2006).

6. F. S. Greenspan and D. G. Gardner, *Basic and Clinical Endocrinology,* 7th ed. McGraw-Hill's AccessMedicine (accessed October 26, 2006).

7. L. W. Way and G. M. Doherty, *Current Surgical Diagnosis and Treatment,* 11th ed. McGraw-Hill's AccessMedicine (accessed October 26, 2006).

8. F. C. Brunicardim, D. K. Andersen, T. R. Billiar, D. L. Dunn, J. G. Hunter, J. B. Matthews, R. E. Pollock, and S. I. Schwartz, *Schwartz's Principles of Surgery,* 8th ed. McGraw-Hill's AccessMedicine (accessed October 26, 2006).

9. V. Fuster, R. W. Alexander, and R. A. O'Rourke, eds., *Hurst's The Heart,* 11th ed. McGraw-Hill's AccessMedicine (accessed October 26, 2006).

10. L. M. Tierney, S. J. McPhee, M. A. Papadakis, eds., *Current Medical Diagnosis & Treatment 2006.* McGraw-Hill's AccessMedicine (accessed October 26, 2006).

11. J. E. Tintinalli, G. D. Kelan, J. S. Stapczynski, O. J. Ma, and D. M. Cline, *Tintinalli's Emergency Medicine: A Comprehensive Study Guide,* 6th ed. McGraw-Hill's AccessMedicine (accessed October 26, 2006).

12. D. C. Eaton and J. P. Pooler, *Vander's Renal Physiology,* 6th ed. McGraw-Hill's AccessMedicine (accessed October 26, 2006).

13. L. L. Brunton, J. S. Lazo, K. L. Parker, I. L. O. Buxton, and D. Blumenthal, eds., *Goodman and Gilman's The Pharmacological Basis of Therapeutics,* 11th ed. McGraw-Hill's AccessMedicine (accessed October 26, 2006).

part 2

Foundations of Communication, Assessment, and Critical Care

9

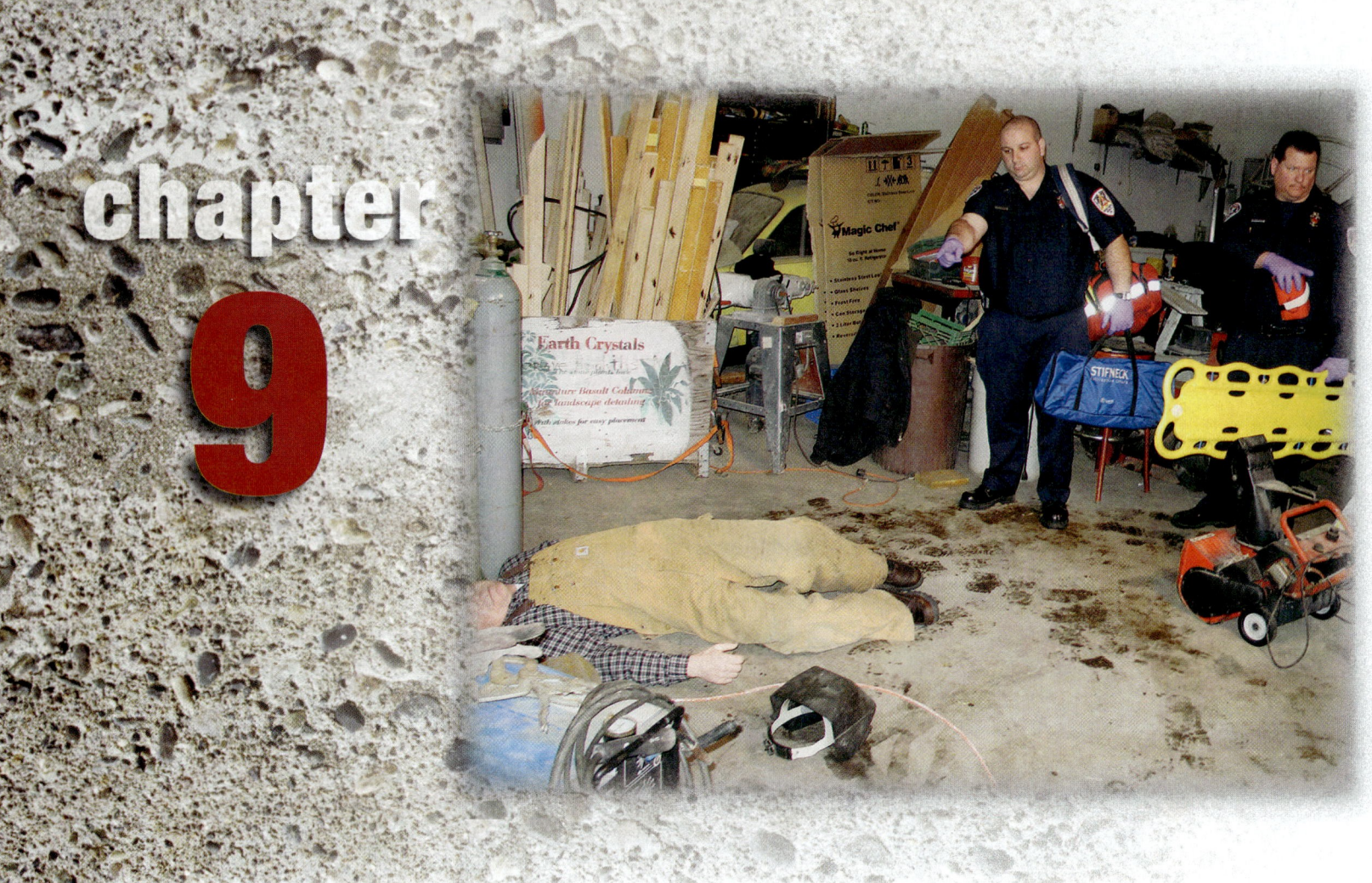

Safety and Scene Size-Up

*"**L**ife for him was an adventure, perilous indeed, but men are not made for safe havens. The fullness of life is in the hazards of life."*

—Edith Hamilton, *The Great Age of Greek Literature,*
referring to Aeschylus

Need To Know

▶ Your personal medical history and immunization status. Immunizations should be updated according to risk and the availability of vaccines.

▶ How to apply and safely remove personal protective equipment (PPE).

▶ How to reduce the possibility of exposure while dealing with contaminated patients.

▶ How to ensure the safety of a scene throughout the EMS call, prior to entering and while on scene.

▶ While paramedics should avoid placing themselves at risk, they should also be familiar with techniques to limit their risk of injury.

▶ The five elements of the scene size-up: (1) scene safety, (2) number of patients, (3) mechanism of injury or nature of illness, (4) body substance isolation (BSI) and PPE precautions, and (5) additional resources assessment.

▶ **Do**	▶ **Ask**
• Update your medical history and vaccination status. • Ensure proper PPE is available at the beginning of every shift, and don proper PPE before every patient contact. • Make sure you wash your hands following every patient contact, and disinfect your equipment and supplies appropriately. • Ensure the safety of every scene before entering. • Employ tactics that minimize the risk of injury.	• Your physician and employer about appropriateness and availability of vaccines. • Your EMS system managers and employers about PPE equipment and protocols in your service. • Your employer about interfacing with police, fire, and other agencies that are available to make the scene safe for EMS. • About educational opportunities to learn techniques for personal protection. • For law enforcement if there is any suspicion that the scene is unsafe to enter.

Introduction

Throughout your career in EMS, safety must be your first consideration in any response (Box 9-1). Danger comes in many forms. Both the scene and the patient present hazards to be addressed. This chapter will discuss ways to address dangerous or violent scenes.

The first consideration is the simplest: Paramedics must protect themselves from exposure to any contamination or hazard from the patients they treat.

In February 2003, the index case of what eventually became a North American outbreak of SARS was diagnosed in Toronto. In March, the cases were epidemiologically linked to a SARS outbreak that occurred in China in 2002.[4] Eventually, 224 people were diagnosed with SARS, and 38 people died. The SARS outbreak in Toronto proved extremely challenging for the city's EMS system, their providers, and medical directors (Figure 9-1). Fortunately, large scale public health emergencies like this are unusual. However, EMS personnel must be constantly vigilant for all biohazards and for signs of possible public health risks and prepared to respond appropriately to reduce the risk of injury or illness to themselves or the spread of the problem to others. Though many of these individual emergencies are covered specifically in other chapters, there are certain universal precautions and preparations that

BOX 9-1 Sobering Facts

Unlike the fire and police service, no national statistics are available to measure just how many EMS providers are killed or injured in the line of duty while providing prehospital care. However, a brief review of the literature provides a few concerning statistics that speak to the danger of the job:

• The National EMS Memorial Service paid tribute to 26 EMS workers who were killed in 2005.[1]

• Three EMS personnel were shot to death in 2004 while on duty.[2]

• Sixteen firefighters involved with EMS events were killed in 2003.[3]

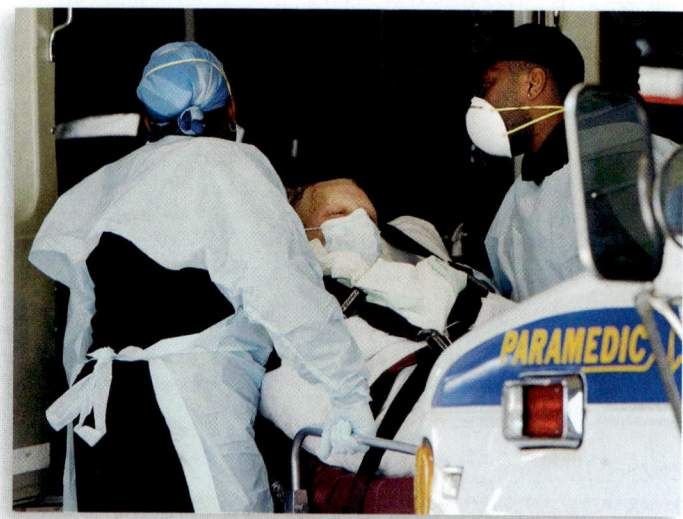

Figure 9-1 The SARS outbreak in Toronto, Canada, severely stressed the workforce of the city's EMS service.

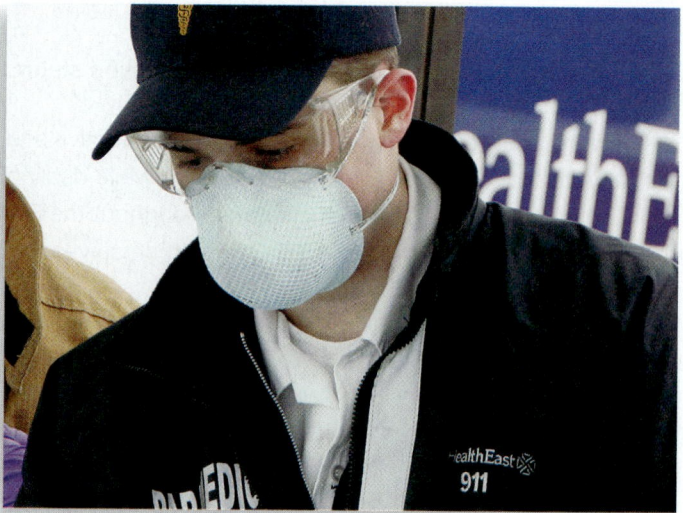

Figure 9-2 Proper PPE is required for every patient encounter.

must be practiced and implemented by paramedics each and every time they treat a patient.

Personal Protection

Perhaps the single most important action taken by a paramedic responding to any scene of a medical emergency is the utilization of appropriate **personal protective equipment (PPE)** to prevent accidental exposure to potentially contaminated bodily fluids from patients. The routine use of equipment such as gloves, masks, eye protection, and gowns, when appropriate, will minimize the risk of exposure and possible infection from a wide variety of infectious organisms including bacteria and viruses (Figure 9-2). Also, paramedics should receive all available immunizations against infectious agents such as influenza, hepatitis, and tetanus (Figure 9-3). DOT 1-8.28, 1-2.43, 5-11.52, 5-12.10

CONNECTIONS Chapter 2: The Well-Being of the Paramedic has more information and tips on how to stay healthy.

The proper use of PPE is critical in many public health emergencies. Proper training, fit testing, and storage of equipment such as particulate filtering (i.e., N-95) masks, gloves, shoe covers, powered respirators, gowns, hoods, and eye protection are essential, as these items will likely be utilized in cases of infectious outbreaks, chemical releases, bioterrorist attacks, or radiation releases. Protection for both the paramedic and the patient must be taken into consideration. Local protocols and guidelines will mandate which elements of PPE are to be utilized for a given situation. DOT 1-2.30, 1.3-8, 1-3.10

The performance of many routine paramedic procedures requires the use of protective equipment.

Basic and advanced airway management techniques such as suctioning, ventilating, and intubation require the use of gloves and eye and face protection from splashes of saliva, mucus, vomit, or blood. Bleeding control and management of open wounds with spurting blood requires the use of gloves, eye and face protection, and perhaps gowns to prevent the uniform from becoming soiled by splashes. Emergency child birth requires gloves, gowns, and face and eye protection from splashes of blood, amniotic fluid, and urine. Administering medications and starting an IV require the use of gloves and techniques that prevent the introduction of pathogens into the blood stream of the patient. DOT 1-8.14, 1-8.33, 2-1.80, 1-2.15

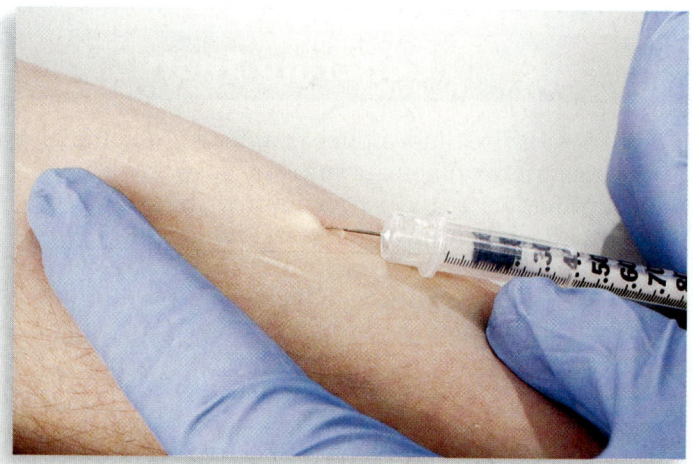

Figure 9-3 Paramedics should receive mantoux (PPD) testing at regular intervals as well as get vaccinated against hepatitis and other contagious diseases.

Working in the Gray Zone

As a paramedic, you serve as a role model for other members of the health care team. Always wear your PPE and use body substance isolation (BSI) precautions. Junior EMS providers may erroneously think that being splashed with blood is a badge of honor. Ensure you provide a good model for them by encouraging them to comply with rules and regulations for using PPE. DOT 4-4.77, 5-11.53

If the use of agents of mass destruction is suspected, EMS personnel must be familiar with the use of appropriate PPE for the suspected agent and the administration of injectable antidotes such as atropine and pralidoxime. Depending on the protocols of the EMS agency, these drugs may be used only for self-administration and protection of EMS personnel, or they may be administered on a larger scale to other rescuers or the public. The paramedic must be familiar with the protocols for proper use of these antidotes and, in the case of large scale incidents, must know where they are stored, how they are released for use, and to whom they are given.

CONNECTIONS See Chapter 53: Hazardous Materials Incidents for more detailed information on the various levels of PPE during hazmat situations and when each should be used.

Hygiene Measures

A few simple hygiene measures can provide significant protection to patients and paramedics and should be followed regularly. DOT 1-2.31

- Frequent handwashing with antibacterial soap is the most important method of protection. Allow the faucet to run while briskly rubbing your hands together using soap and water as hot as you can stand. A good guide on how long to wash your hands is to sing the "Happy Birthday" song through at a normal pace two times while washing your hands. Turn the faucet off with a paper towel, and use a paper towel to open the door when you leave the room. When soap and running water are not available, hands should be sanitized with alcohol-based hand cleansers. Continue rubbing your hands together until the solution has evaporated, and wash your hands using the appropriate technique as soon as you can. Paramedics should also avoid touching their faces with their hands. **See Skill Sheet 61: Handwashing.**
- Cover your mouth and nose with your arm, not your hand, when coughing or sneezing, or wear a surgical mask or **N-95 mask** when coughing.

- While working with patients, consider covering a patient's mouth and nose with a mask if he or she has respiratory symptoms. This becomes mandatory when epidemic illness is known to exist.
- Provide additional airflow in the patient compartment of the ambulance by opening windows, if appropriate.
- Stay home from work when ill with respiratory illnesses to prevent the spread to others.
- Remove soiled gloves properly. The process for removing sterile gloves should also be used to remove soiled gloves of any kind. Make sure you do not contaminate your skin when removing gloves, and wash your hands immediately. **See Skill Sheet 60: Putting On and Removing Gloves.**
- When non-disposable equipment or supplies have been exposed to body substances, ensure they are properly cleaned, disinfected, or disposed of according to the policies and procedures.

Working in the Gray Zone

Follow the instructions carefully when using disinfectant solutions and cleaning products. Make sure the solutions are reconstituted correctly. Do not use a full strength solution if you are directed to dilute it with water. The CDC has reported that some cleaning and disinfectant solutions are not effective unless they are properly diluted. Also, make sure the solution remains in contact with the surface for the amount of time recommended. If it says to leave it on the surface for five minutes, four and a half is not long enough! DOT 1-2.32

Infectious Emergencies

Though it is necessary to train and prepare for public health emergencies of all types, an infectious disease outbreak is the most common large-scale problem encountered by paramedics. Influenza outbreaks occur to some extent nearly every year. Infectious diseases such as bird flu, SARS, encephalitis, meningitis, *E. coli* infections, or whooping cough also occur in epidemics of varying magnitudes. The typical pattern for flu epidemics is to cycle through a community for 10–12 weeks at a time, up to three times or more, spread apart by 10–12 week intervals.[5] Constant awareness of existing outbreaks and vigilance with regard to new outbreaks are necessary to ensure the health of the paramedic and to decrease the accidental or **iatrogenic** (medically caused) spread of such diseases. DOT 1-3.11, 5-11.52

Protocols are necessary to address issues such as the transmission routes and incubation periods of various infectious agents, isolation, and quarantine techniques. They should discuss which types of exposures mandate either isolation or quarantine for a paramedic and the appropriate standards for decontamination of equipment and vehicles. In cases where decontamination procedures are complex and time-consuming, as in serious airborne diseases such as SARS, agencies frequently have protocols that allow for the transport of stable victims to the hospital by private car with a previously exposed driver after proper evaluation and initial treatment by EMS personnel. Patients transported by ambulance should receive nebulizer treatments or other infectious aerosol-producing treatments only if absolutely necessary.[6]

CONNECTIONS See Chapter 52: Teamwork and Operational Interface, Figure 52-8, which shows a protocol in the form of an algorithm for handling special pathogen situations.

Isolation and Quarantine

The need to quarantine or isolate potentially infected or ill paramedics may seriously decrease the number of EMS staff available to respond to calls for transport or transfer. During the Toronto SARS outbreak, 850 paramedics had 1,166 potential exposures to SARS, resulting in 436 medics being placed in a 10-day home quarantine. During quarantine, the paramedics had to wear N-95 respirators continuously. By the time the first outbreak passed, 62 paramedics developed SARS-like illnesses. During the second phase of the outbreak, 200 more paramedics were quarantined.[4] Removing paramedics from duty requires re-deployment of available personnel and places significant stress on the remaining EMS staff.

It is generally better to err on the side of being overly cautious and suspicious and use PPE when treating and transporting patients during a time of public health emergencies, especially very early in the course of the incident. A high index of suspicion and vigilance on the part of the paramedic can prevent the spread of illness or contamination and prevent further problems.

Managing Risk of Personal Injury

Proper Lifting and Moving Techniques

The physical nature of our work puts us at risk of injury. Being in good physical condition and using proper body mechanics can reduce the risk of injury. For instance, when performing a lift:

- Keep your body as close to what you are lifting as possible, keeping your arms tucked in close to your body. For added strength, grasp objects such as

railings so your hands are positioned with the palms facing up instead of the palms facing down.

- Bend at the knees instead of the waist, and keep your back straight with your legs shoulder-length apart.
- Avoid turning or twisting when lifting.
- Know your limitations, and call upon additional help when the weight to be lifted exceeds your lifting ability.
- Communicate clearly and move on three-counts to ensure weight is evenly distributed among the crew doing the lifting.
- Work out a code, such as "stop-stop-stop" that when used by any person performing the lift, results in immediate cessation of the lift, placement of the patient directly on the ground, floor, or other surface, and removal of the weight from the person signaling "stop." This can prevent a minor muscle strain injury due to improper lifting technique from becoming a career-ending injury.

When reaching:

- Avoid reaching more than 15–20 inches beyond the trunk of your body.
- Lean forward from your hips to avoid bending your back.
- Avoid twisting while reaching.

When pushing or pulling:

- Keep elbows bent with arms close to your body.
- Keep the weight close to your body between your waist and shoulders.
- If the weight is lower, push or pull from your knees.
- Avoid pushing and pulling over your head.

Street Secrets

Staying in shape is an important part of injury prevention. As we get older, we need to work harder at conditioning our muscles to protect them from injury when stressed. Chapter 2: The Well-Being of the Paramedic contains helpful information on diet, sleep, and exercise, which provide a prescription for healthy living.

Safety While Driving

Driving Habits

Operating an ambulance in emergency mode is dangerous (Box 9-2). Other drivers may not hear or see an oncoming ambulance until the unit is very close. This can startle the person, causing him to stop in his lane of traffic or swerve out of the way into oncoming traffic or into a ditch. Any individual operating an emergency

BOX 9-2   Ambulance Crash Statistics

- There were an estimated 36,398 crashes involving ambulances between 1988 and 1997.
- Just under 23,000 persons were reported injured and 360 persons were killed in these crashes.
- Almost 1% of the ambulance crashes involved a fatality.
- Unrestrained occupants riding in the patient compartment accounted for over 50% of ambulance crash fatalities.
- 72% of fatalities occurred to occupants riding in the patient compartment, yet only 40% of total occupants rode in the patient compartment.
- Just under 44% of reported incapacitating injuries occurred to occupants riding in the patient compartment, while only 12% of total occupants rode in the patient compartment.
- If involved in a crash, unrestrained ambulance occupants were 3.8 times more likely to be killed and 6.5 times more likely to be severely injured than those wearing occupant restraints.

Source: L. R. Becker, E. Zaloshnja, N. Levick, L. Guohua, and T. R. Miller. "Relative Risk of Injury and Death in Ambulances and Other Emergency Vehicles" *Accident Analysis and Prevention* 35 (2003) 941–948. Elsevier Science Ltd.

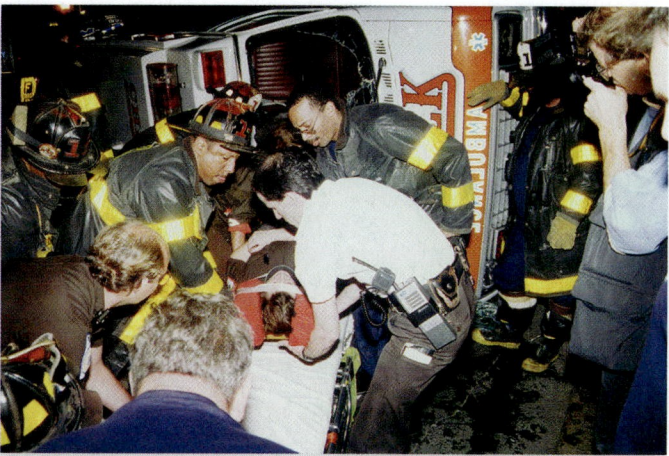

Figure 9-4   Ambulance crashes are a danger to personnel and patients alike.

vehicle must exercise "due regard" for the health and safety of the public. EMS providers have been charged with manslaughter when found guilty of operating an ambulance in an unsafe manner, causing an accident and the death of crew members, patients, or bystanders.[7] DOT 1.2-14

Intersections are particularly dangerous. Even when an ambulance is moving through an intersection and it has a green light and the right of way, it is dangerous and crashes have happened. DOT 1-2.13d

Escorts are not safe. An escort situation occurs when an emergency vehicle, such as a police car for example, leads an ambulance through traffic. The problem with escorts is that once the lead vehicle passes, the drivers who moved out of the way often pull back into traffic unaware that another emergency vehicle is coming along from behind. DOT 1-2.13a

The use of lights and sirens is called "operating in emergency mode." Light and siren use is currently under investigation by several researchers who are trying to determine if it is safe or necessary. Some states, such as Maryland, have laws that mandate an ambulance must have lights and/or sirens on while loaded with patients of a specific priority, but the law also allows the unit's headlights to be the lights that are used. Other states leave the decision up to the discretion of the team leader on the call or have a protocol in place that provides guidance. DOT 1-2.13, 8-1.6

Multiple agency responses involve numerous emergency vehicles traveling to the same location. Paramedics must be constantly alert to the possibility of other responders crossing their path, particularly at intersections.

When it is your turn to drive, do so defensively. Most vehicles you will drive in your paramedic career have a primary function of accommodating bulky equipment, a supine patient, and an emergency crew. This function dictates that these vehicles be large and have high centers of gravity. Unfortunately, their squared-off design also means the driver has large areas of "blind spots" as well. These characteristics do not lend themselves to high speed maneuverability, good stopping ability, or safe operating conditions. Therefore, it is important for you to be in a defensive driving mode at all times and especially when operating in an emergency driving mode since this represents the time of greatest risk for a collision (Figure 9-4).[8]

Street Secrets

Another cause of injuries in the back of the ambulance is loose equipment. Always make sure that equipment is stowed or secured before the ambulance moves. This will not only prevent injury but also protect your heavy, delicate equipment.

Seat Belt Use

A recent study conducted in three EMS services showed that paramedics do not consistently wear seat belts, regardless of where they are sitting within the vehicle.[9] The back of the ambulance can be a difficult place in

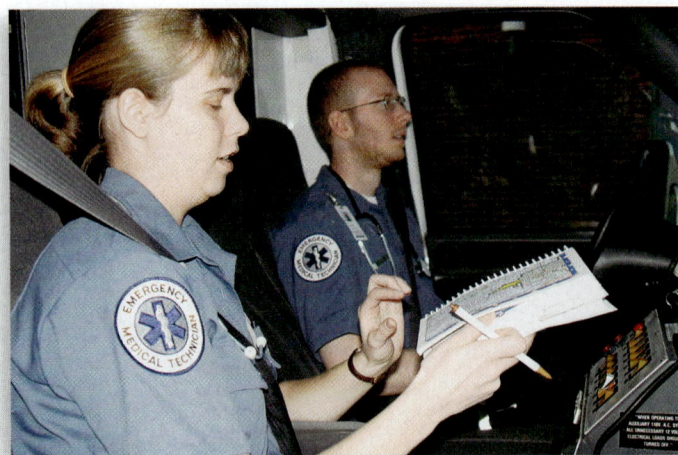

Figure 9-5 The law calls for seatbelts used by all ambulance personnel and our passengers. Studies have shown that injury is reduced with seatbelt use.

which to work when trying to wear a seat belt; however, this study also showed that there were many times that crews were not wearing seat belts while in the front of the ambulance. DOT 1-2.12

As a paramedic, you will be spending large amounts of time in an ambulance. Much of the time the operation of the unit will be in emergency mode, which increases the risks for collision.[8] It is wise to wear a seat belt every time you are in an ambulance (Figure 9-5). It may be appropriate to ask the driver to pull over to the shoulder of the road if you feel you need to be temporarily moving around inside the back of the ambulance to assess or treat the patient.

Working in the Gray Zone

Paramedics responding to calls in ambulances are certainly at no less a risk than drivers in general and are at a higher risk when running lights and sirens. The literature suggests that paramedics and patients in the back of the ambulance are most at risk for injury and have the lowest compliance for seat belt use.

Scene Size-Up and Safety

The scene size-up occurs prior to ever touching the patient (Box 9-3). Much of the size-up can occur before ever setting foot outside of the ambulance. The scene size-up is used to determine if the scene is safe to enter. The safety size-up is also performed continuously throughout the time EMS is on the scene. Ensuring a safe scene is one of the primary responsibilities of the

BOX 9-3 Elements of the Scene Size-Up

- Is the scene safe?
- How many patients are there?
- What is the mechanism of injury or nature of the illness?
- Does every team member have the appropriate personal protective equipment and clothing, including BSI?
- Do we need any additional resources for this situation?

EMS crew. They have a responsibility for personal safety, crew safety, and patient and bystander safety. This section discusses important safety concerns and considerations of the scene size-up. Additional information on the scene size-up will be covered in later chapters. DOT 1-1.31, 1-1.38

The scene size-up assessment begins upon receipt of dispatch information. As you respond to the call, continue to take in information such as the weather, driving conditions, and what is observed on the way to the call; all of this contributes to the size-up. Arriving on the scene, there may be hazards or multiple patients that will mean calling in additional resources such as police, hazmat crews, rescue personnel, etc. The scene should always be determined to be safe before medical personnel enter or approach the patient. All scenes, whether they are at motor vehicle crashes, in an open field, or in an apartment, will have to be observed for safety and the need for additional resources. DOT 3-3.1, 3-3.4, 1-2.13b, 1-2.11

Street Secrets

The only scene that is truly safe is the one you are driving away from after having completed your assignment. Never let down your guard, even for one minute, on any scene. Always continuously reassess that the scene is safe and is remaining so throughout your time on the scene.

Approaching the Scene

When responding to calls that involve motorized vehicles, particularly on roadways that continue to have traffic flow, you will need to consider several things regarding your personal safety. Always consider your visibility to others. Standard approaches

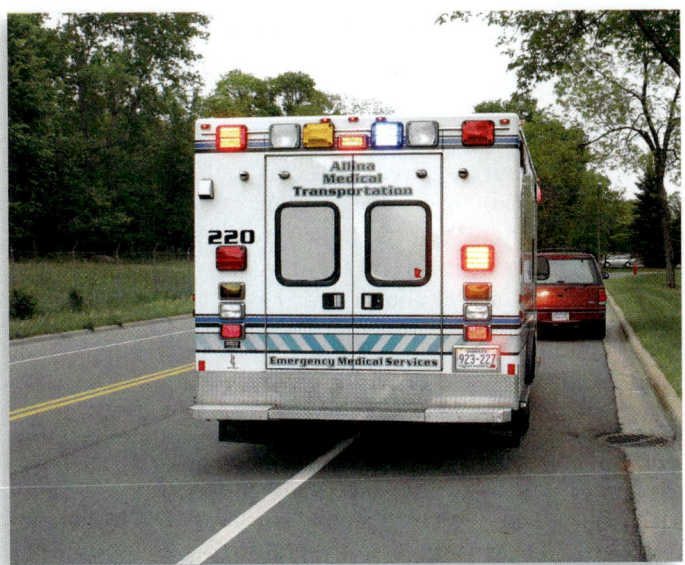

Figure 9-6   This illustrates what approaching traffic sees if the ambulance is positioned properly. The paramedic, the equipment, and the vehicle in the crash are essentially blocked by the correct position of the ambulance which is stopped approximately one to two vehicle lengths behind the work area and offset by a half-vehicle width towards the direction that approaching traffic would need to veer to avoid this scene (in this case, to the left). Note that all warning lights are on.

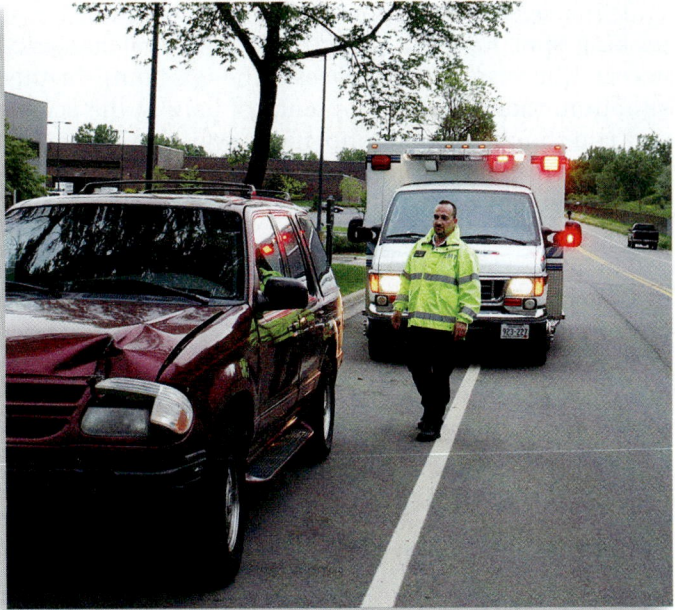

Figure 9-7   This illustrates the view from the front depicting the "corridor of safety" for EMS personnel to work within due to the offset position of the ambulance. Note that warning lights are on and the paramedic has a highly visible, reflective vest on for increased safety. In a night operation, all forward lights (headlights, spotlights, and take-down lights) should be utilized for illumination of the scene.

should include use of all emergency lighting and your personal use of high visibility reflective outerwear over your uniform. Position the ambulance and other public safety vehicles on the scene to provide a "zone of safety" in which to work. A typical strategy is to position the ambulance between the crash scene and oncoming traffic to provide some protection. Figures 9-6 and 9-7 show some common strategies for vehicle positioning. DOT 8-5.2a, 3-3.5, 3-3.3, 1-2.11, 1-2.13e, 1-2.12

The use of cones and flares can help identify the emergency scene. Do not place flares near spills or puddles of liquid or use them if odors are detected in the area of the incident. Law enforcement officers may also provide assistance with directing traffic around the scene. DOT 8-3.21c

CONNECTIONS   Chapter 53: Hazardous Materials Incidents discusses vehicle staging during hazmat operations. Refer to that chapter for additional information.

Approaches to Potentially Dangerous Calls

As an emergency paramedic, you will be called on to respond to a multitude of different situations. Some of these have a higher risk for violent encounters than others. These may include calls such as domestic dis-

turbances, assaults in progress, shootings, stabbings, and calls to addresses where violence has occurred in the past. When responding to these types of calls, you should obtain as much information as possible prior to entering the scene, and never enter the scene until you are certain that the scene is safe. Your employer should have specific policies in place to guide your responses in these situations, and most will have you stage away from the incident until law enforcement officers arrive and report that the scene is under control. DOT 8-5.6c

Street Secrets

The time to request additional help is before you ever exit your vehicle. A visual sweep of the incident can reveal hazards, and the need for more ambulances or other resources can be quickly determined. Call for additional resources before you enter the scene because once you enter you may be too busy or, if the scene becomes dangerous, unable to call. DOT 3-3.10

Approaching a Structure

When responding to calls within a structure, it is often thought that the best place to be is directly in front of the address for ease of patient transport. In fact, when multiple agencies respond, often they will leave a parking spot for EMS directly in front that has easy **access** (the way in) and **egress** (the way out). In this situation, there is already plenty of help at the scene, and you should take that spot if it is available. However, if you are responding alone or are the first unit to arrive, take a moment to evaluate the address before parking directly in front of the scene. DOT 8-3.21a

In most cases of an emergency, the response by EMS is expected and welcomed. Often the front door will be open and lights will be on, or there may be a bystander waiting to greet you upon your arrival. If, however, you approach an address that looks suspicious, you should confirm the address before exiting the vehicle or approaching the scene. If it is the correct address and you are concerned that the address may harbor a potentially dangerous situation, it is probably wise not to park directly in front since you then represent an easy target. DOT 3-3.1, 3-3.2

It may be safer to park beyond the address and approach the scene from the side instead of directly from the front. Approaching the address from the side allows you to evaluate things such as loud noises coming from within, signs of violence like broken windows, or dangerous dogs in the yard. It also places you in a position that most people will not expect you to approach from and will allow you a safer retreat if necessary. DOT 3-3.1, 3-3.2

Additionally, when approaching a structure, it is a good idea not to stand directly in front of windows and doors, if at all possible. You may wish to knock on the door and announce your arrival while standing to either side of the door. When the door opens, if there is a surprising situation on the other side, the door frame may allow you some means of cover or concealment. If the door is open upon your arrival, pause at the doorway to assess the situation beyond before entering. Also, it is usually a good idea to announce your arrival prior to entering a room to avoid surprising the occupants with an unannounced and unexpected entry.[10] DOT 8-5.2c

Nice to Know

Cover protects you from view as well as provides a barrier to stop projectiles such as knives or bullets. **Concealment** provides visual protection, but it does not provide an appropriate barrier to stop projectiles. For example, standing behind a bushy shrub can provide concealment, but standing behind a brick wall can provide cover and concealment.

Approaching a Scene at Night

Darkness brings issues of visibility. First, your visibility to others is decreased, so you should remember to use emergency lighting and wear reflective clothing. When working in high risk areas (such as on a busy roadway), you should consider using every available warning light and device at your disposal. You may also wish to consider positioning an emergency vehicle at the scene in such a way that it may offer a crash barrier to other vehicles (see Figures 9-6 and 9-7). It is much better to sacrifice a vehicle than to sacrifice a life. DOT 3-3.1, 3-3.2, 8-3.21d

Additionally, your ability to perceive potentially dangerous situations is limited because your vision is compromised as well. A working flashlight carried on your duty belt should be mandatory. Make use of all available lighting such as vehicle "take-down" or "alley" lights, headlights, and available spotlights to illuminate a scene. DOT 8-3.21b

Street Secrets

Never allow a patient to move into a position that blocks your egress route. Keep an eye on your partner as well as the position of the patient and bystanders. Never allow a patient to leave your sight, even under the pretense of getting medication or information from another room. Accompany the patient and alert your partner when you leave the room.

Paramedic Awareness at Potentially Violent Scenes

Throughout your EMS career, you will be at risk for personal injury by people and situations. Your personal safety and the safety of your partner are a priority. The most important concept associated with personal safety is not so much a tactic to be practiced as it is a condition of alertness and awareness of every situation and scene. Maintaining awareness of all that goes on around you, perceiving possible threats, and attending to them or employing proper tactics should be a full-time part of your job. DOT 8-5.2

Street Secrets

You are worth two paramedics on every call that you are on. If you become injured while on a scene, it will take two more paramedics to replace you! One will be needed to care for the patient that you had to abandon because of your injury, and the other will have to care for you.

Awareness Color Coding System

There is a simple color coding system to explain awareness that was originally described by Colonel Jeff Cooper, a nationally recognized self-defense expert.[11] These color codes have nothing to do with the present-day color code for national security. Rather, they describe a spectrum of awareness that is taught in many law enforcement academies. This system is useful for any person who encounters dynamic and potentially dangerous situations on a routine basis, and it certainly is applicable to the EMS profession.

Cooper describes four levels of awareness and when each should be maintained. A fifth level has been added by many EMS practitioners. Each level is described (Figure 9-8).

- Condition White
- Condition Yellow
- Condition Orange
- Condition Red
- Condition Black

The concept of awareness is not something that you are born with. It is something that you must learn and continue to practice since it is a degradable skill. From now on in your EMS career, each time you go to work, your sense of awareness is something that you need to put on along with your uniform. DOT 8-5.2b, 8-5.6a, 8-5.6b

Personal Protection Tactics

Now that you know the importance of awareness, you should also become familiar with certain tactical practices that can aid in your safety and survival. Like awareness, these practices are not natural instincts and must be practiced all of the time. They cannot help you if you do not employ them in advance. Most of these practices are adapted from law enforcement teachings.

It is important to remember that many EMS professionals function in a uniformed position with a public service agency. Uniforms will come with patches and often with badges. Duty belts can have clusters of equipment around the waist that may look to a drug- or alcohol-impaired individual like a law enforcement officer's handcuffs and gun. The ambulance will show up at emergency scenes displaying warning lights and blaring a siren. Both law enforcement officers and EMS professionals are subjected to potentially violent behavior on a regular basis, so these principles and practices apply with equal importance to both.[12]

Use of Body Armor

Depending on the agency you work for, the use of body armor may be optional or required. If body armor is an option and you have elected to wear it, do so consis-

tently. Not only is it protective against projectiles and assaults, but it also may give some protection in blunt force trauma such as a motor vehicle crash, an area of high relative risk for the EMS professional. There have been cases throughout the country of EMS crews being shot at or shot.[13] It is not always clear if the EMS crew was the intended target or the unfortunate subject caught in the crossfire. It is clear, however, that if wearing body armor is available to you and you operate in an area that is at risk for this type of danger, you should take advantage of the protection that it offers.

Street Secrets

Never allow wearing body armor to encourage you to enter a scene that you would not enter if you were not wearing body armor. It should never entice you to take risks.

Use of Identifiers

Consider your personal identity something to be guarded. Do not make it easy for patients and bystanders to find you outside of your professional environment. Use your first initial and last name or just your last name on your badge or name tag. Keep your home phone number unlisted, and do not disclose it to patients. Guarding your home address and other personal information is obvious, and if someone asks to be able to contact you later, provide them with the address of your employer. Lastly, avoid using your home address when registering for your professional credentials. Instead, consider using the address of your employer. Much of your credential information is considered public information and can easily be searched for and found online through the Internet.

Personal Appearance

Your appearance to the public should always be professional. The uniform should always be clean and neat. There are some aspects of your appearance, however, which are not covered by your uniform and can represent personal safety problems for you. Long hair gives people something to grab onto and can be a dangerous problem. People with dementia at the nursing home can grab hair just as readily as a violent patient at a bar fight. Dangling jewelry from ears or other pierced sites on the body are at-risk to be grabbed and should not be worn while on duty.

Although it is convenient to hang a stethoscope around the neck, it also gives someone a method with which to grab and choke you. Anything worn around the neck, identification lanyards and neckties, should include a breakaway type of attachment.

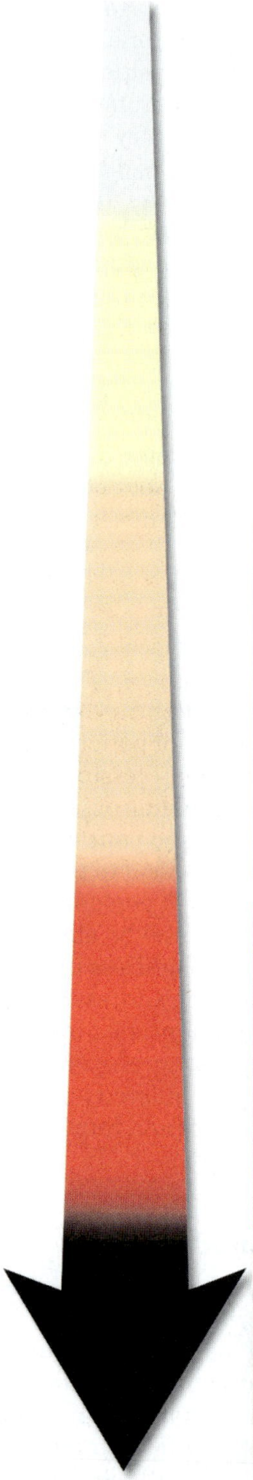

Condition white

Condition white represents complete lack of awareness of your surroundings and possible threats. The person in condition white would be unable to react to any threat because he or she would never notice it in the first place (e.g., the victim who tells you, "I never saw what hit me" was in condition white because he was never aware that the violent person was standing right next to him). This is the condition that most people operate in all of the time. It is never an appropriate operating condition for the EMS professional.

Condition yellow

This is a state of relaxed but constant alertness and readiness. In this state, you are always aware of your environment. You are watchful and constantly evaluating what is occurring within your area of control, such as a new person who has entered into your scope of view. Anyone or anything that enters into your area of control should trigger your mental radar to view it as a potential threat until you have had a chance to assess it. When your mental radar identifies these possible threats, your state of awareness should escalate to condition orange. It is possible to maintain condition yellow for an indefinite period. While on duty, you should never go below condition yellow.

Condition orange

Condition orange is a heightened state of alertness with a very narrow focus. You have now identified a specific potential threat. As you constantly interpret what is going on around you (never lose sight of the big picture just because a single potential problem has presented itself), a plan of action is also forming if certain predictable events occur (e.g., if that person with his hands in his pockets approaches me, I will ask him to stop and show me his hands before I will allow him to advance further; if he does not stop, I will retreat and seek safety). In this condition, you prepare yourself mentally to resolve whatever conflict is at hand. This is a high threat condition, and you can maintain this condition for perhaps a few hours, but not indefinitely. If the threat becomes real (the person advancing on you disregards your requests to stop), you must escalate to condition red. If you have evaluated the threat and deem it to be non-threatening (the person advancing on you is actually coming foward to offer you important information about your patient), you can de-escalate down to condition yellow and maintain vigilance.

Condition red

Condition red is the readiness for fight-or-flight. This is not panic, but rather a condition where you know that a definite threat has presented itself, and you must be ready to act or someone will get hurt (e.g., a person with a knife is advancing on you shouting threats; you now must either retreat or engage since doing nothing would guarantee harm to yourself or someone around you). In condition red, your biggest obstacle will be reaction time. By preplanning your actions, you will have likely eliminated that problem. Your response in condition red is based more on training, adrenalin, and available resources. Often, you do not ever have to do anything physical in this condition since many situations resolve themselves, in which case you would de-escalate down through condition orange and back to yellow. Although you may not have had to physically do anything at this condition, the key is that you were mentally ready and would have physically been ready and able to act had the situation demanded it.

Condition black

The fifth condition, or condition black, is not part of Cooper's original color codes. However, some professionals will refer to this, tongue-in-cheek. Condition black is blind panic. The goal of the EMS professional is to never enter condition black because if you do, it means that you have failed at proper awareness of your situation and are likely fighting for your life. In this condition, fear takes over and you will likely not be able to form a rational interpretation or response to the situation at hand. It is highly likely that someone (possibly you) will be injured or killed in this situation.

Figure 9-8   Colonel Jeff Cooper's spectrum of awareness.

Carefully consider where you choose to keep items that have the potential to be used against you in a violent confrontation. Keep potential penetrating and impact weapons (scissors, sharps, pens, flashlights, portable radio, etc.) in a lower cargo pant pocket to keep them away from easy reach of others. For items worn on your duty belt, consider keeping them on your hips, especially on your strong side (for example, on your right hip if you are right-handed, and vice versa). Items worn here are usually provided with some means of protective cover due to your natural arm and elbow position and are more difficult for others to grab and take away. Your strong side should also have the added protection of being furthest from a potential assailant if you practice the "bladed interview stance" as described below. DOT 8-5.4, 8-5.8a–d

Observation of Hands

Cultural and social practices usually require that you look people in the eye when you greet them. However, as an EMS professional, your interaction with people while on duty will generally not be of a social nature. While it is fine to have eye contact upon greeting someone, it is imperative that you learn the skill of observing someone's entire body during your interaction with him or her, paying particular attention to his or her hands. Hands may be used by others as weapons or as a means to conceal potentially dangerous items. It is acceptable to ask patients and bystanders to keep their hands in view during your interaction.

Nonverbal Cues

Learning to pay attention to nonverbal cues indicating escalation of anger or aggression can provide you with advance warning of potentially violent persons. This chapter is not meant to be a complete tutorial on the range of human behavior, but there are some obvious and universal cues that precede aggression.

CONNECTIONS Chapter 10: Therapeutic Communications and History Taking provides more information on communication techniques.

Nonverbal cues of aggressive behavior include:

- Raised voices
- Agitated movements
- Quickly rising from a seated position
- Pacing back and forth like a caged animal
- Clenched or balled up fists
- Hands raised in a threatening manner

When actions such as this occur, you should be formulating a plan that includes attempts at placating the person's behavior as well as providing for your own protection or escape. You should be in condition red at this time. DOT 8-5.3, 8-5.4a–c

Interviews

As a paramedic, you will spend a lot of time talking with people. They may be patients, family members, or bystanders. Keep in mind that these people are strangers

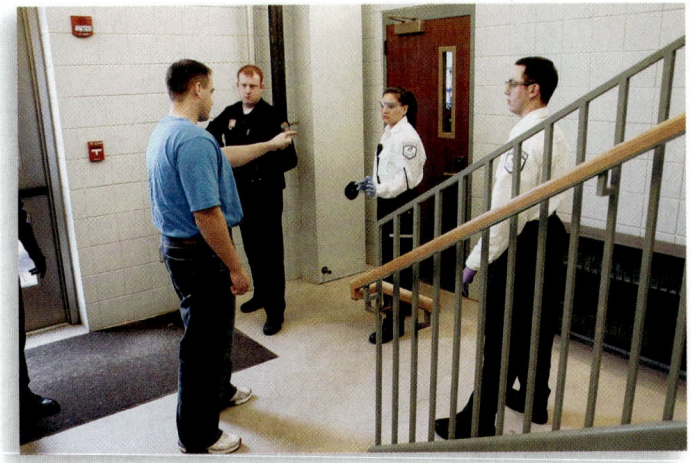

Figure 9-9 A patient's behavior can change rapidly, and your reactionary gap may be too small, as shown here. A bladed stance, an escape route, additional personnel, and police assistance can help you survive a dangerous encounter.

who may not necessarily be happy to see you or to be in the situation they are in. They may not be able to distinguish you from law enforcement personnel, so it is wise to practice a tactical interview process until you have established some rapport. The tactical interview process involves maintaining a safe distance between yourself and the person you are interacting with until you can determine whether he or she represents a threat to you. This distance is often known as the "reactionary gap" (see Figure 9-9).

The **reactionary gap** for a person holding an edged or sharp object is a minimum of 21 feet. It is approximately 7 feet for a person with empty hands. What this means is that it takes at least this amount of distance for you to react to some type of threatening act from this person to avoid personal injury. In addition to maintaining a reactionary gap until you ascertain a person's intent, you should consider taking a "bladed stance" when initially interviewing someone.

A **bladed stance** involves slightly widening your stance and standing at an angle of approximately 45 degrees to the interviewee. This position improves balance and center of gravity and allows for a quicker exit because you are already partially turned away from the person. Your "strong side" should be pointed away from the person (this would be your right-hand side if you are right-handed, and vice versa). Keep sharp objects and potential weapons on the strong side of your belt or body; that way they are furthest from any person that you are interviewing when you assume the bladed stance (Figure 9-10).[14]

Also remember to position yourself between the patient and your egress route; do not let them cut you off from your exit. If you and your partner are interviewing two patients, you may wish to position

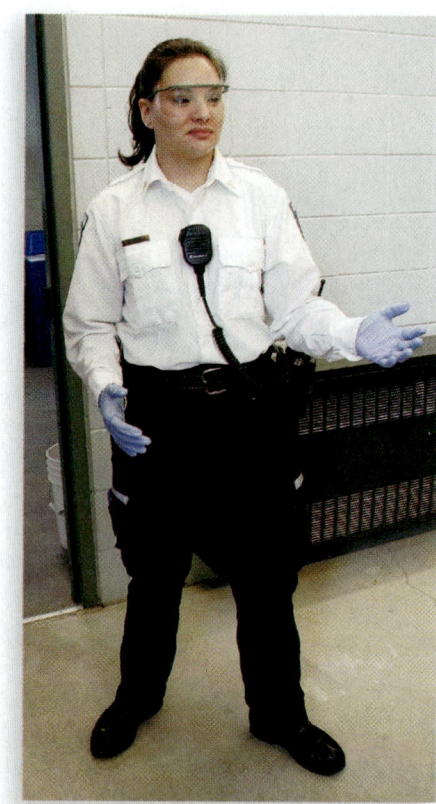

Figure 9-10   A paramedic assuming the bladed interview stance.

yourselves so you and your partner can maintain eye contact and the patients or bystanders cannot readily see each other.

Contact and Cover

The concept of **contact and cover** is taught to law enforcement officers but has excellent applicability to the EMS professional.[10] This concept assumes that you are working with a partner. This simple practice is for you to be either the "contact" member or the "cover" member of your EMS team, and your partner will assume the duties of the role that is unfilled. The role of the contact member is to make contact with the person at hand, whether that is a patient, a bystander, or a witness. The cover member's role is to provide a watchful eye over the contact member as well as the entire scene, monitoring potential threats that enter or exit the scene and maintaining responsibility for ensuring team safety. It is the cover member's responsibility to alert the contact member to any potential problems before they arise or to assist the cover member with any problems once they have occurred. The contact member is responsible for patient care. The cover member is responsible for continued scene safety. The cover member should never get so distracted as to lose sight of the big picture that is occurring. DOT 8-5.8Aa

Summary

This chapter has described some of the risks inherent in the EMS profession. Although awareness is important, the emphasis is on preparation. Paramedics must prepare themselves to minimize risk at every level. Proper immunizations and proper PPE will help protect paramedics and their families from diseases they may be exposed to. Ensuring scene safety includes training in techniques to minimize the risk of injury and developing good observation skills and communication techniques. These are priorities for every paramedic to ensure a safe and productive career.

Notes

1. National EMS Memorial Service: Quick Facts and Statistics. Press/Media Information webpage, http://press.nemsms.org/stats.htm (accessed February 7, 2006).
2. Information from the National EMS Memorial Service, http://www.nemsms.org/notices04.htm (accessed July 1, 2005).
3. U.S. Fire Administration. *Firefighter Fatalities in the United States in 2003* (Washington, DC: August 2004).
4. Mona R. Loutfy, Alexis Silverman, and Andrew Simor. *Toronto Emergency Medical Services and SARS* (September 2004), Center for Disease Control, Emerging Infectious Diseases. http://www.cdc.gov/ncidod/EID/vol10no9/04-0170.htm (accessed April 15, 2005).
5. John M. Barry, *The Great Influenza: The Epic Story of the Deadliest Plague in History* (Viking Press, 2004).
6. John Hick MD, "Department of Health and EMS Regulatory Board," in *EMS Special Pathogen Guide* (St. Paul, MN: MDH, MN EMSRB, 2004).
7. Bell v. Community Ambulance Service Agency for Northern Des Moines County (579 N.W.2d 330). Motorist brought action against ambulance driver, ambulance service, and townships which utilized service, for injuries sustained in collision with ambulance.
8. C. A. Kahn, R. G. Pirrallo, and E. M. Kuhn. "Characteristics of Fatal Ambulance Crashes in the United States: An 11 Year Retrospective Analysis," *Prehospital Emergency Care* 5.3 (2001): 261–269.
9. Laura Bultman et al. "Buckle Up! EMS Use of Seat Belts." Abstract. *Prehospital Emergency Care* 9 (2005).
10. Shawn Watson. "In-Progress Call Responses." *Minnesota Center for Criminal Justice and Law Enforcement. Law Enforcement Integrated Practicum*. St. Paul, MN: Center for Criminal Justice and Law Enforcement, 2004.
11. Tom Givens, "States of Awareness, The Cooper Color Codes." *American Tactical Shooting Association* (May 2004). http://www.teddytactical.com/SharpenBladeArticle/4_States%20of%20Awareness.htm (accessed March 20, 2005).
12. Jonathan S. Smith, "Responders at Risk: Surviving Violence in the Streets." *Diss. United States Fire Academy* (1998). http://www.usfa.fema.gov/pdf/efop/efo29053.PDF (accessed March 20, 2005).
13. M. Spivak, "Hurting Those Who Save: Violence Against EMS Providers." *Emergency Medical Services* 27(5)(1998): 26, 28, 59.
14. Shawn Watson, "Defensive Tactics," *Minnesota Center for Criminal Justice and Law Enforcement. Law Enforcement Integrated Practicum*. St. Paul, MN: Center for Criminal Justice and Law Enforcement (August 2004).

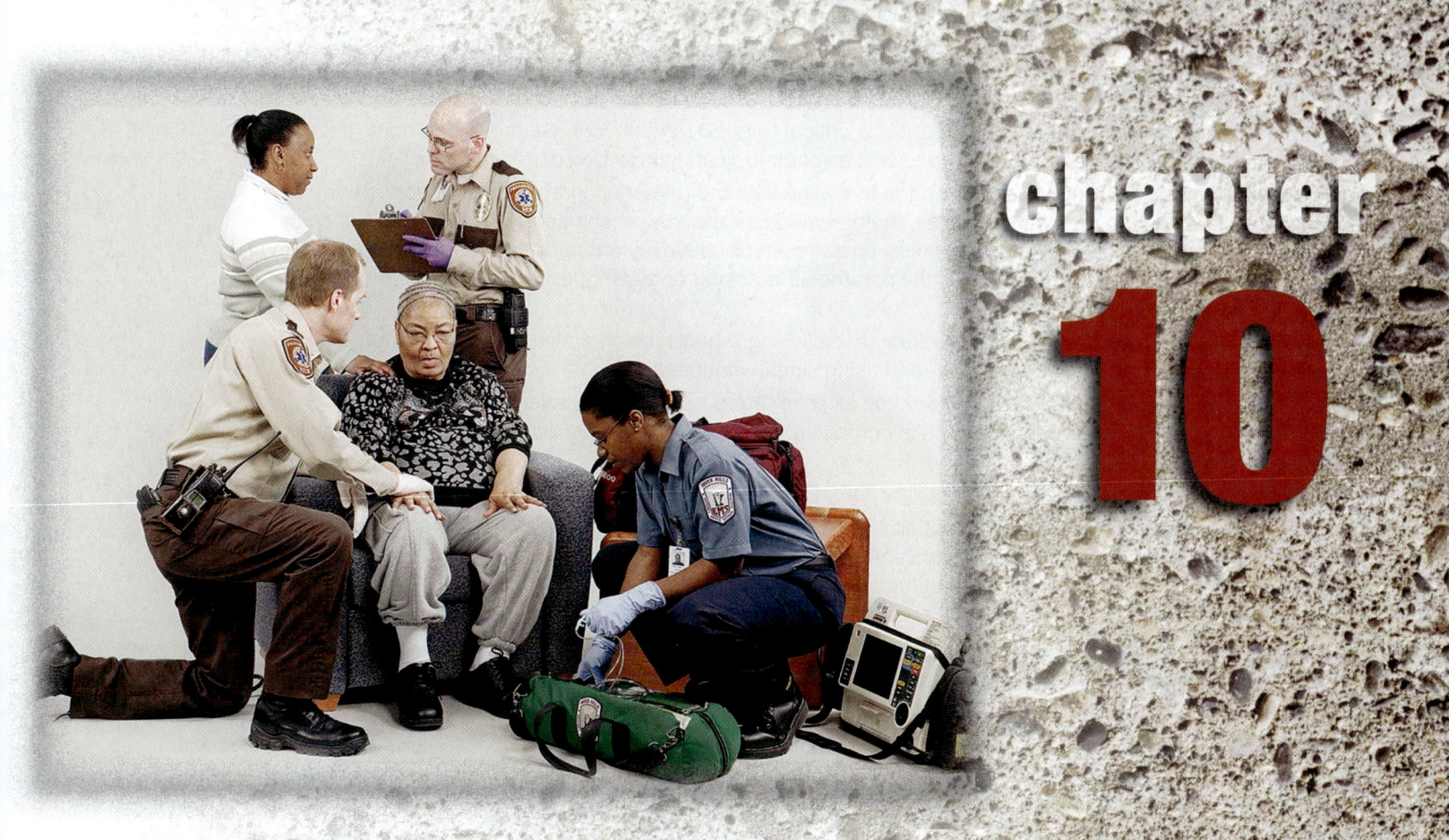

Therapeutic Communications and History Taking

"*Listen, or your tongue will make you deaf.*"

—Native American Proverb

Need to Know

▶ Communication, which is a two way process, is critical to good patient care. Gathering the right information from the patient is just as important as communicating in a therapeutic manner.

▶ The EMS interview is composed of two parts that align with the primary survey and secondary survey of patient assessment. In the primary survey, the paramedic is ensuring scene safety, determining the chief complaint, assessing level of consciousness, ensuring an open airway and proper breathing, and checking for circulation. In the secondary survey, the paramedic is asking detailed questions about the patient's condition and history.

▶ Key elements of medical interviewing include: establishing rapport, using active listening, demonstrating empathy, asking open-ended questions, and using simple language.

▶ Essential information that must be gathered on all encounters includes the patient's biographical information (age, name, address etc.), chief complaint, history of the present illness, pertinent past history, medications, and allergies.

▶ Review and be familiar with the memory aids: OPQRST, SAMPLE, PACE, and LEAPS.

▶ In the case where a patient is *sick,* attention should focus on the primary survey and relevant and pertinent elements of the secondary survey. Some information in the secondary survey may need to be obtained en route or deferred altogether if the patient requires rapid intervention.

▶ DO	▶ ASK
• Remain alert; think of safety as a continuum throughout the call • Start right: introduce yourself, make a good first impression, look the part, be professional • Actively listen to crew members, first responders, bystanders, and your patient • Treat others as you would want to be treated • Read nonverbal behavior for clues about severity/location of symptoms • Use nonverbal behavior to communicate respect and caring • Watch for patients escalating toward aggressive or violent behavior or for withdrawal or disinterest • Use verbal judo principles. The goal is to generate voluntary compliance: Listen, Empathize, Ask, Paraphrase, and Summarize (LEAPS), and consider the PACE: problems, audience, constraints, and ethical issues • Gather medication information and, if possible, take medications with you to the hospital • Take notes and record your observations • Minimize the amount of time spent on scene, but maximize the value of the time you are there by being organized	• Obtain permission before assessing or treating the patient • Ask the patient's name and how he or she would like to be addressed • Ask open-ended questions so the patient can fully explain the problem • Use the acronym OPQRST (Onset, Provocation/Palliation, Quality, Region/Radiation, Severity, Time) to focus your questions on pain or problems • Use the acronym SAMPLE (Symptoms, Allergies, Medications, Past History, Last oral intake, Events) to focus on pertinent history questions

Introduction

The way that you approach a patient, obtain a medical history, and establish good communication not only results in the gathering of vital information, but also, just as importantly, can result in the patient feeling better and trusting you.

Most of medicine and medical education has traditionally underemphasized the art of therapeutic communication, and communication skills in general.[1,2] Instead, medical practitioners have been taught to look for scientific symptoms and use measurable test values to diagnose and treat patients. The focus has been on a mechanical process to collect relevant biomedical information. The medical interview is often viewed by some as unreliable and imprecise because it does not involve measurable criteria such as blood pressure or heart rate. Many clinicians choose to focus on the results from physical tests instead of listening to the patient.[3,4]

Contrary to the traditional approach just described, evidence suggests that effective interviewing can yield precise and reproducible information leading to an accurate diagnosis and that communication is a key determinant in patient satisfaction, earlier recovery, and better quality of life.[3,5,6,7,8] Excellent communication between a patient and a caregiver that is patient-centered gives the patient an increased sense of control over the situation. The classic components of effective communication in western culture are active listening, eye contact, allowing choices, and appropriate touch and nonverbal communication.[9] DOT 1-9.18, 1-9-19

Street Secrets

A prerequisite to good communication skills is having an awareness of personal biases. Upbringing and social, cultural, economic, educational, and spiritual influences have shaped how you see the world and your patients. Being aware of perceptions is the first step in being able to relate with less bias toward a patient. DOT 1-9.13

Communication is the exchange of information between two people. It can be in the form of verbal and nonverbal messages.[10] A message is encoded by the person sending the information and decoded by the person receiving the information. Whether verbal or nonverbal, the patient is "telling his or her story" from the moment you can first observe the individual and throughout your contact. This is true even when you or your partners are not speaking to the patient. DOT 1-9.1, 3-5.1

The actions and behavior of an EMS provider are forms of nonverbal communication. Something as simple as wrapping a blood pressure cuff around an arm may seem like an innocent action you have done a hundred times. However, every time you touch a patient, or perform any kind of task, the way that you approach that task will communicate your intentions, emotions, and values. If you wrap the cuff carelessly and without warning, perhaps even bumping the patient's elbow or roughly yanking on his or her sleeve to clear a space for the cuff, you could be communicating a lack of respect or disregard of the patient's comfort. Although you may have meant no offense, even simple actions may unintentionally distress the patient. This chapter will provide tips and techniques helpful in allowing you to put your best foot forward when therapeutically communicating with patients. DOT 1-9.17

The Science behind a Great Interview

Hospital and clinic-based medicine relies on biomedical and laboratory tests to guide the diagnosis and treatment of patients, but these tests are usually unavailable in the prehospital setting.[3] By gathering objective, precise, specific, and reproducible information, the paramedic becomes one of the most accurate "instruments" in the ambulance.[3]

Precision

In the scientific process, precision relates to the degree with which a measurement is clustered around a mean value (or average finding). The more precise the measurement, the more tightly grouped those values will be. The more imprecise, the more scattered those values will be. For example, in a medical interview basic information begins with the patient's own words. If those words tightly describe the patient's "real" problem, then the measurement will be precise. Incomplete histories or wide variations and inconsistencies in the patient's story make the interview less precise and, therefore, less useful.

Mistakes and errors in measurement are introduced when the patient's complaints are vague and random or when the paramedic makes assumptions, listens poorly, or lacks attention to detail. For example, a patient who says "I just want to die" may be describing suicidal thoughts, severe pain, embarrassment, or simple exhaustion. Clarifying that complaint with more detail is essential in order to discover the patient's true problem.

Sensitivity and Specificity

Other criteria used to better judge the quality of a measurement are degree of sensitivity and specificity. These concepts are easily misunderstood, but their meaning is important in the evaluation and interpretation of information. Both concepts help pinpoint the likelihood that a patient is exhibiting a particular condition.

The **sensitivity of a test** relates to the proportion of people who truly have a particular disease identified by the test. If 98% of all patients with a stroke have trouble reading an eye chart, that test would be more sensitive in determining stroke than if only 45% of stroke patients had blurred vision.

The **specificity of a test** relates to its ability to "rule out" or dismiss the problem. In this case, if blurred vision was limited to patients with stroke, the specificity would be high. However, blurred vision can be caused by many other things including drug use, foreign bodies, or diseases such as macular degeneration or glaucoma. Therefore blurred vision as a symptom is not just limited to stroke patients.

A symptom may be very sensitive (most people having a heart attack experience chest discomfort)[11,12] but not specific (chest discomfort is caused by many different problems, and only 20% of patients with chest discomfort are in fact found to have a heart attack).[13] Few tests in medicine approach 100% sensitivity and specificity, and individual symptoms are definitely not a reliable way to form a working diagnosis in the field. A complete history or the "whole story" often contains most of the information needed for an accurate assessment.[14]

Reliability

Experienced providers often can be heard complaining that the patient changes his or her story on arrival to the emergency department. The reliability of information relates to how similar the results will be when the test, in this case the interview, is performed by someone else. Since human interaction is complex, it should be noted that patients will have different degrees of comfort openly admitting personal information to healthcare professionals. Also, interactions that take place between one provider and a patient may not have the same level of intimacy or disclosure with another provider. Gender, appearance, age, and economic, social, sexual, cultural, and healing preferences are only some of the reasons why patients may react differently to different healthcare workers. DOT 1-9.13

Other issues with reliability include the patients' perception of their symptoms. Patients can often dismiss a symptom as unrelated. For example, a pregnant woman who has a headache and blurred vision may think these symptoms are totally unrelated to her high blood pressure and newly swollen ankles. However, after the first medical person to interview her has asked questions about the two issues, she may see the connection and answer differently when the next person asks.

Starting Off on the Right Foot

It is essential to create a positive relationship, so the patient has confidence and trust in your care.[15,16] The initial moments of contact are a critical time to make a good impression, establish rapport, and demonstrate competence.

Research suggests that a paramedic has only 10 seconds from the initial contact with the patient to establish a strong relationship.[15] The ability to be friendly, professional, clinically competent, and empathetic is nonverbally communicated in those first seconds. Always introduce yourself and your crew to the patient, obtain his or her name, and make eye contact. Even though the patient typically understands that you are there to assist, ask his or her permission to both assess and treat him or her (Figure 10-1).

Before the First Word Is Spoken …

Many of the elements that will set the tone for the initial interaction with the patient happen before a single word is spoken. From the moment the dispatcher describes

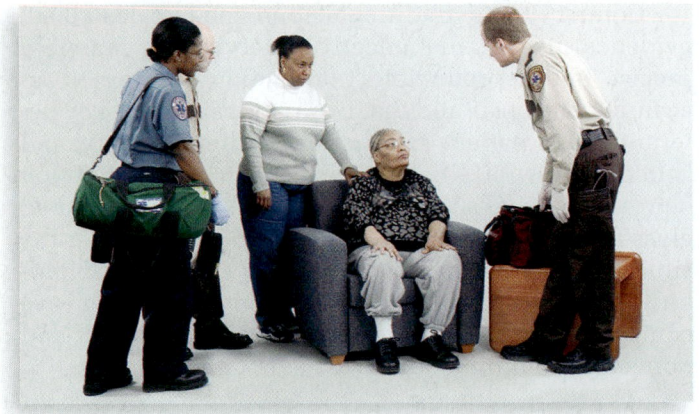

Figure 10-1 Always approach your patient from the front and introduce yourself.

that you are "on the way" and will "be there quickly," to the sound of the siren coming down the block, the patient is beginning to form an opinion of who you are and how helpful you will be. Remember too that many patients may have had unpleasant interactions with EMS or other public safety agencies in the past that may affect their impressions of you. Also, some patients are under a lot of stress, are in pain, or are fearful, so they may not be on their best behavior from the start.

Initial communication with the patient is nonverbal. The manner of approach and entrance to the scene sends a message. For example, parking on the patient's lawn, entering his home without knocking, or tracking mud onto a clean carpet can communicate disrespect before the first word is ever exchanged. A simple smile, eye contact, and a look of concern will demonstrate genuine compassion and caring.

Make Eye Contact

Eye contact is encouraged to establish good rapport; however, it should be noted that in some cases, eye contact has a lot more meaning. Do not be offended if some patients do not look you in the eye. In many Asian cultures, eye contact is disrespectful, especially if the other person is perceived to be in a superior position.[17] Eye contact may also be impolite such as in the Appalachian culture[17] and the Navajo culture, where it is considered a sign of disrespect. Prolonged eye contact in any culture can signal aggression or hostile intent, especially if the person is squinting or looking repeatedly at a particular body part.[18] You should take precautions if any patient is intently staring at someone for any period of time as this can signal previolent behavior.

CONNECTIONS See Box 46-5 in Chapter 46: Patients with Special Challenges for more on eye contact with individuals with autism.

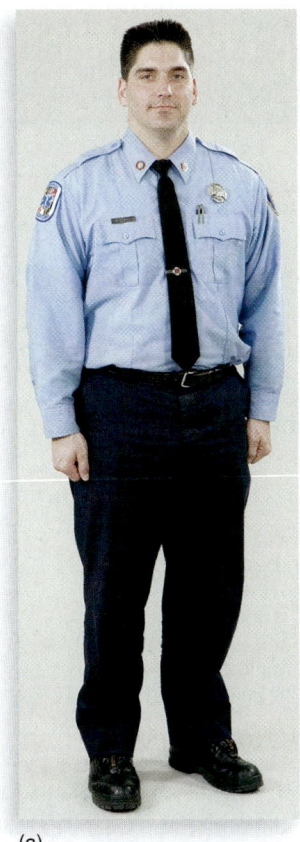
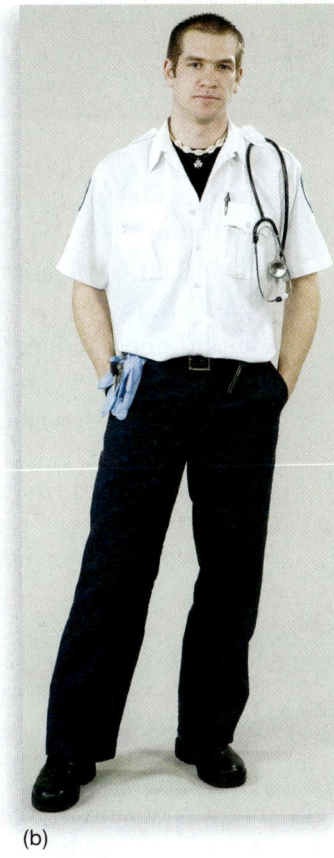

(a)

(b)

Figure 10-2 Make a good first impression (a) by wearing a clean, pressed uniform. Avoid jewelry, body piercings, and casual clothes (b).

As described in Chapter 2, it is important to take emotional stock of your own experiences and maintain a healthy balance between feeling compassion and remaining separate from the patient's emotion. It is, after all, the patient's "emergency," and you must be able to separate your own sadness and fear from the patient's. Managing each call, one at a time, and realizing that there are things you can control and things that are out

The Uniform Appearance

Physical appearance and dress send a strong message. Casual clothing, dangling earrings, prominent ruffles[19] and overly fashion-trendy clothing worn by a caregiver can create a negative impression on patients.[19] Looking as generic and clean-cut as possible can help start you off on the right foot (Figure 10-2). Box 10-1 lists some elements that can help you look professional.

Demonstrate Empathy

To a large extent, your ability to perform an accurate assessment, effectively communicate with a patient, and simply help a patient feel better, depends on your empathy skills. The essence of **empathy** has been described as the ability to see these patients as they see themselves.[20] Empathy is a form of understanding, both intellectually and emotionally.[3] It is different than compassion or sympathy. Sympathy is more like feeling sad or sorry for someone. Compassion implies a desire to alleviate someone's distress. Demonstrating empathy shows patients that you have a concern for their well-being beyond their physical injuries (Figure 10-3).[21]

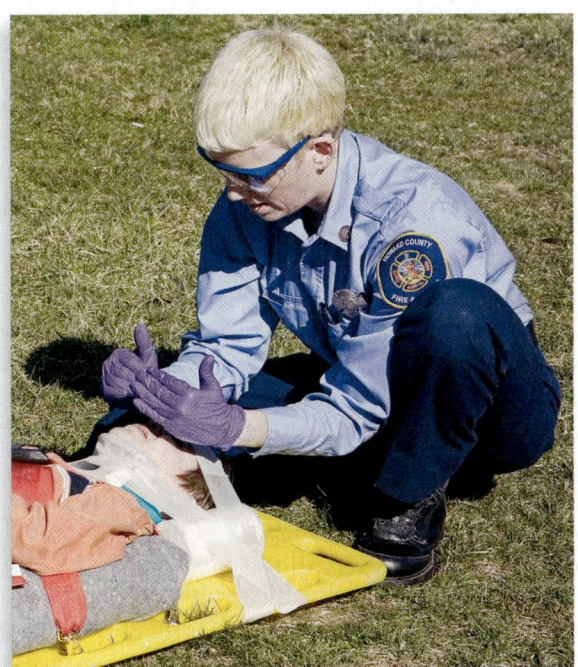

Figure 10-3 This boy was bothered by the bright sunshine. The paramedic shielded his eyes to help him feel more comfortable.

of your control is very important. You will not be able to stop disease, save every life, or make everyone feel better. You will, however, be able to take each work day as a new opportunity to help your patients and serve the community.

Actively Listen to the Patient

Active listening is a core communication skill and one of the most important skills for a paramedic to master. Active listening is interactive and requires that the paramedic pay attention to both the content and the emotions the patient is expressing. Key components of active listening are being attentive, letting the patient talk, making eye contact, and noting discrepancies in how the patient is talking and what is really being said.

As the patient concludes his or her comments, restate, or *paraphrase* what you have heard using a summary or fewer words. Paraphrasing is important to test your understanding of what the patient has said, and it helps clarify what you think you heard.[37] For example, consider the following interaction:

Paramedic: Mr. Johnson, we would like to take you to the hospital for further evaluation and treatment of your back pain.

Mr. Johnson (looking away): *I really hate hospitals, and I'm tired of being in pain. I just got out of that hospital yesterday. They already know me over there. I really don't want to go to the hospital again, and I just want you to take the pain away.*

Paramedic: I'm sorry to hear that you've been having trouble managing your pain. Being in pain for this long can be an awful thing to live with.

Mr. Johnson (in a louder voice and looking away): *I just want to lie here and try to hold still. They can't help me feel better; I'm sorry I called you. I should never have tried to lift that cabinet without any help. I'm so stupid! All of the times before this I've been able to drive myself in to the emergency room, and they always took good care of me. But this last time I just couldn't get comfortable. I think it's a tumor and not a muscle spasm. The pain just grabs me and squeezes and doesn't let up.*

Paramedic: I can see that you are getting frustrated and upset. We want to help you feel better, and staying on the floor without moving is only going to cause more pain. Besides, you can't stay there forever. Please allow us to help you get up. Why do you feel that this is a tumor?

The interaction above demonstrates the importance of listening for both the subject matter and the emotions behind the message. If the patient does not feel that you

BOX 10-2 Active Listening Strategies

- Attentiveness
- Paraphrasing
- Clarifying
- Perception verification
- Summarizing
- Helpful open-ended questions:
  - "Can you tell me more about that?"
  - "Can you describe what you have been feeling?"
  - "What did you notice?" "Tell me what the pain is like?"
  - "How has your health been in the past?"

  DOT 1-9.4

Adapted from J. L. Coulehan, and M. R. Block, *The Medical Interview: Mastering Skills for Clinical Practice*, 4th ed. (Philadelphia, PA: FA Davis Company, 2001) 46.

have understood his problem and the severity of his pain, he is likely to continue to get angry as he gets more frustrated. This patient needs reassurance and needs to know that you heard his concerns. Clarifying why he feels the next hospital visit will end poorly is the first step toward understanding his reluctance to go to the hospital. His theory about the origin of the pain is important to note and explore. This may lead to more information he has not yet shared but also may redirect the patient into less overwhelming reasons for his pain, such as muscle spasm. Box 10-2 lists active listening strategies. DOT 1-9.20, 3-5.7

Silence can also be a useful technique during an interview. It may seem uncomfortable to sit there in silence, but remaining quiet and letting the patient talk will encourage him or her to continue speaking. DOT 3-5.7 **See Skill Sheet 63: Verbal Communication.**

Be Objective and Avoid Premature Interpretation

Objectivity involves stripping away any beliefs or preconceived ideas so that you can focus on what the patient is actually saying and experiencing. Consider this interview by a paramedic:

Paramedic: Hello Ms. Smith, what is troubling you today?

Ms. Smith: *I'm feeling weak and dizzy.*

Paramedic: OK. I see by your medical tag on your wrist that you are a diabetic. When was your last meal?

Ms. Smith: *I can't keep anything down, so I haven't been eating well. I keep vomiting what I eat. I just feel dizzy when I sit up or use the bathroom.*

Paramedic: When was the last time you checked your blood sugar?

Ms. Smith: *Ten minutes ago, it was 120. I've been having a lot of very dark diarrhea so I've been checking it often.*

Paramedic: What kind of insulin do you take?

Ms. Smith: *Humalog™. I haven't taken any today. I'm just so dizzy when I sit up; I'm worried I will black out when I need to go to the toilet again.*

Paramedic: OK. Try to relax. Let's check your sugar again. How often do you have episodes of low blood sugar?

This interview excerpt shows how easily a caregiver can get focused on one aspect of the patient's history and ignore important information about symptoms that the patient is describing. This type of behavior is called **tunnel vision.** It can quickly lead down the wrong path and result in an incorrect assessment and incorrect treatment and can waste valuable time.

CONNECTIONS Tunnel vision is described in detail in Chapter 5: Clinical Decision-Making

In this scenario, because this patient has a history of diabetes, the paramedic is investigating what he thinks is the most likely cause of the symptoms. The information he is gathering is being used only to support or refute his theory that the patient has a low blood sugar. Not only is he asking narrow questions, but he is also not listening to the patient. The patient is explaining a series of symptoms and events that may point to dehydration, a heart attack, gastrointestinal bleeding, and a number of other problems. Consider how this interview could be improved in the following way:

Paramedic: Hello Ms. Smith, what is troubling you today?

Ms. Smith: *I'm feeling weak and dizzy.*

Paramedic: Can you tell me more about your dizziness?

Ms. Smith: *Yes, I only get it when I stand up or bear down on the toilet. I've been having diarrhea all day.*

Paramedic: Diarrhea is not fun; I'm sorry you are going through that. When and how often have you been having episodes of diarrhea?

Ms. Smith: *Since yesterday. My stomach started hurting, then my stools started looking dark. I really think I'm having a bad case of food poisoning from some old cereal I ate a week ago.*

Paramedic: OK. It sounds like your stools have been loose and dark. Can you tell me more about the color, how dark are they?

Ms. Smith: *They look black and tarry.*

Paramedic: Are they still in the toilet so I could see them?

Ms. Smith: *No, I flushed. I just feel terrible when I sit up.*

Paramedic: I'm sorry you are feeling sick. We are going to take good care of you.

Ms. Smith: *Thanks.*

Paramedic: I see you are a diabetic. How are you managing your diabetes today?

Ms. Smith: *My blood sugars have been running in the 120s; I'm checking it constantly because I can't seem to keep any food down.*

Paramedic: Sounds like you have been watching this very closely. Good job.

This second interview allowed the patient to tell her story and quickly yielded very appropriate information about her condition. Listening to the patient, following up on important statements, and clarifying what you think you have heard will help you stay objective and accurate.

In the case listed above, considering the patient's diabetic status and getting a detailed account of the latest blood sugar and oral intake is very important. It is part of a complete and thorough history. The critical difference between the first and second interviews with Ms. Smith is that in the second interview, the paramedic has not made the assumption that the problem is related to the patient's diabetes.

Verbal Judo for EMS Responders

George Thompson, a former police officer and now a consultant and author, offers street-smart tactics to help manage difficult patient interpersonal situations successfully. His book is a valuable tool for the field paramedic. Verbal judo teaches that the goal of each contact is to generate voluntary compliance. "It is a gentle method to engage in tactical communication" writes Thompson who has made a life goal to teach and propagate the following ideals:[20] DOT 1-9.2, 1-9.3

1. **"Always maintain a professional face, but never strive to save your personal face."** Your professional "face" is the demeanor, poise, attitude, and behavior that make you a paramedic. Your personal face is your ego and the image of yourself that you hope others will see. Be careful not to make your patients look dumb.

2. **"Follow the golden rule: Treat others like you want to be treated."** Treating others as you want to be treated will help you temper your response to inappropriate behavior.

3. **"Be careful to distinguish between reasonable resistance and severe resistance."** Let go of the small

stuff, and ignore behavior that does not significantly detract from your main goal: good patient care and prompt transportation to a medical facility.

4. **"Every encounter is unique."** Imagine that every patient you treat is someone who is different, special in his or her own way, and dangerous in another way.

5. **"You alone have a responsibility to create rapport."** Don't expect others to become pleasant, cooperative, or compliant.

6. **"Check your assumptions."** Whether you are confirming what you think you just heard a patient say or double checking the address of a call you are responding to, *assuming* that you know will only lead you to make mistakes.

7. **"Use adrenalin, don't be ruled by it."** When fear or excitement is running rampant in your blood, it is vital that you maintain composure and stay focused on your mission.

8. **"Respond to people, don't react."** Responding implies a measured and deliberate purpose in answering someone while reacting implies less forethought and a certain level of external influence, without really knowing what will happen next.

9. **"Flexibility equals strength: Rigidity equals weakness."** Find alternative ways to talk to patients, appeal to their senses, and find creative solutions to problems.

10. **"Avoid depersonalization and abstraction. Be specific and deal with people as individuals."** Your service is to people, not to their disease or injury.

11. **"Use positive feedback when you least feel like it."** Fight the internal urge to be cynical and to defend yourself from seemingly personal attacks, and turn the other cheek when a patient has clearly tried to insult you.

12. **"Use self talk."** While you are in the middle of an unpleasant contact, keep repeating to yourself some of the simple elements of the PACE and LEAPS acronyms:

PACE

P **Problem** Define the issue(s) or situation that requires attention.

A **Audience** Consider who you are speaking with, their belief system, values, and current state of mind.

C **Constraints** Take into account and then work around obstacles and limitations; accomplish what is realistic.

E **Ethical presence** Maintain a professional demeanor, and do what is right for your patient.

LEAPS

L Listen
E Empathize
A Ask
P Paraphrase
S Summarize

13. **"It's not enough to be good; you've got to look good and sound good."** Imagine that every patient contact has a hidden camera, and your choice of words and actions can and will be questioned if things go wrong.

14. **"Remember that patients can say whatever they want as long as they do what you say."** This is especially true of patients whose behavior is altered by alcohol, drugs, medical conditions, or a psychiatric illness. The patient's aggressive behavior is not aimed at you personally.

Interviewing Pitfalls

Just as verbal judo is a way to encourage good communication, certain behaviors will be counterproductive in establishing a positive relationship with a patient. Behaviors to avoid include:[21]

- *Providing false reassurance.* Reassuring patients is good; giving false hope, however, leads patients to mistrust you and the healthcare system in general.

- *Giving unwanted advice.* Instead of giving advice, try to involve patients in the problem-solving process and lead them to the answers themselves.

- *Avoid using your authority.* Avoid the temptation to use your authority to send a message of: "The paramedic knows best." Patients may not feel comfortable saying it, but they may feel inferior, inadequate, and that you are "talking down" to them. This also promotes dependency and discourages patients from taking responsibility for their own choices. DOT 1-5.8

- *Using euphemisms or avoidance language.* Use direct language in a respectful and gentle way. This will help the patient and family confront bad information in a more real and therapeutic way.

- *Using professional jargon.* When working with patients, it is best to use language that is easy to understand. Medical terminology is usually not appropriate for these interactions. DOT 3-5.27

- *Using leading or biased questions.* You will get more information if you ask open-ended, nonbiased questions. Be sure to ask one question at a time, and only one person should interview the patient at a time. Asking multiple questions at once may result in unclear answers and confusion.[1]

■ ***Talking too much and interrupting.*** Listen to your patients. If you allow them to talk about their illnesses, you are likely to learn more about the exact reasons they are seeking care and will be more able to help them. Interrupt only if it is critical that you redirect or clarify information.[1] DOT 1-9.5, 1-9.14, 1-9.16

The Scene Size-Up

Prearrival Dispatch and Bystander Information

Potential sources of information include the person dispatching the call and the bystander on the scene. Treat this information with caution, and do not be misled. This information is often only as reliable as the person who provided it in the first place, but it can be helpful in determining if the patient is *"sick"* or *"not yet sick."* If the dispatcher, responder, or bystander has significant medical training, he or she will report the most important information he or she has obtained. Care should be taken not to ignore or only to half-listen to these other health care professionals. Listening to a quick report will often help to determine if the patient is in critical condition and may save valuable time. DOT 3-5.22

Scene Safety

Scene safety is always of paramount importance, and it supercedes all other considerations. The reality is that a scene is never 100% safe. The scene of a highway crash may be outside the path of traffic, until a speeding driver inadvertently veers into the scene. An electrical wire might seem perfectly insulated and without current, until sparks suddenly fly. Even without environmental hazards, the smallest and most gentle patients can quickly alter their behavior and become aggressive.

Scene safety considerations exist on a continuum throughout the EMS call. All scenes should be considered extremely hazardous, and even when things might seem stable, maintain a level of alertness such as condition yellow or orange as discussed in Chapter 9. Safety is a concern that should permeate the entire call. DOT 3-3.51, 5-12.10

CONNECTIONS Chapter 9: Safety and Scene Size-Up has additional information on alertness levels, scene safety, and tips for ways to assess and maintain a safe working environment.

Your Presence on the Scene

Scene presence is another way to immediately begin building a good rapport with your patient. "Presence" refers to the ability to project a sense of self-confidence and show that you are at ease with the situation.[9] Nonverbal behaviors can help project this sense of presence. An upright, alert posture communicates that you are present and ready to serve. Slouching or appearing tired will communicate disinterest and a lack of ability.[16] DOT 1-9.3, 1-9.6

Respecting and "Violating" Personal Space

The distance maintained between the paramedic and patient and how the patient is initially approached affect communication. Although there are variations between cultures, as a general rule, the closer two people position themselves at the beginning of their interaction, the more friendly they appear to be.[18] Consider your distance and position from the patient as you begin speaking. Are you towering over someone who is sitting down? This might create a power relationship in which the patient must physically look up to you, and it may create a feeling that you are judging him or her or that you believe you are superior.

Be sure to approach your patients from the front and try not to startle them. Generally (in the United States), 18 inches to 4 feet is considered personal space. Four to 12 feet is considered a social distance, and more than 12 feet is considered a public distance.[9] Take into consideration that within a distance of 10 feet, your ability to react, defend yourself, and flee is greatly diminished.

CONNECTIONS Personal space changes from one culture to the next. Chapter 48: Patients from Diverse Cultures has more information on how various cultures prefer to interact. DOT 1-9.21, 3-5.6

Reading Body Language

Watch your patient's body language as you approach. Consider extending a hand for a friendly greeting handshake. If the patient's eyes narrow or she frowns, it is likely she is defensive or even aggressive towards you. Regardless of the distance at which your interaction begins, once it is established, changes in that distance can clue you in to what your patient is feeling or thinking. If the patient is ambulatory and moves away, it is likely that the patient is not interested in what you are saying or is becoming resistant. If you or the patient leans in and the distance is decreased, it is likely that something important or personal is going to be said. When distance between you and the patient begins to narrow, be alert for signs of aggression and potential violence.[18] Table 10-1 provides some hints for reading body language.

Paramedics often, by necessity, must conduct interviews and physical assessments while in close contact

TABLE 10-1   Reading Body Language

Body Part	Neutral	Resistant	Aggressive
The eyes	Eyes wide open making eye contact	Wandering gaze, less eye contact, disinterested	Narrowed, focused look, prepared to strike
The head	Resting, balanced at center	Leaning back	Leaning forward
The arms	Fully extended, relaxed at the side	Folded across chest (can also mean insecurity and fear)	If sitting, they are above the table
The hands	Palms outward, relaxed	Shifting around	Clenched fists, or opening and closing
The feet	Weight evenly distributed, facing forward evenly	Weight distributed toward the back	Leaning forward on the balls of the feet

Adapted from R. R. Rail, *The Unspoken Dialog: Understanding Body Language and Controlling Interviews and Negotiations* (Kansas City, MO: Varro Press, 2001) 18–38.

with a patient. You are often within striking distance of the patient and inside his or her personal space. You will have little, if any, reaction time to protect yourself. To minimize the danger, position yourself so you are a smaller target: take a bladed stance—shoulder and hips turned, and keep your weight on your back leg so you can easily turn and flee. Make sure your partner or another responder has kept an open escape (egress) route, and avoid remaining too long in locations that do not have an easy way out.

Practice the principles of contact and cover discussed in Chapter 9. As one of you approaches and interacts with the patient, the other maintains a close eye on the environment and patient/provider interaction. Each provider should maintain condition yellow or orange whenever in close proximity to the patient. **Review Skill Sheet 65: Patient Restraints (also see Step-by-Step 65: Physical Restraints).**

CONNECTIONS Refer back to Chapter 9: Safety and Scene Size-Up to review material on the bladed stance and staying in condition yellow or orange at all times.

Nice to Know

Only in very specific circumstances, such as when entering a Muslim mosque or Mormon temple, will you be required to remove your shoes. Remaining culturally aware of the social norms at your scene is vital.

Obtaining Consent for Care and Treatment

In the initial moments of the patient-paramedic interaction, it should become clear that the patient is requesting and consenting to care. Consent can be obtained verbally by deliberately asking if the patient would like you to examine or treat him or her. More often, consent is communicated in a more subtle way, as the patient begins to describe his or her problem and willingly talks to you and allows the assessment. It is important to get an initial sense of whether or not the patient is capable of consenting by assessing the patient's mental status. **Skill Sheet 64: Documentation is also a helpful resource.**

CONNECTIONS Remember that when a patient does not consent to treatment, it is important to document this. In addition, determine if the patient is competent and capable of withholding consent. Chapter 4: Legal Issues explores consent and refusals.

In some cultures, paramedics may need to adjust the initial communication strategy to address someone other than the actual patient to receive approval to speak to and approach the patient. This adjustment is essential to show respect for the patient, their family, and their culture, even if the paramedic feels uncomfortable. Such a show of respect will usually win trust and improve the flow of the call.

Nice to Know

The communications company AT&T has an interpreter service, available through subscription, so ambulance services and public safety agencies have almost immediate access to interpreters for virtually every language that may be encountered in the prehospital setting. **Skill Sheet 62: Communication Challenges– Interpreter Services has more information.**

CONNECTIONS Chapter 3: Professional Ethics and Chapter 4: Legal Issues describe which patients can and cannot directly express consent. Situations with children and vulnerable adults require different approaches as the patients' guardians may need to consent for care. Chapter 48: Patients from Diverse Cultures discusses how specific cultures approach illness.

Maintain Patient Privacy

Protect the patient's privacy as much as possible. This may mean asking others to step out of the room, drawing a curtain or door partially shut, or simply asking the patient to step into the ambulance for a more quiet and safe environment. Patients can be reluctant to answer some questions, especially about the use of drugs or alcohol and pregnancy. They may also be unwilling to disclose their past medical history in front of others. Create a private, yet safe situation for the patient to talk.

Other physical factors can make communications less effective. These include lighting, noise levels on the scene (from televisions, vehicle engines, and other noise), and distracting equipment.[22] DOT 1-9.15

Street Secrets

It is best to begin very formally by addressing patients using the title Mr., Miss, or Mrs. and then their last name. Early on, it is important to ask patients for a name they prefer to be called. Some patients will quickly correct you and request a more relaxed use of their first name or a nickname. You should default to using a formal tone if the patient does not request something different.

Biographical Data

Make every attempt to collect the full name, address, phone number, age, birth date, gender, ethnic origin, and occupation of the patient. Insurance information and a signature permitting the ambulance service to bill insurance companies directly is considered standard information for systems that bill for services rendered. Make sure HIPAA laws are followed and the identity and privacy of the patient are safeguarded.

Forming the General Impression

A general impression, conducted immediately prior to initiating the primary survey helps identify life-threatening problems quickly. If the patient is able to speak clearly and distinctly, the airway is open and probably not obstructed. The patient's speech pattern can give you an immediate idea of level of consciousness and if there is any difficulty in breathing. If the patient speaks only in one or two word sentences or seems out of breath, dyspnea is likely present.

Nonverbal communication is also an important clue to determine how sick the patient may be. For example, a child who is holding perfectly still, drooling, and not crying may be focusing intently on breathing or keeping his or her airway clear. A man who is not moving and is wincing and holding pressure on a deformed limb is obviously in pain.

Assessing Mental Status

The findings of the initial interview help assess mental status. Once again, speech content and patterns are a clue. The speed of conversation, logical flow of ideas, clarity of thought, and comprehension of questions can help identify the patient's orientation and cognitive ability. The paramedic may be able to observe the patient's level of orientation by listening to the context of the patient's conversation. However, it is often necessary to ask the patient to confirm the date and location where he or she is and to identify by name a person known to him or her.

Nice to Know

The volume that a person uses to speak can be an indicator of how important he thinks his message is. Watch for an escalation in volume if the patient is becoming aggressive or previolent. The patient may feel like you are not listening to him, and communication may be breaking down.[18]

Special consideration should be given to children and geriatric patients who may not know specific dates, locations, or the people they are with. In these cases, it is valuable to confirm with a family member or caregiver if the patient is functioning at his or her baseline level of orientation. Patients who cannot hold their attention on the interview, appear forgetful, or cannot track the subject of the conversation should be carefully assessed.

Patients may try to cover up for their lack of knowledge or be embarrassed by their altered level of functioning. Do not be misled or distracted by humor or a sudden change of topics. Patients who fail to accurately report two or more of the following—person, place, and time—are considered impaired.[23] These patients should be considered *sick* until more information is available to explain the change. DOT 1-9.8, 1-9.11

Primary Survey (Initial Assessment)

Much is happening in the first seconds of the paramedic-patient interaction while the scene size-up is occurring. The very next phase of patient assessment is to perform the primary survey. During the **primary survey** the paramedic quickly determines if the patient requires life-saving interventions. Further questioning during the primary survey is accompanied by an assessment and status of the airway, breathing, and circulation (ABC). Questions during this time should be linked directly to the ABC assessment.

CONNECTIONS Chapter 14: Patient Assessment describes the components of patient assessment that include the primary and secondary surveys.

Secondary Survey (Focused Assessment)

The **secondary survey** is performed after the primary survey. In the case where the patient is *sick,* scene time must be minimized by gathering only essential elements before transporting the patient. If the patient is critical and scene time must be minimized, consider taking a witness, family member, or other person aware of the history with you to the hospital. In an emergency, it may only be possible to gather a bird's-eye view of things. The patient's chief complaint, history of the present illness, allergies, and medications may be the only things obtained before leaving the scene.

The need for rapid treatment and transportation must be weighed against the benefit of collecting valuable information from interviews at the scene. Time may be well spent gathering medications and determining key elements of the current history. Looking around the scene may provide valuable clues to the problem the patient is having. The receiving hospital depends on the eyes and ears of the paramedic to bring key information that will help appropriately treat the patient.

There is little scientific evidence to suggest what the optimal amount of prehospital scene time should be. As a general rule, scene times should be as short as possible, with the goal of less than ten minutes for trauma or for any patient who is obviously *sick.*[24] Several studies have shown averages of 11 minutes to 23 minutes on the scene of serious trauma patients.[25,26,27] Similarly, scene times during possible acute myocardial infarctions have been shown to average 16–25 minutes.[28,29] For patients who are not critically ill or injured, it is best to expedite transport without compromising a thorough assessment and appropriate interventions.

The Complete Patient History

Subjective and Objective Findings

The purpose of gathering a thorough history is to collect information, past and present, which is pertinent to the assessment and treatment of the patient. Traditionally, what the patient *says* is considered the **subjective** portion of your assessment and involves the patient's report of symptoms. This implies that it cannot be seen, felt, heard, or even verified by the paramedic. Take the information at face value as there is a limited ability to substantiate the information.

Although both the history and physical examination involve detailed observation of the patient and a degree of objectivity, the history is focused on information that is reported to you by others, including the patient. The physical examination is "objective" data that is seen, heard, and touched by the healthcare team.

The subjective assessment includes the patient's reason for calling, the description of his or her symptoms, past history, pertinent negatives (things the patient denies that help exclude potential diagnoses), and any self-care measures utilized. Even when a patient shows you medication bottles, this information is still considered subjective because you cannot assume that the patient has been taking the medication as prescribed (also termed "compliant").

In contrast, the physical examination is an **objective assessment.** The paramedic is looking, listening, and feeling for physical signs. Remember that no single vital sign or assessment finding typically represents all that is wrong with the patient. A complete assessment is important, so all the findings can be compared and evaluated in relationship to each other.

This concept can be difficult to grasp. If the pain is reproduced on palpation, it is appropriate to document in the physical exam that "tenderness" exists after palpation. "Tenderness" is defined as "pain upon pressure".[30] Pain alone is a symptom and should be documented as part of the history of the patient's present illness.

Defining the Problem: The Reason for Seeking Care (Chief Complaint)

If the patient did not call for help, it is important to determine who initiated the request for assistance and the reason for doing so. The next step is to determine the reason care is being sought. This reason is traditionally called the **chief complaint.**

Working in the Gray Zone

Recently, some have advocated not using the term "chief complaint" as it implies that the patient is a "complainer."[21] It may also be misleading. For example, if the patient is "complaining" of "difficulty breathing," but the cause of this difficulty is a gunshot wound to the chest, reporting "difficulty breathing" can mislead other caregivers. While a change in standard terminology may be coming, the term "chief complaint" is used in this text and will be seen in the field and across the medical literature for quite some time.

The reason for seeking care is traditionally documented in the patient's own words, in quotes, exactly as the patient states it. Studies show that patients usually have more than one primary complaint. To conduct a more patient-centered interview, it is best to let the patient describe what is wrong.[31]

Many practicing paramedics may fear being on scene for long periods of time as the patient rambles on about a small problem. Although no research has been performed on the best techniques in the prehospital setting for gathering information about the patient's chief complaint, we can learn from the experiences of other healthcare providers. One study from a clinic showed that patients, when not interrupted, never took more than 150 seconds to tell their full stories to the physicians caring for them.[32] A different study showed that physicians tend to interrupt the chief complaint within the first 18 seconds of the patient beginning to describe the problem and that this technique led to more closed-ended questions and a prolonged process for actually hearing the chief complaint.[33] DOT 1-9.4

Following an opening question such as "What is wrong today?" the paramedic should help the patient "fill in" details of the story by asking a series of targeted questions. It is important to encourage free expression while helping the patient focus on the important or pertinent details. Do not let the patient wander too far off course.[21] In cases where the patient has a long history of chronic illness, it may be necessary in the emergency setting to limit the interview to symptoms that are new or have changed recently. This might help clarify the reason for seeking care at the time the ambulance is called. DOT 1-9.14

Taking notes is essential to avoid asking the patient questions repeatedly (Figure 10-4). Most patients will understand that you are doing so as part of the performance of your duties. They will most likely appreciate not having to repeat themselves if you forget the details you have previously gathered. DOT 3-5.4, 3-5.5

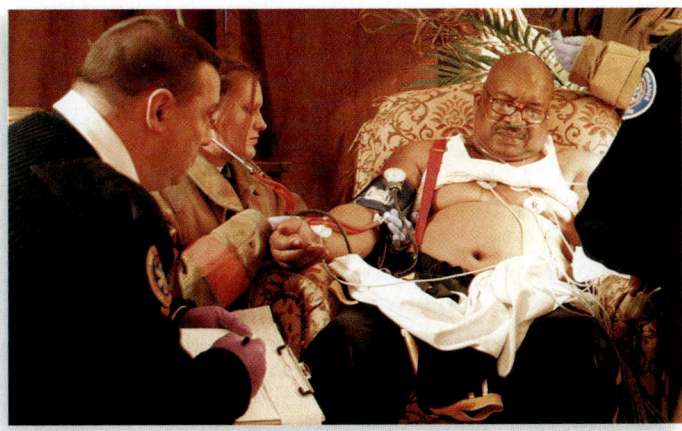

Figure 10-4 Assign one crew member to take notes at each scene.

History of the Present Illness

Medical interviews in the prehospital setting usually begin in a more open and general way and quickly narrow to bring out important details necessary to care.[9] Once the chief complaint is revealed, it may be necessary to ask specific, pointed questions to quickly determine the potential for danger to the patient. Symptoms should be explored, taking particular care to address the "where," "what," "when," and "why" of the problem.

Classic questions that help clarify the attributes of a symptom are best summarized by this acronym:

OPQRST

O Onset This refers to the events that were occurring when symptoms started. Was the patient resting? Doing physical work? In a stressful situation? Did the symptom come on suddenly or gradually over a period of time?

P Provocation or palliation This refers to anything that makes the symptoms worsen or improve, including any interventions performed by the patient.

Q Quality This refers to the nature or character of the symptom or pain. Is the pain dull, burning, or sharp? Is it constant, or does it come and go?

R Region or radiation This refers to the location of the symptom and where it is referred or radiates to. For example, if the patient knows it is gall stones and his shoulder aches, this is referred pain. Radiated pain begins in one location and moves along a path to another part of the body. Chest pain can begin behind the sternum and radiate up the arm and into the jaw.

S Severity This is the patient's self-assessment of a pain level on a scale from 0–10 (0 being no pain; 10 being the worst pain ever experienced by this patient).

T Time This refers to the time of onset of the first symptoms. It can also be helpful to determine when symptoms significantly worsened.

Street Secrets

Nonverbal communication can also help you assess the severity and location of pain. A patient who is guarding her abdomen, curled in a fetal position, and unable to sit up is showing you where and how much she is hurting. Another patient who is also complaining of abdominal pain and is pacing, smoking a cigarette, and yelling at her child for trying to steal a cookie is also showing you a lot about the severity and setting of her pain.

Pertinent Negatives

Just as important as discovering what symptoms are present is observing the noticeable absence of symptoms typically expected for a certain disease process. For example, a patient may say, "I just can't catch my breath." Further questioning to determine if the patient has chest discomfort is helpful to differentiate between a cardiac event versus a respiratory event. Another example would include asking the patient who is complaining of a headache if he or she has blurred vision, a recent traumatic injury, or weakness in the extremities. This would be helpful to rule out a stroke or cerebral hemorrhage.

Pertinent Past History

In a primary care setting, a physician or nurse will typically obtain a full history. This usually includes a thorough interview that uncovers childhood illnesses, accidents or injuries, obstetric history, past surgeries, hospitalizations, immunizations, sleep patterns, diet, tobacco and alcohol use, religious and cultural beliefs, social and economic factors, and daily life issues. DOT 1-9.13

In the EMS setting, there is limited time to explore all of the patient's previous history. While you may touch on several of the elements mentioned previously, this will be after the essential past history is properly explored. The acronym SAMPLE is helpful to simplify the essential elements of a pertinent past medical history for the prehospital setting.

SAMPLE History

S **Symptoms** Determine what the patient is experiencing and feeling as part of the illness or injury.

A **Allergies** Determine what medications and other substances the patient reacts to or is allergic to.

M **Medications** Ask about medications, including over-the-counter and herbal remedies that the patient is actively taking. If the patient is noncompliant with the prescribed regimen, this should be noted in the patient care report.

P **Past History** Ask about chronic illnesses and recent surgeries.

L **Last oral intake** Determine the last time the patient had anything to eat or drink.

E **Events** Ask what occurred leading up to the request for assistance.

The order in which this information in the SAMPLE history is collected does not need to match the acronym. The complete interview often does not have to occur only on the scene. Information may be collected throughout the transport of the patient, and transport should not be delayed if information can be gathered while en route to a hospital. Whenever possible, every one of the elements in SAMPLE and OPQRST should be collected and reported to the receiving care provider at the hospital.

Street Secrets

Ask the patient who reports an allergy to a medication to describe the reaction he or she experiences. Many patients believe that side effects, such as an upset stomach after taking aspirin, represent an allergy. Do not dismiss the patient's statement but rather document the type of reaction that the patient is reporting. In some cases, the benefit of a medication may outweigh the adverse reaction that it causes the patient. Consult with medical direction before administering any medication that the patient reported having an adverse reaction to.

Street Secrets

Occasionally a patient on a prescribed medication used to treat a chronic illness will report she has "no" medical problems. Ask her what she takes each medication for. Some patients may erroneously believe that they no longer have the underlying condition because it is controlled by medication. For example, the patient on an antihypertension medication might believe she no longer has "hypertension" because it is controlled by the drug and her BP reading is always within the normal range when she has it taken at the doctor's office.

Dealing with Uncooperative Patients

Paramedics typically expect patients to follow the traditional role of sick people and be willing and passive recipients of medical care.[34] "Good" patients are those who give information completely and honestly, accept the help that is offered, do not overly complain about their illnesses, and then follow the advice offered to them. Patients who do not conform to this expectation are often labeled difficult or uncooperative.[35]

In reality, some patients do not welcome help, and new EMS responders may experience difficulty when first encountering such patients.[36] Many patients are overwhelmed by emotions, pain, stress, and crisis. They are not only focused inward on themselves, but they are also not necessarily happy to see a paramedic walking through their doors. Anger, frustration, and hostility are common emotions vented by patients. Add intoxication or an altered mental state to an already unfortunate situation, and the result can be patients who do not really care about who is trying to help them.

The following are some of the difficulties routinely encountered while interviewing patients in the medical setting:

- Patients who are afraid, anxious, and angry about their illnesses or injuries
- Patients who have altered mental status from hypoxia, chemicals, or psychiatric impairments
- Patients who have vague complaints or ramble on about unrelated issues
- Patients who are lonely and are calling for comfort, compassion, and human contact
- Patients who do not seem to conform to the norms of society or who choose a lifestyle that is different from what is considered acceptable
- Melodramatic (also called "histrionic") or exaggerated descriptions by patients with whom it is difficult to assess the truthful severity of their symptoms
- Aggressive and violent patients who want to attack emergency responders
- Demanding patients who expect unreasonable accommodations and attention
- Patients who are in police custody who may be trying to fake symptoms to get out of jail

No single technique or solution exists for handling patients in each of these difficult cases. One standard approach is to remind yourself that the only reason you are present in that situation is that it was your turn to respond on a call. Try not to take personal offense at their behavior. Never allow yourself or your team to be assaulted or battered, but also do not let patients push your buttons. Being aware of your own biases and emotional triggers is important so that you do not get frustrated and drawn into a confrontation with a patient.

Some general tips for dealing with difficult situations include the following:

- Avoid making promises that you cannot keep
- Focus the patient on his or her own responsibility; do not let him or her shift responsibility to you
- Remain calm, gentle, and firm
- Stay focused on the patient's health issues, and avoid dealing with police, familial, or other matters that are not related to the patient's healthcare needs and that you cannot control
- Identify and reward the patient's strengths, even if you do not feel like being positive
- Try not to argue or contradict the patient; stay focused on the goal of your interaction: treating and transporting the patient
- Clarify your understanding of the patient's beliefs
- Do not ignore behavior that is dangerous or unacceptable; immediately confront and de-escalate threatening behavior

Again, there is no magic formula for interviewing an uncooperative patient. Experience is sometimes helpful, but the new graduate should not necessarily equate street experience with increased skills and abilities. In one study from the nursing profession, nurses with more patient care experience actually communicated poorly when compared with newer nurses who recently finished a training program.[37] Patience, courage, continuous improvement, and flexibility are key to gradually improving your ability to appropriately manage uncooperative patients. DOT 1-9.7, 1-9.9, 1-9.10

Summary

Medical interviewing is one of the most important steps in gathering all of the information needed to treat the patient effectively.[3] Individual symptoms are small elements of data to collect and use in assessing the patient. They are no different than lab values, vital signs, or ECG tracings.

No one single piece of information is enough to tell you what is wrong with the patient. Focus first on any information that reveals the presence of a life-threatening problem or that confirms that the patient is unstable or sick. As the patient is stabilized and transport has begun, additional history and information can be gathered.

Gather information from any source that is available. The patient, family, friends, first arriving responders on the scene, and primary caregivers are all potential sources for information. Don't discount nonmedical bystanders, such as a neighbor or even a mail carrier, who may have valuable insight into the situation. Nursing home charts, recent discharge papers, or doctor's visit bills might give you a clue about the patient's recent medical history. If the paramedic does not gather the information available on the scene, the rest of the healthcare team may never know there are additional issues.

While this chapter has focused on communication and the gathering of a thorough patient history, it is important to note that integration of the interview with the physical exam and treatment is essential for good patient care. In the field, everything is happening at once. While one person, usually the team leader, is asking questions and communicating with the patient, the partner might be taking vital signs or preparing the stretcher for transport.

Communicating with patients is partly about the science of gathering medically relevant information and partly about the art of using good communication skills to make people feel better and accept your care. It is a challenge to achieve a balance between rapidly gathering critical information and encouraging and empowering the patient to participate in their treatment. Even experienced providers struggle to achieve this balance as they improve and learn with every patient encounter.

Notes

1. N. Jarrett and S. Payne, "A Selective Review of the Literature on Nurse-Patient Communication: Has the Patient's Contribution Been Neglected?" *Journal of Advanced Nursing* 22(1) (1995): 72–78.

2. G. Makoul and T. Schofield, "Communication Teaching and Assessment in Medical Education: An International Consensus Statement," *Patient Education and Counselling* 37 (2) (1999): 191–195.

3. J. L. Coulehan and M. R. Block, *The Medical Interview: Mastering Skills for Clinical Practice,* 4th ed. Philadelphia, PA: FA Davis Company, 2001.

4. P. E. O'Gara, "Therapeutic Communication Part 1," *Accident and Emergency Nursing* 12 (3) (July 2004): 166–172.

5. S. Chant, T. Jenkinson, J. Randel, and G. Russell, "Communication Skills: Some Problems in Nursing Education and Practice," *Journal of Clinical Nursing,* 11(1) (January 2002): 12–21.

6. M. Stewart and D. Roter, *Communicating with Medical Patients* (Newbury Park, CA: SAGE publications, 1989), pp. 16–20.

7. M. Stewart, "Effective Physician-Patient Communication and Health Outcomes: A Review," *Canadian Medical Association Journal* 152 (9) (1995): 1423–1433.

8. S. A. Lewin, Z. C. Skea, V. Entwistle, M. Zwarenstein, and J. Dick, "Interventions for Providers to Promote a Patient Centered Approach to a Clinical Consultation (Chochrane review)" in *The Cochrane Library, Issue 1* (Update Software, Oxford, 2002).

9. K. B. Dernocoeur, *Streetsense: Communication, Safety and Control* (Redmond, WA: Laing Communications Inc., 1996), pp. 56–84.

10. Merriam-Webster Dictionary, http://www.m-w.com/ (accessed August 12, 2005).

11. J. Tintinalli, *Emergency Medicine, A Comprehensive Study Guide,* 6th ed. (New York: McGraw-Hill, 2004), pp. 344–346.

12. Braunwald, *Heart Disease: A Textbook of Cardiovascular Medicine,* 6th ed. (Philadelphia, PA: W. B. Saunders Company, 2001), pp. 1128–1130.

13. V. Fuster, R. W. Alexander, and R. A. O'Rourke, *Hurst's The Heart,* 11th ed. (New York: McGraw-Hill, 2004), chapter 52. Clinical Aspects, http://www.accessmedicine.com/content.aspx?aID=251098 (accessed May 29, 2005).

14. E. C. Rich, T. W. Crowson, and I. B. Harris, "The Diagnostic Value of the Medical History," *Archives of Internal Medicine* 147 (1987): 1957–1960.

15. K.V. Iserson, "Critical Leadership," *Journal of Emergency Medicine* 4(4) (1986): 335–340.

16. R. E. Rakel, *Rakel: Textbook of Family Practice,* 6th ed. (Philadelphia, PA: W. B. Saunders Company, 2002), p. 234.

17. J. Giger and R. Davidhizar, *Transcultural Nursing: Assessment and Interventions,* 3rd ed. (St. Louis, MO: Mosby, 1999).

18. R. R. Rail, *The Unspoken Dialog: Understanding Body Language and Controlling Interviews and Negotiations* (Kansas City: Varro Press, 2001).

19. D. K. Gjerdingen, D. E. Simpson, and S. L. Titus, "Patients' and Physicians' Attitudes Regarding the Physicians' Professional Appearance," *Archives of Internal Medicine* 147 (1987): 1209.

20. G. J. Thompson and J. B. Jenkins, *Verbal Judo, The Gentle Art of Persuasion* (New York: Quill–HarperCollins Books, 2004).

21. C. Jarvis, *Physical Examination and Health Assessment,* 3rd ed. (Philadelphia, PA: W. B. Saunders Company, 2000).

22. United States Department of Transportation, National Highway Traffic Safety Administration, *Paramedic: National Standard Curriculum—Preparatory 1: Therapeutic Communication: 9; Declarative II—C.*

23. C. Goetz, *Textbook of Clinical Neurology,* 2nd ed. (New York: Elsevier, 2003), 537 www.mdconsult.com (accessed August 13, 2005).

24. NAEMT, *PHTLS Basic and Advanced Prehospital Trauma Life Support,* 5th ed. (St. Louis, MO: Mosby, 2003), p. 268.

25. M. C. Gratton, R. A. Bethke, W. A. Watson et al., "Effect of Standing Orders on Paramedic Scene Time for Trauma Patients," *Annals of Emergency Medicine* 20 (1991): 1306–1309.

26. M. Ochs et al., "Paramedic-Performed Rapid Sequence Intubation of Patients with Severe Head Injuries," *Annals of Emergency Medicine* 40(2) (August 1, 2002): 159–67.

27. H. Frankel, "The use of TRISS methodology to validate prehospital intubation by urban EMS providers," *American Journal of Emergency Medicine* 15(7) (November 1, 1997): 630–632.

28. L. Karagounis, S. K. Ipsen, M. R. Jessop et al., "Impact of Field-Transmitted Electrocardiography on Time to In-Hospital Thrombolytic Therapy in Acute Myocardial Infarction," *American Journal of Cardiology* 66 (1990): 786–791.

29. D. Perina, "Acute Myocardial Infarction in the Prehospital Setting," *Emergency Medicine Clinics of North America,* 19 (2) (May 2001).

30. D. Venes, *Taber's Cyclopedic Medical Dictionary,* 19th ed. (Philadelphia, PA: FA Davis Company, 2001).

31. C. Teutsch, "Patient-Doctor Communication," *The Medical Clinics of North America* 87 (2003): 1115–1145.

32. H. B. Beckman, R. M. Frankel, and J. Darnley, "Soliciting the Patients Complete Agenda: A Relationship to the Distribution of Concerns," *Clinical Research,* 33 (1985): 714A.

33. H. B. Beckman and R. M. Frankel, "The Effect of Physician Behavior on the Collection of Data," *Annals of Internal Medicine,* 101 (1984): 692–696.

34. T. Parson, *The Social System* (Glencoe, IL: Free Press, 1951).

35. M. Shattell, "Nurse-patient interaction: a review of the literature," *Journal of Clinical Nursing,* 12(6) (September 2004): 714–722.

36. K. Dernocoeur, "The 'We Save Lives' Myth" in *The Best of JEMS: Timeless Essays from the First 15 Years* (St. Louis, MO: Mosby Lifeline, 1996).

37. C. D. Tamparo and W. Q. Lindh, *Therapeutic Communications for Health Professionals,* 2nd ed. (Clifton Park, NY: Delmar Thomson Learning, 2000), pp. 2–16.

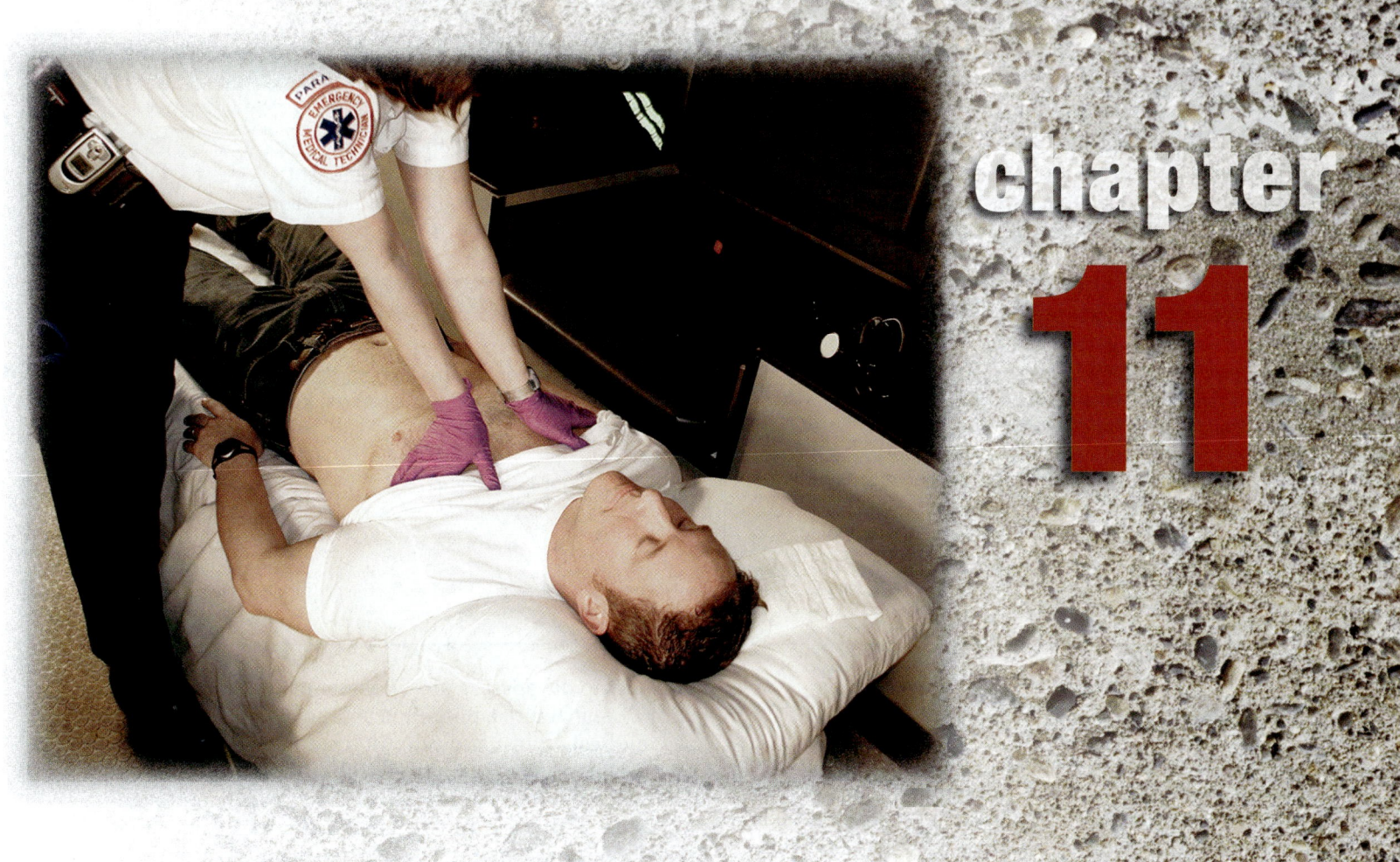

The Normal Physical Examination

"Our body is a well-set clock, which keeps good time, but if it be too much or indiscreetly tampered with, the alarm runs out before the hour."

—Joseph Hall

Need to Know

▶ The normal findings associated with a physical examination.

▶ How to relate normal findings of the physical examination to normal physiological processes.

▶ Understand which tests and evaluations are appropriate for emergency situations and which represent tests and evaluations that help expand your understanding of the human body, but do not add any value to managing a patient in an emergency situation.

▶ Do	▶ Ask
• Compare the vital signs and physical exam findings for your patient with the normal values. • Repeat assessment and perform continuous monitoring in order to detect subtle changes taking place, as vital signs and physical exam findings are dynamic. • Perform physical examinations often, even for minor injuries or illnesses. This will help sharpen your appreciation of "normal" and will improve your ability to quickly detect "abnormal" situations.	• Ask enough questions to get the appropriate amount of information to make good decisions regarding patient care.

Introduction

This chapter introduces you to techniques used to assess physical findings and provides essential information about *normal* findings. While the remainder of this textbook will discuss *abnormal* findings in great detail, the focus of this chapter is to explain the building blocks of the physical exam and what you should expect to see when someone is *not* sick or seriously injured.

The physical assessment of the human body focuses on clinical findings that you can touch, see, hear, and smell. These are considered **objective findings** since they can be observed, evaluated, and recorded in a factual and impartial manner by the examiner. In healthcare, physical signs are considered part of a complete patient assessment and are equally as important as a patient's history. To form a complete and accurate picture of a patient's medical problem, you gather the subjective symptoms that a patient or family member report and use the physical exam to investigate, confirm, or rule out the causes of an illness or the results of an injury suggested by the subjective information. While symptoms that a person reports in a history cannot be seen by an external, impartial observer, the physical exam can be a great help to formulate a complete picture of a patient's problem. DOT 3-2.4

As a paramedic you will use sight, sound, touch, and smell to detect objective findings related to the patient's physical condition. You will also use both basic and advanced equipment to extend your examination techniques. The diagnostic tools available in the prehospital setting have continued to improve as advances in technology and medicine continue. It is important, however, to remember that the most important examina-

tion tools you possess are your hands, eyes, nose, and brain! Long before a patient is able to get an x-ray of his or her chest, your hands should be able to feel unequal chest rise, and your stethoscope should be able to detect diminished lung sounds. It is important not to get focused on technological instruments and forget that simply looking, touching, and listening to a patient will give much of the essential information needed to guide patient care.

Skill Sheets 32 and 33 describe the elements of the primary and secondary surveys, respectively (also see Step-by-Steps 32 and 33). The following Skill Sheets are also cited in this chapter: Skill Sheet 31: Trauma Scoring; 34: Chest Pain Assessment; 35: Dyspnea Assessment; 76: Traumatic Brain Injury Assessment; 37: ECG Acquisition (also see Step-by-Step 37); 26: Blood Glucose Assessment (also see Step-by-Step 26); 29: Orthostatic Vital Signs (also see Step-by-Step 29); 25: Arterial Pulse Locations; 36: Abdominal Assessment, and 12: Pulse Oximetry (also see Step-by-Step 12). Review these as you read this chapter to help sort out which skills and assessments should be performed during each survey.

Beginning Right

During the physical exam, you will perform a variety of techniques, some of which may be invasive and embarrassing to a patient (Figure 11-1). To be successful, it is critical that you establish a trusting relationship with the patient immediately. The patient has to be able to trust that you, a complete stranger, are looking out for his or her best interest. Keep in mind the roles professional appearance, demeanor, and empathy play in setting the tone for positive communications.

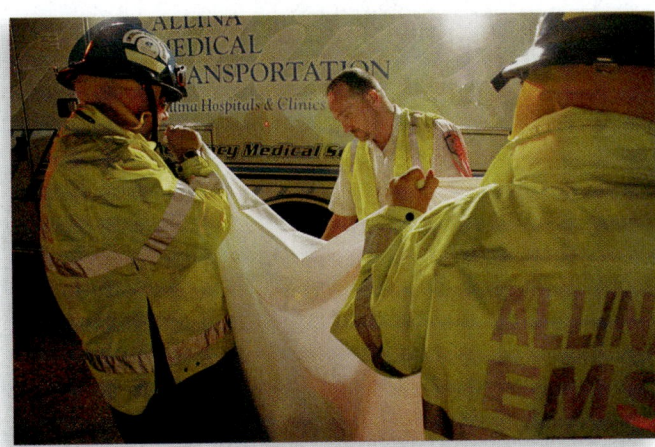

Figure 11-1 Protect the patient's privacy by using sheets to screen the patient from bystanders' prying eyes.

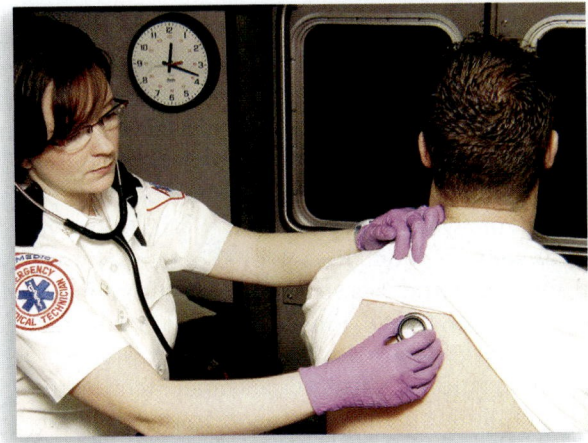

Figure 11-2 Auscultation should be practiced often.

CONNECTIONS Chapter 10: Therapeutic Communication and History Taking discuss specific communication techniques.

General Techniques

Since the beginnings of EMS, the paramedic has been considered a **physician extender.** Out-of-hospital emergency care in the United States evolved in such a way that nonphysicians were educated to perform some procedures such as chest decompression and surgical airway techniques that previously only licensed physicians were allowed to perform. Physician oversight of the EMS profession remains a critical component of the profession, and as a result, the EMS professional is able to continue to perform these dangerous skills under the on-line or off-line direction of the physician medical director.

As physician extenders, paramedics on the scene are the eyes, ears, and hands of the physician.[1] The point is that you will use your senses to detect both normal and abnormal findings and will need to communicate these findings to the physician continuing to care for the patient. In addition to sight, sound, and touch sensation, the sense of smell can also provide valuable clues about the patient's condition. DOT 3-2.1, 3-2.2

Using Sight to Inspect

Using sight to identify findings during a physical examination is called **inspection.** This is often done first during the examination of the body as it is often the least obtrusive to the patient although it does require removal of clothing and visualizing the skin.

Using Sound to Hear or Auscultate

The sounds a patient's body makes can be categorized into two groups: audible sounds and auscultated sounds. **Audible sounds** are those noises that can be heard by the examiner without a stethoscope. Examples of audible sounds include stridor, the noisy inspiration emanating from partial obstruction of the throat, or snoring secondary to an airway partially blocked by the patient's tongue.

The technique of using a stethoscope is called **auscultation.** Auscultated sounds are quiet enough that a stethoscope must be used to hear them. Examples of auscultated sounds are lung sounds, bowel sounds, heart tones, and Korotkoff sounds associated with blood pressure. Auscultation is a skill that requires repetition and practice to perform with accuracy (Figure 11-2).

Nice to Know

Korotkoff sounds are the arterial pressure sounds heard during blood pressure measurement using a stethoscope applied over the brachial artery. They are used to determine the systolic and diastolic blood pressure readings. Dr. Korotkoff, a Russian physician, introduced the auscultation method for obtaining blood pressure in 1905.

Street Secrets

Clean your stethoscope often! Research shows that the diaphragm of a stethoscope can harbor significant levels of bacteria such as *Staphylococcus aureus*.[2] As you apply this frequently used tool from one patient's chest to the next, without properly cleaning it, you may be moving contagious diseases from patient to patient. Immediate and frequent cleaning will reduce the possibility of cross contamination of patients with an infected stethoscope.[3,4] Don't forget to clean the ear pieces, too.

Using Touch to Palpate

A paramedic uses his or her hands to feel for a variety of conditions. **Palpation** is the term used to describe the technique of applying mild to moderate pressure to specific areas and parts of the body to detect abnormalities such as tenderness (pain upon palpation), deformity, or swelling. In addition to palpation, you can use your sense of touch to feel for skin temperature, wetness, and other findings such as the location and quality of a peripheral pulse. Finally, there are several techniques that are specific to the patient complaint or topographical location, such as percussion or tactile fremitus. These techniques are covered later in this chapter.

Using the Sense of Smell

A patient may emit certain odors that can be detected by the paramedic. For example, a slightly sweet acetone smell detected when the patient exhales may indicate diabetic ketoacidosis or chronic alcoholism. A recent ingestion of alcohol or some types of foods may be detected. Toxic ingestions or absorptions may cause odors to emanate from the mouth or skin. Poor hygienic habits may be readily apparent. A gastrointestinal bleed has a very unique odor associated with the mixture of blood and digested gastric contents mixed with feces. Other smells can be unmistakable signs of a specific illness that can aid you in assessing the patient.

Vital Signs

Vital signs are the specific measurements of a patient's ventilatory and circulatory status,[5] and they are primary concerns of the prehospital care provider. It is essential to determine vital signs early during the evaluation of the patient and repeat them often (Figure 11-3). Subtle changes in the patient condition can go unnoticed unless frequent vital sign monitoring is occurring. Vital sign readings may change in one direction or another; for example, a steady increase in pulse and respiration can signal that shock is worsening. Using vital signs to detect changes in patient condition is called **trending.**

DOT 3-2.32, 3-2.33, 3-3.49

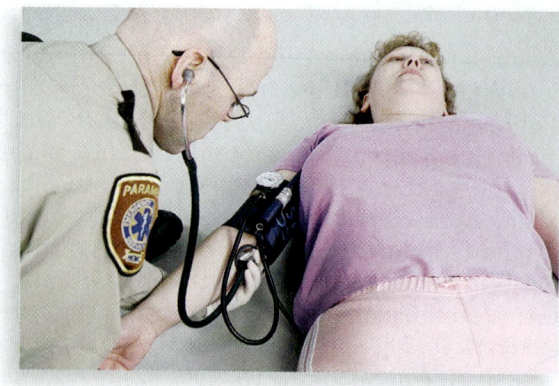

Figure 11-3   Vital signs should be checked often.

TABLE 11-1   Normal Vital Signs for Adults

Breathing	Respiratory rate: 12–20 cycles per minute Rhythm: regular, rhythmic Character: unlabored and effortless in any position
Circulation	Heart rate: 60–100 BPM Rhythm: regular, rhythmic Character: normal, equal forces throughout the body, pulses located in all nine standard areas
Perfusion	Blood pressure: 120/80 mmHg, adequate to maintain perfusion to the brain

The measurements traditionally called vital signs assess the heart (rate, rhythm, and character), respirations (rate, rhythm, and character), and the blood pressure. Over time more diagnostic instruments and tests have come into the prehospital setting, and these are becoming standard additions to the "vital signs." Things such as 3, 4, and 12 lead-ECG tracings, Glasgow Coma Scale (GCS) scoring, glucose levels, skin color, temperature and condition, and pulse oximetry and capnography readings are all gaining acceptance as additional vital signs. Other medical advances are bringing additional measurement devices to the field setting as well. The future may include sonography, dopplers, blood gas analysis, etc. For purposes of simplicity, the traditional vital signs are discussed here. The additional signs listed above are briefly covered later in this chapter and are discussed in detail in other chapters of this book. Table 11-1 lists the normal values for vital signs for adult patients. **Skill Sheet 29 and Step-by-Step 29: Orthostatic Vital Signs review the procedure for conducting an orthostatic assessment on patients who appear to be in shock or suffering from hypoperfusion.**

Respirations

The human body depends upon its ability to transport oxygen into and remove carbon dioxide from its cells to function effectively and efficiently. The structures and organs of the respiratory system perform the vast majority of this function without conscious thought and with little effort. As the body senses even the slightest change in oxygenation and metabolic waste levels, the respiratory system almost immediately attempts to compensate for those changes.[6] Therefore, it is a fundamental vital sign that should be noted with great care. When assessing a patient's respirations, note the rate (the number of breaths taken in a minute), rhythm, depth, and character. Character includes both the depth of breathing and the effort, or work, of breathing. **Skill Sheet 35: Dyspnea Assessment has additional assessment information.**

Rate

The respiratory rate is one of the most important vital signs, yet it is often one that is either estimated or is taken in a cursory fashion. Careful and repeat measurement of the respiratory rate can often provide early clues about a patient and possible deterioration. Ideally, the number of breaths a patient takes in 30 seconds should be counted and then multiplied by two to calculate the rate per minute. In most cases, providers count only the number of breaths for 15 seconds and multiply by four. While less accurate, the latter method provides a close approximation of the actual rate. DOT 3-3.18

The average resting respiratory rate of an adult varies from 12 to 20 cycles per minute.[6,7] An occasional sigh is normal. It may seem intuitive and easy to be able to estimate respiratory rate at a glance; however, casual estimation of the rate has been shown to be inaccurate and should not be a part of any prehospital provider's practice. It is sometimes helpful to observe the stomach move up and down when counting the respiratory rate.

Street Secrets

The respiratory rate is one vital sign that the patient can consciously alter. In order to capture a true respiratory rate, begin with counting the pulse rate. After an appropriate amount of time for the pulse (typically 15 or 30 seconds with a regular rhythm or a full 60 seconds with irregularity), keep your hand on the pulse and switch your attention to counting respirations. The patient will be unaware you are counting the respiratory rate, and you are more likely to obtain a true reading.

Rhythm

When things are normal, the patient's respiratory rhythm should be regular, with an equal rise and fall of the chest. Note if there is any irregularity with the rhythm—does it speed up and slow down? Is it irregular? These may be signs of either a primary or underlying problem.

Depth

The adult typically inhales about 500 mL of air and exhales the same amount in each tidal volume.[6] This is a relatively small volume of air due to the high efficiency of the respiratory system. Again, remember that normal respirations are quiet and without effort. Therefore, the depth of normal respirations will be neither deep nor shallow and may be difficult to determine at a glance.

Effort

The body uses a combination of both the diaphragm and intercostal muscles to breathe normally. If oxygen demand rises, the respiratory rate and depth will increase first, using these structures. If this is not enough, other accessory muscles such as the sternocleidomastoid, and internal intercostals will be used to assist in

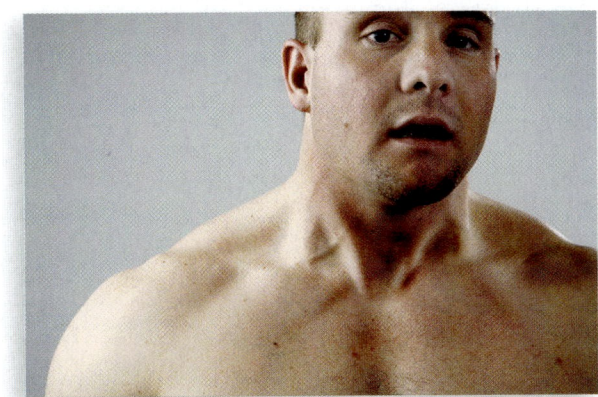

Figure 11-4 You may observe supraclavicular retractions during inspection of the neck. Supraclavicular retractions are always an abnormal finding.

moving air into and out of the lungs more quickly (Figure 11-4). Under normal conditions, the patient should be able to speak in full sentences with minimal respiratory efforts and should be able to breathe easily in any position: sitting, standing, or lying.

CONNECTIONS Refer to Chapter 7: Anatomy Overview and Chapter 12: Airway Management, Ventilation, and Oxygenation for more information on respiration.

Pulse

When the left ventricle of the heart contracts, blood is forcefully squeezed out of the chamber and into the systemic circulation, causing a pressure wave to occur in the arteries. This pressure wave causes the arterial walls to briefly expand and then recoil, forcing blood through the arteries. You can feel the pressure wave by gently pressing down on an artery as it passes over a firm base such as a bone. Assessing the quantity and quality of these pressure waves is called determining the patient's pulse. DOT 3-3.22

When assessing the pulse, determine the rate, rhythm, and character. Character describes the quality or force of pulsations as well as comparing the relative strength of the pulsations at the various pulse sites on the body.

There are nine major **pulse points** in the human body (Figure 11-5). They are named for the arteries where they are found.[6] Of these, the most common site used to assess for the patient's pulse is at the radial side of the wrist (Figure 11-6). Other common sites include the brachial, carotid, femoral, and dorsalis pedis arteries. **Skill Sheet 25: Arterial Pulse Locations provides additional information.**

When locating the radial pulse, press down on the artery with mild pressure, using the pads of your index and middle finger. Try not to use your thumb since it may have its own pulse that could be mistaken for the

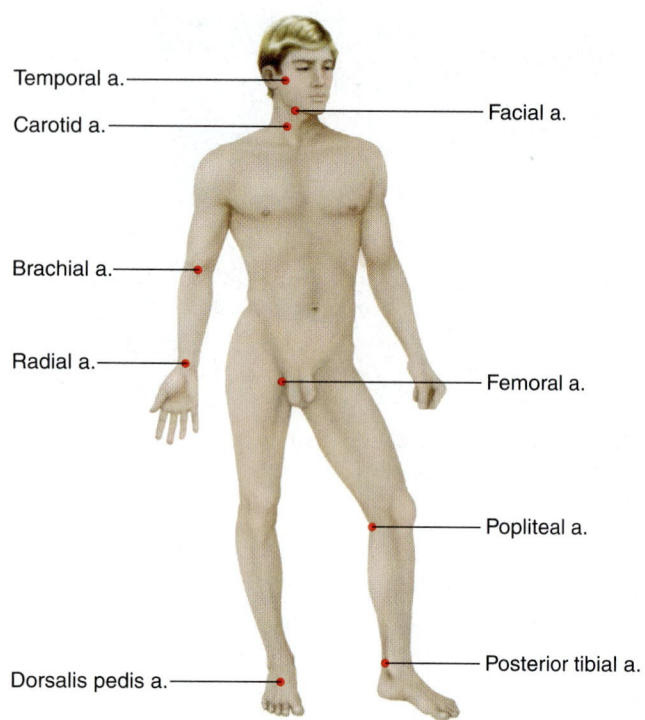

Figure 11-5 The nine pulse points.

patient's pulse. Do not press down too hard, as this temporarily closes the artery off from further blood flow and the pulsations stop. At the same time, pressing too lightly may result in not feeling the pulse at all. Palpating for a carotid or femoral pulse may require more pressure, as these sites are located deeper within the tissues.

Once you find the pulse, determine the following characteristics.

Rate

The pulse rate is measured by counting the number of pulsations felt during a 15 second period and multiplying by four to calculate the number of beats per minute.

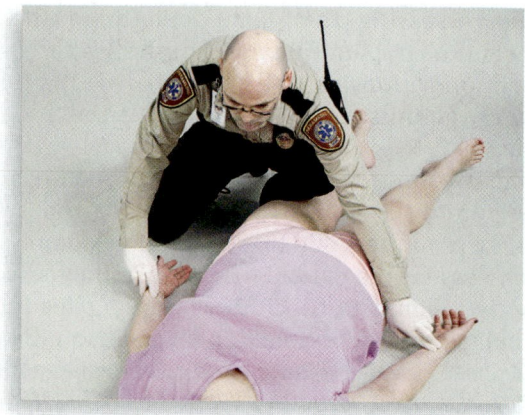

Figure 11-6 The radial arteries in the wrist are common pulse locations. Assess them simultaneously and compare them to each other. They should have equal force and rates.

This technique should be limited to regular heart rates only. If irregular, count the rate for 30 (and multiply by two) or a full 60 seconds. The normal resting heart rate of an adult is between 60 and 100 beats per minute.

Rhythm

Normally, the rhythm should be regular, with no skips or premature beats. Some patients may present normally with sinus arrhythmia, which is a rhythm that slows down slightly with inhalation and speeds up slightly with exhalation. Other patients may experience chronic atrial fibrillation, which results in an irregularly irregular rhythm.

Strength and Quality

The character of the pulse is found in its strength, or quality. It should be neither weak nor excessively strong. A weak or thready pulse indicates poor circulation to that artery. A strong or bounding pulse indicates excessive force being generated by the left ventricle.

CONNECTIONS Pulse characteristics are described in full detail in Chapter 29: Cardiology.

Street Secrets

Bear in mind that in order to be able to judge pulse strength, the pressure you use to palpate must be correct—not too light and not too firm. It takes a long time feeling pulses the right way to be able to differentiate between "normal" and "abnormal."

Blood Pressure

As part of maintaining homeostasis, the body will do whatever it can to maintain an optimal pressure gradient so that adequate blood flow to the tissues and organs is maintained. This pressure gradient is evaluated by measuring blood pressure. Blood pressure is a result of a combination of factors including heart rate, stroke volume, blood volume, and the relative diameter of the peripheral arteries.[6] Blood pressure by auscultation is measured using a **sphygmomanometer** (BP cuff) and stethoscope. It can also be palpated by using only the sphygmomanometer.

CONNECTIONS Chapter 8: Physiology Overview explains blood pressure in detail and describes the interrelationship between blood pressure and cardiac output.

Normal systolic pressure is defined as less than 120 mmHg, and normal diastolic pressure is less than 80 mmHg.[8] Blood pressures of 140 mmHg systolic over 90 mmHg diastolic are considered hypertensive.[9] In some cases, the mere presence of a health care worker can elevate someone's blood pressure.[10]

There are a surprising number of factors that can affect the accuracy of blood pressure measurement. Incorrect bladder size (as opposed to cuff size), improper patient or arm positioning, as well as poor cuff and stethoscope placement can all contribute to an inaccurate blood pressure measurement.[9,11]

Blood Pressure by Auscultation

The American Heart Association has released standards for obtaining accurate blood pressures. Their "gold standard" of blood pressure management involves using an appropriately sized cuff (the bladder is 80% length and 40% width of the arm circumference), removing the clothing around the upper arm, placing the cuff at 2–3 cm above the antecubital fossa, and supporting the arm. For every inch your cuff moves above or below the level of the heart, you may find as much as 2 mmHg variation due to hydrostatic pressure changes. Readings obtained with the cuff below the level of the right atrium, especially with the arm hanging down, will be higher and may be off as much as 10 mmHg or more. Inflate the cuff 30 mmHg above the point at which the radial pulse disappeared. Deflate at a rate of 2–3 mmHg per second. The reading at the point that Korotkoff sounds (thumps) are first heard in your stethoscope represents the systolic pressure. The point at which the sounds disappear represents the diastolic reading. Document the position the patient was in when the blood pressure was taken. A supine position reading is normally 8 mmHg higher than sitting.

Street Secrets

When watching the needle on the gauge drop, watch the needle so that it pulsates approximately three times in each 10 mmHg increment as it drops. This is a good speed of deflation and should allow you to obtain the best reading.

Blood Pressure by Palpation

Blood pressure may also be measured by palpation of the radial artery during the deflation of the blood pressure cuff. This technique is useful if the ambient environment is too noisy to hear the sounds with the stethoscope. With the BP cuff properly positioned and deflated, begin the process by first locating the patient's radial pulse. The BP cuff is inflated until the radial pulse can no longer be felt. Add 30 mmHg more pressure to the BP cuff before starting to deflate. The pressure in the cuff is then slowly released until the radial pulse can be felt again. The reading at the point the pulse is first felt correlates with the systolic pressure. Only the systolic pressure is measured with

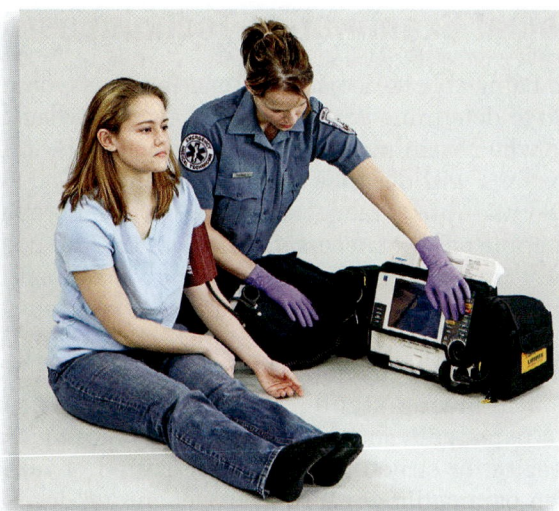

Figure 11-7   An automated blood pressure monitor. These are often built into other devices such as ECG monitors.

this technique. Blood pressure by palpation has been shown to be relatively accurate compared to an auscultated blood pressure.[12] Palpated blood pressures are within 8–10 mmHg of auscultated blood pressures.[9,11]

In addition to manual sphygmomanometers, there are a variety of electronic and automated blood pressure monitors on the market for both professional and home use (Figure 11-7). Finger-based devices have been shown to be inaccurate.[9]

Working in the Gray Zone

Comparing apples to apples

As a healthcare provider, the blood pressure you report may be used later to make serious decisions about the patient care plan. While it is sometimes difficult to get an accurate blood pressure due to the unpredictable prehospital setting, it is important to perform this technique exactly the way other health care professionals perform it. Hopefully, this will yield results that can be an apples-to-apples comparison with future measurements.

Research to date has shown some differences between blood pressures from one arm to another. Unfortunately, in the studies so far, the differences have not been consistent, reproducible, or predictable.[13] The current theory is that it may be normal to find a small difference between blood pressures in both arms. Nevertheless, whenever time permits or the situation indicates the need, you should measure the blood pressure in both arms since detecting a difference may signal a disruption in the aorta, such as an aortic aneurysm, or an arterial occlusion in one extremity.[9]

Physical Examination Techniques

Before being able to detect abnormal findings, you must be able to determine what is *normal,* that is, what is expected when examining that part of the body. The following sections will describe these normal findings. However, normal runs a range, and what may be normal for **most** people may not necessarily be normal in **all** people. The best way to determine what is indeed normal is to perform as many physical examinations as possible on as many patients as possible to recognize the various findings that comprise the normal physical examination.

The following section describes normal observations a paramedic should note when examining a specific region or structure. It is not assumed or implied that the paramedic will use every technique described in this section on every patient encounter. Tests and evaluation techniques provided in the tables and boxes represent nice-to-know information.

Tests and evaluations found in the tables aid in your understanding of the human body, but they may not be appropriate assessments to perform on very sick patients.

Mental Status

Mental status can be assessed grossly by checking the level of consciousness and using the following mnemonic:

AVPU score

A Awake, eyes open, and appearing to be relating appropriately to the surroundings

V Verbal, appearing unconscious or asleep upon approach but easily arousable when asked to "wake up"

P Painful, unconscious and not responding to a verbal command but waking up when a painful stimuli is applied

U Unresponsive, not responding to voice or strong painful stimuli

Normal appearing patients will be awake and alert to their surroundings. They should know who they are, where they are, and have a general sense of the time of day and date. The Glasgow Coma Score (GCS) is a quantifiable tool that assesses level of consciousness based upon how the patient responds to the environment and external stimuli. It assesses consciousness in a similar manner to the AVPU, and it also assesses the appropriateness of the patients' verbal and motor responses. A normal score on the GCS is 15. Assessing the cranial nerves is not normally performed in the prehospital setting, so it is a nice-to-know skill. DOT 3-2.3, 3-2.55, 3-2.56, 3-3.12

Working in the Gray Zone

Whenever using an acronym or abbreviation, it is important to know exactly what each letter stands for so that other healthcare providers can later reference your assessment. The letter "A" in the AVPU scale is referenced in several leading emergency medicine textbooks and is defined as "Alert" without further explanation.[14,15] The term "alert," however, is sometimes used to imply that the patient is *oriented,* which may not be necessarily true. A better term that may be applied here is *"awake,"* which accurately describes the patient's state of consciousness without implying just how oriented he or she is.[16] Since there is no absolute industry standard, it is best to use more descriptive language when describing someone's level of consciousness.

CONNECTIONS Skill Sheets 31: Trauma Scoring and 76: Traumatic Brain Injury Assessment have more information on neurological assessments Chapter 20: Head, Face, and Neck Trauma has detailed information on the AVPU and GCS scores.

Examination Organized by Body Region

Overall Appearance

The body should generally be symmetrical from side to side. The patient should be able to move with ease and fluidity and stand upright without assistance in supporting weight or balance. Personal hygiene and attire will vary from patient to patient based upon socioeconomic issues such as culture, finance, and ethnic background; however, the patient should appear well-nourished, weight-to-height proportionate, and appropriately dressed for the season of year and the weather.

Skin Signs

The skin is the most easily accessible organ of the human body. It acts as a barrier to infection, an insulator/radiator of heat and cold, and a primary sensory organ. The skin is well vascularized and, therefore, is sensitive to internal pulmonary and circulatory changes. Because of its accessibility and sensitivity to physiologic changes, the skin provides immediate information to the paramedic. DOT 3-2.6, 3-2.7

Inspect the skin and note the condition of the hair and nails. Look specifically at the areas of the skin that are the thinnest and most susceptible to perfusion levels. These include the fingernail beds, the lips, and the mucous membranes of the mouth and underside of the eyelids (Figure 11-8).[7] In addition, these areas do not contain melanin, the substance that gives skin its

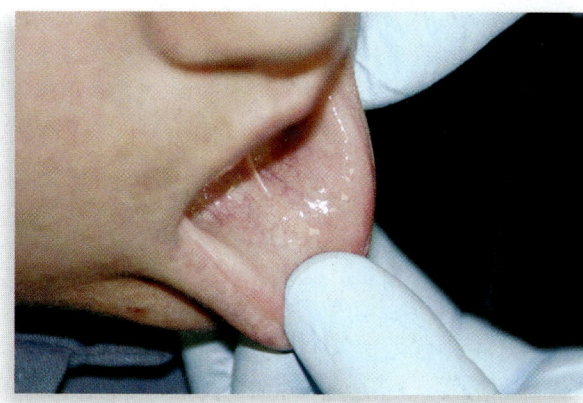

Figure 11-8   Examine the inner lip and gum to see if the patient has cyanosis. The normal appearance is pink. Note the blue veins present. This is more noticeable in light-skinned individuals, and it is also a normal finding.

pigmentation. Therefore these areas should generally appear pink in color. DOT 3-2.5

A second condition of the skin is its temperature. The body generates heat as part of normal metabolic

Nice to Know

The 1 Minute Cranial Nerve Exam

Evaluate all 12 cranial nerves with this series of simple tests:

1. Ask patient to close eyes, smell a common thing (alcohol prep), and identify the odor.
2. Light penlight, ask patient to hold head still, and ask patient to track the light with his or her eyes as you move light around head in an "H" pattern.
3. Ask patient to clench teeth. You palpate the masseter and temporal muscles for tone.
4. Test sensation at forehead, chin, and each cheek.
5. Ask patient to smile and show clenched teeth.
6. Ask patient to open and say "Ahhhh" and watch uvula move.
7. Test gag reflex with tongue blade.
8. Test balance with Romberg test. Ask patient to stand up straight with feet together. Close eyes and observe for sway. Patient should not move if normal.
9. Test hearing by leaning in close and whispering a simple sentence like "Can you hear me?"
10. Ask patient to shrug shoulders upward while you push downward and rotate head to left and right while you put gentle counter pressure on each side of the face. DOT 3-2.57, 3-2.58

processes. The body regulates its ability to retain or lose heat partially by shunting blood either away from the skin or toward it, respectively. This is accomplished by constriction or dilation of the capillary beds located in the dermal layer. Therefore, as blood moves away from the skin, not only will the skin pale, but it will also begin to cool. Conversely, if blood moves toward the skin, it will become flush and warm.

The external environment affects peripheral skin areas as well. Cool or cold ambient temperatures will cause the skin to naturally blanch as the peripheral capillary beds constrict. Because of this response, feeling the forehead or arms for skin temperature may be inaccurate.[17] Placing the back of your hand against the chest or under the axillae may provide a more accurate assessment of the body's temperature.

The third measurement of the skin is its condition. Under typical environmental conditions, the skin should be dry to the touch. If the ambient temperature or body becomes warm, the skin will begin sweating (diaphoresis). This response helps expose water (sweat) to air and, through evaporation, helps cool the body. If the body experiences hypoperfusion, as in shock, the sympathetic response will cause sweat glands to secrete fluid, causing diaphoresis.

CONNECTIONS   For an in-depth look at hypoperfusion, read about shock in Chapter 13: Shock Overview.

Head

The top and sides of the head should be smooth and symmetrical from side to side. Facial structures should also be symmetrical, without tenderness to palpation. Upon command, facial expressions such as a grimace, smile, or lifting of the eyebrows should be equal on both the left and right sides. Speech should be easily understood, without slurring or mumbling. DOT 3-2.8, 3-2.9, 3-2.10

Eyes

When gently pulling on the upper or lower eyelid, note the color of the conjunctiva (Figure 11-9). It should be moist and pink. In the alert patient, the eyes should be spontaneously open and face in the same direction (known as a *conjugate gaze*). They should move in tandem, and the patient should be able to gaze in all directions without difficulty. The patient should not complain of blurred vision or double vision (diploplia). The cornea of the eye should appear clear, and the sclera of the eye should look white in color. The following Nice to Know box lists some additional tests to consider which might be required for an emergency assessment in life-threatened patients. **See also Skill Sheet 28: Nystagmus Assessment.** DOT 3-2.11, 3-2.12, 3-2.13, 3-2.14

Examine the pupils using a penlight. Larger sources of light such as flashlights should be avoided. Although

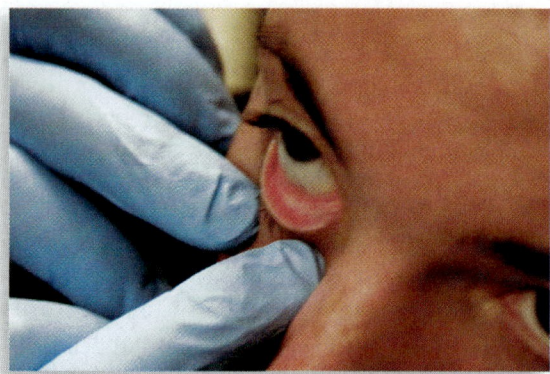

Figure 11-9   Pull down the lower lid, and inspect the conjunctiva. It should be moist and pink. Be very careful not to touch the surface of the eye with your gloved hands as debris or powder can cause irritation. Also be very careful not to touch your face with your gloved hands. Eye infections can be very contagious.

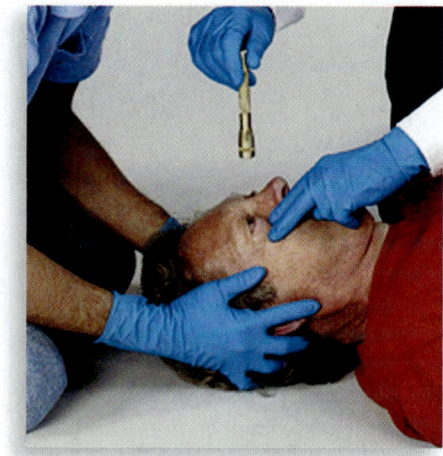

Figure 11-10   Rather than shining the light directly into the eye (as shown here), it should be directed in from the lateral side, and ask the patient to look at a distant object.

Nice to Know

Additional Visual Assessments

Visual field-confrontation (to assess peripheral vision)

Sit in front of patient. Cover one eye, and you cover your opposite eye. Extend your arm out to your side. Slowly bring your arm in toward the midline. Hopefully the patient will see your hand at the same time you do. Do in all four quadrants: LEFT, RIGHT, UP, and DOWN.

Accommodation test

Place an object at least 14 inches away from the eyes centered between the eyes. Ask patient to focus on the object (eyes will not be crossed at this point), and then ask patient to follow the object as you move it toward the tip of the nose. The patient should cross his or her eyes, and the pupils should constrict as the object comes closer to the nose. If this is normal and the eye constricts and dilates as normal, report as PERRLA (Pupils equal, round, and reactive to light and accommodation) on the patient care report (PCR).

Corneal reflex

If patient's eyes are open spontaneously, gently touch a soft cloth to outer lower portion of the eye. Patient should blink when this occurs. If unconscious and the eyes are closed, hold eye open and watch for lid twitching when the eye is stroked in the same location.

not a common prehospital procedure, in certain situations, an ophthalmoscope may be used to inspect the interior aspects of the eye. Using a penlight, shine the light into the eye from the side while asking the patient to look at a distant object (Figure 11-10). This helps to avoid a "near reaction," where the pupil will constrict normally as it tries to focus on any object near it.[7] Observe the following points when examining the pupil of each eye:

- ***Equality.***   The pupils should be relatively equal in size. In some patients, it is normal to have one eye noticeably larger than the other, a condition known as anisocoria. It is not clear how common this condition is in the general population although one estimate is that about 20% of the population normally have pupil inequalities of less than 0.5 mm.[7,18]

- ***Round.***   The pupils are circular in shape. The lens in a normal pupil is clear.

- ***Reactivity.***   Shining a beam of light into a pupil should cause it to constrict briskly as it attempts to reduce the amount of light entering the eye almost immediately (direct reaction). The brisk reaction should be equal in both eyes. In addition, both pupils should react when light is shined into just one (consensual reaction).[7]

- ***Extraocular muscle movement.***   Movement of the eyeball is controlled by the extraocular muscles. Normally, the muscles of both eyes work together so that they move equally and at the same time. Eye motion should be evaluated by having the patient look up, down, right, left, up and to the right, and up and to the left, all performed while keeping the head immobile.

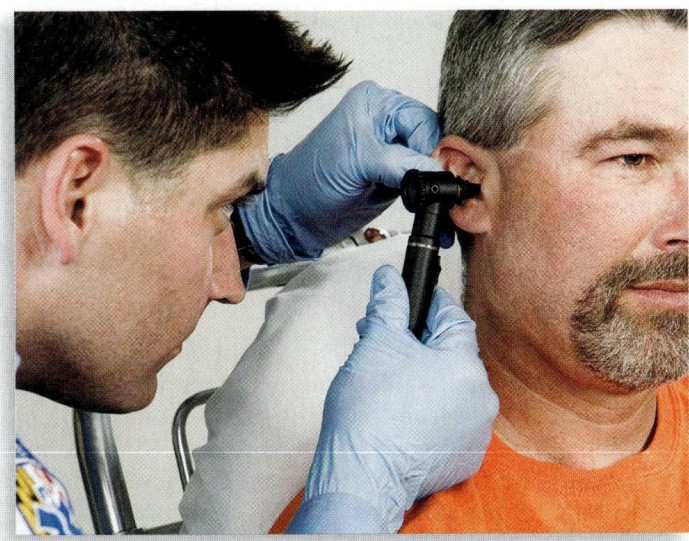

Figure 11-11 An otoscope is used to inspect the ears. Pull the ear gently towards the back of the head to get the best view.

Examining these aspects of the pupils in this order will provide the acronyms:

PERRL: Pupils that are Equal, Round, and Reactive to Light

PEARL: Pupils are Equal And Reactive to Light.

Ears

The ears should be free of any fluid drainage. The patient should be able to hear clearly, equally on left and right, and throughout a wide tonal range (low to high frequency sounds). If an otoscope is available, the eardrums should appear round and flat, not swollen or sunken (Figure 11-11). Cerumen (ear wax) is expected, and it can appear white, yellow, red, or brown/black in color. DOT 3-2.15, 3-2.16, 3-2.17

Nose

The nose should be free of obstructions or fluid drainage, such as blood. Rhinitis (nasal congestion and inflammation) may be expected for a person experiencing common airborne allergies such as pollen. DOT 3-2.18, 3-2.19

Mouth

Ask the patient to open his mouth and extend his tongue. The tongue should project straight out, without deviating to the side. The tongue and oral mucosa should be moist and pink in color. Teeth should be present in the numbers appropriate to the age group. It is normal to observe patients with artificial fillings in their teeth. Dentures and dental implants are examples of dental appliances that are used to compensate for a

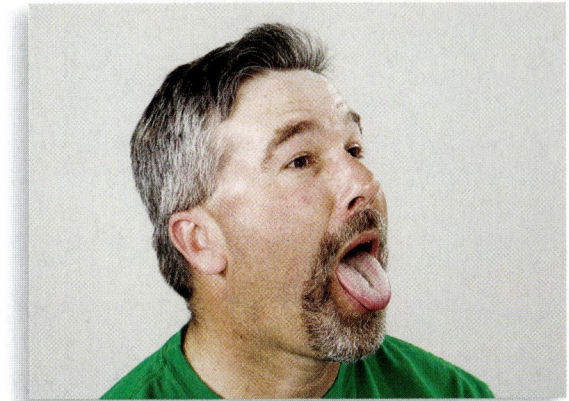

Figure 11-12 Inspect the pharynx and tonsils.

loss of teeth. The patient's breath should be free of any obvious odor other than perhaps halitosis (bad breath). DOT 3-2.20, 3-2.21

Upon command, the patient should be able to open and close his or her mandible without difficulty. The temporomandibular joint (TMJ) should not click or otherwise make any sounds when the jaw is opened and closed (Figure 11-12). The pharynx, or back of the throat, should also be moist and pink in color. Tonsils, located on the right and left sides of the pharynx, may be visible if not previously removed surgically.

Neck

Loosen any clothing and inspect the neck for symmetry (Figure 11-13). Note any unusual masses, swellings, or openings (stoma). Check to see if a "medic-alert" identification tag or emblem is present. DOT 3-2.22, 3-2.23, 3-3.50

The act of normal breathing should not involve the neck muscles, nor should any sounds associated with breathing be heard from the neck region. The jugular neck veins should be flat when the patient is either sitting or standing. There may normally be jugular venous distension when the patient lays supine. The trachea should be located in the midline. DOT 3-2.24, 3-2.25, 3-2.35, 3-2.36

Palpate for carotid pulses. Assess only one side of the neck at a time. Press hard enough to find the pulse yet not enough to reduce blood flow to the head. The pulse should be strong without vibrations. A humming vibration, described as a "cat purring"-like sensation, felt at the carotid artery is called a **thrill.** This is not a normal finding, and is a sign of cardiovascular disease.[7] DOT 3-2.36, 3-2.37

Auscultate the lateral-anterior regions of the neck. Breathing should be clear and quiet. Place the diaphragm of the headpiece of the stethoscope against the carotid arteries and note whether or not any unusual sounds exist, such as **bruits** (a murmur-like sound).[7] Bruits result as atherosclerotic plaque builds up and are not considered a normal finding.

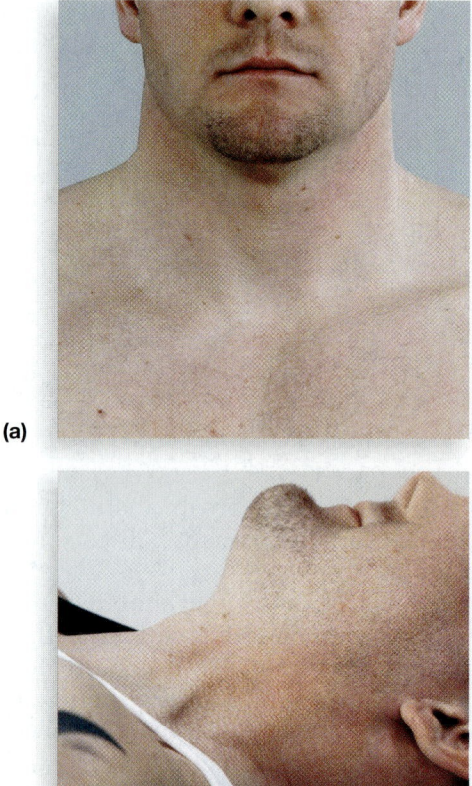

(a)

(b)

Figure 11-13   (a) Inspect the neck for signs of dyspnea or increased work of breathing. (b) The neck veins may appear slightly distended normally, but they should be soft to the touch when palpated.

Anterior Chest

With key structures and organs such as lungs, heart, and major blood vessels located in the chest, it is critical to evaluate this area carefully, even in the absence of trauma. The Nice to Know box at the end of this section provides additional assessments to perform on the chest that are not considered emergency assessments. **Skill Sheets 34: Chest Pain Assessment and 35: Dyspnea**

Assessment have additional assessment information. DOT 3-2.24, 3-2.29, 3-2.30, 3-2.31

Inspection.   Expose the chest while maintaining the patient's modesty. Inspect the chest for symmetry and general shape. Note any bruises, masses, swelling, or signs of surgical interventions. The chest should rise and fall symmetrically without effort during respirations. Normal breathing does not involve accessory muscles such as the internal intercostal muscles.

Auscultation.   With the patient supine or sitting, auscultate the lung fields bilaterally and symmetrically, to make comparisons from one side to the other. Normal lung sounds should be difficult to hear initially since there should be no restriction to airflow. They should be clear of any unusual noises, such as wheezes, crackles, rubbing, or moaning type sounds. Lung sounds should be heard throughout the entire lung field, from the area just below the clavicle down to the last rib, along the mid-axillary line. DOT 3-2.28 **See Skill Sheet 27: Chest Auscultation.**

CONNECTIONS A more detailed description of lung sounds and auscultatory sites can be found in Chapters 12: Airway Management, Ventilation, and Oxygenation and 28: Pulmonary.

Heart Tones.   As the heart pumps blood to both the pulmonary and systemic circulatory systems, heart valves open and close to keep the blood flow unidirectional. Optimally, the patient should be lying supine during auscultation of the heart tones, however, other positions are acceptable. Even under ideal conditions, heart tones may be difficult to hear well.

Palpation.   Palpate the chest wall for tenderness or deformity. Gently press against the lateral chest walls, and ask the patient to take a deep breath. Then, using the lateral aspect of your palm, press against the sternum, and ask the patient to take another deep breath (Figure 11-14). This technique will help you avoid

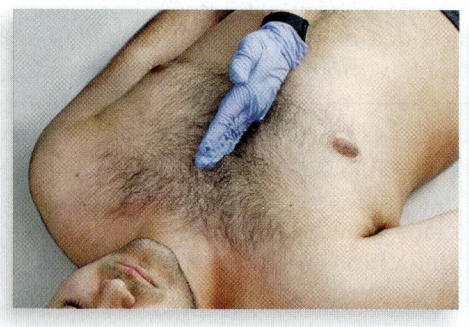

(a)

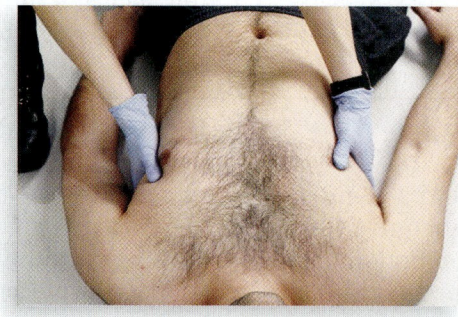

(b)

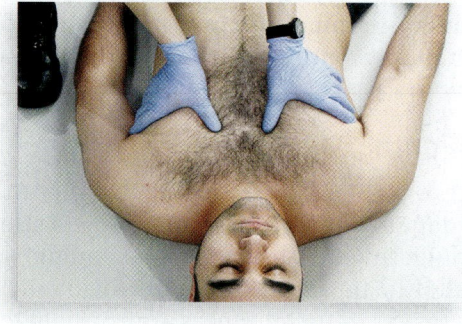

(c)

Figure 11-14   (a) Palpate the center of the sternum while looking for instability or crepitus. (b) Press your hands to each side of the chest and observe the patient breathe. (c) Both sides should move equally and effortlessly.

Nice to Know

Additional Chest Assessments and Tests

Excursion

Find C-7 (most prominent vertebra) and count down to T-10. Place hands on the back parallel to tenth rib with thumbs within an inch of each other. Ask patient to inhale deeply. Thumbs should be symmetrically spread by 3–5 cm.

Tactile fremitus

With hands on posterior chest wall, ask patient to say "99" over and over. You should feel the vibrations of the chest wall while this is done.

Bronchophony

While auscultating the chest, ask the patient to repeat "99" over and over. It should be muffled and indistinct. Clearly heard words indicate fluid or consolidation is present in that part of the lung.

Whispered pectoriloquy

While auscultating, ask patient to whisper "99" over and over. You could also ask the patient to whisper "one, two, three" over and over. It should normally be muffled and indistinct. Clearly heard words indicate fluid or consolidation is present in that part of the lung.

Egophony

While auscultating, ask the patient to repeat the letter long E (EEEEE). If you hear "A" instead of "E," it indicates fluid or consolidation is present in that part of the lung.

PMI (Point of Maximal Impulse) assessment DOT 3-2.38, 3-2.39

This is the left ventricle apex and is felt best with a reclining patient with the head elevated around 30 degrees, but it can be palpated in other positions as well. At the fifth intercostal space medial to the midclavicular line is the PMI. Observe for pulsations in this area. If you cannot see pulsations, ask patient to exhale and hold his breath.

Normal (S_1 and S_2) heart sounds assessment (lub-dub)[7] DOT 3-2.38, 3-2.39

S_1: Auscultate at the fifth intercostal space at the left sternal border. This is the tricuspid valve. Listen at the PMI to hear the mitral valve. These are the AV valves. (This is the "lub" sound of the "lub-dub.")

S_2: Auscultate at the second intercostal space right sternal border for the aortic valve. The second intercostal space left sternal border is the pulmonic valve. These are the semilunar valves. (This is the "dub" sound of the lub-dub.)

Abnormal heart sounds DOT 3-2.38, 3-2.39

Splitting: The mitral and aortic valves close slightly before the tricuspid and pulmonic. If you hear this, it will be two sets in either or both of the S_1 and S_2 heart sounds. A split S_1 sounds like "la-lub," and a split S_2 sounds like "da-dub." Splitting S_2 during inspiration is normal in healthy children and young adults. Expiratory or persistent splitting suggests abnormality (dilated ventricle). Listen at the apex of the heart (PMI) for this.

S_3: Ventricular gallop results from dilated ventricle (hypertrophy). The sound is "lub-dub-dee," and it sounds like "Kentucky."

S_4: Atrial gallop results from blood being pushed into an overloaded ventricle. Sound is "dee-lub-dub," and it sounds like "Tennessee." Listen at the apex (PMI) with patient lying on his or her left side.

---

touching the breasts of a female patient. No pain should be elicited in either maneuver. DOT 3-2.40

Percussion   Percussion of the chest, while difficult to perform in the usually noisy prehospital environment, is a technique that can elicit valuable additional information in certain circumstances, such as an air-filled cavity of a tension pneumothorax or the denseness of lung tissue that is filled with infection. DOT 3-2.26, 3-2.27

Sound contains energy that causes it to vibrate at a certain frequency. The medium sound travels through can either impede or facilitate its transmission. For example, imagine a snare drum. If the drum is filled with air, tapping the skin of the drum would produce a tight, relatively high-pitched sound. However, if the inside of the drum was filled with some sand, the sound would fall in pitch, and the resulting sound would be lower and duller. If you continued to add sand into the drum, the duller the sound would become.

Translate that example into the human body and the concept is the same. An air-filled organ such as the lung would produce a certain "sound" or *resonance* when the surface of the chest is tapped hard enough to send sound waves into the body. If the lung was filled with fluid, such as blood, the resulting sound would be lower than that of a normal lung, or hyporesonant. If the chest cavity were filled with trapped free air, percussing that chest would result in a high-pitched, or hyperresonant sound.

Posterior Chest

Remember that the upper back of the patient is the posterior chest cavity. As such, if the patient is sitting upright, it is easiest to complete the entire chest exam before moving on to the abdomen, rather than waiting for the back examination. In particular, ongoing auscultation of the lungs should be conducted, extending the examination from the anterior chest to the posterior of the chest. Again, listen carefully from side to side in an orderly pattern to determine equality of lung sounds as well as any adventitious (abnormal) noises. It may be easier to determine whether or not wheezes or crackles are present through auscultation of the posterior chest because there is generally less muscle and fat in the back when compared to the front of the chest (Figure 11-15). Percussion may also elicit certain findings of increased density due to blood or infection, as previously described. DOT 3-2.25

Abdomen

During the abdominal exam, ideally the patient should lay supine with both feet flat on the surface and knees bent.[7] This relaxes the abdominal muscles and also presents the abdominal organs and other structures in their most normal positions. Expose and inspect the abdominal wall for any masses, swelling, bruises, or other discoloration. Note any distension. **Skill Sheet 36: Abdominal Assessment provides more assessment information.** DOT 3-2.41, 3-2.42, 3-2.43, 3-2.44

The abdomen can be visually divided into four major quadrants (Figure 11-16). Palpate the abdomen in the four quadrants, using the flat part of your hand. When palpating, imagine pressing deep enough to feel "through" the abdominal wall to touch the actual organ. The abdomen should be soft and nontender in all quadrants. Note any masses that may be felt during palpation. It is possible to palpate the lower margin of the liver in the right upper quadrant during a normal exam.

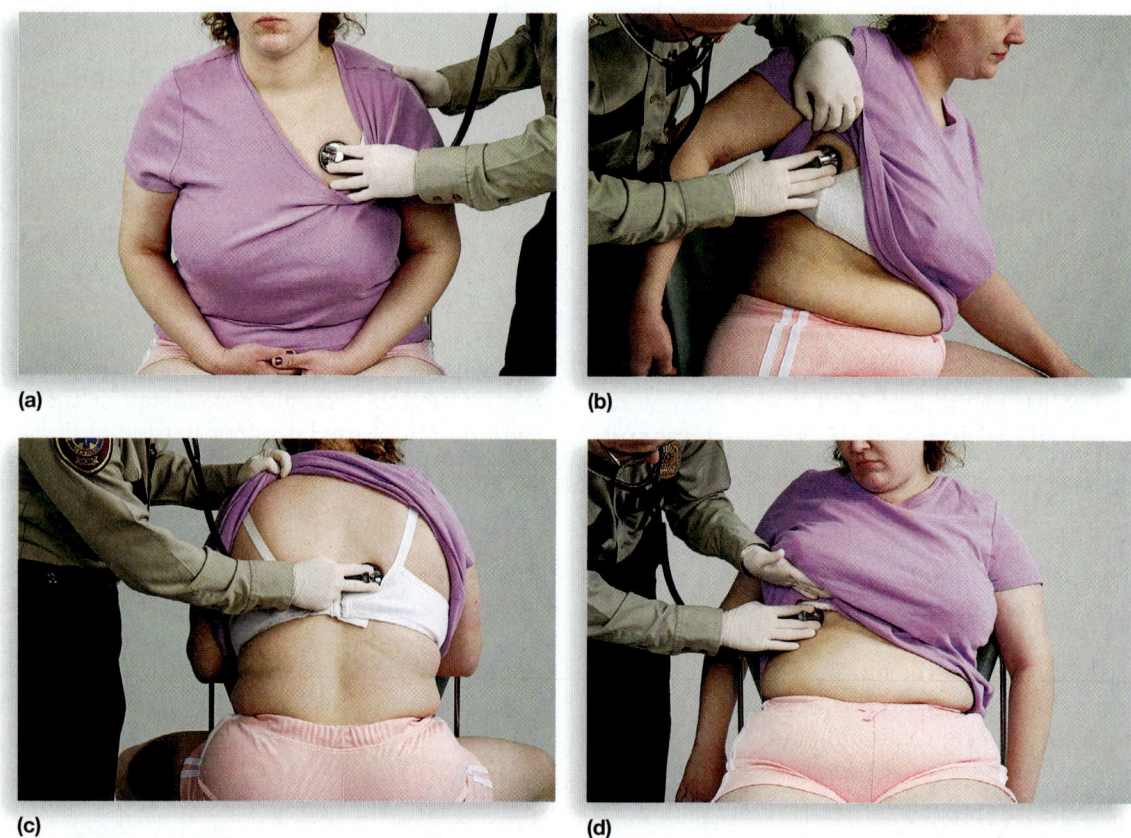

(a)   (b)   (c)   (d)

Figure 11-15   (a) Because there is more tissue and body fat on the anterior of the chest, auscultation on the anterior chest wall may produce less pronounced sounds than the posterior chest wall. (b) Listen in the midaxillary line to hear the purest lung sounds that are not contaminated by sounds transmitted from the trachea and bronchi. (c) Auscultation performed on the posterior surface may yield louder sounds because of less tissue between the skin and the lung. (d) Use the back of the hand to lift the breast out of the way during auscultation.

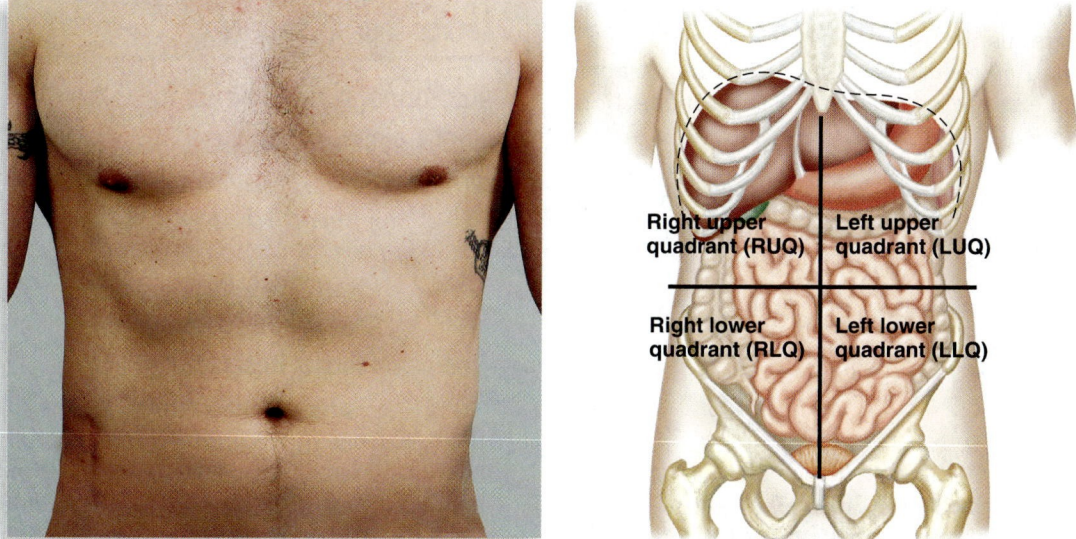

Figure 11-16   The abdomen can be divided into four quadrants, two upper and two lower.

Nice to Know

Abdominal Reflex Assessment

Lightly stroke each side of the abdomen above and below the umbilicus with an irregular object like a reflex hammer, broken cotton swab, or split tongue blade. Muscles will contract, and the umbilicus will deviate (move) towards the stimulus. The absence of this reflex **could** indicate a central or peripheral nervous system disorder. If the patient is not very "ticklish," you may find that you need to stroke more towards the lateral aspect of the abdomen.

find initially, with practice you should be able to note their presence easily. DOT 3-2.45

Inspection of the genital area is not normally performed in the prehospital setting unless it has direct bearing on the chief complaint. For example, a woman in active labor may be examined in order to determine whether birth is eminent. A patient who was sexually assaulted may need visual inspection to rule out bleeding or lacerations. If inspected, the genitalia should appear uninjured and be free of strong odors or discharges. The skin color should be appropriate to the patient but may appear darker than the other skin on the body. The inner surface of the labia of female patients should be pink and moist. Hair may or may not be present on male and female patients depending upon the developmental age of the patient and also depending upon hygiene habits. DOT 3-2.46, 3-2.47, 3-2.48

Auscultation of abdominal sounds will usually not provide a significant amount of information to the emergency care provider.[15] Your care and treatment of patients with abdominal complaints will remain the same whether sounds are present or absent.

Pelvic Area

Expose the pelvic area while maintaining modesty. Inspect the area for any masses, swelling, or bruising. Note any unusual discharge from the penis or vagina. Palpate the femoral pulses. They are located in the "crease" where the thigh meets the abdomen and where the proximal femur region meets the hip region in the pelvis (Figure 11-17). Although they may be difficult to

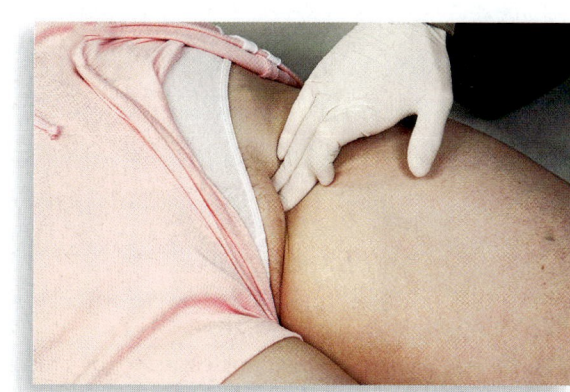

Figure 11-17   The femoral pulse is located deep in the inguinal area.

Anus and rectal examinations are not normally conducted in the prehospital setting. However, certain circumstances, such as rectal bleeding or sexual assault, may necessitate examining this area. Visual inspection of the area is typically all that is required in the prehospital setting. Muscle tone check of the rectal sphincter, which is performed to check for spinal cord injury, is typically not performed in the prehospital setting. DOT 3-2.49, 3-2.50

CONNECTIONS Chapter 36: Urology and Chapter 41: Obstetrics and Gynecology have additional information on examining the genitals and anus.

Lower Extremities

Expose and inspect the legs. While most people's legs are actually slightly unequal in length, it is generally unnoticeable. Note the color and turgor of the skin. Palpate each leg individually for any masses, swellings, deformity, or tenderness. Palpate the popliteal pulse, located behind the knee, and the dorsalis pedis and posterior tibial pulse in the foot and ankle. The popliteal artery may be more difficult to locate due to a greater amount of connective tissue surrounding the artery (Figure 11-18). The Babinski test and reflex assessment are described in the following box. These examinations are not necessary in the emergent situation. DOT 3-2.51, 3-2.52, 3-2.53, 3-2.54

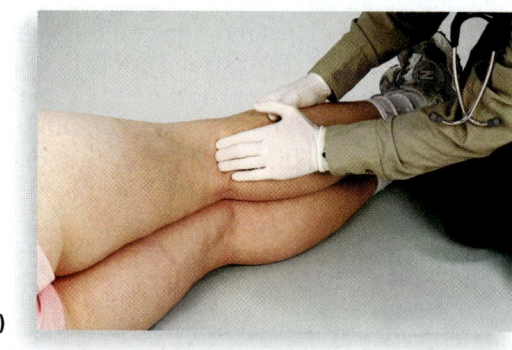

(a)

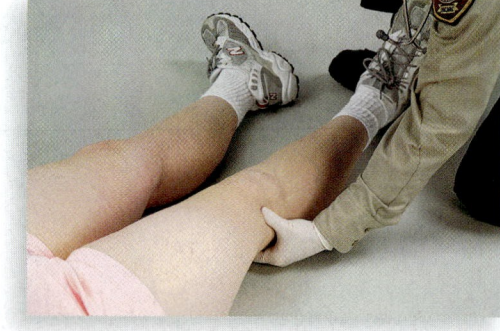

(b)

Figure 11-18   (a) Palpate for the popliteal artery by pressing deep on the posterior of the knee. (b) Wrap your fingers around to the posterior side of the straightened knee and press deep to feel the popliteal artery.

Nice to Know

Additional Assessments for Extremities
Reflex Assessment

Strike a slightly flexed tendon with a reflex hammer. When the nervous impulse is sensed, it stimulates a muscle contraction. The extremity may jerk. This can be performed in each joint space on the extremities.

Babinski Plantar Response

Stroke the lateral aspect (outside edge) of the sole of the foot from the side of the heel up and across the ball of the foot. A positive Babinski response occurs if the patient pulls the great (large) toe towards the knee (dorsiflexes) and the other toes fan out. This response indicates a CNS lesion (problem), except in infants where this is a normal finding.

Street Secrets

Because of its depth inside the musculature, the popliteal pulse is often difficult to palpate. Try to flex the knee slightly and circle the knee with both hands so the fingers meet midline in the back. Press the fingertips of both hands deep into the popliteal fossa.

Gently grasp a toe and ask if the patient can feel your touch. Place the fingers of one hand together, place this flat surface against the sole of the patient's foot, and ask her to push down on them. The patient should be able to comply without difficulty. After inspecting and palpating the other leg, compare the sensory, motor, and perfusion of both legs. They should be equal.

Street Secrets

Having difficulty determining whether the patient's pulse is really there? Take your time. Each patient can be just a little different; explore the area where you think the pulse should be. Vary the pressure of your fingers as well; sometimes pressing a little too hard can compress the artery to the point where it cannot expand as the pressure wave passes through.

Upper Extremities

Expose and inspect each upper extremity for any obvious masses, swelling, or bruises. Palpate each arm for tenderness or deformity. Unlike the leg, peripheral

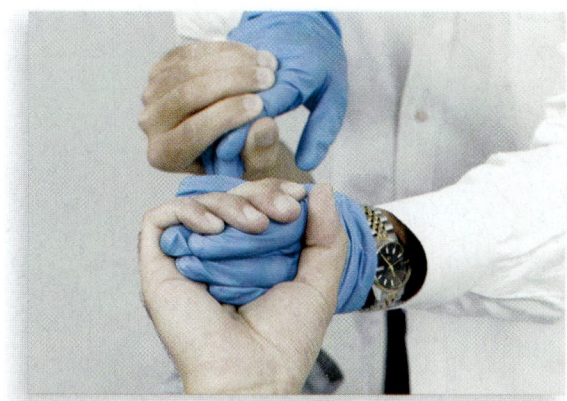

Figure 11-19   The patient should be able to squeeze equally with both hands.

pulses in the arms, such as the radial and brachial pulses, are usually easier to locate. Squeeze the distal tip of a finger for several seconds to blanch the site. Release the pinch and check for capillary refilling. The blanched area should become pink again within 2–3 seconds. Environmental conditions such as cold weather may increase capillary refilling time dramatically. DOT 3-2.51, 3-2.52, 3-2.53, 3-2.54

CONNECTIONS   Refer to Figure 13-3 in Chapter 13: Shock Overview to see capillary refill in an infant.

When squeezing the patient's finger, ask if he can feel that sensation. Compare the patient's perception with the other extremity; they should be equal. When each arm exam is completed, ask the patient to grasp your fingers with each hand (Figure 11-19). The patient should be able to squeeze your fingers with equal strength.

Back

Expose the back and inspect for symmetry. Observe if there is any unusual curvature of the spine. Note any bruises, swelling, masses, or discoloration. Palpate the back to determine any areas of tenderness or edema. Auscultate the posterior chest for lung sounds.

Prehospital Monitoring Devices

In addition to the information provided by the hands-on physical examination, information about normal and abnormal conditions is obtained by the application and use of a variety of monitoring devices.

As technology continues to advance, electronic monitoring devices become smaller, lighter, and more user-friendly. As a result, the portability and opera-

bility of these devices often make them very effective for monitoring out-of-hospital patients. This section does not intend to fully explore every possible device that is available to EMS providers. It describes the more commonly used pieces of equipment available today. DOT 3-4.1

Electrocardiograph (ECG) Monitor

The portable **electrocardiograph** was first used by out-of-hospital care providers in Ireland in the 1960s.[19] Today's ECG monitors are lighter and more durable than their predecessors. In addition to monitoring the patient's basic ECG, these machines often come equipped to monitor more complex 12 leads and have capabilities to monitor blood pressure, pulse rate, oxygen saturation (oximetry), and carbon dioxide levels in expired air (capnography).

CONNECTIONS   Chapter 29: Cardiology will describe the actual production of ECGs in greater detail. Skill Sheet 37: Applying Leads and Multifunction Pads has information on obtaining ECG tracings and monitoring the ECG.

Pulse Oximetry

Pulse oximeters provide a fairly reliable, portable, and noninvasive method to assess a patient's oxygenation in the prehospital environment (Figure 11-20).[20] Typically, a sensor probe is placed on a finger, but probes are also available for earlobes, an infant's foot, or even the nose.[21,22] Wherever it is placed, it must be on a fairly thin-skinned area so that the device can pick up the pulse below the skin surface. **Skill Sheet and Step-by-Step 12: Pulse Oximetry.**

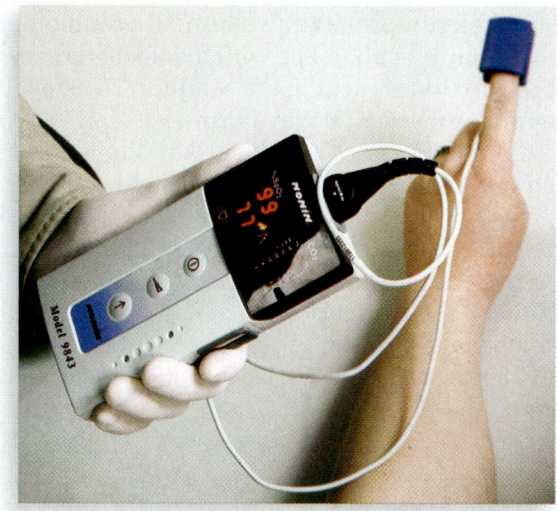

Figure 11-20   Pulse oximetry is often referred to as the fourth vital sign. This model displays the heart rate along with the pulse oximetry reading.

Street Secrets

To obtain the most accurate pulse oximetry reading, ensure that you place the probe on a finger or toe that is free of any nail polish or synthetic nails, and place the probe on an extremity that does not have an IV or a blood pressure cuff, if possible.

Pulse oximeters use a process called spectrophotometry in which red and infrared lights are emitted from the device. With each pulse, the device measures how much of the two lights is absorbed. Hemoglobin that is oxygenated absorbs more infrared light while hemoglobin without oxygen absorbs more red light. The computer within the device then calculates the percentage of oxygenated blood (SpO_2). For example, a reading of 95% on a pulse oximeter means that an estimated 95% of hemoglobin at that pulse site is saturated with oxygen.

Street Secrets

Note that SpO_2 is not equal to SaO_2. SaO_2 is a laboratory measurement that calculates the amount of oxygen saturation in an arterial sample of blood.

Capnography

A key element to the body's ability to maintain homeostasis is its ability not only to bring in oxygen but also to expel excess levels of carbon dioxide. Therefore, the value of being able to measure how adequate the patient's ventilatory status is functioning is tremendous. **Capnography** is a technique that continually measures carbon dioxide levels in exhaled air. As the patient exhales, a probe draws a small volume of that air into a sampling chamber which detects the amount of carbon dioxide present in the sample.[14] The resulting capnograph provides a waveform that can be interpreted not only for how much carbon dioxide is being exhaled but also for how effective the exhalation itself is in terms of releasing carbon dioxide. Typical values of exhaled carbon dioxide range from 35 to 45 mmHg.

CONNECTIONS A more detailed description of capnography and the interpretation of capnograph waveforms can be found in Chapter 12: Airway Management, Ventilation, and Oxygenation.

Glucometer

Critical organs of the body, such as the brain, depend not only on oxygen as a primary energy source but also on the amount of glucose available to the cells.

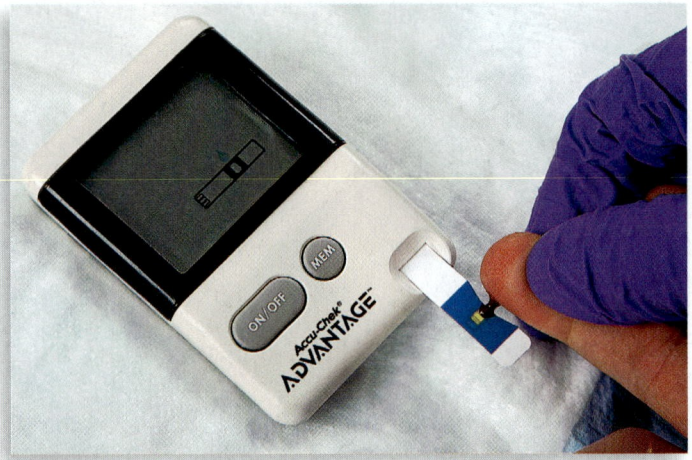

Figure 11-21 Portable glucometers are used to test blood sugar and have been shown to be very accurate.

Glucometry is the method of evaluating blood glucose levels. Hand-held **glucometers** are available to prehospital personnel (Figure 11-21). They are reliable and easy to use. **Skill Sheet 26 and Step-by-Step 26: Blood Glucose Assessment explain the procedure.**

Glucometers measure blood glucose levels either using capillary blood via a fingerstick or venous blood obtained during venipuncture either when inserting an IV or when obtaining blood for laboratory testing. Either method appears to provide reasonable readings of blood glucose levels as compared to full laboratory testing, although glucometers that use capillary blood to measure glucose levels may be more accurate.[23,24] Be careful, however, to not inadvertently mix testing methods with blood sample type. In other words, do not use venous blood if the glucometer requires a capillary blood sample (Box 11-1).

BOX 11-1 \ Point-of-Care Lab Tests

The glucometer is one example of **point-of-care** testing. This is different from laboratory-based testing procedures where measuring techniques often follow a rigid protocol to ensure consistency of test results. While laboratory results may be more accurate than their point-of-care counterparts, they can take a significant amount of time to obtain. In urgent or emergent conditions such as those found in an EMS system or Emergency Department, the advantage of significant time savings using point-of-care testing may outweigh the more accurate findings of laboratory testing.

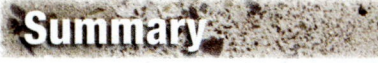
Summary

The human body is a wondrous work—more sophisticated than any machine that has ever been built. Using the physical examination techniques of inspection, palpation, and auscultation, as well as noting abnormal odors, the paramedic will assess the patient for changes from normal, indicating a disease process. With practice, the techniques of physical examination will become easier to perform and will provide critical clues to the critically ill or injured patient.

Notes

1. N. Caroline, *Emergency Care in the Streets,* 2nd ed. (Boston: Little, Brown and Co, 1983).

2. K. J. Kennedy, D. E. Dreimanis, W. D. Beckingham, and F. J. Bowden, "Staphylococcus Aureus and Stethoscopes," *Medical Journal of Australia* 178(9) (May 2003): 468.

3. R. C. Parmar, C. C. Valvi, P. Sira, and J. R. Kamat, "A Prospective, Randomised, Double-Blind Study of Comparative Efficacy of Immediate Versus Daily Cleaning of Stethoscope Using 66% Ethyl Alcohol," *Indian Journal of Medical Sciences* 58(10) (October 2004): 423–30.

4. C. H. Guinto, E. J. Bottone et al., "Evaluation of Dedicated Stethoscopes as a Potential Source of Nosocomial Pathogens," *American Journal of Infection Control* 30(8) (December 2002): 499–502.

5. S. Bobes and D. Bobes, "The Prehospital Physical Assessment," in *Prehospital Emergency Care Secrets* (Philadelphia: Hanley and Belfus, 1998).

6. G. A. Thibodeau and K. T. Patton, *The Human Body in Health and Disease,* 4th ed. (St. Louis, MO: Elsevier/Mosby, 2005).

7. L. S. Bickley and P. G. Szilagyi, *Bates' Guide to Physical Examination and History Taking;* 8th ed. (Philadelphia, PA: Lippincott Williams & Wilkins, 2003), p. 24.

8. A. V. Chobanian et al., Joint National Committee on Prevention, Detection, Evaluation, and Treatment of High Blood Pressure; National Heart, Lung, and Blood Institute; National High Blood Pressure Education Program Coordinating Committee, "Seventh Report of the Joint National Committee on Prevention, Detection, Evaluation, and Treatment of High Blood Pressure: the JNC 7 complete report," *Hypertension* 42 (2003): 1206–1252.

9. P. G. Pickering et al., "AHA Scientific Statement: Recommendations for Blood Pressure Measurement in Humans and Experimental Animals Part 1: Blood Pressure Measurement in Humans," *Hypertension* 45(2005):149–152.

10. T. G. Pickering, White Coat Hypertension, in J. L. Izzo and H. R. Black, eds. *Hypertension Primer,* 3rd ed. (Dallas, TX: American Heart Association, 2003).

11. F. A. McAlister and S. E. Straus, "Evidence Based Treatment of Hypertension: Measurement of Blood Pressure: an Evidence Based Review," *British Medical Journal* (2001):908–911.

12. D. Evans and B. Hodgkinson, "Information Sheet: Best Practices for Vital Signs," http://www.joannabriggs.edu.au/best_practice/bp8.php#anchor30291869 (accessed April 24, 2005).

13. D. Lane, M. Beevers, N. Barnes, J. Bourne, A. John, S. Malins, and D. G. Beevers, "Inter-Arm Differences in Blood Pressure: When Are They Clinically Significant?" *Journal of Hypertension* 20(2002):1089–1095.

14. J. Marx, *Rosen's Emergency Medicine: Concepts and Clinical Practice,* 5th ed. (St. Louis: Mosby, Inc., 2002).

15. J. E. Tintinalli, G. Kelen, and J. S. Stapczynski, *Emergency Medicine: A Comprehensive Study Guide,* 6th ed. (New York, NY: McGraw-Hill Companies, 2004). www.accessmedicine.com (accessed February 6, 2006).

16. Current Emergency Diagnosis & Treatment; Section II Management of Common Emergency Problems—Chapter 10: The multiply injured patient? Emergency Treatment of Specific disorders: Head Trauma, www.accessmedicine.com (accessed February 6, 2006).

17. A. H. Ilsley, A. J. Rutten, and W. B. Runciman, "An Evaluation of Body Temperature Measurement," *Anaesthesia Intensive Care* 11(1) (February 1983):31–9.

18. E. Eggenberger, "Anisocoria," http://www.emedicine.com/neuro/topic479.htm (accessed May 6, 2005).

19. J. F. Pantridge and J. S. Geddes, "A Mobile-Intensive Care Unit in the Management of Myocardial Infarction," *Lancet,* 2(1967): 271.

20. L. Teoh, A. Epstein, B. Williamson et al., "Medical Staff's Knowledge of Pulse Oximetry: A Prospective Study Conducted in a Tertiary Children's Hospital," *Journal of Paediatrics and Child Health* 39 (2003): 618–622.

21. J. M. Cairo and S. P. Pilbeam, *Mosby's Respiratory Care Equipment,* 7ed. (St. Louis, MO: Mosby, 2004).

22. E. A. McConnell, Performing Pulse Oximetry, *Nursing* 29(11) (November 1999):17.

23. A. Kulkarni, "Analysis of Blood Glucose Measurements Using Capillary and Arterial Blood Samples in Intensive Care Patients," *Intensive Care Medicine* 31(1)(2005): 142–145.

24. G. Kumar, "Correlation of Capillary and Venous Blood Glucometry with Laboratory Determination," *Prehospital Emergency Care* 8(4)(2004): 378–383.

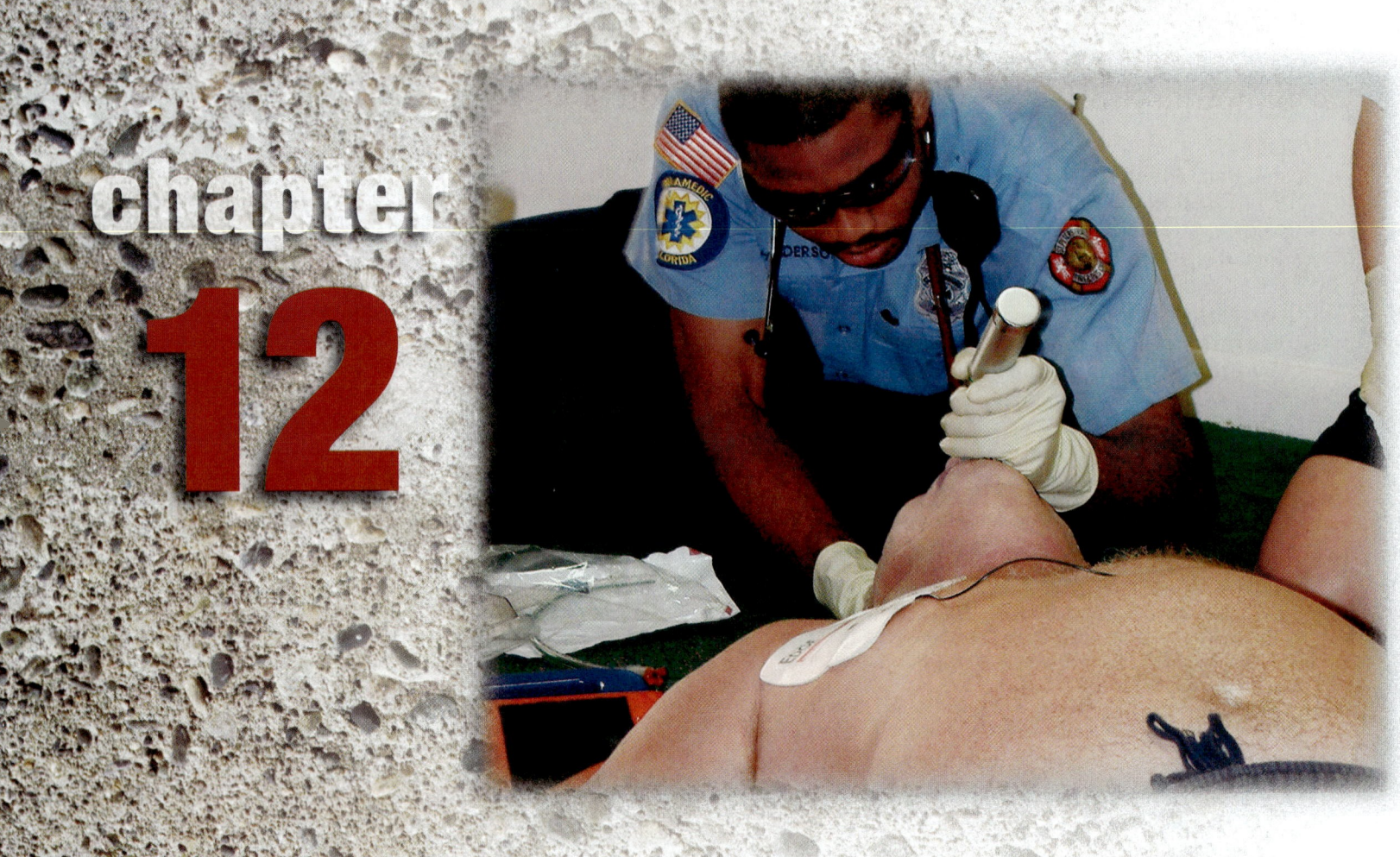

Airway Management, Ventilation, and Oxygenation

"If you don't have an airway, you don't have a patient."

—Attributed to every EMS instructor

Need to Know

▶ The airway is the starting point of the oxygen lifeline. Assuring an open airway is always the first step in caring for a patient.

▶ The UPPER airway begins at the lips and nose and ends at the vocal cords. The LOWER airway begins at the vocal cords and ends at the alveolar-capillary membrane.

▶ Always be alert to potential airway obstruction caused by the position of the patient.

▶ Air moves in and out of the airway and lungs (ventilation) to interface across the thinnest barrier: the pulmonary capillary membranes. It is here that gas exchange (respiration) takes place.

▶ Blood flowing out of the heart through the aorta typically has an oxygen saturation of 97% or more (on pulse oximetry) with a PaO_2 between 80 mmHg and 100 mmHg (on arterial blood gas analysis). Venous blood returning to the heart usually has an oxygen saturation of around 75% and a PaO_2 of around 40 mmHg. A PaO_2 of about 60 mmHg will generally cause a red blood cell (RBC) oxygen saturation of around 90% (SpO_2) on the pulse oximeter.

▶ Normal inhalation (an active process) of air happens because of the negative pressure generated by the diaphragm moving down and the intercostals muscles expanding the ribs. The inhalation phase is normally a little shorter than the exhalation phase (a passive process) of a ventilation cycle.

▶ In patients with circulatory problems, such as shock, dehydration, or cardiac arrest, raising pressure inside of the thorax through assisted ventilation can **dramatically** decrease venous return and thus greatly decrease cardiac output, worsening shock. Therefore, the EMS provider must understand that ventilating patients too fast (with a bag-mask) can drop blood pressure and worsen circulatory collapse in unstable patients.

▶ An airway can become obstructed from a wide variety of causes including blood, broken teeth, food, vomitus, saliva, foreign bodies, and the tongue.

▶ Sick

- Cardiac arrest and traumatic brain injury require airway management by intubation very early in patient care.
- If initial airway management techniques such as supplemental oxygen are not successful, try positive pressure ventilation and then progress to intubation.
- Pulse oximetry readings of 90% or less indicate severe hypoxia (at sea level).
- Capnography should be monitored on every intubated patient. CO_2 readings are normal when they are around 40 mmHg.

▶ Not Yet Sick

- Most patient situations require the focus to be on airway positioning and supplemental oxygen administration via simple adjuncts and devices.
- Pulse oximetry readings above 95% are within the normal range.
- Pulse oximetry readings between 91–95% (at sea level) indicate the patient is mildly hypoxic and the airway and breathing should be assessed thoroughly while supplemental oxygen is administered.
- Make sure the airway is patent and take steps to ensure that it remains patent.
- Assess the effectiveness of every airway device and take corrective action when things are not working.
- Ask If the patient has ever required intubation or hospitalization for the current problem to help you determine potential severity.

Introduction

Assessing and assuring an open airway and ventilation are two of the most important and sometimes challenging tasks that a paramedic will have.[1,2] Without a way for air to enter and move in and out of the lungs, human life is immediately compromised. It is no surprise that airway and ventilation skills are an extensive and vital part of paramedic education and practice.[3,4,5] DOT 2-1.1

This chapter will begin with a basic overview of airway and ventilation anatomy and physiology. A discussion of ventilation and perfusion follows the trip down the airway. The exchange of oxygen and carbon dioxide at the capillary beds is described, along with respiration and ventilation abnormalities. Respiratory cycles, volumes and capacities, respiratory patterns, and breath sounds are also discussed. After establishing a basic understanding of the structures and mechanics involved, we will focus on the most common conditions that may compromise the airway and breathing. The chapter ends with a discussion of how to assess and manage the airway and describes some common airway adjuncts and devices.

Basic Emergency Medical Technicians (EMTs) entering paramedic education programs should have a working knowledge of simple, noninvasive airway maneuvers, adjuncts, and ventilatory techniques. It is important to note that these basic skills alone have been shown to be effective in managing most airway problems.[6,7] This is a very important point that is easily overlooked as you learn new and more advanced invasive skills. Performing basic airway skills flawlessly is the first, and possibly the most important, step to becoming a skilled *advanced* care provider.[7] DOT 2-1.2

Entire books have been written regarding airway skills in the prehospital environment.[8] This chapter will necessarily focus on general assessment and management skills. Please review the skills checklists in the manual that accompanies this text, and practice airway and ventilation skills frequently in training. Nowhere in your training is the saying, "Perfect practice makes for perfect performance" more true. A single mistake in the placement or confirmation of placement of an advanced airway may result in the preventable death of your patient. Your approach, therefore, should be calm, calculated, and systematic and should provide continual reassessment of redundant checks to assure proper placement and patency of the patient's airway. **See all airway Skill Sheets (1–24, 84, 85, 88, and 90) and Step-by-Steps 1–7, 9, 11–14, 18, 19, 21–24.**

The Need for Oxygen

Each cell of the body is a tiny furnace creating the molecules for life. In every one of the billions and billions of cells making up our bodies, microscopic forges burn brightly from the instant of conception until the moment of death in the process that is called life.

Oxygen is required for this enzymatic "burning" that takes place inside of the cells, and carbon dioxide (CO_2) and water are produced by this "fire of metabolism." It may be said that the CO_2 produced is the "smoke of metabolism." This enzymatic consumption of high energy materials taking place inside of cells is called **respiration.**

> In medicine the patient's respirations are thought of as being the rate and the quality of breathing, and this is true.

The respirations seen are directly connected to the state of the enzymatic "respiration" going on inside the cells of the body. Air movement by the patient during ventilation directly reflects the burning of the cellular fire of metabolism in respiration.

Street Secrets

Always remember that the air movement by a patient is a window into the cells of the patient in both sickness and in health. All you have to do is look at the patient to see the process in action. The challenge is to ALWAYS look.

During human development, a complex web of interconnections is woven to bring oxygen to the cells for the burning of substrate. To bring oxygen to the cells and to remove CO_2, air moves in and out of the lungs via the airway under the control of intercostal muscles and the diaphragm. The discussion of air movement begins by thinking about the path by which air moves into the body.

Airway Anatomy and Physiology

A Trip down the Airway

Air movement requires an airway. The human airway begins at the mouth and nose and proceeds down a complex pathway to end at the alveolar-capillary membrane. The next few pages will explore concepts about the airway to set the stage for how to approach the evaluation and management of the patient's ventilation. The airway is divided into two parts: the upper airway, which begins at the lips and nose and ends at the vocal cords, and the lower airway, which begins at the vocal cords and proceeds to the alveolar-capillary membrane (Figure 12-1) DOT 2-1.3, 2-1.4

Upper Airway Anatomy

The upper airway has fixed portions, such as the nose and hard palate, and mobile portions, such as the mouth, lips, tongue, and soft palate (Figure 12-2). The fixed portions of the nose are affected very little by the movement of air and are stable platforms for air movement through the airway. The nasal structures generally help maintain a solid and reliable path for air movement while, at the same time, filtering out large particles and humidifying the inspired air. Trauma to the nose, however, can compromise these functions. Nosebleeds **(epistaxis),** for example, can cause hemorrhage into the airway. Facial fractures can obstruct the nasal passages, causing this portion of the airway to be unstable with associated bleeding into the airway and potential aspiration into the lungs. DOT 2-1.55

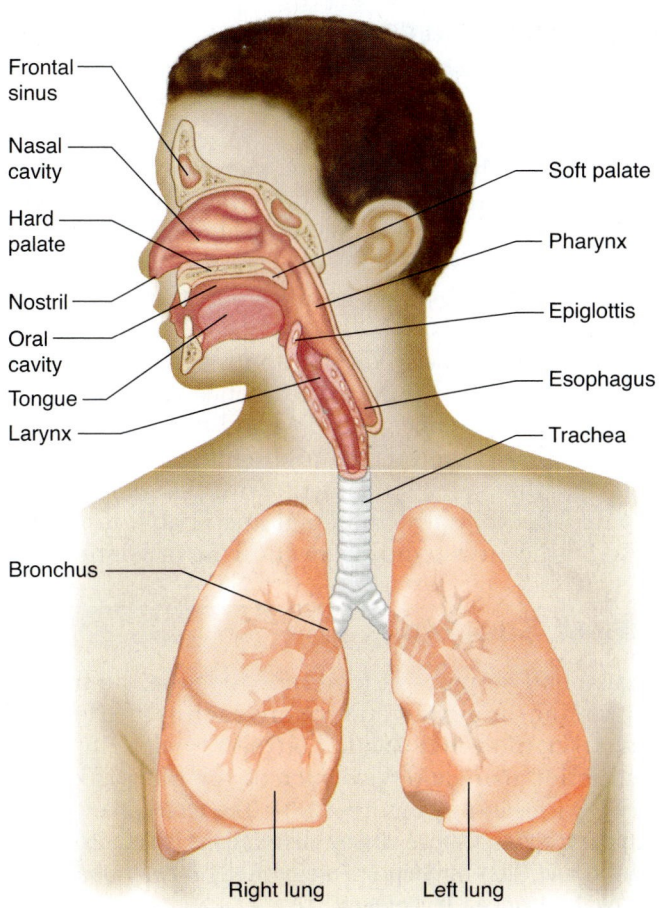

Figure 12-1   The human airway.

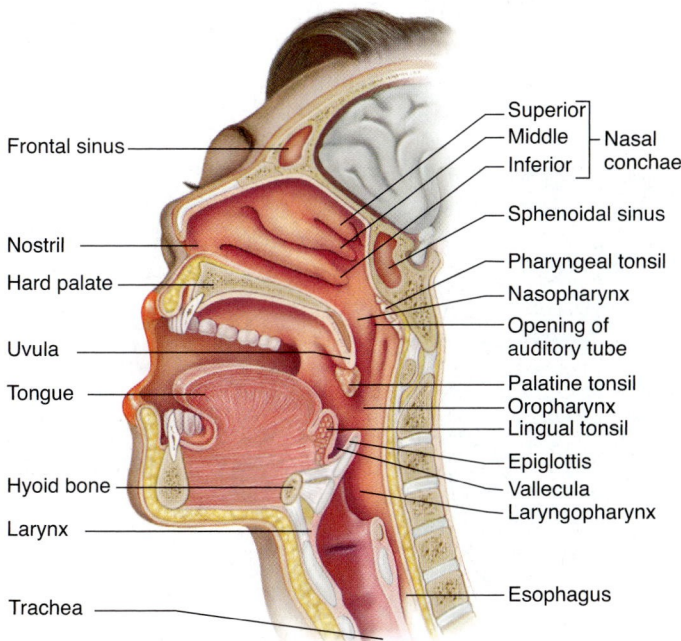

Figure 12-2   The upper airway.

Street Secrets

Blood in the airway can cause potential airway compromise in several ways: (1) It can block passage of air causing a frank obstruction; (2) it can result in aspiration pneumonia within the lung if it is inhaled; and (3) if it enters the stomach, it can irritate the lining of the stomach, resulting in vomiting and further potential airway compromise via aspiration of gastric contents or foreign body obstruction.

The Mouth and Tongue

The mouth and tongue are the most mobile parts of the airway.

- ***The jaw:***   The jaw **(mandible)** is a mobile bone that has hinges (called the temporomandibular joint or TMJ) on both sides just below the ear. People vary as to how wide their jaws will open, making airway management different from patient to patient. Small jaws can provide real challenges in airway management because of the inability to provide a sufficiently wide opening to allow the passage of rescue airways.

- ***Lips:***   The lips are soft structures that may be opened using various motions in order to gain access to the airway. Injuries to the lips may cause bleeding into the airway. Dry or swollen lips may make opening the airway difficult, and dry lips may require lubrication to allow optimal airway opening or to assist in the placement of airway adjuncts and devices.

- ***Inside the mouth:***   The inside of the mouth (called the **oropharynx**) is made up of the hard palate at the top and the jaw at the bottom. The hard palate runs from the back of the upper teeth posteriorly until it terminates just in front of the posterior pharynx. There the **soft palate** begins, which is a flap of skin

Nice to Know

The word "pharynx" refers to the open portion of the alimentary canal (GI tract) between the inside of the lips and the top of the esophagus. The use of "pharynx" as a suffix attached to words like hypo-, laryngo-, naso-, oro-, etc. indicates the open area in proximity to each of these structures or locations. The glottis is also an opening, but this special opening is found within the soft tissues just under the epiglottis, right above the vocal cords, and it marks the entrance into the lower airway.

lying just below the inferior and posterior portions of the nasal structures. The soft palate marks the end of the superior area known as the **nasopharynx.** The soft palate curves around to both sides of the posterior pharynx behind the tonsils.

- ***The tongue:***   The tongue is a soft, pliable structure made of muscle and covered with lingual tonsil and salivary gland tissue. It attaches to the floor of the mouth and the back of the mandible. When a patient is lying on his back, the tongue tends to fall backward into the back of the mouth and against the soft palate, potentially obstructing the airway. "Snoring" is a sound made by the motion of the tongue and soft palate as a result of partial airway obstruction. Indeed, when someone snores while sleeping, this indicates a partial airway obstruction. This can be indicative of risks to the airway in some people, a condition known as "obstructive sleep apnea."

Because of its mobility and its tendency to fall backward when a patient is supine, the tongue is the most common cause of airway obstruction.

- A rescuer must be aware of this potential obstruction and must be prepared to manage it, either through repositioning the patient's head and jaw or by inserting one of several devices used for lifting or bypassing the tongue. The **oropharyngeal airway (OPA)** or oral airway is a curved plastic device which, when properly placed, holds the tongue off of the back of the pharynx. A nasopharyngeal airway (NPA) or nasal airway is placed through the nose, through the nasopharynx, and into the pharynx, lifting the tongue forward off of the posterior pharynx. Mastering the use of these devices is essential.

Transition between the Upper and Lower Airways

The Throat

Humans breathe air and consume food. Both move through the upper part of the airway above the vocal cords. However, both actions cannot occur at the same time. The throat is an important location because both the GI tract and the airway split apart from each other in this location.

The junction between the upper and lower airway is the **glottis.** The opening to the trachea lies just anterior to the opening to the esophagus, and it is present when the vocal cords are relaxed and open. This presents a great risk that stomach contents, during vomiting, can be inhaled. Normally, the epiglottis is able to quickly close off the airway during swallowing or vomiting.

Street Secrets

Occasionally a piece of food may lodge in the trachea, obstructing the airway, and actions such as the Heimlich Maneuver, or even the actual physical dislodging of the obstruction using a device such as the Magill Forceps, may be lifesaving (Figure 12-3). **The technique for using Magill forceps to remove airway obstructions is detailed in Skill Sheet 6 and Step-by-Step 6: Foreign Body Airway Obstruction Removal-Advanced Techniques.**

The Hypopharynx

Just at the back of the tongue is the area where the opening of the gastrointestinal tract, called the esophagus, and the opening of the trachea meet. This area is called the **hypopharynx.** You should be familiar with the anatomy and the appearance of the hypopharynx

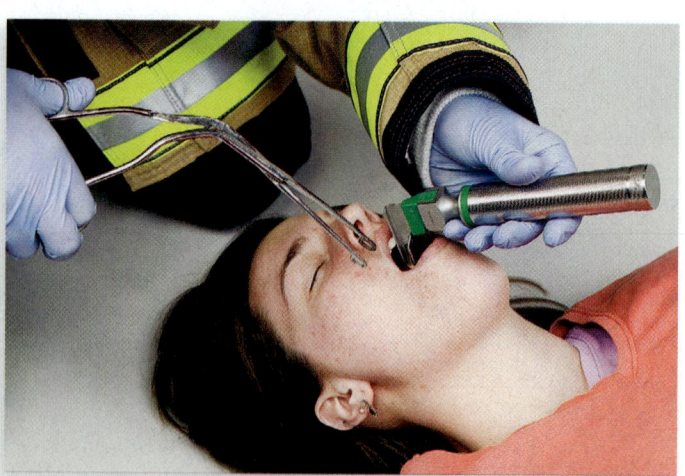

Food trapped in airway

Figure 12-3   If an obstruction can be visualized with direct laryngoscopy, the Magill forceps may be a useful tool to grasp and remove the object.

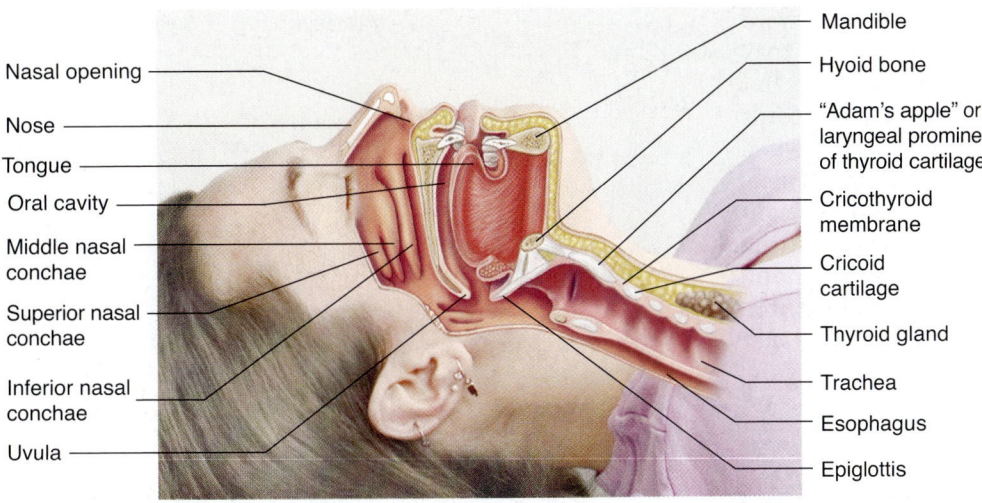

Nasal opening

Nose

Tongue

Oral cavity

Middle nasal conchae

Superior nasal conchae

Inferior nasal conchae

Uvula

Mandible

Hyoid bone

"Adam's apple" or laryngeal prominence of thyroid cartilage

Cricothyroid membrane

Cricoid cartilage

Thyroid gland

Trachea

Esophagus

Epiglottis

Figure 12-4 A good understanding of the hypopharynx is essential for the paramedic. Basic and advanced airways are placed in this area to maintain open airways.

because of the need to be able to perform various emergency procedures which are essential to critical care (Figure 12-4). An example of such a procedure is endotracheal intubation, which will be discussed later in this chapter.

The Glottis and Epiglottis

The glottis is guarded by a somewhat stiff, cartilage-containing flap of tissue, called the **epiglottis.** During swallowing, the epiglottis covers the opening of the glottis to prevent material from getting into the trachea. In front of the epiglottis is a small pouch, called the **vallecula,** and to either side of the vallecula are small recesses called the **pyriform sinuses.** It is useful to know about the pyriform sinuses because occasionally objects can get caught in the pyriform sinuses, such as a nasogastric tube during insertion.

Street Secrets

The vallecula is of particular interest to the paramedic since it is the site where a curved laryngoscope blade is inserted during visualization of the vocal cords for either clearing the airway or for endotracheal intubation. In contrast, a straight laryngoscope blade is inserted directly *over* the epiglottis and lifts the epiglottis to allow direct visualization of the tracheal opening.

Larynx and Associated Structures

The two vocal cords sit within the **larynx.** The larynx can be located by finding the "Adam's Apple" on the front of a patient's neck. This structure is the **thyroid cartilage.** The vocal cords lie just inside the top of the thyroid cartilage and run across the top of the airway to a pair of tiny, pivoting cartilages called the **arytenoids** (Figure 12-5).

As the arytenoid cartilages turn, tiny cartilages attached to their ends, called corniculate cartilage, tighten the vocal cords, changing the pitch of the voice. The arytenoids can be seen during endotracheal intubation as the posterior attachments of the vocal cords, and they are useful landmarks to visualize during this procedure.

Vocal Cords

Vocal cords are mobile, living tissue. When viewed through a laryngoscope, they usually appear as white bands seen on either side of the airway (Figure 12-6). The

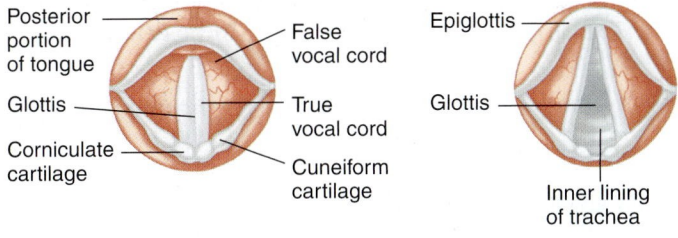

Posterior portion of tongue

Glottis

Corniculate cartilage

False vocal cord

True vocal cord

Cuneiform cartilage

Epiglottis

Glottis

Inner lining of trachea

(a) Vocal cords closed

(b) Vocal cords open

Figure 12-5 Anatomy of the vocal cords.

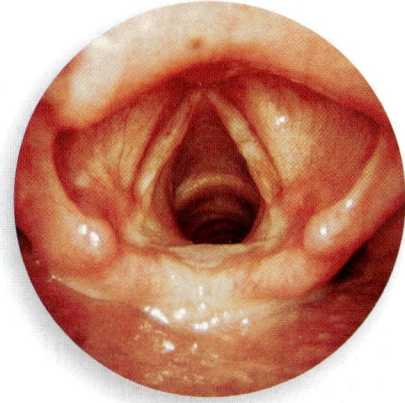

Figure 12-6 Vocal cords viewed through a laryngoscope.

cords are actually thick folds of tissue that turn inward from the inside of the larynx. However, the cords may exhibit a number of conditions that can pose problems for airway management. During allergic reactions, the cords can swell and obstruct the airway. Burns, such as when flame or steam is inhaled, can make the cords swell also.

The vocal cords can go into spasm, becoming tight and closing off the airway. This can occur during some airway procedures or even with use of paralytic medication given to assist endotracheal intubation. **Laryngospasm** can rapidly result in death if not managed appropriately (Figure 12-7).

Working in the Gray Zone

Laryngospasm

Laryngospasm can be disconcerting, particularly if it is triggered during airway management techniques such as an intubation attempt. Treatment of laryngospasm includes providing positive pressure ventilation with a bag-mask unit with 100% oxygen or administering intravenous lidocaine (1.5 mg/kg). If laryngospasm persists and hypoxia develops, succinylcholine (0.25–1 mg/kg [usually the lower dose range]) should be given (if your protocol allows) to relax the laryngeal muscles and allow controlled ventilation. The large, negative intrathoracic pressures generated by a struggling patient during laryngospasm can result in the development of negative pressure pulmonary edema, even in healthy young adults.[9]

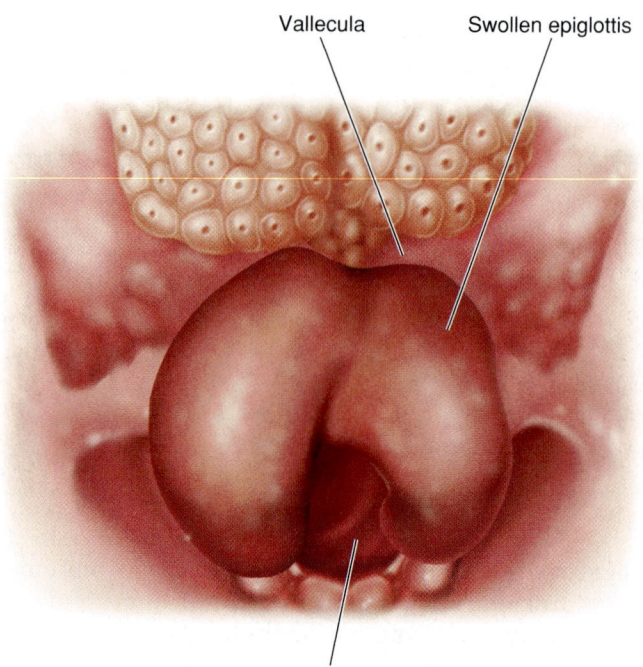

Vallecula   Swollen epiglottis

Partially obstructed glottic opening

Figure 12-7   Laryngoscopic view showing a red, edematous epiglottis and glottic area with marked airway compromise in an adult with epiglottitis. Attempting prehospital intubation on a patient such as this could be very difficult and can worsen swelling or cause extensive bleeding. This is a true airway emergency, and the patient that is breathing on his own should be transported rapidly without laryngosopic visualization of the airway. If the airway should become compromised, advanced airways such as needle cricothyrotomy can be used.

The Lower Airway

The lower airway begins at the undersurface of the vocal cords at the top of the trachea. It continues down through the tracheobronchial tree to the alveoli. This is the portion of the airway where gas exchange (respiration) takes place.

Trachea

The trachea has semicircular, ring-shaped cartilages that are like stiff plastic within the wall of the trachea itself. These cartilages look like the letter "C." The cartilages are lined up along the length of the trachea, one on top of the other, with a small band of muscle separating each one. The opening of the "C" portion of the cartilages is oriented to the back of the trachea next to the esophagus. These cartilages keep the airway open at all times, unless the airway is somehow damaged, such as in swelling of the vocal cords, an obstruction by a foreign body, or direct trauma to the trachea causing a crushing collapse of the cartilages.

Street Secrets

In the average-sized adult, the distance from the teeth to the vocal cords is about 15 cm. The distance to the **carina** is about 25 cm. The distance to where the tip of the endotracheal tube should be placed is about 20 to 22 cm from the teeth. Multiple methods must be used to confirm ET placement.

The Trachea and Espohagus Compared

The structures of the trachea and the esophagus are different. The esophagus may be thought of like the inner tube of a bicycle tire. It is soft and collapsible. In its usual state, the esophagus is indeed empty and collapsed, closed at the top and the bottom by the upper and lower esophageal sphincters, respectively. If a rescuer were to insert a tube into the esophagus, attach a syringe to the tube, and try to pull back air, resistance would be met, and the syringe would not pull back. This is because the esophagus collapses around the inserted tube, and no air can move in.

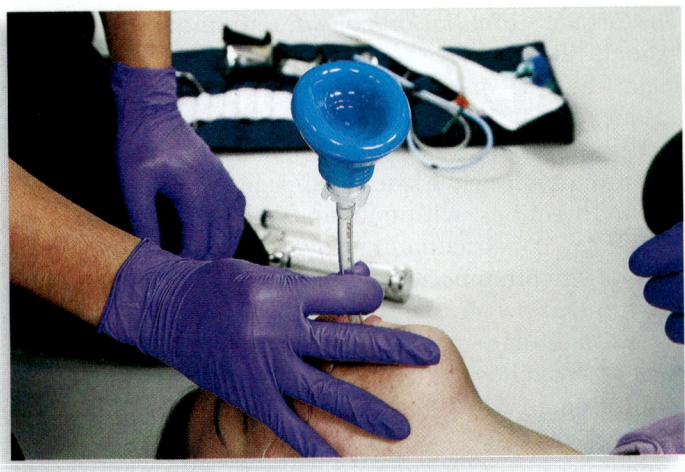

(a)

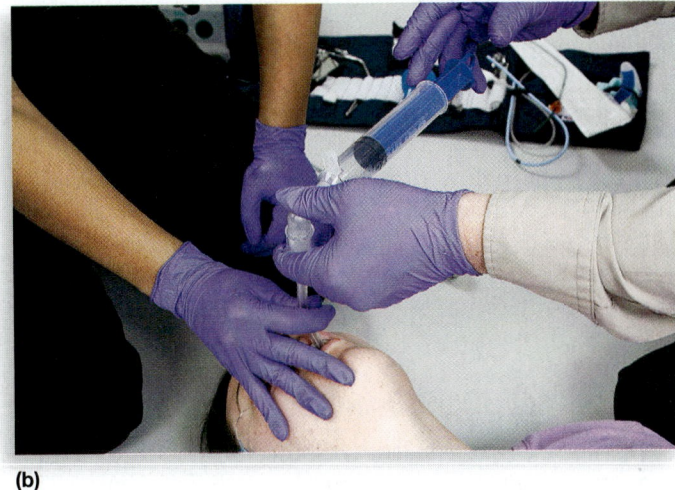

(b)

Figure 12-8 (a) This Tubecheck® is not re-inflating and therefore shows a possible esophageal intubation. (b) The Positube® plunger should be pulled halfway and observed. If it is drawn back, this could indicate a vacuum was created due to esophageal collapse and may indicate an esophageal intubation. Do not pull the plunger all the way out. This will not permit you to observe whether a vacuum was formed.

Street Secrets

During endotracheal intubation, one of the confirmatory steps is to use an esophageal detector device (EDD). These devices are designed to test what has just been described above. When an endotracheal tube is in the trachea, pulling back on the device will not be met with any resistance. This is because the cartilages prevent the airway from collapsing around the device when air is pulled through the tube by the syringe. If the endotracheal (ET) tube is in the esophagus, however, pulling on the EDD should collapse the esophagus and either prevent the plunger from being withdrawn or keep the bulb compressed due to the suction holding it (Figure 12-8a and b). There is little evidence, however, to suggest that these devices actually work the way they are intended. False readings are possible if there is emesis or if there are secretions occluding the airway.

Cricoid Cartilage

Beneath the thyroid cartilage is a small ring of cartilage called the **cricoid cartilage.** This ring is the only continuous piece of cartilage in the trachea. It does not have the "C" shape like the other rings. Between the thyroid and cricoid cartilages is a small space called the **cricothyroid membrane** (Figure 12-9).

This small membrane is the site used to create a surgical opening or needle puncture in order to access the airway in the setting of an upper airway obstruction. It is important to note, however, that this technique should only be used for obstructions that are located ABOVE the cricothyroid membrane.

Examples of indications to consider performing a needle cricothyrotomy would be in the setting of

persistent laryngospasm, laryngeal edema, laryngeal trauma, obstruction of the upper airway due to a foreign body, tongue swelling, or inability to otherwise provide an airway in a patient requiring ventilation.

An intravenous needle attached to a high flow oxygen source can be inserted through the membrane, removing the trochar (metal needle) and leaving the catheter inside of the tracheal lumen to administer jet insufflation of oxygen directly into the airway. This procedure is called **trans-laryngeal jet insufflation.** There are a number of commercial devices available for the rapid performing of a cricothyrotomy, and they will be discussed at the end of this chapter. **The procedure for**

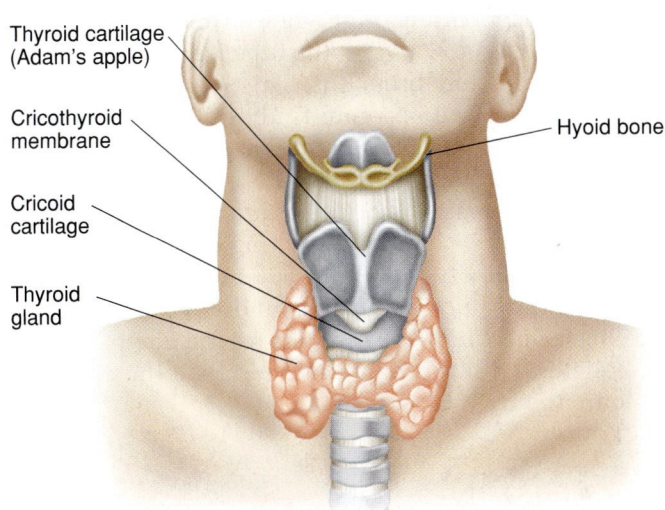

Thyroid cartilage (Adam's apple)

Cricothyroid membrane

Hyoid bone

Cricoid cartilage

Thyroid gland

Figure 12-9 The cricoid cartilage is the most inferior of the laryngeal cartilages.

needle cricothyroidotomy is outlined in detail in Skill Sheet 19 and Step-by-Step 19.

Street Secrets

The area just below the cricoid cartilage is the area of the trachea commonly damaged by trauma, such as from a steering wheel in a car crash or from a gunshot wound, because this portion of the neck is exposed in the front of the patient.

The Left and Right Bronchi

In the middle of the front of the chest is the breast-bone, or **sternum.** The sternum has two main parts: The **manubrium,** which is the smaller upper portion, and the **body,** which is the longer lower portion. At the distal tip of the sternum is the **xiphoid process.**

The junction between the manubrium and the body of the sternum is called the **sternal angle of Louis,** or **sternal angle** for short. This is an important anatomical landmark. It is at this level that the trachea divides into right and left passages called **main-stem bronchi.** The point of this splitting is called the **carina.** Also at this level is the top of the aorta as it exits the heart.

It is important to understand the airway anatomy because an endotracheal tube that is inserted deeper than this point will go into one of the main-stem bronchi, which is too far for the tube to be placed. The right main-stem bronchus angles downward at a more verti-cal angle than the left main-stem bronchus which tends to swing leftward in a less vertical angle. Thus, objects falling down the trachea, including aspirated material, *tend* to fall into the right main-stem bronchus.

Street Secrets

Right main-stem intubation: When an endotracheal tube has gone too far downward, the tube *tends* to move into the *right* main-stem bronchus. This is only a tendency, though, and not an absolute finding. If breath sounds were assessed PRIOR to the intubation attempt and af-terward they are diminished or absent on the left side, consider right main-stem intubation as the most likely cause. This can be fixed by deflating the balloon on the ET tube and slowly pulling back on the tube while lis-tening for the return of breath sounds on the left side of the chest. Once the breath sounds return, compare them for equality with the right side, reinflate the cuff, and resecure the ET tube.

Bronchioles

Proceeding down the main-stem bronchi are further divisions of the airway into smaller diameter passages.

The primary bronchi branch into **secondary (or lobar) bronchi** then **tertiary (or segmental) bronchi,** and ulti-mately they become the tiny **bronchioles.** By the time the airways have divided to this level, they no longer have cartilage in their walls but are flexible muscular tubes. The bronchioles have smooth muscle running in two dif-ferent directions within their walls: circular muscle, which can constrict and narrow the passage, and longi-tudinal smooth muscle, which can open these small air-ways and allow air to move in and out more freely.

Bronchiolar smooth muscle is important in the set-ting of bronchospastic disorders such as asthma and emphysema. When the circular, smooth muscle con-stricts, it causes resistance to air flow OUT of the alveoli, which results in air trapping within the tiny air cells out in the periphery of the lung. This leads to overinflated lung tissues that are unable to exchange air in and out, and it leads to hypoxia.

Alveoli

At the end of the airway circuit is the alveoli. Alveoli, or the alveolus if speaking of the singular unit, look very much like clusters of grapes on a stem. **Alveoli** are mi-croscopic air sacs, and the walls of these air sacs are the thickness of a single cell. Capillaries from the pulmo-nary circulation surround the air sacs, allowing gas dif-fusion through the alveolar-capillary membrane. The capillaries are in very close proximity to the alveoli, so gasses do not have far to go to diffuse from one environ-ment to the other.

Alveoli are so tiny and their walls are so thin that they would naturally collapse due to the surface ten-sion of the tiny amount of moisture that is found within them. Laplace's Law (Box 12-1) describes a

---

BOX 12-1   Laplace's Law

Laplace's Law states that the pressure within a spher-ical structure with surface tension is inversely pro-portional to the radius of the sphere. As the radius of the sphere decreases, the pressure on the sphere in-creases. So, small alveoli will generate larger pres-sures inside and would empty into larger alveoli. Surfactant reduces the surface tension found within the alveoli, causing the membranes of the alveoli to stabilize and resist collapsing and transferring their volume into larger alveoli.

Laplace's Law: $P = 2T/r$,

where "P" is the pressure in the alveolus, "T" is the surface tension in the alveolus, and "r" is the radius of the alveolus.

condition within the alveoli that prevents this from occurring. It states that the pressure inside of the alveoli actually increases as the radius gets smaller. This law explains that the smaller alveoli, in their higher pressure state, should shunt the air inside of them into larger alveoli and then collapse, but they in fact do not do this because of a special chemical. The cells within alveolar membranes and smaller bronchioles (named "type II alveolar cells") manufacture a chemical called surfactant. **Surfactant** is slippery and soapy, and it breaks up the surface tension inside of the alveoli, which allows them to remain open. This enables even the smallest diameter alveolus to remain open to permit air exchange.

CONNECTIONS Surfactant is first produced toward the end of uterine life for the fetus. Premature infants can thus be deficient in surfactant, causing respiratory distress due to the collapse of their alveoli. More information on this occurrence can be found in Chapter 42: Neonatology.

The Alveolar Capillary Membrane

The very end of the air movement circuit is the alveolar membrane. Oxygen, carbon dioxide, nitrogen, and other gasses diffuse across the alveolar membrane, through the tiny amount of interstitial fluid between the membrane and the pulmonary capillary bed, and directly across to the capillary membrane. The direction of the diffusion is based upon the areas of higher pressure created due to the presence of each gas. If more oxygen is in the alveoli than in the capillaries, then oxygen diffuses into the blood from the alveoli. If more CO_2 is in the capillaries than in the alveoli, then CO_2 diffuses into the alveoli from the capillaries. The close proximity of all of these structures facilitates the easy passage of gasses between them.

Lower airway diseases such as asthma and pneumonia impair the patient's ability to ventilate, resulting in an inability to oxygenate the body. The upper airway is intact in this process. This creates a "breathing" problem not an "airway" problem. In severe cases, a large amount of a patient's total body work is devoted to breathing. These patients should be assessed for fatigue. They position themselves upright to maximize their mechanical advantage for breathing. It is important not to force these patients to lie flat.

Ventilation and Pulmonary Perfusion

The Physiology of Air and Blood Movement

The lungs are like sponges with tiny holes. The natural size of the lungs would be about the size of a human fist if all of the holes were allowed to collapse. Human lungs are kept inflated by the surface tension between the smooth outer surface of the lungs (the visceral pleura) and the smooth inner surface of the inside of the chest wall (the parietal pleura) (Figure 12-10). The **visceral pleura** adhere directly to the lung, and the **parietal pleura** adhere directly to the inner surface of the thoracic cavity. **Pleural fluid,** which is secreted by the pleura, lubricates the two linings, so friction does not develop as the lungs expand and collapse during a respiratory cycle.

Negative Pressure Inside of the Normal Thorax

When you look at the chest of a patient, you are looking at an anatomical region composed almost entirely of "negative pressure." This means that, compared to

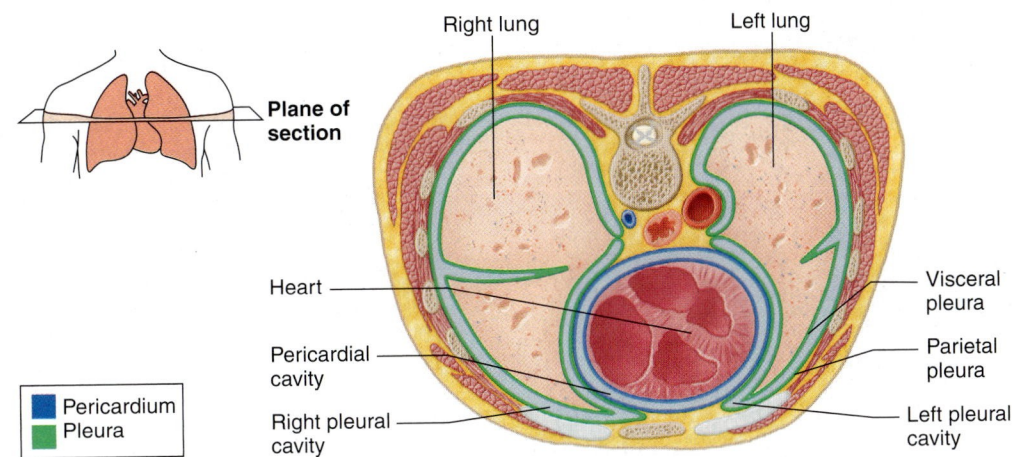

Figure 12-10 Lungs are kept inflated by the surface tension between the visceral pleura and the parietal pleura.

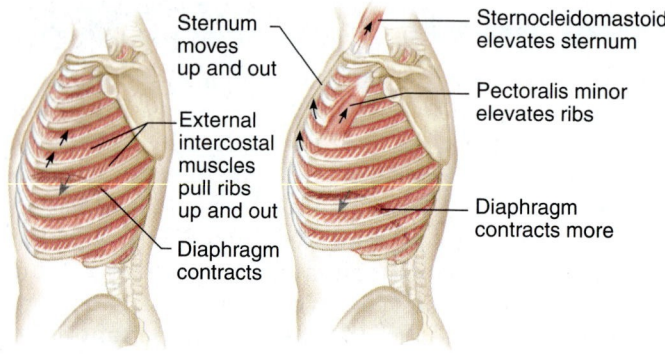

(a) Early inspiration   **(b) Peak inspiration**

Figure 12-11   The muscles used in respiration.

atmospheric pressure, the pressure reading inside the chest is slightly below the atmospheric reading. This is an important concept to understand.

The lungs stay expanded because negative pressure in the pleural space keeps them "pulled open," or inflated.

The muscles of respiration bring air into the lungs because they expand the size of the chest (Figure 12-11). During inspiration, the diaphragm, at the bottom of the thoracic space, pulls downward (contracts) and the intercostal muscles attached to the ribs move outward, similar to a bellows used to blow air on a camp fire as they are pulled open to take in air. All of these actions increase the size of the thorax by up to several liters during inspiration, making the pressure inside of the

thoracic spaces more negative (until air begins to rush in) (Figure 12-12). This negative pressure literally sucks air into the nose and mouth and on into the tracheobronchial tree.

Nice to Know

Prove the concept of "negative pressure" to yourself. Close your mouth and attempt to inhale without letting any air move into your nose. Notice how your cheeks collapse under the negative pressure being created by the diaphragm and intercostals muscles.

Pulmonary Circulation

Deoxygenated blood moves from the right atrium to the right ventricle, then to the pulmonary arteries. It moves on through smaller branches of the pulmonary arterioles and ultimately reaches the pulmonary capillary network. Here it interfaces with air in the alveoli across the alveolar-capillary membrane. Oxygen diffuses into the blood, and CO_2 is released by the blood and diffuses into the alveoli. Then this newly oxygenated blood moves out of the pulmonary capillaries into the pulmonary veins, into the left atrium and left ventricle, and out through the aorta to supply oxygen to the metabolic fires of the cells (Figure 12-13).

The flow of blood into the chest is woven intricately together with air movement. The heart and much of the great vessels also are located inside of the thorax, and

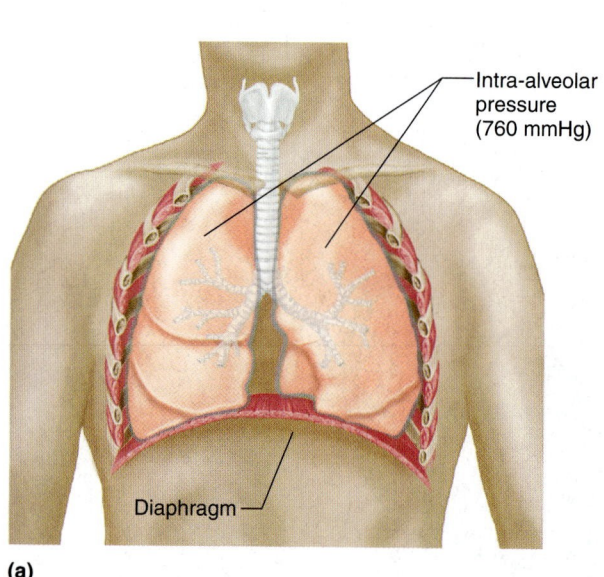

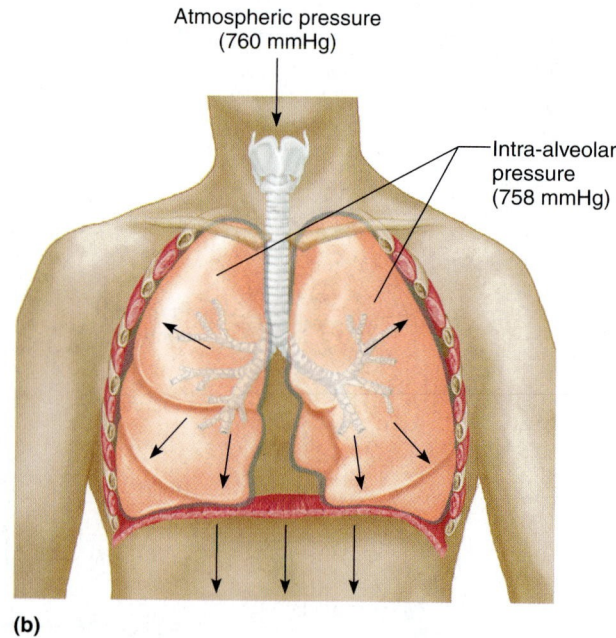

(a)   **(b)**

Figure 12-12   Normal inspiration. (a) Prior to inspiration, the intra-alveolar pressure is 760 mmHg. (b) It decreases to about 758 mmHg as the thoracic cavity enlarges and atmospheric pressure forces air into the airways.

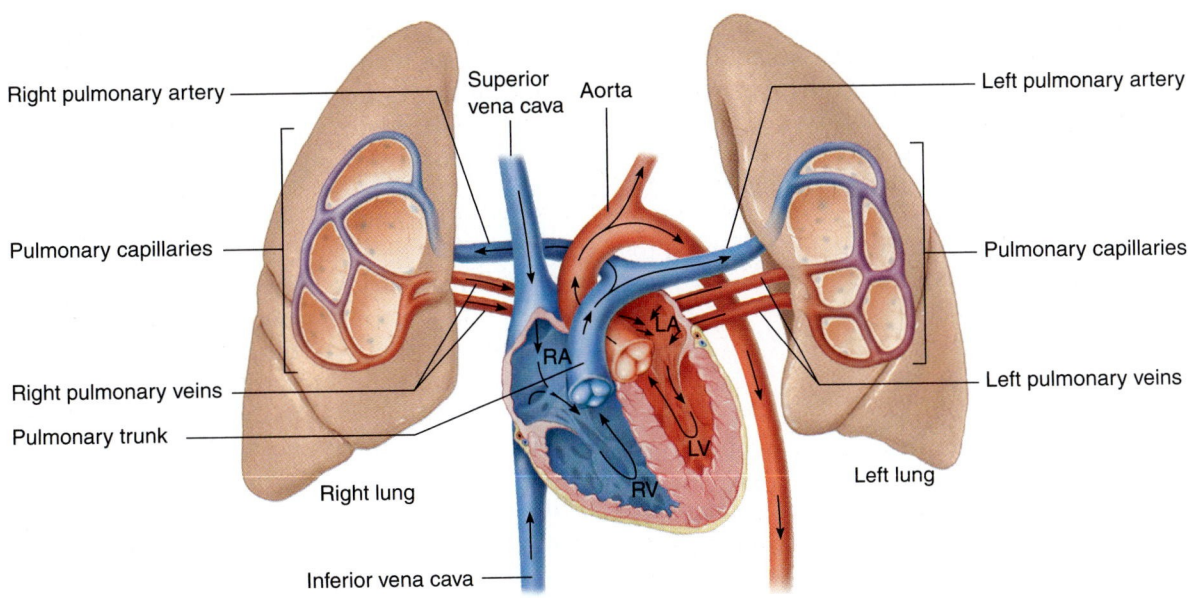

Figure 12-13 Pulmonary circulation.

movement of the diaphragm up and down and the intercostals muscles in and out cause pressure changes that affect these major parts of the circulatory system. DOT 2-1.7

The Role of the Heart

The heart is a pump. Like all pumps, the heart has an "intake" cycle and an "output" cycle. In the average-sized adult, the heart takes in about a half of a cup of blood (roughly 70 mL) on the "intake" (or venous) side with each beat, and it pumps out about a half a cup of blood with each beat on the arterial side through the aorta. The heart only pumps out what it gets back.

The formula for blood pressure is essential to fully understand the impact of capnography, the discussion of which will follow shortly:

Blood pressure = Cardiac output (CO) × Peripheral vascular resistance (PVR)

This means that the pressure inside of the arterial system is directly controlled by how fast the heart beats, by how much blood it moves each time that it beats, and by the constriction, or tone, in the small arteries (called arterioles) in the periphery of the arterial system, found just before the capillary network.

Negative Thoracic Pressure and Blood Return

The heart pulls blood into the atria by negative pressure.

This is an extremely important concept to understand because it impacts so many critical body functions.

After the heart has emptied during the systolic contraction, as it reopens during diastole, it refills and literally sucks blood into the ventricle. This negative filling pressure is very small, about the amount of negative pressure that it takes to suck water into the mouth through a straw. The five quarts of blood that are circulated by the heart each minute are pulled back toward the heart one beat at a time, through negative pressure, just as if the heart were sucking on a straw.

Negative Pressure Helps Breathing and Pumping

The bellows mechanism of the lungs and the blood flow of the heart are tied tightly together. When the diaphragm moves down during inhalation, the pressure inside of the chest becomes more negative. So, when we inhale, we make the pressure inside of our chest cavities more negative, pulling air into the tracheobronchial tree.

This negative pressure from breathing has a similar effect on the heart.

When we inhale and make the pressure inside of the chest more negative, we also pull more blood into the right side of the heart, increasing cardiac output transiently.

Breathing as a "Negative Pressure" Action

It may be said that breathing is a negative pressure activity in normal humans. More specifically, normal inhalation of air happens because of the negative pressure generated by the diaphragm moving down and the intercostal muscles expanding the ribs. When the diaphragm moves down, this action fills the lungs with air throughout the lung fields, opening all areas of the lungs. Blood, of course, is a fluid, and gravity tends to pull blood downward toward the bases of the lungs. Normal negative pressure breathing is able to open the lung fields in all areas including where blood is tending to flow through the lungs due to gravity.

What Is the Problem with Positive Pressure?

When someone becomes acutely ill, a number of actions may be performed in an attempt to help the patient, which are not always good for the physiology of the movement of air and blood in the patient. During cardiac arrest, you press on the patient's chest to try to move blood, and this alters the intrathoracic pressure. If the person is not breathing well, you may take a bag-mask unit, form a tight mouth seal with the mask, and use the bag to blow air into the lungs. Alternatively, you might take a Combitube™ or an endotracheal tube, place it in the patient's airway, and then use a bag to force air into the lungs. Using a bag to force air into the lungs, either with a mask or through the use of tubes inserted into the airway, is called **assisted ventilation.** You do these procedures because these are the only treatments that you have available for these conditions, and your medical protocols indeed call for you to do these.

However, both chest compressions and assisted ventilation, if not performed properly as described in this text, can alter the pressure gradient inside the chest, leading to changes that worsen perfusion and cardiac output.

Assisted ventilation is the use of a device to push air into a patient's lungs to improve the delivery of oxygen and the removal of CO_2. If improperly performed, it actually decreases venous return and affects cardiac output, thus decreasing cerebral perfusion pressure in the brain, and affecting other vital functions that are delicately balanced. Improperly performed chest compressions do not allow for the generation of adequate pressure to enhance the perfusion of the coronary arteries. (See Chapter 29 for a complete discussion on proper chest compressions.) Whenever assisted ventilations or chest compressions are being performed, the rescuer providing them must focus on that task only to ensure a proper rate and depth are used.[10,11,12,13,14,15]

These actions create a positive pressure within the thorax, which is **normally a negative pressure environment.**

It is vital that the EMS provider understands that all of the above procedures—bag-mask ventilation, ET ventilation, other forms of assisting ventilation, and chest compressions—use positive pressure to blow air into the lungs or to move blood during cardiac arrest.

As mentioned above, the heart pumps out the blood that it gets back, and the heart brings blood back by sucking it back because of a slight negative pressure. When air is blown into a patient's lungs during assisted ventilation, this action raises the pressure inside of the thorax, thus decreasing venous return to the heart. In patients with normal circulation, such as in patients undergoing routine surgical procedures under anesthesia, assisted ventilation usually has very little negative effect on blood return to the heart and thus on cardiac output. However, in patients with circulatory problems, such as shock, dehydration, or cardiac arrest, raising pressure inside of the thorax through assisted ventilation can *dramatically* decrease venous return and thus greatly decrease cardiac output, worsening shock.

The Impact of Positive Pressure Ventilation

Assisted ventilation is also called **positive pressure ventilation, or PPV.** Each breath takes a few seconds to push into the patient and to allow for the chest wall to recoil. The more breaths that are pushed into a patient through PPV each minute, the more time that is spent with the condition of higher pressure in the airways. Faster ventilation, therefore, results in increased pressure within the thorax. Box 12-2 discusses some other situations to consider.

Therefore, the EMS provider must understand that bagging patients too fast can drop blood pressure and worsen circulatory collapse in unstable patients.

Current understanding of cardiac arrest, for example, suggests that it may be possible to utilize the chest compressions as a "two stroke" procedure.[1] Press on the chest to move blood forward, and then relax the chest wall to allow the ribs to recoil and prepare for the next compression. New research has indicated that the recoil of the chest wall can be utilized to "return the inside of the chest to a negative pressure state" during chest recoil, if only briefly. Returning the inside of the thorax to negative pressure can cause more blood to return to the heart so that it can be pumped out on the next compression.[1]

This returning of the chest transiently to negative pressure can be accomplished through using a

BOX 12-2 Clinical Scenarios: Avoiding Overventilation

The EMS provider must carefully consider the fact that while it is very important to assist patients in the setting of breathing difficulties, especially during cardiac arrest when the patient is not breathing, pushing too much air into the lungs too quickly can raise intrathoracic pressure, decrease blood return to the heart, decrease cardiac output and blood pressure, and possibly decrease the chance of survival.

A good example of this point is a patient with emphysema. Smoking destroys lung tissue. Over time, the alveoli become progressively damaged, and the ability to exchange oxygen and carbon dioxide is greatly reduced. However, another insidious event occurs, as well, late during the course of emphysema. The small blood vessels of the lungs also become damaged, and it becomes harder for the right side of the heart to pump blood through the lungs. This condition is called **pulmonary hypertension.**

The right ventricle is a low pressure pump. When it becomes more difficult for the right ventricle to pump blood through to the lungs, it becomes thicker and damaged. Over time, the right side of the heart begins to fail. This means that the negative pressure by which the right side of the heart sucks blood back to fill itself for the next pumping action also fails.

When a patient with severe emphysema becomes acutely ill, the EMS provider must remember that the right side of this patient's heart may be failing. This may be manifested by distended neck veins (the blood has difficulty getting into the heart so it backs up into the veins, and the neck veins are the most obvious ones that the provider will see). If the provider applies a high minute ventilation rate to this patient, then this action may raise pressure inside of the chest enough that the right side of the heart cannot suck blood back strongly enough to maintain cardiac output. Thus blood pressure falls.

The rescuer must remember that the heart pumps out what it gets back and that certain patients are very sensitive to overventilation, which can decrease venous return and drop blood pressure.

Another example is a patient with tension pneumothorax. In this setting, air has leaked out of the lung tissue into the pleural space. When the diaphragm contracts, it pulls more air out of the lung into the pleural space, and when the diaphragm relaxes, it compresses the air in the pleural space. Finally, a point is reached in which positive pressure develops inside of the affected pleural space. This positive pressure decreases venous return and thus drops blood pressure, causing shock. This patient needs to have the positive pressure released promptly or shock leads to cardiac arrest. Now the provider can also understand why going *first* to endotracheal intubation on such a patient to provide positive pressure ventilation could drop blood pressure even more.

It is useful to consider cardiac arrest a moment further. In the setting of cardiac arrest, whether due to ventricular fibrillation (VF), pulseless ventricular tachycardia (VT), asystole, or pulseless electrical activity (PEA), the heart has failed as a pump. The heart is no longer able to suck blood back to fill its chambers for the next output stroke. Since the heart is only able to pump out what it gets back, circulation is obviously very poor during cardiac arrest. The tendency for the EMS provider is to try to give the patient a lot of oxygen to make up the deficit. This is usually done through assisting ventilation with a BVM, Combitube, or ET tube. However, giving rapid breaths will raise intrathoracic pressure, decrease venous return, and lower cardiac output even further. Indeed, new American Heart Association standards for 2005 recommend lower ventilation rates for patients in circulatory collapse.[16]

device that will resist the flow of air from moving into the airway for a tiny instant, creating a small amount of negative pressure within the airway as the chest recoils. Such a device, the "Impedance Threshold Device," has shown great promise for cardiac resuscitation and is currently being tested in a major international study to quantify the actual value of this intervention for patients in cardiac arrest (Figure 12-14).[2]

Pulmonary Perfusion

It is across the alveolar-capillary membrane that O_2 and CO_2 move (Figure 12-15). At the level of the alveolus, air movement meets circulation. The alveolar-capillary membrane is a microscopically thin barrier. The alveoli are such tiny air-containing chambers that they would tend to collapse, if not for surfactant. Thus, oxygen must travel through the surfactant and epithelial cells of the

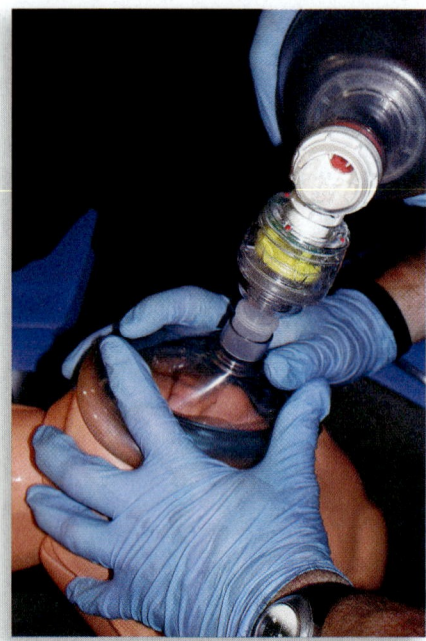

Figure 12-14 The ResQpod® Impedance Threshold device is being used here with a simple mask. If a mask seal is maintained with the device on during chest compressions, air is restricted from entering the lungs, negative pressure is increased, and venous return to the heart is increased. The device has red timing lights that assist rescuers in ventilating at a proper rate. It can also be used with an endotracheal tube.

BOX 12-3 Partial Pressure

Air that we breathe is a mixture of gasses. The total pressure of the atmospheric air, called **atmospheric pressure** is about 760 mmHg. Each gas in the mixture makes up part of this 760 mmHg, and the **partial pressure** of each gas making up the total is derived from the percentage of each gas in the mixture. Thus, oxygen is about 20% of the mixture of gasses in the atmosphere. The partial pressure then of oxygen is $760 \times 20\% = {\sim}150$ mmHg. The partial pressure of CO_2 in the atmosphere is $760 \times .03\% = {\sim}0.2$ mmHg. The reason that the partial pressure of oxygen in arterial blood is not the same as that of the atmosphere is because of the increase of water vapor in the inhaled air added by the structures of the upper airway (about 47 mmHg). This reduces the partial pressure of oxygen from about 150 mmHg in the outside air to about 100 mmHg down in the alveoli.

alveoli, through the interstitial fluid, and on through the wall of the pulmonary capillary to reach the blood cells passing through the lungs. CO_2 must take the reverse path to be excreted.

The process of gas exchange at the alveolar-capillary membrane is very quick in normal tissue, resulting in equilibration of the gasses in the alveoli with the gasses in the blood moving through the lungs. Therefore, arterial blood being pumped out of the heart has about the same level of gasses that are found in the alveoli, with a **partial pressure of oxygen** in the blood (called PaO_2) of between 80 and 100 mmHg and a partial pressure of CO_2 (called $PaCO_2$) of about 40 mmHg (Box 12-3).

Diseases can affect the alveolar-capillary membrane. Smokers destroy the walls of their alveoli, reducing gas diffusion area. Diseases such as Goodpasture's syndrome create inflammation of the alveolar-capillary membrane, reducing diffusion. Since the alveoli are

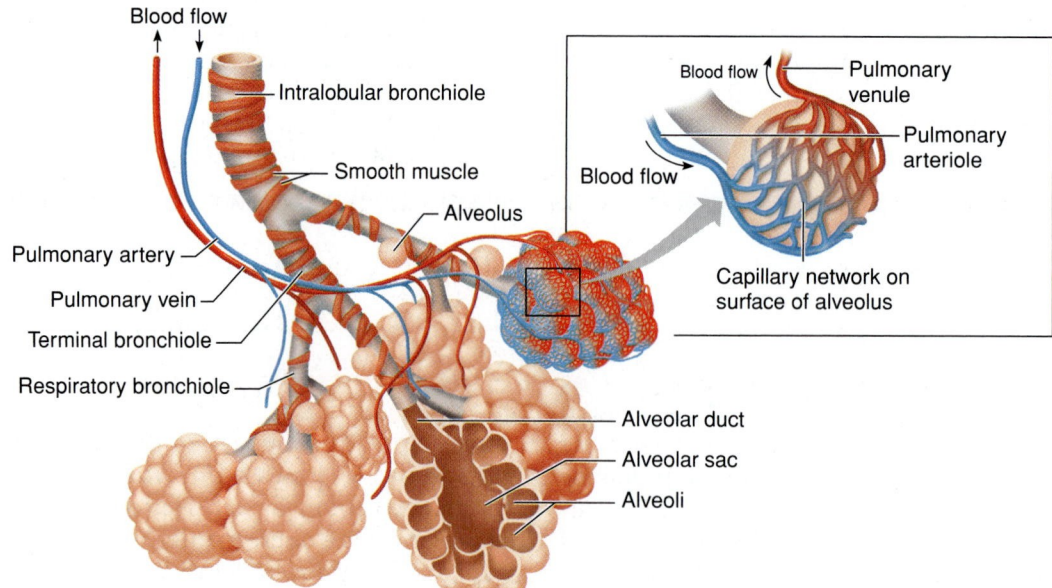

Figure 12-15 The respiratory tubes end in tiny alveoli where air movement meets circulation and gas exchange occurs.

like small holes in a sponge, these holes may collapse, producing a condition called **atelectasis,** permitting blood to pass from the right side of the heart to the left side of the heart without meeting air for gas exchange due to this collapsed diffusion space.

Congestive heart failure can cause increased back pressure from the left side of the heart, causing fluid to leak into the alveoli, a condition called **pulmonary edema.** Acute Respiratory Distress Syndrome, or ARDS, may occur when alveoli become damaged by inflammatory cells in the body, resulting in alveolar wall swelling and leaking, with fluid collecting within the alveoli. All of these conditions, then, can result in decreased gas diffusion across the alveolar-capillary membrane affecting respiration.

Respiratory System Controls

Chemoreceptor Regulation of Ventilations

The cells of the body consume a small amount of oxygen each minute—about 250 mL per minute in the resting state (or about 3.5 ml/kg/min)—and they produce about 175 mg of CO_2 (2.5 mg/kg/min) each minute. The brain has built-in sensors called **chemoreceptors** in the medulla and in the carotid artery that monitor CO_2 and pH levels. If CO_2 increases, this lowers pH. These sensors detect this lowering of pH and give feedback to the brain. From this feedback, the brain decides how fast and how deep a person needs to breathe to provide enough oxygen and to remove the CO_2 (Figure 12-16). DOT 2-1.17

CONNECTIONS Chapter 31: Endocrine, Electrolytes, and Acid/Base discusses pH and related concepts in more detail.

The brain is more sensitive to changes in pH and CO_2 than to changes in oxygen levels in regard to regulating ventilation. The oxygen levels are monitored in chemoreceptors in the carotid arteries and in the aorta. In conditions of shock, the amount of oxygen found by these receptors is lower, and this will stimulate ventilations. Over time, patients with severe lung disease such as emphysema begin to retain CO_2 and become conditioned to both a higher level of CO_2 as well as to lower levels of oxygen. This state is referred to as the hypoxic drive.

Normal and Hypoxic Drives

As mentioned, the brain controls the rate and depth of ventilation as it monitors oxygen and CO_2 levels in the blood. Thus, the levels, of oxygen and CO_2 drive

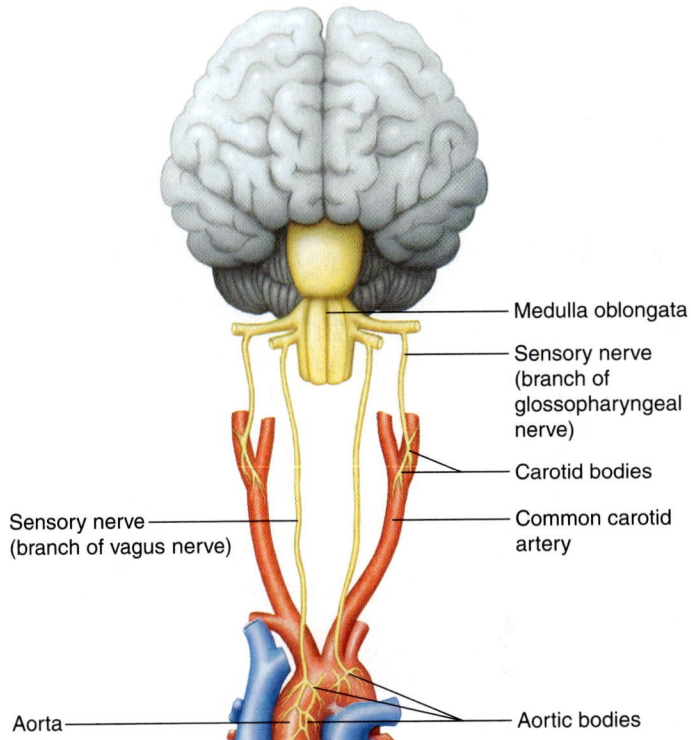

Figure 12-16 The brain decides how fast and deep a person needs to breathe by interpreting signals from the chemoreceptors.

respirations. So, if a patient's oxygen level goes down, this stimulates deeper and faster respirations. If a patient's CO_2 level goes above normal (called **hypercarbia**), this also stimulates respirations. Interestingly, in emphysema patients where the lung tissue has been progressively destroyed, toward the end of the disease process, the level of CO_2 begins to rise above normal. This occurs because it is more difficult to excrete CO_2 from the damaged lung tissue.

Over time, the elevated levels of CO_2 become tolerated by the brain. Thus, the patient with advanced emphysema loses the elevated CO_2 drive for respirations, and this patient depends upon the low oxygen or **hypoxic drive** for respirations to stimulate breathing. This means that the rescuer must be careful about applying too much oxygen to a patient with very advanced emphysema, as this may abolish the "last drive" for ventilation that the patient may have.

This doesn't mean that such a patient should not have supplemental oxygen.

Indeed, supplemental oxygen may be lifesaving to patients with emphysema exacerbations. However, the rescuer must remember that if oxygen is applied to a patient in the late stages of emphysema, then the patient must be observed carefully regarding the rate and depth of ventilations to make sure that adequacy of ventilation is being maintained by the patient.

Street Secrets

When supplemental oxygen is used, monitor the patient closely. Many emphysema patients are already on home oxygen. Ask what setting they typically use, and if they appear to be mentating well and their skin color and vital signs are near their normal baselines, they may not need high flow oxygen, but perhaps they will be comfortable with supplemental oxygen given via a nasal cannula. If supplemental oxygen is being administered and these patients begin to complain of numbness or dizziness, consider a decrease in the liter flow and monitor them closely. It may be normal for them to have pulse oximetry readings in the high 80s or low 90s. Ask the patients if they know their normal values as many do know this information.

Hypoxia and Hypoxemia

Hypoxia is a term that means that the patient is not carrying enough oxygen in the blood to the cells in the body. Hypoxia can be caused by many conditions, from asthma to emphysema to tension pneumothorax to airway obstruction. A low reading on pulse oximetry—assuming that the machine is working properly—is very suggestive that the patient is hypoxic, and steps must be taken to correct this, such as applying supplemental oxygen, assisting the patient with breathing, and looking for a cause through a thorough examination. DOT 2-1.16, 2-1.26

Hypoxemia is a low level of oxygen in the blood. Oxygen is carried on the red blood cells. Hypoxemia can lead to hypoxia, meaning a lack of oxygen circulating and available from the blood can lead to a general low oxygen state throughout the body. The terms do not mean the same thing, but they are often used interchangeably. These concepts will be discussed in more detail later in this chapter. DOT 2-1.16

Gases within the Blood

Gases are transported within blood throughout the body. Oxygen is moved from its "plentiful" location within the lungs to the areas of relative oxygen deficit, namely the cells of the body, where it is being consumed. CO_2 is taken from the cell, where it is created, to the lungs to be excreted.

As far as the carrying of oxygen and CO_2 goes, blood has two basic components: erythrocytes (red blood cells [RBCs]) and plasma. Very little oxygen and CO_2 can be carried by plasma. About 3 mL of oxygen per liter of blood, and about 8% of CO_2 being transported is actually dissolved in the plasma of blood. However, the RBC is designed to carry oxygen. When all available receptors are bound to oxygen, the hemoglobin molecule is said to be saturated. Totally saturated blood can carry about 20 mL of oxygen per 100 mL of blood, meaning that RBCs are very efficient carriers of oxygen.

Oxygen in the Blood

Hemoglobin actually has four binding sites for gasses, two pair for oxygen molecules and two pair for CO_2. Each type of site is different, which means oxygen binds to the oxygen site and carbon dioxide to carbon dioxide. Interestingly, the poison gas carbon monoxide (CO), which is created during combustion or fires in the setting of insufficient oxygen, is carried on the hemoglobin molecule in the same place that oxygen is carried. CO binds to hemoglobin many times more readily, in fact over 250 times better, than oxygen and can literally drive oxygen off of the RBC. This poisons the body and starves cells for oxygen. DOT 2-1.13

Oxyhemoglobin Dissociation Curve

Hemoglobin has specific characteristics that affect how it binds with oxygen. When the RBCs move to areas of the body with low oxygen concentration, such as in the tissues of the body, hemoglobin rapidly unloads the oxygen that it is carrying. Then, in areas of higher oxygen concentration, such as in the lungs, hemoglobin rapidly binds to oxygen. The binding characteristics of oxygen are represented graphically by the **oxyhemoglobin dissociation curve** (Figure 12-17). This graph

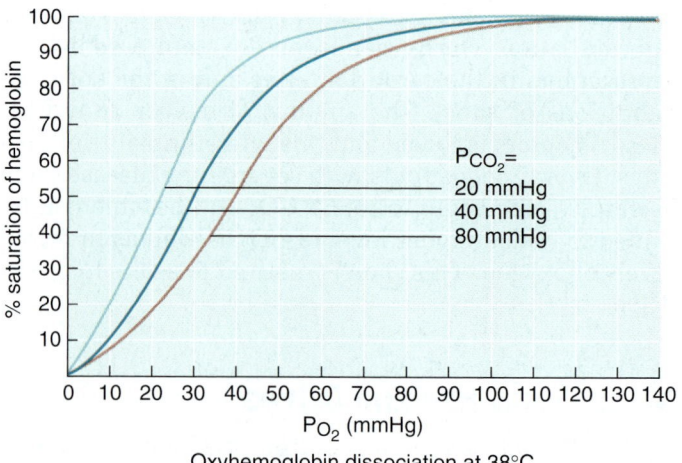

Oxyhemoglobin dissociation at 38°C

Figure 12-17 The oxyhemoglobin dissociation curve.

shows the relationship between oxygen binding to hemoglobin and releasing to body tissues. The factors that influence the binding include the hydrogen ion (pH) concentration, CO_2 tension (concentration), temperature, and 2,3-diphosphoglycerate (2,3-DPG) concentration. The effects of each of these factors, the discussion of which is beyond the scope of this text, shifts the curve either to the left or the right.

When the curve shifts rightward, the oxygen-hemoglobin dissociation curve lowers oxygen affinity, and O_2 displaces from the hemoglobin and moves into the tissues. When the curve shifts leftward, hemoglobin has an increased affinity for O_2, and it binds more strongly and is less inclined to move off and enter the tissues. Normally the curve is shifted leftward in the alveolar-capillary membrane in the lungs (allowing binding) and is shifted rightward in the capillaries of the tissues of the rest of the body. An increase in pH, CO_2 tension, or 2,3-DPG concentration all lead to a rightward shift.[17]

Measuring Partial Pressures of Gasses in Blood

Tests and devices have been created to monitor O_2 and CO_2 levels in the blood. Box 12-4 lists the partial pressures of the primary gasses found within the atmosphere and the lung. DOT 2-1.8

Arterial Blood Gasses (ABGs)

Blood samples can be drawn to measure the partial pressure of O_2 (PaO_2 or PvO_2) and CO_2 ($PaCO_2$ or $PvCO_2$). **Partial pressure** measures the percentage of gas dissolved in the plasma of the blood, not what is actually being carried on the hemoglobin of the RBC. Oxygen in the plasma is not as readily available for use by the tissues as oxygen carried on the hemoglobin molecule. So, the PO_2 measured in this **blood gas analysis** (called ABG analysis) may give a misleading estimation as to the amount of oxygen present. ABG analysis utilizes either arterial blood (Pa), which is not obtained in the prehospital setting, or venous blood (Pv), which reveals less accurate results. Portable blood gas analysis monitors are in use in some prehospital environments, particularly critical care transport teams, but they are not commonly found on ambulances. DOT 2-1.9, 2-1.10

Nice to Know

Remember that the PaO_2 measures the oxygen that is carried by the plasma, NOT the oxygen that is carried by hemoglobin. So, patients who have lost a great deal of blood which may have been replaced with IV fluids such as saline or Ringer's lactate may show a normal or increased PaO_2, especially if the patient has been placed on supplemental oxygen. However, the patient's ability to carry oxygen will have been substantially reduced because of the loss of RBCs and the hemoglobin contained within them.

Pulse Oximetry (SpO_2)

Pulse oximetry is a test that looks at the saturation of RBCs with oxygen (SpO_2), and it is a better predictor of the total amount of oxygen being carried by the blood to the cells than ABG analysis. EMS personnel now routinely monitor pulse oximetry to determine the patient's oxygen saturation as one measure of the adequacy of the patient's ventilatory status.

Blood flowing out of the heart through the aorta typically has an oxygen saturation of 97% or more with a PaO_2 of between 80 and 100 mmHg. Venous blood returning to the heart usually has an oxygen saturation of around 75% and a PaO_2 of around 40 mmHg. A PaO_2 about 60 mmHg will generally cause an RBC oxygen saturation of around 90%.

BOX 12-4 Relative Concentrations of Gases

The concentrations of the mixtures of gasses in air change as air moves into the lungs.

Gas	In the Atmosphere	In the Lungs
Nitrogen	78.6%	About 75%
Oxygen	21%	About 14%
Carbon dioxide	<1%	About 5%
Water vapor	~6%	About 6%

Working in the Gray Zone

As a student, a test score of 90% is cause for celebration. In patient care, a pulse oximeter reading of 90% is not a good finding. Although there are not currently any evidence-based recommendations regarding pulse oximetry readings, the consensus at this point seems to point to "normal" readings being above 95%; mild to moderate hypoxemia is noted between 91–95%, and severe hypoxemia is noted below 90%. Remember, a pulse oximeter reading (SpO_2) of 90% *may* indicate that the PaO_2 is around 60 mmHg, which by definition is **hypoxemia.**

Oxygen Levels and Pulse Oximetry

As discussed previously, the brain closely monitors the levels of oxygen and CO_2 in the blood, modifying the rate of breathing and the depth of each breath to control these levels. Like the brain, you can "see" the amount of oxygen carried by the hemoglobin molecules inside of the red bloods cells (RBCs) in the blood by looking at the patient's appearance and performing simple tests like pulse oximetry and capnography.

A **pulse oximeter** is a device that forces a certain frequency of light through thinner parts of the body, such as the finger, causing the area to glow at a certain electromagnetic frequency. This glow is measured and indicates, specifically, how saturated the hemoglobin is with oxygen. So, 100% saturation on a pulse oximeter indicates that the RBCs are completely saturated with oxygen. Room air, carrying about 20% oxygen, usually provides enough oxygen to saturate a normal person's RBCs to a level of 95% or better, usually above 97% if no damage exists to the air exchange mechanism at sea level.

As patients ascend to higher altitudes, oxygen saturation will diminish. It is important to understand what normal oxygen saturation is for specific altitudes. Below 95% saturation at sea level strongly indicates that something is wrong with the patient's air exchange mechanism, whether there is an obstruction at the epiglottis from a foreign body (airway obstruction) or an air exchange problem at the alveolar-capillary membrane (such as with congestive heart failure when fluid in the alveoli actually prevents air exchange). A pulse oximetry reading of 95% or below at sea level is a strong indication of the need for prompt transport of the patient to an appropriate facility for evaluation. A pulse oximetry reading below 90% indicates that a significant emergency is present regarding this patient's air exchange, requiring prompt transport to an emergency receiving facility.

Working in the Gray Zone

The EMS provider must ALWAYS remember that pulse oximetry indicates how much oxygen is being carried in the RBCs of the blood. Pulse oximetry does NOT indicate how well the oxygen is actually being "burned in the fire of metabolism" by the cells, nor is it telling you if the patient has an adequate number of RBCs in his or her blood. Pulse oximetry gives a rough estimate of "what amount of oxygen is on the RBCs" but not how much is actually being used. Because CO binds to the same sites as oxygen, carbon monoxide gives a false pulse oximetry reading.

Carbon Dioxide in the Blood

CO_2 is produced by the "burning" of carbohydrate by the cells as well as the buffering of acids in the cells. CO_2 is produced through the following chemical relationship:

$$\text{Oxygen} + \text{Carbohydrate} \longleftrightarrow CO_2 + H_2O.$$

Carbonic anhydrase is an enzyme that converts the CO_2 in the following manner:

$$CO_2 + H_2O \longleftrightarrow H_2CO_3 \longleftrightarrow H^+ + HCO_3^-.$$

Thus, CO_2 is rapidly converted to HCO_3^- (bicarbonate) in the cells and in the blood stream, and it is as bicarbonate that about two thirds of the CO_2 is actually carried within the RBCs. Carbonic anhydrase is found in many tissues in the body, creating a **buffer system** that permits the precise control of pH, which is the acid concentration in the body fluids and within cells.

Nice to Know

This buffering system, the carbonic acid (H_2CO_3) equation, is referred to as the **chemical buffering system** of acid base balance. It works the fastest, nearly instantaneously, of the three buffering systems that buffer hydrogen ions and carbon dioxide. Respiratory buffering is the next fastest, typically clearing the body of acid within a few minutes. The slowest system, renal buffering, can take hours or days to restore normal acid/base balance.

Acid/Base Balance.   Cells can only function normally within a narrow range of pH in the body. Thus, the process of breathing and cellular respiration is directly involved with the control of the acid/base concentration in the blood and the body fluids. The interchange of CO_2 with bicarbonate produces a direct interaction between the CO_2 being produced by the cells to be excreted in the lungs *and* with the acid/base buffer system of the body.

Since bicarbonate can combine with acid in the body, which is represented as hydrogen ion protons (or the symbol H^+), the equation can be reversed, causing the formation of CO_2 and H_2O from this combination. In this way, bicarbonate in the blood, body fluid, or cells can combine with excessive acid in these areas to produce CO_2 and H_2O. The excessive CO_2 can then be removed from the body, or "blown off," in the lungs while the H_2O is excreted as urine.

Air movement plays a direct role in the excretion of excess acid that may be formed and in the control of the pH of body fluids.

Acidotic patients, such as those in diabetic ketoacidosis, often present with rapid, deep, and labored respirations (called **Kussmaul's respirations**) as they attempt to rid the body of the excessive CO_2 being generated that is creating acidosis.

Capnography

"Capnos" means smoke. Studying **capnography** in humans, then, is thinking about the smoke from the fire of metabolism. In EMS there is now a wide availability of devices that measure and display capnography as either a waveform or numeric representation. This equipment measures CO_2 as it is exhaled from the airway.

Capnography will serve as a critical link between ventilation and perfusion. Therefore, it provides clues to the circulatory status and whether or not respiration is taking place at the cellular level.

CO_2 is excreted by cells as a waste product of metabolism and from the buffering of acidosis. CO_2 is returned through the venous circulation to the lungs where it is exhaled. On breathing in, very little CO_2 is in the airway since what is inhaled is outside air. CO_2 is only found in a concentration of 0.03% in outside air, which for your purposes here is essentially zero. On the other hand, normal CO_2 in the circulatory system is about 40 mmHg in a healthy person. So, were you to measure this in a graphical way, you would see that during inhalation, with air moving from the outside into the body, measured CO_2 would be around "0," and during exhalation the waveform would climb quickly to about 40 mmHg. This may be plotted on a graph, with the height of the wave being the measurement of CO_2 in the airway and the time of the measurement reading from left to right (Figure 12-18).

Since it is read during the respiratory cycle, the reading is referred to as an **end-tidal CO_2** reading, or **ETCO_2.** A review of the waveform is important to understanding what the reading actually means.

There are four phases represented on a normal capnogram waveform. Phase I is the **respiratory baseline.** It represents the end of inspiration. The rapid vertical rise of the left side of the wave is Phase II. This is termed the

ascending phase and represents the initiation of expiration. Phase III, the **alveolar plateau,** starts with exhaled air that is mixed between bronchi and bronchioles, and at the far rightward portion of Phase III, it represents the concentration of CO_2 from the alveoli. This is the true "end-tidal" value of the reading. Phase IV is the **descending phase** representing the inspiratory limb. Each wave, from Phase I through IV, is a representation of a single respiratory cycle (Figure 12-18).

The **capnograph** transmits a beam of infrared light through the exhaled gas sample and senses the difference between the amounts of light transmitted versus that absorbed (by the CO_2) and calculates the partial pressure of CO_2. This value is averaged over a number of breaths, and the value for end-tidal CO_2 is displayed.[18] When measured from an arterial blood gas, a normal value for $PaCO_2$ is between 35 and 45 mmHg. Under normal conditions in healthy patients, there is a small gradient between $PaCO_2$ and $ETCO_2$ of less than 6 mm.[19] For patients with cardiac or respiratory disease, the gradient can be much higher, making the correlation between $PaCO_2$ and $ETCO_2$ much less accurate. Despite this lesser accuracy, it is valuable to follow the trend in $ETCO_2$ with changes in disease severity and with treatment. Normal values for $ETCO_2$ are an average of 38 mmHg with a range from 35 to 45 mmHg.

Working in the Gray Zone

Colorimetric CO_2 Detection Devices

CO_2 is an acid. Colorimetric CO_2 detectors use paper specially treated to change color in the presence of acid. When CO_2 is present, the detector turns from a purplish color to a yellowish-brown color. The paper should turn color within about six assisted ventilations. It turns yellow after exposure to 2% to 5% $ETCO_2$, which is equivalent to 15 to 38 mmHg PCO_2. There is no color change and the filter paper remains purple with an $ETCO_2$ level that is less than 0.5% which is equivalent to less than 4 mmHg PCO_2. If the paper remains purple, it indicates CO_2 is not being excreted. The problem with colorimetric devices is that they are sensitive to temperature extremes, humidity, and aging. If vomit or airway secretions get in the device, the reading may be unreliable. The devices do not function for a very long period of time, and once the chemical within the paper is used up, the color tends to stay where it is and then slowly fades away. **Colorimetric capnometers** are useful for general readings such as when assessing for proper ET tube placement, but they are not accurate enough when precise determinations are necessary.[20]

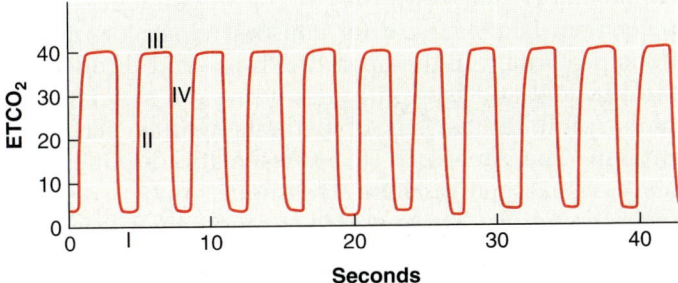

Figure 12-18 A normal capnogram waveform.

Why Measure CO₂?

Measuring CO_2 in the airway achieves three important goals:

1. The appearance of CO_2 in the airway in a wave form indicates that air is moving through the airway. This means that the airway circuit is intact and ventilation is taking place. Sudden loss of the capnography wave form could indicate that the airway circuit failed. This can happen, for example, when an endotracheal tube is dislodged.

2. The shape of the waveform tells a great deal about how "open" the lower airways are. A normal capnography waveform has an almost square shape to it. The waveform of a patient experiencing an asthma attack has more of a curve to the left-hand edge of the wave, which if you recall, represents Phase II, the initiation of exhalation. Exhalation is obstructed during an asthma attack, and thus the CO_2-rich air coming from the alveoli moves more slowly out of the lungs, producing a "shark fin" appearance to the waveform. Treatment of the patient with bronchodilators can result in the "squaring up" of the waveform with loss of the "shark fin" appearance (Figure 12-19).

3. The height of the CO_2 wave during exhalation gives the rescuer a look into the CO_2 production by the cells, the delivery of CO_2 back to the lungs, and the rate of ventilation. In normal circulation, CO_2 production and the regular rate of breathing at rest give rise to a level of about 40 mmHg of CO_2 in the blood, and this is the level that is excreted by normal lungs when it is measured through capnography during exhalation.

Capnography Waveforms During Circulatory Collapse

When circulatory collapse occurs, such as in cardiac arrest, oxygen delivery is reduced to the cells, oxygen consumption falls, CO_2 production decreases, and CO_2 delivery to the lungs through the pulmonary arteries falls. So, when a rescuer measures waveform capnography in such a patient, a low level of CO_2 can mean one of two things:

1. Since only 175 mg of CO_2 is made each minute, a low level of CO_2 may mean that the patient is being bagged too fast, "blowing off" the CO_2 that is being produced, and reducing the height of the wave.

2. A patient who was previously exhaling a normal level of CO_2 but is now blowing out less CO_2 during exhalation *may* be going into worsening circulatory collapse because CO_2 output is now falling.

The rescuer who finds that a patient's CO_2 level is low should first make sure that the patient is not being overventilated. The rescuer should then assess the patient for development of circulatory collapse, such as shock of any cause or cardiac arrest.

> Sudden loss of the capnography waveform is indicative of either the airway becoming dislodged or the patient developing cardiac arrest.

Capnography as a Predictor of Overventilation

As mentioned, the level of exhaled CO_2 may be a strong indicator of overventilation by the rescuer. Remember that positive pressure ventilations can lower venous return. Thus, the rescuer who is assisting ventilation should use the level of exhaled CO_2 as a guide to how fast to ventilate the patient. If a patient in cardiac arrest is exhaling a CO_2 level of 10 mmHg, for example, then the rescuer should slow the rate of ventilations until the CO_2 level rises to at least above 20 mmHg, accompanying this slower ventilation rate with fast and deep cardiac compressions to optimize circulatory status.

Capnography gives the rescuer a window into the metabolic status of the patient that has never been available in EMS before. The immediate changes that occur with capnography give sensitive indicators to the status of the airway and to the patient's circulatory status. Only through a careful understanding of the relationship between capnography, the adequacy of the airway, and the circulatory status of the patient can the rescuer truly assess the condition of a critically ill patient.

In addition to assessing metabolic states, the use of capnography for confirmation of endotracheal tube placement is a standard for anesthesiology for intubations performed in the operating room and throughout the hospital and is rapidly becoming the standard for prehospital intubations of patients with a perfusing rhythm. The American Heart Association defines primary visual confirmation techniques but recognizes their limitations and requires secondary confirmation techniques, such as capnographic waveform devices.[21] Studies of prehospital intubations report unrecognized misplaced intubation rates of 8% to as high as 25%.[22]

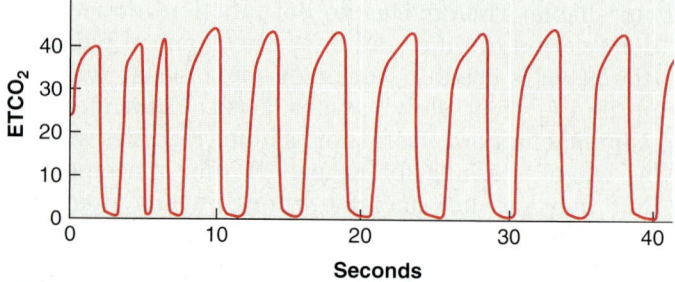

Figure 12-19   A shark fin capnogram typical of asthma.

DOT 2-1.73

A recent study compared unrecognized prehospital endotracheal intubation rates between patients continuously monitored with end-tidal CO_2 devices and patients not continuously monitored.[23] They found the rate of unrecognized misplaced intubations in the group without continuous monitoring to be 23.3% while the rate for the continuously monitored group was zero.

Continuous $ETCO_2$ capnographic monitoring should be implemented as the standard of care for confirmation of prehospital intubation in perfusing patients.

The National Association of EMS Physicians recommends capnography for intubation confirmation in perfusing patients in its position paper: Verification of Endotracheal Tube Placement Following Intubation.[24] It notes that the presence of an $ETCO_2$ waveform "provides compelling evidence of endotracheal placement." One caveat, given the results reported in the previous study with a miss rate of 25% (in one-third of the misses, the ET tube was located above the vocal cords in the hypopharynx), the capnographic waveform should be coupled with the ET tube placed and maintained at an adequate depth (usually 21–23 cm for adult males and 19–21 cm for adult females).[23]

Gas Exchange during Circulatory Collapse

When an individual is not stressed, around 5 liters of air are moving into and out of the lungs each minute. This is achieved through moving a 600 mL tidal volume about every eight seconds or a 500 mL volume every six seconds. It can be generally stated that the depth of breathing is what controls the amount of oxygen that is delivered. This is because deeper negative pressure breaths open more alveoli and expose these alveoli to blood moving through the pulmonary capillary network.

The rate of breathing is generally what controls the amount of carbon dioxide that is removed. This is because CO_2 diffuses much more readily through the alveolar-capillary membrane and is excreted more quickly by the lungs. Thus, raising the rate of ventilation tends to raise the rate of CO_2 elimination, and raising the depth of ventilation tends to improve oxygenation.

When someone collapses in cardiac arrest, circulation quickly begins to fail. Pressure in the aorta is what moves blood forward to the cells, and when the heart stops pumping, pressure in the aorta quickly falls. When this occurs, delivery of oxygen to the periphery of the body fails since the heart is unable to pump blood out. Therefore, since little oxygen is being utilized, little CO_2 is being made by the "fire of metabolism." Since little CO_2 is being made by metabolism, then the rate of ventilation can be slower.

The *rate* of ventilating a patient is tied directly to the need to eliminate carbon dioxide. In settings of circulatory collapse, especially cardiac arrest, little CO_2 is being returned to the lungs, and thus the *rate* of ventilation can be lower.

Positive pressure breathing, given with a bag-mask, laryngeal mask airway (LMA), Combitube™, or ET tube to assist ventilation, raises intrathoracic pressure and thus decreases venous return, which may drop the patient's cardiac output and hence blood pressure. The more positive pressure breaths given per minute, that is, the faster the *rate* of positive pressure ventilation, the higher the pressure inside of the chest is raised.

Do not ventilate the patient more than needed because this may drop the patient's blood pressure, especially if the patient is already in shock!

Once again, patients in shock are very susceptible to raising intrathoracic pressure through overventilation.

Respiratory-Ventilation Abnormalities
The Meaning of Cyanosis

It is no silly analogy to think generally of the ventilation and circulation of the body as, "air goes in and out, and blood goes round and round." As discussed above briefly, RBCs contain hemoglobin (HGB). HGB is an iron-containing protein that carries oxygen and carbon dioxide. Also, remember that about two-thirds of the CO_2 carried by RBCs is carried as bicarbonate, which is rapidly converted back to CO_2 for exchange in the lungs.

Blood turns a "pink" color when exposed to oxygen. Look at your own fingernail beds right now and see how pink they look. This is oxygenated blood. When blood becomes "deoxygenated," it takes on a blue color. Look at the veins of your forearm, and you will see the blue color of blood in the veins. As the amount of oxygen in the blood drops, a bluish tint develops. The areas where this is noted first include the nail beds, the conjunctiva of the eyes, the lips, and the tongue. As cyanosis worsens, the skin will appear bluish gray.

Remember that the average person has about 15 grams of hemoglobin per 100 mL of blood carried in RBCs. If the patient starts bleeding for some reason, then the amount of hemoglobin per 100 mL of blood drops as fluid volume is replaced with IV fluids (or from retained fluid by the kidneys as they attempt to maintain intravascular volume). For cyanosis to be detected, the patient must have at least 5 grams of hemoglobin per 100 mL of blood present to "turn blue" in the absence of enough oxygen. Someone bleeding to death may not have enough blood left to turn blue in the setting of hypoxia. It is critical to give supplemental oxygen at high flow through a nonrebreather mask to attempt to deliver as much oxygen to the patient as possible.

Reasons for Cyanosis

Cyanosis is a condition that occurs due to decreased oxygen getting into the RBCs passing through the lungs. Since the lungs are an organ in which air in the airway is exchanged across the alveolar-capillary membrane with blood moving through the lungs, it follows that a patient can be cyanotic for two reasons: Air may not be exchanging well in the airway, or blood may not be moving well through the lungs. Both reasons are important causes of cyanosis, and both must be considered by the rescuer. DOT 2-1.26

Airway obstruction decreases the amount of air moving through the airway, and it decreases the amount of oxygen that is exchanged in the lungs. Examples of causes of airway obstruction include foreign bodies, trauma to the face or neck, and infections involving the airway. Asthma can obstruct the flow of air through the airway, and emphysema can both obstruct the flow of air as well as prevent air exchange due to alveolar damage. Severe pneumonia can prevent air exchange due to reduced air movement across the affected alveolar-capillary membrane.

Cyanosis can also occur due to conditions which decrease blood flow through the lungs. Tension pneumothorax, cardiac tamponade, massive pulmonary embolism, and severe congestive heart failure diminish blood flow into the thorax and result in less oxygen getting into the blood, producing cyanosis.

Finally, cyanosis does NOT occur from elevated CO_2 levels. A change in CO_2 does not cause the blood to turn different colors. Thus, a patient with severe emphysema who is a CO_2 retainer due to severe lung damage, may improve in color with supplemental oxygen and appear better. However, since this patient may still have an elevated CO_2 level and may be in danger of ceasing to breathe due to CO_2 "narcosis," giving supplemental oxygen to such a patient requires close monitoring.

Respiratory Depression

Respiratory depression occurs when the respiratory rate is slow for a prolonged period of time or if chest wall expansion is inadequate to inflate the lungs, resulting in a lack of adequate perfusion. It can be caused by injury, CNS depression, drugs, or certain medical conditions where the patient's ability to compensate is challenged due to fatigue.

Respiratory Insufficiency

Respiratory insufficiency is noted with the failure of the respiratory system to maintain adequate ventilation or perfusion of the lungs. It is often difficult to distinguish between respiratory depression and insufficiency and it really is not important to correctly label which condition is present. What is more important is to recognize that there is a problem and to work quickly to take corrective action to prevent further deterioration of the patient. Either condition, left undetected or uncorrected, can lead to respiratory failure.

Respiratory Failure and Arrest

Respiratory failure is characterized by decreasing respiratory effort, depth, or adequacy of breathing. If uncorrected, respiratory failure leads to respiratory or cardiopulmonary arrest. There are two basic types of respiratory failure: oxygenation failure and hypercapnic (or ventilation) failure. Oxygenation failure is characterized by hyperventilation and is noted by an inability to take adequate amounts of oxygen into the lungs. Hypercapnic, or ventilation, failure occurs as the result of increased arterial tension due to high carbon dioxide levels within the blood. Acid/base imbalances result with both types of respiratory failure, and if uncorrected, quickly lead to death. **Respiratory arrest** is the cessation of breathing. It can also describe the gasping agonal respirations that occur at a very slow rate (one to three per minute) that are incompatible with life.

Ventilation Perfusion Mismatch

Each of these ventilation and respiratory abnormalities can lead to an imbalance between ventilation (V) and perfusion (Q), called **V/Q defect,** V/Q mismatch, V/Q abnormality, or shunting. The comparison between ventilation and perfusion is referred to as the V/Q ratio. The ratio of pulmonary alveolar ventilation to pulmonary capillary perfusion is measured and expressed in units, with the optimal ratio of 1:1. V/Q defect can occur with two basic abnormalities: (1) where one or more areas of the lung receive ventilation but blood flow into the tissues is inadequate to allow for the exchange of gasses across the alveolar-capillary membrane or (2) where there is adequate blood flow but inadequate ventilation. Assessing peak flows are more helpful than pulse oximetry, capnography, or other methods of respiratory assessment in evaluating V/Q defect. However, peak flow assessment is not performed routinely in the prehospital setting. DOT 2-1.11

Respiratory Cycles, Volumes, and Capacities

Minute Ventilation

The **minute ventilation rate** is the measured amount of air that is exchanged with each breath. It is calculated as the tidal volume times the respiratory rate. These components will be discussed further.

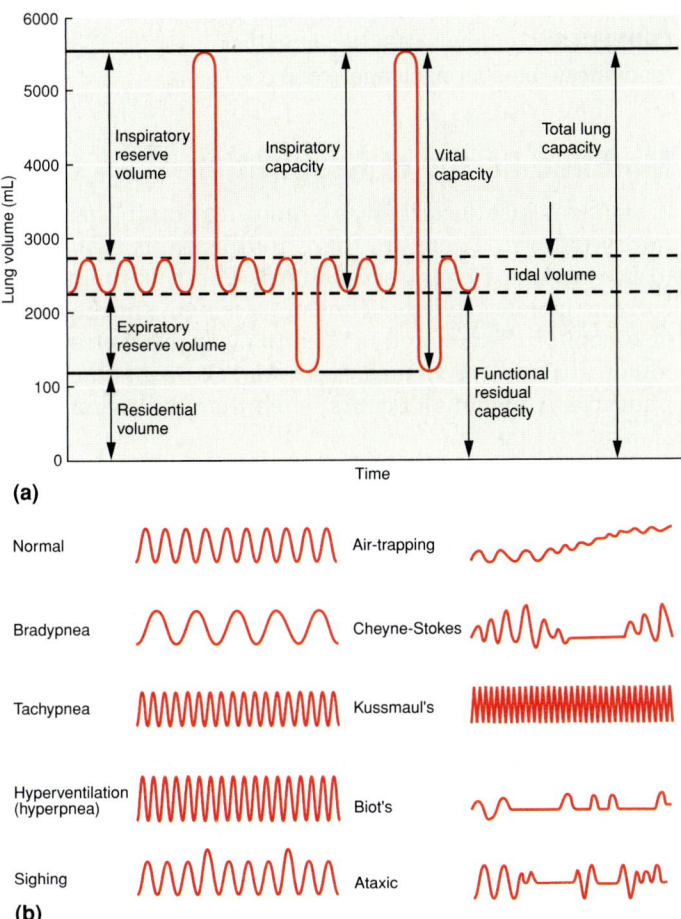

(a)

(b)

Figure 12-20 Respiratory volumes and patterns. (a) This part shows the various components that make up respiratory volumes and lung capacities. (b) This part demonstrates normal and abnormal respiratory rates and patterns.

A spirometer is a device used to measure the volume of air inhaled and exhaled and the respiratory capacity. This volume is measured in liters. **Total lung capacity (TLC)** is the measurable volume of air in the lungs after a maximum inhalation has occurred (Figure 12-20). TLC can be affected by a number of factors including diseases such as COPD, emphysema, asthma, and black lung or by trauma (pneumo- or hemothorax), congestion and infection, thoracic restriction, bronchiolar obstruction, or edema.

Tidal volume (VT) is the volume of air moved into and out of the lungs with each inhalation and exhalation of a respiratory cycle. To prevent under- or over-inflation of the chest, the volume inhaled and exhaled over time must remain equal. Decreased tidal volumes occur as the result of many pulmonary and neuromuscular diseases. To compensate and maintain adequate alveolar ventilation, an increased respiratory rate must occur. Decreased VT and rate is associated with respiratory center depression and is noted with brainstem

lesions (injury) or CNS depression due to drug use. The **minute volume** is determined by multiplying the minute respiratory rate by the average tidal volume. **DOT 2-1.19**

Following a normal inhalation, additional air may be drawn into the lungs forcibly. This volume may be measured also, and is called the **inspiratory reserve volume (IRV)**. Following a normal exhalation, additional air can be forcibly expelled from the lungs. This is called the **expiratory reserve volume (ERV)**. Reductions in the volume of IRV and ERV are noted for patients with restrictive pulmonary diseases. During times of stress or episodic flare-up of disease, these patients frequently have an inability to compensate for inadequate ventilation due in part to the decreased IRV and ERV. The **inspiratory capacity (IC)** is determined by adding the IRV and VT together. The IC measures the total volume drawn into the lungs with a nonforced breath (VT) plus the total that can be forcibly drawn into the lungs (IRV).

Some air always remains in the lung fields at the end of exhalation. The volume of air remaining at the end of the maximal, forced exhalation is measured as the **residual volume (RV)**. Decreases in RV may be noted with infections or diseases, such as pneumonia, that occlude many alveoli. Abnormal increases in RV lead to air trapping and chronic hyperinflation of the chest wall as noted with asthma, emphysema, and bronchial obstruction. For these patients, more ventilation is required to adequately maintain the normal gas concentration in the lungs. An increased VT, rate, and work of breathing are often necessary to maintain adequate ventilation, leaving little room for compensatory mechanisms during times of stress. The **functional residual capacity (FRC)** is the measurement of the total amount of air forcibly exhaled (ERV) plus the reserve volume (RV), which is the amount of air remaining in the lungs following this forcible exhalation.

The largest volume, the **vital capacity (VC),** is the measurement of complete expiration following the deepest inspiration. The equation is

$$VC = IRV + VT + ERV$$

The VC in adults varies; it is increased with height, and it decreases with age. The VC of a woman is generally less than that of a similarly sized man. A decrease in VC can be found in any patient with loss of healthy lung tissue that is normally capable of distending in response to airflow.

Two important components of respiratory function that are not measurable by spirometer are the volume of **dead space gas (VD)** and **alveolar ventilation (VA).** With the average tidal volume of 500 mL, the volume of VD is approximately 150 mL. This small amount of air, found in the open spaces of the respiratory system such as the trachea, bronchi, and larger bronchioles, does not participate in the exchange of gasses and is simply oc-cupying the available space in the respiratory system. The VA, which is approximately 350 mL, is the volume of air that comes into contact with the alveolar-capillary membrane surfaces and does participate in the exchange of gasses between the lung and blood. Hypoventilation can result from decreased VA, and hyperventilation can result from increased VA.

Dead space can be further defined as the anatomic dead space and the physiologic dead space. Normally the volume of the dead space is 150 mL. This is the **anatomic dead space** and represents the normal dead space volume. Certain disease conditions, such as em-physema, result in the formation of scar tissue, some of which is no longer available for gas exchange. This area takes away from the alveolar ventilation volume and means less air is reaching the healthy parts of the lung for perfusion. This dead space is called the **physiologic dead space.**

Respiratory Patterns

Alternations in Respiratory Efforts

Normal minute ventilation usually results in a slight, periodic buildup of CO_2. The brain senses this slight buildup and tells the diaphragm and intercostal muscles to increase the tidal volume of a breath from time to time to handle the buildup. This increased volume breath is called a **sigh,** and this is why we sometimes take occa-sional deeper breaths at rest.

During exercise, the amount of oxygen needed for metabolism and the amount of carbon dioxide produced by the cells greatly increases. This means that more air must be moved by the lungs during ex-ercise to bring to the cells the necessary oxygen and to remove the excreted CO_2, so during exercise, both the ventilation rate and the tidal volume increases, and thus the minute ventilation increases.

Various forms of illnesses cause alterations in min-ute ventilation. In the setting of shock, the brain may perceive that it is not receiving enough oxygen and will increase the rate and depth of ventilation. Patients ex-periencing acidosis for various reasons will rid the body of excess CO_2 by increasing ventilation. This lowering of CO_2 causes the buffering equation discussed above to shift to the left, combining bicarbonate with acid and producing more CO_2, which is then blown off in the lungs. DOT 2-1.12

Differently sized human bodies require different amounts of oxygen delivery and CO_2 removal, so one would expect that tidal volumes and rates of ventilation would be different by age groups. Babies move much smaller amounts of air with each breath, and their rates of ventilation are higher.

CONNECTIONS   Chapter 43: Pediatric Patients lists respiratory rates for each age group.

Modified Forms of Respiration

A sigh was just described as a modification in the respi-ratory pattern. There are four modifications that occur to the normal respiratory pattern. These happen typi-cally as isolated events. They are a cough, sneeze, sigh, or hiccough. The **cough** is used to clear debris from the lower airways. A **sneeze** clears debris from the naso-pharynx. A **hiccough** occurs when the diaphragm has a spasm. DOT 2-1.18

Normal and Abnormal Respiratory Patterns

When assessing respiratory patterns, consider three char-acteristics: rate, depth, and regularity. Eupnea indicates easy normal breathing that has a regular pattern. These patients have adequate airflow and tidal volumes to sus-tain normal body functions and processes. DOT 2-1.20

Tachypnea describes an increased respiratory rate. Tachypnea can be caused by a number of factors: fever, pneumonia, respiratory acidosis, respiratory insuffi-ciency, some poisonings and drugs (such as aspirin overdose or stimulant use), and lesions to the respira-tory center in the brain. If tachypnea is caused by fever, expect to see an increase of around four breaths per minute for each degree of temperature rise. It is impor-tant to assess if tachypnea is due to compensation for a failure of another body system so that you can take cor-rective action, if necessary.

Although tachypnea can offer an injured or ill pa-tient some compensation, it also has a deleterious effect. It is important to understand that the breath you just took into your lungs does not go directly to the alveoli. The molecules first mix with air that is being exhaled as they begin to move into the bronchi and distal air-ways. The next respiratory cycle moves it deeper into the bronchioles, and eventually it reaches the alveoli. Think of this like a flight of stairs. It takes several steps to get down and several to get back up. A tachypneic respiratory system cannot completely exchange air, re-sulting in hypoxia and hypoxemia. "Dirty air" can be trapped in the distal airways while "fresh air" is moved quickly in and out of the tracheo-bronchial tree but does not reach the alveoli. The result is a patient with inad-equate ventilation. This patient may require some level of ventilatory support to control rate and depth of ven-tilation in addition to oxygen administration to prevent further deterioration.

Bradypnea is a slower than normal respiratory rate. It may be caused by narcotic or sedative drugs, tumors, alcohol, metabolic disorders, respiratory system decompensation, fatigue (particularly in pediatric patients), and brain injury. Mild bradypnea is normal in certain stages of sleep. **Apnea** is the absence of respirations. It may be episodic or periodic. Periods of apnea longer than 15 seconds should not be tolerated in the critical care transport situation. These patients require resuscitative efforts or ventilatory support.

Any patient with sustained tachypnea or bradypnea should also be assessed for evidence of hypoperfusion (shock), and corrective action should be taken immediately. Treatment includes oxygenation, ventilation support, the use of airway adjuncts such as the oropharyngeal or nasopharyngeal airway, suction to clear secretions, positioning of the patient to facilitate better ventilation, and advanced invasive airway interventions such as intubation or the use of a ventilator.

In addition to the respiratory rate, the depth of respiration should always be assessed. While minimal chest rise is normal in unstressed supine patients, it is not normal in severely injured or hypoxic patients. **Hyperpnea** is noted when excessively full respiration occurs. The term hyperpnea does not indicate a rapid respiratory rate although tachypnea may also be present. You would expect to see some degree of hyperpnea in acutely ill or injured patients that are experiencing high levels of pain.

Several abnormal respiratory patterns have been described which present as alterations to the respiratory rate, depth, or regularity (see Figure 12-20 page 238).

Cheyne-Stokes Pattern

Cheyne-Stokes pattern is described as a cyclic pattern of increased respiratory rate and depth with periods of apnea. Following the period of apnea, the patient begins breathing with slow shallow breaths that increase in both rate and depth until apnea occurs. It may be caused by increased intracranial pressure, hypoxia secondary to congestive heart failure, renal failure, meningitis, or drug overdose. Otherwise healthy individuals may breathe in a Cheyne-Stokes pattern following exposure to altitude or with hyperventilation syndrome. Acidosis, particularly when due to carbon dioxide levels, may cause a Cheyne-Stokes pattern as well.

Biot's Breathing

Biot's (ataxic) breathing is similar to Cheyne-Stokes, but unlike Cheyne-Stokes, the pattern is irregular. While Cheyne-Stokes has repeating patterns of gradual increases concluding with apnea, three patterns occur in Biot's: (1) slow and deep, (2) rapid and shallow, and (3) apnea without any predictability of which pattern will follow. Biot's can be seen with meningitis, increased intracranial pressure, and central nervous system dysfunction. It often indicates lesions higher in the respiratory center than Cheyne-Stokes patterns.

Kussmaul's Respiration

Kussmaul's respiration is fast and deep without any periods of apnea. The rate is greater than the normal respiratory rate expected for each age group. Breathing sounds are often labored with periods of deep breaths punctuated by sighs. Kussmaul's pattern may indicate metabolic acidosis, diabetic ketoacidosis, or renal failure and is generally noted with conditions causing severe acidotic states.

Apneustic Breathing

Apneustic breathing is noted with lesions in the respiratory center of the brain. The patient exhibits a prolonged, gasping inspiration followed by an extremely short, ineffective expiration. The respiratory rate is between one and two breaths per minute. Over a period of several minutes of ineffective exhalation, the patient's chest may hyperinflate. This respiratory pattern results in severe hypoxemia and if uncorrected, rapid death.

Central Neurogenic Hyperventilation

Central neurogenic hyperventilation occurs as very deep, rapid respiratory rates of 40–60 breaths per minute. It is found in association with midbrain lesions or dysfunction. Generally, patients exhibiting central neurogenic hyperventilation are comatose with Glascow Coma Scores less than eight. These patients require intubation and ventilatory assistance. Because of the excessively rapid respiratory rate, good air exchange does not occur within the alveoli, and the patient can quickly become acidotic if not managed appropriately and aggressively.

Street Secrets

In patients who are breathing normally, both the abdomen and the chest will expand and contract simultaneously. During inhalation, the chest rises and the abdominal girth expands. Patients with upper airway obstruction often have **paradoxical respirations.** When inhaling, the chest will rise, but the abdomen contracts as the patient works harder to create negative pressure to pull air into the lungs. When the patient exhales, the chest wall falls, but the abdomen rises as the patient increases intra-abdominal pressure to boost exhalation. Often, simple jaw thrusts or placement of oral or nasal airways will reverse paradoxical respirations.

Hyperventilation Syndrome

Hyperventilation syndrome is noted with an increase in both rate and depth of respiration. Hyperventilation may be due to exertion, fear, anxiety, fever, hepatic coma, acid/base imbalance, or lesions of the midbrain. A respiratory rate between 20 and 30 per minute in the adult is classified as moderate hyperventilation. A prolonged respiratory rate greater than 30 per minute is considered severe, and ventilatory support is often necessary to prevent decompensation. Hyperventilation syndrome is often due to a state of respiratory acidosis that is caused by increased retention of carbon dioxide despite adequate intake of air. This state is often a difficult one to compensate for, even by healthy patients. Caution must be exercised to adequately assess for the underlying cause of hyperventilation prior to initiating any corrective treatment. Oxygen should never be withheld from a patient exhibiting signs or symptoms of hypoxia or hypoxemia.

Working in the Gray Zone

Although hyperventilation can be seen as a response to respiratory acidosis, it can also cause respiratory alkalosis if hyperventilation occurs as the result of anxiety.

A hyperventilation state may be induced in a patient who is intubated or is receiving ventilatory support. Closely monitor vital signs, pulse oximetry reading, capnography, mental status, and skin color of any patient who is receiving ventilatory support. Hyperventilation is no longer recommended by the American Neurological Association as a treatment for increasing intracranial pressure but is recommended for patients who are exhibiting signs of herniation syndrome. See Chapter 20: Head, Face and Neck Trauma for additional information on the use of hyperventilation with intracranial pressure.

Obstructive Breathing

Obstructive breathing is noted with patients who have prolonged expiratory phases due to increased airway resistance. Patients with chronic lung diseases, like COPD, often breathe with their lips pursed in an effort to maintain **positive end expiratory pressure** or **PEEP.** For patients with healthy lung tissue, during exhalation, the elastic alveoli almost completely collapse as they empty. The presence of surfactant and the elasticity of the alveoli allow for rapid re-expansion with the next breath. For patients with inelastic lungs or with diseases that decrease the production of surfactant, the alveoli can collapse, and the walls can adhere to each other, preventing re-expansion. PEEP is a method of maintaining enough residual volume in the alveoli so that they do not completely empty and collapse during exhalation.

During periods of obstructive breathing, hyperinflation of the chest occurs if exhalation time is not proportionate to inhalation time and air remains trapped within the lungs. In an attempt to compensate, respiration becomes shallow. **Continuous positive airway pressure (CPAP)** is similar to PEEP. Both PEEP and CPAP maintain pressure in the airway and alveoli at the end of the exhalation phase. For patients on ventilatory support, PEEP and CPAP may be provided by the ventilator.

Normal and Adventitious Breath Sounds

Normal Breath Sounds

During normal breathing, the exspiratory phase of the respiratory cycle is slightly longer that the inhalation phase. Specific sounds heard upon auscultation of the lungs are named according to the location of the airflow within the tracheo-bronchial tree. **Tracheal sounds** are heard over the trachea and are primarily heard around the manubrium of the sternum. **Bronchiovesicular sounds** are heard over the mainstem bronchi, which are located below the manubrium and to the left and right of the center of the sternum. **Vesicular sounds** are heard over the lung fields.

When auscultation is performed in the midaxillary line, the purest vesicular sounds are heard. For auscultation of the anterior chest wall along the sternum between the second and fifth intercostal spaces, a combination of bronchial and vesicular sounds are heard and are properly named bronchiovesicular. Sounds which might otherwise be classified as normal that are heard in an unexpected area of the chest wall can indicate an abnormal condition. In other words, tracheal sounds should not be heard in areas you normally hear bronchiovesicular sounds. This abnormality may be due to an illness or injury.

Adventitious Sounds

Adventitious sounds are abnormal breath sounds heard in addition to, or in place of, normal lung sounds. They are often grossly characterized as "wet" or "dry." Wet lungs indicate some degree of pulmonary edema. Dry lungs have restricted airflow due to mechanical obstructions such as constriction, mucous plugs, or foreign bodies that have been aspirated. Adventitious sounds heard over the lung fields in the axillary line are either bronchial, diminished, or absent. Adventitious breath sounds are generally further categorized into two gross categories: crackles or wheezes. Wheezes are further divided into monophonic (having one sound) or polyphonic (many sounds).

Wheezes

A **wheeze** is a high pitched musical sound that is caused by high velocity air flow through a very narrowed or constricted airway. Wheezes can be heard during both phases of the respiratory cycle and may be heard audibly without a stethoscope. Wheezes often begin during the exhalation phase and then are heard during both phases as air is trapped and airflow decreases. Monophonic wheezes indicate that a single area of the lung is affected while polyphonic wheezes mean numerous sites are involved. A wheeze is the lower airway equivalent of rhonchi.

Crackles

Crackles and wheezes are heard as air flow is restricted due to narrowing of structures or blockage by mucopolysaccharide (mucous) plugs, blood, fluid, infection, or other form of debris. A **crackle** is generally heard on inspiration and presents as a discontinuous bubbling noise. The term crackle is preferred over the term rale by the American Thoracic Society because it is more descriptive of the actual sound that is heard. Fine crackles are generated as air moves through the distal bronchiole and alveoli that contain secretions. There are generally numerous sounds heard with crackles. They present as a popping sound created as the alveoli rapidly pop open once the pressure in the distal airway is high enough for the air to flow into the alveolus. The lower pitched rumbling of the **course crackle** is heard in the larger bronchi or trachea and is caused by air traveling through larger masses of debris.

Rhonchi

Rhonchi are heard primarily in the bronchi and larger airways. Rhonchi are often more pronounced with the expiratory phase of respiration. When limited to the bronchi and lower portions of the trachea, they may be eliminated by coughing. The sound of rhonchi is produced by rattling vibrations as air flows through mucous or around an obstruction.

Stridor

Stridor is produced during inspiration when a foreign body, infection, swelling, disease, or trauma occurs within or immediately above the glottic opening. Stridor can produce a loud high-pitched sound, particularly when it occurs in pediatric patients.

Pleural Friction Rub

A **pleural friction rub** is due to an infection or inflammation that has caused the visceral or parietal pleura to stop secreting pleural fluid. This fluid is necessary to lubricate the linings, so the lungs can freely move within the expanding and contracting thorax. Without this fluid, friction causes the tissues to become irritated and inflamed and often results in stabbing pain with breathing or any stretching movement by the thorax.

Percussion and Palpation "Sounds"

Resonance is the sound vibration quality that can be heard with percussion (tapping) on the chest wall or during phonation (speaking). There are three types of transmitted breath sounds that can be assessed using very simple vocal **fremitus** techniques; they are bronchophony, egophony, and whispered pectoriloquy. **Bronchophony** is easily assessed by auscultation of the chest wall while asking the patient to say the number "99" over and over again. When heard over normal, healthy lung tissue, the sound will be unintelligible. Over areas of injured lung, the sound transmits easily, and "99" is heard distinctly.

To assess **egophony,** ask the patient to sustain the letter "e" while you listen to the chest wall. With normal lung tissue, the letter "e" is heard, but with areas of consolidated lung tissue, the letter "a" is heard with a distinct nasal quality. Another test for consolidation is to ask the patient to whisper the numbers "1, 2, 3" over and over again. This test, called **whispered pectoriloquy,** yields an easily understood sound with consolidation but cannot be understood through normal lung tissue.

CONNECTIONS Table 11-4 in Chapter 11: The Normal Physical Examination lists and describes each of these assessments.

Airway Diseases Overview

Airway Obstruction

The airway can become obstructed at many levels, from the mouth all the way down to the smallest airways. The tongue is the most common cause of airway obstruction. Patients with altered mentation who are placed in a supine position often have the relaxed tongues fall back and partially or completely obstruct the upper airways. Trauma to the face, for example, could mechanically obstruct the nasal passages, the mouth, or both. The tongue might swell for a variety of reasons. Infections, mentioned earlier, can cause potentially life-threatening airway blockage. Foreign bodies, including food, teeth, vomitus, etc., can affect both the upper and lower airways, possibly completely obstructing the upper airway, resulting in death, or obstructing only a portion of the lower airway, resulting in blockage of only part of the air movement path. DOT 2-1.25

Airway Obstruction Signs

Signs of upper airway obstruction include both sounds and appearances. Obstruction of the flow of air can cause a high-pitched, raspy sound commonly during inspiration which is called **stridor** and is also associated with snoring. Lower grade obstruction produces stridor on inhalation. When stridor is heard both on inhalation and exhalation, this suggests a very high grade of obstruction. DOT 2-1.24

Working in the Gray Zone

It is important to determine whether the airway obstruction is partial or complete. If it is partial, the patient is able to move some air into the lungs despite the presence of the foreign body. If the airway is partially obstructed and the patient has good air exchange, transport the patient for treatment in the hospital setting. If the air exchange is poor, treat the patient as if there is a complete obstruction and use the abdominal thrusts/chest thrusts to try to clear the airway. DOT 2-1.23

Patients who are conscious may grasp their throats. They may stick out their tongues and make exaggerated arm movements to get your attention. If completely obstructed, they will not be able to speak or talk, otherwise stridor may be present. The movement of the diaphragm and intercostal muscles in attempting to move air causes other signs:

- The area just above the top of the sternum—called the suprasternal notch—may sink in during inhalation, which is called **retraction** (Figure 12-21).
- Retractions may also be seen in the intercostal muscles.
- The "accessory muscles" that are attached to the chest, such as the neck muscles (sternocleidomastoids), will be used to assist in moving the chest wall.
- The work of breathing—both the rate and the quality—will be obviously increased unless the patient is near collapse.
- Cyanosis may appear, manifesting initially in the periphery, such as the nail beds, and then later on the skin of the extremities, torso, and head and neck. Cyanosis of the tongue may be seen also.

Potentially Life-Threatening Airway Infections

The diseases in this section are overviewed. Chapter 28: Pulmonary discusses these diseases in more detail and includes discussing how to assess and treat these conditions.

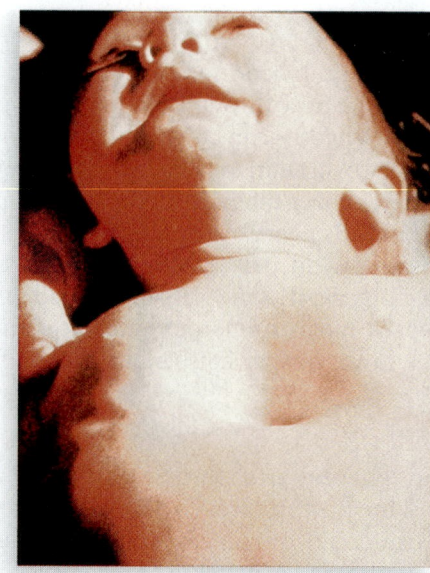

Figure 12-21 Retractions are a sign that the diaphragm and intercostal muscles are aiding respiration. EMSC Slide Set (CD-ROM), 1996. Courtesy of the Emergency Services for Children Program, administered by the U.S. Department of Health and Human Services's Health Resources and Services Administration, Maternal and Child Health Bureau.

The area under the tongue can become infected with bacteria and possibly obstruct the airway, a condition called **Ludwig's angina.** Abscesses can form beside or behind the tonsils, called peritonsillar abscesses, which can threaten the airway. Tonsils can become infected and swell so much that they can obstruct the airway. The posterior pharynx can develop abscesses, called "retropharyngeal abscesses," which can block air movement.

The epiglottis, which covers the opening of the airway, can become infected with bacteria or virus, often developing symptoms very quickly and threatening airway obstruction.

CONNECTIONS Epiglottitis is a viral infection that can cause rapid airway compromise, particularly in children. Chapter 43: Pediatric Patients discusses epiglottitis in detail.

The trachea can become infected by both bacteria and viruses. Bacteria include staphylococcus, which can produce a condition called **tracheobronchitis,** a potentially very serious condition most commonly occurring in children. Viruses can infect this area of the trachea causing a condition called **croup,** in which the lining of the trachea will swell and at least partially obstruct the flow of air.

Less likely to be immediately life-threatening are infections of the bronchi and smaller airways. **Bronchitis,** an infection or inflammation of the main bronchi and some of the smaller branches, is rarely life-threatening though certainly coughing may be severe. Infection can damage these airways, though, causing a condition called **bronchiectasis,** which is dilation of one or more bronchi due to injury from infection. This can result in a collection of mucus distal to these bronchi with pneumonia and sepsis.

The bronchioles can become infected, usually with viruses. Most commonly affected by this condition are babies and small children. The tiny airways become inflamed, secrete mucus into the airway, and become spastic, producing wheezing. This condition is usually not serious, but it may be. Always examine all patients carefully, especially children, and note the work of breathing. Any patient that is breathing fast is sick and must be promptly transported to the closest appropriate facility. Serious mistakes have been made by rescuers in the past who have failed to transport an apparently healthy, smiling playful baby who had an elevated respiratory rate.

Pneumonia is a condition of infection and inflammation in distal sections of the lung including small airways and alveoli. A host of bacteria, viruses, and other pathogens can cause pneumonia, and many of the different pathogens have rather unique characteristics. Streptococcus pneumoniae (S. pneumo) has long been one of the most severe killers of humans and is one of the leading causes of death in nonindustrialized nations.[4] When nations become industrialized, heart disease and cancer take over as the leading killers, followed by pneumonia.

Pneumonia is usually treatable with antibiotics and supportive care, but it may also be fatal due to spread of infection through the blood stream (sepsis), damage to lung tissue, and the release of toxins into the body. In the setting of sepsis, shock may develop, resulting in death.

Alveolar Disease

Fluid inside of the alveoli, such as occurs in congestive heart failure and pneumonia, can reduce gas diffusion through the alveoli, lowering blood oxygen levels and raising CO_2 levels. Emphysema, from smoking and other causes, destroys the walls of alveoli, reducing the surface area that allows for gas diffusion.

The lung may be injured from low perfusion states such as hemorrhagic shock, septic shock, and cardiac arrest. The injury can show up as decreasing oxygen levels and raising CO_2 levels due to direct injury to the alveoli. The syndrome is called acute respiratory distress syndrome (ARDS), and it may rapidly lead to respiratory insufficiency and death.

Obstructions to Pulmonary Blood Flow
Pulmonary Embolism

Blood clots may form in veins throughout the body. Especially likely to form blood clots are the veins of the pelvis and of the lower extremities. Most commonly, these clots remain in the veins where they form, producing a wide range of symptoms including pain and swelling.

Perhaps the greatest danger of blood clots forming in veins is that they will break loose and travel through the circulatory system, back to the right side of the heart and be pumped into the blood vessels of the lungs, obstructing flow of blood to some portion of the lungs. These clots that lodge in the lungs are called **pulmonary emboli (PE)**. Most commonly, these clots are tiny and have few if any symptoms.

However, a large PE can cause serious problems, including death. A PE can be so large as to nearly completely obstruct the flow of blood into the pulmonary artery from the right ventricle, sitting in the middle of the outflow tract; this is called a saddle embolism. Such conditions are often quickly fatal and can be a cause of sudden death syndrome. If such a patient can be revived, prompt removal of the embolus by some measure—including thrombolysis (clot dissolving drugs) or prompt surgical removal—may be lifesaving.

CONNECTIONS A massive PE is one of the differential diagnoses in the management of cardiac arrest due to Pulseless Electrical Activity. Chapter 29: The Cardiac Emergencies and Chapter 28: The Respiratory Emergencies have additional information on this condition.

A smaller PE may cause myriad findings, from acute shortness of breath to tachycardia to chest pain. In the elderly, the only finding might be confusion or altered mental status. Younger patients commonly will have **pleuritic chest pain,** which is a sharp, stabbing pain worsened by breathing.

Tension Pneumothorax

If air leaks from the lung (or through a hole in the chest wall) into the pleural space, then air collects within the pleural space, causing some measure of collapse of the lung on the affected side. Remember that the lung is kept inflated by the surface tension between the surface of the lung (visceral pleura) and the inside of the chest wall (parietal pleura). If only a little air leaks out into the pleural space, then the collapse of the lung on that side may be quite small. If a lot of air leaks out, then the lung on that side may collapse completely. The collapse of a lung to either a greater or lesser degree without positive pressure building up in the pleural space is called a **simple pneumothorax.** Simple pneumothorax can occur spontaneously, especially in smokers, and it usually doesn't cause much problem other than pain and perhaps some shortness of breath.

If air continues to leak out into the pleural space from the lung or through the chest wall and cannot be released, pressure can build up inside the affected side. This positive pressure completely collapses the lung on the affected side and pushes the vascular structures in the center of the chest (called the "mediastinal structures") to the opposite side (as well as compressing and compromising the opposite lung). This increased pressure prevents filling of the heart from the venous side. Decreased filling of the heart, as mentioned above, causes decreased cardiac output and hence decreased blood pressure. Thus, a **tension pneumothorax** causes shock and can quickly result in death because of its obstruction to blood flow through the heart and lungs.

Since blood is moving poorly through the lungs during a tension pneumothorax, air exchange with blood is decreased and oxygen levels drop. This results in cyanosis, which will be discussed later in this chapter. Since blood is not moving well out of the venous circulation, neck veins become distended.

CONNECTIONS Chapter 21: Thoracic Trauma also discusses tension pneumothorax and cardiac tamponade.

Cardiac Tamponade

The pericardium is a double thickness sac that loosely surrounds the heart. It is wrapped around the heart, and the innermost layer is adhered directly to the heart. The outermost layer does not adhere to the heart but instead surrounds the heart like a sac. The two layers are attached together to the base of the heart where the aorta arises from the heart. The space between the pericardium and the heart is called the pericardial space, and usually only a tiny amount of fluid, secreted by the pericardium itself, is found in this space.

The pericardial space can fill with various fluids, though, and this can cause acute or even life-threatening illnesses. The pericardium can become infected, resulting in inflammation and the secretion of excess amounts of fluid into the pericardial space. Metastatic cancer can spread to the pericardium, causing fluid from the cancer to accumulate in the pericardial space. Penetrating trauma to the heart can cause bleeding into the pericardium.

In all of these situations, if this fluid cannot escape from the pericardial space, pressure builds up around the heart. If further accumulation of blood or fluid occurs into the pericardium, the heart becomes compressed and cannot fill, thus cardiac output drops and shock occurs. Since the heart cannot fill and pump forward, blood accumulates in the veins, and the neck veins become distended. Since blood cannot be moved well through the lungs, gas is not exchanged well, and cyanosis and respiratory distress result.

Congestive Heart Failure (CHF)

CHF results from the inability of the heart muscle to pump the blood that is in the blood vessels. This can occur because the heart muscle is weak. CHF may develop after a heart attack, when muscle damage occurs. It can also occur acutely from volume overload, when too much intra-venous fluids may have been given to a patient. It may occur because the heart is beating too fast to allow for adequate filling time, such as with some cardiac dysrhythmias or with a metabolic problem called thyroid storm.

Whatever the cause, CHF causes obstruction to forward blood flow. Back pressure from the left side of the heart involves the pulmonary veins causing fluid to leak out into the alveoli. This reduces air exchange and causes hypoxia and cyanosis with respiratory distress. If the right side of the heart fails as well, then blood backs up into the veins, causing neck vein distension, and peripheral edema develops.

CONNECTIONS Chapter 29: Cardiology discusses congestive heart failure; Chapter 31: Endocrine, Electrolytes, and Acid/Base discusses thyroid storm.

Airway Assessment

Positioning the Airway Is Key

The paramedic must always be alert to potential airway obstructions due to patient positioning.

Whenever a patient is laid supine, the jaw may relax backward, the tongue may fall toward the posterior pharynx, and the airway can become partially or fully obstructed.

Also, when a patient is supine, material from the oral or nasal pharynx can fall backward into the airway and be aspirated. Examples of aspirated material include vomitus, broken teeth, and blood from facial or oral injuries. Aspiration is a very serious problem because of both obstruction and the possibility that aspirated contents will later cause an infection in the lungs and result in pneumonia. Aspiration can cause serious illness or death and should be prevented if at all possible.

The tongue can also cause airway obstruction for other reasons. A condition called **angioedema** causes the tongue to swell dramatically, potentially obstructing the upper airway. Angioedema can occur from allergic reactions to stimuli such as bee stings, food, and medications, or it can also occur due to a particular reaction to a type of medication called "angiotensin converting enzyme inhibitors" (ACE inhibitors). Such swelling can occur quickly, and rapid action may be required by the rescuer to prevent airway obstruction and death.

CONNECTIONS See Chapter 32: Allergies and Anaphylaxis to review anaphylactic reactions and angioedema.

Opening the Airway

The head and neck are extremely mobile. Because of the movement of the head and neck, the passage of air through the airway can be affected greatly by head

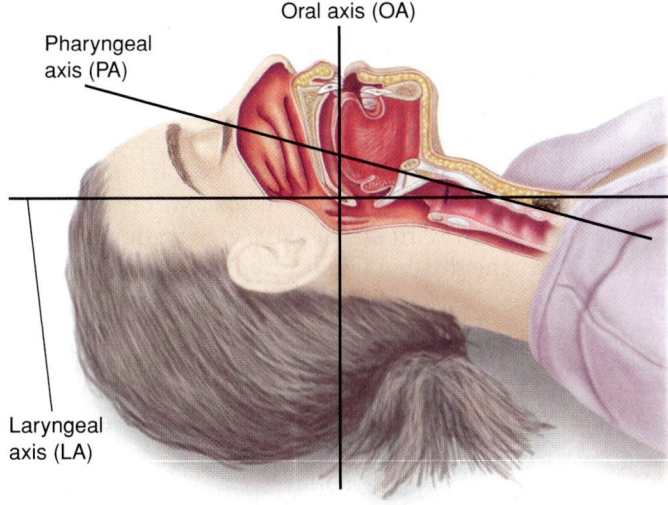

Oral axis (OA)
Pharyngeal axis (PA)
Laryngeal axis (LA)

(a)

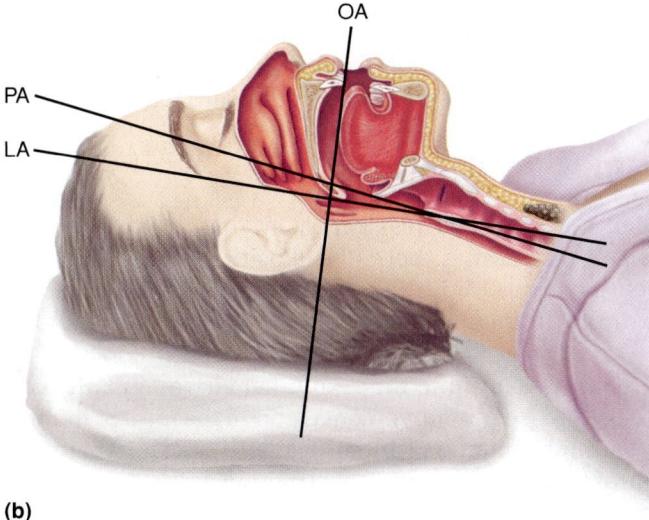

OA
PA
LA

(b)

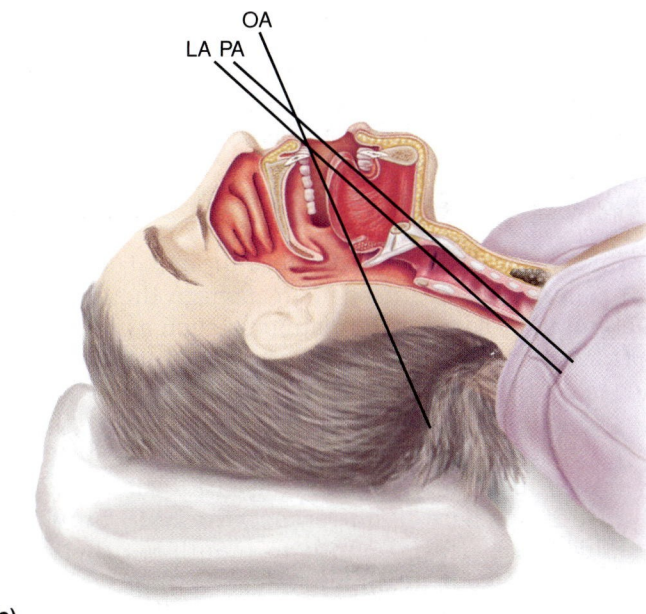

OA
LA PA

(c)

position. If the head is flexed forward at the neck, the soft palate can move forward onto the tongue, obstructing the airway. Extending the head backward tends to pull the soft palate away from the tongue, opening the airway. Therefore, the positioning of a patient to provide optimal air flow through the airway tends to be with the patient supine and with the head extended on the neck. The motion of air in this position can be improved even further by tilting the neck forward very slightly in relation to the chest while maintaining extension of the head on the neck. This is the same position that you use when you are "sniffing the air," with the head high and nose extended but the neck held forward slightly on the chest. This is the **sniffing position** and is usually the optimal position in which to place a patient in preparation for visualizing the larynx for endotracheal intubation (Figure 12-22). DOT 2-1.27

Working in the Gray Zone

The sniffing position in adults is maintained by placing a small pile of padding under the head, one to two inches, depending upon the size and proportion of the head. In contrast, pediatric patients have heads of much greater proportion compared to their body size. Padding placed under their heads would compromise their airways. Children need one to two inches or more of padding placed under their bodies, starting at the shoulders. This places their airway in the best position. DOT 2-1.5

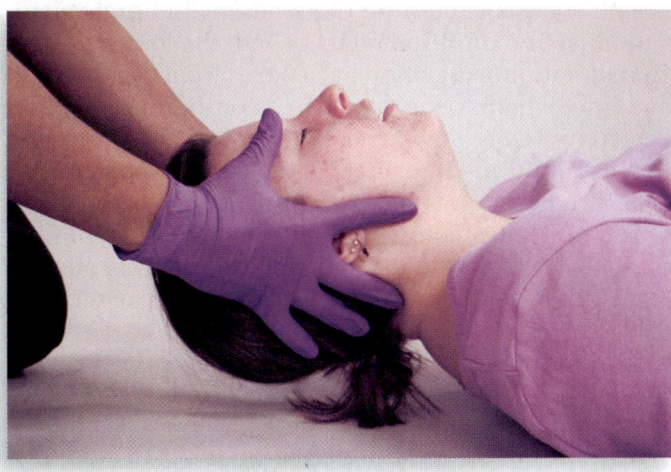

(d)

Figure 12-22 (a) The normal positioning of the three axes (oral, pharyngeal, and laryngeal). By raising the head (b) and extending the head (c) you bring these axes into alignment, shorten the distance, and make a straighter line from the teeth to the glottic opening. (d) Proper positioning of the airway in a sniffing position is one of the keys to successful airway maintenance. The head may require elevation of as much as 10 cm off the floor or bed.

Breath Sounds Assessment Techniques

Breath sounds are best evaluated while the patient is taking slow deep breaths through an open mouth. Be aware of the patient's comfort while you are assessing breath sounds. If you rush the patient through the process, you may cause the patient to begin to hyperventilate or exacerbate any dyspnea.

There are two factors in the generation of the sound that is heard during breath sound assessment: (1) the distance the source of the sound is from the chest wall and (2) the pathway the sound takes as it travels through the tracheo-bronchial tree. The distance the sound is traveling is affected most by the overall body mass of the patient. You would expect to hear a difference in breath sounds between an obese and a normal body weight patient.

The whirling pathway, or **vortices,** is the flow pattern the air takes as it travels through the lungs. This pathway can be affected by injury or blockage, thus altering the sounds you appreciate as you assess the lungs. **Consolidation** is a form of blockage and occurs when areas of lung tissue become firm and inelastic. Consolidation is generally due to pneumonia. **Atelectasis,** or collapsed lung tissue, prevents the affected area of the lung from adequately exchanging oxygen and carbon dioxide. Breath sounds typically are diminished in areas with consolidation or atelectasis. Chronic disease states involving the bronchi, bronchioles, and alveoli can also cause permanent alterations in breath sounds or affect the sounds only during episodes of disease flare up. DOT 2-1.14

Sound Duration, Pitch, and Intensity

Breath sounds should be assessed for duration, pitch, and intensity. **Duration** refers to both the length of time an inspiration/exhalation cycle takes from beginning to end and whether the process is continuous or interrupted by coughing, wheezing, or other disruption. Breath sound **pitch,** or frequency, is described as high or low. Low pitch is the normal finding. The intensity of sound is affected by air flow rate, constancy of flow throughout inspiration, patient position, and site selected for auscultation.

Auscultatory Sites

When performing breath sounds, the auscultatory sites selected will affect the sound heard. Whenever possible, compare one side of the chest wall directly to the opposite side. Use bony landmarks like the ribs to ensure that you are listening to the same site on each side of the chest wall. The goal for auscultation of the lungs in critical situations is to listen to each of the five lobes of the lungs to get a baseline assessment of patient status (you can review the five lobes of the lung by turning back to Figure 7-49 on page 122). This can be accomplished by listening in as few as six places on the anterior chest

wall. A complete assessment may include listening to as many as 18 sites on the anterior, posterior, and lateral chest wall and is generally not required in the prehospital setting. The sites commonly chosen to assess lung sounds are (1) second intercostal space midclavicular line, (2) fifth intercostal space midaxillary line, and (3) seventh intercostal space posterior axillary line.

For the patient with an invasive airway device such as an endotracheal tube, Combitube™, laryngeal mask airway, or other device, listen over the epigastrium and sternal notch as well as the six recommended sites on the anterior chest wall. This is done to assess for proper airflow and placement of the device.

Document the sites chosen for auscultation in your patient care report as well as the status (patency, appearance, and integrity) of any airway management devices. In addition to periodic monitoring of breath sounds during an assessment of the ABC status, an auscultatory assessment should be performed immediately upon your arrival to the patient's side, with any gross patient movement, and immediately prior to turning the patient over to other members of the healthcare team.

Primary Survey

When assessing the respiratory system, begin with the basics by assessing the ABCs. Position the patient and open the airway with the head-tilt chin-lift or modified jaw thrust, if trauma is suspected. Determine whether the airway is open and clear. You may need to look-listen-and-feel to determine this. An open airway is indicated by easy and free air movement through the nose or mouth. This air movement is generally silent. Listen for snoring sounds indicating partial obstruction from the tongue; gurgling sounds indicating the accumulation of secretions, saliva, blood, or vomitus; or stridor indicating narrowing of the airway from swelling or foreign material. An airway adjunct may be necessary to maintain an open patent airway. Suction and positional changes may be required to assist with patency as well (Figure 12-23).

Street Secrets

During the scene size-up, determine what additional BSI precautions are needed to manage the airway. If suctioning or aggressive treatments such as intubation are necessary, make sure you wear eye protection and a face mask while performing these skills. DOT 2-1.21

Develop the habit of carrying a CPR barrier device at all times. There is no reason why EMS providers should *ever* perform mouth to mouth ventilation if a barrier device is available. Many EMS providers no longer perform even mouth to mask ventilation because they ensure they always respond to the patient's side

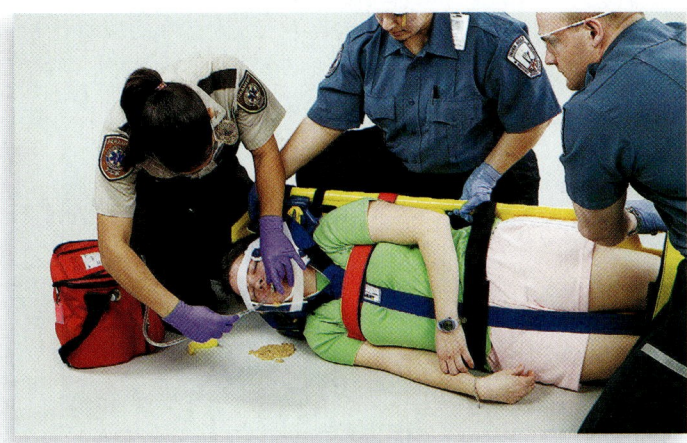

Figure 12-23 If spinal precautions are needed, the patient should be properly immobilized and rescuers should be prepared to turn the patient onto his or her side if necessary.

with the equipment they need to begin resuscitation immediately. This means that at a minimum a bag-mask device, portable suction, and gloves should be carried into each scene. DOT 2-1.43a, 2-1.43c

Secondary Survey

During your visual examination of the airway, note the presence of any structural abnormalities in the mouth or nose, unusual breath odors, or dental devices. Take note of any medications, disease processes, or trauma that might compromise respiration or ventilation. As you assess breathing, take note of the rate, rhythm, depth, and character of respiration. Observe the tidal volume to determine if it is adequate to maintain perfusion.

Visualize the chest wall. Look for symmetrical rise and fall with each respiratory cycle. Look at the skin for tunneled catheters, nitroglycerin, or other medication patches or indwelling devices such as pacemakers, implanted defibrillators, chest tubes, or medication delivery devices. Note any bruising, edema, or the presence and location of crepitus or subcutaneous emphysema. Examine any dressings on the chest wall and determine if they are dry and intact. Measure any drainage that is being collected and note its color and consistency.

Assess for sufficient oxygenation of the patient by using the pulse oximeter, end-tidal CO_2, and ECG monitoring. Because the function of the cardiac and respiratory systems are so closely linked, assessment of circulation is important to develop a complete clinical picture of your patient. Assess blood pressure and pulses as well as skin color, temperature, and capillary refill time. Mental status is also an important consideration as hypoxia directly affects mental status and level of consciousness.

As you auscultate the chest, remember to provide a pace that is comfortable for the patient. Ask him or her to breathe through an open mouth and refrain from talking while you assess airflow, and be sure to compare breath sounds from one side of the chest wall to the other. Perform any vocal or tactile fremitus assessments that are necessary to get a good baseline.

Ensure that any airway adjunct or ventilatory device is intact and working properly. Monitor it closely, and be ready to troubleshoot the device if you detect problems.

Aeromedical Transport Considerations

Altitude-induced pressure changes can occur during travel by helicopter or fixed-wing aircraft. You may need to reassess air filled spaces, such as the balloon of an ET tube, and fill them with fluid instead of air to prevent altitude-related pressure change problems from occurring during transport. You should monitor your patient closely for evidence of dyspnea or the development of an air embolus during air transport.

Airway Adjuncts, Devices, and Techniques

The following airway management and assessment techniques have been discussed in detail previously in this text:

- Techniques for opening the airway and assessing its patency
- The role in vital signs and the physical examination in assessing ventilation and respiration
- Auscultation of breath sounds and inspection, palpation, and percussion
- Utilization of pulse oximetry and capnography

This section describes some additional techniques, airway adjuncts, and equipment that have not been described in detail. Many of these devices have Skill Sheets that accompany them.

Initiation of Ventilation for Patients Requiring Assisted Ventilation

A useful guide for providing assisted ventilation in a patient who requires it is to use about the same minute ventilation as is normal for the patient at rest. For the average adult, this is about 5 liters of air per minute. This ventilation is achieved through a "one hand squeeze" on the bag-mask (which is about a 700 mL breath) at a rate of one every eight seconds or so (Figure 12-24). This is considerably slower than most rescuers typically ventilate critically ill patients, yet restraining the rate of ventilation is necessary to avoid raising intrathoracic pressure and possibly decreasing venous return. Aufderheide has studied this extensively, noting that, even with careful training, rescuers have a strong tendency to overventilate

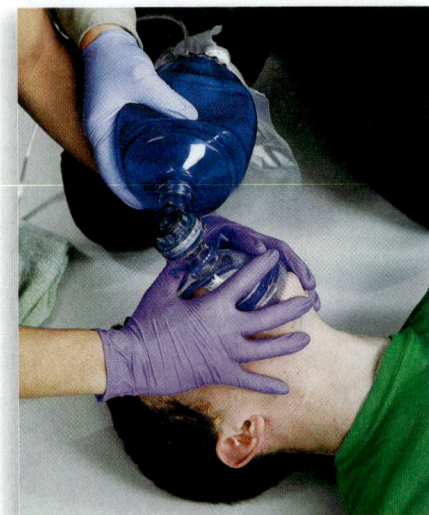

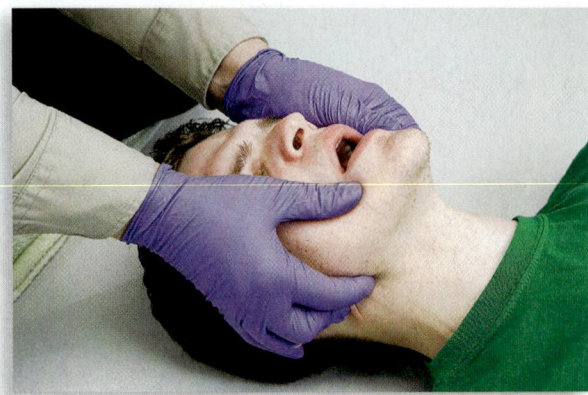

Figure 12-25   Proper placement of fingers is important when performing a jaw thrust. Note the position of the middle, index, and thumb fingers.

Figure 12-24   Adult bag-masks are designed for one-handed use. A typical bag holds approximately 1500 mL of air. Only 500 mL are needed to properly ventilate. If a rescuer uses both hands to nearly empty all the air into a patient's lungs, the rescuer may be delivering too much volume. Over-ventilation and hyperventilation should be avoided. Use one hand to squeeze the bag.

patients.[12] He has also outlined the risks of hyperventilation during cardiac arrest on the patient's circulatory status.[13] Ventilation should be adjusted based on clinical response, blood pressure (if the patient is not in cardiac arrest), and capnography readings (see below).

The Decision to Use More Aggressive Devices

The decision to intubate, or for that matter utilize any aggressive airway technique such as an LMA or a surgical airway, involves three principles: (1) failure of airway maintenance or protection, (2) failure of ventilation or oxygenation, and (3) anticipated clinical course for further treatment.[5]

The patient's airway obstruction may be relieved by a simple BLS measure such as a jaw thrust and the insertion of a nasopharyngeal airway (Figure 12-25). Snoring respirations may immediately cease once the tongue is repositioned and the ventilation effort is sufficient. For example, the anticipated clinical course of a seizure is a self-limited, postictal period (unless status epilepticus occurs). In all of these cases, the management should be supportive and minimally invasive. Intubation in these situations is unnecessary and may result in harm.

If the anticipated clinical course leads you to suspect further deterioration, such as in the case of status epilepticus or seizures of suspected intracranial hemorrhage from a stroke or trauma, intubation should be strongly considered. If an obstruction is located at the glottis and it cannot be removed with abdominal thrusts or Magill

forceps, a surgical airway may be the next appropriate step. Protocols can help guide some of these clinical decisions but so should experience and maturity. DOT 2-1.29

Suction

The application of suction clears secretions, vomitus, and blood from the patient's airway. Suction will help maintain a patent airway and will also prevent aspiration of material that may harm lung tissue. There are two main types of suction, manual and mechanical. Both types have advantages and disadvantages. DOT 2-1.30, 2-1.32

Manual devices include the Laderal V-Vac® suction and the Repro-med's Res-Q-Vac. Other manual devices can be as simple as a turkey baster. The goal of these devices is to remove the fluids when mechanical suction devices are unavailable or nonfunctional. DOT 2-1.31

Mechanical suction devices on board the ambulance include wall-mounted units and portable devices that can be brought to scenes where they can be of immediate use. On some units, the amount of suction can be adjusted. All devices are equipped with a canister which accumulates the suctioned fluid. Mechanical suction devices can also vary by the type of suction tips (catheters) which are used based on what type of secretions are present and what type of airway is in place.

Rigid tip catheters are used most commonly when patients are not intubated to remove large volumes of fluid from the upper airway in a short amount of time. They can also remove larger pieces of debris from the airway than the soft tip catheters. Soft tip catheters are most commonly used for patients that are intubated as they can be placed down the endotracheal tube. DOT 2-1.33

The biggest complication that can occur with suctioning comes with prolonged suctioning of the patient. Patients who need suctioning are often hypoxic to begin with, and prolonged suctioning can cause increased hypoxia. Therefore, suctioning should be limited to 15 seconds or less. DOT 2-1.34, 2-1.35

The procedures for suctioning the upper and lower airways differ. The upper airway equipment should be as clean as possible, but sterility is not required. Lower airway suctioning requires the use of sterile catheters. In order to keep the catheter free from contamination, sterile gloves should be worn during the procedure. **Skill Sheet 60 describes the techniques for putting on and removing gloves.** DOT 2-1.38, 2-1.36

Working in the Gray Zone

Prolonged Suctioning

The purpose of suctioning is to remove foreign matter from the airway so it does not enter the trachea and cause an obstruction or aspiration pneumonia. Every second the suction unit is operating is a second the patient is being deprived of air, but it is also a second that obstructions are being removed. When the patient's pulse oximetry is being monitored, it can help provide you with information valuable to performing suction. If you note the pulse oximeter reading is dropping, stop suctioning and ventilate the patient for 30–60 seconds before another suction attempt occurs.

Oropharyngeal Airway (OPA)

The oropharyngeal, or oral, airway (Figure 12-26) is a device used to help maintain a path for air movement by keeping the tongue off of the back of the pharynx. It is made of plastic, and it comes in a variety of sizes. By touching the tongue, hard palate, and soft palate, it can stimulate a gag reflex, and it should only be used in patients who have a decreased level of consciousness. It can also be used along with an ET tube to provide a "bite block" to prevent damage to the ET tube in the event of a seizure or other jaw clenching occurance. DOT 2-1.6, 2-1.37, 2-1.42

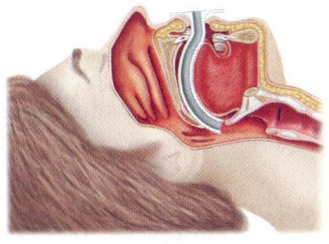 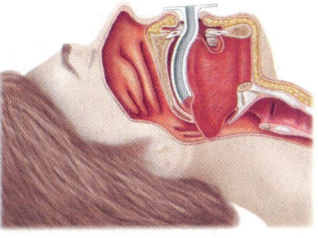

(a)   (b)

Figure 12-26 (a) A properly placed oropharyngeal airway is one of the best tools to maintain an open airway. (b) If the airway is too small, the device can cause the tongue to obstruct the airway.

Nasopharyngeal Airway (NPA)

The **nasopharyngeal airway (NPA)** is a soft, flexible adjunct which is inserted into one of the nostrils, passing over the back of the soft palate into the pharynx, lifting the tongue slightly, and opening the airway. It is used in spontaneously breathing patients to assist in maintaining a patent airway. The airways come in a variety of sizes and lengths, from 17 cm to 20 cm long and from sizes 12 to 36 French. The airway is contraindicated in nasal hemorrhage, for patients on anticoagulant medication, and in the setting of basilar skull fractures. DOT 2-1.37, 2.1-42

Complications include that the airway may stimulate gagging or vomiting. This may be controlled either by removing the airway or by pulling it back out slightly. Also, the nasopharyngeal airway may not completely control the airway, and the patient's head-tilt position (or jaw thrust or lifting of the chin) may require adjustment. Finally, a distinct advantage to this airway is that bag-mask ventilation can usually be accomplished easily with this airway in place.

Supplemental Oxygen Administration

Oxygen Cylinders

Oxygen cylinders must be handled and stored carefully. The gas is under tremendous pressure (a full tank has a pressure of over 2000 PSI). Oxygen can explode and is very flammable. The metal tanks can rupture, creating an extremely hazardous situation. The tanks must undergo periodic testing to ensure no hairline cracks have developed in the canisters. DOT 2-1.47

Regulators must be used to reduce the high pressure from the tank to a working pressure that will allow the gas to be delivered to the patient. The regulator has a gauge to identify the liter flow and volume remaining in the tank. Oxygen cylinders and regulators have a special configuration, called a **pin-index system,** which prevents the regulator from another type of gas from being used on an oxygen cylinder. It also prevents oxygen regulators from being used on other types of gas cylinders. This safety system prevents the accidental mixing of the gases which could lead to an explosion or fire. DOT 2-1.48

Oxygen can dry out mucous membranes. A humidification unit can be attached to most regulators to help keep this from happening. Humidification is provided by forcing the oxygen to flow through sterile water. As the oxygen creates bubbles, some of the water is vaporized. The patient inhales this water vapor, and it helps moisten his or her airways. Humidification is not very practical in the prehospital setting for several reasons. Most units are positional, meaning they must be in an upright position or they will spill or get mixed into the

IV tubing. The reservoir for the water is a breeding ground for bacteria, so it must be changed between each patient. DOT 2-1.50

Nonrebreather Mask

A variety of devices allow for the administration of supplemental oxygen. A standard choice is the **nonrebreather mask,** or **NRBM.** This device should be used with an oxygen liter flow between 10/12–15 LPM. This device works best when the patient has a patent airway and a normal, or near normal, respiratory rate and depth. The mask should be fitted to the face, so there is minimal or no leakage around the sides of the mask. The reservoir bag should be observed to determine if the patient has adequate ventilatory rate and depth. The reservoir bag should collapse no more than halfway with each breath. If the patient is collapsing it all the way, consider increasing the liter flow of oxygen, or assess the patient for the need for further airway management. Pulse oximetry and end-tidal CO_2 can also provide helpful information in monitoring the device's effectiveness. The **fraction of inspired air** (or **FIO_2**) that may be delivered by this device is nearly 100%. DOT 2-1.15, 2-1.51

Cannula

The **nasal cannula** allows for a less restrictive delivery of oxygen. The FIO_2 is substantially lower than the NRBM. The liter flow when using the cannula is set between 0.5 and 6 LPM, and the actual flow rates available are limited to what is available via the oxygen tank regulator. Room air contains 21% oxygen (it has an FIO_2 of 21%). A nasal cannula with a 1 LPM oxygen flow rate delivers 24% oxygen. Each additional 1 LPM increases the FIO_2 by 4%, so a 2 LPM flow rate delivers 28% oxygen, and a 3 LPM flow rate delivers 32% oxygen, etc. up to 6 LPM that delivers 44% oxygen. DOT 2-1.15

The American Heart Association research reports that some cardiac patients may benefit from lower flow rates and has included this information in the management of acute coronary syndrome patients (see Chapter 29: Cardiology for more information). Patients with chronic respiratory diseases such as emphysema may also be better managed through the use of nasal cannula oxygen.

Simple Face Mask

The simple face mask is not commonly encountered in the EMS setting. It looks virtually identical to a NRBM, but it does not have a reservoir bag. Also, the openings in the side of the mask are fully open to allow the mixture of room air with the air delivered through the oxygen

tubing. The FIO_2 of simple masks cannot reach much higher than 60%, even when the liter flow rate is 10 or 12 LPM. Flow rates higher than this are unnecessary because the patient is not inspiring fast enough to use the oxygen being delivered at rates greater than 10–12 LPM.

Venturi Mask

The **Venturi Mask** allows for a precise delivery of a set FIO_2 reading. There are a variety of mask styles, but they all have in common the need to assemble the correct pieces or dial in the correct setting to attain the desired oxygen concentration. The Venturi effect is a law from physics that explains gas movement law. It describes how two gasses can be mixed, by introducing one gas into the flow of another, to achieve a precise concentration. The Venturi mask uses this principle to mix room air into the openings in the side of the mask to deliver a precise concentration to the patient. Assembling the equipment is relatively easy as each piece is marked with the liter flow to use from the tank to achieve the desired FIO_2 written on the piece of equipment.

These masks are used by chronically ill patients who require close supervision of their oxygen intake. An emphysema patient, for example, may need a precise balance between continuous oxygen delivery and CO_2 elimination to avoid CO_2 narcosis and apnea. The Venturi Mask will deliver the precise amount of oxygen, as determined by the pulmonologist and physician. The patient most likely will have this equipment in the home. It is acceptable to use the patient's equipment, if your protocols allow this, since this has been prescribed for the patient's use.

Blow-By Oxygen Administration

Blow-by is a method of oxygen delivery that allows the FIO_2 level of the environment immediately surrounding the patient's mouth and nose to be increased without the stress of forcing the patient to wear a mask or cannula. Blow-by is commonly used in infants and children (Figure 12-27), but it can also be used on adults. The precise FIO_2 cannot be calculated when using blow-by, so the patient must be monitored closely. If no improvement is noted and hypoxia is suspected to be the reason the patient is not improving, other measures such as a mask or cannula must be considered.

Flow Restricted Oxygen-Powered Ventilation Device

The flow restricted oxygen-powered ventilation device (FROPVD), formally called the "demand valve," is a device that is attached directly to the regulator on the oxygen cylinder. This device is triggered by depressing a button.

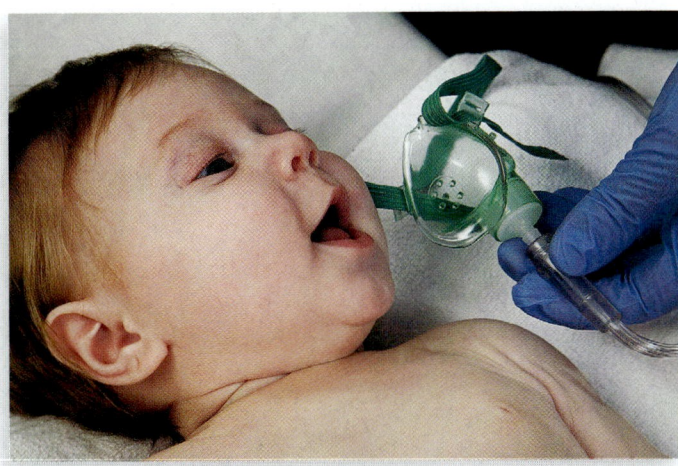

Figure 12-27 When administering blow-by oxygen, it may be helpful to have an assistant or a calm parent hold a mask near a child's face. Scented lip balm can be useful if the child is old enough to understand and desire "flavored oxygen."

Upon triggering the device, oxygen flows out of the device under a pressure of approximately 40 pounds per square inch, or PSI. This pressure provides positive pressure, but the pressure is greatly reduced from earlier models of the device which provided around 110 PSI. The lower pressure device is unlikely to cause pressure-related trauma to the lungs, called **barotrauma.** Even though these de-

vices utilize safer pressures, they can still provide too much positive pressure and cause the same problems as the bag-mask unit. DOT 2-1.43g

Bag-Mask Ventilation

The **bag-mask** is a standard device for assisting ventilation. To be used correctly, it requires training and practice. Its use requires a correct seal of the mask on the airway as well as proper positioning of the patient's airway. Failure to do both of these can result in inadequate ventilation.

The traditional bag-mask technique involves using the weakest part of the hand to lift up the chin and mandible. This is effective in most cases, but even the strongest hands tend to fatigue quickly. Appropriate bag-mask ventilation can be sustained longer and more comfortably if the thumbs are used to position the mask and the remaining four fingers lift the jaw (Figures 12-28 and 12-29). DOT 2-1.43d

Two or three rescuers may perform the bag-mask technique. When two rescuers are performing the technique, one rescuer maintains the airway in an open position by using two hands and the other rescuer can perform a one handed squeeze with one hand and perform the Selleck maneuver with the other, or a third rescuer can perform the Sellick maneuver. Regardless of whether one hand or two are used to squeeze the bag-mask, the appropriate volume should be delivered. The

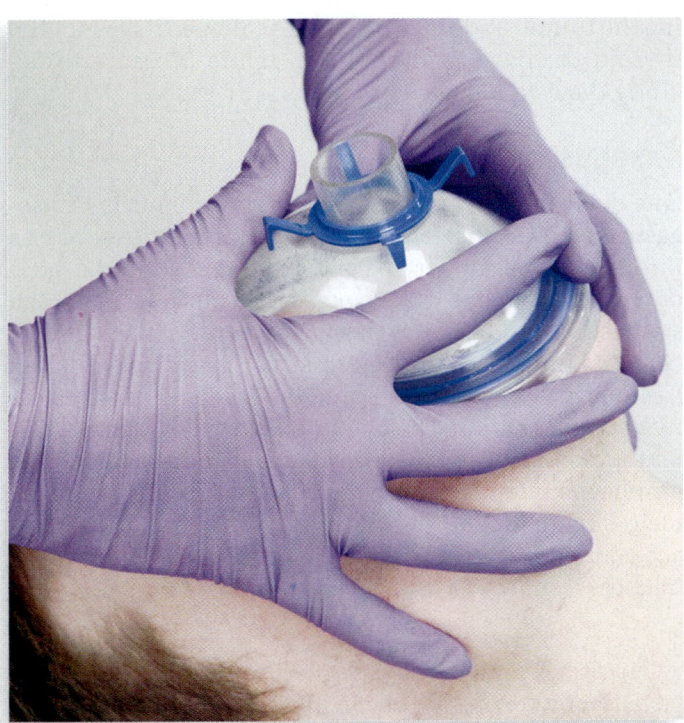

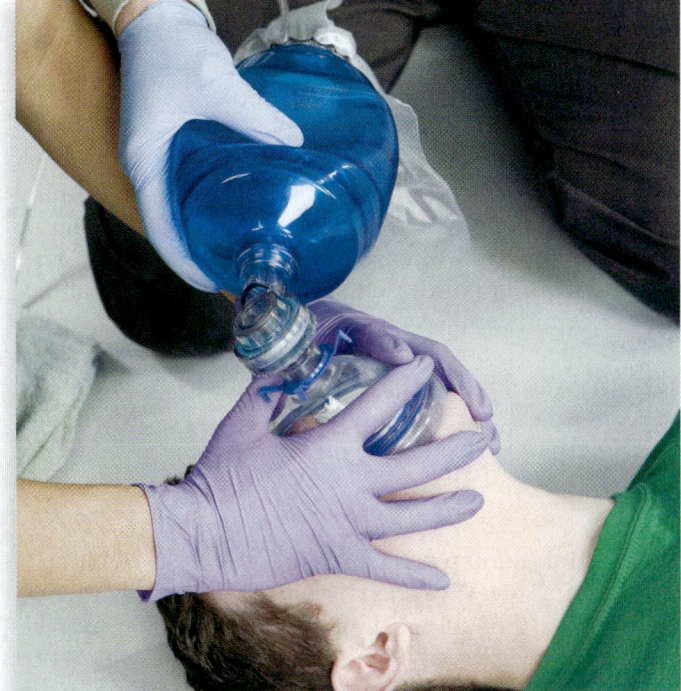

Figure 12-28 Demonstration of the traditional bag-mask technique. This method uses the weakest part of the hand to lift up the chin and mandible and allows for early fatigue.

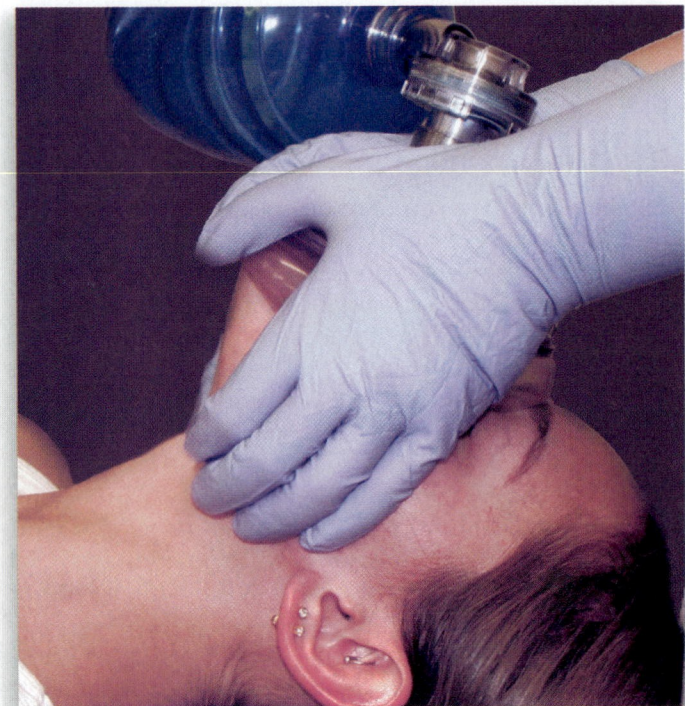
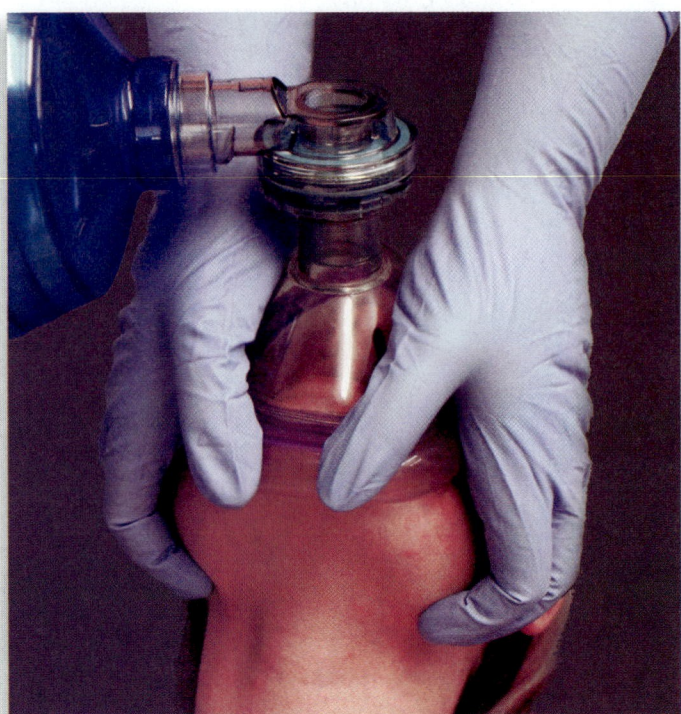

Figure 12-29   Demonstration of the alternate bag-mask ventilation technique, using the thumbs to position the mask and the remaining four fingers to lift the jaw. This method uses the strength of the hands to maintain mask position and is less prone to early fatigue.

squeeze should be rhythmic and slow, and it should stop as soon as the patient's chest begins to rise to avoid over-inflating and causing a positive pressure state within the chest. DOT 2-1.43e, 2-1.43f, 2-1.44

As discussed, the appropriate ventilation rate and volume must be achieved for this device to work properly. Excessive ventilation rates and depths can have a disastrous impact on cardiac output and coronary and cerebral perfusion.

The bag-mask can be used with or without the use of oxygen. In the early moments of resuscitation it may be appropriate to use the bag-mask without oxygen in order to quickly provide one to two breaths. Once an open airway is confirmed, the bag-mask ventilations may continue, and oxygen should be attached as soon as possible. The bag-mask with room air delivers only 21% oxygen. The bag-mask with a 10–15 LPM flow of oxygen, a reservoir bag, and a good mask seal delivers an FIO_2 of 100% oxygen.

Sellick Maneuver

The **Sellick maneuver** should be utilized on patients with altered levels of consciousness requiring assisted ventilation to decrease the amount of air that may be blown into the esophagus and stomach as well as to decrease the risk of vomiting and aspiration. If the Sellick maneuver is used, it should not be stopped until an invasive airway device such as a dual lumen airway, LMA, or ET tube is placed. This technique is not necessary once an ET tube, LMA, or Combitube™ is placed.

The Sellick maneuver should be performed by placing the thumb and finger on the cricoid cartilage, not the thyroid cartilage, and applying gentle pressure to occlude the esophagus. DOT 2-1.28, 2-1.43e, 2-1.43f, 2-1.62

Nasogastric Tubes

One device that is commonly used on patients is a **nasogastric** or **NG tube.** This device enters the nose, passes through the nasopharynx and posterior pharynx, goes down through the esophagus, and continues into the stomach. The NG tube is designed to empty the stomach contents (including air from gastric distension) or to occasionally deliver material into the stomach (such as activated charcoal for poisoned patients or irrigating fluid for the stomach and bowel). The tube passing through the esophagus often causes the esophageal sphincters to remain slightly open. This may allow esophageal or stomach contents to pass up into the hypopharynx and into the trachea, resulting in aspiration.

The rescuer must always be alert to the possibility that a patient with an NG tube in place has an increased risk of aspiration, especially if the patient has an alteration in the level of consciousness. DOT 2-1.39, 2-1.40, 2-1.41

Nice to Know

If the same tube used for NG placement is passed into the stomach via the oropharynx, the device is called an orogastric, or OG tube. The OG tube may trigger a gag reflex more easily than an NG tube. It is typically not used in conscious patients.

Blind Insertion Airway Device

Blind insertion airway devices (BIAD) are placed into the airway without the aid of equipment such as stylets or laryngoscopes. Older versions of these devices included the **esophageal obturator airway (EOA)**, **esophageal gastric tube airway (EGTA)**, and the **pharyngeal tracheal airway (PTL)**. Most of these devices fell out of common use when intubation entered the picture in the 1980s. Because these devices had a single tube (also called a lumen), placement into the trachea instead of the esophagus was potentially deadly when it was not recognized and corrected.

Combitube™

A modern version of these devices, called the **Combitube™**, is designed with more than one lumen (or airway passage), so once the device is placed, auscultation and visual inspection of the rising chest are used to confirm proper placement. In addition to being called a BIAD, the Combitube™ is also classified as a **dual lumen airway device.** DOT 2-1.64

The Combitube™ provides similar advantages to the endotracheal tube: isolation of the airway, reduced risk of aspiration, and more reliable ventilation than bag-mask alone. The advantage of the Combitube™ over endotracheal intubation is related chiefly to the ease of training.[6,25] Ventilation and oxygenation with the Combitube™ are comparable to those achieved with intubation.[26]

The Combitube™ currently comes in two sizes, "small adult" and "regular adult," and is indicated for teenage and adult patients who must have protected airways. The device is indicated only for the unresponsive patient.

Because of the design of the two lumens, it can be placed into either the esophagus or the trachea. Each lumen has its own ventilation port, and once the tube is placed, assisted ventilations can be performed through either tube, as appropriate. About 90% of the time it is used, the device will enter the esophagus, making the blue-colored tube the appropriate one to use initially to confirm placement. Once breath sounds are heard and the appropriate ventilation port is established, the tube

should be secured. Suction should not be performed through the Combitube™, nor should a colorimetric CO_2 detector be used.

Intubation

As previously discussed, the decision to intubate should be based on three essential criteria: (1) failure to maintain or protect the airway, (2) failure of ventilation or oxygenation, and (3) anticipated need for intubation based on the patient's clinical course and likelihood of deterioration.

A trial of bag-mask ventilation is usually appropriate prior to placement of the ET tube. This is particularly true if the primary reason for an altered level of consciousness is due to hypoxia that, if corrected with supplemental ventilation, results in a return to spontaneous consciousness. Cardiac arrest and traumatic brain injuries with a GCS of 8 or less are two instances when intubation is automatically considered as the primary means of airway control, and patient care moves quickly in that direction. Other times intubation is appropriate are not so obvious.

Aggressive application of intubation when it is not warranted is not appropriate patient care. Mastery of the skill is possible, but maintenance of the mastery level is another matter entirely. The endotracheal tube was once considered the "gold standard" for managing the airway during cardiac arrest. It is now clear that the incidence of complications is unacceptably high when intubation is performed by inexperienced providers or there is inadequate monitoring of the tube once it is placed.[16] A recent study showed that one fourth of endotracheal tubes (ETTs) inserted by prehospital personnel in urban EMS systems were misplaced upon confirmation in the hospital setting.[22]

Intubation, as the optimal airway management technique over other techniques such as bag-mask ventilation, has also come under scrutiny. The addition of out-of-hospital endotracheal intubation (ETI) to a paramedic's scope of practice that already included bag-mask ventilation did not improve survival or neurologic outcome of pediatric patients in an urban EMS system.[7] DOT 1-2.57, 1-2.58

There are several approaches to the conventional intubation procedure, including orotracheal, nasotracheal, and digital. Orotracheal intubation involves insertion of the ET tube through the mouth with the aid of a laryngoscope and stylet. Nasotracheal intubation introduces the tube via the nose, and neither the laryngoscope nor stylet is used. Digital intubation is performed by passing the tube over the curved fingers of the gloved hand. This technique is helpful if the patient is entrapped and a standard approach with the laryngo-scope is not possible. A stylet may be used for digital intubation, but a laryngoscope is not. DOT 2-1.63, 2-1.69

Because patients are found in a variety of environments, unconventional approaches are sometimes needed to perform intubation. **In-line manual stabilization of the neck** should be used if the patient is suspected of having cervical trauma. This approach requires additional people to perform the procedure. As one individual is committed to providing in-line stabilization, another may be performing the Sellick's maneuver, another may be operating the bag-mask device, and still another may be inserting the ET tube. **Rapid sequence intubation** is intubation performed with the aid of sedative and paralytic drugs. It is used for patients who need airway control, but their level of consciousness does not allow for a traditional approach. An example is a combative trauma patient with a severe head injury who has an altered mental status. This patient may require sedation in order to provide airway control. An **upright anterior approach** can be used when the patient is trapped in an upright or sitting position. It requires the rescuer to face the patient while holding the laryngoscope in the right hand. The blade is then placed over the tongue from the front, and the mandible is pulled outward and downward. This approach may be necessary when the patient is entrapped and the only real access is from the anterior side of the patient. DOT 2-1.65, 2-1.69

Once the ET tube is passed, tracheal placement must be confirmed. Begin auscultation over the epigastrium and then verify midaxillary breath sounds on the left and right side, in either order. If breath sounds are heard over the epigastrium and not in the midaxillary sites, esophageal intubation must be presumed, and the endotrachael tube should be promptly removed and bag-mask ventilations resumed. Finally, listen over the sternal notch for airflow to determine if the cuff is inflated appropriately. Air flow in this area, following confirmation of breath sounds, indicates leakage around the ET tube, and a few more milliliters of air should be added to the balloon on the cuff. There are several methods of confirming ET tube placement which are listed in Box 12-5.

Aids in Endotracheal Intubation

The **Mallampati classification** is helpful in determining if an airway may be difficult to intubate. The patient is asked to open the mouth as wide as possible and say "Ahhh" while you look to see how much of the uvula, soft palate, and pillars you see. The more tongue and less of the other structures you see, the more difficult the intubation will be (Box 12-6). One obvious drawback to the use of this criterion is that the patient must be conscious and alert enough to

BOX 12-5   Intubation Confirmation Techniques

Primary Techniques

- Observe the ET tube pass through the vocal cords
- See equal chest rise with positive pressure ventilation
- During auscultation, hear no sounds over the epigastrium, and hear equal bilateral breath sounds
- Observe a positive reading on a esophageal detector device
- Note the presence of CO_2 in the exhaled air during capnography

Secondary Techniques

- Note improvement in the pulse oximeter reading, or note that it does not deteriorate if it is greater than 95%
- Note a positive color change on a colorimetric CO_2 detector (turning from purple to tan, light brown, or yellow within six ventilations)
- Note condensation in the ET tube during ventilations
- Note an improvement of skin color and vital signs

BOX 12-6   Mallampati Classification to Predict the Difficulty of Endotracheal Intubation

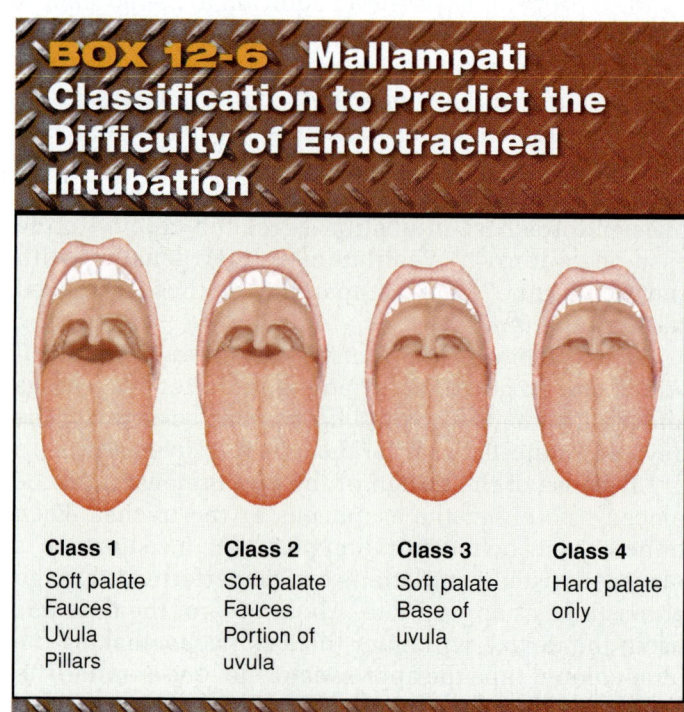

Class 1	Class 2	Class 3	Class 4
Soft palate	Soft palate	Soft palate	Hard palate
Fauces	Fauces	Base of	only
Uvula	Portion of	uvula	
Pillars	uvula		

follow your commands, which probably means the patient is not a candidate for intubation in the prehospital setting. This criteria is helpful in reminding you that airways come in different shapes and sizes and that some are much more difficult to intubate than others. DOT 1-2.61

Gum Elastic Bougie

A useful device during a difficult endotracheal intubation is the **Gum Elastic Bougie** (also known as a Flexguide)® (Figure 12-30).[27] The Bougie can be inserted directly through the vocal cords, and then it serves as a guide wire for ET tube placement. Slide the ET tube, without a stylet, over the Bougie and down into the trachea and then remove the Bougie. The procedure is then completed as normal with confirmation by primary and secondary means.

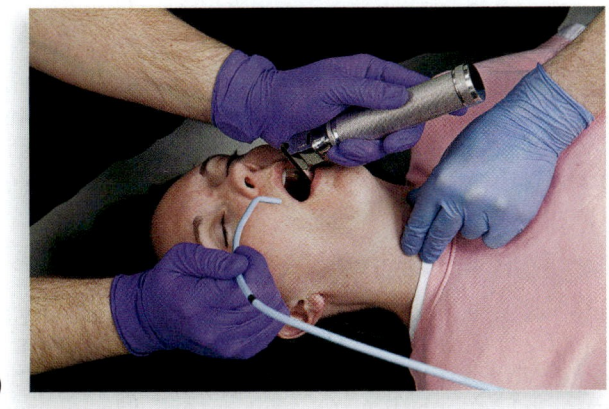

(a)

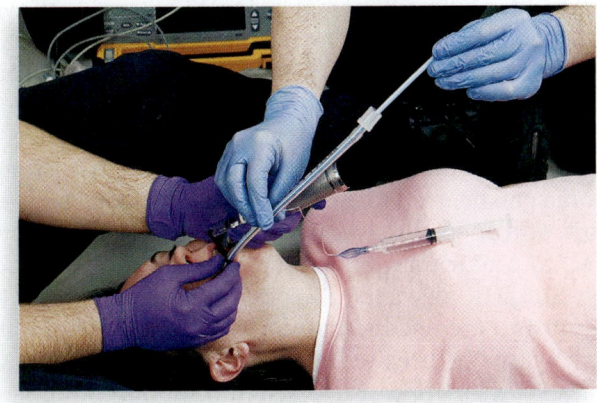

(b)

Figure 12-30 (a) A Flexguide® may be helpful during orotracheal intubation. Once the larynx is visualized, the Flexguide® is passed through the cords. You may be able to feel a "rattle" from the Flexguide® rubbing on the tracheal rings. (b) Once the Flexguide® is in place, an assistant can help thread the endotracheal tube over the guide and into the trachea.

Lighted Stylet

A **lighted stylet** may help illuminate more structures than the light on the ET blade alone.[28] The lightwand has been used successfully for endotracheal intubation and may be especially useful if laryngeal visualization is difficult and there is no evidence of an obstructive lesion of the mouth, pharynx, or larynx.[29]

BURP Maneuver

A common error that occurs during insertion of the laryngoscope blade is that it is inserted too deeply. One technique that avoids this error is to identify the uvula, the epiglottis, and then the arytenoid cartilages as the blade is inserted. If visualization of these structures is difficult, the Sellick maneuver has been the traditional technique to assist in visualization. Recently, however, this procedure has been questioned, and some research studies seem to indicate the procedure may not be as helpful as once thought.[30]

Another option that sometimes aids in visualization is the **BURP maneuver**.[31] The larynx is manually displaced posteriorly (**b**ackward) against the cervical vertebrae, superiorly (**u**pward), and laterally to the right (**r**ightward **p**ressure). This method also has its proponents and detractors.

Finally, **external laryngeal manipulation (ELM)** by the person performing the intubation has also been advocated. In this technique, the intubator moves the trachea into visual position by manipulating the thyroid cartilage. Once good visualization is accomplished, an assistant maintains the position while the primary provider completes the intubation. None of these maneuvers has been shown to be superior to another in the prehospital setting.

Magill Forceps

Magill forceps are a scissor-like device that have a flattened open circle at the tips. The forceps are bent to allow maneuvering inside the mouth. The tip of the forceps can grasp and guide the ET tube or other catheters or tubes inside the mouth.

The forceps can also be used to remove foreign bodies from the glottic opening. Use a laryngoscope to visualize the structures, and then use the Magill forceps to grasp the object and withdraw it from the airway. DOT 2-1.59, 2-1.60

Cut Endotracheal Tube and Meconium Aspirator for Foreign Body Removal

If a foreign body in the airway is lodged past the glottis at the top of the trachea, the Magill forceps may not be able to retrieve it. A cut endotracheal tube attached to a meconium aspirator can be used to try to retrieve the object. The large suction tubing alone is too floppy and cumbersome to try to place into the glottis, but the combination of the meconium aspirator and the ET tube may provide enough stiffness to allow deliberate placement. The combination ET tube and meconium aspirator is also superior to standard suction cathers, even the rigid type, because of the larger size opening on the tube, which may pull the foreign body up into the ET tube.

Laryngeal Mask Airway (LMA)

The **laryngeal mask airway (LMA)** is indicated for assisted ventilation of the patient whose level of conscious is such that a large device in the posterior hypopharynx and supraglottic area can be tolerated. This device comes in several sizes. Unlike the ET tube, this device does not pass through the vocal cords. Instead, it rests over the epiglottis, forming a seal that, if the proper sized device is selected and inserted in the proper location, secures the airway from aspiration.

CPAP/BiPAP

Continuous positive airway pressure, or CPAP, is a procedure used for patients in respiratory insufficiency or failure in order to support ventilations, improve their cardiac and respiratory parameters, and potentially avoid the need to intubate them. In order to apply CPAP, patients must be awake and alert enough to follow commands, have adequate respiratory effort, and have the ability to protect their own airway.[19] Mask CPAP can be applied to various causes of respiratory failure including congestive heart failure, pulmonary edema, COPD, and asthma.

BiPAP is a variation of CPAP. CPAP provides a single level of positive pressure during both inspiration and expiration. Patients in respiratory insufficiency need an adequate level of pressure support during inspiration but a lesser level of pressure to 'stent' the alveoli open on expiration. BiPAP allows the provider to set a separate level of inspiratory positive airway pressure (IPAP) and expiratory positive airway pressure (EPAP). BiPAP machines are more expensive, and there have not been adequate prehospital studies to demonstrate the effectiveness of the device. DOT 5-1.9

Mechanical Ventilators

The bag-mask unit is a manual ventilator. It can provide tidal volume and specific respiratory rates, and with attachments it can also provide positive end expiratory pressure (PEEP). The manual bag-mask has the limits of human operation, and, as discussed throughout this chapter, they can be numerous. If more precise ventilation is required, a mechanical ventilator can be used to provide a fixed tidal volume, respiratory rate, and PEEP.

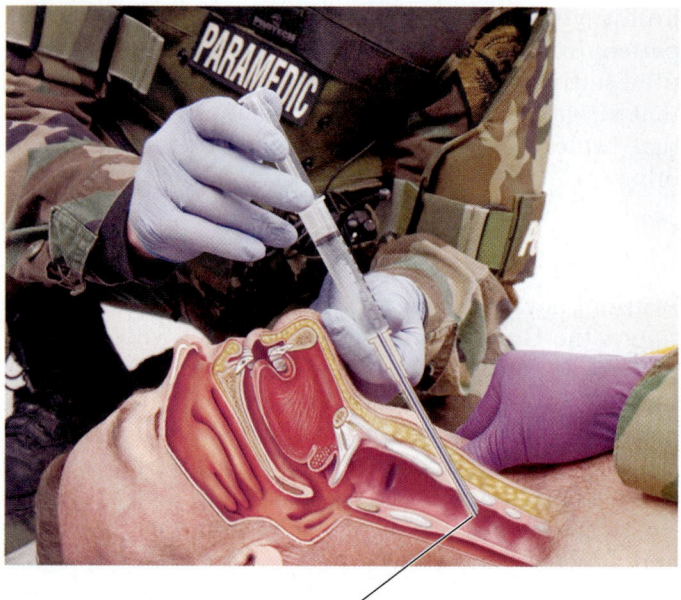

Bevel should face up

Figure 12-31 Needle cricothyrotomy cannula properly placed in trachea.

These devices typically require the patient be intubated or to have a surgical airway such as a tracheostomy in place. These devices are commonly used during critical care intrafacility transports. DOT 2-1.46

Surgical Airways

Surgical airways include **needle cricothyrotomy** (Figure 12-31) and **surgical cricothyrotomy.** The needle cricothyrotomy may be used along with a translaryngeal jet insufflation unit to provide emergency ventilation. The surgical cricothyrotomy allows for the placement of a tracheal tube or provides the means for direct insertion of an endotracheal tube into the trachea. DOT 2-1.72

The surgical opening created in the cricothyroid membrane during the procedure is called a **stoma.** A stoma can be used to ventilate a patient with a bag-mask unit, and special masks can be placed over the stoma as well to provide supplemental oxygen. DOT 1-2.52, 1-2.54

Surgical airways are considered a last resort technique and are used to bypass a problem with the upper airway that is threatening the life of the patient. A surgical airway is appropriate when a foreign body is completely obstructing the glottis, and it cannot be removed with abdominal thrusts or Magill forceps. A surgical airway may be indicated when a patient has severe trauma to the airway, such as with a gunshot wound destroying most of the mandible and soft tissues of the upper airway. In both of these extreme situations, a surgical airway may be the only means to provide oxygen to the patient. DOT 2-1.70, 2-1.71

Summary

This discussion of the movement of air through a patient's body has carefully linked the airway with the circulation of blood because the functioning of these two components is inseparable, so as the rescuer approaches the patient in respiratory distress and finds cyanosis and distended neck veins, the initial approach of giving oxygen and being prepared to assist ventilations is straightforward. However, finding the reason for the cyanosis and distended neck veins, whether it is a tension pneumothorax or advanced pulmonary hypertension due to emphysema, is a challenge.

This work calls for excellence in patient assessment. Patient surveys must be careful and thorough. If the rescuer does not look for distended neck veins during the assessment, then cardiac tamponade or congestive heart failure will probably be missed. If the paramedic does not make "skin color" assessment a part of every single survey, every single time, then the presence of partial airway obstruction might be missed in the unconscious patient.

Paramedics must think carefully which airway adjunct or device is appropriate for each patient encounter. A "one approach fits all" philosophy is not appropriate as patients have varying needs. The "gold standard" should not be providing intubation to secure the airway; the gold standard should be performing an appropriate assessment and determining which airway management approach is appropriate for each individual patient encounter.

The paramedic must understand the processes of ventilation and perfusion and the gasses being circulated around the body. It is critical to understand the relationship created between exhaled CO_2 and the status of a patient's circulation. Monitoring CO_2 levels on an intubated patient is a mandatory procedure and should become as routine as monitoring the vital signs and pulse oximetry. It is mandatory, when CO_2 levels begin dropping in an intubated patient, that the rescuer understand that the patient's circulatory status is worsening and mount an aggressive response to identify and correct the problem.

Airway management is comprised of a series of separate skills that, on the surface, appear not too difficult to master. However, true mastery of airway management lies in understanding of how to use the skills to the greatest benefit of the patient.

Notes

1. H. Wang, D. Kupas, M. Greenwood, et al., "An Algorithmic Approach to Prehospital Airway Management," *Prehospital Emergency Care* 9(2005): 145–155.
2. M. J. Pollock, L. H. Brown, and K. A. Dunn, "The Perceived Importance of Paramedic Skills and the Emphasis They Receive During EMS Education Programs," *Prehospital Emergency Care* 1(1997): 263–8.
3. United States Department of Transportation, National Highway Traffic Safety Administration, "Paramedic National Standard Curriculum, 1998," http://www.nhtsa.dot.gov/people/injury/ems/EMT-P/ (accessed February 25, 2006).
4. D. Vrocher and L. Hopson, "Basic Airway Management and Decision-Making," in *Roberts: Clinical Procedures in Emergency Medicine,* 4th ed. (Philadelphia: W. B. Saunders, 2004).
5. R. M. Walls, "Airway in Rosen's Emergency Medicine," in *Concepts and Clinical Practice,* J. A. Marx, R. S. Hockberger, R. M. Walls, et al., eds., 6th ed. (Philadelphia: Mosby Elsevier, 2006).
6. V. Dörges, V. Wenzel, P. Knacke, and K. Gerlach, "Comparison of Different Airway Management Strategies to Ventilate Apneic, Nonpreoxygenated Patients," *Critical Care Medicine* 31(3)(2003): 800–4.
7. M. Gausche, R. J. Lewis, S. J. Stratton, B. E. Haynes, C. S. Gunter, S. M. Goodrich, P. D. Poore, M. D. McCollough, D. P. Henderson, F. D. Pratt, J. S. Seidel, "Effect of Out-of-Hospital Pediatric Endotracheal Intubation on Survival and Neurological Outcome: a Controlled Clinical Trial," *JAMA* 283(2000): 783–790.
8. G. Margolis, *Paramedic Airway Management* (Sudbury, MA: Jones and Bartlett, 2004).
9. G. E. Morgan, M. S. Mikhail, and M. J. Murray, *Lange Clinical Anesthesiology,* 4th ed. (McGraw-Hill's AccessMedicine Online, 2006) (accessed June 16, 2006).
10. T. P. Aufderheide, Presentation, National Institutes of Health Resuscitation Outcomes Consortium, Chicago, IL, March, 2005.
11. National Institutes of Health Resuscitation Outcomes Consortium, 2004 to present.
12. T. P. Aufderheide and K. G. Lurie, "Death by Hyperventilation: A Common and Life-Threatening Problem During Cardiopulmonary Resuscitation," *Critical Care Medicine* 32(9 Suppl) (September 2004): S345–351.
13. T. P. Aufderheide et al., "Hyperventilation–Induced Hypotension During Cardiopulmonary Resuscitation," *Circulation* 109(16) (April 27, 2004): 1960–1965.
14. K. G. Lurie, T. Zielinski, et al., "Use of an Inspiratory Impedance Valve Improves Neurologically Intact Survival in a Porcine Model of Ventricular Fibrillation," *Circulation* 105(1) (January 1, 2002): 124–129.
15. A. Gabrielli, A. H. Idris, et al., "Alternative Ventilation Strategies in Cardiopulmonary Resuscitation," *Current Opinions in Critical Care* 8(3) (June 2002): 199–211.
16. "2005 American Heart Association Guidelines for CPR and ECC," *Circulation* (Supplement) 112(24) (December 13, 2005).
17. G. E. Morgan, Jr., M. S. Mikhail, and M. J. Murray, *Clinical Anesthesiology,* 4th ed., McGraw-Hill's AccessMedicine (accessed July 11, 2006).
18. SIMS BCI, Inc., *Capnograph Operation Manual,* Catalog Number 1894 (February 2000) p. 5–1.
19. J. Roberts, *Clinical Procedures in Emergency Medicine,* 4th ed. (St. Louis, MO: Elsevier, 2004). http://www.mdconsult.com (accessed July 15, 2005).
20. D. F. Danzl and R. J. Vissers, Chapter 19: Tracheal Intubation and Mechanical Ventilation. In J. E. Tintinalli, G. D. Kelen, J. S. Stapczyski (eds.), *Emergency Medicine:* A Comprehensive Study Guide, 6th ed. New York: McGraw-Hill, 2004, pp 108–118.
21. American Heart Association, "International Liaison Committee on Resuscitation," *Guidelines* 102(2000): 1100–1104.
22. S. H. Katz, and J. L. Falk, "Misplaced Endotracheal Tubes by Paramedics in an Urban Emergency Medical Services System," *Annals of Emergency Medicine* 37(2001): 32–37.
23. S. Silvestri, G. A. Ralls, B. Krauss, J. Thundiyil, S. G. Rothrock, A. Senn, E. Carter, and J. Falk, "The Effectiveness of Out-of-Hospital Use of Continuous End-Tidal Carbon Dioxide

Monitoring on the Rate of Unrecognized Misplaced Intubation Within a Regional Emergency Medical Services System," *Annals of Emergency Medicine* 45(2005): 497–503.

24. R. E. O'Connor and R. A. Swor, "Verification of Endotracheal Tube Placement Following Intubation," *Prehospital Emergency Care* 3(3)(1999): 248–250.

25. D. P. Lefrancois and D. G. Dufour, "Use of the Esophageal Tracheal Combitube by Basic Emergency Medical Technicians," *Resuscitation* 52(2002): 77–83.

26. K. Tanigawa and A. Shigematsu, "Choice of Airway Devices for 12,020 Cases of Nontraumatic Cardiac Arrest in Japan," *Prehospital Emergency Care* 2 (1998): 96–100.

27. P. Jabre, "Use of gum elastic bougie for prehospital difficult intubation," *American Journal of Emergency Medicine* 23(4) (July 1, 2005): 552–555.

28. L. Davis, S. D. Cook-Sather, and M. S. Schreiner, "Lighted Stylet Tracheal Intubation: A Review," *Anesthesia Analgesia* 90(2000): 745–756.

29. F. R. Weis and M. N. Hatton, "Intubation by Use of the Light Wand: Experience in 253 Patients," *Journal of Oral Maxillofacial Surgery* 47(1989): 577–580.

30. J. L. Benumof, "Difficult Laryngoscopy: Obtaining the Best View," *Canadian Journal of Anaesthesiology* 41(1994): 361–365.

31. R. L. Knill, "Difficult Laryngoscopy Made Easy with a 'BURP'", *Canadian Journal of Anaesthesiology* 40(1993): 798–799.

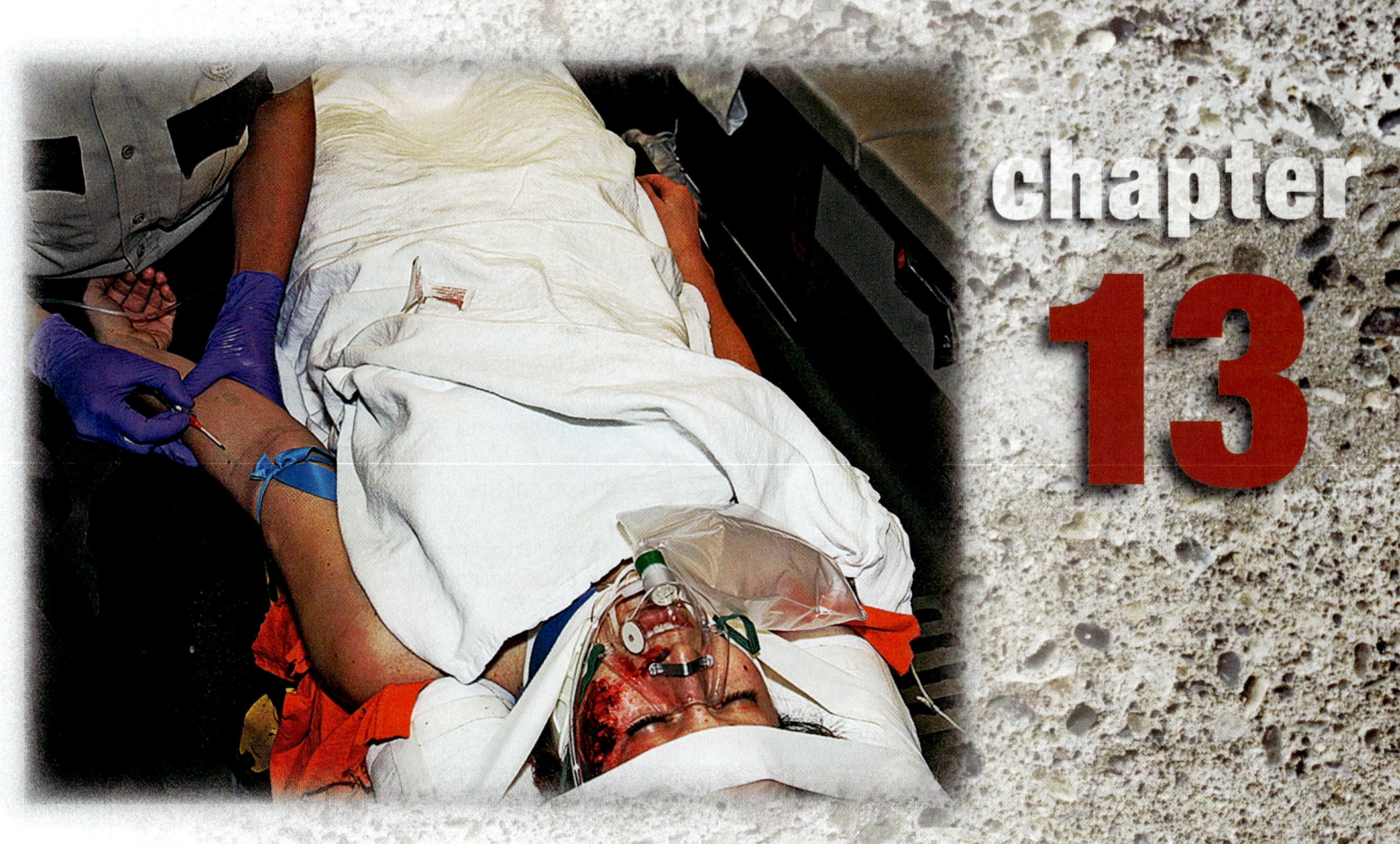

Shock Overview

"Shock is a rude unhinging of the machinery of life."

—Samuel Gross, MD

Need To Know

▶ Shock is a state of inadequate tissue perfusion with reduced amounts of oxygen and glucose being delivered to the body's cells and tissues.

▶ Shock can have high mortality rates and requires rapid intervention.

▶ An intact and functioning heart, circulatory system, and adequate blood volume with the appropriate amount of oxygen and nutrients are required for homeostasis.

▶ Aerobic metabolism is normal. Anaerobic metabolism is not, and it leads to the production of lactic acid and the buildup of wastes in the blood that result in acidosis, organ impairment, organ failure, and eventually death, if untreated.

▶ The sympathetic, parasympathetic, and endocrine systems exert control over the heart and blood vessels.

▶ Shock progresses through three stages: compensated, decompensated, and irreversible.

▶ The patient presentation (signs and symptoms) for shock has some common patterns, but not all patients present with these signs and symptoms, and normal appearing vital signs do not rule out the presence of shock.

▶ Prehospital treatment for shock focuses on airway management (through oxygen administration and ventilation support); hemodynamic support (through controlling additional fluid loss and carefully replacing lost fluid); and rapid transport to the hospital.

▶ Sick	▶ Not Yet Sick
• Watch for the following signs: ill appearance, pale skin, diaphoresis, tachycardia, tachypnea, and signs of poor perfusion, including altered mental status, weak pulses, poor capillary refill, cool mottled skin, and oliguria (i.e., decreased urine output). When these are present, shock is obvious. • The skin of a patient with hypovolemic or cardiogenic shock is often cool, pale, and mottled. • The skin of a patient with distributive shock is often warm and moist. • Progressive bradycardia is an ominous sign and often signals that cardiovascular collapse or arrest is coming. • Patients with unexplained tachypnea should be assumed to be in shock. • Some studies show that hypotension seems to result in higher rates of mortality for hospitalized patients. • Rapid recognition of shock requires immediate integration of the focused history, physical examination, and vital signs.	• Although the incidence of shock is thought to be high, the actual incidence is not actually known. Paramedics should remain suspicious for shock in all patients, regardless of how sick they appear. • The patient may have no obvious etiology (reason) to suggest shock, unless it is caused by trauma. • Vital sign alternations considered "classic" for shock, specifically tachycardia, may or may not be present. If the situation leads you to believe shock is present, take the appropriate steps to ensure it does not worsen. • Pediatric and geriatric patients do not respond to shock in the same manner as adults. • Ask patients what medications they are taking. Remember that some medications regulate electrical and mechanical cardiac function, control fluid volume, or regulate the constriction/dilation of the vascular system, and each of these functions impacts upon the vital signs. • Continuously monitor the patient and be alert for subtle shifts in the vital signs that can signal changes in the patient status.

Introduction

Shock, or **hypoperfusion,** is a common clinical problem encountered by paramedics. It requires rapid recognition and appropriate treatment. Although the incidence of shock is thought to be relatively high, the actual incidence is unknown. It is rarely listed as the primary hospital diagnosis and is commonly hidden among other admission and discharge diagnoses in the medical record. Shock accounts for approximately 1 million emergency department (ED) visits each year and results in an overall mortality rate in excess of 20%.[1] Estimated mortality rates for specific types of shock range from 20% to 90%, and depend primarily on the population studied and the type and severity of the shock state. DOT 4-2.1

Some types of shock have very high mortality rates. For example, approximately 60–90% of the patients who have cardiogenic shock and 30–40% of those with septic shock die within one month of the onset of shock.[2] In addition, the incidence of specific forms of shock (e.g., septic shock) has dramatically increased over the past three decades.[3,4,5,6] DOT 1-6.10, 4-2.16

While **homeostasis** is the normal and dynamic steady state, shock represents a severe disruption in that steady state. It is a complex physiologic process that disrupts cellular metabolism. Shock causes widespread tissue hypoperfusion (i.e., decreased blood flow), resulting in an inability to deliver oxygen and glucose to cells needed to sustain aerobic metabolism (Figure 13-1), thus resulting in decreased venous oxygen levels and metabolic acidosis. If left untreated, shock will proceed to widespread cellular injury, multiple organ dysfunction, organ failure, and then death. As a person remains in an uncorrected shock state, more oxygen is taken from the circulating blood, resulting in a state of "oxygen debt"; the worse the state of oxygen debt, the greater the mortality.[2] DOT 1-6.26, 4-2.15

Every organ, tissue, and system in the body is capable of entering into a shock state. With that in mind, the manner in which shock can be described can take many forms. One of the more common methods of describing shock is to discuss it in terms of the etiology, or cause, of the shock.

Rapid identification and resuscitation of patients in shock is aimed at reversing the cause and normalizing tissue blood flow to improve oxygenation and glucose delivery to cells to prevent morbidity and mortality. The general approach to all patients in the initial stages of shock follows similar principles regardless of the actual cause of the shock. The goal is to preserve the airway, breathing, and circulation; perform appropriate resuscitative measures; and transport the patient quickly to definitive care in the emergency department, trauma center, or other appropriate destination.

Building upon the classic ABCs of EMS resuscitation, shock can be thought of as having a management strategy of **ABCDE**: A = *A*irway, B = *B*reathing, C = optimizing the *C*irculation, D = assuring adequate oxygen *D*elivery, and E = achieving the *E*nd points of a successful resuscitation. The normal end points in resuscitation from shock, as measured in the field setting, are normal blood pressure, heart rate, and urine output, when available, for the patient.[2]

Chapter 8: Physiology Overview discussed basic physiology of the body and described how a body can be in and out of balance. The balance of the body is a delicate thing; when one component is out of balance, it can easily cause other parts of metabolism and regulation to tip out of balance as well. Shock is an example of the body out of balance. The three components required for perfusion include a functioning pump (the heart), an appropriately sized container (the vascular system), and an adequate circulating blood volume with red blood cells capable of carrying oxygen and removing wastes. When one of these three mechanisms fails, either another must compensate or the shock worsens. As you read the overviews of each type of shock, ask yourself, "What part of the perfusion mechanism is out of balance?" and "What must be done to bring the body back into balance?" This will help you understand what is going on and how to correct it. **The following Skill Sheets accompany this chapter: Skill Sheet 42 and Step-by-Step 42: Intravenous Access; Skill Sheet 66 and Step-by-Step 66: Bleeding Control and Shock; Skill Sheet 94: NREMT Bleeding Control/Shock Management.**

Classification of Shock

Shock can be classified into five categories: DOT 1-6.11

1. Hypovolemic shock: due to inadequate circulating blood volume.
2. Distributive shock: due to peripheral vasodilation and maldistribution of blood flow.
3. Cardiogenic shock: due to inadequate cardiac pump function.
4. Obstructive shock: due to non-cardiac obstruction to blood flow.
5. Metabolic shock: due to toxic disruption of cellular function.

Common examples within each category are listed in Table 13-1.

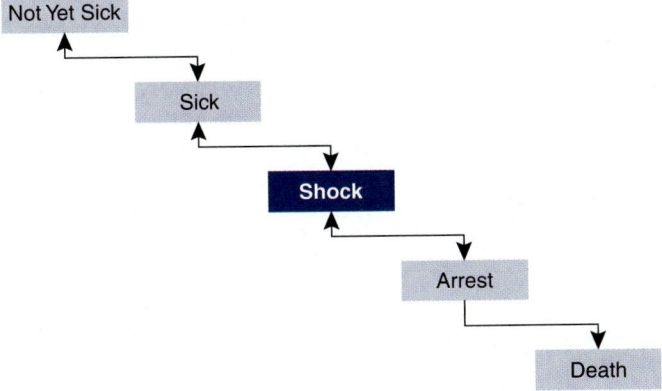

Figure 13-1 Transition states between life and death. Shock is a critical vulnerable state that, if left untreated, will progress to cardiac arrest and death.

TABLE 13-1 Categories and Etiologies of Shock

Category	Etiology
Hypovolemic shock	
Hemorrhagic	Trauma
	Gastrointestinal bleeding
	Vaginal bleeding
	Ruptured abdominal aortic aneurysm
Nonhemorrhagic	Gastrointestinal losses (e.g., vomiting and diarrhea)
	Insensible losses (e.g., burns)
	Sequestration (e.g., ascites)
Distributive shock	Sepsis
	Anaphylaxis
	Spinal cord injury
	Toxic shock syndrome
Cardiogenic shock	Acute myocardial infarction
	Dysrhythmias (e.g., ventricular tachycardia or atrial fibrillation)
	Overdose (e.g., beta-blocker or calcium channel-blocker)
Obstructive shock	Pulmonary embolism
	Cardiac tamponade
Metabolic shock	Carbon monoxide poisoning
	Hydrogen cyanide poisoning
	Hydrogen sulfide poisoning

Hypovolemic Shock

Hypovolemic shock is defined as widespread hypoperfusion resulting from decreased intravascular (blood) volume. This relatively common form of shock is often further subcategorized into **hemorrhagic** and **nonhemorrhagic** groups. DOT 4-2.4

The most common forms of hemorrhage-induced hypovolemic shock are due to trauma. Common causes of nontrauma related hemorrhagic shock include gastrointestinal bleeding, ruptured abdominal aortic aneurysms, and vaginal bleeding (particularly with a ruptured ectopic pregnancy). Nonhemorrhagic forms of hypovolemic shock include gastrointestinal losses from vomiting or diarrhea, insensible losses (e.g, fever in an infant or a prolonged, increased respiratory rate), and **sequestration,** or **"third spacing"** of fluids. Third spacing occurs as fluid leaves the intravascular space and moves into extravascular tissues causing edema. An example of third spacing is seen in patients with a swollen abdomen from leakage of fluid into the peritoneal space. This condition, called ascites, can occur in patents with cirrhosis of the liver and other diseases. DOT 4-2.3

CONNECTIONS Hemorrhagic shock is discussed in more detail in Chapter 19: Trauma and Hemorrhagic Shock. Chapter 29: Cardiology; 31: Endocrine, Electrolytes, and Acid/Base; 34: Gastroenterology; and 41: Obstetrics and Gynecology will also discuss shock.

Distributive Shock

Distributive shock is defined as widespread hypoperfusion due to a *relative* reduction in intravascular volume. The reduction is relative because there is no acute blood loss or fluid loss to account for the hypoperfusion. Instead, it results from peripheral vasodilation and redistribution of circulating blood from the intravascular space into other tissues of the body.[7] Peripheral vasodilation on its own could account for hypotension, but when that is combined with a redistribution of fluid from the vascular space as well, the hypoperfusion can be profound. The most common forms of distributive shock include sepsis, anaphylaxis, central neurogenic (e.g., spinal shock), and toxin-mediated (e.g., toxic shock syndrome). Distributive shock is the final common pathway for most forms of shock:[6] In other words, if any state of shock is untreated, it can degenerate ultimately into distributive shock as fluid leaves the vascular space and the vascular container enlarges from vasodilation.

CONNECTIONS Distributive shock will be discussed in more detail in Chapter 23: Spinal Trauma, 30: Neurology, 32: Allergies and Anaphylaxis, 33: Infectious and Communicable Diseases, and 35: Toxicology.

Cardiogenic Shock

Cardiogenic shock is defined as impaired cardiac output that results in widespread hypoperfusion in the setting of adequate intravascular volume.[5] This form of shock is generally associated with loss of function of more than 40% of the heart's muscle, particularly the left ventricle.[8] Common etiologies include acute myocardial infarction and dysrhythmias. The average time from the occurrence of the acute myocardial infarction to the onset of cardiogenic shock is eight hours.[5] DOT 5-2.112

CONNECTIONS Chapter 29: Cardiology will cover cardiogenic shock in detail.

Obstructive Shock

Obstructive shock is defined as widespread hypoperfusion that results from a condition that obstructs forward blood flow from the heart. Notable examples of this form of shock include pulmonary embolism (in which a large blood clot obstructs blood flow from the heart to the lungs) and cardiac tamponade (in which fluid, commonly blood, accumulates between the heart and the pericardium and reduces blood flow through the heart). Approximately 10% of patients with an acute pulmonary embolism will develop unstable vital signs and will die within the first hour of the event.[9] The most common etiologies of cardiac tamponade include penetrating chest trauma, cardiac rupture from blunt trauma or a massive myocardial infarction, or effusion (fluid collecting from infections).[10]

CONNECTIONS Chapter 21: Thoracic Trauma, 28: Pulmonary, and 29: Cardiology will cover obstructive shock in more detail.

Metabolic Shock

Metabolic shock occurs when poisons interfere with the cells' use of oxygen. Examples of this type of shock include hydrogen cyanide poisoning, hydrogen sulfide poisoning, and carbon monoxide poisoning.[11,12,13] Tissue hypoxia results in all three of these conditions, and metabolism is diverted into anaerobic pathways, leading to the production of lactic acid causing metabolic acidosis. Organ impairment and failure rapidly ensues if the problem is left untreated.

CONNECTIONS Chapter 35: Toxicology will discuss metabolic shock in more detail.

Pathophysiology of Shock

The Body in Balance: What Is Normal?

Normal circulatory function depends on three components: (1) adequate cardiac function (the "pump"); (2) appropriate vascular tone (the "container"); and (3) adequate blood volume (the "fluid"). When one or more of these components fails, shock ensues. **Blood pressure (BP)** is the product of **cardiac output (CO)** and **systemic vascular resistance (SVR)**. SVR is also called **afterload.** Cardiac output is the product of heart rate (HR) and left ventricular stroke volume. **Stroke volume (SV)** is the amount of blood pumped with each contraction of the left ventricle. The quantity of the stroke volume is a function of intravascular volume (preload), systemic vascular resistance (afterload), and myocardial contractility.[14] DOT 4-2.17

Memorize these equations:

$$CO = HR \times SV \text{ and } BP = CO \times SVR$$

CONNECTIONS If these concepts are not clear to you, please review Chapter 8: Physiology Overview.

Cardiac output and vascular tone (two of the three principal determinants of circulatory function and tissue blood flow) are influenced primarily by the combined effects of the sympathetic and parasympathetic nervous systems and the endocrine system.[15] Vascular tone describes the relative degree to which the size of the vascular system is appropriate to maintain blood pressure within the normal range. If the vascular tone is excessive, the vascular system is constricted too much and hypertension may occur; if the vascular tone is low, then the vascular system is excessively dilated and hypotension may develop.

Sympathetic and Parasympathetic Nervous System Balance

The sympathetic and parasympathetic nervous systems are continually active and in general function to balance each other. The degree to which one of the nervous systems functions over the other varies and depends on the clinical condition of the person. In the setting of shock, the sympathetic nervous system dramatically overrides the parasympathetic nervous system in order to help compensate for circulatory impairment. In this setting, the sympathetic nervous system increases the heart's rate and its contractility and causes arterial vasoconstriction in an effort to maintain blood flow to vital organs.[15]

The Body Out of Balance

At the whole-body level, shock induces a series of physiologic responses designed to compensate for inadequate blood flow to tissues. These responses are aimed at maintaining or normalizing blood flow to vital organs in order to maximize the use of oxygen and glucose.

The Initial Nervous System Response

Complex neural (nervous system mediated) and hormonal responses to shock result from decreased arterial wall tension (due to decreased blood flow through arteries). The result of this is stimulation of sensors called baroreceptors, which activate the sympathetic nervous system by stimulation of the **hypothalamic-pituitary-adrenomedullary (HPA) axis** (Figure 13-2). Sympathetic nervous system activation results in an increased heart rate, cardiac contractility, and contraction of peripheral arterioles, resulting in increased systemic vascular resistance. Activation of the HPA axis results in the release of catecholamines (e.g., dopamine, epinephrine, and norepinephrine) from the adrenal medulla, release of

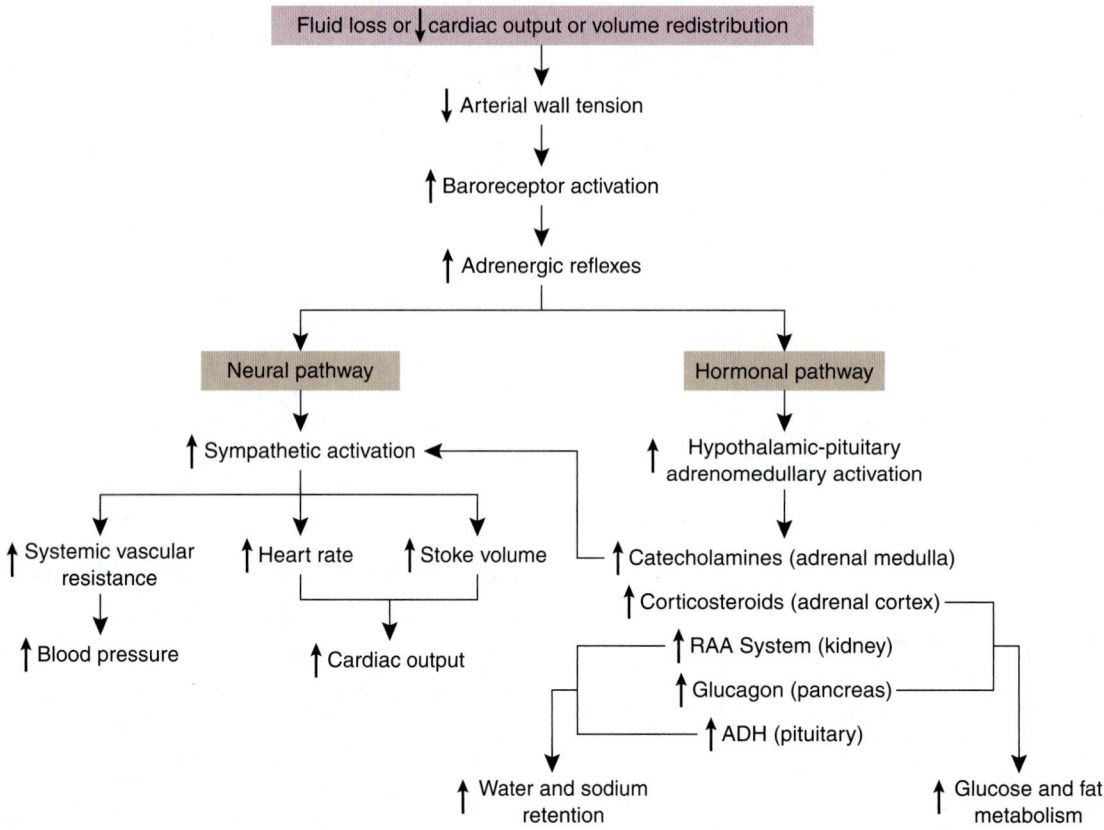

Figure 13-2   Compensatory physiologic mechanisms associated with the shock syndrome [RAA = Renin-Angiotensin-Aldosterone; ADH = Antidiuretic Hormone].

corticosteroids (e.g., aldosterone and cortisol) from the adrenal cortex, release of renin from the kidneys, and the release of glucagon from the pancreas. Catecholamines bind to α- and β-adrenergic receptors and increase cardiac output by increasing heart rate and cardiac contractility (β effects) and blood pressure by increasing vascular smooth muscle contractility (α effects). All of these hormones attempt to compensate for widespread inadequate blood flow by increasing cardiac output, vascular resistance, water retention, and glucose metabolism.[2]

CONNECTIONS   Chapters 8: Physiology Overview and 30: Neurology discuss the nervous system response to illness and injury in more detail.

The Respiratory System Response

The sympathetic nervous system also triggers an increase in respiratory rate. In most circumstances, this results in a decreased tidal volume and increased dead space and overall minute ventilation.[16] The tidal volume is the amount of air drawn into the lungs with each breath. The dead space is the amount of air that is found within the lungs that does not reach the alveoli for gas exchange to take place. Minute ventilation is obtained by multiplying the tidal volume (minus the dead space volume)

times the respiratory rate. The relative hypoxia and subsequent tachypnea result in respiratory alkalosis.

CONNECTIONS   Chapter 28: Pulmonary, and Figure 28-4, page 568, have a complete discussion of all respiratory volumes and capacities.

The Urinary System Response

Aldosterone functions primarily at the level of the renal tubules in the kidney and increases sodium absorption and potassium excretion. This reabsorption induces a comparable osmotic reabsorption of water, thus effectively increasing intravascular volume. Cortisol, another hormone released by the adrenal cortex, is regulated primarily by the hypothalamus and pituitary gland. Cortisol primarily affects carbohydrate, protein, and fat metabolism with the objective of improving nutrient storage and supply to tissues.

Renin-Angiotensin-Aldosterone System

Renin is released from the kidneys and functions as an enzyme that converts angiotensinogen (a protein circulating in the blood) to angiotensin I. Angiotensin I is then converted by another enzyme, angiotensin converting enzyme (ACE), located on the walls of blood vessels, to angiotensin II. This **renin-angiotensin-aldosterone system** plays an important role in maintaining adequate blood volume, blood pressure, and cardiac and vascular function. Angiotensin II has several important physiologic properties including the following: (1) direct vasoconstriction of blood vessels, thus increasing arterial pressures; (2) release of aldosterone from the adrenal cortex, which acts on the kidneys to increase sodium and water retention; and (3) release of vasopressin (also known as antidiuretic hormone or ADH) from the pituitary gland, which acts on the kidneys to increase water retention.

The Endocrine System Response

Glucagon is released from the pancreas and serves to increase blood glucose concentrations (an effect which is exactly opposite to that of insulin). This provides additional nutrient support to tissues. This is particularly important for the brain and heart. These organs have high energy demands, and their energy reserves are low. They are critically dependant upon a continual supply of oxygen and nutrients such as glucose. Neither organ tolerates ischemia very well. When blood pressure falls below 60 mmHg, blood flow to these organs falls and their function deteriorates quickly.[16]

Systemic Inflammatory Response Syndrome (SIRS)

The final unifying feature of all types of shock is the development of **systemic inflammatory response syndrome (SIRS)**.[17] SIRS is the early stage of septic shock. It is characterized by release of proteins into the blood by white blood cells. These proteins are known as cytokines. Examples of cytokines include tumor necrosis factor (TNF)-α, interleukin (IL)-1β, IL-6, IL-8, and IL-10.

This inflammatory process also involves activation of the clotting cascade with the development of disseminated intravascular coagulation (DIC), release of potent chemicals that cause vasoconstriction and vasodilation, and activation of neutrophils (a type of white blood cell).[18,19] High cytokine concentrations result in myocardial dysfunction, altered cellular oxygen utilization, and direct inflammatory injury to the heart and vasculature.[19] In addition, activation of neutrophils promotes their adhering (sticking) to blood vessel walls and triggers the release of toxic reactive oxygen species (free radicals) and proteolytic (protein destroying) enzymes that further damage cells and organs.[20]

Shock at the Cellular Level

At the subcellular level, shock primarily affects the function of mitochondria. Mitochondria are intracellular organelles that serve as the metabolic workhorse for all cells by converting oxygen, glucose, fatty acids, and some amino acids into adenosine triphosphate (ATP),

which is the principal form of energy for all cells.[21] Cells rely on the hydrolysis of ATP for energy. Hydrolysis involves the splitting of the bonds holding ATP together and adding a water molecule. This process allows the released energy to be transferred into other forms to do the work of the cell.

When blood flow is reduced in the setting of shock, mitochondria shift the production of ATP from an oxygen-dependent aerobic process to an oxygen-independent anaerobic process which is not as efficient. Anaerobic metabolism produces ATP at a rate of 5% to 10% of normal and additionally results in the overproduction of the waste product lactic acid.[21] As lactic acid concentrations rise in the cells, the lactate diffuses across cell walls and into the blood, resulting in increased systemic acidosis.[22] DOT 1-6.29

The alterations associated with anaerobic metabolism and lactic acidosis will result in organ impairment if left untreated. Organ impairment is followed by organ failure and death. Unless the underlying problem causing shock results in rapid death, shock tends to evolve sequentially through the following three physiologic stages:[23]

1. **Compensated**
2. **Decompensated**
3. **Irreversible**

The clinical signs and symptoms for varying levels of shock severity are presented in Table 13-2. DOT 4-2.25, 4-2.26, 4-2.27, 4-2.28, 4-2.29, 4-2.30, 4-2.31, 4-2.32, 4-2.33, 4-2.34, 4-2.35, 4-2.36

The Three Stages of Shock

At the outset, shock results in an intricate interplay between neural and hormonal stress responses aimed at maintaining normal or near-normal blood flow. If left untreated, this compensated stage moves imperceptibly into a decompensated stage, resulting in a massive reduction of blood flow, increased lactic acid production, and the development of metabolic acidosis. This leads to the development of the systemic inflammatory response syndrome (SIRS).[23,24] If uncorrected, SIRS leads to multisystem organ failure or disseminated intravascular coagulopathy (DIC). Each stage of shock will be discussed in more detail. DOT 1-6.17, 1-6.21, 4-2.25

The Compensated Stage

Oxygen circulates in the red blood cell attached to the hemoglobin molecule. Each hemoglobin molecule can hold four molecules of oxygen, and each red cell has millions of hemoglobin molecules. If all available hemoglobin molecules are bound with oxygen, the arterial oxygen saturation is 100%.

Oxygen is delivered to the tissues by the flow of blood resulting from the cardiac output. Normally, the

TABLE 13-2 Clinical Signs and Symptoms for Varying Levels of Shock Severity

Signs and Symptoms	Compensated Shock	Decompensated Shock	Irreversible Shock
Heart rate	↑	↑↑	↑ or ↓
Blood pressure	normal or ↑	↓	↓↓
Respiratory rate	↑	↑ or ↓	↓
Skin — hypovolemia	Delayed capillary refill; cool	Delayed capillary refill; cold; cyanotic	Pale; cold; mottled
Skin — distributive	Delayed capillary refill; warm; moist	Delayed capillary refill; cool	Pale; cold; mottled
Level of consciousness	Normal; lethargy; confusion	Combative; unconscious	Coma
Cardiac output	↑	↑ or ↓	↓
Serum lactate concentration	normal or ↑	↑↑	↑↑↑
Systemic inflammatory response	↑	↑↑	↑↑↑

tissues consume about 25% of the oxygen in the arterial blood, and the remaining 75% continues to circulate back to the heart in the venous blood. This provides a great deal of reserve in the event of a problem, but the reserve cannot sustain the body for long.

The first compensatory mechanism that is triggered if the oxygen supply is insufficient to meet the body's demands is an increase in the cardiac output.[2] In the face of actual blood volume loss, the only ways to improve cardiac output are either to increase the heart rate or increase the force of the contraction of the heart. This occurs due to the release of the hormones epinephrine and norepinephrine as discussed earlier. These catecholamine drugs help preserve both cardiac output and blood pressure by causing tachycardia, by increasing the pumping force of the heart, and with vasoconstriction. Blood is also being shunted from some of the areas of lesser need (such as the gastrointestinal [GI] tract and the skin) to preserve the flow to the brain and heart.

Epinephrine and norepinephrine also affect the respiratory system. They cause an increase in the depth and rate of respirations. This results in more gas delivery to the alveoli. Enhanced circulation to the pulmonary circulatory system brings more blood to the lungs, which results in increased diffusion of oxygen into the blood and wastes out of the blood. This can help correct the oxygen saturation deficit experienced earlier and will also cause a respiratory alkalosis as the increased respiratory rate results in decreased CO_2 levels.

Cardiac output = Stroke volume × Heart rate

Blood pressure = Cardiac output × Peripheral vascular resistance

The kidneys receive a hormonal signal to decrease the production of urine. This results in retention of fluid, but it also results in retention of waste products, which adds to the level of acidosis occurring within the blood.

Any of the corrective actions designed to improve cardiac output results in an increase in the overall pressure inside the heart in diastole (the resting state). The blood pressure, which initially drops in response to the blood volume loss or decreased vascular tone, now returns to normal or near normal levels. While both the systolic and diastolic pressures increase, the diastolic pressure often rises more than the systolic, leading to narrowing of the pulse pressure. The **pulse pressure** is the systolic pressure minus the diastolic pressure. For example, the preshock blood pressure can be 120/80, and immediately after a blood loss, the pressure drops to 100/66. Because the bleeding stops, the patient quickly compensates and the pressure rises. Now it can be 110/84. In the first BP reading the pulse pressure was 40 mmHg, in the second it was 34 mmHg, and in the third it was 26 mmHg. DOT 4-2.23

It is important to note that blood pressure will not always fall in response to the development of shock. This is particularly true when there is an increase in peripheral vascular resistance (afterload) in the presence of decreased cardiac output. In this case, the patient will still have tissue hypoperfusion, but the BP evidence is not there.[2] For this reason, there is not a single vital sign that is a reliable indicator of the presence of shock. DOT 4-2.25, 4-2.26, 4-2.27, 4-2.28, 4-2.29

The Decompensated Stage

The physiologic responses noted during compensated shock are a mechanism to protect the body by attempting to normalize blood flow and oxygen and glucose delivery to tissues. Unfortunately, such responses frequently disproportionately overwhelm the protective mechanisms and lead to further tissue injury, as is the result with SIRS. DOT 4-2.24

The body has a limited supply of any given hormone, and once the supply is exhausted, it is gone. If the body is in shock, it is likely that those metabolic pathways are temporarily shut down as the body battles to stay alive.

For example, once the reserve of epinephrine and norepinephrine is gone, the compensation offered by these two agents can no longer occur.

Respiratory alkalosis gives way to metabolic acidosis as acid is built up faster than it can be removed by the respiratory system. The kidneys still retain water to help preserve the blood volume, so filtering of wastes by the kidneys is diminished, adding to additional acidosis. Persistent and progressive hypoxia leads to worsening acidosis, which obtunds (blunts or lessens) cardiovascular and vascular responses to intrinsic compensatory mechanisms and extrinsic therapies aimed at normalizing cardiovascular function.

Many hormones and drugs need a specific pH environment to be effective. Catecholamine drugs such as epinephrine and norepinephrine are known to be ineffective in extremely acidotic environments. The body spirals out of control, and the spiral effect worsens until hemodynamic collapse occurs. The final stage of shock now begins. DOT 4-2.25, 4-2.30, 4-2.31

Street Secrets

It is not always easy to distinguish which stage of shock your patient is in. Monitor all patients closely, and treat them for shock whether it is present or not. Do not wait to find an abnormality such as tachycardia or hypotension to begin treatment for shock. Perform resuscitative stabilization when appropriate, but also remember that many types of shock require aggressive intervention strategies, such as surgery or blood products, that are not available in the out-of-hospital environment. Consider rapid transport as important a treatment as applying oxygen and starting an IV.

DOT 4-2.24, 4-2.30, 4-2.34

The Irreversible Stage

The irreversible stage of shock is as ominous as it sounds. Resuscitative efforts at this stage are unlikely to result in preserving life. The SIRS cascade results in the formation of microemboli, which are microscopic blood clots. These clots block capillaries and prevent the flow of blood through the capillary beds. This, of course, worsens tissue ischemia. As this event occurs in certain areas, vast amounts of tissue can convert from ischemia to necrosis and death. If the particular tissue affected is substantial, it results in multiple system organ failure. DOT 4-2.18

Multiple system organ failure (MSOF) is a common problem associated with critical illness. It is defined as the simultaneous presence of severe dysfunction or outright failure of two or more organs.[16] It can occur in the setting of sepsis, shock, severe inflammatory conditions, and trauma. Some patients who appear to be responding to resuscitation efforts in the field or emergency department will, however, develop multiple

system organ failure and later die in the hospital. SIRS is a common trigger for organ failure. DOT 1-6.12

The kidneys often fail because of the presence of the microemboli and also because of persistent ischemia. The lungs are injured by ischemia and acute respiratory distress syndrome (ARDS) develops.[16] ARDS is also called "shock lung." ARDS leads to non-cardiogenic (non-cardiac-caused) pulmonary edema. As this develops, fluid collects inside the alveoli and increases the distance between the alveoli and the capillaries lining the outside of the alveoli. This leads to difficulty in the diffusion of oxygen and carbon dioxide, worsening hypoxemia and acidosis.

Another possible occurrence, in addition to organ failure, is the development of **disseminated intravascular coagulation (DIC).** As SIRS causes microemboli to form, the clotting factors normally found within the blood are used up. Early in this process, the presence of the clots themselves can lead to fibrinolysis as protective mechanisms break down the clots. The fibrinolytic process is normal and protective under usual circumstances. In this instance, because there are no appreciable reserves of thrombocytes and clotting factors remaining, the fibrinolysis reaction leads to leakage of fluid from the capillaries and bleeding occurs. Many patients have extensive skin and mucous membrane bleeding. Hemorrhage from surgical incisions and venipuncture or catheter sites is also possible. If not treated promptly, the patient will die. Prehospital treatment involves standard shock management, which will be described later in this chapter, and rapid transport. DOT 4-2.32, 4-2.33

Identifying Patients in Shock

The clinical presentation of shock ranges from subtle alterations in organ perfusion to profound hemodynamic collapse (see Table 13-2). Patients who are in shock commonly have no obvious etiology unless the cause is due to trauma.[2] A focused history, physical examination, and assessment of accurate vital signs will help the paramedic recognize shock.

History

Assess the scene and be alert for any mechanism that would suggest trauma. Obtain a history of recent illnesses, allergies, medications, and foods eaten. A history of illness should alert you to fluid volume shifts due to excessive loss (from nausea or vomiting) or may lead you to suspect sepsis, which causes vasodilation and fluid shifting. Some medications cause volume depletion (diuretics), and some depress myocardial contractility (beta blockers and calcium channel blockers). The patient may also have an allergic reaction from a drug or food.

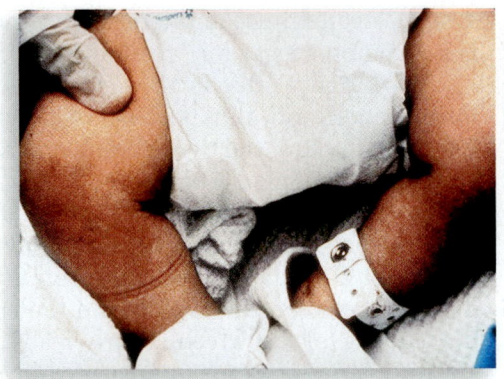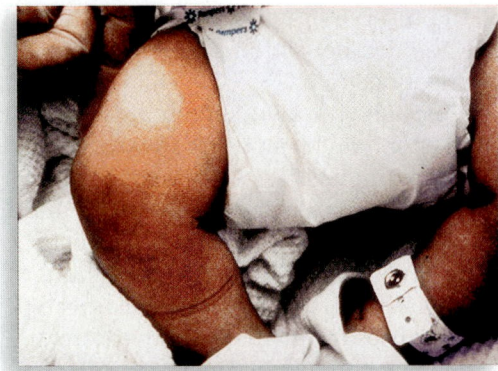

Figure 13-3   Poor capillary refill in an infant. Normal color should return within two seconds following release of pressure.

Physical Examination

As a general rule, patients in shock, regardless of which stage they are in, exhibit a physiologic stress response aimed at compensating for the underlying decrease in perfusion. Clinically, this response is manifested by some or all of the following findings: DOT 4-2.6, 4-2.22

Clinical signs of shock:

- Ill appearance
- Pale skin
- Diaphoresis
- Tachycardia
- Tachypnea

Signs of poor perfusion:

- Altered mental status
- Weak pulses
- Poor capillary refill (Figure 13-3)
- Cool mottled skin (Figure 13-4)
- **Oliguria** (i.e., decreased urine output)

In hypovolemic and cardiogenic shock, the skin tends to be cool, pale, and mottled. In distributive shock, the skin tends to be warm and moist.

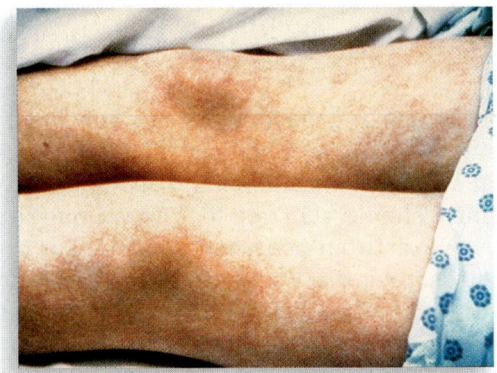

Figure 13-4   Mottled skin in a child indicating poor perfusion.

While the signs just described are considered classic for patients suffering from shock, there are several notable exceptions:

- Ill appearance and altered mental status may be subtle, especially during the early stages of shock (i.e., during compensated shock).
- A patient may appear generally well; thus, a low threshold for suspecting this clinical condition must always be maintained by EMS.

Vital Signs in Shock

Vital signs, although commonly regarded as the most objective measures of hemodynamic status, can be misleading. No single vital sign is diagnostic of shock. Vital signs are insensitive in detecting and assessing the severity of hypoperfusion.[2] At no point should a single vital sign reading drive a treatment plan. Patients are dynamic, and continuous vital sign monitoring is appropriate. The three end points of treatment mentioned earlier are a normalized heart rate, blood pressure, and urine output. Heart rate and blood pressure can be continuously monitored in the prehospital setting. Urine output typically is not.

Heart Rate

Heart rate and blood pressure correlate poorly with overall cardiac function in the setting of shock and often do not reflect the severity of systemic hypoperfusion.[25] In addition, tachycardia represents a manifestation of the compensatory mechanism, but patients in shock may also demonstrate normal heart rates or bradycardia, either due to the use of prescribed drugs (e.g., beta-blockers or calcium-channel blockers) or as a result of profound hypoxemia. In fact, progressive bradycardia (either relative or absolute) in the setting of shock is an ominous sign and a hallmark of impending cardiovascular collapse and arrest.

Clinical studies of patients admitted to the emergency department with hemorrhagic shock have consistently revealed wide ranges in pulse rates, including a

BOX 13-1 Orthostatic Vital Signs Assessment

In addition to assessing vital signs, assessing for **orthostatic** (or **postural**) **vital sign** changes is commonly taught and practiced. Measuring postural vital signs includes measuring the heart rate and blood pressures while the patient is supine, then again one minute after standing. A positive test is generally considered an increase in the patient's heart rate of 30 beats or more per minute, a decrease in the patient's systolic blood pressure by 20 mmHg or more, or the development of lightheadedness. The sensitivity of a postural heart rate increase of 30 beats or more per minute in the setting of large blood volume loss (indicating substantial volume depletion) is 97%; whereas, the sensitivity in the setting of moderate blood loss drops to only 22%.[29] Postural hypotension was found to occur in up to 10% of normovolemic patients less than 65 years of age and in 11% to 30% of normovolemic patients older than 65 years of age.[30,31] In an emergency department study of normovolemic patients, 43% were found to have postural vital sign changes.[32] Severe postural lightheadedness, although demonstrated to be a poor predictor of postural hypotension, is considered the most useful indicator of hypovolemia.[29] Patients with signs of hypovolemia, such as resting tachycardia, and complaints of dizziness upon standing should be presumed to be orthostatic and do not need to have postural vital signs measured in order to prove that they are hypovolemic. Postural vital sign changes have a limited overall utility and, as a general rule, should not be assessed in patients suspected of being in shock. DOT 4-2.24, 3-3.31

substantial proportion of patients with heart rates less than 100 beats per minute. In one study from an urban trauma center, 35% to 44% of hypotensive trauma patients had heart rates less than 100 beats per minute.[26] DOT 4-2.1

Respiratory Rate

Tachypnea, unless profound, is often difficult to identify. It is often the first indicator that the patient is in shock and represents a compensatory physiologic response to the development of a metabolic acidosis. However, tachypnea is often subtle, especially early in this disease course and, as a vital sign, is often merely estimated rather than actually counted. All patients with unexplained tachypnea should be assumed to be in shock until proven otherwise.

Blood Pressure

Blood pressures may also be misleading in shock. Compensated shock is commonly manifested by normal mental status, tachycardia, normal or elevated blood pressure, and delayed peripheral perfusion as demonstrated by delayed capillary refill (see Table 13-2).

This stage of shock may quickly lead to decompensated shock, as manifested by markedly decreased tissue perfusion, altered mental status, and hypotension. An abnormally low blood pressure in the appropriate clinical setting is a clear indicator of shock; however, a normal blood pressure in the setting of suspected shock does not rule it out, and it may reflect compensatory shock which, if left untreated, may quickly progress to a decompensated state. Box 13-1 provides information on orthostatic vital sign assessment.

Working in the Gray Zone

Hypotension kills. Do not wait to observe vital signs deteriorating to begin aggressive intervention for the patient. In a large clinical study of out-of-hospital hypotension, investigators found that nontraumatic hypotension was associated with a significantly higher rate of in-hospital mortality.[27] In this study, a single episode of hypotension prior to hospital arrival conferred a 26% to 32% in-hospital mortality rate; whereas, those patients who were never hypotensive had in-hospital mortality rates ranging from 8% to 11%. In addition, the mortality rate of patients who are hypotensive upon arrival to the emergency department is higher than in those patients who are normotensive when they arrive at the hospital.[28]

Mental Status

Perfusion of the central nervous system is maintained until shock is severe. Obtundation, which occurs as a patient's mental state deteriorates to the point that the patient is virtually unresponsive to the environment, is also an ominous sign.[16]

Pediatric Response to Shock

One of the most important things to remember when assessing a child for shock is that a child can maintain a normal appearance until he or she is in profound shock. Keep a high index of suspicion based upon the mechanism of injury or nature of the illness, chief complaint, history, and physical examination. Any evidence or suspicion of bleeding should be met with prompt transportation and treatment for shock. Infants with simple dehydration from a viral infection can enter into a life-threatening hypovolemic shock state after just a few hours of their illnesses.

Although alterations in vital signs indicating shock are late findings, assessing vital signs in children is still important. Heart rates and blood pressures vary depending on the age of the child. Hypotension exists if the systolic blood pressure is less than 70 mmHg plus twice the age, and for children beyond 10 years of age, hypotension exists if the systolic blood pressure is less than 90 mmHg.[33] Moreover, hypotension in children is typically a late sign, and its development often directly precedes arrest.[34] Finally, respiratory rates also vary with age, but as a general rule, any rate less than 10 or greater than 60 breaths per minute is indicative of impending respiratory arrest in children.

> Children appear to compensate for a long time and then they quickly crash. If the mechanism or history leads you to suspect shock, believe your instincts and treat for shock.

Geriatric Response to Shock

Presentation of shock in the elderly is often extremely subtle. You must have a high index of suspicion when evaluating an elderly patient for possible shock. Such patients do not routinely mount appropriate compensatory physiologic responses and are commonly taking medications that contribute to blunting of their physiologic responses to different types of shock. For example, a patient may be taking beta blocker medication to control blood pressure or help the heart function, and these drugs may prevent tachycardia from developing during hypovolemia.

> The only signs of shock in many elderly patients may be altered mental status or tachypnea.

Prehospital Management of Shock

Paramedic response time to the scene of a patient in shock may impact survival.[35] Although the data are conflicting and more study is necessary, preliminary evidence suggests that paramedic response time of four minutes or less has a positive effect on patient survival. Treatment of shock in the prehospital setting centers on airway management, hemodynamic support, and rapid transport to an emergency care facility. See Box 13-2 for strategies for specific forms of shock.

Prehospital airway management includes providing oxygen and ventilatory support in an effort to maximize the concentration of oxygen in blood in order to improve

the oxygen supply to tissues. Hemodynamic support is primarily provided by infusion of crystalloid solutions, namely isotonic saline. However, specific levels of such therapies will largely depend on the cause and severity of the presenting condition.

In addition, paramedics typically have to rely on a limited history and do not have a lot of diagnostic tools or therapies available to aid in their decision-making process. The goals of treatment of patients in shock center on maximizing oxygenation, normalizing ventilation, and restoring normal perfusion of tissues while expediting the safe transport of the patient.

Working in the Gray Zone

Management strategies considered BLS, such as calming and reassuring the patient and keeping them warm, are critical components of shock resuscitation. Do not forget to provide good BLS-level skills to all shock patients.

General Management Strategies for Shock DOT 4-2.42, 4-2.43

All patients with shock should, at a minimum, be placed on 15 liters of oxygen using a nonrebreather facemask, regardless of the patient's oxygen saturation or degree of respiratory compromise (Figure 13-5). If respiratory failure has occurred or is perceived to be imminent, oxygenation and ventilation should be provided using a bag-mask or via invasive airway management, most commonly by endotracheal tube with end tidal CO_2 monitoring. The objective of this initial therapy is to maximize the concentration of oxygen in blood (either bound to hemoglobin or dissolved in plasma) in order to maximize oxygen delivery to tissues.

Endpoints of oxygen and ventilatory support are a pulse oximeter reading above 93–95%, normal

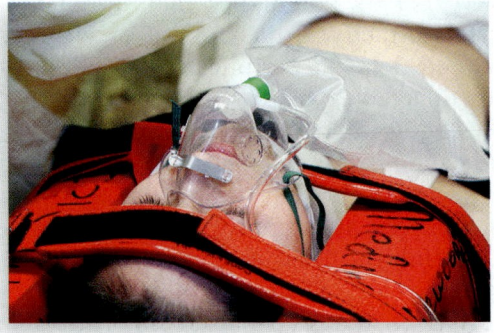

Figure 13-5 All patients with shock should, at a minimum, be placed on 15 liters of oxygen using a non-rebreather face-mask, regardless of the patient's oxygen saturation or degree of respiratory compromise.

BOX 13-2 Prehospital Management Strategies for Specific Forms of Shock

General Management Principles
Airway Support

- Ensure adequate oxygenation using 15 liters by non-rebreather mask or endotracheal intubation in all patients in shock
- Ensure adequate ventilation using bag-mask or endotracheal intubation in all patients in shock

Hemodynamic Support

- Obtain immediate intravenous access using two large-bore (16-gauge or larger) IVs
- Place all patients on continuous cardiac monitoring

Transportation

- All patients in shock should be rapidly transported to an appropriate hospital, and on-scene times should be minimized

Specific Management Principles
Hemorrhagic Shock

- If possible, provide immediate control of hemorrhage (e.g., direct manual pressure, traction for long bone fractures, use of tourniquet for arterial bleeding from extremities)
- Immediate and aggressive use of isotonic saline (20 mL/kg/bolus)
- If extended transport and if available, consider beginning transfusion with packed red blood cells (10 mL/kg)

Non-Hemorrhagic Hypovolemic Shock

- Immediate and aggressive use of isotonic saline (20 mL/kg/bolus)

Septic Shock

- Immediate and aggressive use of isotonic saline (20 mL/kg/bolus)
- If hypotension persists after two saline boluses, consider beginning intravenous vasopressor therapy (e.g., dopamine—starting dose: 10 μg/kg/min)

Anaphylactic Shock

- Immediate intramuscular epinephrine 1:1,000 (0.3–0.5 mL in adults; 0.01 mL/kg in children)
- Immediate and aggressive use of isotonic saline (20 mL/kg/bolus)
- Administer diphenhydramine (25–50 mg in adults; 1.25 mg/kg in children)
- If wheezing is present, administer nebulized albuterol

Cardiogenic Shock due to Acute Myocardial Infarction

- If the patient is in respiratory distress due to pulmonary edema and the blood pressure is >100 mmHg, consider using sublingual nitroglycerin to improve cardiac preload
- If the patient is in respiratory distress due to pulmonary edema and the blood pressure is ≤ 100 mmHg, initiate inotropic therapy (e.g., dobutamine or dopamine)

Cardiogenic Shock due to a Dysrhythmia or Conduction Delay

- Electrical cardioversion for tachydysrhythmias (begin with 25–50J [biphasic] for supraventricular tachydysrhythmias and 50–100J [biphasic] for ventricular tachydysrhythmias and increase energy levels, as necessary)
- Transcutaneous pacing for bradydysrhythmias

Shock due to Pulmonary Embolism

- Immediate and aggressive use of isotonic saline (20 mL/kg/bolus)
- If hypotension persists after two saline boluses, consider beginning intravenous vasopressor therapy (e.g., dopamine—starting dose: 10 μg/kg/min)

Shock due to Cardiac Tamponade

- Immediate and aggressive use of isotonic saline (20 mL/kg/bolus)

---

capnograpy waveforms, and a tan or yellow color on a colorimetric CO_2 detector. If blood gas values are monitored, the $PaCO_2$ reading should be between 35–40 mmHg, the PaO_2 reading above 80 mmHg, and the pH above 7.35.[2]

Concurrently, intravenous access should be obtained with the specific objective of placing one or two large-bore (16-gauge or larger) catheters in the upper extremities (Figure 13-6). Large-bore catheters allow for rapid infusion of fluids necessary for aggressive intravascular

Working in the Gray Zone

Be cautious with the use of positive pressure ventilation as it has been shown to reduce both preload and cardiac output.[2] Positive pressure ventilation can cause barotrauma, which is overstretching or rupture of alveoli from excessively high pressures in ventilation. This can occur from ventilation with either a bag-mask unit or with a flow-restricted oxygen powered ventilation device (or a "demand valve" as it used to be called) or with mechanical ventilation. Hyperventilation is not appropriate in managing patients in shock.

fluid repletion during resuscitation. The importance of placing large-bore catheters increases as the need for aggressive fluid resuscitation increases (e.g., when the patient is hypotensive in the setting of presumed absolute or relative hypovolemia).

A bolus of isotonic crystalloid solution should be given for all patients with a systolic blood pressure below 90 mmHg. Monitor the patient closely during this process and repeat boluses as needed. Patients in mild degrees of hypovolemia should respond to a 20 ml/kg fluid bolus. Medical direction should be consulted per local guidelines. Patients in shock without absolute hypovolemia being the cause, such as cardiogenic shock for example, should have smaller amounts of fluid used. DOT 4-2.37, 4-2.38

Catecholamine vasopressor agents such as dopamine or epinephrine drips can be added to the treatment regimen if the patient is not responding to fluid resuscitation. They may also be used initially when the patient's condition contraindicates the use of fluid resuscitation.

Working in the Gray Zone

How much fluid to give to a shock patient is still under investigation. We know that too much washes out blood clots, causes hemodilution, and can cause pulmonary edema. We also know that too much fluid when the problem is not fluid loss, as in cardiogenic shock, can be deadly. Work closely with your medical director to keep abreast of the updates regarding fluid resuscitation.

If urine output is monitored, the goal of therapy is to achieve an output of over 0.5 ml/kg/hour.

Keep the patient warm. After removing clothing to perform the patient assessment, cover the patient up with sheets and blankets. Turn up the heater in the ambulance (Figure 13-7). Remember, you may be appropriately dressed for the weather, so you may feel warm in the ambulance with a coat on. The undressed shock patient will not be warm unless you take steps to conserve body heat.

In addition, all patients in shock should be placed in a supine position, and should have continuous electrocardiographic monitoring. Clinical evaluation and vital signs will guide the initial therapies provided by paramedics prior to arrival at the hospital.[2]

All patients with compensated shock should be placed on oxygen, have one or two intravenous lines established, and should be transported emergently to the hospital. Those with decompensated shock require oxygen (and ventilatory support, as needed), intravenous access, and specific therapy aimed at improving or restoring perfusion to vital organs.

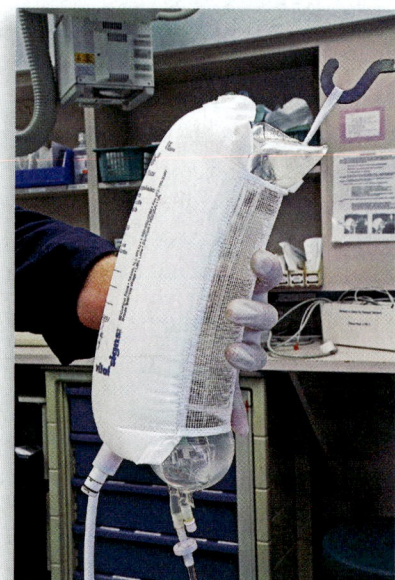

Figure 13-6   Pressure infusers can help infuse fluid more rapidly into patients who are hypotensive.

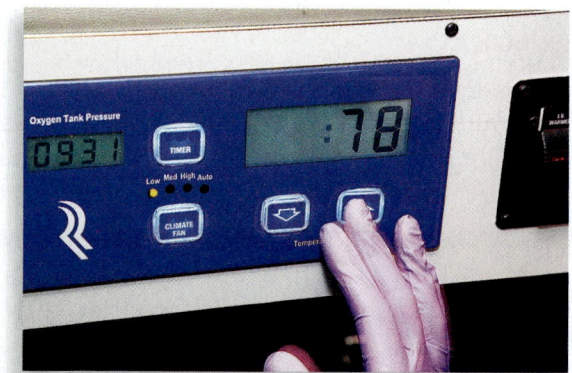

Figure 13-7   Keep the patient warm by turning up the heat in the ambulance.

Summary

Shock is commonly encountered in the prehospital setting. Shock is a state of inadequate tissue perfusion with reduced amounts of oxygen and glucose being delivered to the body's cells and tissues and impaired removal of wastes that are building up.

The signs and symptoms of all types of shock have some common patterns, but not all patients present with these signs and symptoms, and the presence of normal appearing vital signs does not rule out the presence of shock. Recognizing patients with shock is often challenging but relies primarily on a focused history and physical examination, including assessment of valid vital signs.

Although shock has many different classes, the initial treatment for shock follows similar strategies with each type of shock. Other management strategies will depend largely on the underlying etiology of the shock syndrome. If left untreated, shock progresses through three stages: compensated, decompensated, and irreversible. Prehospital treatment for shock focuses on airway management, hemodynamic support, and rapid transport to the hospital.

Notes

1. J. A. Kline, "Shock," in *Rosen's Emergency Medicine: Concepts and Clinical Practice*, 5th ed., Marx, ed. (St. Louis: Mosby, 2002).

2. E. P. Rivers, R. M. Otero, H. Nguyen, "Approach to the Patient in Shock." In J. E. Tintinalli, G. D. Kelen, J. S. Stapczynski (eds.) *Emergency Medicine. A Comprehensive Study Guide* (6th ed.), New York: McGraw-Hill. 2004, pp 219–224.

3. G. S. Martin, D. M. Mannino, S. Eaton, et al., "The Epidemiology of Sepsis in the United States from 1979 Through 2000," *New England Journal of Medicine* 248(2003): 1546–1554.

4. A. P. Wheeler and G. R. Bernard, "Treating Patients with Severe Sepsis," *New England Journal of Medicine* 340(1999): 207–214.

5. R. M. Califf and J. R. Bengtson, "Cardiogenic Shock," *New England Journal of Medicine* 330(1994): 1724–1730.

6. A. Sauaia, F. A. Moore, E. E. Moore, et al., "Epidemiology of Trauma Deaths: a Reassessment," *Journal of Trauma* 38(1995): 185–193.

7. D. W. Landry and J. A. Oliver, "The Pathogenesis of Vasodilatory Shock," *New England Journal of Medicine* 345(2001): 588–595.

8. D. L. Page, J. B. Caulfield, J. A. Kastor, et al., "Myocardial Changes Associated with Cardiogenic Shock," *New England Journal of Medicine* 285(1971): 133–137.

9. J. L. Carson M. A. Kelley, A. Duff, et al., "The Clinical Course of Pulmonary Embolism," *New England Journal of Medicine* 326(1992): 1240–1245.

10. D. H. Spodick, "Acute Cardiac Tamponade," *New England Journal of Medicine* 349(2003): 684–690.

11. K. R. Hardy, and S. R. Thom, "Pathophysiology and Treatment of Carbon Monoxide Poisoning," *Clinical Toxicology* 32(1994): 613–629.

12. R. Gracia and G. Shepherd, "Cyanide Poisoning and its Treatment," *Pharmacotherapy* 24(2004): 1358–1364.

13. R. P. Smith and R. E. Gosselin, "Hydrogen Sulfide Poisoning," *Journal Occup Med* 21(1979): 93–97.

14. R. M. Berne and M. N. Levy, *Cardiovascular Physiology*, 6th ed. (St. Louis: Mosby Year Book, 1992).

15. A. C. Guyton, *Textbook of Medical Physiology*, 8th ed. (Philadelphia: W. B. Saunders Company, 1991).

16. R. V. Maier, "Approach to the Patient with Shock." In *Harrison's Principles of Internal Medicine* (16th ed.). D. L. Kasper, E. Braunwald, A. S. Fauci, S. L. Hauselr, D. L. Longo, J. L. Jameson (eds). New York: McGraw-Hill. 2005, pp. 1600–1605.

17. R. C. Bone, "Towards a Theory Regarding the Pathogenesis of the Systemic Inflammatory Response Syndrome: What We Do and Do Not Know About Cytokine Regulation," *Crit Care Med* 24(1996): 163–172.

18. P. K. Kim and C. S. Deutschman, "Inflammatory Responses and Mediators," *Surgical Clinics of North America* 80(2000): 885–894.

19. P. O. Nystrom, "The Systemic Inflammatory Response Syndrome: Definitions and Aetiology," *J Antimicrob Chemo* 41(1998): A1–A7.

20. M. Wahle, T. Greulich, C. G. Baerwald, et al., "Influence of Catecholamines on Cytokine Production and Expression of Adhesion Molecules of Human Neutrophils in Vitro," *Immunobiology* 210(2005): 43–52.

21. A. L. Lehninger, D. L. Nelson, and M. M. Cox, *Principles of Biochemistry*, 2nd ed. (New York: Worth Publishers, 1993).

22. N. I. Shapiro, M. D. Howell, D. Talmor, et al., "Serum Lactate as a Predictor of Mortality in Emergency Department Patients with Infection," *Ann Emerg Med* 45(2005): 524–528.

23. R. S. Cotran, V. Kumar, and S. L. Robbins, *Robbins Pathologic Basis of Disease*, 5th ed. (Philadelphia: W.B. Saunders Company, 1994).

24. J. C. Marshall, "Inflammation, Coagulopathy, and the Pathogenesis of Multiple Organ Dysfunction Syndrome," *Crit Care Med* 29(2001): S99–S106.

25. C. C. Wo, W. C. Shoemaker, P. L. Appel, et al., "Unreliability of Blood Pressure and Heart Rate to Evaluate Cardiac Output in Emergency Resuscitation and Critical Illness," *Crit Care Med* 21(1993): 218–223.

26. D. Thompson, S. L. Adams, J. Barrett, "Relative Bradycardia in Patients with Isolated Penetrating Abdominal Trauma and Isolated Extremity Trauma," *Ann Emerg Med* 268(1990): 268–270.

27. A. E. Jones, I. G. Stiell, L. P. Nesbitt, et al., "Nontraumatic Out-Of-Hospital Hypotension Predicts Inhospital Mortality," *Ann Emerg Med* 43(2004): 106–113.

28. A. E. Jones, L. S. Aborn, and J. A. Kline, "Severity of Emergency Department Hypotension Predicts Adverse Hospital Outcome," *Shock* 22(2004): 410–414.

29. S. McGee, W. B. Abernethy, and D. L. Simel, "Is This Patient Hypovolemic?" *JAMA* 281(1999): 1022–1029.

30. W. L. Ooi, S. Barrett, M. Hossain, et al., "Patterns of Orthostatic Blood Pressure Change and Their Clinical Correlates in a Frail, Elderly Population," *JAMA* 277(1997): 1299–1304.

31. I. Raiha, S. Luntonen, J. Piha, et al., "Prevalence, Predisposing Factors, and Prognostic Importance of Postural Hypotension," *Arch Intern Med* 155(1995): 930–935.

32. J. Koziol-McLain, S. R. Lowenstein, and B. Fuller, "Orthostatic Vital Signs in Emergency Department Patients," *Ann Emerg Med* 20(1991): 606–610.

33. "Pediatric Advanced Life Support," *Circulation* 102(Suppl I) (2000): 291–342.

34. M. F. Hazinski and R. M. Barkin, "Shock," in *Pediatric Emergency Medicine—Concepts and Clinical Practice*, 2nd ed. (St. Louis: Mosby, Inc., 1997).

35. P. T. Pons, J. S. Haukoos, W. Bludworth, et al., "Paramedic Response Time: Does It Affect Patient Survival?" *Acad Emerg Med* 12(2005): 594–600.

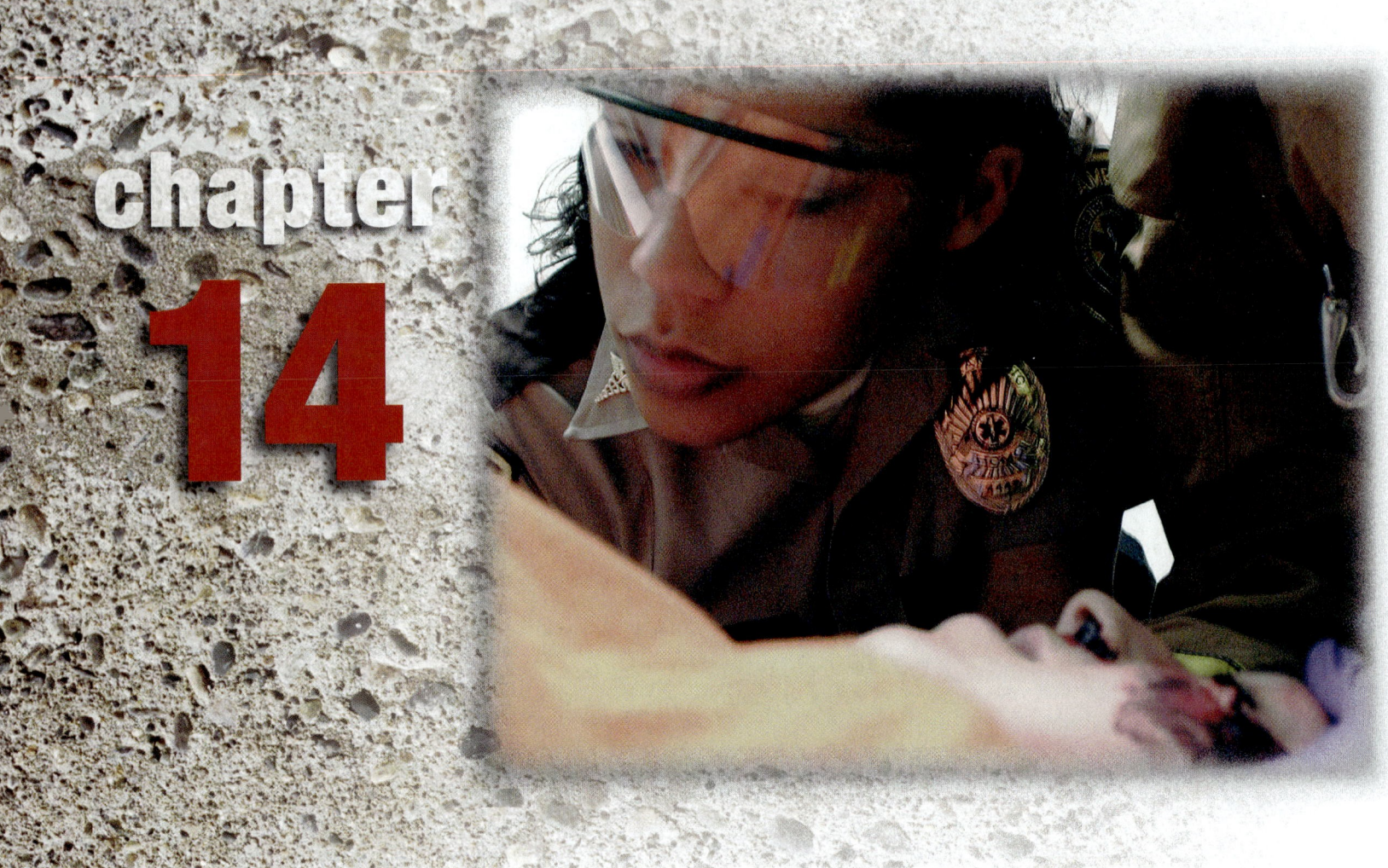

Patient Assessment

"Our bodies communicate to us clearly and specifically, if we are willing to listen to them."

—Shakti Gawain

Need to Know

▶ The paramedic's primary goal in the management of the prehospital patient is to assess, recognize, and treat life-threatening conditions immediately.

▶ The scene size-up is always the first survey conducted for every patient encounter.

▶ The primary survey provides a logical and efficient pathway to identify and manage critically ill or injured patients during the first few minutes.

▶ The secondary survey of a patient will be tailored to the patient's needs based upon whether the patient is sick or injured and whether the patient is conscious or unconscious. It may include performing a head to toe assessment or an assessment focused on a specific region of the body and obtaining vital signs and a history.

▶ The paramedic has to rely upon physical findings and the information provided by the environment and bystanders to determine the underlying conditions that caused a patient to become unconscious or altered.

▶ A patient who has experienced a major injury will need to be evaluated quickly yet accurately. Speed is of the essence in the management of the critical trauma patient. However, do not overlook the possibility of a hidden yet serious condition in the patient who appears to have only a simple, minor injury.

▶ The paramedic must evaluate carefully how to best assess the patient based upon factors that are found in the scene size-up and primary survey.

▶ The patient assessment does not ever finish. Ongoing evaluation of the patient includes the response to treatment, identifying trends in the overall patient condition, and continues all of the way to the hospital.

▶ Do	▶ Ask
• Begin every patient assessment with a scene size-up. • Perform an initial assessment on every patient. • Determine which components of the complete secondary survey should be performed based upon the primary survey findings. • Conduct appropriate ongoing assessments on patients as needed.	• Ask appropriate questions to gather the history (SAMPLE) or to assess pain (OPQRST).

Introduction

Much of the work you will perform as a paramedic can be broken down into two key components: (1) assess and (2) treat sick and injured patients. One could argue that patient assessment is the more important of these two components since you will not be able to treat patients appropriately if you do not first assess and recognize their problems.

To rapidly and accurately assess a patient you will need to hone your skills as a trained observer, use good clinical judgment, and not rely solely on instruments such as the stethoscope, ECG monitor, and pulse oximeter. Success as a competent paramedic will depend upon the ability to collect comprehensive and accurate data about the patient's condition. If assessment skills are sharp, then considering the possible underlying causes for the patient's problem and any life-threatening causes can be accomplished quickly and effectively.

Chapter 11 describes the elements that make up a normal physical examination. The chapter also points out that it is not appropriate to perform each assessment technique on every patient encounter. There must be a balance between gathering information and providing appropriate treatment. A logical and systematic approach to patient assessment will help maximize the speed and accuracy of care.

The basic approach to patient care can be sorted into four distinct components: scene size-up, primary survey, secondary survey, and ongoing assessment.

Box 14-1 has more information on the names of the various components of patient assessment.

The **scene size-up** should always precede any other assessment, and it should be conducted on every call. Virtually every patient situation will demand a **primary survey** (also called the **initial assessment**), and it typically includes all of the elements outlined in this chapter. Based on the conclusions and findings of the primary survey, the **secondary survey** will be started on scene, delayed, performed while the patient is en route to

> ### BOX 14-1   Patient Assessment Terminology
>
> Numerous terms have been used over the years to describe the various components of the assessment process. The terms ABCs, ABCDEs, *primary survey,* and *initial assessment* refer to the process of acquiring the general impression, level of consciousness, and assessment and treatment of any immediate life threats involving the airway, breathing, and circulation. The terms *focused assessment* and *rapid trauma assessment* describe some or all of the steps used to assess a patient in somewhat more detail for potential life-threatening problems. *Secondary survey, detailed assessment, detailed physical examination,* and *head-to-toe examination* describe a very detailed and complete examination from the top of the head to the toes. Ongoing assessment involves reassessment of all or parts of the primary and secondary surveys and focused re-evaluation of pertinent exam findings. For consistency, this text will use: scene size-up, primary survey (interchangeable with initial assessment), secondary survey, and ongoing assessment. This approach follows conventional medical tradition and meets the DOT Paramedic National Standard Curriculum goals.[1]

the appropriate medical facility, or it will not be conducted at all. The **ongoing assessment** represents monitoring activities that occur throughout the patient interaction. An ongoing assessment is conducted as necessary to evaluate the response to treatment and the need for new or different treatment and to monitor the patient status.

CONNECTIONS This chapter ties together the elements of assessment presented in Chapter 10: Therapeutic Communications and History Taking, Chapter 11: The Normal Physical Exam, and Chapter 5: Clinical Decision Making. If you have not read those chapters already, you may want to do so before continuing. This chapter draws on the information presented within those chapters as it explains the components of the patient assessment.

Sick and Not Yet Sick

The term **sick** refers to a "critical" state as it applies to both traumatically injured and medically ill patients. For simplicity, "sick" is used for both conditions. Sick patients have poor vital signs, evidence of shock, or a clinical presentation suggesting that their life is at risk if they do not see a physician very soon. In some cases the patient is so sick that resuscitation efforts must begin before he or she can be taken to the physician. A person

with a dangerously low blood sugar level, allergic reaction to a bee sting, a critical burn, or several long bone fractures is an example of a "sick" patient. DOT 3-4.2

Determining that a patient is sick should be done as quickly as possible, generally within the first minutes of contact. This early determination will help guide a rapid and aggressive life-saving approach for those patients who are in imminent danger of losing their lives. It also identifies the need for beginning the transport as soon as possible.

Some patients are obviously **not sick.** They call for an ambulance for a variety of reasons, and a routine or nonemergent transport is all that is required. These patients will still receive an assessment, but they may or may not receive any treatment at the hands of the transport team. They still need to be monitored throughout the transport and receive compassionate and professional patient care and a continuous ongoing assessment. Great caution must be exercised in labeling patients "not sick" because patient status can change quickly, and an unaware paramedic may be caught off guard when assuming a not sick patient is stable when the patient may not be.

> The patients who are between "sick" and "not sick" can be the most difficult for both experienced and novice paramedics to handle.

The term **not yet sick** describes the patients in between sick and not sick. These patients are not yet showing signs of severe, immediate life-threatening conditions but are sufficiently ill or injured as to require a watchful eye and continual reassessment. Throughout this chapter examples of sick and not yet sick conditions are presented as the various components of patient assessment are discussed.

Overview of Patient Assessment

The essentials of a patient assessment are broken down into four elements:

1. **Scene size-up**
2. **Primary survey**
3. **Secondary survey**
4. **Ongoing assessment**

The NHTSA Department of Transportation (DOT) National Standard Curricula for both EMT-Basic and paramedic training describe four general methods of patient assessment that are based on two basic parameters: whether the patient is experiencing an injury due to trauma or symptoms associated with an illness, and whether the patient is conscious and responsive enough to be interviewed or too altered in mental status to be a reliable source of information.[1] The four pathways that are shown in Figure 14-1 organize and develop key pieces of information about the patient's condition.

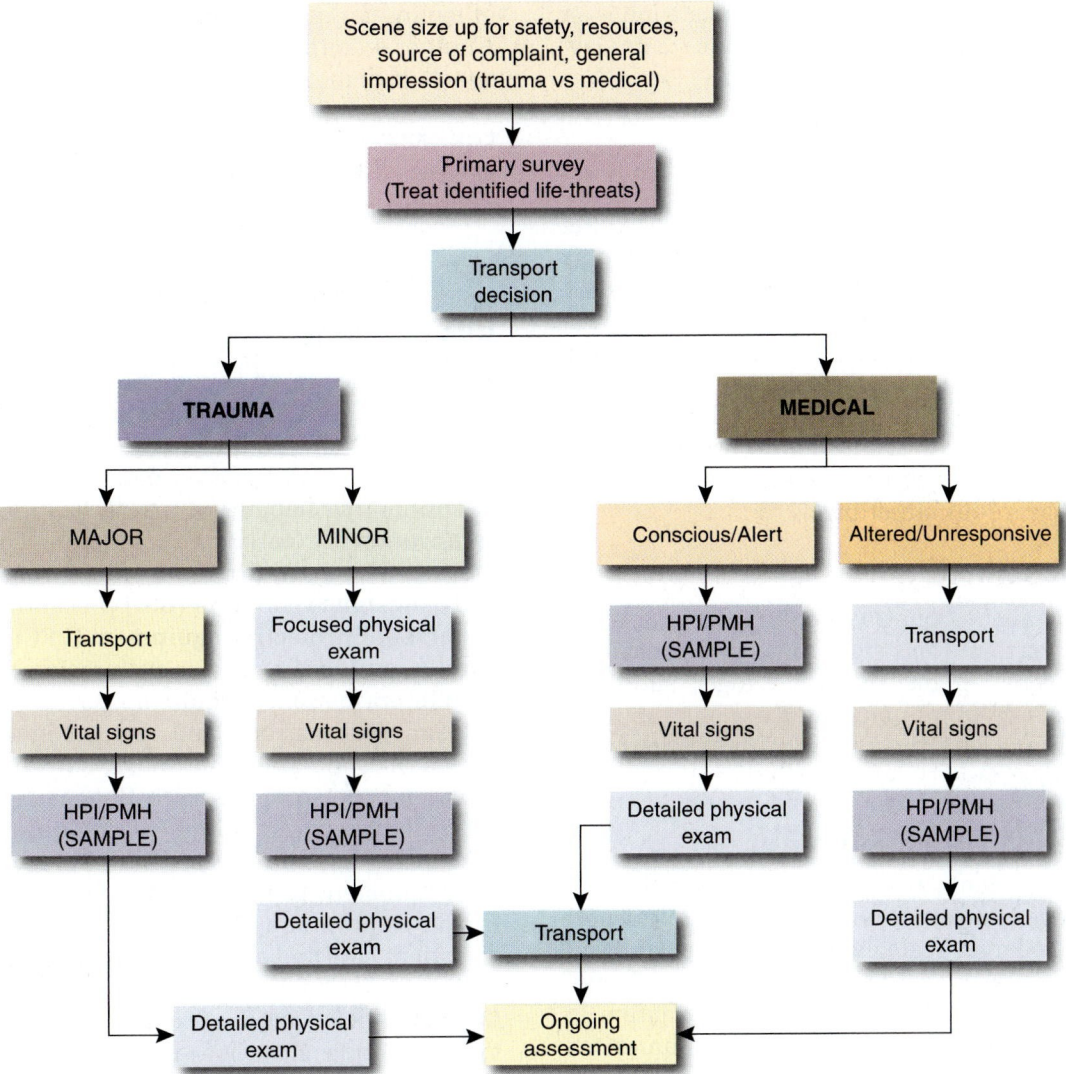

Figure 14-1 This algorithm shows an approach of assigning patients to one of four pathways. Don't feel compelled to do so. Keep an open mind during the primary, secondary, and ongoing assessments. (HPI = history of present illness, PMH = past medical history)

Although this approach provides structure and a logical flow of events, care must be exercised in using this tool. This approach may inadvertently create an artificial situation in which a paramedic feels compelled to "assign" patients into one of these pathways in order to conduct an assessment. The process outlined in this text takes a more open approach to the primary and secondary survey that is similar to the one utilized by physicians. **See the following Skill Sheets for detailed descriptions of assessment skills, including Skill Sheet 10: End Tidal Capnography; Skill Sheet 12: Pulse Oximetry (also see Step-by-Step 12); Skill Sheet 25: Arterial Pulse Locations; Skill Sheet 26: Blood Glucose Assessment (also see Step-by-Step 26); Skill Sheet 27: Chest Auscultation (also see Step-by-Step 27); Skill Sheet 28: Nystagmus Assessment; Skill Sheet 29: Orthostatic Vital Signs (also see Step-by-Step 29); Skill Sheet 30: Prehospital Stroke Evaluation (also see Step-by-Step 30); Skill Sheet 31: Trauma Scoring; Skill Sheet 32: Primary Survey (also see Step-by-Step 32); Skill Sheet 33: Secondary Survey (also see Step-by-Step 33); Skill Sheet 34: Chest Pain Assessment; Skill Sheet 35: Dyspnea Assessment; Skill Sheet 36: Abdominal Assessment; Skill Sheet 37: ECG Acquisition (also see Step-by-Step 37; and Skill Sheet 76: Traumatic Brain Injury Assessment.**

The Scene Size-Up

Prehospital emergency situations present in their own environments. You must carefully take note of the various findings of the scene, both for your own information as well as for other healthcare providers in the continuum of care. The scene size-up gives valuable insight as to the nature of illness, mechanism of injury, and possible need for additional caution and resources. Elements of the size-up include: safety assessment, determining the number of patients, mechanism of injury (MOI)/nature of illness (NOI) assessment, body substance isolation (BSI) and protective equipment assessment, and additional resource assessment. With the exception of the safety assessment, which starts every call and is an ongoing issue, the remaining elements of the scene size-up can be performed in any order. DOT 3-3.1, 3-3.2, 3-3.3, 3-3.4

Dispatch Information

The emergency medical dispatcher (EMD) is usually the first to be in contact with the patient or someone calling on the patient's behalf. As such, information that is gleaned from the caller through the use of established dispatch protocols may generate useful information about a critical incident, even before the arrival of emergency medical providers on the scene.[2,3] In addition to clinical information about the patient, the EMD may also identify and relay scene safety issues to the responding field crews such as potential violence, weapons, or other hazardous situations.

Safety Assessment

Scene safety is always one of your first priorities. Be aware of your surroundings at all times and constantly formulate "escape" plans in case danger suddenly appears. The safety of you and your crew is the most important, followed by the safety of the patient and bystanders. DOT 3-3.5, 3-3-51

Determine the Number of Patients

The number of patients at a scene will determine the number and type of emergency personnel and transport units needed. In larger scale events such as mass casualty incidents, it is critical to estimate the number of injured persons quickly and relay that information to dispatch so that appropriate support and resources can be sent to the scene. DOT 3-3.8

CONNECTIONS Chapter 54: Special Events and Mass Gatherings provides further details about large-scale incidents.

MOI/NOI Assessment

Quickly determine whether the patient's primary complaint is due to a traumatic or medical event. The **mechanism of injury (MOI)** associated with trauma may be readily apparent, as in the case of a motor vehicle crash or an assault. The **nature of the illness (NOI)** is often more difficult to discover from the scene survey alone although certain clues such as medication bottles or in-home medical devices may provide early clues. DOT 3-3.6, 3-3.7, 3-3.52

Be careful not to make the distinction between trauma and medical incidents "black and white." There are times when both types of complaints exist. For example, an older female falls down a flight of stairs, breaking her arm and injuring her hip. It may appear to be purely trauma at first glance, but subsequent questioning of family reveals that the patient complained

of feeling faint, and then she lost her balance and fell. Another example is the driver who because of a heart attack or diabetic emergency crashes his car.

CONNECTIONS Chapter 18: Mechanism of Injury provides greater detail of the forces involved in various types of mechanisms of injury.

BSI, PPE, and Protective Equipment Assessment

The potential to be exposed to blood, saliva, emesis, and other body fluids is high; therefore the paramedic must wear standard body substance precautions whenever entering a scene. EMS personnel run the same risk of contracting hepatitis B as do hospital-based health care workers.[4] Nearly every patient encounter requires the use of gloves. Some situations require additional **body substance isolation (BSI)** precautions and the use of **personal protective equipment (PPE)** such as gowns, goggles, and face masks or even respiratory protection.

Car crash scenes require approved outerwear that is cut and tear resistant and padded in the appropriate places, like the knees and elbows, to protect the body from injury. Respiratory protection may be required if the EMS crew discovers it is at a hazardous materials scene, has already become exposed, and is found within the hot (contaminated) zone. It is better to enter the scene wearing the appropriate PPE and BSI than become involved in patient care and realize that you are not protected.

CONNECTIONS Additional infection control information is found in Chapter 2: The Well-Being of the Paramedic and Chapter 33: Infectious and Communicable Diseases. Appropriate gear for the various zones of a hazardous materials incident is discussed in Chapter 53: Hazardous Materials Incidents.

Additional Resources Assessment

Certain scenes may require additional personnel, specialized equipment, or expertise in order to be brought under control. For example, a hazardous materials team may be needed to mitigate a toxic spill. The police may be required to assist with restraining a patient. Additional personnel may be necessary to assist with a difficult extrication down a flight of narrow stairs. Again, identifying these needs early and communicating them to dispatch is important so that the appropriate resources are sent as quickly as possible. DOT 3-3.10

Look for Environmental Clues

Environmental conditions may either directly or indirectly affect the patient's medical situation. They include such factors as ambient temperature, humidity, time of day, and season. For example, a homeless person who is continuously exposed to even mildly cool, wet conditions may present with altered mental status secondary to hypothermia.

The location of the incident may provide additional clues. For example, a worker who becomes suddenly ill while working in an industrial environment may be exposed to workplace hazards, such as chemicals, and may be sick for completely different reasons than a person who began feeling ill at home.

Other environmental clues about a patient's underlying health include the presence of medical equipment. As healthcare continues to develop in sophistication and complexity, more patients are being cared for outside of the hospital environment. Medical equipment can range from medication bottles and insulin syringes to home oxygen generators, ventilators, and medication pumps. The presence of these items at a scene may provide valuable background information about the patient's current complaint.

The patient's environment may also contain other, more subtle clues about health considerations. Evidence of smoking may provide information about a significant risk factor in many respiratory and cardiac diseases. Limited food or drinking water sources within an apartment or home may be a clue to nutritional disorders. Other examples include the following:

- Poor sanitary conditions and excessive filth.
- Urine or feces found in basins, bottles, or on the floor.
- The presence of flies, maggots, or other insect infestation.
- Too many people living within the home, making it overcrowded.

Organizing the Scene Size-Up Findings

Organize your scene observations as you receive them. Consider access and egress safety routes out of the scene if danger were to suddenly appear. Call for additional resources early so they will be available to you as quickly as possible. Consider if any of your observations have an impact on your patient's condition. Finally, remember to reassess your scene often. Conditions can change on a moment's notice, and you do not want to be caught by surprise. DOT 3-3.9

The Primary Survey (Initial Assessment)

Perhaps one of the greatest hallmarks of a paramedic is the ability to rapidly recognize a patient who is sick. Experience will help in the acquisition of this essential skill.[5] However, even beginning paramedics must rapidly identify, and intervene with life-threatening emergen-

cies. This is accomplished through a rigorous approach to the **primary survey,** or **initial assessment.** The primary survey is designed to rapidly identify real or potential life-threatening conditions and institute immediate care to slow, stop, or even reverse those conditions. DOT 3-3.54

The Pathophysiology behind the Primary Survey

The purpose of the primary survey is to detect and treat any problems threatening the airway, breathing, and perfusion status. The body must maintain a steady flow of oxygen to its tissues as well as eliminate waste products in order to continue functioning effectively. The mitochondria of the cells are the actual "powerhouses" of life itself; by combining sugar and oxygen in a complex series of reactions, these organelles produce the energy required for all metabolic processes. A reduction in energy output by the mitochondria literally places metabolism at risk. Therefore, the body must adequately ventilate, oxygenate, and perfuse itself if cell, organ, and body function are to be maintained (see Box 14-2).

CONNECTIONS Chapter 8: Physiology Overview discusses perfusion, ventilation, and oxygenation in detail.

Formulate a General Impression

Look closely at the patient to get an "overview" of the level of distress as you approach the patient. Determine if the patient is conscious, awake, and looking at you or gazing off into the distance. Look at the skin, and note if it is pale and sweaty or flushed and dry. Note the body position, sitting or supine, and whether or not it is relaxed or tense. Look at the facial expression for signs of anxiety or stress. This initial "across the room" impression of how "sick" the patient appears helps set up your approach to the rest of the primary survey. DOT 3-3.11, 3-3.53

Street Secrets

Compare the dispatch information to the environment and initial impression to determine if the whole story is fitting together. If the story does not match, move your alertness level from condition yellow to orange or higher, and continue to monitor scene safety closely. The alertness levels color codes are discussed in Chapter 9: Safety and Scene Size-Up.

Establish the Need to Manually Stabilize Cervical Spine

Based on findings determined by the scene size-up, it should become rapidly apparent whether the patient has sustained a traumatic injury. In these situations,

BOX 14-2   **A Closer Look: Oxygen, Glucose, and Aerobic Respiration**

Why are glucose and oxygen so important to human life? Simply put, these two molecules are put to use by the cell to produce adenosine triphosphate (ATP), the primary energy unit that powers cellular processes. Simple organisms can generate most of their ATP without oxygen through **glycolysis,** where a glucose molecule is broken down into two pyruvate molecules. Some ATP is produced this way but not enough to power more complex human cells. Our bodies take those pyruvate molecules through a two part process, known as **aerobic respiration,** to generate significantly more ATP. Part one is known as the *Krebs cycle,* where the pyruvate is converted through a series of steps into a variety of different compounds. Along the way, compounds such as CO_2, H^+, and high energy-containing molecules such as $NADH_2^+$ and $FADH_2$ are released, and more ATP is produced (Figure 14-2).

Part two of aerobic respiration uses an **electron transport chain** to take the $NADH_2^+$ and $FADH_2$ molecules and convert them to NAD^+ and FAD. In doing so, a significant amount of ATP and hydrogen ions are produced. The hydrogen ions combine with oxygen to produce water, which is also used by the body. If oxygen is missing or is too scarce, hydrogen will accumulate, and the electron transport chain will fail to produce ATP. Ergo, we can't live without oxygen!

Aerobic respiration

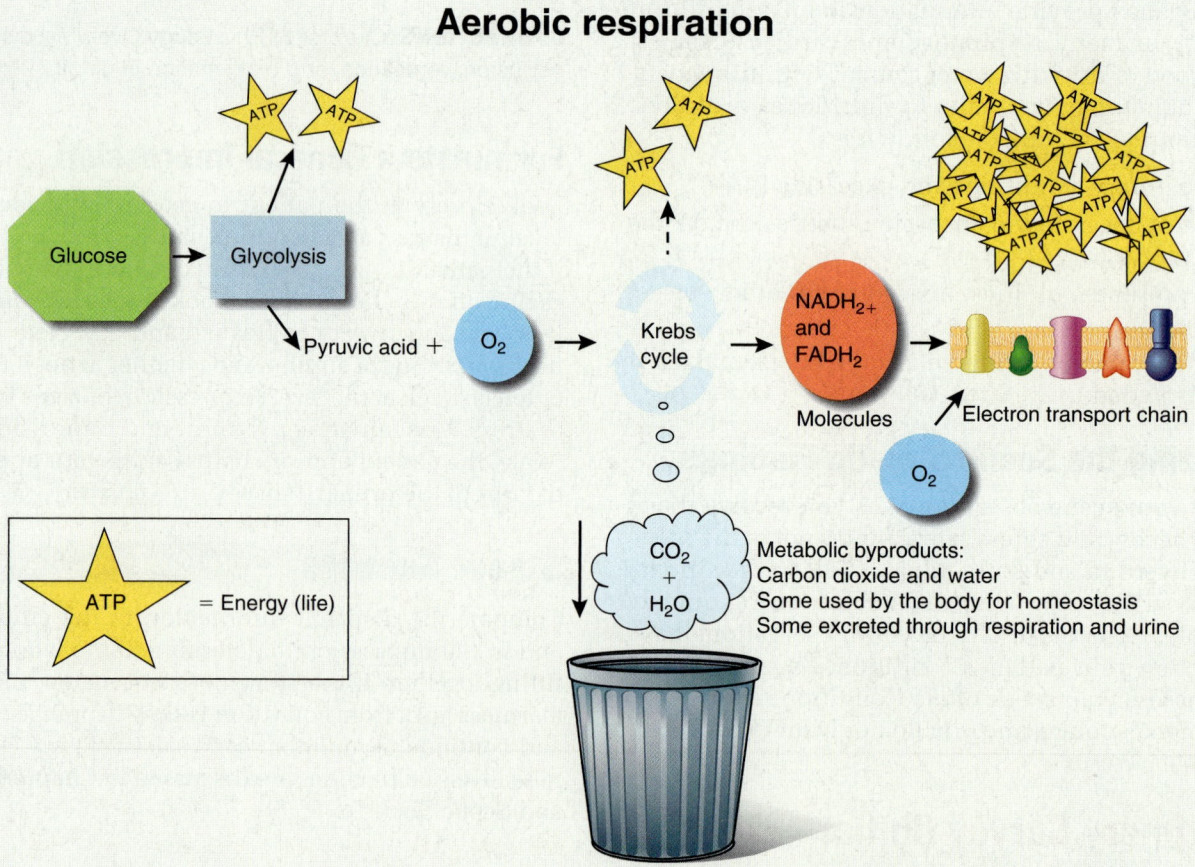

Figure 14-2   Glucose and oxygen are essential to energy (life). Glucose is broken down first by glycolysis and generates energy (ATP stars); the oxygen combines with pyruvic acid and, through the Krebs cycle, produces a little bit more energy, along with the metabolic byproducts, carbon dioxide and water. When energy containing molecules are "fed" into the electron transport chain with more oxygen powering it, *much* more energy is produced. This is why glucose and oxygen are essential to life.

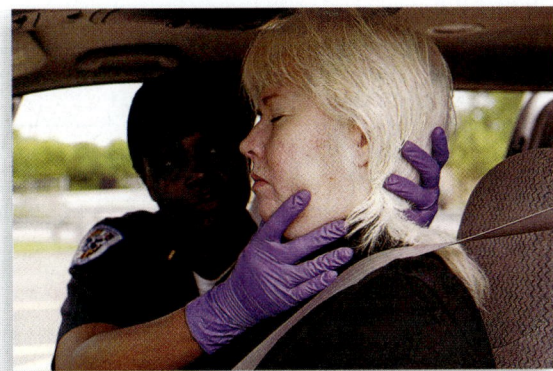

Figure 14-3 Rescuer stabilizing the cervical spine from the side.

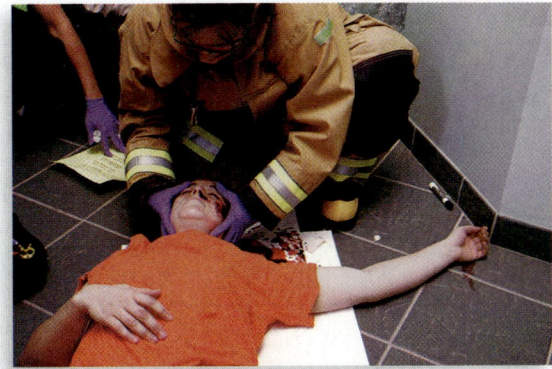

Figure 14-4 Rescuer holding cervical spine on a supine patient from above the head.

you may need to first stabilize the cervical spine and protect the patient from potential further injury as you begin assessing airway, breathing, and circulation. Maintain a high index of suspicion and institute manual cervical spine stabilization if there is any possibility of injury; in other words, if a mechanism of injury involving the spine even remotely exists, manually stabilize the head in a neutral alignment immediately. If further investigation eliminates the possibility of cervical spine injury, then stabilization can be discontinued. DOT 3-3.16, 3-3.17

Working in the Gray Zone

Standards for when to apply spinal immobilization and when to remove it from consideration have recently come under scrutiny. Selective immobilization of the spine is discussed in Chapter 23: Spinal Trauma.

Cervical spine stabilization may begin simply by telling the awake patient *not* to nod or shake his head while another EMS provider gets into position to manually hold the head. For the patient who has an altered mental status or is unresponsive, it may be necessary to reposition the head into a neutral in-line position. Move the head gently and, if resistance is encountered, stop movement and hold the head in that position until additional assessments can be performed (Figures 14-3 and 14-4).

Establishing Responsiveness

Establishing the patient's level of responsiveness will help to establish the basic parameters of oxygenation, ventilation, and perfusion. The use of the AVPU scale during the primary survey can rapidly identify the patient's level of consciousness by determining how a patient responds to some form of stimulus: DOT 3-3.12, 3-3.13

AVPU Scale

A Alert (or Awake)
V Verbal
P Pain
U Unresponsive

These four basic levels of responsiveness comprise the **AVPU** scale. Note that there is no description on *how* alert the patient is or the level of orientation. In the primary survey, only a basic level of consciousness is assessed to rapidly establish the patient's baseline. A more precise measurement of mental status is conducted during the focused physical exam (covered later in this chapter).

Pediatric patients, especially those of toddler age and younger, present communication challenges unique to their age group. Evaluating their initial level of consciousness may need to be adjusted for these differences. Chapter 43: Pediatric Patients will cover assessment approaches to this special population. You should also review Chapter 44: Geriatric Patients to learn about the communication challenges associated with the older segment of the population. DOT 3-3.14, 3-3.20, 3-3.23

Street Secrets

The **Glasgow Coma Score (GCS)** has traditionally been applied to trauma patients to assess their responsiveness. This tool can be used on medical as well as trauma patients. **Skill Sheet 31: Trauma Scoring describes the elements of the exam.**

A: Establishing Airway Patency

Patency of the airway refers to the lack of obstruction encountered when air passes from the outside environment into the lower airway. It also describes the ability of the patient to maintain the airway in an

TABLE 14-1   Potential Airway Obstructions and Immediate Interventions

Potential Obstructions	Signs	Immediate Interventions
Emesis, blood, lower airway secretions	Gurgling	Lateral positioning; finger sweep, mechanical suctioning
Foreign body	Stridor	Abdominal thrusts; Magill forceps, suction
Tongue	Snoring, grunting	Lateral positioning; head tilt, chin lift; modified jaw thrust; oropharyngeal airway insertion
Soft tissue edema, inflammation	Grunting, stridor, drooling	Careful positioning of patient (sitting if necessary)

Working in the Gray Zone

Several EMS textbooks use an **ABCDE** method of describing the primary survey, with "D" meaning disability, or impairment of neurologic function and mental status, and "E" indicating "expose and re-cover."[6,7] The expose and re-cover step reminds the paramedic to remove clothing to visualize the body and then cover the patient up to preserve body heat, privacy, and modesty. While this might be a convenient mnemonic to remember, it also implies that checking for mental status comes *after* checking for airway, breathing, and circulation. This text advocates checking for mental status as you first encounter patients, even before you first touch them.

open and clear state. Under normal conditions, there should be no obstructions impeding air flow, and little or no sounds should be heard with normal respirations. Upper airway obstruction may cause **stridor,** a harsh raspy sound that can be heard without a stethoscope during inspiration. Other obstruction sounds include grunting, snoring, or gurgling. If such an obstruction exists, the primary survey is interrupted, and action is taken immediately. Table 14-1 lists some causes of airway obstruction and the rapid interventions that should be performed to correct each of them. DOT 3-3.15, 3-3.21

B: Establishing Breathing Status

Respiratory effort and rate are fundamental measurements of ventilation. It is not easy to observe how effectively a patient is breathing because of minimal movement in the chest (see the Gray Zone box on page 283). A person at rest will mostly use the diaphragm to breath to move an average of 500 mL of **tidal volume** into the lungs with each breath. During normal, unstressed breathing, diaphragmatic movement is hardly noticeable. Carefully observe both the chest and abdom-

inal areas of the body to look for movement in either location. You may need to remove outer layers of clothing to be able to observe chest wall movement. DOT 3-3.18, 3-3.19

As you observe respirations, take note of the patient's position as well. A patient who needs to sit upright in order to be comfortable breathing is trying to increase lung expansion during inspiration. A patient who needs to lean over and support her weight on her hands and arms is in a **tripod position;** this position allows the weight of the chest to be distributed off the diaphragm (Figure 14-5). A person in respiratory distress will also tend to instinctively place his head and neck into a natural **sniffing position** and even flare his nostrils in order to increase airflow. However, lower airway obstruction, such as occurs with bronchospasm from asthma, obstructive pulmonary diseases, or smoke inhalation, may still cause the patient to **hypoventilate,** despite these positional changes.

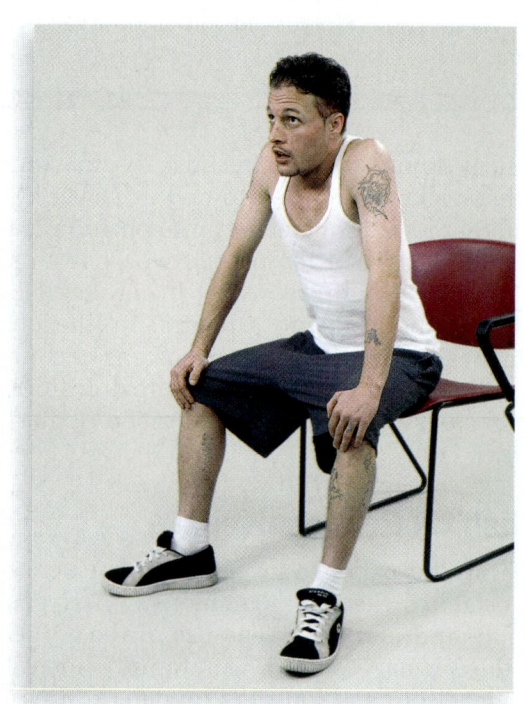

Figure 14-5   Tripod positioning.

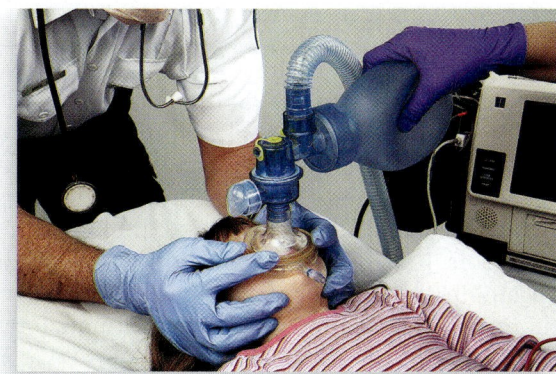

Figure 14-6   Assist ventilations with a bag-mask.

An increase in respiratory rate, or **tachypnea,** may be the first indication of a potentially serious condition. **Hypoxia,** or low levels of oxygen in the bloodstream, may be the cause. The rate increase may be subtle, so listen carefully for unusually short sentence structures as the patient pauses to take additional breaths. Providing supplemental oxygen early will increase the concentration of this gas in the alveolar space, causing it to diffuse into the bloodstream at a faster rate and at a higher concentration. This may help to slow the rate of breathing, helping the patient to conserve energy.

A slow rate of respiration (**bradypnea**) is a sign of impending **respiratory failure.** Once the body can no longer compensate for its condition, it cannot further respond to the abnormal oxygen and carbon dioxide levels in the bloodstream. As a result, the contraction of the diaphragm and accessory muscles fatigue and slow down. A slow respiratory rate in a patient who is altered or unresponsive requires immediate ventilatory management with a bag-mask and supplemental oxy-

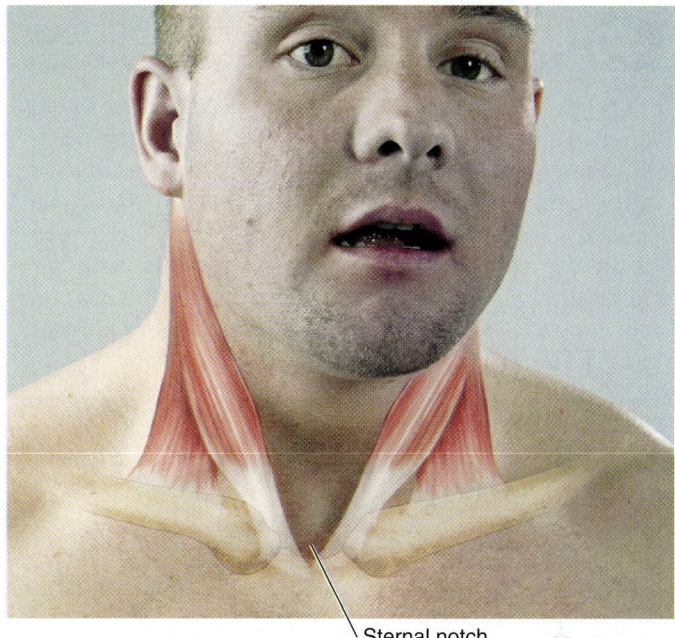

Sternal notch

Figure 14-7   Sternal notch retraction and accessory muscle use.

gen (Figure 14-6). When you identify severe respiratory distress or failure in a trauma patient, quickly expose the patient's neck and trunk area. Identify and manage an open neck/chest wound, and a tension pneumothorax immediately, as both of these conditions are immediately life-threatening.

Street Secrets

One way of assessing dyspnea is to observe the speech pattern. A person in extreme respiratory distress may not be able to move enough air to speak in full sentences. They may use two or three words at a time to answer your questions and have to stop several times when speaking a full sentence. The absence of these behaviors is also telling. Your patient may *feel* short of breath, but speak in full sentences in a loud voice. These full sentences may be an indication that the patient is in fact moving appropriate volumes of air. In this case, you should consider other reasons why the patient feels short of breath, such as a cardiac condition.

In summary, carefully observe the rise and fall of the anterior trunk to estimate respiratory rate, listen to hear if sentence structure is appropriate in length, and note the patient's body positioning and whether any accessory muscle use is evident (Figure 14-7). You may have to expose the chest and neck to observe these areas more closely for accessory muscle use.

Working in the Gray Zone

Though earlier textbooks have stated that the presence of a radial pulse indicates a systolic blood pressure of at least 80–90 mmHg, there is little evidence supporting this statement.[11] In the context of the initial assessment, the presence of a radial pulse indicates a blood pressure that is at least high enough to generate a pulse wave in these distal tissues. Its absence should prompt you to seek a more central pulse quickly.

C: Establishing Cardiovascular Status

Pulse Assessment

Feel for a radial pulse. Many practitioners gently reach for the radial pulse site immediately upon introducing themselves to the patient. If the patient appears sick, assess the radial and carotid at the same time and compare their force of pulsation. DOT 3-3.22

The pulse rate and quality are noted in a rudimentary manner; at this point, just check to see whether the pulse appears "normal," "too fast," or "too slow." This determination is enough to establish the initial perfusion status. If, during this assessment, the patient has a faint, rapid radial pulse or poor skin signs such as pallor or cyanosis, lay the patient supine or lateral recumbent, and try to raise the legs 12 inches or more above the level of the heart. Placing the patient in this **"shock position"** helps reduce workload on the heart and increases preload pressure back to the right atrium.

Be careful not to place patients who are struggling to breathe into positions they do not want to be in—particularly the supine position. Medical patients who are conscious should be allowed to select a position that is most comfortable for them. Encouraging this **position of comfort** will help them maintain some control over their care and help maintain a cooperative attitude towards your team.

Assess the Skin

In addition to quickly obtaining a heart rate, skin temperature baseline can also be established. Check skin color, temperature, and condition. Normal skin will be "pink," warm, and dry. Abnormal findings include pale, cool or cold, clammy (cold and damp), diaphoretic, hot, flushed, or cyanotic skin. Mottled skin color indicates perfusion problems as some capillary beds are well perfused, poorly perfused, or not perfused at all in the same location on the body. This condition signals a very sick patient. DOT 3-3.25, 3-3.26, 3-3.27

Bleeding Assessment

Another part of the circulatory status check is to discover major, external, life-threatening bleeding and recognize clues indicating internal hemorrhage. As with any primary survey problem, if major external bleeding is discovered, the primary survey should be interrupted and the bleeding should be controlled. If major internal hemorrhage is likely, the urgency of transport to an appropriate destination increases significantly. DOT 3-3.24

It is important to interrupt the performance of the primary survey for life-threatening problems only. Your objective should be to *control* external bleeding, not fully bandage and dress the wound. Your partner or other team member can maintain pressure on the wound while you continue with the remainder of the primary survey. Bandaging non-life-threatening wounds should be delayed until the primary survey is complete.

Applying the Sick or Not Yet Sick Philosophy

As you move through each phase of the patient assessment, it is important to keep asking yourself, "Is this patient 'sick'?" This keeps the focus on recognizing the potential for severe illness or injury and taking a proactive approach to rapidly intervene. Sometimes the answer is obvious—the patient who is apneic and pulseless is "sick." But sometimes signs of severe illness can be subtle. For example, you note a slight increase in respiratory rate combined with beads of perspiration building on the patient's upper lip. These may be the first signs of decreased perfusion, indicating someone who is "sick." Early intervention may prevent this patient from deteriorating further. See Box 14-3 for a list of injuries and findings that are always treated as "sick."

Transport Decision

Take a moment at the end of your primary survey to consider your transportation options. There are several key questions to be answered: DOT 3-3.28

1. Does the patient consent to transport, or do you need to encourage the patient to accept help?
2. How will the patient be extricated from the scene?
3. How quickly should the patient be extricated?
4. How quickly should the patient be transported to the facility?
5. To which facility should the patient be transported?

As expected, the majority of these decisions can be made based upon the findings of the primary survey. The more serious the patient presentation is, the more likely the need for immediate transport.

BOX 14-3   "Sick" Conditions

Here are some specific injuries that must be treated as "sick" as soon as they are discovered in the assessment of the trauma patient:[12] DOT 3-3.29

- Unconsciousness — unstable airway
- Severe difficulty breathing or apnea
- Tension pneumothorax
- Open pneumothorax (sucking chest wound)
- Massive bleeding
- Severe head trauma with altered mental status
- Multiple long bone fractures
- Obvious signs of shock

For the medical patients, the following are complaints or findings that must be treated as "sick" when identified:[13]

- Obvious signs of shock
- Altered mental status
- Pain, tenderness, distension, or guarding of the abdomen
- Acute nonmusculoskeletal back pain in patients greater than 60 years old
- Acute chest pain in patients greater than 35 years old
- Profuse hematuria (blood in the urine)
- Major hemoptysis or hematemesis
- Wheezing or crackles in the lungs upon auscultation
- Unexplained diaphoresis

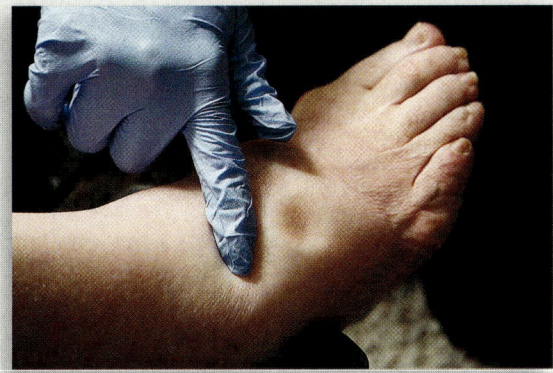

Figure 14-8   Pedal edema. Note the "pit" that remained distal to the index finger.

- Acute, severe headache
- Acute onset of motor weakness, including dysphasia, paralysis, and dysphagia
- Pulseless extremity
- Acute edema to the lower extremities (Figure 14-8)
- Seizures
- Syncope
- Acute neck stiffness with signs of fever
- Immersion event (drowning or near-drowning)
- Lightning strike
- Caustic ingestion or poisoning
- Complicated pregnancy; profuse vaginal bleeding; imminent birth
- Acute scrotal pain

Summarizing the Primary Survey

Organize your primary survey findings to determine how well your patient is ventilating, oxygenating, and perfusing. If there is any indication of a life-threatening problem with the ABCs, correct the problem *immediately.* This patient should also be transported as quickly as possible. The longer the body remains in a hypoperfusing or hypoventilating state, the sicker the patient will become and the harder it will be to recover. DOT 3-3.29, 3-3.30

The Secondary Survey

While the primary survey seeks to find and address any life-threatening conditions, the secondary survey is a more comprehensive assessment of the patient's condition. The purpose is to find any additional injury or illness that was not found during the primary survey.

> The secondary survey is just as important as the primary survey.

Patients who are not yet sick may worsen and become sick, or additional information uncovered in the secondary survey may lead you to reclassify a patient from the not yet sick category to sick, and vice versa. DOT 3-3.40, 3-3.41, 3-3.42, 3-3.43, 3-3.46, 3-3.47

Paramedics may assess for additional information in the secondary survey, often using a variety of diagnostic equipment. The decision to obtain these findings is based upon the chief complaint. For example, you will want to establish the baseline ECG, SpO_2, and perhaps even an end-tidal CO_2 level on a patient complaining of chest pain and shortness of breath.

Common devices include the following: DOT 3-3.44

- Electrocardiogram (ECG), limb-lead based (3- or 4-lead ECG).
- Percent oxygen saturation (SpO_2), using pulse oximetry.
- Blood glucose levels (BGL), using glucometers (glucose monitoring meters).
- Carbon dioxide levels, using capnography.

The Four Approaches to the Secondary Survey

There are four basic approaches to performing the secondary survey. These are based upon the patient presentation and include the following: DOT 3-3.45

1. Assessment of the trauma patient with a major mechanism of injury.
2. Assessment of the trauma patient with a minor mechanism of injury.
3. Assessment of the conscious medical patient.
4. Assessment of the unconscious medical patient.

Assessment of the Trauma Patient with a Major Mechanism of Injury

Early EMS textbooks for both basic and advanced providers focused much of their training on the identification and treatment of seriously injured trauma patients.[14,15] Current-day EMS systems revolve around the concept of quickly transporting critically injured patients to designated trauma centers. Data shows that patients who are transported to appropriate trauma facilities have greater survival from their injuries compared to those transported to a closer, nontrauma facility.[16] DOT 3-3.35, 3-3.36, 3-3.37, 3-3.38, 3-3.39, 3-3.41, 3-3.42, 3-3.43, 3-3.44, 3-3.45, 3-3.46, 3-3.48

The effective management of the injured patient with a major mechanism will depend upon a rapid organized assessment. Time is critical, and every minute that passes for a patient with uncontrolled bleeding in the chest or abdomen increases the likelihood of a poor outcome, and the only place this can be controlled is in the operating room.

CONNECTIONS Chapter 27: Trauma Patients and Trauma Systems reviews the literature that supports the concept of rapid transport of critically injured patients to appropriate trauma facilities reducing morbidity and mortality.[17]

During scene size-up, some clues to the severity of the mechanism of injury may have been noted. The American College of Surgeons committee on Trauma (ACSCOT) has recommended that the following injury mechanisms be considered as major regardless of how the patient initially "looks" upon initial assessment:[18]

Major MOIs

- Ejection from an automobile
- Death of another patient in the same passenger compartment
- Extrication time greater than 20 minutes
- Falls greater than 20 feet (or three times the height of the patient)
- Rollover crash
- High speed auto crash (initial speed greater than 40 mph, major auto deformity greater than 20 inches, intrusion of the damaged vehicle into the passenger compartment greater than 12 inches)
- Auto versus pedestrian or auto versus bicycle with significant impact (greater than 5 mph)
- Pedestrian thrown when hit or run over
- Motorcycle crash greater than 20 mph or with separation of rider from the motorcycle

If the MOI is major, assess the critical areas of the body *quickly* in order to locate potential injury sites. Your assessment begins at the head and systematically covers the central trunk of the body, followed by the extremities, and finally the back. It is not designed to find every single injury and determine every detail; rather, it determines major injury patterns using the combination of inspection, palpation, and auscultation.[17] Pay close attention to the head, trunk, pelvis, and hips as fractures and injuries to these locations often indicate life-threatening problems are present. Look for the conditions outlined in Table 14-2.

The ACS recommends that the following injury patterns should direct a transport decision to a trauma facility:[18]

Direct transport to trauma facility

- Penetrating injuries to head, neck, torso, or extremities proximal to elbows and knees
- Flail chest
- Combination of trauma with burns
- Two or more proximal long bone fractures
- Pelvic fractures
- Open or depressed skull fractures
- Paralysis
- Amputation proximal to wrist and ankle
- Major burns

Measure the patient's vital signs quickly in order to establish the patient's physiologic baseline. Rapid

TABLE 14-2   **Secondary Survey by Body Region**

Body region	Looking for	Body region	Looking for
Head	Deep lacerations, deformity of face and skull, abnormal pupil response, potential airway obstructions, facial edema	Upper extremities	Decreased/absent pulses, deep lacerations, swelling, hematoma, crepitus, deformity, decreased motor and sensory response
Neck	Jugular venous distention (JVD) (see Figure 14-9), deep lacerations, subcutaneous air, point tenderness of the spine	Back/flank/buttocks	Point tenderness along spine, deep lacerations, contusions, discoloration
Anterior chest	Tenderness, crepitus, subcutaneous air, asymmetrical breathing, flail chest, abnormal breath sounds, contusions, deep lacerations, accessory muscle use during breathing, impaled objects		
Abdomen/pelvis	Tenderness, guarding, rigidity, contusions, deep lacerations, eviscerations, impaled objects, crepitus		
Lower extremities	Decreased/absent pulses, shortening/rotation of leg, deep lacerations, swelling, hematoma, deformity and crepitus, decreased motor and sensory response		

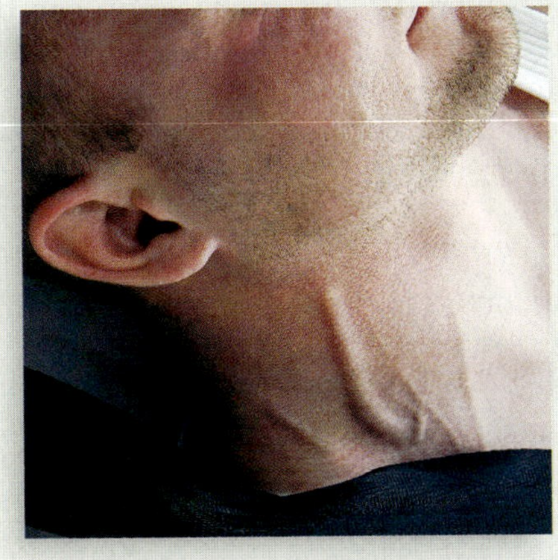

Figure 14-9   Jugular venous distention (JVD).

transport is paramount in the critically injured patient, and a precise and complete measurement of vital signs may not be necessary beyond the initial assessment (presence versus absence and fast versus slow) performed during the primary survey.[17] However, an early assessment of the pulse rate/quality, respiratory rate/depth, and systolic blood pressure should be completed shortly after the primary survey.

The American College of Surgeons has developed a series of physiologic parameters for transport to a trauma center.[18] These physiologic parameters appear to accurately identify trauma patients who need intervention at a trauma facility. They include the following:

Physiologic parameters for direct transport to a trauma center

- Glasgow Coma Scale Score less than 14, OR
- Systolic blood pressure less than 90, OR
- Respiratory rate less than 10 or greater than 29, OR
- Revised Trauma Score less than 11 (Trauma scores are discussed in Chapter 18: Mechanism of Injury).

Packaging for urgent transport begins either during or immediately after the primary survey and treatment of life-threatening conditions. It requires careful coordination among the rescue team. It is not unusual to have additional personnel assist during this process; for example, two or more rescuers may be preparing to immobilize the patient on a long backboard while the paramedic is decompressing the tension pneumothorax and another responder is preparing the back of the ambulance by setting up airway and IV equipment and supplies. Training and practice among team members is essential to maximize the efficiency of movement to the trauma center.

Working in the Gray Zone

At some time you may have learned about a "rapid trauma assessment." Since its introduction in the national standard curriculum, instructors have debated about the exact intent of the term. Is it performed during or after the initial assessment? Is it performed before or after transport begins? Is it designed to identify life-threatening conditions? Because of these unresolved questions, the authors of this textbook have chosen to stay true to the original intent of the primary survey of the trauma patient.

Once en route with a critical patient, perform the secondary survey as time and resources permit. For example, if the patient's airway or breathing status is compromised, you may not be able to obtain the patient's medical history. Conversely, if several rescuers are assisting you during transport, you may be able to complete the survey. The secondary survey includes the SAMPLE medical history, a complete set of vital signs, and a detailed physical examination.

SAMPLE is a mnemonic that can be used to remember the components to ask to quickly elicit a patient's past medical history. This information can be critical to the care of the patient. For example, patients with known heart disease or diabetes face more challenges in recovering from their injuries than do patients without these diseases.[17]

SAMPLE: Past medical history

S Symptoms and signs. A quick mental review of these can help you focus follow-up or clarification questions as you gather information.

A Allergies to medications. This includes over-the-counter (OTC) as well as prescribed medications.

M Medications. These include prescribed, OTC, homeopathic, and herbal remedies.

P Past medical history. In addition to chronic conditions, such as hypertension and diabetes, a prior history of injuries to the same body region as the current event may also be important to record.

L Last Meal. This may be important to note, especially for the patient who may require surgical intervention as part of his care.

E Events that lead up to the current condition. This reminds the paramedic to determine what happened to the patient that resulted in the current traumatic injury.

The DCAP-BTLS acronym may be helpful in remembering key elements of assessment in musculoskeletal injuries.

DCAP-BTLS

D Deformity
C Contusions
A Abrasions
P Penetrations or Punctures
B Burns
T Tenderness
L Lacerations
S Swelling

TABLE 14-3 Detailed Head-to-Toe Examination

Body region	Looking for
Head	Deformities, contusions, abrasions, punctures, burns, tenderness, lacerations, swelling (DCAP-BTLS), blood and/or clear fluid leaking from the nares or ear canals, missing teeth, temporal mandibular joint (TMJ) pain
Neck	DCAP-BTLS; medical alert tag
Anterior chest	DCAP-BTLS; full auscultation of lung fields
Abdomen/pelvis	DCAP-BTLS
Lower extremities	DCAP-BTLS; pulse, motor and sensory function
Upper extremities	DCAP-BTLS; pulse, motor and sensory function
Back/flank/buttocks	DCAP-BTLS
Skin	Color, temperature, condition, and capillary refill time

The detailed physical examination is a precise, head-to-toe examination of the patient. It may take several minutes to complete a detailed examination. It is conducted only as time allows. Beyond the findings associated with the primary survey the detailed physical examination looks for conditions in every part of the body as outlined in Table 14-3. Time permitting, stabilization and further care should be provided. For example, minor wounds should be dressed, and simple closed fractures of long bones should be splinted.

In summary, the trauma patient with a significant mechanism of injury can be assessed in the following manner:

1. Conduct a scene size-up to determine mechanism of injury.
2. Perform a primary survey to identify and manage major life-threatening injuries. Make a transportation decision (including destination and when to begin).
3. Rapidly assess the major body areas to identify potential life-threatening injuries not found during the primary survey.
4. Measure initial vital signs to establish baseline.
5. Package and begin transport, if not already started.
6. Conduct a SAMPLE medical history to determine the patient's past medical history that might compound the injuries.

7. Perform a detailed physical examination as time permits.

8. Continuously conduct an ongoing assessment to detect any changes in condition, or to assess response to treatment.

Assessment of the Patient with a Minor Trauma Mechanism

A minor trauma mechanism generally does not cause enough force to seriously injure the patient. For example, a boy falling off his bicycle will probably not experience anything more serious than cuts and bruises and the occasional fracture of a long bone or wrist. However, you must *carefully* and fully consider the mechanism of injury before deciding that it is indeed minor in nature. If the boy falls off his bicycle and strikes his unhelmeted head against the roadway, he may very well experience a life-threatening brain injury. In fact, the majority of bicycle-related deaths occur as a result of traumatic brain injury.[19]

DOT 3-3.34, 3-3.40

It is also possible that a patient's past medical history or medications can complicate a seemingly minor traumatic event. For example, if a patient is taking anticoagulant (blood-thinning) medication for a heart condition, even the most minor trauma could cause bleeding that cannot easily be stopped. This is especially true in elderly patients who have an impaired ability to compensate for blood loss, low blood pressure, or exposure to heat and cold. The elderly and patients with debilitating bone illnesses may break major bones in their bodies with only minor force. Therefore, it is important to consider all aspects of the mechanism of injury before deciding its severity.

Once the mechanism of injury is determined to be minor and the primary survey is complete, perform a physical examination that focuses on the injury site. The DCAP-BTLS mnemonic, described above, is a helpful memory aid while performing this assessment. If an extremity is injured, carefully confirm that circulation distal to the injury site is not compromised and that the motor and sensory response is intact.

After the focused physical examination, a full set of vital signs should be obtained as well as the SAMPLE medical history. If time permits or the paramedic chooses, a complete head-to-toe physical exam may also be performed. In summary, the trauma patient with a minor mechanism of injury can be assessed in the following manner:

1. Conduct a scene size-up to determine mechanism of injury.

2. Perform a primary survey to identify and manage major life-threatening injuries.

3. If the scene size-up indicates that the mechanism of injury carried little force and the primary survey reveals a patient with little or no distress, perform a focused physical assessment of the presenting minor injuries.

4. Measure initial vital signs to establish baseline.

5. Package and transport.

6. Conduct a SAMPLE medical history to determine the patient's past medical history (PMH) that might compound the injuries.

7. As time permits, perform a detailed secondary physical examination to make sure no other injuries exist.

8. Assess the patient continuously looking for any changes in condition or the response to treatment.

Assessment of the Conscious Medical Patient

For the conscious medical patient, early history taking is an important first step. A significant amount of information can be gained quickly through a well-organized line of questioning. There are several mnemonics that are useful in gathering the **history of present illness (HPI)**. A common one is **OPQRST**, which is used to assess the complaint of pain or discomfort, follows:

DOT 3-3.32

OPQRST

O **O**nset: What were you doing when the pain or discomfort began?

P **P**rovoke/**P**alliate: Is there anything that makes it feel worse or better? Does pressing on it make it better or worse?

Q **Q**uality: Can you describe the pain or discomfort?

R **R**adiate: Where is the pain or discomfort? Does the discomfort travel anywhere? Are there any other symptoms related to your primary complaint?

S **S**everity: How severe is the pain or discomfort?

T **T**ime: When did the pain or discomfort begin? What has it been doing over time?

When a patient reports pain in a particular location, consider the possibility that this pain may be referred. Figure 14-10 illustrates how different organs can signal pain in an area that is completely different from where the problem originates. A myocardial infarction may present with pain in the left arm, and a kidney stone may present itself as pain in the flank area.

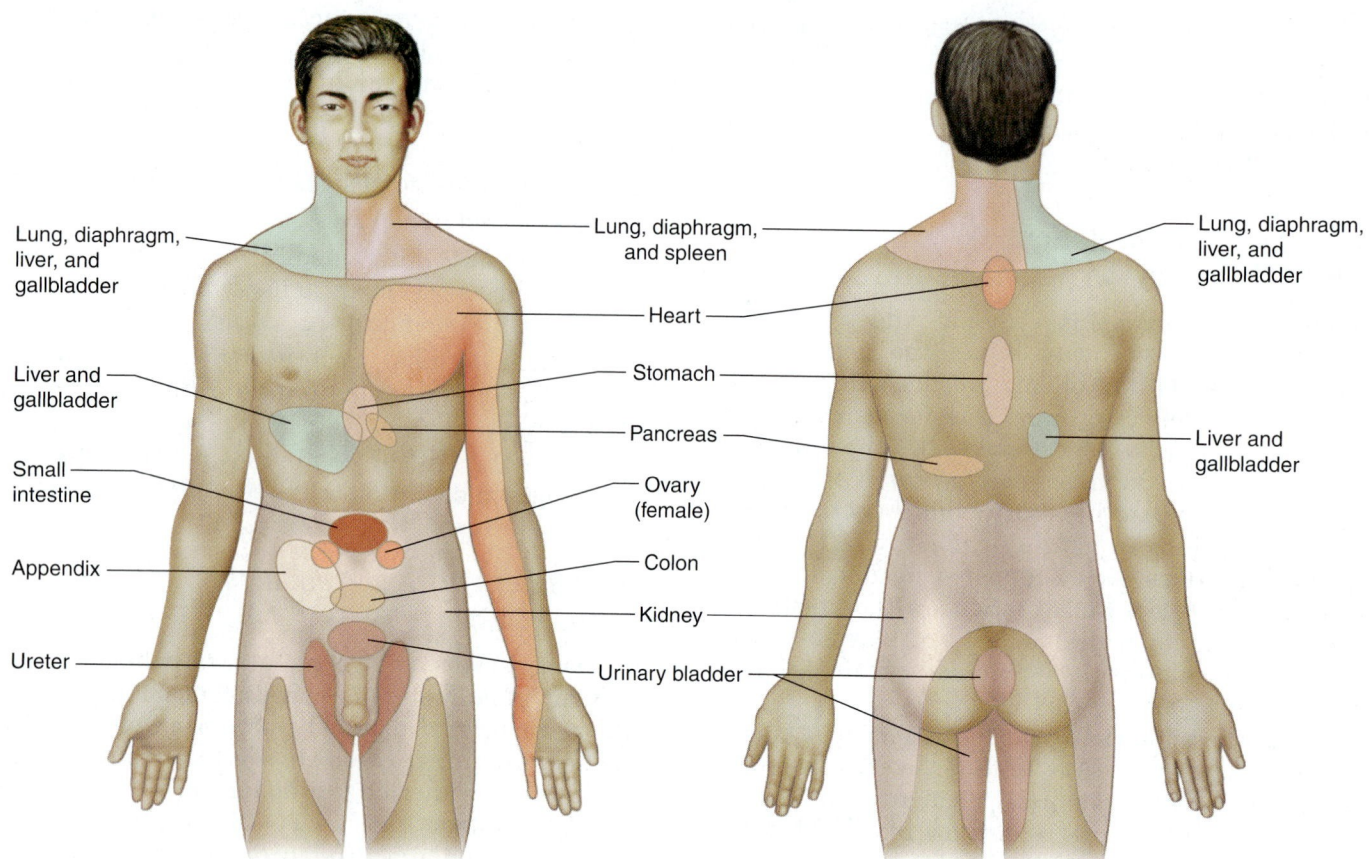

Figure 14-10   Sites of referred pain.

Street Secrets

Referred pain can be difficult to assess. Appendicitis for example can present with peri-umbilical pain or shoulder pain, (See Chapter 34: Gastroenterology for a discussion on referred pain) and a myocardial infarction may present as neck or epigastric discomfort. While charts are helpful to map where particular nerve bundles may transfer a painful sensation, you should keep an open mind. Maintain a high index of suspicion, and look for life threats first. For example, abdominal pain in a person over the age of 30 should be considered a myocardial infarction before you decide it is "just indigestion." Shoulder pain after trauma should be considered a ruptured spleen before it is considered a "stiff muscle." Your job is to suspect the worst-case scenario until a physician can further investigate and diagnose the problem.

While you may not ask these questions in the exact order, the mnemonic is a helpful way to remember them. Another helpful mnemonic, PASTE helps to organize the questions related specifically to shortness of breath:

PASTE

P **P**rovoke, **P**rogression: What was happening when the shortness of breath began? Has it gotten better or worse?

A **A**ssociated Chest Pain: Do you have any chest pain?

S **S**putum, color and amount: Are you coughing? Is there any sputum? What color is it? How much?

T **T**ime, **T**rauma, **T**emperature: How long have you been short of breath? Do you have a fever? Have you fallen or otherwise been hurt?

E **E**xertion, **E**xercise tolerance: Does activity make the shortness of breath worse?

CONNECTIONS Review Chapter 10: Therapeutic Communications and History Taking for more detailed information about information gathering. Remember that a confident, empathetic communication approach will provide a wealth of information about a patient's medical condition and history in a short period of time.

The second part of history taking is soliciting the patient's past medical history (PMH). It is normal to suspect that some part of the patient's medical history is contributing to the current event. The mnemonic, SAMPLE, described earlier in this chapter, can be used to recall the elemental questions. It is important to remember that these questions are not the only ones you will ask; they serve as the foundation for a more thorough and detailed history-taking procedure.

Either during or immediately after history taking, obtain a complete set of vital signs. The first set of vital signs will establish the patient's baseline. As reassessment occurs, trends in the patient's condition can be determined. This information can be valuable to the hospital that is continuing to care for the patient. DOT 3-3.2

The detailed physical examination will begin with a focused physical examination of affected body systems as soon as baseline vital signs are established. Inspect, auscultate, palpate, and percuss as appropriate. Basic findings to determine during a focused medical examination are summarized in Table 14-4. All of the conditions described in Table 14-4 will be covered in detail in their respective chapters.

Think of each of the major body systems as you complete the head-to-toe exam. These systems are interconnected and form a complete picture of the patient. For

TABLE 14-4 Examination Findings for a Conscious Medical Patient

General	Patient position (sitting, supine, or standing; relaxed, tense, tripod, pacing)		Tender chest wall
	Unexplained diaphoresis		Unusual shape of chest; any discoloration or bruising
	Pale or cyanotic skin color		Any pain response during palpation
	Unusual warmth or coolness of skin temperature	Abdomen	Distension
	Sensory acuity (sight, sound, sensation)		Rigidity or guarding
			Unusual masses
Head-Eyes-Ears-Nose-Throat (HEENT)	Pupil size, shape, equality, and response		Unusual discoloration
			Ascites
	Facial symmetry		Needle marks
	Abnormal weakness of facial muscles		Colostomy appliance
			Pain upon palpation
	Dysphasia, dyskinesia		Hematochezia/melena
	Any unusual discharge from nares, ears, mouth	Pelvis	Incontinence of urine
			Hematuria
	Missing teeth, poor oral hygiene		Priapism
	Hematemesis, hemoptysis	Lower extremities	Weak, asymmetric, or absent distal pulses
	Any odor from the mouth		
	Lingual (tongue) trauma		Unusual motor weakness or sensory loss (hemiplegia, hemiparesis)
	Edematous tissue		
Neck	Jugular venous distension versus flat neck veins while supine		Pedal edema
			Needle marks
	Medical condition identification tags		Open sores
			Deep vein tenderness
	Masses or lesions	Upper extremities	Weak, asymmetric, or absent distal pulses
	Accessory muscle use		
	Nucchal rigidity		Unusual motor weakness or sensory loss (hemiplegia, hemiparesis)
	Pain upon movement		
	Bruits		
	Palpable lymph nodes		Needle marks
Chest	Adventitious lung sounds		Medical alert bracelets
	Unequal lung sounds	Back/flank	Sacral edema
	Intercostal retractions		Unusual discoloration
	Sternal notch retraction		Posterior lung sounds
	Evidence of internal pacemaker, automated implanted cardiac defibrillator (AICD), or catheters implanted under the skin		Incontinence of feces
			Sores
			Pain upon palpation/acute onset of flank pain

example, when evaluating a patient with chest discomfort, you should do the following:

- Visualize the chest for symmetry and any unusual deformity, shape, or bruises (musculoskeletal system).
- Palpate the chest wall for tenderness and whether or not the pain is reproducible (musculoskeletal system, respiratory system).
- Auscultate lung sounds (respiratory system).
- Auscultate heart tones (cardiovascular).
- Visualize the neck for jugular venous distension (cardiovascular).
- Palpate the sacral region of the back and lower extremities for edema (cardiovascular).
- Palpate the abdominal cavity for tenderness (GI pain referring to the chest cavity).

In summary, the conscious medical patient should be assessed in the following manner:

Assessing the conscious medical patient

1. Perform a scene size-up to find any environmental clues to the patient's condition.
2. Conduct a primary survey to identify and treat any life-threatening conditions.
3. Elicit a history of the present illness (HPI).

4. Measure baseline vital signs (may be done concurrently with HPI) and a detailed head-to-toe exam as time permits.
5. Perform a focused physical exam (may be done concurrently with HPI).
6. Finalize a transport decision (may be completed prior to now).
7. Continually assess the patient as conditions warrant.

Assessment of the Unconscious Medical Patient

A patient who has a severely altered level of consciousness or is unconscious will be unable to provide reliable information about complaints or medical history. Assessing the unconscious medical patient requires a different approach than the conscious medical patient. After the primary survey, a rapid head-to-toe physical examination is performed in the secondary survey. During this exam, the paramedic should assess for the findings listed in Table 14-5. DOT 3-3.33

Either during or immediately after the rapid medical examination, baseline vital signs should be obtained. It will be particularly important to determine

TABLE 14-5 **Examination Findings for an Unresponsive Medical Patient**

Head-Eyes-Ears-Nose-Throat (HEENT)	Pupil size, shape, equality, and response		Unusual discoloration
	Any unusual discharge from nares, ears, mouth		Ascites
			Needle marks
	Hematemesis, hemoptysis		Colostomy appliance
	Any odor from the mouth		Hematochezia/melena
	Lingual trauma (tongue)	Pelvis	Incontinence of urine
	Edematous tissue		Hematuria
			Priapism
Neck	Jugular venous distension	Lower extremities	Weak, asymmetric, or absent distal pulses
	Flat neck veins while supine		Pedal edema
	Medical condition identification tags		Needle marks
	Masses or lesions		Open sores
Chest	Adventitious lung sounds	Upper extremities	Weak, asymmetric, or absent distal pulses
	Evidence of internal pacemaker/AICD or implanted catheters or devices		Needle marks
			Medical condition jewelry
	Unusual shape to the chest; discoloration or bruising	Back/flank	Sacral edema
	Any pain response during palpation		Unusual discoloration
Abdomen	Distension		Posterior lung sounds
	Rigidity or guarding		Incontinence of feces
	Unusual masses		Sores

oxygenation levels, carbon dioxide retention, and blood glucose levels as soon as possible as these problems could be the cause of unconsciousness. Use the mnemonic AEIOU-TIPS to help recall possible causes of unconsciousness.[12]

AEIOU-TIPS

A Alcohol, acid/base disorders, arrhythmias

E Encephalopathy, endocrine disorders, electrolyte disorders

I Insulin issues (hypo- or hyperglycemia)

O Opiates

U Uremia

T Trauma, tumor, thermal insult (hypothermia)

I Infection, intracerebral vascular disorders

P Poisonings, psychogenic shock (fainting)

S Seizures

Interview the family, friends, or bystanders for history or other pertinent information (Figure 14-11). Recognize that the information may be of limited usefulness, especially if third-party reporters are not familiar with the patient's background. Use mnemonics such as OPQRST and SAMPLE to guide the questioning. Search the immediate surroundings for prescription medications, recreational drugs, medical records or devices, and any other information that might provide a clue to the patient's condition.

For unconscious medical patients, the decision when to transport will most likely have been determined during the primary survey. A decision must be made when to stop performing assessments on the scene and when to begin transporting the patient. Experience in handling patients will help you develop the sense of when it is appropriate to "load and go" and when it is appropriate to "stay and play." Once transport has started, ongoing assessments should be performed often.

In summary, the altered or unconscious medical patient can be assessed in the following manner:

Assessing the unconscious medical patient

1. Perform a scene size-up to find any environmental clues that point to the patient's condition.
2. Perform the primary survey to identify and reverse any life-threatening conditions. Determine when to begin transporting.
3. Rapidly perform a focused physical exam of the patient to identify other potentially life-threatening conditions.
4. Measure baseline vital signs (may be done concurrently with rapid head-to-toe exam).
5. Elicit an HPI and PMH from bystanders and the environment.
6. Continuously assess the patient with an ongoing assessment while transporting.

The Ongoing Assessment

As the call progresses, an ongoing assessment of the patient's condition should be performed continuously. Repeated primary surveys should be done on an ongoing basis in patients who are borderline in terms of their airway, breathing, or circulatory status. Vital signs are reassessed every few minutes and after each intervention. The more critical the patient's condition, the more frequent the need to reassess in order to closely monitor for changing trends. DOT 3-3.48, 3-3.60

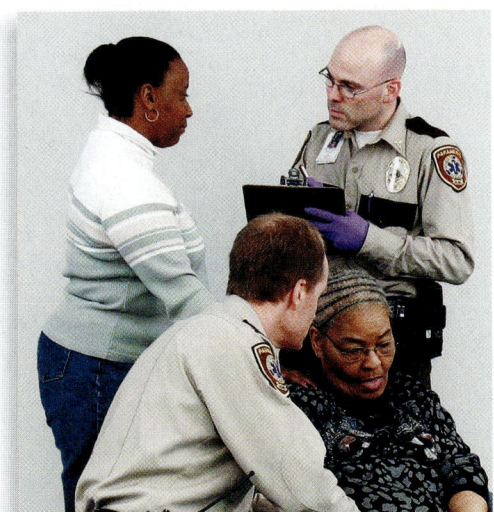

Figure 14-11 Family members can be an important source of information about the patient's medical history and present illness when a patient is unable to speak.

Working in the Gray Zone

The DOT National standard curriculum recommends that a patient's vital signs be assessed every 15 minutes, and for patients who are critically ill, vital signs are taken every five minutes. The philosophy in this book is that these numbers are arbitrary and may inadvertently cause the paramedic to think that he should **only** assess the patient's condition at these intervals. It makes more sense to look at your patient "early and often." If you see a change in symptoms or condition, reassess your patient quickly. If nothing is immediately apparent, keep a constant and vigilant eye.

Summary

The skill of patient assessment is not easy to do well. When patient assessment is approached in a systematic and logical fashion tailored to the mechanism of injury or nature of the illness, it is more likely to contain the appropriate mix of assessment and treatment. The experience of talking with and listening to the patient, combined with the practice of using your sense of sight, sound, touch, and smell, will result in a logical, efficient, and effective approach to the assessment.

Notes

1. Emergency Medical Technician Paramedic: National Standard Curriculum (EMT-P). United States Department of Transportation. http://www.nhtsa.dot.gov/people/injury/ems/emt-p/index.html (accessed August 9, 2006).

2. G. Kallsen, "The Use of Priority Medical Dispatch to Distinguish Between High- and Low-Risk Patients," *Annals of Emergency Medicine* 19.4(1990): 458–459.

3. A. Heward, "Dispatch System Affect Cardiac Arrest Detection?" *Emergency Medicine Journal Online.* http://emj.bmjjournals.com/cgi/reprint/21/1/115 (accessed July 24, 2006).

4. G. Rischitelli et al., "The Risk of Acquiring Hepatitis B or C Among Public Safety Workers," *American Journal of Preventive Medicine* 20.4 (2001): 299–306.

5. P. Benner, "Using the Dreyfus Model of Skill Acquisition to Describe and Interpret Skill Acquisition and Clinical Judgment in Nursing Practice and Education," *Bulletin of Science, Technology & Society* 24.3 (2004): 188–199.

6. B. E. Bledsoe, R. S. Porter, and R. A. Cherry, *Essentials of Paramedic Care* (Upper Saddle River, NJ: Prentice Hall, 2003).

7. M. J. Sanders, *Mosby's Paramedic Textbook,* 3rd ed. (St. Louis, MO: Elsevier Mosby, 2005).

8. E. A. Hooker, D. J. O'Brien, D. F. Danzyl, et al., "Respiratory Rates in Emergency Department Patients," *Journal of Emergency Medicine* 7 (1989): 129–132.

9. Z. V. Edmonds, W. R. Mower, L. M. Lovato, et al., "The Reliability of Vital Sign Measurements," *Annals of Emergency Medicine* 39 (2002): 233–237.

10. P. B. Lovett, "The Vexatious Vital: Neither Clinical Measurements by Nurses nor an Electronic Monitor Provides Accurate Measurements of Respiratory Rate in Triage," *Annals of Emergency Medicine* 45.1 (2005): 68–76.

11. Charles D. Deakin and J. Lorraine Low, "Accuracy of the Advanced Trauma Life Support Guidelines for Predicting Systolic Blood Pressure Using Carotid, Femoral, and Radial Pulses: Observational Study," *British Medical Journal* 321 (2000): 673–674.

12. J. E. Tintinalli, G. Kelen, and S. Stapczynski, *Emergency Medicine: A Comprehensive Study Guide,* 6th ed. (USA: McGraw-Hill Companies, 2004).

13. A. Dalton et al., *Advanced Medical Life Support,* 2nd ed. (Upper Saddle River, NJ: Pearson Publishing, 2003).

14. American Academy of Orthopaedic Surgeons, *Emergency Care and Transportation of the Sick and Injured* (Rosemont, IL: AAOS, 1973).

15. N. Caroline, *Emergency Care in the Streets* (Boston, MA: Little, Brown and Co., 1979).

16. E. Hannan et al., "Physiologic Trauma Triage Criteria in Adult Trauma Patients: Are They Effective in Saving Lives by Transporting Patients to Trauma Centers?" *Journal of the American College of Surgeons,* 200(4) (2005): 584–592.

17. Prehospital Trauma Life Support Committee, NAEMT, *Prehospital Trauma Life Support,* 5th ed. (St. Louis, MO: Mosby, 2003).

18. Committee on Trauma, American College of Surgeons, *Resources for Optimal Care of the Injured Patient* (Chicago, IL: 1999).

19. Insurance Institute for Highway Safety, "Fatality Facts 2003: Bicycles," http://www.hwysafety.org/safety%5Ffacts/fatality%5Ffacts/pdfs/bicycles.pdf (accessed July 15, 2005).

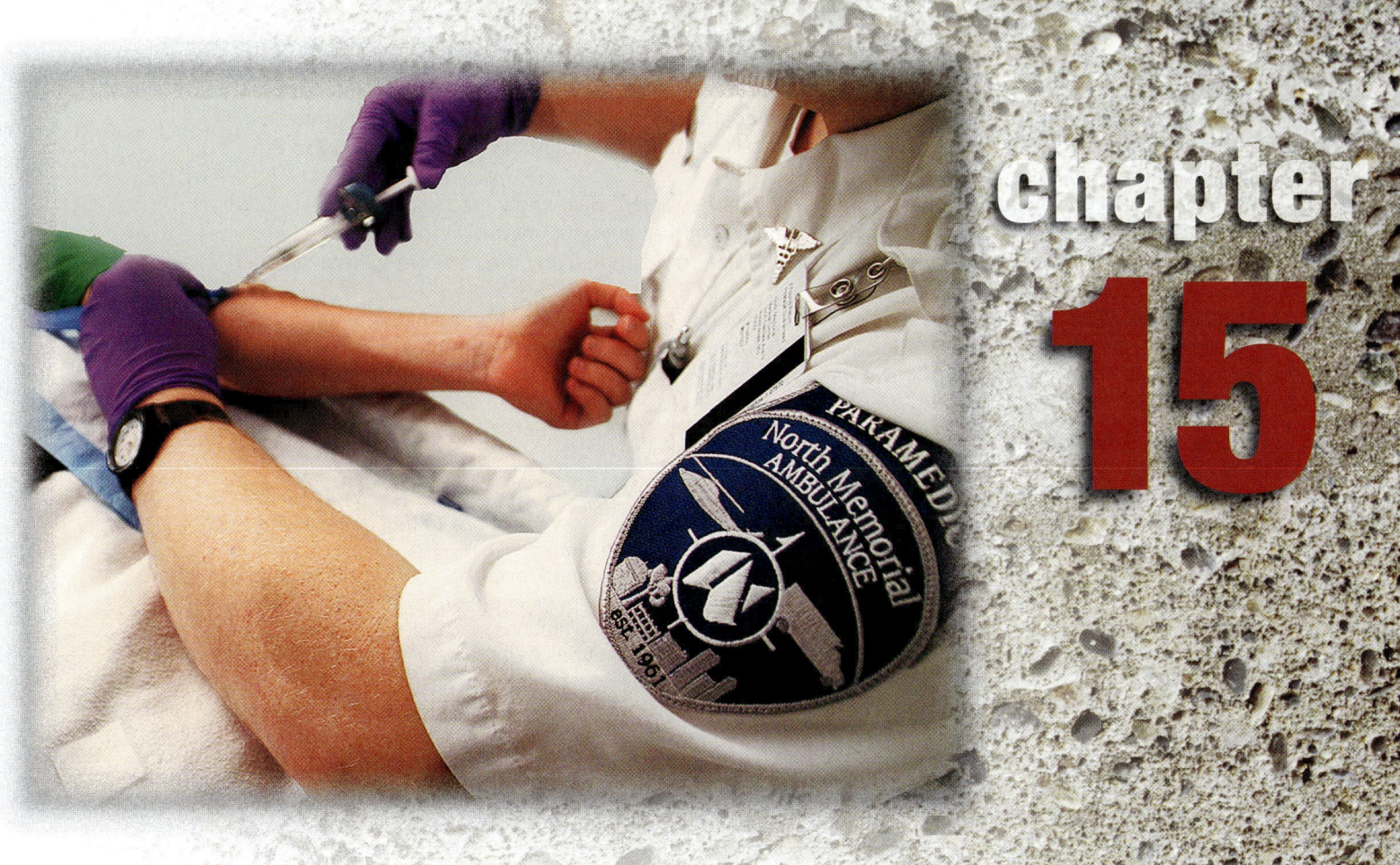

Pharmacology

"The desire to take medicine is perhaps the greatest feature which distinguishes man from animals."

—Sir William Osler

Need to Know

▶ Medication administration is an important skill for paramedics. In order to do this properly, the paramedic needs to possess a basic understanding of the responsibilities and scope of management pertinent to the administration of medications.

▶ The paramedic should understand that drugs have many names and should know the classes of medications that are commonly administered by paramedics or that are encountered in their patients.

▶ The paramedic should appreciate that drugs interact with the body (particularly the nervous system) and with other drugs.

▶ Paramedics should also appreciate that special consideration is given for medication administration to certain groups of patients such as the chronically ill, pediatric, geriatric, and pregnant patients because of physiologic differences found in each of these patient groups.

▶ Do	▶ Ask
• Perform a thorough history and physical examination to ensure the correct gathering of information, synthesizing of the field impression, and developing/implementing the treatment plan. • Determine if the patient is sick or not yet sick as this can make the difference in what, when, and if a drug is used and may determine which dose or route is appropriate. • Follow the medication "rights": the right patient, right drug, right dose, right route, right time, and right (write) documentation as you intervene with medication. • Reassess the patient, and ensure proper documentation following medication administration.	• SAMPLE history questions to determine allergy and medication history. • About prescribed, over-the-counter, herbal, and recreational (illegal or nonprescribed) drugs as well as compliance with medication regimens. • If the patient has had the medication before and if there were any adverse reactions.

Introduction

Pharmacology is the study of drugs. A pharmacist spends years learning about medications. This educational process includes an in-depth study of chemistry, biology, microbiology, pathophysiology, and anatomy. A pharmacist's interaction with a patient generally occurs following a doctor's diagnosis and recommendation for drug therapy. Paramedics spend far less time learning about drugs although they interact with patients directly and are expected to assess the patient and then determine what medication is appropriate for treatment. Often this process is independent of direct physician involvement. In order to perform this job effectively, paramedics must understand the indication, contraindication, classification, and dosage of all medications they are authorized to use in their systems. They also need to know medications commonly used by their patients. Paramedics should have a healthy appreciation of the nature of drugs and how they interact with the body and each other.

The field of pharmacology has many sub-specialties including pharmacokinetics, pharmacodynamics, pharmacogenetics, pharmacogenomics, and others. Pharmacogenetics and pharmacogenomics study the unique family responses to medication which are linked to DNA coding and genetics.[1] It is important to remember that a patient may experience an unusual reaction to a drug because of genetic characteristics, but in-depth understanding of these principles may not be helpful for paramedics. DOT 1-7.1, 1-7.20

Pharmacokinetics and Pharmacodynamics

Pharmacokinetics and pharmacodynamics study how drugs are processed by the body and are the subsets of pharmacology that are important to paramedics. Paramedics treat patients with a variety of medical and traumatic conditions that affect the metabolic processes of the body, so understanding how drugs move around in the body and are processed is very important.

Pharmacokinetics explores how drugs are delivered to, and removed from, affected organs. It includes how drugs are processed in the body through absorption, distribution, metabolism, and excretion. All of these processes occur as drugs pass across cell membranes and move throughout the body. The most important considerations in the pharmacokinetic process are the drug molecule size and shape, **solubility** in water and lipids (oily fats), ability to bind to tissue proteins, and how much a drug is **ionized.** Solubility describes how readily or easily the drug is able to combine with substances such as water or oil. Membranes contain a lipid bilayer, so if a drug is highly water soluble but not very fat soluble, it may not easily pass into a cell unless it is somehow assisted. Ionization describes how much of a drug has been altered through the gain or loss of electrically charged particles (ions). Ionizing a drug changes it into a metabolite.

All of these considerations represent potential barriers to the pharmacokinetic processes.[2] For example, if a drug molecule is too large, it may only be able to enter a cell through a special channel or by attaching to a specific receptor that has the ability to alter the cell membrane to allow passage. If the drug is highly water soluble, it will not easily pass through a membrane because cell membranes are composed of a lipid bilayer that will not easily bind to water. **Pharmacodynamics** studies how drugs interact with the living tissues in the body. DOT 1-7.19, 1-7.20

A drug is any substance that, once introduced into the body, results in a change in the patient. This change can take many forms: it can stop a process from happening, start a process, alter a process, or change the speed at which a process occurs. Drugs can enhance or suppress body systems as well as affect metabolism.[1] Although there are drugs that interact with every body system, organ, tissue, and process, nearly all the drugs used by paramedics interact with the nervous, endocrine, cardiovascular, or respiratory systems. DOT 1-7.14

Drugs come from plants, animals (including bacteria and other microbes), humans, rocks and minerals, and man-made synthetic sources. Box 15-1 lists some common medications, the sources they come from, and some vehicles used to enhance their delivery to tissues. **Vehicle** is a term used to describe a substance added to a drug preparation to provide for or enhance delivery of the drug to the body tissues. The vehicle may make absorption by the tissues easier or allow the drug to be delivered by a different route.

How Drugs Enter the Body

Drugs can enter the body through a variety of ways including ingestion, injection, absorption, and inhalation.

Ingestion

The **ingestion** route introduces drugs to the body by swallowing or eating, so the drug enters the bloodstream by absorption from the gastrointestinal (GI) tract. This absorption can occur through any part of the GI tract including the esophagus, stomach, small intestine, or colon. Drugs sometimes receive a special coating to ensure absorption from a specific location within the GI tract. An **enteric coating** is one such example. Enteric-coated pills do not break down much in the stomach, which can be helpful for patients with ulcers or sensitive stomachs. Drugs in pill, caplet, and capsule forms are generally meant to be ingested. Many liquid forms

BOX 15-1 Some Common Medications and Their Sources or Vehicles

Plants

Aspirin: willow tree
Digitalis: foxglove plant
Haldol Deconoate Injection: vehicle—sesame oil
Atropine: belladonna plant
Atrovent: soya lecithin, soybeans, and peanuts

Animals

Insulin: bovine (beef), equine (horse), and porcine (pork)
Streptokinase: bacteria

Humans

Insulin: DNA and rDNA
Blood clotting factors: blood plasma

Rocks & Minerals

Calcium: clam shells

Synthetic

Alupent: vehicle—chlorofluorocarbons (CFCs)

such as syrups and suspensions can be ingested as well. Glucose paste is another example of an ingested medication. DOT 1-7.3, 1-7.16

Injection

Injection involves placing a medication through the skin into an underlying structure such as the vascular system, muscle, bone, organ, joint, or other tissue or structure. Injection is a common route for administration by the paramedic because it results in rapid, and in some cases, immediate placement of the drug into the bloodstream. Medications for injection are found in sterile packaging and require special handling to prevent the introduction of infection into the body during the act of injection (Figure 15-1). The process of handling medications that require the maintaining of sterility is called **asepsis.**

CONNECTIONS Asepsis means without germs or pathogens (disease-causing agents). Performing procedures with an aseptic technique means the paramedic is focused on preventing the introduction of pathogens into the body by using very careful techniques and maintaining all equipment and supplies free from contamination. Injections and asepsis are covered in detail in Chapter 16: Medication Administration and IV.

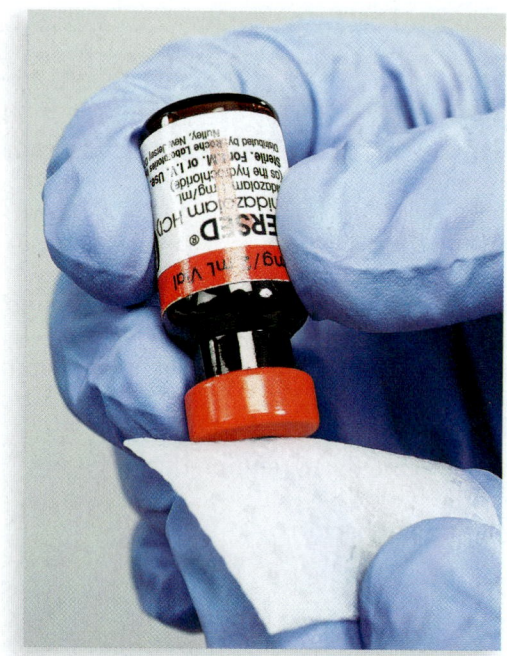

Figure 15-1 If a vial is being used more than once, after the seal has been broken, it should be wiped clean with an alcohol prep before drawing up the medication.

Absorption

Absorption occurs when a medication moves through the skin or mucous membrane into the body cells, tissues, organs, and structures underneath. It can also occur by bringing a medication into contact with a body orifice or structure such as the gum, ear, eye, vagina, or rectum. Nitroglycerin can be absorbed through the skin via a paste or through a dermal patch, as well as through the mucous membranes under the tongue.

Inhalation

Inhalation occurs when a drug is inhaled into and absorbed from the lung. An albuterol inhaler is an extremely fine powdered drug that is aerosolized and inhaled into the lungs or is turned into a fine mist when the liquid form of albuterol is nebulized as a result of oxygen flowing from a tank.

Medication Route Classification

Ingestion, injection, absorption, and inhalation are most correctly, although not frequently, considered sub-routes for medication administration. Medication routes can be classified into one of two categories: enteral or parenteral. See Box 15-2 for more information.

Enteral Route

The **enteral route** brings a drug into the body via the gastrointestinal tract. Therefore, any drug introduced via the mouth, rectum, or anywhere in between is using the enteral route. This includes, oral, buccal (cheek), sublingual (under the tongue), direct introduction of a drug into any portion of the gastrointestinal tract (nasogastric or orogastric), or rectal. Drugs introduced in this manner undergo absorption into the bloodstream and generally pass through the liver and lungs prior to reaching their target tissue (see Box 15-2). DOT 1-7.17

Nice to Know

Some pharmacology reference books place **topical** administration into a category separate from enteral and parenteral. This text has placed the topical route as a subcategory of the parenteral route.

Parenteral Route

Drugs introduced into any other part of the body are following the **parenteral route** and include intravenous, intraosseous (into the bone), intrathecal (into the spinal cord canal), intramuscular, intradermal (into the skin), subcutaneous (under the skin, above the muscle), or absorbed topically through the skin, vagina, nose (nasal), eye (ocular), ear (otic), or respiratory system. Drugs can also be introduced directly into specific organs or tissues of the body through surgical implantation or via direct injection into a specific tissue (see Box 15-2). DOT 1-7.17

CONNECTIONS Chapter 16: Medication Administration and IV describes the techniques of administration of medication via the various routes available to the paramedic.

Comparing the Routes of Administration

Whether a drug is administered via the enteral or parenteral route will depend upon many factors. The enteral route is generally the easiest or most accessible, but the enzymes, acids, and processes of digestion may alter the chemistry of certain medications, making them less effective. Insulin is an example of this. If insulin is ingested, it will be inactivated in the stomach and will not be available for use by the cells.

The taste of a drug may make the enteral route undesirable. Additionally, some drugs are so toxic that they should only be placed directly into contact with the tissues they are supposed to interact with. Chemotherapy drugs, for example, are often very toxic, and it is less toxic to the patient to deliver the drugs directly into the cancerous tissue instead of allowing them to circulate throughout the entire body. It is important to remember that any route of administration eventually results in the introduction of the drug into the entire

BOX 15-2 Medication Administration Routes

Enteral

Buccal: placed in contact with the cheek (also a topical route)

Sublingual: placed under the tongue (also a topical route)

Rectal: introduced into the rectum past the anal sphincter (also a topical route) (Figure 15-2)

Oral: swallowed

Nasogastric or Orogastric: placed directly into the stomach via a tube passed through the nose or mouth

Parenteral

Intravenous: injected directly into the vein

IV bolus: a single dose of medication given at one time interval at a specified speed of IV push delivery

IV drip: a continuous infusion of a small amount of medication given over a defined period of time to allow for slower introduction to the body

Intra-arterial: injected directly into an artery

Intramuscular: injected directly into the muscle tissue

Subcutaneous: injected through the skin and placed above the muscle

Intradermal: injected between the dermal and epidermal layers of the skin

Nebulized: inhaled into the lungs

Intraosseous: injected into the peripheral circulation through a bone

Intrathecal: injected into the spinal cord canal

Topical

Skin: absorbed through the skin

Via mucous membranes:

Intranasal: sprayed on nasal mucosa

Buccal: placed in contact with the cheek inside the mouth

Sublingual: placed under the tongue

Rectal: placed into the rectum of the colon

Intraotic: placed into the ear

Intraocular: absorbed through the mucous membranes of the eye

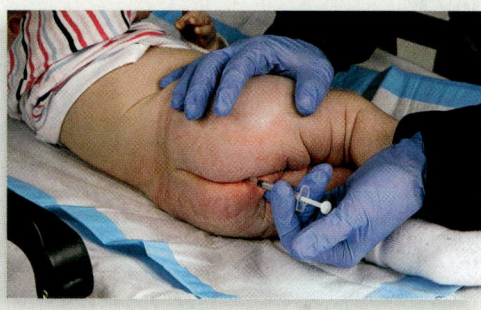

Figure 15-2 When establishing an IV is difficult, such as when a child is actively seizing, Valium™ (diazepam) can be administered rectally.

body, but different routes of administration can control the speed of this process.

Absorption

Absorption describes the rate at which a drug leaves the site of administration and how readily this process occurs.[2] The rate (speed) of absorption varies by the route of administration. Many drugs utilized by paramedics need to reach their target tissues quickly and exert their effects rapidly. The intravenous (IV) route allows direct placement of a drug into the bloodstream for rapid circulation and, therefore, is one of the fastest routes of administration. The IV route actually circumvents the absorption process by placing the drug directly into the circulation.[2] The enteral routes are some of the slowest routes for absorption. Box 15-3 lists the speed of absorption by route of administration. DOT 1-7.14

Absorption is also affected by factors other than the route of administration. Recall that absorption is also affected by how readily a route functions. If a patient is in profound shock, circulation will be impaired in the periphery of the body; therefore, blood circulation will be slower than normal from the arms and legs. For this patient, a drug administered via the subcutaneous or intramuscular routes will have delayed absorption with slower distribution to the central circulation as blood has been shunted away from these tissues in order to maintain vital perfusion. In cardiac arrest, for example, drugs given IV in a peripheral vein may take as long as one to two minutes to reach the central circulation with the standard chest compressions of CPR.[3]

As a drug is introduced into the body, it is absorbed through or across tissues and distributed throughout the body. The most common route to move a drug is to circulate it via the bloodstream. Nearly every cell in the body comes into direct contact with a capillary in the vascular system, so a drug traveling in the bloodstream will eventually reach a target site. The brain, liver, and kidney are highly perfused organs, so they

BOX 15-3 Comparison of Routes and Rate of Absorption

Absorption Rates From Fastest to Slowest Routes

Fastest Routes

Intravenous*
Intraosseous*
Intra-arterial*

Very Rapid Routes

Nebulized
Intrathecal
Intramuscular (depending upon the drug and site selected)
Sublingual (depending upon the drug)

Rapid Routes

Subcutaneous (depending upon the drug and site selected)
Intradermal
Intraocular
Intranasal
Rectal

Slower Routes

Buccal
Nasogastric or orogastric
Intraotic
Topical via skin absorption
Oral

*While not technically considered *absorbed,* these routes allow for immediate placement of a drug into the circulation.

BOX 15-4 Effects of Disease and Conditions on Drug Concentrations and Response

Renal Disease: Filtration via the kidneys is a common means of elimination of drugs from the blood. If a drug is excreted primarily via the kidneys and increased circulating blood levels are associated with toxic effects, the dose should be reduced for patients with renal disease. Sotolol and lidocaine (both antidysrhythmics) are examples of drugs excreted via the kidneys.

Hepatic Disease: The liver detoxifies many drugs. Hepatitis and liver disease reduce the efficiency of this process. The analgesic (pain reliever) meperidine needs extensive hepatic metabolism to remove it from the body.

Heart Failure and Shock: During heart failure and shock, cardiac output is altered to preserve blood flow to the brain and heart and shunted (diverted) from the peripheral circulation. When this occurs, more drug will be presented to the brain and heart, and less will be delivered to the arms and legs. The kidneys may be triggered to slow the elimination of water and wastes through filtration, resulting in an increased plasma level in the circulating blood.

Drug Use in the Elderly: Even in the absence of renal disease, elimination via kidney filtration may be reduced by 35–50% in elderly patients. Elderly patients may also have altered sensitivity to drugs resulting in greater or lesser effects than younger patients. Elderly patients may have multiple drug regimens prescribed by several physicians, increasing the potential for interactions and adverse effects. The elderly may also have many disease processes resulting in impaired hepatic or renal function.

Source: Kasper, et al. eds. *Harrison's Principles of Internal Medicine,* Volume 1, 16th ed., (New York: McGraw-Hill, 2005), pages 19–20.

quickly receive drugs circulating in the blood. The muscles, skin, fat, and viscera receive drugs at a slower rate and may require several minutes to several hours before receiving a circulating drug.[2]

Distribution

Like absorption, distribution of drugs can be affected by impaired body systems (Box 15-4). Any problems or impairments to circulation will result in slowed distribution. This includes renal or hepatic diseases, shock, and problems with the circulatory, cardiac, or nervous systems.[1] DOT 1-7.11, 1-7.14

Drugs continuously undergo physical or chemical processes (called metabolism), resulting in changes to the drug. Passage of a drug through the liver and the renal (kidney) circulation results in chemical alterations to the drug and in elimination of some of the drug from the body. This is called the first pass effect.[2] A specific type of metabolism, referred to as biotransformation, takes place in the liver where drugs are altered into metabolites of their original state. (The biotransformed metabolite may be the active form of the medication and what the tissue really needs, but it may be too unstable a compound to administer in that state.) Bioavailability describes the amount of drug that is available for the body to use following biotransformation and the first-pass events.

The Bioavailability of Medication

Bioavailability can be altered for two reasons: (1) Absorption is reduced, and (2) elimination occurs prior to entering the systemic circulation.[1] Alterations to bioavailability result in a decreased amount of circulating drug available for use by the target tissues. The **half-life** is the amount of time it takes for half of the drug to be eliminated from the body through use at the target site and also from elimination. This results in reduction of the plasma concentration of the drug by 50%.[4] This amount of time will vary between drugs and will determine how frequently the drug needs to be administered to the patient.

The Therapeutic Index

As a drug is researched, scientists determine the actual amount of drug required to give to an average patient that will result in the desired effects with the smallest amount of toxicity or side effects. The **therapeutic index (TI)** for the drug is determined by balancing the amount of drug needed to provide the desired effect compared to the toxicity and side effects. A dose is calculated through observation of the desired effects for 50% of the patients taking the drug. This dose is called the median effective dose, or ED_{50}. The median lethal dose (LD_{50}) is calculated through computer modeling and animal experimentation. It measures the point where half of the animals experimented upon die with a given dose. The TI is calculated by developing a ratio between the LD_{50} and the ED_{50}.[2] DOT 1-7.9

The therapeutic index (TI) is sometimes called the **therapeutic window.** This window provides insight into the closeness of the relationship between the optimal dose for a drug and the potential overdose or under dose. The smaller the "window," the easier it is to leave the therapeutic range and enter into either the dangerous **overdose state,** with too much drug being administered, or the **underdose state,** if not enough is given. The TI window is small for some drugs like digitalis, lidocaine, and phenytoin. Digitalis (a cardiac drug) and phenytoin (for epilepsy) require frequent monitoring of blood concentrations to prevent accidental overdose and under dose. Lidocaine, for cardiac emergencies, may require a reduced dose or a longer period of time between repeat administration if the patient is known or suspected to have renal disease to prevent toxicity from occurring. If the patient is in heart failure, the rate of clearance (or elimination) of lidocaine is reduced by about 50%, and the distribution of lidocaine to the tissues is also reduced, so therapeutic levels can be achieved at about half the normal dose in these patients.[1]

Clearance (Elimination)

Clearance is the measurement of the body's ability to eliminate the drug. If a drug is not used up by the body, it needs to be metabolized or eliminated to avoid damaging cells or tissues due to toxicity. Clearance can be altered in the presence of disease processes such as hepatic or renal disease. It can also be affected if the body is forced to conserve and retain fluids to correct imbalances such as those seen with shock. In these cases, because elimination is reduced, the halflife time is increased or prolonged. Dosages must be adjusted to compensate for these situations. The American Heart Association algorithms for treating cardiac patients have taken this into consideration, and drugs such as lidocaine include dosing ranges for special patient situations.[3] DOT 1-7.10, 1-7.14

Drugs can be excreted (eliminated) from the body via several systems. As long as it is functioning, the liver will continue to break down any drug not used by the target tissues until what remains is a harmless chemical. This process is called **detoxification.** Drugs can also be eliminated from the body when exhaled as waste gas from the respiratory system. The renal and gastrointestinal systems help by eliminating some drugs in either urine or feces. Less common routes of elimination include sweat, emesis (vomit), tears, and breast milk.[1,2]

Receptors

The **receptor** is the site within an organism that is available for interaction with chemicals such as drugs. Proteins form the greatest number of drug receptors in the body. Examples of protein receptors are found on hormones, growth factors, enzymes for critical regulatory and metabolic pathways, and in neurotransmitters (which are explained later in this chapter).

Receptors function as a site to allow drugs to bind to them, and then they may change the function or behavior of the tissue, organ, or system they are attached to.[2] The term **affinity** describes the degree to which the chemical forces of attraction exist between the drug and the receptor site. The stronger the force of attraction, the greater the affinity that exists between the molecules. For example, the carbon monoxide molecule has an extremely high affinity for hemoglobin, in fact, higher than the affinity of oxygen for hemoglobin. If you had an equal amount of oxygen molecules and carbon monoxide (CO) molecules, and they were both exposed to the hemoglobin protein in the red blood cell, 256 CO molecules would bind to the hemoglobin for every single oxygen molecule attaching to the hemoglobin.

Receptor Efficacy

Efficacy is the process of change that occurs as the result of drugs binding to a receptor. The more a desired effect occurs following binding, the higher or greater the efficacy. In the oxygen and carbon monoxide example just described, the efficacy is considered low because CO binding is damaging and potentially lethal to the patient. On the other hand, in order to reverse morphine's depressant effects on the central nervous system, a high efficacy is seen with the binding of naloxone to the receptors to which morphine normally binds. In this case, this binding is strongly desired, so efficacy is considered high. DOT 1-7.14

Agonists and Antagonists

Naturally occurring chemicals found within the body that bind to receptors are known as **endogenous agonists.** Drugs that bind to receptors and then mimic the effects normally seen with that receptor are called **agonists.** Epinephrine given via injection binds to the same receptors as the epinephrine produced within the body and exhibits the same effects, so injectable epinephrine is an agonist of naturally occurring epinephrine.

Drugs which bind to receptors that then inhibit (or prevent) the binding of the endogenous agonist are classified as **antagonists.** These compounds may produce a desired effect simply by inhibiting the action of the agonist. For example, naloxone and morphine both compete for the same receptors. When naloxone binds (it has the greater affinity for the receptor), the effect is to prevent or reverse the respiratory depression caused by morphine. Therefore, naloxone is a narcotic antagonist. Other types of agonists exist although it is not critical paramedics know specifics about these. Figure 15-3 provides additional information on agonists and antagonists.

Street Secrets

Drugs such as naloxone work very well at antagonizing the effect of morphine and its derivatives. In the case of a heroin overdose, it can reverse respiratory arrest or failure, but if the patient is a chronic user (addict), its use may also cause the patient to enter into immediate narcotic withdrawal. Only enough naloxone should be given to restore respirations. It is not necessary to completely waken the patient, which can result in an out of control patient, or put them into withdrawal.

Synergistic Effects

Drugs bind to receptors through all the known types of chemical bonding: ionic, hydrogen, hydrophobic (water "hating"), van der Waals, and covalent.[2] If a drug binds to a receptor that serves a function common to most cells, then the effects of that drug will be widespread. If several drugs act together at the same receptor, this binding may result in additive, synergistic, or inhibitory responses in the cells. DOT 1-7.14, 1-7.21.

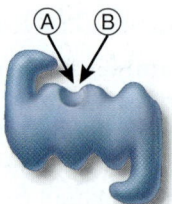

(a) Competitive

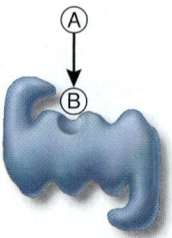

(b) Pseudo-irreversible

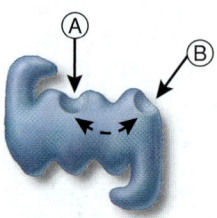

(c) Allosteric

Figure 15-3 This text describes receptors from a superficial perspective. In fact, there are many complex interrelationships between drugs and receptors. (a) Shows how two drugs compete for a bonding site. (b) Shows how some bonds are nearly permanent while most are reversible. Some binding, like that seen in the allosteric bond (which means binding occurs at a site other than the normal site) shown in part (c), results in the promotion or inhibition of other bonds within the same compound.

A **synergistic effect** occurs when the final effect seen with the administration of two drugs is greater than the sum of the administration of each drug. In other words, the response is amplified, so instead of 1 + 1 = 2, 1 + 1 = 3. DOT 1-7.21

Receptor Functions

Receptors serve two functions: **ligand** binding or message propagation. A ligand is an ion or molecule that is a component of a larger substance. A protein bound within the membrane of a cell is an example of a ligand. Message propagation occurs as the receptor allows the passage of an electrical or chemical signal from one cell or molecule to another. For example, a message may transmit from one nerve to the next from the fingertip all the way to the brain.

Regulatory actions of receptors are exhibited directly on cellular targets, effector proteins, or transducer molecules. All three sites play an intermediary role in

BOX 15-5   Receptor Types

Enzyme Receptors

Cell surface protein kinases: A kinin is a protein found in the blood that exhibits its effects primarily on cell surface proteins on smooth muscles. A kinase destroys a kinin. Receptors with other enzymatic activity: Current research is discovering extracellular ligands, the function of which is not well-known.

Ion Channel Receptors

Plasma membranes contain ligand-gated ion channels. These receptors alter the cell's membrane potential or ionic composition to allow the opening or closing of the channels.

G Protein-Coupled Receptors

GTP-binding regulatory proteins are transducers which convey signals on to another protein. It is estimated that about one-half of all nonantibiotic prescription drugs attach to G proteins.

Transcription Factor Receptors

These receptors regulate the transcription of specific genes. This occurs through the transfer of phosphate from one compound to another (phosphorylation), association with another cellular protein, or by binding to a metabolite or cellular regulatory ligand. These bindings can serve a negative regulatory role or activate or inhibit the transcription of genes from DNA.

Cytotoplasmic Second Messengers

In a chemical reaction pathway, cyclic AMP is signaled from another source to trigger a reaction. This reaction can move to another pathway or continue in the current pathway. Cyclic AMP acts as a "second messenger" to influence each pathway directly or by altering metabolism or sharing intracellular targets.

Source: J. G. Hardman, and L. E. Limbird, eds., *Goodman and Gilman's The pharamacological basis of therapeutics,* 10th ed. (New York: McGraw-Hill, 2001), pages 34–36.

cellular signaling to effect metabolic activities. Box 15-5 lists common receptors. You should be familiar with the various receptor types; however, it is not important to memorize the physiology involved in each of the receptors and their binding process.

Classifying Receptors

Drug receptors traditionally have been classified on the basis of the effect they exhibit or on the potency of their agonistic or antagonistic activity. For example, acetylcholine effects mimicked by a drug like muscarine (that are also selectively antagonized by atropine) are termed "muscarinic" effects. Norepinephrine-like effects on the sympathetic nervous system, which are mimicked by drugs such as epinephrine or dopamine, are called "sympathomimetic." The accuracy of this classification system is continuously being altered as new receptors and receptor subtypes are identified or additional drug mechanisms and side effects are revealed.[2] This makes it difficult for all members of the healthcare team, including physicians, to keep up with the changes. It also makes it more important for paramedics to learn the major classifications of medications instead of focusing on memorizing each discrete medication. DOT 1-7.9

If you understand a medication by its classification, you should be able to critically think through expected effects and side effects and know what the medication is used for. If you take a "memorize each drug as it comes along" approach, you will have to update and change your formulary continuously as medications come and

go, and you may not recognize relationships that exist between drugs in the same class.

Neurotransmitters

Drugs work on the body by stopping, starting, or altering a process, thereby affecting or maintaining the homeostatic balance.[2] This frequently occurs from drugs interacting directly with the nervous system, which controls body processes, and other systems. Messages carried via a nerve move from one nerve cell to the next by either chemical or electrical means. Drugs work in the nervous system by binding to the ends of a nerve cell in the junction between the cells. This junction is called the **synapse** (Figure 15-4). Drugs found in the synapse are called neurotransmitters. **Neurotransmitters** allow the transmission of the nerve impulse (or message) across the synapse to continue either along the nerve back to the brain or out towards the target organ or tissue. Neurotransmitter drugs can permit, alter, or prevent (block) message transmission. If these drugs permit message transmission, they can either speed it up or slow it down. DOT 1-7.13

Drugs with an electrical charge in their atomic structures are **ionic.** These drugs, such as calcium, potassium, sodium, magnesium, and phosphate, provide electrical transport for messages (as well as numerous other important functions).

Chemical transport occurs via other drugs which are not ionic. Chemical transport works by allowing or

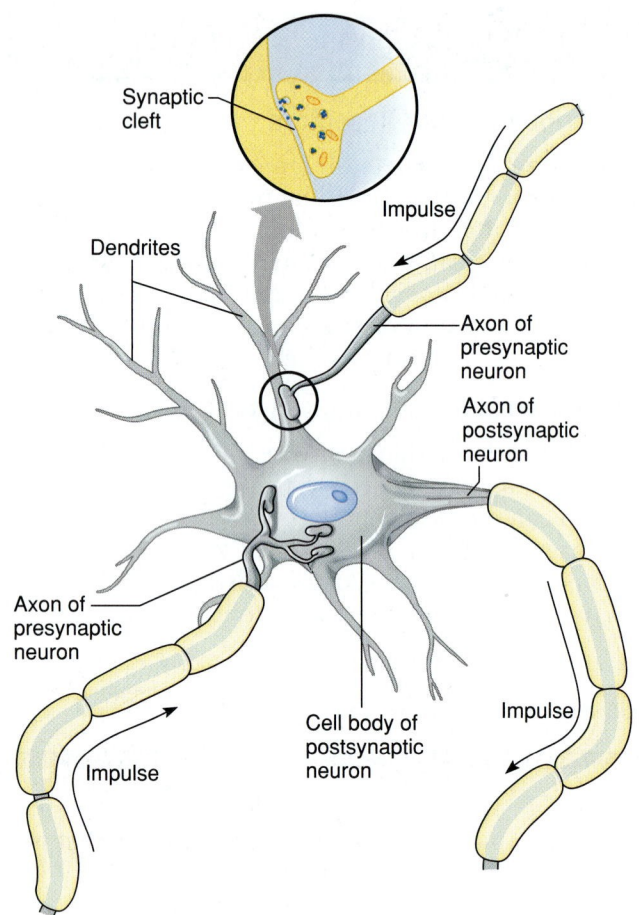

Figure 15-4   The nerve synapse. The distal portion of the dendrite is referred to as a receptor because it receives the impulse stimulus (message) from the axon of the other nerve.

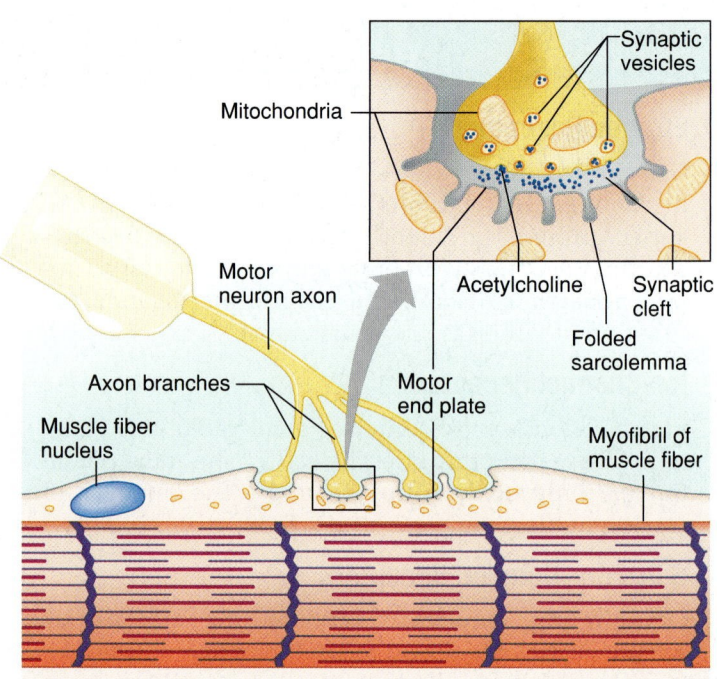

Figure 15-5   The neuromuscular junction functions in a similar manner to a nerve-to-nerve junction.

preventing the nerve impulse message from being transmitted. If binding and transport occurs, the message can pass through the synapse. If binding or transport is not allowed, the message will not cross the synapse and will not be transmitted further.

If a nervous impulse message is at the end of the nerve fiber, it may pass to a muscle cell instead of another nerve. This junction is similar to a synapse in function, but it is called the neuromuscular junction (Figure 15-5). Drugs found in this location are still called neurotransmitters. Both chemical and electrical neurotransmitters are in the neuromuscular junction.

Homeostasis and Balance

The body requires constant regulation in order to remain in balance and stay alive. Homeostasis is the name for this process of regulation. The nervous and endocrine systems are primarily responsible for regulating homeostasis.[5] The nervous system plays a key role by functioning as the control center (see Figure 15-6).

The endocrine system provides the chemicals (hormones) needed to turn on and off the various systems. These two systems control the communication network between all body cells, tissues, and organ systems. Drugs can be used to enhance or suppress the endocrine and nervous system by affecting the receptors within each system, thus impacting homeostasis.

Pulling the Concepts Together

A receptor is the part of a cell or organism that combines with a drug. Drugs are distributed throughout the body via circulation of the blood and are delivered to their target sites through various methods of transport, including active transport, osmosis, and diffusion.

Tables 15-1, 15-2, and 15-3 provide information on receptors, neurotransmitters, and the effects generated following stimulation or inhibition of several of the important receptors. Research is revealing more information on receptors, and our understanding of the interrelationships between each of these components is expanding at a rapid rate. With all of this information, it is difficult for the paramedic to keep up with the changes and focus on concepts pertinent to clinical practice. Table 15-4 provides summaries of key receptors, neurotransmitters, and effects of special interest to paramedics. These receptors were chosen because of the physical presentations they manifest with stimulation or inhibition and with the effects noted in the cardiovascular and respiratory systems.

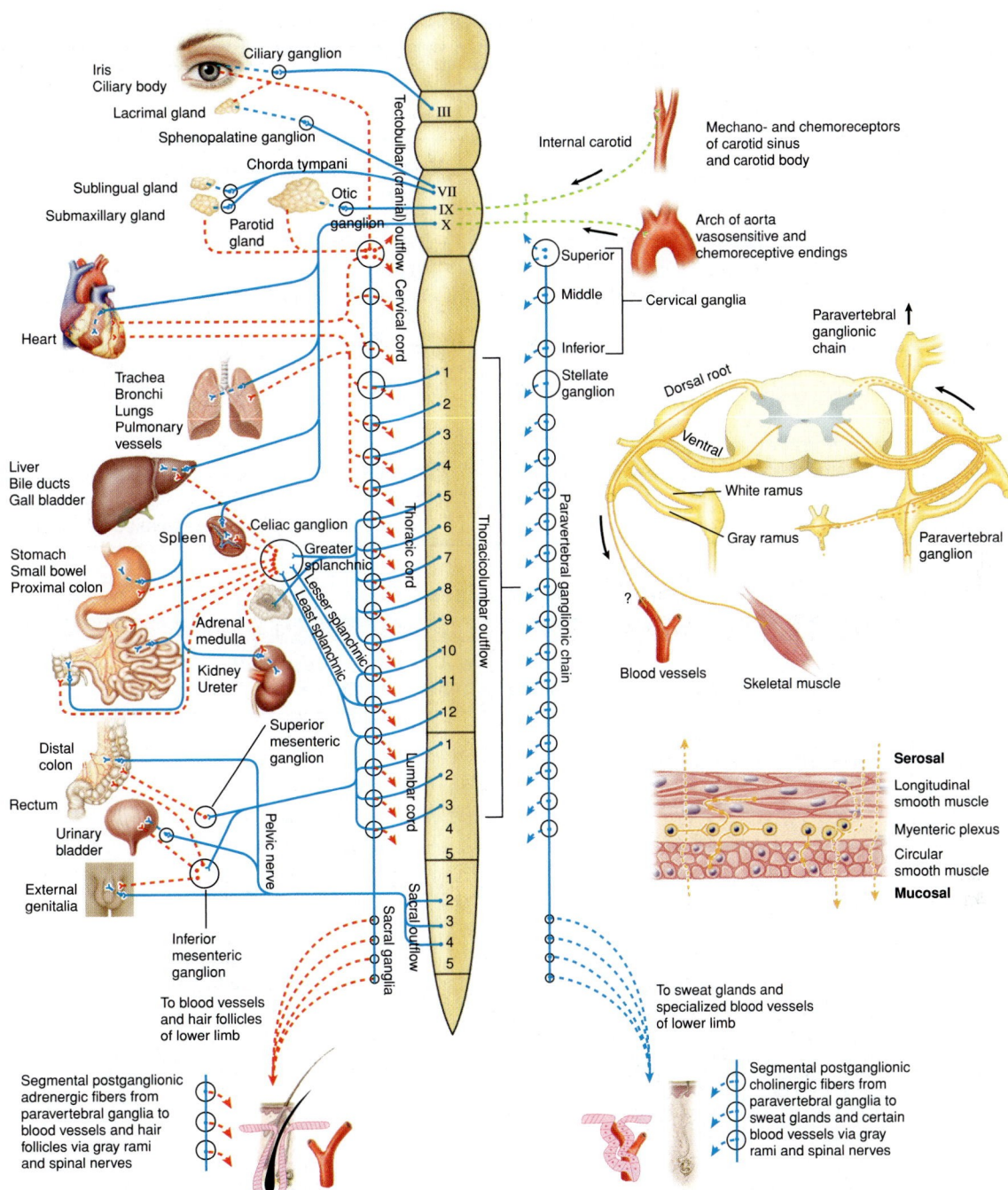

Figure 15-6 The autonomic nervous system in greater detail. The blue lines show the parasympathetic innervation, red lines show sympathetic innervation, and green show visceral afferent nerves. Note the sympathetic and parasympathetic nerves that extend to the major organs.

Drug Names and References

Some drugs require a prescription from a healthcare professional, such as a physician, nurse practitioner, physician assistant, or dentist, who is licensed to write them. Some healthcare professionals have limits on which drugs they are allowed to prescribe related specifically to their areas of clinical practice. A licensed dentist, for example, can prescribe certain pain control medications (analgesics and anesthetics) and some antibiotics. DOT 1-7.2, 1-7.5

Drug preparations that contain doses of medication that do not have too many harmful side effects are often available without a prescription. These drugs are classified as **over-the-counter** or **OTC** medications. Even though their sale does not require a prescription,

TABLE 15-1   **Summary of Autonomic Receptors, Neurotransmitters and Effects**

System	Location and Type of Receptor	Neurotransmitter(s)	Effect Generated
Sympathetic (adrenergic)	Preganglionic	Acetylcholine	Transmits message from nervous system to postganglionic fibers
Sympathetic (adrenergic)	Postganglionic	Norepinephrine Epinephrine Dopamine	Pupil constriction, (+) inotropic, (+) chronotropic, constriction of select arterioles (muscles, gut, skin), dilation of select arterioles (lungs, brain, heart), increased respiratory rate, increased blood pressure, urinary retention, decreased activity in gut (may lead to vomiting)
Parasympathetic (cholinergic)	Preganglionic	Acetylcholine	Transmits message to postganglionic (cholinergic) nervous fibers
Parasympathetic (cholinergic)	Postganglionic	Acetylcholine	Pupil dilation, (−) inotropic, (−) chronotropic, dilation of most arterioles, contraction of bronchial musculature, increased activity in gut, decreased blood pressure

TABLE 15-2   **Responses of Effector Organs to ANS Impulses**

Organ System	Sympathetic Effect[a]	Adrenergic Receptor Type[b]	Parasympathetic Effect[a]	Cholinergic Receptor Type[b]
Eye				
Radial muscle, iris	Contraction (mydriasis)++	α_1		
Sphincter muscle, iris			Contraction (miosis)+++	M_3, M_2
Cilliary muscle	Relaxation for far vision[+]	β_2	Contraction for near vision+++	M_3, M_2
Lacrimal glands	Secretion+	α	Secretion+++	M_3, M_2
Heart				
Sinoatrial node	Increase in heart rate++	$\beta_1 > \beta_2$	Decrease in heart rate+++	$M_2 \gg M_3$
Atria	Increase in contractility and conduction velocity++	$\beta_1 > \beta_2$	Decrease in contractility++ and shortened AP duration	$M_2 \gg M_3$
Atrioventricular node	Increase in automaticity and conduction velocity++	$\beta_1 > \beta_2$	Decrease in conduction velocity: AV block+++	$M_2 \gg M_3$
His-Purkinje system	Increase in automaticity and conduction velocity	$\beta_1 > \beta_2$	Little effect	$M_2 \gg M_3$
Ventricle	Increase in contractility, conduction velocity, automaticity and rate of idioventricular pacemakers+++	$\beta_1 > \beta_2$	Slight decrease in contractility	$M_2 \gg M_3$
Blood vessels (arteries and arterioles)				
Coronary	Constriction+; dilation++	$\alpha_1, \alpha_2; \beta_2$	No innervation	—
Skin and mucosa	Constriction+++	α_1, α_2	No innervation	—
Skeletal muscle	Constriction; dilation ++	$\alpha_1; \beta_2$	Dilation (?)	—
Cerebral	Constriction (slight)	α_1	No innervation	—
Pulmonary	Constriction+; dilation	$\alpha_1; \beta_2$	No innervation	—
Abdominal viscera	Constriction+++; dilation +	$\alpha_1; \beta_2$	No innervation	—
Salivary glands	Constriction+++	α_1, α_2	Dilation++	M_3
Renal	Constriction++; dilation++	$\alpha_1 \alpha_2; \beta_1, \beta_2$	No innervation	
(Veins)	Constriction; dilation	$\alpha_1, \alpha_2; \beta_2$		

(α = alpha receptor, β = beta receptor, M = muscarinic receptor)

TABLE 15-2 (*continued*)

Organ System	Sympathetic Effect[a]	Adrenergic Receptor Type[b]	Parasympathetic Effect[a]	Cholinergic Receptor Type[b]
Endothelium			Activation of NO synthase	M_3
Lung				
Tracheal and bronchial smooth muscle	Relaxation	β_2	Contraction	$M_2 = M_3$
Bronchial glands	Decreased secretion, increased secretion	α_1 β_2	Stimulation	M_3, M_2
Stomach				
Motility and tone	Decrease (usually)+	$\alpha_1, \alpha_2, \beta_1, \beta_2$	Increase+++	$M_2 = M_3$
Sphincters	Contraction (usually)+	α_1	Relaxation (usually)+	M_3, M_2
Secretion	Inhibition	α_2	Stimulation++	M_3, M_2
Intestine				
Motility and tone	Decrease+	$\alpha_1, \alpha_2, \beta_1, \beta_2$	Increase+++	M_3, M_2
Sphincters	Contraction+	α_1	Relaxation (usually)+	M_3, M_2
Secretion	Inhibition	α_2	Stimulation++	M_3, M_2
Gallbladder and ducts	Relaxation+	β_2	Contraction+	M
Kidney				
Renin secretion	Decrease+; increase++	$\alpha_1; \beta_1$	No innervation	—
Urinary bladder				
Detrusor	Relaxation+	β_2	Contraction+++	$M_3 > M_2$
Trigone and sphincter	Contraction++	α_1	Relaxation++	$M_3 > M_2$
Ureter				
Motility and tone	Increase	α_1	Increase (?)	M
Uterus	Pregnant contraction;	α_1		M
	Relaxation	β_2	Variable	
	Nonpregnant relaxation	β_2		
Sex organs, male	Ejaculation+++	α_1	Erection+++	M_3
Skin				
Pilomotor muscles	Contraction++	α_1		
Sweat glands	Localized secretion++	α_1		
	Generalized secretion+++			M_3, M_2
Spleen capsule	Contraction+++	α_1	—	—
	Relaxation+	β_2	—	
Adrenal gland	Secretion of epinephrine and nonrepinephrine			N $(\alpha_3)_2(\beta_4)_3$; M (secondarily)
Skeletal muscle	Increased contractility; glycogenolysis; K^+ uptake	β_2	—	—
Liver	Glycogenolysis and gluconeogenesis+++	α_1 β_2	—	—
Pancreas		α		
Acini	Decreased secretion+	α	Secretion++	M_3, M_2
Islets (β cells)	Decreased secretion+++	α_2	—	
	Increased secretion+	β_2		
Fat cells	Lipolysis+++;	—	—	
	(thermogenesis)	$\alpha_1, \beta_1, \beta_2, \beta_3$		
	Inhibition of lipolysis	α_2		
Salivary glands	K^+ and water secretion+	α_1	K^+ and water secretion+++	M_3, M_2

(α = alpha receptor, β = beta receptor, M = muscarinic receptor)

(*continued*)

TABLE 15-2 (*continued*)

Organ System	Sympathetic Effect[a]	Adrenergic Receptor Type[b]	Parasympathetic Effect[a]	Cholinergic Receptor Type[b]
Nasopharyngeal glands	—		Secretion++	M_3, M_2
Pineal glands	Melatonin synthesis	β	—	
Posterior pituitary	Antidiuretic hormone secretion	β_1	—	
Autonomic nerve endings Sympathetic terminals Autoreceptor	Inhibition of NE release	$\alpha_{2A} > \alpha_{2C}$ (α_{2B})		
Heteroreceptor	—		Inhibition of NE release	M_2, M_4
Parasympathetic terminal Autoreceptor	—		Inhibition of ACh release	M_2, M_4
Heteroreceptor	Inhibition ACh release	$\alpha_{2A} > \alpha_{2C}$		

(α = alpha receptor, β = beta receptor, M = muscarinic receptor)

Source: From Pharmacological Basis of Therapeutics, Goodman and Gilman, 10. Copyright McGraw-Hill Companies, Inc. Reprinted with permission.

[a]Responses are designated + to+++ to provide an approximate indication of the importance of sympathetic and parasympathetic nerve activity in the control of various organs and functions listed.

[b]Adrenergic receptors: α_1, α_2, and subtypes thereof, β_1, β_2, β_3. Cholingergic receptors: nicotinic (N), muscarinic (M), with subtypes 1–4. When a designation of subtype is not provided, the nature of the subtype has not been determined unequivocally. Only the principal receptor subtypes are shown. Transmitters other than acetylcholine and norepinephrine contribute to many of the responses.

TABLE 15-3   **Characteristics of Subtypes of Cholinergic Receptors**

Receptor (Primary Receptors Subtype)*	Main Synaptic Location	Membrane Response	Molecular Mechanism	Agonists	Antagonists
Skeletal muscle (N_M) $(\alpha_1)_2\beta_1\varepsilon\delta$ adult $(\alpha_1)_2\beta_1\gamma\delta$ fetal	Skeletal neuromuscular junction (postjunctional)	Excitatory; endplate depolarization; skeletal muscle contraction	Increased cation permeability (Na^+; K^+)	ACh Nicotine Succinylcholine	Atracurium Vecuronium *d*-Tubocurarine Pancuronium α-Conotoxin α-Bungarotoxin
Peripheral neuronal (N_N) $(\alpha_3)_2(\beta_4)_3$	Autonomic ganglia; adrenal medulla	Excitatory; depolarization; firing of postganglion neuron; depolarization and secretion of catecholamines	Increased cation permeability (Na^+; K^+)	ACh Nicotine Epibatidine Dimethyl-phenylpiper azinium	Trimethaphan Mecamylamine
Central neuronal (CNS) $(\alpha_4)_2(\beta_4)_3$ (α-btox-insensitive)	CNS; pre- and postjunctional	Pre- and postsynaptic excitation Prejunctional control of transmitter release	Increased cation permeability (Na^+; K^+)	Cytisine epibatidine Anatoxin A	Mecamylamine Dihydro-β-erythrodine Erysodine Lophotoxin
$(\alpha_4)_5$ (α-btox-sensitive)	CNS; Pre- and postsynaptic	Pre- and postsynaptic excitation Prejunctional control of transmitter release	Increased permeability (Ca^{2+})	Anatoxin A	Methyllycaconitine α-Bungarotoxin α-Conotoxin IMI

(N = nicotinic receptor, α = alpha receptor, β = beta receptor, γ = gamma receptor, δ = delta receptor, ε = epsilon receptor)

Source: From Pharmacological Basis of Therapeutics, Goodman and Gilman, 10. Copyright McGraw-Hill Companies, Inc. Reprinted with permission.

*Nine individual subunits have been identified and cloned in human brain, which combine in various conformations to form individual receptor subtypes. The structure of individual receptors and the subtype composition are incompletely understood.

TABLE 15-4   **Summary of Clinically Important Receptors: Location and Effect**

Important Receptor Location	Type	Effects
Arterioles	Alpha 1 (sympathetic)	Primarily vasoconstriction with some vasodilation
Veins	Alpha 2 (sympathetic)	Primarily vasoconstriction with some vasodilation
Heart	Beta 1 (sympathetic)	Increased chronotropy, contractility, automaticity, and conduction velocity
Lung	Beta 2 (sympathetic)	Tracheal and bronchial muscle relaxation (dilation)
Fat / heart	Beta 3 (sympathetic)	Not well defined or understood
Skeletal muscle	Nicotinic (parasympathetic)*	Skeletal muscle contraction
Peripheral nerves	Nicotinic (parasympathetic)*	Cell depolarization and secretion of catecholamines
Central nerves	Nicotinic (parasympathetic)*	Control of neurotransmitter release
Autonomic ganglia	Muscarinic 1 (parasympathetic)	Depolarization of cells
Heart	Muscarinic 2 (parasympathetic)	Slow automaticity at atrioventriculer (AV) node, decreased contraction force, decreased conduction velocity
Glands and smooth muscles	Muscarinic 3 (parasympathetic)	Secretion and contraction
Heart	Muscarinic 4 (parasympathetic)	Slow automaticity at AV node, decreased contraction force, decreased conduction velocity
CNS	Muscarinic 5 (parasympathetic)	Depolarization of cells
Blood vessels (located throughout the body on smooth muscles and many organs)	V1 receptors (triggered from nicotinic, histamine [H1], dopamine [D1 and D2], and many other receptors)	Release of vasopressin with potent vasoconstriction and water retention (increases BP)

Source: Goodman and Gillman.

*Nicotinic (parasympathetic) receptors are subdivided into eight alpha and three beta subtypes which are not delineated here.

they are drugs nonetheless, and their misuse can result in illness or death.

Herbal remedies are derived from plants and are often classified as "food" instead of medicine and, therefore, are not regulated by the FDA. It is important to remember that anything taken by a patient that affects body functions or processes should be considered a drug.

Paramedics should always ask patients about their use of prescription, nonprescription OTCs, and herbal remedies when obtaining the patients' histories.

Drugs have several names by which they are known. The **official name** is the name listed in official government publications like the United States Pharmacopeia (USP) or National Formulary (NF). The official name usually has the initials USP or NF following the drug name. The Federal Drug Administration allows only licensed facilities and registered pharmacists to manufacture drugs for use in the United States, and only these individuals can legally own the USP book, which contains compounding ("recipe") information for the drugs listed within the document. Hospitals and approved medical facilities have versions of these documents for their use. DOT 1-7.2

The **chemical name** describes the exact chemical structure of the drug. Since this is written in chemical terms, it can be very long. The chemical name is derived from a council composed of members from pharmaceutical manufacturers, the American Medical Association, the American Pharmaceutical Association, and the United States Pharmacopeial Convention.[2] Knowing the chemical and official name of a medication is not required for the paramedic.

A drug manufacturer will often shorten the chemical name or create a variation of it to develop the **generic name.** The manufacturer will also select the name its company will use when it sells the drug. This name is the **trade name.** Because it is trademarked, no other manufacturer is allowed to use that same name to market the drug. Some drugs, like acetaminophen or aspirin, become so associated with their trade names (Tylenol™ or Bayer™) that all similar medications are referred to by that name, even though other manufacturers are selling the drug with another name. Two other names for the trade name are **brand name** or

TABLE 15-5 Medication Names

Chemical Name	Official Name	Generic Name	Trade Name
(3B, 5B, 12B)-3- ((O-2, 6-dideoxy-B-D-ribohexoopryanosyl-(1-4)-2,6-dideoxy-B-ribohexopyranosyl) oxy)12,14-dihydroxy-card-20(22)-enolide	digoxin tablets, USP	digoxin	Lanoxin™, Digitex™
Pyrazino (1,2:1,6)pyrido(3,4-b)-indole-1,4-dione, 6-(1,3-benzodioxol-5-yl)-2,3,6,7,12,12a-hexahydro-2methyl-, (6R,12aR)-	tadalafil	tadalafil	Cialis™
(bicyclohexyl)-1-carboxylic acid, 2-(diethylamino)-ethylester hydrochloride	dicyclomine hydrochloride USP	dicyclomine	Bentyl™

Source: Physician's Desk Reference (PDR), 59th ed. 2005. Montvale, NJ: Thomson PDR.

proprietary name. Table 15-5 has examples of drug names for three common medications. Because some drugs have many trade names, it is important for paramedics to know the generic and common trade names for medications they will encounter in their clinical practice. DOT 1-7.2

Medications also come in many forms. Table 15-6 lists the most common forms and characteristics of each.

Several reference books are published annually which list the most commonly prescribed medications in the United States. These books can be very helpful and are recommended. One such book is the *Physician's Desk Reference* (or PDR). This reference includes actual-size photographs of many medications. Drugs are listed in different colored indexes, by manufacturer (white pages), by generic and trade

TABLE 15-6 Medication Forms

Form Name	Characteristics
Powder	Powdered solid, may come in a variety of colors
Tablet	Compressed powder with a precise dose, generally swallowed but could be crushed and added to liquid
Enteric coated tablets	Tablets with special coating to allow for absorption from the intestine instead of the stomach
Capsule	Powder compressed and placed inside a gelatinous coating. The coating allows for easier swallowing, prevents the drug from being tasted when taken, or allows for targeted absorption within the gut.
Caplet	Compressed powder-shaped like a capsule with a smooth texture on the outside to facilitate easier swallowing and passage into the gut. May contain a thin coating of starch or other product to prevent tasting of the medication
Gelcap	Capsule filled with liquid medication
Lozenge (or troche)	Hard medication with sugary vehicle for sucking
Suppository	Medication placed into a vehicle of cocoa butter or other easily melted substance for placement into the rectum or vagina for absorption
Solution	Medication dissolved in a liquid so that no particles are present and the medication is equally dispersed throughout
Suspension	Large particle medications placed into a liquid which do not completely dissolve that need to be agitated (shaken) to redisperse the medication
Syrup	Water-based (aqueous) solution with sugar or artificial sweetener added to disguise the taste
Elixir	Flavored medication containing water and alcohol to improve solubility of the medication. The medication is sweetened with natural or artificial sweeteners
Extract	Highly concentrated solutions created by evaporation of materials from plants. Often these are used in syrups to create compounds
Tincture	Similar to extracts, but evaporated in alcohol solutions
Spirits	Medications which are volatile aromatics, are placed in alcohol, and may be diluted with water
Emulsions	Water and oil mixtures of medication and vehicle that result in globules of medication surrounded by the vehicle. Vigorous shaking is required to disperse the medication.

name (pink pages), and by product category (blue pages), making finding information faster and easier. The information from the medication package insert forms the bulk of the information contained within the PDR. This reference is available in several formats including an interactive electronic version, through the internet, and in print. To be most effective, any reference should identify a medication's generic and trade name, classification, indication, dose, route of administration, and any precautions or special considerations.

Patient Medication Rights

The Department of Transportation (DOT) National Standard Curricula (NSC) for Paramedics describes six patient rights.[6] The NSC includes in these "rights" the right patient, drug, dose, route, time, and documentation. In this text, we expand upon this concept to include three additional "rights" that are critical thinking elements. Box 15-6 lists the medication "rights" recommended for the paramedic along with a description of each.

Before giving any medication, you should determine if the circumstances are appropriate for the patient to receive the medication at that time. Sometimes administration of a medication, although indicated by protocol or standing order, should be withheld until other treatment options are explored.

Example 1. A cardiac patient may present with a dysrhythmia resulting in tachycardia and premature ectopic beats. You should understand that there are antidysrhythmic medications that will suppress ectopic beats but that hypoxia can also cause ectopic beats. You should, therefore, ensure the hypoxia is treated with oxygen (which is also a drug) prior to initiating antidysrhythmic medications. DOT 1-7.26

Example 2. For a patient experiencing bradycardia, it is important to determine whether or not the patient has serious signs and symptoms associated with the bradycardia before deciding to administer medications. For example, if the patient has stable vital signs and the transport time is relatively short, the paramedic may elect to monitor the patient closely and expedite the transport instead of remaining in the field to provide drug therapy.[3]

Example 3. If the patient has respiratory distress and is wheezing, but the history and physical exam suggest a cardiac problem may be the cause instead of asthma, it may or may not be appropriate to use a medication like albuterol since it has cardiac stimulating effects. Instead, drugs that promote diuresis or that shift fluid between the body compartments may be more appropriate.

In each of the three examples discussed, the paramedic will need to rely upon a careful history, the

---

BOX 15-6 Medication Rights

* **Right patient:** If assisting the patient with prescribed medications, ensure they are prescribed the medication prior to using it. If using a medication from your stock, ensure it is given with the right indications and circumstances.
* **Right drug:** Perform confirmation at least three times that the correct drug is being used, and repeat any drug order when it is received via online direction.
* **Right dose:** Calculate the dose based upon patient weight, or use the recommended dose by protocol, standing order, or physician direction. Make sure the medication you have is the correct strength or is diluted properly.
* **Right route:** Select correct route of administration consistent with online or offline medical direction.
* **Right time:** The drug is given at the correct time it should be given. Also, observe correct dosing intervals if multiple doses are administered.
* **Right documentation:** Vital signs are assessed pre- and post-administration (every time the drug is given); time of administration is charted as well as dose, route, and patient response. Indicate if drug was administered via standing order or from online direction.

Right technique: Confirm the drug is not expired, tampered with, or otherwise not usable (discolored or particulates noted in the fluid). The drug is given at the appropriate speed of push rate if administered via injection. Also included here is consideration for the correct administration techniques and the maintenance of asepsis with the use of uncontaminated supplies and proper techniques.

Right circumstances: Knowing when to give and when to withhold the administration of a medication. Confirm that no contraindications exist for using the drug (such as allergies).

Right indication: Physical exam findings and history indicate that the use of that drug is appropriate.

Note: *DOT-recommended patient rights.

physical examination, and critical thinking skills to ensure that the best care possible is provided to the patient. DOT 1-7.27

Classifying Medications

There are several strategies for arranging medications into classes. One method classifies them by the body system or disease process they treat, for example cardiac, respiratory, or gastrointestinal drugs. Drugs can also be classified by the chemical groups they are related to. Examples include benzodiazepines, xanthine derivatives, or nitrates. Drugs can also be classified by the receptor to which they bind. Parasympathetic blockers, adrenergic drugs, and dopaminergic agents are examples. DOT 1-7.4, 1-7.23

Other examples of classification methods include the Controlled Substances Act of 1970. It classified drugs likely to cause addiction into five schedules with schedule I being drugs that are highly addictive and

TABLE 15-7   **AHA Classes of Recommendations for Drug Therapies**

Class I
Benefit >>> Risk Procedure/treatment or diagnostic test/assessment should be performed/administered.
Class IIa
Benefit >> Risk It is reasonable to perform procedure/administer treatment or perform diagnostic test/assessment.
Class IIb
Benefit ≥ Risk Procedure/treatment or diagnostic test/assessment may be considered.
Class III
Risk ≥ Benefit Procedure/treatment or diagnostic test/assessment should not be performed/administered. It is not helpful and may be harmful.
Class Indeterminate
Research is just getting started Continuing area of research No recommendation until further research (e.g., cannot recommend for or against)

Source: "Guidelines 2000 for Cardiopulmonary Resuscitation and Emergency Cardiac Care International Consensus on Science." Suppl: *Circulation* 102(8) August 22, 2000.

that have no medical use to schedule V, which includes drugs with low likelihood of addiction. Historically, AHA guidelines placed antidysrhythmic cardiovascular medications into four different classes sorted by the type of blocking they provided: sodium channel blockers, beta blockers, potassium channel blockers, and calcium channel blockers. The 2000 AHA guidelines (Table 15-7) changed to a new method—a classification standard based upon the strength of clinical evidence for the recommendation for use of a drug or therapeutic intervention. The 2000 strategy is that the stronger the evidence is judged to be, the stronger the recommendation for use of that medication.[3] This classification strategy has persisted with the 2005 AHA guidelines. Table 15-8 includes information on drug classes as well as the names of some of the medications commonly found in each class.[7] DOT 1-7.4, 1-7.6, 1-7.7, 1-7.8, 1-7.9

What Paramedics Need to Know about Drugs

There is not a single comprehensive list of medications used across the United States by paramedics.[7] In fact, some states do not even use a consistent list within their own regions, counties, or parishes. There are, however, some commonalities noted across the country. For example, most states follow the recommended guidelines described in the algorithms for managing cardiac patients from the AHA. Although many drugs are available for use by the paramedic, there are thousands of drugs that are not. DOT 1-7.18

Classes of Medications

Paramedics need to know classes of medications commonly used in order to properly manage their patients. Within each class, paramedics should know the indications for using the most common drugs in that class. An **indication** is the situation or circumstance when a particular drug should be used. As discussed previously, a paramedic should understand when a drug is indicated and when it should not be used, even if it is indicated. DOT 1-7.31

Street Secrets

Some generic drugs grouped together in the same class have common suffixes. Some examples include: ACE Inhibitors (-pril), Angiotensin Antagonist (-sartan), Sympatholytics (-in, -ine), Antihyperlipidemics (-statin), Beta Blockers (-olol, -alol), Calcium Channel Blockers (-ipines), Diuretics (-ide), Tricyclic Antidepressants (-amine, -yline), and Opioids (-one, -ine).

(*text continues on page 320*)

TABLE 15-8   Common Prehospital Drug Classes

Note: This list is derived from several sources and represents a cross section of medications reported to be used in prehospital EMS systems in the United States. Not every drug class is listed here nor is every drug within each class listed. Consult with your Medical Director for a complete listing of all medications on your formulary.

Drug	Trade name	Action
ACLS MEDICATIONS: Drugs found within the current American Heart Association (AHA) Advanced Cardiac Life Support (ACLS) algorithms		
Antidysrhythmic: Drugs that prevent, treat or suppress irregular heart rhythms		
Adenosine	Adenocard	Slows AV conduction time
Amiodarone	Cordarone, Pacerone	Prolongs action potential in Phase III
Lidocaine	Xylocaine	Anesthetic; stabilizes membranes; depresses action potential phase 0
Procainamide	Pronestyl, Procanbid	Stabilizes membranes; depresses action potential phase 0
Catecholamine/sympathomimetic: Drugs that stimulate the sympathetic nervous system, directly affecting the cardiovascular and respiratory systems		
Epinephrine 1:10,000, 1:1,000	Adrenalin	Stimulates alpha- and beta-adrenergic receptors
Isopreterenol	Isuprel	Stimulates beta-adrenergic receptors
Inotrope: Drugs affecting the inotropic state (contraction forces) of the cardiovascular system		
Digoxin	Lanoxin	Inhibits sodium-potassium ATPase
Epinephrine 1:10,000	Adrenalin	Stimulates alpha- and beta-adrenergic receptors
Vasopressor: Drugs that cause constriction of the vascular system		
Dopamine		Stimulates alpha- and beta-adrenergic and dopaminergic receptors
Dobutamine		Stimulates beta-adrenergic receptors
Epinephrine 1:10,000		Stimulates alpha- and beta-adrenergic receptors resulting in vasoconstriction
Norepinephrine	Levophed	Stimulates alpha- and beta-adrenergic receptors
Vasopressin	Pitressin	Acts like ADH; directly stimulates smooth muscle V1 receptors, resulting in vasoconstriction
Calcium channel blocker: Drugs that affect the cardiac and vascular systems by blocking the calcium ion		
Diltiazem	Cardizem	Inhibits calcium ion influx into vascular smooth muscle and myocardium, relaxing smooth muscle, decreasing peripheral vascular resistance, dilating coronary arteries and prolonging AV node refractory period
Verapamil	Calan, Isoptin, Verelan	Inhibits calcium ion influx into vascular smooth muscle and myocardium
Parasympatholytic: Drugs that block the parasympathetic nervous system, particularly the vagus nerve, which results in an effect similar to sympathetic stimulation		
Atropine		Antagonizes acetylcholine receptors (anticholinergic)

(continued)

TABLE 15-8   (*continued*)

Drug	Trade name	Action
Mineral/electrolytes: Drugs that provide needed ions and minerals or, by their presence, block other ions or minerals		
Calcium Chloride		Essential component and participant in physiologic systems and reactions
Magnesium Sulfate		Participates in physiologic processes
Sodium Bicarbonate		Ion important for regulating acid/base balance
Endocrine/metabolic enhancing agent: Drugs that promote positive endocrine and metabolic functions		
Vasopressin	Pitressin	Acts like ADH; directly stimulates smooth muscle V1 receptors, resulting in vasoconstriction
ANALGESICS: Drugs that control pain and or suppress the nervous system		
Nonsteroidal antiinflammatory agent		
Ibuprofen	Motrin	Exact mechanism of action unknown; inhibits cyclooxygenase and lipoxygenase and reduces prostaglandin synthesis
Ketorolac	Torado	Exact mechanism of action unknown; inhibits cyclooxygenase and lipoxygenase and reduces prostaglandin synthesis
Narcotic		
Butorphanol	Stadol	Binds to various opiate receptors, producing agonist and antagonist effects (opioid agonist-antagonist)
Fentanyl	Sublimaze	Binds to various opiate receptors, producing analgesia and sedation (opioid agonist)
Meperidine	Demerol	Binds to various opiate receptors, producing analgesia and sedation (opioid agonist)
Morphine sulfate		Binds to various opiate receptors, producing analgesia and sedation (opioid agonist)
Nalbuphine	Nubain	Binds to various opiate receptors, producing agonist and antagonist effects (opioid agonist-antagonist)
Other analgesic		
Acetaminophen	Tylenol	Analgesic mechanism of action unknown; antipyretic effect via direct action on the hypothalamus heat-regulating center
ANAPHYLAXIS: Drugs that stop or prevent allergic reactions, including anaphylactic shock		
Epinephrine 1:1000		Vasopressor via stimulation of alpha- and beta-adrenergic receptors resulting in vasoconstriction, has antihistamine-like effects
Diphenhydramine	Benadryl	Antagonizes central and peripheral H1 receptors (nonselective antihistamine)
Hydroxyzine	Atarax, Vistaril	Antagonizes central and peripheral H1 receptors (nonselective antihistamine)
ANESTHETICS: Drugs that decrease uncomfortable sensations by inhibiting nerve function		
Topical anesthetic		
Benzocaine	Hurricaine	Inhibits ionic fluxes, increasing depolarization threshold

TABLE 15-8 (*continued*)

Drug	Trade name	Action
Cetacaine		Benzocaine: inhibits ionic fluxes, increasing depolarization threshold, Butamben: No info Tetracaine: stabilizes neuronal membranes, inhibiting nerve impulses (ester)
Lidocaine topical gel	MANY!!!	Inhibits ionic fluxes, increasing depolarization threshold
Procaine	Novocain	Stabilizes neuronal membranes
Proparacaine	Alcaine Ophthalmic	Stabilizes neuronal membranes, inhibiting nerve impulses (ester)
Tetracaine		Stabilizes neuronal membranes, inhibiting nerve impulses (ester)
Local anesthetic		
Procaine	Novocain	Stabilizes neuronal membranes
Proparacaine	Alcaine Ophthalmic	Stabilizes neuronal membranes, inhibiting nerve impulses (ester)
Tetracaine		Stabilizes neuronal membranes
Inhaled agent/gas		
Nitrous oxide		Anesthetic and induction agent; allows for rapid absorption of other inhaled anesthetics
ANTIANGINAL AGENT: Drugs that stop anginal discomfort and pain by improving oxygenation of affected tissues		
Nitroglycerin	NitroBid, Nitro-Quick, Nitrostat	Stimulates cGMP production, resulting in vascular smooth muscle relaxation
Nitroprusside	Nitropress, Nipride	Directly dilates peripheral vessels
ANTICOAGULANT: Drugs that interfere with the clotting mechanisms at various points in the pathway		
Heparin		With antithrombin III and heparin cofactor, inhibits thrombin and Factor Xa and inhibits conversion of fibrinogen to fibrin
Warfarin sodium	Coumadin, Jantoven	Inhibits vitamin K-dependent coagulation factor synthesis (II, VII, IX, X, proteins C and S)
ANTICONVULSANTS: Drugs that stop or prevent seizure activity		
Anticonvulsant agent		
Fosphenytoin	Cerebyx	Modulates neuronal voltage-dependent sodium and calcium channels
Phenobarbital		Alters sensory cortex, cerebellar, and motor activities; produces sedation, hypnosis, and anesthesia, also classified as a barbiturate
Phenytoin	Dilantin, Phenytek	Modulates neuronal voltage-dependent sodium and calcium channels
Benzodiazepine		
Diazepam	Valium, Diastat	Binds to benzodiazepine receptors; enhances GABA effects
Lorazepam	Ativan	Binds to benzodiazepine receptors; enhances GABA effects
Midazolam	Versed	Binds to benzodiazepine receptors; enhances GABA effects

(*continued*)

TABLE 15-8 (*continued*)

Drug	Trade name	Action
ANTIEMETICS: Drugs that stop or suppress vomiting		
Droperidol	Inapsine	Exact mechanism of action unknown; antagonizes dopamine and alpha adrenergic receptors (butyrophenone)
Prochlorperazine	Compazine	Exact mechanism of action unknown; selectively antagonizes dopamine D2 receptors (phenothiazine)
Promethazine	Phenergan	Antagonizes central and peripheral H1 receptors (nonselective antihistamine)
Hydroxyzine	Atarax, Vistaril	Antagonizes central and peripheral H1 receptors (nonselective antihistamine)
ANTIHYPERTENSIVES: Drugs that maintain blood pressure at near normal values through a variety of actions		
Antihypertensive		
Clonidine	Catapres	Stimulates alpha2-adrenergic receptors (centrally-acting antihypertensive)
Diazoxide	Hyperstat	Relaxes peripheral arteriole smooth muscle; increases serum glucose
ACE inhibitor		
Enalapril	Vasotec	Inhibits angiotensin converting enzyme, interfering with conversion of angiotensin I to angiotensin II
Captopril	Capoten	Inhibits angiotensin converting enzyme, interfering with conversion of angiotensin I to angiotensin II
Calcium channel blocker		
Nifedipine	Adalate, Procardia	Inhibits calcium ion influx into vascular smooth muscle and myocardium
Vasodilator		
Nitroprusside	Nipride, Nitropress	Directly dilates peripheral vessels
ANTIHYPOGLYCEMICS: Drugs to treat low blood sugar levels		
Dextrose		Provides glucose needed for cellular metabolism
Glucagon		Converts hepatic glycogen to glucose
Oral glucose paste		Provides glucose needed for cellular metabolism
ANTIPLATELET AGENTS: Drugs that interfere with the platelet portion of the blood clotting mechanism		
Acetylsalicylic acid or Aspirin	MANY exist	Exact mechanism of action unknown; inhibits prostaglandin synthesis producing analgesic, antiinflammatory, antipyretic effects; irreversibly inhibits platelet aggregation (salicylate)
ANTITOXICOLOGICS: Drugs to treat or counteract poisonings and other toxicologic emergencies		
Anticholinergic		
Atropine	AtroPen	Antagonizes acetylcholine receptors (anticholinergic)
Antidote		
Cyanide antidote kit: Binds with cyanide		

TABLE 15-8   (*continued*)

Drug	Trade name	Action
Methylene Blue		Accelerates reduction of methemoglobin to hemoglobin; at higher doses, weakly oxidizes hemoglobin to methemoglobin which binds cyanide
Physostigmine		Reversibly binds to and inactivates acetylcholinesterase (anticholinesterase)
Pralidoxime auto injector	Protopam	Reactivates cholinesterase
BETA BLOCKERS: Drugs that block beta receptors of the sympathetic nervous system		
Esmolol	Brevibloc	Selectively antagonizes beta1-adrenergic receptors
Labetalol	Normodyne and Trandate	Selectively antagonizes alpha1-adrenergic receptors; antagonizes beta1- and beta2-adrenergic receptors (selective alpha and nonselective beta blocker)
Metoprolol	Lopressor and Toprol XL	Selectively antagonizes beta1-adrenergic receptors
Propranolol	Inderal	Antagonizes beta1- and beta2-adrenergic receptors (nonselective beta blocker)
DIURETICS: Drugs that promote diuresis (urine) production and/or excretion		
Diuretic		
Mannitol	Osmitrol	Elevates glomerular filtrate osmolarity (osmotic diuretic)
Loop diuretics		
Bumetanide	Bumex	Inhibits loop of Henle and proximal and distal convoluted tubule sodium and chloride resorption
Furosemide	Lasix	Inhibits loop of Henle and proximal and distal convoluted tubule sodium and chloride resorption
FIBRINOLYTICS: Drugs used to stop blood clots from forming or enlarging or that aid in destroying clots that have formed		
Alteplase	Activase	Converts plasminogen to plasmin, promoting fibrinolysis (tissue plasminogen activator)
Antithrombin III	Thrombate III	Forms covalent bond with thrombin
Heparin		With antithrombin III and heparin cofactor, inhibits thrombin and Factor Xa and inhibits conversion of fibrinogen to fibrin
Reteplase	Retavase Of	Converts plasminogen to plasmin, promoting fibrinolysis (tissue plasminogen activator)
Tenecteplase	TNKase	Converts plasminogen to plasmin, promoting fibrinolysis (tissue plasminogen activator)
Urokinase	Abbokinase	Converts plasminogen to plasmin, promoting fibrinolysis (thrombolytic)
GASTRIC DECONTAMINANTS: Drugs used to bind or eliminate toxic substances that are ingested		
Toxicological agents		
Activated Charcoal		Binds to toxins, inhibiting GI absorption
Ipecac		Centrally and locally induces vomiting

(continued)

TABLE 15-8   (*continued*)

Drug	Trade name	Action
INDUCTION AGENTS: Drugs used to promote a comatose or unconscious state for the purposes of performing medical procedures or controlling pain and discomfort		
Analgesic		
Ketamine	Ketalar	Produces analgesia
Barbiturate		
Methohexital	Brevital	Alters sensory cortex, cerebellar, and motor activities; produces sedation, hypnosis, and anesthesia
Thiopental	Pentothal	Alters sensory cortex, cerebellar, and motor activities; produces sedation, hypnosis, and anesthesia
Benzodiazepine		
Midazolam	Versed	Binds to benzodiazepine receptors; enhances GABA effects
Hypnotic		
Etomidate	Amidate	Produces hypnosis
Opiate		
Fentanyl	Sublimaze	Binds to various opiate receptors, producing analgesia and sedation (opioid agonist)
NARCOTIC and BENZODIAZEPINE ANTAGONISTS: Drugs that compete for narcotic or benzodiazepine receptors in order to antagonize (block) their effects		
Flumazenil	Romazicon	Antagonizes benzodiazepine receptors
Naloxone	Narcan	Antagonizes various opiate receptors (opioid antagonist)
Nalmefene	Revex	Antagonizes various opiate receptors (opioid antagonist)
NASAL DECONGESTANTS: Drugs used to dry up mucous membranes to improve breathing		
Oxymetazoline nasal	Afrin	Stimulates smooth muscle alpha-adrenergic receptors
Phenylephrine nasal	Neo-Synephrine	Stimulates smooth muscle alpha-adrenergic receptors
NEUROLEPTICS: Drugs used to relax the patient or place them in an altered state of consciousness		
Antipsychotic		
Chlorpromazine	Thorazine	Exact mechanism of action unknown; selectively antagonizes dopamine D2 receptors (phenothiazine)
Haloperidol	Haldol	Exact mechanism of action unknown; selectively antagonizes dopamine D2 receptors (butyrophenone)
Droperidol	Inapsine	Exact mechanism of action unknown; antagonizes dopamine and alpha adrenergic receptor (butyrophenone)
PARALYTICS: Drugs that block ACH receptors, resulting in temporary paralysis of muscles to facilitate the performance of medical procedures like orotracheal intubation **NEUROMUSCULAR BLOCKING AGENTS (NMBA)**		
Depolarizing NMBA		
Succinylcholine	Anectine	Stimulates motor endplate acetylcholine receptors

TABLE 15-8 (*continued*)

Drug	Trade name	Action
Nondepolarizing NMBA		
Mivacurium	Mivacron	Antagonizes motor endplate acetylcholine receptors
Pancuronium	Pavulon	Antagonizes motor endplate acetylcholine receptors
Vecuronium	Norcuron	Antagonizes motor endplate acetylcholine receptors
POSTPARTUM AGENTS: Drugs given follow the delivery of a baby to assist the mother in recovery		
Oxytocin	Pitocin	Unknown
RESPIRATORY AGENTS: Drugs used to treat respiratory emergencies. In the prehospital setting, this often means medications used to stop a problem (rescue) via bronchodilation versus preventing a problem from starting **BRONCHODILATORS (All drug classes listed here provide bronchodilation)**		
Beta2-Selective adrenergic: (Which target the beta2 receptors in the lungs)		
Albuterol	Proventil, Ventolin	Stimulates beta2-adrenergic receptors
Terbutaline	Brethine	Stimulates beta2-adrenergic receptors
Nonselective adrenergic (which must be observed for possible cardiac and vascular effects)		
Epinephrine	Adrenalin	Stimulates alpha- and beta-adrenergic receptors, causing vasoconstriction and relaxing bronchial smooth muscles
Epinephrine (Inhaled)		Stimulates alpha- and beta-adrenergic receptors, reducing mucosal secretions and relaxing bronchial smooth muscles
EpiPen Autoinjector and EpiPen Jr		Stimulates alpha- and beta-adrenergic receptors, causing vasoconstriction and relaxing bronchial smooth muscles
Metaproterenol	Alupent	Stimulates beta2-adrenergic receptors
Racemic epinephrine	Micronephrin	Stimulates alpha- and beta-adrenergic receptors, reducing mucosal secretions and relaxing bronchial smooth muscles
Combination agents: Sympathomimetic and Parasympatholytic		
Albuterol / Ipratoprium Combination	Duoneb (Nebulizer) Combivent (Metered dose inhaler)	
Methylxanthine		
Aminophylline		Exact mechanism of action unknown; increases cAMP; antagonizes adenosine receptors
Parasympatholytic		
Ipratoprium	Atrovent	Antagonizes acetylcholine receptors, producing bronchodilation
STEROIDS: Drugs used to treat inflammation through inhibition of immune system responses. Drugs used to suppress immune system responses in the case of allergies.		
Dexamethasone	Decadron	Antiinflammatory mechanism of action unknown; produces multiple glucocorticoid and mineralcorticoid effects
Hydrocortisone	Cortef	Antiinflammatory mechanism of action unknown; produces multiple glucocorticoid and mineralcorticoid effects
Prednisone		Antiinflammatory mechanism of action unknown; produces multiple glucocorticoid and mineralcorticoid effects

(*continued*)

TABLE 15-8 (*continued*)

Drug	Trade name	Action
Methylprednisolone sodium succinate	Solu-Medrol	Antiinflammatory mechanism of action unknown; produces multiple glucocorticoid and mineralcorticoid effects
TOCOLYTICS: Drugs used to suppress premature labor		
Magnesium Sulfate		Participates in physiologic processes, can also be given to stop seizure activity during eclampsia
Terbutaline	Brethine	Stimulates beta2-adrenergic receptors (selective beta agonist) which stops labor contractions
VASOPRESSORS: Drugs used to control hypotension by causing vasoconstriction		
Adrenergics, Sympathomimetics, Cathcholamines		
Dobutamine		Stimulates beta1-adrenergic receptors
Dopamine		Stimulates alpha- and beta1-adrenergic and dopaminergic receptors
Epinephrine		Stimulates alpha- and beta-adrenergic receptors
Norepinephrine	Levophed	Stimulates alpha- and beta1-adrenergic receptors
VITAMINS AND ELECTROLYTES: Drugs used as supplemental therapy of naturally occurring vitamins or minerals to enhance or regulate metabolism or other body functions		
Calcium Chloride		Essential component and participant in physiologic systems and reactions
Calcium Gluconate		Essential component and participant in physiologic systems and reactions
Magnesium Sulfate		Participates in physiologic processes
Potassium Chloride		Participates in physiologic processes and contributes to the acid/base balance
Sodium Bicarbonate		Increases serum bicarbonate, raising or restoring pH to normal levels
Thiamine		Participates in physiologic processes, believed to assist in carbohydrate metabolism

Contraindications

Contraindications for use of a medication are also important to know. A **contraindication** identifies when a drug should not be used. The most common contraindication for a medication is **hypersensitivity** (also known as allergy). Pregnancy is a contraindication for many medications. Contraindications are described as either absolute or relative. An absolute contraindication describes conditions when a drug should never be used. Hypersensitivity (allergy) is always an absolute contraindication. A relative contraindication is a situation that causes the paramedic to consider carefully whether the benefits associated with giving the medication outweigh the possible risks associated with giving it. The drug aspirin is given for suspected heart attacks, but if the patient has a bleeding ulcer or takes warfarin sodium (a blood thinner), aspirin use should be considered carefully as these are relative contraindications for its use. Ipratropium (a parasympathetic blocker used for respiratory distress) is derived from peanuts, so patients allergic to nuts and soybeans may have a reaction to this medication.

Street Secrets

When patients tell you they are allergic to a medication that you need to give them, inquire what reaction actually occurs. Some patients misunderstand an adverse reaction, thinking stomach upset means they are allergic to the medication. Hives, facial flushing, itching, swelling, loss of consciousness, etc. are all possible findings with an allergic reaction. Refer to Chapter 32: Allergies and Anaphylaxis for a complete description of signs and symptoms. If the patient really needs the medication and the description given does not sound like a true allergy, consult with medical direction and seek advice about administering the drug. Do not administer any drug that the patient reports an allergic reaction to until you consult with online direction.

Medication Storage and Handling Considerations

Paramedics should know about special storing and handling considerations for medications. The Institute for Safe Medication Practices (http://www.ismp.org/) is a nonprofit organization supported by grants, charitable donations, and contributions that focuses on medication safety issues, including handling and storage. It posts FDA and JCAHO (the federal hospital accreditation agency) alerts and also has a bimonthly newsletter available through subscription called *ISMP Medication Safety Alert!*

The United States Pharmacopeia (USP), as the official public standards-setting authority for all prescription and over-the-counter medicines, dietary supplements, and other healthcare products manufactured and sold in the United States, has published guidelines for the storage and handling of drugs in emergency medical services vehicles. The guideline is available from the USP website (http://www.usp.org) in a supplement called *Revisions in the Second Supplement to USP28 – NF23*. The name of the section is PF30 (6), p. 2118, and the title is "Storage of Drugs in Emergency Medical Services (EMS) Vehicles." DOT 1-7.22

In addition to these guidelines, the insert from the medication package or some drug references will identify the temperature range required for storing a medication. Insulin requires a low storage temperature to prevent it from breaking down while mannitol (an extremely hypertonic osmotic diuretic) will crystallize if exposed to temperatures that are too low. The paramedic should also know if a medication must be kept out of intense light, like sunlight. Nitrates like nitroglycerin and nitroprusside are light sensitive and must be stored out of direct light even though they come in amber-colored glass vials. Some medications, such as amiodarone (a cardiac antidysrhythmic) must be handled very carefully when mixed, as rough handling can result in so much foam forming in the vial it is unusable.

It is also important for the paramedic to know and adhere to any special safeguarding considerations for securing medications carried on the ambulance. Many EMS systems keep all of their drugs secured in locked compartments while others may only lock up narcotics or drugs known to be at high risk of theft or misuse in their system. Often, drug logs are required to track the handling or custody of medications between shifts. Disciplinary actions and even criminal charges can result if medication is lost or stolen. DOT 1-7.22

CONNECTIONS Chapter 4: Legal Issues discusses the legal implications of diverting drugs. Drug diverting behavior is when paramedics provide drugs to the public outside of approved protocol situations. An example of drug diversion is handing out aspirin (which in EMS is used for cardiac patients) to a patient from a motor vehicle crash who is refusing transport but complaining of a headache. Another example is when a paramedic provides a vial of naloxone to a family member of a chronic narcotic user, so they have an antidote for the next overdose. Regardless of how well-intentioned this behavior may be, it is inappropriate.

Disposal of Unused Medication

There may also be special regulations regarding the proper disposal of leftover or unused medication, particularly the controlled substances such as narcotics. The paramedic may be required to dispose of any unused, leftover medication in the presence of a witness. The protocol for this procedure may require that the witness be a healthcare professional not directly connected with the EMS system, such as a nurse in the emergency department. The witness may also be required to sign a log entry attesting to the disposal of the medication. Disciplinary action and even criminal charges can result if medication is improperly disposed of or if the process is incorrectly documented. DOT 1-7.22

Street Secrets

Many paramedics have learned to prepare only the dose they need to administer in the IV, particularly if they are giving the drug in a moving unit. They "waste" excess drug from the prefilled syringe by squirting it into the trash can and then they have the exact dose remaining in the syringe. This is helpful in preventing accidental overdose from injecting too much drug, particularly when the roadway becomes bumpy. It is not recommended to prepare the syringes in this manner when you have to waste the remaining unused drug.

Recommended Dosages

The paramedic should know the dose for all medications carried on the ambulance. Dosages can vary slightly across the United States although some organizations, such as the AHA, provide recommendations for dosages in their algorithms. In addition to the approved protocol dose, it is helpful to be aware about an acceptable dosing range as well. Physicians providing on-line medical direction are required to know the ranges established for their jurisdiction, but some EMS systems allow the physician to order a dose that is outside that listed in the paramedic's standing order or protocol. If the paramedic is familiar with the dosing range for a medication, it will make it easier to follow the physician direction. For example, many jurisdictions give 0.3 mg of epinephrine via injection for an allergic reaction. This is also the dose found in the epinephrine AutoInjector™ prefilled syringe cartridge. Per a commonly utilized online resource (Epocrates Rx), the acceptable range for a single injection of epinephrine is 0.1–0.5 mg SC (every 10–15 minutes) with an alternate dose of 0.1–0.25 mg IV (of 1:10,000 solution) over 5–10 minutes.[8]

Street Secrets

Make a handy quick reference of all your drug dosages by recording this information on a 3 × 5 piece of cardstock or an index card. Include the route and speed for administration and also if on-line permission is needed to administer the drug. Laminate the card and keep it in your pocket.

Routes of Medication Administration

Paramedics should be familiar with the various routes allowed for administration of the medications they carry. Local protocols may restrict the administration route even though there may be many that are recommended by the manufacturer and acceptable per FDA standards. Paramedics should also be familiar with less commonly used routes of administration in case they receive a physician order for administration outside of their protocol route. Box 15-2 (on page 299) lists common routes of administration used by paramedics. DOT 1-7.16

Many medications in a paramedics' formulary are administered via intravenous (IV) bolus. A **bolus** is a single dose of medication that is given at one time to a patient. Regardless of the amount (or volume) of drug given, each drug has an appropriate speed at which it should be given. For example, adenosine is given via rapid push because the drug bolus needs to remain "together" and reach its target site quickly to be effective. If it is given as a slow push, it will be diluted in the blood and will not work.

Dextrose is very caustic to body tissues and viscous (thick), so it should always be administered via slow IV push with frequent aspiration during the procedure to ensure the IV is still patent. DOT 1-7.30

Street Secrets

Despite the speed of injection of a bolus of medication, the paramedic should always ensure the patency of the IV by aspirating prior to injecting any medication. This is crucial because drugs injected into the tissues instead of the bloodstream could have a detrimental effect on the patient. Absorption of the drug may be delayed, and the drug could injure the tissues. To aspirate, the paramedic first pulls back a little on the plunger of the syringe, creating negative pressure in the IV and resulting in the drawing of approximately 1–2 mL of blood back through the catheter hub and into the IV tubing. Seeing blood will confirm that the IV line is intact (the line is patent), and the medication will be delivered directly into the vein. The blood can be immediately injected back into the patient along with the medication. Chapter 16: Medication Administration and IV provides additional information on medication administration.

Drug Interactions, Precautions, and Special Considerations

Drug interactions can occur without warning or can follow predictable patterns. A **drug interaction** arises between two medications or can occur between medications and certain foods.[2] The interaction could result in one or both drugs forming a toxic substance, inactivation of one or both drugs, or increased effects of one or both drugs. In order to minimize the possibility of drug interactions, paramedics should perform a thorough history to include a listing of all prescription and nonprescription medications the patient is taking. Asking about over-the-counter medication (OTCs), herbal remedies (including "teas" and anything placed on the skin or inhaled as smoke), and vitamin supplements should be included in the interview. Some patients will disclose the use of "recreational," nonprescribed, or illegal drug use if you inquire in a nonjudgmental manner. Often this knowledge is important in your care and treatment plan for the patient. DOT 1-7.21

Paramedics should know about medication **precautions** or **special considerations.** A precaution or special consideration is additional information about a medication that does not fall into the category of interaction or contraindication. This may include the order two medications should be administered or describe an effect that may be seen following administration of the drug. For example, when EMS systems used ipecac and activated charcoal as ingested poison antidotes, it was important not to administer the charcoal before the ipecac because the charcoal would absorb and inactivate the ipecac.

Pre- and Postmedication Administration Procedures

Prior to administering a medication, the paramedic should obtain a history of past medical conditions and prescription and nonprescription medication use and allergies. Clues to underlying medical conditions can be gathered by identifying classes of all the medications used by the patient. This can help focus the paramedic on specific signs or symptoms or alert them to otherwise "abnormal" findings in a physical exam. For example, beta-blocker medications taken to regulate the electrical conduction system and pumping force of the heart can also cause a slower than expected heart rate in a patient with hypovolemia from trauma. DOT 1-7.12, 1-7.28, 1-7.29

Vital signs should be obtained before and after the administration of a medication. An assessment should be performed of the body regions or systems affected by the drug before and after administration. The patient should be monitored to see if the desired effects have been achieved and, when appropriate, if repeat administration is necessary. Appropriate documentation should be made in the patient care report including vital signs and history and physical exam findings before and after drug administration. It should also include the name of the drug, strength (if appropriate), time of administration, dose, and route. It is also important to record the patient's response to the medication. DOT 1-7.25, 1-7.27

Summary

Medication administration is an important skill for paramedics. In order to do this properly you need to possess a basic understanding of the responsibilities and scope of management pertinent to the administration of medications. You should appreciate that drugs interact with the cells of the body by binding to receptors.

It is important for you to learn about classes of medications instead of focusing on memorizing lists of generic and trade names of the drugs in the formulary. You should know the classes of medications commonly used by your patients. When you think of medications in terms of their class, you will begin to link drugs with disease processes and medical conditions.

Knowing the indications, contraindications, dosages, routes of administration, and precautions of all drugs carried in your EMS system is also critical. It is important to follow all pre- and postadministration procedures such as obtaining a history and performing a physical examination and following it up with proper documentation.

Notes

1. D. L. Kasper et al., eds., *Harrison's Principles of Internal Medicine,* Volume 1, 16th ed. (New York: McGraw-Hill, 2005).
2. J. G. Hardman, and L. E. Limbird, eds., *Goodman and Gilman's The Pharamacological Basis of Therapeutics,* 10th ed. (New York: McGraw-Hill, 2001).
3. American Heart Association, "Guidelines 2000 for Cardiopulmonary Resuscitation and Emergency Cardiovascular Care," Circulation (Supplement), 102, (8) (August 2000).
4. J. Tintinalli, *Emergency Medicine. A Comprehensive Study Guide* 6th ed. (New York: McGraw-Hill, 2004).
5. Kasper et al., eds., *Harrison's Principles of Internal Medicine* Volume 2, 16th ed. (New York, McGraw-Hill, 2005).
6. DOT Curricula. Objective number 1-8.11, page 4 of Module 1-8.
7. J. S. Lubin, T. R. Delbridge, K. J. Rinnert, and T. E. Platt, "Evolution of Statewide EMS Drug Formularies and Regulations," *Prehospital Emergency Care* 9(2005): 176–180.
8. "Epinephrine," http://rxonline.epocrates.com/(accessed August 22, 2006).

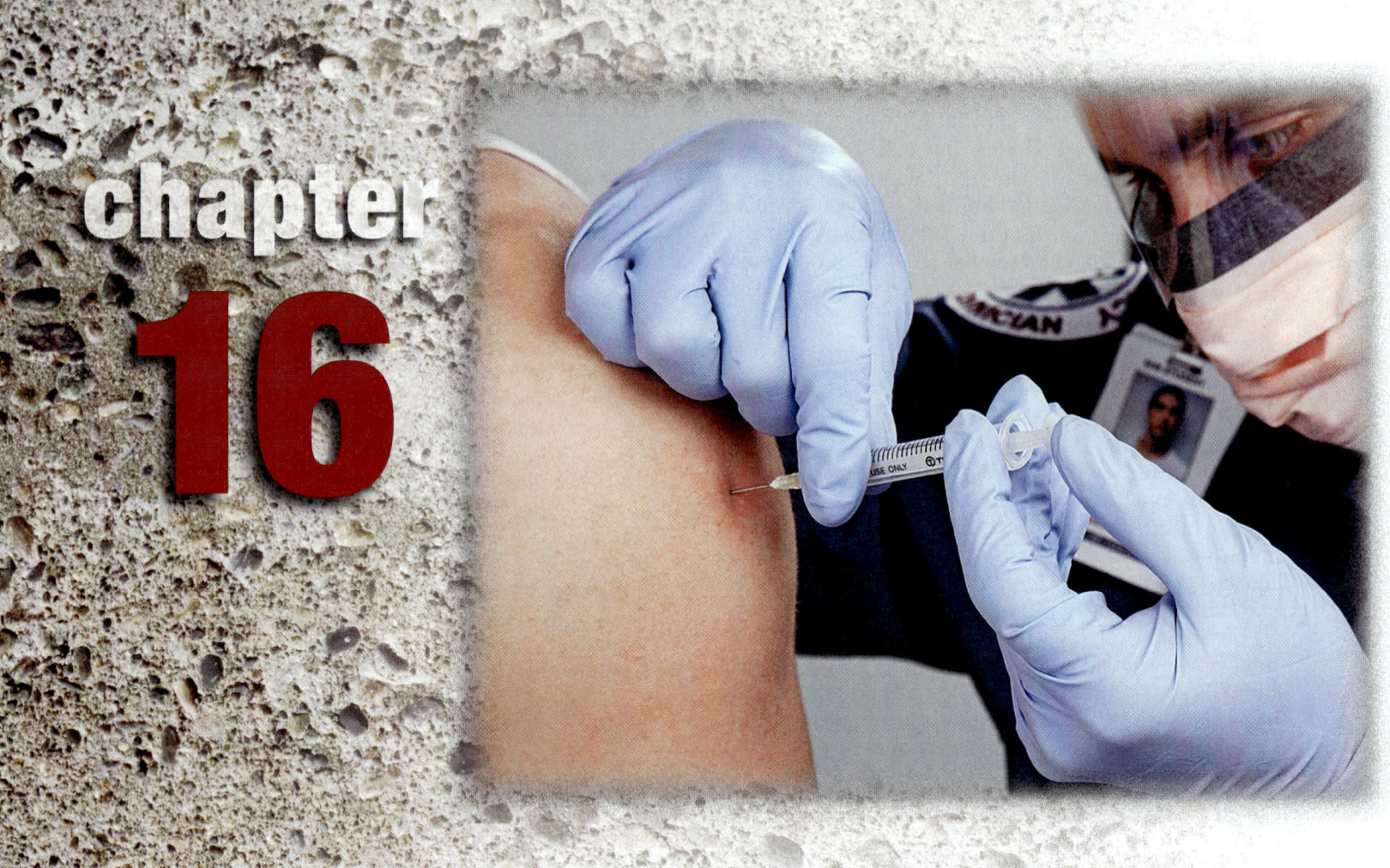

chapter 16

Medication Administration and IV

"Poisons and medicine are oftentimes the same substance given with different intents."

—Peter Mere Latham

Need to Know

▶ How to perform a drug calculation. (Detailed discussion of drug calculations can be found in Chapter 16 of the companion student workbook.)

▶ The proper method to prepare a medication for administration.

▶ The indications, contraindications, precautions, and interactions for all medications in the paramedic's formulary.

▶ How to safely and properly access all approved administration routes.

▶ Safe administration techniques, which include maintaining asepsis, preventing complications or problems with the various administration routes, and proper disposal of contaminated materials.

▶ Performing all required preadministration assessments and procedures including history, physical examination, vital signs, and other monitoring devices information. (And knowing when any of these must not be done because of the severity of the emergency.)

▶ What authorization is required for administering each medication and whether it is through on-line or off-line medical control.

▶ The expected therapeutic effect for all medications used in the prehospital environment.

▶ The potential side effects and complications for all medications used in the prehospital environment.

▶ Postadministration follow-up procedures, including proper documentation, patient reassessment, and monitoring.

▶ Do	▶ Ask
• Check each medication at least three times before giving it to the patient.	• About allergies and drug interactions the patient has experienced before administering any medication.
• Ensure the vital signs have been assessed before and after each medication administration.	• About medications the patient is currently taking (as well as over-the-counter or herbal remedies and any illicit drugs).
• Document medication administration appropriately.	
• Ensure all biological hazardous materials are disposed of in the proper receptacles.	

Introduction

Medication in the prehospital environment is administered by a variety of routes, and each route requires a specific administration technique. You are responsible for ensuring that the correct dose is administered, which may require mathematical conversions or calculations. As discussed in the previous chapter, it is important to understand the indications, contraindications, precautions, and interactions for all medications in your formulary. Safe administration techniques are required which include maintaining the cleanliness of all supplies and equipment (called asepsis), preventing complications during administration, and properly disposing of contaminated materials. You should also understand the expected therapeutic effect for all medications used in the prehospital environment.

Prior to administering any medication, you should collect enough information through history taking and from the physical examination to ensure a correct assessment is made, and the proper therapy is selected. Administration of medication requires authorization from medical direction governing what, where, when,

why, and how it may be used. This permission may take the form of off-line written protocol and standing order or require real-time on-line physician direction via telephone, radio, or satellite consultation. Postadministration follow-up procedures include reassessing and monitoring the patient for effects, both beneficial as well as detrimental. Proper documentation is critical to ensure the patient is followed up appropriately in the hospital setting and to close the loop on the procedure for the paramedic. This chapter will discuss all of these aspects of medication administration. DOT 1-7.12

Medication Skill Sheets include: 42: Intravenous Access (also see Step-by-Step 42); 43: Intravenous Access Using Saline Lock (also see Step-by-Step 43); 44: Phlebotomy; 45: Intraosseous Access and Drug Administration (also see Step-by-Step 45); 46: Umbilical Vein Cannulation; 47: Central Line Access for Fluids and Drug Administration; 48: Intravenous Drug Bolus (also see Step-by-Step 48); 49: Intravenous Drug Infusion (also see Step-by-Step 49); 50: Intramuscular Drug Administration (also see Step-by-Step 50); 51: Intranasal Drug Administration; 52: Nebulized Drug Administration (also see Step-by-Step 52); 53: Subcutaneous Drug Administration (also see Step-by-Step 53);

54: Sublingual Drug Administration; 55: Endotracheal Drug Administration; 56: Eye Drop Drug Administration; 57: Oral Drug Administration; 58: Rectal Drug Administration (also see Step-by-Step 58); 59: Autoinjector Drug Administration Device; 89: NREMT Intravenous Therapy; and 91: NREMT Pediatric Intraosseous Infusion.

General Guidelines of Medication Administration Responsibilities

The responsibilities associated with medication handling and administration parallel the primary paramedic responsibilities discussed previously. These responsibilities come directly from the DOT curricula and include preparation, response, scene assessment, patient assessment, recognition of injury, management, appropriate disposition, treatment and transport, patient transfer, documentation, and return to service.[1] This order, although identified as pertinent for a standard patient interaction, provides an appropriate plan for medication administration as well, so it will serve as the template for this chapter.

Preparation and Response

Before responding to any emergency, ensure that all necessary medications are stocked at the appropriate number, are in date, and are in good condition. Your governing body will provide a list of approved medications for your individual service's **formulary.** A formulary is the listing of medications approved for use along with pertinent information for each drug on the list.

Read the accompanying literature from the medication package box (called the package insert) to determine if there are any special storing or handling requirements. Some medications require storage within a specific temperature range or out of direct sunlight. For example, most injectable medications should not be frozen or stored for long periods of time in temperatures above 90°F. Another example involves the injectable form of nitroglycerin. It should be administered only in glass bottles using special tubing that accompanies the drug. Nitroglycerin tablets should not be exposed to sunlight or the bottle kept open for too long.[2] DOT 1-8.10

Check all expiration dates on a regular basis. Medication and most sterile supplies, like IV catheters and tubing, have expiration dates. To make it easier to check for expiration, mark the box clearly with the expiration date or circle the date on the container. Be careful not to obscure information on the container if you do this. Put those medications that are expiring soonest closer to the front of the storage compartment to ensure they are used first.

Expiration checks should be frequent and should follow agency guidelines (Figure 16-1). Some services require a thorough count and expiration date check with the change of every shift while other services may require weekly, monthly, or a spot check to verify an intact seal

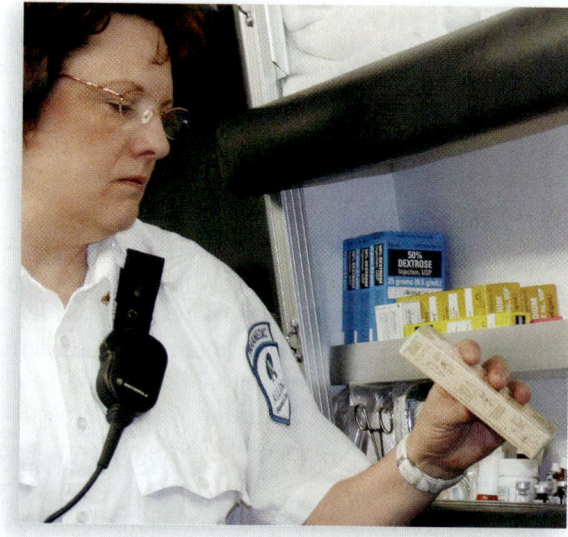

Figure 16-1 Check the expiration date of all medication and sterile supplies at the start of every shift or on the schedule required by your service.

remains on a storage cabinet or container. It may be possible to rotate medications that are close to expiring out of your stock and replace them with fresher ones. For an ambulance service closely aligned with a hospital, this may be easier to do than for an independent service.

Some services store drugs at risk for theft or misuse (such as narcotics) with a higher degree of security than other medications (Figure 16-2). This may include the use of a custody log or special counting procedure. It may also include storage in a special location or control and custody by the most senior member of the healthcare team. Box 16-1 describes the procedures for handling narcotics. DOT 1-7.22

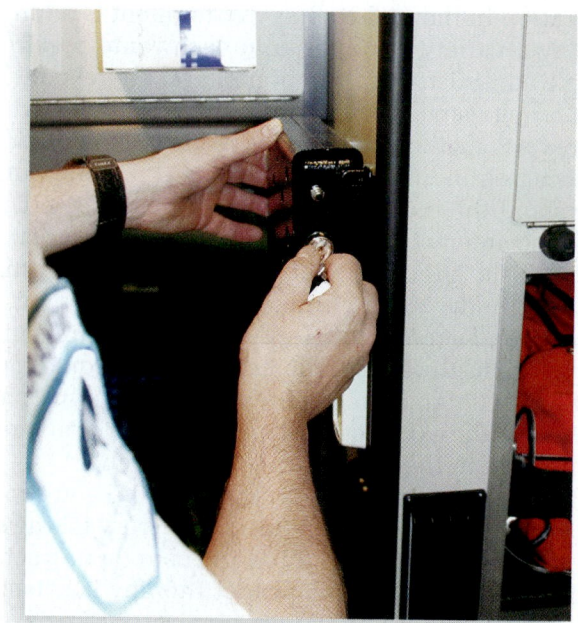

Figure 16-2 Some medication requires additional security measures.

BOX 16-1   Narcotic Drugs

Narcotic administration requires that paramedics follow specific local, state, and federal regulations. It is necessary that paramedics ensure that all narcotics are accounted for at the beginning and end of their shift and that they are secure throughout the shift. Make sure all custody logs are signed and maintained as per protocol. DOT 1-8.10

In addition to preparing the ambulance to respond to patients, paramedics should be ready to respond by being familiar with the protocols and standing orders for all the medications used in their system. Know the pediatric and adult doses as well as all approved routes for administration. Paramedics should understand the indications, contraindications, precautions, and special considerations for each drug. Make a pocket card with the dosages and routes of administration to keep as a reference.

Street Secrets

When marking medication containers with expiration dates, make sure you put the correct month and year of expiration on the box. If the medicine expires on an exact date, for example March 3, 2009, it is better to write 02/09 on the box than 03/09. The 02/09 date will ensure the drug is rotated out of stock prior to the actual expiration date. For expiration dates with just the month and year listed, the last day of the month is considered the expiration date. In this case, a drug with August 2010 could have 08/10 written on the box.

CONNECTIONS Refer to Chapter 15: Pharmacology for more information on medication indications, contraindications, precautions, and special considerations.

Make sure the appropriate supplies are available to prepare and administer every medication in the formulary. This includes having an adequate number of the various sizes of syringes and needles and any solutions needed to dissolve powdered drugs into liquid form.

Pay particular attention to the supplies and equipment used by the facilities that routinely receive your patients. Your ambulance service may interact with medical facilities that support a combination of "needle-less" and "latex-free" environments, which could result in the need to maintain many different sets of supplies. Needle-less equipment and supplies are designed to minimize the possibility of accidental needle stick by replacing some components with special fittings that eliminate the need for needles. Although this equip-

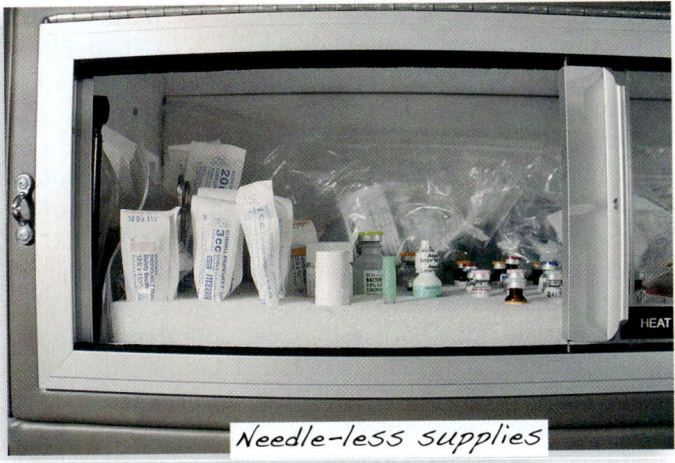

Needle-less supplies

Figure 16-3   Needle-less and latex-free supplies should be clearly labeled and stored separately.

ment makes a safer working environment, it is not compatible with needles. Attempting to use a needle in a needle-less system will contaminate or damage it.

Latex is a natural rubber product derived from tree sap. Many people are allergic to the protein in latex, and there have been some fatalities from anaphylactic reactions caused by latex exposure. Between 5% and 17% of all healthcare workers are estimated to be allergic to latex. The estimated rate of latex allergy in children is 1 in 10,000.[3] Some EMS systems and other healthcare settings are moving away from using latex-containing equipment and supplies (Figure 16-3). Care must be exercised not to cross contaminate these supplies with latex-containing products. Separate storage areas are usually required.

Scene Assessment, Patient Assessment, and Problem Recognition

Size up the scene and look for clues. Before administering any medication, ensure you have completed a thorough scene assessment. As you enter a private residence, look at the door frame or window for a sticker that indicates medical information may be located inside (Figure 16-4). Many EMS services and

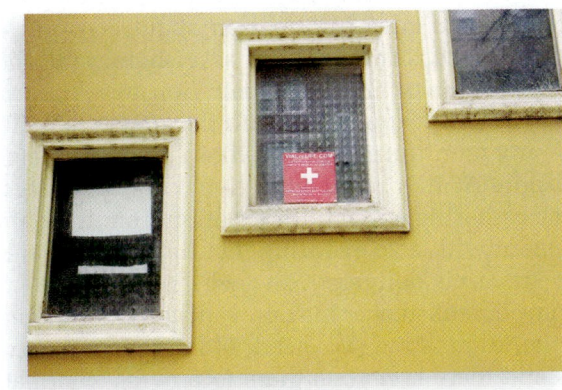

Figure 16-4   Look for clues that the patient has medical information stored somewhere on the scene.

health departments have programs so patients can make medication information available in a consistent location. The refrigerator door is a common location for many of these programs. DOT 1-8.25, 1-8.26

Look around for medication bottles. They could be anywhere in the home including the kitchen, bedroom, bathroom, or living room. Don't forget to look for over-the-counter (called OTCs) and herbal preparations. Be alert for drug paraphernalia and any signs of medication misuse or abuse.

Determine if the patient has been **compliant** with the prescribed dosing regimen. The term compliant describes whether or not a patient has adhered to the medication dosing regimen prescribed by the physician. A noncompliant patient is not taking the medication as prescribed. One study found a 76% discrepancy rate in adherence to dosing regimens between the medications the patients were actually taking and those prescribed by their physicians.[4] This study observed that over three-fourths of all people taking a prescription medication were not taking it according to the directions. Some patients were taking too much (overdosing) or too little (under dosing) or taking it at the wrong time of day (for example in the morning instead of evening) or under the wrong circumstances (for example, with meals instead of on an empty stomach).

Street Secrets

In addition to asking patients if they are compliant, another EMS provider can count pills or measure quantities of medication while you stay with the patient. This permits a comparison between the number of pills that should be missing based on the prescription date versus the number actually missing to help assess medication compliance. This may be necessary if the patient is on a medication that requires continual dosing in order to maintain life or health. Antipsychotic and antidepressant medications are two examples, but blood pressure and cardiac medications are just as important to take regularly.

Before administering any drug, you should obtain a history that includes information about allergies and medications. Perform a patient assessment and obtain vital signs. Begin oxygen administration, as appropriate, and start an intravenous line with the appropriate fluid. Attach any monitoring devices like a pulse oximeter or ECG leads. At this point in patient care, you need to balance gathering enough information from the patient assessment with also ensuring that timely intervention and treatment is delivered. DOT 1-7.26, 1-7.27

Some circumstances may prevent you from gathering all of the information you need. If the patient is unconscious and there is no one there to provide information to you, document this in the patient care report. If the situation is life-threatening, as when the patient is in cardiac arrest, you may not be able to determine if the patient has allergies to all of the medications you are going to administer. You should ask bystanders and family members if the person has any allergies or takes any medication, but seeking this information should not delay treatment.

CONNECTIONS Chapter 10: Therapeutic Communications and History Taking describes techniques that may be helpful in obtaining information from patients and bystanders.

Management and Appropriate Disposition

Once the need for medication use is identified, you must gather the supplies and equipment you need to perform the administration. Collect all the materials together, including the medication and extra supplies in case something becomes contaminated or is not appropriate for use. For example, as you prepare the supplies to administer an injection, you attach a needle to a syringe and set it on a sterile field (the inside of a sterile dressing package) while you open and cleanse the top of the medication vial. The syringe rolls off the paper and you are concerned it is contaminated and now cannot be used. Because you had some extra supplies near by, you can quickly set up a new syringe. (A more thorough discussion of aseptic technique follows later in this chapter.) DOT 1-8.25, 1-8.26

Determine if the final destination for your patient has any impact upon your treatment decision. You may decide not to administer a medication that takes 15 to 20 minutes to begin working if the destination is less than five minutes away, particularly when you know other medication options are available once the patient reaches the hospital. Consider the need to obtain on-line physician consultation in situations like this. Asking for clarification may be appropriate, even when there is a standing order already in place.

Confirm whether on-line or off-line medical direction is needed for permission to administer the medication. Perform the patient "rights."[1] If the patient is conscious, in addition to obtaining consent for treatment, you should discuss any side effects the patient may experience once the medication is administered (Box 16-2). For example, a patient with crushing substernal chest pain may have a headache and dizziness as a natural side effect (caused by dilation of blood vessels and the lowering of blood pressure) after nitroglycerin administration. If the patient is prewarned this could happen, it may reduce his anxiety when it occurs. DOT 1-8.11

CONNECTIONS See Chapter 15: Pharmacology, Box 15-6 (page 311) for a description of the patient "rights" that are identified in the DOT curricula.

BOX 16-2   Indications and Contraindications

An **indication** is the reason a drug is given. For example, albuterol is indicated for a patient with respiratory distress and a history of asthma. A **contraindication** is a reason a drug should not be administered. Hypersensitivity (allergy to a drug) is always an absolute contraindication to its use.[5] Pregnancy is often a relative contraindication to the use of many medications.[6] A **relative contraindication** means there is not enough evidence to absolutely confirm the medication is safe to administer in that particular circumstance, so caution must be used. Patients with certain diseases, such as heart or kidney disease, often have relative contraindications with medicines that could stress that particular organ. For example, drugs that increase blood pressure should be used with caution in cardiac patients.

Medical control may override a relative contraindication if the physician determines that the risk in giving the medication is outweighed by the benefit the patient may receive. An example of this is when a physician orders the use of epinephrine to treat a severe allergic reaction in a patient who is seven months pregnant. The use of epinephrine may cause the onset of premature labor, but if the patient dies from the allergic reaction, the baby may also die. Medical control should always be consulted if a relative contraindication exists.

Treatment and Transport

Prepare the medication for administration. Always check to confirm that the right medication is being administered. DOT 1-8.14

In the pharmacy profession, this check is routinely performed three times. The first time is when the medication is selected from the storage area. The second check is made prior to opening the container (for example, before drawing the dose from the vial, reconstituting the powder, or assembling the prefilled syringe). The third check occurs immediately before giving it to the patient. Often, each check is performed by a different person, and many times there is a log maintained of one or more of the checks. All of these measures add quality control to the process which helps minimize mistakes.

The EMS environment can emulate this system by (1) repeating back the drug name and dosage when received during online consultation, (2) carefully reading the medication name before taking it out of the box, and (3) asking another member of the patient care team to verify the name on the medication container.[7]

Administer the medication following the patient rights, but also use the appropriate procedures and guidelines to ensure safety (Table 16-1). Paramedics are routinely at risk of exposure to blood and body fluid, so it is important to always take appropriate body substance isolation (BSI) precautions (Figure 16-5). The exact type of BSI required will vary with the procedure being performed or the patient's condition. At a minimum, every EMS provider should wear gloves during every patient encounter. The greater the risk of exposure from splashing or uncontrollable circumstances, the more additional BSI precautions are required. Types of BSI equipment include gloves, goggles, a mask to cover the mouth, a combination face mask with eye shield, and a gown. Respiratory precautions with a particulate mask may be required if a potential pathogen is airborne. DOT 1-8.14

Preventing Exposure to Infectious Agents

A contaminated needle stick is a common way in which healthcare providers are exposed to infectious diseases.[6] A 1998 survey of 3,162 emergency medicine residents found that over 50% reported having at least one occupational exposure to blood during their training, and over 70% of the exposures were from a needle stick or sharp object.[8]

There have been a few studies conducted regarding EMS workers and exposure to blood or potentially contaminated bodily fluids and infectious agents. One study, published in 1993, evaluated the frequency of exposure to patients with hepatitis B virus (HBV) and human immunodeficiency virus (HIV) in the city of Portland, Oregon.[9] During the two year time frame the

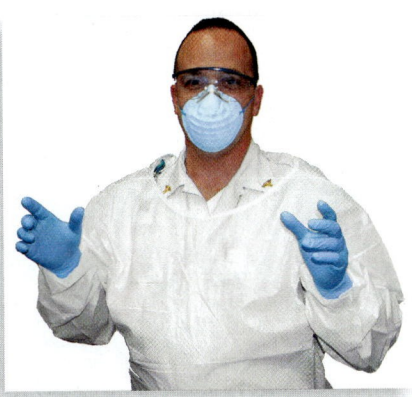

Figure 16-5   BSI precautions should be observed any time you have a potential to be exposed to pathogens, including medication administration.

TABLE 16-1 **Medication Administration**

See the following Skill Sheets for step-by-step instructions for each method of administration

Skill Sheet name	Skill Sheet number		Skill Sheet name	Skill Sheet number	
Blood Draw Using Vacutainer and Leuer Adapter	44		Eye Drop Drug Administration	56	
Blood Draw Using Syringe	43		Intramuscular Drug Administration (also see Step-by-Step 50)	50	
Intraosseous Access and Drug Administration (also see Step-by-Step 45)	45		Nebulized Drug Administration (also see Step-by-Step 52)	52	
Intranasal Drug Administration	51		Intravenous Drug Infusion (also see Step-by-Step 49).	49	
Intravenous Drug Bolus	48		Nebulized Drug Administration (Nebulized Mask)	52	
Central Line Access for Fluids and Drug Administration	47		Nebulized Drug Administration (Pipe)	52	
			Oral Drug Administration	57	

TABLE 16-1 (*continued*)

Skill Sheet name	Skill Sheet number		Skill Sheet name	Skill Sheet number	
Rectal Drug Administration	58		Intravenous Access Using Saline Lock (also see Step-by-Step 43)	43	
Sublingual Drug Administration	54		Autoinjector Drug Administration	59	
Subcutaneous Drug Administration	53		Putting on and Removing Sterile Gloves	60	
Intravenous Access (also see Step-by-Step 42)	42		Handwashing (also see Step-by-Step 61)	61	
			Endotrachael Drug Administration	55	
			Umbilical Vein Cannulation	46	

study was conducted, 256 exposures were documented. The rate of exposure compared to the call volume was 4.4 exposures per 1,000 patient contacts. Fourteen (5.5%) of the exposures were needle sticks, 15 (5.9%) were eye splashes, 8 (3.1%) were mucous membrane exposures, 38 (14.8%) were exposures to nonintact skin, 120 (46.9%) were exposures to intact skin, and 61 (23.8%) were respiratory exposures. Forty-eight of those individuals (including 64% of the needle stick injuries) were treated and followed for signs of infection. While all of the EMS workers were vaccinated against HBV, 26% of those who were exposed during the study actually tested with inadequate HBV titres at the time of their exposures. This means that while they believed they were adequately immunized, their blood work showed they were not within the recommended levels of antibody protection.

Accidental sticks can occur during the use of glucometers as well. The glucometer is the device used to check the blood sugar level. It requires a drop of blood for the test. The blood is most frequently taken from the fingertip, but it can also come from the IV needle or IV site if fluid or drugs have not been infused.

One study examined the frequency of accidental sticks while using glucometers among 477 EMS providers in one EMS system. The study compared the incidence of injury from spring-loaded lancets and nonspring-loaded lancets.[10] The **lancet** is the needle-like device that pricks the finger of the patient so a drop of blood can be obtained for the glucometer. The spring-loaded lancets would quickly pierce the skin and then retract into the device, eliminating the protrusion of the needle, while the nonspring-loaded lancets had a portion of the needle tip remaining exposed once they were used. The incidence of needle stick injuries decreased from a rate of 16 per 954 EMS workers per year to two per 477 EMS workers per year when the use of spring-loaded lancets was instituted in that EMS system.

In another study, EMS workers in three U.S. cities with high AIDS incidence were observed to determine the frequency and type of exposure the workers encountered in their daily work.[11] In an eight-month period of time, EMTs and paramedics were interviewed when they returned to their stations following an EMS call to determine if they were exposed to blood or body fluids. A total of 165 shifts were surveyed with a total of 2,472 patients attended to by the crews. Sixty-two blood contacts were reported by the EMS providers: One was a needle stick, and 62 were skin contacts. The team then surveyed the receiving hospitals to determine the HIV status of the patients transported to them. The three hospitals participating in the survey reported HIV rates among those patients at 8.3, 7.7, and 4.1 per 100 patients. The conclusion of that study is that EMS workers regularly encounter blood contacts, most of which are skin contacts, but because the HIV status is unknown for most patients, EMS providers should always practice universal precautions.

Continual vigilance for safety is crucial to minimize occupational exposure to blood and body fluids. Hand and skin washing, needle-less devices, proper immunizations, and focus on universal precautions all help minimize the risks to EMS providers.

Street Secrets

Minimize the possibility of accidental needle stick due to vehicle movement by performing all injections or IV's while the ambulance is not moving whenever possible. If patient transport has begun, gather and prepare the equipment while the ambulance keeps moving. When ready, ask the driver to pull over and stop for a minute while you perform the venipuncture. Once the flash is obtained, if the road surface is relatively smooth, the driver can go while you finish securing the line.

CONNECTIONS Chapter 9: Safety and Scene Size-Up has additional information on BSI precautions.

Handwashing

Handwashing is the most important form of BSI precaution for a healthcare provider. Hands should be washed in tepid water before and after each patient contact as well as after handling contaminated equipment. Exposed skin should be examined carefully for small cuts or abrasions, and these should be covered with an occlusive dressing to prevent accidental exposure from splashed blood. It has been proven in many studies that hand and skin washing is the best method of controlling the spread of pathogens.[12] **See Skill Sheet 61: Handwashing.**

Disposal of Contaminated Material

All equipment and items that have come in contact with blood or body fluids must be treated as potentially infectious and be disinfected or disposed of properly. A **biohazard container,** called a **sharps container,** is specifically designed for disposal of needles and anything capable of piercing the skin (Figure 16-6). In the United States, these devices are rigid containers that are red in color and labeled with a warning about the contents. Sharps containers come in a variety of sizes and shapes. Used nonsharp materials like gloves or face masks should be disposed of in an appropriate biohazard receptacle. These storage devices may be red or yellow and often carry warning labels as well. DOT 1-8.14, 1-8.24

Patient Transfer

Upon arrival at your destination, give a verbal and written report directly to the individual assuming patient care. The report should include the following information:

- The patient presentation upon your arrival, including level of consciousness and amount of distress the patient was having.

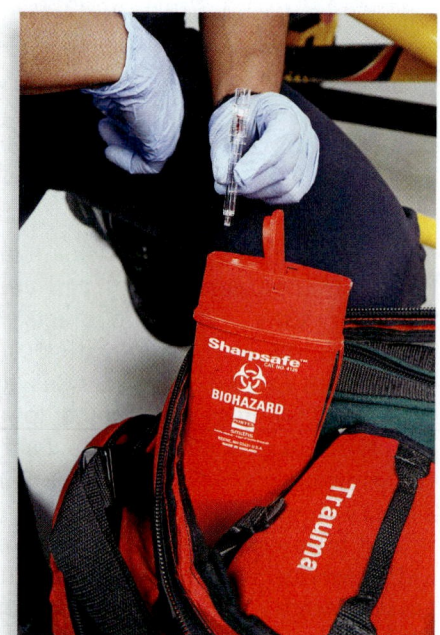

Figure 16-6 Sharps containers and biohazard bags should be used to properly dispose of contaminated sharp instruments and equipment.

- The physical examination and history findings leading to your decision to give the medication, including copies of ECG tracing, monitoring device printout, and vital signs prior to the medication administration.
- The name of the drug, dose, strength, route, and time it was administered.
- A description of the patient's response to the medication, including vital signs postadministration and reassessment findings.
- If on-line direction or any other permission was required prior to medication administration, include the name of the physician ordering the medication. This can be especially important if the receiving facility (and physician) is different from the consulting physician.
- If the medication dosing regimen requires repeat administration, inform the receiving facility when the next dose is due, so they may, at their discretion, continue administering the medication.

CONNECTIONS Chapter 17: Documentation and Communication details information on performing a radio consultation. Please consult that chapter for additional information.

Documentation

Appropriate documentation in the patient care report includes the drug name, time administered, dose, strength/concentration (if appropriate), route, and site of administration. Time of administration is very important to include in the report, especially if the drug can be repeated. The vital signs of the patient as well as their response to the medication should also be recorded.

Administration of narcotics or other controlled substances requires that the paramedic follow specific local, state, and federal regulations. It is necessary that paramedics ensure that all narcotics are accounted for at the beginning and end of their shift and that they are secure throughout the shift. Make sure all custody logs are completed as per system protocols. Dispose of any unused medication by following agency requirements. Obtain the signatures of any person who witnesses the disposal of medication in either the patient care report or the medication custody log from the ambulance.

CONNECTIONS Chapter 17: Documentation and Communication details information on what elements are important to capture for the patient care report. Given the number of medication errors occurring throughout all aspects of healthcare, documentation of medication administration is especially important. Please consult this chapter for additional information.

Return to Service

Replace used drugs, supplies, and equipment before returning to service. To ensure the correct medication is obtained, confirm the drug name three times just as when it is given to the patient. Label the expiration date on the new box using the method previously described. Store the new medication in the appropriate location, so those drugs expiring soonest will be chosen first. Complete any logging procedures required to document that the drug was used and replaced appropriately.

Medical Asepsis during Medication Administration

Medical asepsis means the medical environment is free of pathogens. Pathogens are disease-causing organisms such as viruses, bacteria, fungi, spores, etc. The setting for patient care is often contaminated with many of these pathogens, and the patients are susceptible to infection, particularly if they have chronic diseases or traumatic injuries. DOT 1-8.12, 1-8.13, 1-8.14, 1-8.24, 1-8.28, 1-8.30, 1-8.31, 1-8.32, 1-8.33, 1-8.43

Paramedics perform many procedures on patients that place them at an increased risk of infection. Initiating an intravenous line, drawing blood, dressing open wounds, medication administration, needle thoracostomy (chest decompression), and endotracheal tube placement are just a few of the skills that invade the body, exposing it to possible infection. Pathogens are found not only in the environment around us but also in and on us. It is important to keep our environments and ourselves as clean as possible to decrease the potential spread of infection. The use of sterilization procedures, disinfectants, and antiseptics can help in this process. DOT 1-8.12

Sterilization means that the environment or equipment is free of all forms of life, including bacterial spores, which are very difficult to kill. Extreme heat from steam under pressure **(autoclaving)**, dry heat, or ethylene oxide gas are the only three acceptable methods for sterilization, so not all equipment is capable of being sterilized.[13] Also, human tissue is not capable of being sterilized. It is nearly impossible to have a sterile environment and keep objects sterile in the prehospital setting, so medically clean techniques are the accepted standard of care. **Medically clean** means handling sterile equipment in such a way as to prevent contamination The technique used to prevent infection is called **aseptic.**

All equipment used to initiate an IV, to penetrate into the skin (such as a scalpel used for a surgical airway), or that is introduced into the body (like an endotracheal suction catheter) is sterile. The upper portion of the chamber of the IV tubing (called the **spike**) that is introduced into the IV solution should not be

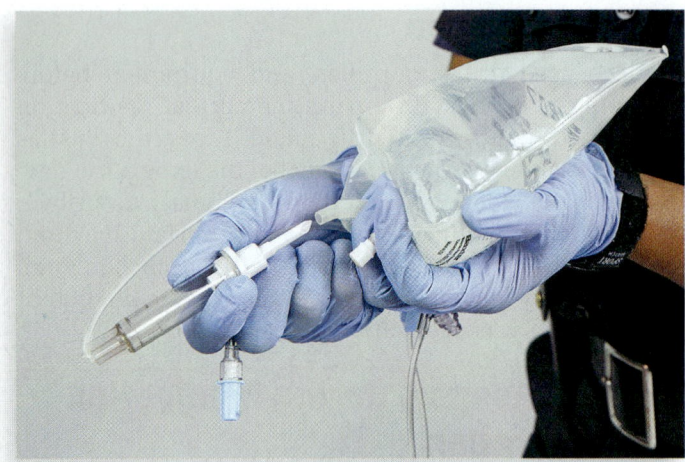

Figure 16-7 Join the heels of your hands to stabilize yourself and ensure that the flashchamber insertion spike and the newly exposed IV spike port are not touched. The two ends of these devices should remain sterile.

contaminated. The portion of the IV tubing that is placed inside the hub of the catheter should not be touched (Figure 16-7). The IV catheter should be handled carefully, so it is not contaminated once the protective cover has been removed. The portion of the needle and the catheter that enters the skin should not be touched or come into contact with any surface prior to insertion. In this fashion, all of these various pieces of equipment are kept as clean as possible.

Prior to performing any incision or puncture into the skin, the patient's skin should be cleansed with either 70% alcohol or 2% iodine in 90% alcohol. In the operating room setting, if the skin is prepared (cleaned) for one minute using either of these two solutions, it is just as effective in controlling wound infection as the traditional surgical procedure of scrubbing for 5–10 minutes using povidone-iodine.[13]

Disinfectants are cleansing agents that are toxic to living tissue, while **antiseptics** are cleansing agents that are nontoxic to living tissues. Thus, equipment should have disinfectants used on them, and antiseptics are used on patients to cleanse sites for drug administration. Disinfectants and antiseptics are capable of destroying or inhibiting the growth of most microorganisms. The most common antiseptics used in IV initiation and drug administration are alcohol and iodine.[13] DOT 1-8.13

Follow package guidelines when using all disinfectants and antiseptics. This means maintaining exposure of the disinfecting solution with the contaminated surface for the proper amount of time in order for disinfection to occur. It also means mixing the disinfectant solution correctly. Some disinfectants come in concentrated form and require mixing with water prior to use. Surprisingly, to be most effective, many of these chemicals must be diluted appropriately for optimal cleaning power. In some cases, using a full strength solution is not as effective. The Department of Labor's Occupational Safety and Health Administration (OSHA) and the Environmental Protection Agency (EPA) work together to investigate and approve the labeling of all chemicals used for cleaning, disinfection, and sterilizing as they pertain to healthcare worker safety. In addition to these two groups, the Centers for Disease Control and the Food and Drug Administration all work together to set standards regarding bloodborne pathogens.[14]

The actual amount of time required for proper handwashing is not clear, even in the surgical setting in the hospital.[13] A two-minute scrub with soap and warm water seems to be adequate, provided there is attention paid to the fingertips and nail beds. These areas are known to contain the greatest numbers of bacteria on the hands. The best cleaning product to use on skin is one containing chlorhexidine or one of the iodophors. Alcohol foam can be used as a temporary cleansing agent if soap and water is not available.

Biohazard Exposure Plans

It is required by law that all medical organizations have a biohazard exposure plan in place and that employees are familiar with the process to follow if they are exposed.[15] If you are exposed to blood or body fluid, immediately wash the affected area with soap and water. If soap is unavailable, irrigate with copious amounts of water. Immediately contact your supervisor, medical director, infection control officer, or other designated individual as necessary to implement the exposure plan. Make sure all appropriate documentation is completed, including an incident report of the situation.

Summary

Administering medication is a fundamental part of being a paramedic. Proper techniques need to be followed to ensure proper delivery of the medication to the intended target organ. You should follow the primary paramedic responsibilities of preparation, response, scene and patient assessment, recognition of medical problem, patient management, appropriate disposition, treatment and transport, patient transfer, documentation, and return to service to ensure you cover all the responsibilities associated with medication administration.

Notes

1. Emergency Medical Technician Paramedic: National Standard Curriculum (EMT-P), United States Department of Transportation (www.nhtsa.dot.gov/people/injury/EMS/EMT-P/index.htm) (accessed August 24, 2006).
2. Clinical Pharmacology Copyright © 2005 Gold Standard.

3. G. E. Morgan, M. S. Mikhail, and M. J. Murray, *Clinical Anesthesiology,* 4th ed., McGraw-Hill's AccessMedicine (accessed August 23, 2006).

4. S. E. Bedell et al., "Discrepancies in the Use of Medications: Their Extent and Predictors in an Outpatient Practice," *Archives of Internal Medicine* 160(14) (2000): 2129.

5. L. C. Grammer et al., "Drug Allergy and Protocols for Management of Drug Allergies, 3rd ed., Part II, General Principles of Prevention of Allergic Drug Reactions," *Allergy Asthma Proceedings* 25(2004): 267.

6. J. E. Tintinalli, G. D. Kelen, J. S. Stapczynski, O. J. Ma, and D. M. Cline, *Tintinalli's Emergency Medicine: A Comprehensive Study Guide,* 6th ed., McGraw-Hill's AccessMedicine (accessed August 23, 2006).

7. J. C. Morey, R. Simon, G. D. Jay, et al., "Error Reduction and Performance Improvement in the Emergency Department Through Teamwork Training: Evaluation Results of the MedTeams Project," *Health Services Research* 37(2002): 1553.

8. C. H. Lee, W. A. Carter, W. K. Chiang, et al., "Occupational Exposures to Blood Among Emergency Medicine Residents," *Academy of Emergency Medicine* 6(1999): 1036.

9. E. Reed, M. R. Dava, J. Jui, K. Grellman, L. Gerber, and M. O. Loveless, "Occupational Infectious Disease Exposure in EMS Personnel," *Journal of Emergency Medicine* 11(1) (January–February 1993): 9–16.

10. W. F. Peate, "Preventing Needlesticks in Emergency Medical System Workers," *Journal of Occupational Environmental Medicine,* 43(6) (June 2001): 554–557.

11. R. Marcus, P. U. Srivastava, D. M. Bell, P. S. McKibben, D. H. Culver, M. H. Mendelson, R. J. Zalenski, and G. D. Kelen, "Occualtional Blood Contact Among Prehospital Providers," *Annals of Emergency Medicine* 25(6) (June 1995): 776–779.

12. D. L. Kasper, E. Braunwald, A. S. Fauci, S. L. Hauser, D. L. Longo, J. L. Jameson, and K. J. Isselbacher, eds., *Harrison's Principles of Internal Medicine,* 16th ed., McGraw-Hill's AccessMedicine (accessed August 23, 2006).

13. L. W. Way, and G. M. Doherty, *Current Surgical Diagnosis and Treatment,* 11th ed., McGraw-Hill's AccessMedicine (accessed August 23, 2006).

14. OSHA website: http://www.osha.gov/pls/oshaweb/owadisp. show_document?p_table=INTERPRETATIONS&p_id=20789

15. Occupational Safety and Health Standards, *Bloodborne Pathogens, Regulations (Standards-29 CFR),* http://www. osha.gov/pls/oshaweb/owadisp.show_document?p_table= STANDARDS&p_id=10051.

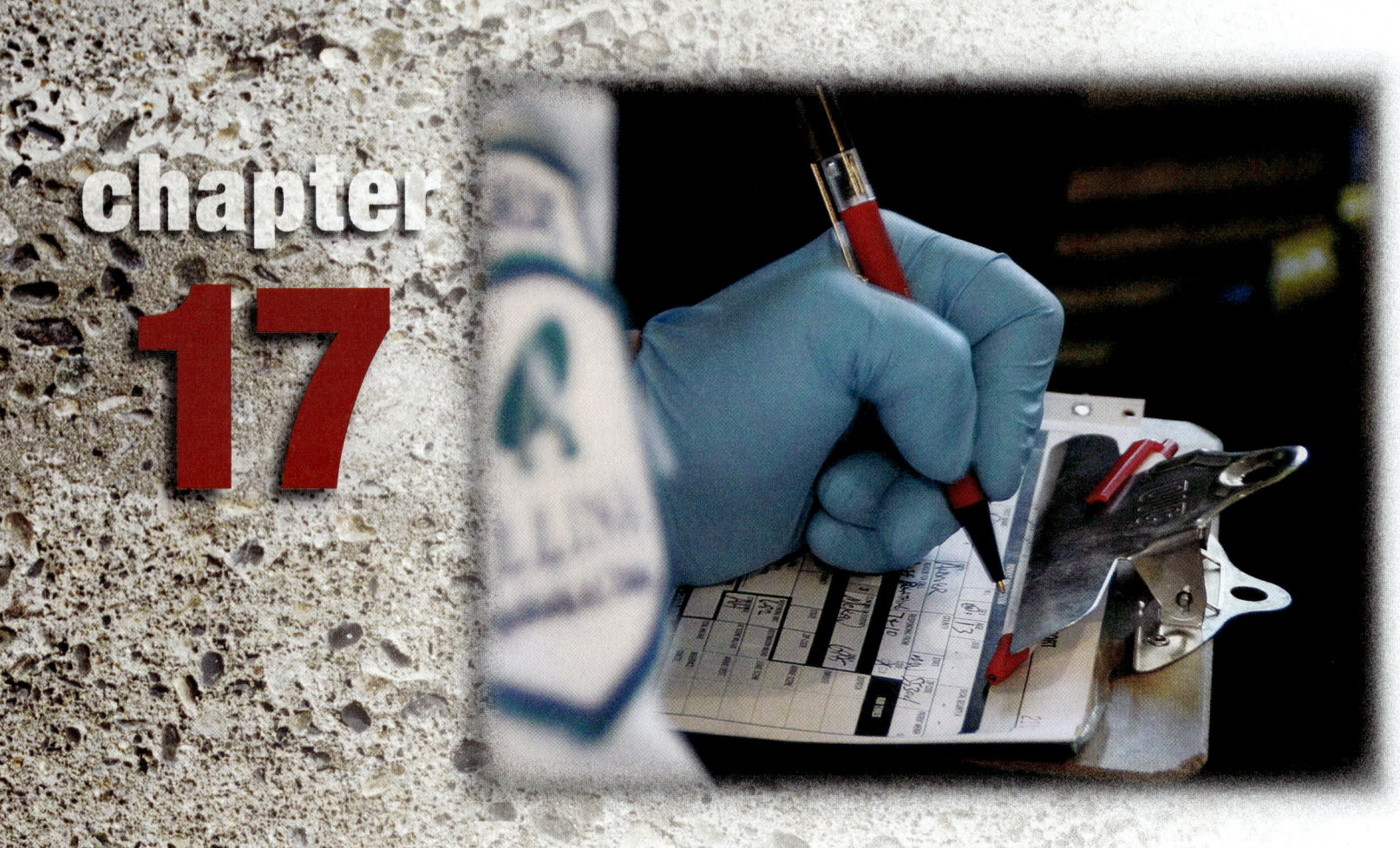

chapter 17

Documentation and Communication

"Though we name the things we know, we do not necessarily know them because we name them."

—Homer W. Smith

Need to Know

▶ Report writing and radio reporting are critical skills that are just as important as starting IVs and giving medication.

▶ Written reports and recorded on-line consultations are legal documents that can be called into evidence. They should be concise and professional.

▶ A common phrase used to describe medical documentation is: "If you did not write it down, you did not do it." Review your reports carefully to ensure all of the assessments and care you provided are reflected in your documentation and that your care reflected the standard of care and your protocols.

▶ The quality of your written documentation and verbal communication conveys your level of professionalism to other members of the healthcare team.

▶ Do	▶ Ask
• Look up the spelling of words that are not familiar. • Use common words to convey your meaning as you learn more complex medical terminology. A simply worded, accurate report is preferred to one that is poorly written, containing lots of medical terminology and jargon, especially if it is incorrectly used.	• Your employer or supervisor if they have a list of approved abbreviations that you can use in your written reports. • Your employer which format they want your reports written in and if they have samples of well-constructed reports that you can review if the format is unfamiliar. • Your partner to read over your report before you submit it for the patient's medical record.

Introduction

Written documentation and verbal communication are critical skills for paramedics to master. The **patient care report (PCR)** is a permanent record of events that transpired on the ambulance call. These documents can be used in the days and weeks that follow to provide information to the hospital staff that continues to care for the patient. They can also be used later to reconstruct the call for court cases. DOT 3-5.1, 3-5.2

During the call, the verbal report informs the receiving facility a patient is coming. It also connects the physician at the consultation center or receiving facility (or both) with the paramedic on scene. This can be helpful when patient care is complicated or an appropriate destination is unclear or must be coordinated between facilities. Paramedics use on-line medical consultation to ask for orders for treatment and/or medication and to seek advice on patient care. DOT 3-5.1, 3-5.2

Both written and verbal radio reports reflect our level of professionalism to other members of the medical community. These skills should be considered of equal importance with any other skill performed by paramedics. **Skill sheets that complement this chapter include Skill Sheet 62: Communication Challenges—Interpreter Services, Skill Sheet 63: Verbal Communications, and Skill Sheet 64: Documentation.**

Documentation

Documentation is written, factual evidence that reflects patient care during the patient encounter. Documentation is the core principle of professionalism and accountability. Your documentation should not be governed by a "minimum standard." The phrase **minimum standard** implies that something is equal to mediocre; it represents the opposite of excellence. The patient care report (PCR) should reflect high levels of professionalism and convey to the other members of the medical profession that EMS is worthy of their respect. An unfortunate crossover to prehospital medicine from other healthcare professions is the legal crisis of medical litigation, and to endure as a profession, prehospital providers need a working knowledge of the fundamental principles of documentation. The basic knowledge and skill of a proper documentation process ultimately creates a protective, legally defensible report. Providers must write prehospital reports with the jury that may potentially review the PCR in mind. Your reports serve as your testimony and your defense, and, conversely, they may be used as primary evidence against you, your crewmembers, and the agency or jurisdiction you represent in the event of litigation against you.

Your PCR should not be a legal handicap—it should be your legal shield.

The foundation of documentation begins with a simple, systematic, written account of the prehospital encounter. It includes the assessment (including pertinent scene size-up information, medical history, vital signs, and physical examination), treatment, and continued reevaluation of the patient based on a standardized protocol or standard of care. The final component of strategic documentation reflects the final disposition of the patient. This puts an end cap on responsibility for the patient and the inherent liability that comes with patient care.[1]

Prehospital documentation is defined by specific expectations: agency requirements, jurisdictional considerations, state obligations, local parameters, and certification or licensure responsibilities, with each of the preceding citations even further defined by HIPAA (Health Information Portability Accountability Act) constraints. DOT 3-5.14

Professional Accountability through Documentation

You will protect yourself through **strategic documentation**. As with all medical professional careers, an excellent report-writing standard is promoted in order to clearly document your assessment and actions as well as to protect you and defend your actions in the event of an accusation of professional misconduct or malpractice. Such an accusation may take the form of an administrative complaint or a serious legal claim of wrongdoing or negligence. An attorney evaluating a complaint of negligence may be dissuaded from litigation by a runsheet that is well-written, all-inclusive, and promotes a professional stance. Conversely, a poorly written patient care report may implicate you in certain circumstances. Your documentation may reveal an omission of required treatments, violations of the protocol, or simply the lack of vital and supportive documentation.[1]

CONNECTIONS Chapter 4: Legal Issues discusses malpractice and negligence.

Elements of a Well-Written Report

You bear the responsibility to ensure your report is accurate and complete. Proofread your prehospital report before you turn it in. Does it convey an accurate word picture of the prehospital events? The patient care report should promote graphic imagery involving the senses of sight, touch, smell, and hearing. The reader of the report should be able to visualize what you saw, feel what you palpated, discern the sounds you heard, and be sensitive to the scents you were exposed to. The report should allow the reader to

appreciate your decision-making and the rationale supporting the protocol and treatment plan you followed. Through your report writing, the reader should "witness" the prehospital scene as though they were actually present on the call. DOT 3-5.8, 3-5.10, 3-6.16, 3-6.22

The document and information contained in the PCR constitutes medical evidence and is a permanent part of the patient's medical record, retrievable for an indefinite period of time through varied information storage banks.

Who Has Access to Your PCR?

Medical professionals involved with the patient after you transfer care will read the report. These medical professionals may be physicians, nurses, respiratory therapists, physical therapists, social workers, and other allied health professionals with the purpose of gathering facts from the prehospital component of care. However, there are other professionals, who may be nonclinical in nature, who also have a prospective interest in the facts revealed in your documentation. Their interest may stem from a financial drive, a legal drive, or a combination of both. These nonclinical professionals may include billing agents; insurance auditors; local, state or federal investigators; risk managers; EMS administrators; police officers; detectives; forensic specialists; attorneys; expert witnesses; and even jurors (Figure 17-1). DOT 3-6.1

Documentation Is Evidence— A Legal Record of the Incident

Your documentation is deemed credible written testimony, judged to be reliable and truthful simply because it was recorded either contemporaneously or immediately following the patient encounter. Its factual credibility is enhanced when the report itself is timely,

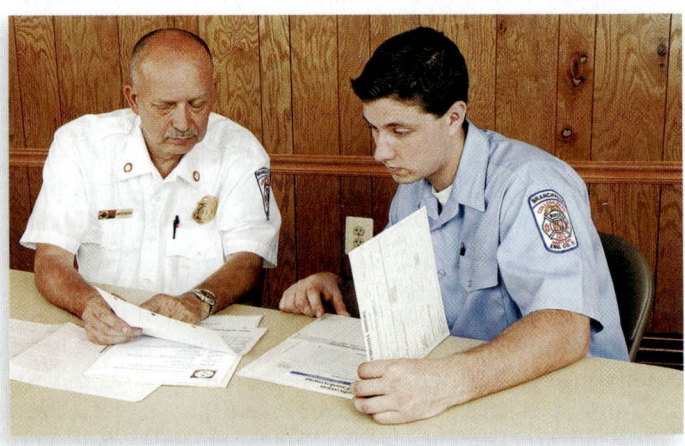

Figure 17-1 Supervisors and administrators will review your reports for completeness and accuracy.

concise and accurate, organized, properly punctuated with words correctly spelled, and puts forth an overall impression of professionalism. DOT 3-5.11, 3-6.11, 3-6.12

Form and Content of Strategic Documentation

A well-written report reflects the EMS provider's education, competence, and level of professionalism. Meticulous record keeping with treatment documentation clearly reflective of the accepted protocol is a provider's best defense and self-protection in the event of official inquiries, formal and informal criticism, or potential legal action.

The documentation system has to meet the clinical demands of the on-the-street providers, the information need of subsequent healthcare providers, the needs of the accounting department for billing, and possibly legal requirements if liability issues are raised. The provider must determine what factual information is to be included in the runsheet and how the facts will be presented; the presentation form and the content presented by the format are the essential foundations for strategic documentation. While there are other theories on healthcare-related documentation, the three organizational strategies cited below represent the professional standard for presentation of the facts through prehospital documentation.[1] DOT 3-6.5

Hallmarks of a Well-Written PCR

The hallmarks of a well-written report include the following:

1. A professional documentation standard for presentation of the facts.
2. A strategic format for management of the facts (form and content).
3. Respect for the prehospital provider's accountability and sole responsibility of proper documentation, not simply with regard to the patient, but with consideration for all crewmembers involved, the sponsoring agency or jurisdiction, and the overseeing medical director. DOT 3-5.8, 3-5.10

There is a direct correlation between provider training and education, level of expertise and experience, personal and professional commitment, and the ability to construct a high-quality, descriptive prehospital report. The form or format is simply a framework to work within. It is the foundation on which to build your written testimony, and it dictates the way your facts are displayed. It compels you to organize the information in the framework and ultimately yields a credible report. A functional format streamlines the documentation process through centered organization, the use of focused acronyms, the protocol as a template for documentation of treatment, and presentation of all of the facts in a clear and concise manner.

Working in the Gray Zone

Many EMS agencies and systems have implemented spinal immobilization policies or protocols that are based on critical evaluation of select criteria indicating the need for spinal immobilization. One study, however, demonstrated extremely poor documentation of these criteria in a system that implemented such a protocol.[2] Failure to provide adequate documentation indicating the reasons for not placing spinal immobilization in a patient subsequently found to have a spinal injury can lead to serious financial consequences for both the paramedic and the EMS agency.

Organizational Framework for the PCR

Poor organization of the facts in the report leaves a poor impression of the provider and possibly a poor impression of the care provided. Simply put, if your report skips from fact to fact, repeats, or shifts back and forth in time, it scatters the factual information and presents a disorganized word picture.

> A substandard report often is equated to substandard care.

A well-organized report leaves a positive impression and reflects positively on the professionalism of the provider. A framework keeps your documentation focused and organized; the use of organizational acronyms within the foundation framework further ensures that the presentation of your facts is focused and organized. There are commonplace secondary acronyms that keep the facts focused and organized and literally serve as prompts for required information.

Two commonplace frameworks used for strategic documentation are presented in the form of acronyms—CHART and SOAP (or SOAPIER)—that by design make the layout of the framework a relative fill-in-the-blank template for data. These framework layouts can be used in conjunction with or in lieu of a narrative-style written report.

Whether or not the CHART approach or one of the various SOAP approaches is adopted is often up to the jurisdictional medical director or administrator. Both formats describe the identical information required in a prehospital report. Each format also incorporates the secondary organizational tools: SAMPLE (a valuable and complete history-taking tool), OPQRST (for evaluating the chief complaint, injury and illness, and first aid interventions prior to your arrival), DCAP-BTLS (physical assessment parameters with regard to injury), and lastly TTFN (final disposition and transfer of care accountability, which includes mutual aid services, support services, or the receiving facility).[1]

CONNECTIONS Chapter 14: Patient Assessment contains full descriptions and additional information on the SAMPLE, OPQRST, and DCAP-BTLS mnemonics.

The CHART Framework. The **CHART** framework uses the acronym CHART, as in "charting" or documenting, in writing the patient care report. CHART is a straight forward, simplistic acronym effectively employed by all levels of emergency medical technician (Figure 17-2). It is practical and easy to recall:

CHART Framework

C "Chief complaint" of the patient or the reason EMS was summoned

H History (using the SAMPLE mnemonic)

    S Symptoms (using the OPQRST mnemonic)

        O Onset

        P Provocation or Palliation

        Q Quality

        R Region or Radiation

        S Severity

        T Time

    A Allergies

M Medications

P Past and pertinent medical history

L Last oral intake

E Event leading up to the injury or illness

A (Physical) Assessment (utilizing one of the following approaches)

- Head to toe approach
- System by system approach
- Primary and secondary assessment approach

R Rx Treatment (following a protocol template)

- Detailed listing of the treatment in accordance with the accepted protocol
- Evaluation or response to each element of treatment

T Transport and Transfer (Utilizing the TTFN acronym)

- To: who received the patient and at what facility
- Time: of transfer of care to the receiving facility
- Fluids: type and volume of any fluids or medications received by the patient
- Necessary status update: on the patient condition

The SOAPIER Framework. The acronym **SOAPIER** is also an organized format used for constructing patient care reports. There are several variations of this format: SOAP, SOAPE, SOAPIE, and SOAPIER are all utilized in EMS narrative report writing.

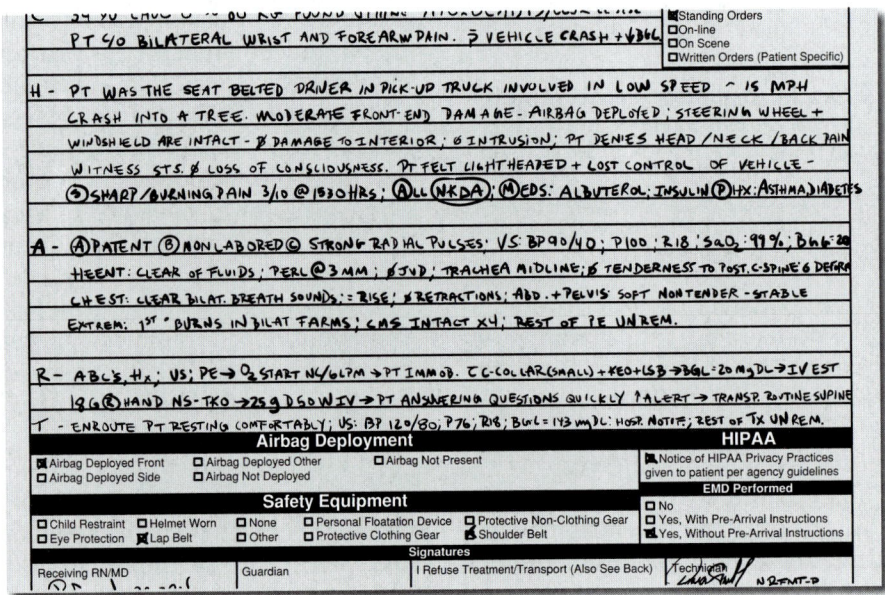

Figure 17-2 A PCR in the CHART format.

SOAPIER Framework

S Subjective Information: "Chief Complaint" and Patient History

  S Symptoms (use OPQRST mnemonic)

  O Onset

  P Provocation and Palliation

  Q Quality

  R Region or Radiation

  S Severity

  T Time

  A Allergies

  M Medications

  P Past medical history

  L Last oral intake

  E Event leading to injury/illness

O Objective Information: Physical Assessment appropriate for the patient

  • Head to toe approach

  • System by system approach

  • Primary and secondary assessment approach

A/P Analysis of assessment and protocol to be used

I/E Implementation of protocol/evaluation of treatment

  • Chronological listing of treatment provided based on accepted protocol

  • Evaluation or response to each element of treatment

R Report (utilizing the TTFN acronym)

  • To: who received the patient and at what facility

  • Time: of transfer of care to the receiving facility

  • Fluids: type and volume of any fluids or medications received by the patient

  • Necessary status update: on the patient condition

Subjective and Objective Information

Some EMS providers have difficulty distinguishing between **objective information** and **subjective information.** *Ob*jective notations are *ob*served: Objective data are generally observable clinical signs and symptoms, physiologic data, technology-derived data, among other observable data. When documenting objective findings, avoid vague or non-measurable phrases; instead, choose to write descriptive observations or measurable comparatives to identify trends and relative condition of the patient. DOT 3-6.8

Subjective notations reflect information provided by the patient or family member, that which they state or express, such as the chief complaint(s) and information regarding past medical history, medication history, allergies, etc. **S**ubjective information can be remembered as **s**poken by the patient, family member, bystander, or additional source. Unless the subjective information you collect stems from the patient or a direct witness, such as a family member or bystander, or additional source, a provider should avoid subjective documentation. The documentation reflective of your observations, treatment, and evaluation, as well as final disposition of the patient, should be as objective and factual as possible.

Working in the Gray Zone

As discussed in Chapter 5: Clinical Decision-Making, prehospital providers do not officially diagnose; however, to be broadly relevant to a given set of subjective symptoms and objective observations, all of your protocols are based on working diagnoses. There is a very slim line between diagnosing, which can be construed as practicing medicine as would a physician, and formulating a functional assessment and approach toward appropriate treatment.

Avoiding Biased Information

Biased information is considered prejudicial information, born of preconceived judgment or opinion by the provider; it too is subjective based on past experience. Though prior life experiences (in or out of the prehospital arena) may evoke a certain attitude, a runsheet should not reflect the provider's personal or professional bias, whether it is positive or negative. Your negative bias may lend itself to a complaint of libel. As described in Chapter 4: Legal Issues, libel is a written communication that is defamatory, discrediting, or damaging to the patient's character. Simply put, personal or professional prejudice is unprofessional and may be a source for administrative or legal controversy. DOT 3-5.9

Recording Pertinent Negatives

It is crucial to record pertinent negatives on the patient care report. **Pertinent negatives** are critical findings (or more accurately nonfindings) from the assessment or history provided by the patient. They are items that are generally present for a given disease process that are not present in the current patient's presentation. Examples of pertinent negatives include the absence of chest pain during a cardiac event, the absence of dizziness or lightheadedness in a patient with hypoglycemia, and the absence of tachycardia in a patient with a significant loss of blood from an external bleed. The recording of pertinent negatives provides evidence that a thorough history was performed, and it provides valuable information to the receiving health care professionals. When pertinent negatives are not recorded, it may convey the impression that an incomplete assessment or history was performed. DOT 3-6.19

Traditional Narrative Format

The narrative format is the most traditional form of documentation; it is durable and crosses over all lines of healthcare related documentation and has been a timeless documentation practice. Traditional narratives, when unstructured, can be the source of a fragmented collection of disjointed facts, creating an erratic word picture and an incomplete and incompetent-appearing medical record. This open-ended style of documenting takes more time to construct than the succinct SOAPIER or CHART format. Retrieval of pertinent facts or tracking specific details is burdensome for the reader who must review the entire narrative or large portions of the information, as there is no segmental division of the data with the narrative style runsheet. DOT 3-6.14

The Opening Statement of the PCR

All formats should be preceded by an opening statement that sets the scene for the reader. The opening statement should answer the following queries: who, where, what, and why. A predesigned handwritten report layout may include fill-in-the-blank categories, or a computerized report layout may utilize drop down boxes to accommodate this basic information.

Make sure that your opening statement matches the rest of your documentation.

- **Who:** identifies the emergency medical service unit arriving on the scene. Somewhere in the documentation, every provider and every responding unit should be recorded. The "who" element may also provide general demographic information about the patient, including patient name, age, gender, address, insurance information, next of kin, or date of birth. DOT 3-6.4
- **Where:** provides descriptors for the word picture of the on-scene setting and environment in which the patient was found. The descriptor "where" contributes to an appreciation for the overall landscape of the call. It can also provide information directly connected to the on-scene time. For example, if the patient was entrapped in a crashed motor vehicle at the base of a hill 40 feet from the road, a longer than usual scene time could be expected as the patient is extricated and transported up to the roadway.

- **What:** answers the query of the general patient situation regarding the illness or injury. It describes what the provider discovered or saw, smelled, felt, or heard on arrival. It may describe the general appearance or demeanor of the patient. In certain circumstances, the "what" overlays the "where" descriptor.
- **Why:** may reflect anecdotal information provided by the patient, family members, or bystanders regarding how the patient was injured or displayed illness. In general, it is not necessary to document the reason for dispatch; if documented, it should be separate from the patient's chief complaint, as it may differ from the patient's chief complaint or true nature of call, and it may not provide factual, objective, or accurate information regarding the patient encounter.

The reason for dispatch is not a necessary part of the patient's legal medical record; however, it is imperative to record the patient's chief complaint as part of the legal medical record.

Informants such as the patient, family member, or bystander are valuable sources of information and should always be quoted and their relationships to the patient identified. The "why" of the accounting pertains to the patient's chief complaint and is further detailed in the body of the report as the subjective portion of the SOAPIER, historical portion of CHART, or as symptom-related information in both the SOAPIER and CHART formats. DOT 3-6.15

Content Issues

Legibility in Written Communication

Legible handwriting is important. It speaks to clear presentation of the facts. A well-organized report can send an overshadowing message of incompetence if the handwriting is not legible (Figure 17-3). You must remember that a runsheet is an extension of your hands-on care. Illegible handwriting may be construed as substandard hands-on patient care. If you have poor penmanship, use all capital letters or block printing on your runsheet, and proofread to make sure it is legible. DOT 3-5.9, 3-5.10

Street Secrets

It is always a good idea to have another member of your crew proofread your report for content, spelling, and legibility. It is much easier to amend a report before it is officially submitted and becomes a part of the patient record.

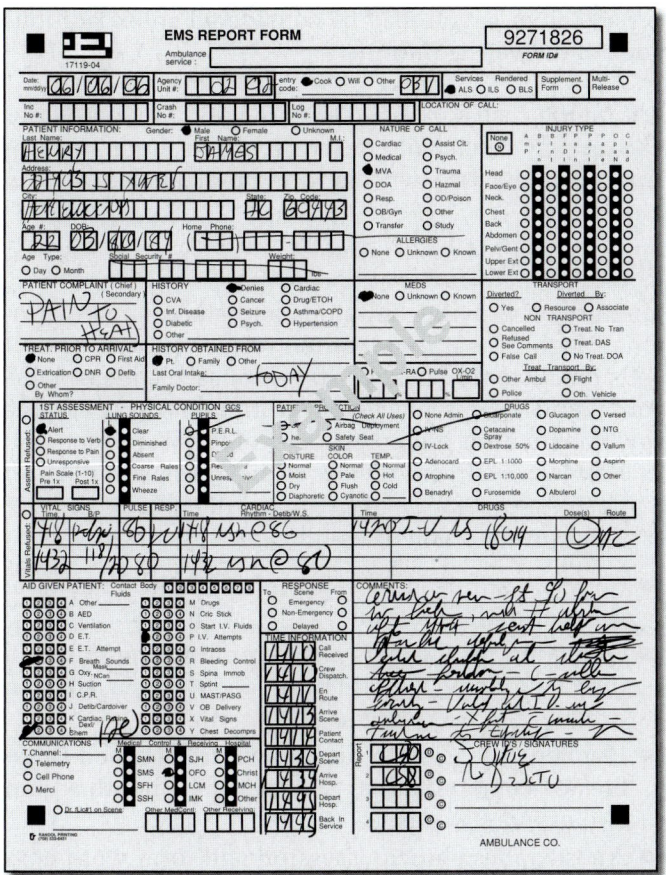

Figure 17-3 Poorly written reports reflect badly on you.

Many EMS systems utilize documentation forms that copy to several pages simultaneously or that can be scanned into document readers. Legible documentation also pertains to properly marking any double-copy or triple-copy runsheet checkboxes and darkening or coloring in data entry circles. As with the handwritten word, proper completion of this form of written communication is paramount. Use firm pressure when writing by hand. A true and accurate report may be compromised through stray or inconsistent markings. Utilize the correct writing instruments to complete the reports. Black or blue ink is generally preferred for legal documents such as PCRs, but some of the documents that are scanned by optical readers require the use of a number two pencil.

Mechanical Correctness in PCRs

You are judged by the mechanical aspects of your report. The mechanics of transferring the facts of the call into the runsheet are important. Spelling, sentence structure, proper capitalization, punctuation, and the use of proper English are required. Because your runsheet is an extension of your care, a runsheet that is

mechanically substandard leaves a poor perception of the care provided to the patient, or it may be construed as a general lack of intellect. Knowing the application of simple, basic writing skills, proper mechanics, punctuation, and correct spelling reflects a professional and knowledgeable provider on the prehospital report. DOT 3-6.2, 3-6.7

Nice to Know

Information collected on the PCR can be used for research purposes. It is important to collect as much information as possible and that this information be accurate. Legislators can use the information in deciding where to spend taxpayer money on prevention programs or in the crafting of safety laws. State EMS officials can use the information to determine quality assurance standards, set benchmarks, and track compliance with standards and regulations. Researchers can use it to test the effectiveness of treatments or to develop new treatments. Many of these processes are dependant upon the information collected by street-level providers, and their outputs are only as good as the information we input into the system. DOT 3-5.12

Mechanics of Standard English

Conversational English frequently differs from the rules of Standard English. The spoken word, conversational English, often reflects regional variances, expressions, and **colloquialisms.** Colloquialisms are terms or phrases that only have meaning within their own culture. Examples of colloquialisms in EMS include referring to the ambulance as a "bus," "unit," or the "office." Unless directly quoting (by using quotation marks) the patient, patient's family, bystander, or other informant, the use of proper English is required.

Mechanics of Sentence Structure

Write in complete sentences whenever possible; however, when this practice is not possible, sensible phrases and bulleted items will suffice. A phrase is a brief expression and can contribute important detail. A bulleted item is a brief communication that gives essential detail. Examples of phrases include *Pt. was AAOx3 in NAD* (which means "the patient was awake; alert and oriented to person, place, and time; and in no apparent distress") and *FROM of all extremities noted* (which means "full range of motion was found in all of the extremities upon assessment"). Make sure only approved abbreviations are used in the PCR.

Mechanics of Spelling

Misspelling and the misuse of words can put forth an inaccurate report or word picture of the prehospital encounter. Misspellings and misused words in assessment, descriptors, or historical information can mislead the reader and interfere with proper communication and continuity of care. Computer-generated runsheets frequently provide for spelling checks and the ability to correct misspelled words. Providers employing handwritten runsheet forms must strive for correct spelling. Availability of a medical dictionary is beneficial for those who have difficulty spelling properly. DOT 3-6.6

CONNECTIONS   Refer to Chapter 6: Medical Terminology for tips on spelling medical terms.

Mechanics of Diction

Diction reflects the proper usage of words that may sound alike but are spelled differently and possess a dissimilar definition that gives way to a different meaning or presentation of the word picture. Examples are the words *their, there,* and *they're;* the words *right, rite,* and *write;* and the words *to, too,* and *two.* For each example, the words sound the same but have different definitions.

Words need to convey the intention and meaning of the writer. Be sure to make suitable word choices when writing a narrative. Improper word choices can mislead the reader and create confusion about the true facts.

Jargon and Slang Terminology

As mentioned previously, jargon has no place in the patient care report. **Jargon** can be defined as a hybrid language of technical terminology, characteristic of a special activity or group. Like colloquialisms, the meaning of jargon is generally appreciated by those belonging to the group, such as prehospital providers, but not to the medical community at large. DOT 3-5.4, 3-6.3

Jargon is often understood by those who routinely converse with prehospital providers, such as emergency physicians, nurses, respiratory therapists, physical therapists, social workers, and other allied health professionals who practice in the emergency department. It is used frequently during the verbal report from the prehospital provider to the emergency department staff as a mode of conversational English; it serves the purpose of expediting the verbal report and is visually descriptive and literal in nature.

One aspect of prehospital jargon is to improperly utilize nouns as verbs. For example: in lieu of reporting that the, "patient had a 'brand name' cervical collar placed . . . ," the prehospital provider may simply state that "the patient was 'c-collared.'" The practice of conversing in jargon may be considered an expeditious mode of delivering information.

While the casual verbal communication that includes jargon may be visually descriptive and literal, it is inappropriate for the written legal medical record.

Punctuation

Punctuation provides for stops and starts of conversational English as it is converted to the written word; it lends character to your words, emphasizes ideas, joins words, and relates pieces of information in a useable way. Punctuation promotes focus of the word picture.

Below is a cursory review of the purpose and use of applicable punctuation marks that will enhance the professional presentation of a prehospital document:

- Commas are used to separate items in a series of three or more items.
- Quotation marks mark the beginning and end of a direct quotation, certain titles, and words used in an exceptional way such as slang terms.
- Hyphens are used to divide words (between syllables or compounds) at the end of a line; they join two or more words.
- Apostrophes show possession and form word contractions.
- Colons are used to indicate that a block of information or a series of ideas follows.
- Parentheses are used to enclose an explanation or qualification.

Abbreviations and Symbols

The use of proper abbreviations and the utilization of symbols minimize documentation time, enhance the readability of your information, and decrease the problem of misspelled words. A proper abbreviation or approved symbol is one that is formally recognized by the professional community and so commonly accepted and used in a particular profession that it does not require additional explanation. The proper abbreviation or symbol must be used in the proper context, cited properly within the sentence, and be used in lieu of the complete word or object it represents. As with prehospital jargon and slang, there are prehospital-associated abbreviations and symbols.

Prehospital agencies and jurisdictions should maintain an approved listing for providers to utilize. In addition, the JCAHO (Joint Committee on Accreditation of Healthcare Organizations) provides a listing of medical terms, symbols, and abbreviations that are found to cause documentation confusion and errors.[3] This list, (Table 17-1) called the "Do Not Use" list, is updated on an annual basis. It is a good resource and

TABLE 17-1   JCAHO Do Not Use List

Official "Do Not Use" List*		
Do Not Use	**Potential Problem**	**Use Instead**
U (unit)	Mistaken for "0" (zero), the number "4" (four) or "cc"	Write "unit"
IU (International Unit)	Mistaken for IV (intravenous) or the number 10 (ten)	Write "International Unit"
Q.D., QD, q.d., qd (daily)	Mistaken for each other	Write "daily"
Q.O.D., QOD, q.o.d, qod (every other day)	Period after the Q mistaken for "I" and the "O" mistaken for "I"	Write "every other day"
Trailing zero (X.0 mg)†	Decimal point is missed	Write X mg
Lack of leading zero (.X mg)		Write 0.X mg
MS	Can mean morphine sulfate or magnesium sulfate	Write "morphine sulfate" Write "magnesium sulfate"
MSO_4 and $MgSO_4$	Confused for one another	

*Applies to all orders and all medication-related documentation that is handwritten (including free-text computer entry) or on preprinted forms.

†**Exception:** A "trailing zero" may be used only where required to demonstrate the level of precision of the value being reported, such as for laboratory results, imaging studies that report size of lesions, or catheter/tube sizes. It may not be used in medication orders or other medication-related documentation.

Additional Abbreviations, Acronyms, and Symbols (For <u>possible</u> future inclusion in the Official "Do Not Use" List)		
Do Not Use	**Potential Problem**	**Use Instead**
> (greater than)	Misinterpreted as the number "7" (seven) or the letter "L"	Write "greater than"
< (less than)	Confused for one another	Write "less than"
Abbreviations for drug names	Misinterpreted due to similar abbreviations for multiple drugs	Write drug names in full
Apothecary units	Unfamiliar to many practitioners Confused with metric units	Use metric units
@	Mistaken for the number "2" (two)	Write "at"
cc	Mistaken for U (units) when poorly written	Write "mL" or "milliliters"
μg	Mistaken for mg (milligrams) resulting in one thousand-fold overdose	Write "mcg" or "micrograms"

should be used by EMS. Strictly adhere to the list in order to avert misunderstandings. Resist the temptation to create your own "working list" of abbreviations and symbols. DOT 3-6.3

Timeliness in Documentation

Documenting while in a moving vehicle is a challenge for any provider; however, it does not provide a viable defense for substandard written communication (Figure 17-4). An alternative to attempting to document legibly while careening down the road would be to simply take notes while en route and transcribe the

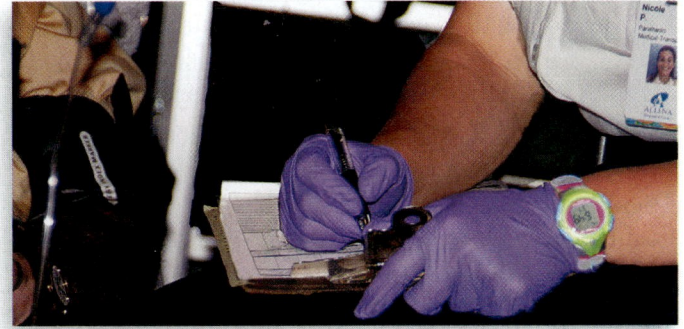

Figure 17-4   Whenever possible, try not to write your reports in the back of a moving ambulance.

information onto the formal report in the hospital setting. This plan of action also accommodates the fact that runsheets must be completed in a timely manner, when the facts of the call are most readily recalled.

> The call is not complete until the runsheet is complete.

More importantly, most local, state, or federal agencies have written requirements stipulating the timely handover of written documentation (after verbal reporting) on the transfer of patient care. Your commitment and responsibility to the patient does not end until the obligation of written communication is completed.

An appropriate accounting of all aspects of time in the prehospital arena is critical. You must record the following:

- Times pertinent to the performance of the call
    - The time the call was received in the dispatch center.
    - The time your unit was alerted or dispatched for the call.
    - The time your unit began responding to the call (the time you left the station, left your staging area, or began responding while on the road).
    - The time your unit arrived at the scene of the incident.
    - The time initial contact was made with the patient.
    - The time your unit left the scene en route to a receiving facility.
    - The time your unit arrived at the receiving facility.
    - The time your unit returned to service.
    - The time your unit returned to the station.
    - If you are cancelled when en route or diverted to another destination and do not complete the call you were initially dispatched for, document that time as well.
- Record medication administration time.
- Record the time each time vital signs are obtained.
- Record the time specific procedures like beginning CPR, initiating a medication drip, or pronouncing death are performed.

There is another factor of time that is frequently forgotten that must be addressed. Arrival time at the hospital does not constitute the time of transfer of care. It is virtually impossible to transfer care at the very moment in time you arrive at the hospital. Your transfer of care time is exactly that, the time you transfer responsibility and liability to the receiving qualified provider. This generally takes place *after* the patient is physically

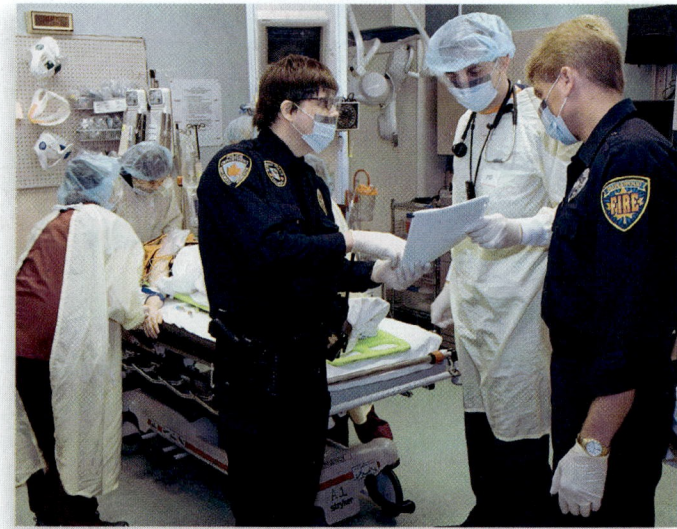

Figure 17-5   Transfer of care occurs after you have physically transferred the patient and after you have given a verbal report to the receiving staff.

transferred from your stretcher onto a hospital bed and *after* a verbal report is provided to the receiving staff member (Figure 17-5).

Street Secrets

Consider a daily routine of synchronizing all prehospital timekeeping pieces, from the communication division to each piece of monitoring equipment and personal timekeeping pieces such as wristwatches. One minute spent synchronizing timepieces may minimize documentation discrepancies.

Accuracy in Documentation

Accurate reports are those that exemplify precise and comprehensive recording of the facts of the call, including pertinent patient information, quality physical assessment, treatment provided, evaluation of treatment, and transfer of the patient to another qualified healthcare provider (this may be in the prehospital setting or in the emergency room).

To accurately relay treatment services provided to a patient, providers must become adept at using the actual protocol as a template for documentation. Literally, itemize throughout your report the assessment findings that support treatment decisions, based on the protocol, and the respective evaluation of treatment. Your runsheet must accurately show that you followed the accepted protocol, thereby adhering to the standard of care. Itemizing your treatments, as the protocol dictates, can refute questions about whether or not the care provided to the patient was consistent with the standard of care.

Accurate transcription of factual detail is another technical point reflecting professionalism in written word. Often, there is more than one location within the same runsheet that factual information is housed. One study of violent injury documentation demonstrated that 29% of paramedic run reports had internal documentation inconsistencies.[4] These documentation inconsistencies can cause significant difficulties for the paramedic if called to testify in a court case. DOT 3-6.14

While it may sound like a simplistic mistake, providers have inadvertently interchanged qualifiers such as right with left, distal with proximal, inferior to superior, and even medial with lateral. With a lapse in time from the date of the incident, writing of the report, and questions about the accuracy of the facts as transcribed in your runsheet, you may not be able to accurately state which qualifier correctly represents the patient situation.

Precise versus Concise

Strategic documentation that is concise warrants brevity, which means it should be direct and to the point. Every word should be sharply relevant to the word picture described. Distinctive writing qualities create an accurate word picture that is crisp and clear in the mind of the reader.

While computerized documentation claims to be an advancement and advantage in healthcare medical recordkeeping, it creates some disadvantages as well. The individuality of some situations cannot always be captured in a "one size fits all" box or field on a computerized document. The "drop down" boxes or specified "fields" for information can force an inaccurate response because some chief complaints, assessments, and responses to treatment cannot be described within the forced parameters. As a result, the documentation is not forthright and factual. Fortunately, many of these documents have an open area, often located in the "narrative field," that is the place to properly account for factual information that cannot be accommodated or reported in other sections of the PCR. DOT 3-6.17

Evaluation Checklist

Proofread your end product. Request that your crewmembers proofread the end product (it legally protects them also). Is the word picture comprehensive? Are the (organizational) acronym prompts for detailed information complete? Are there spelling errors? Is the punctuation correct? Does the runsheet factually reflect the patient encounter? Is it free of errors and erroneous detail (error of commission) or is there factual information that was inadvertently omitted (as an error of omission)? DOT 3-6.9, 3-6.10, 3-6.18

Providers must account for **erroneous documentation,** legally defined as errors of commission and errors of omission.

Corrections (deletions or additions) should *never* be made on any copy of the original record *after* it is released to the receiving facility; this constitutes tampering with a medical record and may be deemed criminal activity.

If the error of omission is realized *before* the runsheet is forwarded to the receiving facility, a timely notation may be added to the runsheet after the conclusion of the document as space allows. If there is inadequate space or the error of omission is realized *after* forwarding of the document to the receiving facility, a supplemental form should be submitted as soon as possible. Cross-reference the initial document in case the two are separated. Include the incident number, date and time, and patient name on the supplemental form. Copies of each of the documents must be forwarded to each of the required and receiving entities. DOT 3-6.20, 3-6.21

Street Secrets

Make sure you comply with jurisdictional requirements when filing a supplemental PCR document. This may involve notifying your supervisor, Medical Director, state EMS official, or other individuals of the discrepancy. Inform your partners of the discrepancy as well, so they are kept in the loop.

Informed Refusal

Many legal issues involving prehospital care revolve around refusal situations.[5] For the optimal legal protection, each refusal should be an **informed refusal.** When patients decline services, the refusals must be legal, intentional, educated, and knowledgeable.

CONNECTIONS Refer to Chapter 4: Legal Issues for more information on informed consent and informed refusal.

Patients who have the legal and mental capacity and possess adequate decision-influencing information have the legal right to accept or refuse your offer of treatment or transport. Each of these three elements of informed refusal must be thoroughly documented in the patient care report: DOT 3-6.13

1. **Legal capacity** references the legal age of majority in a given state or jurisdiction. Documentation showing the patient's age (date of birth or age in chronological years) must be provided and is generally accounted for in the demographic data.
2. **Mental capacity** cannot be solely defined by a patient's mental ability (or disability) or cognitive or intellectual challenge. Consideration must be given for the possible physiological interferences that may

temporarily or chronically disable or limit a patient's mental capacity (hemodynamic instability, physical and emotional trauma, hypoxia, illness, injury, or chemical influence by toxicological agent, drugs, or alcohol). Documentation reflective of the level of consciousness and orientation to person, place, time, and situation speak toward mental capacity. Written descriptions of behaviors that are either co-operative or uncooperative (and beyond) are reflective of mental capacity as well.

3. **Adequate information for decision-making** includes an offer of services commensurate with the patient situation, including full disclosure of the risks and benefits of specific treatments, an offer of transportation to an appropriate facility, and the risks or consequences of the refusal of treatment or transport. The information offered by the paramedic regarding treatment or transport should be based on patient history, presentation of the injury or illness, physical assessment, and protocol.

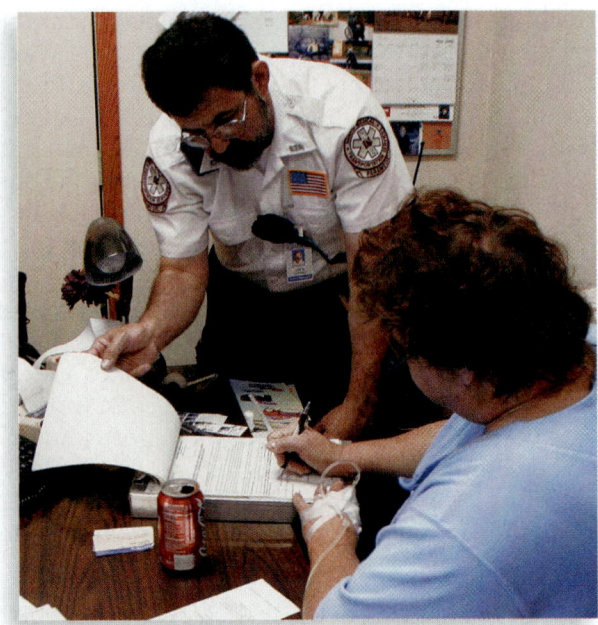

Figure 17-6 Patients who refuse care need to sign that they understand the implications of their refusal.

Working in the Gray Zone

Several studies have documented that all too often, paramedics fail to appropriately document many of the criteria necessary to show that the patient was competent to refuse care and was appropriately informed of risks and benefits of refusing.[6,7] In the largest study of its kind, looking at approximately 2,700 such patients, over one-third of the reports were inadequately documented. Specifically, of those records deemed to be inadequate, half of them did not document the risks of refusal; one-third did not document patient vital signs; and one-fifth did not describe the patient's mental status.

The patient's chief complaint and historical information must be relayed in the refusal of care report; the physical assessment, to the extent it was performed, must be documented; the proposed treatment, including any elements of treatment provided, consistent with the protocol, must be recorded; and the expression of refusal by the patient must be included as well. Providers must document in the written evidence that the patient's informed refusal was indeed against the provider's medical advice. The documentation must specifically cite advice, guidance, or recommendations for treatment or transport. More importantly, it must cite (within your level of expertise) the reasonable, foreseeable risks or complications of the refusal as discussed with the patient.

When offering this information, use language that patients understand. Do not speak in the language of medical terminology or use jargon they cannot

understand. It is also important to have patients state back to you their understanding of the advice given and their understanding of the risks or complications of refusal. This practice of having patients recite and reflect their understanding is an effort to avert any misunderstanding and allows for the clarification of questions. When the process is conducted in this manner, it holds patients (or their representatives) accountable for their decisions.

These discussion points should be well documented, as the provider will customarily be requesting the patient's (or their representative's) signature on the document (Figure 17-6). A witness's signature is merely an acknowledgment that the patient (or representative) actually signed the document; it does not make any other implications or imply an agreement of any kind.

Street Secrets

If the patient refuses to sign and there is not another bystander on the scene, ask someone other than a member of your crew to sign the refusal form. This could be someone from another ambulance, a fire department representative, or a law enforcement officer who is also on the scene. Make sure whoever signs also legibly prints their name, records their relationship to the patient (or unit or badge number), and includes contact information. Since refusal of care forms are often separate from the standard PCR, make sure you cross reference the refusal form in the patient care report and document that it was signed against your advice (if applicable).

Cancellation of Services

If the EMS provider is canceled en route to a call, the provider must generate agency approved documentation indicating the canceling authority and the time of the formal cancellation. This means that the provider is accountable for a working knowledge of who holds authority to cancel emergency medical service providers in a given situation. Also, if providers are canceled after arrival to the scene of an injury or illness, the canceling authority must be cited as well as the time of the cancellation and mitigating circumstances of the cancellation. If the provider does not initiate a patient-provider relationship with a patient, the documentation should specifically state that there were "no patient contacts made."

If a patient contact was made, the provider is obliged to document an informed refusal report.

It is important to properly determine who maintains authority to cancel the emergency medical service providers, as in this situation you have arrived at the site, made a cursory assessment of the scene, but are accepting the refusal of your service at the request of one in authority. This has the potential to kindle a legal or, to a lesser degree, ethical dilemma for some providers.

Verbal Reports

Verbal reports take many forms: reports to other EMS providers, consultation with on-line medical direction, and communication with medical staff at the receiving facility. Each of these forms of communication takes on a slightly different character, but a theme of them all is the need for a concise, accurate exchange of information between each of the individuals involved. DOT 3-5.5

Verbal Report to Other EMS Providers

EMS providers frequently exchange information in the midst of treating a patient. Whenever care is transferred from one provider to the other, the following key pieces of information must be exchanged:

- Pertinent patient demographic information: name, age, weight, DOB, etc.
- Chief complaint or reason for the transport.
- Current medical and mental condition and if this represents a change from their normal baseline.
- Description of their medical history or traumatic injuries.
- List of current medications and allergy history.
- Orders from the sending or receiving facility (if appropriate). This may include the need to stop a medication infusion during transport and consult the receiving facility if there is a significant change in the patient status or the destination (room number and unit) of the patient upon arrival at the receiving facility.
- A list of assessments performed, including vital signs and SAMPLE history.
- A list of treatments rendered and the patient's response to the treatment.
- Any information deemed critical for the receiving provider to know, for example, where the parents of a pediatric patient are and if they are meeting the child at the receiving facility, if the patient has an ongoing infection or has a compromised immune system, or if the patient has received medication and when the next dose is due.

Sometimes care is transferred from an ALS provider to a BLS provider. When this occurs, the ALS provider should carefully assess if this is appropriate. For example, a patient with a sprained ankle may be appropriate for a BLS unit to transport following an ALS assessment. If, however, the patient reports a cardiac history and an episode of unexplained syncope immediately prior to the fall that caused the ankle injury, this patient should not be transferred to BLS level care.

In the event that care is transferred to a BLS provider, the ALS provider should provide a verbal transfer of care report like the one outlined above. The ALS provider should complete a patient care report documenting the assessment, any treatment (ALS or BLS level) provided, and the reason the patient was transferred to BLS level care. If any ALS level care is rendered, the patient should not be transferred to a BLS level care team.

The BLS level provider's understanding of the situation should be assessed, and any questions should be answered before care is transferred. If, upon discussion with the BLS provider, any question exists in the ALS provider's mind of the capability of the BLS team to manage the patient, the ALS provider should continue patient care. If an incorrect decision is made, a charge of abandonment may result.

The Radio Report (Consultation with On-Line Medical Direction)

Standing orders allow EMS providers on the scene to operate within an established framework and define the standard of care allowed in the prehospital setting. This framework clearly describes the boundaries that exist between off-line and on-line medical control. Off-line medical control occurs via the written protocols and standing orders that EMS providers follow that do not require real time permission. By virtue of the written protocol, permission is granted to perform the procedure following the correct assessment.

Many protocols have a point where continued or additional treatment requires consultation with or confirmation by an on-line consultation, or it represents a

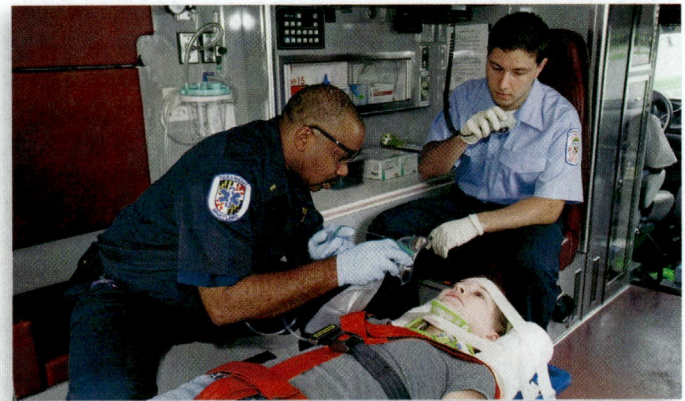

Figure 17-7 You may have to confer with a physician before providing additional care.

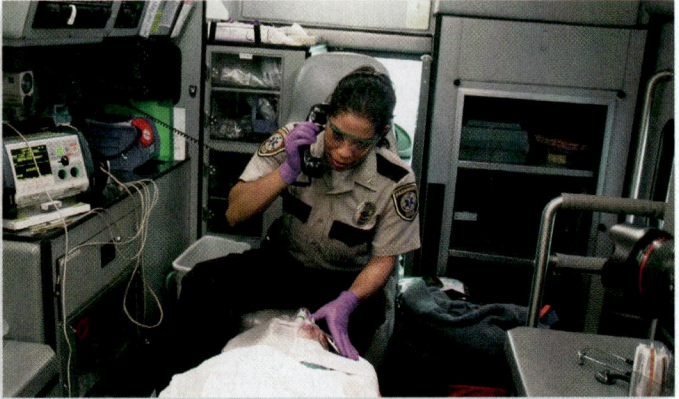

Figure 17-8 Repeat orders back to the physician to ensure that you have understood them correctly.

point in the continuum of care where decisions could branch off in one direction or another. At these points, the jurisdictional, regional, or state medical director, designated state EMS official, or official committee has established the place within protocol care where direct medical consultation by a physician is required prior to any additional care (Figure 17-7).

Sometimes the EMS provider on scene needs guidance or support in decision making. This can occur at times other than those specified within the protocols. In these situations, consultation is not only appropriate; it is encouraged. Professional paramedics know when it is appropriate to seek guidance from the physician on-line and are willing to do so because it is in the best interest of providing good patient care.

Consultations with hospitals may be recorded. Consultations that are managed through a 9-1-1 center or dispatch center usually are recorded. Always consider any communication performed through a radio, telephone, computer, telemetry device, microwave, satellite, or other technology to have been recorded and to be available for access at a later time. DOT 3-5.13

Radio consultations should contain the following elements: DOT 3-5.24

- Name of unit calling and, if appropriate, your name.
- Confirmation that the person the paramedic is speaking with is the appropriate individual to render advice, provide medical direction, or approve requests for medication or treatment by the paramedic. Obtain the physician's name if orders are issued.
- ETA (estimated time of arrival) to the receiving facility and patient priority.
- A concise description of the initial impression of the patient upon your arrival on scene, including any care that was rendered prior to your arrival.
- Description of the age, sex, and weight of the patient.
- Level of consciousness of the patient.
- Level of distress of the patient.

- Vital signs, assessment findings, and history information.
- Treatments provided so far (including oxygen, IV, glucometer reading, medications administered, ECG reading, stabilization of fractures, immobilization, needle decompression, etc.) and the patient's response to the treatment.
- Any requests you have (treatments or medications that require medical direction).
- Ask the physician for any questions or orders.
- Repeat back to the online physician any orders or requests to confirm your understanding (Figure 17-8). DOT 3-5.7

Street Secrets

Some jurisdictions allow nonphysician hospital staff to receive a consultation. In most cases, these individuals are permitted to obtain information only (which is the primary reason for a majority of the consultations performed); they are not permitted to grant permission for treatments or medications. If this is the case in your jurisdiction, begin the consultation by asking for a physician. State you are seeking permission for a treatment or medication. This will prevent you from having to repeat your consultation to the physician. DOT 3-5.6

Verbal Report to Staff Person at the Receiving Facility

Upon arrival at the receiving facility, report to the appropriate staff person to begin the transfer process. In some cases, you will be met by a team that is receiving your patient, and in others, you approach the charge nurse or the nearest staff member and announce your arrival. Often, there is a common staging area that the patient is placed in until the receiving facility is ready to receive the patient. Make sure at least one member of your team remains with the patient at all times until the transfer of care is complete. If permitted, assist the receiving facility in transferring the patient from your stretcher to their bed. As previously discussed, your liability continues until such time as the receiving facility has officially received the patient and resumes care. DOT 3-5.23

Working in the Gray Zone

The staff member receiving your report will either continue to care for the patient where you left off, will ask questions to clarify the information you provide, or may begin all over again. As you build trust with those receiving your patients, there will be more reliance upon the information you provide, provided it is helpful to them. If the receiving staff member chooses to dismiss you before you can give a report, do not be offended by their behavior. Handle them with the therapeutic communication techniques described in Chapter 10, and take pride in the fact that you advocated appropriately for the patient. Gently ask them if they would like to receive a report from you, and if they decline, walk away without displaying unprofessional behavior. DOT 3-5.6

A concise report should be given to the person receiving care. It should include the following:

- Description of the chief complaint or reason for the transport.
- SAMPLE history, vital signs, and physical examination findings.
- Information of any treatments rendered and the patient's response to the treatments.
- Time of administration of any medications and information of when the next dose would be given if the drug is to be continued.
- Time when any critical events occurred. Examples include when spontaneous circulation returned, when CPR was initiated, when chest decompression was performed, when the baby was born, when the symptoms first began, when the 12-lead ECG tracing was obtained, etc.
- Turn over any medical records and HIPAA compliance documents that were sent with the patient, and document this transfer in your patient care report.

- Turn over any patient effects that are in your custody (jewelry, clothing, wallet, purse, cell phone, etc.), and document this transfer in your patient care report.
- Ask the staff person if they have any questions. DOT 3-5.7

Summary

Written documentation, transfer of care reports, and radio reports bear as much importance as the skills performed directly to the patient. When preparing and evaluating the patient care report, remember that these documents represent the care you provided, and they serve as a testimonial to your professionalism. Your report should be a reflection of your adherence to the standard of care and accepted protocol. It should be organized, legible, mechanically correct, properly punctuated, timely, and fortified with concise and accurate details of the patient encounter. Verbal communication also reflects your professionalism. Attention should be paid so that verbal reports are organized and concise. They should pass on the information required for the receiving provider to continue to care for the patient without having to reconstruct your assessment and history gathering efforts. Radio consultations should be concise and brief, providing the information you know the physician needs to see the patient through your eyes, so that you can obtain the advice or order that you need to provide optimal levels of patient care.

Notes

1. D. Graham, *The Missing Protocol—A Legally Defensible Report* (Ashton: Clemens Publishing, 1999).
2. A. M. Pennardt and W. J. Zehner, Jr., "Paramedic Documentation of Indicators for Cervical Spine Injury." *Prehospital Disaster Medicine* 9(1)(1994): 40–43.
3. http://www.jointcommission.org/PatientSafety/DoNotUseList/ (accessed April 11, 2006).
4. L. A. Boergerhoff, S. G. Gerberich, A. Anderson, L. Kochevar, and L. Waller, "Out-of-Hospital Violence Injury Surveillance: Quality of Data Collection," *Annals of Emergency Medicine* 34(6)(1999): 745–750.
5. J. Weaver, K. H. Brinsfield, and D. Dalphond, "Prehospital Refusal-of-Transport Policies: Adequate Legal Protection?" *Prehospital Emergency Care* 4(1)(2000): 53–56.
6. B. S. Selden, P. G. Schnitzer, and F. X. Nolan. Medicolegal Documentation of Prehospital Triage. *Annals of Emergency Medicine* 19(5)(1990): 547–551.
7. D. C. Cone, D. T. Kim, and S. J. Davidson, "Patient-Initiated Refusals of Prehospital Care: Ambulance Call Report Documentation, Patient Outcome, and On-Line Medical Command," *Prehospital Disaster Medicine* 10(1)(1995): 3–9.

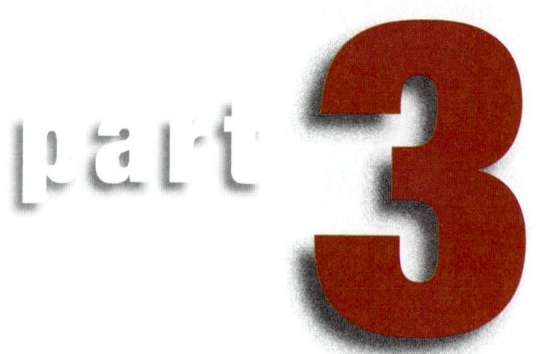

part **3**

Trauma

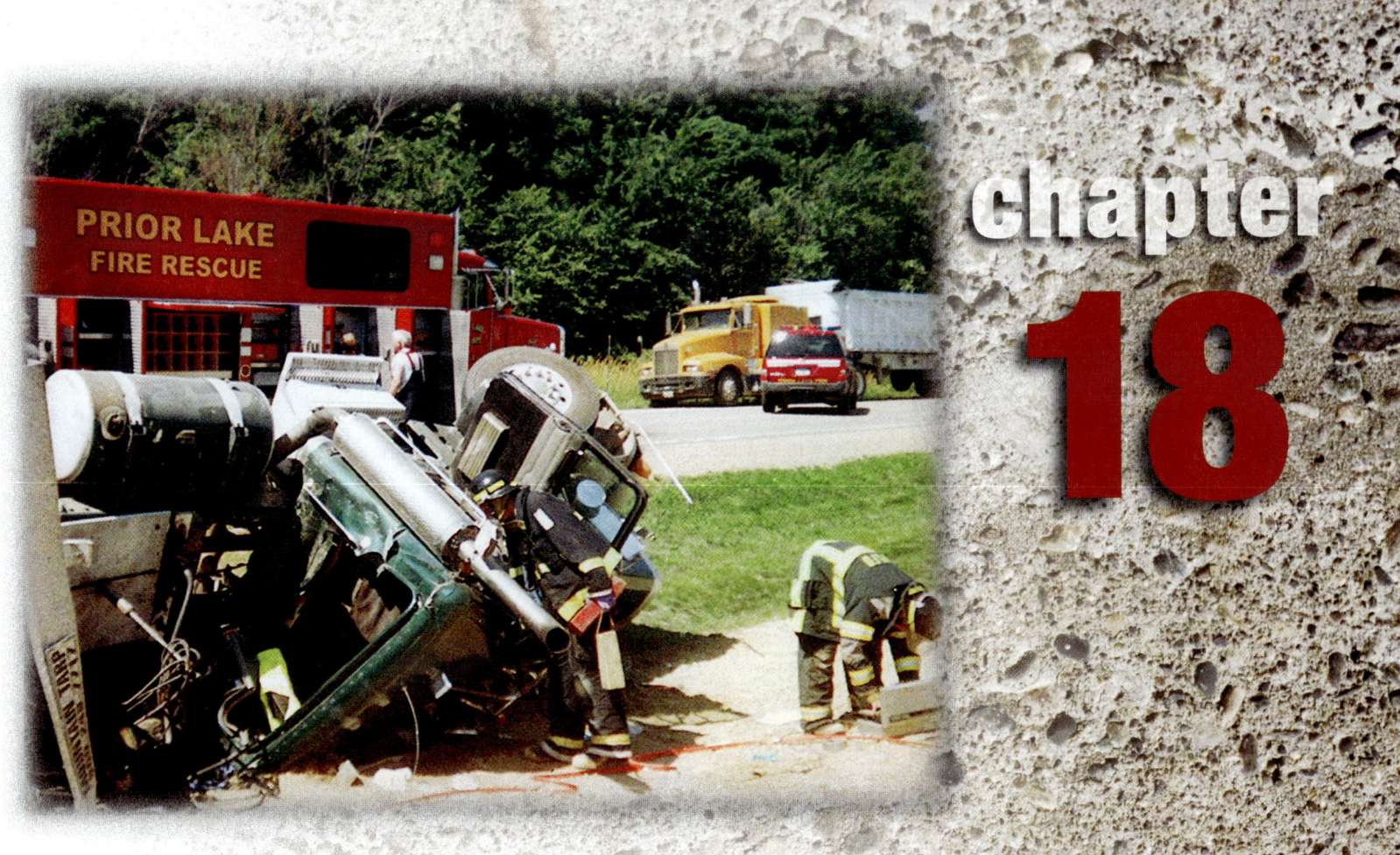

Mechanism of Injury

"*G*ravity explains the motions of the planets, but it cannot explain who set the planets in motion. God governs all things and knows all that is or can be done."

—Sir Isaac Newton

Need to Know

▶ Consider that there is an underlying injury that you cannot see. Learn the various injury patterns associated with the mechanism of injury, and apply this knowledge on every trauma call.

▶ Predictable patterns emerge based upon the type of trauma, age of the patient, and general health status of the patient. The very young and the very old generally do not fare as well as other patients, given equal types of forces applied to their bodies.

▶ Work = force acting over a distance (a measure of energy)
   • Kinetic energy (the energy possessed by an object in motion) = $(1/2)mv^2$ (m = mass [weight], v = velocity [speed]). This is a component of Newton's first law.
   • Potential energy = mass (weight) $\times$ force of gravity $\times$ height.
   • Force = mass $\times$ acceleration (Newton's second law).

▶ Do not remove impaled objects. The only exception is when it interferes with the performance of CPR or other lifesaving treatment.

▶ Sick	▶ Not Yet Sick
• The patient who says "I am going to die" often is right. • Abnormal vital signs are ominous and should be addressed immediately. Low BP and a fast pulse rate are bad findings (it indicates advanced shock). High BP and a slow pulse is a very bad finding (it often indicates increasing intracranial pressure). • Pediatric and geriatric patients do not follow the same "rules" regarding their response to trauma. They often have worse outcomes to injuries that seem less significant. Monitor them closely and be on the alert for clues for hidden injuries.	• The finding of normal vital signs does not mean the patient is "not sick." Look for clues to hidden injuries, and use your understanding of kinematics to predict injury patterns. • Check the pulse and blood pressure frequently as they may change quickly and without warning. • Screaming patients have an open airway, breathing, and circulation, so continue to triage all the patients, then concentrate on the most serious. Do not let obvious injuries or screaming patients distract you from performing a thorough assessment. Always check and manage ABCs first, and repeat your assessment of the ABCs often. • Inspect the scene closely to uncover clues to the mechanism. • Even when the situation seems to be an obvious trauma, remember to also ask the patient about signs and symptoms of medical illness. Certain medications, for example, will cause altered vital signs that represent the "baseline" for the patient.

Introduction

Unintentional injuries are the leading cause of death in the United States for patients between the ages of one and 44 years (95,795 deaths from 2001 to 2002).[1] This figure does not include homicide, suicide, or other violent means that when added to the total increase the number dramatically. For example, in 2002 over 161,000 Americans were fatally injured.[2] More than 500,000 people are nonfatally injured riding bicycles annually and in 1999, 750 bicyclists died in crashes, and over 95% of those who died were not wearing helmets. Motor vehicle crashes (MVCs) remain the 10th leading cause of traumatic death (Figure 18-1). For 16- to 17-year-old drivers, the risk of fatal crashes increases with the number of passengers. Males ages 16 to 35 are among those at highest risk for traumatic injuries and death from accidents and violence. Having a gun in the home increases the likelihood of homicide nearly threefold and of suicide fivefold. Alcohol and drug use are associated with increased risk of violent death.[3]

Each year between one in three and one in four Americans are injured severely enough to seek medical care resulting in a total of 23 to 28 million visits to emergency departments and other medical facilities. The economic burden just from motor vehicle-related deaths and injuries is enormous, costing the United States more than $150 billion each year.[4]

Traumatic injury occurs when the body is exposed to more energy than its tissues and organs can tolerate. The way in which this energy is transferred to the body relates to the laws of physics. Kinetic energy plays a role as objects in motion transfer energy to other objects they come in contact with. This transfer of energy is not always easily identified. Many times the energy transfer is noted by obvious detectable signs: a hole in the skin,

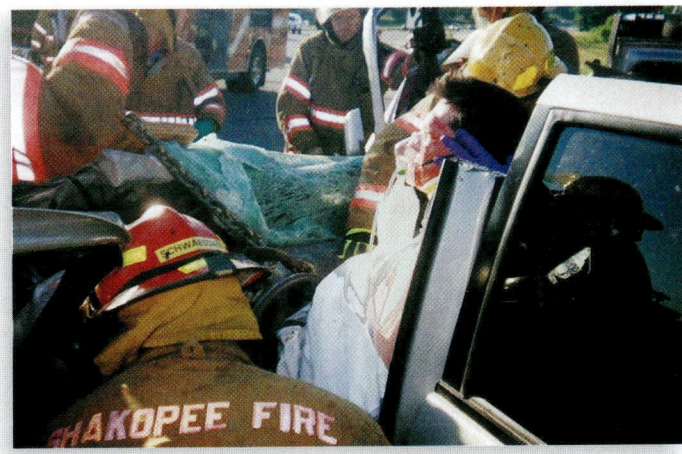

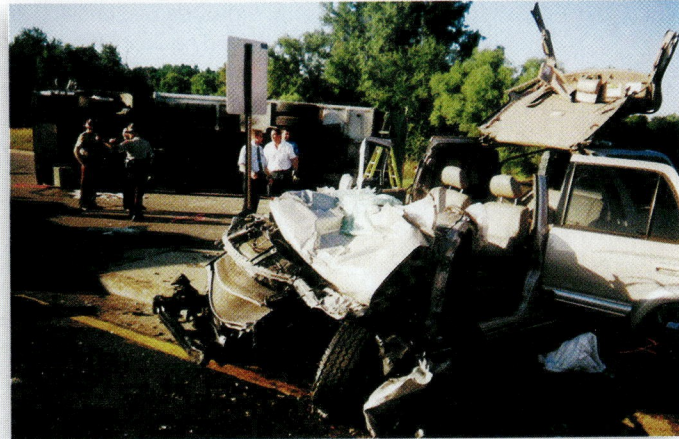

Figure 18-1   What injuries do you suspect?

a bruise, or even complaints of pain at a specific location. However, many times injuries cannot be seen externally or the patient is unable to tell you where the pain is coming from. In these cases, you have to look for clues but also remain suspicious because of your knowledge of predictable patterns of injury gained from understanding kinematics. The greater the force applied to the body, the more damage that is present, whether it

is obviously visible or not. These forces can cause such life-threatening problems as liver laceration, a torn aorta, cavitation injury from gunshot wounds, and hemorrhage. EMS professionals must have a basic understanding of not only the injury but also the mechanism of its cause. **Kinematics** is the study of trauma and what the forces of energy do to the body. DOT 4-1.12

> The greater the force that is applied to the body, the more damage that is present, whether it is visible or not.

Modern principles of the management of injury prevention and treatment of traumatic injury are based upon concepts developed by William Haddon, Jr. in the late 1960s. At that time, the goal was to develop a better way to assess traffic safety by using public health measures. The measurement techniques that came from this research allowed for improved analyses of the countermeasures needed to avoid injury. **Haddon's Matrix** (Table 18-1) resulted from this research. This matrix looks at the precrash, crash, and postcrash phases of injury and correlates (matches) them with factors that are potentially changeable (Table 18-2).

Haddon's group defined a crash as any force exerted on a body tissue as a result of some event. The **agent of injury** is usually some form of energy, for example mechanical, thermal, electrical, radiation, etc. This energy is transmitted to the host (the patient) through a vehicle (an object such as a car, a metal fragment, or some other moving object) or a vector (some micro- or macro-organism). The pathway the energy takes is consistent with each mechanism, and it affects body organs and tissues in a similar manner with each different age group.

These initial concepts have evolved over the years and now include a third dimension that allows for measurable outcome data relative to the intervention points.[5] In other words, the most recent enhancements look at the effects various treatments have on patient outcome and survival. All of this together has allowed for

TABLE 18-1   **Haddon Matrix**

The host column refers to the person at risk of injury. The agent of injury is energy (for example mechanical, thermal, electrical) that is transmitted to the host through a vehicle (inanimate object) or vector (person or other animal). Physical environments include all the characteristics of the setting in which the injury event takes place (for example a roadway, building, playground, or sports arena). Social and legal norms and practices in the culture are referred to as the social environment.[3]

	Factors	Host	Agent/Vehicle	Physical Environment	Social Environment
Phases	Precrash				
	Crash				
	Postcrash				

TABLE 18-2 Haddon Matrix Applied to the Problem of Rural Traumatic Cardiac Arrest Transport to Appropriate Level of Care

	Factors	Host (Rural/remote Communities)	Agent/vehicle Transport	Physical environment (Rural/remote home)	Social environment (community norms, policies, rules)
Phases	Preevent (before arrest starts)	Teach risk assessment and means to decrease risk of traumatic events.	Redistribute advanced care medical personnel.	Augmented 9-1-1 systems. Mobile phone company incentives for rural towers. Cell phones with 9-1-1 GPS.	Improve efforts to educate community members regarding trauma risks and prevention strategies.
	Event (during cardiac arrest)	Teach 9-1-1 medical dispatch to all rural communities. Teach aspects of trauma care including aspirin, oxygen, and AED usage.	Design vehicles with improved capabilities for transport.	More reliable first responder airway devices.	Fund the EMS departments adequately to provide personnel and equipment for more rapid response and advanced training.
	Postevent (after arrest occurred)	Provide first-aid, hemorrhage control, and CPR training to all family members.	Design community for improved access to needed advanced interventions.	Distribution of aeromedical evacuation system.	Aggressive recruitment of specialty care into rural environments.

AED = Automated External Defibrillator, ALS = Advanced Life Support, CPR = Cardiopulmonary Resuscitation, GPS = Global Positioning System

interpretation of traumatic events and prediction of injuries and injury patterns based on mechanism of injury (kinematics). This has resulted in developing prevention, intervention, and treatment strategies. **See Skill Sheet 31: Trauma Scoring and Skill Sheet 83: NREMT Patient Assessment Trauma.**

The Cause of Damage to the Body from Trauma

The most important concepts to understand about mechanism of injury are anatomy (discussed in Chapter 7), the transfer of energy to the body, and how the body responds to that transfer. The complex interactions of these factors combine into predictable injury patterns.

In a traumatic event there may be more than one patient. Each patient is viewed as a separate set of injury patterns, even when the injury is caused by a direct interaction between the two patients. An example would be when the rear-seat passenger is thrown forward into the driver when their vehicle is hit head-on. Another example would be when two riders are in a four-wheel sports vehicle crash, and the helmeted driver is thrown into the handlebars while the nonhelmet wearing second rider is thrown to the side.

Motor vehicle crashes are often described in terms of a three collision model.[6] This model, although fairly simplistic, is a good reminder that the patient absorbs and

transfers energy at least three times during a crash. The first collision occurs when the vehicle comes into contact with a moving or stationary object that alters the initial direction of movement. The alteration of direction of movement results in a transfer of energy between the two objects. This transfer results in the second collision. This occurs as the vehicle occupant continues to travel in the original direction the energy was traveling, striking the interior of the vehicle or other object. The third collision occurs as the organs within the patient strike the inside of the body compartment in which they reside. At this point, the patient has stopped moving in the original direction, but their organs still have not. DOT 4-1.5

Motorized vehicle crashes generally have three collisions:

- Crash 1: The vehicle strikes an object
- Crash 2: The patient strikes the vehicle or other object
- Crash 3: The organs within the patient strike the inner surfaces of their body cavity.

An example of the three collision model is seen when a car strikes a tree. The car stops, recoils, and bounces backward, or it is deflected in another direction, but the driver is still traveling in the forward direction. The driver's chest strikes the steering wheel and the forehead strikes the windshield. The heart and lungs are still moving forward, and they strike the inside of the thoracic cavity, impacting with the bones and muscles of the rib cage, while the brain strikes the inside of the skull. The aorta, the upper portion of which is held firmly in place by ligaments, is torn in the process, and the patient dies from hemorrhage, or the brain is bruised and a traumatic brain injury results, which can also be fatal.

The concept of "anatomy" should be viewed from the perspective of the vehicle as well as in terms of the structures making up the human body. When a car hits a pole head-on, the component parts, or "organs" of the car, will have similar types and directions of force applied to them. They will absorb or transfer energy until all of the energy of the velocity is dissipated. Depending upon how the car is engineered, this energy transfer can be vectored (or moved) away from the passenger, resulting in less damage to the patient. Predictable injury patterns emerge because we are familiar with the forces and types of energy exerted upon both the passengers and the vehicle.

Look at the anatomy of a gunshot injury as another example. In this example, multiple crashes are described. As the trigger is pulled, the striking of the firing pin by the hammer is one energy expense (Crash 1). The firing pin striking the bullet casing is another energy expense (Crash 2). The firing pin igniting the gunpowder is another energy expense (Crash 3). The gunpowder explosion propels the bullet at a high rate of speed, and this is another expenditure of energy (Crash 4). The bullet striking the skin causes a release of energy to those tissues (Crash 5) as well as the shock wave transmitted through the underlying tissues (Crash 6). The bullet continues into the patient, having the same interaction with body organs (Crash 7 to infinity depending on the energy needing to be expended), until all the energy that was imparted to the bullet by the gun is now expended on the patient. The underlying crashes need to be understood as part of the treatment of traumatic injury.

A bullet or other projectile causes damage as it imparts energy to tissue. The maximum amount of damage that may be caused by any type of projectile is related to the projectile's mass and its velocity as demonstrated by the following equation:

Speed kills $Energy = \frac{1}{2}\ Mass \times Velocity^2$

The critical component of this equation to remember is that velocity (speed) is squared. When speed is doubled, the mathematical result is a quadrupling, or a multiplying by four times, of the force! The speed of the projectile is critically important. Perhaps it is even more important than the size of the object in determining damage potential. This makes sense if placed in the following context: Would you rather be struck by a semi truck moving at 5 miles per hour or a compact sports car moving at 75 miles per hour? Remembering that speed

quadruples the amount of force is important in the prehospital setting. You need to consider the speed (high-powered versus low-powered) rather than focusing on the caliber of the bullet.

Street Secrets

There are many considerations, in addition to velocity, for determining the severity of trauma. A semi truck that rolls over you at 5 miles per hour with the tire stopping on your chest will just as likely kill you as the compact sports car striking you at 75 miles per hour as you cross the street. The gunshot wound from a high powered rifle may not be fatal if it passes straight through the flesh of the outer thigh, but if a low velocity gunshot travels medially and strikes the femoral artery high in the thigh, it is likely to be fatal due to rapid, uncontrollable arterial bleeding. Keep the concept of velocity in context, and use it to assume that the patient has hidden injuries even if they do not appear initially injured upon your arrival on the scene.

Newton's Laws Explained

Sir Isaac Newton's three laws of motion form the basis of injury kinetics and are the foundation of **kinematics** (the science of trauma energy).

Newton's First Law   The Law of Inertia: A body at a constant state remains at that constant state until some outside force acts upon it.

This first law explains that a body at rest will remain at rest, and a body in motion will remain in motion until acted upon by some outside force that is trying to make it change direction. DOT 4-1.6

Why does the sudden starting or stopping of motion result in trauma and damage? A principle of physics states that energy cannot be created or destroyed, but it can be changed in form, and it is this change in form that results in damage to the body. The inertial motion in these accidents is a form of energy, so when the motion starts or stops, the energy must be transformed to another form of energy. This force may assume thermal, electrical, chemical, radiant, or mechanical forms. However, the form of energy most often produced by the sudden change in motion or deceleration occurring in a motor vehicle is mechanical.

Kinetic energy is a function of the weight of an object and its speed. Kinetic energy is a property of a moving object or particle and depends not only on its motion but also on its mass (size). The kind of motion may be **translation** (or motion along a path from one place to another), rotation about an axis, vibration, or any combination of motions. Translational kinetic energy of a body is equal to one-half the product of its mass and the square of its velocity, or the formula we already discussed: **KE = ½ mass × velocity²**. The name of the unit of energy described in the meter-kilogram-second system is the "joule." A two-kilogram mass (something weighing 4.4 pounds) moving at a speed of one meter per second (slightly more than two miles per hour) has a kinetic energy of one joule.

When a person gets in a car, the car will stand still until the driver presses the accelerator, and energy is imparted from the engine to make it move. The car will keep moving until another force is applied that makes it stop. The amount of force required to make it stop is explained by Newton's second law:

> **Newton's Second Law**   The Law of Acceleration: Force = Mass × Acceleration

This law applies to both **acceleration** (speeding up) and **deceleration** (slowing down). The second law states that the rate of change of momentum of a body is equal to the resultant force acting on the body and that this force needs to be in the same direction the original force was traveling. The physical meaning of this law is that objects interact by exchanging momentum, and they do this via applied force. This law is often described by the formula, force = mass × acceleration. An example would be when a speed skater in a relay race lines up behind a teammate and pushes the person in front so they can go a little faster than their opponent. The first skater was moving along very fast, but the second one, coming from behind, adds additional energy to the first, propelling him faster down the ice.

If the driver in our previous motor vehicle example hits a brick wall at 55 miles per hour, the car (and the person in it) will be subjected to greater forces than if they were traveling at 10 miles per hour. After the car is stopped by the wall, the person is stopped by the car. (Remember the three collision idea discussed earlier.)

It is at this point that the person experiences Newton's third law of motion:

> **Newton's Third Law**   Law of Reciprocal Actions: For every action, there is an equal and opposite reaction.

In other words, as the person pushes against the steering wheel and windshield of the car, those objects push back with equal force against the person. The way that different forces involved in an accident transfer energy is the explanation of the injury or damage that is imparted to the objects and patients involved in the collision. The energy is not lost when the vehicle above is stopped, only converted to another form that dissipates through the patient and surroundings.

Car companies consider Newton's Laws when they are designing a vehicle. Restraint systems such as seat belts, lap belts, and airbags hold the patient in place and absorb energy. Rollover bars prevent the vehicle from crushing the patient. Vehicles have crumple zones and shock absorbing bumpers that absorb energy in a collision. All of these safety features allow the dissipation of the forces to be more gradual and dispersed throughout the body of the vehicle instead of the body of the occupant.[7]

It is estimated that it requires 50 Newtons (N = kg · m/s²) of force to penetrate the skin, 255 N to penetrate the temporal region, and 540 N to penetrate the parietal region. The estimated force of an average knife attack is somewhere between 1000 and 2000 N, which is more than sufficient to enter the skull.[8]

Blunt Force Trauma

Blunt trauma is caused as the body absorbs energy. It may result in obvious or hidden injuries. Motor vehicle crashes, falls, and sports injuries account for the majority of blunt trauma.[3] In the United States there has been a steady decline in the number of motor vehicle crash deaths per mile driven, but it still remains the tenth leading cause of death. Restraint systems such as seat belts protect against serious injury and death, but at least one-fourth of adults and one-third of teenagers do not use seat belts routinely. Air bags provide protection for adults; however, they do not protect small children.[9]

Blunt trauma is a major cause of vascular injury. It occurs most often from fractures or joint dislocations. Fractures of large heavy bones can cause cavitation forces similar to high-velocity bullets. There can be extensive damage to soft tissues, neurovascular injury, and edema, all of which can interfere with blood flow.

Blunt thoracic aortic injury (BTAI) is a serious traumatic injury with high mortality. It is associated with high-speed modes of transportation. Autopsy data from fatal BTAI cases showed 57% of the patients died at the scene or upon arrival to the hospital, and 37% of the remaining patients died during the first four hours in the hospital. Blunt injury to the abdominal aorta is uncommon, but it has been reported from lap seat belt trauma. Blunt carotid artery injuries have mortality rates between 30% and 50%, and over 50% of the survivors have permanent, severe neurological deficits. There is a 70% incidence of cervical spine injuries in these patients as well. Traumatic injury to the meningeal artery in the brain has a 50% mortality rate. The popliteal artery (found behind the knee) and the brachial artery (found in the upper arm crossing through the elbow joint) are particularly susceptible to injury.[10]

Blunt trauma can result in severe head trauma as well. Any patient with head trauma and a Glasgow Coma Score (GCS) of three to eight is at high risk for significant traumatic brain injury. These patients require aggressive airway intervention and management that may include

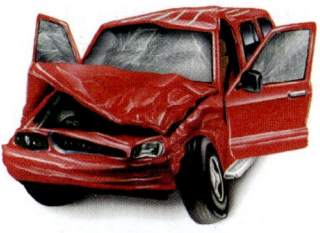

Frontal

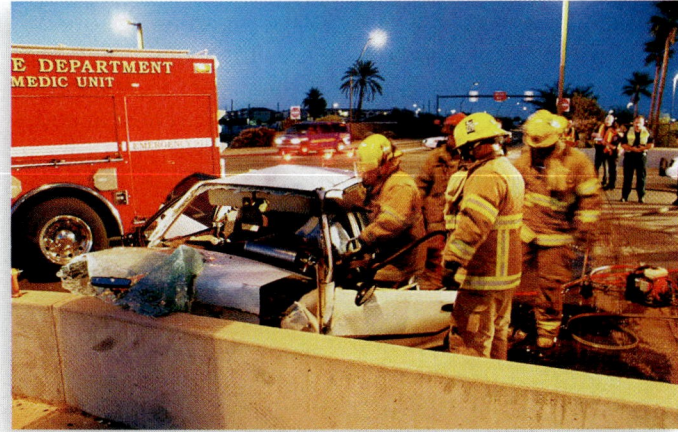

Figure 18-2   Head-on crash—car hitting cement barrier.

intubation, sedation, pharmacological paralysis (if they are semiconscious and combative), or hyperventilation if signs of cerebral herniation develop.[11]

CONNECTIONS Chapter 20: Head, Face, and Neck Trauma discusses the management of traumatic brain injured patients.

Blunt trauma produces injuries by two mechanisms—deceleration and compression. These two traumatic forces produce predictable injury patterns in each of the following types of motor vehicle accidents: head-on or frontal impact, rear impact, lateral (or side) impact, rotational impact, and rollover. Each type of trauma will be discussed. DOT 4-1.7, 4-1.8, 4-1.9

Head-On or Frontal Impact Collisions

Head-on impacts result in forward motion being stopped abruptly (Figure 18-2). When this occurs in a motor vehicle accident (e.g., a car hitting a brick wall), the first collision occurs when the car impacts the brick wall, resulting in damage to the front of the car. The amount of damage noted to the car can be used to help estimate the speed the car was traveling at the time of impact. A more severely damaged car was probably moving at a higher velocity and will probably contain more severely injured victims. When the vehicle suddenly ceases forward motion, the unrestrained (and even the restrained) body continues to move forward and will follow one of two possible pathways for the second collision: down and under or up and over the dashboard. DOT 4-1.7, 4-1.8, 4-1.9

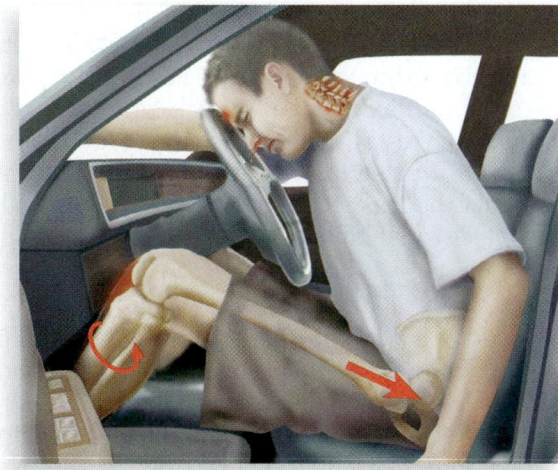

(a)

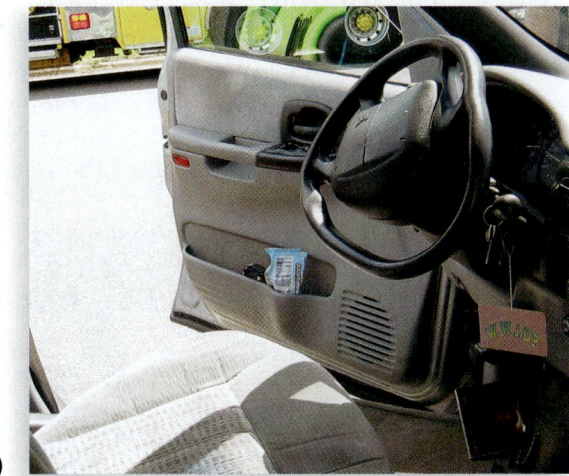

(b)

Figure 18-3   (a) Injuries from down and under path. (b) Bent steering wheel from a down and under path.

Down and Under Pathway

With the down and under path, the occupant continues to travel downward into the seat and forward into the dashboard or steering column. The knees strike the dashboard; the upper leg absorbs most of the impact; therefore, these victims can have dislocated knees, fractured femurs, and a fractured pelvis or dislocated hip bones (Figure 18-3). Prehospital personnel should focus not only on the knees where the impact occurred but also on the femur and the lumbar and thoracic spine for injuries. Since the energy that caused the knee injury had to transfer somewhere, all three parts of this classic knee-femur-hip injury pattern should be considered. DOT 4-1.7, 4-1.8, 4-1.9

After the knees impact, the upper body bends forward into the steering wheel or dashboard. The patient can have compression injuries to the anterior chest, which can produce broken ribs or sternum, anterior flail chest, pulmonary contusion, and myocardial contusion or, if low on the chest wall, rupture the solid organs in the abdomen such as the liver or spleen. After the anterior chest wall stops, the organs continue moving forward, and the third collision occurs. The head may also be a point of impact. When the head stops its forward motion, the momentum of the torso must be absorbed. Hyperextension or hyperflexion of the neck produces severe angulation, often resulting in dislocation of the vertebrae. If the neck hits the steering wheel or the steering column, the larynx may be crushed, or if the face strikes the wheel or windshield, facial bones may be fractured.

Up and Over Pathway

In the up and over path, the body is thrown up and over the steering wheel into the windshield or inside roof of the car. The head is usually the lead point in this type of collision, crashing into the windshield and sustaining scalp lacerations, skull fractures, or cerebral contusions or hemorrhage (Figure 18-4). The dome of the skull is fairly strong and may absorb the impact without fracturing, but then the tissues underneath absorb the energy. The cervical spine is more flexible and cannot tolerate the pressure of the impact without significant angulation or compression. In-line absorption of the impact

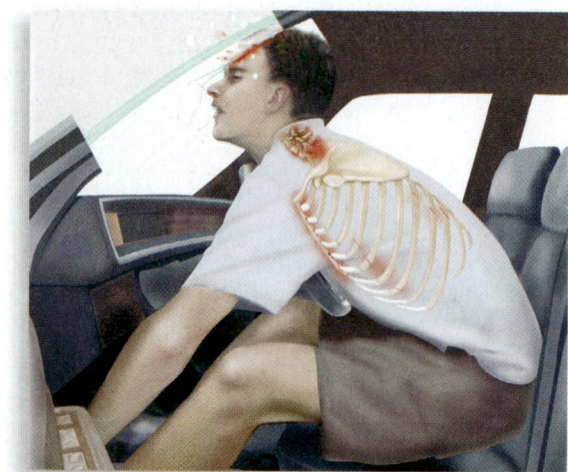

(a)

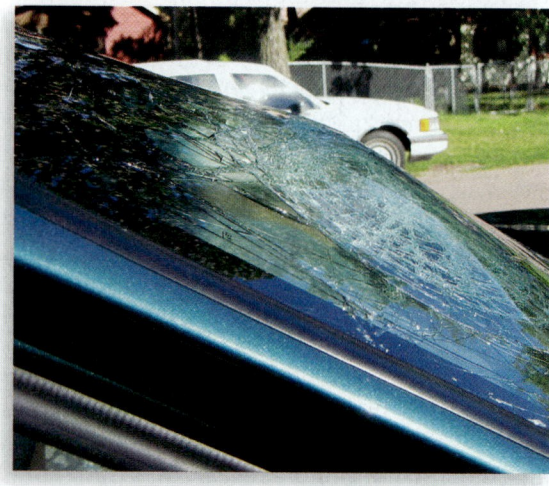

(b)

Figure 18-4   (a) Injuries from up and over path. (b) The passenger in this car sustained head, neck, and scalp injuries. Note the indentation of his head in the windshield.

leads to a compression fracture of the cervical spine. Flexion (a chin to chest motion) or hyperextension (tipping the head back) may cause cervical spine injury and significant damage to the soft tissues of the neck. Hyperextension or hyperflexion of the neck produces severe angulation, possibly resulting in a fracture or dislocation of the vertebrae, and direct compression crushes the vertebrae. Either can result in an unstable spine that can compress the spinal cord in the spinal canal. If the throat strikes the steering wheel or the steering column, the larynx may be crushed, just as the facial bones will fracture if this is the point of impact. DOT 4-1.7, 4-1.8, 4-1.9

Like the down and under pathway, the chest or abdomen typically impacts the steering wheel, resulting in similar injury patterns as described previously. The knees or femur may strike the bottom of the steering wheel, or the feet and lower legs may strike under the dash or become tangled in the foot pedals. The patient may have rib fractures, flail chest, cardiac contusion, pulmonary contusion, aortic tear, lacerated liver, or a ruptured spleen.

Rear Impact Collisions

Rear impact collisions occur when the vehicle is hit from behind (Figure 18-5). In this collision, the energy of the impact is transferred into acceleration motion. The front car moves ahead like a bullet shot from a gun, as does everything in contact with the car. This can result in the head and neck hyperextending causing classic "whiplash" from stretched or torn neck muscles, tendons, and ligaments or vertebral and spinal cord damage. If the car strikes another car or object head-on or the driver slams on the brakes and stops suddenly, the occupants are then thrown forward and demonstrate the impact characteristics of a frontal collision (either down and under or up and over). The accident then involves two impacts: rear and frontal. The double impact increases the chance of injury. The provider should take this into consideration when dealing with this type of accident and should look for two sets of injuries—those caused by the rear impact and those caused by the frontal impact. DOT 4-1.7, 4-1.8, 4-1.9

Seat belts and shoulder harnesses are active restraint devices. This means they require the vehicle occupant to actually put them on, and they must be placed correctly to be most effective. Many people either do not use the devices or use them incorrectly. Incorrectly used devices (too loose or worn at the wrong part of the body) can cause injury as well. Many of the traditional passive restraint devices like airbags work best in frontal and rear impacts. Side impact devices are in development, and many automobiles now have such devices as well.

Lateral or Side Impact Collisions

Lateral impacts occur when a vehicle is struck from the side (Figure 18-6). Injury occurs as the door, post,

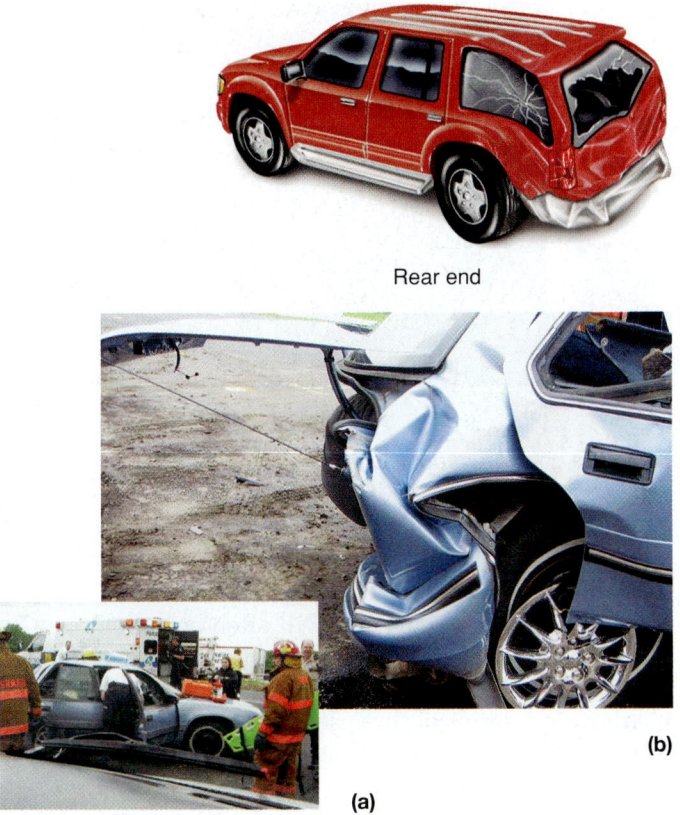

Rear end

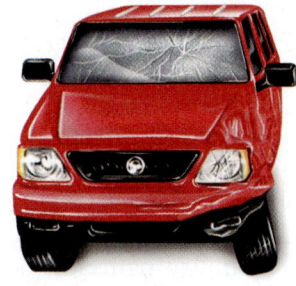

(b)

(a)

Figure 18-5   Rear impact. (a) Vehicle that was struck from rear. (b) Close-up of rear-end damage.

Lateral

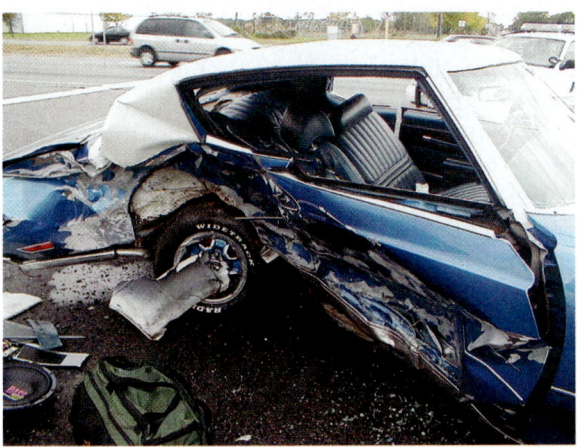

Figure 18-6   Lateral or side impact collision; the passenger sustained a liver laceration with significant internal bleeding.

or other interior structure of the car, such as the arm rest, impacts directly on the occupant. The proper use of seat belts will reduce the severity of injury. Because of the lap belt, when the occupant begins lateral motion along with the car, they are "pulled" away from the side of the car. The upper body or head may still strike the car interior. The major areas of injury in a lateral impact are the chest wall, pelvis, and head/neck. As the chest receives the impact, lateral compression injuries result, fracturing the ribs on the side of the impact. This may produce a lateral flail chest, pulmonary contusion, or a ruptured liver or spleen. In the United States, occupants on the driver's side are vulnerable to splenic injuries since the spleen is a left-sided organ, whereas those on the passenger side most often receive injury to the liver. If the victim's arm is down at the side, it absorbs the impact and transfers the force to the humerus, the clavicle, and the chest wall. The pelvis or femur is also commonly injured. The wing of the ilium (pelvis) can be pushed in, fracturing the pelvis anteriorly and posteriorly. Finally, the head is jerked laterally as the body moves out from under it. The result may be tears or strains of the ligaments and supporting structures of the neck. Fractures of the spine are more common with lateral collisions than with rear collisions. Injury to the spinal cord in this type of impact may result in neurological deficit. Head or scalp injuries may also be present. DOT 4-1.7, 4-1.8, 4-1.9

If there are other passengers in the vehicle, they may be thrown into each other. For example, a car is struck on the passenger door, and neither occupant is restrained. The person in the passenger seat will be hit by the door on the right and the driver on the left. The driver will hit the passenger on the right and, depending upon the rotational force, may strike the steering wheel or car interior roof or be recoiled into the door on her side. Passive side impact restraint systems are more difficult to place into the structure of the vehicle, and the logistics of developing activating systems for those devices are more difficult to design, but progress is being made, and many vehicles do have such devices in place. Seat belts and shoulder harnesses are available in every vehicle being manufactured and still offer the best protection.

Rotational Impact Collisions

Rotational impacts occur when one corner of the car—usually the front quarter—strikes an immovable object or one that is moving slower or in the opposite direction. Following Newton's first law of motion, this part of the car will stop while the rest of the car continues its forward motion until its energy is completely expended. This will result in the car rotating around the point of impact. Rotational impacts result in injuries that are a combination of those seen in head-on and lateral impacts. Often, the patient nearest the point of rotation will have the greatest amount of injuries

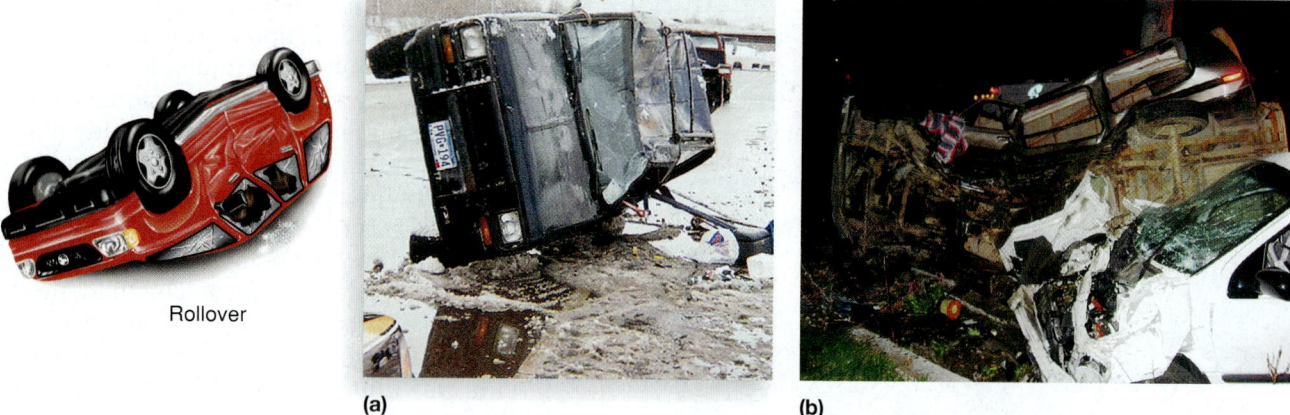

Rollover

(a)   (b)

Figure 18-7 Rollover collisions. (a) The male driver who rolled this car into a ditch was found unconscious and was trapped for 55 minutes during extrication. (b) The full-size, brown minivan was struck on the driver's side by the white minivan, which was fleeing from police at high speed. The brown van (shown here in its resting position) was pinned against a tree. Two patients were trapped, requiring extrication.

because much of the energy will be transferred directly through them as it is dissipated throughout the rest of the vehicle. DOT 4-1.7, 4-1.8, 4-1.9

Rollover Collisions

During a rollover, the car may impact many times at many different angles, as will the occupants and their organs (Figure 18-7). Injury and damage may occur with each one of these impacts. It is almost impossible to predict the injuries these victims may receive although this should raise the provider's index of suspicion to a high level. If the patient was thrown from the vehicle, the patient has a much greater chance of sustaining fatal injuries. Unrestrained patients within a vehicle receive multiple collisions as they tumble around inside the vehicle, striking the vehicle, hitting other passengers, or having debris inside of the vehicle strike them. DOT 4-1.7, 4-1.8, 4-1.9

Automobile-Pedestrian Collisions

In addition to motor vehicle crashes, there are predictable patterns of injury that occur with other mechanisms of injury, specifically automobile versus pedestrian collisions and falls from heights. Knowledge of these patterns can help the paramedic look for specific injuries that might otherwise remain unrecognized when patients have complaints of greater pain elsewhere.

A collision between a motor vehicle and a pedestrian generally produces two patterns of injury, depending on whether the pedestrian is an adult or a child. The injury patterns will vary as a result of the height of the individual struck as well as response differences between adults and children when they realize the impact is about to occur. In most cases, when an adult realizes that a collision is imminent, the adult will attempt to evade the crash by trying to turn away. This often results in lateral body

impact. In contrast, children will often become frozen in place and be struck while facing the oncoming vehicle, causing frontal body damage. In both cases, the injuries result from a series of three sequential collisions.

Adults will usually first be struck by the bumper of the vehicle, which will, in most cases, cause injury to the lower leg or knee. This initial collision will cause the victim to fall toward the hood of the vehicle, initiating the second strike, which usually involves the pelvis, abdomen, and chest. The head and neck may also be injured, depending on the ability of the patient to protect the head with their arms. This second collision may also result in the patient being tossed up onto the hood and the head and neck striking the windshield. Finally, the pedestrian is usually then thrown off the vehicle as the driver begins to brake, resulting in additional injury, particularly to the head and neck.

Children, on the other hand, present with a somewhat different injury pattern. Because of the child's smaller height, the first collision often occurs at the level of the femur or pelvis and, since the patient is usually facing the oncoming vehicle, may involve both lower extremities. This is rapidly followed by the thorax and head striking the hood of the motor vehicle, causing injury to these parts. Sometimes the child will then be thrown from the vehicle as will an adult; however, often because of their smaller size, they will instead fall down in front of the moving vehicle and be dragged underneath or run over, causing additional injury to all involved body parts.

Falls from Height

Falls from height also can result in injury from one or more impacts. While there is no specific height measurement that clearly indicates the likelihood of significant injury, an injury can certainly occur with falls from a very low height (even less than one foot). The American

College of Surgeons committee on Trauma (ACSCOT) has recommended a general rule that if the patient fell from a position that was greater than 20 feet or three times the individual's height, there is significant likelihood of serious injury.[11] Therefore, a responding paramedic should always attempt to determine the actual height of the fall to anticipate the potential injuries.

In addition to the height of the fall, the paramedic should also evaluate the likely position that the patient landed in. Specifically, did the patient land prone, supine, headfirst or feet first? Patients who land either prone or supine will usually have multi-system injuries as multiple areas of the body impact the ground. Therefore, head, spine, truncal, and orthopedic injuries can all be seen in these cases.

Patients who land headfirst will present with head and spinal injuries in particular and may have trauma to other areas of the body once those parts impact the ground. Finally, those patients who land feet first also usually sustain a series of collisions resulting in a predictable pattern of injuries. When the feet strike the ground, fractures of the calcaneus or ankles generally result. As the momentum of the body continues downward, forces act to fracture the femurs, hip bone, or pelvis. Then the trunk of the patient will usually bend at the waist, often causing spinal fractures and possibly an intra-abdominal injury. The patient often will subsequently attempt to brace their fall with their outstretched arms, causing fracture to one or both of the upper extremities. Finally, the head will strike the ground, causing possible head and cervical spine injury. DOT 4-1.11

Penetrating Trauma

Penetrating trauma may be seen alone or in combination with blunt trauma. The most frequent cause of penetrating trauma in America is injury from a firearm. In 2003, there were 29,730 deaths related to firearms in the United States.[7] Penetrating trauma can happen accidentally (as during a fall onto an object or during an explosion, motor vehicle crash, tornado, or hurricane) but can also be the result of a deliberate act with a firearm, knife, box cutter, axe, ice pick, screwdriver, or glass fragment. As in blunt trauma, an understanding of the mechanism behind the injury is vital to anticipating the severity of injury. This section will provide a brief review of ballistics, special considerations based upon the location of injury, some forensics tips, and some patient management pearls. DOT 4-1.10, 4-1.11

Location of Injuries

Specific penetrating trauma to organs and anatomic locations are discussed elsewhere in this text, so we will not go into depth here. Understand that when a certain anatomic location is affected, the way to look at the injury is to think about predictable patterns of injury.

Ask yourself
- What organs are in this area?
- What systems do those organs regulate?
- What can deflect the missile?
- Where will it deflect?
- What vital signs, if any, may change based on these patterns of injury?

Penetrating wounds to the chest and abdomen often result in exsanguination, or the loss of blood from the vascular system. The presence of blood in the peritoneum can also cause hemorrhagic shock, abdominal pain or tenderness, rigidity, or a sensation of dread and doom. When enough blood is present in the peritoneum, it may be visible on the surface of the abdomen as a bluish discoloration. This finding is known as **Cullen's sign.** Although usually a late sign, if the problem is recognized quickly and the patient is treated quickly, there is a good outcome.

Patients with respiratory distress, tachycardia, and absent breath sounds on the side of a gunshot wound, stab wound, or chest wall **ecchymosis** (discoloration and bruising) with hypertympany upon percussion should be suspected of having tension pneumothorax. If upon percussion the patient has dullness, or nonresonance, assume hemothorax is present.[9] Both injuries require rapid transport and intervention.

Delayed mortality comes from complications such as hepatic failure, renal failure, and bowel necrosis due to lack of blood flow caused by hypovolemia and ischemia (lack of oxygen). Bowel contents (food or fecal matter) can leak from a damaged gastrointestinal organ, causing chemical irritation or bacterial contamination. When a patient with such an injury presents for treatment late in the course of the injury, they are often quite ill and may be in septic or hypovolemic shock from the untreated blood loss or intra-abdominal infection. Palpation tenderness and rebound often identify the need for surgery, and the patient is commonly promptly transported to the operating room for exploration. These patients will require significant amounts of fluid during the resuscitative phase and early surgical intervention. The volume of hemorrhage required to produce severe hypotension in a young healthy 70-kg patient is over 2 liters.[9]

In stabbings, the spleen is the most commonly injured organ because it is solid and on the left side, and most assailants are right-handed.[12] In penetrating injuries to the neck, hypotension may be from hypovolemia, tension pneumothorax, cardiac tamponade, or damage to the sympathetic chain of the nervous system.

Penetrating trauma to the extremities requires continual reassessment throughout transport. Vascular injury is assessed by evaluating the pulse distal to the injury. If time permits, the injured extremity should also be assessed with a blood pressure cuff and the reading compared to the unaffected extremity. This is true for the leg as well as the arm, and the cuff can be placed on the lower arm or leg as well as the upper arm or leg. Inflate the cuff until the pulse is no longer palpable. Slowly release the cuff while continuing to feel for the pulse in that same location. Document the number when the pulse is again felt representing the systolic blood pressure. Repeat the same procedure on the unaffected extremity, and use this for comparison. If they are more than 10% different, you have detected vascular compromise. This is probably the most sensitive screening tool for detecting vascular injury for the out-of-hospital setting.

Street Secrets

It is helpful to mark the location of palpable pulses with a pen or marker. This allows for quick repeated measurements even in a moving vehicle. It can also be helpful in determining whether compromise of circulation is present, as this site will be the one used consistently to monitor for trends.

The palpation method of blood pressure assessment is adequate for gross changes but will become less useful as the injury worsens and the pulses are no longer palpable. Capillary refill testing is not a reliable tool in recognizing vascular compromise as it is rarely indicative of anything when the patient is in temperature extremes, has significant hypovolemia, or has significant swelling. It is insensitive (not accurate) and will falsely reassure the provider approximately half of the time.[9] Extremities with penetrating trauma that have pulses present intermittently are at high risk for arterial injury. It is always vital to assess pulse, sensation, and motor function both before and after splinting an injured extremity.

Street Secrets

There is no contraindication to the use of analgesic medication in patients with penetrating trauma other than hypersensitivity or allergy to the selected medication. They will often require significant amounts of narcotics to control their pain.

Ballistics

Bullets or other projectiles cause damage as energy is transferred to tissue. The maximum amount of damage caused by any type of projectile is related to the projectile's mass and velocity and matches Newton's equation that was previously discussed:[5]

$$\text{Energy} = \frac{1}{2}\,\text{Mass} \times \text{Velocity}^2.$$

As a bullet strikes tissue, it crushes the tissue in front of it, creating a temporary tunnel that expands to create a larger tunnel, called a **cavitation wave,** and then collapses into a smaller pathway, called the permanent cavity. The **permanent cavity** is the remaining wound once the projectile has passed through the body.

Some of the energy of the projectile is expended in making this permanent cavity; however, it also sends a ripple of energy through the tissues as it passes through the body. This energy causes damage to the surrounding tissue by compression, deformation, and shear forces, creating the temporary cavity. The temporary cavity can be up to 30 times larger than the diameter of the bullet itself.[5] The higher the velocity of the projectile, the greater the size of the cavitation tunnel. After the bullet has passed through, the temporary cavity snaps closed, but the tissue, which now seems to have returned to its normal location, may be severely damaged and non-viable (Figure 18-8). Of course, many other factors, in addition to mass and velocity, alter the amount of damage done by a penetrating object: type of projectile used (whether it is designed to fragment, peel apart, explode on impact, etc.), type of tissue it passes through, the path of the projectile, and even the clothes it passes through. For example, an intact peritoneum does not preclude intraabdominal injury. There have been multiple case reports of victims with injuries to the spleen or intestines from a bullet that never penetrated the peritoneum. The damage is due to the temporary cavitation caused by a bullet passing near the organ.[13]

Nice to Know

High-powered rifles launch a projectile greater than 1000 meters per second whereas a .45 caliber handgun generally launches its projectile at 300 meters per second. Skin penetration requires a bullet velocity between only 45 and 60 meters per second, and even slow projectiles can produce significant damage.[14]

Most bullets are made of lead and encased in a harder metal shell, called a jacket, which is typically made of copper. The copper jacket prevents the softer lead from deforming when fired. Most military bullets have a "full metal jacket" that also prevents the lead from deforming when striking tissue. This prevents the bullet from slowing quickly and allows it to penetrate more deeply, often passing completely through the victim. These types of bullets generally cause less damage (relative to where they penetrate and how close the patient is to the gun when it is fired) than bullets that do not have a full metal jacket.

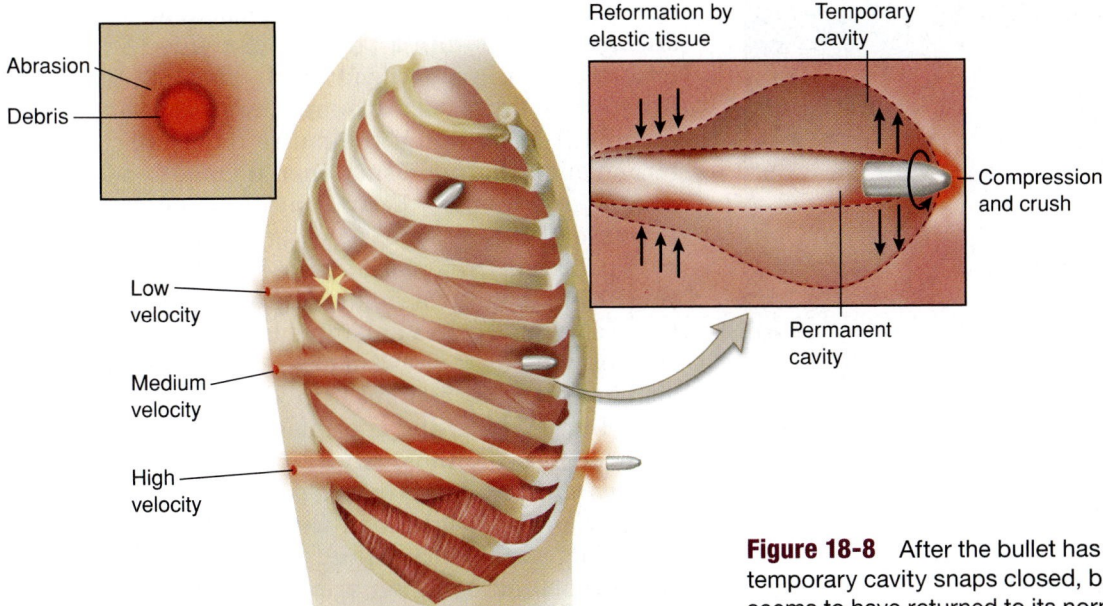

Figure 18-8   After the bullet has passed through, the temporary cavity snaps closed, but the tissue, which now seems to have returned to its normal location, may be severely damaged and nonviable.

Soft point or hollow point bullets leave a portion of the lead exposed, allowing the bullet to deform on contact with tissue (Figure 18-9). The bullet fragments and deforms into a blunt mushroom-shaped projectile that can leave a permanent cavity 2.5 times larger than the original bullet and a much larger temporary cavitation cavity. These bullets often do not penetrate as deep, but they can cause far more damage. Most hunting ammunition is of this variety.

A good analogy to bullet ballistics can be found with the sport of diving. A diver that enters the water in a streamlined position causes little splash and goes much deeper before stopping. However, a diver that performs a belly flop makes a much bigger splash and does not go far beneath the surface before his descent stops.[9] By definition, bullets that pass through a body retain some of their kinetic energy, thus allowing them to continue to travel onward. In contrast, bullets that remain within the body have transferred all of their kinetic energy to the victim, potentially causing greater damage.

Knife wounds, arrow wounds, and other nonballistic penetrating injuries are similar to gunshot wounds in many respects. The knife creates a permanent cavity from the blade; however, there is a much smaller temporary cavity as the energy of the strike is dissipated. Because of the slower speed during penetration, the damage to surrounding tissue is less extensive.[15] Accordingly, stabbing victims generally have a better prognosis than shooting victims. In most penetrating trauma, the primary determinant of outcome is the location of the wound and the structures impacted along the pathway.

Working in the Gray Zone

A study analyzing 862 patients undergoing emergency thoracotomy at a trauma center yielded only 3.9% neurologically intact survivors, and there were no survivors in the group of patients who presented with blunt trauma and no vital signs in the field. Patients with stab wounds to the chest (and vital signs in the field) had the greatest rate of survival at 23%.[9]

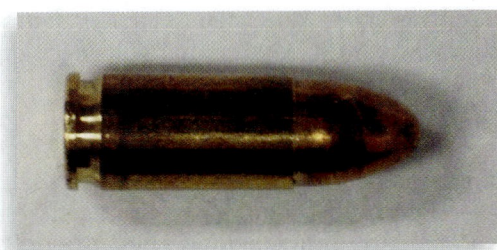

Figure 18-9   This bullet is an example of the type that will flatten, mushroom, or expand upon impact, causing greater tissue change.

Managing Penetrating Trauma

In some ways, the management of penetrating trauma is not very different from the management of any other patient, whether traumatically injured or presenting with a medical problem. However, the few differences that do exist may mean the difference between life and death. The first important thing to do is to assess scene safety. It does the patient little good if you become a patient yourself. Always make sure there are no more uncontrollable

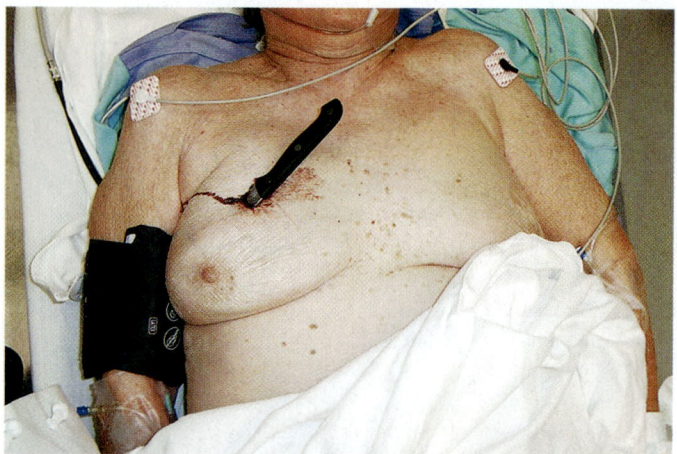

Figure 18-10   Penetrating trauma. The impaled object should be left in place as shown here.

threats to the victim or yourself before entering the scene. Anytime a victim has a penetrating wound, you must consider it to have resulted from a violent act by an assailant until proven otherwise. Make sure law enforcement has secured the scene and they remain present until you leave. Even if the patient is in a motor vehicle crash, a gunshot wound may have been the cause of the crash.

If the impaled patient has the object still in place, leave it in place (Figure 18-10). Efforts should be made to prevent a rescuer or the patient from removing it. Never remove an impaled object unless medical direction has ordered it or consented to it. Removing the object may cause further damage, lead to the destabilization of the patient, or make it harder for the surgeon to treat the patient. The object may be tamponading (compressing) a hematoma or a bleeding vessel. The object should be secured in place with tape and supported as necessary. The patient will be transported immediately to the operating room for removal in an environment most likely to be able to control any bleeding associated with the impalement.[9]

Street Secrets

Towel rolls, tongue depressors, wadded up gauze pads, and lots of tape make the best support for an impaled object. The fire department or rescue squad can often shorten the impaled object, for example, if the patient fell onto a long metal bar at a construction site. This may help you stabilize and support the object better. Be careful as vibrations or heat generated from the cutting process and loud noise from the tools can add to anxiety and pain. You may have to restrain the patient to keep him from attempting to remove the object.

As in any patient care situation, the ABCs should be assessed rapidly. The patient should be given supplemental oxygen ſrnd ventilatory support. Exposure is important to assure that all wounds are identified. If

there is no contraindication, the patient should be allowed to remain in a position of comfort. If the patient must be immobilized but is bleeding profusely from a mouth or neck wound, the patient should be immobilized and then the entire device and patient turned on the side and suctioned frequently to prevent airway compromise. Early control of the airway (for example with sedated or paralyzed intubation) should be considered, even in the awake and alert patient. The concern is that dynamic distortion of the airway may occur as a result of an enlarging hematoma. This is not always evident by physical exam, and there may be no visible external hematoma or change in voice. If airway distortion is occurring and is progressing, the chance of successfully intubating the patient decreases with each passing minute. Any interventions that are undertaken should be performed with appropriate sedation and analgesia. In the setting of a head, neck, or eye wound, patient agitation or performing the Valsalva's maneuver may raise arterial or intracranial pressure enough to dislodge a stable clot and increase bleeding.

If the patient has significant bleeding, it should be controlled with direct pressure. Never try to clamp a bleeding vessel in the field. Nerves and major blood vessels tend to be located adjacent to one another. While clamping a major vessel, it is likely that a major nerve can be damaged, leading to significant morbidity. Tourniquets should be avoided in all but the most extreme cases. Tissue that surrounds a penetrating injury has already been injured by the forces that create the temporary cavity, but it may still be viable. If the tissue is hypoperfused and made more hypoxic by the application of a tourniquet, the chances that the tissue will survive are decreased. Tourniquets are only used if the patient is at risk for immediate exsanguination from the extremity wound. Even extremity amputations are best managed by direct pressure and not by a tourniquet.

Working in a Crime Scene

One of the challenges in managing penetrating trauma is that, in addition to the injuries, you also must be alert that you may be working inside a crime scene and everything there is potential evidence. Be careful as you walk around the scene. Do not let crime scene management (which is a law enforcement task) distract you from patient care, but be aware that your very presence complicates their investigation. Accommodate the law enforcement officers as much as you can, but again, do not compromise patient care in the process. Most likely you will leave all soiled supplies (like dressings, IV packaging, etc.) on the scene where you used them. The officers may also request as evidence any clothing or personal effects removed from the patient. Avoid contact with the media that may be on the scene, and refer them directly to law enforcement or to your public information officer if present.

Nice to Know

Crime Scene Tips

- While stabilizing the patient must be foremost in your mind, do your best to avoid disturbing the scene or altering evidence. If this cannot be avoided, make sure to tell the police exactly what was changed about the crime scene and which member of the health care team did it.

- Do not throw anything away, no matter how bloody or dirty it is, as potentially everything may be used for evidence. Leave all packaging materials and used supplies such as gauze, on the scene for photographing and cataloging by the crime scene investigators.

- When removing clothes, do not cut through bullet holes, slashes in the fabric, powder burns, or other things that may be needed as evidence. When removing clothes, be alert for bullets or other projectiles that may be loose under the clothing.

- Do not pick up projectiles with forceps, as the metal may scratch the projectile and interfere with ballistic analysis. Immediately contact law enforcement officers if you find any ballistic materials or weapons on the scene.

- Document what the patient or others present at the scene may say, but avoid questioning them about the incident (except of course for SAMPLE survey information). This may lead to a lot of time spent in court as a witness.

- If the patient is stable, try to allow the police to ask a few questions prior to transport; however, do not delay transport for prolonged questioning as your "apparently" stable patient may suddenly deteriorate.

- Finally, try not to conjecture or make statements about what has happened. As a medical person, you are seen as an authority figure and other people, including the police, will document what you say. Avoid speculating on which wounds are entrance wounds and which are exit wounds, as they are often difficult to distinguish and require a forensic exam to confirm. These comments can become problematic.[16]

At a crime scene, it is important to get as much information as possible and record factual observations in the patient care report. Perform a standard physical exam and obtain a SAMPLE history. Include the following information if it is available in your report: what the patient was injured with, how many wounds are noted, how far the object entered into the body, where the body was entered, and if the injuries passed all the way through.

If the weapon was a knife, ice pick, etc., record how long the blade or point was. If the weapon was a gun, record what kind of gun, whether it was high-powered or low-powered, what kind of ammunition was used, and how far away the patient was from the shooter. All of these things have a bearing on the type of injuries you should expect and may assist the criminal investigators later. The Nice to Know box to the left has some additional crime scene tips.

Miscellaneous Trauma

Blunt and penetrating trauma make up the majority of all traumatic injury and total lives lost every year.[17] There are other forms of trauma that can contribute significantly to morbidity and mortality, and these include crush injuries, thermal injuries, and blast injuries. Each of these subsets of injury contains components of the blunt and penetrating mechanisms with very specific differences. It is these differences that warrant their discussion separately. **DOT 4-1.11**

Less-Than-Lethal Weapons

In recent years the law enforcement community has actively sought to develop effective means of controlling hostile, belligerent, or altered suspects without resorting to lethal force. Much of this grew out of the 1960s when law enforcement came under intense scrutiny for its use of force to control race riots and other protests. Today there are several devices in use that you should be familiar with. You may see patients who have had these devices used on them. The injuries, while usually minor as intended, occasionally can be lethal.[18]

The first class of weapons is **impact munitions.** These weapons are meant to strike and incapacitate a person without killing them or causing serious bodily harm. In the 1970s, the U.S. military developed the bean-bag round. This is a 12-gauge shotgun shell containing a synthetic bag filled with lead pellets. While in the shell, the bag is tightly wadded. Upon firing, it should unfold into a square-shaped projectile, which, upon striking its target, will disperse its energy over a larger surface area. In theory, this should knock down or incapacitate the subject without penetrating the body. There are several variations on this theme. Some are fired from shotguns, and some are fired from other specially designed guns.

By and large, these devices usually work as designed, but there are reports of the bags failing to open and basically becoming a slug. This has led to penetrating thoracic injury and, on occasion, death.[18]

Another less-than-lethal device, which has recently gained popularity with police departments, is the **Advanced Taser.** This is a device that resembles a gun but fires two metal probes with 4-mm barbs on their ends that are designed to attach to a subject's skin or clothing. The probes are fired at over 160 feet per second by compressed nitrogen. They are connected to the Taser by long insulated wires that allow the device to deliver rapid pulses of 50,000 volts of electricity in five-second pulses. This device grew out of earlier handheld stun guns and an earlier model of the Taser. The electricity causes the subject to lose voluntary neuromuscular control and fall to the ground. From the paramedic's standpoint there are three issues to consider.[19,20]

- First, the barbs will be impaled into the subject's body. They are only 4 mm and can usually be removed easily. However, it is important to know local protocols as to who can remove them and under what circumstances they can be removed.

- Second, there have been rare instances of cardiac arrest in patients who have been Tasered. If a paramedic discovers on primary survey that a patient is in cardiac arrest, then appropriate ACLS measures should be taken as discussed in Chapter 29.[18,19]

- Third, if called to evaluate a Tasered patient, take into account that the patient likely fell and do an appropriate trauma evaluation, including cervical spine immobilization if indicated. No formal studies exist to guide an evidence-based recommendation for care. But until evidence is available, there is enough reason to suspect that the patient who was Tasered received significant enough trauma to warrant evaluation in the emergency department.

CONNECTIONS   Pepper spray and other similar nonlethal chemicals are discussed in Chapter 35: Toxicology.

Amputation

These injuries are combinations of blunt and penetrating injuries and involve shearing and crushing forces (Figure 18-11). First, try direct pressure to stop the bleeding so as not to worsen underlying damage. Bring

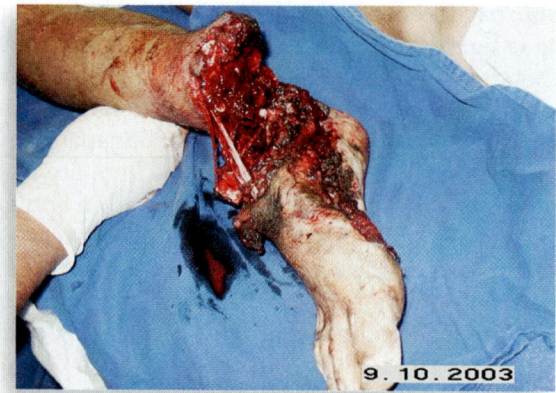

Figure 18-11   A 22-year-old man with traumatic amputation caused by a gear.

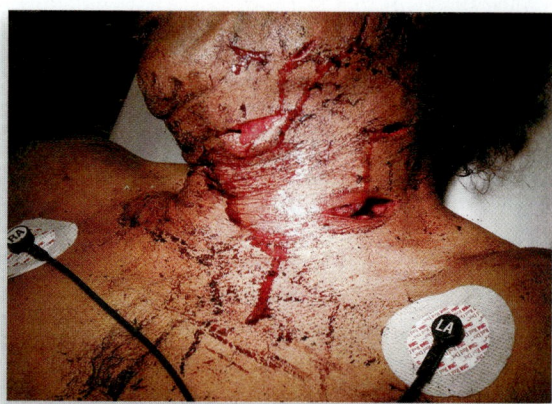

Figure 18-12   This pit bull attack demonstrates how animal wounds can be combination injuries: penetrating (tooth punctures), blunt (the tossing around of victim), and crush injury (the crushing bite of the jaws) are all noted in this patient.

the amputated part into the receiving facility if it can be easily located. Do not delay transport of the patient in order to look for the amputated body part. Other responders can remain on the scene to look for the amputated part while you rapidly transport the patient to the trauma center. Keep the amputated tissues cool and wrap the cut ends of the amputation with saline moistened dressings. Do not place them directly on ice or in water. Tourniquets are seldom needed to treat amputations in nonmilitary combatant situations when EMS providers have adequate personnel present to attend to the patient.

Crush Injury

Crush injury commonly occurs in the setting of blunt trauma (Figure 18-12). Crush injury results from a compressive force that causes cellular disruption with immediate cell **lysis** (meaning destruction). These dead cells release their internal contents into the local area, which in turn stimulates inflammatory responses. This increases the blood flow into the surrounding tissues, resulting in edema in the affected area. This cascade of events contributes to **crush syndrome,** which can lead to tissue death or patient death. Systemic manifestations of crush injuries include **rhabdomyolysis** (the muscle cells that break down and release their protein, which damages the kidneys), electrolyte abnormalities, acid/base abnormalities, hypovolemia, and acute renal failure.[21] As the time from entrapment lengthens, ischemia worsens and more intracellular components leak out, causing worsening inflammation, ischemia, necrosis, and pain. Many times this occurs within the first hour after the injury and can manifest quickly upon removal of the compressive forces.

When a body is crushed, the tissues directly involved become ischemic. The ischemia is localized and remains so because there is decreased or absent blood flow into that area. The tissues distal to the ischemic area are not perfused and can also become ischemic, releasing intracellular components.

A life-threatening problem arises when the person is extricated and some blood flow is restored. As soon as the compressive force is removed, the intracellular components and built up tissue wastes can now be flushed into the circulating blood volume. This causes a significant concentration of waste products released into the systemic circulation all at one time. The end product of the entire process is that the waste can lead to significant hypovolemia and shock severe enough to cause cardiac arrest.[22] Many specialists advocate early fluid resuscitation (2–3 liters) during the extrication phase and even the use of a bicarbonate infusion (via IV drip) while the patient is still entrapped.

Another condition, called **compartment syndrome,** is the culmination of crush injury and crush syndrome worsening. (There are other causes of compartment syndrome, such as burns and electrical injuries, although the end result is the same: compressive forces inside a closed space.) In crush injury, the tissue is compressed, forces cause direct cellular damage, and waste products cause edema and local tissue reactions. As these cause worsening edema at the site, there is edema in the underlying structures as well. These underlying structures are anatomically contained in nonexpansile compartments, which means they are not as elastic as other soft tissues around them and are less able to accommodate dramatic changes in their size.

An example is seen with muscle and its surrounding fascia. The fascia is tough and rather inelastic and will not stretch significantly if the muscle inside begins to swell. When the muscle becomes ischemic from a compressive force, it swells from edema. As the edema worsens, it causes more ischemia, which, in turn, causes more compression because the compartment is closed (sealed and inelastic). Eventually, the compartment pressure becomes higher than tissue perfusion pressure in that area, and necrosis begins as capillary blood flow stops. This can happen with minimal symptoms.[23] The assessment must be ongoing and frequent in patients with a high likelihood of this injury pattern.

There are several signs to monitor continuously in patients with crush injury to watch for the development of compartment syndrome:

Signs of compartment syndrome
- Pain
- Paresthesia (loss of sensation)
- Paresis (paralysis)
- Pallor
- Pulselessness

Severe pain noted with passive motion of the fingers or toes on the affected limb is one sign that compartment syndrome may be occurring. This is the most sensitive finding and often is the first to occur. **Paralysis** (no motor movement) and **paresthesia** (sensations such as numbness, prickling, tingling, etc.) are late findings in the development of compartment syndrome. They commonly manifest as a loss of two-point discrimination or vibratory sensation and the inability to move the fingers or toes of the affected area. The two-point discrimination test is described below.

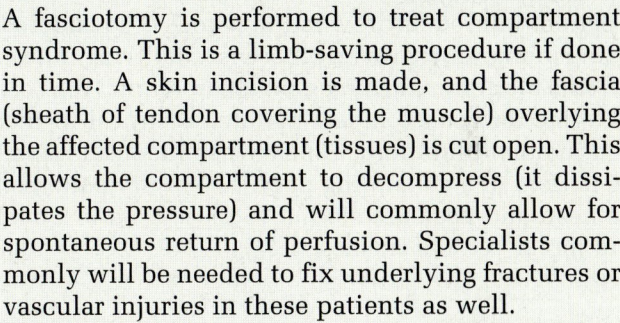

Nice to Know

A fasciotomy is performed to treat compartment syndrome. This is a limb-saving procedure if done in time. A skin incision is made, and the fascia (sheath of tendon covering the muscle) overlying the affected compartment (tissues) is cut open. This allows the compartment to decompress (it dissipates the pressure) and will commonly allow for spontaneous return of perfusion. Specialists commonly will be needed to fix underlying fractures or vascular injuries in these patients as well.

Pallor (paleness or blanching of the skin) will also occur late. It is due to decreased perfusion and will commonly begin distally with the nail beds looking dusky (gray) or bluish. Pulselessness of an extremity is also a very late finding.[24] Loss of pulse more likely indicates an acute arterial injury causing obstruction and no forward flow of blood into the area. This will cause more ischemia, leading to more edema, leading to worse perfusion and a spiraling of the process as it continues. Document the time the pulse is lost, and contact the receiving facility with an update on this change. The physician will have a limited amount of time in which to intervene in order to restore pulses, salvage the tissue, and save the extremity.

Two-Point Discrimination Test

The integrity of each digital nerve may be evaluated using either a blunt-tipped caliper or an unfolded paper clip to test **two-point discrimination.** The two points of the testing instrument are held apart at a measured distance. The examiner alternates between touching the skin with one or two points, and the patient is asked to identify how many points he or she was touched with. The points may be either touched (static two-point discrimination) or longitudinally moved (moving two-point discrimination) against the skin on either the radial or ulnar side of the finger. The points should be pressed against the finger until the skin just begins to blanch. The two-point discrimination value is the smallest distance between the two points that the patient can correctly detect in two out of three trials. Because of the increased sensory cues provided by movement, moving two-point discrimination will usually have a value less than or equal to static two-point discrimination. Static two-point discrimination is normal if the patient can detect two points when the distance is less than 7 mm, impaired if 7 to 14 mm, and absent if 15 mm or more.

Diving Injuries

A patient injured or drowned in a pool is considered a diving injury until proven otherwise. In diving injuries, extreme blunt trauma forces are focused upon the cervical spine and cause injury patterns identical to those seen in other blunt force injury when the head impacts the bottom of a swimming pool. The injury patterns to the head and neck are similar to those seen in up and over motor vehicle crashes.

Blast Injuries

Blast injury is an extremely violent form of both blunt and penetrating trauma. The blast wave consists of a shock wave (high pressure) followed quickly by an air wave (air movement with force).[25] Explosive forces in blasts cause injury by four mechanisms: primary, secondary, tertiary, and quaternary.

Primary injuries are the direct effects of the blast itself and are pressure related. The energy from the pressure causes a sudden, massive increase in air pressure that is easily transmitted through the atmosphere, and primarily causes compressive damage anywhere the compressive force is applied to air-filled spaces in the body (lungs, stomach, sinuses, and ears). Thus, the injuries caused include rupture of the eardrum, pneumothorax and pulmonary contusion, and stomach or bowel rupture.

Secondary injuries are mostly penetrating (but can be blunt) as these are the injuries from the projectiles thrown in the blast that strike the victim.

Tertiary injuries result from the blast throwing the patient some distance. Most of these injuries are blunt trauma unless the patient is impaled onto an object.

Quaternary injuries are those injuries or complications sustained from being in close proximity to the blast that are triggered or caused by the blast. These do not fit in the above three categories, but they include complications of underlying medical problems (acute myocardial infarction or delivery of an infant secondary to the stress of event), burns (from associated fires), and exposure to toxins (burning buildings release toxins or materials in an explosion).[26] See Table 18-3.

Pregnancy

Pregnancy contributes to trauma in many unique ways, the most obvious being that there are two patients instead of one. Significant trauma complicates 6–8% of all pregnancies. The most common cause of blunt abdominal trauma is motor vehicle crashes and accounts for about 70% of acute injuries. Up to 5% of pregnant women sustaining apparently minor traumas experience uterine abruption. One study identified that 31% of traumatic injuries in pregnant patients were due to intentional injuries, and most studies cite rates of domestic violence during pregnancy at 4–8%. Fetal mortality rates in penetrating abdominal trauma are as high as 70%. While the overall rate of maternal visceral injuries from trauma is 19–38%, there is still a 60–90% chance of fetal injury.[9]

The fetus can be injured in all of the same ways as the mother in spite of the amniotic fluid cushion it is in. The **gravid** (pregnant) uterus can actually protect some of the mother's internal organs and change injury patterns of blunt and penetrating injuries. Unfortunately, the gravid uterus can also be the site of significant injury in the mother.

Blunt trauma, especially to the abdomen, can result in a partial or complete tearing away of the placenta from the uterine wall. This injury is called a placental abruption. This is the result of the blunt forces being translated into shearing forces, removing the placenta from its uterine attachment.[27] Partial abruptions can produce significant amounts of blood loss in the uterus, causing signs and symptoms of shock even with minor appearing trauma. The internal organs of the mother are also shifted into other areas of the abdomen, which may lead to temporary changes in physical location of the organs as the uterus enlarges and takes up more space. This can cause increased forces to act upon the diaphragm, vena cava, or other structures in the abdominal cavity.

At a molecular and cellular level, the mother's metabolism changes throughout the pregnancy; therefore, her stress responses are different. The mother has a relative increase in blood volume in the later stages of pregnancy; however, there is a relative anemia present because the plasma volume portion increases the overall blood volume but the amount of cellular components is not increased as much. The mother may not show signs of shock immediately, but the fetus will be under tremendous stress and will possibly be hypoxic.

TABLE 18-3   The Effects and Injury Patterns Associated with the Different Categories of Explosions[9]

Category	Characteristics	Body Part Affected	Types of Injuries
Primary	Unique to high-order explosives (defining supersonic overpressurization wave) and results from the impact of the overpressurization wave with body surfaces.	Gas-filled structures are most susceptible Lungs, GI tract, and middle ear	Blast lung (pulmonary barotrauma) TM rupture and middle ear damage Abdominal hemorrhage and perforation Globe (eye) rupture Concussion (TBI without physical signs of head injury)
Secondary	Results from flying debris and bomb fragments	Any body part may be affected	Penetrating ballistic (fragmentation) or blunt injuries Eye penetration (can be occult)
Tertiary	Results from individuals being thrown by the blast wind	Any body part may be affected	Fracture and traumatic amputation Closed and open brain injury
Quaternary	All explosion-related injuries, illnesses, or diseases not due to primary, secondary, or tertiary mechanisms. Includes exacerbation or complications of existing conditions.	Any body part may be affected	Bums (flash, partial, and full thickness) Crush injuries Closed and open brain injury Asthma, COPD, or other breathing problems from dust, smoke, or toxic fumes Angina Hyperglycemia, hypertension

Source: "Explosions and Blast Injuries: A Primer for Clinicians," http://www.cdc.gov/masstrauma/preparedness/primer (accessed November 21, 2005).

Pediatric Patients

Head injury is the most frequent cause of traumatic death in children. MVCs are the leading cause of death in children over the age of one, accounting for 37% of all deaths due to trauma. MVCs are also the most frequent cause of injury in children. Alcohol use by the driver is a factor in almost 25% of these crashes. Suffocation is the most common cause of trauma death in children under the age of one. Other leading causes of death in children include drowning, fire and burns, and firearms. Death rates for boys over the age of five are twice the rate for girls. Children who are economically disadvantaged are 2.6 times more likely to die from trauma. Homicide accounts for 25% of all pediatric deaths. Infants are 10 times more likely to die from homicide than children ages five to nine. Rates of death for children have declined over the past 10 years in the United States for all categories except for firearms, suffocation, and poisoning.[9]

Pediatric Response to Trauma

Children do not respond to trauma in the same manner as adults. Their head is proportionately larger and their nervous system is less well developed, resulting in imbalance in the center of gravity. Their ability to compensate for shock is less driven by catecholamine stimulation than adults, and they have less cardiac reserve. The internal organs of children are less well protected by bony structures than those of adults. Their immune systems are less mature and not as efficient as those of older patients. They have less ability to compensate for environmental factors such as heat and cold than adults do because they have a relatively larger body surface area when compared to their overall mass.

Ideally, children should be transported to trauma centers that specialize in the care of pediatric patients. Table 18-4 lists the indications for transfer to a pediatric trauma center. Children need different criteria to identify the threshold for transport to pediatric trauma centers. For example, falls from heights as low as 27 inches (0.68 meters) can cause serious injury, especially if the child lands on a hard surface.[28] Intracranial injuries are frequently associated with these low-level falls.[29]

Even though children do not respond to trauma as do adults, the priorities for managing injured children do not differ from those of adults. Life-threatening situations compromising the ABCs are treated during the primary survey. Tasks to perform during this survey include airway management, cervical spine stabilization, placement of IV or IO (intraosseous) lines for fluid resuscitation or medication administration, and

TABLE 18-4 **Indications for Transfer to a Pediatric Trauma Center**

Mechanism of injury	Ejected from motor vehicle
	Fall from low- or higher-level height
	Prolonged extrication
	Death of another occupant in motor vehicle
Anatomic injury	Multiple severe trauma
	Spinal fractures or spinal cord injury
	Amputations
	Severe head or facial trauma
	Penetrating head, chest, or abdominal trauma

Source: J.E. Tintinalli, G.D. Kelen, J.S. Stapczynski, O.J. Ma, and D.M. Cline, *Tintinalli's Emergency Medicine: A Comprehensive Study Guide,* 6th ed. (McGraw-Hill's AccessMedicine, Table 252-4).

exposure of the child. All other conditions and problems are identified and managed during the secondary survey.

Airway management requires an understanding of pediatric anatomy that is age specific as well as a familiarity with BLS and ALS airway management techniques. Cervical spine immobilization requires application of an appropriate amount of padding under the shoulders and along the length of the body to account for the large occiput (Figure 18-13). Since no studies have been completed to date that enable EMS providers to reliably predict which children require immobilization, it should be utilized often with mechanism of injury alone triggering its use. Spinal pain, tenderness, significant multiple system trauma, severe head or facial trauma, significant distracting injury, and altered mental status along with trauma should all be considered appropriate mechanisms to trigger the use of spinal precautions.[30] A properly fitting rigid collar should be used. The head should be secured to an appropriately sized pediatric immobilization de-

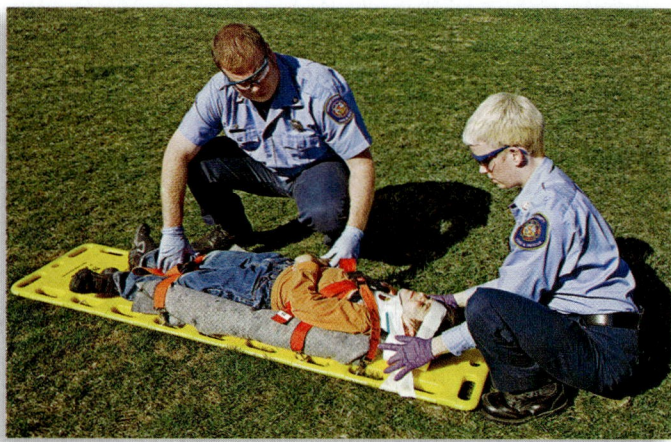

Figure 18-13 For cervical spine immobilization in children, place padding under the shoulders and along the length of the body to account for the large occiput.

vice. In the event that the device is too large, padding should be added to prevent lateral movement of the child in the event the device is log rolled.

All trauma patients should receive supplemental oxygen. Breathing assessment should include identification of inadequate oxygenation and ventilation. Signs of hypoxemia include cyanosis, mottling, agitation, poor capillary refill, bradycardia, and low pulse oximetry readings. Signs of inadequate ventilation include tachypnea, nasal flaring, grunting, retractions, stridor, and wheezing. Breath sounds are easily transmitted across the entire chest wall, so breath sounds should be auscultated in the midaxillary line. If signs of inadequate oxygenation do not improve rapidly with the administration of high-flow oxygen, positive pressure ventilation and perhaps intubation are indicated.

The classic presentation of tension pneumothorax in a child is absent breath sounds and tympany on palpation on the affected side, the chest wall fixed in an expanded position, hypotension, and jugular vein distension. Needle decompression should be performed in a manner identical to the adult patient, using a smaller gauge needle or catheter. The classic presentation of massive hemothorax includes absent breath sounds and dullness to percussion on the affected side, poor to absent chest wall motion with ventilation efforts, and hypotension. Rapid transport is the most appropriate treatment, and needle decompression is not indicated in this patient. An open pneumothorax in a pediatric patient is treated identically to the adult, with application of an occlusive dressing and monitoring for the development of a tension pneumothorax.[9]

During the circulatory assessment, signs of shock may be identified. Signs of shock include tachycardia, cool extremities, weak peripheral pulses, prolonged capillary refill beyond three seconds, altered mental status, and low urine output. Capillary refill is fairly unreliable and is often affected by hypothermia. Treatment for shock includes crystalloid fluid boluses of 20 mL/kg. Depending upon protocol, up to three 20 mL/kg boluses may be attempted in children in shock who do not have cardiac abnormalities.

Traumatic cardiac arrest in pediatric patients has a poor outcome. A small percentage of children in traumatic arrest from penetrating chest or abdominal trauma may survive, provided the time of arrest is short. In children with arrest from blunt trauma, the outcome is always death.[31] Most children in traumatic arrest have asystole or PEA, and standard ACLS algorithms should be followed during rapid transport to the hospital.

Cardiac tamponade or aortic rupture is extremely rare and usually fatal.[32] Children with cardiac tamponade who survive to reach the hospital alive present with Beck's Triad, just as adults do. **Beck's Triad** includes the findings of muffled heart tones, jugular

TABLE 18-5 Glasgow Coma Scales for Infants and Children/Adults Total = E + V + M

Infant Glasgow Coma Scale					
Eye opening (E)		**Verbal response (V)**		**Motor response (M)**	
Spontaneous	4	Coos, babbles	5	Obeys	6
Reaction to speech	3	Irritable cry	4	Localizes	5
Reaction to pain	2	Cries to pain	3	Withdraws	4
No response	1	Moans, grunts	2	Flexor response (decorticate)	3
		No response	1	Extensor response (decerebrate)	2
				No response	1
Child/Adult Glasgow Coma Scale					
Eye opening (E)		**Verbal response (V)**		**Motor response (M)**	
Spontaneous	4	Oriented	5	Obeys	6
Reaction to speech	3	Confused	4	Localizes	5
Reaction to pain	2	Inappropriate words	3	Withdraws	4
No response	1	Incomprehensible sounds	2	Flexor response (decorticate)	3
		No response	1	Extensor response (decerebrate)	2
				No response	1

vein distension, and severe hypotension. Prehospital treatment for both conditions is the same as for adults, with the primary treatment being recognition and rapid transport to an appropriate (preferably pediatric) trauma center.

Vascular access in traumatically injured children is difficult. Ideally, two lines should be placed, so medication can be given simultaneously with volume resuscitation efforts. Intraosseous (IO) line placement should be considered early in the process as all medications and fluids, in the same volume and concentration, can be given in the IO site as well as the IV site. Studies have shown that the speed with which medications and fluids enter the central circulation from the IO site is virtually identical to that of the IV.

Determining Disability in Pediatric Patients

Disability in children is assessed using a modified **Glasgow Coma Scale** (Table 18-5). As with adults, lower GCS scores are associated with increased mortality. The GCS score of eight, which is the threshold for intubation in adult patients, holds for children as well. Children with scores less than eight also appear to benefit from intubation.[33] Cranial nerve assessment and evaluation of the pupils should be performed as well as assessment of the motor strength of each limb. Gross strength is all that needs to be assessed during the primary survey.[9]

The final component of the initial assessment is exposure. The child is first exposed to identify any injuries that have so far escaped detection, and the assessment ends with the child being covered with sheets or blankets to conserve and preserve body heat. Children chill easily, and an injured child can rapidly lose body heat, even on a warm day. Children should be kept covered, and, if possible, IV fluids should be warmed before infusion. Actively bleeding wounds or penetrations will direct the priority of resuscitation during the primary survey. Bleeding is controlled in the same manner as for adults.

Pediatric trauma scores can help identify children who need more experienced care. Two commonly used scores are the **pediatric trauma score,** or **PTS** (Table 18-6), and the **revised trauma score,** or

TABLE 18-6 Pediatric Trauma Score (PTS)

	−1	+1	+2
Size (kg)	<10	10–20	>20
Airway	Unmaintained	Maintained	Normal
Systolic blood pressure (mmHg)	<50	50–90	>90
Level of consciousness	Comatose	Altered	Awake
Wounds	Major open	Minor open	None
Skeletal trauma	Open/multiple	Closed	None

Source: McGraw-Hill's AccessMedicine, Tintinalli, Table 252-2.

TABLE 18-7   Revised Trauma Score (RTS)

Number	Glasgow Coma Score	Systolic Blood Pressure	Respiratory Rate
4	13–15	>89	10–29
3	9–12	76–89	>29
2	6–8	50–75	6–9
1	4–5	1–49	1–5
0	3	0	0

Source: McGraw-Hill's AccessMedicine, Tintinalli, Table 252-3.

RTS (Table 18-7). These scores include physiologic information, such as blood pressure and respiratory rate, as well as anatomic variables, such as level of consciousness. Higher numbers on either score are associated with a higher likelihood for survival. A child with an RTS of less than 12 or a PTS of less than 8 should be taken to a pediatric trauma center.[34]

Geriatric Patients

The age category for "geriatric" varies somewhat, and it is important to scrutinize the age ranges used. Typically, statistics citing an age category are clarified to include the age range involved. Age-related changes occur in posture, balance, motor strength, coordination, and reaction time that put the elderly population at greater risk for trauma. In addition, changes in tissues and organ systems as well as chronic diseases make it more difficult for elderly patients to recover following injuries. Decreased visual acuity, hearing loss, and increased memory loss may make it more difficult for an elderly person to recognize or avoid environmental hazards.

Falls

Falls are the most common cause of injury in patients over the age of 65, with 50% of those who fall doing so repeatedly. In the United States, these falls result in over 9,500 deaths each year. Syncope has been implicated in many geriatric falls. Syncope can occur secondary to venous pooling, dysrhythmias, autonomic nervous system disease, hypoxia, hypovolemia, anemia, or hypoglycemia. Chronic medication or alcohol use can contribute to falls. Sedatives, antihypertensives, antidepressants, diuretics, and hypoglycemic agents are the most common causes.

Most of the falls occur on level surfaces and occur from a standing height. These falls are called "ground level falls," and they often result in orthopedic injuries of the wrist, hip, and vertebra. About 1% of falls

result in hip fractures that overall have a 20% mortality rate.[3] Many of these falls occur in residential settings such as nursing homes. Twenty percent of fatal falls in the age group over 85 occur in nursing homes.[9]

Chronic subdural hematoma should be suspected in elderly patients with new neurological signs, particularly **obtundation** (dullness to pain or sensations) or a change in personality. Headache is an uncommon presentation for chronic subdural hematoma in geriatric patients. There may be no history of trauma in these patients.[3]

Fifty percent of those individuals who fall are unable to get up without assistance.[35] Patients who are unable to get up from a fall are at-risk for dehydration, hypothermia, electrolyte imbalance, pressure sores, and rhabdomyolysis. Prevention strategies should be aimed at diminishing the amount of medications taken; improving strength and balance, gait training; and improving bone density through vitamin D and calcium supplements.[36] There is also some evidence that vitamin D supplementation may even help prevent falls.[37]

Assistive devices such as canes and walkers, when used correctly, can prevent falls. Patients should have phones at floor level, portable phones, or radio call systems that can be worn on the patient's clothing or around the neck in order to provide easy access to call for help in the event of a fall. Hip protectors have been shown to dramatically decrease the incidence of fractures from falls (by as much as 80%), but the devices are cumbersome and poorly tolerated by many elderly persons.[3]

Figure 18-14 presents an algorithm for evaluating elderly patients who have fallen.

Motor Vehicle Crashes

Motor vehicle crashes result in a high fatality rate for the elderly. MVCs are the second leading mechanism of injury sending elderly patients to trauma centers. Twenty-two percent of all pedestrian automobile fatalities occur in the 65 and older group. There is a 53% fatality rate among these patients.[9]

Burns

Burn center admissions by elderly patients account for 13–20% of all admissions. This group has the highest rate of fatality of any age group. Most burn injuries result from careless activity in the home. The most common causes, in order of frequency, are smoking, cooking, and scalds in the tub. The **Baux Index** is a simple but highly predictive tool for mortality for burn injuries.

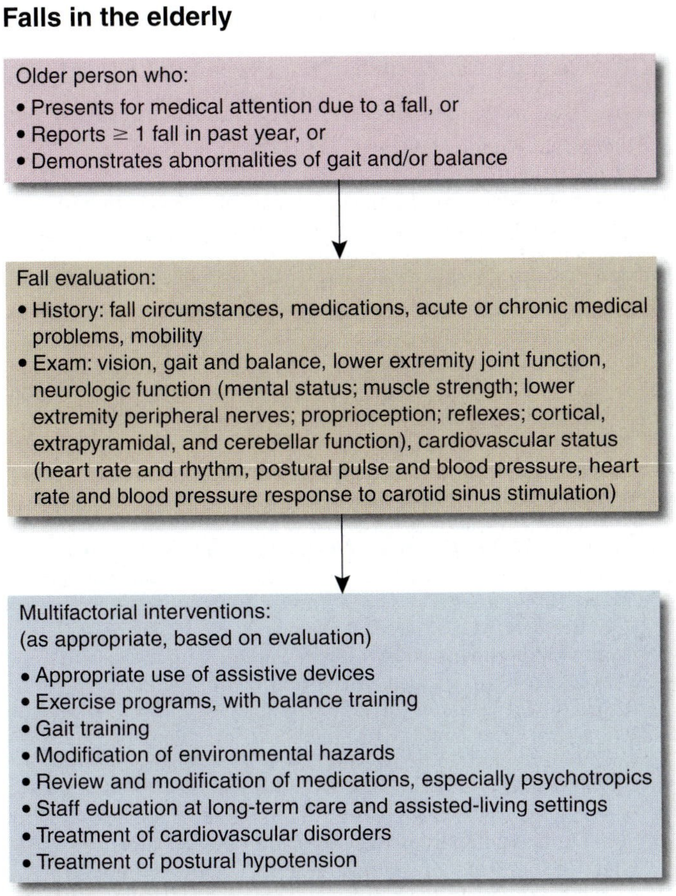

Falls in the elderly

Older person who:
• Presents for medical attention due to a fall, or
• Reports ≥ 1 fall in past year, or
• Demonstrates abnormalities of gait and/or balance

Fall evaluation:
• History: fall circumstances, medications, acute or chronic medical problems, mobility
• Exam: vision, gait and balance, lower extremity joint function, neurologic function (mental status; muscle strength; lower extremity peripheral nerves; proprioception; reflexes; cortical, extrapyramidal, and cerebellar function), cardiovascular status (heart rate and rhythm, postural pulse and blood pressure, heart rate and blood pressure response to carotid sinus stimulation)

Multifactorial interventions:
(as appropriate, based on evaluation)
• Appropriate use of assistive devices
• Exercise programs, with balance training
• Gait training
• Modification of environmental hazards
• Review and modification of medications, especially psychotropics
• Staff education at long-term care and assisted-living settings
• Treatment of cardiovascular disorders
• Treatment of postural hypotension

Figure 18-14 Algorithm for evaluating falls in the elderly.
Source: From "Current Practice Guidelines in Primary Care," 2006, by Ralph Gonzales and Jean Kutner. Copyright © The McGraw-Hill Companies, Inc. Reprinted with permission.

Baux Index
Add the age of the patient and the total body surface area burned (including relatively minor burns) to get a prediction of chance of dying. For example, if the patient is age 65 and has 10% total body surface area burned, the patient has a 75% chance of dying from the burn.

Geriatric patients with Baux Index scores greater than 70% usually do not survive, even with aggressive management of their injury by the burn center.[9]

Elder Abuse and Violence

Violent assaults account for 6% of all trauma center admissions for geriatric patients. The elderly are often seen as ideal targets. Use of ethanol (drinking alcohol) by the assailant or victim has been found to be present in a majority of all fatal assaults. The incidence of elder or parent abuse is on the rise as well and should be suspected with the same attention that pediatric abuse

and assault receives.[9] Clues to physical and psychological abuse, exploitation, and neglect include the patient's appearance, recurrent medical visits, missed appointments, suspicious physical findings, and implausible explanations for injuries.[3]

Summary

Traumatic injury results from the reaction of the body to the energies imparted upon it. Both speed and mass kill, but of the two, speed is the more deadly component of the equation. As an object travels faster, the amount of kinetic energy it has to release increases exponentially. Stopping that speed abruptly leads to transferring the energy into something else; unfortunately, it may be the patient whose organs and tissues cannot tolerate it.

The forces of energy do not always leave immediately visible signs on the patient. Many times these forces act at sites below the skin surface, in underlying organs and systems. Fortunately, these underlying injury patterns are predictable with critical evaluation of the mechanism of injury. High levels of suspicion can lead to the early initiation of treatment strategies, and early intervention may improve patient outcome under appropriate conditions.

Scenes of traumatic injury can give a prehospital provider an adrenalin boost. They can be horrific and graphic, leaving you to marvel at how the human body can sustain such damage and still be alive. In other situations, you can size up the scene and wonder why you are not seeing a more severely injured patient based upon the condition of the surroundings. Remember the importance mechanism and kinematics play in injuries. Looking at how the car came to rest, what tools the rescue squad is using for extrication, and even the position of the patient are all important to evaluation of the mechanism of injury.

By understanding the injury patterns produced by the mechanism of trauma, you can be alert to certain injury patterns. Anticipation of these injuries will lead to quicker recognition and result in treatment measures being initiated before obvious signs or symptoms develop. Understanding the mechanism will keep you one step ahead of the patient's vital signs because you will already be treating the suspected underlying injuries.

Understanding the mechanism behind both blunt and penetrating trauma is important in trying to predict which wounds the patient may have sustained. Obtaining as much information as possible about the wounding mechanism is a vital adjunct to your normal history and examination. By combining the visible wounds with the history you obtain, you can do a reasonable job of anticipating the patient's injuries and instituting early management.

Notes

1. "10 Leading Causes of Death, United States 2001–2002, All Races, Both Sexes" (http://webapp.cdc.gov/sasweb/ncipc/leadcaus.html) (accessed November 18, 2005).

2. "2002 United States, All Injury Deaths and Rates per 100,000 All Races, Both Sexes, All Ages" (http://webapp.cdc.gov/sasweb/ncipc/mortrate10_sy.html) (accessed November 18, 2005).

3. M. A. Papadikis and S. J. McPhee, eds., 2006, *Current Consult: Medicine* (McGraw-Hill's AccessMedicine, Quick Access). (accessed August 23, 2006).

4. "Community-Based Interventions to Reduce Motor Vehicle-Related Injuries: Evidence of Effectiveness from Systematic Reviews," http://www.cdc.gov/ncipc/duip/mvsafety.htm (accessed August 23, 2006).

5. R. A. Santucci and Y. Chang, "Ballistics for Physicians: Myths About Wound Ballistics and Gunshot Injuries," *Journal of Urology* 171 (April 2004):1408–1414.

6. National Association of Emergency Medical Technicians, *Prehospital Trauma Life Support,* 6th ed. (St. Louis, MO: Elsevier Mosby, 2007, p. 38).

7. "Life Expectancy Hits Record High," *National Vital Statistics Reports* 53(15)(February, 28, 2005).

8. D. G. E. Caldicott, A. Pearce, R. Price, et. al., "Not Just Another 'Head Lac' . . . Low-Velocity Penetrating Intra-Cranial Injuries: A Case Report and Review of the Literature," *Injury,* 35(2004): 1044–1054.

9. J. E. Tintinalli, G. D. Kelen, J. S. Stapczynski, O. J. Ma, and D. M. Cline, *Tintinalli's Emergency Medicine: A Comprehensive Study Guide,* 6th ed. (Mcgraw-Hill's AccessMedicine) (accessed August 23, 2006).

10. G. M. Doherty and L. W. Way, *Current Surgical Diagnosis and Treatment,* 12th ed., McGraw-Hill's AccessMedicine (accessed August 23, 2006).

11. Committee on Trauma, American College of Surgeons *Resources for Optimal Care of the Injured Patient* (Chicago, IL: American College of Surgeons, 1999).

12. K. L. Eckert, "Penetrating and Blunt Abdominal Trauma," *Critical Care Nursing Quarterly* 28(1) (January–March 2005): 41–59.

13. O. P. Sharma, M. F. Oswanski, and P. W. White, "Injuries to the Colon From Blast Effect of Penetrating Extra-Peritoneal Thoraco-Abdominal Trauma," *Injury* 35(2004), 320–324.

14. L. C. Haag, "Falling Bullets: Terminal Velocities and Penetration Studies" (Wound Ballistics Conference, Sacramento, California, April 1994).

15. M. Dickinson, "Understanding the Mechanism of Injury and Kinetic Forces Involved in Traumatic Injuries," *Emergency Nurse* 12(6) (September 2004), 30–34.

16. J. M. Wick, "Don't Destroy the Evidence!," *AORN Journal* 72(5), (November 2000): 807.

17. "2002 United States, Years of Potential Life Lost (YPLL) Before Age 65, All Violence-Related Injury Deaths, All Races, Both Sexes" (www.cdc.gov) (accessed August 23, 2006).

18. D. de Brita, K. R. Challoner, A. Sehgal, W. Mallon, "The Injury Pattern of a New Law Enforcement Weapon: The Police Bean Bag," *Annals of Emergency Medicine* 38(2001): 4.

19. A. Bleetman and R. Steyn, "Introduction of the Taser into British Policing: Implications for UK Emergency Departments: An Overview of Electronic Weaponry," *Emergency Medicine* 21(2004): 136–140.

20. Taser International, Electronic Press Kit, www.taser.com/documents/TASER_press_kit.pdf (accessed May 31, 2005).

21. O. S. Better, "Rescue and Salvage of Casualties Suffering From the Crush Syndrome After Mass Disasters," *Military Medicine,* 164(5) (1999):366–369.

22. D. Ron, U. Taitelman, M. Michaelson, et al., "Prevention of Acute Renal Failure in Traumatic Rhabdomyolysis," *Archives of Internal Medicine,* 144 (1984):277–280.

23. M. Michaelson, "Crush Injury and Crush Syndrome," *World of Surgery* 16(5) (1992):899–903.

24. D. Gonzalez, "Crush Syndrome," *Critical Care Medicine,* 33 Suppl (2005): S34–S41.

25. R. G. DePalma, D. G. Burris, H. R. Champion, and M. J. Hodgson, "Blast injuries," *New England of Medicine.* 352(13) (March 31, 2005):1335–42.

26. "Explosions and Blast Injuries: A Primer for Clinicians," http://www.bt.cdc.gov/masstrauma/explosions.asp (accessed November 21, 2005).

27. J. D. G. Neufield, "Trauma in Pregnancy." In J. A. Marx, ed., *Rosen's Emergency Medicine Concepts and Clinical Practice,* 5th ed. (St. Louis, MO: Elsevier Mosby, 2002, pp 256–266).

28. G. E. Bertocci, M. C. Pierce, E. Deemer, et al., "Using Test-Dummy Experiments to Investigate Pediatric Injury Risk in Simulated Short-Distance Falls," *Archives of Pediatric & Adolescent Medicine* 157(2003):480.

29. J. A. Murray, D. Chen, G. C. Velmahos, et al., "Pediatric Falls: Is Height a Predictor of Injury and Outcome?" *American Surgeon* 66(2000):863.

30. M. A. Eleraky, N. Theodore, M. Adams, et al., "Pediatric Cervical Spine Injuries: Report of 102 Cases and Review of the Literature," *Journal of Neurosurgery* 92(1 Suppl) (2000):7.

31. A. A. Sheikh and C. B. Culbertson, "Emergency Department Thoracotomy in Children: Rationale for Selective Application," *Journal of Trauma* 34(1993):322.

32. R. Karny-Jones, E. Hoffer, M. Meissner, et al., "Management of Traumatic Rupture of the Thoracic Aorta in Pediatric Patients," *Annals of Thoracic Surgery* 75(2003):1513.

33. J. R. White, Z. Farukhi, C. Bull, et al., "Predictors of Outcome in Severely Head-Injured Children," *Critical Care Medicine* 29(2001):534.

34. J. P. Marcin and M. M. Pollack, "Triage Scoring Systems, Severity of Illness Measures, and Mortality Prediction Models in Pediatric Trauma," *Critical Care Medicine* 30(11) (2002):S457.

35. M. A. Papadikis and S. J. McPhee, *Current Consult: Medicine* McGraw-Hill's AccessMedicine, Quick Access (accessed August 23, 2006).

36. American Geriatrics Society, British Geriatrics Society, and American Academy of Orthopaedic Surgeons Panel on Falls Prevention, "Guidelines for the Prevention of Falls in Older Persons," *Journal of American Geriatrics Society,* 49(2004):664.

37. H. A. Bischoff-Ferrari et al., "Effect of Vitamin D on Falls, a Meta-Analysis," *Journal of the American Medical Association* 291(2004):1999.

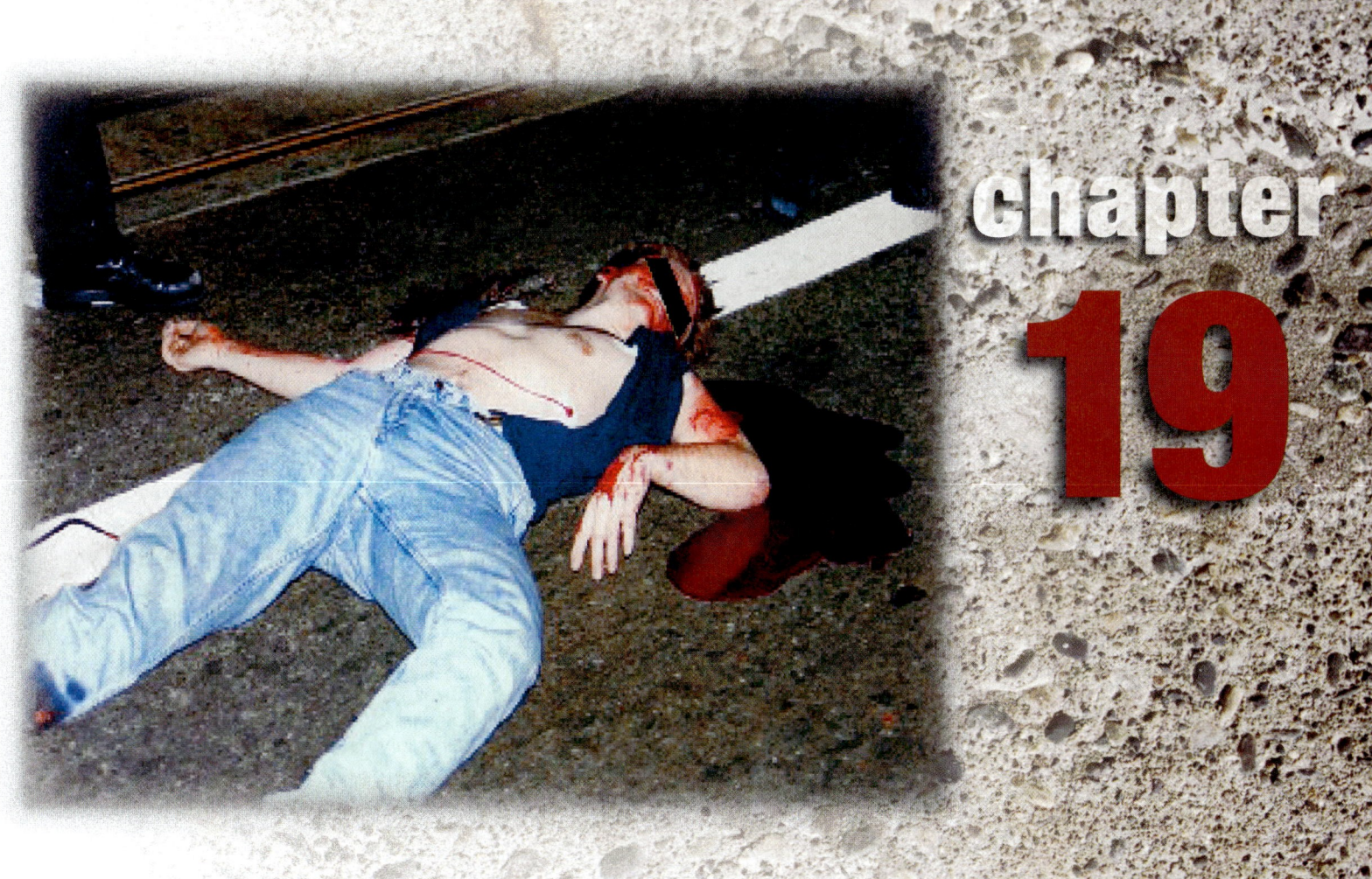

Trauma and Hemorrhagic Shock

"The Patient's Rule: It's not a matter of life and death—it's more important than that."

—Anonymous

Need to Know

▶ Hemorrhage affects the ability of cells to use normal aerobic metabolism, and ischemia quickly develops. Anaerobic metabolism begins as tissue perfusion drops off. Anaerobic metabolism is inefficient and results in worsening cellular ischemia.

▶ Blood loss can affect any component of blood pressure. It results in a decrease in stroke volume, and the hormones that are released in response to bleeding result in an increase in heart rate or an increase in vasoconstriction.

  • Blood pressure = Cardiac output (CO) × Peripheral vascular resistance (PVR)
  • Cardiac output = Stroke volume (SV) × Heart rate (HR)

▶ Shock has three stages: compensated, uncompensated, and irreversible. Treatments can be given at any stage in the process, but the lowest mortality rates occur when shock is stopped before the patient decompensates.

▶ Sick

- Hemorrhagic shock has signs and symptoms that are considered "classic" presentations: anxiety, restlessness, altered mental status, tachycardia, tachypnea, pallor, cool and clammy skin, cyanosis, and hypotension. However, patients do not necessarily manifest these signs, and an absence of these signs does not rule out the possibility of shock.
- Patients with any suspicion or evidence of hemorrhagic shock should be transported to a trauma center immediately for further evaluation and follow up.
- Patients typically begin to develop signs of shock when blood loss reaches 10–15%.
- Treat shock aggressively. Treatments may include bleeding control, oxygen, ventilatory support, fluid resuscitation, cardiovascular support with catecholamines and vasopressures once fluid resuscitation is complete, calming and reassuring the patient, conserving body heat, and rapid transport.

▶ Not Yet Sick

- Patients can compensate for blood losses of up to 10% without any obvious signs or symptoms.
- Perform a thorough scene size-up and evaluation of the mechanism of injury. This helps gather information that can lead you to suspect certain injury patterns or help explain the patient's response to hemorrhage.
- Follow the ABC (or ABCDE) order when performing the initial assessment.
- Find out about medication use and past medical history, and be alert for how medication and disease processes affect hemorrhagic shock.

Introduction

Shock is a complex clinical entity in which there is inadequate oxygen and nutrient delivery to tissues leading to a cascade of events that, if left untreated, ultimately results in death. This inadequate perfusion (also called **hypoperfusion**) may be the result of a number of mechanisms. They may be generally classified as cardiogenic shock, in which the output from the heart is inadequate to meet tissue needs; distributive shock, caused by peripheral vasodilation and maldistribution of blood; neurogenic shock, in which alterations in vascular tone due to sympathetic injury result in poor tissue perfusion; and hemorrhagic shock (or hypovolemic), in which there is inadequate blood volume to provide tissue perfusion. DOT 1-6.10, 1-6.11, 4-2.5

A **normotensive** individual has a blood pressure that is adequate for perfusion to all organs and tissues of the body. A **hypotensive** individual has lost perfusion to nonessential areas of the body and has maintained perfusion to the vital organs like the brain, heart, and lungs. Often, the patient displays the classic signs or symptoms for shock, and if uncorrected, death will occur. As shock worsens, the patient will begin to lose perfusion to the vital organs as well. DOT 4-2.37

The layperson's definition of a person "in shock" is someone who is seriously ill who may die. Like many nonmedical descriptive definitions, this one is very

accurate. Even when treated aggressively, shock identifies an individual with a high potential for mortality. One study found that patients with septic shock have mortality rates of 30–45%, and patients with cardiogenic shock have mortality rates ranging from 60–90%.[1]
DOT 4-2.1, 4-2.16

This chapter will focus on shock related to traumatic causes. Shock that accompanies trauma is caused primarily by acute blood loss (hemorrhage). Cardiogenic, distributive, and neurogenic shock are discussed in other chapters.

Skill Sheets that complement this chapter include Skill Sheet 66: Bleeding Control and Shock (also see Step-by-Step 66), Skill Sheet 67: Bleeding Control with a Tourniquet (also see Step-by-Step 67), Skill Sheet 72: Rapid Extrication, Skill Sheet 81: MAST/PASG Application, Skill Sheet 83: NREMT Patient Assessment Trauma, and Skill Sheet 94: NREMT Bleeding Control/Shock Management.

Hemorrhage

Hemorrhage is the loss of blood from the vascular system. It results from a break in blood vessels, with the loss of blood outside of the circulation. The concepts behind hemorrhage are fairly simple and follow the basic laws of fluid dynamics with some caveats: Larger holes in vessels result in greater hemorrhage; larger vessels bleed faster than smaller ones; and vessels under higher pressure (arteries) bleed faster than vessels with lower pressure (veins). These principles result in the classic first step for bleeding control (called **hemostasis**) where pressure directly applied on a bleeding site compresses the vessel and closes the hole. When pressure on a vessel stops the bleeding, normal regulatory mechanisms have the opportunity to build a clot in the affected tissues that will prevent further blood loss. DOT 4-2.5

Blood is rich in platelets and clotting factors that adhere to many surfaces including vessel walls, sterile bandages, and dressing materials. Conditions that impair the patient's intrinsic ability to clot (including things like medication, hypothermia, liver disease, leukemia, or chemotherapy) may cause increased hemorrhage. Finally, the vessels themselves vary, with arteries having muscular fibers that, when triggered to do so, result in spasm and contraction of a vessel, which can help stop bleeding. Veins typically do not have these muscles and are more likely to bleed continuously if left untreated.

Clinically, blood loss does not have to be externally visible. Hemorrhage may be internal, like that found with bleeding into the peritoneum, the thorax, or the retroperitoneal space. This can occur following trauma. With fractures of the long bones of the extremities, bleeding can occur into the surrounding soft tissues as well. Internal bleeding may result in some visible clues like swelling or discoloration of the skin as **hematoma** (literally "blood tumors") or **ecchymosis** (bruising) developing.

Physiology of Blood Loss

In understanding the body's response to blood loss, a brief review of the maintenance of blood pressure is in order. Chapter 8: Physiology Overview has more detailed descriptions of these key concepts. Please consult that chapter if more information is desired.

The key determinants of blood pressure are **cardiac output** (amount of blood delivered by the heart) and **peripheral vascular resistance** (resistance to flow as produced by the blood vessels, primarily the arterioles, against which the heart must pump). Cardiac output is determined by the **stroke volume** (volume of blood ejected each time the ventricle contracts) and **heart rate** (beats per minute). DOT 4-2.2

Stroke volume is directly impacted by the amount of blood returned to the heart from the venous circulation (**preload**) and the force of contraction of the ventricle. The peripheral vascular resistance (PVR, which is also called **afterload**) varies according to the amount of sympathetic nervous system (SNS) tone and is modified by catecholamine hormones secreted by the efferent nerve fibers of the SNS. The more catecholamine present, the greater the SNS-stimulating effects. All of these relationships and interrelationships can be expressed as:

- Blood pressure = Cardiac output (CO) × Peripheral vascular resistance (PVR)
- Cardiac output = Stroke volume (SV) × Heart rate (HR)

As the body strives to maintain blood pressure, events that affect one parameter, result in changes in the other. Blood loss, for example, results in a decrease in stroke volume. To maintain a constant blood pressure, the body acts to increase the peripheral vascular resistance and increase the heart rate. With a decrease of peripheral resistance due to spinal cord injury (the "message" to constrict cannot get through from the brain), the normal response results in a concomitant increase in HR (because a nerve travels from the brain directly to the heart, so the "increase the heart rate" message does get through) although patients are often still hypotensive.

CONNECTIONS For more information on neurogenic shock read Chapter 30: Neurology.

The rate of hemorrhage impacts the degree of physiologic change. The goal of this compensatory mechanism is to preserve adequate tissue perfusion for vital organ function. Rapid hemorrhage demands rapid changes in vascular tone and heart rate, manifesting as vasoconstriction and tachycardia. More gradual hemorrhage allows more time for the body to compensate. This occurs most commonly through movement of fluid from the extracellular space into the vascular tree. As a result, vascular tone and heart rate changes are minimal until the reserves found in the extracellular space are depleted.

Tachycardia, when present in patients suspected of shock, should be a strong indication for shock. Other signs and symptoms that may be present will be discussed as well. Unfortunately, patients do not always present with the signs or symptoms we believe represent the "classic" presentation of shock, and this could lead to missed opportunities for treatment. Understanding clinical manifestations of the changes that occur, whether detectable signs are present, is vital in appropriately managing patients in shock. DOT 4-2.6

Street Secrets

Medications can affect the vital signs and shock signs a patient has during acute blood loss. For example, blood thinning medications like aspirin, warfarin sodium, and antiplatelet medications inhibit the formation of clots, which leads to longer bleeding times and makes it more difficult to stop bleeding. Beta blocker medications regulate the force of cardiac contractions, improving the pumping action of the heart, but they also regulate the heart rate, which is not easily overridden, even when the brain tries to stimulate the heart directly into becoming tachycardic. Other medications have side effects that prevent the patient from sweating very much or that keep the patient somewhat dehydrated, so the common finding of diaphoresis may not be present. All of these situations can cause the patient not to present with the "classic" shock signs even if they are in shock.

Cellular Pathophysiology

The goal of blood pressure is to provide adequate perfusion to the body so that oxygen and nutrients may be delivered to cells and waste products removed. These essential functions occur in the capillary beds of the vascular system. Perfusion at the arteriolar end of the capillary (the proximal end) delivers fluid, oxygen, and nutrients to the interstitial spaces (Box 19-1). The interstitial space surrounds all cells and is used for subsequent transport of materials across cell walls. At the venous end of the capillary (the distal end), fluids, CO_2, and other waste products of cellular metabolism diffuse into the vasculature where they are returned to the

BOX 19-1   Perfusion

Perfusion is the delivery of oxygen and nutrient-rich blood to each cell of the body and the removal of waste products from the cellular environment via this circulating blood. The term *adequate perfusion* indicates that this process is functioning properly. Inadequate perfusion means that some part of the process is not working appropriately. The body can often adjust, or compensate, for minor problems with perfusion, but when the problem overwhelms the body's coping mechanisms, shock results.

lungs, liver, and kidneys for excretion or further processing for recovery of their components. DOT 4-2.17, 4-2.18, 4-2.19, 4-2.20, 4-2.21, 4-2.22, 4-2.23

Anaerobic Metabolism

In the situation when the normal mechanisms fail, either by inadequate flow of blood to tissues or inadequate oxygen delivery, cells shift from aerobic metabolism (with maximal production of energy in the form of ATP) to anaerobic metabolism (with inadequate ATP production and an increase in lactic acid production). The body's ability to adjust to, compensate for, or even correct these problems results in the development of the various stages of shock.

Understanding the impact of inadequate blood flow to cells and the physiologic response of the body is the focus of much clinical research on hemorrhagic shock. In the early stages of blood loss, the perfusion to tissue becomes compromised. Remember, perfusion is a two-way process, with nutrients being delivered and wastes being removed. The vascular tree works to maintain vital organ perfusion to the brain, heart, and kidneys. During inadequate blood flow, compromise occurs first to the skeletal muscles and the visceral organs. The result of this decreased flow to cells is the transition from aerobic to anaerobic metabolism, with lactic acidosis occurring at the cellular level.

Lactic Acidosis

The body's normal response to the abnormality of anaerobic metabolism is first to convert lactic acid to lactate. Lactate is then transported via the blood to the liver where it is neutralized, as it is further metabolized to bicarbonate and water. Early on in this process, bicarbonate is fairly easily handled by the intrinsic buffering capacity of the circulation. When more severe abnormalities occur and tissue perfusion worsens, the amount of lactic acid production increases. At this time, the ability of the body to process lactate becomes overwhelmed, resulting in metabolic acidosis. DOT 4-2.15

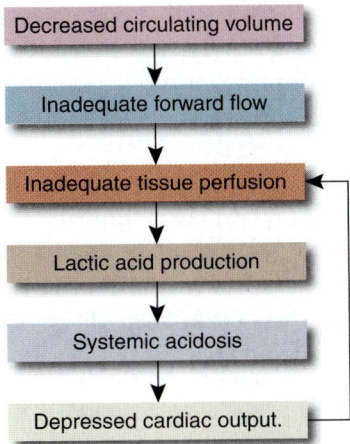

Figure 19-1 If uncorrected, shock spirals out of control.

Acidosis results in myocardial irritability, which causes dysrhythmias, decreases cardiac output, and depresses cardiac contractility. All of this is due to suboptimal myocardial muscle cell function from the abnormal cellular pH level. These cardiac effects further decrease peripheral blood flow, creating a spiral of worsening shock, which if uncorrected could lead to irreversible shock. Figure 19-1 illustrates this process.

Acidosis and energy depletion affect the sodium-potassium ATP pumps that maintain the balance of ions inside and outside the cell (called ion gradients) and also affect cell wall integrity. When cell wall integrity is compromised, it leads to the loss of chemicals and contents from within the cell, or it permits the entry of undesired chemicals into the cell. As acidosis persists and cell wall integrity further deteriorates, the result is cellular death.

Systemic Inflammatory Response Syndrome (SIRS)

Another important pathway in the worsening shock state is the activation of a **systemic inflammatory response (SIRS)** reaction which results in the release of inflammatory mediators like cytokines, arachidonic acid metabolites, free radicals, etc. These inflammatory mediators result in worsening, or exacerbation, of shock. See Chapter 13: Shock Overview for a more complete discussion of the SIRS process.

Compensated versus Uncompensated Shock

Adapting to Fluid and Blood Volume Loss

The ability to adapt to blood loss and shock is a crucial physiologic mechanism for survival. **Compensated shock** occurs as the body adjusts to the fluid loss and organ perfusion is maintained. At the peak of this process, if no additional support comes to the body to allow it to transition back to aerobic metabolism, the patient will slide into the **decompensated shock** state. If the decompensated state is uncorrected, **irreversible shock** results in death. DOT 4-2.12, 4-2.13, 4-2.34

The response to a mild fluid deficit is a gradual one. When there is inadequate blood flow to the kidney, the receptors in the kidney increase the production of the hormone renin, which stimulates release of increased amounts of the hormone aldosterone from the adrenal cortex. Aldosterone causes increased salt and water reabsorption in the kidney, which allows the body to retain fluids instead of excreting them.

As the brain identifies a fluid deficit, it produces antidiuretic hormone (ADH), which further stimulates free water reabsorption in the distal tubule of the kidney. The brain also stimulates a feeling of thirst, which leads to increased fluid intake that allows for more water absorption. DOT 4-2.30, 4-2.31

Total Body Water

This mechanism, though helpful, is clearly not adequate to respond to the fluid needs of the body after a significant insult like a gunshot wound to the abdomen. **Total body water** (TBW) is divided into two functional fluid compartments: the extracellular (ECF) and intracellular (ICF) spaces (Table 19-1).[2] Extracellular fluid comprises approximately one-third of TBW, and intracellular fluid makes up the other two-thirds. Extracellular water makes up an average of 20% of the **total body weight** and is divided between plasma (5% of total body weight) and interstitial fluid (15% of total body weight). Intracellular water makes up approximately 40% of the total body weight, with the greatest amount

TABLE 19-1 Total Body Water

	Percent of body weight	Typical volume	
		Woman (120 lb [55 kg])	Man (154 lb [70 kg])
Total body water	50–60	28 L	42 L
Intracellular fluid	35–40	20 L	28 L
Extracellular fluid	15–20	8 L	14 L

of water in the intracellular compartment found within the skeletal muscle mass.

Fluid shifts after traumatic blood loss must be rapid in order to maintain vital organ perfusion. Extracellular fluid (which is 20% of the TBW) serves as an important reserve supply for the blood stream.[3] The ECF shifts rapidly to the intravascular space to compensate for acute blood loss. As blood loss continues, the ability of the ECF to maintain adequate flow and forestall shock becomes exhausted. Without fluid resuscitation, the body loses its ability to further counteract shock, resulting in a spiral toward irreversible shock and death. DOT 4-2.30, 4-2.31, 4-2.32

The Importance of ECF in Staving Off Shock

The importance of the ECF in this mechanism is illustrated in the early work of Wiggers et al., which measured the clinical outcome of laboratory animals in response to blood loss.[4] These researchers bled animals to varying levels of blood loss. The blood was removed into a reservoir, resulting in a period of hypotension and shock. They then transfused the removed blood back to the animals and observed them for response. When the blood loss was around 10%, the animals were able to tolerate the period of hypovolemia because their blood pressures returned to normal quickly, and virtually all the animals survived.

As the amount of blood loss increased to around 25%, even though the animals returned to a normal blood pressure after their blood was returned, they deteriorated over the next few hours and had an 80% mortality rate. Wiggers identified these animals as reaching a point of irreversible hemorrhagic shock at which the body was unable to correct or compensate for the insult of acute blood loss despite resuscitation attempts. The mechanism proposed as responsible for this is the rapid shifting of the fluids from the reinfused blood back to the depleted ECF space, which resulted in a continued decreased intravascular volume and actually worsened shock. DOT 4-2.30, 4-2.31

These experiments identified that blood loss alone is not the only element in the development of shock and that fluid shifts and fluid resuscitation of the extracellular space are crucial to stave off irreversible shock. They showed that fluid resuscitation using an isotonic (balanced) salt solution (essentially normal saline) helped dramatically reduce the mortality associated with acute blood loss.[4] Fluid resuscitation of the patient in shock will be discussed later in this chapter.

Pathophysiology of Vital Organ Failure

Development of irreversible shock occurs as shock progresses and depends greatly on the severity of the initial insult and the ability of the body to withstand the physiologic insult. For example, a young patient with normal cardiac function and no coronary disease is able to tolerate longer periods of low cardiac flow compared to an older patient with preexisting disease.

Multiple System Organ Failure

The myriad clinical effects of shock result in cell death. If uncorrected, they progress rapidly to multisystem organ failure (MSOF). As tissue blood flow decreases due to peripheral vasoconstriction and hypovolemia, the cells are said to be in an **ischemic phase.** DOT 1-6.12, 4-2.19

As ischemia worsens, sludging of blood moving through the capillary beds begins to occur. This further decreases blood flow to the organs and tissues. **Capillary sludging** results in the formation of microscopic-sized blood clots, called **microemboli.** This event is called the **capillary stagnation phase** because little blood flow is occurring and little perfusion or circulation of nutrients and wastes is occurring. The microemboli further clog up the vascular beds, worsening circulatory compromise. This process uses up the available clotting factors and leads to the development of a systemic hemorrhagic state known as **disseminated intravascular coagulopathy,** or **DIC.** As the capillary beds become more hypoxic, the sphincter muscles relax and the remaining contents that are not formed into microemboli move out of the capillary bed. This stage is termed the **washout phase.** Unfortunately, the components of the blood that continue to circulate are filled with toxins and are not functioning efficiently. DOT 4-2.20

Capillary sludging in the liver and kidney can cause hepatic or renal failure, which may or may not be reversible. Sludging can also result in disruption of the capillary beds in the lungs, which leads to capillary leak, fluid extravasation (leakage out of the vascular bed) into the lung tissue, and the development of either **acute respiratory distress syndrome (ARDS)** or **noncardiogenic pulmonary edema.** Either condition further worsens the shock state by increasing systemic hypoxia. Sludging of the capillaries in the viscera can lead to bowel necrosis and results in sepsis and acidosis. Injury to any single organ, or any combination of organs, can be a terminal event for the patient. DOT 4-2.19-4-2.21

The Initial Assessment of the Shock Patient

It is important to gather as much information as possible prior to your interaction with the patient because the mechanism of the incident will have specific implications. However, this should not delay the face-to-face assessment of a potentially critical patient. If resources allow, allocate on-scene resources to the gathering of information from bystanders and to further evaluation of the mechanism of injury while the initial assessment is performed. DOT 4-2.7, 4-2.8, 4-2.42, 4-2.43, 4-2.44

Upon completion of the initial assessment and initial treatment interventions, a decision regarding transport and patient destination is made. Immediate removal from the scene may be required, or a decision may be made to remain on the scene a little longer to perform additional assessments or treatments.

The discovery of a patient in any stage of shock represents a life-threatening emergency, and transport should be started as quickly as possible. DOT 4-2.33

The secondary survey is typically performed at this time, but it may be done on the scene or while en route to the hospital. The secondary survey is a head-to-toe evaluation of the patient designed to look at each region of the body and each body system. It includes repeat attention to all elements of the initial assessment.

CONNECTIONS Chapter 14: Patient Assessment describes the surveys appropriate for injured patients.

Penetrating trauma produces far different injuries than blunt trauma. For instance, penetration of the thorax or abdomen can cause life-threatening internal hemorrhage. If the object is still present in the body, any movement may result in additional trauma to the tissues. Removal of the object from the body may result in increased bleeding as the object may actually be providing tamponade pressure against a damaged blood vessel and preventing aggressive bleeding. Blunt trauma can also cause internal hemorrhage, particularly if it is in the thorax, abdomen, or pelvis. External hemorrhage from a limb injury can be substantial, particularly if it is in a difficult to control location like a joint. The differences between blunt and penetrating trauma will directly affect the care that is required for the patient. DOT 4-2.3, 4-2.35

Once direct evaluation of the patient begins, it is best to follow the structured assessment of the ABCs. Each component of the ABCs must be sequentially assessed and managed. In this initial phase of patient care, management of the ABCs is limited to situations and conditions that, if uncorrected, will result in additional deterioration of the patient. Any life-threatening problem noted during the ABC assessment, even if it is successfully corrected, deserves continued attention and monitoring. As the patient is stabilized and additional assessments are performed, any other problems found are further evaluated, and the decision to treat will be made based upon many factors (Box 19-2).

Skill Sheet 72: Rapid Extrication and Skill Sheet 83: NREMT Patient Assessment Trauma are helpful resources.

Airway

The initial assessment of all patients begins with airway assessment. Patency of the airway must be established prior to proceeding with the evaluation. If the airway is

BOX 19-2   The Initial Assessment: ABC versus ABCDE

Classic EMS education has focused on the initial assessment of the patient centered on the airway, breathing, and circulation, or "the ABCs." The last ten years or so have added additional elements onto the initial assessment to include a brief assessment of the nervous system (which added a "D" for disability) and the reminder of the need to expose the patient in order to more fully assess the patient (which added an "E" for exposure). Regardless of whether you think of the initial patient assessment phase as the "ABC" assessment, or the "ABCDE" assessment, the basic principles remain consistent for each:

- Quickly evaluate the patient for life-threatening problems (this evaluation should take 90 seconds or less to perform if it is uninterrupted by treatments)
- Treat only those problems that worsen the patient's condition and threaten their life *right now*
  - Prioritize the other problems and treat them later as time and resources permit
- Always perform the assessment in the ABC or ABCDE order to ensure a consistent, thorough assessment is performed
- Do not interrupt this assessment until it is done unless you need to treat a life-threatening problem (delegate the treatment if resources allow)
- Complete the entire assessment before you stop

not patent, the patient is unable to maintain an open and clear airway without some level of assistance. This may require airway opening and positioning, suctioning, or the insertion of airway adjuncts to maintain patency. Cervical spine stabilization must be provided for any patient with possible cervical spine injuries. The jaw thrust maneuver should be used to open the airway in these patients. The need for suction should be assessed if any foreign matter such as blood or vomit is noted on the mouth or nose. If the patient is able to speak, the airway is likely patent, and the initial assessment can continue.

Breathing

The assessment for the adequacy of breathing includes evaluation for respiratory effort and a gross determination of rate and volume. It is not necessary at this point to obtain an actual respiratory rate. It may be necessary to visualize the chest, particularly if penetrating injuries are suspected, as these injuries have implications for breathing.

All critically injured patients should have supplemental oxygen administered with the patient closely monitored for response. If the patient's ventilatory efforts are not adequately maintaining oxygenation (as measured by pulse oximetry, end-tidal CO_2, or as observed as altered mental status, cyanosis, or dyspnea), more aggressive management may be required. Ventilation can be supplemented by using the bag-mask unit to control respiratory rate and depth, or by introducing invasive airway adjuncts like the endotracheal tube, Combitube, PTL airway, LMA airway, or other approved device. The use of oxygen-powered ventilation devices like the flow restricted demand valve remain controversial and have largely fallen out of use in many prehospital settings.

As previously mentioned, assessment of breathing during the initial assessment phase includes identification of injuries to the chest wall or abdomen that may impact breathing mechanics. For instance, if rib fractures or a flail segment are identified, gas exchange in the lungs may be significantly affected, and these patients may require ventilation support in addition to supplemental oxygen.

Circulation

Evaluation of circulation is especially important in patients who are potentially suffering from hemorrhagic shock. The patient's skin color and pulse should be checked along with an evaluation for external bleeding.

As a general rule, patients who have lost a significant amount of blood will often appear pale or ashen whereas a generalized pink coloration of the skin is indicative of a normovolemic patient. However, it is important to remember that the patient who looks "normal" initially may have ongoing occult bleeding and suddenly deteriorate within a matter of minutes.

The carotid and radial pulses can be checked simultaneously and compared for rate, rhythm, and quality. If neck or head trauma prevents palpation of the carotid pulse, the femoral pulse should be examined. As with the breathing assessment, a gross determination of the rate and quality is all that is necessary, and an actual heart rate is not required at this time.

> A patient who has significant hemorrhage will often have a weak or thready and rapid pulse.

Tachycardia due to acute blood loss should result in a regular rate, so an irregular pulse should alert the care provider to a dysrhythmia that could be the result of a new injury or a preexisting problem. DOT 4-2.36

Assessment of circulation is not complete until potential sources of hemorrhage are examined and

BOX 19-3 When to Control External Bleeding

Although control of external hemorrhage technically falls under "C" (circulation), it is certainly appropriate and desirable to stop external hemorrhage immediately upon discovery. As you approach the patient and note severe external bleeding, you can place your gloved hand on the wound while you begin assessing the level of consciousness and the airway. As other resources arrive to assist, you can transition hemorrhage control to these resources while you continue the initial assessment.

controlled (Box 19-3). Significant amounts of blood can leak into internal cavities (most commonly the thorax and abdomen or pelvis areas) or be external to the body. If the body is not examined directly for open wounds at this time, be sure to squeeze the patient's clothing and then observe the gloves for blood. As soon as possible, remove all clothing and visualize the skin directly for injuries or signs of internal bleeding. Methods of hemorrhage control for external bleeding will be discussed later in the chapter. **Skill Sheets 66: Bleeding Control and Shock (also see Step-by-Step 66) and 67: Bleeding Control with a Tourniquet (also see Step-by-Step 67) discuss bleeding control, as does Skill Sheet 94: NREMT Bleeding Control/Shock Management.** DOT 4-2.29

Disability

Evaluation of neurologic disability is required for the assessment of any critically ill patient. The goal of the neurologic portion of the initial assessment is to establish a baseline for the patient's level of consciousness. The most common reporting schemes are the AVPU method or the Glasgow Coma Scale (GCS) which are covered in depth in Chapters 11 and 14 for AVPU and 20 for GCS. During the initial assessment, the AVPU will provide a quick assessment of consciousness only. Later, assessments with the GCS will quantify the level of consciousness (Box 19-4).

In the setting of hemorrhage or hemorrhagic shock, nonfocal neurologic disability can be an indication of declining or low blood pressure. For example, when a patient who is being treated for hemorrhagic shock becomes abruptly confused or less responsive, you must consider hypotension as a probable cause for this change. A conscious patient can report on the sensory pathway by stating if a touch on the hands and feet is felt. A patient can also be asked to move the fingers and toes to assess gross motor response. Observing the ability to follow these simple commands will also add information about the patient's mental status.

BOX 19-4   Using AVPU Instead of the GCS in the Initial Assessment

The AVPU assessment is a brief tool that simply provides an initial impression of the gross level of consciousness. AVPU stands for Awake, Verbal, Painful, and Unresponsive, and it indicates only when the patient opens the eyes and seems awake. The further into the assessment you must go, the more concerned you should be that there is a problem for the patient. In other words, a patient responding to a loud voice is, for the moment, considered in better neurologic shape than the patient who does not respond to verbal stimulation.

The AVPU tool does not assess the quality of the interaction of the patient with the paramedic. In other words, it will not tell you the patient is confused or that thought patterns are altered, but it will tell you that the patient is awake.

During the initial assessment, this information will guide you in your assessment without distracting you from finishing the remainder of the initial assessment. Once the initial assessment is complete, it may be appropriate to immediately perform a GCS assessment (particularly if a traumatic brain injury is suspected), or another body system may be the focus of your concern.

Exposure

Patients who are victims of either penetrating or blunt trauma should be fully exposed if possible. Although attention must be taken to avoid delaying transport, this is an important step to avoid missed sources of bleeding. Treatment of hemorrhaging patients begins with preventing further blood loss. Care must be taken to examine all aspects of the chest, abdomen, and extremities (especially those with noticeable deformities). Examination of the patient's back is usually difficult because of concern for cervical spine injuries or perhaps limited resources to perform the assessment. This should be deferred until adequate spinal immobilization can be maintained for examination of the patient's back, but it should be balanced with the need to manage and treat the patient.

A blood sweep of the posterior-lateral aspect of the patient's thorax and abdomen or examination of the patient's clothing and surroundings can detect significant blood loss from the posterior aspect of the patient. Use caution when placing hands in areas that cannot be visualized prior to insertion. Make note of the surface the patient is lying on, and use extreme caution if sharp objects are suspected. Once the skin is inspected, quickly cover the patient to avoid hypothermia and to protect the patient's privacy and dignity.

Street Secrets

Covering the long back board with a blanket or sheet also helps conserve body heat. Although they are "BLS" skills, maintaining body heat and preventing further loss of heat are important shock management treatments.

Features of Internal and External Hemorrhage

The ability to differentiate between internal and external hemorrhage has implications in the treatment of patients with hemorrhagic shock. Although this determination may seem simple, often it can be quite difficult in certain conditions and environments encountered in the out-of-hospital setting. DOT 4-2.9, 4-2.10

Direct observation of the patient and scene can be helpful in identifying external hemorrhage. An overview of the scene can identify pooled blood or other evidence of external hemorrhage associated with the patient. Depending on the mechanism of injury (e.g., ejected driver involved in a motor vehicle collision), such findings may be far removed from the patient. Also, complete or near-complete exposure is required to rule out external hemorrhage. Brisk, arterial, or pulsatile bleeding can rapidly result in hemorrhagic shock. Methods to control such bleeding will be discussed later.

Internal hemorrhage can be much more elusive, especially with the limitations in the out-of-hospital evaluation process. Many tools used to identify internal hemorrhage, such as nuclear imaging and CT scans, are not available in the prehospital setting, so a high index of suspicion is required.

Injuries to the thorax can easily result in life-threatening hemorrhage. Injuries to the thorax may be identfied during the primary or second survey. Pneumothoraces and other penetrating chest wounds from isolated or multiple rib fractures often have an associated hemothorax. These injuries are typically easy to identify when clothing is removed. Patients who have significant chest deformities will often be hemodynamically unstable because of poor lung mechanics and potentially life-threatening bleeding into the thoracic cavity. Other less subtle findings of simple rib fractures or a small flail segment may go unnoticed if the patient is breathing at a shallow depth and has other injuries. These injuries, if missed on the primary survey can be uncovered in the

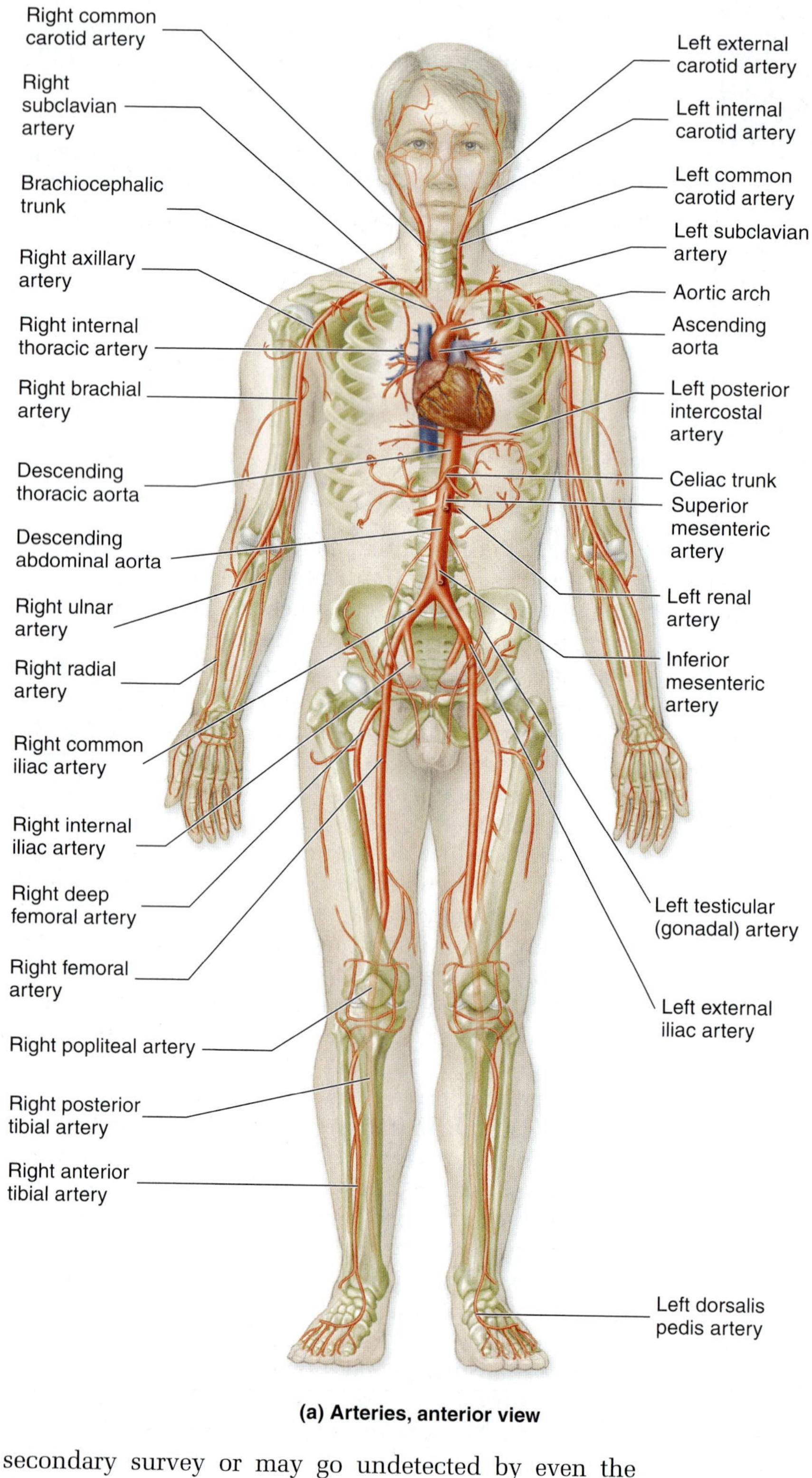

Right common
carotid artery

Right
subclavian
artery

Brachiocephalic
trunk

Right axillary
artery

Right internal
thoracic artery

Right brachial
artery

Descending
thoracic aorta

Descending
abdominal aorta

Right ulnar
artery

Right radial
artery

Right common
iliac artery

Right internal
iliac artery

Right deep
femoral artery

Right femoral
artery

Right popliteal artery

Right posterior
tibial artery

Right anterior
tibial artery

Left external
carotid artery

Left internal
carotid artery

Left common
carotid artery

Left subclavian
artery

Aortic arch

Ascending
aorta

Left posterior
intercostal
artery

Celiac trunk

Superior
mesenteric
artery

Left renal
artery

Inferior
mesenteric
artery

Left testicular
(gonadal) artery

Left external
iliac artery

Left dorsalis
pedis artery

(a) Arteries, anterior view

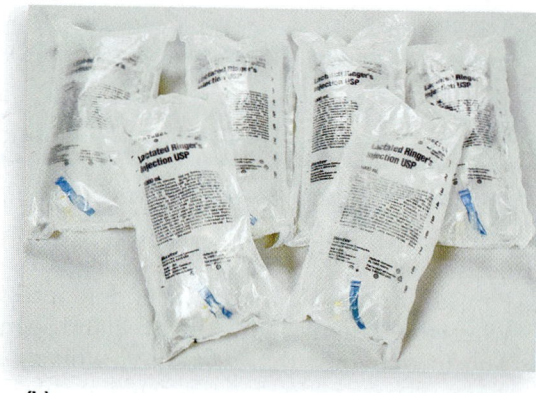

(b)

Figure 19-2   (a) The arterial system. (b) These six liters of IV fluid represent the average volume of blood in an average-sized adult.

hepatic (liver) or splenic (spleen) injury. Ecchymosis over the inferior abdominal wall is associated with intestinal injury. In motor vehicle crashes, this injury is often seen from seat belts and is even called the **seat belt sign.**

Pelvic fractures can cause life-threatening hemorrhage, and significant bleeding should be assumed in any patient that appears to have a pelvic fracture. Bleeding from pelvic fractures can be into the abdominal cavity or into the soft tissues of the pelvis, abdominal wall, back, and perineum.

Degrees of Shock

Classes of hemorrhage are defined based on volume of blood lost (see Figure 19-2 and Table 19-2).[5] These classes are most useful to emphasize the fact that significant blood loss can occur before the patient is symptomatic or changes in hemodynamic parameters are detectable. In summary, Class I hemorrhage describes a patient that is asymptomatic while Class IV hemorrhage applies when the amount of blood volume lost is sufficient to be life-threatening without immediate resuscitation. Classes II and III represent grades of shock along the continuum. DOT 4-2.4

Initial Treatment of Hemorrhage and Hemorrhagic Shock

Recent studies in trauma care have supported treatment of hemorrhagic shock based upon the mechanism of trauma and

secondary survey or may go undetected by even the trauma center team until x-ray, CT scan, or nuclear study is performed.

Abdominal trauma can cause significant internal hemorrhage. An obviously rapidly distending abdomen can be an indication of bleeding into the peritoneal cavity, but there can be more subtle signs. For instance, physical evidence of low, anterior, or lateral rib fractures should suggest the possibility of either

TABLE 19-2 Estimated Fluid and Blood Losses*
Based on Patient's Initial Presentation

	Class I	Class II	Class III	Class IV
Blood loss (mL)	Up to 750	750–1500	1500–2000	>2000
Blood loss (% blood volume)	Up to 15%	15%–30%	30%–40%	>40%
Pulse rate	<100	>100	>120	>140
Blood pressure	Normal	Normal	Decreased	Decreased
Pulse pressure (mmHg)	Normal or increased	Decreased	Decreased	Decreased
Respiratory rate	14–20	20–30	30–40	>35
Urine output (mL/hr)	>30	20–30	5–15	Negligible
CNS/mental status	Slightly anxious	Mildly anxious	Anxious, confused	Confused, lethargic
Fluid replacement (3:1 rule)	Crystalloid	Crystalloid	Crystalloid and blood	Crystalloid and blood

*For a 70-kg man.

The guidelines in Table 2 are based on the "3-for-1" rule. This rule derives from the empiric observation that most patients in hemorrhagic shock require as much as 300 mL of electrolyte solution for each 100 mL of blood loss. Applied blindly, these guidelines can result in excessive or inadequate fluid administration. For example, a patient with a crush injury to the extremity may have hypotension out of proportion to his or her blood loss and requires fluids in excess of the 3:1 guidelines. In contrast, a patient whose ongoing blood loss is being replaced by blood transfusion requires less than 3:1. The use of bolus therapy with careful monitoring of the patient's response can moderate these extremes.

whether the hemorrhage is controllable or uncontrollable in the field. Specifically, it is necessary to determine whether the patient's shock state is secondary to internal (uncontrollable) or external (controllable or uncontrollable) hemorrhage. This differentiation will be important as it determines treatment methods and goals. DOT 4-2.10

Transport Decisions

Immediate transport to a trauma center or suitable hospital is one of the main goals of the out-of-hospital management of trauma victims. The emphasis on timely transport and brief scene times is because expeditious definitive treatment is the most important parameter in determining morbidity and mortality of trauma patients. For instance, patients with signs or symptoms of internal hemorrhage must be assumed to have uncontrollable bleeding. These injuries can only be treated with operative management. Therefore, no delay should occur in transporting these patients to an appropriate facility, optimally a trauma center, to manage their problems.

Treatment Goals

First, the ABCs must be assessed, and any life threats discovered should be quickly treated. Remember, any patient who is believed to be in shock is potentially in a life-threatening state, so rapid transport is indicated. The patient must be immobilized for transport with appropriate spine precautions maintained during any procedures. Hemorrhage must be stopped (or slowed if stopping is not possible), and the treatment of shock must be initiated. DOT 4-2.12, 4-2.13, 4-2.14

The resuscitation of a patient in hemorrhagic shock depends largely upon whether the site of bleeding is controllable or uncontrollable. Finally, regarding the

severely traumatized or unstable patient, no on-scene interventions (beyond attempts to correct ABC life threats) should delay transport.

Prevent Ongoing Blood Loss

If the source of external hemorrhage is identified, the primary goal becomes preventing further loss of blood from the injured tissue, vessel, bone, or the affected area. The duration of ongoing hemorrhage is correlated with increased mortality.[6] Therefore, early intervention to control the bleeding is always indicated.

Bleeding Control with Direct Pressure, Pressure Dressings, and Pressure Points

The most important first step toward hemostasis is the application of direct pressure to the site of the wound (Figure 19-3). There are multiple methods of applying

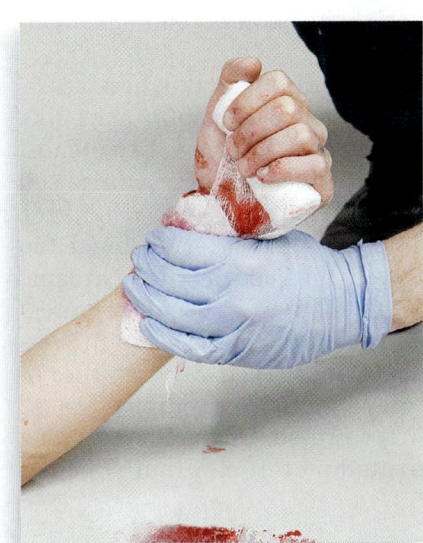

Figure 19-3 Direct pressure is the first method to use to control external bleeding.

BOX 19-5 Dressings and Bandages

Dressings are sterile cotton pads placed directly over a wound that absorb blood and provide a surface on which the blood clot can form. Excessive amounts of dressing material on the wound actually lessen the pressure that is applied to the wound, which results in delays in obtaining hemostasis. **Bandages** are used to provide additional pressure to a wound or to hold the dressing material in place. They do not have to be sterile since they are not in direct contact with the wound.

direct pressure to a wound: direct manual or digital pressure, direct manual or digital pressure over gauze, or the use of pressure dressings to maintain pressure on the site of bleeding. Several studies have attempted to determine which method is most effective.

The most common form of hemostasis is to apply pressure over gauze pads (Box 19-5). This method is often effective. Two recent studies have evaluated the use of direct manual pressure for bleeding from the femoral artery after cardiac catheterization. Although these studies did not investigate situations that would occur in a prehospital setting, the findings are still illustrative of the efficacy of direct manual pressure. One study randomized patients to either the use of direct manual pressure or to the use of one of two devices designed to maintain pressure either by mechanical clamp or pneumatic pressure.[7] Manual pressure was found to be more effective when the time of compression required to control bleeding, patient discomfort, and hematoma size were evaluated. Similarly, another study of postcardiac catheterization patients revealed that manual compression was associated with shorter time to hemostasis when compared to mechanical clamping.[8]

Pressure points are areas of the body where an artery is either lying close to the surface of the skin, like in the neck, or is found directly over a bone, like in most other locations. These are the places where a pulse can be felt when fingertip pressure is applied. When this area is compressed, it pushes the artery against the bone, limiting blood flow to the distal or "downstream" region of that portion of the body. The use of compression at pressure points to stop bleeding is controversial, and there are no data in the medical literature to support its use. If a paramedic is to attempt pressure point compression, direct pressure over the bleeding site should always be attempted first. Finally, use of pressure points can have some negative consequences. For instance, improper compression could occlude venous return but not the arterial supply to the limb, which could worsen bleeding. Also, finding the pulse to compress in a hypotensive patient can be quite difficult. Searching for the pressure point could divert the attention away from the proven treatment of direct compression.

Street Secrets

Sometimes the application and inflation of a BP cuff just proximal to the site of bleeding can provide circumferential pressure (without creating a tourniquet effect) that can allow the flow of blood into the extremity to slow enough that the combination of direct pressure and the BP cuff can stop the bleeding. Do not overinflate the BP cuff; the patient should not complain of numbness, tingling, or pain from the use of the cuff. Also, do not remove the cuff once it is applied.

Although effective, manual pressure to achieve hemostasis does have its limitations. First, the pressure must be maintained at all times until the bleeding is stopped, and stopping the pressure to check if the bleeding has stopped can cause it to resume at a faster rate.

Constant pressure is often difficult to maintain in the prehospital setting, especially when the patient is being moved. Also, depending on the patient's other injuries and condition, it may be difficult to devote one person to maintaining pressure on the site of bleeding. During these situations, pressure dressings can be utilized to maintain pressure on the bleeding site. This can be achieved by applying a small stack of sterile 4 × 4 gauze pads (approximately four to eight, depending on the size and depth of the wound) and wrapping them with an elastic bandage or roller gauze. Two EMS providers are required to perform this skill as one needs to maintain pressure directly on the wound while the second rescuer wraps the bandage. A recent case series reports the efficacy of pressure dressings in achieving hemostasis of wounds considered life-threatening.[9] In some rare circumstances, the bleeding is too brisk or the bleeding site is too large (for example, large, deep bleeding abrasions or degloving injuries) or inaccessible for direct pressure to be effective.

Tourniquets

Despite the use of tourniquets for centuries, their present-day use is controversial. The earliest form of a tourniquet was the "stick and cravat" device, where a circumferential dressing was tied around a stick, and then the stick was turned to tighten the dressing until the bleeding stopped. Once hemostasis was attained, the stick was secured in place.

With **tourniquets,** blood loss is stopped by compressing the artery proximal to the bleeding wound. Tourniquets that are commonly used today employ either a ratchet system, pneumatic bladder, or strapping system to apply compressive force to the extremity (Figure 19-4). Recently, a retrospective analysis of 550 patients treated for hemorrhage outside the hospital was performed.[10] This study found that 91 patients (16%) had tourniquets applied, and 78% were effective in controlling hemorrhage. Further analysis revealed that upper extremity bleeding was controlled better with tourniquets than bleeding from the lower extremities.

Another study published interesting and conflicting results when it examined a group of patients injured while clearing land mines after the first Iraq War.[11] This is a retrospective study of 68 patients with traumatic amputations. The first 18 patients were treated with tourniquets; however, clinicians realized that the tourniquets were not effectively controlling bleeding. Subsequently, only compression dressings were used on the next 50 patients. The study found that mortality rates were improved (3/18 versus 1/50), and less blood loss was observed (initial hemoglobin 8.6 g/dl versus 10.5 g/dl). Therefore, the conclusion was made that compressive dressings are more effective.

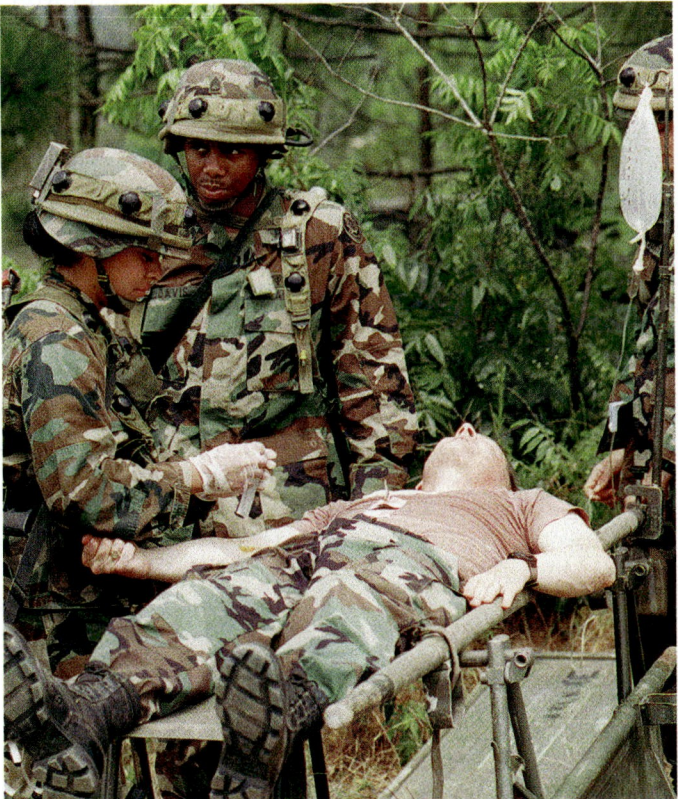

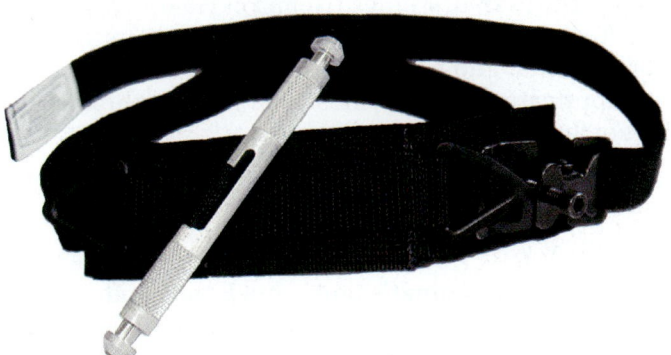

Figure 19-4 This style of tourniquet is currently in use by the military. Reports from the field indicate there are varying degrees of success with the use of tourniquets.

Working in the Gray Zone

In the prehospital setting, blood loss is measured by estimation only and a few studies have shown that EMS providers are not very accurate in their assessments of blood loss. Fortunately, shock is treated as potentially life-threatening, and management is aggressive, regardless of the estimated loss. In the hospital setting, blood loss is quantified by measuring the hemoglobin levels of the patient. Normal values for hemoglobin are established by weight and sex. The hemoglobin level of the patient is compared with their normal expected value, and a more accurate assessment of actual lost volume is made.

Another group of physicians acknowledge that there is still significant controversy and many unanswered questions regarding the use of tourniquets, but they conclude that clinicians can rely on several simple guidelines.[12] First, tourniquets are effective and lifesaving in certain situations. Second, bleeding can reoccur if the tourniquet is released. Third, repair of the injured limb or vessel (salvage procedures) can be attempted two to six hours after tourniquet application. Finally, amputation should be performed (prior to release of the tourniquet) of any limb to which a tourniquet has been applied for more than six hours.

Although few will argue with the efficacy of tourniquets for controlling hemorrhage, often the complications are significant. Several reports describe both permanent and transient nerve palsies resulting from the use of tourniquets in the operating room.[13,14,15] Also, pathophysiologic effects and complications after the release of tourniquets have recently been described.[16] Tourniquet application leads to decreased blood flow and eventual necrosis or death of all tissues distal to the tourniquet. These processes cause inflammation and the release of cellular contents that can circulate throughout the body once the tourniquet is removed, causing metabolic derangements. Therefore, the use of tourniquets should be reserved for truly life-threatening extremity bleeding that persists despite all other efforts.

Hemostatic Devices and Agents

A recent advancement in the treatment of hemorrhage has been the development of agents and devices that are easily stored, transported, and applied to wounds to stop ongoing bleeding. Several of these agents are currently on the market and available for use out-of-hospital (Figure 19-5).

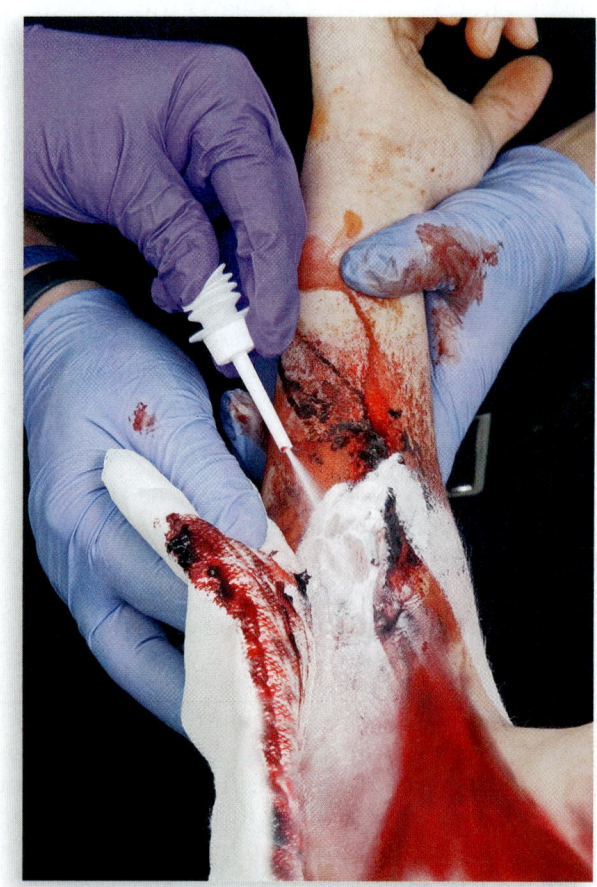

Figure 19-5 TraumaDex™ (shown above), HemCon™, and QuikClot™ are additional blood control agents that are showing varying degrees of success. Additional research is needed to determine when and if they are useful.

A microporous polysaccharide hemosphere (MPH) compound is sold as TraumaDEX™ (Medafor, Inc., Minneapolis, MN). This agent absorbs water and other inactive substances in blood, which then concentrates the clotting factors that are present in the wound.[17] TraumaDEX™ is a powder that is poured into the wound from a small, single-use, plastic cylinder. TraumaDEX™ has been shown to be effective in treating minor or moderate bleeding.[18] One unpublished study also found that TraumaDEX™ effectively stopped bleeding of superficial skin wounds on healthy volunteers.[19]

Mineral zeolite powder (sold as QuikClot™, Z-Medica, Newington, CT) functions similarly to MPH since it absorbs water and concentrates clotting factors at the wound to stop bleeding.[17] QuikClot™ is inert and nonallergenic, but the absorption of water can elevate the local temperature to 42 to 44°C which is several degrees above the normal body temperature of 37°C.[20] QuikClot™ is also a powder that is poured directly on the wound from a single-use envelope. QuikClot™ has been issued to U.S. Navy corpsmen serving in Iraq since 2003.[17] Anecdotal reports of battlefield use have indicated that QuikClot™ is not effective, but one author found that QuikClot™ decreased hemorrhage in an animal model with a lethal groin injury.[17,20] Future studies are needed to support or refute the efficacy of this agent.

Chitin, an algae-derived polysaccharide biopolymer, and **chitosan,** a closely related product to chitin, have been used to manufacture dressings designed to limit bleeding.[17] These substances are believed to attract cells necessary for the clotting process and cause vasoconstriction in the affected vessels.[21] Chitin dressings appear to be effective for minor to moderate bleeding, but evidence supporting its use for severe bleeding is varied.[22,23,24,25] Chitosan dressings have been found to be more effective than chitin dressings for increasing survival and decreasing blood loss of severe hemorrhage.[26] The United States Army has issued chitosan dressings (HemCon Hemorrhage Control Technologies, Lake Oswego, OR) to its Special Forces units, and anecdotal reports indicate successful application and hemostasis for life-threatening hemorrhage.[17]

Pneumatic Anti-Shock Garment (PASG) or Military Anti-Shock Trousers (MAST)

The modern **pneumatic anti-shock garment (PASG)** was used extensively during the Vietnam War; subsequently physicians and surgeons quickly began using the device to treat hemorrhagic shock in civilians (Figure 19-6). Since that time, the indications for and the effectiveness of the device have been repeatedly debated. DOT 4-2.39, 4-2.40, 4-2.41

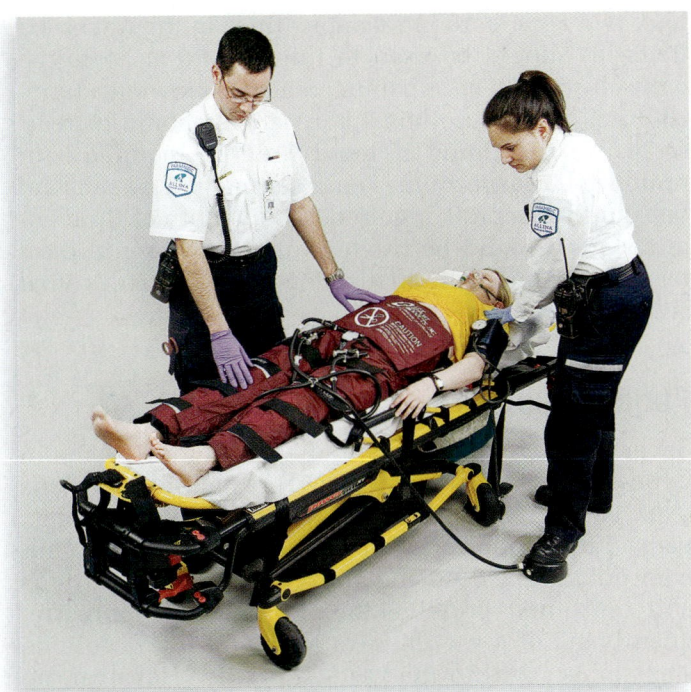

Figure 19-6   The use of the PASG (MAST) device is controversial.

The PASG functions by three different but often simultaneous mechanisms. First, application of the PASG causes vascular compression that mimics an increase in peripheral vascular resistance.[27] Secondly, the PASG can tamponade (compress and control) active external hemorrhage if the device overlies the site of hemorrhage.[28] Finally, the PASG can stabilize pelvic fractures, thus limiting further blood loss.[29]

Although many studies have been performed to evaluate the use of the PASG, none are conclusive. Specifically, two studies of trauma patients found no difference in condition upon arrival or survival between groups of patients treated with or without the PASG.[30,31] One study, however, did indicate that survival was greater for severely hypotensive patients treated with the PASG.[32] Importantly, at least two studies have shown that use of the PASG can increase mortality, especially for patients with thoracic trauma.[33,34] These findings are also supported by animal studies which found that if the PASG was inflated directly over the site of bleeding (i.e., pelvis and abdomen), there was improved survival. However, if the source of hemorrhage was in the chest, survival was decreased.[35]

Overall, based on a review of current literature, the following guidelines can be made.[35] Applying the PASG to patients with hemorrhagic shock can be harmful if the source of bleeding is in the thorax. In a hypotensive patient with abdominal trauma, the PASG may be of benefit. Finally, the PASG has the greatest potential in those patients with severe hypotension (unobtainable by BP assessment or with a thready pulse). In 1997, the National Association of EMS Physicians published a position paper reflecting these findings.[36] **Skill Sheet 81: MAST/PASG Application describes the application of this garment.**

Correct placement of the device is necessary for optimal effect. The upper edge of the PASG should be at the level of the last rib. The garment should be wrapped so that there is maximum Velcro™ to Velcro™ contact, which means that the uninflated garment may appear loose on some patients. This is important, however, as a lot of pressure is placed on the Velcro™ closures when the garment is inflated, and slippage of contact could occur if it is not wrapped correctly.

Once correct placement of the PASG is confirmed, inflation can begin. The leg compartments may be inflated first or simultaneously with the abdominal compartment. The abdominal compartment alone must never be inflated prior to the leg compartments as venous pooling in the legs can occur.

The compartments should be inflated to a level that results in an improved blood pressure. Each compartment has a manometer to monitor the pressure applied by the PASG, and the valves will vent when excessive pressures occur. Compartment pressures greater than 80–100 mmHg should be avoided, and venting often results when pressures reach 110 mmHg.[35]

During long transports, environmental effects can result in alteration of the compartment pressures.[35] For instance, increased temperature will cause an increased pressure within the compartments. Also, decreased atmospheric pressure can cause increased compartment pressures. Although most civilian air medical transports occur at an altitude that is not associated with a marked fall in atmospheric pressure, this property needs to be considered during high altitude aeromedical transports. The patient's vital signs and compartment pressure need to be monitored continuously during transport.

Deflation of the PASG can cause significant hypotension and should therefore be avoided in the out-of-hospital setting. Ideally, the PASG is only deflated when definitive treatment can be provided (i.e., surgical repair of the bleeding source). However, prolonged inflation of the PASG is not without consequences. Ischemia of the lower extremities and even compartment syndrome associated with the use of the PASG has been reported.[37]

Volume Resuscitation

The key to adequate and appropriate volume resuscitation in trauma patients is to approach these patients as a heterogeneous group instead of attempting to apply a single treatment to all.[38] To accomplish this, the prehospital provider needs to answer three questions: Is the hemorrhage controllable or uncontrollable? What is the mechanism of injury (blunt or penetrating trauma)? Is the patient in shock or showing signs of hypotension?

DOT 4-2.11, 4-2.28, 4-2.37

The State of Hemorrhage Control

If bleeding is controlled, volume resuscitation is recommended if there is evidence of shock (altered mental status, hypotension, or poor peripheral perfusion).[38] Fluid should be administered in small boluses to a total volume that reverses the signs of shock. If hemorrhage is not controllable, the only measure to take is rapid transport while continued efforts are made to control the bleeding.

The Implications of the MOI

The recommendations for volume resuscitation of uncontrolled hemorrhage depend on the mechanism. For patients with continuing uncontrollable bleeding, you must determine the mechanism of injury. A large study of hypotensive patients resulting from penetrating torso injury found that those treated with aggressive volume resuscitation prior to operative intervention had a higher mortality and complication rate as compared to patients who were given their fluid resuscitation at the time of surgical repair.[39]

The proposed mechanisms for these results are that increased blood pressure results in more brisk bleeding, dislodgment of newly formed blood clots, and dilution of clotting factors in circulation.[38,39,40] Therefore, the current recommendation is to obtain intravenous access and administer fluids at low maintenance rate or **KVO,** which stands for **"keep the vein open."** In the event that the patient becomes unstable and is approaching circulatory arrest, volume resuscitation can be attempted but is unlikely to provide much benefit.[38]

The Degree of Shock

There is no compelling evidence to support aggressive fluid resuscitation in shock patients; however, the recommendation for volume resuscitation to reverse the signs of trauma still stands.[38] Paramedics must resist over-resuscitation in trauma patients to avoid causing pulmonary edema, which can increase the patient's mortality. Conversely, in patients with suspected head trauma, it is especially important to support their blood pressure with fluids as necessary to provide adequate cerebral perfusion. In the setting of profound volume loss, two large-bore intravenous lines in the upper extremities should be used to infuse fluid at an initial bolus dose of 20 mL/kg. Immediately following administration of the fluid bolus, the patient should be reassessed to determine if more fluid is required. For prolonged transport times or in settings where substantial fluid infusion is required, the quantity of fluid administered should be titrated to the patient's clinical response, namely, normalization of the patient's vital signs. DOT 4-2.11

Fluid Selection

Several intravenous fluids can be used for patients in hypovolemic shock, including crystalloid solutions (e.g., saline, lactated ringers), blood products (e.g., packed red blood cells), or blood substitutes (e.g., human polymerized hemoglobin).[41,42] Colloid solutions and the blood protein albumin are used more frequently in Europe with the rationale that more volume stays longer within the vasculature.[43,44] However, no definitive research has demonstrated superiority of one resuscitative fluid over another, and because isotonic crystalloid solutions are the only fluid type routinely carried on ambulances, initial intravascular volume replacement should be performed with isotonic saline or lactated ringer's solution.[45,46,47] Since crystalloid fluid is inexpensive, nonantigenic, and readily available, it will likely remain the mainstay of therapy in the United States for the foreseeable future.

CONNECTIONS Chapter 20: Head, Face, and Neck Trauma discusses fluid resuscitation guidelines for patients with brain injuries.

Special Considerations for Fluid Resuscitation

For a patient with existing cardiac and respiratory disease, or if the patient has any disease process that requires fluid restriction (for example a dialysis patient), the patient should receive the bolus of fluid in several divided doses with continuous evaluation of the vital signs and clinical response during the treatment. For example, if the patient weighs 75 kg, at 20 mL/kg, the total dose of normal saline to infuse is 1500 mL (or 1.5 liters). The patient should receive 250–500 mL infused over 5–10 minutes, then the vital signs should be reassessed and 250–500 mL more can be given until vital signs improve or evidence of respiratory distress or pulmonary edema begin to develop. Early access to on-line medical direction is appropriate for these patients.

Summary

Hemorrhage and shock caused by trauma is a situation that all paramedics will treat during their careers. Although definitive treatment often requires surgical intervention, several interventions are effective and can be delivered in the out-of-hospital setting. The treatment of shock is an evolving science, and attention must be paid as treatment modalities are updated to reflect newer recommendations in patient management.

Notes

1. E. P. Rivers, R. M. Otero, and H. B. Nguyen, "Approach to the Patient in Shock," in J. E. Tintinalli, G. D. Kelen, and J. S. Stapczynski, *Emergency Medicine: A Comprehensive Study Guide* (New York: McGraw-Hill, 2004).

2. F. C. Brunicardi, D. K. Andersen, T. R. Billiar, D. L. Dunn, J. G. Hunter, J. B. Matthews, R. E. Pollock, and S. I. Schwartz, "Chapter 2: Fluid and Electrolyte Management of the Surgical Patient." *Schwartz's Principles of Surgery,* 8th ed. McGraw-Hill's AccessMedicine (accessed August 23, 2006).

3. M. A. Papadikis and S. J. McPhee, eds., "Chapter 42: Fluid, Electrolyte, and Acid-Base Emergencies." *2006 Current Consult: Medicine.* McGraw-Hill's AccessMedicine, Quick Access (accessed August 23, 2006).

4. G. T. Shires, P. C. Canizaro, and C. J. Carrico, "Shock," in S. I. Schwartz, G. T. Shires, F. C. Spence, and E. H. Storer, *Principles of Surgery* (New York: McGraw-Hill Books, 1979).

5. American College of Surgeons Committee on Trauma, *Advance Trauma Life Support for Doctors-Student Manual,* 6th ed. (Chicago: American College of Surgeons, 1997).

6. G. Regel, M. Stalp, and U. Lehmann, et al., "Prehospital Care, Importance of Early Intervention on Outcome," *Acta Anaesthesiologica Scandinavica* 110 (1997): 71–76.

7. K. G. Lehmann, S. J. Heath-Lange, et al., "Randomized Comparison of Hemostasis Techniques After Invasive Cardiovascular Procedures," *American Heart Journal* 138(6) (1999): 1118–1125.

8. A. Simon, B. Bumgarner, et al., "Manual Versus Mechanical Compression for Femoral Artery Hemostasis After Cardiac Catheterization," *American Journal of Critical Care* 7(4)(1998): 308–313.

9. S. A. Naimer and F. Chemla, "Elastic Adhesive Dressing Treatment of Bleeding Wounds in Trauma Victims," *American Journal of Emergency Medicine* 18(7)(2000): 816–819.

10. D. Lakstein, A. Blumenfeld, et al., "Tourniquets for Hemorrhage Control on the Battlefield: A 4-Year Accumulated Experience," *Journal of Trauma* 54(5Suppl) (2003): S221–225.

11. J. Pillgram-Larsen and S. Mellesmo, "[Not a Tourniquet but a Compressive Dressing. Experience From 68 Traumatic Amputations After Injuries From Mines]," *Tidsskrift for Den Norske Laegeforening,* 112(17)(1992): 2188–2190.

12. J. Navein, R. Coupland, et al., "The Tourniquet Controversy," *Journal of Trauma* 54 (5Suppl) (2003): S219–220.

13. I. D. Kornbluth, M. K. Freedman, et al., "Femoral, Saphenous Nerve Palsy After Tourniquet Use, a Case Report," *Archives of Physical Medicine and Rehabilitation* 84(6) (2003): 909–911.

14. A. Landi, A. Saracino, et al., "Tourniquet Paralysis in Microsurgery," *Annals of the Academy of Medicine Singapore* 24(4Suppl)(1995): 89–93.

15. E. Savvidis and K. Parsch, "[Prolonged Transitory Paralysis After Pneumatic Tourniquet Use on the Upper Arm]," *Unfallchirurg* 102(2)(1999): 141–144.

16. A. Wakai, J. H. Wang, et al., "Tourniquet-Induced Systemic Inflammatory Response in Extremity Surgery," *Journal of Trauma* 51(5)(2001): 922–926.

17. K. King, "Hemostatic Dressings for the First Responder: A Review," *Military Medicine* 169(9)(2004): 716–720.

18. F. Murat, M. Ereth, et al., "Evaluation of Microporous Polysaccharide Hemospheres as a Novel Hemostatic Agent in Open Partial Nephrectomy: Favorable Experimental Results in the Porcine Model," *Journal of Urology* 172(3)(2004): 1119–1122.

19. M. Ereth, Y. Dong, et al., "Microporous Polysaccharide Hemospheres Provides Effective Topical Hemostasis in a Human Modified Bleeding Time Incision Model," Annual Meeting of the American Society of Anesthesiology, September 2002. http://www.nataonline.com (accessed July 2003).

20. H. Alam, G. Uy, et al., "Comparative Analysis of Hemostatic Agents in a Swine Model of Lethal Groin Injury," *Journal of Trauma* 54 (2003): 1077–1082.

21. Y. Ikeda, L. H. Young, et al., "Vascular Effects of Poly-N-Acetyl-Glucosamine in Isolated Rat Aortic Rings," *Journal of Surgical Research* 102 (2002): 215–220.

22. D. Kulling, J. N. Vournakis, et al., "Endoscopic Injection of Bleeding Esophageal Varices with Poly-N-Acetyl Glucosamine Gel Formulation in the Canine Portal Hypertension Model," *Gastrointestinal Endoscopy* 49 (1999): 764–771.

23. D. J. Cole, R. J. Connolly, et al., "A Pilot Study Evaluation of the Efficacy of a Fully Acetylated Poly-N-Acetylglucosamine Membrane Formulation as a Topical Hemostatic Agent," *Journal of Surgery* 126 (1999): 510–517.

24. M. W. Chan, S. D. Schwaitzber, et al., "Comparison of Poly-N-Acetylglucosamine with Absorbable Collagen and Fibrin Sealant for Achieving Hemostasis in a Swine Model of Splenic Hemorrhage," *Journal of Trauma* 48 (2000): 454–458.

25. A. E. Pusateri, H. E. Modrow, et al., "Advanced Hemostatic Dressing Development Program: Animal Model Selection Criteria and Results of a Study of Nine Hemostatic Dressings in a Model of Severe Large Venous Hemorrhage and Hepatic Injury in Swine," *Journal of Trauma* 55 (2003): 518–526.

26. A. E. Pusateri, S. J. McCarthy, et al., "Effect of a Chitosan-Based Hemostatic Dressing on Blood Loss and Survival in a Model of Severe Venous Hemorrhage and Hepatic Injury in Swine," *Journal of Trauma* 55 (2003): 177–182.

27. J. Ali and K. Duke, "Timing and Interpretation of the Hemodynamic Effects of the Pneumatic Anti-Shock Garment," *Annals of Emergency Medicine* 20 (1991): 1183–1187.

28. S. L. Wangensteen, R. M. Ludewig, et al., "The Effect of External Counterpressure on Arterial Bleeding," *Surgery* 64 (1968): 922–927.

29. L. M. Flint, A. Brown, et al., "Definitive Control of Bleeding from Severe Pelvic Fractures," *Annals of Surgery* 189 (1979): 709–716.

30. W. H. Bickell, P. E. Pepe, et al., "Effect of Anti-Shock Trousers on the Trauma Score: a Prospective Analysis in the Urban Setting," *Annals of Emergency Medicine* 14 (1985): 218–222.

31. W. H. Bickell, P. E. Pepe, et al., "Randomized trial of Pneumatic Anti-Shock Garments in the Prehospital Management of Penetrating Abdominal Injuries," *Annals of Emergency Medicine* 16 (1987): 653–658.

32. C. G. Cayten, G. M. Berendt, et al., "A Study of Pneumatic Anti-Shock Garments in Severely Hypotensive Trauma Patients," *Journal of Trauma* 34 (1993): 728–735.

33. K. L. Mattox, W. H. Bickell, et al., "Prospective Randomized Evaluation of Anti-Shock MAST in Post-Traumatic Hypotension," *Journal of Trauma* 26 (1986): 779–786.

34. B. Honigman, S. R. Lowenstein, et al., "The Role of the Pneumatic Anti-Shock Garment in Penetrating Cardiac Wounds," *Journal of the American Medical Association* 266 (1991): 2398–2401.

35. R. E. O'Connor and R. M. Domeier, "An Evaluation of the Pneumatic Anti-Shock Garment (PASG) in Various Clinical Settings," *Prehospital Emergency Care* 1(1) (1997): 36–44.

36. R. M. Domeier, R. E. O'Connor, et al., "Use of the Pneumatic Anti-Shock Garment (PASG)," *Prehospital Emergency Care* 1(1) (1997): 32–35.

37. C. Chisolm and D. Clark, "Effect of the Pneumatic Anti-Shock Garment on Intramuscular Pressure," *Annals of Emergency Medicine* 13 (1984): 581–587.

38. P. E. Pepe, V. N. Mosesso, and J. L. Falk, "Prehospital Fluid Resuscitation of the Patient with Major Trauma," *Prehospital Emergency Care* 6 (2002): 81–91.

39. W. H. Bickell, M. J. Wall, et al., "Immediate Versus Delayed Fluid Resuscitation for Hypotensive Patients with Penetrating Torso Injuries," *New England Journal of Medicine* 331 (1994): 1105–1109.

40. W. H. Bickell, S. P. Bruttig, et al., "The Detrimental Effects of Intravenous Crystalloid after Aortotomy in Swine," *Surgery* 110 (1991): 529–536.

41. S. A. Gould, E. E. Moore, D. B. Hoyt, et al., "The First Randomized Trial of Human Polymerized Hemoglobin as a Blood Substitute in Acute Trauma and Emergent Surgery," *Journal of the American College of Surgeons* 187 (1998): 113–120.

42. F. A. Moore, B. A. McKinley, and E. E. Moore, "The Next Generation in Shock Resuscitation," *Lancet* 363 (2004): 1988–1996.

43. I. Roberts, "Human Albumin Administration in Critically Ill Patients," *British Medical Journal* 317 (1998): 235–240.

44. D. Cook and G. Guyatt, "Colloid Use for Fluid Resuscitation: Evidence and Spin," *Annals of Internal Medicine,* 135 (2001): 205–208.

45. M. M. Kraus, Y. Horn, and D. Gross, "The Combined Effect of Small Volume Hypertonic Saline and Normal Saline Solutions in Uncontrolled Hemorrhagic Shock," *Surgery, Gynecology & Obstetrics* 174 (1992): 363–368.

46. O. Chiara, P. Pelosi, L. Brazzi, et al., "Resuscitation from Hemorrhagic Shock: Experimental Model Comparing Normal Saline, Dextran, and Hypertonic Saline Solutions," *Critical Care Medicine* 31 (2003): 1915–1922.

47. M. M. Kraus, "Controversies in Shock Research: Hypertonic Resuscitation—Pros and Cons," *Shock* 3 (1995): 69–72.

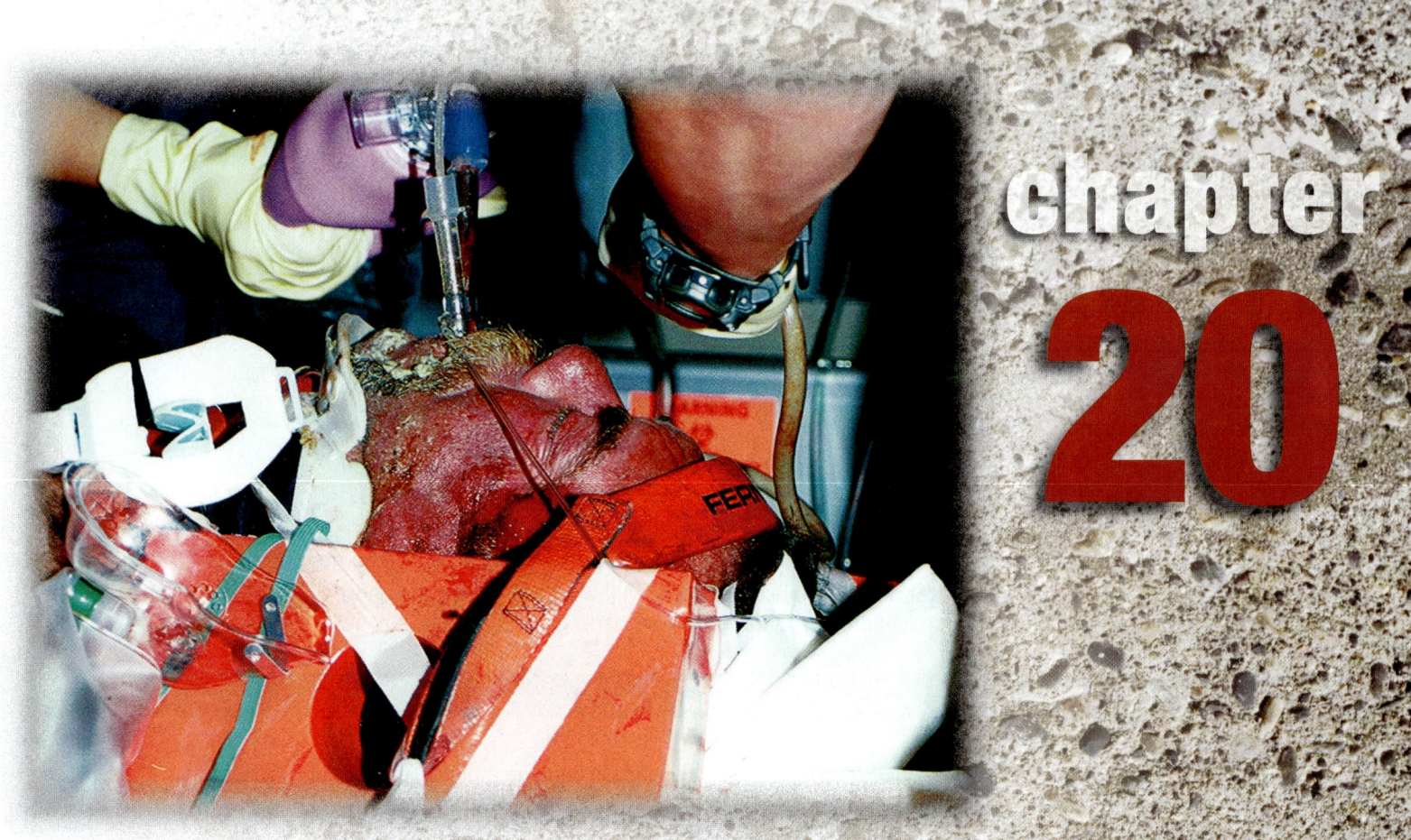

Head, Face, and Neck Trauma

"**E**stimated amount of glucose used by an adult human brain each day, expressed in M&Ms: 250."

—*Harper's Index,* October 1989

Need to Know

▶ Traumatic brain injury (TBI) is one of the leading causes of death and disability in the United States.

▶ Suspect a spinal injury any time a patient presents with a head injury, and take appropriate cervical precautions as necessary.

▶ Head injuries have a wide range of severity. Objective evidence of severe injuries includes decreased level of consciousness, abnormal flexion or extension of limbs (posturing), unequal pupils, extreme hypertension or hypotension, and respiratory depression.

▶ The Glasgow Coma Scale (GCS) is an important tool for assessing the severity of traumatic brain injuries.

▶ Appropriate field management of an individual with traumatic brain injury is critical. Oxygenation, ventilation, and prevention and treatment of low blood pressure and low pulse oximetry readings are critical to prevent secondary brain injuries.

▶ Assessment of the patient that is impaired due to mood-altering substances (such as alcohol or drugs) may be very difficult. The use of alcohol and drugs may also increase the possibility of brain injury. Alcohol- or drug-intoxicated patients, even those who think they are not injured severely, should be evaluated in the emergency department or trauma center.

▶ Facial injuries and bleeding can cause significant airway compromise, and patients can rapidly decompensate.

▶ The neck is full of important vessels (carotid and vertebral arteries and the jugular veins), the esophagus, and trachea, which, due to their vulnerable anatomy, can be easily injured.

▶ Sick	▶ Not Yet Sick

• Hypertension in the face of a traumatic brain injury (TBI) indicates the TBI is worsening because the intracranial pressure (ICP) is rising.
• Hypotension in the face of a severe TBI is an ominous finding. Maintain systolic BP > 90 mmHg.
• Treat pain and nausea as both can raise ICP.
• Herniation is suspected when the following triad of signs are noted:
  • Unilaterial OR bilateral fixed and dilated pupils and unresponsive to light (also known as blown pupils)
  • Patient is unconscious and unresponsive to painful stimuli
  • Patient is showing decerebrate posturing OR has flaccid paralysis
• If an eye injury is present, bandage and protect both eyes.
• Consider the psychological impact from soft tissue injuries to the face.
• Administer enough IV fluid to keep the blood pressure > 90.
	• Check blood sugar to make sure hypo- or hyperglycemia is not complicating the problem.
	• Assess a SAMPLE history and determine what impact medications or past history have on traumatic injuries.
	• Perform a cranial nerve assessment as time permits.
	• Assess oxygenation and ventilation status and make corrections as appropriate to keep the pulse oximeter reading above 95%.
	• Protect the airway and titrate ventilations as appropriate. Use ETCO$_2$ and pulse oximetry monitoring when available.
	• Prepare for TBI patients to be combative and for complications from emesis.
	• Practice the GCS score often so you become very familiar with it. A GCS score can be taken on every patient until you are confident in using it.

Introduction

Brain injury is the most common cause of traumatic death and disability. Two types of brain injuries occur: primary and secondary. The primary brain injury is often preventable with the use of safety equipment and practices. EMS has a role in prevention activities as EMS providers promote safety in general and safe practices in driving, sports recreation activities, and fall prevention in the elderly. Secondary brain injuries occur following the primary injury if the patient becomes hypotensive or hypoxic. Education of EMS providers as to the nature of the TBI (traumatic brain injury) and prevention strategies has the potential to drastically reduce the number and severity of secondary injuries occurring in the prehospital setting.

Other injuries to the head occur besides TBI. The soft tissues and relatively thin bones of the face can easily be damaged with trauma. The neck, mouth, and airway are vulnerable to both blunt and penetrating trauma with edema and foreign bodies (including blood) causing obstruction and affecting breathing. The nose may be injured and may compromise the airway in the process. The eyes are vulnerable to injury as well when the actual globe is penetrated, the surface is scratched, or a foreign body is embedded. The bony structure supporting the eye in the skull is vulnerable to fracture as well. The soft tissues of the ear can be avulsed and the delicate ear canal, inner ear, and tympanic membrane (eardrum) can be damaged by penetrating trauma or blast waves during explosions.

This chapter explores the injuries that can occur to the brain, face, and skull as a result of blunt or penetrating trauma. **Skill sheets that pertain to this chapter include Skill Sheet 1: Airway Positioning and Maneuvers (also see Step-by-Step 1); Skill Sheet 8: ALS Airway Adjuncts; Skill Sheet 19: Needle Cricothyroidotomy (also see Step-by-Step 19); Skill Sheet 28: Nystagmus Assessment; Skill Sheet 31: Trauma Scoring (includes Glasgow Coma Scale); Skill Sheet 66: Bleeding Control and Shock (also see Step-by-Step 66); Skill Sheet 68: Seated Spinal Immobilization (also see Step-by-Step 68); Skill Sheet 69: Standing Spinal Immobilization; Skill Sheet 70: Supine Spinal Immobilization (also see Step-by-Step 70); Skill Sheet 71: Helmet Removal (also see Step-by-Step 71); Skill Sheet 76: Traumatic Brain Injury Assessment; Skill Sheet 80: Eye Irrigation; Skill Sheet 83: NREMT Patient Assessment Trauma; Skill Sheet 92: NREMT Spinal Immobilization (Seated Patient); and Skill Sheet 93: NREMT Spinal Immobilization (Supine Patient).**

Head Trauma

Traumatic brain injury (TBI) is a term that specifically refers to injury of the brain as opposed to that of the external structures of the head and will be the term used to describe conditions of brain injury in this chapter. Traumatic brain injuries are a common cause of disability and death in the United States.[1] The scope of traumatic brain injury varies from minor to severe, and the clinical presentation of these injuries can vary over time as the injury evolves. DOT 4-5.35, 4-5.38

TBI is somewhat unique in that it involves two components of injury: one that the paramedic can do nothing about (except of course to work toward preventive measures), *primary injury;* and the other that it is critical to do something to prevent, *secondary injury.* Primary injuries occur at the time of impact and result from bruising, bleeding, or shearing of the brain. Secondary injuries are potentially preventable and treatable problems such as hypotension or hypoxia, which can lead to additional brain injury if not prevented, treated, or reversed immediately when detected.[2]

Paramedics have a unique role in the treatment and management of TBI patients, as outcomes are based on prompt recognition of the primary injuries and prevention of secondary injuries. Appropriate initial management of these patients is critical to TBI survival and minimizing long-term disability.

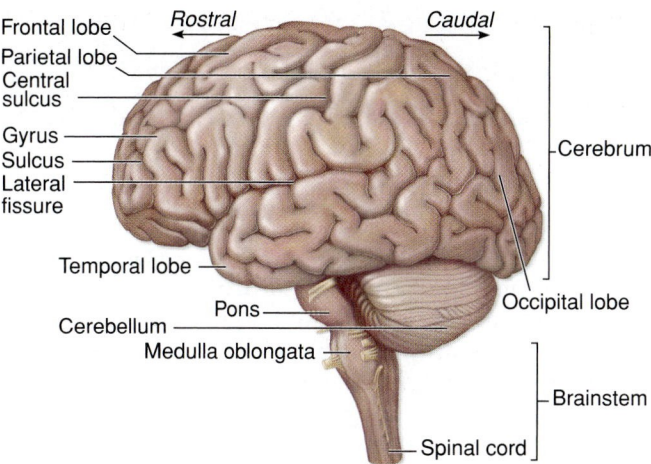

Figure 20-1 The anatomy of the brain. The three main parts are the cerebrum, the cerebellum, and the brainstem.

Epidemiology

There are approximately 1.5 million traumatic brain injuries in the United States each year. Of these, it is estimated that one million patients will be evaluated and released from the emergency department; 230,000 will be admitted to the hospital; and 50,000 people will die. An additional 70,000–90,000 people will be left with permanent neurologic disability.[3]

TBI is common at any age but is more frequent in adolescents and young adults, and those older than 75. Men are twice as likely to sustain a TBI as women. The leading causes of TBI in the United States are motor vehicle collisions, followed by acts of violence and falls. Firearms are the primary cause of death from TBI.[4] DOT 4-5.35

Anatomy and Physiology of the Brain

The brain is encased in the skull and is somewhat free-floating within the surrounding cerebrospinal fluid. The brain has three coverings: the inner covering that is basically adhered to the brain itself (pia mater), a middle covering (arachnoid mater) under and around which run a network of small arteries and veins, and the outer covering (dura mater) that is located against the skull and under which lies a large system of bridging veins. The brain is constantly bathed in an electrolyte-rich fluid called **cerebrospinal fluid (CSF)** that runs underneath the arachnoid layer.

The brain itself can most simply be divided into three parts: the cerebrum, cerebellum, and brainstem (Figure 20-1). The **brainstem** is the lower extension of the brain that connects to the spinal cord. It is responsible for the basic functions of survival (breathing, blood pressure) and arousal. It is also the pathway through which all tracts relaying information from the brain to the spinal cord must run. Most **cranial nerves**

BOX 20-1   Areas of the Brain and What Each Controls

Frontal lobe → Personality
Parietal lobe → Motor and sensory function
Temporal lobe → Speech
Occipital lobe → Sight
Cerebellum → Fine motor coordination
Hypothalamus → Endocrine function
Reticular activating system → Consciousness
Medulla → Respiratory and cardiac function

Nice to Know

Mean arterial pressure (MAP) is the best reflection of true blood pressure, and is calculated as 1/3 systolic blood pressure + 2/3 diastolic blood pressure
 Intracranial pressure (ICP) is the amount of pressure within the skull. Normal ICP is <15 mmHg.[6]
 Cerebral perfusion pressure (CPP) is the pressure needed to maintain blood flow to the brain and is defined as the MAP minus the intracranial pressure (ICP). The minimum CPP for normal function is 70 mmHg.

also originate in the brainstem. The **cerebellum** is located in the back of the brain and is responsible for coordination of movement and balance. The **cerebrum** is the upper brain and is responsible for higher functioning. It is further broken up into anatomic lobes, all of which are responsible for different functions such as motor, sensory, visual, and memory (Box 20-1). DOT 4-5.36

The brain has a very high metabolism rate in comparison to other organs in the body. It consumes 20% of total body oxygen and 25% of total body glucose, which is impressive considering it accounts for less than 2% of total body weight. Ninety-five percent of the brain's function requires aerobic (oxygen requiring) metabolism.[5] The body is able to maintain this high metabolic rate in the brain by sensing and regulating the blood flow to the brain in spite of fluctuating whole body blood pressure via a process called autoregulation. This maintains a relatively constant **cerebral perfusion pressure (CPP).** Blood flow to the brain is shown in Figure 20-2.

When the brain is injured, there is a risk of increasing the **intracranial pressure (ICP).** Within the skull there are three main components that influence ICP: blood, brain, and CSF. Not surprisingly, there is not much room for expansion within the skull, since the skull is a compartment with a fixed amount of space. If there is an increase in size of any one of the components of ICP, the others will need to give up their place. Cerebral edema is a common cause of increased ICP in TBI patients. Edema is caused by leaky cell membranes from damaged cells within the brain. ICP is also increased with any type of hemorrhage into or around the brain.[7] DOT 4-5.39, 4-5.40

As ICP increases, CSF is displaced initially into the spinal canal. If the ICP continues to rise, the brain itself will begin to be squeezed. Since the tissue of the brain is spongy, this can be tolerated to a point. Beyond this point, the tissues of the brain will begin to be damaged.

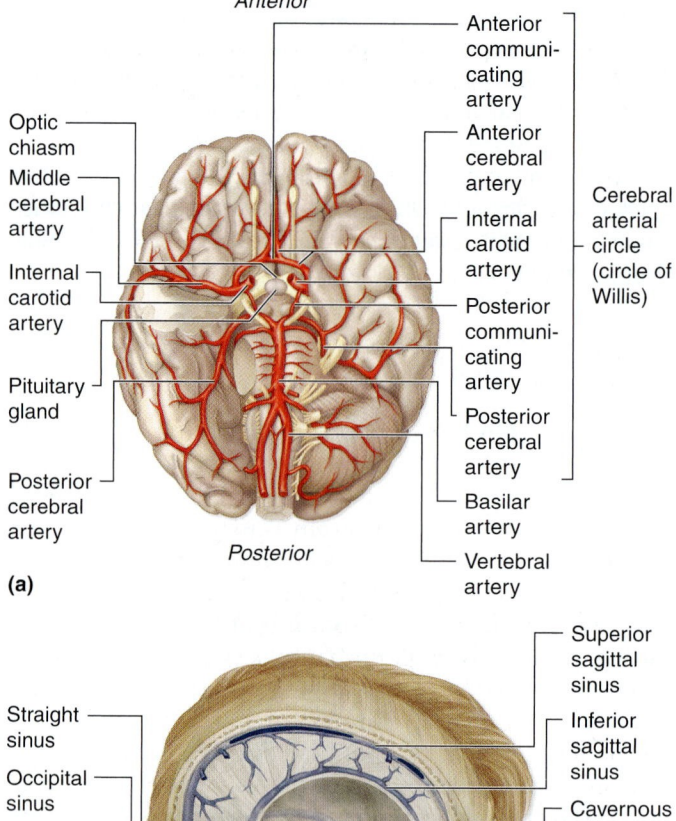

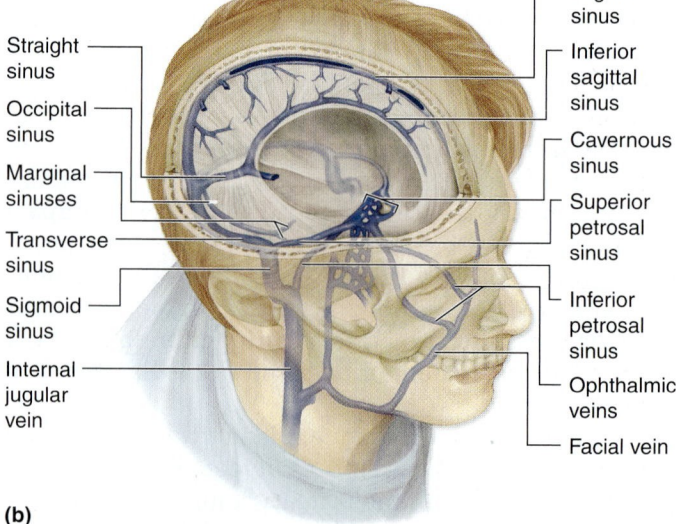

Figure 20-2   The blood supply to the brain. (a) Arteries of the brain, inferior view. (b) Cranial and facial veins.

Nice to Know

As ICP increases beyond 15 mmHg, autoregulation is lost, and CPP is dependent exclusively on blood pressure, which is why it is critical to keep blood pressure up in these patients.[8]

Portions of the brain will eventually be squeezed through various openings in the skull resulting in **herniation**.[8] When the brain herniates, assuming there are no additional man-made holes in the skull (such as bullet wounds), the only direction it can go is down, either through the tentorium (which is a fibrous shelf that supports the cerebrum) or through the foramen magnum at the base of the skull, injuring the brainstem by forcing it into the spinal canal. The foramen magnum is already occupied by the brainstem, and as the rest of the brain is pushed down, it compresses the brainstem. Because the brainstem is in control of the reflexes of life (breathing, heart rate, etc.), this is most often a terminal event (fatal).

One of the signs of impending or ongoing herniation is pupillary changes. One large fixed pupil in an unconscious patient indicates herniation until proven otherwise.

Pupillary responses are based on input from parasympathetic and cranial nerves that originate near the brainstem. In the most common type of herniation (uncal), the third cranial nerve (oculomotor nerve) is compressed on the side of the herniation, and the pupil on that side will dilate and become nonreactive to light while the pupil on the other side should continue to function normally. Other types of herniation are less common and lead to compression of another portion of the brainstem (the pons), leading to pinpoint pupils.[9] DOT 4-5.37

CONNECTIONS Chapter 30: Neurology describes the 12 cranial nerves in detail and provides an illustration.

Focal areas of injury to the brain can lead to focal areas of motor dysfunction. Generally, injuries to one side of the brain lead to motor findings on the opposite side of the body. All tracts from the brain to the spinal cord run through the brainstem. If there is a disruption of these tracts, this may lead to **posturing,** which is involuntary reflexive movements. **Decorticate posturing** is characterized by abnormal flexion due to a lesion higher in the brain, and has a slightly better prog-

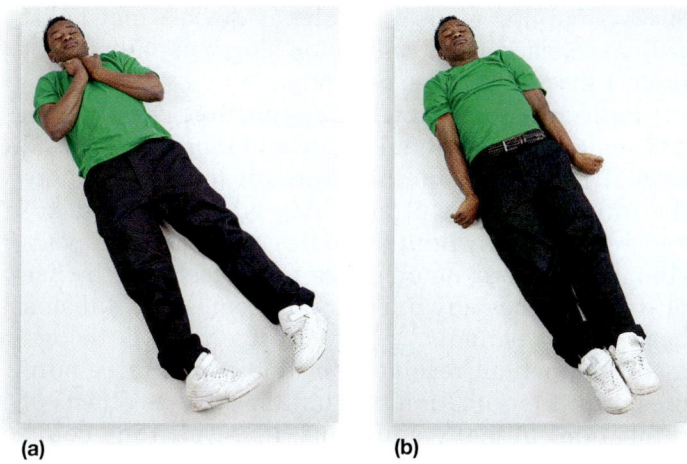

(a)　　　　　　　　　　**(b)**

Figure 20-3　(a) Decorticate posturing. (b) Decerebrate posturing.

nosis. **Decerebrate posturing** is abnormal extension due to a lower brain injury, and has a poor prognosis (Figure 20-3).

Primary Survey

The mechanism of injury can provide valuable clues about the possibility of a head or facial injury. The surface that the patient's head struck, or was struck by, may provide a clue about the potential underlying injury. Harder surfaces and heavier objects are more likely to cause internal damage, even when no other external injury is visible. Commonly, the initial impact to the head causes the first injury and is described as the **coup** (from the French term "blow"). A second impact may occur to the brain when it strikes the inside of the skull on the opposite side of the impact (**contrecoup**). DOT 4-5.38

Airway

As with any patient, the initial focus of the primary survey should be the airway. Patients with TBI are at high risk for airway compromise. Altered level of consciousness, vomiting, clenched jaws, and facial trauma are common causes for increased risk of airway compromise. Adequate oxygenation in these patients is critical; therefore, a patent airway is key. Patients with a severe head injury, GCS < 8 (the GCS scoring criteria is outlined in the Disability section on page 402), are considered to be unable to protect their airway and are at great risk for aspiration.[10] Intubation is a common method for securing the airway in a compromised patient.[11] Other airway adjuncts include the laryngeal mask airway (LMA), or oral airway. Keep in mind that only tracheal intubation is considered a "definitive" airway, and that while other airway devices may assist with oxygenation and ventilation, they generally do not protect the patient from aspiration.[11]

Performing endotracheal intubation can cause a transient decrease in pulse rate and increase in intracranial pressure. Administration of lidocaine before the intubation attempt may help minimize these adverse effects. Only limited studies in humans are available, and there is no evidence to suggest that the use of lidocaine has any effect on outcomes of intubated head injury patients.[12,13,14,15] Most protocols recommend the patient receive lidocaine one to three minutes prior to intubation to blunt the adverse effects of intubation. In many situations, this wait time could be deleterious to the patient's condition, so the decision to use lidocaine must be weighed carefully. You should consult your local protocol to determine if premedicating head injured patients with lidocaine is a standard of care in the EMS system in which you work. DOT 4-5.46

In patients with suspected airway obstruction, a jaw thrust is the initial maneuver of choice to open the airway, as nearly all head injured patients are at great risk for cervical spine injury as well. If the obstruction is caused by the tongue, this action will likely take care of the problem. Because of the high risk for aspiration, one must be suspicious of a foreign body such as food, teeth, or glass. Attempts at removal of a suspected foreign body include suction or direct visualization of the airway with laryngoscopy with removal by suction or McGill forceps. Airway compromise can also be caused by edema or hematoma due to laryngeal injury.[21]

Vomiting is a common symptom of TBI, and those who do not have a definitive airway in place are at great risk for aspiration.[22] Be ready to turn these patients on their side while still observing spinal precautions and have suction equipment at hand. Aggressively treat nausea with intravenous antiemetic agents if approved for use in your EMS system. If the patient seems at high risk for vomiting, make sure they are not fitted with a tight oxygen mask, so the vomit will have an exit route and keep suction ready.

Breathing

Depending on the area of the brain injury, patients with TBI can have variable alterations in their breathing mechanics and may be breathing too fast **(hyperventilating),** too slow **(hypoventilating),** or not at all **(apneic)** (Box 20-2).

Working in the Gray Zone

There is considerable controversy surrounding the use of prehospital intubation in the severely brain injured patient. While it seems logical to want to oxygenate, ventilate, and control the airway via tracheal intubation, many recent studies have reported either no benefit to this practice or evidence of worse outcomes in those individuals who were intubated in the prehospital setting, even when the studies controlled for severity of injury.[16,17,18,19] A meta-analysis of studies on prehospital intubation in TBI patients also shows that patients have worse outcomes.[20]

The reasons for these findings are unclear. All of the studies have been retrospective, so there may be some bias that cannot be accounted for. It is unlikely that intubation itself is harmful, but there are a number of potentially harmful events surrounding intubation. Oxygen desaturation, aspiration, and increased intracranial pressure during intubation are harmful to the TBI patient. Intubation increases scene time and, potentially, time to "definitive care." After intubation, there is the possibility for unrecognized tube dislodgement or esophageal intubation. Also, unrecognized hyperventilation in the TBI patient can lead to cerebral ischemia not only by constriction of the blood vessels in the brain but also by a build-up of pressure in the chest from the positive pressure ventilation, which can lead to decreased venous return of blood from the rest of the body and thus decreased cardiac output of blood to the rest of the body (i.e., the brain).

Those patients who would seem to be good candidates for prehospital intubation are those who will have a long transit time, are unable to be adequately ventilated or oxygenated with bag-mask, or are at significant risk for aspiration. During and following the procedure, care needs to be taken to prevent secondary injury from hypoxia (one cause is desaturation during prolonged intubation attempts without ventilation), hyperventilation, and aspiration.

While there will certainly be more research in this field in the future, these findings highlight the concept of "first do no harm." Prehospital intubation is known to be a life-saving procedure in some patients, but the evidence seems to point to worse outcomes in the TBI patient.

BOX 20-2 Oxygenation and Ventilation

Oxygenation and *ventilation* are two different things. **Oxygenation** refers to the introduction of oxygen from the lungs to the circulation. **Ventilation** is the removal of carbon dioxide from the circulation to the lungs and out of the body. Just because someone is oxygenating well does not mean they are ventilating well. Retention of carbon dioxide (hypercarbia) can be just as devastating as hypoxia. Oxygenation is easily measured with pulse oximetry, but for ventilation, you either need an end-tidal carbon dioxide (ETCO$_2$) detector, if available, or you will need to rely on your lung exam to ensure the patient is exhaling effectively. Chapter 12: Airway Management, Ventilation, and Oxygenation explains these concepts in detail. DOT 4-5.47

Hyperventilation can be a direct result of neurological damage, or it can be one of the mechanisms of the body to compensate for increased intracranial pressure. The opposite effect may also occur. The injured brain may slow breathing down or stop it altogether. This can be devastating as the brain is further deprived of oxygen.

Evidence-based guidelines put out by the Brain Trauma Foundation show that patients with a documented episode of prehospital hypoxia (defined as oxygen saturation <90%) have significantly poorer outcomes than those who were not hypoxic.[23]

Because of this, guard against both hypoxia and hyperventilation. Oxygen saturation should be kept above 95% if possible, and, if the patient is not breathing, you should breathe for the patient with the bag-mask 10–12 times per minute. If the patient is intubated, use an end-tidal carbon dioxide (ETCO$_2$) detector to guide (titrate) your ventilations.

CONNECTIONS End tidal CO$_2$, capnography and advanced airway maneuvers are described in Chapter 12: Airway Management, Ventilation, and Oxygenation.

As a general rule, most patients with suspected TBI should be given supplemental oxygen. If supplemental oxygen and repositioning do not reverse hypoventilation, hypoxia, or apnea, more aggressive intervention will be necessary.

Working in the Gray Zone

Increased carbon dioxide (CO$_2$) levels cause blood vessels in the brain to dilate. This leads to greater blood volume in the brain, leading to increased intracranial pressure (ICP) and worse patient outcomes. Decreasing levels of CO$_2$ create the opposite effect. Blood vessels will constrict, thus decreasing intracranial pressure. At face value, this sounds like the right intervention when the desire is to preserve the contents within the valuable space of the cranium. For years, this theory led to the common practice of hyperventilating patients with TBI, but no study ever showed this to improve patient outcome.[24,25,26] DOT 4-5.41

Recent studies show that this vasoconstriction due to hyperventilation leads to decreased cerebral blood flow and can lead to cerebral ischemia (brain cell death). It may still be helpful in theory to use very brief, mild hyperventilation to decrease ICP in the setting of impending brain herniation. A normal CO$_2$ level is around 40 (35–45 is a commonly reported range for many laboratory studies); mild hyperventilation (conservative treatment) is considered decreasing the CO$_2$ level to 35. A more aggressive approach is to allow the CO$_2$ to range between 30–35 mmHg.[27] Check with your medical director and protocol to determine the desired number or range for your EMS agency. DOT 4-5.42

Although one should be able to tell on physical exam if the patient is hypoventilating, it is quite difficult to know exactly how poorly the patient is breathing. Given the harm that abnormal CO$_2$ levels can produce, the emerging standard of care appears to be the prehospital use of end-tidal CO$_2$ detectors, especially in those who are receiving assisted ventilation. DOT 4-5.46

Circulation

Hypotension from any cause is devastating to patients with TBI. Numerous studies have shown that hypotension is a reliable predictor of poor outcome in TBI patients.[28,29]

Just one episode of prehospital hypotension can increase the risk of death and permanent disability significantly.[30]

Aggressive blood pressure control is therefore necessary in TBI patients. DOT 4-5.46

All patients with severe TBI should have at least one IV line inserted, and those with hypotension should have two. The brain has a very high rate of metabolism, so even a brief episode of hypoperfusion can result in significant injury. Aggressive IV hydration is the mainstay of prehospital treatment of hypotension.

Hypotension as a direct result of isolated TBI is usually a late sign and is due to the swelling brain herniating out of the skull and into the spinal canal. This causes neurological effects such as vasodilation, which in turn leads to hypotension. Brain herniation is often a terminal event.

> You should suspect hypotension if you see unilateral pupillary dilation or the patient begins to posture.

Posturing is an abnormal involuntary contraction of the limbs. The arms can flex inward (towards the core), termed "decorticate posturing," or extend outward, termed "decerebrate posturing". If brain herniation is occurring, one may also see hypertension and a slowing of the pulse (bradycardia). This is one of the only times when managing the patient with mild hyperventilation is thought to be beneficial. DOT 4-5.42, 4-5.43

Street Secrets

The combination of bradycardia and hypertension is called **Cushing's reflex** and is indicative of impending brain herniation.

Hypotension, in most cases, is much more likely to be caused by injuries other than brain trauma. Bleeding into or around the brain cannot cause enough loss of blood to cause a patient to be hypotensive from blood loss alone, except in very small children. As many as 60% of head injured patients are victims of multiple trauma;[31] therefore, sources of blood loss causing hypotension, other than TBI, should be aggressively sought out and addressed.

TBI patients are also subject to dysrhythmias (irregular heart rhythms). Virtually any cardiac dysrhythmia can occur in these patients and cause instability. These dysrhythmias can be due to hypoxia, electrolyte imbalance, or direct cardiac injury. Therefore, they should be treated according to standard ACLS protocols in the same way as nontrauma patients with arrhythmias.

Disability

This text has emphasized that the components of the primary survey include assessment of airway, breathing, and circulation. Chapter 14: Patient Assessment also discusses that some prehospital providers are taught to use ABCDE to guide their primary survey.

Management of the TBI patient benefits from the ABCDE approach instead of just the ABC approach. When D and E are attached to ABC, a brief and focused neurological exam is performed on all suspected TBI patients during the primary survey. The main components that are added to the ABC assessment focus on assessing the level of consciousness, orientation, and pupillary response and determining the Glasgow Coma Score (GCS).

Assess the Level of Consciousness.   Evaluating the patient's level of consciousness, and how it changes for better or worse over the time that you are with the patient, is the single most important part of the neurologic assessment.

Patients who present initially awake and then become confused, unable to follow commands, or comatose are at much greater risk of having a serious TBI compared to patients who initially had a loss of consciousness or were confused but now are awake and following your directions.

Determining the **level of consciousness (LOC)** of someone who has just sustained a head injury may be difficult, especially in the presence of complicating factors such as alcohol ingestion, mood-altering substances, or trauma. It is best to make simple observations about the patient's ability to follow commands, to recognize the surroundings, and to describe the events that led to the injury and the moments before and after the event. Words such as lethargic, stuporous, or semiresponsive may be commonly used but are not as helpful as a simple description.[32]

One method of assessing the LOC is to first ask the patient to open their eyes. If the patient complies, ask the patient to perform a simple task like, "Show me two fingers." When a patient follows your simple command, the patient is demonstrating motor response as well as an ability to receive and process information. If the patient fails to open the eyes, perform a painful stimulus like pinching the shoulder or rubbing the sternum to see if pain will illicit spontaneous eye opening.

The Glasgow Coma Scale.   The GCS is a score that was devised in 1974 by Teasdale and Jennett to give an objective measurement to the level of consciousness.[33] It is a simple test for the initial assessment of level of consciousness and is repeated to determine improvement or deterioration from the initial assessment (Box 20-3). The three components are based on eye, motor, and verbal responses.

When calculating the GCS, the patient's *best response at the time of the assessment* is what should be scored. For example, if you apply a sternal rub to wake the patient, who then grumbles incomprehensible sounds, you immediately do it a second time. If the

BOX 20-3   Glasgow Coma Scale

Best Eye Response (4)

1. No eye opening
2. Eye opening to pain
3. Eye opening to verbal command
4. Eyes open spontaneously

Best Verbal Response (5)

1. No verbal response
2. Incomprehensible sounds
3. Inappropriate words
4. Confused
5. Orientated

Best Motor Response (6)

1. No motor response
2. Extension to pain
3. Flexion to pain
4. Withdrawal from pain
5. Localizing pain
6. Obeys Commands

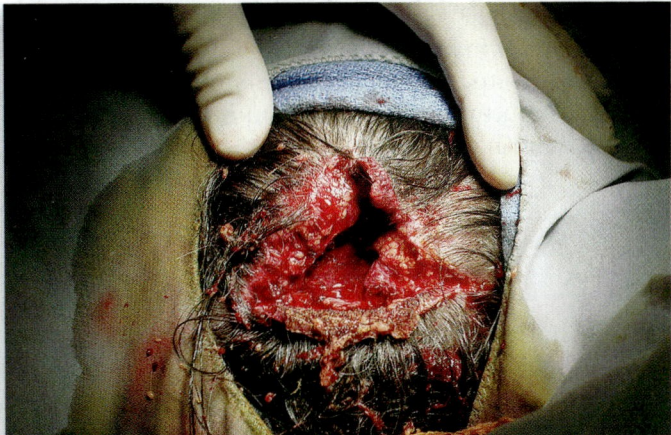

Figure 20-4   Deep laceration of the head and scalp.

Secondary Survey

After performing the primary survey and stabilizing any problems noted, begin the secondary survey.

On the head, eyes, ears, nose, and throat (HEENT) exam, look for external evidence of head trauma. Lacerations should be dressed; if they are actively bleeding, a pressure dressing should be considered. You may palpate the scalp, feeling or looking for signs of a skull fracture, keeping in mind that aggressive palpation over a skull fracture is essentially going to be pushing on the underlying brain, which is to be avoided (Figure 20-4). Look and feel for signs of midface instability. This can be done by placing gloved fingers inside the mouth and giving gentle anterior traction on the upper jaw (maxilla) to see if it moves. Palpate over the cheekbones and mandible (jaw) for other evidence of facial fractures. Look at the ears to see if there is blood or pinkish (blood-tinged) CSF leaking out of the ear canals. This is evidence of fracture at the base of the skull.[37] DOT 4-5.51–4-5.53

All of the cranial nerves should be tested to evaluate their function, comparing right and left sides for any abnormalities. Finally, a sensory and motor exam of the extremities should be performed, looking for any deficits or abnormal responses. The cranial nerve assessment and sensory and motor examination tips are described in Chapter 14: Patient Assessment.

patient then tells you to "Knock it off!," the patient should get a "4" or "5" under verbal, not a score of "2". If, however, the patient's status changes from a GCS of "14" on-scene to a "9" a few minutes later during the ride to the hospital, this should be documented as two separate scores with the time each assessment was taken recorded as well. It is important when giving the verbal report to mention from what areas of the scale points were lost (i.e., "GCS is 11" is not as helpful as "GCS is 11; patient is confused and opens eyes to pain").

A GCS of three is the worst (and lowest) possible score, and a 15 is the best. A low initial prehospital GCS score is predictive of poor outcome.[34] Patients with improvement of the GCS score from the scene to the emergency department of greater than two points are more likely to have better outcomes than those with no change in the GCS.[35] DOT 4-5.45

Pupillary Response.   Pupillary response is another important component to the neurological exam. Unilateral pupillary dilation or unresponsiveness is suggestive of brainstem herniation. Other abnormal findings suggestive of intracranial injury include pinpoint pupils, bilateral pupillary dilation, and gaze deviation to one side.[36] The following section provides more details on pupillary response.

Street Secrets

Remember to check *blood sugar* in any patient with altered mental status—even if you think you know the cause. Make this a consistent habit in your assessment as you will often "awaken" a "comatose" head injured patient who in reality passed out from hypoglycemia and then struck the head. Failure to recognize hypoglycemia can lead to brain damage that is every bit as severe and permanent as TBI.

The rest of the evaluation of the head injured patient is not different than that of any other trauma patient. As stated earlier, up to 60% of head injured patients are the victims of multiple trauma, so you must be vigilant in seeking out other injuries.

Working in the Gray Zone

While normal saline (NS) and lactated ringers (LR) have been the mainstay in prehospital treatment of hypotension for TBI patients, there is now a new possibility: hypertonic saline (HTS). The normal concentration of sodium (Na) in the blood is 0.9%. NS is also 0.9% NaCl whereas HTS is 3% NaCl. In addition to the actual volume infused, HTS actually pulls fluid into the vascular space via its osmotic effect, as opposed to NS where a great deal of it is lost out of the blood vessels by the same process. This osmotic effect of HTS may also be beneficial in TBI because it reduces brain swelling (cerebral edema) and thus, intracranial pressure.[38,39]

Although HTS sounds promising, only one study regarding use of HTS in the prehospital setting for TBI has been published and showed similar outcomes to those receiving NS. More information on it is sure to come in the future.

Working in the Gray Zone

Hyperthermia has been shown to increase the brain's metabolic demands and worsen neurological outcome after insult. Armed with this information, there has been discussion about induction of hypothermia to improve outcome in TBI. It is known that hypothermia increases perfusion and oxygenation to the brain and decreases intracranial pressure. There are relatively few human trials of induced hypothermia in patients with TBI. The data are quite limited and appear mediocre with the studies showing minimal to no improvement in outcome in patients with mild induced hypothermia (32–33°C). Selected populations may have improved outcome, but these have not been well delineated, and more studies are needed to clarify a true improvement in outcome. In patients with multiple trauma and sources of bleeding, hypothermia is likely to be harmful as it will inhibit clotting. More information on this subject is sure to come.[5,40,41]

Specific Brain Injuries

Cerebral Contusion

Contusions (bruises) are one of the most frequent types of TBI.[9] Contusions most frequently occur in the subfrontal cortex, in the frontal and temporal lobes, and occasionally in the occipital lobe. Contusions may occur directly at the site of blunt trauma (coup) or on the opposite side as the contrecoup injury. An intracerebral hemorrhage can develop days after a significant blunt trauma, and often these injuries occur at the site of the contusion. DOT 4-5.48, 4-5.57, 4-5.59

Initially, the patient with a cerebral contusion is unconscious. Edema that surrounds the contusion may cause fluctuations in the level of consciousness, and seizures can develop. Patients must be carefully monitored for neurological deterioration. As the edema progresses, herniation can occur.[42] DOT 4-5.54–4-5.56

Intracranial Hemorrhage

Intracranial hemorrhage is a potentially devastating form of traumatic brain injury. There is not only primary injury from the initial damage to the neurons but also secondary injury from the accumulation of blood and interstitial edema (i.e., the fluid leaking from damaged cell membranes). As previously described, the skull is a tight, fixed space with very little room for expansion. As blood accumulates, the brain gets squeezed out of the way, leading to compression of neurons, decreased blood flow, and edema as the cells die. Types of hemorrhage are based on location of the bleeding and include epidural, subdural, subarachnoid, and intraparenchymal. It is difficult to distinguish the type of hemorrhage in the prehospital setting, but some historical clues and exam findings may lead you to suspect one over another.

Epidural Hematoma

Epidural hemorrhage is bleeding into the epidural space of the brain, which is a potential space that lies between the inner surface of the skull, and the dura mater, a covering of the brain (Figure 20-5). Although an epidural hemorrhage can occur with any injury, it classically occurs with blunt trauma to the side of the head, fracturing the temporal or temporoparietal bone. The skull is thinner in that location, and a large vessel (the middle meningeal artery) runs directly underneath it. If this artery is lacerated, it can release arterial blood into the epidural space. The blood accumulates rapidly under the arterial pressure. Although these patients can have immediate and rapid decompensation, the classic presentation is a brief loss of consciousness from trauma followed by a period of lucidity, varying from a few minutes to a few hours; then rapid and severe decompensation with

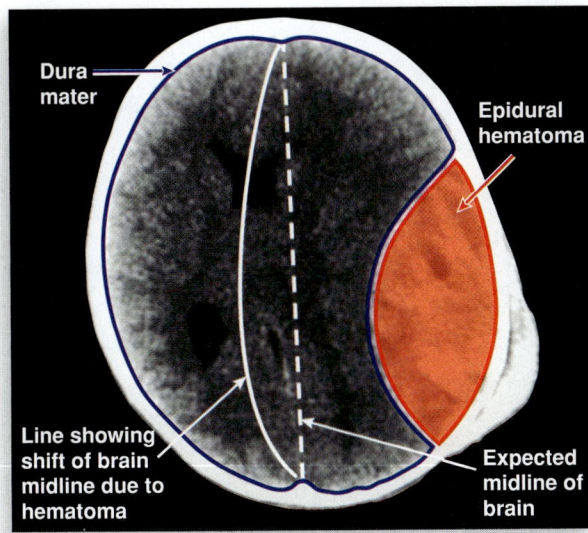

Figure 20-5   Epidural hematoma.

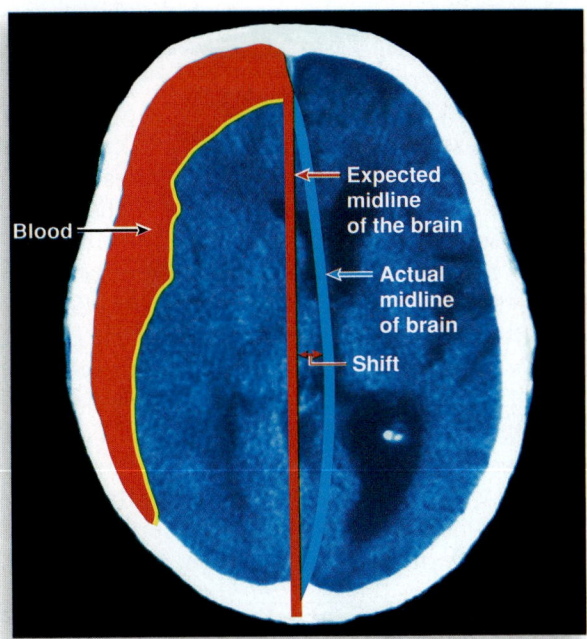

Figure 20-6   Subdural hematoma. Blood is under the dura; the shape of the collection follows the contours of the brain.

headache, vomiting, and loss of consciousness.[43] The **lucid interval** is the period of time when the patient awakens from unconsciousness with sometimes little to no signs of obvious damage. Many times these patients are erroneously assumed to have a "concussion" instead of an actual intracranial bleed.

Field treatment is directed at maintaining an adequate airway and blood pressure, preventing any secondary insults, recognizing and treating signs of increased ICP and herniation, and rapid transport to an appropriate destination. Definitive care involves surgical evacuation of the expanding hematoma and hemorrhage control.

Subdural Hematoma

Subdural hemorrhage is bleeding into the space between the outer (dura mater) and inner coverings (arachnoid mater) of the brain (Figure 20-6). There are many veins that run through this space, and they are susceptible to tearing. Most subdural hemorrhages present as a slow, steady decline after a head injury. They are more common in the elderly. They most often manifest within 48 hours of injury but can occur rapidly or have a delayed presentation over a period of weeks following the initial trauma as the blood slowly accumulates under venous pressure. Field treatment goals are identical to those of patients with epidural hemorrhages.

Street Secrets

A trick to remember that epidural bleed is faster and more immediately life-threatening is that it involves an artery. Subdural bleeds are Slower (starts with an S) and involve venouS blood.

Subarachnoid Hemorrhage

Subarachnoid hemorrhages (SAH) (between the inner coating of the brain, and the brain itself) and **intraparenchymal hemorrhages (IPH)** (within the brain) occur from either direct damage to a vessel or traumatic rupture of an already existing aneurysm. SAH most often presents with global neurological dysfunction (i.e., confusion, lethargy, coma) whereas IPH may present with either global or focal neurologic findings. Focal neurologic deficits are abnormal neurologic findings in those parts of the body specifically controlled by the area of the brain that has been damaged by the IPH.

Diffuse Axonal Injury

Diffuse axonal injury (DAI) is a significant TBI injury caused by deceleration that results in shearing forces on the connections within the brain. Following the initial assessment of this patient, perform a rapid transport while following the procedures outlined for severe TBI patients. These patients generally will not regain consciousness and remain in a persistent vegetative state.[44] Mortality is very high with DAI. DOT 4-5.48, 4-5.50

Concussion

Minor TBI and concussions are likely a spectrum of the same disease. Minor TBI has classically been described as patients who have an initial GCS of 13–15. However, those with GCS of 13 are more likely to have significant brain injury on further evaluation and are considered by some to be in the "moderate" TBI category. DOT 4-5.49

Nice to Know

Cerebrospinal fluid (CSF) leaks may be evident with a fractured skull and noted as clear or pink rhinorrhea (nasal or ocular secretions). If CSF is present in the clear secretions, a dextrose stick test may be positive for glucose. Use the glucometer to perform this test. Another test, called the "halo" test, is performed by placing the bloody fluid on filter paper (a coffee filter or a fibrous paper towel works well) and a "halo" or double ring may be seen as the blood and CSF separate as they dry. The CSF, which is not as viscous (thick), will spread out beyond the blood and will form a second ring outside the blood that looks like a "halo." A word of caution—do not delay transport or consider conducting these tests a priority. The reliability of both of these tests has been questioned.[45]

Concussion is a temporary and brief interruption of neurological function after head trauma.[8] Concussion syndromes can vary in severity and symptoms but are, by definition, reversible and do not lead to permanent structural damage.[46] There may or may not be a loss of consciousness. The patient may report feeling dazed or seeing stars, have nausea and vomiting, have a significant headache, or may be repeating comments or questions that have already been answered (this is called **perseverating**). In addition, many patients often have no recollection of the events leading up to or occurring immediately after the incident causing their concussion. This is referred to as **retrograde** and **antegrade amnesia,** respectively. Symptoms generally resolve within 6 to 24 hours although many patients report prolonged difficulty with concentrating, forgetfulness, and difficulty sleeping, lasting weeks to months. Treatment is supportive.

Special Situations

Helmets

It has been shown that helmet use reduces rates of head injury. A report from the CDC shows that motorcyclists not using helmets are 2.9 times more likely to sustain brain injury than those who do use them.[47] Bicyclists who utilize helmets have an 80% risk reduction of head injury (Figure 20-7).[48] There is little published in the way of evidence-based guidelines regarding helmet removal in the head or neck injured patient. If the patient has lost consciousness or has a compromised airway, at a minimum the face mask, if not the entire helmet, should be removed to permit rapid intervention if necessary. DOT 4-5.61

There is controversy in the EMS community regarding need for removal of the helmet in patients that do not have an airway compromise. In athletes with shoulder pads, it is not recommended to remove the helmet unless

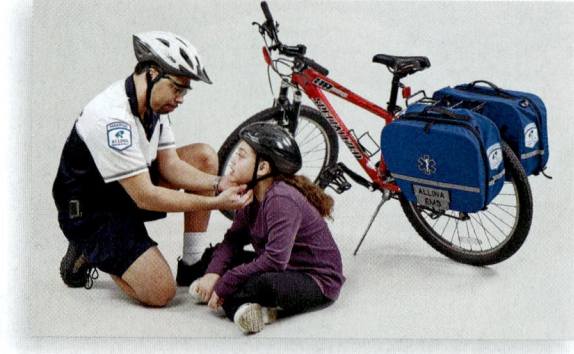

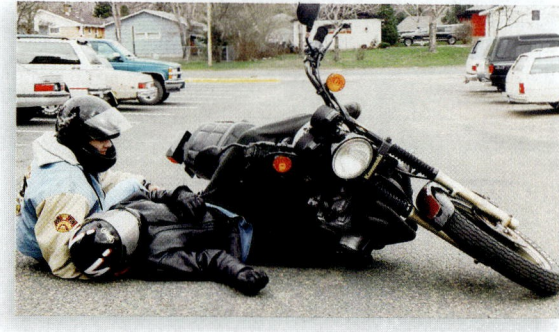

Figure 20-7 (a) Paramedics should advocate wearing properly fitting helmets whenever possible. (b) Full face motorcycle helmets greatly decrease head injuries.

absolutely necessary, as the shoulders elevate the body and keep the spine in line with the head that is elevated by the helmet. Removal of the helmet will result in hyperextension of the neck. If it is necessary to remove the helmet in the case of an airway emergency, coordination between two or three rescuers is necessary in order to stabilize the head and neck during this risky maneuver, as well as place appropriate padding to support the head.

In athletes and other patients who do not have shoulder pads, the helmet is likely to cause neck flexion when the patient is placed on a long spine board. If neutral alignment of the spine will be compromised, the helmet should be removed. **Skill Sheet 71 and Step-by-Step 71: Helmet Removal describe helmet removal techniques.** DOT 4-5.60, 4-5.62

Alcohol Intoxication

Alcohol intoxication and head injury are a common combination. Acute and chronic alcohol abuse can lead to hemodynamic and respiratory depression; dehydration, due to its diuretic effects; impaired clotting mechanisms; and blood-brain barrier disruption.[49]

CONNECTIONS To review the effects of alcohol intoxication see Chapter 35: Toxicology.

These physiologic effects have the potential to exacerbate the degree of injury in these patients.[50] Alcohol also acts as a CNS depressant and can mask clinical symptoms. Because these patients have an unreliable neurological exam that prevents clinical clearance of injury, they should be assumed to have spinal and intracranial injury until proven otherwise. Patients who are obviously intoxicated are not capable of providing an informed refusal of care, and law enforcement assistance should be sought if the patient is uncooperative. These patients should be transported to the closest appropriate hospital as they should be evaluated by a physician.

Facial Trauma

Incidence of Facial Injuries

Up to 60% of all patients with severe facial injuries also have multisystem trauma. Twenty to fifty percent of all patients with facial trauma also sustain concurrent brain injury, especially those with upper face and midface fractures. These patients have a great potential for airway compromise. Falls are an important cause of facial injury in the very young and the elderly. Most research shows no increased incidence in cervical spine injury in patients with facial trauma. However, cervical injury should be considered for all patients with significant trauma, particularly if maxillofacial fractures have occurred. Factors that increase the likelihood of the combination of cervical and brain injury include MVCs and older aged patients.[51] DOT 4-5.1

The cause of facial trauma varies between urban and rural areas. Penetrating trauma and assault-related injuries are more common in urban areas while motor vehicle crashes and sports and recreational injuries are more common in the rural areas. Fractures of the nose and mandible are the most common facial injuries seen in nontrauma center hospitals. In trauma centers midface and zygomatic injuries are more frequent.[9]

Domestic violence, elder abuse, and child abuse often result in facial trauma of varying severity. Facial injury accounts for the majority of emergency department visits related to domestic violence. As many as one-fourth of women with facial trauma are victims of domestic violence.[52] If a woman has an orbital trauma fracture, the likelihood that sexual assault or domestic violence was the cause is 30%.[53] DOT 4-5.3, 4-5.7

Anatomy and Physiology of the Face

The face is made up of a number of bones (Figure 20-8). The midfacial bones tend to be quite thin and can be fractured easily. The face also has a vast supply of blood vessels and nerves to support its complicated and delicate movements. These can also be easily injured with any facial trauma.

The nose is uniquely susceptible to injury by virtue of its prominent location on the face. Nasal fractures and nosebleed (epistaxis) are common injuries. Injury to the lips, teeth, and tongue is also a common occurrence. It is particularly important to evaluate for the potential of aspiration of a fractured tooth or obstruction of the airway from dentures or blood. DOT 4-5.2, 4-5.6

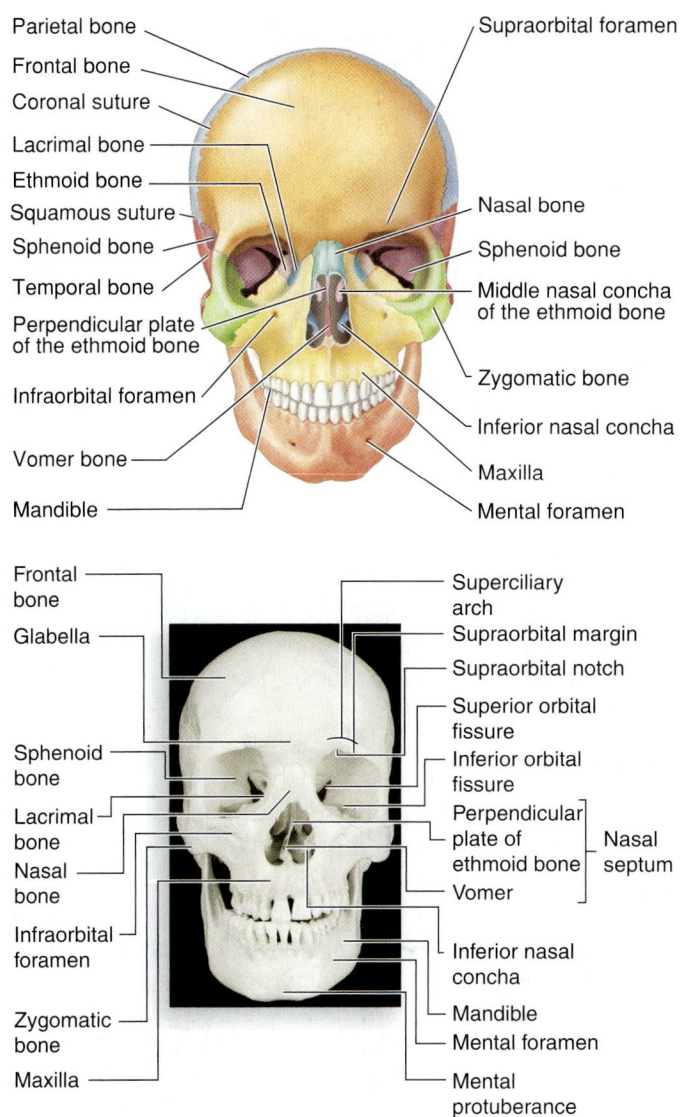

Figure 20-8 The bones of the face.

The eyes are highly sensitive and obviously important; while they are well protected by the bones of the orbit, they are also susceptible to injury in facial trauma (Figure 20-9). Blindness occurs in 0.5–3% of patients with facial injuries. It is associated with LeFort II and III fractures as well as zygoma fractures (see Figure 20-11). Motor vehicle crashes and gunshot wounds are the most frequent cause of vision loss.[54] DOT 4-5.4

Primary Survey

Airway

Significant facial trauma can cause airway compromise, either from anatomic disruption of normal supporting structures or from bleeding into or around the airway. Positioning of the patient, depending on their injuries, can be important in maintaining airway patency by altering anatomy or gravity. Although it is standard practice to make the trauma patient lay down, it may be

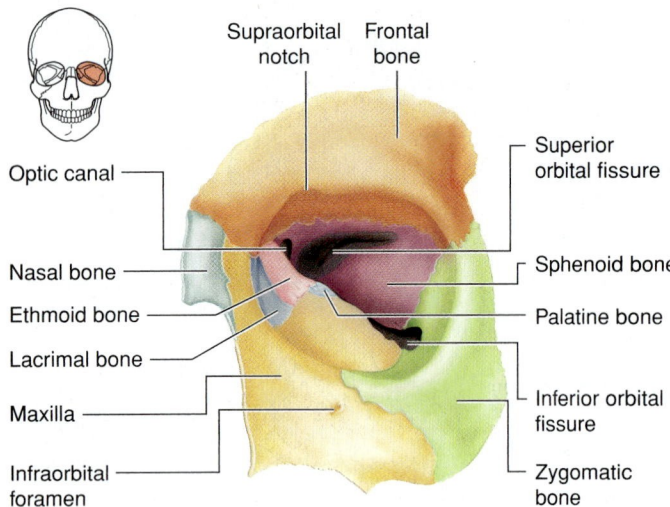

Figure 20-9   The bones of the orbit.

necessary to immobilize and transport a patient in a sitting position with a half backboard, and c-collar to ensure that fluids, blood, or loose tissue do not obstruct the airway. DOT 4-5.8, 4-5.9

Breathing

Monitor and provide ventilatory support as outlined in the primary survey section previously.

Circulation

The face is extremely well vascularized. Although facial bleeding is not often life-threatening, it can be significant. Good IV access should be obtained in any patient with significant bleeding, and IV fluids should be administered to prevent hypovolemia (Figure 20-10).

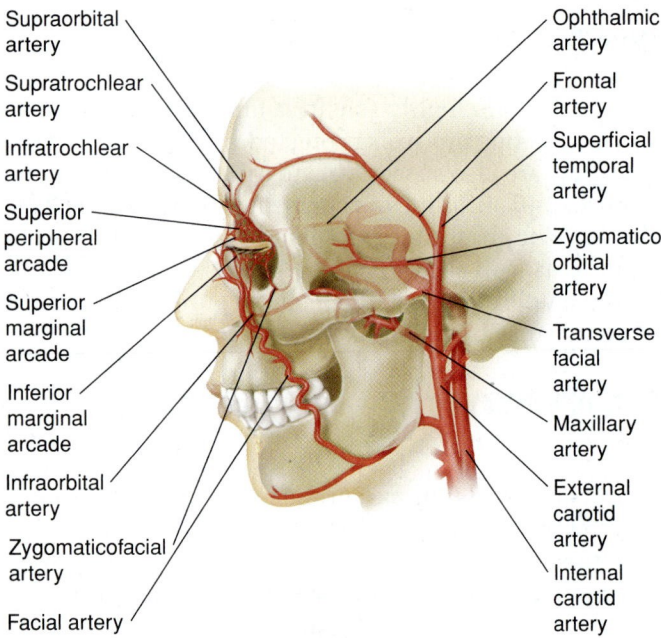

Figure 20-10   The blood supply of the face.

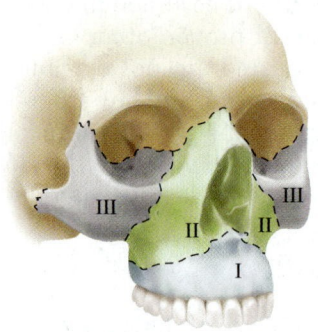

Figure 20-11   LeFort fractures.

Disability

Due to the close proximity of the face to the brain, always be aware of the potential for brain and spinal cord injuries in these patients. Apply a c-collar if indicated, and perform a brief neurological exam.

Specific Facial Injuries

Facial Fractures

Facial fractures can range from inconsequential to major. The most significant of these are the **LeFort fractures** (Figure 20-11). They are classified as LeFort I, II, or III and involve injury to bones on both sides of the face. LeFort I is a fracture through the floor of the maxillary sinuses, II goes through the maxillary sinuses, and III goes through the orbits.[37] These injuries cause the midface to be unstable; as the bony attachments have been disrupted, only tendons and muscles keep the various portions of the midface and lower face attached to the skull. This can lead to a sagging of the midface or significant underlying soft tissue injury and can cause potential airway obstruction. These injuries can be suspected by gentle traction on the maxilla or hard palate. However, it is unlikely that this procedure will be performed in the prehospital setting.

Other common fractures include the zygoma (cheekbones), orbital walls or floor (these bones are extremely thin), as well as the mandible (jaw).

Mouth Trauma

The most common mechanism of injury in mouth injuries is falls.[9] Sporting injuries, fights, and motor vehicle collisions account for most of the remainder (Figure 20-12). Injury to the maxillary central incisors accounts for 70% of dental injuries. Management of dentoalveolar trauma depends on the extent of tooth and alveolar involvement, the degree of development of the apex of the tooth, and the age of the patient. DOT 4-5.30

Total displacement of a tooth from its socket, called an **avulsion,** accounts for up to 16% of all injuries to teeth. It is necessary to reimplant avulsed permanent

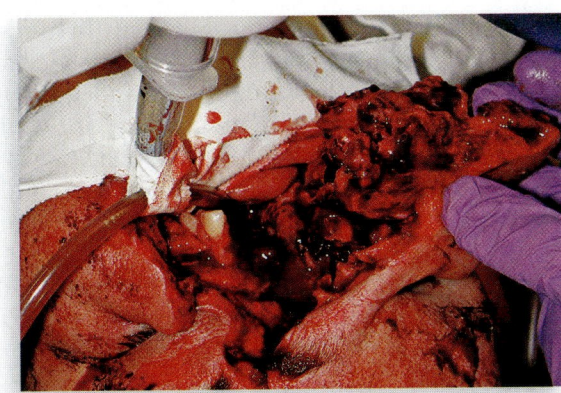

Figure 20-12   Victim of a motorcycle crash. Facial trauma was caused by striking a guardrail while wearing an open-face helmet.

teeth as soon as possible. Reimplantation is possible if performed within 20 to 30 minutes. To minimize this time, ideally, the patient or healthcare provider at the scene should reimplant the tooth. The tooth should be rinsed with sterile normal saline, sterile water for irrigation, or tap water to remove debris. Never scrub the tooth manually as this diminishes the likelihood of successful reimplantation. Care should be taken to handle only the crown portion of the tooth, and it should be reimplanted immediately into the socket. If this is not possible, or if the risk of aspiration is high, such as in a child or a patient with a decreased level of consciousness, then the tooth should be transported with the patient to the hospital. Acceptable transport media include isotonic solutions such as Hank solution, sterile saline, and milk. Commercial preparations of Hank solution such as Save-A-Tooth™ (TPS, Biologic Rescue Products, Inc., Pottstown, PA) are available and come with a useful transport container as part of the system.[55,56] DOT 4-5.31 – 4-5.34

Traumas to the soft tissues of the oral cavity are common. Use direct pressure to control any external bleeding from the mouth. Utilize suction as necessary to control secretions and blood. Use airway adjuncts to help maintain an open patent airway, and provide oxygen and ventilatory support as needed. If bleeding is not controllable, airway management may require intubation or surgical or needle cricothyrotomy.

Nasal Trauma

Traumatic fracture of the nose is the most common of the head and neck fractures. It is often associated with septal fractures and epistaxis.[9,57,58] Although frequently the result of battery, a broken nose is often not life-threatening. Significant functional impairment and physical disfigurement may result if a displaced fracture is not treated promptly.[58] The patient often presents with pain, **periorbital ecchymosis (raccoon's eyes)**, displacement of the nose, and crepitus. DOT 4-5.20

Edema following the injury is often extensive. The delicate bone structure of the nose fractures easily, and concomitant breakage of nasal blood vessels can cause bleeding that can range from trivial to profuse. A flow of copious clear fluid from the nose following head trauma may signify leakage of cerebrospinal fluid through a fracture at the base of the skull. Epistaxis can also occur spontaneously without precipitating trauma.

Young children are prone to insert small foreign bodies into the nose, causing irritation, bleeding, and the potential for aspiration of the offending object into the lower respiratory tract. More cases of nasal trauma in children are the result of accidental sports injury and play rather than from fights or battery. However, it is estimated that between 30% and 50% of all pediatric abuse victims present to the emergency department with maxillofacial injuries including fractured noses.[58]

Manage lacerations, contusions, or other superficial trauma to the nose with gentle pressure for bleeding control and standard wound care. Foreign bodies in the nose should be left in place and the patient transported to an appropriate receiving facility. Removal may require specialized equipment, and inappropriate attempts at extrication in the field may cause inadvertent aspiration of the object.[9]

In 90% of the cases, bleeding originates from the rich vascular network of Kiesselbach's plexus.[9] Because of its relatively exposed position along the anterior wall of the septum, irritation caused by dry air, frequent nose blowing, or the insertion of a finger (also called digital trauma) can spark hemorrhage. Nose bleeds in this area are classified as anterior and are readily controlled with digital pressure applied for five to ten minutes.[57] Although packing with nasal tampons or balloons is an effective hospital treatment, it has not been shown to be effective in the prehospital setting, so it is not recommended. DOT 4-5.21–4-5.24

Eye Trauma

Severe eye injuries that can require immediate attention include globe rupture, retinal detachment, hyphema, and retrobulbar hematoma. The globe is a very delicate structure. While it is compressible, it does not take much force to rupture or penetrate the thin cornea. A brief eye exam should include an evaluation of the pupils and visual acuity. The acuity assessment does not need to be specific or involve any equipment or supplies. Simply hold up your hand at a distance of one foot from the patient's face and ask whether the patient can see how many fingers you are holding up, or ask the patient with a more significant injury if shades of light or dark can be seen.

CONNECTIONS   See Chapter 11: The Normal Physical Examination to review the assessment of the pupils.

Globe rupture can be caused by blunt or penetrating trauma to the eye. It usually causes significant pain (especially with movement of the eye) and decreased vision. It can be suspected on exam by noticing a flattened appearing globe (due to the loss of internal fluid) with an irregular pupil and contents or fluid extruding from the globe. It is very important not to place any pressure on the globe as this will cause further extrusion of globe contents; cover it with an eye shield to prevent any inadvertent touching.[37] Treat nausea aggressively, as vomiting significantly increases intraocular pressure (IOP). Though the evidence is mostly anecdotal and theoretical, succinylcholine is contraindicated in patients with globe rupture that require airway management due to an increase in IOP.[59] Resist the temptation to pull out any foreign body from the eye, as doing so can cause further disruption of its contents. Bandage both eyes to prevent **sympathetic eye movement;** this occurs when one eye moves and the other follows.

Traumatic retinal detachment is the separation of the posterior elements of the globe. Patients will present with direct globe trauma (i.e., hit with a racquetball) and either complete or partial loss of vision with floaters, lightning, or wavy lines in their vision. Floaters, lightning, and wavy lines are all descriptions of what patients say they are seeing from the affected eye. Again, prevent unnecessary movement or touching of the eye.

Hyphema is blood in the anterior chamber of the eye (just behind the cornea and in front of the iris and pupil) (Figure 20-13). Small hyphemas can be difficult to detect, especially with the patient lying down. Large hyphemas can look like the pupil and iris are either dark red or black when examined with a light. It is important to keep the patient sitting up, as this will allow the blood to pool at the base of the eye instead of spreading it over the whole field of vision.[60]

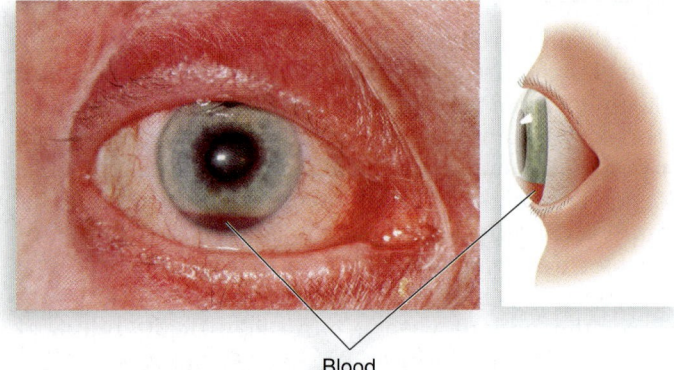

Blood

Figure 20-13   Hyphema is blood in the anterior chamber of the eye, just behind the cornea.

Retrobulbar hemorrhage is bleeding behind the globe. Bleeding into this closed space can be vision-threatening. As pressure builds up behind the eye, it causes compression or stretching of the optic nerve (the one that gives you sight), and it can cause the globe to be pushed out of the orbit. On exam you may notice the globe appears to be bulging from the orbit **(proptosis).** Prolonged stretching or pressure on the optic nerve can lead to permanent loss of vision. Treat nausea and pain. This injury will likely require surgical intervention. DOT 4-5.10–4-5.14

Ear Trauma

Trauma to the external ear is rarely life-threatening, but it can cause significant bleeding and long-term cosmetic harm.[9] Pressure waves generated by significant blunt trauma to the ear can traverse the external auditory canal to rupture the fragile eardrum (tympanic membrane or TM) and cause sudden hearing loss.[58] Blunt trauma is the most common cause of traumatic hearing loss. Motor vehicle crashes are the major cause of blunt head trauma and account for approximately 50% of all temporal bone injuries. Penetrating trauma is relatively rare, occurring in less than 10% of all cases.[58] Penetrating or blunt trauma that fractures the base of the skull can cause bleeding within the middle ear **(hemotympanum)** that likewise compromises hearing and may disrupt the normal sense of balance by damaging the vestibular labyrinth. DOT 4-5.15

As with all patient encounters, the initial assessment of the patient with an ear complaint begins with a focused history while vigilance is maintained for other conditions that may threaten the airway, breathing, or circulation. Obvious trauma to the ear signals a potential for injury to the brain or cervical spine, and the patient must be quickly assessed for signs of trauma to other vital regions such as the neck and upper chest. Blood emanating from the canal may signify TM rupture and, potentially, an underlying fracture of the base of the skull. Copious clear fluid in the canal often represents leakage of cerebrospinal fluid through such a fracture as well. Bleeding from a basilar skull fracture may also fill the mastoid air cells, giving a bluish hue to the bony prominence behind the auricle **(Battle's sign).**[61]

Traumatic ear injuries are managed in the same way as any other soft tissue injury. Save any severed or avulsed portions of the auricle, and transport them with the patient in saline-soaked gauze.[37] When dressing an ear injury, placing a small amount of packing between the ear and the side of the head helps to support the auricle in its natural position. Bleeding or cerebrospinal fluid emanating from the external auditory canal should be absorbed with gauze placed at the opening of the external auditory canal, but the canal itself should never be packed. Similarly, never probe the canal or attempt to remove any foreign body as this may result in canal laceration.[58] DOT 4-5.16–4-5.19

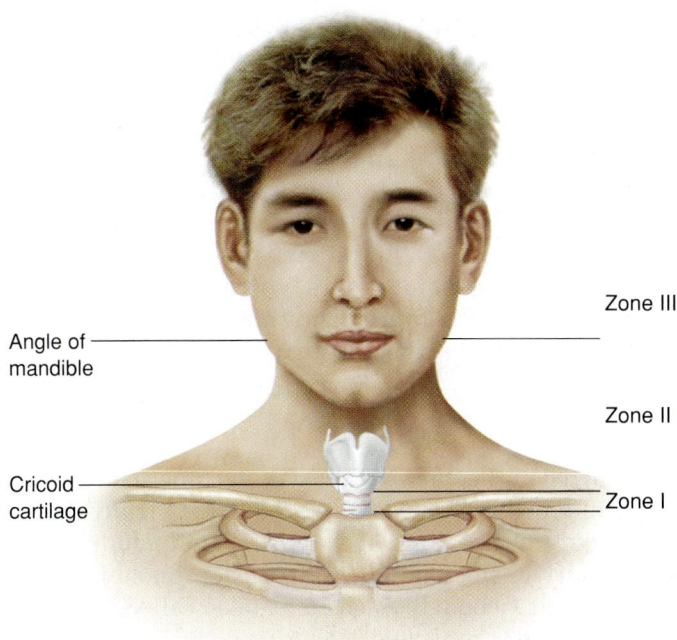

Figure 20-14   Zones of the neck.

Neck Trauma

The neck is a highly vulnerable area of the body. There is little to protect its important structures from traumatic injuries. Important vascular structures include the carotid and vertebral arteries and the jugular veins. One study has linked carotid artery injury to severe facial trauma.[62] DOT 4-7.25

The neck also includes the esophagus, trachea, lower cranial nerves, thyroid gland, brachial plexus, and spinal cord. Only the spinal cord has the luxury of significant bony protection. Penetrating injuries often injure one or more of these important structures and are commonly associated with injuries to other parts of the body as well. Penetrating injuries are more commonly life-threatening than blunt trauma to this area, although blunt trauma can also lead to severe injury.[9]

Anatomy and Physiology of the Neck

The anatomy of the neck is complex and made of many important structures. The neck has classically been divided into "triangles" by anatomists, but clinically it is divided into "zones" in order to guide clinical management (Box 20-4). Zone I extends from the clavicles to the cricoid cartilage, zone II from cricoid to the angle of the mandible, and zone III from the angle of the mandible to the base of the skull (Figure 20-14).[63] The underlying structures of the neck are covered by only a few layers of fascia and a thin muscle called the platysma. DOT 4-5.26

Each side of the neck contains one carotid artery and one vertebral artery that deliver blood to the anterior and posterior portions of the brain, respectively.

Each side also contains one jugular vein (which splits into the internal and external jugular veins) bringing blood back to the heart from the brain. The pharynx, proximally, divides in zone II into the larynx and esophagus, distally. The larynx turns into the trachea in zone I.

Primary Survey

Airway

Airway patency and compromise are of utmost concern in patients with significant neck injuries. Tracheal laceration, laryngeal fracture, and expanding hematomas are some mechanisms for airway compromise. Listen for a hoarse voice and stridor; look for signs of an expanding hematoma (a pulsatile mass), air bubbling out of the wound, tracheal deviation to one side of the neck, and hemoptysis (bloody sputum); and feel for subcutaneous emphysema (air under the skin).

If the airway is clearly in jeopardy, a definitive airway will be required. Orotracheal intubation is often the airway of choice, but in cases of tracheal or laryngeal injury, there is risk for tracheal transection, or the creation of a false passage during intubation.[64] Because of this risk, cricothyrotomy or tracheostomy may be the procedures of choice for securing the airway. These alternative procedures might also be necessary in the case of profuse bleeding into the airway. While this needs to be decided on a case by case basis, airway patency can deteriorate rapidly in the

> **BOX 20-4   Zones of the Neck and Their Contents**
>
> **Zone I:** Vertebral artery, carotid artery, thoracic vessels, lung apex, esophagus, trachea, thoracic duct, and spinal cord
>
> **Zone II:** Vertebral and carotid arteries, jugular vein, esophagus, larynx, spinal cord
>
> **Zone III:** Carotid and vertebral arteries, pharynx, and spinal cord

case of an expanding hematoma or subcutaneous emphysema, and early airway control may be preferred while it is still possible. **Skill Sheet 19: Needle Cricothyroidotomy (also see Step-by-Step 19) outlines performance of this skill.** DOT 4-5.27–4-5.29

Depending on individual anatomy and injuries, airway compromise may be positional, as stated in the facial trauma section. If the patient is insistent on lying in a certain position or sitting up, you may need to weigh the importance of compromising spinal immobilization with that of maintaining the airway.

Breathing

Although it may come as a surprise, the lung apex is actually contained in "zone I" of the neck (see Figure 20-14). Any injury to this zone of the neck may include direct lung injury or pneumothorax. If tension pneumothorax is suspected, needle thoracostomy (also called chest decompression) is indicated.[65]

CONNECTIONS For a review of tension pneumothorax, see Chapter 21: Thoracic Trauma and **Skill Sheet and Step-by-Step 77: Management of Chest Trauma.**

Circulation

Both penetrating and blunt neck trauma can lead to significant injury to the large vessels of the neck.[66] Penetrating injury to these vessels can rapidly lead to exsanguination. One or preferably two large-bore IV's must be started, with fluid boluses given to treat hypotension. The bleeding site must be controlled with direct pressure; do not place a clamp blindly in the neck in an attempt to control bleeding.

Blunt injury to the neck can also lead to arterial dissection of the inner lining of the blood vessel, resulting in occlusion of that vessel. Since the arteries of the neck supply the brain, the clinical appearance is that of a stroke.

Secondary Survey

HEENT

In the neck injured patient, the HEENT exam may be revealing for underlying injuries.

> **HEENT**
>
> **H** Head
> **E** Ears
> **E** Eyes
> **N** Nose
> **T** Throat

The pupil on the affected side may be small (miosis) if the sympathetic chain of nerves, which travels up the neck, is severed (which is significant, as most of its path runs with the carotid artery). Recognizing a small pupil is often difficult as most often the examiner will presume that the other one is dilated. Careful evaluation of reactivity will help differentiate which pupil actually is abnormal. Examine the cranial nerves using the assessment described in Chapter 14. The assessment may indicate either direct injury to the path of the nerve or a disruption in blood flow to the brain. The oropharynx exam may reveal a laceration as the tongue has large arteries (lingual artery) that can be damaged, leading to bleeding into the airway or an expanding hematoma. A zone III injury can also lead to laceration of the tongue, which can swell and obstruct the airway. DOT 4-5.5

Neck

The neck exam is mainly to localize underlying injury.

Look:

- For an expanding hematoma, which will indicate arterial or venous injury. Manual compression of the hematoma will help to lessen its expansion.
- For tracheal deviation. This may indicate an expanding hematoma or collection of subcutaneous air, which is pushing it to one side. It is also a very late finding in a tension pneumothorax and is deviated away from the affected side.
- For air bubbling from a wound. This indicates a tracheal, laryngeal, or lung injury from which air is escaping into the wound. Placement of an occlusive dressing is important in order to prevent air embolism.
- For bleeding. Compression of the bleeding site will help to control it.
- For violation of the platysma (the outermost layer of the neck); this signifies underlying injury until proven otherwise.

Feel:

- For subcutaneous emphysema. This is air under the skin from an underlying injury to the trachea, lung, or larynx. This is called **crepitus,** and will feel like how crispy rice cereal sounds when milk is poured over it.

Listen:

- For a **bruit.** This is the sound of blood rushing through a damaged or leaking artery. This is done by placing your stethoscope over the carotid artery; it sounds like rushing water in conjunction with the pulse. This is performed only if time permits in a stable patient and in a quiet environment.

Neurological

The neurological exam is important in neck injured patients as they have multiple mechanisms for dysfunction. Examination of cranial nerves, as well as peripheral strength and sensation, can indicate direct cranial nerve injury, spinal cord injury, and stroke symptoms due to cerebral ischemia.

Pulmonary

As stated under the primary survey, the lung apex is included in zone I of the neck, and pneumothorax can result from injury to this area. Simple pneumothorax can lead to increased work of breathing, pleuritic pain, and decreased breath sounds on the affected side. Respiratory distress can also result from injury to the phrenic nerve. This nerve originates from C3–C5 and controls the movement of the diaphragm; its injury will cause paralysis of the affected side of the diaphragm.

Summary

Head, facial, and neck trauma lead to a wide spectrum of disease, ranging from minor annoyance to severe life threats. In evaluating and treating these patients, manage the life threats with diligence and caution to prevent secondary injury. Maintain the ABCs by preventing or treating hypotension and hypoxia. Always be thinking one step ahead in your management of stable patients, as they can deteriorate rapidly.

Notes

1. Centers for Disease Control and Prevention, "Traumatic brain injury in the United States; a report to congress" (Department of Health and Human Services, November 25, 2003), http://www.cdc.gov/doc.do/id/0900f3ec8006ca49 (accessed December 10, 2005).

2. American Speech-Language-Hearing Association, "Traumatic brain injury," March 12, 2001, http://www.asha.org/public/speech/disorders/Traumatic-Brain-Injury.htm (accessed December 10, 2005).

3. Traumatic Brain Injury Resource Guide, "Epidemiology of TB," Centre for Neuro Skills, http://www.neuroskills.com/index.shtml?main=/tbi/epidemiology.shtml (accessed December 8, 2005).

4. T. D. Kirsch and C. A. Lipinski, "Chapter 255. Head Injury." McGraw-Hill's (2005). J. E. Tintinalli, G. D. Kelen, J. S. Stapczynski, O. J. Ma, and D. M. Cline, *Tintinalli's Emergency Medicine: A Comprehensive Study Guide*, 6th ed., McGraw-Hill's AccessMedicine (accessed June 2, 2006).

5. J. E. Wright, "Therapeutic hypothermia in traumatic brain injury," *Critical Care Nursing Quarterly* 28(2) (2005):150–161.

6. G. E. Morgan, Jr., M. S. Mikhail, and M. J. Murray, "Anesthesia for neurosurgery," *Clinical Anesthesiology,* 4th ed., McGraw-Hill's AccessMedicine (accessed December 28, 2005).

7. F. C. Brunicardi, D. K. Andersen, T. R. Billiar, D. L. Dunn, J. G. Hunter, J. B. Matthews, R. E. Pollock, and S. I. Schwartz, "Neurosurgery," *Schwartz's Principles of Surgery,* 8th ed., McGraw-Hill's AccessMedicine (accessed December 23, 2005).

8. M. H. Biros, "Head trauma," In *Emergency Medicine: Concepts and Clinical Practice,* 4th ed., P. Rosen, ed. (Minneapolis: Mosby, 1998).

9. J. E. Tintinalli, G. D. Kelen, J. S. Stapczynski, O. J. Ma, and D. M. Cline, "Head injury." *Tintinalli's Emergency Medicine: A Comprehensive Study Guide,* 6th ed., McGraw-Hill's AccessMedicine (accessed December 28, 2005).

10. American College of Surgeons Committee on Trauma, *ATLS Student Course Manual,* 6th Ed. (Chicago, IL: American College of Surgeons, 1997), pp. 65–66.

11. R. M. Walls, "Rapid-Sequence Intubation in Head Trauma," *Annals of Emergency Medicine* 22(6) (1993):1008.

12. N. Robinson and M. Clancy, "In Patients With Head Injury Undergoing Rapid Sequence Intubation, Does Pretreatment With Intravenous Lignocaine/Lidocaine Lead to an Improved Neurological Outcome? A Review of the Literature," *Emergency Medicine* 18 (2001): 453–457.

13. J. J. Brucia, D. C. Owen, and E. B. Rudy, "The Effects of Lidocaine on Intracranial Hypertension," *The Journal of Neuroscience Nursing* 24 (1992): 205–214.

14. R. Lev and P. Rosen, "Prophylactic Lidocaine Use Preintubation: A Review," *Emergency Medicine* 12(1994):499–506.

15. S. F. Reynolds and J. Heffner, "Airway Management of the Critically Ill Patient: Rapid Sequence Intubation, Chest," 127 (4) (April 2005) (accessed January 22, 2006).

16. D. P. Davis, J. Peay, et al., "The Impact of Prehospital Endotracheal Intubation on Outcome in Moderate to Severe Traumatic Brain Injury," *The Journal of Trauma* 58(5)(2005):933–939.

17. J. A. Murray, D. Demetriades, et al., "Prehospital Intubation in Patients with Severe Head Injury," *The Journal of Trauma* 49(6)(2000):1065–1070.

18. G. V. Bochicchio, O. Ilahi, et al., "Endotracheal Intubation in the Field Does Not Improve Outcome in Trauma Patients Who Present Without Acutely Lethal Traumatic Brain Injury," *The Journal of Trauma* 54(2)(2003):307–311.

19. D. P. Davis, D. B. Hoyt, et al., "The Effect of Paramedic Rapid Sequence Intubation on Outcome in Patients With Severe Traumatic Brain Injury," *The Journal of Trauma* 54(3)(2003):444–453.

20. S. Ayan, "Prehospital Endotracheal Intubation in Adult Major Trauma Patients with Head Injury," *Emergency Medicine* 22(2005):887–892.

21. D. C. Bloch and A. H. Murr, "Laryngeal trauma," *Current Diagnosis and Treatment in Otolaryngology-Head and Neck Surgery.* McGraw-Hill's AccessMedicine (accessed August 28, 2006).

22. A. H. Ropper and R. H. Brown, "Craniocerebral trauma," *Adams and Victor's Principles of Neurology,* 8th ed., McGraw-Hill's AccessMedicine (accessed December 23, 2005).

23. E. T. Gabriel, J. Ghajar, et al., "Guidelines for prehospital management of traumatic brain injury," Brain Trauma Foundation, 2000. http://www2.braintrauma.org/guidelines/downloads/btf_guidelines_prehospital.pdf?BrainsTrauma_Session=d275c0a08533c33fb7f76acbd5ab6b9f (accessed December 6, 2005).

24. R. L. Paul, O. Polanco, S. Z. Turney, et al., "Intracranial Pressure Responses to Alterations in Arterial Carbon Dioxide Pressure in Patients with Head Injuries," *Journal of Neurosurgery* 36(1972):714–720.

25. J. P. Muizelaar, A. Marmarou, J. D. Ward, et al., "Adverse Effects of Prolonged Hyperventilation in Patients with Severe Head Injury: A Randomized Clinical Trial," *Journal of Neurosurgery* 75(1991):731–739.

26. Trauma.org. "Control of intracranial hypertension" (May 1, 2001), http://www.trauma.org/neuro/icpcontrol.html (accessed December 7, 2005).

27. D. P. Davis, J. V. Dunford, M. Ochs, et al., "The Use of Quantitative End-Tidal Capnometry to Avoid Inadvertent Severe Hyperventilation in Patients with Head Injury After Paramedic Rapid Sequence Intubation," *The Journal of Trauma* 56(2004):808–814.

28. M. R. Fearnside, R. J. Cook, et al., "The Westmead Head Injury Project Outcome in Severe Head Injury: A Comparative Analysis of Pre-Hospital, Clinical, and CT Variables," *British Journal of Neurosurgery* 7 (1993): 267–279.

29. R. M. Chestnut, L. F. Marshall, et al., "The Role of Secondary Brain Inury in Determining Outcome from Severe Head Injury," *The Journal of Trauma* 34(1993):216–222.

30. A. Marmarou, R. L. Anderson, et al., "Impact of ICP Instability and Hypotension on Outcome in Patients with Severe Head Trauma," *Journal of Neurosurgery* 75(1991):S159–S166.

31. J. H. Siegel, "The Effect of Associated Injuries, Blood Loss, and Oxygen Debt on Death and Disability in Blunt Traumatic Brain Injury, The Need for Early Physiologic Predictors of Severity," *Journal of Neurotrauma* 12(4)(1993):579.

32. P. Pons and V. Markovchick, *Prehospital Emergency Care Secrets: Questions You Will be Asked–at the Scene, in the ED, on Exams,* (Philadelphia, PA: Hanley and Blefus, Inc., 1998), pp. 204–206.

33. G. Teasdale and B. Jennett, Assessment of Coma and Impaired Consciousness, A Practical Scale," *Lancet* 2(1974):81–84.

34. T. L. Massagli, L. J. Michaud, and F. P. Rivara, "Association Between Injury Indicies and Outcome After Severe Traumatic Brain Injury in Children," *Archives of Physical Medicine and Rehabilitation* 77(1996):1125–1132.

35. J. V. Winkler, P. Rosen, and E. J. Alfrey, "Prehospital Use of Glasgow Coma Score in Severe Head Injury," *Emergency Medicine* 2(1984):1–6.

36. J. D. Easton, S. L. Hauser, and J. B. Martin, "Cerebrovascular Diseases," In *Harrison's Principles of Internal Medicine,* 14th ed., A. S. Fauci, E. Braunwald, et al., eds. New York, NY: McGraw-Hill, (1998), p. 2343.

37. K. J. Knoop, L. B. Stack, and A. B. Storrow, "Head and Facial Trauma," *Atlas of Emergency Medicine,* 2nd ed., McGraw-Hill's AccessMedicine (accessed December 27, 2005).

38. J. A. Doyle, D. P. Davis, and D. B. Hoyt, "The Use of Hypertonic Saline in Treatment of Traumatic Brain Injury," *The Journal of Trauma* 50(2)(2001):367–383.

39. D. J. Cooper, P. S. Myles, et al., "Prehospital Hypertonic Saline Resuscitation of Patients with Hypotension and Severe Traumatic Brain Injury," *Journal of the American Medical Association* 291(11)(2004):1350–1357.

40. D. W. Marion, L. E. Penrod, et al., "Treatment of Traumatic Brain Injury with Moderate Hypothermia," *New England Journal of Medicine* 336(1997):540–546.

41. G. L. Clifton, R. Emmy, et al., "Lack of Effect of Induction of Hypothermia After Acute Brain Injury," *New England Journal of Medicine* 344(2001):556–563.

42. M. J. Aminoff, D. A. Greenberg, and R.P. Simon, *Clinical Neurology,* 6th ed., McGraw-Hill's AccessMedicine (accessed June 6, 2006).

43. D. L. Kasper, E. Braunwald, A. S. Fauci, S. L. Hauser, D. L. Longo, J. L. Jameson, and K. J. Isselbacher, eds., "Concussion and Other Head Injuries," *Harrison's Principles of Internal Medicine,* 16th ed., McGraw-Hill's AccessMedicine (accessed December 27, 2005).

44. J. R. Wasserman and R. A. Koenigsberg, "Diffuse Axonal Injury," *Emedicine* (February 24, 2004), http://www.emedicine.com/radio/topic216.htm (accessed December 7, 2005).

45. D. W. Munter and T. D. McGuirk, *Emergency Medicine Atlas,* McGraw-Hill's AccessMedicine (accessed June 4, 2006).

46. U. De Girolami, M. P. Frosch, and D. C. Anthony, "The central nervous system," In *Robbins Pathologic Basis of Disease, 5th ed.,* R. S. Cotran, et al., eds. (Philadelphia, PA: W. B. Saunders Co, 1994), p. 1304.

47. Centers for Disease Control, "Head injuries associated with motorcycle use—Wisconsin, 1991," *MMWR Weekly* 43(23)(1994):423, 429–31.

48. Centers for Disease Control, "Injury prevention and control," *CDC Performance plans* (January 12, 2000). http://www.cdc.gov/od/perfplan/2000/2000xbicycle.htm (accessed December 30, 2005).

49. D. F. Kelly, "Alcohol and Head Injury: An Issue Revisited," *Journal of Neurotrauma* 12(5)(1995):883–890.

50. D. A. Yost, "Acute Care for Alcohol Intoxication," *Postgraduate Medicine* 112(6)(2002):14–26.

51. W. Hackl, K. Hausberger, R. Sailer, et al., "Prevalence of Cervical Spine Injuries in Patients With Facial Trauma," *Oral Surgery, Oral Medicine, Oral Pathology, Oral Radiology, and Endodontics* 92(2001):370.

52. H. A. Ochs, M. C. Neuenschwander, and T. B. Dodson, "Are Head, Neck and Facial Injuries Markers of Domestic Violence?" *Journal of the American Dental Association* 127(1996):757.

53. K. N. Hartzell, A. A. Botek, and S. H. Goldberg, "Orbital Fractures in Women Due to Sexual Assault and Domestic Violence," *Ophthalmology* 103(1996):953.

54. N. Zachariades, D. Papavassiliou, and P. Christopoulos, "Blindness after facial trauma," *Oral Surgery, Oral Medicine, Oral Pathology, Oral Radiology, and Endodontics* 81(1996):34.

55. M. Trope, "Clinical Management of the Avulsed Tooth," *Dental Clinics of North America* 39(1995):93.

56. L. Blomlof, "Milk and Saliva as Possible Storage Media for Traumatically Exarticulated Teeth Prior to Replantation," *Swedish Dental Journal* 8(1981):1.

57. G. M. Doherty and L. W. Way, *Current Surgical Diagnosis and Treatment,* 12th ed., McGraw-Hill's AccessMedicine (accessed September 2, 2006).

58. A. K. Lalwani, *Current Diagnosis and Treatment in Otolaryngology—Head and Neck Surgery.* McGraw-Hill's AccessMedicine (accessed September 2, 2006).

59. J. Robson, A. J. Behrman, and S. Abbuhl, "Globe Rupture," *Emedicine.com.* (July 13, 2005). http://www.emedicine.com/emerg/topic218.htm (accessed January 2, 2006).

60. J. Tang and V. A. DeRamo, "Treating Traumatic Hyphema," *Eyenet Magazine,* American Academy of Ophthalmology (October 2003). http://www.aao.org/aao/news/eyenet/pearls/pearls_oct_2003.htm (accessed January 2, 2006).

61. S. G. Fermin and S. J. Letterle, "Maxillofacial and Neck Trauma," *Current Emergency Diagnosis and Treatment,* 5th ed., C. K. Stone and R. L. Humphries, eds., McGraw-Hill's AccessMedicine (accessed September 2, 2006).

62. R. D. Marciani and S. Israel, "Diagnosis of Blunt Carotid Injury in Patients with Facial Trauma," *Oral Surgery, Oral Medicine, Oral Pathology, Oral Radiology, and Endodontics* 83(1997):5.

63. A. J. Roon and N. Christensen, "Evaluation and Treatment of Penetrating Cervical Injuries," *The Journal of Trauma* 19(1979):391.

64. F. J. Baumgartner, B. Ayers, and C. Theuer, "Danger of False Intubation After Traumatic Tracheal Transaction," *Annals Thoracic Surgery* 63(1)(1997):227–228.

65. D. P. Davis, K. Pettit, et al., "The Safety and Efficacy of Prehospital Needle and Tube Thoracostomy by Aeromedical Personnel," *Prehospital Emergency Care* 9(2)(2005):191–197.

66. D. W. Larsen, "Traumatic Vascular Injuries and Their Management," *Neuroimaging Clinics of North America.* 12(2)(2002):149–169.

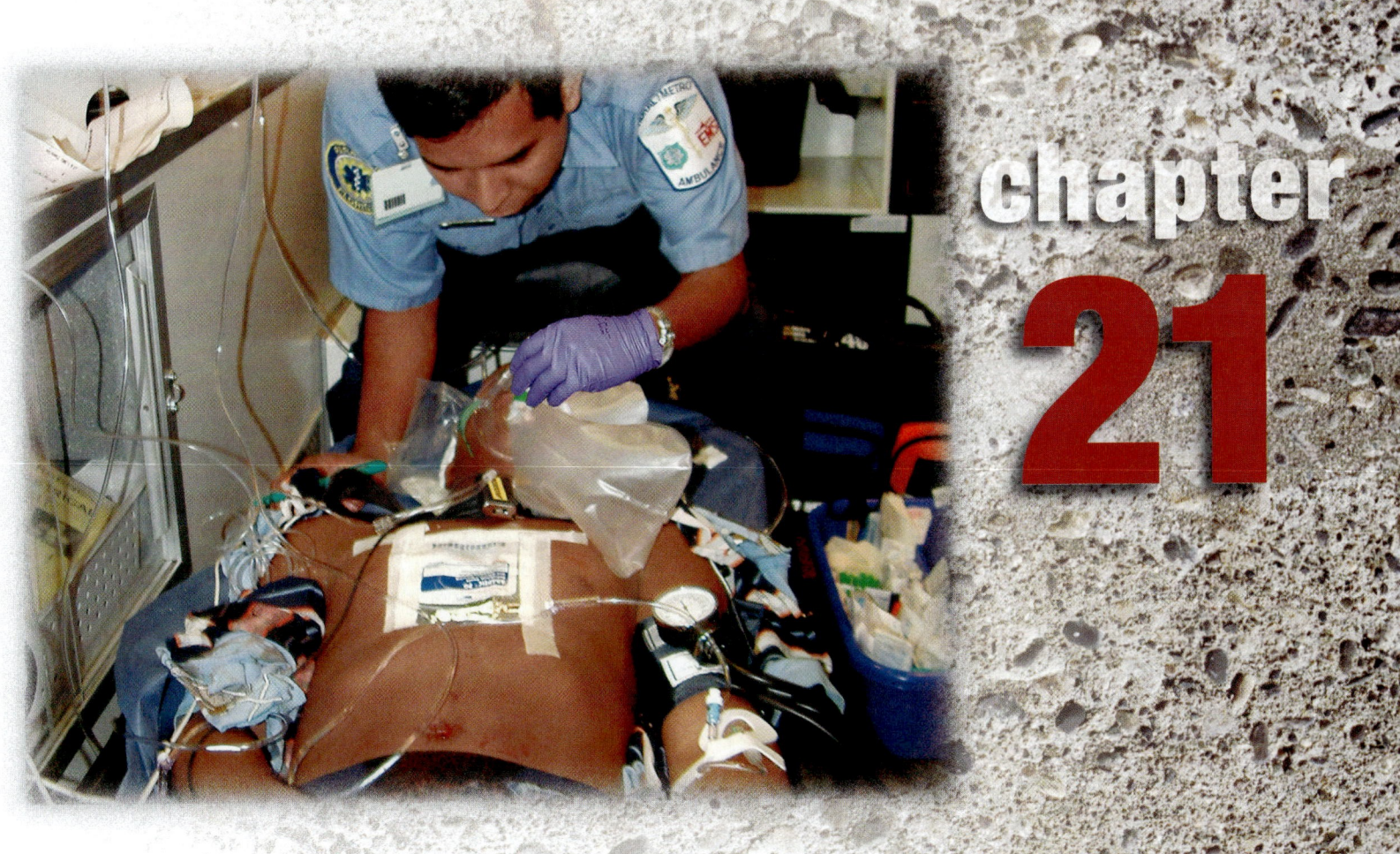

Thoracic Trauma

*"**W**hereat, with blade, with bloody blameful blade, He bravely broached his boiling bloody breast."*

—William Shakespeare, *A Midsummer Night's Dream*, 1595–1596

Need to Know

▶ Because the chest houses vital organs for perfusion and ventilation (heart and lungs), injuries to this area can rapidly become lethal.

▶ Anatomically speaking, any injury between the umbilicus and nipple line should be suspected of having penetrated the chest cavity as well as the abdomen.

▶ Immediately assessing airway and breathing is essential. The goal is to identify life threats such as tension pneumothorax and flail chest.

▶ Absent lung sounds alone equal pneumothorax or hemothorax, or both.

▶ Penetrating trauma to the chest often results in both pneumo- and hemothorax.

▶ The danger with hemothorax is massive bleeding. Each side of the chest can hold up to two liters of blood.

▶ Sick	▶ Not Yet Sick
• Look for signs of tension pneumothorax and perform a needle decompression if a tension pneumothorax develops.	• Use the ECG monitor on every thoracic trauma patient, and watch for cardiac rhythm disturbance.
• Transport rapidly if pericardial tamponade is present. If allowed, a percardiocentesis may be performed. Medical direction should be actively involved in the decision to perform this procedure.	• Worsening dyspnea is a possible indication that a chest injury such as a pneumothorax is changing to a tension pneumothorax.
• Perform bag-mask ventilations to help improve breathing if a flail chest is present.	• Continuously reassess vital signs, recording the readings about every five minutes.
• Absent or significantly diminished lung sounds indicate a very sick patient.	• Frequently ask the patient, "Are you having difficulty breathing?"
• Signs the problem is worsening include:	
• Narrowing pulse pressures	
• Hypotension	
• Pulsus paradoxus	
• With the exception of performing a decompression or placing an occlusive dressing, most thoracic injuries are treated in a similar manner: Recognize the patient is sick, support and monitor the ABCs, and perform a rapid and safe transport to a trauma center.	

Introduction

Trauma to the thorax can cause devastating injuries. A patient with trauma to the thorax who is alert and talking one moment can rapidly deteriorate to the point of cardiopulmonary arrest within a few short minutes. The reason is simple: The thorax houses the cardiovascular system and is the center of the body's mechanism for circulation, air exchange, and oxygen delivery. The various components of this system exist in a delicate balance of carefully regulated interactions. Trauma to the thorax can overwhelm a patient's compensatory mechanisms and seriously impair oxygen delivery to the brain and other organs of the body. Unfortunately, this can happen very quickly, leaving the paramedic with a narrow window of opportunity to recognize an injury and make a meaningful intervention. DOT 4-7.11, 4-7.12

It is critical to understand how the thorax works, how we breathe, and why damage to any given component may compromise a patient's health. Good patient assessment skills are also critical to be able to identify specific injuries to the chest that may require drastic and life-saving interventions in the field. There are 12 potentially deadly conditions connected to the thorax that are listed in Box 21-1.

Street Secrets

Be careful. Patients will not fit neatly into the categories described in textbooks. Memorizing a laundry list of different chest injuries and a set of algorithms to treat them may not be as helpful as using common sense and good clinical judgment.

Skill sheets related to this chapter content include: Skill Sheet 18: Continuous Positive Airway Pressure (also see Step-by-Step 18); Skill Sheet 7: Endotracheal Intubation (also see Step-by-Step 7); Skill Sheet 12: Pulse Oximetry (also see Step-by-Step 12); Skill Sheet 14: Nasal Intubation (also see Step-by-Step 14); Skill Sheet 15: Digital Intubation; Skill Sheet 16:

BOX 21-1 The Deadly Dozen

Major traumatic chest injuries can be deadly. Think of them as the following:

The lethal six (identified in the primary survey)

1. Airway obstruction
2. Tension pneumothorax
3. Cardiac tamponade
4. Massive hemothorax
5. Open pneumothorax
6. Flail chest

The hidden six (identified in the secondary survey)

1. Thoracic aortic disruption
2. Tracheobronchial disruption
3. Myocardial contusion
4. Traumatic diaphragmatic tear
5. Esophageal disruption
6. Pulmonary contusion

Adapted from L. Yamamoto, C. Schroeder, C. Beliveau, "Thoracic Trauma, The Deadly Dozen," *Critical Care Nursing Quarterly* 28 (1) (2005): 22–40.

Endotracheal Intubation in Face-to-Face Position; Skill Sheet 27: Chest Auscultation (also see Step-by-Step 27); Skill Sheet 34: Chest Pain Assessment; Skill Sheet 35: Dyspnea Assessment; Skill Sheet 66: Bleeding Control and Shock (also see Step-by-Step 66); and Skill Sheet 77: Management of Chest Trauma (also see Step-by-Step 77).

Epidemiology

In general, thoracic trauma results in more than 16,000 deaths annually in the United States. Twenty to 25% of traumatic deaths are due to thoracic trauma.[1] Death rates are relatively low once the patient reaches the hospital (~5%) but rise sharply if multiple systems are involved. DOT 4-7.1

The most common cause of blunt thoracic trauma is the motor vehicle crash (MVC). In 2001, 44% of the nearly 98,000 unintentional injuries resulting in death in the United States resulted from MVCs. It is also estimated that the MVC mechanism alone carries a 7% risk of serious thoracic injury.[2] Overall, isolated injuries to the thorax give the patient an approximately 10% chance of dying. However, about one-third of patients will die if two or more organ systems are involved.

Applied Anatomy and Physiology

An understanding of the anatomy and basic physiology of the thorax is essential for the prehospital provider. Here we will briefly review some of the pertinent thoracic anatomy as it relates to chest trauma.[3] DOT 4-7.2

The outer structure and shape of the chest is provided by 12 sets of paired ribs, which are connected posteriorly to thoracic vertebrae 1 through 12. Ribs 1 through 7 wrap around from their respective thoracic vertebrae and connect to the sternum anteriorly through the costal cartilage. These are called the true ribs. Ribs eight, nine, and ten are called **false ribs** as their anterior connection is to the costal cartilage of the seventh rib. Ribs 11 and 12 do not have any anterior attachment at all and thus are called **floating ribs** (Figure 21-1).

Figure 21-1 (a) The thoracic cage. (b) Radiograph of the thoracic cage. The light region behind the sternum is the heart. The diaphragm can be seen at the bottom. See also Figure 7-36 in Anatomy Overview.

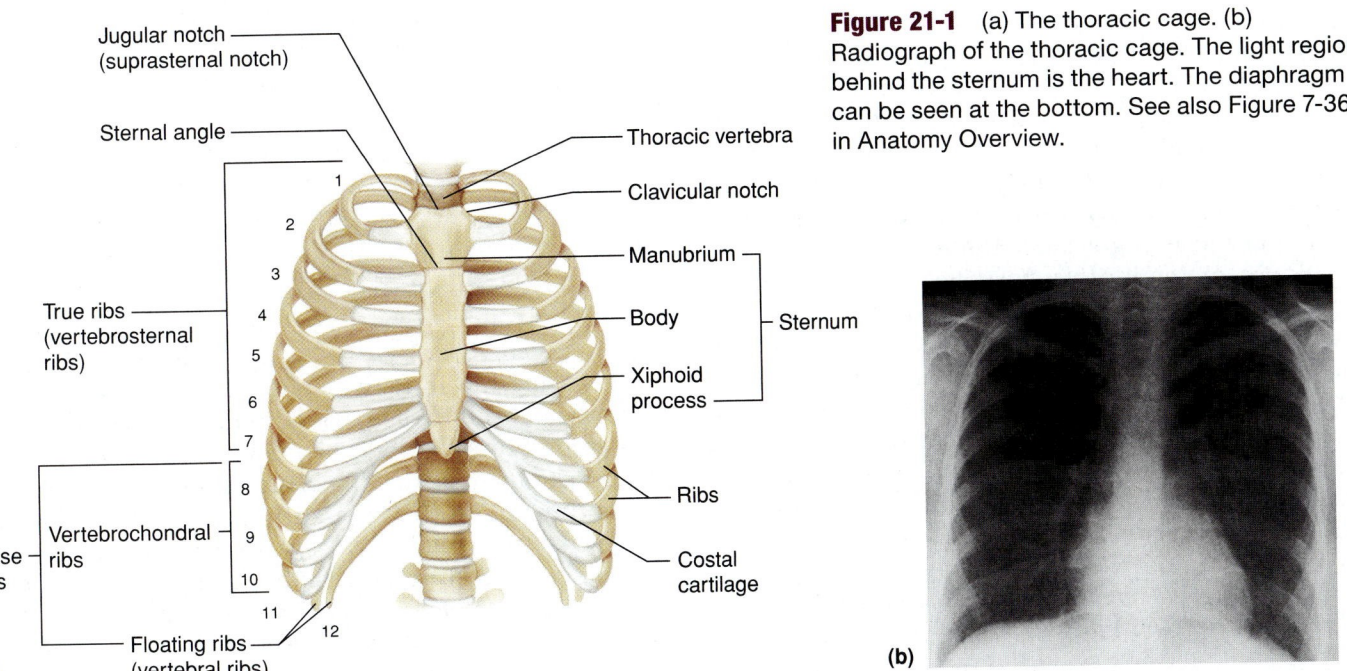

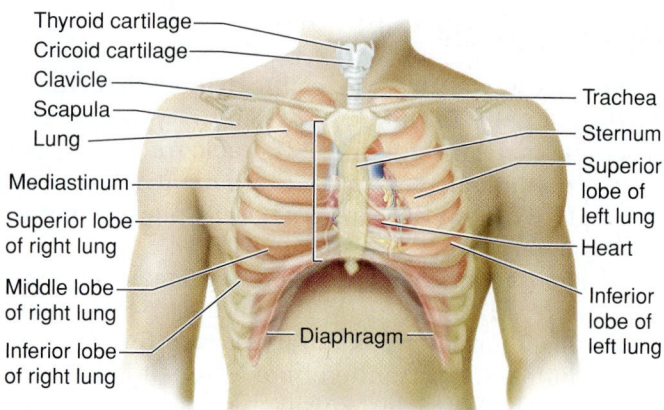

Figure 21-2   The thorax. Each side is called a hemithorax; the space in the middle is the mediastinum.

A neurovascular bundle consisting of the intercostal vein, artery, and nerve runs along the underside of each rib in the intercostal groove.

The thorax is divided into two sides, each called a hemithorax. Each hemithorax contains one lung. The space between the lungs is called the mediastinum. This central area houses the heart, great vessels, esophagus, thoracic duct, and some major nerves, including the phrenic and the vagus (Figure 21-2).

The vascular system is essentially a pair of closed loops with the heart acting as a set of paired pumps simultaneously supplying both circuits. These two loops are the pulmonary circulation and the systemic circulation. Blood from the upper part of the body returns to the heart via the superior vena cava, and that from the lower part of the body returns by the inferior vena cava. This returning blood combines and empties into the right atrium. From the right atrium, the blood enters the right ventricle. During systole, the right ventricle pumps blood through the pulmonary circulation of the lungs to exchange carbon dioxide for oxygen. At the same time, the newly oxygenated blood from the previous cycle returns to the left atrium and then enters the left ventricle. The left ventricle pumps its blood out into the systemic circulation by way of the aorta (Figure 21-3).

The aortic arch gives rise to the vessels supplying the upper extremities (subclavian arteries) and the cerebral circulation (carotid and vertebral arteries) before traveling downward through the thorax into the abdominal cavity. A piece of fibrous tissue called the **ligamentum arteriosum,** which is a remnant of the embryological circulatory system, tethers the aortic arch to the pulmonary artery outflow tract (Figure 21-4). This structure plays an important role in deceleration injuries of the great vessels as will be discussed in the Nice to Know box on page 420.

Each lung is covered by a thin serous membrane called the **visceral pleura.** In direct opposition to this

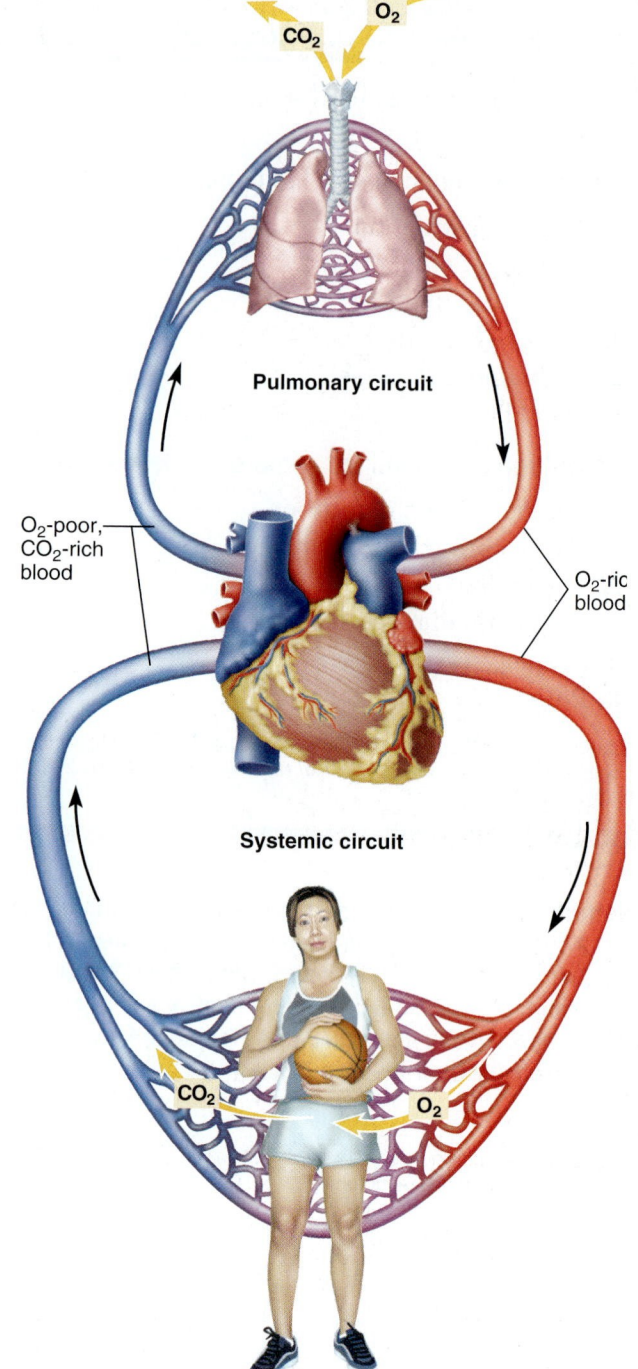

Figure 21-3   The vascular system.

and lining the interior of the chest wall is a similar membrane called the **parietal pleura.** A small amount of pleural fluid lies between these pleura and serves to lubricate them as they move against each other during each breath. More importantly, the intrapleural space acts like two panes of glass with water between them, causing them to stick together. This pleural space is considered a potential space because normally there is really no space at all between the two layers of pleura.

The most important feature of the pleural space is that, by design, it will generate a negative intrapleural pressure of about 3 mmHg when the chest wall expands. The lungs and thoracic cage, therefore, act like a blacksmith's bellows. As their volume is increased, the corresponding negative pressure inside them draws air in through the trachea and the upper airways.

Pathophysiology of Chest Injuries

The two types of forces that cause chest injures are blunt and penetrating. Chapter 18: Mechanism of Injury introduced these two general categories of trauma. Each type of mechanism can be further subcategorized, and a discussion of each type within each category follows below. If you have not already read Chapter 18, you should do so before continuing. DOT 4-7.41, 4-7.42, 4-7.43, 4-7.44

Blunt Trauma

Blunt trauma is commonly divided into three major types of injury. These are shearing, compression, and blast.[2] DOT 4-7.3, 4-7.4

Shearing Forces

Rapid deceleration causes **shearing forces.** The various organs of the thorax and their components are tethered together with fibrous tissues that have varying tensile strength, meaning varying amounts of force are required to tear and damage the tissues. Thus, in response to the application of force to the body and its internal organs, some structures move rapidly and others less so, generating shearing forces between the structures that

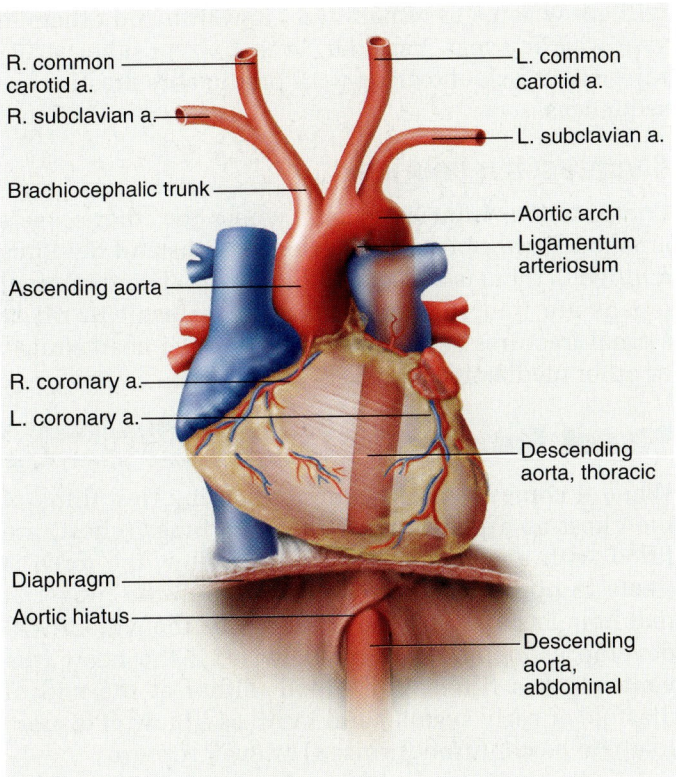

Figure 21-4   Beginning of the aorta. Note the position of the ligamentum arteriosum. (R. = right; L. = left; a. = artery)

However, any injury or illness that allows blood, air, or other fluid to enter between the two pleura can convert this into a true space and compromise a patient's respiratory function.

Working in the Gray Zone

Negative pressure has very positive results! The negative pressure in the chest created when a person expands the chest wall and contracts (drops) the diaphragm is not only necessary to draw air into the lungs, but it may have other important cardiovascular effects as well. Recent research shows that negative pressure in the chest also helps draw venous blood back into the heart.[4,5,6,7,8,9] Blood usually flows back into the heart during diastole (relaxation). This is thought of as a passive process. This very important connection between negative pressure in the chest and enhanced circulation has become an important topic in cardiac arrest research. New devices that impede the flow of air into the lung during recoil of the chest after a CPR compression have been shown to enhance blood flow back to the heart. This may have significant implication for thoracic injuries (such as flail chest and open pneumo-

thorax), when a person cannot create negative pressure in the chest, perhaps leading to compromised blood return to the heart. There are additional implications regarding ventilation. Emergency responders have shown a tendency to hyperventilate patients even after being coached to decrease ventilation rates. This may have detrimental effects in circulation for any patient, not just cardiac arrest or head injury patients.[7]

CONNECTIONS For more information about negative pressure and its role in respiration, review Chapter 12: Airway Management, Ventilation, and Oxygenation; for information regarding cardiac arrest research and new circulatory enhancements to CPR, review Chapter 29: Cardiology, Box 29-25; for information about flail chest and open pneumothorax see pages 426 and 432 of this chapter.

Nice to Know

The aorta is relatively free of attachments to other structures. In a rapid deceleration injury (such as an MVC) shearing forces are most likely to tear the aorta at its point of attachments.

There are only three points of direct attachment: the aortic valve, the ligamentum arteriosum, and the point of entry to the abdomen behind the diaphragm.[10]

In addition, the descending aorta is enclosed in a layer of fibrous tissue that holds it against the adjacent spinal column. When sudden deceleration forces are applied to the body, the heart, ascending aorta, and aortic arch are able to keep moving forward, causing the aorta to tear or shear, most commonly at a point just beyond the ligamentum arteriosum near the junction of the arch and descending aorta (Figure 21-5). This results in rapid exsanguination, and the patient either bleeds to death or an unstable trauma-induced aneurysm forms. This patient is in danger of dying unless surgical repair occurs quickly.

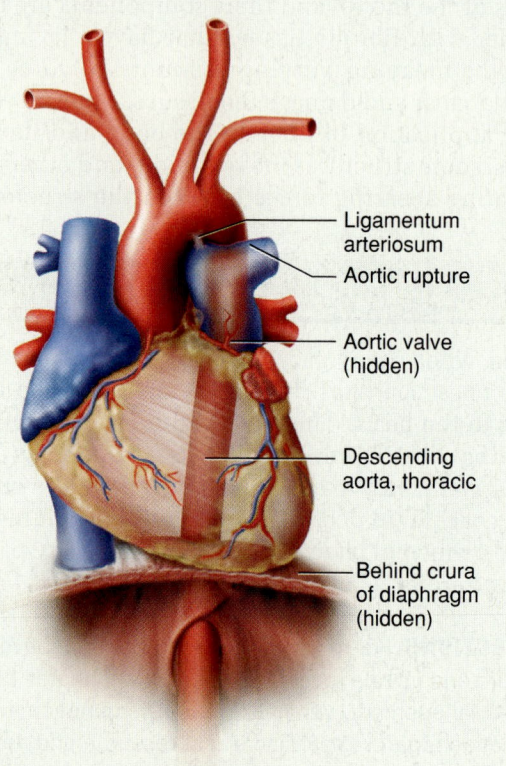

Ligamentum arteriosum

Aortic rupture

Aortic valve (hidden)

Descending aorta, thoracic

Behind crura of diaphragm (hidden)

Figure 21-5   Aortic rupture occurs most often at the junction of the arch and descending aorta.

will allow some to remain tight and firm and others to give way and tear. Vascular, bronchial, or other structures are at risk of tearing with predictably drastic consequences. DOT 4-7.5

Compression Injuries

Compression injuries occur when the thorax gets crushed. If the ability of the ribs to withstand the force applied to them is exceeded, the chest wall and internal organs are injured. Such injuries can result in rib or sternal fractures as well as damage to the heart, lungs, or other mediastinal organs.

Street Secrets

When it comes to blunt compression injuries, think of the chest as a paper bag. When the lungs (chest) are filled with air and receive a direct blow, the force is likely to pop the bag (creating a hole in the lungs). If that hole lets air enter the chest cavity, the patient will develop a pneumothorax. Likewise, if the heart (the ventricles) is filled with blood (either at the end of diastole or early systole) and receives a blow, it is more likely to be contused (bruised) or even rupture.

Blast Injuries

Blast injuries are a combination of compression and shearing, as well as penetrating trauma from flying debris and shrapnel. Air-filled spaces, such as the alveoli of the lungs, are in danger of barotrauma from the overpressurized blast wave.

CONNECTIONS Blast injuries are covered in detail in Chapter 25: Soft Tissue and Muscle Trauma.

Penetrating Trauma

Penetrating trauma can be classified as impaling or projectile. Penetrating injuries, in general, have less mortality than blunt trauma because damage with most penetrations is limited to the actual track of the wound. High-velocity projectiles, of course, are an exception because of the cavitation wave.

Impaling Injuries

Impaling injuries generally entail low-velocity forces such as a stabbing by a knife or falling on a fixed object (Figure 21-6). One of the characteristics of impaling injuries is that their damage is usually limited to the structures located along the object's pathway into and out of the body. If an object is impaled into a patient's chest, the paramedic should not remove it, as this could cause greater injury along the path of the impalement. Additionally, the impaling object may be putting pressure on

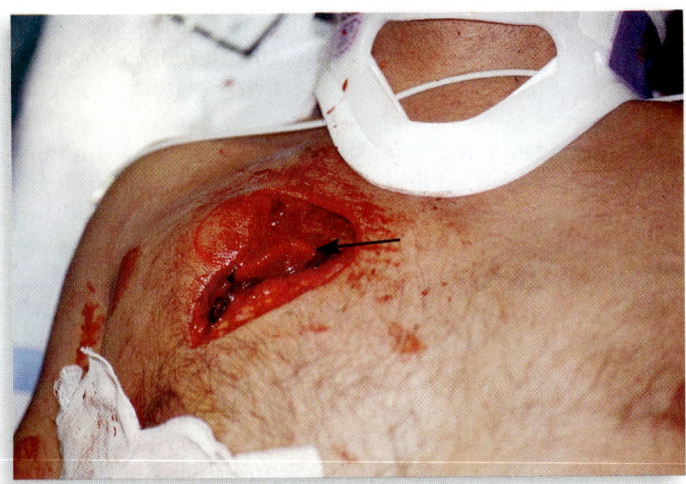

Figure 21-6   This patient was stabbed in the chest. A portion of lung tissue is visibly herniating (arrow).

a bleeding vessel, and removal of the object may actually cause more bleeding. A more detailed review of impaled objects can be found in Chapter 25: Soft Tissue and Muscle Trauma.

Projectile injuries

Projectile injury is caused by any airborne high-velocity object (such as a bullet) that enters the chest cavity. It too will damage anything in its path, but there are two other factors to take into consideration. First, its path is much harder to predict. A bullet may enter at one location and deflect in an entirely different direction (ricochet) after impact with a bony structure. A gunshot wound to the thorax can therefore result in abdominal injury, or vice versa. Second, a high-speed projectile causes cavitation forces to be generated as it tears through the body (Figure 21-7).[11]

When a bullet enters the body, it creates its path of damage called the **permanent cavity.** The permanent

cavity remains after the projectile has passed through the body. A larger temporary cavity is also created when the walls of the permanent cavity are temporarily pushed aside as the bullet travels past them. This temporary cavity can cause stretching and tearing of adjacent tissues, thus increasing the amount of damage beyond the permanent cavity. Chapter 18: Mechanism of Injury has more information on ballistic wounds.

Scene Survey

A great deal of information can be learned about a patient's injuries from the scene survey. After ensuring your own safety, rapidly assess the scene to try to determine the mechanism of injury. Each mechanism of trauma (motor vehicle crash, gunshot wound, fall, or explosion, for example) has unique injury patterns and characteristics. Information about the severity of the injury force (high-speed versus low-speed, height of falls, caliber of gun) and other incident-specific circumstances (landing position of falls, direction of impact, distance from explosion) is crucial. Additionally, make use of witnesses and bystanders to fill in gaps or clarify inconsistencies between the scene presentation and the patient presentation. Not only is all of this information important for the prehospital team, but it is also important to pass pertinent information along to the hospital team.

Working in the Gray Zone

Many EMS systems carry digital or Polaroid™ instant cameras and photograph of the scene showing the mechanism of trauma for the receiving hospital. These images should be safeguarded and treated with as much respect as any private patient information. They should *never* be shared with individuals outside the direct healthcare team taking care of the patient, including the media. If they are going to be used for educational purposes, the patient and any individual who can be identified in the image should sign a consent form allowing the image to be viewed by others.

Primary Survey

The ABCs

As you begin the ABC survey, follow the standard techniques discussed previously in Chapter 14: Patient Assessment. Expose the patient's chest as you begin assessing airway, breathing, and circulation. The basic principles of "look," "listen," and "feel" typically

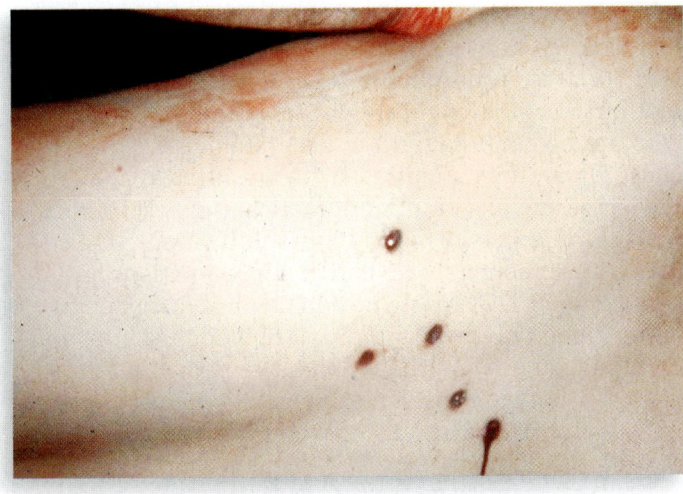

Figure 21-7   Multiple gunshot wounds to the back.

discussed in the context of the airway and breathing assessment are the foundation to evaluate the thorax of a traumatically injured patient as well. Within the primary survey, make a rapid determination about the breathing status of your patient. You need to ensure that the patient is able to move air through their lungs and blood through their heart. Chest injuries may involve the trachea and cause airway obstruction or bleeding into the lungs. Clearing the airway can become a real challenge in these cases. Endotracheal intubation and suctioning may be needed early on. **See Skill Sheet 7: Endotracheal Intubation (also see Step-by-Step 7) and Skill Sheet 16: Endotracheal Intubation in Face-to-Face Position.** DOT 4-7.6

Tension pneumothorax must be detected and treated quickly if it is found. Needle decompression (needle thoracostomy) is described in detail later in the chapter but should be performed as part of the primary survey. **Skill Sheet and Step-by-Step 77: Management of Chest Trauma outlines the performance of needle decompression.**

Initial Assessment of the Neck

Quickly visualize the patient's anterior neck and chest to assess for any difficulty in breathing. Look for signs of distress, which can include retractions of the skin at the sternal notch and between the ribs (intercostal retractions) or shoulder shrugging or positioning in postures such as tripod or sniffing that allow for better breathing. Look for obvious deformities, jugular vein distension, or tracheal deviation.

Tracheal deviation (usually due to tension pneumothorax or a massive hemothorax) can be very difficult to assess by sight alone. It is important to palpate the trachea for signs of deviation. Normally you should feel a person's trachea when you gently put your fingers in the sternal notch. If the trachea has been displaced, you may feel the trachea to one side, or not feel the trachea at all.

When present, tracheal deviation indicates the condition is advanced and the danger of imminent death is great. Conversely, the patient may die from a tension pneumothorax before tracheal deviation ever develops.

Inspect and palpate the chest wall. If you note any asymmetric or asynchronous chest wall motion, then chest wall damage, flail chest, or splinting from pain can be present. Clearly, the finding of any penetrating wounds mandates an exhaustive hunt for additional wounds. Lift the arms and quickly and carefully look at both axillae for hidden wounds. Roll the patient using spine precautions (if indicated) to look for posterior wounds.

Street Secrets

One common misconception is that running a gloved hand under the patient's back to look for blood is a substitute for rolling the patient. Penetrating wounds often have much less bleeding than you might think, leading to a missed injury and inappropriate treatment or triage. Any penetration to the anterior thorax warrants visual examination of the posterior thorax for another penetration wound. Do not be misled into thinking that only a straight through and through pattern is possible. Remember, projectiles can ricochet and change directions, and an entrance in the upper anterior chest can exit from the posterior flank.

Working in the Gray Zone

Reliable signs in tension pneumothorax do not include Jugular Vein Distension (JVD)

A good rule of thumb to differentiate a tension pneumothorax from a simple pneumothorax or hemothorax is to look for signs that pressure is building and compressing the heart and uninjured lung. Look for the following:

- Difficulty breathing (including absent lung sounds on the affected side)
- Hypotension (absent radial pulse)
- Tachycardia (rapid heart rate)

If the patient does not exhibit the three signs listed above, it would be very rare that a tension pneumothorax is present. Other classic signs usually described in a textbook may not be as reliable. Jugular vein distension (JVD) is an unreliable "sign" in a tension pneumothorax as it is often present in supine individuals who are not injured, and to accurately assess it in a chest injury, the patient needs to be sitting at a 30- to 90-degree angle, which is impractical for most trauma patients because of spinal immobilization. It also may be impractical to visualize when a patient has a c-collar on. JVD also depends on having enough circulating blood volume in order to see blood backing up into the jugular veins. A hypotensive patient may not have JVD but may still have a tension pneumothorax. Subcutaneous emphysema may or may not be present as well. Box 21-2 on page 424 has more information.

Initial Assessment of the Chest

Look

Visualize the chest. If you see open wounds, especially any that are bubbling (air escaping from the chest), you should immediately place your gloved hand on the wound and quickly follow with the application of an occlusive dressing.

Feel

Next, palpate the chest wall. Subcutaneous air has a crunching puffed rice cereal feel, suggesting a pneumothorax. Sternal tenderness may suggest a fracture with potential injury to underlying mediastinal structures. Palpate and compress the ribs to help identify fractures and possible pneumothorax or hemothorax. Palpate the back; shoulder blades and shoulders should also be evaluated to assess for other injuries.

Listen

Finally, rapidly auscultate the patient's chest with a stethoscope.[12] In a trauma situation, this can be simple and quick, listening to the lungs bilaterally at the midaxillary line at both the fifth interspace (approximately at the nipple line) and lower at the tenth interspace. The heart can be listened to on both sides of the upper sternum and the apex.[12]

Pneumothoraces and hemothoraces are often associated with impaired breath sound transmission and subsequent decreased sounds. Pulmonary contusion with interstitial fluid may, although rarely in the prehospital setting, be evident by hearing rales. If the heart sounds are very distant or muffled, this may signify a pericardial tamponade.

Continually assess the quality and character of the patient's breathing as needed in thoracic trauma.[12] Normal breathing should be an effortless quiet process with only a soft sound of air moving at the mouth and nose. The normal respiratory rate should be 12–20 respirations per minute. **Tachypnea** is a rate greater than 20 respirations per minute, and its presence can signify anxiety, pain, shock, or metabolic problems. Most significantly, it may be the first sign of compromised gas exchange due to thoracic trauma. **Bradypnea** is a rate less than 12 respirations per minute and can result from the above-listed causes after the patient can no longer compensate or it may develop after a neurological insult. DOT 4-7.7, 4-7.8

Secondary Survey

The importance of a thorough secondary survey cannot be overemphasized in thoracic trauma. The existence of injury to another organ or system in a chest trauma

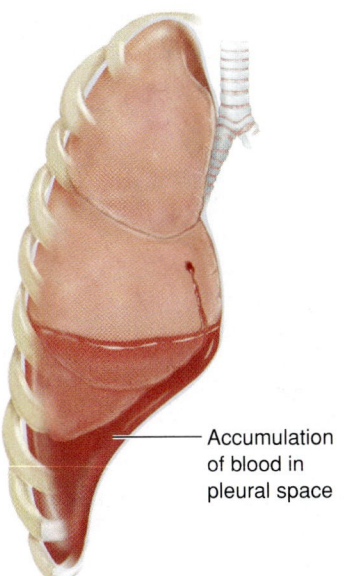

Accumulation of blood in pleural space

Figure 21-8   Hemothorax.

patient significantly increases the chance of the patient dying. Even though the injury to the thorax may be the most obvious one, there may be additional injuries to the head, neck, or abdomen.

Specific Thoracic Injuries

Lung and Pleural Injuries

Pneumothorax and Hemothorax.   If an injury causes a tear in one or both of the lungs, air or blood can enter the pleural space. These conditions are called **pneumothorax** and **hemothorax** respectively (Figure 21-8).[19] They most commonly occur after blunt trauma to the chest during a motor vehicle crash (72.2%) as well as penetrating injury.[13] Recognizing these is vital since they can easily develop into a serious breathing problem.

Very important: Simple hemothorax and pneumothorax are usually not life-threatening and usually do not require prehospital intervention beyond recognition and monitoring. If this accumulation of air or blood begins to compress the unaffected lung or the heart, the situation may become serious and eventually critical. Although confirmation of a pneumothorax must be done with an x-ray, approximately 90% of patients will have chest pain, and 80% will complain of shortness of breath. The severity of their symptoms may depend on the size of the pneumothorax.[14]

Tension Pneumothorax. Within the category of traumatic injury to the lungs, the most serious condition is **tension pneumothorax,** but it is also the most uncommon.

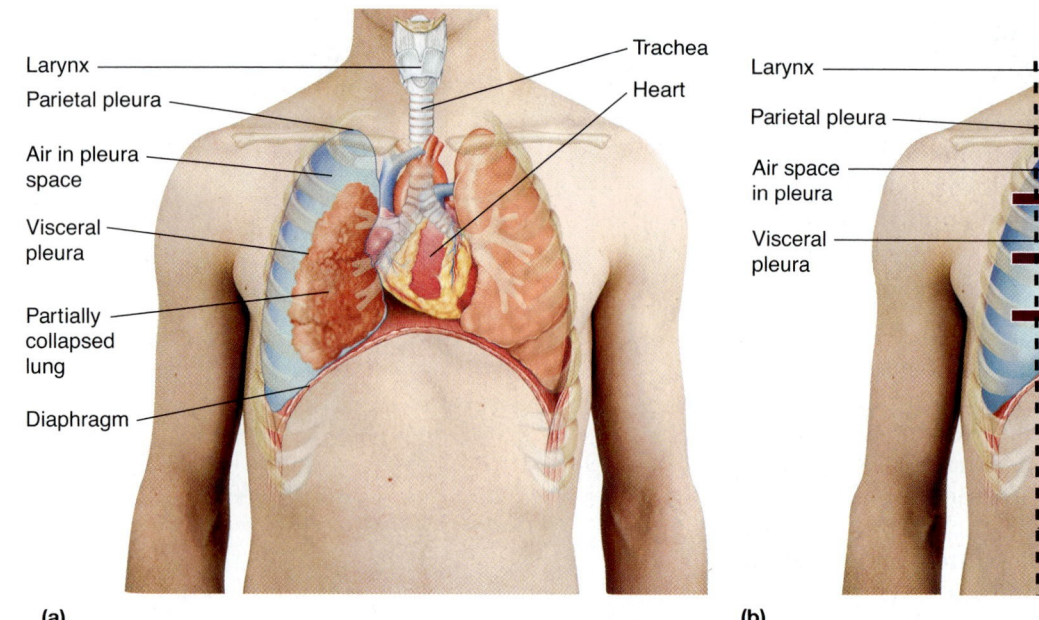

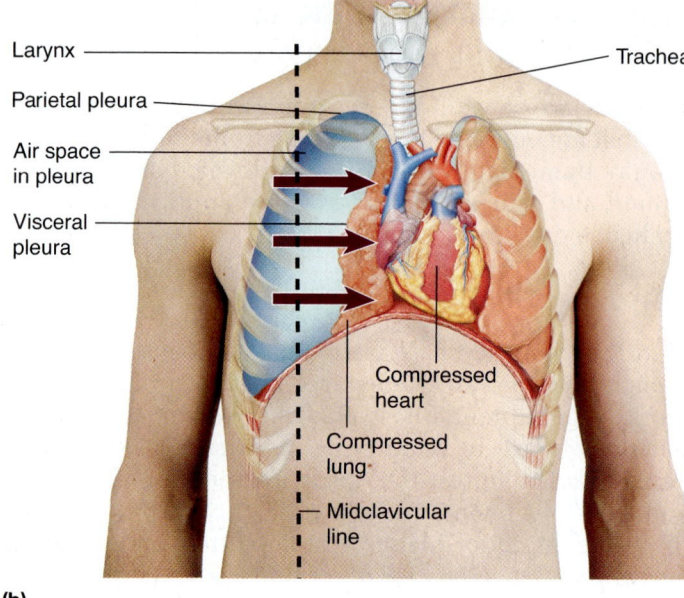

Figure 21-9 (a) Pneumothorax. (b) Tension pneumothorax.

If air is actively entering the pleural space and not able to escape, this condition may trap enough air that it begins to put pressure on the heart, great vessels, and opposite lung. This is known as a tension pneumothorax (Figure 21-9). The expanding pneumothorax can cause progressive collapse of the affected lung and a shift of the structures in the center of the chest (mediastinal structures such as the heart and trachea) away from the affected side. It is thought that this shift effectively pinches off the superior and inferior vena cavae, preventing the return of blood to the heart (preload) and also begins to compress the other lung. Without enough blood returning, cardiac output will also drop. DOT 4-7.13c

Clinical signs suggesting a tension pneumothorax include tachycardia, hypotension, asymmetric breath sounds, and deviated trachea (Box 21-2).

Street Secrets

Endotracheal intubation and positive pressure ventilation have a higher potential of turning a simple pneumothorax into a tension pneumothorax, particularly if the respiratory rate is high and the volume of each breath is excessive. Current recommendations for assisting ventilations using a bag-mask for adults are to provide *no more* than about 10 breaths per minute. CPR compression guidelines recommend "push hard—push fast" but think of assisted ventilation as "go slow—volume is low."

There are only a handful of definitive actions that a paramedic can take in the prehospital setting to save a patient's life. Recognizing and treating a tension pneumothorax is one of them. If a tension pneumothorax is suspected, the affected side of the chest needs to be decompressed. This is accomplished by needle decompression **(needle thoracostomy)** with a large-bore 10–14 gauge angiocatheter or needle. **See Skill Sheet and Step-by-Step 77: Management of Chest Trauma.**

BOX 21-2 Signs and Symptoms of Tension Pneumothorax

- Asymetrical breath sounds (could be absent or diminished on the affected side)
- Difficulty breathing that is worsening (80% of patients have this sign)
- Chest pain (90% of patients have this sign)
- Worsening difficulty in performing bag-mask ventilations
- Hypotension (absent radial pulse)
- Tachycardia (rapid heart rate)
- Drop in pulse oximetry reading
- Pulsus paradoxus (which is very difficult to properly assess in the prehospital setting)
- JVD (*late* finding and unreliable)
- Tracheal deviation (*late* finding)

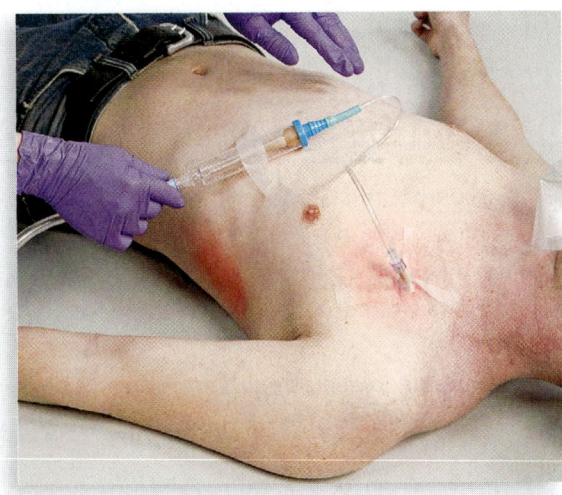

Figure 21-10 Needle thoracostomy with a Heimlich® valve.

The classic location is to insert the needle above the third rib into the second intercostal space at the midclavicular line.[1,15,16,17] The needle is inserted until a rush of air is heard. If done properly, the patient's clinical condition and vital signs should start to improve rapidly. Breathing should improve or, if the patient was already intubated, the patient should become much easier to ventilate. If there is no improvement, immediately look for other problems. DOT 4-7.50a

Needle thoracostomy changes a life-threatening condition of tension pneumothrorax into a more "stable" open pneumothorax. Although any opening in the chest cavity can cause increased difficulty breathing, the small size of the catheter is not considered to be enough to cause a problem.[17] There is no evidence to suggest that using a one-way flutter valve would be beneficial. Trauma-focused continuing education programs such as Prehospital Trauma Life Support recommend not using a one-way valve.[17] The Heimlich® valve is a commercially available device that is meant to allow for air to exit the chest and then to collapse when air tries to reenter into the chest at that site (Figure 21-10).

Street Secrets

In patients who are either obese or very muscular, the anterior approach may be difficult to successfully complete because the needle may not be long enough to enter the pleural space. Be sure to use a catheter that is at least 4.5 cm (2 inches) long, if possible.[19]

Tension pneumothorax may also occur after a penetrating injury to the chest. In the primary survey, you may have identified and treated an open chest wound with an occlusive dressing. If you suspect that air is now building up and causing a tension pneumothorax,

the first and simplest procedure is to simply remove the occlusive dressing. If the wound is still open, lifting the occlusive dressing may be all that is needed to allow for air to escape. If lifting or removing the dressing does not correct the situation, then it may be necessary to perform a needle decompression.

It is also possible that the first catheter you use to perform a needle decompression may become occluded. Catheters used for phlebotomy (venous access) are softer and collapse more easily than catheters designed for performing decompression. Needle decompression catheters can look like the IV catheter but are thicker and longer and may even have tiny wire filaments inside the catheter wall, adding strength and also making them radiopaque (visible upon x-ray).

If signs of tension pnuemothorax reoccur, it may be necessary for you to decompress the chest a second time.[19]

Working in the Gray Zone

Patients with life-threatening tension pneumothorax (TP) may show signs of hypotension or tracheal shift as a late event. More sensitive signs of TP are tachycardia and lack of oxygenation (hypoxemia), as noted by a falling oxygen saturation on a pulse oximeter.[17] Needle decompression (thoracostomy) is rarely performed in the field, and recognition of a TP is difficult in a patient with a normal blood pressure.[18] Consider contacting on-line medical direction for advice on further care. Ideally, with a normal blood pressure, the patient will be stable enough to permit the extra time for the consult, but on-scene time should not be prolonged to perform the consult. As always, you must follow local protocol, but if you believe that your patient has a TP and recognize that the patient is deteriorating (decrease in blood pressure or oxygenation, increased heart rate, and difficulty moving air), performing a needle thoracostomy may be a life-saving procedure. If you are wrong, the risk of having caused more harm to the patient is low compared to the benefit.[19] More importantly, if there is no improvement after decompression, you should immediately suspect other causes for the patient's condition and aggressively search and treat other causes. Document your thought process in your report, and contact your medical director or supervisor to follow up after the incident.

Simple Pneumothorax. A **simple pneumothorax** is a condition in which air has entered the pleural space. The source could be external, such as a stab wound, or it could be internal, such as from a bronchiole ruptur-ing from blunt trauma. Regardless of the mechanism of injury, a patient with a simple pneumothorax is usually relatively stable. The patient will usually complain of some chest pain and have some shortness of breath. DOT 4-7.13a

CONNECTIONS A pneumothorax may also occur spontaneously in adults with healthy lungs. This is likely to be caused by a lung blister (bleb) that can rupture and leak air into the pleural space. Approximately 90% of spontaneous pneumothoraces are in males and smokers or ex-smokers.[20] Tall, thin patients are at greater risk of developing blebs, possibly due to a greater pressure gradient during respiration. Since their chest is larger, more force is needed to draw air in. To read more about pulmonary problems, refer to Chapter 28: Pulmonary.

Open Pneumothorax. An **open pneumothorax** is a wound that allows air to pass unimpeded between the outside and the pleural space with each breath. If this wound is gurgling, it is known as a "sucking chest wound," named for the gurgling sound that can be heard at the wound site as air bubbles through blood. These wounds are often caused by high-caliber rifles, shotguns, or a large object that impales the chest wall.[1,21] With a large wound in the chest wall, the mechanics of respiration are significantly compromised. The nega-tive pressure, which is normally created to inspire air through the trachea, cannot be generated effectively, so it becomes difficult for the patient to fill the lung on the affected side. DOT 4-7.13b

The care of an open pneumothorax is simple but requires care to avoid turning it into a tension pneumo-thorax. Take an occlusive dressing, such as the plastic wrapper from a bandage, and tape it on three sides, leav-ing one side open. This creates a one-way flutter valve system, which allows air to escape but prevents it from further entering the thorax. It is critical that once an open pneumothorax is sealed, the patient is continu-ously monitored for the development of a tension pneu-mothorax.[5,19] Prehospital treatment priorities remain the same except that the paramedic must be even more concerned about the possibility of underlying injuries. Administration of narcotic analgesics can be considered if allowed by medical control. DOT 4-7.15, 4-7.16

Hemothorax. A **hemothorax** is similar to a pneumo-thorax except that blood fills the space in the chest. The blood can come from any number of sources, in-cluding a lacerated intercostal vessel after a rib frac-ture, a stab wound, great vessel transection, or a pulmonary laceration. Hemothoraces rarely, in and of themselves, create a tension condition but they often

> **BOX 21-3 Signs and Symptoms of Massive Hemothorax**
> - Hypotension and obvious shock
> - Pain
> - Tachypnea and shortness of breath
> - Low pulse oximetry reading
> - Tachycardia
> - May have decreased breath sounds
> - Tracheal deviation is a late and unreliable finding

coexist with a pneumothorax. This condition where both injuries exist is called a **hemopneumothorax.** The real danger of a hemothorax is the potential for sig-nificant blood loss (Box 21-3). Each half of the chest can hold as much as two liters of blood.[19] Bleeding on this scale can lead to significant hypotension and shock. DOT 4-7.13d, 4-7.13e

Clinically, patients with any pneumothorax or he-mothorax will likely present with pain, tachypnea, and shortness of breath. There will likely be some evi-dence of trauma to the affected side but not always. It is always important to roll the patient and look for puncture wounds or other trauma to the posterior chest. Breath sounds will likely be decreased on the affected side, depending on the extent of the condi-tion. Tension physiology may cause decreased blood pressure, increased pulse, low oxygen saturation, and, as the wound progresses, tracheal deviation away from the affected side or distended neck veins. DOT 4-7.14

Differentiating between pneumothorax and hemo-thorax is difficult in the prehospital environment. This is a moot point, however, as there is a great deal of over-lap between the two, and the presence of either one represents a significant injury that requires aggressive support and emergent transfer.

In either case, the patient should receive supple-mental oxygen and have intravenous access obtained. As discussed earlier, any open pneumothorax should be appropriately dressed. Signs of tension pneumothorax warrant needle decompression. In patients who have undergone endotracheal intubation, mechanical venti-lation puts them at higher risk for developing a tension pneumothorax because of the positive pressure being exerted.

Pneumothorax poses special problems for patients undergoing air-medical evacuation. All paramedics should be aware of this but especially those who are

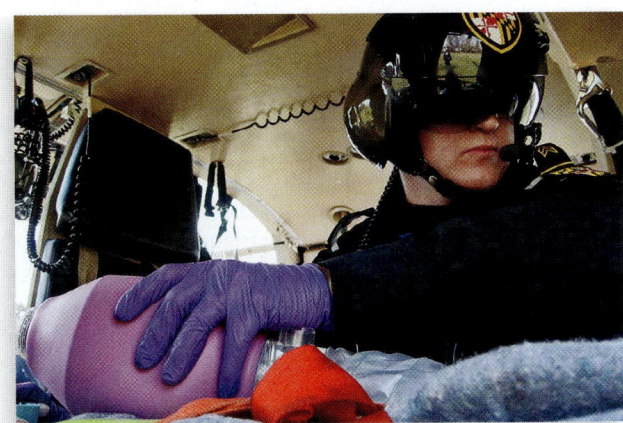

Figure 21-11 Flight crews must monitor for tension pneumothorax.

involved in air transport of critically ill patients. The decreased atmospheric pressure during flight can cause a small pneumothorax to enlarge. Persons on the flight crew should be extra diligent in monitoring for tension pneumothorax and have the equipment available to treat one if necessary (Figure 21-11).

Traumatic Asphyxia. **Traumatic asphyxia** is a rare entity caused when the thorax undergoes a significant compression, forcing blood backwards into the pulmonary system and into the veins of the neck and head.[7] Since the large veins of the head and neck do not have valves, the full force of the blood being pushed in reverse is transmitted to the capillaries of the head, face, and neck, causing blood to leak out into the subcutaneous tissues. Clinically, a patient may present with flushed face; purple discoloration of the head, face, and neck; and bilateral subconjunctival hemorrhages. DOT 4-7.37

There can be quite a range of presentations associated with traumatic asphyxia. Commonly, it is a benign condition that has a dramatic presentation. Occasionally, there can be significant underlying injury, causing the patient to present with severe dyspnea and possibly leading to cardiopulmonary arrest. From the prehospital standpoint, the paramedic should provide supplemental oxygen, protect the cervical spine if indicated, and transport to the emergency department. If the injury was associated with deceleration or a significant blunt force, any of the other injuries described in this chapter may be present, including great vessel injury. DOT 4-7.38, 4-7.39, 4-7.40

Pulmonary Laceration. Any penetrating injury to the thorax can lacerate one or both lungs. Additionally, a blunt injury, which may cause the sharp end of a broken rib to project inwards, can lacerate the lung. Pulmonary laceration causes hemothorax or pneumothorax. In addition to the symptoms and signs of hemopneumothorax, the patient may also present with hemoptysis, which is noted by the patient coughing up bloody sputum coming from the lungs. Pulmonary lacerations are not usually life-threatening by themselves; however, all the other injuries described in this chapter can coexist or may have caused the laceration in the first place. Severe pulmonary lacerations are reported to be present in only about 3% of patients with trauma to the thorax.[7] Prehospital treatment is supportive with an emphasis on early transport.

Pulmonary Contusion. A contusion is the medical term for a bruise. Just as a patient can get a bruise or contusion of the skin and soft tissue, it is possible to contuse the lung. Contusions occur most commonly when the lung is subjected to blunt trauma or a blast injury but can also occur due to the cavitation wave of a high-velocity missile injury.[8] Capillaries and alveolar walls are damaged as a result of the trauma to the lungs. The alveoli in the affected area then fill with fluid and blood and can no longer contribute to the exchange of carbon dioxide for oxygen. The affected portion of the lung is the area called the pulmonary contusion. Clearly, the larger the area of lung that is affected, the greater the degree of respiratory compromise. DOT 4-7.13f

As with most of the pathologic processes discussed in this chapter, patients can present with dyspnea, tachypnea, tachycardia, hypoxia, and possibly cyanosis. Hemoptysis may occur in up to 50% of cases.[1] On exam, decreased breath sounds or rales may be noted. Evidence of concomitant rib fractures and, especially, a flail chest segment should be actively sought. DOT 4-7.14

Pulmonary contusions have been reported to occur in 30–50% of patients with major blunt trauma. Additionally, they coexist with extrathoracic trauma in 87% of patients. They are also the most common major thoracic injury in the pediatric population as the pediatric chest wall is more deformable, affording the lungs less protection.[7]

CONNECTIONS For more information on pediatric pulmonary contusions, refer to Chapter 43: Pediatric Patients.

It usually takes some time for a contusion to fully develop; therefore, it may not be evident in the prehospital setting.

The important thing for you to keep in mind is that thoracic injuries are not static and may worsen as care is being provided.[19]

Pulse oximetry should be checked and documented. Any decrease in oxygen saturation, especially if it occurs despite high-concentration supplemental oxygen, should raise concern for impending respiratory failure. Expeditious transport, frequent patient reassessment, and aggressive respiratory support are your top priorities. DOT 4-7.14, 4-7.15

Tracheo-Bronchial Injuries

Both blunt and penetrating trauma can cause a disruption of the tracheo-bronchial airways. The incidence, however, is relatively rare; only about 3% of patients with chest trauma have a tracheo-bronchial injury. It is, however, associated with a mortality of 30%, and over half of these patients die within an hour of the injury occurring.[7]

Gunshot wounds can injure the airway at any location. Intrathoracic airways are more protected from knife wounds, whereas stab wounds to the neck or upper thorax are more likely to injure the airway.

Blunt trauma may subject the intrathoracic airways to shearing stresses and possible rupture, making airway injury more common there than in the neck. A sudden deceleration will pull the lungs and mediastinum forward while the trachea remains fixed. Obviously this could lead to severe airway compromise if the trachea tears.[5] DOT 4-7.33

Clinically, patients with tracheo-bronchial tree damage will present with significant dyspnea. They may also have dramatic subcutaneous emphysema or hemoptysis. Depending on where the defect is, air may enter into the pleural space, causing a pneumothorax. DOT 4-7.34

As with all injuries to the thorax, supportive treatment and expeditious transport are imperative. With tracheo-bronchial injuries, blind nasotracheal intubation, and even orotracheal intubation with direct laryngoscopy, can be risky. A partial disruption of the trachea could be made worse with the endotracheal tube. The tube may even transect the partially torn trachea and enter into the adjoining soft tissues.[7] If possible, patients should be supported with high-concentration oxygen and a bag-mask until intubation can be performed in the emergency department. Ideally, patients would be intubated with a fiberoptic laryngoscope, which would allow direct visualization of the trachea during the procedure. DOT 4-7.35, 4-7.36

Cardiac Injuries

The heart is arguably one of the best-protected organs in the body, for good reason. Coordinated contraction of the heart depends on a tightly controlled balance of oxygenated blood to supply the myocardium and proper electrolyte balance in the blood. Any direct injury to the heart can compromise this balance and be rapidly fatal.

Working in the Gray Zone

Due to varying definitions in the literature, it is difficult to describe the true incidence of any of these injuries. One study reported that cardiac tamponade was the most common presentation in penetrating chest trauma, being present in 80–90% of stab wounds and 20% of gunshot wounds.[22] Others report it as a rare occurance.[35] The incidence in various studies often does not factor in the cause of death as reported on autopsy, so the true incidence of some of these injuries may be unrecognized. It is important to remember that many cardiac and severe thoracic injuries, such as aortic disruption, are incompatible with life and result in a patient who is dead upon arrival of the EMS care team. True statistics on the prevalence of injuries must also factor in the numbers from autopsy reports in order to reflect the true incidence of occurrence.

Pericardial Tamponade. When the heart itself or a blood vessel in the heart is injured, it may bleed into the sac surrounding the heart (pericardial sac) (Figure 21-12). The accumulation of blood in this sac can cause compression (tamponade) of the heart, and, as a result of this increasing pressure, it will not fill or pump properly. The heart refills its chambers while it rests (diastole). This is a somewhat passive event and requires enough space for the muscle to relax and expand after it has contracted (systole). The problem caused by tamponade is lack of internal space inside the heart chambers caused by the external compression resulting from blood accumulating inside the

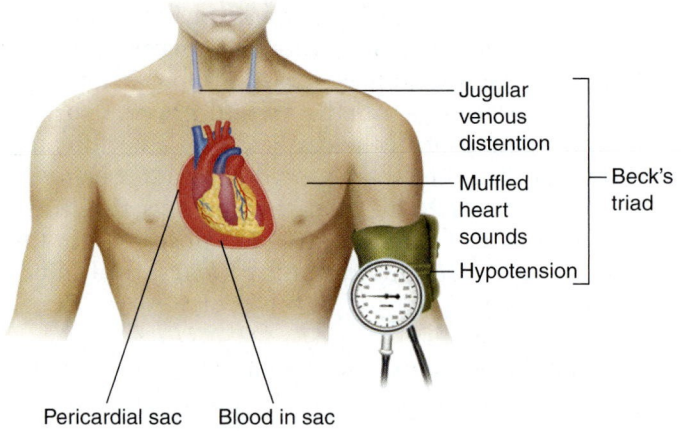

Figure 21-12 Pericardial tamponade.

pericardial sac. As the pressure around the heart increases, the heart will not be able to fill with enough blood to produce a good volume during systole. If the heart cannot pump enough volume, cardiac output will fall, causing the blood pressure to fall also. This is why cardiac tamponade is a life-threatening condition.

One of the ways in which the body compensates for the low cardiac output in tamponade is to speed up the circulation of the little volume it has left. This results in tachycardia. Sympathetic stimulation may cause peripheral vasoconstriction (as with other forms of shock) and may shunt more blood to the vital organs. As more blood is not able to be pumped back out, it will back up and engorge the jugular veins. The amount of blood in the pericardial sac needed to produce symptoms may vary. In the acute traumatic setting, the ability of the sac to stretch is limited.[19] In the acute setting, as little as 60 mL may be enough to produce symptoms of tamponade.[28] On the other hand, it may be possible to hold as much as 200–300 mL before compressing the heart.[12] In chronic conditions, fluid accumulates much more slowly, allowing the sac to gradually expand. Thus, the pericardial sac may be able to accommodate as much as 1 to 2 liters of fluid, but this is rare.

Prehospital recognition of pericardial tamponade may be very difficult. You should maintain a high index of suspicion with any trauma to the chest (Box 21-4).

If blood is accumulating slowly in the pericardial sac, you may be able to see subtle signs that are helpful early on. Tachycardia may be present. As pressure on the heart increases, you may be able to see jugular vein distension (JVD).

BOX 21-4 Signs and Symptoms of Pericardial Tamponade

- Hypotension
- Pulsus paradoxus (which is difficult to assess in the prehospital setting)
- Tachycardia
- Beck's triad:
  - JVD—Kussmaul's sign
  - Narrowing pulse pressure—Kussmaul's sign
  - Muffled heart tones

Note: Beck's triad is a late and ominous sign. One-third of all cardiac tamponade patients have the full triad, and 90% have at least one sign.

Street Secrets

It is possible for anyone to have jugular vein distension when they are supine or in Trendelenburg. Therefore, when a patient is backboarded or has a c-collar in place, the detection of JVD is not very reliable. Instead, observe the patient, if possible, in a sitting position at a 30- to 90-degree angle with the head turned to the side.[12,23] The right side may be easier to observe than the left since it is more directly tied to right atrial pressure.[24]

You may also be able to see a drop in systolic blood pressure during inspiration. This is known as pulsus paradoxus (See Box 21-5). In addition, as pressure continues to increase, and the heart is not able to relax and refill, the diastolic blood pressure may increase. If this occurs and the systolic pressure begins to drop, the difference between the two will decrease. This event is called narrowing pulse pressure. This too is a sign of pressure building around the heart.[26,28]

Nice to Know

Jugular venous pressure and pulsus paradoxus are considered the two **Kussmaul's signs.** This can be very confusing since another clinical finding of a specific abnormal breathing pattern noted with diabetic ketoacidosis is termed Kussmaul's respirations. Chapter 12: Airway Management, Ventilation, and Oxygenation discusses Kussmaul's respiration.

Classically, the clinical features of tamponade include hypotension, jugular vein distention (JVD), and muffled heart sounds (this is known as **Beck's triad,** shown in Figure 21-12). Only one of these signs, hypotension, may be reliable in the prehospital setting (and it may be caused by a wide variety of other etiologies, which must also be considered in the trauma patient). JVD may be absent due to hypotension or unreliable due to positioning. Muffled heart tones may be difficult to auscultate due to ambient noise. This leaves you with few definitive telltale signs of tamponade.

Approximately one-third of patients with pericardial tamponade have all three elements of Beck's triad, but approximately 90% have at least one.[23] Actually seeing all three components of the triad is usually a late and ominous finding.

Suspect pericardial tamponade if you have persistent hypotension, which is resistant to fluid resuscitation. Also suspect it if your patient is pulseless but has electrical activity on the ECG, especially if you have already ruled out the possibility of a tension pneumothorax or corrected hypovolemia.

BOX 21-5 Assessment of Pulsus Paradoxus

Pulsus paradoxus is a drop of 10 mmHg or more in blood pressure that occurs during inspiration.[12,25,26,27] This phenomenon can be observed in many conditions where there is increased pressure inside the chest or airway constriction on expiration: tension pneumothorax, pericardial tamponade, asthma, COPD, croup, and massive pulmonary embolus.[28] Assessment of pulsus paradoxus is best accomplished with an electronic measurement of the arterial pressure by using an in-dwelling arterial pressure monitor observing a drop in the wave form during inspiration.[25,26,28]

Without advanced equipment, it is theoretically possible to auscultate the drop in pressure by using a standard blood pressure cuff. To do this, you should pump up the cuff until no sounds are audible. Release the air very slowly, and stop when you hear the first (systolic) sound (called Korotkoff sound), audible on expiration only. Note the pressure reading and do not continue to deflate the cuff. The sound will normally disappear on inspiration and return on expiration. Deflate the cuff slowly until you hear sounds continuously during both inspiration and expiration. If the difference between the two pressures exceeds 10 mmHg, it is considered pulsus paradoxus.[12,28] One study with attending physicians in a controlled laboratory setting concluded that this measurement may be generally valuable for clinical use, but auscultated measurements were not as accurate as electronic measurements. No studies are available regarding the ability of paramedics to assess this sign. Since rapid breathing and low blood pressures may make the skill harder to perform, you could assume that the technique may be more difficult in the prehospital presentation of pericardial tamponade.

Occasionally, **electrical alternans** may be seen on the cardiac monitor. This is an alternating high and low amplitude QRS complex on the cardiac monitor.[1] As you look at the printed ECG strip or observe the screen in dynamic mode, you will see an undulating wave as the QRS gets taller and then shorter. This occurs as the heart is shifting its axis with inspiration and expiration inside the fluid-filled pericardial sac. DOT 4-7.18

CONNECTIONS To learn more about ECG interpretation, pulseless electrical activity, and axis deviation, turn to Chapter 29: Cardiology.

Pericardial tamponade is a very serious condition that can be rapidly fatal. If it is suspected, the patient must be supported with oxygen, a trial of fluid replacement, and emergent transport to the hospital. DOT 4-7.17a

Pericardiocentesis is a procedure whereby a needle is inserted into the pericardial sac and excess blood or fluid is drawn out with a syringe. The procedure carries a high risk of complications, especially when performed without the aide of advanced diagnostic tools (such as ultrasound).[29,30] The needle may lacerate or puncture the ventricle or lung. In addition, cardiac dysrhythmias can develop. This procedure, when performed correctly in the right situation, is life-saving. You may work in a system where this procedure is performed by paramedics. **Skill Sheet 82: Pericardiocentesis will be provided by your instructor if this skill is approved in your EMS system.** DOT 4-7.20

Blunt Cardiac Injuries. A sudden deceleration of or direct blow to the thorax can cause blunt injury to the heart. There is a continuum of injury that has been described from a simple concussion of the myocardium that results in a benign injury to rupture of the heart wall.[1] In between, patients may have myocardial contusions and myocardial infarctions.

- *Myocardial rupture:* The most devastating of the myocardial injuries is myocardial rupture. This occurs when the heart is compressed with such force that it ruptures. Rupture can occur in the wall of the heart as well as the septum and the valves. These injuries are generally rapidly fatal and are reported to represent approximately 15% of deaths from thoracic trauma.[1] The right atrium is the most common site of the rupture because of its position in the chest and location right behind the sternum.[31] The patient is likely to be in very critical condition and may not have detectable vital signs. DOT 4-7.17c

This condition is difficult if not impossible to distinguish from other catastrophic events (such as pericardial tamponade or torn aorta) without advanced diagnostics (ultrasound, CT) or a thoracotomy. In the prehospital setting, it is important to look for other causes of hypotension (especially reversible causes such as tension pneumothorax, severe blood loss, flail chest, or pericardial tamponade), before adding myocardial rupture as a suspected diagnosis. This is termed a **diagnosis of exclusion,** meaning that all other causes should be considered before deciding that myocardial rupture is considered the working diagnosis. Look for evidence of shock and tamponade when preliminary diagnosis indicates of blunt traumatic injury to the chest.

Definitive treatment for myocardial rupture requires emergency operative repair performed at a trauma center. Rapid transport, fluid resuscitation, airway management, and CPR, if necessary, are the mainstays of care. DOT 4-7.20

■ *Myocardial infarction (traumatic):* With significant trauma to the chest wall and underlying heart, a patient may actually sustain an acute myocardial infarction (AMI).[29,31] If an area of the heart is so damaged that adequate blood flow cannot reach a portion of the myocardium, there may be death of the myocardial cells. Just as with a non-traumatic myocardial infarction (MI), if enough of the heart muscle is involved, the patient can develop cardiogenic shock or develop changes in their ECG rhythm. Common ECG disturbances may include ST-segment elevation, T-wave changes, premature ventricular complexes, and ventricular tachycardia.[32]

CONNECTIONS Chapter 29: Cardiology has more information about cardiac dysrhythmias.

Treatment includes standard advanced cardiac life support measures such as electric defibrillation if necessary and urgent transport. Aspirin should be avoided in trauma patients due to its inhibition of platelet function.[29] DOT 4-7.19, 4-7.18

■ *Myocardial contusion:* Blunt trauma to the chest may also cause a myocardial contusion. This is an actual bruise of the heart muscle. Mechanisms include a sudden direct blow to the chest wall or a sustained compression, which pushes the sternum back against the heart, thus bruising the cardiac muscle.[1] DOT 4.17b

In myocardial contusion injuries, there is actual microscopic damage to the myocardium and blood vessels of the heart. Approximately 73% of patients with myocardial contusion will have external signs of chest trauma.[1] Patients will usually have the same constellation of symptoms (including chest pain and dyspnea) seen in other pathologic states discussed in this chapter. There may or may not be dysrhythmias seen on the cardiac monitor. Additionally, there may be hypotension or sinus tachycardia, which is present in nearly 70% of patients with documented myocardial contusion.[1]

■ *Myocardial concussion:* A myocardial concussion is simply a direct blow to the thorax and transfer of energy, which stuns the heart. This "stunning" of the heart can interrupt the normal flow of electrical activity that regulates the cardiac rhythm. The result can be temporary myocardial irritability, causing dysrhythmia, chest pain, brief loss of consciousness, or transient hypotension. There are usually no lasting effects from this injury.

Penetrating Cardiac Injuries. Patients with gunshot wounds or stab wounds to the thorax should raise the paramedic's concern for injury to the heart itself. Most penetrating injuries to the chest occur from acts of violence.[33,34] The heart lies behind and to the left of the sternum and is surrounded by a fibrous casing called the pericardium. The heart is also slightly turned to the left, so the right ventricle is the most anterior structure and is injured more commonly than the left ventricle.

CONNECTIONS See Chapter 7: Anatomy Overview, pages 117 and 118, for diagrams of the heart.

Penetrating injuries to the heart consist of direct injury to one or more of the heart chambers, laceration of a coronary artery, or bleeding into the space between the pericardium and the myocardium, causing pericardial tamponade. Additionally, the penetrating object may damage one or more of the heart valves.

Laceration of any of the chambers of the heart will cause predictable clinical consequences, which go down one of two clinical paths. The first is the inability of the heart to properly pump blood, which will quickly result in cardiogenic shock. If the wound bleeds into the pleural space, patients may become hypotensive from severe loss of blood volume into the chest. Alternatively, the bleeding may be contained in the pericardial sac, causing pericardial tamponade (see Figure 21-12).[35]

In approximately 75% of cases of stab wounds and 35% of cases of gunshot cardiac wounds, patients survive the operation once they arrive in the trauma center. However, it is estimated that 80–90% of patients with gunshot wounds of the heart do not reach the hospital alive.[38] DOT 4-7.21b, 4-7.21c

Great Vessel Injuries

The thorax contains a number of large, critical vascular structures including the aorta, the superior and inferior vena cava, and the pulmonary veins and arteries. An injury to any of these vessels through blunt or penetrating trauma can have disastrous consequences.

Blunt Trauma to the Great Vessels. It is reported that 80–92% of traumatic aortic injuries (TAI) are due to motor vehicle crashes (MVC), but they can also result from any number of other deceleration injuries.[36] Fifty percent of TAIs are caused by frontal impact collisions, with side impact to the victim's side representing the second largest group. The incidence of TAI is difficult to determine because of differences in the types of injuries that are considered in this category (inclusion criteria) and the way it is diagnosed. In general, reports of TAI vary from 1.2–8% of patients sustaining significant blunt trauma.[36] It has been reported that rupture of the aorta causes immediate death in 75–90% of victims. Thirty percent of those that initially survive will die in 24 hours, and 50% will die within one week.[36] DOT 4-7.22

Because the various blood vessels are tethered to the other structures of the thorax with fibrous tissue at different sites, they are at risk for rupture during deceleration injuries. The most devastating injury is an aortic arch rupture. As previously described, the ligamentum arteriosum tethers the arch in place (see Figure 21-5). Sudden deceleration force can cause the arch to tear just beyond this tethered region. The result is almost always massive fatal hemorrhage. In fact, 80–90% of blunt trauma victims with large vessel trauma (especially the aorta) die at the scene. A patient with blunt trauma who goes into cardiac arrest in the field has a dismal chance of survival. Several studies have put the likelihood of survival after a blunt trauma prehospital cardiac arrest between 0 and 2.6%, and many of the survivors are neurologically impaired.[37] However, the wall of the aorta is made of several layers and sometimes the thin, outermost layer contains the hemorrhage. In these cases, if the injury is diagnosed in time, the aorta can be repaired and the patient will survive. DOT 4-7.21a

Penetrating Trauma to the Great Vessels.   Any penetrating injury, be it a knife or gunshot wound, can puncture a great vessel with the same catastrophic outcome as described above. One important difference, however, is that penetrating injuries are more amenable to repair. Unlike blunt trauma, which may cause diffuse vascular injury at several sites, penetrating trauma tends to have more discrete injuries, which can possibly be repaired surgically.

A trauma patient with penetrating thoracic injuries who has lost vital signs prior to arrival of prehospital personnel is deceased and is not a candidate for resuscitation.[23] Patients who lose their vital signs while in the care of EMS should have CPR started, receive volume resuscitation, and be transported expeditiously to the nearest trauma center.

The receiving facility should be notified as soon as possible so that a trauma team can be ready. In the hospital setting, these patients may be candidates for a resuscitative thoracotomy allowing for temporizing measures such as clamping large bleeding vessels and repairing lacerations to the heart. DOT 4-7.23, 4-7.24

Chest Wall Injuries

As described, the sternum, ribs, and thoracic spine create a protective cage that surrounds the vital chest organs and creates the bellows system that allows for the inspiration and exhalation of air. The whole design of the thorax from the sternum through the ribs to the spine allows for some flexibility, such that the chest wall can often help to dissipate forces of blunt trauma. Obviously, it can only provide so much protection against penetrating injuries.

In evaluating a patient with any of the following injuries, one of the earliest signs to look for will be pain and trouble breathing (dyspnea). All of the structures that make up the chest wall are very well innervated and will cause significant pain if injured. Signs and symptoms include rapid breathing (tachypnea) and an effort on the patient's part to breathe carefully and with less volume (auto-splinting).

Flail Chest.   A significant injury occurs when three or more adjacent ribs are fractured in two or more places. The result is a free-floating segment of the chest wall called a **flail chest** (Figure 21-13). It is estimated to occur in 5–13% of chest wall injuries.[2,39] Patients with a flail chest will complain of significant pain and trouble breathing (dyspnea). They will likely have a much larger area of tenderness than those with an isolated rib fracture. On exam there may be a palpable or visible deformity as a result of the flail segment. Additionally, by watching the patient's respirations, you may notice paradoxical chest wall motion. This is when the flail chest wall segment moves inward during inspiration

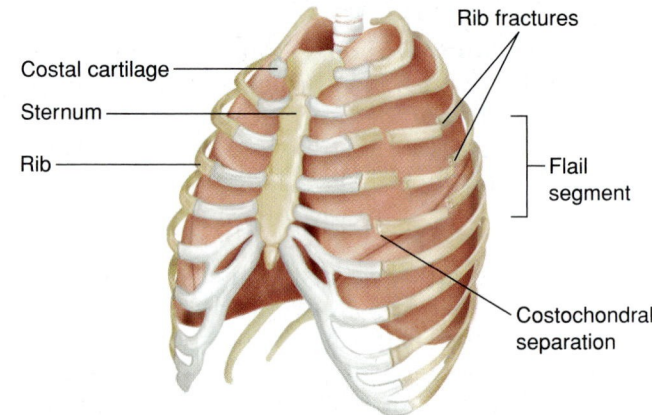

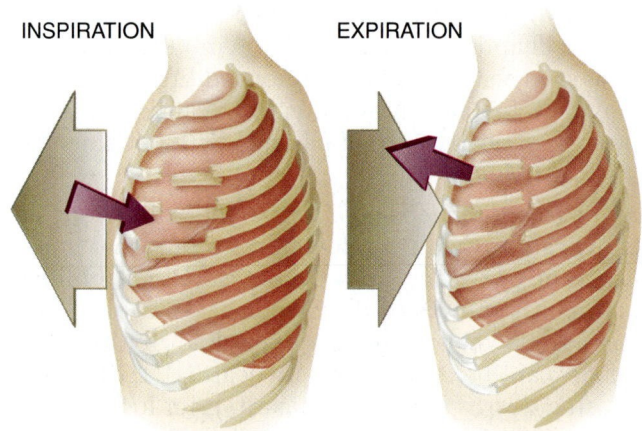

Figure 21-13   A flail segment occurs when three or more ribs are broken in two or more places. The affected section moves in an opposite direction to the rest of the thorax during inhalation and exhalation.

and outward during expiration. As a result of the negative pressure generated during inspiration, the now free-floating flail segment is "sucked" inward, and as the pressure inside the chest increases during expiration, the flail segment is pushed outward. A flail segment is associated with a higher incidence of underlying pulmonary contusion, which increases the chance of respiratory decompensation and failure.[43] DOT 4-7.9b, 4-7.10

Street Secrets

To really see paradoxical movement, the patient needs to have an adequate tidal volume, which will lead to full expansion of the chest wall. In many patients with flail segments, this will obviously cause increased pain, so many of these patients intentionally breathe shallow, quick breaths (auto-splinting), and the paradoxical motion will only be noted when they take a full inhalation or when you begin to perform bag-mask ventilation.

Because a flail segment may seriously compromise the mechanics of breathing, early detection and intervention is very important. Supplemental oxygen should be administered as soon as possible. In more serious cases, the patient may benefit from early assistance with breathing.[29] Many patients that appear to be tolerating the initial flail injury well later develop increasing difficulty breathing as their chest muscles fatigue and the underlying pulmonary contusion increases the work of breathing. Positive pressure ventilation with the bag-mask device is recommended as well as early endotracheal intubation. Ventilation not only assists with oxygenation and lung inflation but may also effectively serve as an internal splint. These patients often require intubation and mechanical ventilation in the hospital if they are unable to maintain their oxygenation.[40]

Continuous positive airway pressure (CPAP) ventilation, if available in your EMS system, can also be utilized.[2] Unfortunately, no prehospital studies are available to guide any evidence-based treatment recommendations. Although CPAP is more commonly thought of as a treatment for respiratory distress in congestive heart failure, it may also be helpful with some lung injuries such as flail chest. For more information about this refer to Chapter 28: Pulmonary and refer to **Skill Sheet and Step-by-Step 18: Continuous Positive Airway Pressure.**

The old recommendation of splinting flail segments with sand bags, strips of tape, or anything that will bind or restrict the chest is no longer supported.[16,29] Any treatment that restricts the ability of the chest to expand may be detrimental to breathing and worsen the patient's condition.

Street Secrets

Pain management may be the secret key to effectively managing the patient with a flail segment. If you can minimize the pain during inspiration, it is possible the patient may breathe more effectively and require fewer aggressive measures.[29]

Rib Injuries. Simple rib fractures are the most common injury in blunt thoracic trauma. The curved shape of each rib gives them some elasticity, but if enough force is applied, they can be broken. Rib fractures signify that force was transmitted to the thorax and that significant injury may have occurred to the underlying organs of the thorax and the upper abdomen. Fractures of the first and second ribs are uncommon since they are protected by the shoulder and other bones.[43] If the impact is strong enough to cause injury to these ribs, other injuries are likely, and mortality is increased by 50%. The fourth through tenth ribs are more likely to be injured and are also more likely to cause injury to the lungs.[43] Fractures of the lower ribs are also associated with injury of those abdominal organs located underneath these ribs. DOT 4-7.9a

Nice to Know

Elderly patients can have significant morbidity with rib fractures. The chance of pneumonia and pleural infections goes up significantly as the number of fractures and age of the patient increases.[44] It is estimated that the risk of death increases 132% for every 10-year increase in age beyond 55 years.[2] There is evidence that even at 45 years of age, however, the risk of serious complications increases with multiple rib fractures. This does not change what should be done in the prehospital arena, but it is important for you to have a sense of the seriousness of the injury. Administration of narcotic analgesics can be considered because it will decrease pain in breathing, which will allow for more effective ventilation. DOT 4-7.12

A patient with rib fractures will complain of significant point tenderness at the fracture site. Increased breathing depth may cause extreme pain, so patients will purposely take shallow breaths (splinted respirations) in order to minimize the pain. DOT 4-7.10

When performing a physical exam, placing your hand over the site that the patient says hurts the most and asking the patient to take a deep breathe will often reveal boney crepitus as the broken ends of the fractured ribs grate against each other. In addition, gentle comparison of the anterior chest wall and on the sides of the chest will often cause increased tenderness at rib fracture sites, allowing the patient to specifically indicate the injury location.

Management of these patients is directed at evaluation for underlying serious injury, maintenance of oxygenation, and pain relief.

Sternal Injuries.   The sternum lies in the midline, anterior to the heart and great vessels and, with the shock-absorbing quality of the ribs, offers a substantial degree of protection to these structures.

Nice to Know

Most fractures of the sternum were thought to be caused by blunt trauma to the anterior chest, commonly caused by automobile crashes. A 1993 study showed that motor vehicle crashes were responsible for 3% of sternal fractures.[41] It has been reported that the number of sternal fractures has gone up by three times since the introduction of the across-the-shoulder seat belts. This is not an endorsement for not wearing a seat belt, however, since overall appropriate restraint decreases mortality significantly.[1] DOT 4-7.9c

A sternal fracture would seemingly be associated with significant internal damage, but studies have shown that this is not usually the case. There may be an associated cardiac contusion, but there is usually not any pulmonary compromise from this injury.[42] Isolated sternal fractures occur most often in postmenopausal women. Isolated sternal fractures have been reported to have only a 0.7% mortality rate and low intrathoracic morbidity.[1] Cardiac contusions occur in only 1.5–6% of cases, and there is no clear association between sternal fractures and aortic rupture.

These numbers aside, it is still difficult to determine the extent of injury in the field. Patients with sternal fracture complain of significant anterior chest pain and dyspnea. In an isolated fracture, dyspnea will likely be due to the pain. Pulse oximetry should be assessed and supplemental oxygen given if it is below 95%. Depending on local prehospital protocol and the patient's vital signs, a narcotic or other analgesic (such as morphine or fentanyl) could be considered.

Other Injuries in the Chest

Esophageal Injuries

The overall incidence of esophageal injury in association with chest injury is very low.[15] The esophagus is a relatively well-protected organ in the thorax, so injuries tend to occur more commonly in the cervical region. A large but older British study which looked at penetrating wounds of the neck, chest, and abdomen found a 0.4% incidence of esophageal injury.[1] This being said, however, if the esophagus is perforated, it can be a catastrophic injury. When oral and gastric secretions leak out of the esophagus into the mediastinum, severe infection, called mediastinitis, can develop. Even with aggressive surgical and medical management, esophageal perforation has nearly a 30% mortality rate.[7] DOT 4-7.29

Any penetrating trauma, especially to the upper thorax and neck, should alert you to the possibility of an esophageal injury. Patients may present with some combination of neck pain, chest pain, pain with swallowing (odynophagia), dyspnea, hypoxia, tachycardia, possibly subcutaneous emphysema, and hemoptysis. They may also have Hamman's sign, which is a crunching sound heard during auscultation with each heart beat as a result of mediastinal emphysema.[45] DOT 4-7.30

Treatment.   The main prehospital considerations are support, rapid transport, and a greater awareness when it comes to airway control. DOT 4-7.31, 4-7.32

Diaphragmatic Injuries

Diaphragmatic injuries are most commonly caused by penetrating trauma.[43]

Street Secrets

Any stab wound below the nipple line or in the mid- to upper abdomen should raise the suspicion that the diaphragm has been violated. Gunshot wounds should raise it even more, as the trajectory cannot always be predicted. Any injury between the nipple line and the umbilicus (belly button) should be suspected to be both an abdominal and a chest injury.

Diaphragmatic rupture in blunt trauma is less common, occurring in only 4–5% of patients hospitalized with thoracic trauma. This rises to nearly 8–10% if there is a fracture of the pelvis.[1] DOT 4-7.25

It is estimated that about 60–70% of normal ventilatory function is dependent on the diaphragm working properly.[1] With a small tear, it is likely that only minimal findings will be seen in the prehospital setting. A rupture of the left side of the diaphragm is more common and may cause abdominal contents to enter the thorax (herniation). Left-sided injuries are associated with injuries to the spleen and can cause bowel and spleen herniation.[46] Larger injuries, however, may lead to significant breathing compromise when abdominal contents herniate into the chest and compress the lung, compromising its function.

Street Secrets

Diaphragmatic injuries can be difficult to detect, even in the hospital setting. If undetected, the abdominal contents can herniate into the chest cavity. If this becomes severe, the involved bowel may become strangulated, or it can compress the mediastinal structures, leading to a tension enterothorax. This can happen early in the course of an injury, but it more commonly happens days, weeks, or possibly years later if undetected.[47,48] If you hear bowel sounds when auscultating the chest, it is a clue to consider diaphragm trauma. Ask the patient about prior traumatic events. DOT 4-7.26

Prehospital diagnosis will likely be very difficult. Auscultation of bowel sounds in the chest would suggest the diagnosis, but, realistically, this will be hard to detect in a noisy environment. Management includes assuring adequate oxygenation, initiation of intravenous access, complete assessment for associated injuries, and rapid transport to an appropriate destination. DOT 4-7.27, 4-7.28

Summary

There is a complex interplay of the organs in the human thorax, and there is great potential for catastrophic cardiopulmonary failure should something cause this system to fail. The mechanisms and types of injuries have been described for the two major mechanisms of injury: blunt and penetrating trauma.

It is easy to "lose the forest for the trees" and become paralyzed into inactivity if one gets too hung up in the details of these conditions. This is not to say that paramedics should not try to learn as much as they can about the various pathophysiologic processes. It is just that when the heat is on, step back and remember that there are two basic questions to answer. First, "Is the patient sick?" If so, then the patient needs aggressive assessment of the ABCs, supportive monitoring, and care and transport to an appropriate facility. The second question is, "Is there a potentially life-saving procedure that I can do in the field?" With regard to trauma, this boils down to assuring a patent airway, breathing support, and decompressing a tension pneumothorax. Taking care of victims of thoracic trauma is challenging, both intellectually and emotionally. At the same time, it can also be very rewarding because, with proper prehospital care, you can make a significant impact on the outcome of patients who have sustained thoracic trauma.

Notes

1. M. Eckstein, S. Henderson, and V. Markovchick, "Thorax." In *Rosen's Emergency Medicine Concepts and Clinical Practice,* J. A. Marx, 5th ed. (St. Louis, MO: Elsevier Mosby, 2002), pp. 381–414.
2. S. Wanek and J. C. Mayberry, "Blunt Thoracic Trauma: Flail Chest, Pulmonary Contusion, and Blast Injury," *Critical Care Clinics* 20 (2004):71–81.
3. K. M. Van De Graaff and S. I. Fox, *Concepts of Human Anatomy and Physiology,* 3rd ed., Dubuque, IA: Wm. C. Brown (1992).
4. K. G. Lurie, K. A. Mulligan, et al., "Optimizing Standard Cardiopulmonary Resuscitation with an Inspiratory Impedance Threshold Valve," *Chest* 113(4)(1998):1084–1090.
5. K. G. Lurie, W. G. Voelckel, et al., "Improving Standard Cardiopulmonary Resuscitation with an Inspiratory Impedance Threshold Valve in a Porcine Model of Cardiac Arrest," *Anesthesia and Analgesia* 93(3) (2001):649–655.
6. K. G. Lurie, T. Zielinski, et al., "Use of an Inspiratory Impedance Threshold Valve Improves Neurologically Intact Survival in a Porcine Model of Ventricular Fibrillation," *Circulation* 105(1) (2002):124–129.
7. T. P. Aufderheide, R. G. Pirrallo, et al., "Clinical Evaluation of an Inspiratory Impedance Threshold Device During Standard Cardiopulmonary Resuscitation in Patients with Out-of-Hospital Cardiac Arrest," *Critical Care Medicine* 33(4) (2005):734–740.
8. R. G. Pirrallo, T. P. Aufderheide, et al., "Effect of an Inspiratory Impedance Threshold Device on Hemodynamics During Conventional Manual Cardiopulmonary Resuscitation," *Resuscitation* 66 (2005):13–20.
9. R. C. Thayne, D. C. Thomas, et al., "Use of an Impedance Threshold Device Improves Short-Term Outcomes Following Out-of-Hospital Cardiac Arrest," *Resuscitation* 67(1)(2005):103–108.
10. R. Drake et al., *Gray's Anatomy for Students* (Philadelphia, PA: Elsevier Health Sciences, 2005).
11. M. L. Fackler, "Civilian Gunshot Wounds and Ballistics: Dispelling the Myths," *Emergency Medical Clinics of North America* 16(1)(1998):17–28.
12. H. M. Seidel, J. W. Ball, J. E. Dains, and G. W. Benedict, "Chest and Lungs," *Mosby's Guide to Physical Examination* (St. Louis, MO: Mosby-Year Book, 1995).
13. R. Ladurner, "Pneumopericardium in blunt chest trauma after high-speed motor vehicle accidents," *The American Journal of Emergency Medicine* 23(1) (January 1, 2005): 83–86.
14. K. Friend, "Prehospital Recognition of Pneumothorax," *Prehospital Emergency Care;* January/March 2000 (1) (January/March 2000).
15. D. Bliss and M. Silen, "Pediatric thoracic trauma," *Critical Care Medicine* 30 (2002):11.
16. R. Fowler and P. E. Pepe, "Prehospital Care of the Patient With Major Trauma," *Emergency Medical Clinics of North America* 20 (2002): 953–974.
17. NAEMT, *Prehospital Trauma Life Support,* 5th ed., (St. Louis, MO: Elsevier Mosby, 2004).
18. M. Eckstein and D. Suyehara, "Needle Thoracotomy in the Prehospital Setting," *Prehospital Emergency Care* 2 (1998): 132–135.
19. E. F. Reichman and R. R. Simon, *Emergency Medicine Procedures* (New York, NY: McGraw-Hill, 2004), pp. 222–224.
20. G. L. Baum, J. D. Crapo, B. R. Celli, and J. B. Karlusky, eds., *Textbook of Pulmonary Diseases,* 6th ed. (Philadelphia: Lippincott–Raven, 1998).
21. E. A. Ullman, L. P. Donley, and W. J. Brady, "Pulmonary Trauma Emergency Department Evaluation and Management," *Emergency Medical Clinics of North America* 21 (2003): 291–313.

22. V. H. Thourani, D. V. Felician, G. Rozycki, et al., "Penetrating Cardiac Trauma at an Urban Trauma Center: A 22 year perspective," *The American Surgeon* 65(9) (1999): 811–818.

23. K. J. Knoop, L. B. Stack, and A. B. Storrow, "Chest and Abdominal Conditions," *Atlas of Emergency Medicine,* 2nd ed., (New York, NY: McGraw-Hill, 2002).

24. D. L. Kasper, E. Braunwald, A. S. Fauci, S. L. Hauser, D. L. Longo, J. L. Jameson, and K. J. Isselbacher, eds., "Physical Examination of the Cardiovascular System." *Harrison's Principles of Internal Medicine,* 16th ed., McGraw-Hill's AccessMedicine (accessed September 2, 2006).

25. G. D. Jay, K. Onuma, R. Davis, M. Chen, A. Mansell, and D. Steele, "Analysis of Physician Ability in the Measurement of Pulsus Paradoxus by Sphygmomanometry," *Chest* 118(2) (August 2000): 348–352.

26. Terri J. Metules, "Cardiac tamponade," *RN* 62(12) (December 1999):26–31.

27. Mary Gavaghan, "Cardiac Anatomy and Physiology: A Review," *AORN Journal* 67(4)(April 1998):802–822.

28. Jennifer Hawley and H. Michael Dreher, "Cardiac tamponade: The pressure's on," *Nursing* 32(4) April 2002:32-1–32-4.

29. J. E. Tintinalli, G. D. Kelen, J. S. Stapczynski, O. J. Ma, and D. M. Cline, *Tintinalli's Emergency Medicine: A Comprehensive Study Guide,* 6th ed., McGraw-Hill's AccessMedicine (accessed September 2, 2006).

30. R. J. Harper, *"Pericardiocentesis." Clinical Procedures in Emergency Medicine,* 4th ed. (Philadelphia, PA: W.B. Saunders, 2004) 305–322.

31. N. T. Feghali and L. M. Prisant, "Blunt Myocardial Injury," *Chest* 108(1995): 1673.

32. A. D. Neal, "Blunt Thoracic Trauma," http://www.trauma.org/ thoracic/bluntthoracic.html (accessed November 17, 2005).

33. C. Bartlett, "Clinical Update: Gunshot Wound Ballistics," *Clinical Orthopaedics and Related Research* 1(2003):28.

34. M. Fackler, "Gunshot Wound Review," *Annals of Emergency Medicine* 28(1996):194.

35. T. G. Buchman, B. L. Hall, and W. M. Bowling, "Thoracic Trauma." In *Emergency Medicine: A Comprehensive Study Guide,* 6th ed., J. E. Tintinalli, G. D. Kelen, J. S. Stapczynsti, O. J. Ma, and D. M. Cline, eds. (New York, NY: McGraw-Hill, 2004), pp. 1595–1613.

36. W. E. Baker and J. Wassermann, "Unsuspected Vascular Trauma: Blunt Arterial Injuries," *Emergency Medical Clinics of North America* 22(2004):1081–1098.

37. NAEMSP Standards and Clinical Practice Committee and the ACS Committee on Trauma, "Guidelines for Withholding or Termination of Resuscitation in Prehospital Traumatic Cardiopulmonary Arrest," *Journal of the American College of Surgeons* 196 (2003):106–112.

38. J. R. Macho, R. E. Markison, and W. P. Schecter, "Cardiac Stapling in the Management of Penetrating Injuries of The Heart: Rapid Control of Hemorrhage and Decreased Risk of Personal Contamination," *The Journal of Trauma* 34(1993):711.

39. J. LoCicero and K. L. Mattox, "Epidemiology of Chest Trauma," *The Surgical Clinics of North America* 69(1989):15.

40. G. C. Velmahos, P. Vassiliu, and L. S. Chan, "Influence of Flail Chest on Outcome Among Patients with Severe Thoracic Cage Trauma," *International Surgery* 87(2002):240–244.

41. J. G. Brookes, R. J. Dunn, and I. R. Rogers, "Sternal Fractures: A Retrospective Analysis of 272 Cases," *The Journal of Trauma* 35(1993):46.

42. J. R. Sadaba, D. Oswal, and C. M. Munsch, "Management of Isolated Sternal Fractures: Determining the Risk of Blunt Cardiac Injury," *Annals of the Royal College of Surgeons* (England) 82(3)(2000):162.

43. R. F. Wilson, "Trauma," In *Textbook of Critical Care,* 2nd ed., W. C. Shoemaker, et al., eds. (Philadelphia, PA: W.B. Saunders, 1989).

44. J. B. Holcomb, N. R. McMullin, R. A., Kozar, et al., "Morbidity From Rib Fractures Increases After Age 45," *Journal of the American College of Surgeons* 196(2003):549–555.

45. M. Duncan and R. K. H. Wong, "Esophageal Emergencies: Things That Will Wake You from a Sound Sleep," *Gastroenterology Clinics of North America* 32(4)(December 2003) 1035–1052.

46. G. Haciibrahimoglu et al., "Management of Traumatic Diaphragmatic Rupture," *Surgery Today* 34(2004):111.

47. L. L. Kaw, B. M. Potenza, R. Coimbra, et al., "Traumatic Diaphragmatic Rupture," *Journal of the American College of Surgeons* 198(4)(April 1, 2004):668–669.

48. B. McCann and A. O'Gara, "Tension Viscerothorax: An Important Differential for Tension Pneumothorax," *Emergency Medicine Journal* 22(2005):220–221.

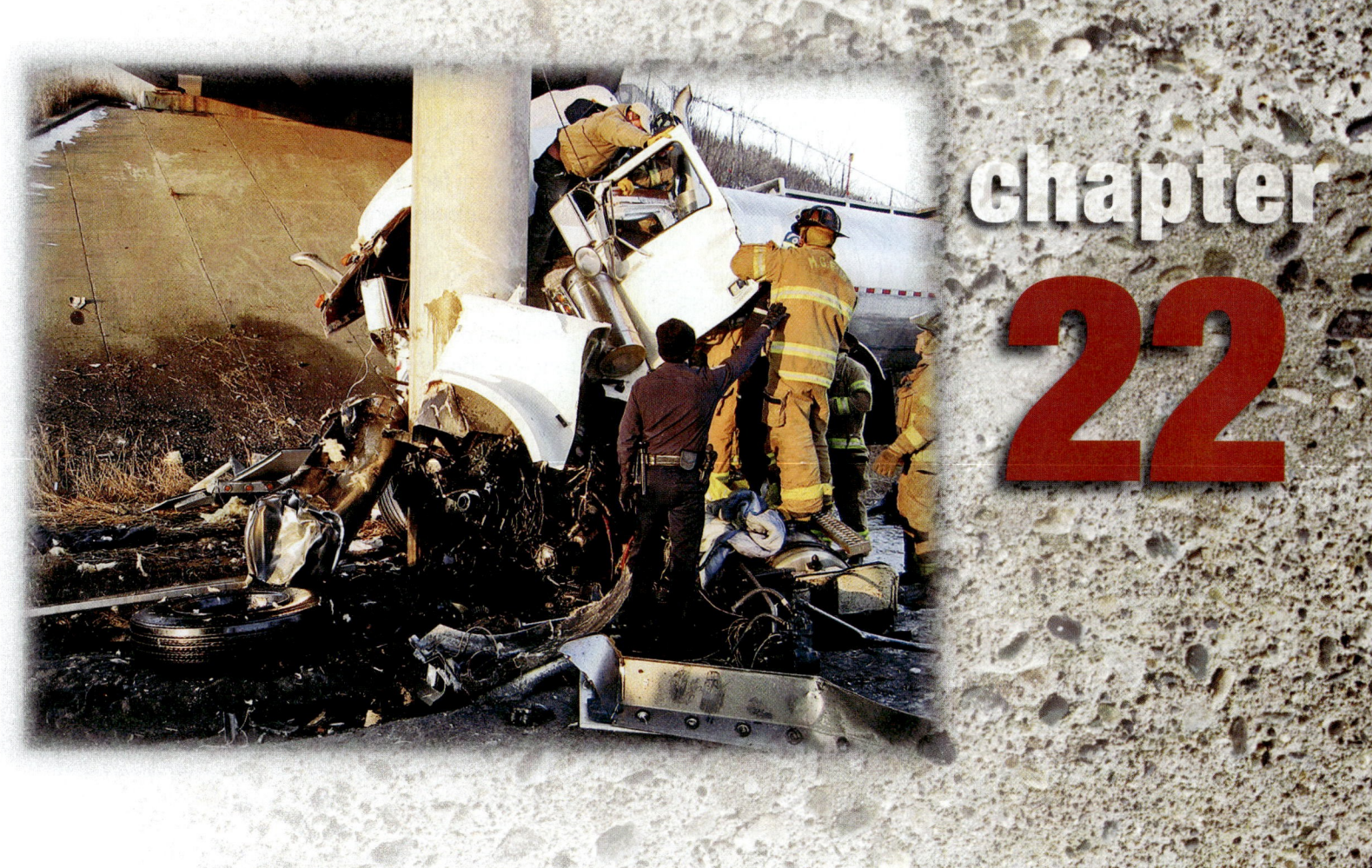

Abdominal Trauma

*"**W**ounds leading into the different cavities of the body are very common . . . . These wounds become more or less dangerous, according to the mischief done to the contents of the cavity into which they penetrate."*

—J. Hunter, 1794

Need to Know

▶ The abdomen possesses a substantial surface area that is largely unprotected by the boney skeleton, allowing for frequent injuries by both blunt and penetrating trauma.

▶ Solid, vascular organs, especially the spleen and liver, are most often injured and can bleed significantly.

▶ Penetrating trauma to the body between the nipple line and the umbilicus should be considered to have injured both the thorax and abdomen until proven otherwise.

▶ Abdominal bleeding is difficult to assess; large amounts of blood can pool in the abdominal cavity before being detected. A high index of suspicion must be maintained.

▶ Failure to identify and rapidly intervene in abdominal trauma may lead to increased mortality.

▶ Shock from internal bleeding is a high priority emergency. Ideally, the presence of shock will be detected in the primary survey. If so, the decision to perform rapid transport will be made immediately. If it is not present, the decision to begin transporting should be made as soon as intra-abdominal injury is suspected.

▶ Sick	▶ Not Yet Sick
• Any patient presenting in shock is very sick, and rapid transportation to a trauma center is needed.	• Increasing agitation with mild tachycardia can indicate internal bleeding is present.
• Rigidity or distension indicate a significant amount of blood has collected in the abdomen.	• Guarding indicates possible abdominal injury is present. Watch the patient closely.
• Eviscerations are significant injuries, but they may not be life-threatening unless they are bleeding significantly (which is rare). Cover eviscerations with an occlusive dressing and keep it warm. Keep the legs flexed to prevent stress on the abdominal wall.	• Survey the scene to uncover clues about the mechanism.
	• Watch the abdomen for signs of internal bleeding; increased girth can indicate blood is collecting. A simple tape measure placed around the abdomen can be used to measure the size and watch for changes.
• Administer IV fluids to maintain a systolic blood pressure of 90 mmHg. Do not force the pressure much higher as it can cause additional bleeding.	• Ask the OPQRST questions to focus the questions about pain. Ask patients to rate pain on a one-to-ten scale, and seek medical direction for permission to provide pain-relieving medications.

Introduction

Trauma is the top killer of Americans age one to 44 years and is surpassed only by cancer and heart disease in those age 45 years and over.[1] Abdominal trauma often poses a particular challenge for both diagnosis and treatment in the field.[2] Injury severity can vary greatly. The evaluation is often complicated by the coexistence of other signs of serious trauma— such as injuries to the head, chest, or pelvis.[3] The evaluation may also be confounded by anxiety, agitation, intoxication, or unconsciousness.[4] Detection of abdominal injuries is crucial because unrecognized abdominal injuries may have an associated mortality rate of up to 50% or more.[5] DOT 4-8.1

In the case of severe abdominal trauma, threats to life are most frequently related to bleeding. There are five areas where enough blood can collect to result in a fatal outcome: the thorax, peritoneum (anterior abdominal cavity), retroperitoneum (posterior abdominal cavity), pelvis, and externally or spilled onto the ground.[3] The abdomen is a large enough container that it has the capacity to hold a person's entire blood volume.[6] DOT 4-8.4

Street Secrets

Consider any injury between the nipple line and the lower pelvis to be both a thoracic and abdominal wound until proven otherwise.[7]

Abdominal trauma, as with other forms of trauma, is categorized into the two types of mechanism of injury: blunt and penetrating. In the case of blunt injury, the main concern is hidden bleeding. Since a young adult can lose up to 50% of their circulating blood volume internally and have no symptoms, it is possible that the only sign of injury is tachycardia and, later on, hypotension.[6] DOT 4-8.3, 4-8.4

In the case of penetrating trauma, the injuries are often more easily identified. While the risk of profuse active bleeding is still a concern, it is more likely that the visual cue of the penetrating wound will help identify the problem. Attempt to determine the depth of penetration. If the weapon or object is available, look it over to help make this determination.

Less frequently, abdominal injuries causing diaphragmatic injury, bowel perforation, or traumatic pancreatitis may cause respiratory distress from abdominal distension, direct irritation or compression of the lung, or splinting secondary to pain. At times, the airway may also become compromised as a result of vomiting food or blood (hematemesis).[3,4] DOT 4-8.3

Morbidity and mortality rates in severe injuries increase with delay to surgical intervention.[8] Your main goal with abdominal trauma is to have a high index of suspicion for internal bleeding and the development of shock, and to rapidly transport the patient to an appropriate facility. During transport, the goal is to begin to reverse hemodynamic instability that may result from hemorrhage in the abdomen, as well as appropriate bandaging of any open abdominal wounds.[2] **Skill Sheets that relate to this chapter include Skill Sheet 36: Abdominal Assessment; Skill Sheet 66: Bleeding Control and Shock (also see Step-by-Step 66); and Skill Sheet 83: NREMT Patient Assessment Trauma.**

Applied Anatomy and Physiology

Anatomy

It is unlikely that you will be able to make a diagnosis of an organ-specific injury in the field. This can, at times, be extremely difficult, even in the hospital following sophisticated imaging studies.[6,9] However, knowledge of the location of abdominal organs, as well as possible signs associated with these injuries, can increase your suspicion, even in the presence of subtle cues (Figure 22-1). DOT 4-8.2

As described in Chapter 12: Airway Management, Ventilation, and Oxygenation, the structures involved with respiration move within the chest during inspiration and exhalation. The muscular diaphragm, which separates the abdominal and thoracic cavities, moves from approximately the fifth intercostal space where it comes to rest at the end of expiration to as low as the bottom of the costal margin at the lateral ribs at the end of inspiration. Because of this wide area for movement, it is often difficult to determine if an injury that is sustained between the umbilicus and the nipple line involves the thoracic or abdominal cavity or both.

Regions of the Abdomen

Simply speaking, the abdomen includes everything from the diaphragm down to the pelvic bones, between the anterior abdominal wall and the vertebral column (see Figure 22-1).

CONNECTIONS   Refer to Plates A, B, and C at the end of Chapter 7: Anatomy Overview for more detailed images of the abdomen on pages 136–138.

The abdomen is divided into four quadrants: right upper quadrant, left upper quadrant, left lower quadrant, and right lower quadrant. Referring to the abdomen by quadrants is the usual convention.

Another strategy that dates back to the early 1900s divides the abdomen into nine sections of equally sized pieces that resemble a tic-tac-toe board.[10] Horizontally, each section is referred to as a zone. The upper margin of these zones is drawn through the ninth ribs where they join the costal cartilage. The lower zones' inferior border is drawn across the top of the iliac crests in the pelvis. The center section is over the belly button and is called the **periumbilical region.** Immediately above this and just inferior to the xiphoid is the **epigastric region;** the **suprapubic region** (sometimes called **hypogastric**), is just below the periumbilical region and is just superior to the symphysis pubis. The left and right lateral (side) sections are called the hypochondriac (top); lumbar (middle) and inguinal (or iliac) are the lower sections[4] (Figure 22-2, page 441).

Street Secrets

In the real-life setting of clinical practice, the three center vertical regions of the nine abdominal sections are more commonly used: epigastric, periumbilical (for umbilical), and suprapubic (for hypogastric). The terms on each of the sides are rarely used. If you choose to use them, other healthcare professionals may mistake the term "hypochondriac," which has several meanings. The descriptions of the nine regions are included in this text because of their existence, not because of their common use.

Organs in the Abdominal Cavity

Intraperitoneal Structures. The peritoneum is the largest serous membrane in the body and contains many folds and pouches. It covers over and contains many organs of the body. In males it is a closed sac, and in females it is closed except for where the fallopian tubes pass through it. **Intraperitoneal structures** are found inside the peritoneum. These include the liver, spleen, stomach, small bowel (with the exception of the duodenum), colon, gallbladder, and female reproductive organs.

Retroperitoneal Structures. The **retroperitoneal cavity** is a fold of the peritoneum, which in essence creates another compartment. Organs within the retroperitoneal

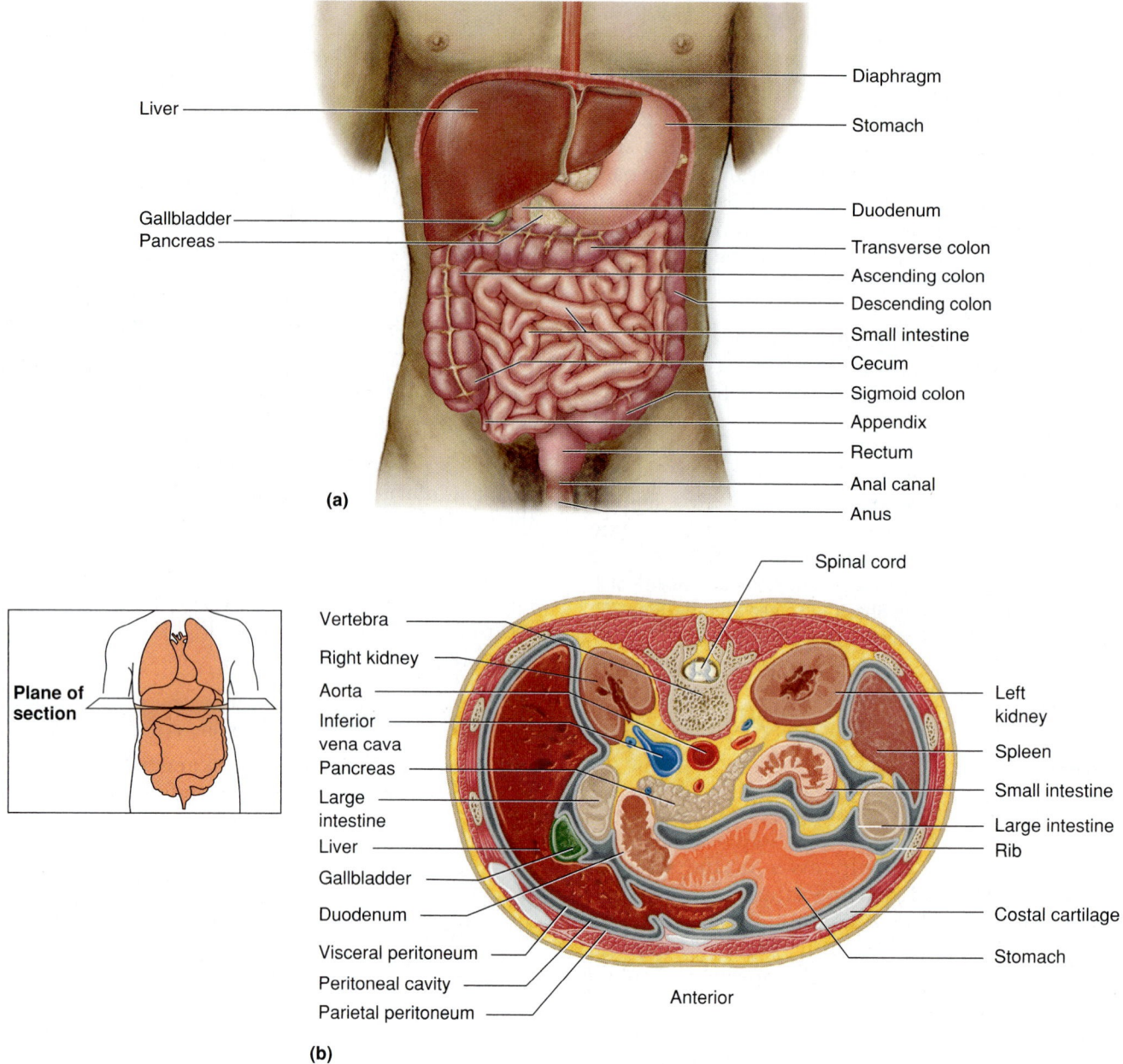

Figure 22-1 Knowledge of the location of the structures and organs of the abdomen will help you interpret clues to injuries to the abdomen. The abdomen includes everything from the diaphragm to the pelvic bones.

space include the duodenum, pancreas, major abdominal vessels (inferior vena cava (IVC) and abdominal aorta), kidneys, and ureters (Figure 22-3). Injury to these organs may result in life-threatening blood loss (aorta, IVC); leakage of enzymes, urine, or bowel contents (pancreas, kidneys, ureter, duodenum); or back pain, as fluids accumulate in the retroperitoneal space.

Solid and Hollow Organs. The abdomen contains both solid and hollow organs. This is an important differentiation, as injury to these two types of organs may produce different signs and symptoms, and the

severity of these injuries is usually quite different. DOT 4-8.13, 4-8.19

The **solid organs** of the abdomen include the following:

- Liver
- Spleen
- Kidneys
- Pancreas

These organs are highly vascularized, meaning they have a rich blood supply. The primary concern with injuries to these organs (mainly the liver and spleen)

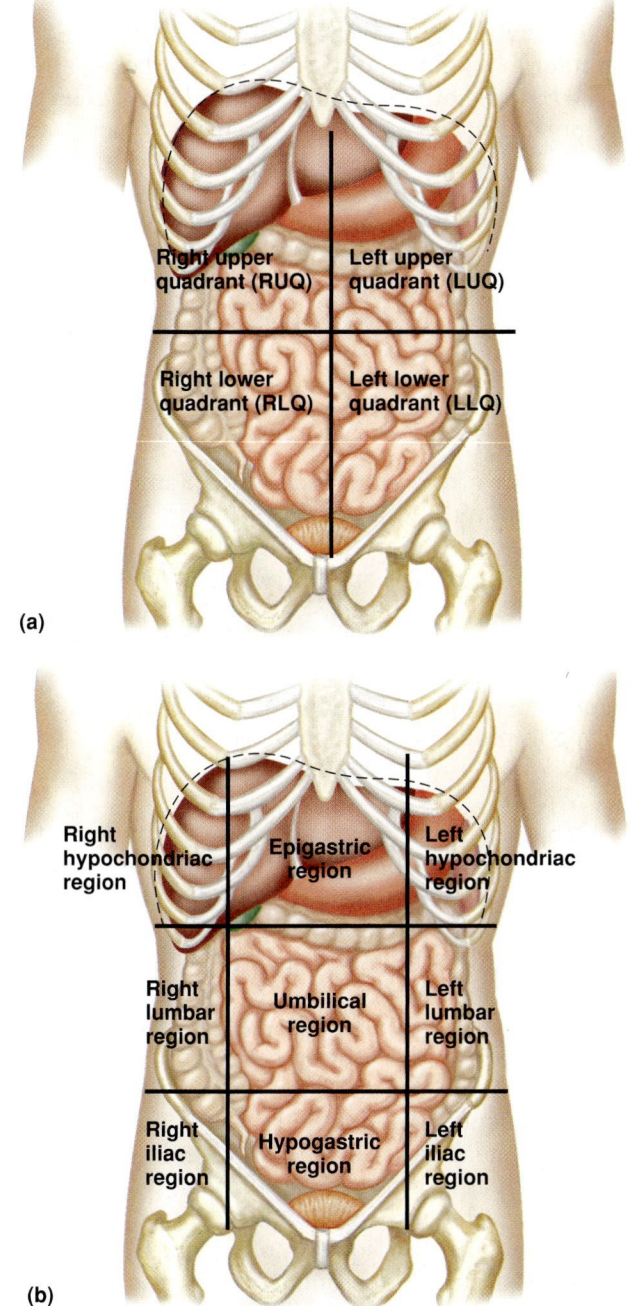

(a)

(b)

Figure 22-2 (a) In describing the location of organs within the abdominal cavity, it is typically divided into four quadrants. (b) Another older and less commonly used method divides the abdomen into nine regions resembling a tic tac toe board.

is the potential to cause substantial or even fatal blood loss.[11] DOT 4-8.14

Hollow visceral organs in the abdominal cavity include the following:

■ Stomach
■ Small bowel
■ Colon
■ Gallbladder

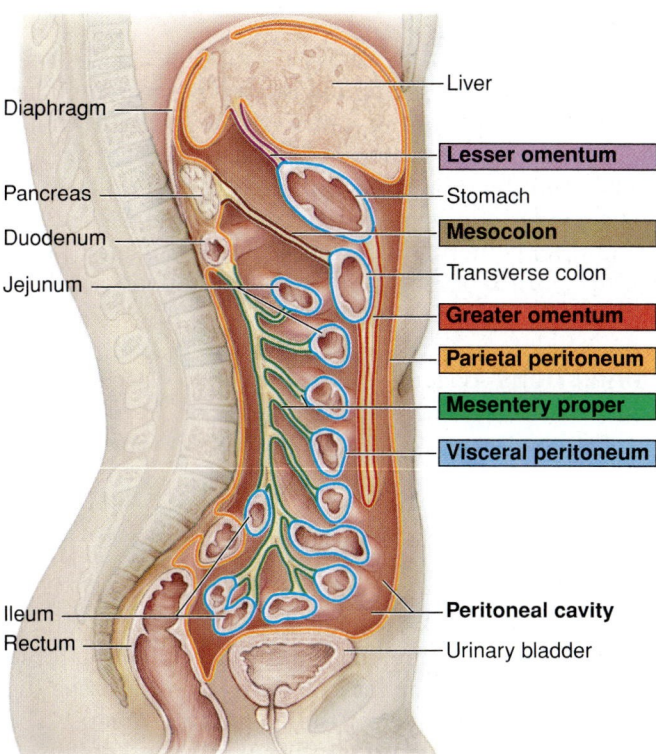

Figure 22-3 Viewed laterally, the abdominal contents can be viewed from the diaphragm down to the pelvic organs. The delineation between the intraperitoneal (anterior) and retroperitoneal (posterior) organs can be seen.

■ Ureters
■ Urethra
■ Fallopian tubes
■ Uterus
■ Urinary bladder

While these organs also may bleed if injured, the blood loss is rarely life-threatening. More commonly, damage to hollow organs creates a serious problem for the patient when the contents (acid, bacteria, partially digested food, and stool) are released into the abdomen. Apart from local irritation to the surrounding tissues (peritonitis), if not discovered and repaired in a timely manner, this leakage can lead to life-threatening septic shock. Although serious, these injuries are rarely immediately life-threatening; they become so if not detected and repaired.[4,6] DOT 4-8.20

CONNECTIONS The organs of the abdomen and retroperitoneum belong to several different systems and provide a variety of functions that are discussed in the medical portions of the text as diseases of each organ system are explored. This chapter will focus on the pathophysiology of injury sustained from blunt and penetrating trauma.

Pathophysiology

Abdominal trauma is divided into two types: blunt and penetrating. Penetrating injury results in disruption of the skin while blunt does not. This differentiation aids in the identification of possible injury patterns. Do not forget the possibility that both types of injuries may exist simultaneously. For example, a victim may be assaulted with a baseball bat then subsequently stabbed with a knife. DOT 4-8.5

CONNECTIONS Chapter 25: Soft Tissue and Muscle Trauma describes specific injuries, such as lacerations, avulsions, etc., that soft tissues sustain from blunt and penetrating trauma.

Blunt Trauma

Blunt trauma often results from a direct blow, causing compression, shearing, deceleration, or crushing forces to the patient.[1] Injury may also result from forces that cause an internal shift of the abdominal organs. This happens most frequently at the point where organs attach to less mobile structures, such as ligaments or blood vessels.[2,4] DOT 4-8.1, 4-8.3, 4-8.33

CONNECTIONS Since abdominal trauma can be hard to detect, careful review of the mechanism of injury is needed. More information on MOI can be found in Chapter 18.

Blunt trauma is the most common mechanism of abdominal trauma encountered in the United States.[4] It also carries a greater mortality than does penetrating trauma. This is thought to be because of the difficulty in detecting hidden injuries and the frequency of having multisystem trauma associated with abdominal trauma (Table 22-1).[4,8,28]

Motor vehicle crashes (MVCs) are the most frequent cause of blunt abdominal trauma in the U.S.[26] An auto striking a pedestrian, direct blows to the abdomen, and falls also represent mechanisms associated with significant injury. Prior to leaving the scene of an MVC, it is important to take note of the amount of damage to the car; the type of collision (rollover, head on, rear impact, side impact, sudden stop from a single vehicle versus tree, etc.); location of impact on the car versus the patient's position; whether the patient was wearing a seat belt and what type; whether airbags deployed; deformity to the steering wheel; starring of the windshield, which would suggest the patient struck it; and any prolonged extrication time to remove the entrapped patient from the vehicle. DOT 4-8.39

Street Secrets

A picture is worth a thousand words. Some ambulance services and individual EMS providers carry photographic cameras (Polaroid or digital) to quickly snap a picture of the mechanism of injury. The pictures can be left in the patient's chart as part of the medical record or deleted as soon as the appropriate caregivers have observed the mechanism. A note of caution: Photos may be considered a part of the medical record; care should be taken to protect patient privacy.

All of these considerations can be vital information, as higher energy mechanisms have increased likelihood of severe injury and should be relayed to hospital personnel.[4,26,30] Likewise, the height of a fall is important, as falls from greater than 20 feet (or three times the height of the patient) are associated with increased likelihood for intraabdominal injury.[29] This being said, significant injuries are sometimes seen in cases with seemingly insignificant trauma.[12]

The reduction of abdominal injuries, as well as overall mortality, may be accomplished by universal seat belt usage as well as multiple airbags (driver, passenger, rear seat, etc.) in vehicles.[13] Although increased seatbelt use has also increased the frequency of some types of injuries, such as intestinal and mesenteric injuries as well as certain spinal fractures, the overall incidence and severity of the majority of serious injuries have decreased.[29]

CONNECTIONS Undeployed airbags may pose a threat to you during extrication. Visit Chapter 51: Rescue Awareness for a more in-depth review of this potentially hazardous situation.

In the case of blunt abdominal trauma, the spleen is the most frequently injured organ, followed by the liver.[1,4,26]

It is not uncommon for one of these organs to be injured in isolation; however, they also frequently occur in combination with other injuries. Injury to more than one

TABLE 22-1 Patterns of Blunt Abdominal Trauma

Direct impact	Organ affected
Right lower rib fractures	Liver, gallbladder, right kidney
Left lower rib fractures	Spleen, left kidney
Mid epigastric contusion	Duodenum, pancreas, small bowel mesentery
Lumbar transverse process fracture	Kidney, ureter
Anterior pelvic fracture	Bladder, urethra

Source: V. Markovchick, and P. Pons, *Emergency Medicine Secrets,* 3rd ed. (Philadelphia, PA: Hanley & Belfus, 2003).

organ in the abdomen has been shown to carry an increase in mortality.[14] The small bowel is the most commonly injured hollow organ, followed by the colon and rectum, duodenum, and stomach.[4,15,16,26]

Penetrating Trauma

Penetrating trauma is the result of direct injury to tissues as the offending object passes through or as energy released from the penetrating object is transmitted through the tissues. DOT 4-8.1, 4-8.3, 4-8.39

Stab wounds are considered low-velocity wounds. They occur nearly three times more frequently than do gunshot wounds and often appear straightforward.[6] They may, however, be misleading given the possibility that the entrance wound may appear small and innocuous yet result in a large amount of internal damage (the size of the blade and trajectory should be taken into account).[17] It is easy to underestimate the degree of damage done. In addition, a large proportion of these victims are under the influence of drugs or alcohol, which may further complicate the evaluation.[4,26]

The liver is the most frequently injured organ in stab wounds, followed by the small intestine, diaphragm, and colon. This pattern is largely accounted for by the large surface area of these organs.[1]

At times, the opening from a stab wound or laceration may be large enough to expose internal structures or even lead to evisceration. The patient may also be impaled on an object with the object remaining in place. DOT 4-8.30

Gunshot wounds, like stab wounds, cause direct tissue injury. In addition, they may cause secondary injury due to energy transmission from the bullet or from fragmentation of the bullet or bone it has struck. Thus, it is possible for organs or vasculature to be injured without the bullet ever coming in direct contact with them.[6] Although they occur less frequently than do stab wounds, gunshot wounds account for up to 90% of the mortality due to penetrating trauma.[4]

Shotguns and handguns typically produce medium-velocity injuries, while high-powered hunting rifles and military-type weapons produce high-velocity injuries, resulting in more significant energy transmission and secondary injuries. In addition, the resultant damage to the body is also affected by the distance of the victim to the weapon as well as the trajectory.[2,4]

The most frequently injured organ in gunshot wounds is the small bowel followed by the large bowel, liver, and major vascular structures. Frequently, multiple organs are damaged with this particular type of trauma.[1] DOT 4-8.24

Mortality related to penetrating abdominal injury is affected by the wounding agent, the specific organs injured, the number of organs injured, as well as the severity of the organ injuries.[1]

Before leaving the scene of a penetrating trauma, take detailed information about the weapon and estimated blood loss. This may become important, as the bleeding may have slowed significantly upon arrival at the hospital, potentially leading hospital personnel to underestimate the need for urgent blood transfusion.[4]

CONNECTIONS It is extremely difficult to estimate blood loss. See Working in the Gray Zone, Chapter 19, page 389, for more information on blood loss.

Solid Visceral Injuries

Injuries to the solid visceral organs, such as the liver, spleen, kidneys, and pancreas, can cause substantial blood loss, with the potential to cause rapid development of tachycardia and hypotension.[4,26] DOT 4-8.14, 4-8.35

Along with these findings, rapid blood loss can cause skin and mental status changes consistent with shock. In older patients, these findings may develop rapidly or may actually be blunted due to chronic use of certain medications (for example, beta-blockers). In younger patients, on the other hand, substantial blood loss may result in only minimal signs or symptoms, so the care provider must remain ever vigilant.[18] While many patients with serious injuries may have significant pain or signs of abdominal distension, others may have an apparently insignificant exam or other painful injuries, such as significant orthopedic injuries or chest trauma that may distract them from the abdomen. This may lead both the patient and examiner to underestimate the extent of abdominal injuries.[5] DOT 4-8.15–4-8.17

Nice to Know

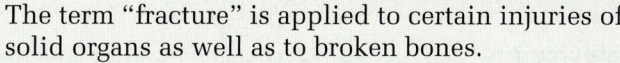

The term "fracture" is applied to certain injuries of solid organs as well as to broken bones.

It is crucial always to keep in mind that hypovolemic shock may result from substantial internal blood loss without obvious external signs. Quick action is critical in dealing with potential solid organ injuries, as mortality related to delayed treatment of hemorrhage is high. Solid organ injuries are seen in both blunt as well as penetrating trauma.

Hollow Organ Injuries

Hollow viscera (which is the plural form of viscus, which refers to internal organs in the trunk of the body) include the stomach, small bowel, colon, gallbladder, ureters, urethra, fallopian tubes, uterus, and the urinary bladder. Injuries to these organs may occur in the setting of blunt trauma when a sudden rise in intra-abdominal pressure causes the hollow viscus to rupture. Having a full stomach or bladder at the time of the injury or impact may increase the risk of rupture. Injuries may also occur in the setting of direct trauma as a result of a penetrating injury. DOT 4-8.17

Injuries to such organs typically result in abdominal contamination from leaking contents as well as blood loss. Stomach and intestinal enzymes, acid, and bacteria are rapidly irritating, often causing the peritoneal signs of abdominal pain, an acute onset of symptoms, and peritoneal irritation within hours of the time of the injury.[6] Urine, which is usually sterile, escaping into the retroperitoneum, on the other hand, may not cause symptoms for days. Injuries to the stomach and intestines frequently have associated bleeding from mesenteric injuries caused from shear tearing forces while bladder injuries almost always cause hematuria (blood in the urine), which will likely be undetected in the prehospital setting.[19] DOT 4-8.18, 4-8.35

Retroperitoneal Injuries

Retroperitoneal structures include the pancreas, duodenum, kidneys, abdominal aorta, inferior vena cava, ureters, and the urinary bladder. Injuries to the nonvascular structures are often subtle, with few or no symptoms upon initial presentation in the prehospital setting.[20] The main vessels that supply major organs of the abdomen are also subject to injury and can cause significant hemorrhage. DOT 4-8.10, 4-8.11, 4-8.35

Injuries to the great vessels of the retroperitoneum—the abdominal aorta and the inferior vena cava—can be devastating. These vessels have the potential to release the patient's entire blood volume into the retroperitoneum or, in the case of penetrating injury, into the abdominal cavity in a matter of just a few minutes. DOT 4-8.11, 4-8.21, 4-8.22, 4-8.23

CONNECTIONS See Chapter 21: Thoracic Trauma for more information on injury to the great vessels of the thorax.

Penetrating trauma is by far the most common mechanism of injury to these vessels in the abdomen, accounting for 90–95% of the injuries.[21] Major injuries to either of these vessels commonly results in death prior to arrival of the patient to the hospital or even the arrival of EMS to the scene. At times, due to the location of the bleeding or the fact that the bleeding is slow enough to allow for partial clotting, the retroperitoneum may actually allow enough pressure to build up to allow for tamponade at the site of injury, which acts to slow or even stop the bleeding.[22]

Unfortunately, due to the difficulty in gaining easy surgical access to these retroperitoneal vessels, many patients, even if they survive long enough to reach the operating room, do not survive surgery.[21] The most common signs of this injury are profound tachycardia and hypotension, consistent with hypovolemic shock. At times, abdominal distention or a contusion over the back, flanks, or abdominal wall may be seen.[22] DOT 4-8.29, 4-8.31

One recent study reported pancreatic injury was most commonly associated with blunt injuries.[23] In the case of blunt trauma, it typically results from the body of the pancreas being compressed against the vertebral column—often when the patient strikes the upper abdomen against a steering wheel or handle bars. These injuries may cause immediate or, more frequently, delayed symptoms. Symptoms are often a result of the release of digestive enzymes into the surrounding tissues or through some degree of autodigestion of the pancreas itself. In this type of injury, the patient typically complains of epigastric pain or pain in the mid-back directly posterior to the epigastrium and may have nausea or vomiting.[20]

Bladder and renal injuries may present with pain, typically over the suprapubic region or the back and flanks. Sometimes blood may be noted at the opening of the urethra, indicating the likelihood of a urethral tear.[6]

Diaphragmatic Injuries

The diaphragm is the upper boundary of the abdomen. During expiration, the top of the diaphragm can rise as high as the nipple line or approximately the fourth to fifth intercostal space.[24] Diaphragmatic injuries are difficult to detect and rarely occur. Suspect a diaphragmatic injury if there is penetrating trauma to the upper half of the abdomen.[6] DOT 4-8.10, 4-8.11 4-8.35

In approximately 5% of blunt abdominal trauma, the diaphragm is injured.[9] In this case, the injury is usually due to an abrupt compressive force to the abdomen that ruptures the diaphragmatic muscle and forces abdominal organs into the chest.[6]

The patient may present with respiratory distress or may be asymptomatic. If the defect in the diaphragm is large enough, abdominal contents may actually herniate through into the chest cavity. If this occurs, you may note decreased breath sounds and may even hear bowel sounds in the chest (Figure 22-4).

Pain and Other Symptoms of Abdominal Injury

Liver and splenic injuries often cause pain directly over the injured organs, in the right upper and left upper quadrant, respectively. If injuries to these or other organs result in bleeding that irritates the diaphragm, pain is often referred to the shoulder on the same side as the irritation. This referred pain is called **Kehr's sign**.[25]

Bowel injury often results in periumbilical pain but can also cause diffuse pain in the case of peritonitis, resulting from bowel contents being spilled into the peritoneum. Pain referred to the groin may signal a retroperitoneal injury. Pain in the mid-back may be a sign of pancreatic damage while tenderness at the posterior and inferior borders of the ribs where they meet the spinal column suggests the kidneys as the possibly injured organ.[4]

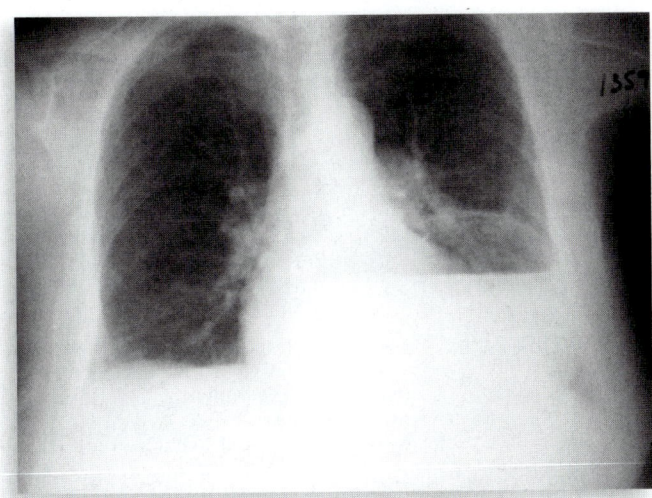

Figure 22-4 This x-ray image shows a ruptured diaphragm with the stomach herniated into the left chest. Abdominal contents protruding into the chest cavity will impair breathing and can damage the organs that have pushed through the diaphragm.

It is important to remember that abdominal contents may be injured not only as a result of injury directly to the abdomen but also due to trauma to the lower chest, flank, back, and buttocks.[17]

The Scene Size-Up

Survey the scene prior to contact with the patient. The mechanism of injury will give you many clues about the potential for an abdominal injury. If the mechanism is blunt, look for clues about the cause (e.g., bat, fists), protective equipment (e.g., seatbelts, lap or shoulder belts, airbag), or damage to the location where the patient's body first collided (side door intrusion, steering column, handlebars). Penetrating trauma may involve impalement, low-velocity weapons (e.g., knives), or high-velocity weapons (e.g., firearm). DOT 4-8.38

After scene safety is considered, if a weapon is involved, the type of weapon and consideration of whether or not the wounds are self-inflicted are important. Police should be at the scene or called to the scene of any trauma caused by the use of a weapon, regardless of type. For example, a tire iron swung in anger is just as much a weapon as a handgun. If a suicide attempt is suspected, ensure the weapon is secure and does not pose a risk to the EMS team. DOT 4-8.7, 4-8.12

Primary Survey (Initial Assessment)

As with any other traumatic condition, the condition of the airway, breathing, and circulation are the first priorities. If the mechanism indicates potential for spinal injury, precautions should be taken. Blunt injury to the abdomen may cause rupture of the diaphragm and

impair the patient's ability to breathe. Thorough assessment of the patient's breathing is essential. Watch for signs of respiratory distress. Carefully inspect the chest, observing rate and depth of chest expansion, intercostal retractions, symmetry, and use of accessory muscles.

The immediate threat to life in abdominal trauma is undetected bleeding. Studies show that delays in discovering active bleeding lead to increased mortality.[6,26] As one of the first advanced-level caregivers to evaluate the patient, you have an important role in alerting hospital staff if you suspect abdominal trauma.

Injuries to the solid organs, the liver and spleen, along with the major vasculature of the abdomen, the abdominal aorta and inferior vena cava, have the potential to bleed large volumes in a very short period of time. Pay particular attention to the patient's vital signs for evidence of tachycardia or hypotension. As part of the primary survey, carefully assess the patient's heart rate and the character of the pulse (strong, weak, or thready).[27]

Less common presentations of severe abdominal injuries that affect the primary survey are also possible. The airway may become compromised secondary to vomiting as a result of gastric trauma. Difficulty breathing may be present secondary to abdominal contents herniating into the chest cavity, as might be the case with rupture of the diaphragm. Abdominal distension may restrict normal diaphragmatic function and also cause breathing impairment.[3] DOT 4-8.34, 4-8.36

Treatment includes clearing the airway, or definitive airway management such as intubation, if needed. Difficulty breathing from diaphragmatic injury may require ventilatory support. Oxygen should be administered to keep SpO$_2$ saturations above 95%. All patients with an abnormal finding in the primary survey should be rapidly transported to a trauma center with adequate diagnostic and surgical capabilities.[28] DOT 4-8.32

During transport, you should place two large-bore IVs, and if the patient is hemodynamically unstable (blood pressure less than 90 mmHg), start fluid replacement with crystalloid fluids (most commonly normal saline or lactated Ringers).[29] Your target blood pressure is between 90 and 100 mmHg.

Secondary Survey

The speed with which the secondary survey is completed and the optimal location to perform it depend upon the situation. If the patient is hemodynamically unstable, the secondary survey will be performed en route to the hospital, if time permits. In stable patients, it is important to be thorough, and the survey may be performed on the scene or in the ambulance. It should be thorough, however, because it is possible to find something unexpected on exam that may change the course of your management or the ultimate destination of transport.

Working in the Gray Zone

How useful are bent steering wheels in predicting abdominal injuries? One recent study points to the need for a careful assessment of the steering wheel after a motor vehicle crash.[30] This study looked back (retrospectively) at eight years of crash data (from 1995 to 2002). It confirmed a direct correlation between the degree of steering wheel damage and injuries to the thorax and abdomen. Severity of steering wheel damage was directly correlated with severity of thoracic injuries in drivers and with abdominal injuries in passengers (Figure 22-5).

The authors of this study theorize that when the driver's chest strikes the steering column, the abdomen is protected from further injury. This study helps emphasize the importance of carefully inspecting the steering wheel at the scene of a crash. It also points to increasing your suspicion of abdominal injuries in passengers of a vehicle that sustained steering wheel damage.

Airbag deployment was also considered a factor in predicting severity of injury. More research is needed to discover if the airbag itself is the cause of further injury or if frontal collisions (when airbags are deployed) result in more severe injuries.

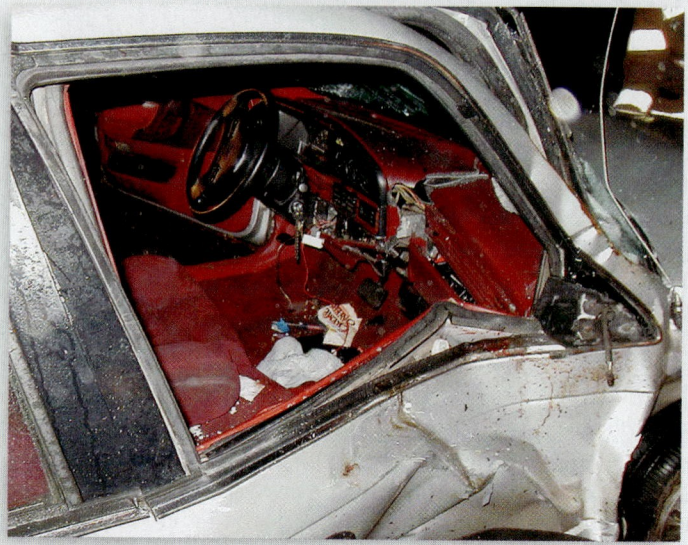

Figure 22-5   In this vehicle crash you can see the break in the dashboard as it was pushed upward. The passenger's head struck the right upper corner, pushing the windshield outward.

Abdominal Evaluation after Blunt Trauma

All trauma patients should undergo an abdominal examination as a part of the secondary survey. If other serious injuries exist, such as head, chest, or orthopedic injuries, you should be suspicious for coexistent abdominal trauma. Keep in mind that if the patient is intoxicated with drugs or alcohol or has a head injury, the evaluation will be even more difficult.[31] DOT 4-8.6

The examination of the abdomen should begin with inspection for obvious, visible signs of injury, such as distention; wounds; obvious external blood loss; abrasions or contusions and ecchymosis to the abdomen, lower chest, flanks, and back. DOT 4-8.9

The **seat belt sign** is a contusion seen over the chest and abdomen where the seat belt rested. This should raise the suspicion for injury to intraabdominal organs caused from compression between the seat belt and the vertebral column.[32] (Figure 22-6)

The mainstay of the abdominal examination is direct palpation. Watch for pain with palpation (documented as *tenderness* on your care report). Location of this pain, distention, guarding, masses, and rigidity are the most useful signs.

Remember that blood is initially not an irritant to the peritoneum, so bleeding may still be occurring even if the patient does not feel it. Also, the abdomen can accommodate a significant amount of blood (1.5 liters in the average adult) without causing signs of distension.[2] Maintain a high index of suspicion for bleeding in the abdomen when a trauma patient has unexplained shock or shock seemingly out of proportion to injuries, even with a "normal" abdominal exam.[6]

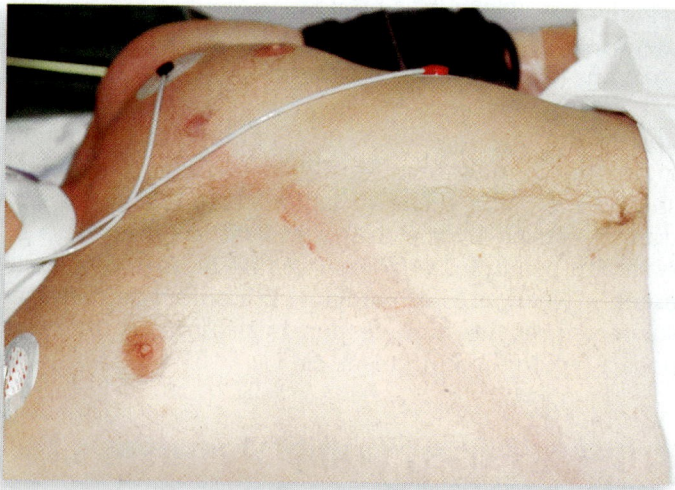

Figure 22-6   Abrasions on the chest and abdomen indicate the placement of a shoulder harness and seat belt at the time of impact. This indicates the potential for injuries to the organs beneath the abrasions.

Street Secrets

Always make an attempt to ask the patient which area is most tender prior to palpation. You should then start palpating the abdomen in the quadrant furthest from this location, approaching the painful region gradually and gently. This allows for the most accurate exam possible, as the patient is not immediately distressed from palpation of an extremely painful location.

Working in the Gray Zone

Are auscultation and percussion useful assessments for abdominal trauma? There is no research to support the use of bowel sounds in the prehospital setting. An attempt to auscultate bowel sounds in a quiet and nonemergent environment may be useful as their absence may signal injury. Absent bowel sounds, however, do not rule in an injury and present bowel sounds do not rule out an injury, thus making this test an *insensitive* finding. Performing this assessment in the prehospital setting is of questionable value and it should not be performed if the patient is potentially unstable.

Percussion of the abdomen is another examination technique that has not been studied in the prehospital setting. Percussion may be helpful to assess for the presence of bleeding. A dull tone may indicate fluid (possibly blood) when compared to a more tympanitic tone (indicating air or less dense structures). Again a quiet and nonemergent environment is needed, and the exam is not definitive.

As discussed previously, a normal physical examination of the abdomen does not rule out injury. Do not delay transport of a patient with obvious serious injuries or bleeding for this exam. Repeated examinations performed by the same examiner, evaluating for interval change, can increase the potential for detection of injury.[8]

Abdominal Examination after Penetrating Trauma

The physical examination in penetrating trauma is focused on inspecting the abdomen for open wounds, impaled objects, and eviscerations. The trajectory of the weapon is frequently difficult to determine both in stab wounds and gunshot wounds, leaving the possible extent of injury unknown. Because the depth of the wound is frequently difficult to ascertain, based upon the location of the wounds and your knowledge of

the underlying organs, presume that there is an intra-abdominal injury and manage the patient accordingly.

The basic principle of the abdominal examination in patients with penetrating injury is the same as outlined previously. Inspection (including the back) is the first and probably most important step as it focuses further examination techniques. All wounds that may have penetrated the abdomen should be identified.

On occasion, while examining the abdomen and back for penetrating wounds, it is apparent that a wound has penetrated because intraabdominal contents are found to be protruding out of the wound (**evisceration**). In these cases, rapid transport is appropriate, but do not stop the initial assessment to begin treating the evisceration. You can and should instruct a crewmember to begin applying a moist occlusive dressing; however, it is not important for you to stop the primary survey to apply the dressing. Palpating the abdomen of patients with penetrating injury is often not helpful as the abdomen will usually be tender to palpation in all four quadrants just because of the wound, whether or not there is a significant associated intraabdominal injury.[6]

Penetrating wounds have a high rate of intra-abdominal injury. In addition to the potential injuries to any of the organs mentioned above, direct injury to the major vasculature of the abdomen, including the abdominal aorta, inferior vena cava, and the vasculature supplying the major organs, is a significant concern.[1]

Management

Prehospital management of severe abdominal injuries, regardless of the actual source of the injury or bleeding, is as follows: DOT 4-8.8, 4-8.37

- Rapid assessment
- Identification as a high-priority sick patient
- Administer high-concentration oxygen to maintain the SpO_2 at greater than 95%
- Packaging for transport
- Transport to a trauma center with immediate surgical capabilities
- Control obvious bleeding
- Dress open wounds
- Secure any impaled objects
- Treat shock aggressively with fluids, titrating the amount of fluid given to a systolic BP of 90–100 mmHg[4]

In the case of evisceration of abdominal organs, handling exposed structures more than necessary should be avoided (Figure 22-7). Do not attempt to replace them into the abdominal cavity. Cover the evisceration with moist, sterile dressings or an occlusive dressing. Cover that dressing with additional soft, light padding to help

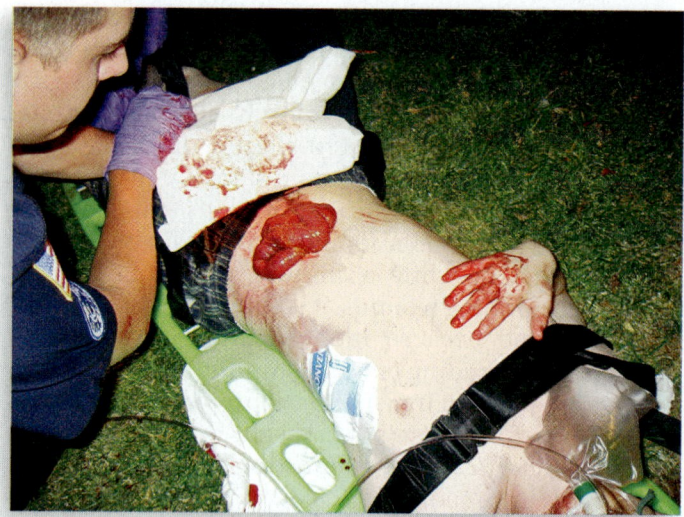

Figure 22-7 Handle exposed structures as little as possible. Do not attempt to replace them into the abdominal cavity. Cover with moist, sterile dressings or an occlusive dressing. Cover that dressing with additional soft, light padding to help maintain body heat.

maintain body heat. Avoid using dry dressings directly on the wound and eviscerated organ as these may adhere to the wound, causing problems for the surgical team. Sterile saline should be used to keep the dressing moist, which decreases evaporation and decreases drying of the organs.[2,33] If the organs dry, they likely will die and will require surgical removal.

If not already done, start two large-bore IV's and initiate fluid replacement.[29] The source of the bleeding in "closed" abdominal trauma, whether obvious or not, as well as in cases of "open" abdominal trauma is treated the same way: by replacing fluids. In addition, apply a dressing and pressure over any wound that is actively bleeding.

No definitive treatment for internal bleeding injuries is possible in the prehospital environment as their management will require further diagnostic tests and possibly surgery. Avoid giving the patient anything by mouth as this may precipitate vomiting either now or later. Keep a portable suction device ready for use in the event that the patient vomits. Obtain medical direction if IV narcotics are needed for pain control.[29]

It is important to remember that most severe abdominal injuries causing hemorrhage can be definitively controlled only in the operating room. Survival of the patient may be directly related to the time from injury until surgical control of the bleeding in the operating room—so any delay in transport may impact survival. Therefore, presenting to a hospital with a trauma surgeon immediately available may make the difference between life and death.[36] While en route, continue frequent examinations as a seemingly stable

Working in the Gray Zone

The use of the pneumatic anti-shock garment (PASG), or MAST trousers, has been a controversial topic. As of this writing, use of the PASG has been listed as acceptable with uncertain efficacy for severe traumatic hypotension (where a pulse may be palpable but no blood pressure is obtainable).[34] It is considered inappropriate for penetrating thoracic injury, diaphragmatic rupture, abdominal evisceration, and pregnancy. Check your local protocols and follow the orders of your medical director.[35]

patient's status can change quickly. Notify the receiving facility of the patient's impending arrival, so appropriate staff have time to assemble with any needed equipment.

Nice to Know

In the past, most patients with high suspicion for significant abdominal injury were taken directly to the operating room for an exploratory laparotomy; however, a shift in treatment strategies has occurred. Now even significant injuries may be treated nonoperatively with selective embolization of the blood vessel supplying the site of bleeding by an interventional radiologist, or, at other times, these injuries are managed with simple observation.[1] As such, evaluation in the emergency department has evolved to include more imaging and assessment modalities, such as bedside ultrasound, CT scanning, diagnostic peritoneal lavage, or even serial abdominal exams and observation.[18]

If the patient is hemodynamically unstable at presentation or becomes so during the observation period and the source of the bleeding is felt to be in the abdomen, the patient is then typically taken to the operating room for exploration and repair.[37]

Summary

Abdominal injuries are deadly if they are hidden and not discovered in a timely manner. Often life-threatening injuries exist with minimal or no outward signs. You should remain vigilant and maintain a high index of suspicion to give the patient the highest possible chance of survival. Any injury between the nipple line and the umbilicus has the potential of involving both the chest and the abdomen and requires a thorough evaluation in the emergency department. Being familiar with the anatomical location of abdominal organs and combining this knowledge with careful observation of the mechanism of injury can help predict injuries and potential severity.

Prehospital care for abdominal trauma focuses on rapid assessment and transportation to the appropriate trauma-receiving facility. Open abdominal wounds should be dressed and intravenous lines should be established once transport has been initiated.

Notes

1. S. R. Todd, "Critical Concepts in Abdominal Injury," *Critical Care Clinics* 20(1)(2004):119–134.

2. National Association of Emergency Medical Technicians, *Prehospital Trauma Life Support,* 5th ed. (St. Louis, MO: Elsevier Mosby, 2005).

3. J. E. Tintinalli, G. D. Kelen, J. S. Stapczynski, O. J. Ma, and D. M. Cline, "Abdominal Injuries." *Tintinalli's Emergency Medicine: A Comprehensive Study Guide,* 6th ed., Mcgraw-Hill's AccessMedicine (accessed September 2, 2006).

4. J. A. Marx, ed., *Rosen's Emergency Medicine Concepts and Clinical Practice,* 5th ed. (St. Louis, MO: Elsevier Mosby, 2002).

5. P. C. Ferrera et al., "Injuries Distracting from Intraabdominal Injuries after Blunt Trauma," *The American Journal of Emergency Medicine* 16(2)(1998):145–149.

6. J. E. Tintinalli, *Emergency Medicine, A Comprehensive Study Guide,* 6th ed. (New York, NY: McGraw-Hill, 2004): 1614.

7. A. Hirshberg et al., "Double Jeopardy: Thoracoabdominal Injuries Requiring Surgical Intervention in Both Chest and Abdomen," *The Journal of Trauma* 39(1995):229–231.

8. C. K. Sung, "Missed Injuries in Abdominal Trauma," *The Journal of Trauma* 41(1996):276–282.

9. M. Blaivas, "Bedside Emergency Ultrasonographic Diagnosis of Diaphragmatic Rupture in Blunt Abdominal Trauma." *The American Journal of Emergency Medicine* 22(7)(November 1, 2004):601–604.

10. H. Gray, *Gray's Anatomy* (Philadelphia, PA: Running Press, 1974):895.

11. J. D. Richardson, "Changes in the Management of Injuries to the Liver and Spleen," *Journal of the American College of Surgeons* 200(5) (2005):648–669.

12. G. C. Velmahos et al., "'Insignificant' Mechanism of Injury: Not to be Taken Lightly," *Journal of the American College of Surgeons* 192(2)(2001):147–152.

13. M. Sochor, "National Highway Traffic Safety Administration (NHTSA) notes. Knee-Thigh-Hip Injuries in Frontal Crashes," *Annals of Emergency Medicine* 46(2)(August 1, 2005): 168–169; discussion 169–171.

14. A. K. Malhotra, R. Latifi, T. C. Fabian, et al., "Multiplicity of Solid Organ Injury: Influence on Management and Outcomes after Blunt Abdominal Trauma," *The Journal of Trauma* 54(2003):925–929.

15. D. D. Watts and S. M. Fakhry, "Incidence of Hollow Viscous Injury in Blunt Trauma: An Analysis From 275,557 Trauma Admissions from the EAST Multi-Institutional HVI Trial," *The Journal of Trauma* 54(2003):289–293.

16. S. M. Fakhry, D. D. Watts, and F. A. Luchette, "Current Diagnostic Approaches Lack Sensitivity in the Diagnosis of Perforated Small Bowel Injury: Analysis from 275,557 Trauma Admissions from the EAST Multi-Institutional HVI Trial," *The Journal of Trauma* 54(2003):295–305.

17. J. P. Pryor et al., "Nonoperative Management of Abdominal Gunshot Wounds," *Annals of Emergency Medicine* 43(3)(2004): 344–353.

18. M. Blaivas, P. Sierzenski, and D. Theodoro, "Significant Hemoperitoneum in Blunt Trauma Victims with Normal Vital Signs and Clinical Examination," *The American Journal of Emergency Medicine* 20(3)(2002):218–221.

19. N. S. Xeropotamos, V. E. Nousias, H. V. Ioannou, and A. M. Kappas, "Mesenteric Injury After Blunt Abdominal Trauma," *European Journal of Surgery* 167(2)(2001):106.

20. R. H. Emmerick and S. R. Petersen, "Evaluation of Pancreatic Injury after Blunt Trauma," *Annals of Emergency Medicine* 27(1996): 658–661.

21. J. Asensio et al., "Visceral Vascular Injuries," *The Surgical Clinics of North America* 82(1)(2002):1–20.

22. R. J. Mullins, R. Huckfeldt, and D. D. Trunkey, "Complex and Challenging Problems in Trauma Surgery: Abdominal Vascular Injuries," *Surgical Clinics of North America* 76(4)(1996): 813–832.

23. L. S. Kao, E. M. Bulger, and D. L. Parks, "Predictors of Morbidity after Traumatic Pancreatic Injury," *The Journal of Trauma* 55(2003): 898–905.

24. V. Markovchick and P. Pons, *Emergency Medicine Secrets,* 2nd ed. (Philadelphia, PA, Hanley & Belfus, 2006) p. 426.

25. H. S. Bjerke, "Splenic Rupture," http://www.emedicine.com/med/topic2792.htm (accessed October 24, 2005).

26. R. Sikka, "Unsuspected Internal Organ Traumatic Injuries." *Emergency Medical Clinics of North America)* 22(4) (November 1, 2004): 1067–1080.

27. J. Pryor, "Shock, Hemorrhagic," http://www.emedicine.com/MED/topic2115.htm (accessed October 18, 2005).

28. J. A. Weinberg, K. McKinley, S. R. Petersen, et al., "Trauma Laparotomy in a Rural Setting before Transfer to a Regional Center: Does it Save Lives?" *The Journal of Trauma* 54(2003): 823–828.

29. B. R. Boulanger and B. A. McLellan, "Blunt abdominal trauma," *Emergency Medical Clinics of North America* 14(1)(1996): 151–171.

30. C. D. Newgard, "Steering Wheel Deformity and Serious Thoracic or Abdominal Injury Among Drivers and Passengers Involved in Motor Vehicle Crashes." *Annals of Emergency Medicine* 45(1) (January 1, 2005): 43–50.

31. T. A. Amoroso, "Evaluation of the Patient with Blunt Abdominal Trauma: An Evidence Based Approach," *Emergency Medical Clinics of North America* 17(1)(1999):63–75.

32. H. J. Asbun et al., "Intra-Abdominal Seatbelt Injury," *The Journal of Trauma* 30(1990):189–193.

33. L. J. Kaplan, "Abdominal Trauma, Penetrating," http://www.emedicine.com/emerg/topic2.htm (accessed October 24, 2005).

34. R. M. Domeier et al., "Use of the Pneumatic Anti-Shock Garment (PASG)." Position paper by the National Association of EMS Physicians, Prehospital Emergency Care, 1(1) (January/March 1997): 33–35.

35. New York State Department of Health Bureau of Emergency Medical Services, "Medical Anti-Shock Trousers, advisory no. 97-04," http://www.health.state.ny.us/nysdoh/ems/policy/s97-04.htm (accessed October 18, 2005).

36. D. Demetriades et al., "Trauma Deaths in a Mature Urban Trauma System: Is 'Trimodal' Distribution a Valid Concept?" *American College of Surgeons* 201(2005):343–348.

37. P. R. Miller et al., "Associated Injuries in Blunt Solid Organ Trauma: Implications for Missed Injury in Nonoperative Management," *The Journal of Trauma* 53(2002): 238–242.

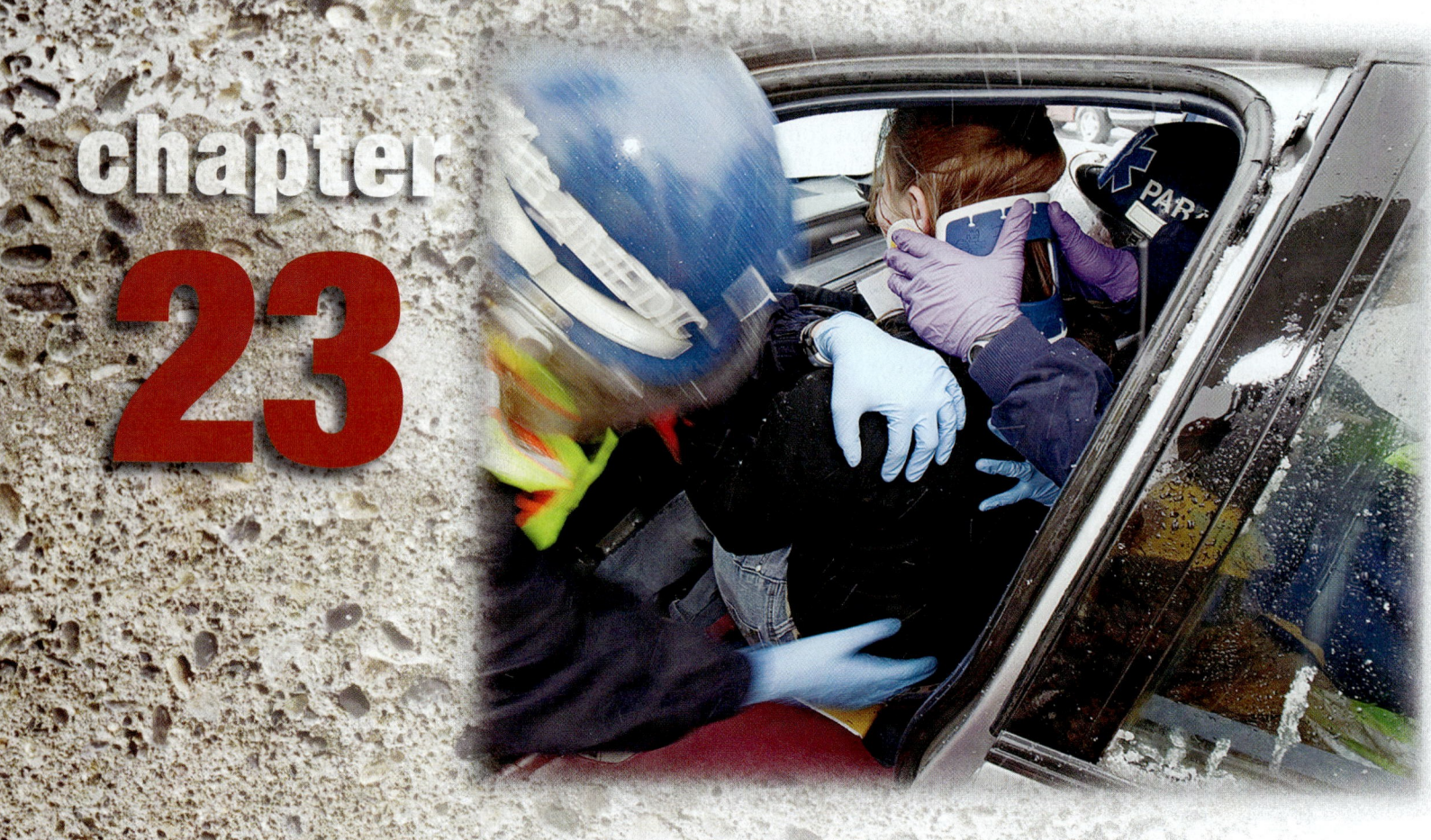

Spinal Trauma

"*The whole problem with the world is that fools and fanatics are always so certain of themselves, but wiser people so full of doubts.*"

—Bertrand Russell

Need To Know

▶ Suspected spinal cord injuries are a frequently encountered EMS complaint, but the actual incidence of spinal cord injuries is dramatically less than suspected. However, because it is virtually impossible to determine if an actual injury exists in the out-of-hospital setting, it is best to treat the potential spinal injury with stabilization and immobilization.

▶ A recent focus on some of the "side effects" of spinal immobilization (even when properly performed) has lead to the development of criteria for ruling out potential injuries. Early research evidence seems to indicate that if used properly, such criteria can be effective.

▶ Perform a thorough pulse, motor, and sensory assessment before and after immobilization.

▶ When the patient has a spinal injury, the condition of the patient may change, for worse or better. Always use care and caution when stabilizing and immobilizing these patients. Remember that they may not feel pressure, pain, pinching, or other sensations if they have a nervous system injury, so you have to monitor them carefully and continuously.

▶ There is a difference between spinal shock and neurogenic shock. The terms are not interchangeable nor are the signs and symptoms or cause.

▶ Sick	▶ Not Yet Sick
• A high spinal injury affecting the upper cervical vertebra or upper portion of the spinal cord can affect ventilation and respiration, thus making the spinal injury a high priority. • Spinal shock and neurogenic shock are not common findings, even with spinal cord injured patients. Suspect any patient with low blood pressure as having hypovolemia before assuming spinal or neurogenic shock is present. • Determine where on the body the patient notices a loss of sensation or movement, and mark the skin. Perform repeat assessments to determine if the injury is worsening.	• Spinal stabilization begins during the ABCDE assessment, but the actual assessment, immobilization, and treatment of spinal injuries does not usually involve a life-threatening situation. • Frequently ask the patient if there are any changes in sensation or motor. Sensations that change from tingling and numbness to burning indicate a need for additional assessment as does a sudden inability to "feel" or move an extremity or part of the body. • Immobilization equipment should be applied so that movement is restricted, but it should not increase pain, cause undue discomfort, or compromise respirations or circulation. Continually ask the patient if devices are too tight or if they are causing rubbing or friction, and loosen or add padding as needed. • Determine if there are any distracting injuries, neurological complaints, or impairments (alcohol, drugs, or head injuries) present before deciding whether to immobilize a patient. • Perform an ABCDE primary survey instead of just an ABC primary survey. Remember, "D" means disability, which applies primarily to the nervous system. • Perform a thorough pulse, motor, and sensory assessment before and after immobilization.

Introduction

The magnitude of the impact that spine trauma has on healthcare in the United States is staggering. The initial evaluation and treatment of spine injuries often occurs in the prehospital setting. This is a tremendous undertaking as it has been estimated that 1.9 to 2.4 million patients are immobilized by prehospital personnel for suspected spine injury each year.[1] Unfortunately, the effects of spinal injuries extend well beyond the acute event, as there are estimated to be 11,000 new spinal cord injuries each year, with healthcare costs attributable to these injuries exceeding 7.7 billion dollars.[2,3] Similar monetary expenses and effort are directed toward the initial evaluation of patients with suspected spine injury. It has been estimated that 800,000 screening cervical spine radiographs (x-rays) are ordered each year at an annual cost of $180 million.[4]

All of this effort is generated in the face of data demonstrating that the actual incidence of injuries to the spine is relatively low; only 2% of patients evaluated for an injury to the spine end up having a fracture. On the other hand, none of these statistics take into account patients who die at the scene as a result of their spinal injuries. DOT 4-6.1

The actual incidence of spine injuries is difficult to calculate. It has been estimated that the incidence of spinal cord injuries is approximately 40 cases per million.[2] Males are injured four times more often than females. Since 1973, the average age of patients when a spinal cord injury occurs is 33. It is interesting to note a recent demographic trend that shows the age when spine injury occurs is increasing. In the time period from 1973 to 1979, the average age was 28.9 years whereas in the 2000 to 2003 period, it was 38 years.[2]

The mechanism of injury resulting in injuries to the spine has been fairly consistent over the past three decades. Acute spinal cord injury is caused by blunt trauma 85–90% of the time, and penetrating trauma accounts for 10–15% of all injuries.[5] For blunt trauma, motor vehicle crashes are the most common etiology, representing 45.6% of all spinal injuries.[2] Less common etiologies include falls (19.6%), violence (17.8%), and sports-related injuries (10.7%). The most common cause of penetrating wounds of the spine is gunshots, with a small minority caused by stab wounds.[6]

Most spinal injuries involve the upper spine, and greater than 54% of spinal injuries are found in the cervical area. Within the cervical spine, fractures are localized to either the upper or lower vertebral bodies. One large study found that the most commonly fractured vertebral body was the second cervical vertebra (24%).[7] The next most common areas of injury were the sixth and seventh vertebrae. In comparison, the combined incidence of trauma to the rest of the spine constitutes the remaining 45% of spinal injuries.[2] After the cervical region, the next most common regions to be injured are the thoracolumbar junction, the thoracic region, and the lumbar segments.[8]

Applied Anatomy

CONNECTIONS Refer to Chapter 7: Anatomy Overview, Figures 7-29 and 7-30, for additional information on the anatomy of the spine.

Vertebral Body

The basic element of the spinal column is the **vertebra.** Each vertebra consists of a body, lamina, pedicle, transverse process, and spinous process (Figure 23-1). The bulk of the vertebra is the body. It appears ovoid and cylinder-shaped and is covered on each end with cartilage. Posterior to the body is the vertebral arch, which is comprised of two pedicles and two lamina. The

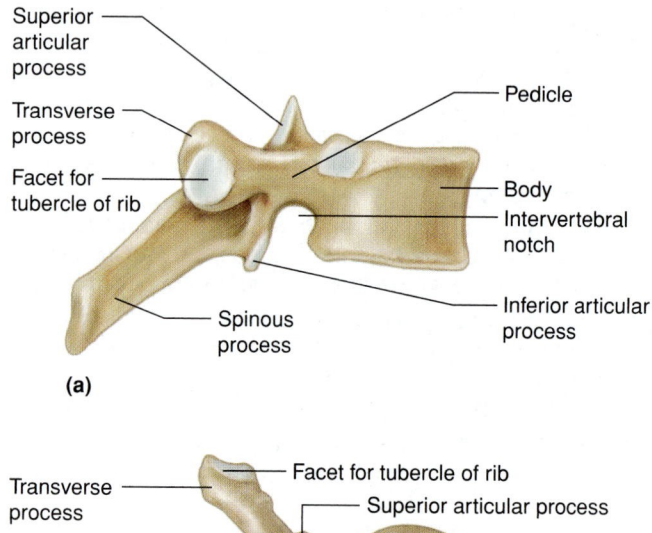
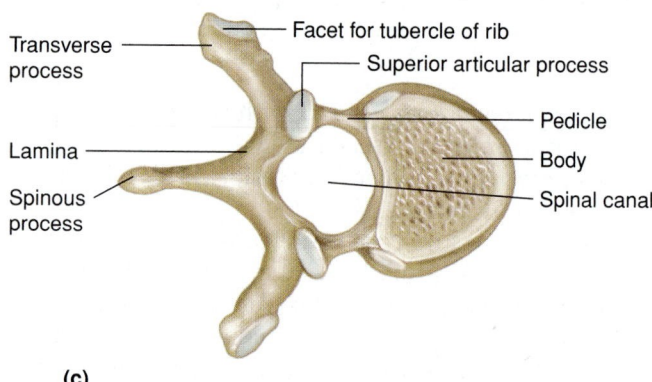
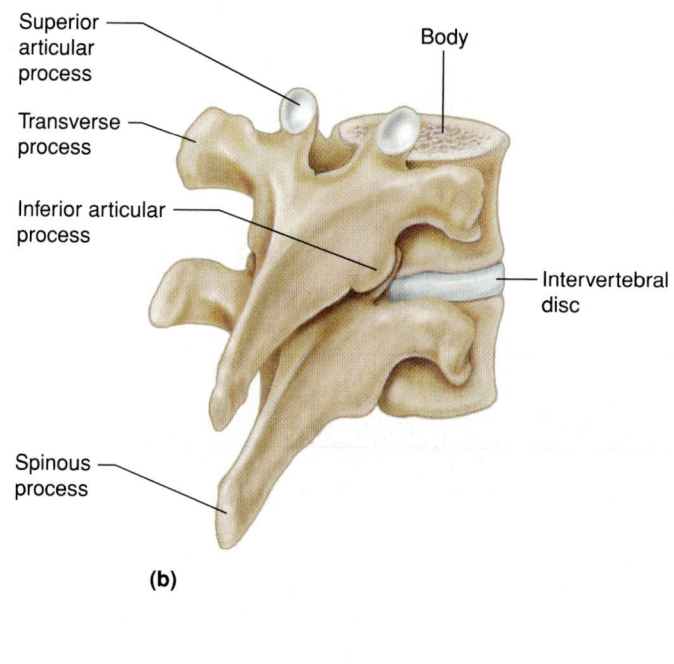

Figure 23-1 Appearance of typical vertebrae.

fusion of the vertebral arch and body comprise an extremely important anatomic area, which is the vertebral canal. The importance of the vertebral canal is that it houses and forms a protective barrier for the spinal cord. DOT 4-6.2

Spinal Column

The normal **spinal column** consists of 33 vertebrae aligned one on top of another (Figure 23-2). The upper seven vertebrae comprise the **cervical spine.** The next twelve vertebrae constitute the **thoracic spine** (and there is one vertebra for each pair of ribs in the thoracic cage), and the five vertebrae below this make up the **lumbar spine.** The remaining nine vertebrae are fused into two separate segments called the **sacrum** and the **coccyx,** and they form the posterior, or back, of the pelvis. The cervical, thoracic, and lumbar vertebrae are united to those above and below by a **fibrocartilaginous** (meaning "composed of fibrous cartilage") **intervertebral** (meaning "located between the vertebrae") disk and a number of ligaments.

The mobility of a normal spine is due to the compressibility and elasticity of the disks, which allow movement of the vertebrae upon each other. When the disks are misaligned, ruptured, or otherwise damaged, the result is pain, difficulty in moving, and perhaps compression to the spinal cord or nerves. A dense

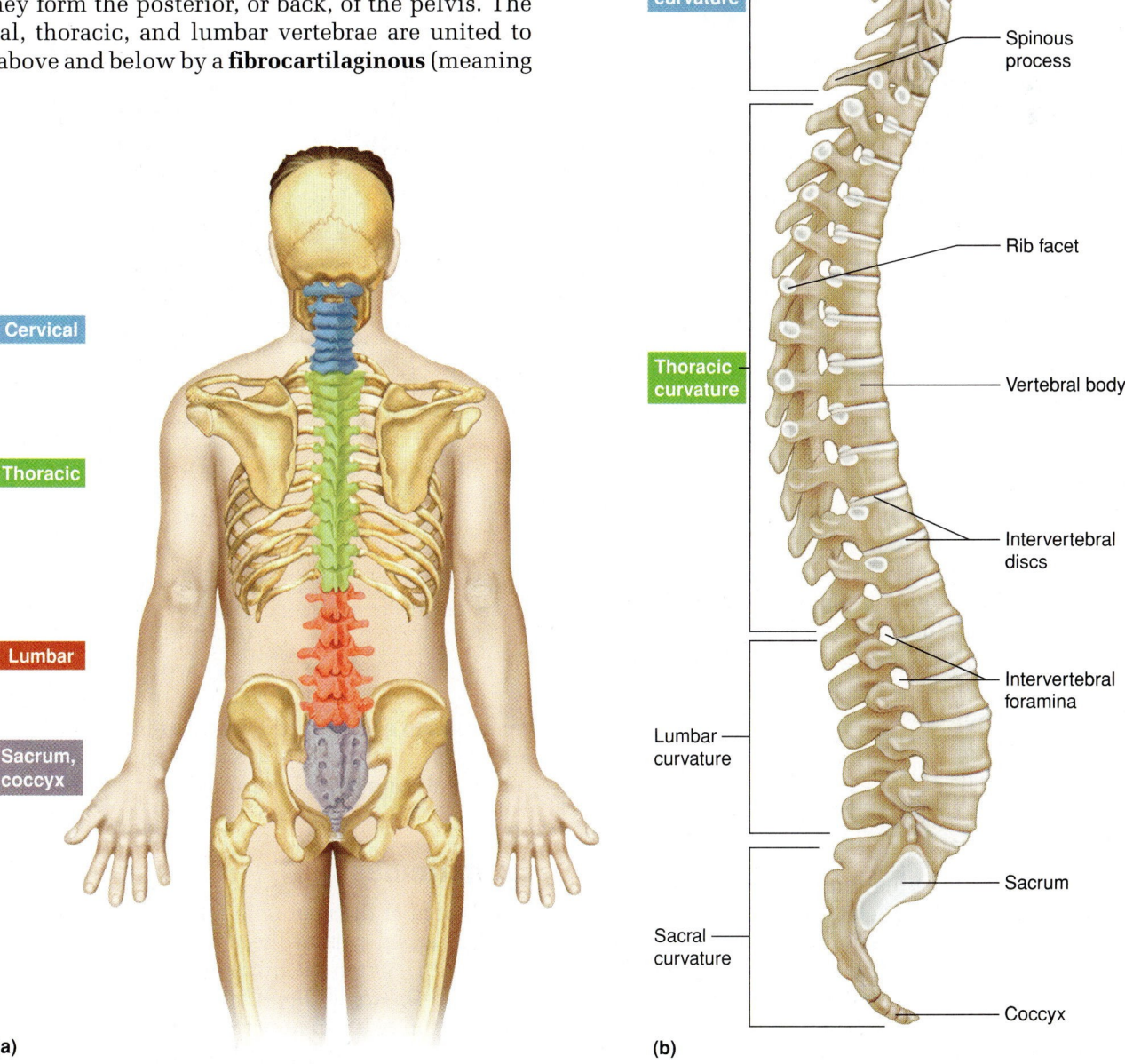

(a)   (b)

Figure 23-2 (a) Appearance of the vertebral column. (b) Thirty-three individual vertebrae make up the spinal column: seven cervical, twelve thoracic, five lumbar, five sacral, and four coccyx.

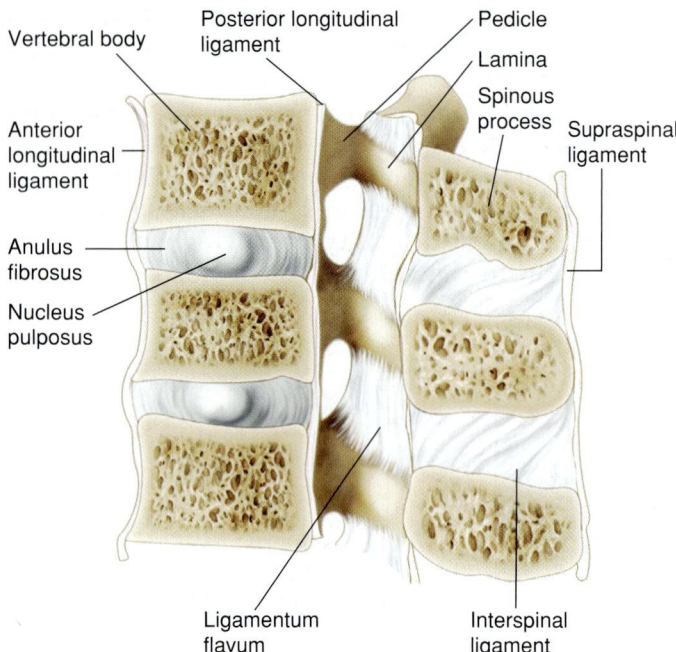

Figure 23-3   Ligaments of the anterior and posterior column. A dense network of ligaments and muscles provide strength and stability to the spinal column.

network of ligaments and muscles surround the vertebrae to provide stability along the length of the spinal column and to provide protection to the spinal cord (Figure 23-3).

Spinal Cord

One of the functions of the spinal column is to provide bony protection for the spinal cord. The **spinal cord** is one of the two parts of the central nervous system, with the other part being the brain. Relatively speaking, the spinal cord has a fairly basic function: to carry messages back and forth between the brain and body. The spinal cord originates from the base of the brain and almost immediately exits the base of the skull as it enters the vertebral canal of the first cervical vertebra (Figure 23-4). While it is actually shorter than the spinal column itself, its length varies a little from person to person. It generally ends between the second and third lumbar vertebra in the lower back.

The ability of the spinal cord to relay neurologic information (in the form of electrical impulses) to surrounding muscles and tissues in the torso and extremities is the job of individual nerve roots. **Nerve roots** are branches off the spinal cord that leave the spinal column through each intervertebral space. In total, there are 31 nerve roots that originate from either side of the spinal cord. The significance of this anatomic arrangement is that each nerve root provides neurologic function and

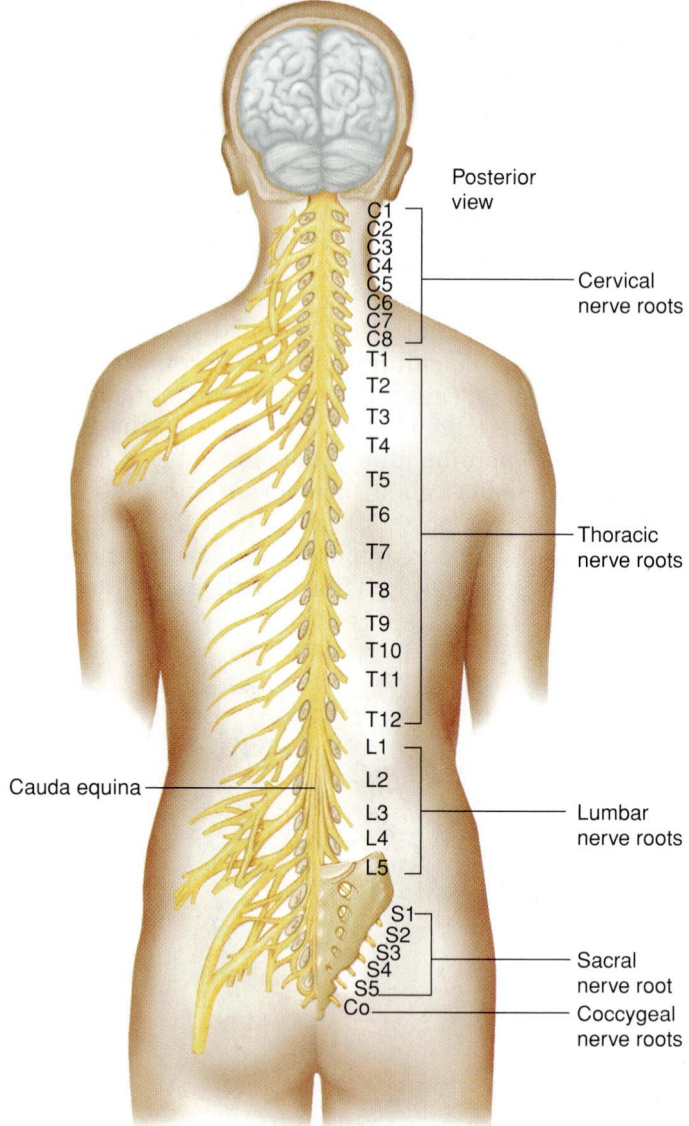

Figure 23-4   The spinal cord exits from the base of the brain and ends between the second and third lumbar vertebrae.

sensation to a very specific area of the body. The actual area of skin sensed by a single one of these roots is called a **dermatome** (Figure 23-5).

Dermatomes

Knowledge of the anatomic distribution of dermatomes is an essential part of the neurologic evaluation of patients with a potential spine injury. Armed with knowledge of dermatomes, healthcare providers can pinpoint the location of a spinal cord injury based on the dermatome where the transition between normal and abnormal function and sensation occurs (Box 23-1). For instance, a patient with a spinal cord injury may relate

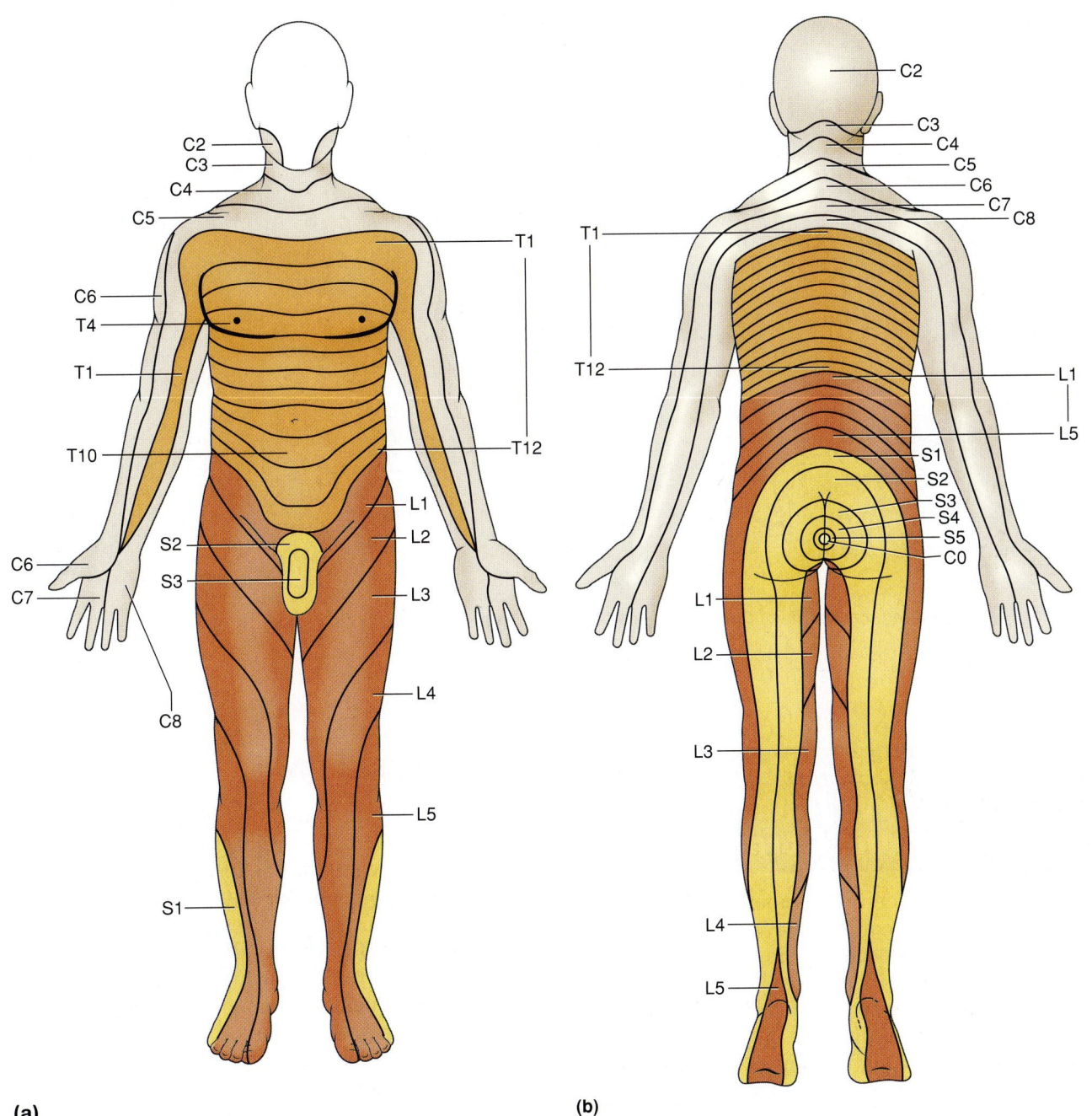

(a)

(b)

Figure 23-5   Dermatomes describe the areas of the body served by each of the 31 nerve roots emanating from the spinal cord.

that they are able to feel an examiner touch their skin at the umbilicus (belly button), but they cannot feel below that point. Knowledge of dermatomal anatomy enables the examiner to predict that the approximate level of the spinal cord injury is the tenth thoracic vertebra. DOT 4-6.3

The actual anatomy of the spinal cord itself is very complex, but knowing some of the basic anatomy can be helpful. In general, each side of the spinal cord can

be divided into **anterior** and **posterior "horns."** The **lateral horns** are projections on each side of the midline (Figure 23-6). In general, the posterior horns receive the incoming sensory fibers that transmit pain, temperature, and vibration. The anterior horn is the area where nerves that ultimately go to muscles originate. Therefore, the anterior horns are primarily responsible for motor function that controls movement. The muscles of the arms and legs are controlled by the anterior horns. DOT 4-6.3

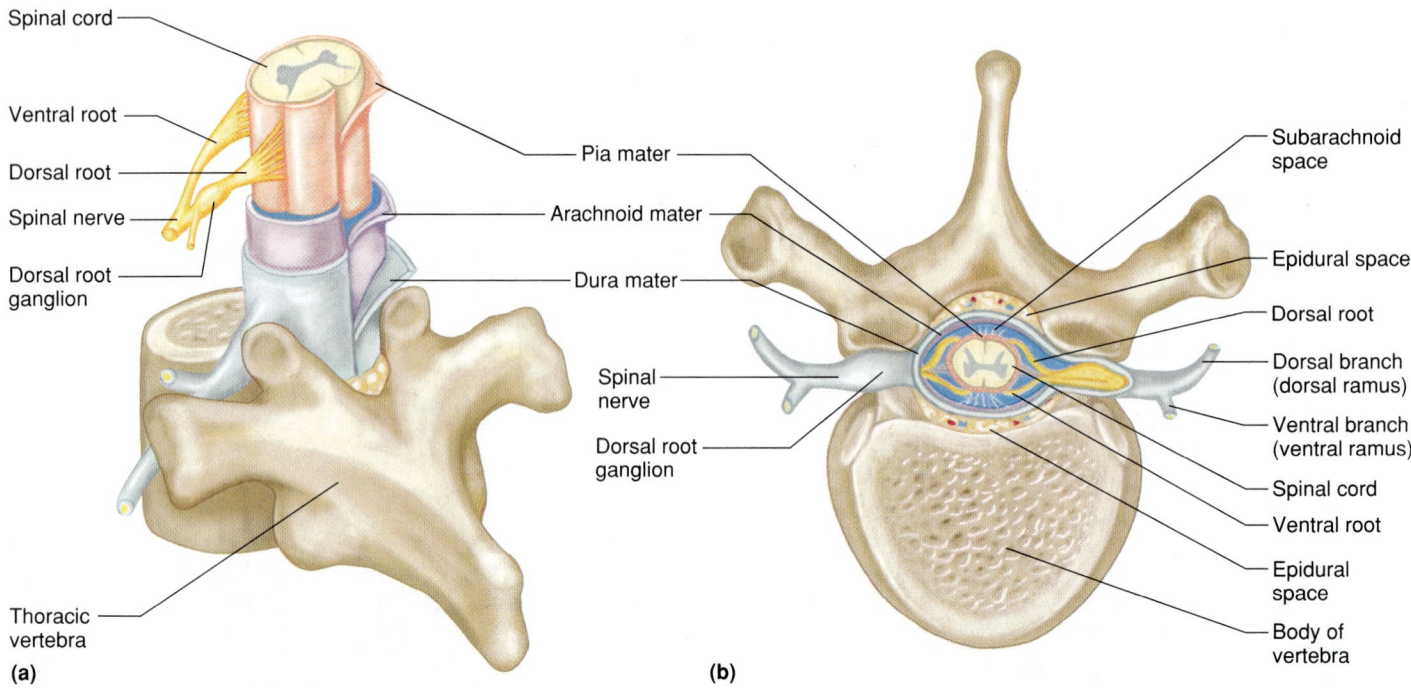

Figure 23-6 Cross-sectional anatomy of the spinal cord and nerve root.

Performing an assessment to pinpoint injury to a specific dermatome or nerve is a level of sophistication that is not always necessary in the prehospital setting. Often the identification of an injury is difficult enough, so pinpointing exactly which nerve is injured is even more difficult. However, as you gain experience in evaluating patients with neurovascular injuries, it will be helpful to the receiving facility if you have been tracking the evolution of the injury as well as suspecting one is present. Let's use the patient from the text as an example: You report that your patient had sensation at the belly button upon your arrival on scene, but you noted that upon repeat assessment 10 minutes later, the patient had lost sensation in that area. Upon arrival at the hospital, you report that the patient now has lost sensation below the nipple line. This information, along with an approximate time line can be valuable to the neurosurgery team treating the patient, as it helps them determine the progression of the injury.

Pathophysiology

One of the primary functions of the spine is to provide stability to the erect (upright) human body while at the same time allowing for flexibility in an infinite number of postures and angles. Equally important, it is a protective bony column that houses the spinal cord and provides support for the skull. The spine's ability to successfully perform these functions is a constant battle between its structural elements (bones, ligaments, cartilage) and the external forces. The cervical spine is at particular risk for any applied abnormal force as it carries the weight of the head. The most common types of externally applied forces include vertical compression, flexion, extension, rotation, and distraction. DOT 4-6.4, 4-6.5, 4-6.10

Vertical Compression

Vertical compression is a force applied to either the top or bottom of the spine, which is directed along the length of the spine (Figure 23-7). When the force is applied to the top of the cranium, it is called an **axial load.** Common mechanisms of injury for vertical compression injuries include falls, diving accidents, or any trauma to the top of the head, such as being struck by a falling object, hitting the windshield, or helmet-to-helmet football injuries. A number of specific fracture patterns in

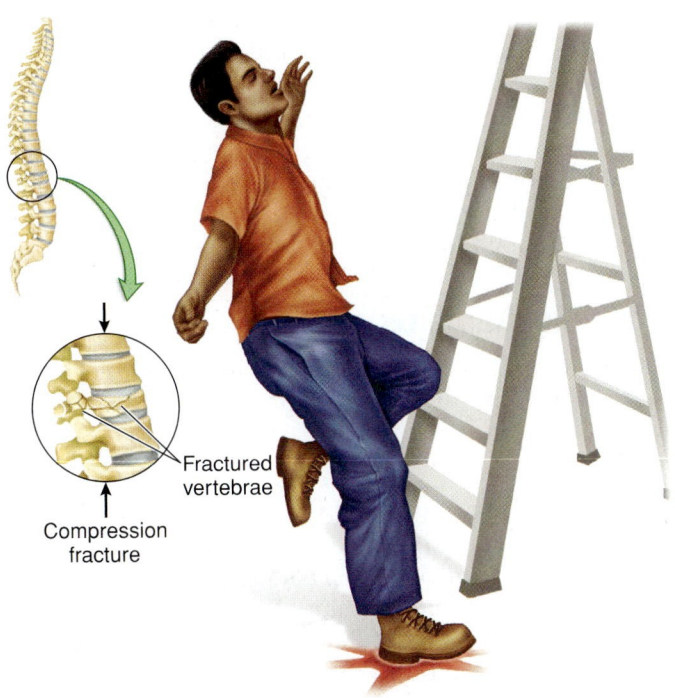

Figure 23-7 Illustration of compression mechanism and the associated injury pattern.

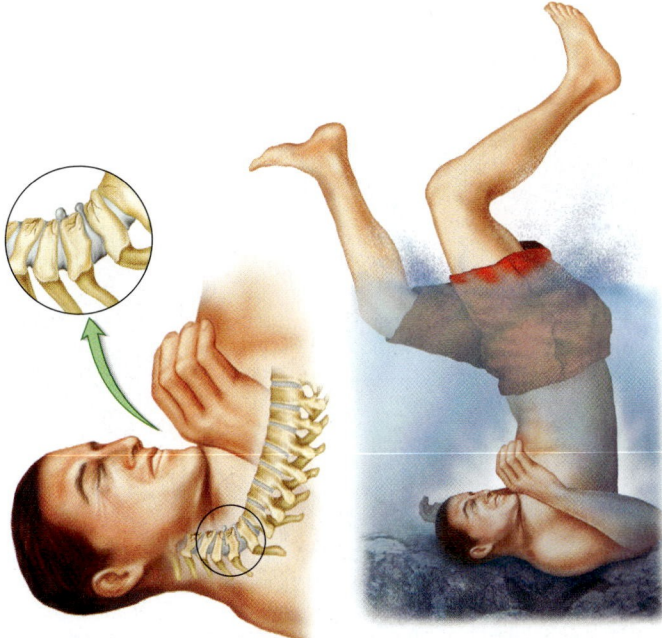

Figure 23-8 Illustration of flexion mechanism of injury and associated injury patterns.

the upper and lower spine are associated with vertical compression.

In the lumbar spine, the vertical compression forces are directed towards the middle aspect of the vertebral bodies. When these forces exceed the ability of the vertebrae to resist them, the vertebral body shatters outward from within. This is called a **burst fracture.** This type of injury commonly occurs when someone falls from a height landing on the feet or buttocks. A similar mechanism occurs in the upper spine, but it is directed toward the C1 and C2 vertebrae. In this case, the ring of C1 is pushed down on the body of C2, resulting in a break in the ring of C1. This pattern is called a **Jefferson fracture,** and it is usually a very unstable injury with high mortality.

Recall that C2 is the most commonly fractured vertebra.

Flexion

Flexion injuries occur when a force causes part of the spine to move forward relative to the rest of the spine (Figure 23-8). Extreme movement of this type causes compression of the anterior aspects of the spine and abnormal opening of the posterior aspects of the spine. In most cases, the posterior ligaments remain intact, so the end result is a fracture to the anterior aspect of the vertebral body, called a **wedge fracture** or **compression**

fracture. A more severe outcome is a **subluxation,** or movement, of one vertebral body on the one immediately below or above. This abnormal movement is a result of complete disruption of the supporting ligaments and can be associated with spinal cord injury. Common mechanisms of injury resulting in flexion injuries include rapid acceleration/deceleration motor vehicle accidents or trauma directed to the posterior aspect of the skull from a fall or an assault.

Extension

The forces associated with extension injuries can be thought of as almost the exact opposite of those occurring with flexion. Thus, extension injuries cause compression of the posterior elements of the spine and abnormal opening of the anterior aspect of the spinal column. In particular, the head and spine are pushed backwards, or in a posterior direction, relative to the torso (Figure 23-9). This occurs with mechanisms of injury such as a rear-end motor vehicle accident or instances when abnormal forces are directed towards the face or forehead and includes falls, motor vehicle accidents, or assaults. Many of the injuries associated with an extension force are stable, with the exception being bilateral fractures of the pedicles of the second cervical vertebra. Although this pattern of injury is called a **Hangman's fracture,** there are a number of mechanisms that can cause it.

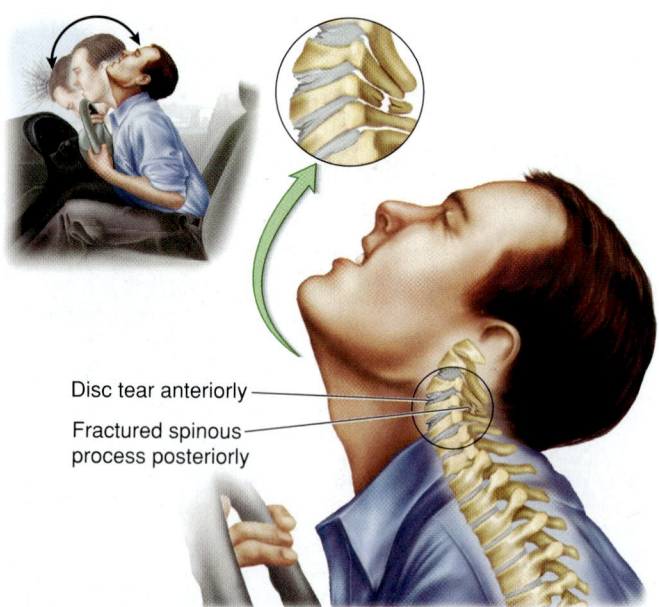

Disc tear anteriorly

Fractured spinous process posteriorly

Figure 23-9   Illustration of the extension mechanism of injury and the associated injury patterns.

Rotation

Rotation injuries occur when forces cause one side of the vertebral column to act as a fulcrum against which the opposite side turns (Figure 23-10). In many instances, rotation is a part of other mechanisms such as flexion or extension although it can also be an isolated force, causing spinal injury.

Distraction

Distraction injuries result from part of the spine maintaining a fixed position while the adjacent area of the spine is pulled in the opposite direction. The classic mechanism is a hanging injury where two vertebrae are pulled apart, resulting in injury to the spine and spinal cord. This injury is similar to the extension injury

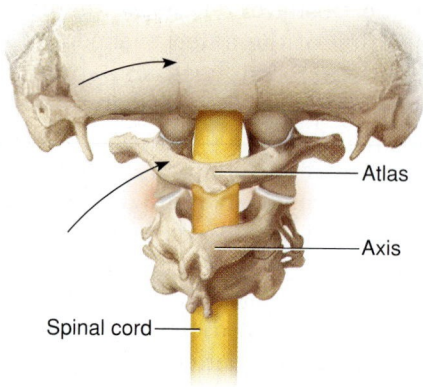

Atlas

Axis

Spinal cord

Figure 23-10   Illustration of rotation mechanism of injury and the associated injury pattern.

previously described, except in this case, one part of the spine is fixed while the other is pulled away. Distraction injuries can occur as a result of playground accidents, accidental hangings, or motor vehicle crashes. Picture this injury: A child is sticking her head between horizontal bars on a piece of playground equipment when she slips, and then dangles as her body is pulled away from her trapped head.

Other Mechanisms

Less common forms of spine trauma include direct blunt injuries, penetrating injuries, and electrical accidents.
DOT 4-6.10

Blunt Trauma

Blunt trauma can affect not only the spinal column resulting in a fracture, but it can also lead to damage of the spinal cord. This can take many forms, including acute injuries involving **hematoma** (blood collection in the tissues) within or around the cord, **transection** (a right angle, or lateral, shearing force) of the cord, or **impingement** (pinching) of the cord from bony fragments or intervertebral discs. Signs or symptoms of blunt injury to the spine, in particular those to the spinal cord, may not present acutely but may develop over time.[9] This probably results from an inflammatory response and edema formation in a specific area of cord contusion, but the mechanisms involved in this process are still being studied.

Penetrating Trauma

Penetrating trauma can be the result of gunshot, stabbing, or missile injuries. It can be due to direct trauma to the spine or distant sites of entry with involvement of the spine. In some cases, there will be complete transection of the spinal cord. In others, there will be partial involvement of the spinal cord or nerve roots. Additionally, some high-energy missiles may result in blast fragments or concussive forces, causing damage to the spinal cord.

Electrical Injuries

Electrical injuries from either a lightning strike or electrocution can cause injury to the spine. These can be due to direct injury to the spine and spinal cord from high-voltage electrical current resulting in violent contraction of the muscles of the body. Other mechanisms of injury are more difficult to pinpoint. More than likely, there is a direct injury to the spinal cord from electrical trauma, but the onset and pathogenesis are not clearly understood.[10]

CONNECTIONS Chapter 26 discusses burn trauma, including electrical injuries.

Types of Injuries

Injuries to the spine are notable on two counts. First, the scope of injuries is limited to the categories of sprains and strains, fractures, dislocations, and spinal cord injuries. Secondly, patients rarely have injuries isolated to a specific injury category, as there is significant overlap of the categories. Consequently, while there is discussion on each type of injury as a specific entity, in fact, patients can have a number of different types of spinal injuries. Therefore, multiple injuries should be considered for any given patient. DOT 4-6.7, 4-6.10

Primary versus Secondary Injuries

The discussion of traumatic brain injuries (from Chapter 20) made a key point to focus on the prevention of secondary injuries due to hypoxia or hypotension following primary injuries. What is true for the brain in this regard is also true for the spinal cord; both primary injuries and secondary injuries can occur. Primary injuries occur as the traumatic event causes compression, stretching, or laceration of the spinal cord.[11] Secondary cord injuries occur minutes, hours, days, or weeks later as the primary injury evolves. **Spinal cord ischemia** has been suggested as the principle cause of secondary injury although other mechanisms such as edema may also exist.[8,11,12] Ischemia can be caused by many things. The blood supply to the cord is not very substantial and can be disrupted easily by trauma to the spinal arteries or a clot that forms in a large regional vessel supplying the spinal arteries. General systemic hypotension and shock can cause a low blood flow state to the cord, even if the arterial system is intact.

Although EMS providers will likely not see the development of secondary spinal injury in the field, it is important to realize that the injury can continue to evolve. Gentle handling of suspected injuries is critical as is evaluation following significant mechanism of injury, even if the patient denies any signs or symptoms of injury. An incomplete lesion can evolve to become a complete injury, or the level of injury can become higher because of cord changes that occur during the secondary injury.[5] DOT 4-6.16 and 4-6.17

Sprains and Strains

Sprains and strains are terms used to describe injury to ligaments, muscles, and tendons. Often they are thought of as being interchangeable terms, but in fact, they relate to different structures. **Sprains** involve injury to supporting bone ligaments, and **strains** involve the tendons of muscles. (Remember that ligaments attach bone to bone, and tendons attach muscle to bone.) Sprains and strains occur as a result of violent contraction or excessive forcible stretch from essentially any nonpenetrating mechanism of injury. Twisting, bending, flexing, and stretching are all movements that can cause sprain or strain injuries. Another common term used by the lay public to describe sprains and strains of the cervical spine is a **whiplash** injury.

In the prehospital setting, it is not important to distinguish between sprains or strains. In part, this is because the diagnosis of a sprain or strain necessitates first excluding the possibility of a fracture. Without having access to x-ray or other sorts of imaging, this is not possible. Another reason why it is not important to differentiate between them is that the treatment for each is identical in the prehospital setting: stabilize the spine (followed by immobilization if indicated by the assessment findings), perform a standard ABCDE assessment, treat any life-threatening or high priority injuries first, assess the injury site, and transport the patient for further evaluation and treatment. Pain management may be appropriate as well.

Fractures

A fracture involves the disruption of one or more bony elements of the spine. Most commonly, they involve the upper and lower vertebrae, but any aspect of the spine can be affected.[7] In general terms, spinal fractures can either be classified as stable or unstable. From a purely clinical perspective, this distinction is nearly impossible to make, especially in an out-of-hospital setting lacking diagnostic equipment. Therefore, the definitive assessment of spinal fractures is accomplished by imaging, either using plain radiography (x-ray) or computed tomography (CT). Additionally, because it is difficult to assess these injuries, it is better to be conservative in the approach, assume an injury exists, and immobilize appropriately.

The most common type of spinal fracture is a wedge-shaped compression fracture. In isolation, they are stable fractures, but if accompanied by ligament injury from a severe flexion mechanism of injury, they can be very unstable (Figure 23-11). Another common bone injury is a spinous process fracture. It typically results from blunt trauma to the posterior aspect of the neck, and if it is the only injury, it is considered to be stable. Other injuries, such as a fracture of the ring of the first cervical vertebra (also known as a Jefferson fracture) or fractures of the other vertebrae, can often appear intact on plain film radiography but in fact, represent a very unstable fracture (Figure 23-12). It results from an axial load to the top of the skull from such mechanisms as diving into a shallow pool or pond.

> One of the most important points to remember is that not all spinal fractures result in spinal cord injury, and, similarly, not all spinal cord injuries are associated with a fracture.

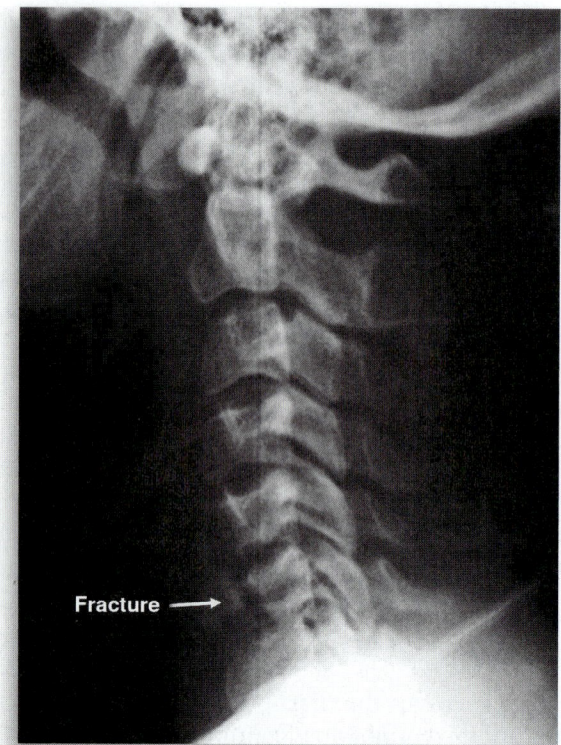

Figure 23-11 Radiograph of patient with a fracture of the vertebral body. A severe flexion mechanism caused this fracture, and it resulted in a very unstable injury.

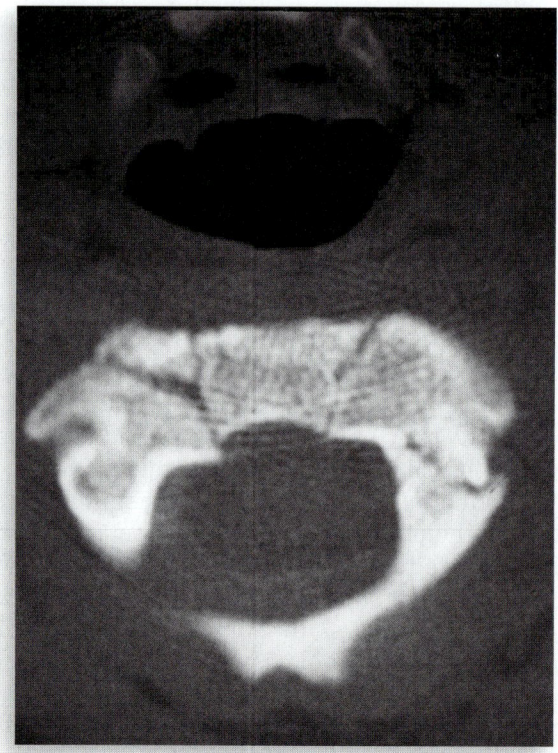

Figure 23-12 CT scan radiograph demonstrating a very unstable, comminuted (multiple pieces) fracture of the second cervical vertebra.

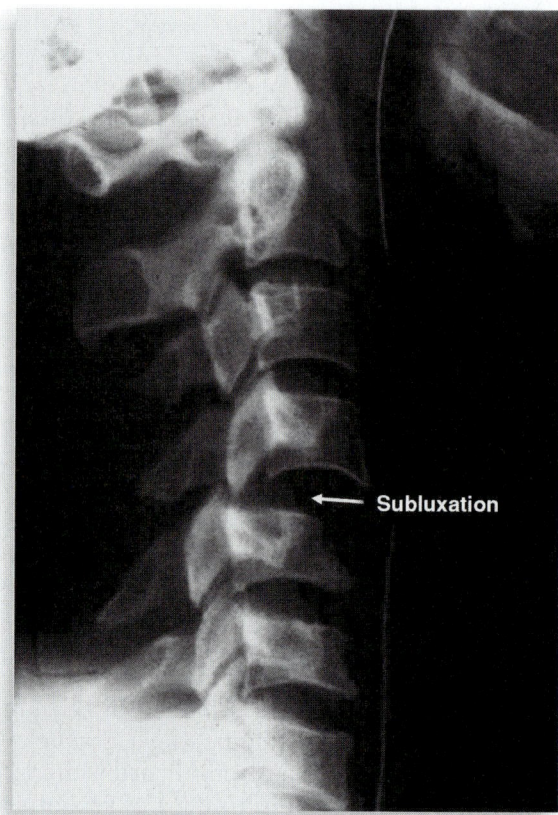

Figure 23-13 Radiograph demonstrating dislocation or subluxation of one vertebra on another. This is a very unstable injury that commonly is associated with spinal cord injury.

Therefore, all patients with suspected spine injury should be considered to have a fracture until proven otherwise by some form of imaging.

Dislocations

Trauma to the spine can also result in improper alignment or **dislocation** of one vertebra on another (Figure 23-13). This occurs when the ligaments are completely disrupted, so they no longer provide structural support for the bony vertebrae. These are very unstable injuries, and if gross misalignment of the spinal column is detected, clinically the patient will likely also have an associated spinal cord injury.

Spinal Cord Injury

Spinal cord injury can occur from a number of different mechanisms of injury and can take many different forms. For instance, complete cord disruption can occur in the patient with a severe flexion injury that causes disruption of the ligamentous structures, or partial cord damage can occur after impingement (pinching) caused by a bony fragment in a severely fractured vertebrae. The most important aspect of evaluating for spinal cord trauma is to be able to recognize the presence of any symptoms or signs that suggest the possibility of spinal cord injury. In addition, it is helpful to distinguish between complete and partial injuries and to be able to appreciate complications that occur in conjunction with these injuries. DOT 4-6.13

Complete spinal cord injuries occur when there has been transection of the cord at a specific vertebra level. A **transection** is an injury that goes all the way through the cord, in effect severing it into two pieces. As a result, the patient will have complete absence of motor and sensory function below the level of the injury. This includes loss of pain, temperature, vibratory (sensing touch or movement on the skin), and position (being aware of where a body part is in relation to the rest of the body) sensations as well as movement. The prognosis for recovery of function in a patient with a complete spinal cord injury is poor, and rarely do patients experience significant improvement in function after the extent of the injury is determined. If the injury occurs below the level of the cervical spine, the upper extremity motor and sensory functions remain intact, so the patient is **paraplegic.** While this is a devastating injury, there is typically a substantial difference in quality of life if patients have upper extremity and torso neurologic function. If the injury occurs above the fourth cervical vertebra, the patient will have no motor function of the arms and legs and is therefore **quadriplegic.** DOT 4-6.13

There are a number of issues specific to the patient with a complete spinal cord injury that are extremely important to prehospital evaluation and treatment. First, the muscles of the diaphragm are controlled by the nerves originating at the fourth cervical vertebra. If the spinal cord injury occurs at or above this level, there will be little or absent diaphragm motor function, leading to hypoventilation or apnea. Second, a complete spinal cord lesion (injury) leads to loss of sympathetic tone below the level of the lesion, which results in **neurogenic shock** (see Box 23-2). The patient presents with hypotension but also has dry, warm skin, normal capillary refill, and a paradoxical bradycardia. While neurogenic shock may be considered to be the etiology of hypotension in a patient with a complete spinal cord injury, many patients will have other injuries causing hypotension, such as blood loss. Consequently, in the field, the trauma patient with hypotension should be considered to have hemorrhagic shock and managed as such, even when the findings suggest a complete spinal cord injury. DOT 4-6.8, 4-6.9

The other end of the spectrum from complete spinal cord injuries is that some patients will have partial injuries that will only affect a certain part of the cord and only certain functions. As a group, these injuries are called partial or incomplete spinal cord injuries, and they generally fall into one of three categories: anterior, central, and Brown-Sequard. The most common

BOX 23-2 Classic Neurogenic Shock

Classic **neurogenic shock** presents as hypotension; dry, warm skin; normal capillary refill; and bradycardia. This is because the injured spinal cord cannot carry the message from the brain to the adrenal glands, signaling them to release epinephrine to counterbalance impending shock. Therefore, the typical sympathetic response of tachycardia, tachypnea, vascular constriction, and shunting, and all the other compensating mechanisms designed to preserve cardiac output and maintain blood pressure, are not seen in these patients. Suspect neurogenic shock if the patient reports any loss of sensation, function, or movement, but always rule out hemorrhagic shock first. DOT 4-6.13

mistake made by medical providers caring for these patients is to assume that because some neurologic function remains, there is no possibility that the spinal cord was actually damaged; therefore, no precautions are taken. DOT 4-6.19

Anterior Spinal Cord Injuries

Anterior spinal cord injuries can occur from direct trauma to the anterior cord or injury to the anterior spinal artery resulting in ischemia to the cord. Because motor and pain sensory neurons are located in the anterior aspect of the spinal cord, patients will present with loss of pain and motor function below the level of the injury (Figure 23-14). The posterior spinal cord function

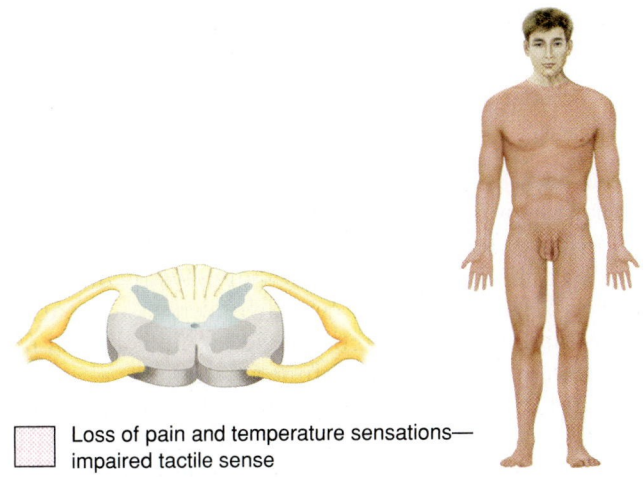

Loss of pain and temperature sensations— impaired tactile sense

Figure 23-14 Spinal cord tracts that are injured in an anterior cord syndrome.

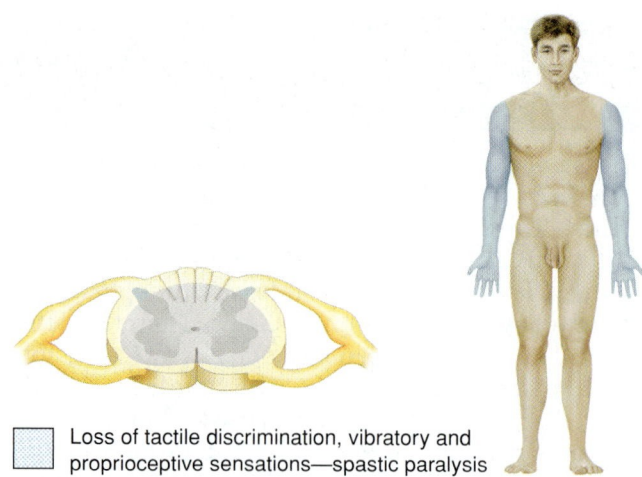

Loss of tactile discrimination, vibratory and proprioceptive sensations—spastic paralysis

Figure 23-15 Spinal cord tracts that are injured in the central cord syndrome.

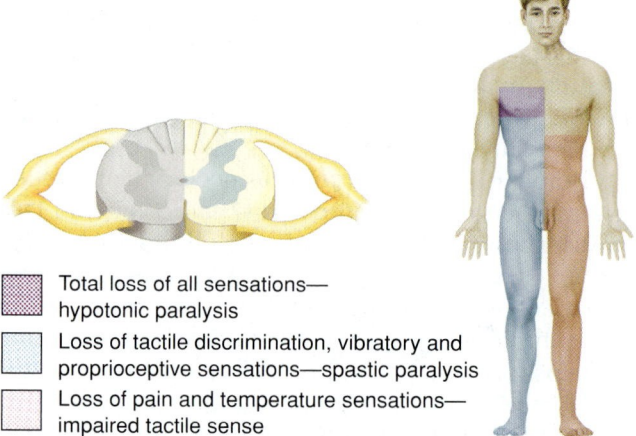

Total loss of all sensations— hypotonic paralysis

Loss of tactile discrimination, vibratory and proprioceptive sensations—spastic paralysis

Loss of pain and temperature sensations— impaired tactile sense

Figure 23-16 Schematic of an injury at the T4 level in a patient with the Brown-Sequard syndrome.

will be preserved in patients with this injury, so their position and vibratory sense will be preserved. DOT 4-6.13

Central Spinal Cord Injuries

Central spinal cord syndrome is usually seen in patients with narrowing of the spinal canal associated with conditions such as degenerative spine disease, congenital stenotic ("narrowed opening") canal, or acute trauma with bony fragments causing damage or intervertebral disc herniation (protruding out of its position). The characteristic findings of this syndrome result because the central portion of the cord is affected more than the periphery (outer aspect). Clinically, patients present with variable sensory loss but with abnormal motor findings that are more pronounced in the upper extremities than the lower extremities (Figure 23-15). The explanation for the motor findings found in central cord syndrome is that the motor fibers for the upper extremities are located more medially or centrally in the corticospinal tract than those for the lower extremities, which are more peripheral. DOT 4-6.13

Brown-Sequard Cord Injuries

The **Brown-Sequard syndrome** is a unique, partial spinal cord syndrome that involves injury to a lateral half of the cord. Classically, this occurs with penetrating injuries that result in transection of one side of the spinal cord. This syndrome can also occur as a result of blunt trauma, tumor, and disc disease. The clinical presentation is that of a motor function deficit on the side of the injury and a sensory (pain and temperature) deficit on the opposite side (Figure 23-16). The basis for these neurologic findings is that the motor fibers cross over from one side of the spinal cord to the other in the medulla whereas the sensory fibers cross over one or

two segments above the level where they exit the spinal column. DOT 4-6.13

Nice to Know

Another condition involving the spinal cord is **Spinal Cord Injury Without Radiographic Abnormality,** or a **SCIWORA.** This occurs in children who have demonstrable injury to the spinal cord by magnetic resonance imaging (MRI) but who have normal imaging of the bony structures of the vertebral column. Diagnosing this is not possible in the prehospital setting, but you may encounter this term during your interaction with other healthcare team members.

Differentiating Neurogenic Shock from Spinal Shock

Pathophysiology of Neurogenic Shock

The autonomic nervous system (ANS), which maintains the body's systems, has two divisions: sympathetic and parasympathetic. The anatomy of the ANS is complex.

CONNECTIONS Chapter 7: Anatomy Overview, Chapter 8: Physiology Overview, and Chapter 30: Neurology contain additional discussions of the nervous system.

The outflow portion of the sympathetic nervous system starts with neuron cell bodies located in the lateral gray horns of the first thoracic vertebra to the second lumbar segments or, in some cases, extending to the third lumbar segments. These cells are controlled by the hypothalamus of the brain, but they are located along the spinal cord. The sympathetic trunk is located on each side of the entire length of the vertebral column. Sympathetic fibers that innervate the heart arise primarily from the second to fourth thoracic segments.

The anatomy of the parasympathetic nervous system is very different. The majority of the parasympathetic nervous system is carried along the cranial nerves, which arise directly from the brain. They may pass near the spinal cord but do not necessarily travel as a portion of the cord. There is a small portion of the parasympathetic nervous system that involves the second to fourth sacral segments of the spinal cord, but this is along the inferior portion of the cord. The portion of the parasympathetic division that innervates the heart originates from the vagus nerve (cranial nerve X), again arising directly from the brain.

Recalling this information will help you understand why neurologic shock affects the body in the manner it does. If the cord is injured high in the cervical area, the surviving connection is from the parasympathetic nervous system, so bradycardia is more likely than tachycardia.

Spinal Shock

The American Spinal Injury Association defines a **complete neurologic lesion** as the absence of sensory and motor function below the level of injury.[13] This includes loss of function to the level of the lowest sacral segment. In contrast, a lesion is **incomplete** if sensory, motor, or both functions are partially present below the neurologic level of injury.

Spinal shock (or **areflexia**) refers to the temporary loss of spinal reflex activity that occurs below a near-total or total spinal cord injury.[14] This generally resolves within 24 to 48 hours, but it can remain for weeks, months, or years. At the point in time that spinal shock resolves, the true extent of the injury can be determined and lesions can be identified.

Below the lesion is the loss of control of autonomic function. Vasomotor tone, sweating, and **piloerection** ("goose bumps") in the lower parts of the body are temporarily abolished. Systemic hypotension may be severe and contribute to spinal cord damage. The lower extremities lose heat if left uncovered, and they swell if they are placed in a dependent position. The skin becomes dry and pale, and ulcerations may develop in time over bony prominences in response to pressure. The sphincters of the bladder and the rectum remain contracted to some degree, and there is passive distention of the bowel, retention of feces, and absence of peristalsis, so bowel sounds will be silent. The signs of spinal shock are listed in Box 23-3.[15]

BOX 23-3   Signs of Spinal Shock

- Elevated blood pressure (early sign)
- Pounding headache
- Bradycardia (may be a relative slowing so that the heart rate is still within the normal range)
- Profuse sweating above the level of the lesion, especially in the face, neck, and shoulders, or possibly below the level of the lesion
- Piloerection or goose bumps above or possibly below the level of the lesion
- Cardiac dysrhythmias, atrial fibrillation, premature ventricular contractions, and atrioventricular conduction abnormalities
- Flushing of the skin above the level of the lesion, especially in the face, neck, and shoulders, or possibly below the level of lesion
- Blurred vision
- Appearance of spots in the patient's visual fields
- Nasal congestion
- Feelings of apprehension or anxiety over an impending physical problem
- Minimal or no symptoms, despite a significantly elevated blood pressure (silent autonomic dysreflexia)

Neurogenic Shock

Neurogenic shock, by contrast, is not due to a loss of spinal reflex activity but is due to disruption of sympathetic outflow that leaves unopposed vagal tone. If you recall from the pathophysiology description at the beginning of this section, the sympathetic nervous system fibers are closely associated with the cord, and the parasympathetic fibers are not. When the sympathetic division is disrupted, the parasympathetic division remains intact and operates without the normal balance found between the two. For this reason, neurogenic shock is characterized by hypotension, warm, dry skin, and bradycardia. The presence of bradycardia is not universal. The loss of the vasoconstrictor impulses results in increased vascular capacitance (the container dilates), decreased venous return, and decreased cardiac output.[16] Because sympathetic tone is lost, the body cannot redirect blood from the periphery to the core, there is an excess loss of heat from the skin, and hypothermia can develop.[17]

The symptoms of neurogenic shock typically last from one to three weeks.

The anatomic level of the injury to the spinal cord influences the likelihood of both the development and severity of neurogenic shock. Any injury above T1 is capable of disrupting the spinal tracks that control the sympathetic nervous system. Any injury between T1 and L3 has the potential to disrupt sympathetic outflow. The higher the level of injury in this zone, the more likely or severe neurogenic shock will be. Incomplete cord injury can also cause neurogenic shock.

In a study of patients with blunt cervical spine and cord injury, neurogenic shock alone was believed to be responsible for 69% of the cases of shock. In another study of penetrating spinal injury (at various anatomic levels), neurogenic shock was responsible for only 22% of all cases of shock.[18] For both studies, hypovolemia was the next most common cause of shock in blunt trauma and the primary cause in penetrating trauma.

> Neurogenic shock should not be presumed to be the cause of shock until all other possible sources of shock—particularly hemorrhage—have been ruled out.[19]

Evaluation and Assessment

In the overall evaluation and assessment of trauma patients, attention directed toward the spine (beyond simple stabilization) follows other primary survey priorities. After the scene size-up, evaluating and managing threats to the ABCs is the next priority. Only after these aspects of care have been completed should the evaluation of the spine and other secondary aspects of the exam commence. DOT 4-6.14, 4-6.15, 4-6.18

When a spinal injury is suspected (often based upon mechanism), you or another team member should place your gloved hands on each side of the head to start the stabilization process. This should be maintained until such time that immobilization of the head via an appropriately sized cervical collar and immobilization device is provided or the possibility of cervical injury is ruled out and cervical stabilization is discontinued.

Evaluating the Need for Spinal Immobilization

There are two main goals for the assessment and evaluation of the spine. The first is to identify patients at risk for spinal injury, and the second is to determine the current extent of injury. Historically, much of what has become standard practice in prehospital care with respect to identifying patients at risk for spinal injuries is based on intuition and individual preference rather than evidenced-based medicine. As a result, the vast majority of trauma patients are placed in cervical spine precautions in the field only to then have to undergo radiological imaging in the emergency department.

TABLE 23-1 Criteria for Clearing Cervical Injuries in the Emergency Department

According to NEXUS low-risk criteria, cervical spine radiography can be omitted for trauma patients only if they exhibit *all* of the following criteria:
No posterior midline cervical spine tenderness
No evidence of intoxication
Normal level of alertness
No focal neurologic deficit
No painful distracting injuries

Source: J. L. Larson, *Tintinalli's Emergency Medicine,* "Chapter 272: Injuries to the Spine." McGraw-Hill's AccessMedicine (accessed June 7, 2006). From "Emergency Medicine," by J. Tintinalli et al. Copyright © The McGraw-Hill Companies, Inc. Reprinted with permission.

The previously subjective nature of evaluating for spinal injuries has now been challenged by a number of studies that offer another approach. For instance, two recently published, very large studies assessed whether or not predetermined indicators could predict the necessity of radiographs in patients presenting to the emergency department with suspected spinal injury.[20,21] The result of the studies (Table 23-1) is a critical-thinking decision process consisting of several criteria, which use both historical and physical exam findings to identify patients who are and are not at risk for spinal injury. The ramifications of using decision rules such as these are potentially great as it has been estimated that they can decrease the ordering of x-rays by up to 50%.[22] Equally impressive results have been reported when explicit decision rules for the assessment of spinal injury have been adopted in the community emergency medicine setting.

Similar decision rules have been investigated for use in the out-of-hospital setting.[23,24,25,26,27] With the caveat of concerns for evaluating patients at the extremes of age, these studies suggest that if decision rules are rigorously followed in the prehospital setting, selective immobilization is possible.

Working in the Gray Zone

Before implementing a personal practice of selectively immobilizing spinal injuries in the field, consult with your medical director. Actions such as this must be protocol-driven. Although some strong scientific studies appear to indicate this is a viable skill, there is still a huge issue of liability and challenging convention. Review the literature and talk with your medical director. Find systems that selectively immobilize c-spines in the field, and ask if they will share their protocol.

BOX 23-4   Signs and Symptoms of Spinal Cord Injury

- Anesthesia below the level of the lesion.
- Altered sensations and motor function involving a single area of the body or a single or both limbs (upper or lower) or limited to one side of the body or the other.
- Deformity, edema, ecchymosis, muscle spasm, or tenderness at the injury site on the spine.
- Neck muscle pain and tenderness, hoarseness, or dysphagia if the cervical spine is involved.
- Diaphragm paralysis may occur in high cervical injuries that results in dyspnea and hypoventilation. If the injury is higher, apnea can result.
- Priapism or decreased or absent rectal sphincter tone.
- Muscle tone may be normal, increased, or decreased, and tremors may be present. Grip strength may be diminished.
- Alterations in sensation include feelings of hot, cold, numbness, tingling, pain, or no sensation at all.

Evaluating for Spinal Injury

The first component of the evaluation of patients with the potential for cervical spine injury is determining who should be considered for evaluation. Those who should be considered for evaluation are any patients with trauma above the clavicles or who have a history of being subjected to a high-energy mechanism of injury.

One of the reasons pinpointing an injury of the nervous system is difficult is that each patient presentation is unique. There are common signs and symptoms found with spinal cord injuries and nervous system damage, and these are summarized in Box 23-4. DOT 4-6.6

Consider spinal precautions in any patient who has a history of being subjected to high-energy transfer, trauma above the clavicles, and

1. Midline c-spine tenderness or deformity
2. Any neurological abnormality or deficit
3. Any patient where history or physical exam is unreliable
4. Extremes of age

The patient should be evaluated for deformity or tenderness. Any deformity or tenderness would indicate the need for continued spinal stabilization followed by immobilization and a neurological exam. Most studies have evaluated for tenderness of the spine by palpating over the midline. However, many spine injuries may not necessarily produce midline tenderness but rather result in paraspinous muscle spasm, causing pain and tenderness more laterally. Therefore, serious consideration for a spinal column injury should also be given to any patient who complains of lateral neck pain or tenderness.

It is important to consider if there are any distracting injuries that might divert the patient's attention from a spinal injury. An example would be a patient with a painful angulated fracture of the lower arm, focusing his attention on that injury and not recognizing that his neck also hurts. In addition to distracting injuries, look to see if the patient's mental status is unimpaired. If the patient has drugs or alcohol in his system, has a significant head injury, or has hypoxia from an injury, he may not be able to feel pain or use good judgment when interacting with you.

Gross neurological deficits are usually clearly evident in the conscious patient by simple clinical observation or by conducting a cursory physical exam that tests for movement and sensation. A positive finding is an ominous sign for potential spinal injury and should prompt an in-depth neurologic assessment, which focuses on motor and sensory function and reflexes. Any alteration in mental status will make it more difficult to detect neurologic deficits related to a spinal cord injury.

Motor Examination

Motor abnormalities can best be appreciated by remembering that nerve roots controlling movement are localized to specific vertebral levels (refer back to Figure 23-5). For instance, the spinal injured patient who presents with apnea can be presumed to have a cord injury above the level of C4, which is the level that controls diaphragm function. An injury to the C5 level of the spinal cord would result in the inability to shrug the shoulders. Elbow flexion and extension are lost due to injuries at the C6 and C7 levels, respectively. Injuries or lesions at C8 or T1 cause loss of finger flexion. From T2 through T12, intercostal and abdominal muscles are affected.

In the lower half of the body, spinal cord injuries at L1 to L2 will affect the patient's ability to flex at the hip. Adduction (movement towards the body center, or midline) and abduction (movement away from the midline) of the hip are controlled at L3 and L4, correspondingly. The patient's ability to dorsiflex (lifting the toes upward and flexing the ankle) the foot is hampered with an injury or a lesion at L5, while plantar flexion (bending the foot downward extending the ankle) is affected at S1 and S2 vertebral levels. Lastly, rectal sphincter tone is lost with injury at the S2 to S3 level, so the patient may be incontinent and may defecate involuntarily.

Sensory Examination

The sensory exam provides other meaningful clues to possible spinal cord injury as well as to its extent. When an area of diminished sensation is located, two separate tests should be conducted. Since the patient is more sensitive to the onset (start) of a stimulus rather than its terminus (when it stops), testing should begin in the area with decreased feeling and move upward. First, a soft stimulus, such as the corner of a gauze pad, should be stroked lightly across the skin to delineate the area without sensation. The same test should be performed again using a more noxious stimulus, such as a pen, to test pain receptors. Be careful not to scratch or cut the patient. This pairing of strong and weak sensation ensures that both the anterior and posterior spinal tracts are evaluated. Establishing and physically identifying a **line of demarcation** between areas of positive and negative findings is vital when trending the progression of a sensory deficit. Since a progressive worsening of symptoms will track upwards from baseline, any clinician treating the patient can recognize deterioration in the patient's presentation.

Reflexes

Finally, although not commonly performed in the field, provoking a deep tendon reflex might also lend some objective information to the physical exam since loss of movement or sensation is generally considered to be an effort-dependent or subjective finding. Loss of bicep reflex indicates a lesion at the level of C6, tricep reflex is lost at C7, patellar reflex is lost at L4, and achilles reflex is lost at S1.

Subtleties in the physical exam are many times more difficult to appreciate in the field setting, but patients with suspected spinal injury should be evaluated as early as feasibly possible to provide a baseline assessment. Examination and subsequent documentation of motor, sensory, and reflex findings have the potential to provide significant diagnostic information that can lead to early and appropriate treatment of a patient with a spinal injury. Also, a complete exam documents neurologic findings before, during, and after immobilization.

Penetrating Trauma

Patients presenting with mechanisms of injury that involve a missile or other penetrating object present a unique situation. In part, this is because the trauma is rarely isolated to one area, such as the spine. A gunshot wound that traverses the neck or a stab wound to the back puts many structures at jeopardy. Consequently, rarely is the spinal column or cord the sole structure injured or at risk. In fact, in many instances, treatment of the other sustained injuries (for example the trachea or neck vessels) is hindered if the patient is immobilized. A number of studies have looked at this select population, and guidelines have been developed that call for immobilization only if the patient with penetrating neck or back trauma has neurologic symptoms.[28,29] Otherwise, in the awake and oriented patient with penetrating spine trauma and normal spinal cord function, immobilization has not been shown to be necessary, and, as discussed, it may hinder treatment efforts.

Spinal or Neurogenic Shock

The evaluation of patients who present in shock is difficult, regardless of whether the presentation occurs in the prehospital or in-hospital setting. Spinal and neurogenic shock are no different in this regard. Patients with hypotension should be suspected of having hemorrhagic shock until proven otherwise, even with a suspected complete spinal cord injury.

Confounding Situations

As described briefly before, if the physical exam or history is unreliable, the patient should have spinal stabilization and immobilization. A patient can be considered to be unreliable for a number of reasons. For instance, if someone is under the influence of an intoxicant, particularly alcohol, they cannot be assessed reliably. Significant injury, particularly long-bone fractures, may be sufficiently distracting as to render a physical exam unreliable.[30] In patients where a language barrier exists, questions about subtle neurologic symptoms may not be understood. Altered mental status, particularly secondary to head injury, may also prevent a reliable history or exam. An intubated trauma patient should be assumed to have a spinal injury until proven otherwise. Finally, patients emotionally traumatized or otherwise unstable secondary to the incident or other factors may not be reliable enough to fully cooperate with an evaluation of the spine. DOT 4-6.9

Patients at the extremes of age present a unique assessment problem for care providers evaluating for a spine injury (Figure 23-17). The pediatric patient can be very difficult to evaluate because, developmentally, a child may not be able to communicate symptoms. As well, an anxious or crying child may not cooperate with the physical examination.

An elderly patient with suspected spine trauma can also present challenges. Changes in bone density put an older patient at greater risk for injury to the spine, therefore lower energy mechanisms should prompt concern for a fracture in the geriatric patient.[31] Alterations in an older patient's mental status may also put the care provider at

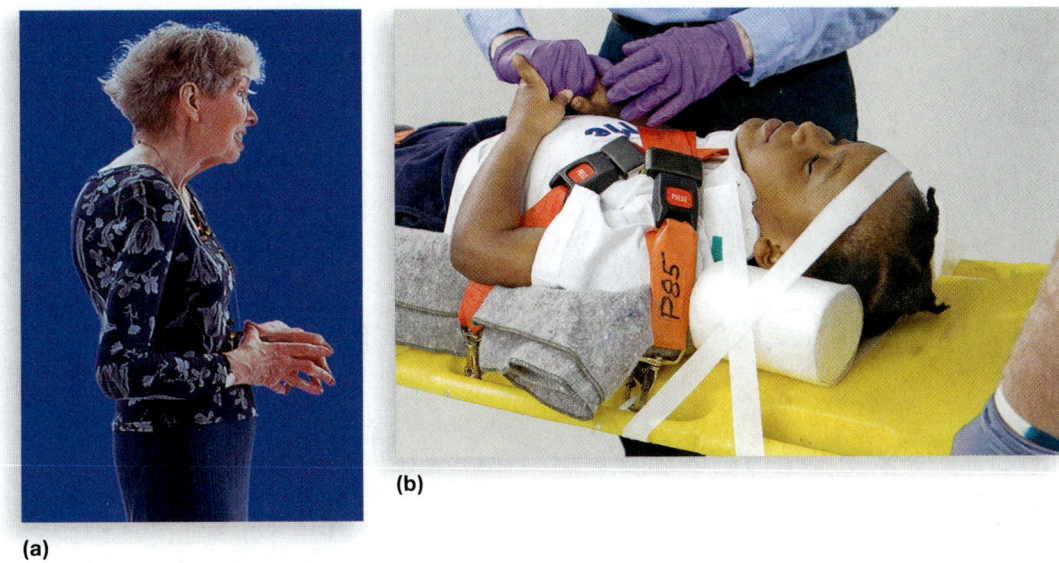

Figure 23-17   Spinal immobilization should be done with consideration for the patient's anatomy. (a) Elderly patients with pronounced kyphosis will need to have padding to support them in a comfortable position. (b) Pediatric patients with head larger in proportion to the body will need to have the shoulders padded.

a disadvantage, but when the patient is alert, oriented, and cooperative, physical exam and historical screening criteria are still reliable in the geriatric patient.[32]

Treatment of Spinal Injuries

Stabilization

The fundamental treatment for actual, or suspected, spinal injury is stabilization, followed by immobilization. In the prehospital setting, immobilization is useful in a number of important circumstances. Specifically, it may prevent a stable injury from becoming unstable. Also, it may prevent neurologic injury in the patient with an unstable injury but who presents neurologically intact. Lastly, there are reports of patients with unstable injuries and neurologic injury whose symptoms resolved with in-line stabilization.[33] The various stabilization and immobilization techniques are described here. **Applicable stabilization and immobilization techniques are outlined in the following Skill Sheets: Skill Sheet 68: Seated Spinal Immobilization (also see Step-by-Step 68); Skill Sheet 69: Standing Spinal Immobilization; 70: Supine Spinal Immobilization (also see Step-by-Step 70); Skill Sheet 72: Rapid Extrication; Skill Sheet 92: NREMT Spinal Immobilization (Seated Patient); and Skill Sheet 93: NREMT Spinal Immobilization (Supine Patient).** DOT 4-6.11, 4-6.12

Manual Stabilization

The cooperative patient without gross neurological impairment or diminished level of consciousness can effectively stabilize his or her own cervical spine simply by not moving. If resources are limited and the coopera-

tive patient is not being manipulated (see Box 23-5), these patients can be instructed not to move about.

Manual stabilization of the cervical spine is best performed by lightly grasping the frontal and occipital regions of the skull. This position allows for a cervical

BOX 23-5   Which Is First: Move into Neutral Alignment or Stabilize the Spine?

Whenever possible, perform a quick assessment (by inspection and palpation) of the head and neck in the position found, prior to movement of the head and neck into the neutral alignment. If ABCDE compromise is suspected or unknown, a thorough assessment for neurologic signs may not be possible prior to moving the patient into position to correct problems identified during the ABCDE assessment. Remember, completing the primary survey has priority! Whenever possible, use one rescuer to try to stabilize the head and neck before another (or several) rescuers move the patient into a neutral alignment or supine position for assessment. If significant resistance is met, pain increases with movement, or the patient complains of new or increasing neurologic symptoms, it may be appropriate to stabilize the patient in a position other than neutral. Alert the receiving facility to this situation, and remember to document this in the patient care report.

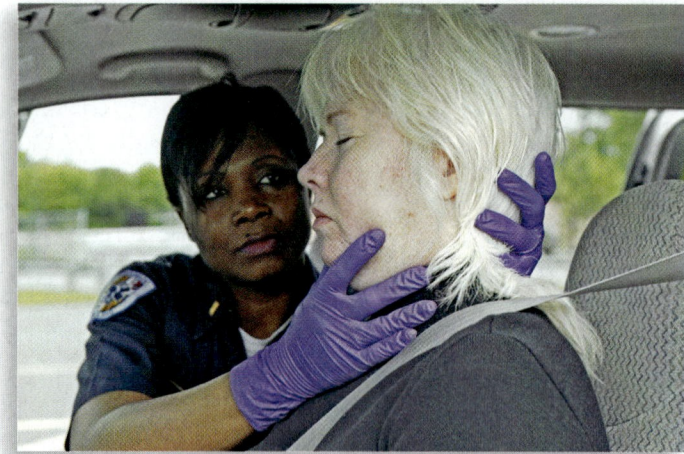

Figure 23-18   Manual in-line stabilization performed while the care provider is at the side of the patient.

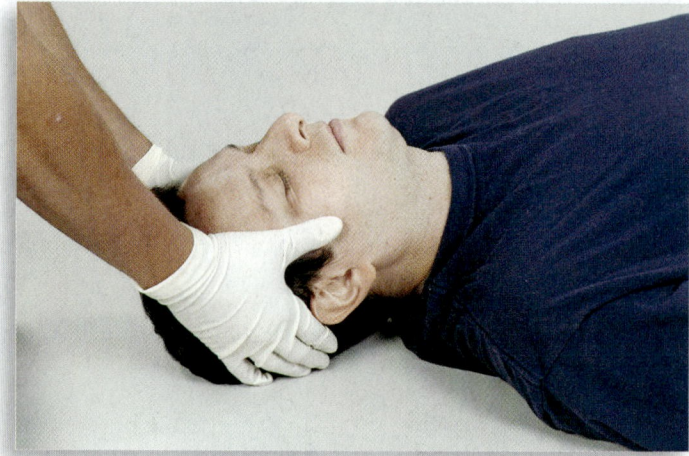

Figure 23-19   Manual in-line stabilization performed on a supine patient.

collar to be placed while the manual stabilization is maintained. While this can be done from any position, keep in mind that the goal is to keep or return the head in a neutral position. Communicate frequently with your patient during the procedure. Manual stabilization should be maintained until a more definitive form of stabilization is in place. It is only a temporary measure.

While manual stabilization with neutral repositioning is appropriate for the initial care of most patients with the potential for spine injury, there are certain cases where it is contraindicated. In particular, patients who experience severe pain, have resistance to movement, or develop or have an increase in neurologic symptoms should not undergo repositioning. Also, if there is severe misalignment of the head or if airway compromise develops, repositioning may need to be deferred.

There are two common approaches to manual stabilization and neutral repositioning in the patient who is sitting or standing. The first is with the care provider facing the patient, and an alternative is to approach the patient from the side (Figure 23-18). The patient who is supine requires an alternative approach to manual stabilization and neutral repositioning since the care provider is usually situated at the top of the patient's head (Figure 23-19).

Stabilization with the Log Roll Technique

The most commonly used method for moving a patient onto and off of a long spine board or from a prone to supine position is the log roll. Although it has come under scrutiny for allowing lateral movement of the lumbar spine, when properly executed, the patient's spine will be kept in a neutral position while the rest of their body is moved as a single unit.[34]

Once the decision has been made to log-roll the patient, adequate personnel should be assembled. In most instances, this procedure requires four care pro-

viders. Larger or uncooperative patients may require even more resources. Before any move is executed, a plan should be formulated as to which direction to roll the patient, and this should be communicated to the team performing the move. Factors that may affect the move include unstable or unsafe scenes, weather, terrain, placement of immoveable objects, or injuries involving one side of the patient. The care provider at the patient's head has the best field-of-view and should control the steps of the procedure. There is not a lot of literature regarding which movement is superior for positioning the patient on the board—lateral or vertical movement to align the patient. The team should ensure there is no compromise to alignment of the spine when the patient is moved.

Street Secrets

Evaluating and treating a patient who is in the prone position is exceedingly difficult. Consequently, if a trauma patient is found facedown and unresponsive, there should be no delay to prepare for a log roll maneuver: the patient should be moved as a unit as carefully as possible to a supine position so that life-threatening conditions can be addressed. Time and steps can be saved if a long board can be placed next to the patient, with the back quickly assessed prior to rolling the patient, so that the patient is log-rolled onto the adjacent board.

Cervical Collar Application

There are a tremendous number of commercial cervical collars available, yet there seems to be little that distinguishes one from another.[35] More than anything else, it is important to be familiar with the device you will be using in your practice.

Selecting the right size of collar for a particular patient is important as there is not one collar that is designed to fit every size and shape neck. Most popular brands not only target the pediatric or adult patient but also have small, medium, and large size collars of each type. Also, many are adjustable to allow additional attempts to attain a proper fit. Keep in mind that some smaller stature, adult patients may be fitted better using a "pediatric" collar. A correctly placed cervical collar should limit motion while not interfering with the patient's airway or circulation. While the device should fit snugly against the mandible, it should not inhibit the patient from talking or opening their mouth. Also remember that once the collar is applied, it should be reassessed to determine that it is properly sized and fitted. Despite the variability encountered in choosing a brand and size of collar for an individual patient, the method for application is consistent.

Short Spine Boards

Short spine boards are primarily used to immobilize the neck and back of patients who are sitting upright or are in a confined space. A simple short board can be used in combination with a cervical collar and tape to provide intermediate immobilization although there are many commercial devices that include all the necessary equipment. In studies comparing various devices, short boards provide increased stability compared to a collar alone, but there does not appear to be one that is clearly superior to the others.[36,37]

Long Spine Boards

Long spine boards are one of the most commonly employed pieces of equipment in the prehospital setting. While they can be used in the non-immobilized patient as a lifting and moving device, more often they are used in conjunction with a cervical collar to provide definitive immobilization for transport. There are many different types of rigid backboards available with none clearly better than the others. Commercial cervical immobilization devices are available that may be pre-attached to the long board. Regardless of which long backboard is being used, the technique is similar for its application.

When used properly, long, rigid spine boards have been shown to provide a significant degree of immobility for the spine, but there are also complications that can result from their use. Specifically, they can be uncomfortable, can lead to the development of pressure sores, and can restrict ventilatory capacity.[38] Most of these adverse effects can be averted by repositioning, adding padding, being attentive to the tightness of the stabilization straps, and removing the patient from the board as soon as is clinically indicated.[39,40]

Street Secrets

Always secure the body first, followed by the head. This is important in the event that the patient requires log-rolling. Experience teaches paramedics to have suction equipment ready at all times, but occasionally this lesson is forgotten. If the patient begins vomiting while you are immobilizing and suction is not handy, you need to quickly log-roll the patient to sweep the mouth and allow drainage. If you have secured the head but not the body, you will lose neutral alignment as the patient's body slides when you perform the log roll.

Nice to Know

A common practice in early paramedic education was to use sandbags to immobilize the head and neck. Since there were no other devices available and much of EMS was partnered with the fire service, sandbags were readily available even though they weighed a lot and were often too big or very dirty. Now that properly sized lightweight commercial products are available, many with hook and loop (Velcro™), tacky, or sticky attachments, use of items such as sandbags or liter-size IV bags is not a good idea.

Special Circumstances

Immobilization in Water

Management of the trauma patient who is in water may be very difficult and is potentially dangerous to the provider. Only those care providers specially trained in water rescue techniques should ever enter the water. Those who work in or around the water routinely practice these techniques on simulated patients who are partially or completely submerged. Special equipment is required as many standard items found on the ambulance do not float. A backboard with enough positive buoyancy to float with a patient loaded to it is ideal—especially when working in deep or moving water.

As with other extrications, getting to the patient and managing the airway is the first priority. Attempt to keep the patient's head in a neutral position. A throwable flotation device, such as a ring buoy, can be put under the patient's shoulders and aid the rescuer in keeping the patient in proper position and slightly above the surface of the water. A cervical collar should be applied whenever possible. With a calm or unconscious patient found in deeper water, the floating position may be maintained while the patient is guided to the edge of a pool, to a boat, or to a shallow area where the rescuer can stand. If the patient is pulled forward by both feet (with a rescuer holding the head and neck stabilized in the rear) the patient will tend to remain in a more neutral spinal alignment.

A backboard, even one with significant positive buoyancy, can be pushed below the surface of the water and floated under the patient. The board should then be allowed to surface under the patient in a position that has the patient centered on it. A word of caution—backboards that are not specifically designed for maritime use may float until a patient is affixed to them and then promptly sink or roll to one side or another. Be prepared with enough help and resources to take care of the patient properly. Once removed from the water, the patient can be secured and transported properly.

Pediatric Patients

Pediatric patients offer numerous challenges, not only in their assessment but also in their treatment. One key factor is the anatomical difference in children compared to adults, particularly those differences noted in infants or very young toddlers.[41] Proportionately, they have a much larger occiput (head) than adults. Because of this, when placed on a backboard without any padding, their head tends to flex forward with their chin moving towards their chest. In addition to moving out of a neutral alignment, this position may lead to airway occlusion. Children are more flexible and have greater mobility of the spine because of their level of development. They have less rigid ligaments, shallow (smaller, less defined) angulations of facet joints, immature development of neck muscles, and incomplete ossification of the vertebrae leading to "softer" bones.[41] The end result is that, while the incidence of spinal trauma is lower in pediatric patients than adults, the injuries they sustain are much more severe and more commonly involve the cervical spine.[42]

While pediatric collars are available, an ill-fitting collar is less preferable to using towel rolls, trauma pads, or other items on hand to prevent movement of the head. Once that has been accomplished, securing the patient for transport may require more ingenuity or utilization of a commercial device specifically designed for pediatric patients. Make sure the child is kept warm, and provide padding from the edge of the child to the edge of the immobilization device so the child does not slip under the straps.

Helmet Removal

The helmeted patient provides the prehospital provider with a dilemma—to remove or not to remove the helmet. Partial helmets that cover the top of the head and attach by chin straps, such as those used for biking, rollerblading, or other non-motorized sports are easily removed. Helmets fully enclosing the patient's head, such as those

for riding a motorcycle, skiing, or sports such as football, are much more difficult to manage.

If the helmet interferes with assessment or treatment of the patient in any way, particularly in airway management, it should be removed. At a minimum, stable patients should have their chin straps and facemasks removed, providing the correct equipment to do so is available. The helmet itself can be kept on until radiographs have been obtained.[43] The only other instances where the helmet should be removed in the prehospital setting are when the helmet is so loose that adequate spinal immobilization cannot be obtained with the helmet in place or if the helmet prevents immobilization for transport.[43,44]

Placement of a cervical collar is frequently difficult in the helmeted patient, but using tape, straps, and bulky dressings has been shown to provide adequate immobilization.[45]

Presence of Neurologic Findings

When neurological deficits are present, a number of factors should be considered. Symptoms can progress, and the clinician must be vigilant in reassessing the patient. Additionally, patients with spinal cord injury may not be able to sense pain; therefore, they may not be able to appreciate when extrication or treatment is worsening their symptoms.

CONNECTIONS See Chapter 20: Head, Face, and Neck Trauma for more information on neurologic complications.

Obvious Spine Deformity

There are some cases where circumstances may prevent moving the patient's head into a neutral position or may require treatment without a cervical collar. In these instances, using towel or blanket rolls in an attempt to prevent further manipulation of the head or spine may be necessary. If the treatment exacerbates (worsens) neurological findings, resistance is noted with attempts to move the head, or the patient reports increased pain, the procedure should be halted and the course reevaluated. When completing the patient care report, be sure to fully explain the reasons why the procedure was modified.

Thick, Short Neck

Some patients may not fit into a cervical collar. Obese, short necked, or thick necked individuals may not fit into a commercial cervical collar or immobilization device. In such cases, malpositioned or ill-fitting cervical collars can occlude the airway or prevent the patient from ventilating properly. If no cervical collar can properly fit the patient, tape and towel rolls, a blanket, or an alternative item may be used in its place.

Intubation Approach

Orally intubating the suspected spinal trauma patient can be difficult for a variety of reasons. A cervical collar may inhibit the patient's mouth from opening completely, thus obscuring landmarks from view. By opening the collar and having an assistant hold manual, in-line stabilization, the jaw will be able to fully extend to facilitate a better view. It is important to realize that manipulation of the head can cause unwanted movement, and care should be taken not to move the spine. Another provider can perform the Sellick maneuver (also called cricoid pressure) to help move the glottis into view. In certain cases where the oropharynx cannot be accessed, blind nasotracheal intubation may be a better option.

Impaled Objects

Impaled objects may present substantial difficulty in treating patients suspected of having spine injuries. Unless the impaled object occludes the airway or prevents CPR, it should not be removed, but in most instances of isolated penetrating trauma, cervical immobilization is not necessary.[28,29] If spinal injury is suspected and the object protrudes from the posterior aspect of the patient, spinal immobilization and keeping the patient's head in a neutral position can be accomplished by placing the patient in a lateral recumbent position. This position can be supported with pillows and blankets. An alternative solution may entail cutting a long object before attempting immobilization.

Pharmacologic Therapy

Spinal Cord Injury

While methylprednisolone (Solu-Medrol) is thought to have some benefit in reducing inflammation in spinal cord injuries (and therefore to provide some long term benefit in functional outcome), its use in the prehospital setting is controversial, and, unless specifically directed by local protocol, it should not be considered. An extenuating circumstance would be systems that regularly face long transport times, as the benefit of steroids in spinal cord injuries is found if they are initiated within eight hours postinjury.[46] A more beneficial pharmacological intervention should include pain management or sedation of the uncomfortable or combative patient.

DOT 4-6.11, 4-6.12

Neurogenic shock may require excessive volumes of fluid to restore normal hemodynamics. Boluses of 20 mL/kg are standard for fluid resuscitation in the prehospital setting, but in the case of a 90-kg (198-lb) patient, the initial bolus is nearly two liters of fluid, and this may not be enough. Seek medical direction early in the process of providing fluid resuscitation if you believe large volumes will be required. Maintain the systolic blood pressure at 90–100 mmHg (or 85–90 mean arterial pressure). Dopamine can be added if the patient is not responding to fluid boluses.[16]

Nice to Know

Once hemorrhage has been ruled out *hospital treatment* may include the use of potent vasoconstrictor medications such as dopamine, phenylephrine, or norepinephrine to augment vascular resistance. Medical practice guidelines indicate that the use of vasoconstrictors is typically of short duration, lasting between 24 and 48 hours.[16] These patients are also closely monitored in the hospital for the development of cardiac dysrhythmias and hypotension that can occur up to 14 days after the injury.

Spinal or Neurogenic Shock

Hypotension in the prehospital setting should rarely, if ever, be attributed to neurogenic shock. Box 23-6 describes the treatment for neurogenic shock. Other causes of shock, such as ongoing blood loss, cardiac tamponade, or a tension pneumothorax, should be the focus of therapy. Also, the hypotension related to spinal shock usually responds to fluid boluses or Trendelenburg positioning, so the presence of persistent hypotension after these maneuvers in the patient with a

BOX 23-6 Treatment for Neurogenic Shock

1. Perform the scene size-up and ABCDE primary assessment and assign a transport priority.
   a. Provide neutral alignment and cervical spine stabilization for the primary survey and then immobilization sometime after the primary survey is complete.
   b. Assess "D" and "E" because of the potential neurologic compromise.
2. Give fluid resuscitation with isotonic crystalloids. Maintain mean arterial pressure at 85–90 mmHg.
3. Carefully search for and treat (if possible) causes of hypotension and blood loss.
4. Transport patient to trauma center (or spinal center if available).

Adapted from *Tintinalli's Emergency Medicine*, Table 35-1 Treatment of Neurogenic Shock (McGraw-Hill; AssessMedicine,) (accessed June 8, 2006).

complete spinal cord injury should prompt the search for an alternative source of the low blood pressure.

Transport

The immobilized patient should be properly secured to the stretcher or cot to prevent sliding or movement during transport. Take care to communicate with your patient about the transport. Fear of the injury, adrenalin rushing through the blood stream, and facing a moving ceiling while riding backwards may be disconcerting, and nausea may develop. Suction equipment should be readily available.

The transport of the spinal injured patient is urgent, but it may not be emergent, meaning the injured spine requires prompt attention, but it is typically not a life-and-death situation. Transportation of these patients should be prompt but performed gently with a minimum of additional movement applied to the spine. If the patient is not immobilized correctly, additional injury may result. DOT 4-6.8, 4-6.27, 4-6.28

Documentation of Care

In addition to the standard elements for every patient care report, the spinal injured patient's report should contain the following additional information: DOT 4-6.36, 4-6.37, 4-6.38

- The position the patient was found in, a description of the scene, and any pertinent information describing the what, where, when, and how of the environment and incident. Include a photo of the mechanism if possible.
- What you assessed during your physical exam and the results of your assessment. Make sure you identify the condition of the patient before and after stabilization and if there were any changes as a result.
- Provide a time line of events. This is particularly important if there is a change in sensation or motor response or a change in the location of any deficits.
- Substantiate any reasons causing a deviation from your standard protocols. If neutral alignment was not possible because of excessive pain, another injury that complicated movement, or any inability to reposition the patient, note the reasons in the report.

Summary

Suspected and actual spine trauma is a common prehospital presentation whose care requires an in-depth knowledge of the common mechanisms of injury, musculoskeletal and nervous system anatomy, and pathophysiology. Neurogenic and spinal shock can

occur in the prehospital setting, but more common reasons for shock (for example, hypovolemia from uncontrolled hemorrhage) typically exist before neurogenic shock should be considered the cause.

The prehospital care provider can use established methods of care that include a number of techniques for immobilization. A properly immobilized patient will not only be less likely to experience injury from untoward movement but will also have their chances of worsening an existing injury minimized.

Notes

1. R. M. Domeier, R. W. Evans, R. A. Swor, E. J. Rivera-Rivera, and S. M. Frederiksen. "Prospective Validation of Out-of-Hospital Spinal Clearance Criteria: A Preliminary Report," *Academic Emergency Medicine* 4(1997):643–646.
2. A. B. Jackson, M. Dijkers, M. J. Devivo, and R. B. Poczatek. "A Demographic Profile of New Traumatic Spinal Cord Injuries: Change and Stability Over 30 Years," *Archives of Physical Medicine and Rehabilitation* 85(2004):1740–1748.
3. M. J. DeVivo, "Causes and Costs of Spinal Cord Injury in the United States," *Spinal Cord* 35(1997):809–813.
4. J. R. Hoffman, D. L. Schriger, W. Mower, J. S. Luo, and M. Zucker, "Low-Risk Criteria for Cervical-Spine Radiography in Blunt Trauma: A Prospective Study," *Annals of Emergency Medicine* 21(1992):1454–1460.
5. J. E. Tintinalli, G. D. Kelen, J. S. Stapczynski, O. J. Ma, and D. M. Cline, "Neurologic Shock." *Tintinalli's Emergency Medicine: A Comprehensive Study Guide,* 6th ed., McGraw-Hill's AccessMedicine (accessed June 7, 2006).
6. R. I. Zipnick, T. M. Scalea, S. Z. Trooskin, et al., "Hemodynamic Responses to Penetrating Spinal Injuries." *The Journal of Trauma* 35(1993):578.
7. W. Goldberg, C. Mueller, E. Panacek, S. Tigges, J. R. Hoffman, and W. R. Mower, "Distribution and Patterns of Blunt Traumatic Cervical Spine Injury." *Annals of Emergency Medicine* 38(2001):17–21.
8. S. C. Kirsblum, S. L. Groah, W. O. McKinley, et al., "Spinal Cord Injury Medicine. 1. Etiology, Classification and Acute Medical Management," *Archives of Physical Medicine and Rehabilitation* 83(2002):550, 590.
9. J. S. Harrop, A. D. Sharan, A. R. Vaccaro, and G. J. Przybylski, "The Cause of Neurologic Deterioration After Acute Cervical Spinal Cord Injury," *Spine* 26(2001):340–346.
10. S. H. Ko, W. Chun, and H. C. Kim. "Delayed Spinal Cord Injury Following Electrical Burns: A 7-Year Experience." *Burns* 30(2004):691–695.
11. J. W. McDonald and C. Sadowsky, "Spinal Cord Injury," *Lancet* 359(2002):417.
12. C. H. Tator, "Experimental and Clinical Studies of the Pathophysiology and Management of Acute Spinal Cord Injury," *Journal of Spinal Cord Medicine* 19(1996):206.
13. J. E. Tintinalli, G. D. Kelen, J. S. Stapczynski, O. J. Ma, and D. M. Cline, "Spinal Cord Injuries." *Tintinalli's Emergency Medicine: A Comprehensive Study Guide,* 6th ed., McGraw-Hill's AccessMedicine (accessed June 7, 2006).
14. P. P. Atkinson and J. L. D. Atkinson, "Spinal Shock," *Mayo Clinic Process* 71(1996):384.
15. Paralyzed Veterans of America/Consortium for Spinal Cord Medicine, *Acute Management of Autonomic Dysreflexia: Individuals with Spinal Cord Injury Presenting to Health-Care Facilities* (Washington, DC: Paralyzed Veterans of America (PVA), 2001).

16. F. C. Brunicardi, D. K. Andersen, T. R. Billiar, D. L. Dunn, J. G. Hunter, J. B. Matthews, R. E. Pollock, and S. I. Schwartz, "Shock." *Schwartz's Principles of Surgery*, 8th ed., McGraw-Hill's AccessMedicine (accessed June 7, 2006).

17. G. J. Gilson, A. C. Miller, F. W. Clevenger, and L. B. Curet, "Acute Spinal Cord Injury and Neurogenic Shock in Pregnancy," *Obstetrical & Gynecological Survey* 50(1995):556.

18. A. B. Guha and C. H. Tator, "Acute Cardiovascular Effects of Experimental Spinal Cord Injury," *The Journal of Trauma* 28(1988):481.

19. R. I. Zipnick, T. M. Scalea, S. Z. Trooskin, et al., "Hemodynamic Responses to Penetrating Spinal Injuries," *The Journal of Trauma* 35(1993):578.

20. J. R. Hoffman, W. R. Mower, A. B. Wolfson, K. H. Todd, and M. I. Zucker, "Validity of a Set of Clinical Criteria to Rule Out Injury to the Cervical Spine in Patients with Blunt Trauma, National Emergency X-Radiography Utilization Study Group," *The New England Journal of Medicine* 343(2000):94–99.

21. I. G. Stiell, C. M. Clement, R. D. McKnight, et al., "The Canadian C-Spine Rule Versus the NEXUS Low-Risk Criteria in Patients with Trauma," *The New England Journal of Medicine* 349(2003):2510–2518.

22. I. G. Stiell, G. A. Wells, K. L. Vandemheen, et al., "The Canadian C-Spine Rule for Radiography in Alert and Stable Trauma Patients," *Journal of the American Medical Association* 286(2001):1841–1848.

23. R. M. Domeier, R. A. Swor, R. W. Evans, et al., "Multicenter Prospective Validation of Prehospital Clinical Spinal Clearance Criteria," *The Journal of Trauma* 53(2002):744–750.

24. D. G. Hankins, E. I. Rivera-Rivera, J. P. Ornato, R. A. Swor, T. Blackwell, and R. M. Domeier, "Spinal Immobilization in the Field: Clinical Clearance Criteria and Implementation," *Prehospital Emergency Care* 5(2001):88–93.

25. G. Stroh and D. Braude, "Can an Out-of-Hospital Cervical Spine Clearance Protocol Identify All Patients with Injuries? An Argument for Selective Immobilization," *Annals of Emergency Medicine* 37(2001):609–615.

26. T. M. Dunn, A. Dalton, T. Dorfman, and W. W. Dunn, "Are Emergency Medical Technician-Basics Able to Use a Selective Immobilization of the Cervical Spine Protocol? A Preliminary Report," *Prehospital Emergency Care* 8(2004):207–211.

27. R. M. Domeier, S. M. Frederiksen, and K. Welch, "Prospective Performance Assessment of an Out-of-Hospital Protocol for Selective Spine Immobilization Using Clinical Spine Clearance Criteria," *Annals of Emergency Medicine* 46(2005):123–131.

28. Y. Barkana, M. Stein, A. Scope, et al., "Prehospital Stabilization of the Cervical Spine for Penetrating Injuries of the Neck: Is it Necessary?" *Injury* 31(2000):305–309.

29. R. A. Connell, C. A. Graham, and P. T. Munro, "Is Spinal Immobilisation Necessary for All Patients Sustaining Isolated Penetrating Trauma?" *Injury* 34(2003):912–914.

30. A. Ullrich, G. W. Hendey, J. Geiderman, S. G. Shaw, J. Hoffman, and W. R. Mower, "Distracting Painful Injuries Associated with Cervical Spinal Injuries in Blunt Trauma," *Academic Emergency Medicine* 8(2001):25–29.

31. L. D. Bub, C. C. Blackmore, F. A. Mann, and F. M. Lomoschitz, "Cervical Spine Fractures in Patients 65 Years and Older: A Clinical Prediction Rule for Blunt Trauma," *Radiology* 234(2005):143–149.

32. M. Touger, P. Gennis, N. Nathanson, et al., "Validity of a Decision Rule to Reduce Cervical Spine Radiography in Elderly Patients with Blunt Trauma," *Annals of Emergency Medicine* 40(2002):287–293.

33. D. D. Brunette and G. L. Rockswold, "Neurologic Recovery Following Rapid Spinal Realignment for Complete Cervical Spinal Cord Injury," *The Journal of Trauma* 27(1987):445–447.

34. R. A. McGuire, S. Neville, B. A. Green, and C. Watts, "Spinal Instability and The Log-Rolling Maneuver," *The Journal of Trauma* 27(1987):525–531.

35. G. Del Rossi, T. P. Heffernan, M. Horodyski, and G. R. Rechtine, "The Effectiveness of Extrication Collars Tested During the Execution of Spine-Board Transfer Techniques," *The Spine Journal* 4(2004):619–623.

36. J. M. Howell, R. Burrow, C. Dumontier, and A. Hillyard, "A Practical Radiographic Comparison of Short Board Technique and Kendrick Extrication Device," *Annals of Emergency Medicine* 18(1989):943–946.

37. J. R. Cline, E. Scheidel, and E. F. Bigsby, "A Comparison of Methods of Cervical Immobilization Used in Patient Extrication and Transport," *The Journal of Trauma* 25(1985):649–653.

38. I. Kwan, and F. Bunn, "Effects of Prehospital Spinal Immobilization: A Systematic Review of Randomized Trials on Healthy Subjects," *Prehospital Disaster Medicine* 20(2005):47–53.

39. W. H. Cordell, J. C. Hollingsworth, M. L. Olinger, S. J. Stroman, and D. R. Nelson, "Pain and Tissue-Interface Pressures During Spine-Board Immobilization," *Annals of Emergency Medicine* 26(1995):31–36.

40. S. I. DeBoer and M. Seaver, "Big Head, Little Body Syndrome: What EMS Providers Need to Know," *Emergency Medical Services* 33(2004):47–48, 50, 52.

41. C. Roche and H. Carty, "Spinal Trauma in Children," *Pediatric Radiology* 31(2001):677–700.

42. B. Cirak, S. Ziegfeld, V. M. Knight, D. Chang, A. M. Avellino, and C. N. Paidas, "Spinal Injuries in Children," *Journal of Pediatric Surgery* 39(2004):607–612.

43. K. N. Waninger, "Management of the Helmeted Athlete with Suspected Cervical Spine Injury," *The Americal Journal of Sports Medicine* 32(2004):1331–1350.

44. D. M. Kleiner, "Prehospital Care of the Spine-Injured Athlete: Monograph Summary," *Clinical Journal of Sports Medicine* 13(2003):59–61.

45. K. N. Waninger, J. G. Richards, W. T. Pan, A. R. Shay, and M. K. Shindle, "An Evaluation of Head Movement in Backboard-Immobilized Helmeted Football, Lacrosse, and Ice Hockey Players," *Clinical Journal of Sports Medicine* 11 (2001): 82–86.

46. M. B. Bracken, "Steroids for Acute Spinal Cord Injury," *Cochrane Database System Review:* CD001046, 2002.

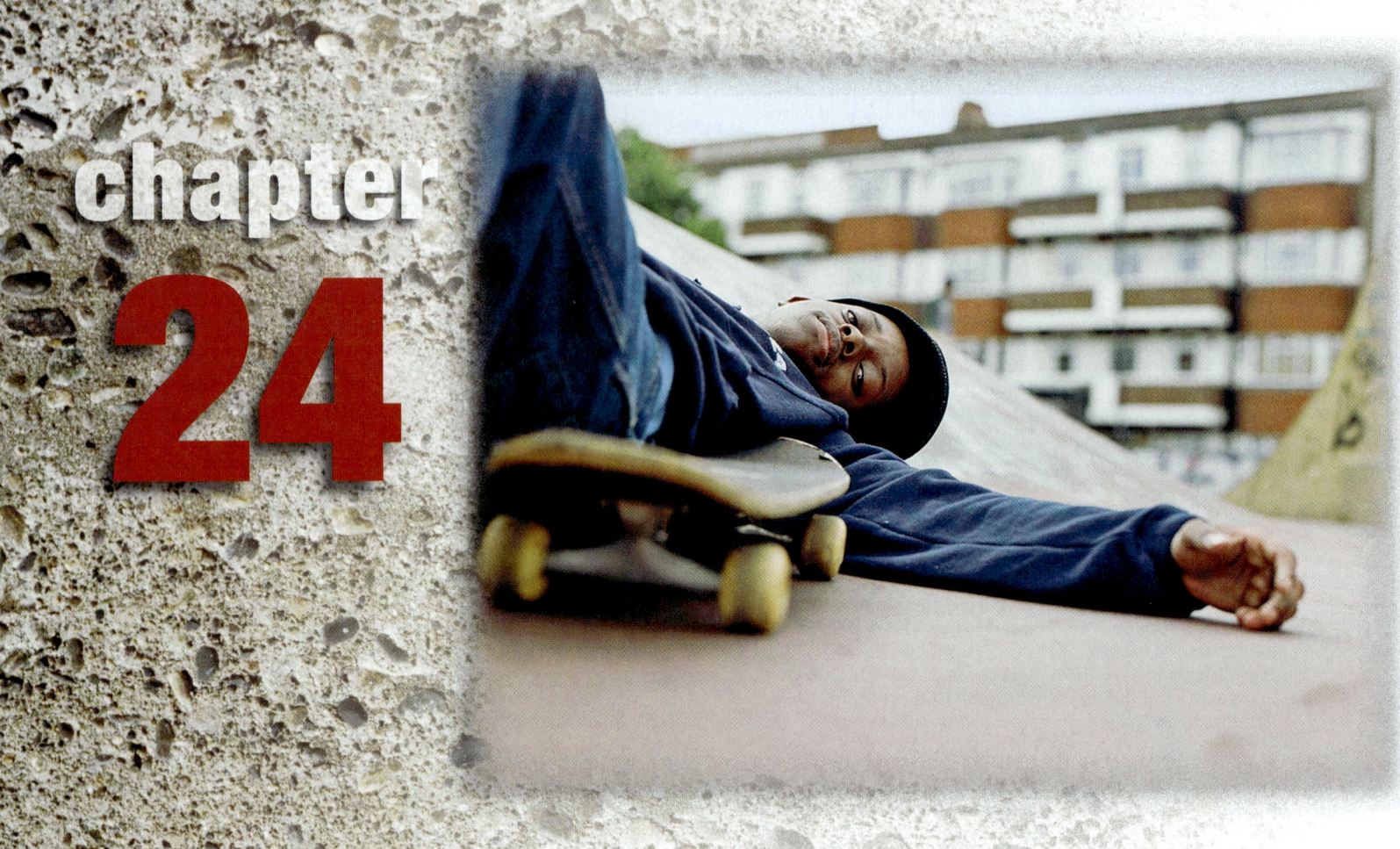

chapter 24

Skeletal Trauma

"*There are a lot of myths about my injuries. They say I have broken every bone in my body. Not true. But I have broken 35 bones. I had surgery 14 times to pin and plate. I shattered my pelvis. I forget all of the things that have broke.*"

—Evel Knievel

Need to Know

▶ Injuries to bones, muscles, cartilage, tendons, and ligaments are common but rarely life-threatening by themselves. During the primary survey, the paramedic should not be distracted by extremity trauma. You must remain alert to the mechanism of injury and the potential for more serious injuries, including hidden injuries. In the presence of life-threatening injuries, extremities are splinted with a whole-body fracture immobilization concept: using a long spine board and straps to immobilize the entire body at once. Transportation of a critical trauma patient should not be delayed to splint a fractured limb.

▶ For patients who appear not yet sick, care focuses on detailed assessment, appropriate splinting, and pain management. Assessment of an injured extremity is focused on evaluating circulation, motor function, and sensation of the injured limb. If these are compromised, the patient is then reclassified as "sick" and must be emergently splinted and transported. Fractures of large long bones, such as the femur, and of the pelvis may cause significant bleeding that is hard to detect. Shock and internal bleeding should be suspected and treated appropriately.

▶ Good documentation and continual reassessment of circulation, motor function, and sensation are essential.

▶ Sick	▶ Not Yet Sick
• Treat the ABC problems before splinting any extremity fractures. Look for threats to life or circulatory compromise in a limb.	• Ask the patient about previous history, including disease, that may lead you to suspect pathologic fractures (osteoporosis, cancer, etc.).
• Pelvic and femur fractures are associated with significant blood loss.	• Look for DCAP-BTLS and the findings for suspected compartment syndrome.
• Treat for shock aggressively and use the long board to splint the patient. Splint other injuries as time permits while en route to the trauma center.	• Realign long bone fractures only if circulation is compromised.
	• Continue to look for hidden injuries and bleeding.
	• Check for circulation, motion, and sensation before and after splinting.
	• Treat the pain with gentle handling, splinting, ice, and positioning of the injured part above the heart (if possible and feasible), and use analgesics.
	• Immobilize and splint injuries on scene before beginning transport.
	• Handle fracture sites gently so closed fractures do not convert to open fractures.

Introduction

A musculoskeletal injury is any injury involving bones, cartilage, muscles, tendons, and ligaments. It is one of the most common types of injury sustained in trauma, second only to soft tissue injuries. Nearly 60 million injuries occur annually, accounting for one in six hospital admissions.[1] They result from the application of significant forces, either direct or indirect, and a variety of mechanisms, such as motor vehicle crashes, falls, violence, and athletic activities.

As of 2001, the Centers for Disease Control and Prevention designated motor vehicle crashes (MVCs) the most common cause of fatal injury and the most common cause of nonfatal injuries (3 million injuries) in people age 15–24 years.[1] Serious MVCs occur more frequently in rural, rather than urban, settings. In people age 65 years or older, falls are the most common cause (63%) of fatal and nonfatal injuries.[1]

Overall, about 48% of all nonfatal injuries are to the extremities. Lacerations account for nearly 26%, sprains and strains for just over 20%, and contusions and abrasions for around 18% of the nonfatal injuries treated at hospital emergency departments. Males are significantly more likely than females to incur both nonfatal and fatal injuries.[1] However, certain musculoskeletal injuries, such as ankle fractures, are more common in elderly females.[2] DOT 4-9.32, 4-9.33

The majority (70–80%) of multisystem trauma patients sustain musculoskeletal injuries.[3] Lower extremity injuries are associated with greater magnitudes of force, more secondary blood loss, and are more difficult to manage in multisystem trauma patients, thereby rendering them more serious. This is especially true of femur and pelvic fractures that have the potential for large internal blood loss and often involve injury to major blood vessels. Upper extremity injuries, though rarely a threat to life, contribute to long-term disability. They account for approximately 1.4 million doctor visits per year and are responsible for 15% of all trauma-related emergency department visits. DOT 4-9.1

While musculoskeletal trauma causes less morbidity and mortality than other types of trauma, such as that to the head, abdomen, and chest, it is often more complicated and may be just as debilitating. These injuries can permanently alter a person's quality of life and ability to work. Injury risks increase in athletes, individuals who engage in risk-taking behaviors such as riding motorcycles, and in the winter months because of cold and ice. Children and the elderly are also at higher risk for many reasons, especially as pedestrians struck by a vehicle. **Skill Sheets that relate to this chapter include Skill Sheet 73: Appendicular Skeleton Splinting and Skill Sheet 74: Traction Splinting (also see Step-by-Step 74).**

Musculoskeletal Terminology

The use of **eponyms** (the naming of conditions and diseases for the physician or scientist who first discovered or classified them) to identify fractures or deformities is falling out of favor. Names such as Colles, Salter, Smith, Barton, etc. are often misused or misapplied to musculoskeletal injuries. It is better to describe the assessment in terms of suspected fractures or dislocations by referring to the correct anatomic location.

Applied Anatomy and Physiology

The musculoskeletal system is comprised of muscles, bones, ligaments, and tendons that work together to give the body its form and function. Any disruption in this continuous, dynamic functional unit causes impairment to the body. DOT 4-9.2

CONNECTIONS Refer to Chapter 7: Anatomy Overview, Figures 7-59, through 7-65, for more illustrations of the musculoskeletal system.

Bones

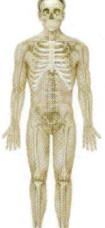

The skeletal system is made up of 206 bones and is divided into the axial and appendicular skeletons (Figure 24-1). The **axial skeleton** forms the central (longitudinal) axis of the body and includes the skull, vertebral column, and bony thorax. The **appendicular skeleton** includes the paired long bones of the body, such as the humerus, radius, and ulna. These attach to the axial skeleton by the clavicle and scapula (commonly referred to as the pectoral girdle). Also part of the appendicular skeleton are the lower extremities, specifically the femur, tibia, and fibular bones that attach to the axial skeleton by the pelvic girdle, which consists of three bones: two innominate bones and the sacrum. The innominate bones are further subdivided into the ilium, ischium, and pubis.

Bones provide the architecture of the body, stabilizing it and protecting the vital organs (e.g., thoracic cage) while simultaneously acting as a point of attachment for tendons, cartilage, and ligaments, which are important for movement. Bones are also responsible for the storage of salts and other metabolic materials as well as the production of red blood cells in the marrow.

Bone Anatomy Overview

Bone contains three types of cells: osteoblasts, osteocytes, and osteoclasts. **Osteoblasts** are the cells that form bone. Once they lay down new bone tissue, the osteoblasts become **osteocytes.** They are imprisoned within the mineralized matrix of the bone, becoming a component of the bone. **Osteoclasts** are cells that reabsorb bone for the purpose of growth and repair. The bone matrix is made up of collagen fibers, proteins, carbohydrate-protein complexes, ground substance, and minerals. Bones are composed of two types of tissue: compact bone **(cortical bone)** and spongy bone **(cancellous bone).** Both types contain the same structural elements, and, with few exceptions, both types are found in all bones. The cortical bone forms the hard outer layer, and the cancellous tissue makes up the inner portion. The cancellous tissue is less densely organized than the compact bone, and it contains the red marrow, which manufactures blood cells. Capillaries pass through both compact and spongy bone. All bones are covered with a **periosteum,** which is a thickened layer of connective tissue. At the distal ends of bone is the **physis,** which includes the **epiphysis** and epiphyseal plate, which is the site of growth in children. Between each epiphysis is the **diaphysis.** The ends of the bone are covered with articular cartilage. The articular cartilage, in conjunction with tendons that provide attachment points for muscles and ligaments that hold adjacent bones together, form joints that allow for movement.

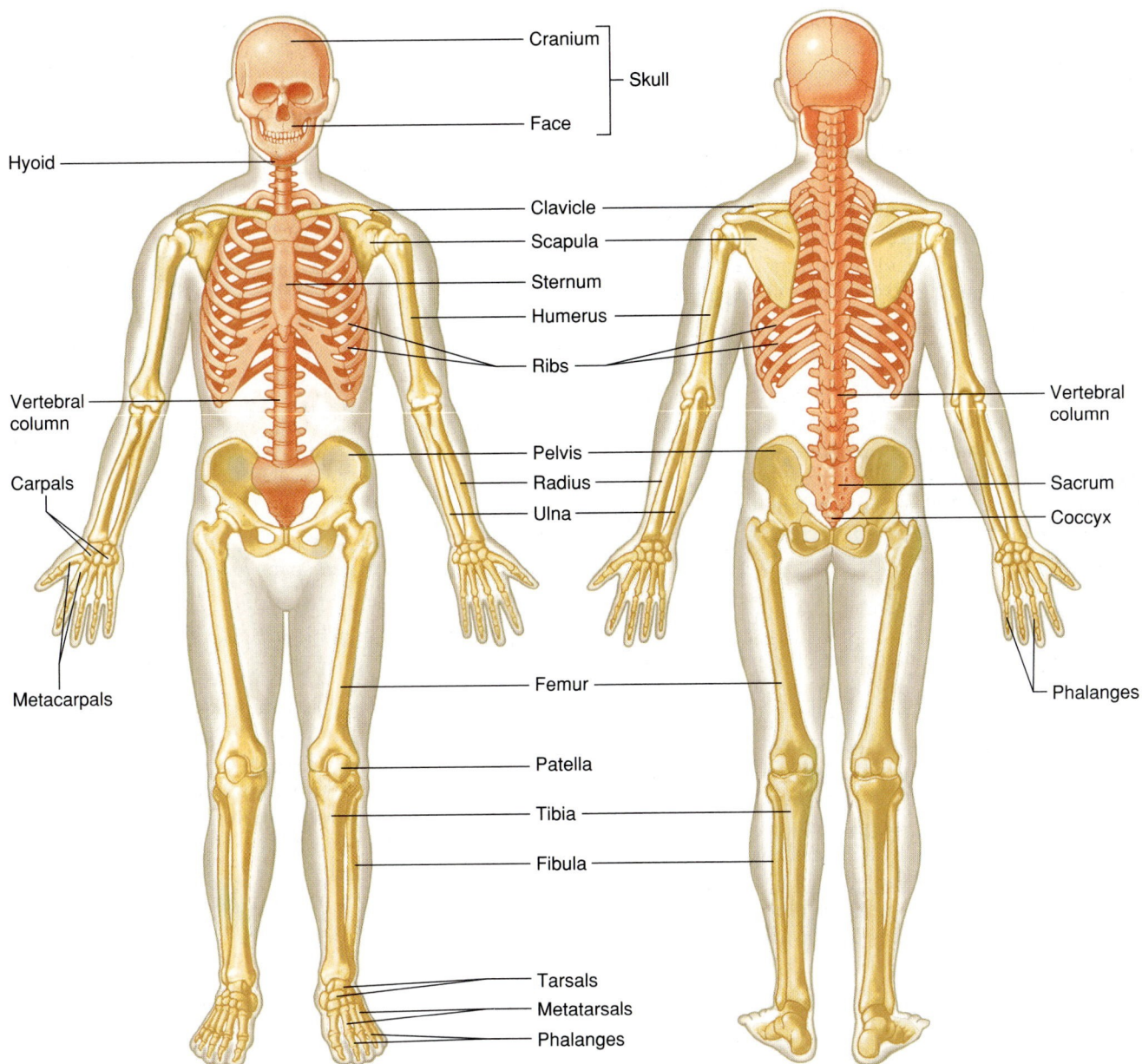

Figure 24-1   The 206 bones of the skeleton are divided up into the axial (shown in pink) and appendicular (shown in brown) skeleton.

Fracture Healing

Healing from fractures can be described as occurring in three phases: inflammation, reparative, and remodeling.[4] Each phase gradually blends into the next until the bone is healed. When a fracture occurs, the microvessels crossing the fracture line are severed, depriving the damaged bone ends of their blood supply. These cells necrose (die) during the next few days, which triggers an **inflammatory response.** This phase is brief, but it creates an environment for the repair to begin. Granulation tissue begins to infiltrate the area, and the **reparative phase** begins. Specialized cells within the granulation tissue are capable of forming collagen,

cartilage, and bone, which are the ingredients of callus. The callus surrounds the fractured bone ends and stabilizes them. With time, the callus becomes densely mineralized. Osteoclasts remove the necrotic cells, allowing for the reabsorption and recycling of some components of the damaged bone. **Remodeling** is the final phase of healing. It can take weeks to years to complete. During this phase, the bone tends to return to its normal shape and contours. The callus is reabsorbed and replaced by new bone laid down following the original lines of stress of the bone. The degree of success of this process is related to a number of factors. Young children have a greater capacity for remodeling than adults, and they suffer less deformity as well, particularly if the bone is not very angulated. Fractures located closer to the epiphysis (but not through it) heal better than midshaft fractures.

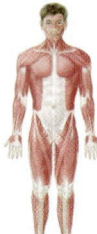

Muscles and Connective Tissue

There are three types of muscles in the body: cardiac, smooth, and skeletal muscle. Cardiac and smooth muscle are discussed in detail in other chapters. This chapter deals specifically with skeletal muscle (Figure 24-2).

CONNECTIONS Cardiac muscle has unique and interesting properties that help sustain life. Read more about it in the cardiology chapter (Chapter 29). Smooth muscle is found in the lower airways, blood vessels, and intestines. Chapters 7: Anatomy Overview, 12: Airway Management, Ventilation, and Oxygenation, and 34: Gastroenterology specifically discuss this type of involuntary muscle.

Skeletal Muscles

Skeletal muscles are the major muscles associated with the musculoskeletal system. They are different from the other muscle types in that they are under conscious, or voluntary control. As the major muscle mass of the body, they provide mobility and support of the skeletal system with assistance from the tendons. There are over 600 skeletal muscles, and each skeletal muscle is a separate organ that is encased by a connective tissue called fascia. The fascia protects the muscle fibers; provides a structure for a network of nerves, blood vessels, and lymph channels; and provides for the attachment of the muscle to the bone.

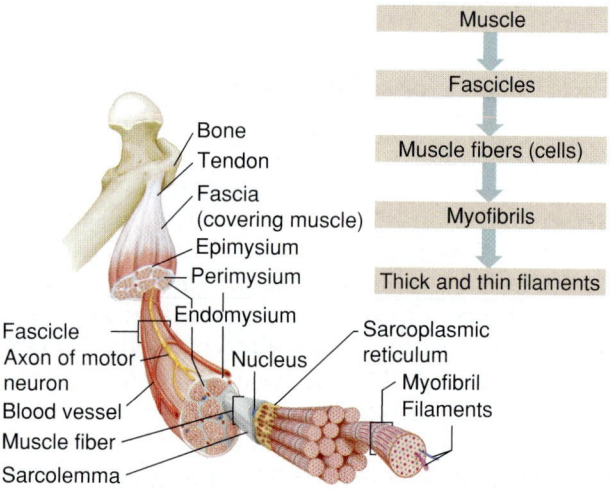

Figure 24-2 The major muscle mass of the body is made up of skeletal muscle. Skeletal muscle is different in that it is under conscious or voluntary control. See Figure 25-3, page 506, for a larger view of this image.

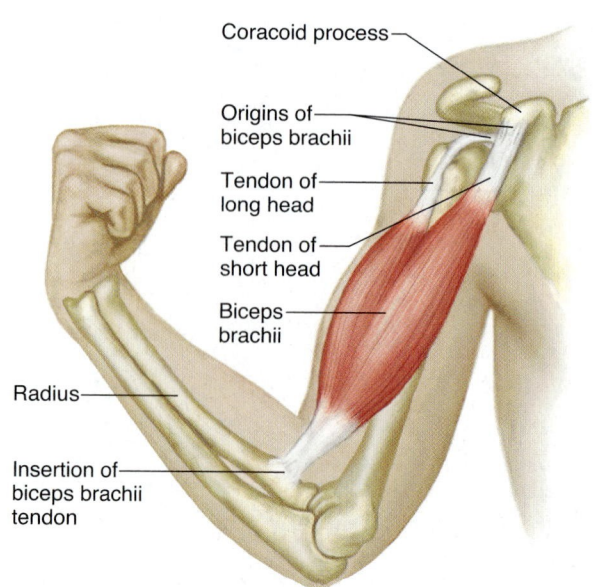

Figure 24-3 Tendons bind muscle to bone providing the power of movement across the joints.

Tendons and Cartilage

Tendons are bands of connective tissue that bind the muscles to bones. Tendons provide the power of movement across the joints (Figure 24-3). **Cartilage** is the connective tissue that covers the epiphysis of joints. Cartilage provides a smooth surface for the articulation of two bones, which allows for movement (Figure 24-4). **Ligaments** are bands of connective tissue that support and stabilize joints by attaching bone to bone. Ligaments provide a means to maintain the proper relationship of two bones and for stability throughout the range of motion of a joint (Figure 24-5). A **sprain** is caused by stretching forces applied to a ligament. A **strain** is caused by stretching forces applied to a tendon. DOT 4-9.34, 4-9.28,4-9.31

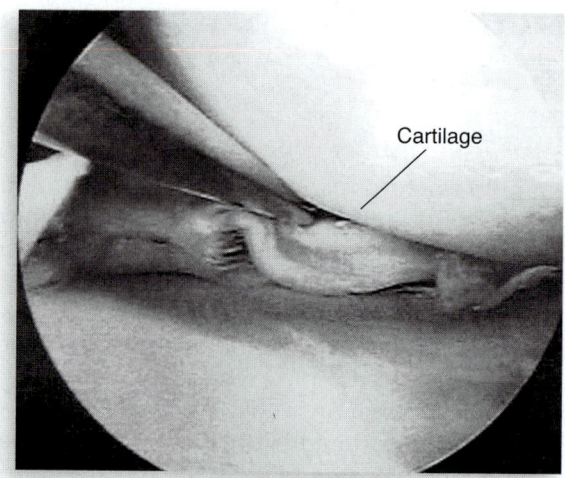

Figure 24-4 Cartilage provides a smooth surface that allows smooth movement in the joints.

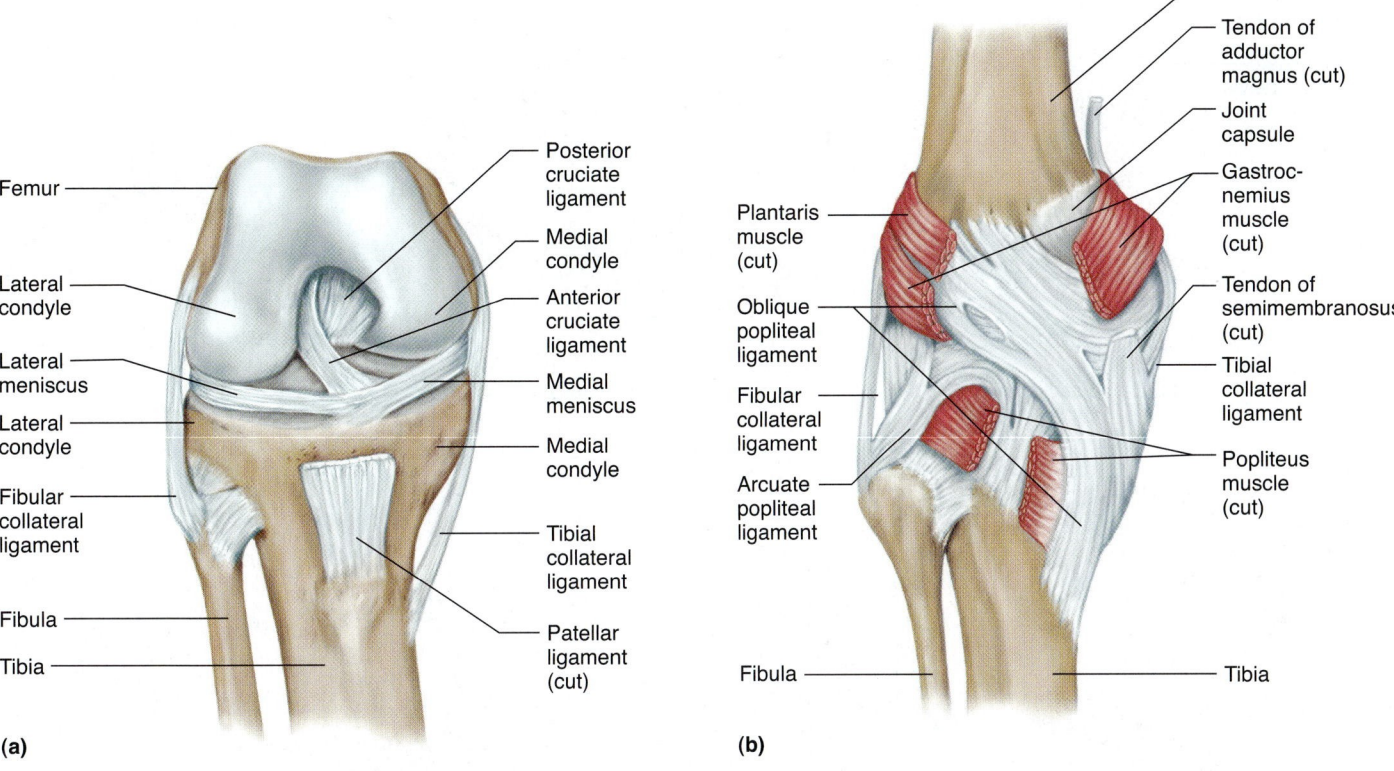

Femur

Lateral condyle

Lateral meniscus

Lateral condyle

Fibular collateral ligament

Fibula

Tibia

Posterior cruciate ligament

Medial condyle

Anterior cruciate ligament

Medial meniscus

Medial condyle

Tibial collateral ligament

Patellar ligament (cut)

(a)

Plantaris muscle (cut)

Oblique popliteal ligament

Fibular collateral ligament

Arcuate popliteal ligament

Fibula

Femur

Tendon of adductor magnus (cut)

Joint capsule

Gastroc-nemius muscle (cut)

Tendon of semimembranosus (cut)

Tibial collateral ligament

Popliteus muscle (cut)

Tibia

(b)

Figure 24-5 Securing the bones of a joint together. (a) Ligaments provide stability to the joints. (b) Tendons allow for movement.

Joints

Joints consist of tissue to bind bones at each junction. Although joints vary in structure and function, they are classified into three main groups: fibrous, cartilaginous, and synovial.

- **Fibrous joints.** Fibrous joints are made of dense connective tissue that provide stability and permit only very slight movement, such as the sutures between the flat bones of the skull. The tibia and fibula in the leg are attached to each other by this type of joint.
- **Cartilaginous joints.** Cartilaginous joints are made up of two bones that are joined together by an intervening segment of cartilage such as the joints found in the spine. The symphysis pubis is another example of a cartilaginous joint. It permits a woman's pelvic bone to shift as she gives birth.
- **Synovial joints.** Synovial joints are fluid-filled to lubricate articulations. Of all the joints, synovial joints are the most common and the most intricate. They are made up of articular cartilage, a joint capsule, and a synovial membrane, which secretes synovial fluid. These joints are classified into six different types according to the movement they

allow. These categories are hinge, pivot, ball and socket, condyloid, gliding, and saddle joints. They allow for all of the various movements of the body including gliding and angular movements, flexion, extension, abduction, adduction, circumduction, and rotation (Figure 24-6).[5]

Injuries to Joints

Joint dislocations occur when there is displacement of the normal articulating ends of two or more bones. A **luxation** is the complete dislocation of a joint. A **subluxation** is a partial or incomplete dislocation of a joint. Either can result in damage and instability of the joint. An example of a subluxation is "nursemaid's elbow" in children in which a forceful pulling motion subluxes the head of the radius, leading to pain and inability to use the arm, but the remainder of the joint (ulna and humerus) is unaffected. The shoulder is the most commonly dislocated joint, followed by the elbow. Suspect a joint dislocation if a joint is deformed or does not move through its normal range of motion. All dislocations can result in damage and instability of the affected joint and may have associated fractures.

DOT 4-9.4, 4-9.23

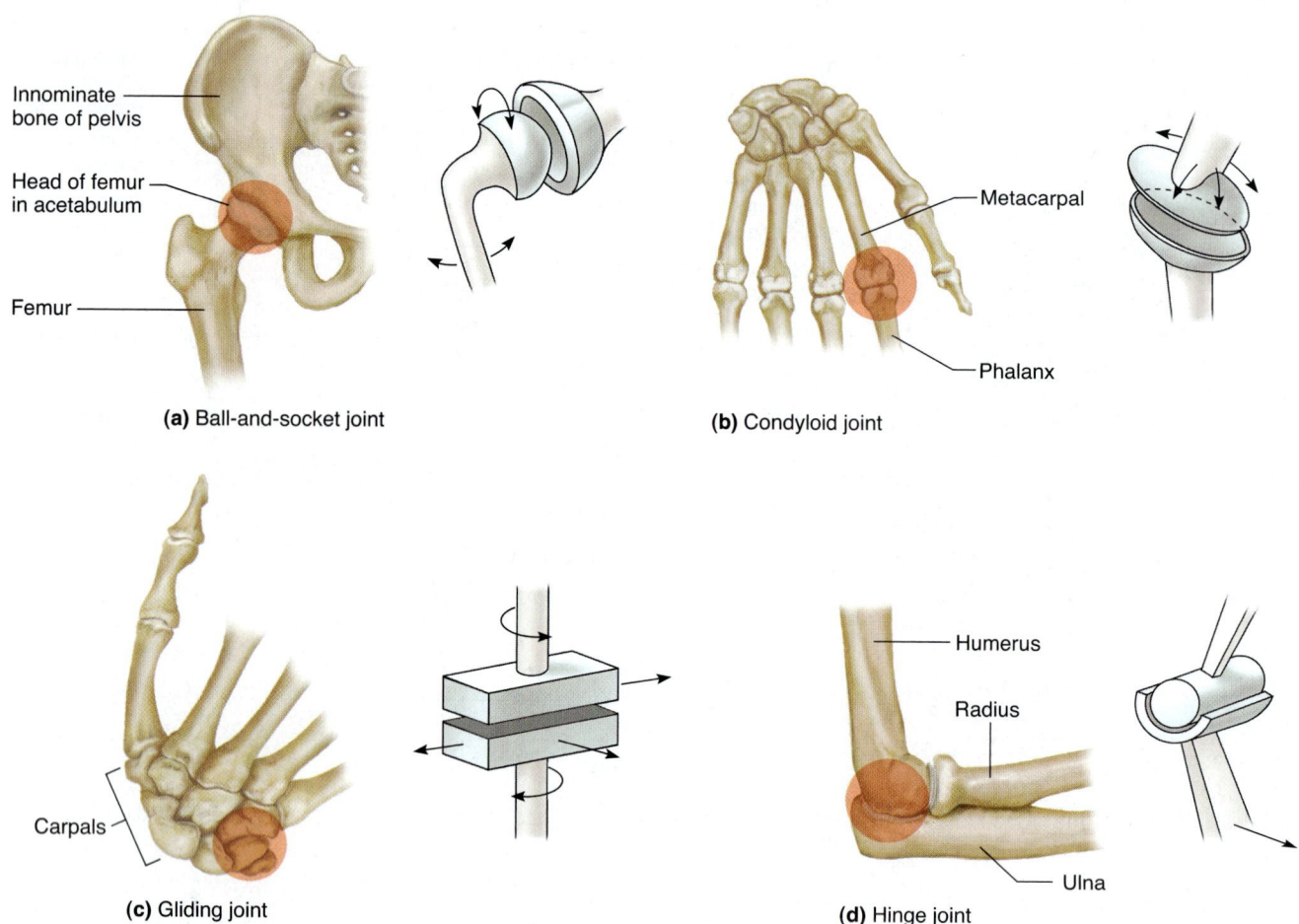

(a) Ball-and-socket joint

Innominate bone of pelvis

Head of femur in acetabulum

Femur

(b) Condyloid joint

Metacarpal

Phalanx

(c) Gliding joint

Carpals

(d) Hinge joint

Humerus

Radius

Ulna

Figure 24-6 Fluid-filled synovial joints, the most common and intricate joints, allow for gliding and angular movements such as flexion, extension, abduction, adduction, circumduction, and rotation.

Dislocations

A joint is dislocated when the articular surfaces (bone ends) that normally meet to form the joint are displaced completely out of contact with each other. A potential complication of dislocation is neurologic or circulatory compromise. The nerves and blood vessels, called the **neurovascular bundle,** that pass by near the joint can be kinked, stretched, or pinched. The longer the process is allowed to continue, the greater the potential for permanent disability. Also, the longer a joint is allowed to remain in a dislocated state, the more difficult it is to reduce. This is believed to be due to edema, muscle spasm, and other tissue changes.[2] The hip carries the added risk of developing avascular necrosis following a dislocation because most of the blood supply to the femoral head is delivered through vessels that emerge from the acetabulum. When the joint is disrupted, circulation to the femoral head is disrupted. The knee is also at great risk following traumatic dislocation as loss of circulation from damage to the blood supply (popliteal artery) of the

lower leg will result in gangrene of the leg and foot. Ischemia of more than four to six hours is associated with poor prognosis for limb salvage.[6] DOT 4-9.4

Reduction

Reduction is the movement of the misaligned bone ends or displaced joint to restore proper alignment. An absent pulse distal to the fracture site or dislocation is a common indication for the need to perform a reduction in the field. Most jurisdictions recognize the need to attempt to realign angulated fractures in order to apply splints and immobilization devices, but care should always be exercised when handling fractures or dislocated extremities.

Joints are often difficult to reduce because of pain, muscle spasm, bleeding or edema. Many joint reductions require the use of sedatives or muscle relaxants, which may not be available in the prehospital setting. Manipulation of a dislocated joint may result in the creation of a fracture/dislocation or may damage the adjacent neurovascular bundle. Generally, joint reduction is not appropriate for the prehospital setting except in extreme circumstances such as wilderness locations or when transport times will be significantly delayed for hours or days. Even then, on-line medical direction may be desirable prior to attempting the procedure.

Because there is no common standard for reduction of deformity, the decision ultimately remains with the medical director and supervisor of the EMS service.[2] Consult with your medical director and know your protocols to determine what, if any, circumstances allow you to perform reductions in the prehospital setting. DOT 4-9.27

Fractures

A **fracture** is a break in the continuity of a bone or cartilage. It typically results from significant forces applied to bones. The bony cortex can be disrupted by a variety of mechanisms, including a direct blow, axial loading, angular forces causing bending, torque (twisting) force, or a combination. The fracture may be complete or incomplete, depending on whether the fracture goes all the way through the bone, as well as open or closed, depending on the integrity of the skin over the fracture site. Fractures are classified by their injury type or by their injury mechanism. DOT 4-9.4

Classification of Fractures by Injury Type

Paramedics are primarily concerned with identifying that a possible fracture exists and then stabilizing appropriately. Besides the obvious state of a fracture being open or closed, paramedics are not required to classify fractures. A description of the various types of fractures is included for information purposes only. DOT 4-9.3

- *Open fracture.* An open fracture is evidenced by any soft tissue wound adjacent to a suspected fracture and is an urgent matter because of its potential for infection. The most dreaded complication of an open fracture is osteomyelitis (infection of the bone) as this may result in months or years of pain, disability, medical therapy, or surgical procedures, and may ultimately result in the need for amputation. The term "compound" for describing an open fracture is dated and is no longer used. Also, an open fracture may have made contact with the skin some distance from the fracture site. It is important to stabilize any fracture with caution to prevent turning a closed fracture into an open fracture (Figure 24-7). Fractures may be open in two ways:
  - From the inside out (such as when a protruding bone fragment pierces the skin, causing a soft tissue injury)

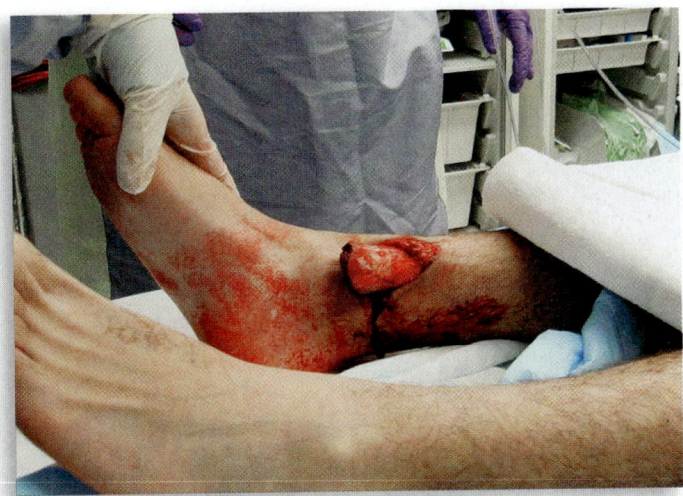

Figure 24-7 Fractures in which broken bone ends break the surface of the skin are referred to as open fractures.

  - From the outside in (such as after a gunshot wound) DOT 4-9.17
- *Closed fracture.* A closed fracture is a break in the bone that has not penetrated through the surrounding soft tissue. It may not be obvious, but the potential for other serious complications such as hemorrhage leading to shock remains the same (Figure 24-8). DOT 4-9.17
- *Incomplete fracture.* An incomplete fracture involves only one side of the bone (e.g., torus or greenstick in pediatrics).
- *Complete fracture.* A complete fracture involves all of the layers of a bone.
- *Displaced fracture.* A displaced fracture is one where there is movement of the two bone fragments away from one another. After x-rays and other imaging studies are obtained, the displacement is subcategorized into minimally, moderately, or completely displaced.
- *Nondisplaced fracture.* A nondisplaced fracture is one where the two fragments remain in alignment with one another. When splinting a fracture, it is important not to turn a nondisplaced fracture into a displaced one.
- *Comminuted fracture.* A comminuted fracture is a fracture that involves several breaks in a bone. Damage is often increased due to the presence of multiple fragments (Figure 24-9).
- *Pathological fracture.* A pathological fracture is a fracture that occurs through diseased bone due to an inherent underlying weakness. Common examples include metastatic (cancerous) lesions, benign bone cysts (such as those sometimes found in the humerus of Little League pitchers), and vertebral compression

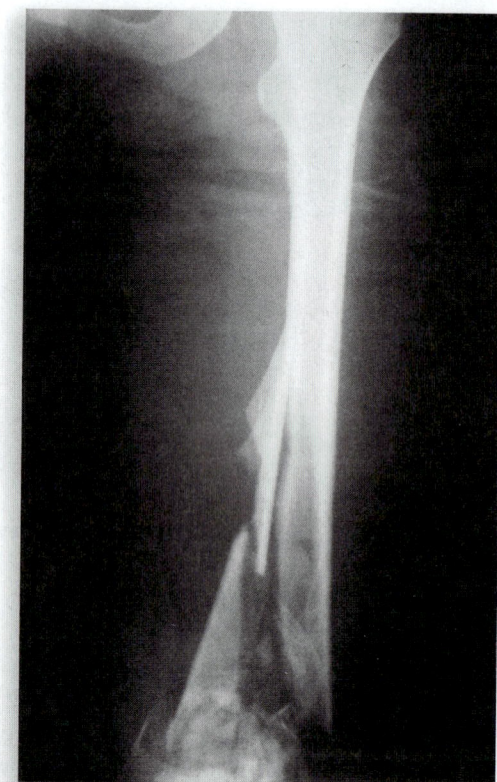

Figure 24-8 When fractures occur that don't feature bone ends breaking the surface of the skin, they are referred to as closed fractures. Angulation may be apparent, but swelling and pain may be the only indication.

fractures in patients with advanced osteoporosis. High suspicion for this type of fracture should be considered when the mechanism of injury seems too minor to have produced a fracture or when a patient has certain risk factors, such as osteoporosis or cancer. In high risk patients, never assume that the mechanism is not enough to produce a significant injury.

- **Stress or "March" fracture.** A stress fracture is a break in a bone, especially those of the foot, ankle, metatarsals, distal tibia and fibula, or femoral neck, caused by repetitive, long-term, or abnormal stress. These often occur after a sudden increase in physical activities, such as running or for soldiers in boot camp (the reason for the name "march"). They are often diagnosed by a physician from the signs and symptoms alone. They are often not very apparent by x-ray.[7]

- **Epiphyseal plate fractures.** The epiphyseal plate is responsible for the elongation of the bone during growth. Some fractures near or through this area can result in alternations in normal growth. It may stop or slow, but it may also speed up. The potential for growth disturbance is related to the number of years the child has left to grow and the pattern of the fracture line through the epiphyseal area.

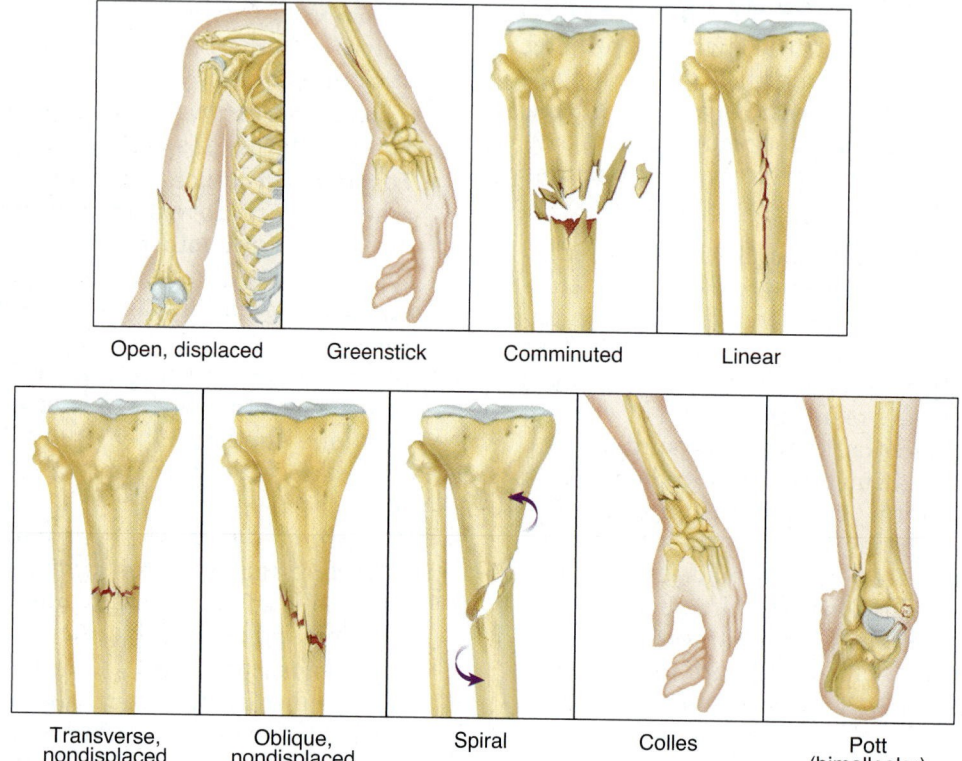

Open, displaced   Greenstick   Comminuted   Linear

Transverse, nondisplaced   Oblique, nondisplaced   Spiral   Colles   Pott (bimalleolar)

Figure 24-9 Bones can fracture in a variety of ways due to a variety of forces. These diagrams illustrate different mechanisms of fracture.

Classification of Fractures by Injury Mechanism

As mentioned in the previous section, paramedics are not required to classify fractures by their mechanism. It is, however, helpful to learn about the types of injuries that can occur to a bone because of the various forces that are applied.

> Painful, swollen, and deformed areas of the body that contain bone should be handled as if a fracture were present; stabilize, immobilize, and transport for further evaluation.

Direct Trauma

Direct trauma results from force applied directly to a bone. Some examples include the following:

- *Nightstick fractures.* This is a linear fracture resulting in two segments. It is usually associated with little to no soft tissue injury.
- *Crush fractures.* This is a comminuted or transverse fracture associated with extensive soft tissue injury and usually results in significant morbidity.
- *Fractures from penetrating injury.* A penetrating fracture can be the result of a high-velocity injury that results in fragmentation of the bone. These fragments go on to form secondary missiles and cavitations causing severe soft tissue injury. Gunshot wounds with associated fractures are an example of these (Figure 24-10). Low-velocity projectiles often result in less fragmentation of the bone.

Indirect Trauma

Fractures from indirect trauma occur as energy is transferred from one body tissue to another. While force is not directly applied to the bone, the energy is transmitted through adjacent tissues resulting in fracture. These injuries include the following:

- *Torus (buckle) fractures.* These fractures are characterized by a buckling of one side of the cortex, usually in the metaphyseal region, and most often result from compressive forces, such as falls on an outstretched arm.
- *Greenstick fractures.* These fractures result from an angular force applied to a long bone that causes a break in the convex side of the cortex and a bowing of the concave side of the cortex.
- *Compression "Y or T" fracture.* These are fractures in which an axial load along the long axis of a bone results in its compression. These are associated with delay or failure of proper growth.

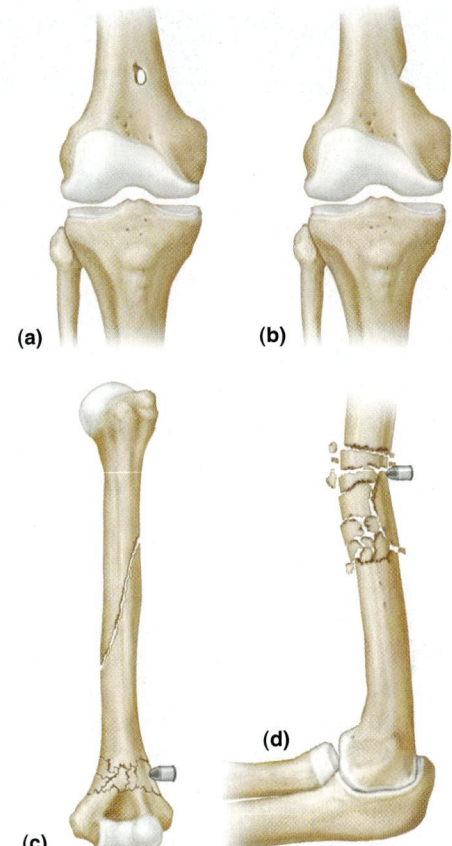

Figure 24-10 Types of fracture patterns created by bullets: (a) drill hole, (b) unicortical, (c) distort spiral, (d) comminuted.

- *Spiral fracture.* A break in a bone that is caused by a rotational force or twisting motion results in a spiral fracture. Pure rotational injuries are rare. When they occur in children and the elderly, they require special attention as they may represent possible abuse.
- *Oblique fracture.* When spiral fractures are associated with an axial load, they break at a slanting angle across the bone, and they are called oblique fractures.

Complications from Musculoskeletal Injuries

Bleeding

The most worrisome complication occurring immediately after a fracture is bleeding. Major hemorrhage is possible at the fracture site or surrounding tissue. Bleeding can be extensive in large long bone fractures such as the femur or the pelvis (Figure 24-11). A typical tibia and fibula fracture can result in as much as 500 mL of blood loss in the first two hours; a femur fracture can

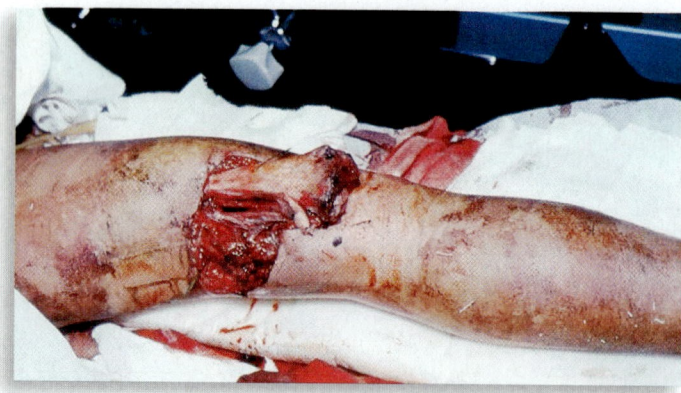

Figure 24-11   Bones can bleed extensively. A tibia can cause 500 mL of bleeding, a femur can lose one to two liters of blood, and the pelvis can lose liters.

result in up to 2000 mL loss (Table 24-1).[8] Hemorrhagic shock may occur secondary to bleeding from a pelvic fracture and is a major cause of death in these patients. Retroperitoneal bleeding is also associated with some pelvic fractures, and up to 6 L of blood can easily be lost in the retroperitoneal compartment.[9] DOT 4-9.18

Large hemorrhage and any other interruption in blood supply due to arterial injury can result in decreased blood flow to the distal extremities as evidenced by weak or absent distal pulses. With any fracture, neurologic injury is also possible. This can lead to alteration in motor and sensory functions. Prompt recognition of injuries, proper splinting, and transport is essential. Delay of greater than four to six hours in the repair of an arterial injury has been shown to significantly increase the incidence of severe complications.[8]

Fat Embolism Syndrome

Fat embolism is relatively common but only rarely causes symptoms.[10] When a long bone is fractured, fat globules can be released into the blood. Fat particles can be found in the pulmonary vascular bed in 90% of patients who have sustained fractures of long bones or undergone joint replacements. **Fat embolism syndrome** can result in neurologic dysfunction, respiratory insufficiency, and petechiae of the axillae, chest, and proximal

TABLE 24-1   Blood Loss Associated with Fracture Types

Fracture type	Amount of blood loss (mL)
Tibia/Fibula	500–1000
Femur	1000–2000
Pelvis	1000–Massive

Adapted from National Association of Emergency Medical Technicians, *Prehospital Trauma Life Support*, 6th ed. (St Louis, MO: Elsevier Mosby, 2006), Table 12-1, p 318.

arms. Fat embolism syndrome characteristically begins 12 to 72 hours after injury but may be delayed for several days. Most patients with fat embolism recover spontaneously in three or four days although a mortality rate of up to 10% is quoted, usually related to the underlying injuries. Treatment primarily involves respiratory support.[11]

Street Secrets

Suspect fat embolism as part of your assessment criteria when you are called to treat a sudden onset of shortness of breath and you find the patient has been treated for a recent significant fracture.

Compartment Syndrome

Compartment syndrome is caused by increased pressure in an enclosed space that leads to compromise of circulation to and function of tissues within the space. It can occur in muscle as the result of swelling from trauma or surgery. The fascia of muscle is relatively inelastic, and pressure from bleeding or edema can build up inside the tissues, compromising circulation. If left untreated, the tissues become ischemic. Severe ischemia for six to eight hours leads to nerve or muscle death.

The lower leg and forearm are the most common locations for compartment syndrome to develop. Pain with passive range of motion of the fingers or toes is thought to be the most sensitive early sign.[12] An immediate surgical procedure (fasciotomy) is indicated to avoid permanent injury. This procedure is not performed by paramedics, so recognition of the problem and rapid transport are the appropriate field treatments.

Late signs of arterial insufficiency caused by compartment syndrome include pain, pallor, paresthesia, and paralysis. If nerve or muscle ischemia has been present long enough, paralysis, paresthesia, and tissue damage has likely occurred. Pulselessness is not reliable as it does not always occur with the late stages of compartment syndrome.

The traditional understanding about compartment syndrome has been that when tissue pressure is greater than arterial pressure, compartment syndrome occurs because circulation is compromised. However, research has shown that compartment syndrome can occur at pressures below arterial pressure, and

compartment syndrome can exist in a pink limb with normal pulses.[13]

The finding of pain out of proportion to the injury, particularly when the fingers or toes are passively stretched by a paramedic, is the best finding for suspecting compartment syndrome.[12]

TABLE 24-2 Associated Complications of Musculoskeletal Injuries

Immediate	Intermediate	Long-term
Bleeding	Compartment syndrome	Reflex sympathetic dystrophy
Neurovascular compromise	Fat embolism syndrome	Contractures
Tissue devitalization		Nonunion
Loss of limb		Avascular necrosis
Instability		Deformities
		Stiffness and arthritis

TABLE 24-3 Commonly Encountered Occult Injuries

Primary injury	Occult injury
Scapular fracture	Rib fracture
	Lung injuries
	Major thoracic injury
Clavicle fracture	Major thoracic injury
Fracture or dislocation of elbow	Brachial artery injury
	Median, ulna, and radial nerve injury
Major pelvic fracture	Abdominal, thoracic, or head injury
	Pelvic vascular hemorrhage
Femur fracture	Thigh hemorrhage
Knee dislocation or displaced tibial plateau fracture	Popliteal artery or nerve injuries
Calcaneal fracture	Spine injury
	Fracture or dislocation of foot
	Tibial plateau fracture
Open fracture	Other nonskeletal injury in 70%

Long-Term Complications

Although encountering long-term complications from fractures is rare in the prehospital setting, proper recognition and treatment in the out-of-hospital setting is the best way to help prevent complications. Complications can include reflex sympathetic dystrophy; Volkmann's ischemic contractures; nonunion (the fracture does not heal properly); avascular necrosis; deformities such as angulation, overgrowth or shortening of a limb; joint stiffness; and post-traumatic ossification or arthritis. Proper splinting techniques and maintenance of circulation are the keys to prevention of many of the complications. See Table 24-2 for associated complications of musculoskeletal injuries.

Associated Injuries

More troublesome than the complications directly associated with fractures are the associated injuries that may be **occult.** Despite a thorough evaluation, these injuries are either missed or not appreciated on initial examination and can be life-threatening. History, physical exam, mechanism of injury, reevaluation, and a high index of suspicion for potentially life- or limb-threatening associated injuries are the keys to trauma care and assessing musculoskeletal injuries. Listed in Table 24-3 are some commonly encountered associated or occult injuries.[2] DOT 4-9.9

Special Considerations

Pediatric Musculoskeletal Injuries

Children proportionally have a greater percentage of cartilage than adults, and their bones are continuously growing (lengthening) at the epiphyseal plates. This flexibility of a child's bone leads to the greater likelihood that children will sustain **greenstick fractures,** partial fractures where there is disruption of a portion of a long bone. In a greenstick fracture, the fractured side can become the site of more rapid growth. Therefore, there is angulation or distortion of the disrupted bone fibers. Luckily, the periosteum of bone is much thicker in children, and its blood supply is plentiful. Children often heal well and rarely require physical therapy. These conditions make initial displacement of the fracture less concerning to the medical provider, allowing for easier closed reductions (nonoperative fracture reduction) and rendering complications uncommon.[14]

CONNECTIONS For more information on pediatric injuries and considerations see Chapter 43: Pediatric Patients.

Geriatric Musculoskeletal Injuries

There are several significant changes associated with aging that put older patients at greater risk of musculoskeletal injuries. There is a progressive decline in both bone mass and strength beginning around age forty years. This leads to more porous, brittle bones and an increased risk for fracture. Weak areas, and consequently common sites of fractures, are the vertebrae, the proximal femur neck, shoulder, and distal radius and wrist. The elderly are also at higher risk for injury because of decrease in muscle strength, coordination, posture, and overall flexibility. DOT 4-9.16

The water content of intervertebral disks decreases with age, resulting in an increased risk of disk herniation and chronic back pain. This is a very common problem that results in a significant loss of productivity and quality of life. Other changes associated with increasing age are a loss of one-half to three-quarters of an inch in stature as the trunk shortens from bone tissue disorders, a gradual arching of the vertebral column, and the ossification of the costal cartilages, making the thorax more rigid and breathing more shallow.

CONNECTIONS   For more information on geriatric injuries go to Chapter 44: Geriatric Patients.

Scene Size-Up

Mechanism of Injury

The mechanism by which an injury occurs may help to predict the type of injury produced. Clear, accurate communication and documentation is critical in conveying injury mechanisms to the hospital staff. If done properly, it can increase the likelihood of discovering occult injuries. For instance, in the case of a motor vehicle crash, the speed and damage to the vehicles, scene fatalities and injuries, and position in which each victim was found should be noted and communicated to the trauma team receiving the patient. Falls require documentation of the height from which the patient fell, the surface landed upon, and the position the patient landed in, as there is a common association of calcaneal fractures, femur and hip injuries, and lumbar spine fractures in these patients. In any injury not consistent with the history, one should consider abuse or other underlying medical conditions.

Penetrating injuries increase the risk of infection, surrounding soft tissue injury, hemorrhage, neurovascular injury, and hemodynamic instability. If a foreign body is impaled, it requires stabilization to prevent damage to neighboring tissues. DOT 4-9.5

Nice to Know

Though some studies have shown that there is little association between mechanism and severity of injury, mechanism of injury can still be used to help predict occult injuries as well as loosely estimate injury severity.[15] Additional concern for injury should always exist in patients with comorbid disease or extremes of age. Substantial injuries in these patients often result from seemingly insignificant mechanisms.

Sports-Related Injuries

Athletic activities are a common source of musculoskeletal injuries. This is especially true of football, soccer, basketball, in-line skating, skiing or snow boarding, wrestling, and rock climbing. These injuries often involve the shoulder, elbow, wrist, clavicle, knee, ankle, foot, or tibia and fibula. In order for these patients to regain normal use of their extremities, the injuries require immediate recognition and treatment. Do not allow an athlete to continue to play on an injured extremity. This places undue stress on it and can lead to even more damage or disability. Have the player rest the injury while a thorough physical exam is conducted. Ice and elevate the injured part to help decrease swelling. After the first 24 hours, the patient may be instructed to alternately apply heat and cold to help increase perfusion to the injured area and speed healing. DOT 4-9.14, 4-9.15

Street Secrets

As a paramedic, you will routinely be called to stand by or respond to sports venues. Often, players, coaches, parents, and athletic trainers are present and may try to influence the patient's decision to continue to play, rest, or accept care and transportation. While those competing interests may complicate your management of these scenes, your responsibility to the patient remains the most important guiding factor in your recommendations and care. Remove the patient from the field of play while you make your assessment, and encourage the game to continue without the injured player. Giving the patient some space and time and letting the coaches and other parties focus on the game will help you make a better unbiased assessment. It is also common to treat underage patients in sports venues. Attempt to reach the parents to obtain consent for treatment and to help guide care and transportation decisions.

Primary Survey

During the initial approach to the patient, do not be distracted by gross musculoskeletal deformities. While these may appear severe and in need of immediate attention, they can easily lead to skipping initial assessments and missing nonobvious, potentially life-threatening injuries. To ensure an optimal outcome, patients with obvious musculoskeletal trauma first require attention to the primary survey and then stabilization of the musculoskeletal system.[16] DOT 4-9.11, 4-9.12

In an organized and efficient manner, evaluate the mechanism of injury. If appropriate, manually stabilize the cervical spine and assess the patient's level of consciousness. The patient's airway, breathing, and circulation take precedence. Address any problems identified during the primary survey with airway adjuncts, oxygen therapy, and resuscitation, if needed. It is important to support the patient's cardiac and respiratory functions while assessing the neurologic status. DOT 4-9.37

Street Secrets

Evaluating the patient's pulses has been considered an aid in rapidly estimating a blood pressure. The presence of a palpable radial pulse indicates that the systolic blood pressure is likely above 80 mmHg; a femoral pulse indicates a blood pressure above 70 mmHg; a carotid pulse, the last pulse lost in hypotension, indicates a blood pressure of at least 60 mmHg. There is little evidence to support these estimates. Blood pressure should always be formally measured.

Do not overlook life- or limb-threatening musculoskeletal trauma, but do not allow a gross but noncritical musculoskeletal injury to distract attention from the comprehensive assessment and stabilization of the patient. To control bleeding in a fractured extremity, apply direct pressure where needed. Always return to the primary survey, and reassess vital signs whenever there is any change in the patient's status.[17] Definitive care for the traumatized patient happens in the hospital. Field management is directed at the rapid transport and delivery of a viable patient.

Appropriate out-of-hospital treatment in life-threatening trauma situations consists of a rapid primary survey, airway and cervical spine control, appropriate respiratory and cardiovascular assistance, the application of a long rigid spine board for whole body fracture stabilization, and immediate transport. For less severely injured patients, complete the primary survey and a full secondary survey as appropriate. Immobilization of injured extremities, as well as administration of appropriate pain management should be completed if time permits. Continue monitoring and reevaluating to prevent overlooking important findings or changes in the patient's status. DOT 4-9.40

Secondary Survey

After completion of the primary survey, address the secondary survey. Evaluate each body system in an organized manner from head to toe. Practicing and performing it in the same fashion each time will help to prevent missed injuries. Careful inspection and palpation may reveal signs common to extremity trauma.

The DCAP-BTLS acronym may be helpful in remembering key elements of assessment in musculoskeletal injuries:

D Deformity
C Contusions
A Abrasions
P Penetrations or punctures

B Burns
T Tenderness
L Lacerations
S Swelling

In addition to the DCAP-BTLS signs, look for crepitus, pain on palpation or movement, decreased range of motion, false movement (unnatural movement of an extremity), and decreased or absent sensory perception or circulation distal to the injury. Communicate effectively with your patient, and explain any splinting procedures before you perform them. DOT 4-9.6, 4-9.8

When conducting a physical exam, note the position in which the patient was found and his or her surroundings. Note the surface the patient is lying on and, if appropriate, the height he or she fell from. Be aware of abnormal skin color changes (e.g., cyanosis or pallor), bleeding (quantify amount), and obvious deformities or dislocations. Compare the injured extremity to the unaffected extremity, noting any differences in pulse, motor or sensory, guarding or self-splinting by the patient.

Evaluation of limb injury for compartment syndrome includes assessment for the following:

Pain on passive movement or palpation (tenderness)—usually the first sign
Pallor of skin (or poor capillary refill or poikilothermia [coolness])
Paresthesia—sensation of pins and needles
Paralysis—loss of motor function, a late and ominous sign
Pulselessness—diminished or absent DOT 4-9.7

Palpate the bony structures, and test for abnormal (reduced or increased) range of motion. Perform sensory and motor testing, and check for pulses both before and after any significant movement or immobilizing because even minor positional changes can result in loss of neurologic or vascular function (Figure 24-12). Use the findings of a thorough assessment to formulate a working assessment, and develop a treatment plan. This may include immobilizing the suspected injury with the appropriate splint. DOT 4-9.41

The basis for identification of musculoskeletal injuries is history, mechanism of injury, and assessment findings. From this information, a field impression can be generated and a plan developed for specific management. For instance, findings of a shortened, externally rotated extremity in an elderly female after a fall may indicate a

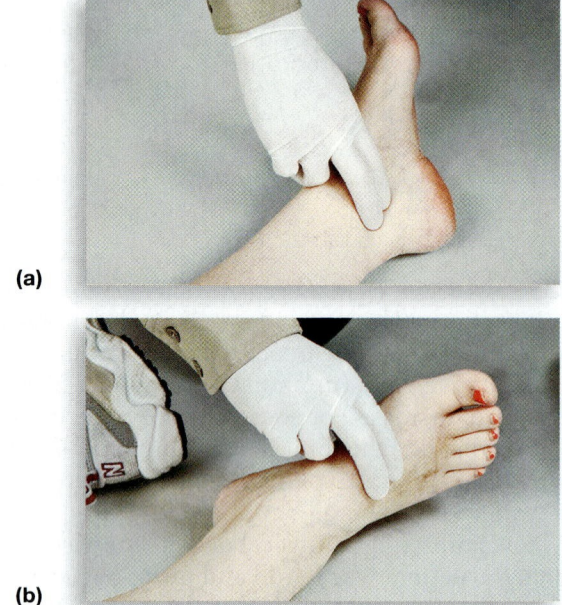

(a)

(b)

Figure 24-12   (a) In any fracture, pulses should be checked on initial exam and again after any significant movement, distal to the injury (b).

femur fracture at the hip. Depending on her vital signs, the paramedic provider may decide that IV fluid administration and splinting with sufficient analgesia is indicated, followed by transport to an emergency department for definitive care. DOT 4-9.20, 9.38, 9.39

Pain Management

The concept of pain management has taken on increasing importance for paramedics and out-of-hospital providers. Previously reserved for patients with chest pain associated with acute coronary syndromes and burn victims, pain management for musculoskeletal injuries and fractures is now a routine part of out-of-hospital care. Although the best pain management is achieved with immobilization, splinting, and ice, serious injuries may require the use of opioid analgesics or other pain medications. This is especially true if you have to move or extricate the patient. DOT 4-9.42

A significant percentage of patients do not receive appropriate analgesia in the out-of-hospital setting, and there is a lack of standard analgesia protocols for EMS systems.[18] One study suggested that younger age was a positive predictor for receiving analgesia, despite injury severity in the elderly. Additionally, the study suggested that patients who receive analgesia from EMS providers receive this medication an average of two hours earlier than patients who do not get it in the field.[18] Inadequate analgesia administration has also been reported in emergency departments in general.[19]

A dose of pain medication is appropriate in the right setting. Patients receiving pain medication can be closely monitored, and some medications (such as opiates) have an antidote (naloxone), which can reverse the medication if the patient has a negative reaction to it. Appropriately used, analgesia should be a part of routine care by EMS just like monitoring vital signs and transporting.

CONNECTIONS One of the most powerful weapons in the paramedic's arsenal against pain and fear is the ability to project a sense of calm and communicate in a therapeutic manner. Review some strategies for putting patients at ease in Chapter 10: Therapeutic Communications and History Taking. You can have a significant impact on a patient's emotional response to a traumatic event by simply de-escalating the scene and forming a trusting and caring bond. Remain compassionate, explain as much as possible to the patient, and be reassuring.[14]

Pain scales are often used to measure the effectiveness of the interventions being performed. Ask the patient to rate their pain on a scale from zero to ten. Zero represents no pain, and ten is the worst possible pain the patient has experienced.[7] In this fashion, the patient's response to the analgesic and ongoing level of pain can be better quantified. See Drug Box 24-1 for more information on medications used for pain management for musculoskeletal injuries.

Opiate analgesics are considered the mainstay of therapy. The most commonly prescribed opioid analgesics are morphine and fentanyl. At their appropriate dosing, both have been shown to be highly effective with a minimal side effect profile. Nitrous oxide and benzodiazepines have also been shown to be useful.[2]

The paramedic must rely on patient perception and also use sound clinical judgment to determine the severity of a patient's pain and the most appropriate way to treat it. Although intra-muscular injection is an acceptable administration route, the medications will be effective more quickly if administered intravenously.[7]

Side effects may include pruritus (itching), hypoventilation, hypotension, or nausea. Morphine is relatively inexpensive, can be titrated to effect, and is longer acting than fentanyl. Fentanyl has been slower to gain acceptance than morphine. Reasons include its higher abuse potential by those with access, a common concern of EMS system medical directors, and the fact that it is shorter acting than morphine. This may be advantageous for services with shorter hospital transport times, such as urban EMS systems or aeromedical services. In addition, one advantage to the use of fentanyl over morphine is that it has a much faster onset of action.

Drug Box 24-1

Medication	Trade name	Class	Half-Life	Routes of administration	Precautions
Morphine	Morphone	Opiate	2–4 hours	PO, IM, IV, SC	• Respiratory depression • Hypotension • Histamine release
Hydromorphone	Dilaudid	Synthetic narcotic	2.6 hours	IV	• Euphoria
Fentanyl	Sublimaze	Phenylpiperidine	1–2 hours	IV	• Truncal rigidity in higher doses
Midazolam	Versed	Benzodiazepine	2.5 hours	PO, IM, IV	• Caution in hypotension
Nalbuphine	Nubain	Synthetic Opiate	5 hours	SC, IM, IV	• Respiratory depression
Nitrous Oxide	Nitronox			Self-Administered Inhaled	• May worsen a pneumothorax or bowel obstruction

Sources: Marx, Rosen's *Emergency Medicine*, 5th ed., Epocrates.com, Physician Drug Reference.

While other choices of opioids, such as meperidine, are available, their side effect profile and potential for abuse are much greater, making them less desirable. Ketorolac, an IV or IM, nonsteroidal antiinflammatory agent, is not as rapid acting as the opioid analgesics, and some orthopedic surgeons do not use it because it has been shown to inhibit bone healing.

Nitronox, which has been used by many EMS systems over the years, is an alternative to opioid analgesia. A premixed combination of oxygen and nitrous oxide, Nitronox, has a fast onset of action, has a short duration of action, and is a combined analgesic and sedative. Nitronox may be desirable in cases where the paramedic does not want to mask the possibility of other distracting trauma from the physician. Nitronox can cause nausea and vomiting and requires patient cooperation in order to self administer the medication via a positive pressure oxygen system. It cannot be used for patients with alteration in mental status, with head injury, or with underlying pulmonary problems or pneumothorax.

Although not directly indicated for the management of pain, benzodiazepines, especially diazepam and midazolam, could be helpful. Benzodiazepines have a relatively safe side effect profile and are among the most effective muscle relaxants available. These are beneficial when treating muscle spasm, as well as helping to provide sedation for fracture and dislocation reduction.

Review your system's protocols for specific medications carried and their indications and dosing.

Management of Fractures

Consider any soft tissue wound next to or near a suspected fracture to be evidence of an open fracture. Open fractures have significant potential for infection, which can cause delays in healing. The manipulation of open fractures should be limited only to what is necessary to relieve neurovascular impairment or to achieve hemorrhage control. There is evidence that the infection rate of open fractures is four times lower in patients that had a sterile dressing applied at the accident scene until the time of wound exploration in the sterile operating room.[20] Of special note are fractures of the tibial shaft, which have the highest rate of infection of all open fractures.[12] DOT 4-9.17

General Fracture Care and Splinting

Splints are an integral and invaluable part of out-of-hospital care of fractures. Providers need to be comfortable with their use. An understanding of the basic principles of proper splinting will help you adapt your care according to the special needs of various situations. This is one area of medicine in which creativity and resourcefulness are very helpful. A paramedic with a bit of imagination should be able to construct whatever type of splint that a patient may require. DOT 4-9.12, 4-9.25

The mainstay of field treatment for musculoskeletal injuries of all types includes controlling external hemorrhage with direct pressure, stabilization, elevation of the affected part above the level of the heart (if appropriate), immobilization, reassessment of pulse, motor and sensory, and sufficient analgesia until transfer to the hospital can occur. It is generally best to immobilize injured joints, and for that matter even significantly angulated fractures, in the position they are found so as not to cause further damage and then to transport the patient to the emergency department for realignment and reduction.

Street Secrets

The rigid long backboard can be used as a "whole body splint" for patients with multiple fractures whose condition does not allow for the application of a splint to each potential fracture site. If this is done, make sure each extremity has an adequate amount of padding applied to prevent movement during transport. Also, consider applying a blanket directly to the long board to provide some additional padding.

Because of the very real potential for an injury to worsen after manipulation, attempt realignment only in the presence of an absent distal pulse or if delayed or prolonged transport is expected. Limb-threatening injuries that require transport for emergent physician evaluation are posterior knee dislocations, dislocations of the ankle, and subcondylar fractures of the elbow. Due to a high risk of complications, never attempt elbow manipulation in the out-of-hospital setting.

Immobilize dislocations in the position found or the position of comfort to ensure good vascular supply and pain reduction. To alleviate swelling, elevate and apply cold packs to the extremity, if possible. The application of cold packs helps to decrease inflammation in the area of injury thereby decreasing swelling and subsequent pain. DOT 4-9.14

Street Secrets

Never apply an ice pack directly to the skin. Always place a cloth between the skin and the ice pack to prevent cold injury from occurring to the skin. Do not place an ice pack directly into the bandage that is wrapped around the wound or fracture site, as this will be difficult to remove later and doing so will compromise the integrity of the dressing or result in excessive manipulation of the splint.

Splint the joints above and below the area of injury to provide the best possible stabilization and limitation of movement (Figure 24-13). Some specific types of fractures, described later in this chapter, have joint injuries or additional fractures that commonly accompany them. The immobilization of open fractures and closed fractures is the same procedure except that open fractures are also covered with a sterile dressing to minimize contamination.

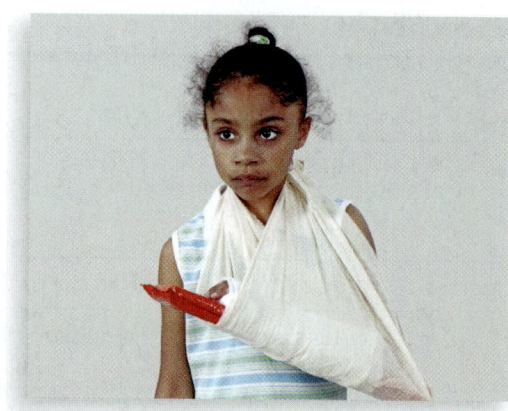

Figure 24-13   Immobilizing joint injuries to include the bone above and the bone below the joint protects the joint from further injury.

Two or more rescuers should stabilize and immobilize injured joints and fracture sites. One rescuer should stabilize the injured part while the other assesses the initial neurologic (sensation and motor) and vascular status. The team can then apply gentle in-line traction to achieve normal anatomical alignment. If resistance is encountered, stop immediately and do not attempt the reduction again. Pain should decrease greatly with proper realignment or reduction. Any increase or excessive pain during the procedure is often indicative of tissue pressure or ischemia and requires urgent correction.[8] Neurovascular deficits and compartment syndrome are possible with any fracture or dislocation and can occur after splinting; therefore, reassess sensation, motor function, and distal pulses before and after any manipulations or patient movement. DOT 4-9.10, 4-9.13

Angled fractures and dislocations may pose significant problems with splinting, patient extrication, and transportation. Consultation with medical control may be warranted before manipulation of these types of injuries.

Types of Splints

As long as the general rules of splinting are met, splinting devices are limited only by the paramedic's imagination and the budget of the department you work for. Typical splints are summarized in Table 24-4. This list is not comprehensive and is meant only to provide examples of some typical devices. The table is divided into five types of splints: rigid, semirigid, soft, pneumatic, and traction.

Some serious musculoskeletal injuries preclude conventional splinting devices. Cravats (e.g., triangular bandages), Velcro™ straps, bandages, and immobilization of the patient on a long spine board may be considered as alternatives.

Traction Splints

There are two types of traction splints, a bipolar frame device and a unipolar frame device. The bipolar

TABLE 24-4   Types of Splinting Devices

Type of splint	Examples	Advantages	Precautions
Rigid	Board splints	Cost effective	Must be padded
Semirigid	Ladder splints Metal sheet splint SAM® splint	Can be shaped to angulations	May not provide enough support
Soft	Pillows, blankets slings, swathe	Cost effective, easily available, produce less pressure	
Pneumatic	Air splints Vacuum splints	See-through, allows for x-ray without removal, lightweight	Must be stored flat, changes in air temperature and atmospheric pressure (such as altitude) can cause splint to overly constrict or lose support
Traction	Hare splints Sager splints	Provide traction, reduce pain, improve circulation	Traction must be maintained, splints should be in good working condition

(Thomas™ or Hare™) traction splint cradles the leg and elevates it off the ground. It uses lengthening shafts to pull a foot and ankle harness against pressure that is applied to the crease of the buttock (Figure 24-14). The unipolar (Sager™) splint does not elevate or stabilize the extremity as does the bipolar traction splint, so one must be careful when moving the patient once it is applied. The Sager™ is designed to be able to pull traction on both legs simultaneously, so a single device can be used if bilateral femur fractures are suspected (Figure 24-15).

Though traction splinting is the best method to care for a hemodynamically stable patient with an isolated midshaft femur fracture, it may not be indi-

cated if the patient also has other serious injuries of the knee, leg, ankle, or foot that preclude harness placement. Open femur fractures may be a contraindication to traction splinting in your jurisdiction, and local protocols should be followed.

A pelvic or hip fracture in conjunction with a femur fracture (in any location on the femur), or a hip dislocation, is a contraindication to using a traction splint of any type. The splint can apply pressure to the fractured pelvis or hip, causing further bone displacement and hemorrhage. The padded proximal end of the Hare splint abuts the ischial tuberosity. The proximal end of the Sager splint rests against the pubic symphysis. These splints cannot be used if a pelvic fracture is suspected because the pressure on the pelvis may further displace a fracture and cause more bleeding.[2]

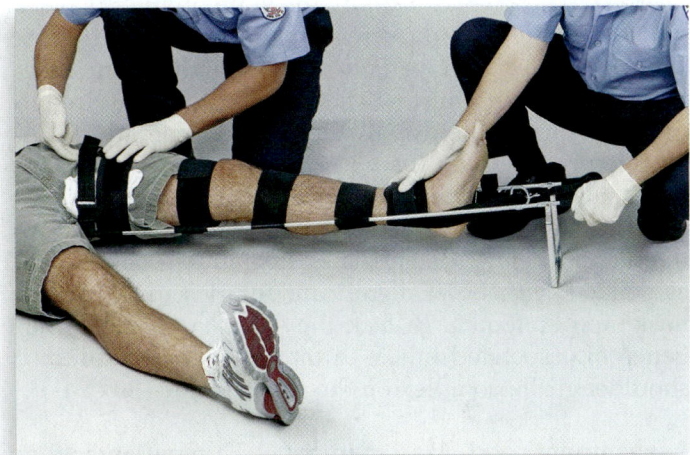

Figure 24-14   Mid-shaft femur fractures are treated with traction splinting to secure the bone ends and prevent further injury caused by motion of the bone ends. Hare™ type or bipolar traction devices are one way of accomplishing this.

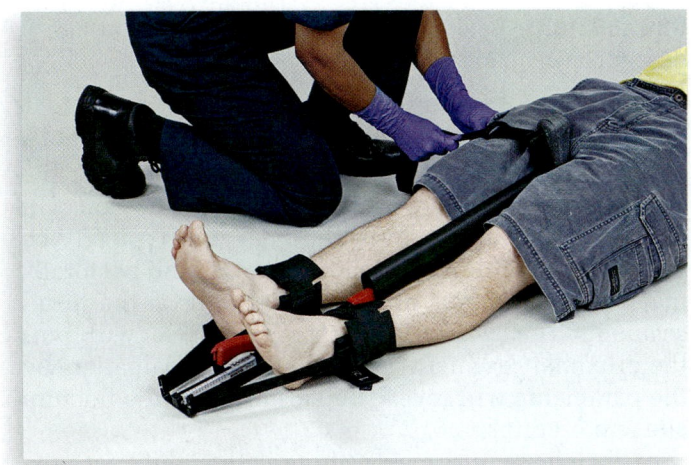

Figure 24-15   Monopolar devices like the Sager™ splint can also be used to stabilize midshaft femur fractures.

Management of Specific Injuries by Location

Upper Extremity

The shoulder girdle serves to attach the arms to the axial skeleton and is the place of attachment for muscles of the arm and chest. Each pectoral girdle has two bones—the clavicle and scapula. Injuries to this girdle frequently result from a fall on an outstretched arm and are common in older adults because of their weaker bone structure.

Clavicle Injuries

The clavicle is the most frequently fractured bone in the body. It is responsible for 87% of all shoulder injuries in zero to fourteen-year-olds and 37% of adults, with an incidence of 198 per 100,000.[21] It is a long, slender, s-shaped bone that lies horizontally just beneath the skin, acting as a brace that holds the upper limbs away from the trunk.

The clavicle serves to transmit forces from the upper limbs to the axial skeleton while providing an attachment site for muscles of the neck, thorax, back, and arm. In addition to falls, fractures can also occur from a direct blow such as that occurring in contact sports. Associated injuries include brachial plexus palsy, vascular injury, rib fracture, and pneumothorax.

There are three types of clavicle fractures; middle third (midshaft) is the most common, then lateral third and medial third. Fractures of the proximal third result from direct blows to the anterior chest and only account for 5% of injuries. Fractures of the middle third account for 80% of injuries and are usually due to indirect forces. Fractures of the distal third account for 15% of injuries and occur because of direct blows to the top of the shoulder. These may be difficult to distinguish from AC dislocations.

CONNECTIONS Refer to Chapter 21: Thoracic Trauma for a description of rib fractures and chest wall injuries.

Assessment and Management. The patient with a clavicular fracture usually complains of pain over the fracture site and holds the arm close to the body. In middle third fractures, the shoulder will typically be slumped forward, down, and inward as the pectoralis major and latissimus dorsi muscles pull on the distal segment. The sternocleidomastoid muscle will pull the proximal fragment upward. Careful palpation by the paramedic will reveal a deformity over the fracture site and crepitus.

Clavicle fractures, even those with significant misalignment, heal well. A simple sling is the preferred treatment.[22] A sling and swathe or the Velpeau bandage

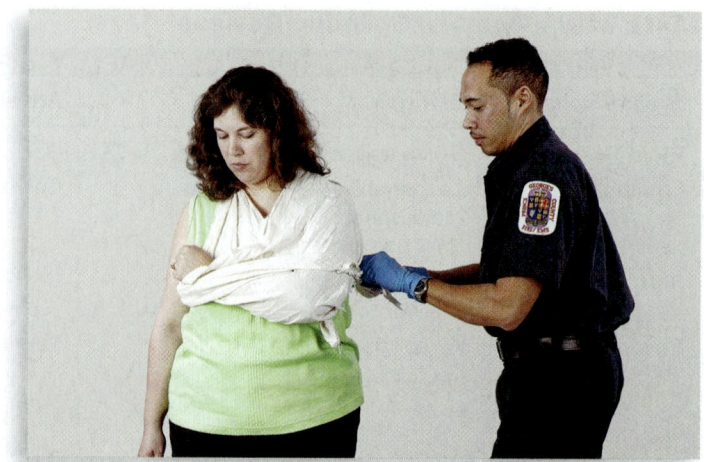

Figure 24-16 Shoulder and clavicular fractures can be controlled with sling and swathe immobilization.

may provide additional comfort for some patients during the first few days of treatment. Caution is encouraged when fractures involve the distal third of the clavicle (Figure 24-16).

Complications. Complications of middle third clavicular fractures are very rare. However, the impact needed to produce distal fractures may drive the clavicle into the thorax, producing rib fractures, pneumothorax, and other internal injuries. If the articular surface is injured, there can be chronic pain due to arthritic changes.

Scapula Injuries

The scapula is a flat, triangular bone that forms the posterior part of the shoulder girdle. The body, spine, and coracoid and acromial processes of the scapula provide attachment sites for numerous muscles and ligaments. Scapular fractures, especially those involving the body or spine of the scapula, result from high-energy trauma such as high-speed vehicle crashes, falls from great heights, or crush injuries. The extreme force required to produce them explains why they account for only 1% of all fractures and less than 5% of all shoulder girdle injuries, having a low incidence of 12 per 100,000 cases.[23] Because of the amount of force required to fracture the scapula, early diagnosis is essential because it is associated with other significant injuries to the chest, neck, and abdomen. In fact, they have a 75–98% incidence of associated injury to the lung, chest wall, and shoulder girdle complex on the affected side (Box 24-1).

Assessment and Management. The patient often presents with the shoulder adducted and the arm held closely to the body. Any movement will cause significant pain. Tenderness, crepitus, or hematoma may be palpable over the fracture site. Once stabilized, treat

BOX 24-1   Injuries Associated with Scapula Fractures

- Rib fractures
- Pulmonary contusion
- Pneumothorax
- Clavicle fracture
- Brachial plexus injury
- Vascular injury (subclavian or axillary vessels)

the patient with appropriate pain medications and ice and support the involved extremity with sling and swath immobilization.

Shoulder Fractures and Dislocations

The glenoid fossa, more commonly referred to as the shoulder socket, is a depression in the scapula that receives the head of the humerus to form the shoulder joint and allows rotation of the arm at the shoulder. When the head of the humerus is displaced away from the glenoid fossa, the patient has sustained a shoulder dislocation.

The glenohumoral (shoulder) joint is the most common dislocation injury.

Dislocations are typically related to overhead trauma when the arm is abducted, extended, and externally rotated. Anterior shoulder dislocation is the most common dislocation. Posterior dislocation can also occur, but it is more rare, which is fortunate, because it is reported that as many as 60% of posterior dislocations are misdiagnosed.[12] Acromioclavicular dislocation is usually caused by a fall on to an outstretched hand. DOT 4-9.24

Sternoclavicular joint dislocation is rare. The mechanism is usually an MVC or sporting injury. Dislocation of the sternoclavicular joint in children is often associated with a fracture.

In anterior fractures or dislocations of the shoulder, the patient often holds the affected arm close to the chest. The lateral aspect of the shoulder appears flat instead of rounded, and a deep depression can be noted between the head of the humerus and the acromion, laterally; this has been coined a "hollow shoulder" and is the empty glenoid fossa. Rotator cuff tears and impingement are common sources for shoulder pain. Patients present with pain and weakness related to attempted active movements with the arm. Posterior dislocations occur in less than 2% of cases.[24]

Shoulder Realignment.   Shoulder realignment generally should be performed by a trained physician. The paramedic may encounter patients who have a chronic reoccurrence of this condition and may request immediate assistance or may even be capable of reducing their own dislocation. There is no evidence to support paramedic field reduction. In most cases, an x-ray is required to rule out complicating fractures. A careful exam for potential neurological and vascular injury is also required. In some cases, such as wilderness areas, off-shore oil platforms, or other remote locations where a paramedic may be stationed, a medical director may elect to train a paramedic to perform shoulder reductions. Many reduction techniques have been described with each reporting similar success rates ranging from 70–96%.[24] DOT 4-9.27

If there are no severe distracting injuries, physician attempts at realigning the displaced shoulder should occur as soon as possible. This is especially true in cases of neurovascular compromise. An analgesic and muscle relaxant are warranted to decrease pain and increase the ease of realignment.

Humeral Fractures

The humerus is the longest and largest bone of the upper extremity. It provides an attachment for many important muscle groups, such as the rotator cuff, that help to stabilize the humeral head within the glenohumeral joint. Most fractures result from direct trauma. These injuries can also result from a direct blow to the lateral aspect of the arm.

Fractures of the proximal humerus occur most often in elderly individuals with osteoporosis. This group is also at risk for neurovascular injuries and rotator cuff tears. The weakened bones and frequency of falls in this group also predispose them to hip fractures. It is always important to determine if the incident was precipitated by a syncopal episode, myocardial infarction, stroke, transient ischemic attack, or seizure.

Fractures of the humerus account for 4–5% of all fractures, with an incidence of 114 per 100,000 at a mean age of 67 years.[25] Children and older, osteopenic patients (females by a 3:1 ratio) often sustain them after a fall onto an outstretched, abducted arm. Older patients are more prone to fracture while younger patients may dislocate or fracture. Middle-aged patients may sustain a combination fracture-dislocation.

Assessment and Management.   These patients present with the arm held close to the body with motion restricted due to pain. Tenderness, ecchymosis, deformity, crepitus, and hematoma are noted over the site of the fracture.

The humerus is often difficult to stabilize and has the potential for severe vascular complications. Therefore, it is important to assess the patient's neurovascular status. If there is any evidence of vascular compromise, provide immediate gentle traction, and apply a rigid splint with a sling and swathe or splint the arm in extension (straight). If there is a potential neck injury, avoid tying a sling around the neck. Apply cold packs to decrease swelling, and provide analgesic medication for pain.

Elbow Injuries

The elbow acts like a hinge joint, allowing the forearm to flex and extend. It consists of three major bones, arteries, nerves, and 22 muscles. Elbow fractures are common in athletes and children, in which they are especially dangerous; they have the potential to result in ischemic contractures with serious deformity of the forearm and a claw-like hand. The usual mechanism of injury for elbow fractures in children is forced hyperextension such as with a **F**all **O**n an **O**ut**S**tretched **H**and **(FOOSH)** or a flexed elbow.

The elbow is the second most commonly dislocated joint in the adult.

Posterior elbow dislocation is by far the most common type of elbow dislocation. Anterior, medial, and lateral elbow dislocations are relatively rare. Dislocation occurs from an axial force applied to the extended elbow. The extremity may appear to be shortened and the elbow flexed. Both collateral ligaments are also disrupted in this injury. Elbow injuries have a higher probability for vascular and nerve damage. Associated complications include laceration of the brachial artery and damage to the radial nerve. DOT 4-9.24

Assessment and Management. Immediately assess the neurovascular status of the extremity. Pay special attention to the brachial artery and function of the radial nerve. Splint the extremity in the position found with a pillow, rigid or padded wire splint, and sling and swathe (Figure 24-17). Reduction of the joint injury should occur in the emergency department or trauma center.

Injuries to the Radius, Ulna, and Wrist

Similar to the pelvis, the anatomy of the forearm should be thought of as a closed ring. This ring is comprised of the radius and ulna and the proximal (wrist) and distal (elbow) joints. A flexible, interosseous membrane connects the radius and ulna, the two bones of the forearm that articulate to form a pivot joint. In conjunction with the pronator and supinator muscles, they allow the palm to turn up (supination) and down (pronation). When the palm is facing up, the radius and ulna are parallel to one another, but when the palm is down, the two bones cross. The radius is located on the thumb side of the forearm when the palm is facing forward. It is shorter than, lateral to, and rotates around the fixed ulna. The ulna is the longer of the two forearm bones and is lo-

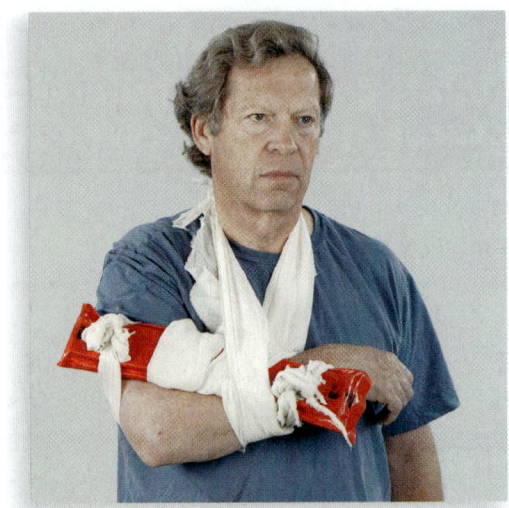

Figure 24-17 Elbow injuries are splinted with padded splints maintaining the elbow in a 90-degree angle unless the angulation prevents this positioning.

cated on the small finger side of the forearm. It is relatively straight and is medial to the radius.

Since these bones work together as a unit, a fracture of one is usually associated with a fracture or dislocation of the other. Fractures of both forearm bones or one bone with a concomitant joint injury are more common than a fracture of either bone by itself. When found, isolated fractures of either bone are typically caused by a focal impact, such as a nightstick injury. Forearm or wrist injuries are common in both children and adults and usually result from a fall on an outstretched arm. Wrist injuries may involve the distal radius, ulna, or any of the eight carpal bones.

Remember that because of the "ring" structure, there is a possibility for more than one fracture site. One consistent combination is a fracture of the ulna shaft and associated dislocation of the proximal radioulnar joint, and another is a fracture of the distal radius with associated distal ulna dislocation. These patients present with an ulnar styloid that is very prominent and tender.

Assessment and Management. As with all extremity injuries, careful assessment of the neurovascular status should be performed before and after any, even minor, manipulation. Splint the arm and wrist with rigid or formable splints in the position found, and apply a sling and swathe. Apply cold packs and elevate the extremity while en route to the emergency department. Most carpal (wrist) fractures occur in the proximal carpal row adjacent to the radius and ulna. The scaphoid carpal bone is the most commonly fractured wrist bone.

Splinting of the hand should include slight wrist extension with the metacarpophalangeal (MP) joints flexed 60 to 90 degrees and the finger joints extended.[12] This position is often referred to as the "position of function" and is important if the splint will remain in place for an extended period of time (four to six or more hours). Compartment syndrome is a possible complication of forearm injuries, so reassess for pain and pulse, motor, and sensation often.

Hand (Metacarpal) Injuries

Metacarpal injuries frequently result from direct trauma during contact sports, violence (fighting), and industrial accidents or crush injuries. A common injury is a boxer's fracture, which results from direct trauma to a closed fist, fracturing the fifth metacarpal bone. These fractures may be associated with large hematomas and open wounds and often have a noticeable deformity with significant pain. They also have a high incidence of nerve and small vessel damage.

Assessment and Management. Assess neurovascular status, splint with rigid or formable padded board splint in position of function, elevate the extremity, and apply a cold pack.

Finger (Phalangeal) Injuries

Finger injuries are common and should not be considered trivial. Serious injuries include thumb metacarpal fractures, any open fracture, or a markedly comminuted metacarpal or proximal phalanx fracture. There are many small, contained spaces in the fingers, leaving them very vulnerable to infection. Loss of hand and finger function can be devastating to daily life activities, causing severe morbidity.

Assessment and Management. Assess neurovascular status, splint with either soft or rigid splints, apply cold packs, and elevate the extremity. Taping the injured finger to an adjacent one ("buddy taping") is an alternative (Figure 24-18).

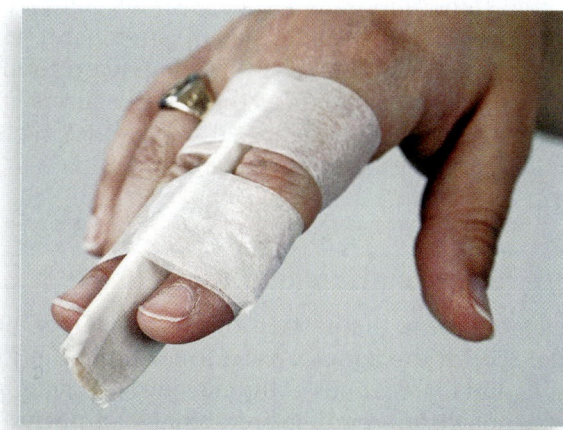

Figure 24-18 Anatomical splinting works best with finger injuries. "Buddy taping" the injured finger to an uninjured finger stabilizes the fracture effectively. (Any rings should be removed as early as possible as subsequent swelling may compromise distal blood flow.)

Finger Realignment. There is no indication for realignment of finger fractures or dislocations or, for that matter, of wrist injuries in the prehospital setting. Many times, the patient is realigned in order to provide a more normal anatomy for positioning on transportation devices. A knee or, to a lesser degree, an elbow injury may need repositioning through the hip or shoulder (hopefully the unaffected joints) in order to facilitate packaging for transport. This is not an issue for the hands and wrists or feet and ankles. The patient can be transported on any stretcher, orthopedic (scoop) stretcher, or long board immobilization device, regardless of the position of the hands or feet. A thin pillow or mound of trauma pads can serve as a soft splint in which to rest the injured hand during transport. DOT 4-9.27

Lower Extremity

Compared with upper-extremity injuries, lower-extremity injuries are associated with greater forces and more significant blood loss. They are more difficult to manage because the patient may present with multiple associated injuries. They are more likely to be life-threatening. The most worrisome injuries are femur fractures and pelvic fractures.

Injuries to the Pelvis

The pelvis is made up of three bones: two innominate bones and the sacrum and coccyx. The innominate bones are further subdivided into the ilium, ischium, and pubis. By the age of 16, the three distinct ossification centers of each innominate, the pubis, ischium and ilium, unite. DOT 4-8.25

The posterior portion of the pelvic ring, with the support of several ligaments, is responsible for most of the pelvis' stability. It transmits much of the force generated by weight bearing across the sacroiliac joint into the lower extremities, while the anteriorly situated pubic symphysis prevents collapse of the ring. Stability of the pelvic ring depends entirely on the strong ligaments that connect the innominate bones to the sacrum. Pelvic stability is defined as the ability of the pelvic ring to withstand physiologic forces without abnormal deformation. The pelvis is important for bearing the weight of the body, serving as the point of attachment for the legs, and protecting the organs in the pelvic cavity. DOT 4-8.25

The pelvic ring contains important genitourinary structures: the bladder, ureters, and urethra, the colon, the reproductive organs in women, and a fetus in a pregnant female, as well as the lumbosacral plexus, the internal and external iliac vessels, and their branches.

Pelvic fractures are among the most serious injuries and account for 3% of all fractures.

About 60% of pelvic fractures result from vehicle-related trauma (automobile, motorcycle, and bicycle),

30% from falls, and 10% from crush injuries, athletic injuries, or penetrating trauma. Pelvic fractures are the third most commonly seen injury in fatalities due to motor vehicle accidents. Complications of pelvic fractures include life-threatening hemorrhage, deformity, neurologic injury, and genitourinary injury. Over the years, mortality rates have varied from 9–20% in the 1970s to 6–10% in the 1980s. Although profound shock is an uncommon presentation early in the injury, patients with pelvic fractures who are hemodynamically unstable upon arrival at the hospital have mortality rates between 40–50%. The overall mortality rate for open pelvic fractures is as high as 50%, compared with 8–15% for closed fractures.[12] DOT 4-8.26

Hemorrhage is the leading cause of death in patients with pelvic fractures, accounting for 60% of all deaths.[21] Most of the blood loss is from the fracture site itself, but it can also be from injured vessels such as the retroperitoneal veins. Only 20% of pelvic fractures are associated with major arterial bleeding. There is a reported average blood replacement of 5.9 units per patient.[12] Retroperitoneal bleeding is unavoidable with a pelvic fracture, and up to six liters can be lost into the retroperitoneal space.[9] DOT 4-8.26

Pelvis Fracture Types

Although a number of classifications for pelvic fractures exist, their complexity and the lack of differences for immediate patient management concerns render them of little significance in the out-of-hospital setting. Still, the history obtained by the paramedic and knowing the mechanism of injury are instrumental in helping the trauma team and orthopedic surgeons predict injury patterns, injury severity, and morbidity or mortality.

The Young-Burgess classification system relates the type of pelvis fracture to the likely mechanism of injury. Lateral compression injuries are typically seen after a broadside motor vehicle collision. Anteroposterior compression fractures are most often noted after head-on crashes. Vertical shear fractures are commonly seen after falls from a height. Lateral compression injuries have the lowest mortality of approximately 13% whereas the other two classes have a mortality of approximately 25%.

Assessment and Management. Care of pelvic injuries centers around hemodynamic stabilization of the patient, securing the fractured pelvis, and rapid transport to a trauma center. Since massive blood loss is possible, two large bore IVs are required with the administration of lactated ringers or 0.9% normal saline administered to maintain a systolic blood pressure between 90–100 mmHg. In addition, provide the patient with high-concentration oxygen. DOT 4-8.28 4-9.11

Once the ABCs are established, evaluate the patient more thoroughly. Consider the possibility for pelvic fractures in all patients who are unconscious after trauma or who have pelvic complaints. On inspection, note bleeding, abrasions, contusions, and deformities. In some cases, deformity may be difficult to visualize, so suspect injury to the pelvis based on mechanism of injury and the presence of tenderness on palpation. Compress the pelvis lateral to medial by pushing inward on the sides of the iliac crests, anterior to posterior by pushing on the symphysis pubis, and anterior to posterior by pushing posteriorly on the iliac crests, and note the presence of pain and tenderness as well as the stability of the pelvic ring. Compression of the pelvis should always be performed gently and preferably only once as it will cause significant pain if a fracture is present. There is no good reason for every caregiver to repeatedly compress the pelvis to "confirm" what someone else has already found, while inflicting pain on the patient each time. Compress the greater trochanters, and determine the range of motion of the hips.[4] DOT 4-8.27

Be aware of characteristic signs that may be of value. These include **Destot's sign,** a superficial hematoma of the scrotum or perineum, blood at the urethral meatus representing urethral or bladder rupture, or rectal or vaginal bleeding from their being punctured by fragmented bone.

While controversial, application and inflation of the pneumatic anti-shock garment (PASG), as per local protocol, may be instituted as an air splint to stabilize the pelvis.[9] An alternative is to wrap and tie a bedsheet around the patient's pelvis in order to stabilize the pelvis or apply a commercial device used to compress and stabilize the pelvis. DOT 4-9.21

Patients with pelvic fractures also require full body immobilization on a long spine board, frequent monitoring of vital signs, and transport to a trauma center. Consider utilizing the orthopedic (scoop) stretcher to move the patient from the ground to the long board to minimize log-rolling movements as these will cause significant discomfort to a patient with a pelvic fracture, particularly if the fracture is unstable.

Hip Fractures and Dislocations

The acetabulum is the portion of the pelvic bone that articulates with the femoral head to form the hip joint. Fractures and dislocations of the acetabulum occur from direct trauma to the area or indirect axial loading through the lower limb. The position of the limb at the time of impact will determine the pattern of injury. Rotation, flexion, abduction, and adduction all affect the nature and location of the fracture. A comminuted fracture of the acetabulum is common.

Dislocation of the Hip.   Traumatic dislocation of the hip joint may occur with or without fracture of the acetabulum or the proximal end of the femur. It is common during the active years and is usually the result of severe trauma, unless there is preexisting disease of the femoral head, acetabulum, or neuromuscular system. DOT 4-9.24

- Posterior dislocation: The head of the femur is usually dislocated posterior to the acetabulum while the thigh is flexed. This can occur during a head-on motor vehicle crash when the driver's knee is driven violently against the dashboard. Significant clinical findings include shortening of the leg, adduction, flexion of the leg at the hip and knee, and internal rotation of the leg. Common complications are fracture of the acetabulum, injury to the sciatic nerve, and fracture of the head and shaft of the femur.

- Anterior dislocation: Anterior dislocation is rarer. It usually occurs when the hip is extended and externally rotated at the time of impact. Associated fractures of the acetabulum and femoral neck are rare. The classic presentation of this injury is a flexed hip, abducted and externally rotated.

Assessment and Management.   In addition to using a well-padded long spine board for comfort during transport, the affected extremity should be splinted with the hip and knee in slight flexion. Neurovascular status of the distal extremity and vital signs should be monitored frequently. Hip reduction is reserved for trained physicians and should be done emergently in the emergency department for patients with dislocations.

Femur Fractures

The femur is the longest and strongest bone in the body and requires considerable force to cause injury. It is divided into many parts including a head, neck (anatomical and surgical), intertrochanteric and subtrochanteric area, and mid-shaft, as well as the condylar and supracondylar parts. If displacement of the fractured bone ends has occurred, the extremity is usually externally rotated and shortened. The patient can often actively move the extremity. Fractures are classified as stable or unstable. Stable fractures include stress fractures and impacted fractures. Unstable fractures are usually displaced or comminuted and can be life-threatening events, particularly in older patients.

Patients with stable fractures may be able to walk with some pain and a limp.

No obvious shortening or deformity is apparent on physical exam with a stable fracture. DOT 4-9.22

Head and Neck Fractures.   Fracture of the femoral neck occurs most commonly in patients over age 50.

Proximal fractures, such as those of the femoral neck and intertrochanteric region, constitute over 90% of hip fractures and are often the result of minimal trauma. The typical clinical appearance is that of a leg that is shortened and externally rotated. A femoral neck fracture after trauma may occur in association with a midshaft femur fracture and, if overlooked, increases morbidity. Injury to the sciatic nerve, superficial femoral artery, and vein are not common with these fractures. Traction splints are contraindicated for use on these types of femur fractures.

Midshaft Fractures.   Fractures of the femoral shaft are relatively uncommon in the young and are usually due to high-energy trauma (motor vehicle crashes and automobile versus pedestrian collisions). Therefore, they often occur along with multiorgan injury as well as pelvis fracture or hip dislocation or fracture. They are a major cause of morbidity and mortality in patients with lower extremity injuries. Unfortunately, in children, these fractures are commonly associated with abuse.

Indirect, violent torsional stress is likely to cause spiral fractures that extend along the bone. Most are closed fractures, but some are open. Open fractures most often result from the bone protruding out from within. Extensive soft tissue damage, bleeding, and shock are commonly present. The most significant clinical features are severe pain in the thigh and deformity of the lower portion of the extremity. Several units of blood can be lost into the thigh with only moderate swelling apparent on exam.

Femoral shaft fractures are more common in the elderly due to age-related factors such as osteoporosis and malignancy causing pathological fracture through an area of bone with metastatic cancer. Any elderly patient presenting with a femoral shaft fracture should warrant a high index of suspicion and work up for a pathologic fracture.

Distal Femur Fractures.   Injuries to the distal femur, such as condylar and epicondylar fractures, very often involve adjacent nerves and the vasculature and are, therefore, important. They may involve the knee, so the use of a traction splint for this fracture is contraindicated.

Assessment and Management.   The powerful thigh muscles surrounding the femur spasm and contract, causing the fractured bone ends to override each other, which leads to significant pain and soft tissue trauma. Patients generally present with shortening of the injured limb and their foot turned outward in external rotation, with possible significant midthigh swelling from hemorrhage. Assess neurovascular status. However, resist attributing hemodynamic compromise solely to an isolated femur fracture because studies have shown that there is a lack of association between isolated femoral shaft fractures and hypotensive shock.[26,27] Maintain awareness for other sources of bleeding, especially with multisystem trauma. DOT 9.18, 9.22

Priority should be given to the ABCs and insuring hemodynamic stability. High-concentration oxygen should be started. Stabilize and immobilize the hip with blankets and cravats. Use a long back board or long padded board splints to stabilize a hip or femur fracture. Only apply a traction splint to a midshaft femur fracture. An orthopedic (scoop) stretcher is a helpful device to transition a supine patient from the ground to a long back board if the log-roll technique is not desirable. Monitor vital signs frequently, and reassess neurovascular status after every manipulation.

Street Secrets

Application of traction splints and other splints should not be performed on the scene if the patient is in obvious shock or has a life-threatening ABC complication that requires continuous attention. Use the long back board to move the patient to the ambulance where traction devices and other splints can be applied as time permits while en route to the trauma center.

Knee Injuries

The knee joint is comprised of the patella, the distal femur, the tibia, the fibula, and numerous soft tissues, ligaments, and tendons. Though it acts primarily as a hinge joint, providing flexion and extension, it also serves to allow slight lateral and medial rotation.

The knee is one of the most commonly injured joints in the body, especially with sports injuries (Figure 24-19). Annually, over one million patients present to the emergency department with complaints of acute knee injuries.[21] Fractures of the knee and fractures or dislocations of the patella commonly result from motor vehicle collisions, pedestrian accidents, contact sports, and falls on a flexed knee. Care must be taken with these injuries, as the popliteal artery is closely related to the knee joint. Vascular injury, particularly with posterior dislocations, is a dangerous complication of knee injuries.

Traumatic dislocation of the knee joint is uncommon and is caused by severe trauma. Do not confuse this injury with patella dislocation. Signs of neurovascular injury below the site of a knee dislocation are an indication for prompt reduction and anatomic realignment of the leg. In most cases of short transport time, the reduction should generally occur in the emergency department or trauma center; however, if transport is prolonged, realignment should be undertaken in the field with appropriate analgesia. Failure to recognize compromise of circulation to the lower leg will result in gangrene of the

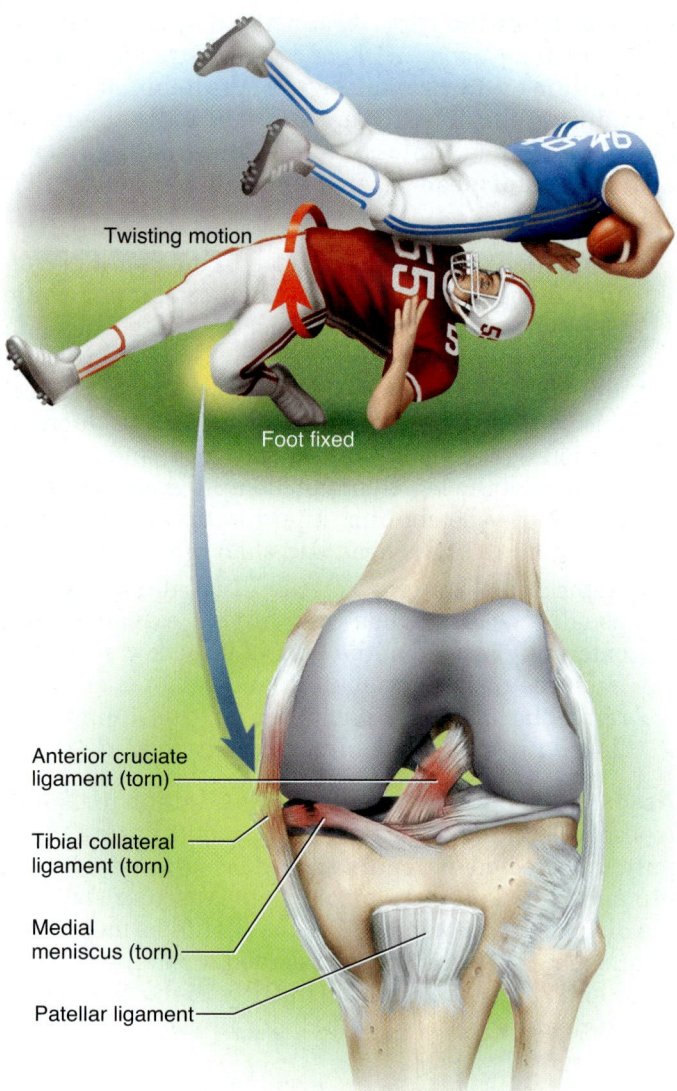

Figure 24-19   Twisting injuries to the knee can result in dislocating patella injuries or torn ligaments. The patella and upper portion of the patellar ligament have been removed to allow the underlying structures to be viewed.

leg and foot. Ischemia of more than six hours is associated with poor prognosis for limb salvage.[6] DOT 4-9.24, 4-9.26

As the largest sesamoid bone in the body, the **patella** assists the quadriceps tendon in extension of the knee. One percent of all fractures in adults involve the patella, but these injuries are less common in children because a thick cartilage surrounds their patella.[21] Transverse fracture of the patella is the result of significant force applied with the knee in a semiflexed position. Swelling of the anterior knee region is caused by **hemarthrosis** (bleeding within the knee joint) and hemorrhage into the soft tissues overlying the joint. Damage to the cartilage is common with trauma to the knee. If displacement of the fracture segments is present, the defect in the patella can be palpated, and active extension of the knee is lost. DOT 4-9.35, 4-9.36

Dislocation of the patella occurs either acutely (from trauma) or episodically. The direction of dislocation is usually laterally. Patella dislocations occur from twisting on an extended knee. They are more common in women.

Assessment and Management. The patient will usually present with marked swelling of the knee from hemorrhage into the joint or effusion and may have a palpable defect in the case of patella fracture, as well as crepitus. Whenever a knee injury is recognized or suspected, examination to exclude other injuries such as femur fractures, acetabular fractures, and hip dislocations must be undertaken.

After assessing the neurovascular status, the leg should be splinted in the position found with a rigid or formable splint that also effectively immobilizes the hip and ankle. Elevation of the extremity should be completed. Perform a rapid transport if there is any circulatory or neurologic compromise.

Spontaneous reduction of a dislocated patella may occur if the joint is extended. Expect hemarthrosis and localized tenderness to remain after the joint reduces itself. DOT 4-9.24

Tibia and Fibula Fractures

The tibia is responsible for supporting 85% of the body's weight while the smaller fibula articulates with the tibia, stabilizing it.[28] Together, these are the most common long bone fractures. They result from either direct or indirect trauma or twisting injury, typically MVCs, falls, pedestrian accidents, or sporting injuries. If associated with a knee injury, popliteal artery trauma should also be suspected because of its anatomical placement in close proximity to the proximal tibia.

Fractures of the proximal tibia (called the plateau) occur as a result of a combination of axial compression and strong medial or lateral load applied to the knee. A classic example is a pedestrian struck by a car. The bumper applies severe force on the side of the knee while the leg is axially loaded and fixed by the foot to the ground. The fracture may be a pure split, a pure compression, or a combination of both. Injuries of the ligaments of the knee are commonly associated with plateau fractures.

Fractures of the shaft of the tibia and fibula occur most commonly in the adolescent and young adult patients.

> Fractures of the tibial shaft have the highest rate of nonunion (not healing) of all long bone fractures and the highest rate of infection of all open fractures.

Low-energy rotational mechanism and high-energy motorcycle accidents commonly cause tibial shaft fractures.

Distal tibial fractures have the greatest number of mechanisms, patterns, and treatment pitfalls. Injuries include low-energy avulsions to high-energy fractures, where the distal end disintegrates within and through the thin layer of soft tissues.

Assessment and Management. Stabilize the leg and assess the neurovascular status. Dress any open wounds carefully with a sterile dressing. Apply a rigid or formable splint to immobilize the fracture site and the joint above and below the injury site. If the patient is supine, elevate the extremity above the heart. Reassess distal motor function, sensory response, and circulation. You may splint the injured extremity to the unaffected leg for increased stability. Compartment syndrome is a worrisome complication of lower leg injuries, so reassess for pain, pulse, motor, and sensation often.

Ankle and Foot Injuries

The ankle consists of three bones, the tibia, fibula, and talus, attached together by ligaments. Stability is provided by the talus, which provides for articulation of the tibia and fibula as well as for dorsiflexion and plantarflexion of the foot.

> Ankle trauma accounts for 3–12% of all emergency department visits and represents the most common reason a patient reports to the ED with a musculoskeletal complaint.

Only 7–36% of the patients will actually have a fracture. The frequency and severity of ankle fractures is increasing as the population ages. Elderly women are the most frequent patients with ankle and foot fracture. Obesity, intoxication, and high-heeled or platform shoes are risk factors for ankle and foot injuries. Motor vehicle crashes also remain a common cause.

Ankle sprain is most commonly caused by inversion of the foot (rolling the sole of the foot medially and the ankle laterally) that occurs with stumbling or tripping on uneven ground. Pain is most commonly found on the anterior and lateral aspect of the joint. The majority of these injuries involve the lateral ligaments, notably the anterior talofibular ligament. Eversion sprains, which occur with rolling the ankle the opposite way, are not common. Dislocation of the ankle joint is much less common because the talus bone cannot be dislocated unless all the ligaments are torn, which requires significant force. DOT 4-9.24, 4-9.29, 4-9.30

Nice to Know

> Sprains occur as joints are stretched and ligaments are damaged. Strains occur as tendons (which attach muscles to bone) are stretched. Joint injuries can result in a combination of both sprains and strains. DOT 4-9.4

Fractures and dislocations of the foot and ankle may result from crush injury, fall from a height, or excessive rotational force. Fractures and dislocations of the ankle often involve more than one bone and several ligaments. The patient usually complains of point tenderness and is hesitant to bear weight on the extremity.

The calcaneus (heel) is the most frequently fractured tarsal (foot) bone. The calcaneus is frequently fractured during a fall from a height. As a result, patients with calcaneal fracture often have other injuries. Ten percent of calcaneal fractures are bilateral (involving both feet), and 10% are associated with comminuted and impaction fractures of the thoracolumbar junction of the spine. Twenty-six percent are associated with other lower extremity injuries.[29]

Assessment and Management.   All suspected fractures of the foot are managed in the prehospital setting in a similar manner. Assess neurovascular status, and apply a formable splint such as a pillow or blanket. Look for signs of other injuries and treat accordingly. If the patient is supine, elevate the foot above the heart. Do not attempt to reduce fractures or dislocations of the ankle unless specifically directed to do so by medical direction. As previously discussed, ankle or foot deformity should not impact your ability to stabilize the patient to a stretcher or long board, nor should it interfere with your ability to transport the patient.

DOT 4-9.27

Toe (Phalanx) Injuries

Injuries to the toes, often caused by "stubbing" the toe on an immovable object, generally do not require much in the way of prehospital management other than pain treatment. Evaluation of neurovascular status is required. Reduction of dislocation or fracture should occur in the emergency department after appropriate imaging has occurred to rule out fractures or other injuries.

Documentation and Reporting Considerations

Use clear, concise, and detailed language to describe your assessment and care. Findings at the incident location may help the emergency department identify potential injuries. Include the following in your report: (1) The position in which the patient was found, (2) estimated amount of blood loss or pooling at the site, (3) areas of exposed bone, (4) open wounds in proximity to obvious or suspected fractures, (5) obvious deformities or dislocations, (6) neurovascular status at the time of initial assessment and after all interventions, and (7) stability of the patient on-scene and en route to the hospital.

Though studies have shown that blood loss estimation by on-scene personnel is not accurate, an attempt at estimating this should be made.[30] Report changes in limb function, perfusion, and neurologic status before and after any intervention (e.g., splinting, fluid resuscitation) or change in stability on-scene or en route. Remember always to document your reevaluation. Note dressings and splints applied, especially if excessive pressure was used over boney prominences that may result in peripheral nerve compression injuries, compartment syndrome, or crush syndrome.

Patient Refusal and Referrals

In cases of non-life- or limb-threatening musculoskeletal injuries, a patient with decision-making capacity may refuse transport to the emergency department. Some patients with minor musculoskeletal injury (e.g., a sprain) may not require or want EMS transport, and a retrospective review has shown some of these transports to be medically unnecessary.[31] To assist a patient in making a transportation determination, evaluate the need for immobilization, radiographic evaluation, physician follow-up versus emergency department assessment, and the presence of distracting injuries.

Studies have shown that 10% of patients may be undertriaged without predefined, nontransport criteria.[32] Therefore, any referral of a patient to their personal physician should be in conjunction with on-line medical control and in accordance with local protocol. Patients not transported to the hospital should receive written advice on how to care for their injury. If available, consider providing a patient instruction sheet, as some studies have shown that only 22% of patients who receive oral instructions will remember them.[33] If there is any doubt about the seriousness of the patient's injury, transport to the emergency department for physician evaluation.

Summary

There are many different conditions affecting the musculoskeletal system. This chapter focuses on traumatic injuries to the musculoskeletal system. Though many of these injuries are not a threat to life, some significant exceptions are pelvic fractures, femur fractures, and multiple fractures. In these situations, the associated hemorrhage is the primary cause of shock and death.

Most musculoskeletal injuries are easily identified by their common signs and symptoms and can be similarly managed with some variation, depending on their severity. It is important to remember to stabilize the patient's airway, breathing, and circulation according to standard trauma protocols before treating isolated musculoskeletal injuries. Due to the higher potential for morbidity and mortality, evaluate and manage head, neck, spine, torso, and pelvis or hip injuries before those of the peripheral musculoskeletal system. Once the ABCs are managed, treat extremity injuries. Depending upon the severity of the injury, this may occur en route to the trauma center.

Goals of management are to stop bleeding by applying direct pressure, cover open wounds, position and immobilize the affected limb along with the joint above and below the injury, carefully monitor the distal neurovascular status, and transport a patient to the emergency department for definitive care. Monitor the patient closely for the development of compartment syndrome, particularly if the injury is to the forearm or lower leg.

Fractures can be managed by immobilizing the extremity with a splint. Joint injuries, such as dislocations, pose a greater risk for neurovascular damage. Therefore, they are typically splinted as found, except in cases of prolonged transport time or distal neurovascular compromise. In these cases, with medical direction, the extremity can be carefully manipulated and splinted in a position that restores circulation. Continuously monitor the patient's stability, and frequently reevaluate neurovascular status, both prior to and after any intervention. Lastly, remember to maintain judicious records and always remain compassionate and professional.

Notes

1. Centers for Disease Control and Prevention, *Morbidity and Mortality Weekly Report: Surveillance Summaries* 53(September 3, 2004): SS-7.
2. J. E. Tintinalli, G. D. Kelen, J. S. Stapczynski, O. J. Ma, and D. M. Cline, "Initial Evaluation and Management of Orthopedic Injuries," in *Tintinalli's Emergency Medicine: A Comprehensive Study Guide,* 6th ed., McGraw-Hill's AccessMedicine (accessed June 9, 2006).
3. C. K. Stone and R. L. Humphries, *Current Emergency Diagnosis & Treatment,* McGraw-Hill's AccessMedicine (accessed June 9, 2006).
4. J. A. Buckwalter, T. A. Einhorn, and J. L. Marsh, "Bone and Joint healing," in *Rockwood and Green's Fractures in Adults,* vol 1, 5th ed., R. W. Bucholz and J. D. Heckman eds. (Philadelphia, PA: Lippincott Williams & Wilkins, 2001), p. 245.
5. Shier, Butler, and Lewis, *Hole's Anatomy and Physiology,* 10th ed. (New York NY: McGraw-Hill, 2004).
6. R. C. Schenck, Jr, and J. D. Heckman, "Injuries of the Knee," *Clinical Symposia* 45(1993): 1.
7. J. A. Marx, ed., *Rosen's Emergency Medicine Concepts and Clinical Practice,* 5th ed. (St. Louis, MO: Elsevier Mosby, 2002).
8. R. F. Wilson, *Handbook of Trauma Pitfalls and Pearls* (Philadelphia PA: Lippincott Williams & Wilkins, 1999).
9. K. J. Knoop, L. B. Stack, and A. B. Storrow, "Extremity Trauma," *Emergency Medicine Atlas,* McGraw-Hill's AccessMedicine (accessed June 9, 2006).
10. G. M. Doherty, "Postoperative Complications," in *Current Surgery,* McGraw-Hill's AccessMedicine (accessed June 9, 2006).
11. A. H. Ropper and R. H. Brown, *Adams and Victor's Principles of Neurology,* 8th ed., McGraw-Hill's AccessMedicine (accessed June 9, 2006).
12. G. M. Doherty and L. W. Way, *Current Surgical Diagnosis and Treatment,* 12th ed., McGraw-Hill's AccessMedicine (accessed June 9, 2006).
13. M. M. McQueen and C. M. Court-Brown, "Compartment Monitoring in Tibial Fractures: The Threshold for Decompression," *The Journal of Bone and Joint Surgery (British),* 76(1966): 99.
14. R. D. Stewart, "Pain Control in Prehospital Care," In *Pain Management in Emergency Medicine,* P. M. Paris and R. D. Stewart, eds. Norwalk, CT: Appleton & Lange, 1988.
15. K. W. W. Lansink, C. J. Cornejo, T. Boeije, et al., "Evaluation of the Necessity of Clinical Observation of High-Energy Trauma Patients without Significant Injury after Standardized Emergency Room Stabilization," *The Journal of Trauma,* 5(2004): 1250–1259.
16. American College of Surgeons Committee on Trauma, *Advanced Trauma Life Support for Doctors,* 6th ed. (Chicago, IL: American College of Surgeons, 1997).
17. C. F. Richards, "Initial Management of the Trauma Patient," *Critical Care Clinics* 20(1)(January 1, 2004): 1–11.
18. C. C. McEachin, J. T. McDermott, and R. Swor, "Few EMS Patients with Lower-Extremity Fractures Receive Prehospital Analgesia," *PreHospital Emergency Care* 6(4)(2002): 406–410.
19. T. Rupp, "Inadequate analgesia in emergency medicine," *Annals of Emergency Medicine* 43(4)(April 1, 2004): 494–503.
20. H. Tscherne, H. J. Oestern, and J. Sturm, "Osteosynthesis of Major Fractures in Polytrauma," *World Journal of Surgery* 7(1983): 80
21. D. A. Della-Giustina and M. Coppola, "Emergency Medicine Clinics of North America," *Orthopedic Emergencies* 17(4)(1999), pp. 873–874.
22. K. Anderson, P. O. Jensen, and J. Lauritzen, "Treatment of Clavicular Fracture: Figure-of-Eight Bandage Versus a Simple Sling," *Acta Orthopaedica Scandinavica* 58(1987): 71–74.
23. J. D. Zuckerman, K. J. Koval, and F. Cuomo, "Fractures of the Scapula," *Instructional Course Lectures* 42(1993): 271–281.
24. J. E. Tintinalli, G. D. Kelen, J. S. Stapczynski, O. J. Ma, and D. M. Cline, "Dislocation of the Glenohumeral Joint," in *Tintinalli's Emergency Medicine: A Comprehensive Study Guide,* 6th ed., McGraw-Hill's AccessMedicine (accessed August 29, 2005).
25. B. Kristiansen et al., "Epidemiology of Proximal Humeral Fractures," *Acta Orthopaedica Scandinavica* 58(1987): 75–77.
26. R. Ostrum, G. Verghese, and T. Santner, "The Lack of Association Between Femoral Shaft Fractures and Hypotensive Shock," *Journal of Orthopaedic Trauma* 7: 338–342.
27. J. Lynch, M. Gardner and B. Gains, "Hemodynamic Significance of Pediatric Femur Fractures," *Journal of Pediatric Surgery* 31(1996): 1358–1361.
28. P. C. Ferrera, S. A. Colucciello, J. A. Marx, et al., *Trauma Management: An Emergency Medicine Approach* (St. Louis, MO: Elsevier Mosby, 2001).
29. J. E. Tintinalli, G. D. Kelen, J. S. Stapczynski, O. J. Ma, and D. M. Cline, *Tintinalli's Emergency Medicine: A Comprehensive Study Guide,* 6th ed., McGraw-Hill's AccessMedicine (accessed June 9, 2005).
30. R. Moscati, A. J. Billittier, B. Marshall, et al., "Blood Loss Estimation by Out-of-Hospital Emergency Care Providers," *Prehospital Emergency Care* 3(1999): 239–242.
31. T. A. Schmidt, R. Atcheson, C. Federiuk, et al., "Hospital Follow Up of Patients Categorized as Not Needing an Ambulance Using a Set of Emergency Medical Technician Protocols," *Prehospital Emergency Care* 5(4)(2001): 366–370.
32. M. Kamper, B. Mahoney, S. Nelson, et al., "Feasibility of Paramedic Treatment and Referral of Minor Illnesses and Injuries," *Prehospital Emergency Care* 5(2001): 371–378.
33. T. A. Schmidt, N. C. Mann, C. S. Federiuk, et al., "Do Patients Refusing Transport Remember Descriptions of Risks After Initial Advanced Life Support Assessment?" *Academic Emergency Medicine* 5(1998): 796–801.

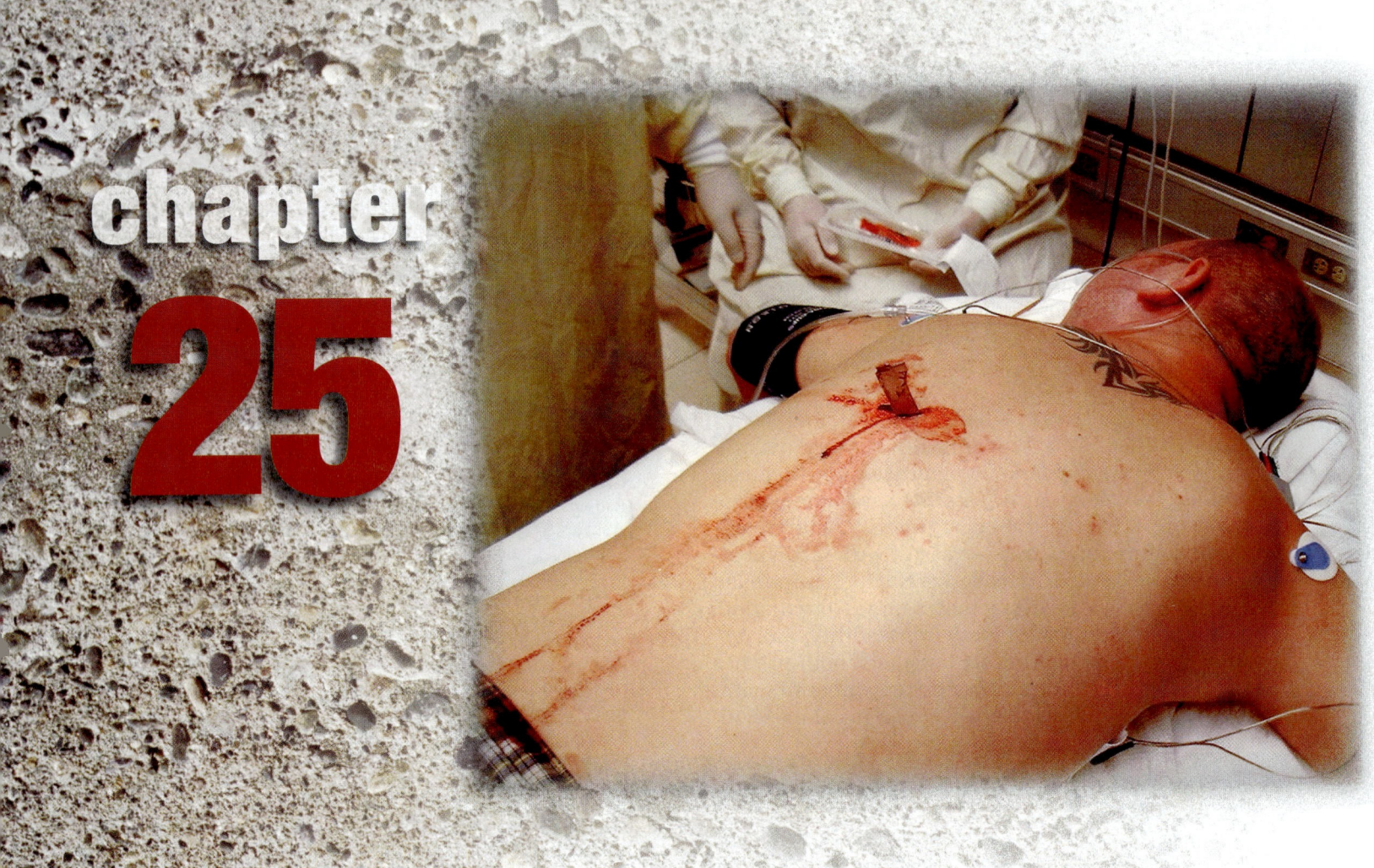

25

Soft Tissue
and Muscle Trauma

"It is a glorious thing to be indifferent to suffering, but only to one's own suffering."

—Robert Lynd

502

Need to Know

▶ The skin is the largest organ of the body. Protection, prevention of water loss, temperature regulation, and self-repair are the most important functions of the skin.

▶ Control of bleeding is the first and foremost priority with any soft tissue injury. Direct pressure applied to the wound is the best method to control bleeding. Tourniquets should be used as a last resort.

▶ Lacerations to the neck should be considered life-threatening. An occlusive dressing should be placed to prevent air embolism. These wounds often require exploration in the operating room, and these patients should be transported to an appropriate trauma center.

▶ Impaled objects should not be removed but rather should be stabilized in place.

▶ Amputations generally do not bleed much. Place the amputated part into a plastic bag and cool with ice. Take care not to freeze the part.

▶ Crush injury, crush syndrome, and compartment syndrome occur when pressure is applied to or builds up within a confined part of the body.

▶ Sick	▶ Not Yet Sick
• Distinguish between injuries that are high-priority requiring rapid transport from low-priority injuries. • Look for hidden injuries/bleeding/life threats or circulatory compromise. Treat ABCs, perform whole-body splinting, and transport emergently • Apply an occlusive dressing to an open wound in the neck to prevent air embolism.	• Ask detailed information about the MOI. • Treat the pain • Do not allow a distracting soft tissue wound to divert your attention and prevent you from performing a complete assessment.

Introduction

Soft tissue injuries involve a wide range of skin and neuromuscular injuries that include everything from a simple scratch of the skin to an impaled object. In most cases, it is rare that damage to the skin results in a life-threatening condition. However, when it does, it is most likely due to the location of the break in the skin and the potential that the injury went deep enough to have caused damage to the underlying structures (such as blood vessels, nerves, or organs). Life-threatening conditions addressed in this chapter include uncontrolled bleeding, amputations, impaled objects, crush injuries, and compartment syndrome. Less serious conditions addressed include wounds to the skin (epidermis and dermis), muscles, tendons, and ligaments (such as sprains and strains).

In the year 2002, the National Center for Health Statistics reported that there were 40.2 million emergency department (ED) visits and 10.9 million outpatient department visits for all injuries in the United States. In 2000, over 8 million traumatic soft tissue injuries were examined in the ED. This accounts for about 7% of all ED visits. The face, scalp, fingers, and hands are the most frequently involved areas of the body. The face and scalp account for approximately 50% of wounds treated in the ED. Approximately 40% of the soft tissue traumatic injuries in adults are caused by blunt trauma.[1] Pediatric patients sustain different wounds than adults. Traumatic wounds on children will more likely be located on the head and are often caused by blunt trauma.[2] DOT 4-3.1

Applied Anatomy and Physiology

The Skin

The skin is the largest (1.6 to 1.9 square meters or 17 to 20 square feet in the average-size adult), thinnest (varies from less than 0.05 cm to slightly more than 0.3 cm in thickness), and one of the most important organs of the body.[3] Along with nails, sweat glands, and sebaceous glands, the skin makes up the integumentary system (Figure 25-1). Protection from the outside environment and infection, prevention of water loss, temperature regulation, and self-repair are the most important functions of the skin. The skin protects the body against injury and invasion of microorganisms (bacteria, fungi, and viruses), other harmful substances, and radiation. The skin also synthesizes vitamin D. Emotional well-being, including one's response to the daily stresses of life, is also reflected in the skin.[4] DOT 4-3.3

The skin has two main layers: the **epidermis** and the **dermis** (Figure 25-2). The epidermis (the outermost layer) is mostly made of dead, flattened, and hardened (keratinized) cells called the **stratum corneum.** These dead cells are continuously sloughed off as they are exposed to the harsh external environment and replaced with other cells coming from the deeper layers.[5] The epidermis has a small amount of living immune cells that help in the protection against pathogens. DOT 4-3.2

CONNECTIONS Chapter 32: Allergies and Anaphylaxis discusses the immune system defense in more detail.

The epidermis is water resistant. It helps keep fluid in the body, except when sweat glands are active and perspiration occurs. The average adult looses 500 mL each day through evaporation from the skin and respiratory passageways during breathing.[6]

Current research indiates that 35 days are required for one complete turnover or regeneration of skin from the innermost level (stratum basale) to the outermost layer (stratum corneum). The epidermal layer has no blood vessels and relies on the dermal layer for nutrition.

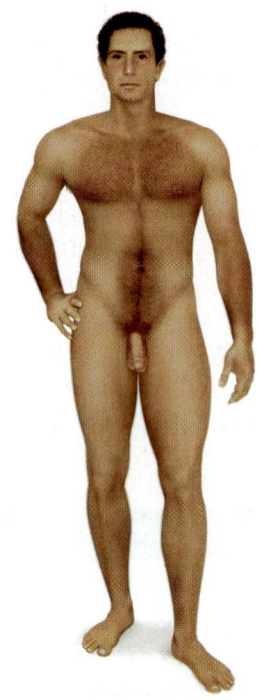

Figure 25-1   The skin contains sensory nerves, holds in body fluids, and protects the body against injury and invasion by microorganisms.

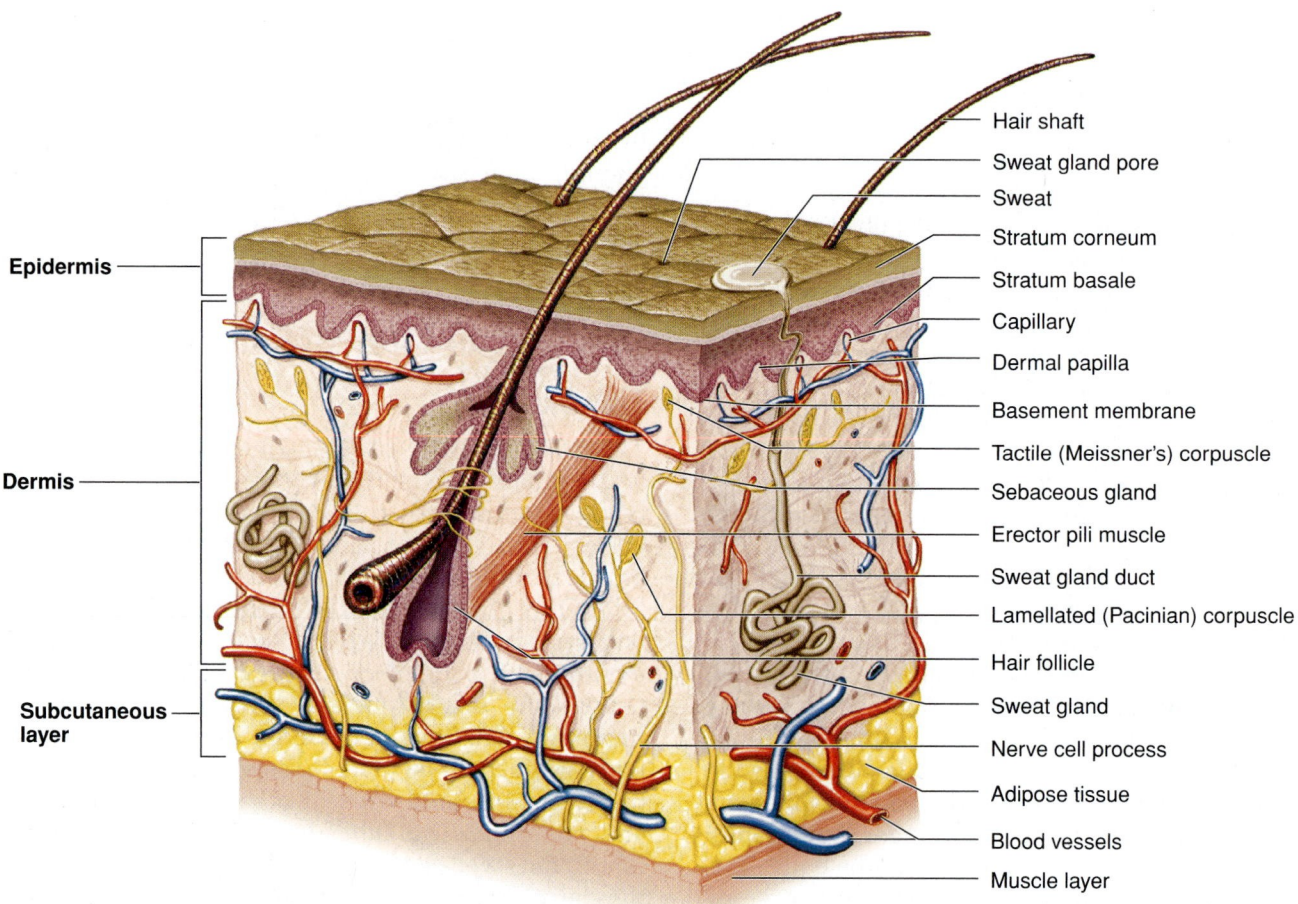

- Hair shaft
- Sweat gland pore
- Sweat
- Stratum corneum
- Stratum basale
- Capillary
- Dermal papilla
- Basement membrane
- Tactile (Meissner's) corpuscle
- Sebaceous gland
- Erector pili muscle
- Sweat gland duct
- Lamellated (Pacinian) corpuscle
- Hair follicle
- Sweat gland
- Nerve cell process
- Adipose tissue
- Blood vessels
- Muscle layer

Epidermis

Dermis

Subcutaneous layer

Figure 25-2   The skin is made up of epidermis, dermis, and subcutaneous layers.

CONNECTIONS In Chapter 16: Medication Administration and IV, subcutaneous medication administration is discussed.

Muscle Tissue

Directly underneath the skin and subcutaneous tissue lies muscle tissue or bone. There are three types of muscles: skeletal, smooth, and cardiac. Skeletal muscle can be controlled by choice and is called voluntary muscle. It is striped (striated) and shaped like a cylinder (Figure 25-3). Skeletal muscle becomes stronger and cordlike where it attaches to bone. At this point, the tissue is called a tendon. Cardiac muscle is involuntary and is also striated. Smooth (visceral) muscle is found in organs and is also involuntary. It can be found in the stomach, intestine, blood vessels, and the respiratory (bronchioles) system.[3,5]

Nice to Know

Muscle Contraction

At the simplest level, muscle contraction occurs when two proteins, **actin** and **myocin,** engage with each other and pull themselves together. This shortens the muscle fiber **(sarcomere)** and effectively creates movement.

Pathophysiology of Hemostasis

Hemostasis is the process by which bleeding is stopped, either by physiological properties of vasoconstriction and coagulation or through the assistance of artificial pressure applied externally by the paramedic's gloved hand.[7] Without the ability to control one's own bleeding, any minor cut or scrape could become a life-threatening event. Hemostasis involves four components: vasoconstriction, platelet aggregation, fibrin formation, and fibrinolysis. Although the processes occur in that general order, the products of each of these four processes are interrelated in such a way that there is a continuum and multiple reinforcements along the way. DOT 4-3.6a

CONNECTIONS See Chapter 19: Trauma and Hemorrhagic Shock for more information on hemostasis.

Vasoconstriction begins almost immediately as arteries, arterioles, and some veins constrict in response to injury. This response helps to reduce bleeding and may even completely stop bleeding, at least temporarily. In addition, the cut ends of larger vessels may retract (through vasospasm), and this also reduces bleeding. This physical reaction to vascular injury occurs rapidly and provides time for the coagulation phase of bleeding control to begin.

Nice to Know

What Is a Blister?

A blister is an accumulation of plasma that has leaked out from damaged blood vessels and formed a fluid-filled pocket between the dermis and epidermis.

The dermis lies beneath the epidermis and is sometimes called the "true skin." It contains hair and hair follicles, sweat glands, sebaceous (oil) glands, sensory nerves, muscles, and pressure receptors.[3] Sweat glands and tiny muscles around the blood vessels in the dermis help regulate body temperature by (1) enhancing evaporative cooling from sweat; (2) bringing more blood to the skin surface to be exposed to cooler air for cooling; or (3) constricting the vessels to shunt blood toward the warm inner body core.

The blood vessels in the dermis are also responsible for skin color changes. When blood is not well oxygenated it will turn blue **(cyanosis)**—think about the difference between the color of venous blood and that of arterial blood. Similarly, if a person becomes frightened and "turns white," their fright has activated the sympathetic system to constrict blood vessels in the dermis. This shunts blood away from the skin and gives the skin a pale appearance. The same mechanism also produces pale skin during shock. On the other hand, the opposite occurs when someone "blushes." In this case, blood vessels dilate, and a person "turns red" or gets a "flushed" appearance.[5]

Nice to Know

You may encounter medication patches (transdermal patches) that are placed directly on the skin. The medication slowly diffuses through the epidermis and is absorbed in the dermis. This allows for a timed release of the drug.

Subcutaneous Tissue

Subcutaneous tissue, also called the **hypodermis,** lies directly under the dermis. It is made of adipose (fatty) connective tissue and is not considered part of the integumentary system. Its extensive network of blood vessels make it an ideal route for medication administration as an injected drug can be carried to the rest of the body quickly by the vascular system. The fatty layer of the hypodermis also acts as a thermal insulation layer and stores energy.[5,6]

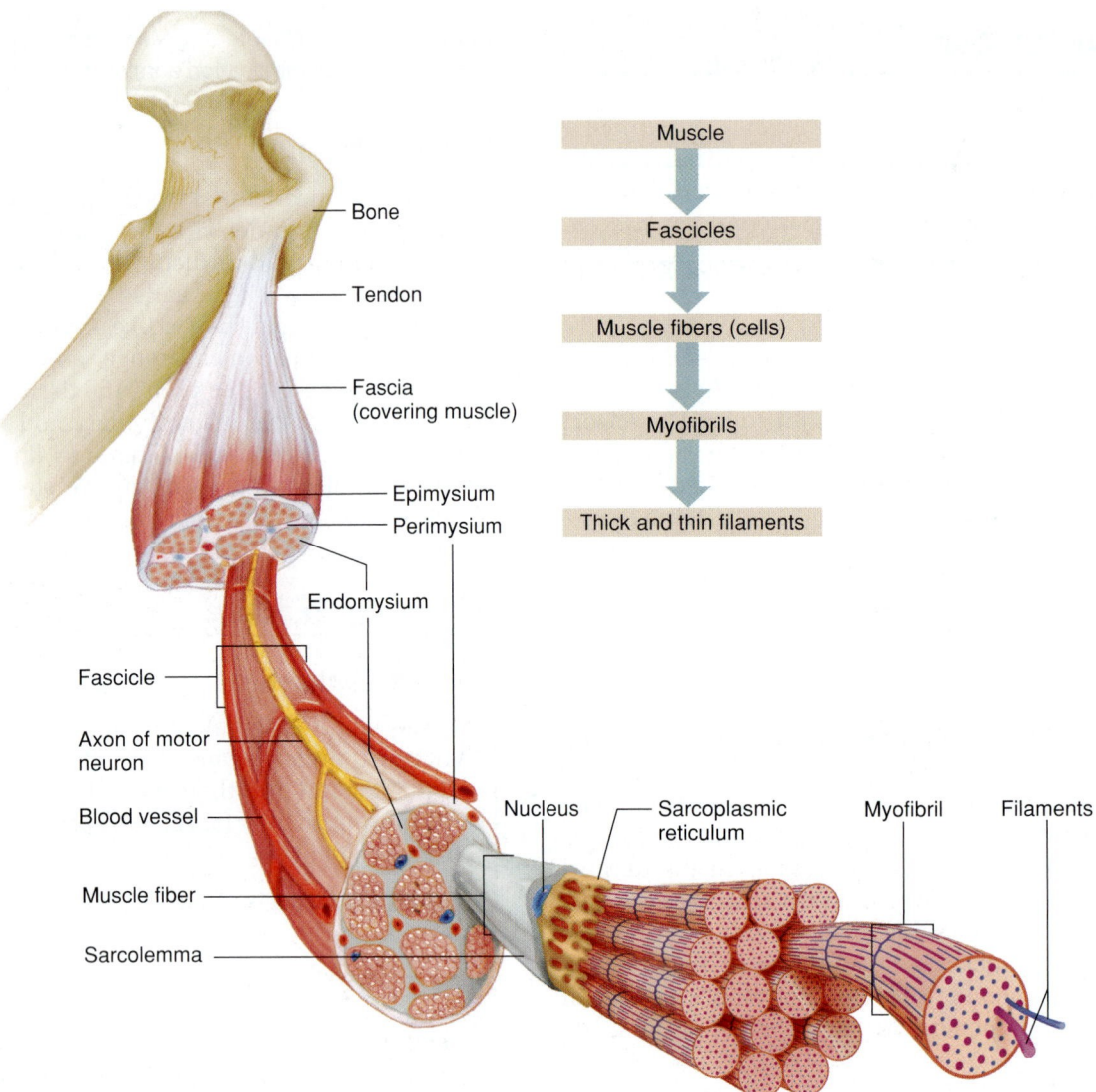

Figure 25-3 Skeletal muscle is voluntary, is attached to bones, and allows for movement. Skeletal muscle cells are cylindrical in shape and striated (striped).

Platelets (thrombocytes) are free-floating structures in the bloodstream. When the platelets come into contact with damaged or injured blood vessels, they swell and change from a smooth slippery shape to a spiked shape. The platelets become sticky and secrete chemicals that activate other platelets to come and join together to form a plug. This process is referred to as **aggregation.** These activated platelets actually stick to one another and form a "platelet plug" at the site of the damage to the blood vessel. This event is referred to as **agglutination** or clumping. If the injury is small, this may be the only control necessary to stop bleeding. If the injury is larger, then coagulation will begin.

The **coagulation cascade** is a complex chemical and biological process used to control bleeding. From initiation of the first signal indicating injury to the vessel, usually less than 30 minutes is required for a blood clot

to form.[5,8] Box 25-1 explains the process in more detail. Fibrin formation is the initial step in this process. Once hemostasis has been achieved, the vessel can be repaired, and the fibrin clot is destroyed **(fibrinolysis)** so blood flow can resume.

Pathophysiology of Wound Healing

Wound healing is divided into several overlapping phases that are defined by the cells that are found in each phase and the biochemical activities that are taking place. A brief description of each phase will be discussed. The three phases are DOT 4-3.6

- Hemostasis and inflammation
- Proliferation
- Maturation and remodeling

BOX 25-1 Casting the Fibrin Net: Coagulation

When a blood vessel is injured, a complex process is set into motion to create a blood clot (Figure 25-4). Basically, a network of protein fibers, called **fibrin,** weave themselves together and trap red blood cells in order to form a plug in the open blood vessel and stop hemorrhage. The blood clot forms in three stages.

Stage I: Injury activates clotting factors that produced **prothrombin activator (PTA).**

Stage II: Platelets, calcium, and PTA activate **prothrombin** to create **thrombin.**

Stage III: Thrombin activates **fibrinogen** and forms the fibrin fibers (the net) that trap other blood cells to form the clot **(thrombus).**

As a paramedic, you will encounter patients who are taking blood "thinners," which are anticoagulants (such as Coumadin or warfarin sodium), or you might give a drug such as heparin or aspirin to a cardiac patient. Coumadin works on the liver to decrease the creation of prothrombin; heparin works as an antithrombin agent. Aspirin interferes with the prostaglandin synthesis (which is a component of clot formation), and drugs such as clopidogrel (Plavix™) inhibit the ability of platelets to aggregate. Fibrinolytics are sometimes used to destroy blood clots. These "clot-busting" drugs (such as tissue plasminogen activator or tPA) work to degrade the fibrin net.[5]

CONNECTIONS To learn more about blood coagulation disorders, see Chapter 37: Hematology; to review the role of aspirin, heparin, and thrombolytics, visit Chapter 29: Cardiology.

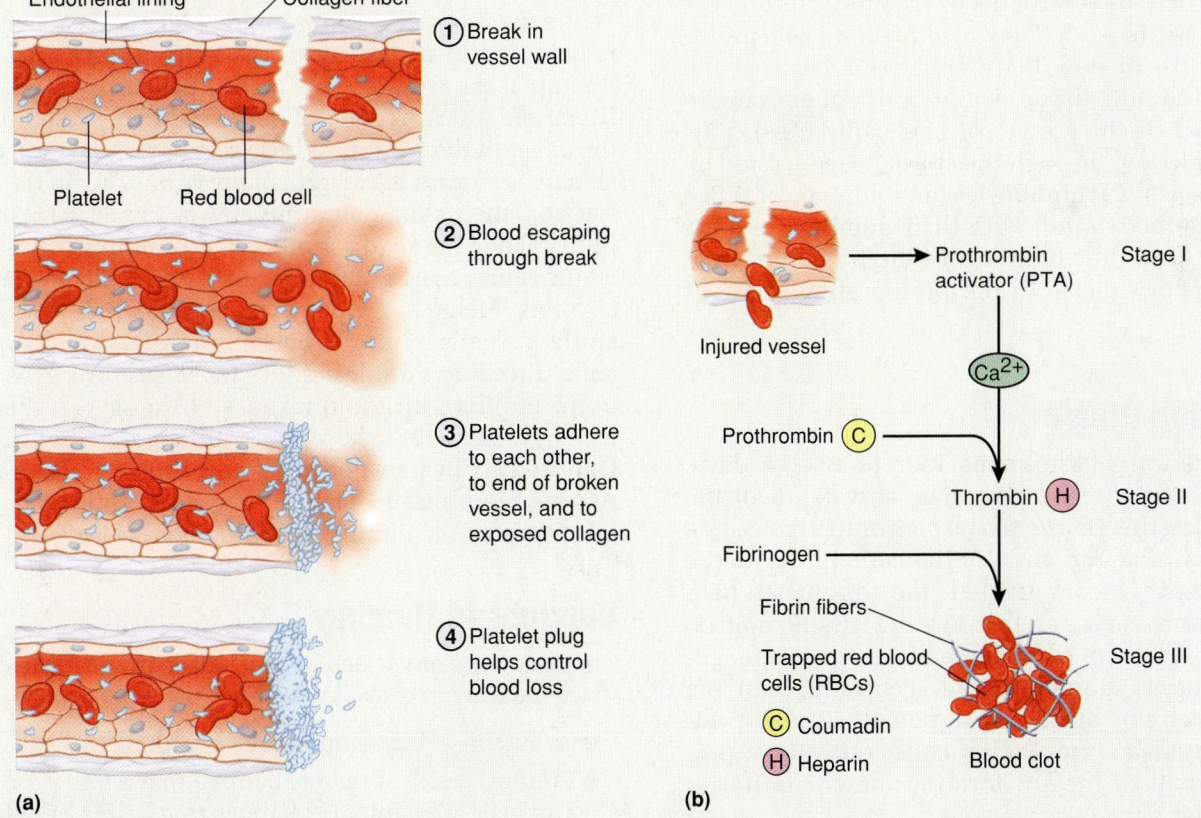

Figure 25-4 Following an injury, a complex process is set in motion that begins with (a) the formation of a platelet plug, followed by (b) fibrin fibers weaving themselves together to form a blood clot in the bleeding vessel.

Hemostasis and Inflammation Phases

Following a soft tissue injury and damage to blood vessels, subendothelial collagen is exposed to platelets. The platelets aggregate, degranulate, and activate the coagulation cascade described above. Many factors such as platelet-derived growth factor, transforming growth factor, platelet-activating factor, fibronectin, and serotonin are released. Hemostasis is reached when bleeding stops. The fibrin clot serves as a scaffold for the migration of white blood cells (WBC) into the wound, which initiates inflammation. Inflammation results in the release of chemotactic factors from the wound site that calls an army of WBCs into the area. This process peaks in 24 to 48 hours and helps to fight off any bacteria that may have contaminated the wound. DOT 4-3.6a, 4-3.6b

The **neutrophils** (one of the white blood cells) that migrate into the area phagocytize (eat) bacteria and tissue debris. These WBCs are replaced by another type of WBC, a macrophage. **Macrophages** are essential to the healing process. They achieve a significant number within 48 to 96 hours. They contribute to the management of microbes by producing oxygen radicals and the synthesis of nitric acid. They also regulate cell proliferation (growth of new body cells), synthesis of the matrix that the new tissue is grown upon, and angiogenesis (which is the growth of new capillaries). This is all accomplished through the substances secreted by the macrophages. **T lymphocytes** (another type of WBC) also infiltrate the wound, with their numbers peaking in one week, and they help bridge the transition from the inflammatory phase to the proliferative phase of healing.

Proliferation Phase

The proliferation phase spans four to twelve days, depending upon the severity, size, and depth of the wound. During this phase, tissue continuity is reestablished. Fibroblasts and endothelial cells infiltrate the healing wound. Once activated, the fibroblasts help synthesize and remodel the healing tissue matrix. **Cytokines** and growth factors released by macrophages help the process along. Lactate accumulates in the wound over time, and it is a potent regulator for collagen synthesis. Endothelial cells continue to proliferate, and they begin forming new capillaries (angiogenesis). DOT 4-3.6c

Collagen is the most abundant protein in the body. Although there are 18 types of collagen, Type I is the major component of the skin matrix, and Type III is prominent and important in the skin repair process. Collagen synthesis is highly dependant upon systemic factors, including an adequate oxygen supply, presence of sufficient nutrients, vitamins and minerals, and the local wound environment having a rich blood supply and being free of infection. A tissue referred to as "ground substance" comprises the granulation tissue found during healing. Fibroblasts synthesize this for the first three weeks of healing.

Maturation and Remodeling

The temporary scar that has formed is now broken down, and the tissue is replaced by stronger tissue. Collagen is broken down by matrix metalloproteinases at a rate nearly as fast as collagen is being synthesized. Fibronectin and collagen Type III were pervasive in the first matrix scaffold. It was replaced by glycosaminoglycans and proteoglycans, which are found in the second matrix. The second matrix is being replaced by collagen Type I. This will be the final matrix for the healing process. The scar continues to remodel matrix two into matrix three for six to twelve months until the wound is totally healed. DOT 4-3.6d, 4-3.6e

Epithelialization

While the internal repair is taking place and each matrix is being built or destroyed, the skin is regrowing over the top of the wound. This occurs primarily by the proliferation and migration of epithelial cells from around the edges of the wound. Within one day of the injury, the skin cells around the margin of the wound begin thickening and then start migrating across the surface of the injury. They undergo a rapid series of mitotic divisions, leapfrogging over each other until the entire surface is covered. Once the wound is covered, the migrating epithelial cells return to their normal shape and appearance, and their mitotic activity increases further as they begin building up the thickness of the layer. After the layer reaches the appropriate thickness, the surface keratinizes (the new dermis is now formed), the process returns to normal metabolic processes, and the epidermis forms as the dermis cells die. DOT 4-3.6c

Barriers to Healing

The following have been identified as providing barriers to the healing process: DOT 4-3.37–4-3.41

- *Infection:* Infection delays healing.
- *Aging:* Most surgeons believe that aging produces intrinsic physiologic changes that result in delayed or impaired wound healing.
- *Hypoxia:* Low-oxygen tension (saturation in the blood) has a profoundly negative effect on all aspects of wound healing. Fibroplasia, although stimulated initially by the hypoxic wound environment, is significantly impaired if hypoxia continues. Optimal collagen synthesis requires oxygen as

a cofactor, particularly for the hydroxylation steps. Increasing subcutaneous oxygen tension levels by increasing the fraction of oxygen (F_iO_2) of inspired air for brief periods during and immediately following surgery results in enhanced collagen deposition and in decreased rates of wound infection after elective surgery.[9,10,11]

- *Steroids:*   Large doses or chronic usage of glucocorticoid steroids reduce collagen synthesis and wound strength.[12] The major effect of steroids is to inhibit the inflammatory phase of wound healing (angiogenesis, neutrophil and macrophage migration, and fibroblast proliferation) and the release of lysosomal enzymes. The stronger the antiinflammatory effect of the steroid compound used, the greater the inhibitory effect on wound healing.

- *Diabetes:*   Diabetes mellitus is the best known of the metabolic disorders that contribute to increased rates of wound infection and failure.[13] Uncontrolled diabetes results in reduced inflammation, angiogenesis, and collagen synthesis. Additionally, the large and small vessel disease that is the hallmark of advanced diabetes contributes to local hypoxemia. Defects in granulocyte function, capillary ingrowth, and fibroblast proliferation all have been described in diabetes. Obesity, insulin resistance, hyperglycemia, and diabetic renal failure all contribute significantly and independently to the impaired wound healing observed in diabetics.[14]

- *Poor nutrition:*   The important role of nutrition in the recovery from traumatic or surgical injury has been recognized by clinicians since the time of Hippocrates. Poor nutritional intake or lack of individual nutrients significantly alters many aspects of wound healing.

Pathophysiology of Soft Tissue Injury

As in many other chapters, the information in this section is presented in the order from worst (most life-threatening) to least serious. This is intended to help the reader prioritize the conditions that are most likely to affect the outcome of a patient and recognize important life threats early on. The types of dressings and bandages that may be used in the prehospital setting are summarized in Table 25-1. DOT 4-3.28, 4-3.46

Closed Wounds

Crush Injury

Crush injury is defined as a mechanism of injury in which skeletal muscle, as well as the overlying skin, subcutaneous tissue, and associated structures such as bones, nerves, and blood vessels, are compressed by

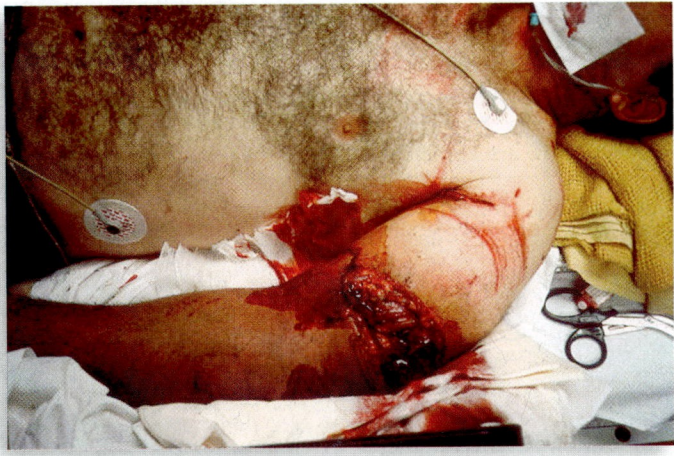

Figure 25-5   Crushing injuries present a cascade of problems that can lead to complications in recovery.

high-pressure forces.[15] Injuries can vary from simple contusions to fractures, rupture of internal organs, lacerations, and hemorrhagic shock (Figure 25-5). **Skill Sheet 79 outlines crush injury management.** DOT 4-3.10, 4-3.12h, 4-3.15a, 4-3.21, 4-3.22a

Crush Syndrome

Crush syndrome is a systemic disorder involving severe metabolic disturbances, resulting from the crush of skeletal muscle. For crush syndrome to occur, the skeletal muscle must be exposed to the high-pressure crushing forces for an extended period of time. The shortest time documented for crush syndrome to occur is four hours.[16] The continual pressure results in minimal or no circulation of blood into the compressed areas, and the tissue undergoes ischemia, followed by necrosis (tissue death). During this time period, a number of toxic substances build up in the crushed tissues. When the pressure is released, the toxins (myoglobin, phosphate, potassium, lactic acid, and uric acid) are released from the necrotic tissue.[15] These toxins can overwhelm the heart (disrupting the electrical system and causing life-threatening dysrhythmias), and the liver and kidneys cannot remove them fast enough to prevent damage. The patient suffering from crush syndrome will present with hypovolemic shock, hyperkalemia, hypocalcemia, metabolic acidosis, acute myoglobinuric renal failure, and perhaps compartment syndrome.[17] Death can occur rapidly in these patients. DOT 4-3.21, 4-3.25, 4-3.23, 4-3.53c

Rhabdomyolosis from Crush Syndrome

A potential complication from crush syndrome is a condition called **rhabdomyolysis.** Rhabdomyolysis results from necrosis of skeletal muscle that can occur for a variety of reasons but in this situation is due to injury

TABLE 25-1 Dressings and Bandages Used in the Prehospital Setting DOT 4-3.35a1–a10, 4-3.35b1–b5

Name	Description
DRESSINGS are applied directly on the wound.	
Sterile	Soft, woven cotton, absorbent fabric placed directly on the wound. It is packaged in a sterile container as single pads or many pads together. Called "sponges" in surgical medicine. This dressing is suitable for placement directly on open wounds.
Nonsterile	Typically made of the same material as the sterile dressings, only it is not sterile. It should not be placed directly on an open wound, but it can be used to add additional absorbent reinforcement for a sterile dressing. In a multiple casualty situation, these may need to be used as the dressing placed in contact with the wound. A note should be made in the patient care report reflecting this.
Occlusive	Nonporous dressing (often plastic) placed directly over a wound to prevent air from entering the wound. It may or may not be clear in color. A sterile surface is optimal. The inner portion of the package from a sterile trauma pad or large sterile dressing is a good source for this type of material.
Nonocclusive	Porous dressing material that allows a wound to "breathe." It may or may not be sterile. Sterile is optimal if it is being placed on an open wound.
Adherent	A dressing that will cling to a wound and close the wound. Tegaderm™ and BioOcclusive™ are examples of adherent dressings. These both happen to be sterile and clear as well. Sterile is best if placed directly on an open wound. This type of dressing may attach to a clot and, upon removal, pull the clot from the wound as well.
Nonadherent	A dressing that is coated with a substance (such as petroleum jelly) or other substance that will prevent it from adhering directly to the wound. Only sterile dressings should be placed directly on the wound, and care must be taken when using these dressings as they may introduce unwanted materials into the wound.
Absorbent	A dressing capable of soaking up blood, pus, or other secretions from wounds. These may adhere to clots and, when removed, pull the clot from the wound, resulting in rebleeding. Only sterile type should be placed in contact with an open wound.
Nonabsorbent	A dressing that is coated, so it will not absorb blood or body fluids. Only sterile type should be placed in contact with an open wound.
Wet	Commercially prepared sterile material can be purchased but its use is governed by prescription as with all medications. Virtually any dressing material described above (with the exception of non-absorbent and occlusive) can be made into a wet dressing with the application of sterile saline. Sterile water is usually not recommended as it is hypotonic and can damage fragile cells inside the wound. Other liquids such as alcohol or iodine should NOT be used to make a wet dressing. Wet dressings are used to provide pain relief for some burns and also to promote healing.
Dry	Dressing materials not provided with additional sterile liquids. Be careful that the dry dressing does not adhere to the wound as removal can result in rebleeding as the clot is torn away. Only sterile dressing should be placed directly on wounds.
BANDAGES are used to hold dressings in place and to help provide pressure to a bleeding wound. These materials do not have to be sterile, but they should be clean.	
Absorbent	Allows for the absorption of blood and body fluids.
Nonabsorbent	Will not allow for the absorption of blood or body fluids.
Adherent	Will stick to the skin without the need for additional measures such as tape to keep them in place. Some elastic bandages and stretchy gauze rolls will adhere to a dressing. Porous skin tape is another example of an adhering dressing material.
Nonadherent	Will not stick to the dressing unless wrapped circumferentially and tucked in or secured with tape. Most elastic bandages and rolls of gauze are nonadherent.
Tourniquet	Device designed to provide circumferential pressure around an extremity to help control bleeding when other measure have not worked. A tourniquet may be made from triangular bandages or strips of cloth, or a commercial device may be used. A blood pressure cuff may also be used if it is monitored closely to ensure it does not deflate.

from the crushing forces. The complications of rhabdomyolysis include acute renal failure (ARF), metabolic derangements, disseminated intravascular coagulopathy (DIC), and mechanical complications (e.g., compartment syndrome or peripheral neuropathy). Acute renal failure is the most serious complication of rhabdomyolysis. Although rhabdomyolysis is thought to account for up to 10% of all cases of ARF, the incidence of this complication in rhabdomyolysis is less clear.[18] It is estimated that between 0% and 50% of patients with rhabdomyolysis develop ARF, with 33% being the most often quoted figure.[19,20,21] DOT 4-3.24

Signs of muscle necrosis and rhabdomyolysis include myoglobinuria, renal insufficiency, markedly elevated creatine kinase levels (a blood test performed in the hospital), and, frequently, multiorgan failure as a consequence of other complications of the trauma. Renal insufficiency from myoglobinuria is caused by tubular damage, resulting from filtered myoglobin that enters and clogs the kidneys once the patient has been released from entrapment.

> It is nearly always associated with hypovolemia, so treating and preventing hypovolemia is recommended to help prevent rhabdomylosis.

When hypovolemia is addressed, normal volumes of urine are produced, and toxic products within the blood are diluted, so there is less impact on the kidneys. Experimental models of severe rhabdomyolysis states in which blood volume and pressure have been maintained within normal values are not associated with acute tubular necrosis. From a practical point of view, however, many patients who sustain crush injuries are also hypovolemic; therefore, oliguric renal failure is often encountered.[22] DOT 4-3.26, 4-3.27

Nice to Know

> Crush syndrome can result from open wounds as well as closed ones. All of the underlying tissues can sustain damage, including the bones, muscles, organs, nerves, arteries, and veins. The skin as well could be lacerated and torn, or broken bones can puncture it from the inside.

Compartment Syndrome

Compartment syndrome is caused by increased pressure in an enclosed space that leads to compromise of circulation and function of tissues within the space. It can occur in a muscle as the result of swelling or hemorrhage from trauma or surgery. The fascia of muscle is relatively inelastic, and the pressure can build up inside the tissues, compromising circulation. If left untreated, the tissues become ischemic. Severe ischemia for six to eight hours leads to nerve or muscle death. DOT 4-2.22c

The lower leg and forearm are the most common locations for compartment syndrome to develop. Pain with passive range of motion of the fingers or toes is thought to be the most sensitive early sign.[23] An immediate surgical procedure, called a **fasciotomy,** is indicated to avoid permanent injury. This procedure is not performed by paramedics, so recognition of the problem and rapid transport are appropriate treatments.

Late signs of arterial insufficiency caused by compartment syndrome include pain, pallor, paresthesia, paralysis, and pulselessness. If nerve or muscle ischemia has been present long enough, paralysis, paresthesia, and tissue damage are likely. Pulselessness is not reliable as it does not always occur with the late stages of compartment syndrome.

The traditional understanding about compartment syndrome has been that when tissue pressure is greater than arterial pressure, circulation becomes compromised and compartment syndrome develops. However, research has shown that compartment syndrome can occur at pressures below arterial pressure.

> Compartment syndrome can exist in a pink limb with normal pulses.[24]

The finding of pain out of proportion to the injury, particularly when the fingers or toes are passively stretched by a paramedic, is the best finding for suspecting compartment syndrome.[23]

CONNECTIONS Compartment syndrome can occur secondary to fractures or dislocations of the bones and joints, particularly those of the lower leg and forearm. Chapter 24: Skeletal Trauma discusses compartment syndrome as it relates to these injuries.

Hematomas

A **hematoma** is a localized collection of blood, usually clotted, in an organ, space, or tissue, due to a break in the wall of a blood vessel. When the injury involves a larger blood vessel, the bleeding can be significant. An injury involving an artery may be so severe as to separate tissue and allow blood to pool into large collections. These hematomas are often very visible in locations such as the face and head due to the very vascular nature of the head, or they may be extremely difficult to identify, such as when they occur in the abdomen or retroperitoneal space. DOT 4-3.8b, 4-3.53b

Important concerns related to hematomas are that as hematomas enlarge, they cause compression of the adjacent tissues. This is particularly important and can become life-threatening when such bleeding involves certain parts of the body, for example, if the hematoma occurs inside the skull and compresses the brain or if it involves the neck, distorting the anatomy of the airway and compressing the trachea. In addition, the hematoma may later become infected and produce sepsis and septic shock.

In most cases, however, a hematoma does not result in a life-threatening problem. Instead, its presence indicates that the patient has sustained an injury, and concern for associated or underlying organ damage is warranted.

Contusion

Contusions, also known as **bruises,** are the result of blunt force trauma and can occur in any part of the body. The bruising is the result of damage to small blood vessels in the area of the injury. Blood leaks from the damaged vessels and causes swelling and reddening at the site of injury. As the leaking blood enters the injury site, the hemoglobin gives up the oxygen molecules it is carrying, and blood cells become dark red and then blue (called **ecchymosis**).[25] Because this process can take up to 24 to 48 hours, prehospital personnel may not initially see any bruising at the site of the trauma. The presence of a contusion can indicate other potential injuries to the patient; therefore, careful evaluation for injury to underlying organs and structures must be performed. Within days, as it heals, the bruise will turn colors. There are no scientific data to support a particular color progression, but there is general agreement that the contusion will initially appear red, black, or purple and will later turn brown, yellow, and green. The speed at which a bruise heals depends on the amount of blood extravasated and the depth and location of the injury.[26]

DOT 4-3.8.a, 4-3.53a

The presence of bruises of multiple ages has been cited as a marker of abuse. Bruises in children, especially those that have a particular pattern such as a hand print, belt buckle, or other objects, may also indicate abuse or assault. Whenever facial wounds are observed on an adult patient, domestic violence must be considered and the proper authorities notified if appropriate. Look for the following signs of domestic violence:

- Most victims have maxillofacial injuries.
- Women are more commonly affected than men.
- Fists are the most common weapon.
- Left side of the face is the most common site of injury.
- Nasal bone is commonly fractured.

CONNECTIONS Chapter 45: The Abused and Neglected discusses this in more detail.

Street Secrets

Estimating the age of a bruise is imprecise. Some bruises may not be visible before 48 hours and, depending on the depth of the bruise, may not show on the surface of the skin at all.

Open Wounds

Open wounds are identified as abrasions, lacerations, incised wounds, punctures, avulsions, amputations, and human or animal bites. Anytime there is a break in the skin as a result of trauma or force and there is bleeding (no matter how minimal—as in capillary bleeding), the patient has sustained an open wound. See Box 25-2 for descriptions and illustrations of open wounds. DOT 4-3.11, 4-3.12j, 4-3.15b, 4-3.50

Tetanus Prophylaxis

All patients treated for any type of open wound (including impaled objects) should be seen by a physician and preventatively treated for the disease tetanus, which is commonly called lockjaw. **Tetanus** is an acute, often fatal, infectious disease caused by the anaerobic, spore-forming bacillus *Clostridium tetani,* an agent that most often enters the body through a contaminated wound. Other portals of entry can include burns, surgical wounds, injection sites of drug users, the umbilical stump of neonates *(tetanus neonatorum),* and the postpartum uterus. Tetanus may begin with muscle spasms in the jaw, difficulty swallowing, and stiffness or pain in the shoulder, back, and neck muscles. Protection against both tetanus and diphtheria can be achieved by vaccination with the Td vaccine. The vaccine is considered to be protective for 10 years, and all adults should receive a booster every 10 years.

Other Wound Complications

There are various medical conditions that can and do complicate wound management. These complications include impaired hemostasis, re-bleeding, and delayed healing.

Impaired Hemostasis

In addition to genetic conditions, such as hemophilia, that interfere with hemostasis and the clotting process, certain medications also impair hemostasis. Aspirin is a powerful inhibitor of platelet aggregation. Patients who are high-risk for heart attack and stroke are prescribed aspirin for just this reason. Aspirin and other

BOX 25-2 Open Wounds

(a) Amputations

An amputation is the removal of part or all of a limb or other appendage from the body. Amputations usually involve the fingers and toes, hands and feet, and arms and legs. Bleeding from these wounds can be fatal if immediate care is not provided. Often, when there is a guillotine type injury with a complete amputation, the blood vessels contract into the tissue, and hemorrhage may be minimal. DOT 4-3.12f, 4-3.53g

Amputations can be described as follows:

A-E amputation = above-the-elbow amputation
A-K amputation = above-the-knee amputation
B-E amputation = below-the-elbow amputation
B-K amputation = below-the-knee amputation

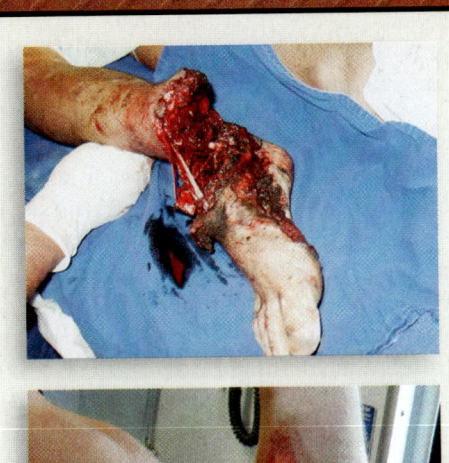

(a)

(b) Abrasions

Abrasions are the rubbing away of the skin through a mechanical process.[7] This wound is the result of friction against exposed skin (i.e., sliding along concrete after falling from a bicycle). If there is any bleeding associated with this wound, it will be capillary bleeding (small droplets of blood are formed). There is usually considerable pain and a high risk for infection with this type of injury. The pain results from the nerve endings being exposed to the air, and the infection risk is from the protective surface of the skin having been scraped away, exposure to opened blood vessels, and debris being ground into the wound. DOT 4-3.12.a, 4-3.53d

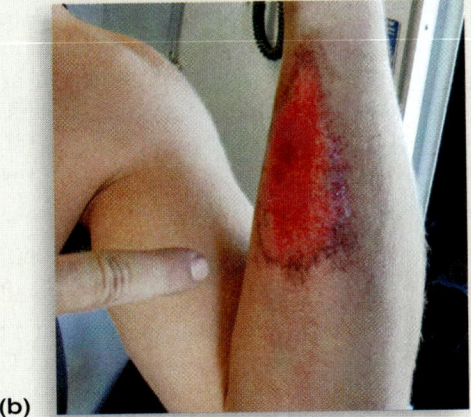

(b)

(c) Lacerations

A laceration is a torn, ragged, mangled wound of the skin.[7] This wound is the result of blunt force. The skin is torn or ripped as the result of blunt trauma or the skin catching on a sharp object and being torn open. Bleeding from these wounds can be very profuse, and the risk of infection is also high. The size of the wound will vary according to the amount of force applied. If the wound is deep enough, lacerations may involve underlying structures such as arteries and veins. Arterial bleeding can be identified by a brighter red and sometimes pulsating rapid blood flow. Venous bleeding is slower and darker. DOT 4-3.12b, 4-3.12c, 4-3.28b, 4-3.28c, 4-3.53e

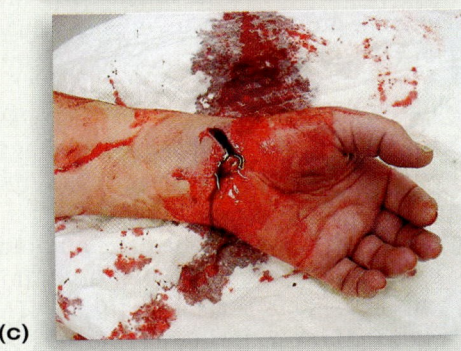

(c)

(d) Incision

An incision is a cut or a wound produced by cutting with a sharp instrument.[7] This wound is the result of a knife or a razor blade type of instrument. The margins of the wound are sharp and regular. Bleeding from these wounds can be profuse because the blood vessels are cut apart and tend to bleed freely. These wounds are also commonly referred to as lacerations

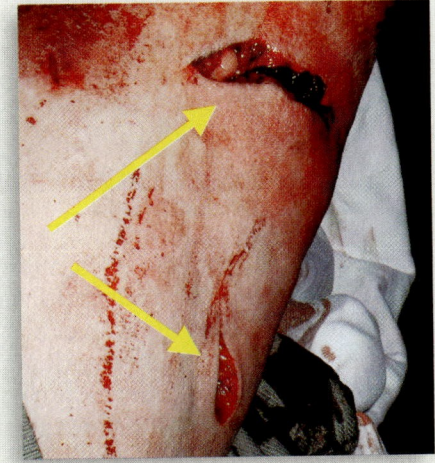

(d)

(*continued*)

BOX 25-2 (continued)

unless they were made as a result of a medical intervention or procedure. DOT 4-3.12g

(e) Punctures

Puncture wounds are the result of a sharp, pointed object being pushed or forced through the skin. Objects such as nails, knives, bullets, needles, and wooden splinters produce puncture wounds. While the entrance wound produced can be small, the tissue damage created can be severe. Punctures can have deep penetration and can result in injuries to tissue and organs beneath the puncture. In addition to deep tissue injuries, puncture wounds have a high potential for infection. In general, puncture wounds are produced when an object enters the skin and is either pulled out (i.e., knife) or goes through (i.e., bullet), leaving an open wound. If the object is still present in the wound, it is considered to be an impaled object. DOT 4-3.53i

(f) Avulsions

An avulsion is the ripping or tearing away of a part of the skin or tissue.[7] An avulsion is an injury involving a flap of skin that has been torn or cut from the body. It typically refers to chunks of soft tissues and does not involve bone, but it could involve cartilage such as flap type injuries to the nose or ear. DOT 4-3.12d, 4-3.53.f

(g) Degloving injury

Degloving injury is a special type of avulsion injury. With degloving, the avulsion is usually circumferential. The force applied to the tissue separates the skin and fat layer down to muscle. The force applied pulls the tissue from the muscle (and sometimes down to the bone) and deposits it as a roll of tissue. (The best example for describing a degloving injury is to push your socks down your leg to your ankle. Don't roll, but push the material down to your ankle. This is degloving, where your sock is skin and fat and your leg is muscle.) Bleeding from degloving injuries can vary from minimal to massive.

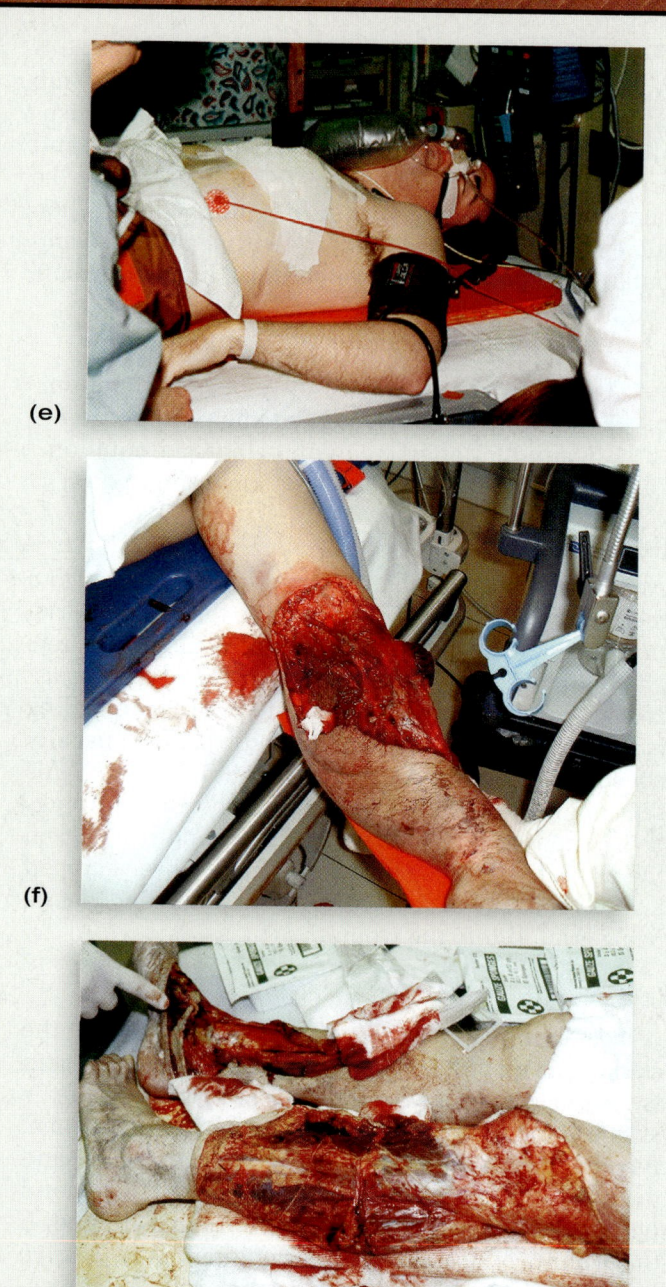

(e)

(f)

(g)

platelet-inhibiting drugs reduce clot formation in the coronary arteries (reducing the danger of heart attack) and cerebral arteries (reducing the danger of stroke). In addition, patients prescribed anticoagulants such as Coumadin® (warfarin) and heparin will have impaired clot formation if they sustain soft tissue injuries.

CONNECTIONS See Chapter 37: Hematology for more information on hemophilia.

Re-Bleeding

Re-bleeding is when bleeding starts again following initial control. This can happen when the patient moves and the clot controlling the hemorrhage is disrupted. This can often be the case when you are treating lacerations of the arms or legs. In these situations, splinting the limb will reduce movement and enhance bleeding control. Bleeding can also resume if bleeding control measures such as direct pressure are not maintained for a long enough period of time or if dressing materials are removed prematurely.

Delayed Healing and Infection

Delayed healing is the result of the body being unable to repair its own wounds due to medical and other physiological problems. Patients that are elderly, are long-term diabetics, are chronically ill, or who suffer from malnourishment are at great risk for delayed healing. Many of these patients have impaired circulation, which impedes the healing process. Often, these patients will develop infections at these delayed healing sites. Drainage from these infections is usually cloudy yellow in appearance and is malodorous. The skin will often be warm or hot to the touch, swollen, reddened or discolored, and painful. Prehospital treatment includes applying nonadherent sterile dressings and protecting the wound from injury or further contamination. The patient should be transported for further evaluation and additional wound care, including antibiotics. The infection can spread to the blood and lead to septic shock. DOT 4-3.39, 40, 41

Nice to Know

The cloudy, yellow drainage from an infected wound is referred to as **purulent drainage.** Yellowish, clear-colored fluid is called **serous** because of its resemblance to blood serum. Blood-tinged fluid is called **sanguinous.**

Decubitus Ulcers (Pressure Injuries)

Decubitus ulcers result from the breakdown of skin and underlying tissue. These wounds are sometimes also called pressure sores. They occur most commonly in debilitated patients who lie in one position in bed, cannot turn on their own, or are not turned often enough. In addition, decubiti may be found in patients with impaired circulation such as the elderly and diabetics. They can form in any patient who is immobile long enough for circulation to the tissues to be compromised. Decubiti can form in any area of the body but are more prevalent over bony prominences or in locations that are pressed into constant contact with another surface. Because of the pressure, there is reduced circulation to the tissue and hypoxic injury leading to necrosis results. These wounds may become infected or may erode into blood vessels and bleed.

Scene Size-Up and Primary Survey

As with any case involving trauma, begin your scene size-up before even reaching the patient. While taking note of any scene safety issue, evaluate the scene and determine the mechanism of injury (MOI). The assessment of patients who sustained soft tissue injuries must begin with immediate life-threatening conditions (airway, breathing, circulation, and severe bleeding). During the primary survey, you may be able to determine quickly if a patient is sick or if the mechanism is significant enough to warrant the need for specialized services at a trauma center. DOT 4-3.33

Scene Size-Up

As you approach the scene, look for anything that will enable you to determine the mechanism of injury. Once you do this, you will be better prepared to predict the injuries your patient may have, the trauma severity, the need for any specialized equipment for extrication, and possible medical conditions your patient may develop.

Be conscious of the scene and possible hazards to yourself, your crew, your patient, and any bystanders. Because soft tissue injuries generally involve body fluids, be certain that everyone involved in responding to the incident is using the appropriate level of body substance isolation precautions.

Primary Survey

If you suspect your patient has been subject to a significant mechanism of injury involving the head and neck, attempt to approach your patient from the front in order to avoid having the patient turn to look at you. As you approach, instruct your patient not to move the head or neck, and instruct a crew member to establish manual cervical in-line stabilization. With a conscious patient, explain everything you are doing and why. This will help alleviate anxiety for your patient and begin to build trust and confidence. If your patient is unconscious, immediately assess airway, breathing, and circulation. Perform a rapid examination for severe, life-threatening bleeding and, if found, correct immediately. Check the patient for signs of adequate perfusion (skin color, temperature, and condition), and assess the patient's capillary refill. While capillary refill is most useful on patients less than four years of age, performing capillary refill examination on an adult will give you an immediate indication of peripheral circulation. Correct all life-threatening conditions, and proceed to the secondary survey. DOT 4-3.5, 4-3.7, 4-3.9

Management of Soft Tissue Injuries

Following the patient assessment, it is time to take care of the soft tissue injuries discovered. The severity of any bleeding will determine if hemorrhage control is attempted immediately or while en route to the hospital. Severe, life-threatening bleeding must be controlled immediately. If the bleeding is not severe, this is a low priority in terms of the patient's needs if other primary survey abnormalities are noted. Once life-threatening conditions have been addressed, you can dress and bandage wounds. This can be performed en route to the hospital in most cases. With high-priority patients, transportation should never be delayed for dressing and bandaging wounds; however, initial attempts to control bleeding must be started prior to moving the patient from the scene. DOT 4-3.10, 4-3.34

Dressing and bandaging wounds has three objectives: DOT 4-3.31

1. The first and most important is to control bleeding.
2. After you have controlled bleeding, dressing and bandaging prevents debris from entering the open wound and keeps it as clean as possible.
3. The final objective is to immobilize the area to prevent additional bleeding.

Improperly applied dressings often will not achieve the desired goals of minimizing exposure to infecting organisms, providing immobilization, and controlling hemorrhage. In fact, improperly applied dressings may, paradoxically, actually increase bleeding. If the bandage is tight enough to block venous outflow from the extremity, venous bleeding from the wound site will increase as blood backs up into the injured extremity and forces the clot to dislodge from the wound. If an excessive amount of dressing and bandaging material is used, the direct pressure applied to the wound will be too diffuse and the dressing will not be tight enough to stop bleeding. In addition, the bulk of the dressing materials will continue to absorb blood, and you may be unaware that bleeding has continued until it emerges through the dressing.

Hemorrhage Control

Apply Direct Pressure

When you are dealing with soft tissue injuries involving hemorrhage, the most effective method to control bleeding is the application of direct pressure.

Placing a sterile dressing directly over the wound and applying pressure with the appropriately gloved hand will control most hemorrhages. Ideally, the amount of pressure applied should not exceed capillary pressure, which is 30 mmHg, and should not impede vascular flow to the distal tissues.[27] Secure the dressing with a self-adherent or elastic bandage to keep the wound closed, and apply constant pressure with the bandage.

After you have secured the dressing, monitor the patient to (1) make sure the bleeding has stopped and (2) make sure the bandage is not too tight, cutting off circulation distal to the wound. A simple pressure dressing applied to a wound for 20 minutes will usually control any oozing that may continue once significant bleeding is controlled.[28] Assess capillary refill time and sensation in the distal portion of the extremity to ensure ischemic injury is not occurring. **The following Skill Sheets outline the step-by-step process for hemostasis: Skill Sheet 66: Bleeding Control and Shock (also see Step-by-Step 66), Skill Sheet 67: Bleeding Control with a Tourniquet (also see Step-by-Step 67), and Skill Sheet 94: NREMT Bleeding Control/Shock Management.** DOT 4-3.31a, 4-3.31b, 4-3.31.c , 4-3.31d, 4-3.31e

Elevate the Wound

If direct pressure alone is not sufficient to control the hemorrhage, simple elevation of the wound above the level of the heart in addition to direct pressure may help slow bleeding.

By elevating the wound site above the heart, the arterial pressure is reduced. In addition, elevation will also increase venous return and reduce swelling that may be present due to trauma. However, do not elevate the injured area if it will result in additional harm to the patient (if an extremity also has a fracture). In addition, be careful when moving extremities as this may compromise the in-line position of the spine.

Compress Pressure Points

If direct pressure and elevation do not control the bleeding, the next step is compression of pressure points.

If you are able to locate a pulse that is immediately proximal to the injury, apply pressure at the pulse site to reduce the flow of blood to the wound site. Maintain this pressure for at least 10 minutes to make sure the bleeding does not continue.

There may be times when bleeding can be very difficult to control. If after application of direct pressure, elevation, and pressure point, the bleeding has not ceased, reassess all of your applications. Make sure that the direct pressure is applied directly over the wound, make sure elevation is maintained, and ensure that the major pressure point has been identified. Note: This technique may or may not be helpful. See Working in the Gray Zone at the top of the next page.

Working in the Gray Zone

Not much support is found in the medical literature for the performance of pressure point pressure in hemorrhage control techniques. Every reference found on hemostasis stated a strong preference for direct pressure, elevation, and pressure dressings, and the application of the tourniquet was reserved as the final effort. Some of the opposition to pressure point utilization included difficulty in finding the particular artery responsible for that area of the skin, the potential damage prolonged compression would cause on tissues distal to the area, and the lack of documented efficacy.[28,29]

Apply a Tourniquet

If bleeding still cannot be controlled and the patient's life is threatened, then a tourniquet must be applied.

The application of a tourniquet is the last option for bleeding control. When the tourniquet is applied, blood flow will stop, not only to the open wound, but also to all tissues distal to the tourniquet. When you apply the tourniquet, it may come down to a choice of "life or limb."

Apply the tourniquet using a cravat or other wide band of material, opened to a width of at least 2 inches wide. DO NOT use narrow bands of material (e.g., rope or wire) as this will also damage the tissue directly beneath the tourniquet. To apply the tourniquet, place it approximately 1–2 inches above (proximal to) the injury. Once the tourniquet has been applied and bleeding is controlled, do not remove the tourniquet except under physician order. Record the time of application of the tourniquet. Monitor the tourniquet (to ensure bleeding does not restart) and the patient continuously en route to the emergency department. Most patients can tolerate the ischemia resulting from the application of a tourniquet for 15–20 minutes.[28] After that, tissues under and distal to the tourniquet begin to suffer ischemia. As a result, the patient will usually complain of increasing pain beyond the tourniquet as the tissues become ischemic. Narcotic analgesia will often be required in cases of longer transport for patient comfort. DOT 4-3.36

In addition to the cravat or a commercial tourniquet band, a blood pressure cuff can also be used as a tourniquet. Apply the blood pressure cuff at the same location you would apply the classic tourniquet. Be sure you have the maximum Velcro to Velcro contact with the cuff and sleeve so the device remains securely fastened. Pump up the blood pressure cuff to 20–30 mmHg above the systolic pressure or to a point where the bleeding stops.[28] Unfortunately, pumping up a blood pressure cuff and maintaining it for bleeding control often results in the Velcro popping off and loss of hemorrhage control. Securing a length of 2-inch tape around the inflated BP cuff can prevent slippage. In addition, all blood pressure cuffs eventually leak air, resulting in a gradual loss of pressure; thus, it is not an ideal tourniquet.

During radio consultation with the emergency department, alert the hospital to the placement of the tourniquet and the time of application. During multiple casualty incidents, place tape on an easily visible part of the patient, (the forehead), and mark it with "TQ" and the time ("1845 hrs") of application. The use of military time will eliminate any question of time of application.

Documentation of the location and approximate size, shape, and condition of the wound is important. This will help other healthcare providers later on but may also be used in court to document the types of injuries a victim may have had. In some police and EMS departments, a photo is taken on the scene and included in the record. DOT 4-3.52

Hemostatic (Blood Stopper) Material

Several products have been developed to control bleeding. These products are composed either of processed cellulose, chitosan (shrimp shell-based material), potato starch, or granulated minerals. While these products are effective in stopping hemorrhage, there are problems that have been identified with several of these items. Products made of biological material are reported to have the potential to induce anaphylaxis in patients. Some products generate an exothermic reaction and produce significant heat (temperatures up to 140°F have been observed) with contact with water or fluids. In addition, a few of the products have up to three steps for application to injury sites. Prices vary for single applications from $6 to $100, and shelf-life varies from six months to indefinite. Products currently on the market include ActCel™, HemCon™, Surgicel™,

Working in the Gray Zone

There is currently little published research on human subjects to support the use of hemostatic agents although there is experience with their use in the military. One study on pigs showed that QuikClot® was more effective than TraumaDex®. This study compared only these two products and showed them both to be superior to simple direct pressure.[30] Other studies have shown that the use of hemostatic agents after surgery may produce necrosis and may delay healing.[31,32] Having the patient apply direct pressure for at least five minutes may be just as effective and may free your hands to continue care.[32]

QuikClot™, and TraumaDEX™. The use of the products in the field setting will vary by individual protocols.

Wound Protection and Decontamination

After bleeding control, the second most important item of patient care is wound cleanliness. The wound should be kept as free of dirt and debris as possible. While it is not necessary to clean every wound prior to bandaging, if there is an extreme amount of contamination, rinse the wound with saline solution. Using either bottled or bagged sterile saline, rinse as much debris as possible from the wound.

After this gross decontamination of debris, apply the bandage to the wound and secure it with self-adherent roller gauze. In many cases, this bandaging of the wound will reduce patient anxiety. Instead of looking down and seeing a severe laceration that is bleeding, they look down and see a neatly wrapped bandage.

Immobilization

The third and final step to bleeding control is immobilization of the limb or area that is injured. While immobilization is usually thought of with fractures, immobilization can play an important role in bleeding control. Immobilization of a limb will help prevent any blood clots that have formed from being disrupted by movement.

As with immobilization of fractures, you will need to monitor the patient's extremity to make sure the bandage or immobilization material is not too tight and that there is continued circulation distal to the wound. The dressing that was applied earlier may have become too tight due to swelling of tissue from trauma to the soft tissue. Monitor the patient for distal pulse, motor function, and sensation.

Pain and Edema Control

After bleeding control, the control of pain and swelling from edema are also very important. Depending on the extent of soft tissue injury, there may be considerable swelling. Swelling can be reduced with the application of cold packs to the injured area. The application of cold packs reduces swelling by reducing the flow of blood into the tissues, which slows the inflammatory response.

Commercially available ice packs or a bag of ice should not be applied directly to the skin. This could cause more discomfort and possibly freeze tissues. Cold packs and ice packs should always be wrapped in a towel or cloth and then applied to the injured area.

Cold application will also assist in pain management. However, if this is not sufficient and the injury is severe enough, the administration of an analgesic or sedative may be indicated. Consult your local protocol for the choice of medication and to confirm whether on-line medical control is required before administering the medication.

Anatomical Considerations for Bandaging

Certain areas of the body lend themselves to bandaging more readily than others. Arms and legs are the easiest to bandage since they are usually straight. When bandaging the extremities, it is appropriate to bandage in a distal to proximal direction.

The difficulty in bandaging the shoulder and chest relates to the amount of area involved. Care must be taken if bandaging the shoulder includes going around the neck, which could potentially compress the airway.

Working in the Gray Zone

Is Wound Care a Paramedic Skill?

Paramedics are trained to approach some of the most complicated and life-threatening conditions that a human being can sustain. Conversely, some of the simple baseline skills that are taught to other healthcare professionals are not included in paramedic education.

Proper wound care is one of those simple skills that is not traditionally taught as part of the paramedic curriculum.[33] In some EMS systems with prolonged transport times or in a situation where you might serve as a primary caregiver (such as the medical officer at an oil platform, ship, or remote location), you may be called upon to clean a wound. Proper cleansing requires additional training. You should be aware of this in case you are working in an environment that will require you to perform these services. This is also important to know in the event a patient is refusing care but has a soft tissue injury. Simple soap and water may not be enough to prevent infection or further complications. EMS responders, when properly trained, are capable of making accurate assessments of which wounds will require further care. One study showed that EMT-basics were capable of determining which wounds would require sutures (stitches).[34] As the scope of practice for EMS expands, it may be possible to work in an environment where minor wound care will be expected, so it is in your best interest to seek out additional continuing education into this area. DOT 4-3.37, 4-3.38

Using self-adhesive bandages to secure dressings will work fine if the patient is standing. However, if the patient is prone or supine, then every wrap of the bandage will require moving the patient. In cases such as this, it would be best to use cravats to secure dressings.

Because of all the contours in the area of the hips and buttocks, bandaging can be difficult. Again, the biggest problem is if the patient is prone or supine. Using cravats will reduce the need to move the patient excessively. Large bulk dressings can be secured with cravats. Bandaging of special needs areas is shown in Box 25-3.

BOX 25-3   Bandaging

(a) Head

Bulk dressings with wide wraps are the usual treatment. It may be possible to visualize small scalp arteries that are bleeding in scalp lacerations, and apply direct pressure to them to control hemorrhage. It is important that bandaging not interfere with the airway, mouth, and nose and allows the patient to open the mouth. Take care when wrapping around the head and under the chin. Wounds involving the ears are also difficult to properly bandage. Placing dressings both behind the ear and over the ear will reduce the need to push the cartilaginous ear back against the head, causing discomfort to the patient.

(b) Neck

Attempts to bandage the neck can cause airway problems. In some situations, it may be necessary to hold direct pressure over the wound rather than wrap a circumferential dressing around the neck and compromise the trachea and airway. Caution must also be used around the carotid arteries and the nearby vagus nerve. Vagal stimulation can result in slowing of the pulse.

Occlusive dressings are appropriate if damage to the veins is suspected.

(c) Elbow

The elbow joint needs to be in the position in which it is going to stay before bandaging occurs. If the elbow is straight when it is bandaged and the joint is then bent, it could cause undo pressure and constriction. Put the elbow in the position it will be in for transport, and then apply the bandages and dressings.

(d) Knee

The knee needs to be in the position in which it is going to stay before bandaging occurs. If the knee is straight when it is bandaged and the joint is then bent, it could cause undo pressure and constriction. Put the knee in the position it will be in for transport, and then apply the bandages and dressings.

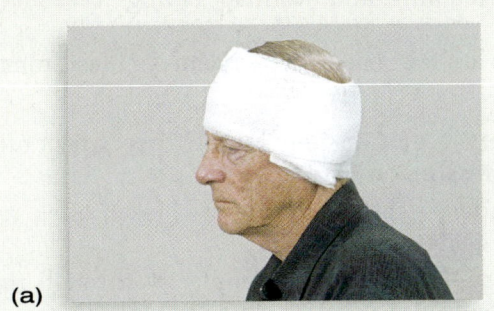
(a)

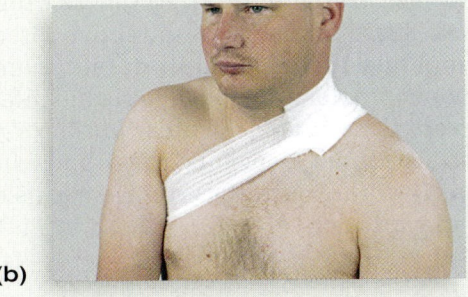
(b)

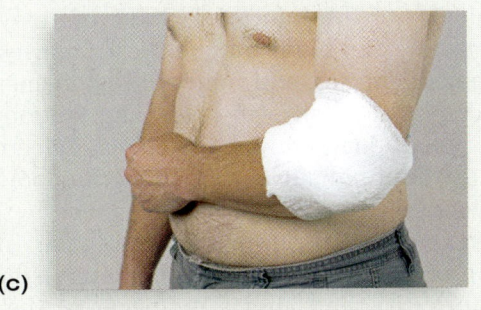
(c)

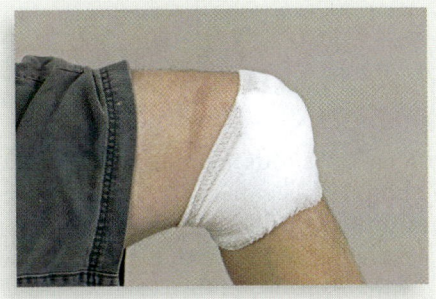
(d)

Management of Specific Injuries

Blast Injuries

Blast injuries result from the detonation of high explosives and the release of large amounts of energy in the form of expanding gasses. These gasses compress and superheat the surrounding air or water so rapidly that a "shock wave" is created. This wave (also called a blast wave) delivers high pressure to any surface it contacts. Damage occurs when the blast wave encounters tissues of different densities, creating differential pressure forces, motion, stretching, and eventual tearing.[1] DOT 4-3.12.i, 4-3.13, 4-3.53j

There are four basic mechanisms of blast injury: DOT 4-3.14a, b, c

- Primary—caused solely by the direct effect of blast overpressure on tissue.
- Secondary—caused by flying objects, often resulting in penetrating injury.
- Tertiary—occurs when people fly through the air and strike other objects, causing blunt injury.
- Quaternary—sustained from being in close proximity to the blast and are triggered or caused by the blast. These do not fit in the above three categories, but they include complications of underlying medical problems (acute myocardial infarction or delivery of an infant secondary to the stress of event), burns (from associated fires), and exposure to toxins (burning buildings release toxins or materials in explosion).[35]

Blast injury victims are likely to be severely injured. This is due to the large surface area of the body impacted by the blast wave, multiple body regions affected, and the complexity of the injuries.[36] Survivors may have both penetrating and blunt trauma. Head injuries, fractures of the extremities, and injury to the organs of the trunk are common. Crush injuries and amputations have also been noted. Pneumothorax is also a concern, and in one study approximately 20% of victims presented with lung contusions.[37,38] DOT 4-3.15

When explosions occur in confined spaces (mines, buildings) or involve structural collapse, there is greater morbidity and mortality because the blast forces are contained and there is often associated crush injury.

Pathophysiology of Blast Injuries

Blast waves cause sudden compression of the structures of the body. This causes "hollow" organs such as the eardrum, lungs, and bowel to rupture in much the same way as a bag inflated with air will pop when it is compressed. Patients may then be struck by flying debris, causing penetrating injury, or they may be physically thrown, striking other objects and sustaining blunt trauma and fractures. DOT 4-3.16, 4-3.17

Specific Blast Injuries

Ears.   The forces transmitted to the inner ear may cause rupture of the eardrum with associated bleeding as well as temporary or permanent hearing loss.[1] DOT 4-4.12, 4-3.18

Street Secrets

If your patient is having trouble hearing you and you suspect that the tympanic membrane has ruptured, the blast force is theoretically serious enough to cause other, more lethal organ injuries. Be alert to more serious life-threatening injuries.[39]

Lungs.   Tearing of pulmonary tissue can result in hemo- or pneumothorax. Blood entry into the large bronchi may compromise airway patency. Air entry into the pulmonary venous system can lead to systemic arterial air embolism.[40] "Blast lung" is the direct consequence of the blast wave and the most common fatal primary blast injury among temporary survivors. Blast lung should be suspected in anyone with dyspnea, cough, hemoptysis, or chest pain following blast exposure.

Bowel.   Bleeding from the gastrointestinal tract can occur into the lumen, the bowel wall, the intraperitoneal cavity, or the extraperitoneal space. In addition to blood loss, tears in the stomach, small bowel, or colon can result in peritonitis.[1]

Other.   Other injuries seen in survivors of explosions occur from missiles, generally causing penetrating trauma; blunt trauma can also result from flying objects.[41] Other miscellaneous injuries can occur including burns, toxic inhalations, and traumatic amputations. Crush injuries will be seen if the victims are caught within the structural collapse.[40] DOT 4-3.15

Treatment for Blast Injuries

The care for patients injured in a blast is centered around the findings and treating specific body regions that have been injured. If the patient's airway is compromised by bleeding or other injury, secure the airway with an advanced airway (endotracheal intubation, dual lumen airway) and be prepared to suction.[1] Inadequate ventilation should be treated with standard care, including positive pressure ventilation (PPV).

Continuous positive airway pressure (CPAP) is described as an option. Unfortunately, there is a chance that positive pressure ventilation will increase the risk of arterial air embolism or pneumothorax. As much as possible, allow patients to breathe on their own. Intervene when patients are unable to adequately ventilate themselves.[1] Lung sounds may present with wheezing due to a potential pulmonary contusion and should be treated with inhaled brochodilators. If blood pressure begins to drop for no apparent reason, suspect intra-abdominal bleeding. DOT 4-3.19, 4-3.20

Impaled Objects

If the object that created a wound is still in the body, the patient is said to have an impaled object. There may be little or no bleeding from an impaled object because the object itself is acting to control the bleeding. Objects can vary in size from a staple gun staple, to an arrow, to a piece of fencing (wooden or metal). The length of the impaled object will determine if it needs to be reduced in size (shortened) for transport to the hospital. Impaled objects should not be removed in the field if at all possible because removal may permit a previously compressed or occluded blood vessel to start hemorrhaging and result in exsanguination.[1,41] DOT 4-3.12e, 4-3.53h

Impaled objects need to be immobilized in place. Large bulky dressings should be positioned around the object to stabilize it. The purpose of stabilization is to prevent additional injury or tissue damage by the object as well as displacement of the object with resulting hemorrhage. The patient needs to be transported to the trauma center with the least movement possible. DOT 4-3.12e

If, however, the object is too large to fit inside the ambulance, (i.e., patient is impaled on fencing) it will be necessary to cut the object. Hand or power saws, an acetylene torch, or bolt cutters may be needed. The patient must be protected from heat and vibration during the rescue operation. You may wish to consider sedation of the patient during such operations, depending on local protocols.

Objects impaled in or around one eye must be stabilized as with any other impaled object. However, with this injury, it is necessary to cover both of the patient's eyes to reduce consensual eye movement.

One rare instance where an object may have to be removed is an object impaled in the central portion of the chest when the patient needs CPR. In this situation, medical consult should be attempted prior to removal. If this is not immediately possible, remove the object and initiate general patient care. Keep in mind that a patient in traumatic arrest has a very poor prognosis.

Working in the Gray Zone

Traditionally, EMS texts suggest that field removal of an impaled object in the cheek is acceptable. There appears to be no evidence to suggest that this is a safe or therapeutic treatment. If the object is not occluding the airway or immediately detrimental to care, then it is best to leave it in place, regardless of where it is impaled. If the object is interfering with the patient's airway and ability to breathe, it must be removed. It should be removed in the direction of least resistance.

Crush Injury

Crush injury, as discussed earlier, occurs when a part of the body is subjected to a high degree of force or pressure, usually after being squeezed between two heavy or immobile objects.[15] Injuries associated with crushing mechanism include lacerations (open wounds), fractures, bleeding, bruising, neurovascular injury, crush syndrome, and compartment syndrome. Crush injury severity depends on the amount and location of tissue involved. It can be minor (the end of a finger crushed between two rollers), or the injury can be extreme (the entire arm or leg crushed under a heavy weight) to fatal (crush of the abdomen, chest, or head). DOT 4-3.25, 22.a

Initial assessment and treatment of life-threatening conditions must always be performed. Bleeding control, bandaging, immobilization, and pain management will vary depending upon local protocols. The debate over the preferred intravenous fluid for volume resuscitation (crystalloid versus colloid solutions) for crush injury or crush syndrome has not been resolved.[11] Local protocol will guide your selection of resuscitation fluid. Morphine (IV or IM) for pain management needs to be considered.

Crush Syndrome

Crush syndrome occurs after crush injury and is a systemic disorder of severe metabolic disturbances resulting from the prolonged crush of skeletal muscle and the release of toxins into the systemic circulation once the patient has been extricated. As mentioned earlier, this toxic cocktail of proteins and chemicals includes myoglobin (muscle protein), phosphate and potassium (from cellular death), lactic acid (byproduct of anaerobic respiration), and uric acid (from protein degradation). Crush syndrome will present with hypovolemic shock, hyperkalemia, hypocalcemia, metabolic acidosis, and acute myoglobinuric renal failure. DOT 4-3.22b

It is important to anticipate the development of crush syndrome and to try to establish IV therapy prior to releasing the patient from the crushing object. It will permit the administration of fluids, analgesia, and drugs for resuscitation or stabilization. Treatment for crush injury must begin immediately upon extrication if it was not started during the extrication process.

Isotonic solutions have a proven safety record, produce a known rise in cardiac output, and are evenly distributed throughout the extracellular space. In addition, isotonic solutions do not draw water out of the intravascular space. Hypertonic solutions have a greater ability to expand blood volume and thus blood pressure and, presumptively, tissue perfusion. The use of hypertonic solutions can cause an osmotic shift of fluid from the intracellular and interstitial spaces to the extracellular compartment. Sodium bicarbonate has been used to help prevent the deposition of myoglobin in the kidneys, leading to renal failure. Local protocols should help guide you in deciding if bicarbonate is to be administered or not.

CONNECTIONS Compartment syndrome is discussed in detail in Chapter 24: Skeletal Trauma. Please consult that chapter for a complete discussion of assessment and management strategies.

Injection Injury

Injection injury is a unique type of soft tissue injury. This type of injury is usually the result of high-pressure liquids, gasses, or sand blasting products (glass beads or sand) being forced through the patient's skin and into the adjacent subcutaneous tissues. This injury commonly occurs with paint spraying equipment, diesel injectors, and hydraulic lines. The injury typically occurs during cleaning or mishandling of equipment.

The injury can be very misleading in the minutes following the initial injury. On early examination, a small puncture wound or no apparent break in the skin may be found. Minimal swelling is present, but swelling and pain increase over time. The injected material tends to spread along fascial planes, so the extent of the injury can be quite misleading and is often subtle on initial presentation.

Vascular compromise can occur directly from compression, secondary to swelling, or from the inflammatory response that the body produces in response to the materials injected. A petroleum-based hydraulic fluid may damage the tissue via chemical disruption of tissue and cells. The chemical itself may alter the body's ability to heal and may cause infection. Delays in treatment can lead to compartment syndrome.[42] Amputation may be necessary if this injury is not recognized and treated appropriately early in its course. Hospital treatment involves immediate surgical debridement and exploration of the full extent of the damage.

Pressure Injuries (Decubitus Ulcers)

As discussed earlier in this chapter, pressure injuries are the result of prolonged compression of the skin and tissues below the skin. In prehospital care, pressure injuries may be created when patients are immobilized to backboards and other similar devices. This damage can be created in an hour or less. Because of this, whenever placing a patient, particularly the elderly, on a backboard or orthopedic scoop stretcher, pad with a blanket before placement.

Care of Specific Wounds

Amputations

Amputations can bleed heavily or bleed minimally. Bleeding control can usually be accomplished with bulky trauma dressings and direct pressure. If this does not control bleeding, then application of a tourniquet is indicated above and as close to the amputation site as possible. Once the tourniquet has been applied, you should not remove it unless directed to do so by an on-line physician. In many cases, the amputated limb can be recovered and transported to the trauma center with the patient. However, do not delay transporting the patient if access to the limb is delayed. Have a second crew find and transport the amputated limb to the trauma center in another unit. Sharp, guillotine type amputations without crush or avulsion damage are the best candidates for reimplantation.[43]

Treat the patient as you would for an open fracture. Handle the injury carefully. Apply gentle pressure to the injury site to stop bleeding. Manage the patient's pain with analgesics. System or regional protocols should be followed with regard to reimplantation center protocols.

Keep the amputated part clean. The amputated limb should be wrapped in a sterile dressing that has been moistened with sterile saline, placed in a plastic bag, and put on ice. An ice pack works best. If real ice must be used, the limb should not come into direct contact with the ice or water. Never use dry ice as this can lead to freezing of the part. The main objective is to keep the tissue cool, which increases the viability of the tissue for reimplantation from six to eight hours to 12 to 24 hours when cold (see Box 25-4).[44]

BOX 25-4 Procedure for Handling Amputations

- Cleanse the wound with sterile saline (NS) or lactated Ringer's (LR). Do not use sterile water.
- Wrap the part in sterile gauze that has been moistened with NS or LR and place into a plastic bag.
- Label the bag or container with the time of injury and fill the container (not the bag with the amputated part) with crushed ice.
- Don't freeze the part.
- Transport the part with the patient if possible, but do not delay transport of the patient to do so.

Considerations for Reimplantation Injuries

Consider all patients as candidates for reimplantation. Reimplantation of amputated limbs has an overall success rate of over 80%.[44] Patients are selected based on age; the presence of preexisting diseases such as diabetes, neuropathy, or vascular disorders; their expected chance of survival; predicted morbidity; and functional outcome. The relative indications for reimplantation are traumatic amputations of almost any part in a child; multiple digits (fingers); individual digits proximal to the distal joint of a finger, the thumb, the wrist or proximal to it; and partial hand (through the palm). Reimplantation of toes and portions of the foot have a low success rate in adults, so some facilities will not even attempt reimplantation.

Face and Neck Wounds

Soft tissue injuries to the face and neck will present special care needs for the patient. Not only is severe bleeding a special problem, but airway compromise with blood, secretions, and other debris will complicate matters as well. Maintaining an open airway is your primary responsibility. Facial and neck trauma may distort physical features and landmarks for intubation. The "golden rule" of intubation is always direct visualization of the glottic opening and vocal cords for tube placement. In cases of severe facial trauma and bleeding, this may not be possible. Once the tube has been placed in what you believe is the trachea, you must be certain that the tube is properly placed by using multiple primary and secondary confirmation methods. DOT 4-3.43a

CONNECTIONS Chapter 12: Airway Management, Ventilation, and Oxygenation describes intubation confirmation in great detail. Confirmation and reassessment of intubation is a critical step in the procedure. It is recommended that you review these procedures frequently. Needle or surgical cricothyrotomy, if system protocols allow, may be the only procedure to ensure the patient has a patent airway. If possible, avoid cutting through neck hematomas that could result in additional severe bleeding. **See Skill Sheet 19: Needle Cricothyroidotomy (also see Step-by-Step 19).**

Cervical in-line stabilization and immobilization must be maintained throughout the prehospital phase of care for trauma patients suspected of spinal injury. Manual opening of the airway by the jaw-thrust maneuver and intubation may take as many as three providers to accomplish when spinal precautions are also required. A fourth provider may be necessary just for suctioning the airway or performing the Sellick maneuver during the procedure.

Once the airway has been opened and the patient is breathing, attention moves to severe bleeding. You may need to avoid direct pressure to skull lacerations if underlying skull fractures are suspected. Here, large bulky dressings need to be applied and secured.

Street Secrets

Open lacerations to the neck add a special danger of air emboli. Cover any large, open neck wound with an occlusive dressing as a precaution to minimize the danger of air aspiration into an open vein. Lacerations to the neck are often explored in the operating room and should be considered a potentially life-threatening problem until proven otherwise (Figure 25-6). DOT 4-3.32

Thorax

The presence of superficial injuries to the thorax may not reveal their true severity to the untrained observer. Injuries to the thorax are likely to cause injuries to the pleura and lungs. Small lacerations may be sufficient to cause a pneumothorax or a hemothorax. Penetrating injuries, such as a stabbing or shooting, can result in pericardial tamponade, penetrating heart trauma, and wounds in the major arteries and veins, esophagus, bronchi, and diaphragm (Figure 25-7).

A complete physical examination, including both anterior and posterior parts of the chest, is necessary. Cleaning blood off these surfaces will be necessary for proper inspection. Be alert for any bubbling

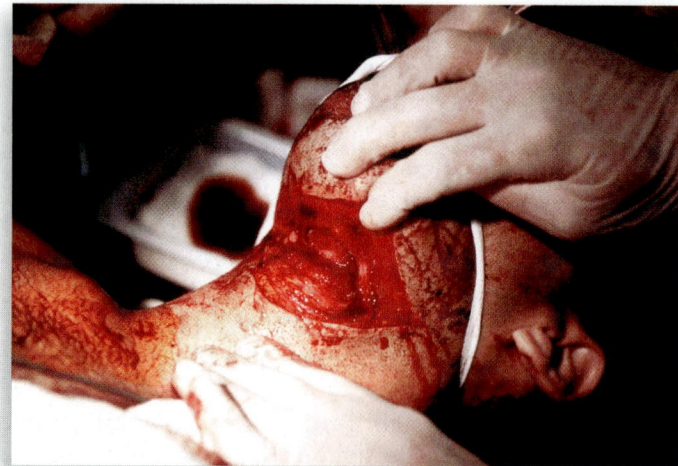

Figure 25-6   Bleeding neck injuries have the potential of substantial bleeding. They should be dressed to control bleeding without impairing the airway.

wounds, subcutaneous emphysema, and crepitation, which would indicate an open pneumothorax. Apply an occlusive dressing that is sealed on three sides, and auscultate every three to five minutes. Watch that the occlusive dressing on the chest does not form a complete seal with blood and convert a simple pneumothorax into a tension pneumothorax. DOT 4-3.32, 4-3.43b

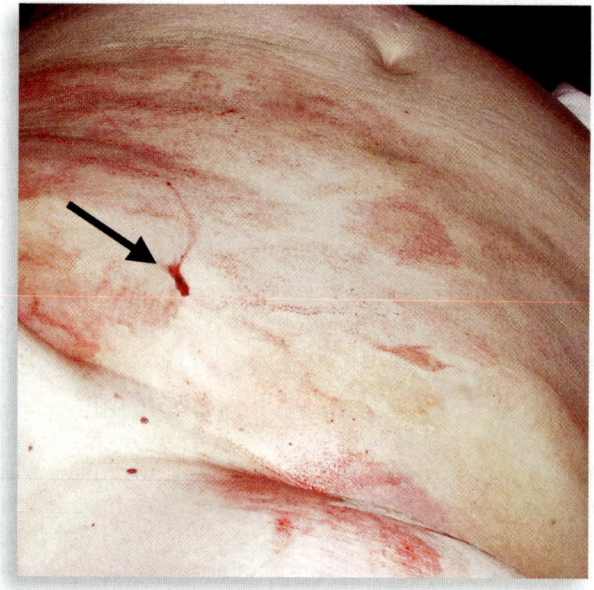

Figure 25-7   A small wound may be the only indication of a life-threatening problem. This 50-year-old woman was stabbed with a butcher knife in the epigastric area. The arrow shows the location of a small stab wound that caused a tension pneumothorax and pericardial tamponade. The patient lived thanks to early prehospital recognition and chest decompression.

CONNECTIONS   Chapter 21: Thoracic Trauma has more information on penetrating and soft tissue injuries to the thorax.

Street Secrets

Patients who have altered mentation, especially those under the influence of alcohol and mood-altering substances, will often not know that they are wounded. If you are treating a patient who may have distracting injuries, has been assaulted, or is simply injured, look carefully for soft tissue injuries, especially in the chest. A small wound may be the only indication of a life-threatening problem.

Abdomen

Blunt and penetrating trauma to the abdominal cavity can result in hollow and solid organ injury. Severe bleeding from lacerations of the liver, spleen, or major arteries and veins and perforation of intestinal organs that will empty digestive material into the abdominal cavity are all life-threatening injuries. The signs and symptoms of internal injuries can be very subtle early in their courses. Eviscerations and other injuries to the abdominal cavity can be very dramatic, but the undetected internal injuries are the ones that will be deadly. Prehospital treatment is supportive, including administration of oxygen, bandaging of wounds, prevention of shock, and transport to an appropriate destination. DOT 4-3.43c

CONNECTIONS   Chapter 22: Abdominal Trauma has more information on soft tissue injuries to the abdomen.

Ongoing Assessment

During the transport to the hospital, continue ongoing assessments of the patient's airway, breathing, and circulation. Obtain additional sets of vital signs to monitor the patient's physical condition. One set of vital signs tells you how the patient was doing at that point in time. A second set of vital signs will tell you the progress of your patient—has the patient responded positively to your treatment or is the patient getting worse? A high-priority patient's vital signs are taken every three to five minutes and a low-priority patient's vital signs are taken at least every 15 minutes. DOT 4-3.42, 4-3.43

All soft tissue injury patients should receive oxygen therapy. High-priority patients should be placed on 15/lpm nonrebreather mask. When soft tissues are injured, the optimal FiO$_2$ is 100%, particularly if significant hemorrhage was present.[1] Fluid resuscitation should be aimed at maintaining perfusion to the brain and vital organs but should not be excessive. Current EMS guidelines for fluid resuscitation, as discussed in various other chapters as well as within this one, recommend titrating to a systolic blood pressure between 90–100 mmHg. DOT 4-3.44, 4-3.45

Summary

Any injury to soft tissue will compromise the protective layer of the body: the skin. A break in the skin will invite bleeding, fluid loss, and infection. Because of the importance of the skin, all injuries must be assessed and properly managed in the field.

Visualization of external wounds may provide the only clue to injuries that are internal and hidden from view. You will not always have discoloration and swelling early on when inspecting patients, so a high index of suspicion is important. Use the assessment of mechanism of injury to help increase your alertness for possible injuries. The patient's response (pain) and careful palpation may also identify a possible trauma site. The goals of soft tissue injury care are hemorrhage control, immobilization, keeping the wound clean of debris, and recognizing which injuries require immediate transportation for physician follow-up.

Notes

1. J. E. Tintinalli, D. G. Kelen, and J. S. Stapczynski, *Emergency Medicine: A Comprehensive Study Guide,* 6th ed. (New York NY: McGraw-Hill, 2004).

2. D. W. Vane and S. R. Shackford, "Epidemiology of Rural Traumatic Death in Children," *Journal of Trauma* 38(1995): 867–870.

3. G. Thibodeau and K. Patton, *Anatomy and Physiology,* 5th ed. 6: Skin and Its Appendages (St. Louis, MO: Elsevier Mosby, 2003).

4. *Handbook of Pathophysiology,* 2nd ed. (Philadelphia, PA: Lippincott, Williams & Wilkins, 2005).

5. B. Herlihy and N. Maebius, *The Human Body in Health and Illness* (Philadelphia, PA: W. B. Saunders, 2000), pp. 93–97.

6. M. McKinley and V. O'loughlin, *Human Anatomy* (New York, NY: McGraw-Hill, 2006), pp. 122–125.

7. *Dorland's Illustrated Medical Dictionary,* 28th ed. (Philadelphia, PA: W. B. Saunders, 1994).

8. D. Shier, J. Butler, and R. Lewis, *Hole's Human Anatomy & Physiology,* 11th ed. (Dubuque, IA: McGraw-Hill, 2007), p. 546.

9. K. Jonson, J. A. Jensen, W. H. Goodson III, et al., "Tissue Oxygenation, Anemia and Perfusion in Relation to Wound Healing in Surgical Patients," *Annals of Surgery* 214(1991): 605.

10. H. W. Hopf, T. K. Hunt, J. M. West, et al., "Wound Tissue Oxygen Tension Predicts the Risk of Wound Infection in Surgical Patients," *Archives of Surgery* 132(1997): 1997.

11. R. Greif, O. Akca, E. P. Horn, et al., "Supplemental Perioperative Oxygen to Reduce the Incidence of Surgical-Wound Infection Outcomes Research Group," *New England Journal of Medicine* 342(2000): 161.

12. H. P. Ehrlich and T. K. Hunt, "Effects of Cortisone and Vitamin A on Wound Healing," *Annals of Surgery* 167(1968): 324.

13. P. J. E. Cruse and R. A. Foord, "A Prospective Study of 23,649 Surgical Wounds," *Archives of Surgery* 107(1973): 206.

14. D. K. Yue, S. McLennan, M. Marsh, et al., "Effects of Experimental Diabetes, Uremia, and Malnutrition on Wound Healing," *Diabetes* 36(1987): 295.

15. Austin G. Rinker, Jr., "Crush Injury: Estimating Skeletal Muscle Damage by the Rule of Thirds," *Emergency Medical Services,* 33(11) (2004): 68–69.

16. M. Michaelson, U. Taitelman, Z. Bshouty, G. Bar-Joseph, and S. Bursztein, "Crush Syndrome: Experience from the Lebanon War, 1982," *Israel Journal of Medical Science* 20(1984): 305.

17. O. Better, "Rescue and Salvage of Causalities Suffering from the Crush Syndrome after Mass Disasters," *Military Medicine* 164(5) (1999): 366–369.

18. J. Veenstra, W. M. Smit, R. T. Krediet, et al., "Relationship Between Elevated Creatine Phosphokinase and the Clinical Spectrum of Rhabdomyolysis," *Nephrology, Dialysis, Transplantation* 9(1994): 637.

19. R. Sinert, L. Kohl, T. Rainone, et al., "Exercise-Induced Rhabdomyolysis," *Annals of Emergency Medicine* 23(1994): 1301.

20. D. A. Feinfeld, J. T. Cheng, T. D. Beysolow, et al., "A Prospective Study of Urine and Serum Myoglobin Levels in Patients with Acute Rhabdomyolysis," *Clinical Nephrology* 38(1992): 193.

21. P. A. Gabow, W. D. Kaehny, and S. P. Kelleher, "The Spectrum of Rhabdomyolysis," *Medicine* 61(3)(1982): 141–152.

22. L. M. Tierney, S. J. McPhee, and M. A. Papadakis, eds., *Current Medical Diagnosis and Treatment, 2006,* McGraw-Hill's MedicalAccess (accessed June 10, 2006).

23. G. M. Doherty and L. W. Way, "Orthopedics," in *Current Surgical Diagnosis and Treatment,* 12th ed., McGraw-Hill's AccessMedicine (accessed June 9, 2006).

24. M. M. McQueen and C. M. Court-Brown, "Compartment Monitoring in Tibial Fractures: The Threshold for Decompression," *The Journal of Bone and Joint Surgery (British)* 76(1996): 99.

25. T. Nowak and A. Handford, *Pathophysiology—Concepts and Applications for Health Care Professionals,* 3rd ed. (New York, NY: McGraw-Hill, 2004), pp. 679–680.

26. W. Lane, "Diagnosis and Management of Physical Abuse in Children," *Clinics in Family Practice* 5(2) (June 2003): 493.

27. J. E. Tintinalli, G. D. Kelen, J. S. Stapczynski, O. J. Ma, and D. M. Cline, "Transfusion Therapy," in *Tintinalli's Emergency Medicine: A Comprehensive Study Guide,* 6th ed., McGraw-Hill's AccessMedicine (accessed June 11, 2006).

28. L. J. Kroot and D. Hurst, "Wound Care," in *Current Emergency Medicine,* McGraw-Hill's AccessMedicine (accessed June 10, 2006).

29. F. C. Brunicardi. D. K. Andersen, T. R Billiar, D. L. Dunn, J. G. Hunter, J. B. Matthews, R. E. Pollock, and S. I. Schwartz, "Hemostasis, Surgical Bleeding, and Transfusion," in *Schwartz's Principles of Surgery,* 8th ed., McGraw-Hill's AccessMedicine (accessed June 9, 2006).

30. H. B. Alam, G. B. Uy, D. Miller, et al., "Comparative Analysis of Hemostatic Agents in a Swine Model of Lethal Groin Injury," *Journal of Trauma Injury, Infection and Critical Care* 54(2003): 1077–1082.

31. R. B. Armstrong, J. Nichols, and J. Pachance, "Punch Biopsy Wounds Treated with Monsel's Solution or a Collagen Matrix: A Comparison of Healing," *Archives of Dermatology* 122(1986): 546–549.

32. D. S. Behroozan, "Surgical Pearl: Patient-Applied Manual Pressure for Hemostasis," *Journal of the American Academy of Dermatology* 53(5) (November 2005): 871–872.

33. J. E. Hipskind, J. M. Gren, and D. J. Barr, "Patients Who Refuse Transportation by Ambulance: A Case Series," *Prehospital and Disaster Medicine* 12(4) (1997): 278–883.

34. D. Hale and K. Sipprell, "Ability of EMT-Bs to Determine which Wounds Can Be Repaired in the Field," *Prehospital Emergency Care* 4(2000): 245–249.

35. "Explosions and Blast Injuries: A Primer for Clinicians," www.bt.cdc.gov/masstrauma/explosions.asp (accessed November 21, 2005).

36. Y. Kluger, "The Special Injury Pattern in Terrorist Bombings," *Journal of the American College of Surgeons* 199(6) (December 1, 2004): 875–879.

37. P. Singer, "Conventional Terrorism and Critical Care," *Critical Care Medicine* 33(1 Suppl) (January 1, 2005): S61-5.

38. S. Wanek, "Blunt Thoracic Trauma: Flail Chest, Pulmonary Contusion, and Blast Injury," *Critical Care Clinics* 20(1) (January 1, 2004): 71–81.

39. E. Levonas, "Blast Injuries," Topic 63, www.emedicine.com/emerg/topic63.htm (accessed November 3, 2005).

40. J. M. Wightman, and B. A. Wayne, "Blast and Crush, Injuries," in *Emergency Medicine: A Comprehensive Study Guide,* 6th ed. (New York, NY: McGraw-Hill, 2004).

41. A. J. Cartwright, K. O. Taams, M. J. Unsworth-White, et al., "Suicidal Nonfatal Impalement Injury of the Thorax," *Annals of Thoracic Surgery* 72(2001): 1364.

42. J. E. Tintinalli, G. D. Kelen, J. S. Stapczynski, O. J. Ma, and D. M. Cline, *Tintinalli's Emergency Medicine: A Comprehensive Study Guide,* 6th ed., McGraw-Hill's AccessMedicine (accessed June 10, 2006).

43. C. K. Stone and R. L. Humphries, "Orthopedic Emergencies," in *Current Emergency Diagnosis & Treatment,* McGraw-Hill's AccessMedicine (accessed June 10, 2006).

44. W. H. Harris and R. A. Malt, "Late Results of Human Limb Replantation: Eleven-Year and Six-Year Follow-Up of Two Cases with Description of a New Tendon Transfer," *The Journal of Trauma* 14(1) (1974): 44–52.

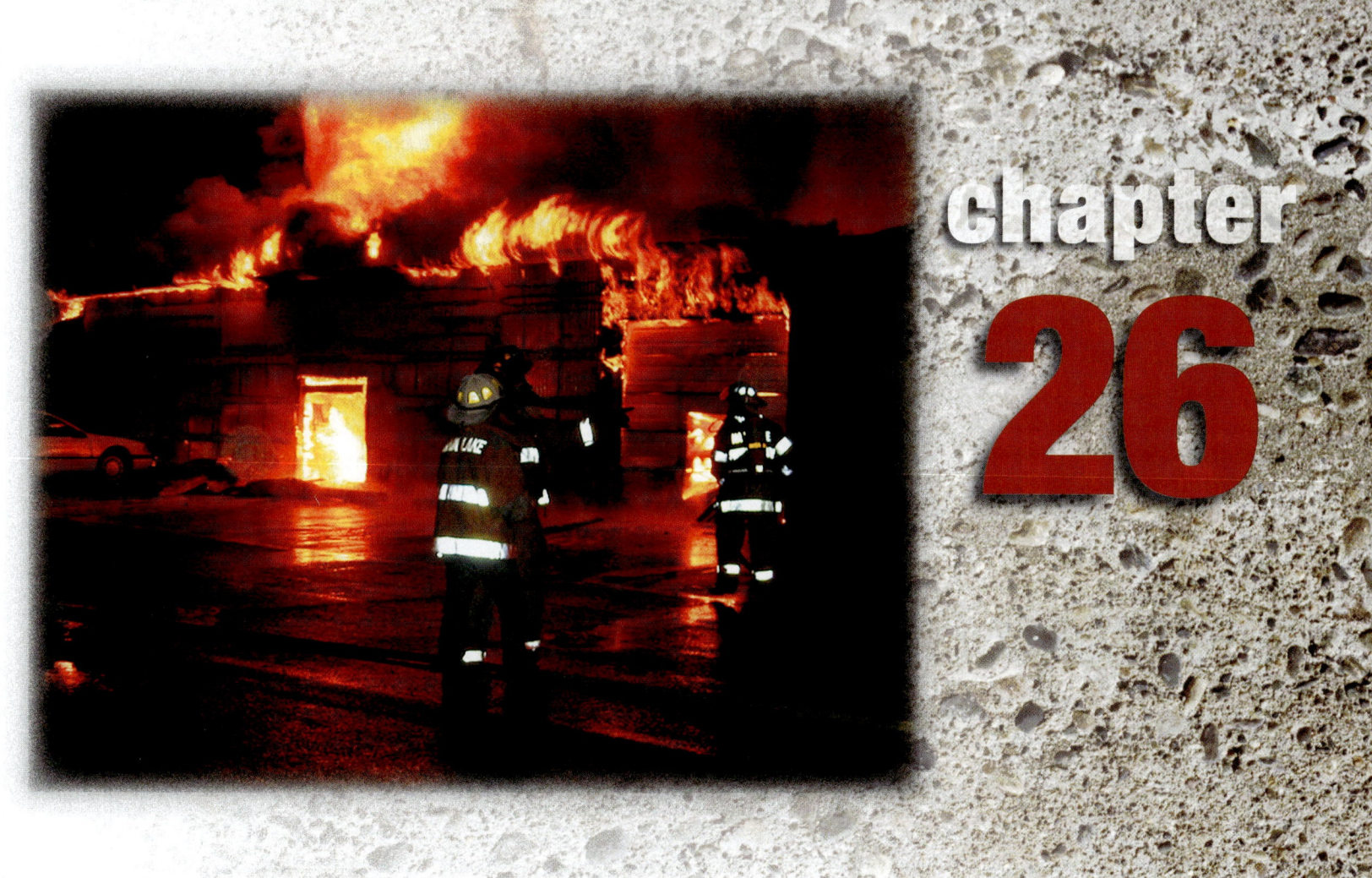

Burn Trauma

*"**B**ehold how great a matter a little fire kindleth."*

—James 3:5, King James Bible

Need to Know

▶ An important consideration in managing burn patients is to ensure that the scene is safe prior to entering and that it remains so throughout the emergency. Even if the patient is seriously injured, it is not appropriate to endanger yourself or members of your crew trying to rescue a patient from a burning environment unless you have the appropriate protective clothing and gear and are trained to do so.

▶ Once the patient is presented to your team for treatment, first stop the burning process by putting water on smoldering clothing. Work quickly so you do not chill the patient.

▶ Perform an initial assessment, and be alert for airway compromise and signs of inhalation injury. If noted, early aggressive airway management is necessary to ensure patient survival. If you find signs of hypovolemic shock (including tachycardia above 130 beats per minute, absent peripheral pulses in non-burned extremities, or low blood pressure) be aware that the cause is NOT the burn.

▶ Always assess the patient carefully for other injuries.

▶ Determine the severity of the burn by applying the rule of nines and following the American Burn Association (ABA) or local protocol criteria to determine the appropriate destination for the patient, whether it is the local hospital emergency department or a burn center.

▶ Sick	▶ Not Yet Sick
• Soot around the mouth and nose, coughing, and wheezing are signs of potential significant inhalation injury. • Large amounts of second and third degree burns; burns to the face, joints, hands, and feet; and elderly burn patients are all critical burns. • Presence of tachycardia, tachypnea, and hypotension indicate shock. Do not assume shock immediately following a burn is caused by the burn. Suspect hypovolemia or some other cause and begin there.	• Alert patients with appropriate responses are likely not significantly sick at this time, but they should be watched closely. • Small isolated extremity burns in young healthy patients are painful but probably not critical. • Obtain information about preexisting diseases and the age of the patient. These factors can have a significant impact upon the final outcome of the patient and are important for the hospital to know. • Determine if the patient sustained a loss of consciousness in the incident. Patients are at risk for more significant burns, inhalation injury, and toxic chemical exposures if they were unconscious in the fire.

Introduction

A burn is a painful and expensive injury to experience as a patient and is difficult and visually disturbing to treat as a paramedic. Burn trauma has a high mortality associated with it, and respiratory complications are common. Scene safety is a high priority when responding to a call involving burn injuries. Each of these issues makes burn trauma a unique category of traumatic injury, deserving special attention. DOT 4-4.71, 4-4.73, 4-4.77

The focus of this chapter is on major burn injuries that should be referred to a burn center. Treatment may take months, and reconstruction may take years. It often requires extraordinary measures to resuscitate these patients in the burn center, and the prehospital care provided is a critical component in this process. Prehospital management can be less difficult if paramedics understand the pathophysiology of the burn process and how it affects the body.

Etiology and Physiology of Burns

Burns are a form of traumatic injury caused by heat, electricity, chemicals, scalds, or radioactivity. **Thermal burns** are caused by contact with flame or extremely hot surfaces on the exterior of the body. **Electrical burns** occur as a result of electrical current flowing through the patient. These burns tend to go deeper than the surface of the skin. **Chemical burns** occur as acids or alkalis of varying pH levels, which are in liquid, solid, or gaseous states, come into contact with external and internal body tissues. How deeply these chemical agents penetrate will vary with differing pH levels. The more acidic a chemical, the more surface damage occurs while the more alkaline the chemical, the more it penetrates deeper into tissues. **Blistering agents** are chemicals that cause burn-like reactions in the body by disrupting cells, tissues, and organs. Blistering agents are also in the WMD (weapons of mass destruction) category. **Scalds** occur as superheated liquids or gaseous steams come into contact with tissues. In the case of scalds, even plain water can result in significant damage or even death. **Radioactive agents** result in destruction at a cellular level. DOT 4-4.11, 4-4.12

CONNECTIONS Chapter 55: Responding to WMD Events has additional information on recognizing and treating WMD agents such as blistering agents.

Many of these causes can also offer significant risk to the responding emergency team, so appropriate precaution should always be taken to avoid contamination and to preserve scene safety. Inhalation injury, with its associated pulmonary complications, is a significant factor in mortality from burn injury (50–60% of fire deaths on the scene are secondary to inhalation injury).[1]

Incidence of Burns

Over 2 million people are burned each year in the United States with approximately one-half burned significantly enough to seek treatment.[2] Over 75,000 people per year are hospitalized, and about 5% die as a result of their burn injuries. This total includes deaths from fires; motor vehicle and aircraft crashes; contact with electricity, chemicals or hot liquids, and substances; and other sources of burn injury. Approximately 30% of the patients who die sustain smoke or thermal damage to their respiratory system. Because it is difficult for an autopsy to distinguish between smoke inhalation and burns as a cause of death, exact statistics are not possible. In the last few decades, the incidence of burn deaths has been on the decline. Overall, burn injury is responsible for approximately 8,000 to 12,000 fatalities in the United States anually.[1]

DOT 4-4.2, 4-4.75

There are many factors that account for death following burns. The age and general state of health of the patient and amount and type of burn all contribute to patient mortality (see Box 26-1). In the 1970s, 50% of all patients with as little as 30% **total body surface area (TBSA)** burned died from their burns. Now patients with 80% TBSA burns account for 50% of all mortality. This means that more patients are surviving

BOX 26-1 Predicting Mortality from Burns

Patients should always be treated aggressively by the paramedic. Many times paramedics with limited experience are surprised when a patient under their care does not survive, especially when they believe optimal care was given. As discussed, survival after a significant burn has a lot to do with the age of the patient and the severity of the burn, so much so that a mortality predictability score was developed. The Baux Score is a "rule of thumb" that calculates mortality by adding the patient's age to the percentage of body surface area burned.[4]

Patient age in years + TBSA of critical burn = mortality percentage

Example:

50 years + 20% burn = a predicted 70% mortality

76 years + 10% burn = a predicted 86% mortality

their burns. Looking at it another way, patients who would have died from smaller burns (say 30%) in 1970 would probably live today, even if they have bigger burns (like 80%). The amount of time patients spend in the burn center has been cut in half over the last 30 years, and almost 95% of all patients admitted to burn centers in the United States survive, with over half returning to preburn levels of physical and social functioning (Box 26-2).[3] DOT 4-4.10

Two categories emerge as the most common age groups for victims of burns: children less than eight years old and young adults (particularly men).[1] The leading cause of burn injury in toddlers and infants is scald burns while thermal burns (flames and heat) are the greatest cause of burns in the young adult group

Working in the Gray Zone

Although tools such as the Baux Score help you understand when patients do not survive injuries that seem minor, it does not permit you to choose which patients you treat and which you do not. This type of tool is for your own emotional well-being and to help you cope with the unpleasantness of losing a patient to a burn injury.

BOX 26-2 Brent Custard

On October 18, 1989, Brent Custard lit a match while an open gas can sat directly in front of him. The fumes immediately ignited and set the entire gas can and Brent on fire. Brent had time to raise his arms and protect his face but quickly collapsed inside his garage, which was now on fire. Thanks to a speedy response by his local fire department and a heroic rescue, Brent was extricated and treated by two Divine Redeemer paramedics and rushed to Regions Hospital, a level I Trauma Center. Brent had third degree burns on over 60% of his body (Fig-ures 26-1a, b). Only days after his admission, he was in the operating room for a bilat-

eral amputation of his legs when his surgeon decided he would wait one more day before amputating his legs. Brent improved gradually and was able to keep his legs, and, thanks to months of meticulous care, protecting him from infections, and skin grafting from cadavers and from his own skin (Figure 26-1c), he made a full recovery. Since his accident, Brent's dream was to become a paramedic. On May 16, 2006, Brent became a Nationally Registered Paramedic (Figure 26-1d). His story shows not only how fire and EMS response can save a life but also how courage, tenacity, and hard work can make dreams come true.

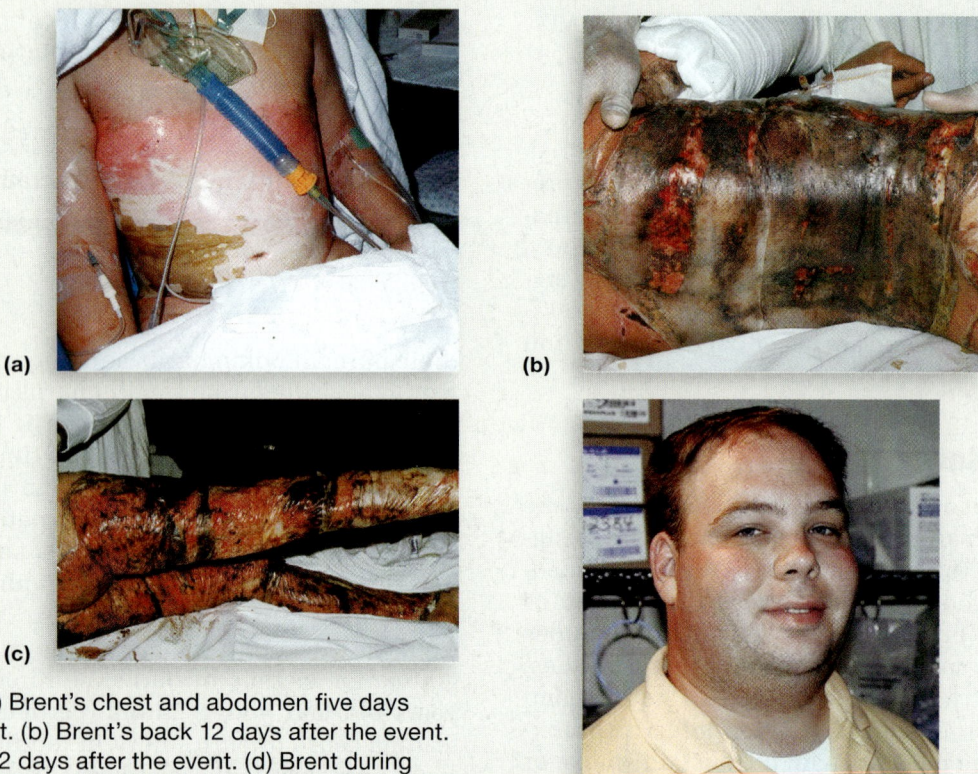

(a)
(b)
(c)
(d)

Figure 26-1   (a) Brent's chest and abdomen five days after the accident. (b) Brent's back 12 days after the event. (c) Brent's legs 12 days after the event. (d) Brent during paramedic school.

(Figure 26-2). Thirty-six percent of burn patients experience burns related to motor vehicle crashes. Over 90% of all burns are preventable, with one half of all burns related to smoking or substance abuse. Most burn injuries occur in the home, and work is the second most frequent site for burn injuries.[5,6] DOT 4-4.15

Burns occurring as the result of war and military action have a different incidence and are not discussed herein nor are their statistics used in compiling the above information. The incidence of burns in military trauma is significant. Between 5% and 10% of military battlefield injuries include burns along with other types of trauma such as gunshot wounds

or blast injuries. Less than 7% of nonmilitary burn patients experience other trauma along with their burns.[1]

Overview of the Severity of Burns

The severity of burns is determined by the following factors:[7] DOT 4-4.1

- **Depth.** Including degree (first–third) or thickness (partial or full thickness).
- **Extent.** Estimate the percentage of TBSA (total body surface area) involved.

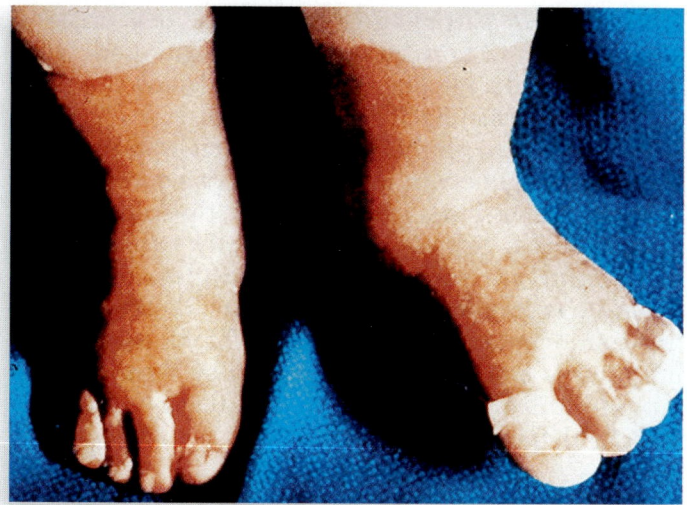

Figure 26-2 Circumferential burns with a clean edge or end to the burn are caused when a child is dipped or lowered into scalding water.

- *Age of the patient.* The very young and very old have poorer outcomes.

- *Area/part of the body burned.* The face, hands, feet, perineum (groin), and deep circumferential burns (which go around the chest, abdomen, or extremities) require special care.

- *Medical history.* Patients with certain diseases (for example diabetes or congestive heart failure) are at higher risk for death.

- *Suspicion of respiratory involvement.* The presence of inhalation injury or respiratory system involvement increases mortality significantly.

Applied Anatomy and Physiology

The Skin

The skin consists of two layers: the epidermis (top layer) and the dermis. The epidermis is of varying thickness on the body. For example, the skin of the forearm is relatively thin; whereas, the skin of the soles of the feet is extremely thick. The epidermis functions as the external barrier between the outside environment and the rest of the body. The outermost cells of the epidermis are actually dead tissue, which transitions to living cells as you go deeper into the body. It is this layer that also gives us our pigmentation or color. The underlying dermis contains structures such as hair follicles, sweat glands, nerve endings, and sebaceous (oil) glands (Figure 26-3).[8]

The skin has several functions. It serves as a barrier to water, vapors, and infection. It regulates body temperature by retaining or releasing heat from the body. It provides protection to underlying body structures. When temperature extremes are placed on or near the skin, the skin can be damaged. Excessively hot, cold, or caustic substances can damage or "burn" the skin. Once this damage occurs, the skin loses its ability to perform its many functions. If the damage has occurred in a superficial manner, the skin may be able to recover, and, once healed, it may be difficult to determine where the injury occurred. If the injury has penetrated beyond the skin, it may go deep into the body and involve the subcutaneous tissues, muscles, bones, organs, the deep vessels (veins and arteries) of the vascular system, and the nerves or other structures of the nervous system.

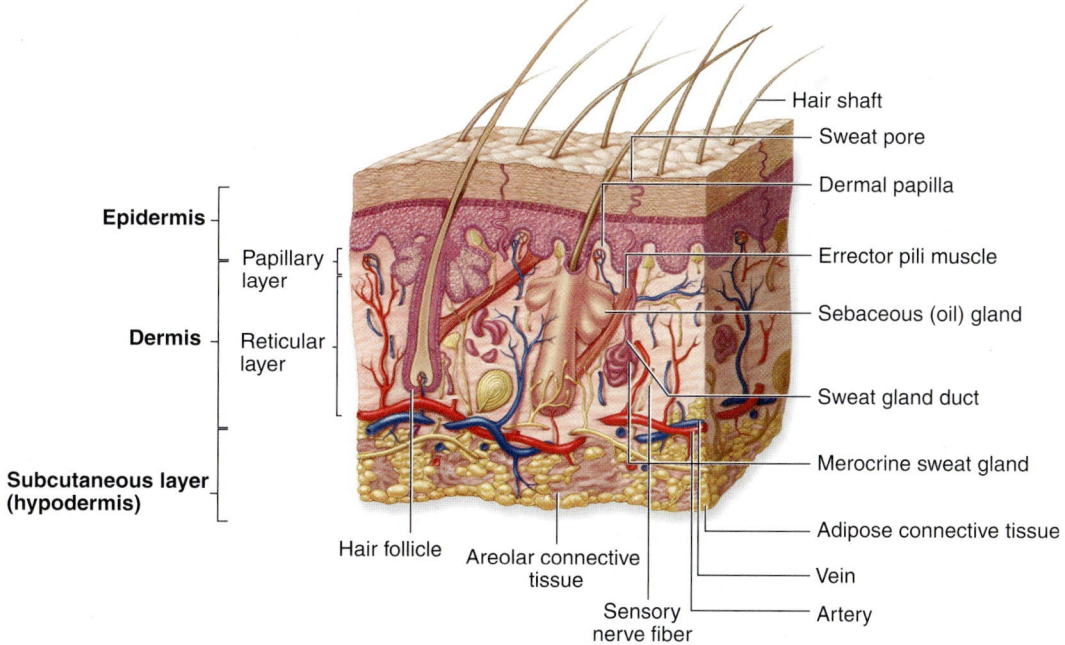

Figure 26-3 The layers of the skin and the structures within the layers.

Classification of Burns by Degree and Thickness

Burns are classified by the depth of the tissues they penetrate (see Table 26-1).[9] This classification gives the "degree" of burn. Each larger number represents a greater depth of penetration. **First degree burns** involve only the outermost layer of skin tissue, the epidermis, and are not life-threatening. DOT 4-4.5

Second degree burns involve the dermal layer, and they are subdivided into categories of "thickness," which will be discussed later.

Third degree burns have penetrated through both layers of the skin (epidermis and dermis) and have extended into the subcutaneous layers.

Fourth degree burns are classified as burns that penetrate deep into the body (such as a burn into muscle and bone). The term **fourth degree burn** has gone out of style and is not currently used by the American Burn Association. What was called fourth degree is now simply referred to as a "deep third degree." Often, deep third degree burns are caused by electricity, direct contact with flame, immersion in burning liquid or burns sustained by individuals who were unconscious in a fire.[1,9]

Burns are also classified by describing their "thickness." First degree burns are also called **superficial**. Second degree burns are referred to as **superficial partial thickness** or **deep partial thickness**, depending upon the depth of the injury. Superficial partial thickness burns are erythematous, blistered, and painful. Deep partial thickness burns look waxy in appearance and may be red or white in color. Third (and fourth) degree burns are both referred to as **full thickness burns.** A first degree burn (for example, simple sunburn) rarely needs a hospital or burn center and is not counted in estimating the amount of burn wounds.[10] In a burn center, partial thickness burns may be either left alone or surgically treated. Most deep burns are surgically removed (debrided), and new skin is grafted over the injury site. Distinguishing between deep and shallow partial thickness burns is not always straightforward, and many burns have a mix of clinical characteristics, making it difficult to classify them precisely.[1] DOT 4-4.5

Determining the Extent of Burn Injury

It is important to determine how much of the body is involved with burns beyond the first degree. Burn size can be determined by estimating how much of the total body surface area (TBSA) is involved. There are three ways to estimate the size of a burn:

1. Rule of nines
2. Rule of the palm
3. Lund and Browder chart DOT 4-4.6

The **rule of nines** has been the traditional method of measurement in the prehospital setting.[1,9] The actual rule of nines is applicable only to adults because infants and children have different body proportions than adults. Modified charts, which are also frequently called "Rule of Nines" charts (because of their similarity in form and function to the adult chart) must be used for children and infants.

The **rule of the palm** is less rigid than the rule of nines and is used for burns involving a small TBSA or for those with a patchy pattern.[1] The **Lund and Browder chart** is more complex than the "rule of nines" and is used primarily by hospitals.

The Rule of Nines

The body of the adult is divided into nine parts, and each portion of the body equals approximately 9% of the total body surface area. The head is 9%, with the face 4%, back of the head 4%, front of the neck 0.5%, and back of the neck 0.5%. The chest is 9%, and the abdomen is 9%. The upper back from the bottom of the neck to the waist is 9%, and the buttocks are 9%. Each arm is 9% total, with 4.5% assigned to the anterior (front) of the arm and 4.5% assigned to the posterior (back) of the arm. Each leg is 18%, with 9% anterior and 9% posterior. The remaining 1% is assigned to the perineum (groin) area. As you can see in the figure, the charts for the child and infant are adjusted for their body proportions as well. Note that in the infant, the head accounts for nearly 20% of the

TABLE 26-1   Burns Classified by Depth

Depth of burn	Signs and symptoms
First degree	Pink to red Slight edema that subsides quickly Pain that is relieved by cooling
Second degree *Superficial partial thickness*	Pink or red Blisters form Edematous and elastic Wound is moist and painful Hair does not pull out easily
Deep partial thickness	Mottled white and red Reddened areas blanch with pressure May be yellowish, but still elastic Sensitive to cold air May or may not be sensitive to touch Hair pulls out easily
Third degree	Color varies from waxy white to brown Reddened areas do not blanch with pressure Not elastic; leathery texture Not painful

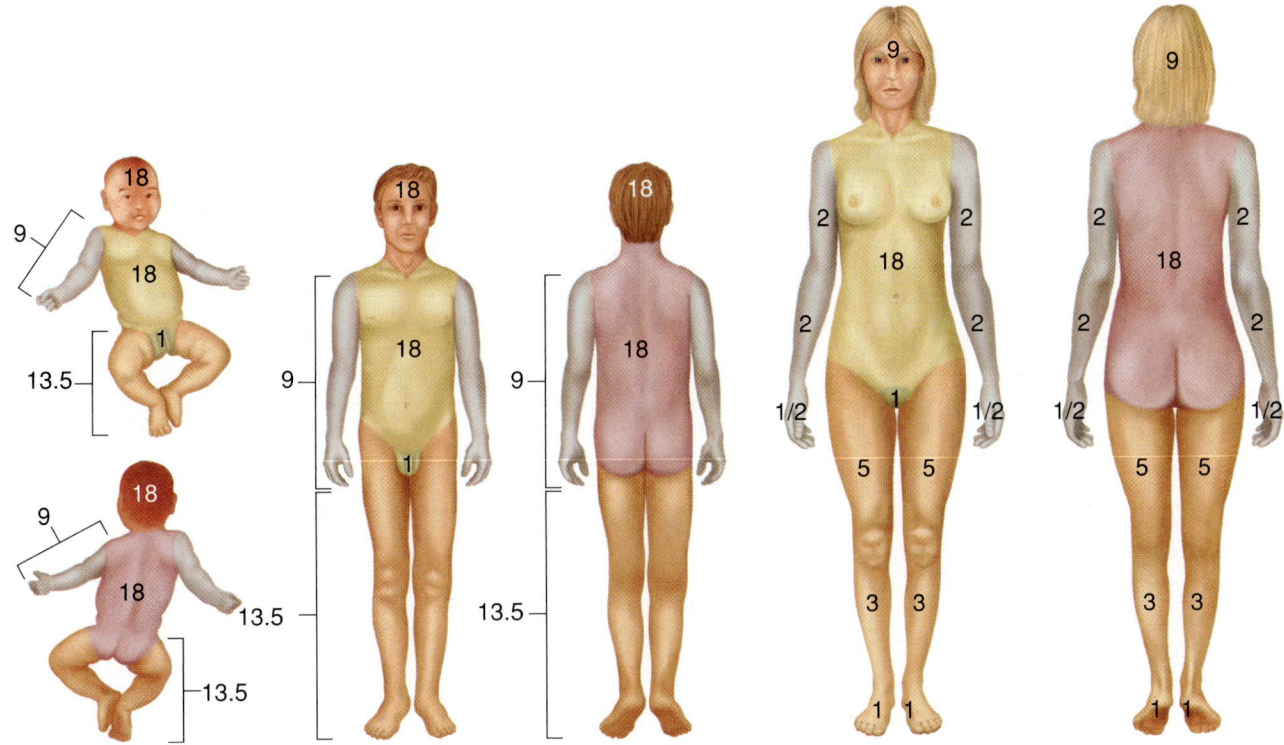

Figure 26-4   The "Rule of Nines" is used to calculate the TBSA (Total Body Surface Area) involved in the burn.

TBSA, so it is important that the correct chart be used for each age group (Figure 26-4). **Skill Sheet 78: Burn Percentage Estimations is a tool that uses the rule of nines for both adult and pediatic patients.**

The Rule of the Palm

The patient's palm (which is the entire hand surface, including the fingers) is estimated to equal approximately 1% of the patient's TBSA. The Rule of the Palm method is best used for evaluating patchy or splatter type burns that are small or isolated[1] (Figure 26-5).

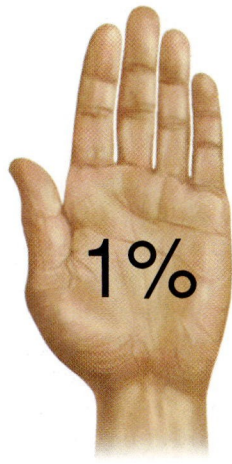

Figure 26-5   The "Rule of the Palm" or "palmar method" uses the palm of the patient's hand to represent 1% of the patient's body surface area in measuring the burned area.

The Lund and Browder Chart

This is the most accurate tool for estimating burn size and is the standard tool utilized in burn centers in the United States (Figure 26-6). It is not practical for use in the prehospital setting because it is time-consuming. It scales burn severity for size and age. Using the drawings on the chart, the burn areas are colored in either red or blue pencils, delineating partial and full thickness burns. The percent TBSA involved is then recorded in the provided spaces on the chart, and an adjusted score is obtained. It is excellent for estimating burn size and, as a result, correct fluid resuscitation needs.[11]

Pathophysiology of Burn Injuries

Basic Pathology of Burn Injuries

A burn injury results from energy transfer from a heat source, cold source, or caustic agent to the body. The depth of injury seen from a burn is proportional to the temperature applied, duration of contact, and thickness

AREA	PERCENT OF BURN					SEVERITY OF BURN		TOTAL PERCENT
	0–1 Year	1–4 Years	5–9 Years	10–15 Years	ADULT	2*	3*	
Head	19	17	13	10	7			
Neck	2	2	2	2	2			
Ant. Trunk	13	17	13	13	13			
Post. Trunk	13	13	13	13	13			
R. Buttock	2-1/2	2-1/2	2-1/2	2-1/2	2-1/2			
L. Buttock	2-1/2	2-1/2	2-1/2	2-1/2	2-1/2			
Genitalia	1	1	1	1	1			
R. U. Arm	4	4	4	4	4			
L. U. Arm	4	4	4	4	4			
R. L. Arm	3	3	3	3	3			
L. L. Arm	3	3	3	3	3			
R. Hand	2-1/2	2-1/2	2-1/2	2-1/2	2-1/2			
L. Hand	2-1/2	2-1/2	2-1/2	2-1/2	2-1/2			
R. Thigh	5-1/2	5-1/2	8-1/2	8-1/2	9-1/2			
L. Thigh	5-1/2	6-1/2	8-1/2	8-1/2	9-1/2			
R. Leg	5	5	5-1/2	6	7			
L. Leg	5	5	5-1/2	6	7			
R. Foot	3-1/2	3-1/2	3-1/2	3-1/2	3-1/2			
L. Foot	3-1/2	3-1/2	3-1/2	3-1/2	3-1/2			

CODE: Blue areas indicate 2*
Red areas indicate 3*

TOTAL

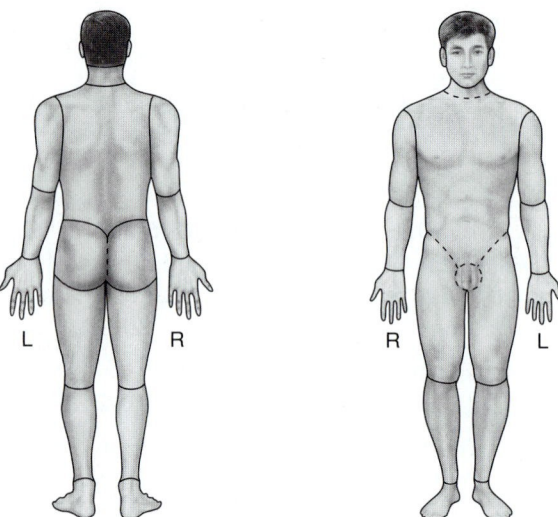

Figure 26-6 The "Lund and Browder Chart," while not practical for use in the field, is a more accurate method for calculating TBSA and is used in hospitals and burn centers.

of the skin where contact occurred.[1] The source of burn injury may be a scald, flame, flash, or direct contact. All sources are discussed in detail later in this chapter. DOT 4-4.3, 4-4.14, 4-4.20

Many factors alter the response of body tissues to these sources of heat. Local tissue conductivity refers to the ability of tissues to withstand the presence of heat. Of all the body tissues, bone is the most resistant to heat accumulation. Lesser resistance is seen in nerves, blood vessels, and muscle tissue.[1]

Burns that do not penetrate all the way through the dermis leave skin organs intact, like sweat glands and hair follicles with sebaceous glands, which can aid in the healing process. When the dead dermal tissue is

removed, the living cells from these remaining structures can move into the surrounding areas to form a new fragile dermal and epidermal layer.[1] Skin appendages vary in depth, and the more that are damaged the less that are available to aid in healing. The longer it takes a burn to heal, the greater the inflammatory response and the more severe the scarring. Burns that heal within three weeks generally have the least amount of scarring and functional impairment.[1]

Burns isolated to the epidermis (first degree) do not blister (Figure 26-7). They become erythematous (red) because the underlying blood vessels become dilated and blood flow into the tissues is increased. The nerves in this area are irritated, and the skin is

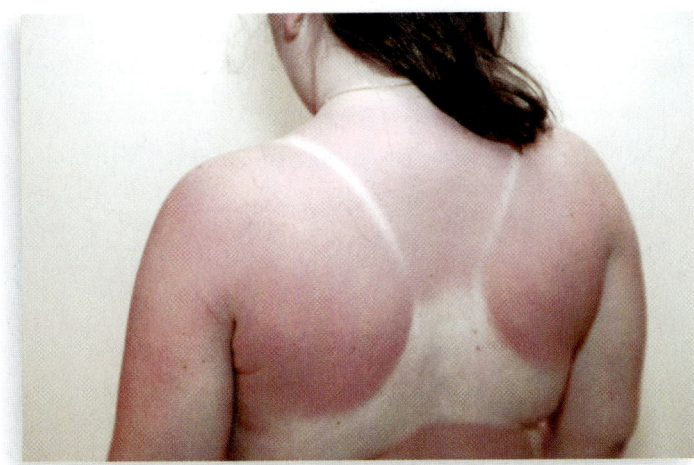

Figure 26-7 First degree burns will present as painful reddened skin without blister formation.

quite painful. Over a period of two to three days, the pain subsides. The dried out epidermis peals away, leaving newly dead dermis tissue in its place to form the new epidermis. There will be no scars with an epidermal burn.[1]

Blister formation is common with second degree burns and serves as a visual distinction between first and second degree burns for the paramedic (Figure 26-8). Because the burn is to the upper layer of the dermis (superficial partial thickness), fluid-filled blisters will form as the damaged tissue responds to the injury. The formation of blisters can be rapid (within minutes of the burn occurring), or they can take 12 to 24 hours to develop. Generally, the deeper the second degree burn, the faster the blisters form. When the blisters are removed, the skin underneath is pink and sensitive to air movement. Superficial second degree

burns will blanch (turn white) when pressure is applied to the skin. They will usually heal within three weeks and usually do not form scars if infection does not occur.[1]

Street Secrets

Never remove blisters or burned tissues adhering directly to the body in the prehospital setting. This tissue may be removed in the hospital or burn center, but it provides some protection to the tissues underneath, so it should not be removed.

Deep partial thickness burns (which are deeper second degree burns) extend into the reticular layers of the dermis (Figure 26-9). The reticular layer is the deepest portion of the dermis and is comprised primarily of interlacing white-colored fibers. As with all burns, burns in this area can occur with varying levels of depth, some partially into the dermis and some almost all the way through the dermis. Areas that are partially involved remain somewhat perfused (therefore, "pink"), and areas that are more completely involved appear white. These burns also blister, but the patchiness from the pink and white colors leads to a mottled appearance. The patient often experiences less pain with this burn than the superficial partial thickness burn because the nerves may be damaged. Capillary refill tests performed on this tissue result in absent or delayed return of color to the tissue. On the second day of injury, the wound is usually white in appearance and dry. If not surgically removed and infection is prevented, these burns generally heal in three to nine weeks. They often heal with scars. If they involve tissues over the joints, scar formation will lead

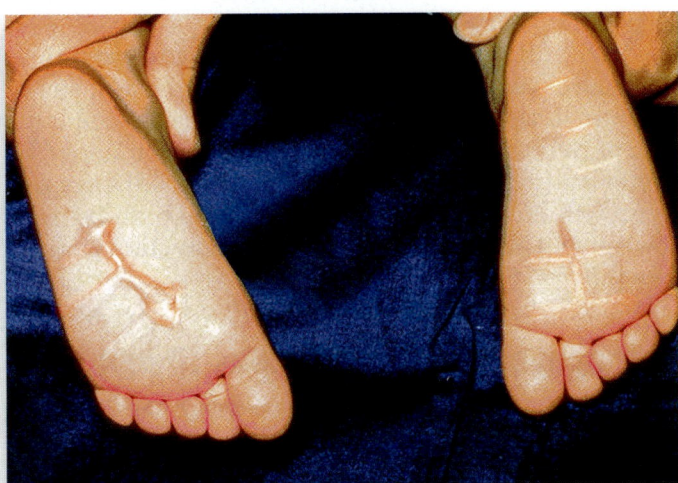

Figure 26-8 Blister formation is the visual distinction between first and second degree burns. (This child's burns should also raise the possibility of abuse.)

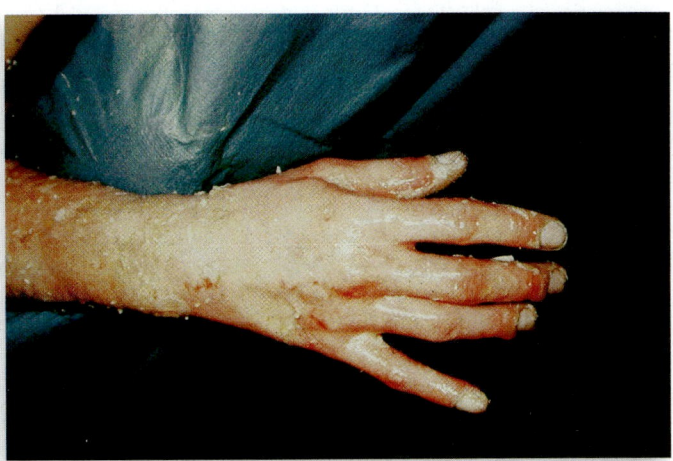

Figure 26-9 Deep partial or second degree burns extend into the reticular layer of the dermis. The most affected areas may become blotchy or whitened.

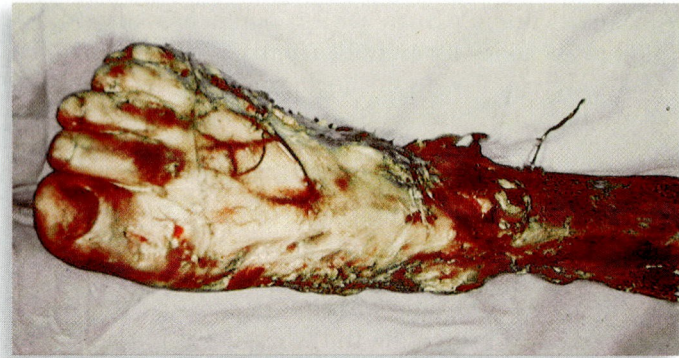

Figure 26-10 Full thickness or third degree burns appear white or waxy, cherry red, charred, or black depending on the source and depth of the burn.

to extremity contractures or limitation in range of motion, therefore, physical therapy is required to preserve function of the extremity.[1]

Full thickness burns (third degree) involve all layers of the dermis and will only heal if grafted, or, if the burn is small enough, it may be able to close from the outside margins inward, from epithelialization of skin outside the wound area (Figures 26-10 and 26-11). This epithelialization process is similar to that described previously for partial thickness burns.

Full thickness burns appear white or waxy, cherry red, charred, black, or leathery, depending upon the source and depth of the burn. Scalds will usually appear waxy and white while flame burns from clothing often look sooty and charred. These burns may or may not have deep blisters present. They feel hard, leathery, and firm and look depressed when compared to the normal skin at their margin. In some cases, clotted blood vessels may be present under the skin, which has taken on a translucent appearance.

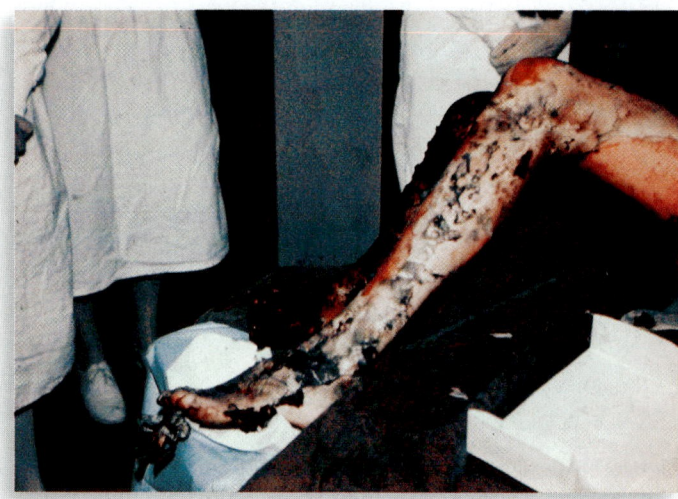

Figure 26-11 Full thickness burn.

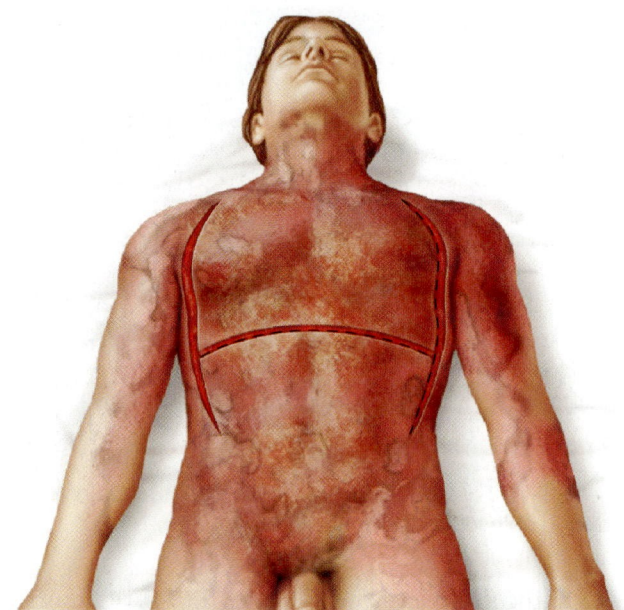

Figure 26-12 Circumferential burns involving the chest can restrict breathing, necessitating a surgical procedure called an escharotomy to allow the respiratory muscles to function.

Because the protein within the skin has unfolded **(denatured)** during heating, eschar scar tissue forms as the skin cools. Eschar is inelastic dead dermis tissue, and over time, it separates from the underlying tissues. If the full thickness burn is circumferential, it can constrict blood flow in the underlying tissues, or, in the case of the chest, it can impair respiratory efforts. A surgical procedure, called an **escharotomy,** can be performed to cut open this tissue to allow the muscles to move and blood to flow (Figure 26-12). Although extremely rare, this procedure could be performed by a paramedic under physician direction, so it is described in Box 26-3.

Each full thickness burn has an area referred to as the **zone of coagulation.**[9] This area is the deepest part of the burn. It is surrounded by a **zone of stasis** (a combination of living and dead tissue), which is surrounded by **erythema** (redness). It is very similar to a bull's eye pattern, with the most severe portion of the burn being in the center. Grafting usually is required to close wounds like this.[1]

Pathophysiology of a Serious (Deep) Burn

Following a deep burn (such as a deep partial thickness or full thickness burn), blood plasma starts to leak out of the capillaries into the surrounding soft tissues (called **third spacing**) as the patient enters into the **systemic inflammatory response syndrome (SIRS).** SIRS consists of changes in the metabolic, cardiovascular, gastrointestinal, and coagulation systems.[1] This

BOX 26-3 Escharotomy

The complications of eschar formation are the result of what occurs in the tissues underlying a third degree (full thickness) circumferential burn. The skin itself looks like it has been tanned, hardened, and leatherized. As edema develops underneath, the circumferential eschar prevents expansion and swelling, so instead it becomes constricting, and blood flow into the tissues is compromised. When it involves the chest, expansion may become inadequate or impossible. It becomes difficult to ventilate the patient even if intubated, and the patient is essentially no longer able to breathe. A chest escharotomy may be a life-sustaining procedure. If considered by the paramedic, consultation with medical direction must be obtained. If at all possible, the patient should receive a bolus of morphine, if conscious, prior to the procedure. The dose for an adult may be 10–20 mg or more, given by slow IV push. In an extremity, as injured tissue under the eschar accumulates edema fluid, it causes compression of muscle and blood vessels, leading to compromised circulation in the extremity.

An escharotomy is an incision made with a scalpel, through the burned, devitalized, dead tissue and just into the layer of fat underneath. In the chest, it is a straight line incision from just below the clavicle in the anterior axillary line to approximately three to four inches below the diaphragm. This is done on both sides of the chest. A horizontal incision connects these two lines just below the diaphragm. A basic "H" is made on the chest. Avoid making the incision through the nipple line. Extremities may require escharotomies as well, but this can be done in the hospital.

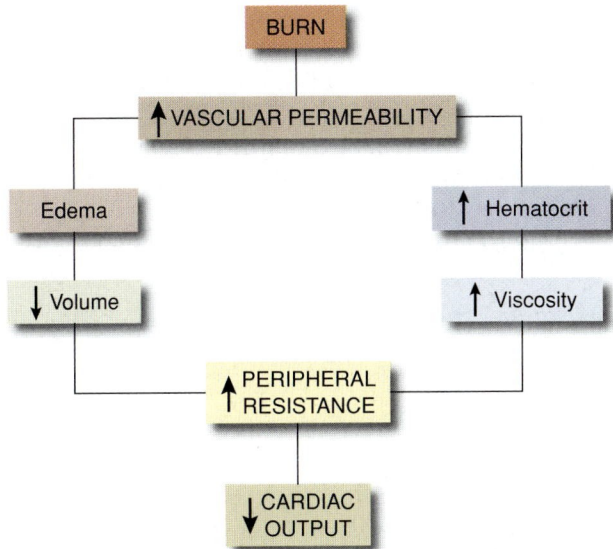

Figure 26-13 Systemic Inflammatory Response Syndrome (SIRS) results from plasma leaving the vascular space and entering soft tissues. This diagram illustrates the burn pathology resulting from deep and extensive burns.

swelling (see Figure 26-13). This initially occurs due to the direct trauma to the tissues. Vascular permeability (the degree to which the fluid within the blood vessels stays there) increases in the blood vessels adjacent to the burned tissues, and plasma levels drop as fluid leaves the blood stream and moves into the damaged tissues. The hormone **histamine** is released in large quantities from dying cells, resulting in increased vascular permeability, which contributes to additional fluid loss from the bloodstream.[1] The hypermetabolic state results in the heart rate increasing in an effort to circulate the remaining blood volume and maintain cardiac output. An adult with a major burn usually has a heart rate of 110–130 bpm.[12]

White blood cells leave the bloodstream to respond to chemical signals from cells that are dying from ischemia (hypoxia, or lack of oxygen) and the toxins collecting in the damaged tissue. Although the volume remaining in the vascular system starts to decrease because of the loss of plasma, the number of red blood cells remains relatively stable. For this reason, the hematocrit (which is the measurement of the ratio of red blood cells to plasma fluid) increases (concentrates) and the blood thickens.[13]

Because of this thickening of the blood, peripheral resistance increases within the vascular bed and maintains a near normal blood pressure immediately after the burn injury occurs. As the blood volume continues to drop, cardiac output eventually starts to fall. (Remember that cardiac output is calculated as the heart rate times the stroke volume.) As cardiac output falls, blood pressure eventually falls as well.

syndrome results in hypermetabolism (with high levels of epinephrine circulating in the blood), increased permeability of cells (they gain or lose electrolytes inappropriately), hemodynamic changes (blood pressure is not regulated properly), and extensive **microthrombosis** (many small blood clots forming and blocking blood vessels). With appropriate fluid and electrolyte resuscitation, the cardiovascular effects of the syndrome largely disappear within 24 to 48 hours following the burn trauma. The exception to this is the hypermetabolic state, which does not completely resolve until the burn is actually healed. DOT 4-4.7, 4-4.56, 4-4.57, 4-4.58, 4-4.59, 4-4.61, 4-4.62, 4-4.63, 4-4.64

Initially in SIRS, the plasma leaves the bloodstream and enters the subcutaneous tissues, resulting in tissue

(Blood pressure equals cardiac output times the peripheral vascular resistance.) Intravascular fluid continues to third space, and the vascular volume decreases further.[1] In this state, the patient appears to be in hypovolemic shock from fluid loss although the total fluid volume has not really dropped. The fact that plasma has shifted from the vascular system to the body tissues causes a type of burn-induced shock.

CONNECTIONS Chapter 8: Physiology Overview describes cardiac output, peripheral vascular resistance, and blood pressure in detail.

The result of all of the SIRS processes is generalized swelling (edema) in the body tissues, particularly in those damaged by the burn. Edema occurs four to six hours after the burn trauma happens. It will reach its maximum in approximately 24 hours.[1]

The bloodstream continues to leak contents, and **hypoproteinemia** results from the loss of protein from the blood.[13] An adequate amount of protein is necessary in order to maintain blood pressure and peripheral vascular resistance. When it is not present in an adequate amount, the blood vessels become more permeable (leaky) and lose even more plasma.

Sodium begins to shift into injured cells.[13] As cells die, their contents are released into the surrounding tissues. Potassium, as the chief intracellular cation, is released from ruptured dying cells, causing hyperkalemia. This can result in cardiac rhythm disturbances. Hypokalemia (low potassium levels) occurs as fluid shifts occur, and the kidneys filter out the excess potassium. The potassium lost from the body is not easily replaced. This can also lead to cardiac rhythm problems. Both conditions do not occur for several hours postburn, so they should not be a concern in the prehospital setting unless transport time is long or delayed.

Patients who do not die on the scene from the burning process may die from the burn if the total body surface area or depth is too great for their body to compensate. Death in the first few hours after the burn is often due to toxic gas inhalation or airway compromise due to edema. As electrolyte imbalances occur, death may also occur. Children, for example, may experience seizures from electrolyte imbalances.[13] Adults may experience cardiac rhythm disturbances from electrolyte imbalances. In the days or weeks following the burn, patients may develop infection, which can lead to septic shock and death. This is the greatest cause of mortality in burn patients who survive the initial insult.[13] One study cites death rates as high as 50% for patients who develop infections from *C. albican* alone.[13]

Types of Burns

Scald Burns

Scalds are the most common cause of burns and are seen most often in children (see Figure 26-2).[1] The most frequent source of scalds is hot water. Water at a temperature of 140°F causes a deep partial thickness or full thickness burn in three seconds. If the temperature rises 16° to 156°F, a deep scald burn occurs in one second.[14] To keep this in perspective, coffee at its freshly brewed temperature is around 180°F. Box 26-4 has more information on temperatures and burns. DOT 4-4.4

With scalds, exposed areas of skin tend to be burned less deeply than clothed areas because the clothing remains in contact with the skin and it retains the heat. Immersion scalds occur when the skin comes into contact with hot liquid by being dipped or plunged and are often deep and severe because the hot liquid remains in contact with the skin for a longer period of time. These burns tend to occur more frequently in children and the elderly who have thinner skin.[1]

Scalds from cooking oil or grease are usually severe as the temperature for both of these substances is generally in the range of 400°F. Tar and asphalt burns are also considered scald burns. These substances are maintained at temperatures between 400 and 500°F. Burns caused by hot tar directly from a storage container are at full temperature and are generally full thickness. Once the tar is spread on the road surface, it has cooled enough for the burn to be partial thickness.[13]

Thermal Burns

Flame burns are the most common injury in adults and the second most common type of burn injury.[1] Damage results from the heat, causing the proteins within the skin to denature (come unfolded), and then when they cool, they refold into the inelastic eschar tissue described earlier. The most frequent causes of thermal burns include (in order of frequency) smoking related fires, improper use of flammable liquids, motor vehicle collisions, and ignition of clothing by stoves and space heaters (Figure 26-14). If bedding or clothing has been on fire, full thickness burns are common. DOT 4-4.4, 4-4.16

Flash Burns

Flash burns are next in frequency after thermal burns.[1] Explosions account for most flash burns. Chemicals such as natural gas, propane, combustible liquids, gasoline, and the like and electrical arcs cause intense heat for a brief duration of time. Unlike scald burns,

BOX 26-4   Temperature Impact Upon Burn Severity

Burn depth is directly related to the temperature of the burning agent and the duration of contact with body tissue. This information applies to adult patients only. Remember that the elderly and pediatric patient would sustain injury sooner than this.

- Below 44°C (112°F), no local damage occurs unless exposure is for a prolonged period.
- At 49°C (120°F), it takes five minutes of exposure to create a full thickness burn. Public buildings are required to set hot water heaters no hotter than this.
- At 52°C (125°F), the exposure time required for a severe burn to result is two minutes.
- At 60°C (140°F), only three to six seconds are required for a severe burn.
- At 70°C (159°F), it takes one second to create a full thickness burn in a healthy adult.

Source: F. C. Brunicardi, T. R. Andersen, T. R. Billiar, D. L. Dunn, J. G. Hunter, J. B. Matthews, R. E. Pollock, and S. I. Schwartz, *Schwartz's Principles of Surgery,* 8th ed. McGraw-Hill Online. (2005).

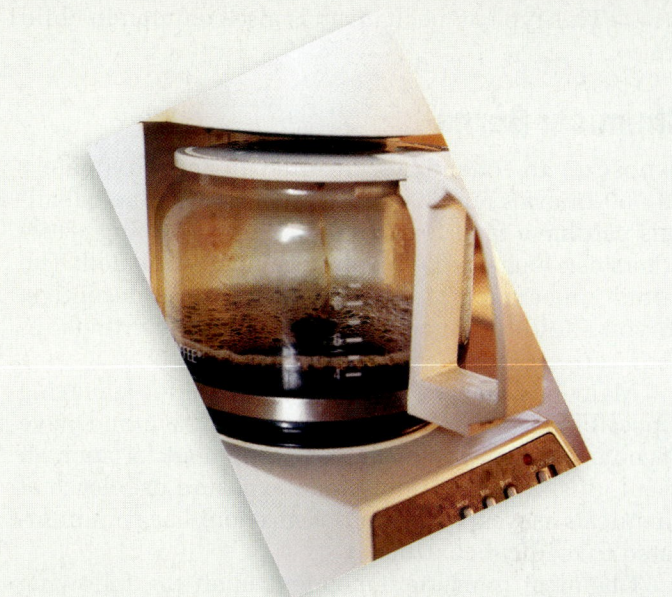

Spilling freshly brewed coffee, at 180°F, is a frequent cause of burns.

clothing is usually protective in a flash burn, unless it ignites, in which case thermal burns may result. Burns are noted on all exposed skin surfaces, with the deepest burns seen on the skin facing the ignition source. Flash burns are often epidermal or partial thickness, but those from electricity or gasoline are generally full thickness and require grafting (Figure 26-15). Extensive damage to the airway should also be suspected in these burns.[1]

DOT 4-4.4, 4-4.83

Contact Burns

Contact burns result from direct skin contact with very hot substances such as metal, plastic, glass, or hot coals. Their size is usually limited to the size of the surface contacted, but they can be very deep (see Figure 26-8). If this burn is the result of an industrial accident, it is common to have associated crush injuries from contact with hot heavy objects. Motor vehicle and motorcycle

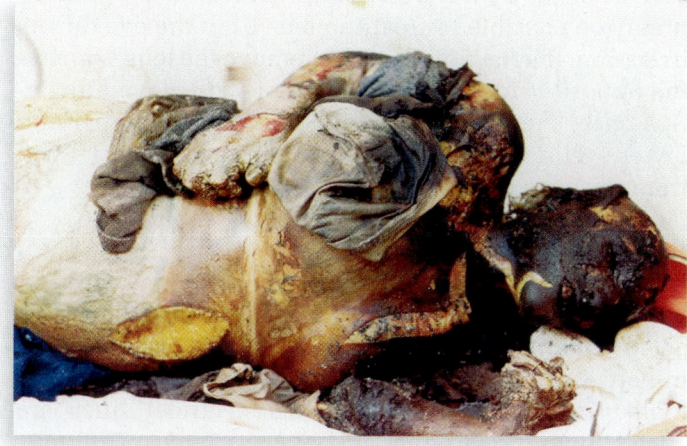

Figure 26-14   Direct contact with flame is the most common injury in adults and second most common burn injury.

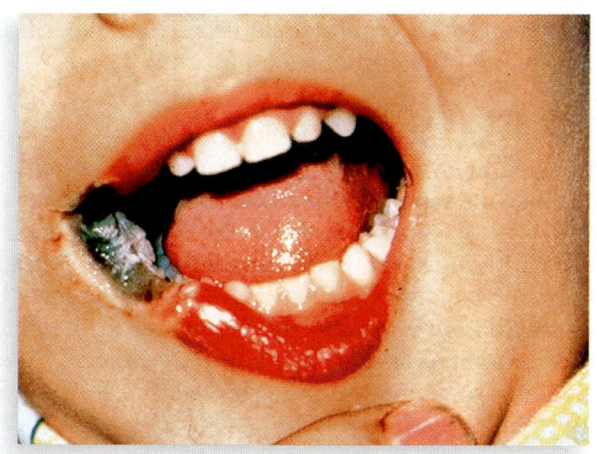

Figure 26-15   A common electrical burn is caused by a child biting into an electrical cord.

crashes may leave a patient in contact with hot motors or exhausts. Contact burns in unconscious or postictal (postseizure) patients are often deep third degree burns.[1] DOT 4-4.4 This type of mechanism is also common in child abuse.

Chemical Burns

Exposure to chemicals results in approximately 60,000 injuries and 3000 deaths a year.[15] Some chemicals can have fatal toxic effects from poisoning while others can damage the respiratory tract if inhaled. The initial appearance of these injuries can be deceptive, so you should assume they are deeper than they appear. DOT 4-4.31, 4-4.32, 4-4.33, 4-4.34, 4-4.35, 4-4.36, 4-4.37

Many hospitals have instituted a plan for managing a possible terrorism-related chemical attack and have decontamination protocols and equipment for such an event. Suspicions of intentional exposure or release of chemicals as weapons or terrorism should be communicated to medical control.

Chemical injury is dependent upon the following factors: the strength and concentration of the chemical, quantity (amount) of agent involved, duration of contact with the patient, the mechanism of action, extent of penetration into the body, and the method it enters the body.[1] Chemicals can enter the body through the skin or mucous membrane by **absorption.** They can be **inhaled** and enter through the respiratory system. They can be **ingested** by swallowing or eating, **injected** with a needle, or enter through a punctured site on the skin.

Chemicals in powder or gaseous form carry a significant risk of inhalation, so look into the nose and mouth of these patients. A chemical burn to the oropharynx might be the only sign of damage to the respiratory system. Gasses such as anhydrous ammonia (used as a fertilizer on farms and in the production of methamphetamine) can damage the respiratory tract, quickly leading to pulmonary edema. Close monitoring and continued reassessment of respiratory status are crucial during treatment and transport of such patients.

Chemical Burns to the Eye

With the advent of more "do-it-yourself" projects at home, the incidence of chemical injuries to the eye is on the rise.[16] Chemical burns to the eye can erode the sclera (white of the eye) and the cornea. Both acid and alkaline substances are caustic, and tissue damage begins immediately upon contact. Exposures to chemicals should be treated as true ocular emergencies.[17] Alkali substances are generally more devastating to the eye.[9] Alkali penetrates the eye while acids burn the surface. Long-term blindness can result if both types of chemicals are not washed quickly and effectively from the surface of the eye. DOT 4-4.31, 4-4.32, 4-4.33, 4-4.34, 4-4.35, 4-4.36, 4-4.37, 4-4.38

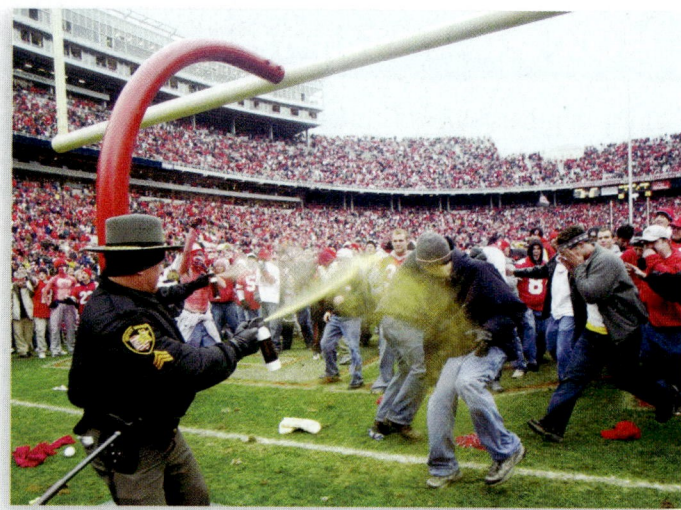

Figure 26-16   Mace or pepper sprays cause intense tearing and irritation of mucous membranes of the mouth and nose. Surrounding tissues may be burned as well.

Patients with caustic chemical exposure will complain of intense pain as well as blurred or diminished vision, photophobia (light sensitivity), or a feeling that a foreign body is present. The eye will be red, and the surrounding tissues may be burned also. Riot control agents and defensive sprays such as tear gas, mace, and pepper spray cause an immediate onset of severe ocular burning, intense tearing, and irritation of the mucous membranes of the nose and mouth (Figure 26-16). These agents may denude (remove) the corneal epithelium and inflame the eye, so they should be treated as chemical exposures as well.[9] DOT 4-4.58, 4-4.63, 4-4.68, 4-4.79, 4-4.82

The presence of contact lenses should be noted. If a contact lens is present, it must be removed to prevent trapping any residual chemical between the lens and the surface of the eye. If attempted removal is too painful, it may be possible to float the lens from the eye during irrigation. If irrigation does not remove the lens, squeeze the opposite sides of the lens either with gloved fingertips or by exerting pressure and closing the upper and lower eyelids. This will bow the lens and break its seal from the cornea.

Electrocution Burns

Scene safety concerns are particularly important with electrical injuries. Ensure all power is off prior to entering any scene involving electrical injuries. Do not be fooled into believing unmoving electrical lines are "dead" lines. Power lines and electrical equipment may be energized and conducting current even when they are not moving. DOT 4-4.39, 4-4.40, 4-4.41, 4-4.42, 4-4.43, 4-4.44, 4-4.45, 4-4.46

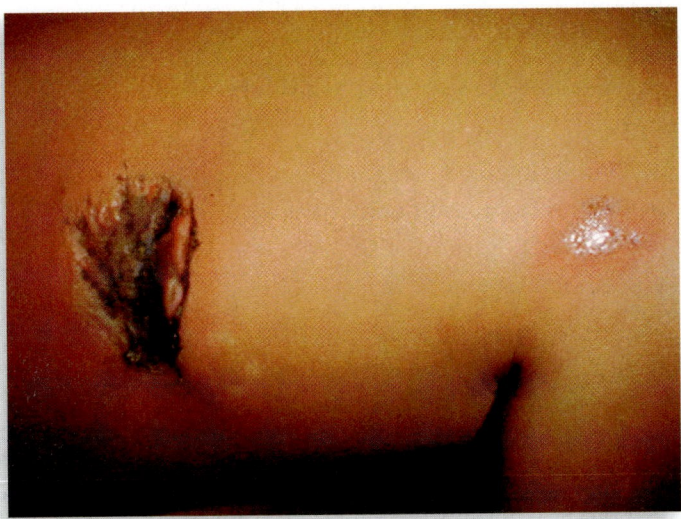

Figure 26-17   The path the current follows through an electrical burn patient can be described by the location of the entrance and exit wounds.

With alternating currents (AC) of 25–300 Hertz (Hz), low voltages (less than 220 Hz) tend to produce ventricular fibrillation; high voltages (greater than 1000 Hz) cause respiratory failure; and intermediate voltages (220–1000 Hz) may cause both. More than 100 milli-Amps (mA) of domestic house AC of 110 volts at 60 Hz is very dangerous to the heart and can cause ventricular fibrillation. In contrast, direct current contact is more likely to cause asystole.[4]

When a person contacts an electrical charge, that charge instantaneously seeks a path out of the body. Electrical injuries may come from direct contact, an arc, or concomitant flame injury.[1] The path of the electric current can often be evaluated by looking for entry and exit burns (Figure 26-17). An entrance wound exists where the electricity enters the body. Exit wounds occur where electricity exits the body. Exit wounds are always third degree. Several points of entry and exit can be found with electrical wounds, so the entire body of the patient should be examined for injury. Remember that electricity penetrates deep into the body and often moves toward and along the nerves and spinal cord.

Contact burns and arcs can reach temperatures up to 2500°C.[1,4] An arc injury is best described as an indirect injury. This is a similar analogy to a car accident. While electrocution can be compared to a head-on collision, an arc burn is similar to being sideswiped. An arc can reach up to 10 feet away from the source. Injury occurs when the victim interrupts the arc. The flame injury occurs when clothes ignite. Musculoskeletal trauma may occur from the tremendous muscle spasm and torque that may occur. Electrically injured patients often fall from heights as well, so spinal injuries and other trauma should be suspected.[1]

Along the path taken by electricity as it passes through the victim, resistance to the flow of the current generates heat and can damage whatever tissue is located between the entry and exit points. The following tissues are listed in the order they offer resistance to the flow of electricity, from low resistance to high resistance: nerves, blood vessels, muscle, skin, tendon, fat, and bone. The difference between alternating and direct current is of little value in the prehospital setting as is the distinction between low (less than 1000 volts) and high (greater than 1000 volts) voltage.[1]

Massive electrical charges with extended contact times can leave limbs blackened and charred. Conversely, extended contact at lower voltages can leave a victim with extensive deep tissue trauma that is not immediately visible externally on the scene. Electrical burns are progressive, and may take from one to three weeks for all the damage to develop.[4] If the charge traversed the chest, at least 10% of the electricity is presumed to have passed through the myocardium (heart). In addition to cooling smoldering clothing, look beyond the visible burn when assessing and treating these injuries and assume substantial internal damage is present.

Radiation Exposure

Every EMS system should have a prehospital plan for evacuation and management of radiation disasters. The hazmat team often takes the lead in managing the emergency. Every hospital is required by the Joint Commission on Accreditation of Healthcare Organizations (JCAHO) to have a protocol regarding receiving, treating, and managing patients from radiation emergencies.[9] DOT 4-4.47, 4-4.48, 4-4.49, 4-4.50, 4-4.51, 4-4.52, 4-4.53, 4-4.54, 4-4.55

The concept of "exposure is not the same as contamination" is an important one to remember. Being present in an environment with radiation does not necessarily mean contamination has occurred. Many people are particularly wary of radiation because of the image portrayed of it in science fiction stories or as a natural consequence of our heightened awareness of terrorism and security issues. However, with the exception of radioactive dust, patients exposed to radiation (which is an extremely rare occurrence) are not hazardous to the EMS team handling them. Chapter 53: Hazardous Materials Incidents and Chapter 55: Responding to WMD Events have more information on radiation.

The United States Department of Energy's **Radiation Emergency Assistance Center/Training Site (REACTS)** began in 1944. REACTS monitors radiation incidents and collects data from around the world. Since 1944, 426 radiation accidents have been recorded worldwide with 133,811 victims. Of these, 3036 were classified as having significant exposure, and 134 victims died. The 1986 Chernobyl accident accounts for the majority of these patients with 116,500 exposed and 28 deaths. The most frequent radiation accident is caused by a high-dose exposure, usually to the hands, by a radiation device. The majority of these incidents occur in industrial settings.[9]

The EMS team may be an active component of the hazmat team, with members actually taking part in the rescue operation, or they may serve a support function and receive and transport patients once they have been decontaminated, if contamination with a radioactive substance has actually occurred. If the issue of contamination or exposure is unknown, then the patient is managed as if contaminated. Appropriate personal protective equipment, respiratory protection, and turnout gear will be identified within the protocol. These guidelines must be strictly adhered to in order to maintain scene safety for all responding EMS providers. Radiation events can only be monitored with special equipment.[9] DOT 4-4.60, 4-4.65, 4-4.70, 4-4.84

CONNECTIONS   More on radiation injury and decontamination can be found in Chapter 53, page 1292, and Chapter 55, page 1320.

Primary Survey

As with all trauma victims, a primary and secondary trauma survey, including assessment of the airway, breathing, and circulation, is required. Immediately following the burn injury, the patient's blood pressure is usually within normal limits or slightly elevated. There is often mild tachycardia (120–130 bpm) with perfusion noted in all extremities, unless that extremity is burned severely. Respiratory rates are usually moderately or significantly increased, depending upon the severity of the burn. The respiratory *effort* is a key issue to assess due to the frequency of inhalation injury and the resulting airway compromise.

Because vital signs are near normal at this stage of the injury, patients with signs of hypovolemic shock immediately after being burned are that way because of blood volume loss.[1] Depending upon the cause of the burn, other traumatic injuries should be suspected and searched for during the trauma patient assessment. For example, if there was also an explosion, look for internal bleeding, potential spinal injuries, and other signs of trauma. Fluid loss from the burn will begin immediately but will not be significant enough to cause hypovolemia and vital sign changes for a few hours.[2]

After initial threats to the airway, breathing, and circulation have been identified and treated, focus on the extent and severity of the burn injury. Burn size, patient age, depth of the burn, and preexisting conditions are the primary determining factors for whether or not a burn will be fatal.[1,3] DOT 4-4.10

Management of Burns

Management of the acute burn injury includes

- Hemodynamic stabilization
- Evaluating for possible inhalation injury
- Preventing loss of body heat
- Estimating wound size
- Pain management

Hemodynamic stabilization will start in the field with intravenous fluid resuscitation. ABA criteria state that the presence of major trauma takes precedence over burn management. Therefore, patients with both burns and major trauma should go to a trauma center first and then be transferred to the burn center once the trauma is stabilized.[13] A generalized approach to management of burn patients is presented first, followed by management of special cases such as inhalation injury and chemical burns. DOT 4-4.13, 4.4-21, 4-4.80

Guidelines for Treating Burn Patients

- Approach these patients in a manner similar to all trauma patients. Perform a thorough scene size-up. Pay particular attention to scene safety. Ensure that the burning process has stopped, and apply sterile or plain water for no more than one minute if the burn is less than 10%.[18] One minute or less total cooling time is recommended to avoid causing hypothermia. Practically speaking, the burning process must be completely stopped, so use your judgment in applying this principle. Remember to use respiratory and eye protection if chemicals are involved. DOT 4-4.74

  - Never apply ice to cool a burn. Frostbite can occur too easily to injured tissue.
  - Dressings may be moistened with sterile water if the TBSA is less than 10%. This is done for patient comfort only. In general, wet or gel dressings for TBSA over 10% are not recommended for use by the ABA.

- Perform a primary survey and treat any problems or immediate threats to life.
- Undress the patient and cover with a dry, sterile (or clean) sheet to preserve body heat.

  - Immediately apply 100% oxygen if the burn occurred in a confined space, there is suspicion of CO poisoning or other toxic inhalation, or if respiratory distress is present.
  - Consider immediate intubation if signs of respiratory distress associated with inhalation injury are present.

- Perform a head-to-toe rapid trauma assessment looking for other injuries.

- Start one or two large bore IVs with an isotonic crystalloid fluid. Lactated Ringer's is the recommended fluid of choice by the ABA.[1]
- Provide pain management if allowed by protocol. Morphine sulfate, a benzodiazepine (such as diazepam or lorazepam), or any of the sedation drugs used for rapid sequence intubation may be considered.
- Transport the patient quickly to the appropriate facility.
- If time permits nonadherent clothing may be removed.
- All jewelry and body piercings should be removed in the field.
- Elevate burned extremities if possible to reduce blood flow into the tissues and help control edema formation. Monitor peripheral pulses.
- Elevate the head of the stretcher if not contraindicated by the injuries. This can improve respiratory efforts.
- Respect the patient's feelings and expressions of stress, pain, fear, cold, and fatigue. DOT 4-4.72

Intravenous Fluid Therapy

Per ABA criteria, immediate IV fluid resuscitation is indicated for the following:

- Adults with burns involving more than 18–20% of TBSA.
- Children with burns involving more than 12–15% of TBSA.

Patients with electrical injury, the elderly, or those with cardiac or pulmonary disease may have a compromised response to burn injury. These patients require meticulous monitoring and may require a modification of fluid requirements. The goal is to give sufficient fluid to allow perfusion of vital organs without overhydrating the patient and risking later complications from circulatory overload. Generally, an isotonic crystalloid solution such as lactated Ringer's is used initially. An IV may not be necessary if there is no other trauma, pain management is not an issue, the wound is small or superficial, and transport time is less than one hour. DOT 4-4.76

A general guideline for fluid resuscitation in the prehospital setting is as follows:

- Adults with 20% TBSA receive 500 mL/hr of Ringer's lactate
- Adolescents (ages five to fifteen) with greater than 15% TBSA receive 250 mL/hr of Ringer's lactate
- Young children (less than five-years-old) with 15% TBSA receive 125–150 mL/hr of Ringers lactate[7]

Nice to Know

Weapons of Mass Destruction: Blister Agents

Per current ABA guidelines, fluid resuscitation for blistering agents is run at maintenance (84–125 mL/hr) levels only, and Ringer's lactate is still the fluid of choice. Physiologically, blistering agent wounds behave similar to a condition called TENS (toxic epidermal necrolysis syndrome), and massive amounts of fluid are usually not necessary to manage these patients. Overhydration can lead to circulatory overload and pulmonary edema.

The Parkland Formula

The **Parkland formula** is used by emergency departments and burn centers to estimate the amount of fluid appropriate for burn patient resuscitation. It is not appropriate for use outside of the hospital setting unless transport times are great or an interfacility transport is being performed. In either situation, medical control guidance should be used. Parkland, along with several other formulas (Evans, Brooke), is used to estimate the amount of fluid to be given in the first 48 hours following the burn trauma. The total amount of fluid is calculated by multiplying the patient's weight and total body surface area burned by the recommended volume of two to four mL of Ringer's lactate. One-half of the fluid is given over the first eight hours. The remaining half of the total required fluid is given over the next 16 hours. In the next 24 hours, another formula is used to adjust fluid volumes based on the response of the first 24 hours. Fluid boluses may be given to achieve a desired urinary output of 50 cc/hr in the adult. Electrical injuries require double the urinary output.

Prehospital Pain Management

Even a small burn can hurt. Narcotics should be given in small, frequent amounts, much like those given for chest pain. The most commonly used prehospital analgesic is morphine. Other common narcotics used include fentanyl, hydromorphone (Dilaudid), or other agents as defined by individual jurisdictional protocols. All medications are given intravenously. The patient is given small amounts frequently because they are in a hypermetabolic state and the drug is metabolized rapidly. Adults may require 20 mg of morphine or more. The dosage of morphine for children is based on weight and is 0.1–0.15 mg/kg.[19] Be prepared with a narcotic antagonist and ventilatory support if respiratory depression, apnea, or hypotension occurs as a result of the narcotic administration.

In the event vascular access is unavailable or inappropriate, inhaled nitrous oxide, if utilized in your EMS system and no contraindications for its use exist, may be another option for pain management. Intramuscular (IM) or subcutaneous (SQ) injections into the skin are contraindicated in extensive burns, even in nonburned skin, because absorption is significantly impaired in the entire body with a TBSA involvement of greater than 30%.

Burn pain can be impressive and may require medication doses exceeding standard EMS guidelines. Medical consultation is typically always available and should be used.[2]

Special Considerations for Children

Not many circumstances can affect healthcare providers as much as a badly burned child (Figure 26-18). While most of the assessment and treatment strategies discussed in this chapter work well with burned children, there are some situations that require further exploring. As with all situations of illness and injury, children are not just little adults. DOT 4-4.9

Between 40% and 70% of pediatric burn injuries are from scalding liquids. A caregiver's statement regarding the mechanism should match the pattern of the burn.[1] Reports of falling into a hot bathtub are suspicious, especially if there are no burns to the chest or head (children are top heavy) or the child is too young or unable to walk. It is estimated that up to 14% of all cases of abused children in the United States involve burns and can come from any socioeconomic class.[20]

It is required by law that all cases of suspected child abuse be reported to the appropriate jurisdictional authority, which may be the police department, a social worker, a child protective agency, or hospital staff. In most states, paramedics, as well as nurses, doctors, teachers, social workers, and police officers, are required to report suspected abuse.

CONNECTIONS See Chapter 45: The Abused and Neglected for more information on child abuse and your responsibilities for identifying and reporting suspected cases.

Treatment of Chemical Burns

Clothing should always be assumed to be contaminated and a threat to prehospital providers and receiving medical facility staff, so it must be immediately removed. As with thermal burns, rings, watches, and other jewelry must be removed to prevent a tourniquet-like effect and restriction of blood flow as edema develops. DOT 4-4.38

A large amount of water flushed over the patient is still the mainstay of initial decontamination. Consider performing this procedure in an area that can contain the runoff water if the chemical is dangerous to the environment. If containment of the runoff is not easily accomplished, dilution of the runoff with additional water is an acceptable alternative. Also consider whether the decontamination operation should be performed by the hazmat or other specially trained decontamination team. Full body decontamination is best performed by trained individuals with special equipment and supplies that can manage the wastewater produced in the process. Contaminated clothing should be placed in double thickness trash bags and surrendered to the hazmat team for further processing.

Dry chemicals should be brushed from the skin before the flushing process begins. Place eye and respiratory protection on both you and the patient, so the chemical cannot enter into the eyes or lungs when brushed away. Then flush the area with copious amounts of water. Once decontamination is complete, the patient should be covered with dry blankets to conserve body heat. If the patient experiences additional burning sensations, irrigation should be continued. The burns should be treated as would any other burn by first monitoring and treating any threats to airway, breathing, and circulation, then treating the burn with the application of dry sterile dressings.

White Phosphorous

White phosphorous is the only chemical for which direct immersion (soaking) in water is recommended as the initial treatment. This provides minimal comfort, but the chemical continues to burn until surgically excised (removed). The hospital will use a 1% copper sulfate solution, which will stain the phosphorus blue to make excision easier. Up until recently, white phosphorous was uncommon outside of industrial settings; however, since it is a component in one of the many

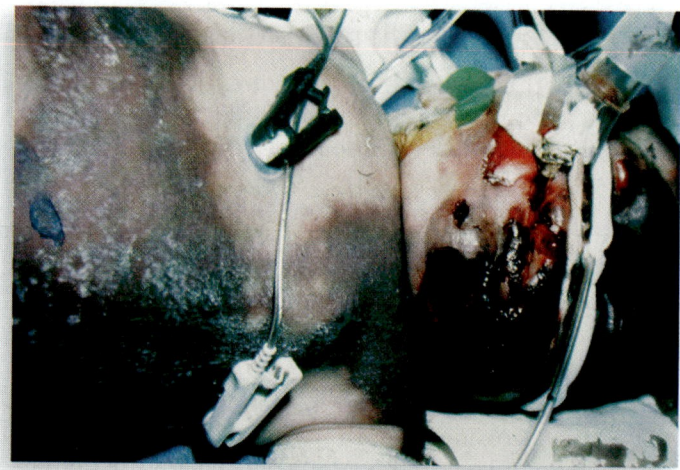

Figure 26-18 Badly burned children present special challenges to responding paramedics.

Nice to Know

Hydrofluoric acid (HF) quickly penetrates the dermis, distributing a large amount of hydrogen and fluoride ions into the tissues. The hydrogen ions cause an acid burn and the fluoride begins to bind with calcium and magnesium. Many chemical plants keep benzalkonium chloride (Zephiran™) 1:750 solution or calcium gluconate 2.5% gel, pads, or permeated gloves as an antidote for topical application after immediate, emergency flushing with water in the event of HF exposure.[21]

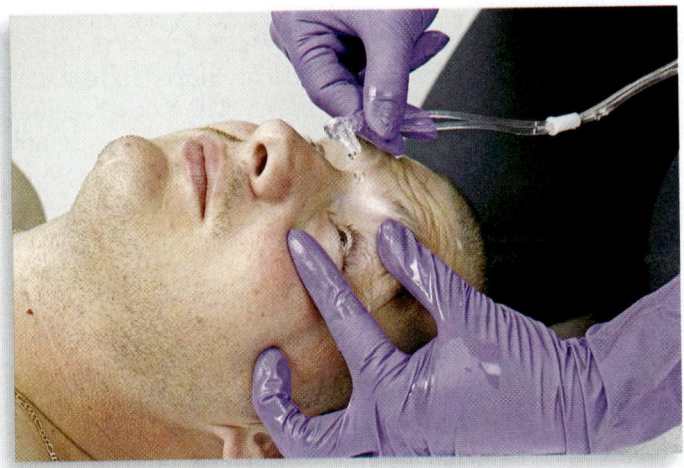

Figure 26-19 When irrigating eyes, if possible, position the head so that the fluid flows medial to lateral, allowing the fluid to run off the face rather than into the other eye.

methamphetamine manufacturing methods, its incidence may be on the rise.

Treatment of Chemical Burns to the Eye

Treatment with copious irrigation of water should begin immediately. Topical anesthetic eye drops may be used to provide symptomatic relief and ease the process of irrigation, if permitted by your local EMS protocols. Lactated Ringer's solution is preferred for irrigation, but normal saline may be used also. A minimum of two liters should be used to flush the chemical from the eye.[17] Flow the fluid through standard IV tubing, and the use of a Morgan lens is recommended. Morgan lenses, however, have a distinct disadvantage for particulate matter, which may become trapped beneath the lens. An alternative is to use a nasal cannula placed on the bridge of the nose and attached to IV tubing for irrigation. This allows flushing from the inner to outer canthus of both eyes simultaneously. Ensure you protect your own eyes and skin from splash contact with the chemical by using proper body substance isolation (BSI) precautions such as eye or respiratory protection. This is particularly important if the chemical is in powder form, as brushing it off the patient can place it into the air, resulting in inhalation. DOT 4-4.77, 4-4.78

Never use any chemical substance or "antidote" other than water or saline to flush the eye. It is often necessary to hold the eyelids open during irrigation because of the natural inclination to close the eyes in response to pain and irritation. A steady stream of irrigating fluid should be directed onto the medial surface of the exposed globe and allowed to run off the lateral aspect of the eye to avoid contaminating the opposite eye (Figure 26-19). If possible, turn the side of the patient's face with the eye to be irrigated downward to facilitate this runoff. Irrigation should be continuous for a minimum of 20 minutes or longer if the chemical is known to be alkaline. If both eyes have been exposed, use the nasal cannula technique to irrigate both eyes simultaneously.

In the hospital setting, determining the pH of the eye will be used to assess if decontamination is complete. In the prehospital setting this is not available, so irrigation should continue if the patient complains of ongoing pain. The use of sedatives or analgesics may also be appropriate to help calm the patient or control pain.[13]

Methamphetamine Production and Burns

Illicit production of methamphetamine (also called "meth") has been increasing across the United States. These laboratories utilize ingredients such as acetylene, gasoline, anhydrous ammonia, white phosphorous, and dozens of other very dangerous chemicals. The manufacturing process (called "cooking") produces highly explosive gasses. Many meth labs are also booby trapped with explosives or devices to injure anyone entering the premises. As you would expect, safety measures and OSHA mandates are ignored during manufacture of this drug, so the number of burn victims from laboratory explosions and fires has increased.

Recently, some surprising facts regarding methamphetamine have been noted. The most surprising is that methamphetamine patients with burns greater than or equal to 40% TBSA die.[7,22] The projected survival rate for this group of patients is calculated at 60%. While research is ongoing for methamphetamine-related burns, it appears that this group requires almost twice the amount of fluid normally calculated for resuscitating burns. This is apparently due to a combination of the use of the drug itself (which increases the metabolic rate) and the exposure to toxins during manufacturing mishaps.

Treatment of Electrical Burns

Treatment modalities for electrical burns follow the guidelines established for all burns. They deserve special attention because the true extent of damage cannot be determined by their initial appearance. Therefore, they should always be assumed to be severe and deep, and burn center transport is required.

If the electrical charge caused cardiac arrest, managing the burn is no longer the priority. The first 20 minutes are the most critical, and resuscitation may be most effective during that time. Generally, if airway, breathing, and circulation were not compromised from the electrical exposure, the heart will continue to work following the electrocution; however, cardiac monitoring should be initiated.

Commonly, electrocution injuries are accompanied by other trauma that is a result of falls, explosions, or massive muscle contractions. Cervical spine stabilization and immobilization with a back board should be automatic. Splint all suspected fractures, and provide wound care. Since the extent of the injury may be hidden, prompt transport is indicated.

Treatment for Radiation Emergencies

Patients with radiation exposure should receive the same care as previously outlined for burn patients. Radiation exposure is usually not immediately life-threatening; however, resuscitation should supersede the need for decontamination. If contamination of the patient is unconfirmed or unknown, the patient should be assumed to be contaminated and undergo decontamination or should only be handled by EMS providers wearing appropriate safety equipment. Most radiation control measures such as decontamination, covering wounds, removing clothing, and so forth will be performed on the scene. The decontaminated patient will then be transferred to the ambulance and transported.[9]
DOT 4-4.47, 4-4.48, 4-4.49, 4-4.50, 4-4.51, 4-4.52, 4-4.53, 4-4.54, 4-4.55, 4-4.60, 4-4.65, 4-4.70

The receiving facility should be notified of the following:

1. Circumstances of the accident or event.
2. Number of victims.
3. Medical condition and physical injuries of the victims.
4. Type and extent of radiologic insult: irradiated, externally contaminated, or internally contaminated.
5. Identification of the radioactive material, if known.
6. If victims were able to be surveyed radiologically in the field.
7. Exposure to other hazardous material that may be chemically toxic or corrosive.

Burns to the Airway and Smoke Inhalation

The majority of deaths from fire are due to smoke inhalation (Box 26-5). Of those burn victims hospitalized each year, approximately 30% have an inhalation injury.[1] Carbon monoxide, thermal injury, and smoke inhalation are three components common to most inhalation injuries.

Normally, the oropharynx, nasopharynx, and upper airway regulate the temperature of inspired air and dissipate any excess heat, even in the presence of fire. However, dissipation of heat within the airway can result in significant thermal injury to the proximal portion of the tracheo-bronchial tree, causing edema and life-threatening airway compromise. Thermal injury manifests immediately as edema, hemorrhage, and ulceration, and the swelling can progress very rapidly. True thermal damage to the lower airway is rare, unless exploding gasses or steam are inhaled directly. When present, these patients often die from untreatable asphyxia.[1] DOT 4-4.23, 4-4.24

Patients with the greatest risk of airway obstruction are those injured in an explosion with burns to the face and upper thorax and also those unconscious in a fire in what is referred to as a "confined space" situation such as a small room. These patients are at greatest risk for airway compromise within the first 24 hours following the injury.[1] Signs of respiratory burn include singed nasal hairs, soot around the nares, carbonaceous sputum (sooty spit), hoarseness, stridor (a sound that occurs during inspiration from an upper airway constriction), and symptoms of respiratory distress.[20] DOT 4-4.25, 4-4.81

Patients suspected of respiratory burns should be intubated at the earliest sign of airway compromise.

Absolute indications for intubation are **increasing hoarseness, stridor,** and **drooling.**[2]

It may be necessary to use advanced airway techniques, including rapid sequence intubation. Use the largest endotracheal tube possible when intubating such a patient given the amount of swelling, as it is easier to ventilate these patients through a larger bore tube. A surgical airway like a cricothyrotomy may be required if intubation is not possible.[1] DOT 3-2.63, 3-4.1, 4-4.26, 4-4.27

Assessment for Inhalation Injury

If the victim was burned in an enclosed area (confined space), there should be a high index of suspicion that smoke inhalation has occurred. Evaluate all patients in closed-space fires for symptoms of carbon monoxide poisoning, which includes headache, visual changes, confusion, irritability, decreased judgment, nausea, ataxia, and collapse. Question the patient about the types of things that might have burned in the room, including the type

Smoke inhalation can be a lethal injury. Despite the fact that smoke and toxic gas inhalation are responsible for more people found dead at fire scenes than the actual fire, much attention is given to those with obvious burns. In order to accentuate the importance of smoke inhalation, a review of history involving some fire disasters is provided. DOT 4-4.22

1. The Coconut Grove Fire, Boston, MA, 1942. "Several hundred perished, many of whom displayed no surface burns. In addition, there were hundreds of unburned or lightly burned patients with severe lung injury."[5]

2. Gothenburg Discotheque Fire, Sweden, 1998. Of an estimated 375 people, 63 died. Of the fatalities 97% had COHb (carboxyhemoglobin) in excess of 30% (normal is 0%, up to 10% for smokers). Ninety-eight percent had lethal doses of COHb. Of the 213 survivors, 158 (74%) had inhalation injuries requiring active treatment.[12]

3. World Trade Center Attack, New York, 2001. Of 790 survivors, 386 had inhalation injuries, 39 had burns.

4. The Station Night Club Fire, Rhode Island, 2003.[23] "All but four of the total deaths (97) occurred in the nightclub itself. The remaining patients died much later, at Burn Centers with family and friends."[24]

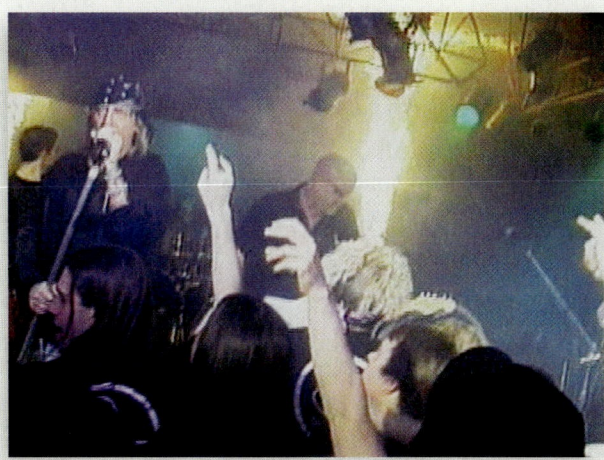

All but four of the 97 deaths at the Station Night Club Fire in Rhode Island in 2003 occurred at the scene.

of carpet, vinyl articles, and synthetics and plastics. This will provide clues as to the type of toxins the patient may have inhaled. Sulfur dioxide and nitrous oxide are toxic agents often present in soot. In the presence of water (as found in the lungs), they form corrosive acids that are extremely toxic. Toxic fumes from burning plastic are more dangerous than smoke. Noxious gasses include hydrogen cyanide, hydrochloric acid, sulfuric acid, and halogens, and even phosgene can result from fires involving furniture, rugs, and the like. DOT 4-4.28, 4-4.29

Ventilation can also be decreased because of noncardiogenic pulmonary edema.[10] When this occurs, it impairs gas exchange as fluid builds up in the lung tissues.

Evaluate the patient for upper body burns, erythema (redness), or blistering of lips, buccal mucosa (the inner cheeks), or pharynx. Assess the quality of air movement in and out of the lungs.

When evaluating for smoke inhalation, think about the following:

- Stridor
- Increasing hoarseness
- Drooling

When noted, consider the need for immediate intubation to prevent loss of airway due to edema:

- Burns occurring in a closed structure or vehicle (smoke)
- Inhalation injuries caused by steam (thermal airway trauma)
- Inhalation injuries involving chemicals

Signs and symptoms of possible inhalation injury include:

- Complaints of dyspnea
- Facial burns
- Singed hair, eyebrows, and nasal hair
- Soot present in the airway and sputum
- Coughing
- Wheezing
- Episode of unconsciousness related to the event
- Burns in the mouth
- Unexplained anxiety and restlessness (assume hypoxia) [2]

Treatment of Inhalation Injury

Treatment modalities for inhalation injuries follow the guidelines established for all burns. They deserve special attention, however, because of the speed with which airway compromise develops following an inhalation injury. Be especially alert to increasing hoarseness, stridor, and drooling as these are indicators for immediate intubation. Suspected respiratory burns or inhalation injuries should always be assumed to be severe, and burn center transport is required. If the burn size exceeds 60% TBSA, especially if it includes the face, early endotracheal intubation is advised. If endotracheal intubation is impossible, a surgical airway (needle or surgical crichothrotomy) may be necessary.[20] **See Skill Sheets 19: Needle Cricothyroidotomy (also see Step-by-Step 19).** DOT 4-4.30

Carbon Monoxide Poisoning

Patients who have inhaled the products of combustion are likely to have sustained carbon monoxide (CO) poisoning. In most cases, it is unknown how much CO may have been inhaled. CO binds with hemoglobin at a rate 250 times greater than oxygen.[11] Not only does CO occupy oxygen receptor sites on red blood cells, but it also has a half-life of four hours in room air. This means that it takes approximately four hours for the total amount of carbon monoxide present to be reduced by one-half. High flow oxygen administered at 12 to 15 liters per minute via a nonrebreather mask can reduce the half-life of CO to 90 minutes or less. Table 26-2 lists the symptoms of carbon monoxide poisoning. Pulse oximetry is misleading in patients suspected of CO poisoning. Carboxyhemoglobin (CO poisoning) results in falsely high readings from the pulse oximeter because the machine determines the presence of oxygen

TABLE 26-2 Carbon Monoxide Poisoning Symptoms

Carboxyhemoglobin level (% of total CO on blood cell)	Symptoms
0–10	Usually none
10–20	Headache, atypical dyspnea
20–30	Headache, concentration problems
30–40	Headache, thinking problems
40–50	Confusion, weakness, syncope
50–60	Respiratory fatigue, seizures
>70	Coma, death

molecules bound to hemoglobin by a colorimetric method, which is fooled by the presence of carbon monoxide. It cannot differentiate if the color detected results from oxyhemoglobin (the normal state) or carboxyhemoglobin. Patients with significant carbon monoxide poisoning are usually treated in a hyperbaric chamber to rapidly remove the carbon monoxide and provide high levels of oxygen; however, the use of hyperbaric chambers to treat CO poisoning is becoming controversial. Recent studies have reported mixed results on its effectiveness.[1] It is important to remember that the priority for care is management of the airway, supplemental oxygen administration, and burn treatment. DOT 4-4.30, 4-4.67

BOX 26-6 Burn Center Referral Criteria

The ABA has identified the following injuries as those requiring referral to a burn center after initial assessment and stabilization at an emergency department:
DOT 4-4.8

1. Partial thickness and full thickness burns totaling greater than 10% TBSA in patients under 10 or over 50 years of age.

2. Partial thickness and full thickness burns totaling greater than 20% TBSA in other age groups those between age 10 and 50.

3. Partial thickness and full thickness burns involving the face, hands, feet, genitalia, perineum, or major joints.

4. Full thickness burns greater than 5% TBSA in any age group.

5. Electrical burns, including lightning injury.

6. Chemical burns.

7. Inhalation injury.

8. Burn injury in patients with preexisting medical disorders that could complicate management, prolong the recovery period, or affect mortality.

9. Any burn with concomitant trauma (for example, fractures) in which the burn injury poses the greatest risk of morbidity or mortality. If the trauma poses the greater immediate risk, the patient may be treated initially in a trauma center until stable before being transferred to a burn center. The physician's decisions should be made with the regional medical control plan and triage protocols in mind.

10. Burn injury in children admitted to a hospital without qualified personnel or equipment for pediatric care.

11. Burn injury in patients requiring special social, emotional, or long-term rehabilitative support, including cases involving suspected child abuse.

Source: American Burn Association, http://www.ameriburn.org/index. html. (accessed November, 2005).

Determining the Need for Transport to Burn Centers

The average size of a burn injury resulting in admission to a burn center is about 14% TBSA. By comparison, burns with 10% or less TBSA involvement account for 54% of all burn center admissions, while 60% TBSA burns account for 4% of the admissions.[2] DOT 4-4.8, 4-4.66

The American Burn Association has identified burn injuries requiring referral to a burn center. These criteria state that burn center transport should occur after the patient has received initial assessment and stabilization at an emergency department. In areas of the country with direct access to burn centers from the prehospital setting, immediate transport to a burn center may be preferred over transport to an emergency department. At least one state protocol recommends that if the burn center is within 60 minutes of the scene and the patient has severe burns with no other trauma obvious or suspected, the burn center should be the initial destination.[1,25] Follow local protocols in making this decision. See Box 26-6 for the ABA burn center criteria.

DOT 4-4.17, 4-4.18, 4-4.19

Summary

The management of burn patients bears striking similarity to management of other critically injured patients: focus on maintaining the airway, breathing, and circulation. Burn patients are particularly susceptible to airway compromise, so special attention needs to be focused on this.

Burn trauma has a high mortality associated with it. Specialty centers for managing burns have been instrumental in decreasing mortality. Although these centers are the optimal place to manage burn patients, the patient should not be transported there until other significant traumatic injuries are attended to by the trauma center.

EMS providers should pay particular attention to scene safety when dealing with burn trauma. Whatever injured the patient—flames, electricity, chemicals, or something else—the same injury may await the medical team that is not tuned in to safety.

Notes

1. F. C. Brunicardi, D. K. Andersen, T. R. Billiar, D. L. Dunn, J. G. Hunter, J. B. Matthews, R. E. Pollock, and S. I. Schwartz, *Schwartz's Principles of Surgery,* 8th ed., McGraw-Hill's AccessMedicine (accessed September 11, 2006).
2. American Burn Association, http://www.ameriburn.org/index.html (accessed September 11, 2006).
3. S. B. Brych, L. H. Engrav, F. P. Rivara, et al., "Time Off Work and Return to Work Rates After Burns: Systematic Review of the Literature and a Large Two-Center Series," *The Journal of Burn Care and Rehabilitation* 22(2001):401.
4. L. M. Tierney, S. J. McPhee, and M. A. Papadakis (eds.), R. Gonzoles and R. Qeiger (online eds.), *Current Medical Diagnosis and Treatment 2006,* McGraw-Hill's AccessMedicine (accessed October, 2005).
5. F. D. Moore, "Then and Now: Treatment Volume, Wound Coverage, Lung Injury, and Antibiotics: A Capsule History of Burn Treatment at Mid-Century," *Burns* 25(1999):733–737.
6. W. Dougherty and K. Waxman, "The Complexities of Managing Severe Burns with Associated Trauma," *The Surgical Clinics of North America* 76(1996):4:923–951.
7. L. R. Schwartz and C. Blalkrishnan in *Emergency Medicine: A Comprehensive Study Guide,* J. Tintinalli et al. (eds.), 6th ed. (New York, NY: McGraw-Hill, 2004), pp. 1220–1223.
8. Gretchen Carrougher, *Burn Care and Therapy* (St. Louis, MO: Elsevier Mosby, 1998).
9. J. E. Tintinalli, G. D. Kelen, J. S. Stapczynski, O. J. Ma, and D. M. Cline, *Tintinalli's Emergency Medicine: A Comprehensive Study Guide,* 6th ed., McGraw-Hill's AccessMedicine (accessed September 11, 2006).
10. Robert Sheridan, (ed.), *Advanced Life Support Course: Instructor's Manual* (Chigaco, IL: American Burn Association, 2001).
11. Robert Gillespie (ed.), *Pre-Hospital Burn Life Support Course,* (Chigaco, IL: American Burn Association, 1991).
12. J. Cassuto and P. Tarnow, "The Discotheque Fire in Gothenburg 1998, A Tragedy Among Teenagers," *Burns* 29(2003):405–416.
13. G. M. Doherty and L. W. Way, *Current Surgical Diagnosis and Treatment,* 12th ed., McGraw-Hill's AccessMedicine (accessed September 11, 2006).
14. A. Moritz, and F. Henriques, "Studies of Thermal Injury II. The Relative Importance of Time and Surface Temperature in the Causation of Cutaneous Burns," *The American Journal of Pathology* 23(1947):695.
15. T. L. Lee-Chiong, "Smoke Inhalation Injury," *Postgraduate Medicine* 105(2)(1999):1–11.
16. P. Riordan-Eva and J. P. Whitcher, *Vaughan & Asbury's General Ophthalmology,* 16th ed., McGraw-Hill's AccessMedicine (accessed September 11, 2006).
17. K. J. Knoop, L. B. Stack, and A. B. Storrow, "Opthalamic Trauma," *Atlas of Emergency Medicine* (New York, NY: McGraw-Hill Online, 2002).
18. National Association of EMTS, *Prehospital Trauma Life Support,* 5th ed. (St. Louis, MO: Elsevier Mosby, 2003).
19. V. Gunn and C. Nechyba (eds.), *The Harriet Lane Handbook, A Manual for Pediatric House Officers,* 16th ed., The Johns Hopkins Hospital (Philadelphia, PA: Elsevier Mosby, 2002).
20. C. K. Stone and R. L. Humphries, *Current Emergency Diagnosis & Treatment,* McGraw-Hill's AccessMedicine (accessed September 11, 2006).
21. Allied Chemicals, "Recommended Medical Treatment for Hydrofloric Acid Exposure," 6/1993.
22. R. Gillespie, ed., *Advanced Burn Life Support Course: Instructor's Manual* (Chicago, IL: American Burn Association, 1994).
23. B. Boodram, I. Torian, P. Thomas, S. Wilt, D. Pollock, M. Bell, and D. Budnitz, "Rapid Assessment of Injuries Among Survivors of the Terrorist Attack on the World Trade Center—New York City, September 2001," *Morbidity and Mortality Weekly Report* 51(01)(2002):1–5.
24. M. J. Dacey, "Tragedy and Response—The Rhode Island Nightclub Fire," *The New England Journal of Medicine* 349(2003):1990–1992.
25. *The Maryland Medical Protocols for Emergency Medical Services Providers* (Baltimore, MD, Maryland Institute for Emergency Medical Services Systems, 2006).

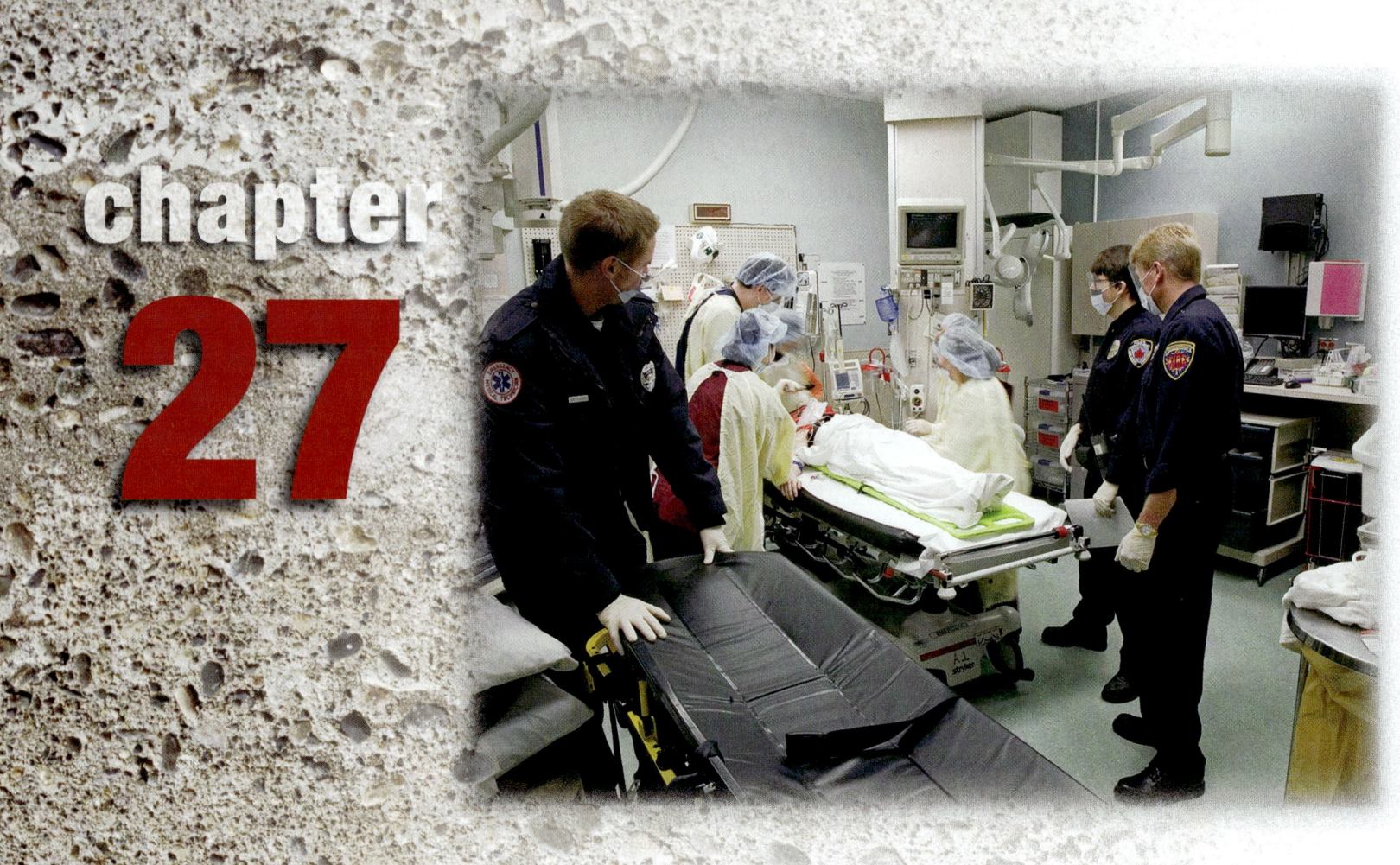

Trauma Patients and Trauma Systems

*"**O**rder is light, peace, inner freedom, self determination: it is power."*

—Henri Frederic Amiel

Need to Know

▶ A paramedic must be able to recognize life-threatening injuries using established criteria and then transport the patient to a trauma center without delaying for unnecessary treatment or evaluation.

▶ Safe response and arrival, and continued situational awareness are keys to good prehospital care and timely intervention.

▶ Patients should be reassessed continually for new, developing, or changing problems.

▶ Paramedics must know how their trauma system is set up and what levels of care are available.

▶ Paramedics must be familiar with the trauma triage system in use in their jurisdiction and where patients should be transported.

Introduction

Taking care of a patient with significant trauma can be one of the most stressful events in a paramedic's career. This applies whether a paramedic has 10 years or 10 days of experience. The scene of a vehicle crash is often chaotic in the initial moments, presenting dangers such as passing traffic, leaking hazardous materials, or inclement weather. Often, the scene is complicated by upset friends and family who can elevate the stress level and distract or interfere with the paramedic who is trying to render care. Finally, the injuries encountered at scenes of trauma have the potential to be grotesque and difficult to forget.

Traumatic injuries and death very commonly happen to young people doing something they enjoy, such as motorcycle riding or boating. Trauma is the leading cause of death in children, the leading cause of death in adults under the age of 45, and the fifth leading cause of death across all age groups of adults.[1] Since trauma predominantly occurs among young and active adults, it is not surprising that trauma has a significant economic impact on society.

The historical development of trauma systems has led to an organized system of response and care, with designations for the various levels of services provided. Level I, II, and III facilities each serve a unique role in a comprehensive trauma system. Along with emergency departments and EMS services, the modern trauma system is designed and equipped to serve the community. Unfortunately, not all areas of the country have a well-established trauma system in place. More work needs to be done before universal trauma system coverage is available for all victims of trauma.[2]

Injury prevention, data collection, and research are important responsibilities of a modern day paramedic. Traumatic events are tragic, but they are even more tragic when the events leading up to the injury were preventable. Injury prevention programs educate the public to dangers that may seem obvious to EMS professionals. Dangers such as not using safety equipment, operating motor vehicles under the influence of drugs or alcohol, or handling firearms in an irresponsible and unsafe manner seem like obvious areas of risk, but they may not be so to the uneducated. Research and data collection help identify these areas of risk as well as provide information on the best medical treatment and clinical practices. Quality assurance allows the system to conduct evaluations in an environment designed to look for solutions to problems rather than just punish those who do not perform to the required standard.

This chapter brings full circle the concepts of patient management discussed in Part 3: Trauma as well as concepts discussed throughout the book on critical thinking (Chapter 5), patient assessment (Chapters 11 and 14) and the history of EMS (Chapter 1).

History of Addressing Trauma

Trauma-related death is not unique to modern society. Since the dawn of man, people have died as a result of unintentional as well as intentional injury. As civilizations evolved, man invented new ways to inflict harm as well new ways to become injured. EMS and trauma systems have primarily developed as a result of lessons learned through the aftermath of armed conflict.

CONNECTIONS Chapter 1: The EMS Profession provides a historical perspective of the development of EMS.

In the early 1960s, America was entering into its fourth war of the century when some medical scholars began to notice the overwhelming number of deaths on U.S. highways. They compared the survival rates between the two environments and discovered better survival on the battlefield than on the highway. In 1966, The National Academy of Sciences, National Research Council published *Accidental Death and Disability: The Neglected Disease of a Modern Society*. Following distribution of this document, the federal government approved the 1966 EMS Act, authorizing the federal Department of Transportation to oversee Emergency Medical Services, and modern EMS was born.

Also during the early 1960s a physician by the name of R. Adams Cowley at the University of Maryland Hospital in Baltimore, Maryland, was studying the impact of trauma on the body. Doctor Cowley believed that if you could rapidly evacuate critically injured patients from the scene of injury to a hospital, just as the U.S. military in Korea and Vietnam were using ambulances and helicopters to evacuate injured soldiers to a surgical field hospital or "definitive care", patients would stand a greater chance of survival. The concept of rapid evacuation of critically injured patients from the scene of injury to a trauma center and the provision of definitive emergency and surgical care within 60 minutes became known as the *Golden Hour.*

In the early days of EMS, federal funding was tied to initiatives to specifically reduce mortality on America's streets and highways. On March 19, 1970, the Maryland State Police Aviation division flew the first civilian medical evacuation (medevac) mission and delivered the patient from the scene to Dr. Cowley's newly created Shock Trauma Center.

Throughout the 1970s and 1980s, states began to develop organized EMS systems; however, trauma system development lagged behind in favor of a focus on cardiac and respiratory emergencies. In 1985, the National Research Council published *Injury in America: A Continuing Public Health Problem,* once again returning the spotlight to the neglected disease of accidental death and disability. Finally in 1990, the federal government passed the Trauma Care Systems and Development Act. The 1990 legislation provided funding for states to develop and plan for statewide organized trauma systems, system implementation, and evaluation.

Trauma Systems

With the funding of the Trauma Systems Development Act and other federal funding sources, states were able to begin to develop and strategically deploy EMS assets and trauma hospitals to allow for prompt treatment of the critically injured. While severe trauma only accounts for a small percentage of the overall number of trauma patients seen in hospitals, access to prompt surgical care can greatly reduce morbidity and mortality in these patients.

The percentage of severely injured may seem small; however, the cost of care and the financial impact is astronomical. For example, there are 1.6 million head injuries per year. Over 800,000 patients receive treatment in emergency departments or outpatient care facilities, with 270,000 patients requiring hospital admission and 52,000 people dying. Of those patients 70,000–90,000 are left with some permanent neurological impairment or disability. Traumatic brain injury costs society more than 30 billion dollars annually.[3] In the face of such great physical, emotional, and economic cost to society, the development of organized trauma care demands a systematic approach. Care of the severely injured requires access to specialized care such as designated trauma hospitals, EMS triage criteria, and strategies to ensure proper resource allocation (Figure 27-1).

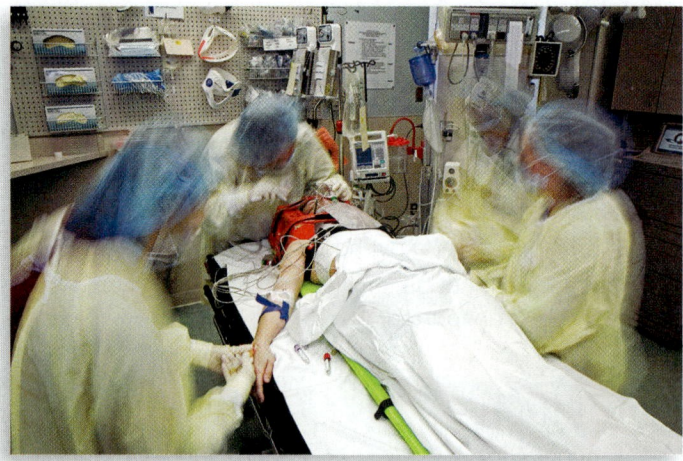

Figure 27-1   Organized trauma systems are comprised of specially trained people in specially equipped hospitals receiving patients from well-trained EMS providers.

CONNECTIONS Chapter 20: Head, Face, and Neck Trauma discusses traumatic brain injuries and provides management strategies to prevent the development of secondary brain injury.

The concept of a trauma system has grown significantly over the years. While many people think of a trauma system as being made up of the ambulance response and the hospital to which the patient is taken, in fact it has become much more. The modern trauma system begins with efforts to prevent traumatic injury in the first place and to provide for easy access to emergency medical care, an efficient EMS response system, an appropriate destination to which to transport the injured patient, the necessary staff and equipment to provide needed care, a comprehensive rehabilitation process to help return the trauma victim to a productive life, the gathering of data so that the efficacy of the system can be evaluated, and ongoing research to improve practices in each of the components.

Trauma Center Designation

Most systems across the country designate trauma centers at one of three levels. A Level I Trauma Center is the highest level resource available. The number and level of centers is often proportionate to the population of the region or the state. Some states use a designation system that follows the requirements of the American College of Surgeons (ACS) criteria for trauma centers. Other areas use a self-designation system that allows the hospital to declare itself a trauma center and apply for verification from the ACS. There are several states across the country that have an all-inclusive approach to trauma center designation, meaning that there are no limits to the numbers of trauma centers. These states use a level I to IV or I to V scale with levels I through III being the same as any

TABLE 27-1   Trauma Center Designations (American College of Surgeons Committee on Trauma)

Level I Regional Trauma Center	Level II Area Wide Trauma Center	Level III Community Trauma Center	Level IV Rural Trauma Center
Specialty referral center located in large urban area with capabilities to treat all types of injury or illness.	Large community hospital equipped to handle the most common types of injury. May refer more complex injury and specialty patients to Level I Centers.	Local community hospital equipped to stabilize and treat common types of injury. Limited surgical capabilities and limited specialty capabilities. Will transfer complex injury to specialty centers.	Rural facilities provide initial evaluation and assessment but most patients are transferred to higher level centers.
24/7 in-house capability for managing all aspects of trauma	24/7 in-house capability for managing most aspects of trauma	24/7 capabilities but not all specialties	

Source: Resources for Optimal Care of the Injured Patient 2006. American College of Surgeons Committee on Trauma (ACS-COT).

other state. Another approach to trauma center designation is to designate trauma centers as well as specialty referral centers such as burn trauma, pediatric trauma, neurotrauma, hand trauma, and hyperbaric centers.

Trauma centers are configured in different ways to receive patients, with the most common model being the hospital emergency department (ED) as the primary receiving unit for trauma patients from the scene. Another configuration involves a separate receiving unit just for trauma located within, or in close proximity to, the emergency department.

It is often difficult for providers to sort through all the requirements to understand the differences between trauma center designations. One common misconception is that all trauma centers are alike. Table 27-1 provides a synopsis of the features of each trauma center designation.

Level I Designation

A **Level I Trauma Center** is the highest level facility. The Level I center is most often located at major university medical centers in large municipalities with large populations. These programs also support resident and fellowship programs for the training of physicians in trauma care. These hospitals are uniquely equipped with a large number of specialty services and mechanisms to care for patients with complex injuries and illnesses (Figure 27-2).

A Level I Trauma Center will have a 24/7 resuscitation unit, operating rooms dedicated to trauma surgery available immediately, critical care units, and in-house (readily available) trauma surgeon staff. In addition, they will have specialty physicians such as emergency physicians, anesthesiologists, orthopedic surgeons, neurosurgeons, radiologists, and critical care intensivists. The Level I Trauma Center will have all the necessary support services such as blood bank, radiology, pharmacy, and laboratory capabilities around the clock. The Level I Trauma Center is often referred to as a regional trauma center, servicing a large portion of a city or state, with the ability to serve as a resource center for EMS as well as other lower level designated trauma centers and hospitals. The Level I Center will see in excess of 1,200 trauma patients a year and is fully committed to providing trauma care.

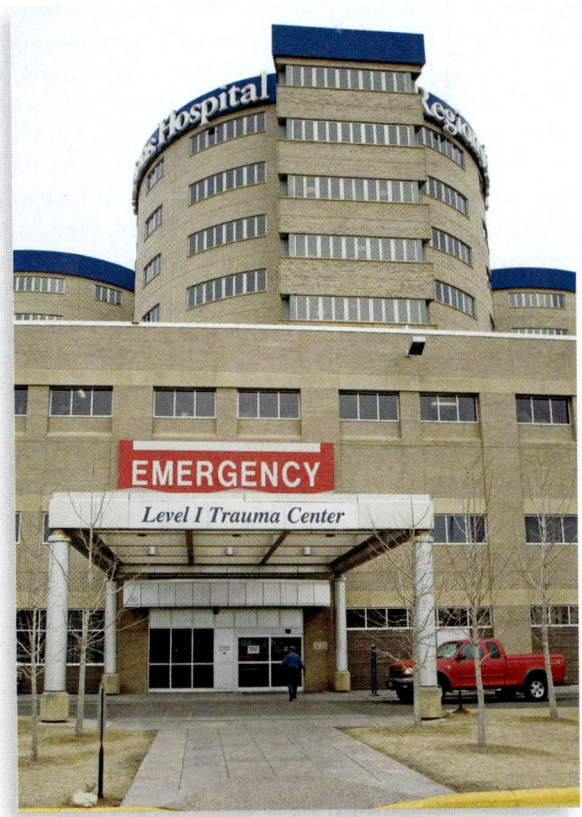

Figure 27-2   The highest level of trauma care is provided by Level I Trauma Centers. These are typically at hospitals affiliated with universities in larger cities.

Level II Designation

The **Level II Trauma Center** is often referred to as an area wide trauma center. The Level II Center will often be a large county or public hospital that may or may not also be a teaching hospital. The center has the majority of resources of the busy Level I Trauma Center but may not have all the specialty physicians available in the hospital around the clock. In some regions, the Level II Center might serve as the primary trauma receiving hospital due to the region's limited resources. The Level II Center is permitted to see less trauma volume than the Level I Center unless there is no Level I Center in the region. The level of commitment and dedicated resources is strong but often not to the same level of intensity as the larger Level I Centers.

Level III Designation

The **Level III Trauma Center** is required to have trauma surgery and orthopedic surgery coverage but not neurosurgery coverage. Often, Level III Centers have the surgical staff on a callback schedule and have trauma trained ED staff begin the resuscitation. They call in the trauma team once they are notified of the transport of a critical patient or the patient arrives at the center. The Level III Center is usually the local community hospital in rural areas and frequently the only hospital in the geographic area. These hospitals are equipped to evaluate and treat most routine trauma patients; however, multisystem trauma and patients requiring specialty services are frequently transferred to larger Level I or II Trauma Centers (Figure 27-3). The Level III hospital, therefore, is often referred to as the community trauma center.

In areas that are more remote and access to care is limited based on population density and resource availability, local hospitals will typically serve as an evaluation and stabilization point for trauma patients before the patients are transferred to larger centers.

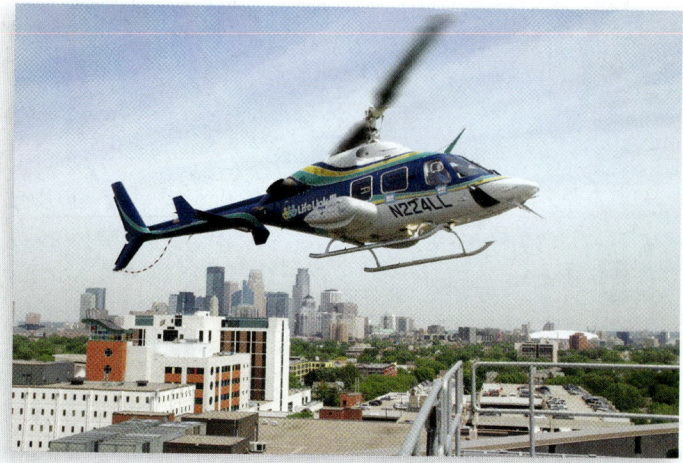

Figure 27-3 Aeromedical programs can move patients from remote hospitals or scenes to trauma centers.

Level IV Designation

The Level IV designation recognizes a rural hospital that can provide initial evaluation of trauma patients but will need to transfer patients to a higher level trauma center.

Injury Prevention

If injury could be prevented, lives could be saved. Organizations such as the American Trauma Society, Mothers Against Drunk Driving (MADD), and Safe Kids Coalition have lead widespread education programs to increase awareness of how injuries occur and how to prevent injuries (Figure 27-4).

Automobile manufacturers have installed seatbelt and passive restraint systems to reduce injury in the event of a collision. The passive restraint systems now include front and side impact airbags as well as head curtains to reduce or prevent devastating traumatic brain injuries. Manufacturers have also developed stronger and more durable car frames with "crumple zones" designed to absorb much of the energy during a crash.

During the late twentieth century, the Department of Transportation lead states to create speed limits and laws to reduce collisions. Studies were conducted to improve the design of highways and safety barriers. Many states began to require the mandatory use of seat belts for vehicle occupants, child safety seats, and helmets for motorcyclists and bicyclists.

Paramedics play a role in educating the public on proper use of safety devices and injury prevention programs to reduce morbidity and mortality. Injury prevention organizations have created programs to promote safety in daily living as well as at play. Paramedics can make a significant impact by supporting these programs as well as by setting a safe example for the public to follow.

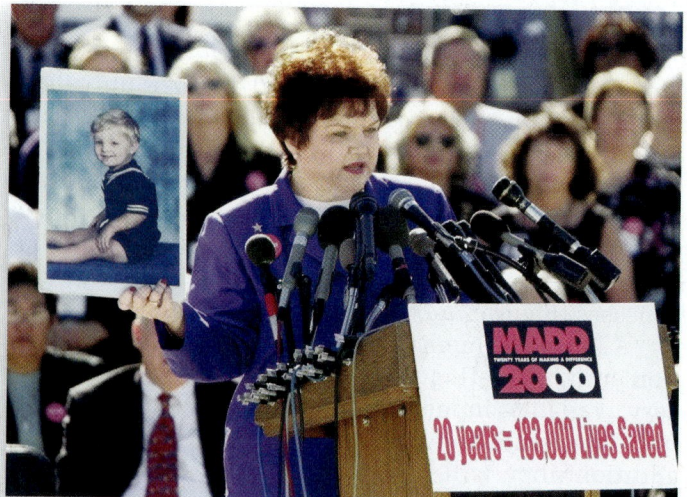

Figure 27-4 An example of injury prevention education is MADD, or Mothers Against Drunk Driving, and its educational programs.

Over the past several decades, there has been a reduction in mortality and morbidity associated with motor vehicle collisions due to education programs, design improvements, and legislative initiatives. There have been major efforts by federal agencies and departments (too numerous to even mention) to promote injury prevention and awareness. Since automobile crashes are the most common cause of musculoskeletal injury and workplace injuries are growing steadily, these organizations have been instrumental in reducing injuries and injury severity. In addition, Emergency Medical Services (EMS) organizations have teamed with various groups in an attempt to increase community safety awareness as well as provide educational courses and training (for example, CPR training programs).

Driving while under the influence of alcohol, the most frequent cause of fatal motor vehicle crashes, accounts for approximately 40% of all traffic fatalities. Laws pertaining to DUI (driving under the influence) regulations have been lifesaving.[4] Other prevention strategies focus around sports training, helmet use, seat belt and child safety seat laws, mandatory airbags in newer vehicles, gun safety laws and education, motorcycle driver education, insurance company accident prevention incentives, and fall prevention.

Data Collection

Data collection is a vital part of any EMS and trauma system. Collecting key data from EMS patient care reports as well as from hospital admission records, police reports, and coroner reports allows epidemiologists, government officials, and clinicians to develop prevention strategies, enhance EMS and trauma system design, and develop clinical practice recommendations for EMS and trauma centers. These data are usually collected in a database referred to as the system trauma registry. The trauma registry is a set of predetermined data points that are collected from the various sources mentioned. The trauma registry serves as a measuring stick for EMS and trauma systems to determine the effectiveness or ineffectiveness of the system and to identify factors that may contribute to an increase or decrease in patient morbidity and mortality.

For example, with the rapid advancement of passive restraint systems and seat belt usage, there have been changes in the injury patterns from motor vehicle collisions. Through the trauma registry, we have seen a reduction in severity of injury to the chest and abdomen when seat belts and airbags are used.

Quality Improvement

While the trauma registry provides a means to measure system performance and examine practice, the application of an enhanced trauma and EMS quality improvement (QI) or quality management (QM) system brings the process full circle. Through continuous review of data, patient reports, and EMS run sheets, QI and QM committees can determine the effectiveness of the EMS system and whether or not agreed-upon standards are being met. The QI and QM committees can make recommendations to revise practices, change EMS protocols, identify areas for improvement, and suggest education programs to ensure the standards are met. Quality improvement is a dynamic, not static, process. It is imperative that all providers embrace the process and become involved to ensure the best possible care is provided to each patient.

Research

Research is a difficult subject for many providers. It often involves complicated mathematical formulas and uses terminology foreign to many. In addition, research takes time, money, commitment, and discipline in order to conduct an effective study. It may be difficult for providers to alter their normal clinical practices in order to take part in studies they do not understand or, worse, think may not prove beneficial to the patient.

Prehospital research has been identified as a vital component in the National EMS Agenda for the Future and the Research Agenda. As prehospital providers, you must embrace research and be willing to evaluate the effectiveness of your clinical practice, discover new and better ways to provide care to your patients, and be willing to identify areas of weakness in your practice or your system to advance the profession of prehospital medicine.

For a variety of reasons, it is not acceptable to simply move emergency department practices from the hospital setting into the prehospital environment. What is effective practice in the hospital may or may not be effective, appropriate, or practical in the prehospital environment. It is only by engaging in research that these questions can be answered and the best practices emerge.

The Golden Period for Trauma Resuscitation

The Golden Hour, mentioned earlier, is the concept that if trauma patients can reach definitive care within an hour of the time of injury, they have the greatest chance of survival. Over the years, the Golden Hour concept has been changed to refer to a **Golden Period** rather than one, 60-minute hour. This is because we now recognize that while some patients may, in fact, have "one hour," others have a shorter time in which to reach definitive care, and some may have a longer period of time. The Parkland Trauma Handbook states that appropriate care in this "golden" time period will increase survival dramatically and possibly improve morbidity.[5] Thus the concept really refers to a window of opportunity in which the patient may survive if quickly managed. The role of the EMS provider is to recognize which trauma patient is sick and, therefore, requiring rapid evacuation to the trauma center. The strategic positioning of trauma centers to ensure that patients can rapidly reach care by ground or air also increases survival.

In trauma, every minute that passes means blood is lost and tissue is deprived of oxygen. Once an injury occurs, activating the EMS system, the response time, extrication measures, and transport all reduce the valuable minutes of the patient's Golden Period.

When communities establish integrated EMS systems, enhanced 9-1-1 and communications mechanisms, EMS education, advanced protocols, and transport policies, valuable time is gained for trauma patients. The key to survival of these critically injured patients is rapid assessment, stabilization, and transport to the trauma center.

In some communities, resources may be limited and distances to trauma centers may be great. In such communities, the deployment of air medical evacuation resources can save valuable time. When making the decision to fly or drive a patient to the trauma center, you as the provider must consider the weather conditions, estimated time of arrival for helicopter, load time, and transport time. If the total time for an air medical response exceeds the estimated time to transport the patient by land, then it may be in the best interest of the patient to transport by ambulance.

Prehospital guidelines, protocols, standards of care, and triage criteria help providers determine which patients would be better served at a trauma center versus the local hospital. Based on certain types of injury, signs and symptoms, and mechanism of injury, trauma triage criteria have been established to guide providers in making critical transport decisions. These criteria are based on clinical research and observations of critically-injured patients.

One of the most critical decisions a provider will make is the decision to continue treatment on-scene or to rapidly transport the patient. As a rule, patients meeting the trauma decision criteria should be rapidly transported to a trauma center with treatment continuing during transport. Certain lifesaving treatments are sometimes required to stabilize a critically injured trauma patient prior to transport. Treatments such as managing an airway, or pleural decompression might be necessary to deliver a viable patient to the trauma center.

As you put together the picture of the carnage that has unfolded prior to your arrival at the patient's side, sometimes all the pieces and assessments do not add up.

Experienced providers often make statements like "something's not right" or "I have a gut feeling" when applying trauma triage criteria. When things do not fit the triage criteria perfectly but you are uncomfortable with something in the patient's presentation, it is always better to err on the side of the patient when it comes to triage destination decisions, and transport the patient to a higher level of care.

This critical thinking process is referred to as "overtriage." **Overtriage** takes into consideration the mechanism of injury and that some injuries are subtle to detect and may not yet have developed the signs and symptoms indicating severe injury. The American College of Surgeons has maintained that it is acceptable to have an overtriage rate as high as 50% to avoid high **undertriage** rates, which may result in a patient being transported to a facility that cannot provide the needed level of care.

Trauma Patients

Initial Approach to the Trauma Patient

Patients who are critically injured have a much better chance of survival if they are rapidly transported to a hospital prepared to deal with traumatic injuries.[6] For this reason, you must become comfortable recognizing which patients are at risk of imminent death due to their injuries and which ones are not yet critical but have the potential to become acute.

CONNECTIONS Chapter 18: Mechanism of Injury discusses mechanism of injury.

The American College of Surgeons guidelines recommend using the primary and secondary survey to quickly identify those patients who need immediate transport.[7,8] Primary survey problems require immediate intervention and should be dealt with *as the team prepares to transport* the patient to the nearest trauma center. In other words, if there is a problem in the primary survey, transport should be expedited, and a team approach is necessary to keep packaging for transport moving along while critical initial interventions are performed. In these cases, delays for on-scene care and procedures (such as starting an IV or applying a limb splint) that do not affect the primary survey should be avoided.

The secondary survey is performed after the primary survey is completed and all related interventions have been performed. In the case of a critical trauma patient, the secondary survey is performed while en route to the trauma center. In addition to an appropriate patient assessment, the secondary survey includes vital signs and taking the SAMPLE history.

A thorough assessment does not mean a slowly performed assessment. The secondary survey is performed as rapidly as possible, especially when there is a significant mechanism of injury or other reason to believe the patient may have multiple injuries that put them at risk for deterioration.

CONNECTIONS See Chapter 11: The Normal Physical Examination and Chapter 14: Patient Assessment for additional information on the elements of patient assessment.

The goal of the secondary survey is to identify all of the injuries affecting the patient that may not have been apparent during the primary survey. While many injuries discovered during the secondary survey may not be immediately life-threatening, the sum of their effects over time can turn a stable trauma patient into a gravely ill patient very quickly. If you encounter involvement of two or more body systems (called **multisystem trauma**), there is much greater potential for rapid deterioration. Examples of significant multisystem trauma include a head injury and an abdominal injury, fractures of major bones combined with tenderness in the chest, or pelvis fracture and an impaled object in the neck. Much of the care and evaluation of the trauma patient is best performed while en route to the hospital to ensure the best chance of a good outcome.

Working in the Gray Zone

It can be challenging to determine which patients need immediate transport to a trauma center and which can safely be transported with less urgency. To help in that process, there are various printed criteria including the Maryland Criteria[8] and the American College of Surgeons Trauma Triage Guidelines.[7,9] These guidelines tend to use abnormal vital signs, mechanism of injury, area of specific injury, or findings on primary survey to help the paramedic decide how to triage a patient. There have also been attempts to utilize scoring systems such as the Prehospital Index.[10] Ideally, these scores and criteria can be very helpful in predicting severe injury and outcome. In reality, it may be too challenging to calculate some of these scores or remember the exact criteria to be used at a real scene. Furthermore, these scores and criteria have not been shown to always predict the most injured patients.[11] Your best bet is to use common sense and the simple criteria provided in this text.

Many paramedics will learn with experience to recognize patterns of injury that put the patient at greater risk of immediate death. While this is a valuable tool for assisting in the decision process, it should not be the only criteria used to decide on the disposition (transport destination) for the patient.[12] Do not be fooled. Even in the absence of major mechanism or serious symptoms, patients can have life-threatening injuries. It is best to err on the side of transporting patients for a complete and thorough evaluation before declaring them injury-free.

Mechanism of Injury

Trauma can result from myriad instruments or mechanisms. Whether the mechanism involves blunt force or penetrating injury, there are certain events that create a higher index of suspicion for underlying injury. For example, when you arrive on the scene of a motor vehicle collision (MVC), you see the aftermath of the collision spread out on the scene. Imagine if you could hit a rewind button and see the events as they occur. The damaged vehicles, eyewitness statements, and patients' statements provide that instant replay. The tire marks indicating the direction the vehicles were traveling, the apparent speed, and degree and location of damage to the vehicle lead you to anticipate certain injury patterns. The mechanism of injury provides information that is useful in determining whether or not to transport the patient to a trauma center (Box 27-1).

During scene size-up, some clues to the severity of the mechanism of injury may have been noted. The American College of Surgeons Committee on Trauma (ACSCOT) has recommended that the following injury mechanisms be considered as major, regardless of how the patient initially "looks" upon initial assessment:[13]

Major MOIs

- Ejection from an automobile
- Death in the same passenger compartment of another patient
- Extrication time greater than 20 minutes
- Falls greater than 20 feet (or three times the height of the patient)
- Rollover crash
- High speed auto crash (initial speed greater than 40 mph, major auto deformity greater than 20 inches, intrusion of the damaged vehicle into the passenger compartment greater than 12 inches)
- Auto versus pedestrian or auto versus bicycle with significant impact (greater than 5 mph)
- Pedestrian thrown when hit or run over
- Motorcycle crash greater than 20 mph or with separation of rider from the motorcycle

BOX 27-1   Trauma Decision Tree for Transport to a Trauma Center

Physiological Signs

GCS less than 8, BP less than 90 (adult) or BP less than 60 (pediatric), or respiratory rate less than 10 or greater than 29

Major Injuries

Flail chest

Pelvic fractures

Penetrating injury to the head, neck, torso, or above the knee or elbow

Two or more long-bone fractures

Rapidly declining GCS

GCS 8–14

Amputation proximal to the wrist or ankle

Mechanism of Injury Factors

Ejection from vehicle

Rollover collision

High-speed crash

Intrusion into passenger compartment

Fall from greater than three times the patient's height

Exposure to blast

Pedestrian struck

Motorcycle crash greater than 20 mph

Comorbidity Factors

Other factors known as comorbidity factors such as age, preexisting medical conditions, and immunosuppressed patients

Getting to the Scene Safely

It is worth a brief discussion about the importance and risk of rapid response to the scene of an injured patient. The premise of timeliness in trauma care has been present since the introduction of the Golden Hour in the late twentieth century.

While paramedics must recognize that timely medical care is important for the trauma patient, they must

Working in the Gray Zone

Do Lights and Sirens Matter?

One study investigated the effect of light and siren use on response time in the rural setting and found that when ambulance crews used lights and sirens to get to a scene, they arrived in 30% less time.[14] There have been other studies attempting to identify a difference in response times using lights and sirens in the urban setting.[15] Each found that there were statistically significant differences in response times. However, even though the use of emergency lights and sirens resulted in statistically faster response times, the clinical significance has not been demonstrated.[16] Specifically, there is no evidence that responding to a scene one or two minutes faster affects patient outcome or survival. Thus, clinical significance must be evaluated in addition to statistical significance. A more appropriate question is whether faster response times improve the survival of the patients. It is one thing to get to a scene quickly, but to make a case for the benefit, it would be interesting to see if the patients actually fared better. This has been studied in several published reports. In 2002, Blackwell and Kaufman, who did not look only at trauma patients, reviewed over 5,000 ambulance runs in an urban setting.[16] They showed little change in patient survival when comparing the response

times of the ambulance that cared for them. Pons and associates evaluated approximately 10,000 patient transports and showed that survival was better only if the ambulance response time was under four minutes.[17] Pons and Markovchick evaluated approximately 3,500 trauma patients and found no difference in survival based on an ambulance response time that was less or greater than eight minutes.[18]

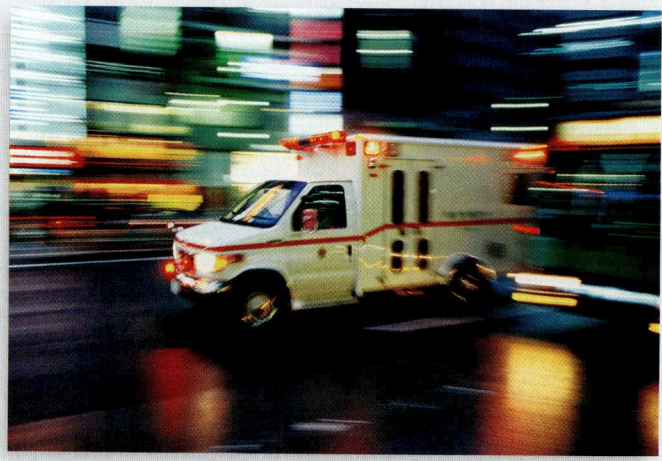

Getting to the patient expediently and safely is the goal of emergency response.

also realize that driving recklessly and taking risks for the sake of time and patient care is unwarranted. While the standard of care is still to drive with warning lights and sirens, driving in control and with caution is the priority.

Staying Safe at the Scene

As a paramedic crew arrives at a scene, they must continuously evaluate scene safety. This starts with information obtained from dispatch regarding the presence of police and fire at the scene and the possibility of hazardous materials. It is good to know how many patients to expect and what the mechanism of injury was. Upon arrival, the crew must assess the area for threats such as traffic, fire, or inclement weather or, in cases of violence, ensure the person causing the violence is no longer a concern. Violence directed against prehospital providers who are tending to patients is rare, but it must still be considered a possibility each and every time.[19]

Unfortunately, prehospital crews must also keep in mind the possibility of terrorism as the cause of the event. That could mean the presence of secondary explosive devices or weapons of mass destruction. Cooperating with police and firefighters at the scene will make the task of assessing risk much more manageable and safe.

Street Secrets

Keep your guard up and senses alert to danger during every response. In order to provide the best patient care, you must keep yourself safe, despite a multitude of dangers that may be present at a scene. Chapter 9: Safety and Scene Size-Up discusses the Awareness Color Coding System. Remember that on virtually every ambulance call, it is appropriate to remain at least in Code Yellow, with a heightened awareness of the environment and scene.

Reducing Scene Time

As we search for ways to reduce the time from injury to definitive care in a hospital, the evaluation of time includes not only the response time and transport time, but also the time spent at the scene treating patients. There has been a shift in the tactics of patient management by prehospital providers over the last few decades. Earlier approaches were based on the idea of "treat at the scene," where providers were armed with knowledge of procedures and the tools to use them, hoping to save the life in the field. This works well for most medical conditions, especially cardiac arrest. With time, the focus changed with the recognition that the true place of definitive care for trauma patients with significant injuries is the hospital (particularly a trauma center).

Now the emphasis in prehospital care has been refined further; paramedics are encouraged to rapidly assess the patient for immediate, reversible, life-threatening injuries and should take steps to correct them in the field prior to initiating transport. If a significant life threat such as a tension pneumothorax or arterial hemorrhage is present, begin treating the patient immediately on the scene. Once all life-threatening injuries have been identified and treated (if possible), the next priority is to prepare for transport, move the patient to a vehicle, and begin transport. All further attempts to correct the primary survey life threat as well as the secondary survey assessments and treatments will be done en route.

Research from two decades ago showed that paramedics doing procedures at the scene often delayed arrival at the hospital, without providing significant benefit to the patient in the form of increased survival.[20] Similarly, a much more recent study investigating prehospital systems in Canada showed that patients cared for by EMTs with only BLS skills had a lower mortality rate than those cared for by paramedics or physicians.[21] This suggests that there may be no direct increase in survival of trauma patients when ALS procedures are performed.

> Delay at the scene to perform procedures does not appear to improve survival.

Therefore, make every effort to minimize scene time. A direct correlation has been shown between shorter prehospital times and decreased mortality of trauma patients.[6]

Reassessing the Trauma Patient

One of the most useful tools for the paramedic is the physical exam. It is an important skill that you can hone with each patient you see. It is the method by which you will identify critical information about your trauma patient. A good physical exam may help identify a subtle discrepancy in lung sounds that could turn into a tension pneumothorax. Keen observation may identify a small wound on a patient's chest that, if unrecognized, may become the fatal stab wound. Unlike training scenarios where moulage and instructors provide hints, in the field you will need to seek out signs of injury.

Performing a good initial assessment and then following that with repeated assessment offers many benefits. It allows you to recognize improvements brought about by interventions and reinforce your medical decision making. It may also provide an early indication of a worsening clinical condition before it becomes life-threatening. Examples are increased bleeding in an injured mouth or progressively worsening shortness of breath that may indicate the development of a tension pneumothorax.

You should reassess continuously, particularly when you believe a patient's condition is worsening. In most trauma cases, a condition that causes a sudden significant change will be found by repeating the primary ABCDE survey. Another look at the airway may show you that the nasal airway is obstructed with blood or vomitus. Listening to the lungs again may indicate the ET tube has shifted into the right mainstem bronchus. Reevaluating the patient's circulation may reveal previously missed bleeding or a progressively distended abdomen.

Traumatic Arrest and Resuscitation Efforts

A difficult situation you will encounter is death from traumatic injury. Statistically, these patients are more likely to be young and healthy, and caring for one may cause you to reflect on your own mortality. After attempting to help someone who has sustained mortal injuries, you may ask yourself whether you gave up too early or missed an important clue that might have made a difference.

Until recently, there had been little guidance for prehospital personnel to rely on when making the decision to terminate resuscitation efforts or not to even initiate them. Unless the situation is one of an injury not "compatible with life," the paramedic needs to make a quick decision to initiate efforts to save someone. Once started, it is even more difficult to stop resuscitative efforts, especially at the scene where the patient's family or friends may be present.

It is well documented that very few patients survive a traumatic cardiac arrest, with reported rates of survival from 0% to 4%.[22,23] With this in mind, paramedics should have protocols for either not initiating or terminating CPR on trauma patients. A recent position paper from the National Association of EMS Physicians provides some simple guidelines to use when deciding whether or not to initiate resuscitative efforts.[24] The authors recommend the following:

Guidelines for Initiating Resuscitation Efforts

- Do not attempt to resuscitate a patient of blunt trauma who is pulseless, apneic, and has no organized electrical rhythm on a cardiac monitor.
- Patients of penetrating trauma have a slightly higher chance of survival, even with the above findings; therefore, attempt resuscitation if

the person is pulseless and apneic, but has spontaneous movement, pupillary reflexes, or a rhythm on the cardiac monitor. Even if attempts are made in this setting, the paramedic should recognize that the likelihood of survival is very low.

Putting It All Together: A Few Minutes with a Medical Director

Emergency medicine providers often argue that the first and most important branch-point in emergency medicine is the question of whether the patient is "sick" or "not yet sick." For this discussion, patients who are "not yet sick" have had a minor mechanism of injury, are stable, and are in no danger of decompensating in the near future. A "sick" patient is just the opposite of this. For them, paramedics need to do something immediately or the patient will decompensate or die. This differentiation seems obvious, but it is not as easy as you might think.

Sometimes paramedics think that if a patient is awake and talking then "everything will be alright." Just because a patient is talking does not mean that the patient will not be dead in a few minutes. That is why in this part of the chapter the discussion will turn to the most critical element of prehospital care—being able to take a step back, take in all the facts that are racing around in your head, and treat the patient even if you do not know what is wrong.

One of the many characteristics of the proactive component of emergency medicine is that it is often practiced with an incomplete set of information. This is not to say that its practitioners from the EMT level through to physicians are ignorant or uneducated. They do know the potential conditions that a patient could have—they just may not yet know the exact condition that a particular patient has before they begin to provide treatment. For instance, if a patient presents with tachypnea, decreased breath sounds on one side, tracheal deviation away from that side, and declining blood pressure and level of consciousness, then that side of the chest needs to be decompressed. Whether that patient has a tension pneumothorax from a stab wound, gunshot wound, or blunt trauma or whether they have one rib fracture or a full flail chest needs to be determined eventually but is not relevant immediately.

You might say, "Okay, that sounds easy enough, but how do I actually do it?" In this regard, emergency medicine is just like any other skill such as playing golf or the guitar. You need to master the fundamentals and keep coming back to them. In basic life support and even the most basic cardiopulmonary resuscitation (CPR) course, the concept of the ABCs is presented. These are airway, breathing, and circulation.

Many readers of this chapter may be saying, "Come on, I've known about the ABCs for a long time; teach me the real secret to taking care of sick patients."

In fact, the ABCs and the vital signs are the secret to taking care of sick patients.

- The components are in that order for a reason, and they are meant to be approached sequentially.
- If there is a problem with any element of the ABCs, you stop right there and fix it.

This may sound overly simplistic, but it is actually quite a powerful statement. It is much easier to dogmatically discuss anatomy, physiology, and the finer points of thoracic pathology when you are in the classroom relaxing with a cup of coffee than it is on the side of the highway at night with a patient who is gasping for air and coughing up blood. An emergency physician approaches a patient exactly the same way an EMT does. Does the patient have an airway? If not, fix it. Is the patient breathing? If not, breathe for them. Does the patient have circulation? If not, do something to correct the situation. As you progress to higher levels of training, you simply acquire more skills and tools with which to fix the problem. The fundamentals, however, remain the same.

The vital signs are the same way. They are called "vital" signs for a reason. What is the patient's pulse? Is it 100 just because of anxiety? Maybe, but what if it goes up to 110 after a few minutes? Is the patient just getting more anxious? Unlikely. You need to search for the cause. The "vital signs" section of a patient care report is not just a series of boxes to be filled in like the date or address box. They are meant to be constantly reevaluated and taken in context of the overall clinical situation.

The evaluation of a patient with thoracic trauma provides a good example. As you approach the scene, look around and absorb as much information as you can about the mechanism of injury. If the mechanism is significant, you will approach the patient with an attitude of "sick until proven otherwise." When you approach the patient, what is your impression after the first 10 seconds? Is the patient alert, oriented, and speaking to you in full sentences? If yes, you can rapidly move into getting vital signs and starting the secondary survey. If no, then a light bulb needs to go off in your head that something needs to be done. The critical thing is to be able to quickly get in the mindset that an action is required. Many "sick" patients will be identified during this first interaction.

Proceed to the ABCs. Is the airway clear? If not, then use an appropriate maneuver to open it while protecting the cervical spine. Use suction as necessary and an oral or nasopharyngeal airway as appropriate.

Now that the airway is open, is the patient breathing? Are they breathing well enough to support life? Remember that apnea is often preceded by a period of inadequate breathing. Just because the patient is making some respiratory effort does not mean that it is enough. You may still need to support them with a bag-mask. Consider nasotracheal or orotracheal intubation if appropriate, and at the very least, administer supplemental oxygen.

Included with breathing is looking at the chest wall and making sure that all the components for respiration are there. If there is a sucking chest wound, close it with a dressing. Is the patient breathing but in severe pain due to blunt trauma? Is there an area of obvious paradoxical motion? If your protocol allows and the patient's blood pressure is reassuring, then give a short-acting narcotic for pain relief.

Intravenous access is important, but, in general, transport should not be delayed while trying to establish access. Remember that the sickest trauma patients need definitive treatment that will be provided only in the hospital not in the back of the ambulance. Once IV access is established, you may consider a fluid bolus. A full discussion of fluid resuscitation is beyond the scope of this section, but suffice it to say that there is growing evidence that overly aggressive fluid resuscitation can be dangerous. One theory is that the increased blood pressure can dislodge clots and lead to increased bleeding. This is an area of active research, and the understanding of prehospital fluid resuscitation will undoubtedly change in the coming years. If a patient is severely hypovolemic, it is prudent to try a crystalloid bolus titrated to improve the patient's mentation and to try to keep the systolic blood pressure at approximately 90 mmHg.[25]

CONNECTIONS Refer to Chapter 13: Shock Overview for further information on fluid resuscitation.

Also included under the circulation section of the algorithm is the control of bleeding. Significant bleeding should be controlled with direct pressure and dressings. Again though, the temptation to spend a great deal of time at the scene putting on elaborate dressings and splints should be avoided. People do not generally die from a broken arm, they die from internal injuries. Keep the scene time as short as possible, and get patients to the hospital.

Summary

Caring for patients who have sustained trauma will be one of the more challenging and adrenalin-producing moments in your career. There is a significant amount of learning that goes into understanding how to provide optimal care to these patients. With attention focused on the basic, important points discussed in this section, you can be assured that you are providing the best care for the patient.

A trauma system is an integrated group of components working together for the good of its patients. As a paramedic, you are an important component of that system. As prehospital providers, you serve as the gatekeepers to the trauma system. Through your assessment and triage decisions, you determine if the patient meets the criteria to be sent to a trauma center or if the patient can be evaluated and treated in the local emergency department. You determine what resources of the system to utilize in the best interest of the patient. You are responsible for determining which patients require helicopter transport and which can be transported by ground. You must determine if a patient would be better served by being transported to a specialty center or higher level trauma center. You also play an important role in prevention efforts designed to minimize morbidity and mortality.

Trauma remains a leading cause of death and disability in society today. As long as people continue to work and play, there will be injuries occurring. It is the paramedic's responsibility to understand the role and functions of all the components of the trauma system and apply them in clinical practice.

Notes

1. *National Safety Council Injury Facts* (Itasca, IL: National Safety Council, 2004), p. 2.
2. *Emergency Medical Services at the Crossroads* (Washington, DC: Institute of Medicine, 2006).
3. *Guidelines for Prehospital Management of Traumatic Brain Injury* (New York, NY: Brain Trauma Foundation, 2000).
4. National Highway Traffic Safety Administration, *Traffic Safety Facts 2001: Pedestrians,* Publication HS-808 772 (Washington, DC: US Department of Transportation, 1998).
5. Miguel A. Lopez-Viego, *The Parkland Trauma Handbook* (St. Louis, MO: Elsevier Mosby, 1994).
6. J. S. Samaplis, "Trauma Care Regionalization: A Process-Outcome Evaluation," *The Journal of Trauma* 46(4) (April 1999):565.
7. *Trauma Evaluation and Management* (Chicago, IL: American College of Surgeons, 1999), p. 41.
8. National Association of EMTs, *Prehospital Trauma Life Support,* 6th ed. (St. Louis, MO: Elsevier Mosby, 2007).
9. J. E. Tintinalli, G. D. Kelen, J. S. Stapczynski, O. J. Ma, and D. M. Cline, *Tintinalli's Emergency Medicine: A Comprehensive Study Guide,* 6th ed., Mcgraw-Hill's AccessMedicine (accessed September 11, 2006).
10. R. J. Bond, "Field Trauma Triage: Combining Mechanism of Injury with Prehospital Index for an Improved Trauma Triage Tool," *The Journal of Trauma* 43(2)(August 1997):283–287.
11. J. R. Plant, "Limitation of the Prehospital Index in Identifying Patients in Need of a Major Trauma Center," *Annals of Emergency Medicine* 26(2)(August 1995):133–137.
12. S. A. Mulholland, "Is Paramedic Judgement Useful in Prehospital Triage?" *Injury* 36(11)(November 2005):1298–1305.
13. Committee on Trauma, American College of Surgeons, *Resources for Optimal Care of the Injured Patient* (Chicago, IL: American College of Surgeons, 2006).
14. J. Ho and M. Lindquist, "Time Saved with the Use of Emergency Lights and Siren While Responding to Requests for Emergency Medical Aid in a Rural Environment," *Prehospital Emergency Care* 3(2)(April–June 1999):127–130.
15. D. J. O'Brien and D. G. Price, "The Effectiveness of Lights and Siren Use During Ambulance Transport by Paramedics," *Academic Emergency Medicine* 9(4)(April 2002):288–295.
16. T. H. Blackwell and J. S. Kaufman, "Response Time Effectiveness: Comparison of Response Time and Survival in an Urban Emergency Medical Services System," *Academic Emergency Medicine* 9(4)(April 2002):320.
17. P. T. Pons, J. S. Haukoos, W. Bludworth, et al., "Paramedic Response Time: Does it Affect Patient Survival?" *Academic Emergency Medicine* 12(2005):594–600.
18. P. T. Pons and V. J. Markovchick, "Eight Minutes or Less: Does the Ambulance Response Time Guideline Impact Trauma Patient Outcome?" *The Journal of Emergency Medicine* 23(2002):43–48.
19. C. C. Mechem, "Injuries from Assaults on Paramedics and Firefighters in an Urban Emergency Medical Services System," *Prehospital Emergency Care* 6(4)(October–December 2002):396.
20. J. P. Smith, "Prehospital Stabilization of Critically Injured Patients: A Failed Attempt," *The Journal of Trauma* 25(1)(January 1985):65.
21. M. Liberman, "Multicenter Canadian Study of Prehospital Trauma Care," *Annals of Surgery* 237(2)(February 2003):153.
22. Z. T. Stockinger, "Additional Evidence in Support of Withholding or Terminating Cardiopulmonary Resuscitation for Trauma Patients in the Field," *Journal of the American College of Surgeons* 198(2)(February 2004):227–231.
23. S. K. Martin, "Blunt Trauma Patients with Prehospital PEA; Poor Ending Assured," *The Journal of Trauma* 53(5) (November 2002):876–880.
24. L. R. Hopson, "Guidelines for Withholding or Termination of Resuscitation in Prehospital Traumatic Cardiopulmonary Arrest," *Prehospital Emergency Care* 7(1)(January 2003): 141–146.
25. R. Fowler and P. E. Pepe, "Prehospital Care of the Patient with Major Trauma," *Emergency Medical Clinics of North America,* 20(2002):953–974.

part 4

Medical Issues

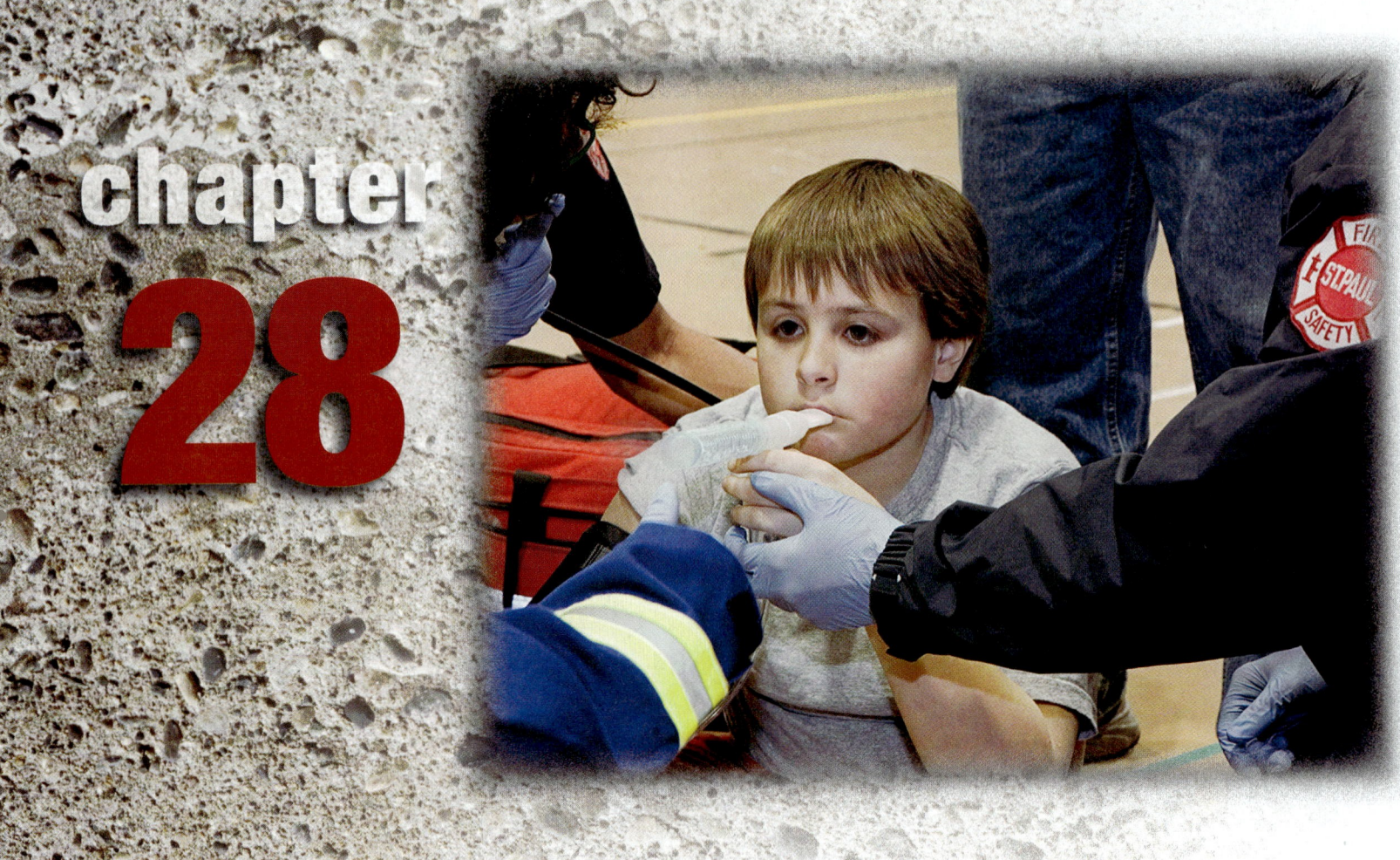

Pulmonary

"*A*nimals live by two principle things, food and breath (spirit, pneuma); . . . of these by far the most important is the respiration, for if it be stopped, the man will not endure long, but immediately dies."

—Aretaeus the Cappodocian [81–138 A.D.]

Need to Know

▶ Respiration involves the delivery of oxygen to the tissues; ventilation involves the removal of carbon dioxide from the body.

▶ The primary survey may reveal life-threatening breathing problems that require rapid intervention before you have a thorough understanding of the disease or illness.

▶ COPD, asthma, and respiratory problems may be difficult to distinguish from cardiac-caused problems.

▶ Diagnosing the root cause of the breathing problem is not as important as properly assessing and making wise treatment decisions.

▶ Wheezing can be caused by many diseases other than asthma and by problems other than respiratory diseases, such as foreign body obstruction and toxic inhalation.

▶ Some chronic respiratory diseases may cause an elevated CO_2 level (by $ETCO_2$ reading) that may need to be tolerated by the paramedic, provided the O_2 reading (by pulse oximetry) is indicating hypoxemia is not present.

▶ Patients with chronic lung disease switch their trigger to breathe from high CO_2 levels, which they will have chronically, to low oxygen levels. Even though hypoxia is the driving factor for these patients to breath, oxygen should never be withheld from any patient who presents in respiratory distress.

▶ Sick	▶ Not Yet Sick
• Any COPD patient with a pulse oximetry less than 90% with signs of respiratory distress should receive oxygen.	• Ask if the patient knows the peak flow values, home oxygen setting, or other factors, to help guide your decision-making process.
• A patient with respiratory complaints who has an altered mental status should be aggressively managed to prevent respiratory failure (which may already be present) or to prevent respiratory arrest.	• Determine if past exacerbations of the patient's conditions have resulted in the need for intubation or hospitalization.
• Any patient with cyanosis has respiratory insufficiency or failure.	• Monitor the patient very closely, taking note of any signs of fatigue as a serious sign of the patient's level of distress.
	• Pulse oximetry readings over 95% are within normal limits.
	• For COPD patients with a normal mental status and no significant respiratory symptoms, a pulse oximetry less than 95% may be normal.
	• $ETCO_2$ readings below 40 mmHg are generally within the normal range.
	• $ETCO_2$ readings less than 45 to 50 may be normal for the COPD patient—particularly if the mental status is good and there are no significant respiratory complaints.

Introduction

Acute respiratory complaints are among the most common causes of prehospital medical calls. The National Highway Traffic Safety Administration (NHTSA) Emergency Medical Services Outcomes Evaluation project analyzed data collected from five states over a one-year period.[1] They found that respiratory distress ranked second in frequency when it came to high-priority prehospital cases. It was also the third most frequent symptom for prehospital pediatric calls. New evidence from the OPALS (Ontario Prehospital Advanced Life Support) research study in Ontario, Canada, has shown how beneficial prehospital interventions in patients with a pulmonary problem can be.[2] Unlike many other areas of prehospital care where there is little evidence to show a benefit to EMS care, respiratory care appears to be emerging as an area where advanced life support makes a significant difference in outcomes.

CONNECTIONS Chapter 43: Pediatric Patients addresses pediatric issues and contains additional information on pediatric respiratory emergencies.

Respiratory distress may be caused by many different illnesses and injuries. Likewise, the care you will provide for these various problems may be markedly different. This chapter will focus on pulmonary *diseases* of medical origin. It is important to note that traumatic injuries to the chest and lungs and cardiovascular disorders most notably heart failure (pulmonary edema), may also present with symptoms of respiratory distress and involve serious pulmonary and ventilatory problems. These problems may be severe, even life-threatening, and should be identified early in your assessment. These problems are addressed in Chapter 21: Thoracic Trauma and Chapter 29: Cardiology.

Treating patients with breathing difficulties can be especially challenging in the prehospital environment. You will have to make rapid assessments and decisions about how to treat a patient who is struggling to breathe. To complicate matters, chronic obstructive pulmonary disease (COPD); pneumonia, and congestive heart failure (CHF) may be very difficult to tell apart from each other in the field. The rate of misdiagnosis of CHF has been demonstrated to be as high as 23–32% in prehospital studies.[3]

Several diseases of the respiratory system are often grouped under the large category of COPD. These include asthma, chronic bronchitis, and emphysema. COPD is estimated to affect 32 million people in the United States and is the fourth leading cause of death in this country.[4] Each of the diseases that make up COPD will be presented in order from the most reversible and acute to the most permanent (less reversible) or chronic. Other pulmonary causes of distress such as pulmonary embolus, acute respiratory distress syndrome (ARDS), lung cancer, and spontaneous pneumothorax will also be discussed. DOT 5-1.1

Diagnosing the root cause of a patient's pulmonary disease may not be as important as properly assessing and making wise treatment choices that will help the patient breathe better, no matter what the final diagnosis may turn out to be. This chapter will address key concepts and clinical factors that will assist you in making the right treatment choices. DOT 5-1.1

Street Secrets

Patients with pulmonary problems typically present with shortness of breath, chest pain, or both. A carefully obtained history (including past medical history and medications), along with specific physical exam findings and selected ancillary tests like breath sounds, will help to more accurately identify the causes and direct treatment for patients experiencing shortness of breath or chest pain.

Applied Physiology

CONNECTIONS For an in-depth review of the anatomy of the upper and lower airway, see Chapter 7: Anatomy Overview. To review normal ventilation, see Chapter 12: Airway Management, Ventilation, and Oxygenation.

The upper airway performs many important functions. First, the upper airway must be patent to allow air to pass to the lower airways in the lungs for oxygenation. As air passes through the upper airway, it is filtered to prevent particles and contaminants from reaching the lower

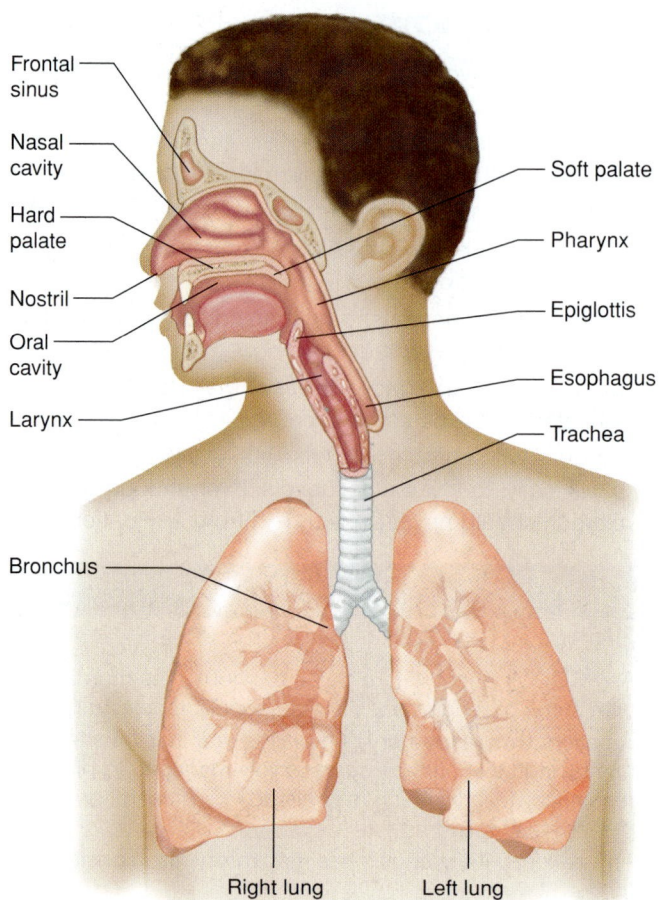

Figure 28-1   The anatomy of the upper and lower respiratory system.

airway. In addition, the mucous membranes of the nasopharynx humidify and warm the air before it reaches the lower airway. Interference with these functions can cause respiratory insufficiency or failure. Any illness or injury that causes partial or complete obstruction of the upper airway will impair air movement and, consequently, oxygenation and ventilation (Figure 28-1). DOT 5-1.2

Obstruction of the lower airways may be caused by mucus plugging or, less commonly, a small foreign body that will obstruct one specific area, impairing but not preventing air exchange completely. In asthma and COPD, partial narrowing caused by bronchospasm at the level of the bronchi and bronchioles can cause wheezing. Other conditions, such as swelling from burns or congestion from heart failure, can cause the alveoli to fill with fluid, impairing oxygenation and ventilation. DOT 5-1.2

Oxygen Delivery and Metabolism

When a patient breathes in, air is transported through the airways and into the alveoli. At this level, red blood cells (RBCs) march end to end through the alveolar-capillary membrane and gas exchange (respiration) occurs. Oxygen molecules basically trade places with carbon dioxide as the RBCs march through in single file. In more scientifically accurate terms, oxygen (O_2) is diffusing across the alveolar capillary membrane. Diffusion, which is addressed in Chapter 12: Airway Management, Ventilation, and Oxygenation, is the process by which molecules move from an area where they have a high concentration gradient to an area of lesser concentration. In the case of the alveolar capillary membrane, there is a large amount of oxygen inside the alveoli and a lesser oxygen concentration in the capillary blood (Figure 28-2). DOT 5-1.3

Hypercarbic and Hypoxic Respiratory Drives

Control of respiration occurs in the brainstem (medulla). Chemical sensing receptors (chemoreceptors), located in the carotid arteries, the arch of the aorta, and in the medulla, sense changes in the partial pressures of oxygen, carbon dioxide (which is acidic), and pH and transmit nerve impulses to the respiratory center to modify respiration as necessary to restore the proper balance (Figure 28-3).

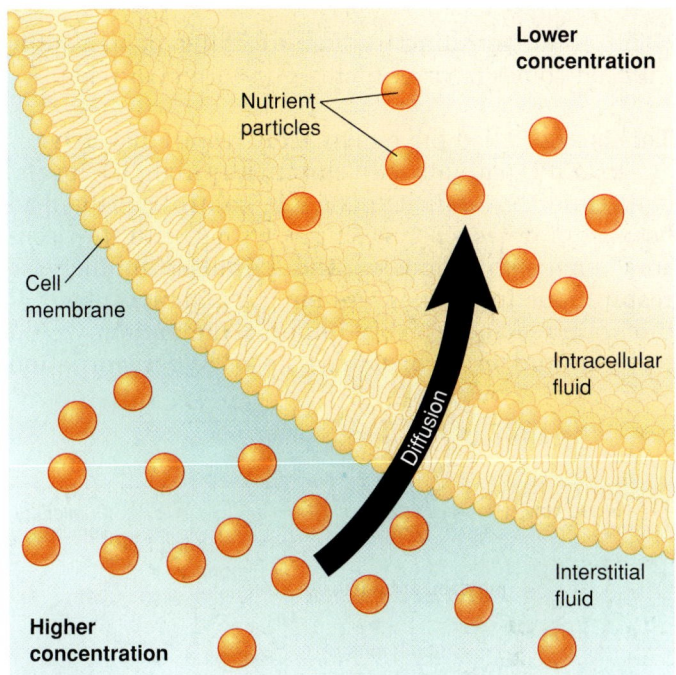

Figure 28-2   Diffusion is the process by which molecules move from an area of high concentration gradient to an area of lesser concentration.

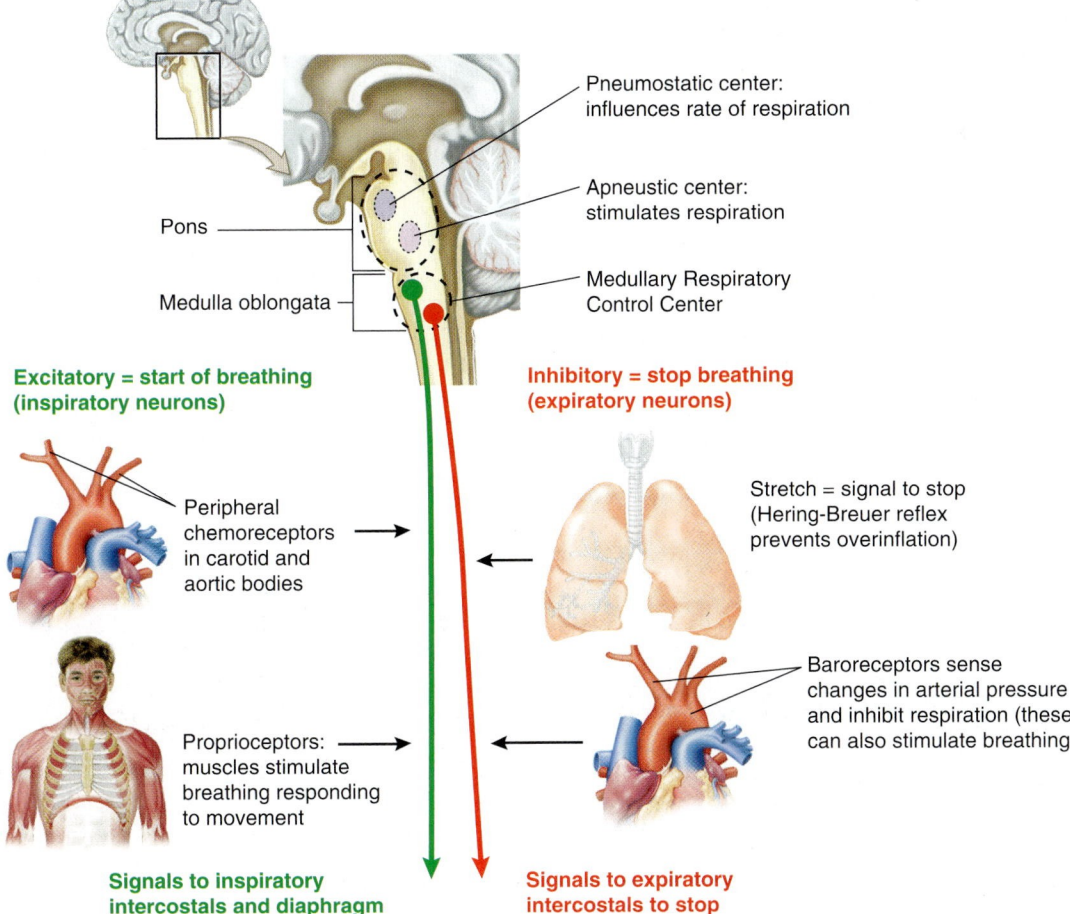

Figure 28-3   The central chemoreceptors within the medullary center respond to changes in CO_2 and pH. Normally, a person is stimulated to breathe when a small increase in CO_2 leads to respiration. The peripheral chemoreceptors in the aortic arch and carotid bodies also respond to decreased O_2 or increased CO_2 and can stimulate breathing.

The dominant stimulus for breathing in a healthy person comes from an increase in carbon dioxide.

This is also called the **hypercarbic respiratory drive.**

In COPD patients with chronically high CO_2 levels, over time the brain adjusts the control mechanism because it detects something is wrong with the "sensors" that continuously send impulses to increase respirations to compensate for the high acid level. If the brain reacted to every impulse, the patient would walk around in a constant state of hyperventilation in an attempt to correct the imbalance. Little by little, the COPD patient's brain adjusts the sensors to pay more attention instead to the concentration of oxygen in the arterial blood. After this change occurs, when the oxygen levels drop (hypoxia), the patient's brain receives a signal to take another breath. The patient is now operating with a **hypoxic drive** instead of the hypercarbic drive. This mechanism will continue to operate for the remainder of the person's life.

DOT 5-1.3

Ventilation

Ventilation results in the elimination of CO_2 from the lungs, thus removing this waste product of cellular metabolism from the body. Ventilation is defined as the process of exchange of air between the lungs and the environment, including inspiration and expiration (Figure 28-4)[5] An objective measure of this is **minute ventilation (MV).** MV is the volume of air exchanged between the environment and the alveoli in sixty seconds. Minute ventilation is calculated as the number of breaths in a minute multiplied by the depth (tidal volume) of those breaths:

$$MV = \text{Respiratory rate (RR)} \times \text{Tidal volume (VT)}.$$

DOT 5-1.3

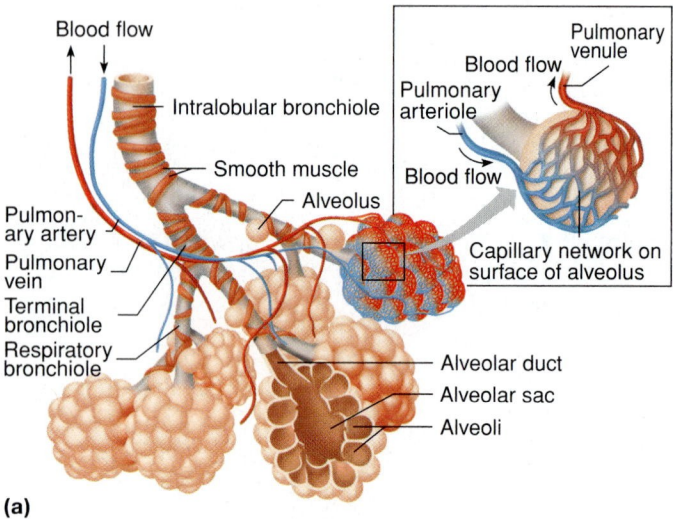

(a)

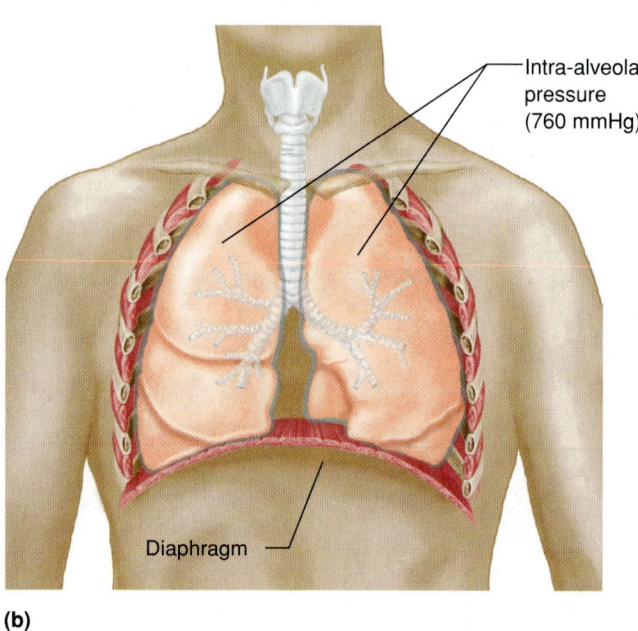

(b)

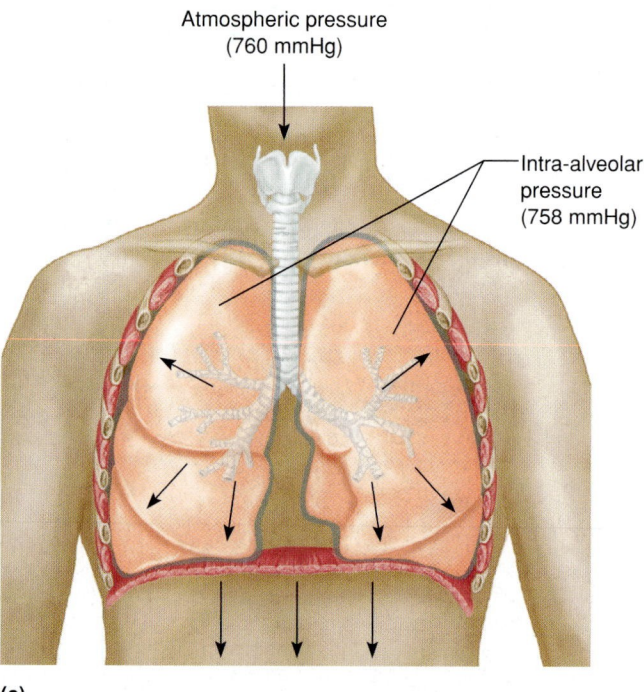

(c)

Figure 28-4 Ventilation is the process of exchange of air between the lungs and the environment. (a) The respiratory tubes end in alveoli, which are surrounded by capillary networks. (b) Prior to inspiration, the intra-alveolar pressue is 760 mmHg. (c) It decreases to 758 mmHg as the thoracic cavity enlarges and atmospheric pressure forces air into the airways.

Working in the Gray Zone

Over the years, EMS providers have been taught to limit the amount of oxygen a COPD patient receives because "too much oxygen may cause the patient to stop breathing." While this may be true when oxygen is administered for a long period of time, the COPD patient who is short of breath needs to be on high-flow oxygen for a while before the patient will potentially stop breathing. It is more accurate to think of the oxygenation of the COPD patient as a system requiring a delicate balance. A small amount of oxygen, such as the quantity delivered by a nasal cannula, can tip the balance between a patient who is oxygen deprived and one who has an adequate amount. Indeed, small amounts of oxygen via nasal cannula are often enough to re-establish the oxygenation balance of a patient with COPD.

Calculating Minute Ventilation

Assume you are treating a patient who is breathing eight times a minute (RR = 8) and that these breaths have a normal tidal volume of 500 mL. Using the MV equation, the actual minute volume is 4 liters.

(MV) is 8 (RR) $\times$ 500 mL (VT) = 4 liters.

This minute volume of 4 liters will normally result in an arterial CO_2 concentration of 40 mmHg.

In order to remove more carbon dioxide, this patient would have to increase the rate or depth of ventilation. Hypothetically, if the patient breathes twice as fast with the same VT, this would double the MV and decrease the CO_2 by approximately one-half of its previous value.

DOT 5-1.3

Nice to Know

A More In-Depth Look at Ventilation

In between breaths, as your body uses oxygen to produce energy, you produce carbon dioxide (CO_2) as a byproduct. It is helpful to think of metabolism as the "fire of life." Metabolic processes burn oxygen and produce "smoke"—CO_2. As CO_2 is produced and accumulates in the blood, it increases the production of carbonic acid, which leads to acidosis. Acidosis, which is a drop in pH, is sensed by the chemoreceptors, which send impulses to the brain to stimulate the body's next breath.

Pathophysiology of Pulmonary Disease

Injury or illness of the pulmonary system may result in insufficient oxygen delivery to critical organs. Both hypoxia and hypercarbia can cause dysfunction of critical organs. In the brain, these conditions are most commonly manifested as an alteration in the level of consciousness.

Hypoxia and Hypoxemia

Hypoxia is the term used to define a reduction of oxygen supply to the tissues. **Hypoxemia** is a state of a low oxygen level in the blood. Hypoxemia will lead to widespread hypoxia if it is not corrected. Diseases, through different mechanisms, result in decreased oxygen delivery to tissues and can cause serious damage to all of the organs in the body.

Hypoxemia is commonly caused by **hypoventilation** (decreased ventilation) but can also be caused by pulmonary disease. (See Box 28-1 for causes of hypoventilation.) Alveoli that are filled with mucous or fluids

BOX 28-1   Causes of Hypoventilation

Depression of the respiratory center
   Narcotics
   Benzodiazepines
   Barbiturates
Disease of the respiratory center
   Infection
   Hemorrhage
   Stroke (cerebrovascular accident or CVA)
Injury of the nerves to the diaphragm (through the spinal cord)
Penetrating spinal cord injury
Diseases of the neuromuscular receptor
Anticholinesterase pesticide poisoning
Nerve agent poisoning
Injuries to the thoracic cage
Trauma with crush injury
Upper airway obstruction
Foreign body
Epiglottitis
Trauma

from swelling or infection impair oxygen and carbon dioxide exchange. Examples of these diseases include pneumonia, congestive heart failure (CHF), and acute respiratory distress syndrome (ARDS).

Oxygen delivery to tissues may also be compromised if blood is prevented from flowing through areas of the lungs. For example, if a clot (thrombus or embolus) lodges in one of the pulmonary arteries (causing a pulmonary embolus), the normal flow of blood will be restricted. This blockage prevents the blood from reaching the alveoli, so the exchange of oxygen and carbon dioxide is impaired, which results in hypoxemia and tissue hypoxia. DOT 5-1.4

Cyanosis

Cyanosis is a bluish discoloration that can be observed in the nail beds or other tissues such as the lips. It results from hemoglobin that does not have oxygen bound to its binding sites. Cyanosis can be described as either central or peripheral in nature. Peripheral cyanosis occurs as the body attempts to shunt the circulating blood volume to the core of the body. Central cyanosis reflects a whole body's lack of adequate perfusion. Generally, the arterial oxygen level must fall to 50 mmHg or below to produce cyanosis. This level of hypoxia is typically associated with a pulse oximetry reading (SpO_2) near 80% (see Table 28-1 and Figure 28-5).[6] The presence of cyanosis signals severe hypoxia.

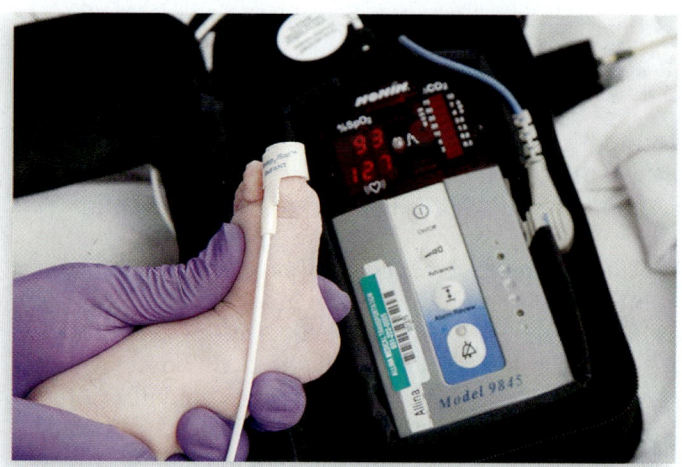

Figure 28-5   Sometimes referred to as "the fifth vital sign," pulse oximetry can assist in identifying hypoxic patients.

Street Secrets

Do not be mislead by a "good" pulse oximeter reading. Patients may be able to compensate for breathing difficulties quite well by increasing the depth and rate of breathing, at least for a while. They may have SpO_2 readings above 95% until they acutely and rapidly decompensate into respiratory arrest. This is especially true of children. If a patient appears to be out of breath, uses accessory muscles to breathe, speaks in short phrases, and has poor lung sounds, trust your assessment regardless of what the monitoring devices are showing.

Certain chronic respiratory problems such as bronchitis affect the patient in an episodic manner, meaning the disease flairs up periodically but there are periods of time when the patient is relatively free of symptoms. These patients tend to exhibit cyanosis more readily than those with a chronic respiratory disease such as COPD, which in the final stage of the disease causes near-constant symptoms of dyspnea. Both diseases will be discussed in greater detail with explanations of why this occurs.

Street Secrets

Keep in mind that an absence of cyanosis does not rule out clinically significant tissue hypoxia. If a patient has hypovolemia from active bleeding, cyanosis may not develop in the skin because there is an overall lack of blood cells.

CONNECTIONS Since hemoglobin is needed to move oxygen in the blood, a decrease in hemoglobin, called anemia, may also result in hypoxia. To review blood disorders, see Chapter 37: Hematology.

TABLE 28-1   Causes of Cyanosis

Central cyanosis	Peripheral cyanosis
Hypoxemia	Reduced cardiac output
Decreased FiO_2*:	Cold extremities
high altitude	Maldistribution of blood
Hypoventilation	flow: distributive forms of
Ventilation-perfusion mismatch	shock
Right-to-left shunt: congenital	Arterial or venous
heart disease, pulmonary	obstruction
arteriovenous fistulas,	
multiple intrapulmonary	
shunts	
Hemoglobin abnormalities	
Methemoglobinemia:	
hereditary, acquired	
Sulfhemoglobinemia: acquired	
Carboxyhemoglobinemia (not	
true cyanosis)	

*FiO_2 = fraction of inspired oxygen

Source: Tintinalli's Emergency Medicine, 6th ed. Section 8: Pulmonary Emergencies, Chapter 62: Respiratory. www.accessmedicine.com.

Hypercarbia

Just as low levels of oxygen can be deadly, so can elevated levels of carbon dioxide (CO_2). The condition of excess carbon dioxide in the blood is termed **hypercarbia.** As mentioned previously, CO_2 is a waste product of cellular metabolism. When a patient has decreased ventilation (hypoventilation), the body cannot rid itself of CO_2 and more and more CO_2 will accumulate in the blood. Acute rises in CO_2 (above 50 mmHg when measured by arterial blood gas analysis) generally represent respiratory failure.

The rising level of CO_2 will have multiple clinical effects. As more carbonic acid is produced, the pH of the blood will drop, causing respiratory acidosis.

Street Secrets

One clinical tool available to paramedics is end-tidal CO_2 monitoring with a capnography unit. Capnography will enable you to detect an acute rise in blood CO_2, which, with appropriate treatment, will prevent extended periods of acidosis. A rise from 40 to 80 mmHg in the end-tidal CO_2 monitor will result in a drop in the pH by approximately 0.2 units, from 7.4 to 7.2 (normally Ph should be 7.35–7.45).[6]

Rising levels of CO_2 will also cause symptoms in the central nervous system. One of the earliest signs is headache. As levels raise further, restlessness, slurred speech, and fluctuations of mood can occur. At even higher levels, carbon dioxide causes disorientation and depression of consciousness similar to that seen with narcotic overdose.[6] This is commonly referred to as **CO_2 narcosis.**

Primary Survey

Patients who are experiencing respiratory distress need a thorough assessment of airway and breathing. As part of your initial assessment, begin by taking a moment to observe the patient's respiratory effort and general appearance. This will help give you a sense of whether the patient is sick or not yet sick.

In your initial approach to the patient, observe the way the patient is sitting. A patient who is sitting bolt upright, leaning forward, propped up on his arms in a tripod position, and appears to be air hungry is sick until you can determine another cause for this posture (Figure 28-6).

Assess the patient's rate and depth of respirations. Rapid and shallow breathing indicates that the patient's breathing is labored. Accessory muscle use (intercostal retractions, sternocleidomastoid contractions), **air hunger,** and one or two word dyspnea (able to speak only one or two words at a time) demonstrate that the patient is sick. Immediately begin providing

Working in the Gray Zone

Partial Pressures of Oxygen and Carbon Dioxide

Normally when working with percentages, the expectation is that 100% represents the full amount of something. In other words, if a pie is carved up into four equally sized pieces, each piece equals 25% of the pie. Gasses dissolved in the blood should not be thought of in this manner. Oxygen and carbon dioxide are separately measured. They do not "add up" to 100% if you sum them together. The normal value for oxygen is 80–100 mmHg, and the normal value for carbon dioxide is 35–45 mmHg. These values are independent of each other when it comes to measuring them. It is possible for each value to be too high or too low, or mixed with one high and the other low. That is one reason why both end-tidal CO_2 and pulse oximetry are important measurements: Pulse oximetry measures respiration, and end-tidal CO_2 measures ventilation.

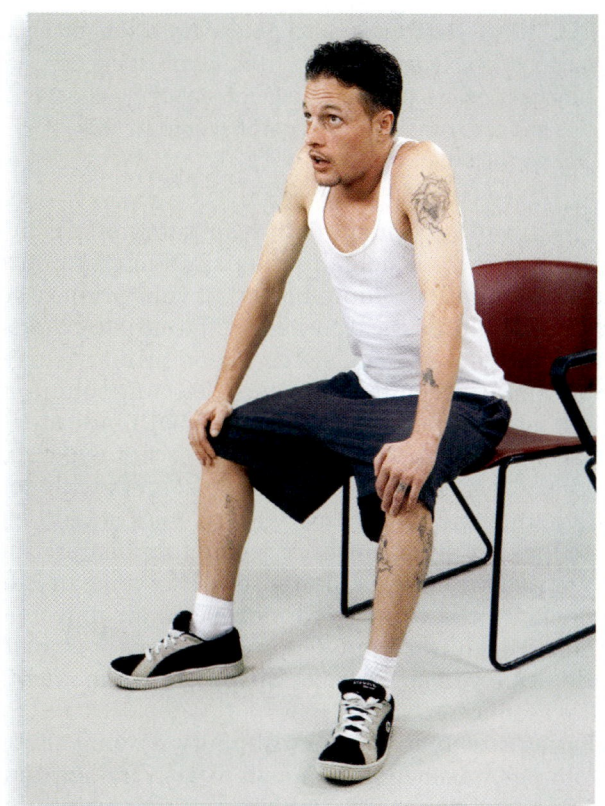

Figure 28-6 A patient presenting in the tripod position is in respiratory distress.

supplemental oxygen and perhaps ventilatory assistance, listen to the lung sounds, and focus your attention on a rapid but thorough assessment of the pulmonary system.

CONNECTIONS   Review Chapter 12: Airway Management, Ventilation, and Oxygenation and 14: Patient Assessment for more information on performing the assessment of airway and breathing.

Your initial priorities are to ensure that the upper airway is in fact open and patent. A quick assessment of the patient's ability to speak and move air is critical. If an obstruction such as mucus or other secretions is found in the upper airway, immediately suction until the airway is clear. Keep in mind that every second you are applying suction is a second you are depriving the patient of oxygen. Balance the need to clear the airway with the need to provide oxygen, and limit the length of time suction is applied. Most references indicate an upper limit of 15 seconds per suction attempt.

Supplemental oxygen should be applied immediately to patients who complain of difficulty breathing. If patients cannot breathe on their own, assist their breathing with bag-mask ventilation. The rate of ventilations should generally be no more than 10–12 breaths per minute (one breath every 6 to 7 seconds).[7]

CONNECTIONS   Refer to Chapter 12: Airway Management, Ventilation, and Oxygenation for a discussion of the dangers of creating a positive pressure environment in the chest and how this impacts venous return, cardiac output, and cerebral perfusion.

Chest wall movement with respiratory efforts does not mean that air is actually moving in and out of the lungs. Auscultation should be part of your primary survey and should be used to help differentiate between the sick and not yet sick states. In the primary survey, you are simply listening to be sure that lung sounds are present on each side of the chest. This will indicate immediately if a lung has collapsed or is not expanding properly. Clear, equal, bilateral lung sounds with good tidal volume and no accessory muscle use should lead you to look for other causes of respiratory distress such as a cardiac problem, acidosis, severe anemia, or other problem. On the other hand, decreased air movement and abnormal lung sounds (such as wheezes or crackles) should lead you to strongly suspect a pulmonary or cardiovascular problem.

Patients who are having difficulty moving enough air volume or exchanging enough oxygen in their lungs "compensate" for these problems by increasing their rate and depth of respiration to increase their minute ventilation. This means that patients may appear to be in a stable condition (good skin color, good oxygen saturation, and good mental status) but in fact may be working very hard to ensure adequate oxygenation. Patients working hard to breathe for an extended amount of time may be very tired when you assess them. Be prepared to support their breathing quickly and consider the placement of an advanced airway.

Asthma

Asthma is a chronic inflammatory disorder of the airways. In susceptible individuals, this inflammation causes recurrent episodes of wheezing, breathlessness, chest tightness, and coughing, particularly at night or in the early morning. These episodes are usually associated with widespread but variable airflow obstruction that is often reversible either spontaneously or with treatment. Asthma also causes an associated **bronchospasm** and increase in the existing bronchial hyperresponsiveness to a variety of stimuli.

Recent research has improved the understanding of asthma. The common factor influencing the lungs and causing the symptoms patients experience with this disease is **inflammation**.[8] This one factor, inflammation, stimulated by many environmental variables, is the common stimulus causing changes in the lung, which create asthma. Among the obstructive respiratory diseases, asthma is the most reversible and the most treatable for the prehospital provider. A single nebulizer treatment will often make an asthmatic breathe better. DOT 5-1.10b

It is important to note that prehospital treatment revolves around alleviating the symptoms and bronchospasm. Because prehospital care generally does not address the root cause of the problem, inflammation, it is important to remember that patients with moderate or severe symptoms should be transported to the emergency department for further evaluation and treatment. DOT 5-1.5

Epidemiology of Asthma

Asthma is a common disease; interestingly, despite intensive treatment and research, its prevalence continues to increase, now affecting nearly 8% of the U.S. population.[9] In all, asthma affects nearly 15 million people, resulting in 470,000 hospitalizations and 5,000 deaths annually. Death rates for asthma are consistently highest among African Americans ages 15 to 24 years and have increased over the past decade.[8] Multiple factors contribute to this mortality including poverty, lack of access to medical care, lack of patient and provider recognition of an acute episode, inadequate treatment, and failure of physicians to prescribe antiinflammatory corticosteroid therapy.[10]

Applied Anatomy and Physiology of Asthma

Normal lung tissue has complex structure and function. The bronchial passages are lined with epithelial cells, cilia, and mucus-producing cells. When small particles or pollutants make their way past the nasopharynx and are deposited in the bronchi, the mucus lining the airways traps the particles so they can be swept upward into the upper airway by the cilia. This mucus in the upper airway may stimulate a cough reflex, which expels the particles from the airway. There is also some passive removal of the particle-filled mucus into the esophagus.

Smoking destroys the cilia lining the airways. Movement of mucus via cilia and the cough reflex are therefore particularly diminished in smokers. This means smokers are at greater risk of developing infections and inflammation.

Also present in the airways are multiple cells that respond when inflammation is present as well as immunoglobulins, proteins, and other substances that mediate the inflammatory response of the lung to a stimulus.

The autonomic nervous system plays an important role in the lung's response to inflammation. Parasympathetic fibers in the vagus nerve innervate the upper trachea and bronchi down to smaller caliber airways. Stimulation of the vagus nerve produces bronchoconstriction in these airways, increases mucus secretions, and causes vasodilation.

Sympathetic innervation is limited in the upper airway but both α (alpha) and β_2 (beta$_2$) receptors are present in bronchial smooth muscle with the frequency of β_2 (beta$_2$) receptors increasing as the airways become smaller.[10] Stimulation of β_2 (beta$_2$) receptors relaxes the smooth muscle in the airways, causing bronchodilation. Albuterol, a β_2 agonist, is one of the most common medications used to treat asthma in the prehospital setting.

Pathophysiology of Asthma

Asthma is an inflammatory disease of the airways with both an acute component as well as a component of persistent chronic inflammation. In the acute, early response, an antigen binds with cells, releasing inflammatory mediators such as **histamine.** The airways are hypersensitive to the presence of many stimuli, not just histamine.

Antigens include environmental allergens (pollen, dust mites, mold, and animal dander), viral respiratory infections, cold exposure, exercise, medications (aspirin and nonsteroidal anti-inflammatory drugs), irritants (tobacco smoke, air pollutants), and food additives (sulfites). In the early phases, inflammation causes airway **hyperresponsiveness,** an exaggerated acute bronchoconstriction response. The clinical effect of the exaggerated response is airflow limitation, manifested by wheezing. At this early stage in the first minutes to a few hours, asthma is most reversible when treated with β_2 (beta$_2$) agonist nebulizations. As the inflammation progresses, the pulmonary vasculature begins to leak fluid. This causes airway swelling. Then mucus is secreted and becomes thickened to the point of causing mucus plugs. Both airway swelling and mucus plugging combine to cause additional bronchial obstruction. These late phase changes are less reversible than the early bronchospasm. The clinical signs of late phase asthma occur within a few hours to days or weeks after the initial stimulus.[8,10] The patient may not clear his respiratory distress and wheezing with treatment and may have only a minimal or partial response to inhaled β_2 (beta$_2$) nebulizations.

CONNECTIONS Paramedics who desire to learn an evidence-based approach to asthma diagnosis and treatment will improve their understanding of this prevalent and severe disease by reading pertinent sections of the Expert Panel Report 2: Guidelines for the Diagnosis and Management of Asthma published in 1997 by the National Institutes of Health as a Clinical Practice Guideline (EPR 2).[11]

Another problem in obstructive diseases is the trapping of air inside the chest. During bronchospasm, the patient will have trouble moving air in and out of the lungs. Since inhalation is an active process (chest wall expands and the diaphragm contracts) and exhalation is a passive process (relaxation of the chest), the asthmatic patient will be more likely to be able to draw air into the chest; however, getting the air out easily or quickly is difficult. Therefore, "trapped" air remains in the lungs at the onset of the next inspiration. It is more difficult to exhale as the narrowed airways do not let air flow out, and exhalation is less powerful than inhalation.

Primary Survey

The initial goals of evaluation for respiratory insufficiency, tiring (inability of the patient to keep up with the work of breathing), and alterations in mentation discussed in primary assessment must be reassessed as part of the more detailed secondary survey.

Asthma patients with a mild exacerbation are short of breath with exertion, generally can speak in full sentences, and can lie down. Conversely, those asthma patients with a severe episode are short of breath at rest, sit upright, and speak only a few words before having to breathe again. Careful auscultation of the lungs performed during the secondary survey may reveal rales or rhonchi, in addition to the wheezes of asthma, suggesting infection (pneumonia) as a factor in the acute attack. Alteration in alertness, such as drowsiness or confusion, indicates severe or worsening asthma in spite of treatment. Diaphoresis in upright asthma patients indicates severe obstruction to airflow.[10] Tachycardia and tachypnea are usually present; patients with a pulse greater than 120 or a respiratory rate greater than 30 have more severe asthma. Refer to Table 28-2 for additional information useful to differentiate the stages of asthma, a classification of the severity of asthma exacerbations.[8]

Particularly ominous signs suggesting impending respiratory failure include asthma patients who complain of shortness of breath but have a "normal" respiratory rate or "quiet" lung exam on auscultation with few wheezes heard. A patient with an acute asthma attack should have an increased respiratory rate. A normal respiratory rate indicates that the patient is getting tired and may progress to respiratory arrest. By the same token, a "quiet" chest with few, if any, wheezes heard on auscultation also suggests that the patient is tiring and not moving adequate amounts of air.

Altered mental status, resulting from asthma, implies inadequate oxygen delivery to, or removal of carbon dioxide from, the brain. This is often manifested by an asthmatic patient who appears to fall asleep whenever he or she is not being stimulated. Altered mentation may compromise airway patency or respiratory effort. Ventilatory support with 100% oxygen should be used. Altered mentation is an indication for endotracheal intubation of the asthmatic patient.[8] Intubation should follow adequate bag-mask ventilation with the goal of improving oxygenation.

Proper technique for ventilation involves slow ventilations, also called "controlled hypoventilation" or "permissive hypercapnia." This slow ventilation is necessary to allow time for the patient to exhale. Ventilation

TABLE 28-2   Classifying Severity of Asthma Exacerbations

	Mild	Moderate	Severe	Respiratory Arrest Imminent
Symptoms				
Breathlessness	While walking Can lie down	While talking Prefers sitting	While at rest Sits upright	
Talks in	Sentences	Phrases	Few words	
Alertness	May be agitated	Usually agitated	Usually agitated	Drowsy or confused
Signs				
Respiratory rate	Increased	Increased	Often > 30/min	
Use of accessory muscles; suprasternal retractions	Usually not	Commonly	Usually	Paradoxical thoracoabdominal movement
Wheeze	Moderate, often only end-expiratory	Loud; throughout exhalation	Usually loud; throughout inhalation and exhalation	Absence of wheezing
Pulse/minute	< 100	100–120	> 120	Bradycardia
Functional Assessment				
Peak Expiratory Flow % personal best or % predicted	$> 80\%$	Approx. 50–80% or response lasts < 2 hours	$< 50\%$	
PaO_2 (room air)	Normal	> 60 mmHg	< 60 mmHg; possible cyanosis	
SaO_2 (room air)	$> 95\%$	91–95%	$< 91\%$	
PCO_2	< 42 mmHg; usually < 35 mmHg	< 42 mmHg	> 42 mmHg; possible respiratory failure	
End-tidal CO_2 ($ETCO_2$)	< 45 mmHg; usually < 35 mmHg	< 45 mmHg	> 45 mmHg; possible respiratory insufficiency or failure	

Source: Adapted from EPR 2 Report, Guidelines for the Diagnosis and Management of Asthma, July 1997 (National Institutes of Health, 1997).

Nice to Know

Other Causes of Wheezing

A common medical saying, "all that wheezes is not asthma," is especially helpful when evaluating the cause of patients' wheezing. Patients with foreign body ingestion (toddlers) or aspiration (geriatric) can manifest wheezing. In these cases, the wheezing will be more focal rather than generalized. Patients with exacerbations of congestive heart failure may have fluid build-up in the lungs. Air movement will be restricted enough that the patients will wheeze or edema will cause bronchospasm. In this case, the "wheezing" may be more prominent in the bases bilaterally.

BOX 28-2   Peak Expiratory Flow Measurement

Peak expiratory flow (PEFR) measurement is recommended both for the patient and for the provider. The PEFR measurement is repeated three times, and the highest value is used. To coach the patient to do a PEFR measurement, perform the following:

1. Move the indicator of the peak flow meter to the bottom of the numbered scale.
2. Instruct the patient to take in a deep breath, filling his lungs completely.
3. Ask the patient to place the mouthpiece in the mouth and seal the lips around it. Instruct the patient not to put the tongue in the hole.
4. Tell the patient to blow out as hard and as fast as possible in a single blow.
5. Write down the number. Reset the flow meter.
6. Repeat the procedure two more times and record the highest of the three values.

When a patient knows personal normal values, you can compare the patient's best effort on these attempts with the patient's personal best effort. Divide the current peak flow measurement by the personal best and multiply by 100 to calculate the percentage of best effort. Values less than 50% of the patient's personal best indicate a severe exacerbation of asthma. Typically, peak flow is not measured on an acute asthma patient in the prehospital setting as most EMS services do not routinely carry a peak flow meter; however, it is a valuable tool, and its use should be considered.

forces air into the lungs, but exhalation still depends on passive relaxation of the chest. If air is being trapped by constricted airways, a longer expiratory phase is critical to allow as much emptying as possible. Too much air trapping may even lead to a pneumothorax, so careful reassessment of lungs sounds is important.

Peak Expiratory Flow Rate Measurement

Using **peak expiratory flow (PEFR)** measurement is an objective indicator of the severity of the asthma attack and the response to treatment administered. Ideally PEFR measurement should be recorded before treatment and then after treatment. Many patients use PEFR as a home monitoring tool, and this then becomes a decision point for seeking ED care. Ask patients if they know their baseline PEFR reading as this can aid in the assessment process. The technique of how to obtain accurate PEFR readings from asthmatic patients is described in Box 28-2. DOT 5-1.9

Secondary Survey

Oxygen should be applied to all asthmatics in respiratory distress. The route of administration, nasal cannula versus mask, depends on which route is best tolerated and whether the patient is receiving a nebulizer treatment at the same time. A patient with a coexisting disease, for example heart disease, or a pregnant patient should have a goal of maintaining oxygen saturation greater than 95%.[8]

Depending upon the severity of the patient's respiratory distress, treatment may be started initially and the history obtained following improvement in symptoms. A patient with moderate or severe asthma may

monitor lung function at home with a PEFR meter (see Box 28-2) and may have a written detailed asthma action plan based upon PEFR results and response to home treatment.[8] The action plan is designed around the patient's personal best peak flow reading and uses that reading to establish three zones (green, yellow, and red), analogous to a stop light. As an example, an asthmatic patient with a personal best PEFR reading of 400 liters per minute (lpm) would have the following zones:

Green (80 to 100% of personal best): 320–400 lpm

Yellow (50 to less than 80% of best): 200–319 lpm

Red (50% or less of best): less than 200 lpm

In the asthma action plan, if the patient became symptomatic, measured the PEFR as 150 lpm (Red zone), and

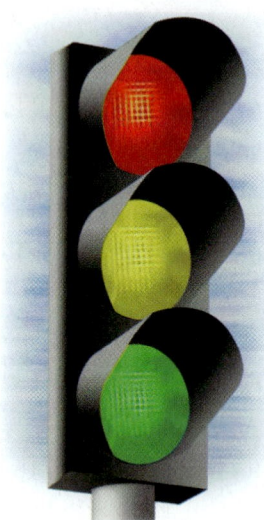

Red zone: less than 200 lpm (50% or less than your best): Call your doctor or go to the ED

Yellow zone: 200–319 lpm (50–less than 80% of best): Use quick relief medicine

Green zone: 320–400 lpm (80–100% of best): Use preventive (anti-inflammatory) medicine

Figure 28-7   An example of an Asthma Action Plan.

BOX 28-3   Risk Factors for Death from Asthma

- Past history of sudden severe exacerbations
- Prior intubation for asthma
- Prior admission to an intensive care unit
- Two or more hospitalizations for asthma in the past year
- Three or more emergency department (ED) visits for asthma in the past year
- Hospitalization or an ED visit for asthma within the past month
- Use of more than two canisters of short-acting inhaled beta$_2$ agonist per month
- Current use or recent withdrawal from systemic corticosteroids
- Difficulty perceiving airflow obstruction or its severity
- Comorbidity, as from cardiovascular disease or chronic obstructive pulmonary disease
- Serious psychiatric or psychosocial problems
- Low socioeconomic status and urban residence
- Illicit drug use (especially inhaled cocaine or heroin)

Source: Adapted from EPR 2 Report, Guidelines for the Diagnosis and Management of Asthma, July 1997 (National Institutes of Health, 1997) and *Rosen's Emergency Medicine: Concepts and Clinical Practice,* 5th ed. (St. Louis, MO: Elsevier Mosby, 2002).

How short of breath are you right now?

0	1	2	3	4	5	6	7	8	9	10

Where 0 = no shortness of breath and 10 = shortness of breath as bad as can be

Figure 28-8   The numeric rating scale for dyspnea.

initiated treatment based upon the plan, but after initiating home treatment, the PEFR reading was 180 lpm (still in the Red zone), the plan would instruct the patient to see the doctor or go to the ED. This could result in a call to 9-1-1 for prehospital treatment and transport (Figure 28-7).

While treatment is administered, obtain a focused history and physical exam. The objective of the brief focused history and physical is identification of a patient at risk for deterioration: respiratory insufficiency, failure, or death. Risk factors for death from asthma are listed in Box 28-3.[8,10] The brief history should focus on the severity of symptoms compared with previous exacerbations using the numeric or visual scale for dyspnea (Figures 28-8 and 28-9), prior intubations, recent treatments or steroid use, compliance with medications, and potentially complicating illness (cardiac disease or COPD).

Treatment of Asthma

There are three principal goals for treating acute exacerbations of asthma:

1. Maintaining oxygenation.
2. Treating bronchospasm by administering beta$_2$ agonists.
3. Administering corticosteroids in the hospital to decrease the associated inflammation.

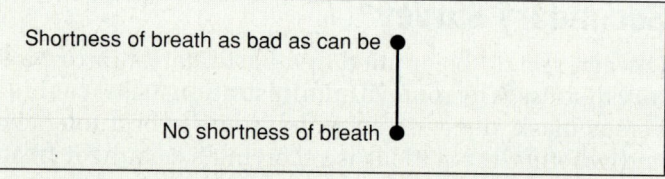

Shortness of breath as bad as can be

No shortness of breath

Patient Instructions: Make a mark on the line that best describes your shortness of breath

Provider Instructions: Measure from the bottom and record distance to mark in millimeters.

Figure 28-9   An example of a visual analog scale for describing dyspnea.

Maintaining Oxygenation

Asthmatics who are very sick, apneic, or unconscious should be treated with immediate bag-mask ventilation with 100% oxygen followed by intubation.[8] Once intubated, ventilation should be directed at improving oxygenation by delivering an oxygen concentration high enough to result in oxygen saturations, ideally above 97% and acceptable above 94%.

At the same time, "controlled hypoventilation," providing a tidal volume of 8–10 mL/kg (approximately 500–700 cc in an averaged-sized adult) at a respiratory rate of less than or equal to 10 breaths per minute minimizes barotrauma.[10] At this setting, as long as oxygen saturations are acceptable, high $ETCO_2$ levels are tolerated. This ventilation strategy minimizes the risk of pneumothorax from high inflation pressures. Elevated pressure inside the chest cavity will also affect venous return to the heart. This is also known as **auto-PEEP**, which causes a reduction in venous return and cardiac output, resulting from too rapid positive pressure ventilation.[12] Ventilating more slowly minimizes this pressure build-up.

Patients with a severe asthma exacerbation may also be candidates for noninvasive continuous positive airway pressure (CPAP) (Box 28-4). Indications for CPAP include rising levels of $ETCO_2$ above 45 mmHg despite treatment; dropping oxygen saturations; exhaustion; and inability to keep up with the work of breathing. Decreasing mental status, however, is a contraindication to using CPAP. When mental status decreases, the patient is in need of more aggressive therapy, and they will most likely not benefit from CPAP at this point. Benefits of CPAP include increasing lung compliance and reducing the work that fatigued respiratory muscles must perform.[10] Drawbacks include barotrauma, although proponents would point out that the barotrauma associated with CPAP is less than would likely occur if the patient were intubated on positive pressure ventilation.

Treating Bronchoconstriction

The second of the three principal goals in treating an acute exacerbation of asthma is to reverse bronchoconstriction by inhaled, short-acting beta₂ agonists.[10] After beginning to address hypoxemia, inhaled beta₂ agonist nebulized medications should be administered. The most common inhaled beta₂ agonist in the prehospital scope of practice is albuterol. It is most effective diluted to a volume of 4 mL with saline. Albuterol is more selective for the beta₂ receptor than beta₁. At lower doses, it causes less tachycardia than other nonselective inhaled beta agonists. Prehospital protocols differ in dosing frequency for albuterol administration. Check your local protocol. DOT 5-1.7

BOX 28-4 Noninvasive Mask CPAP for Respiratory Insufficiency

Some of the more severe asthma attacks do not respond well to treatment with bronchodilators, and the patient develops respiratory insufficiency or failure and requires respiratory support. These patients can generally be recognized by hypoxia (O_2 saturation less than 90%); failure of their vital signs and oxygen saturation to improve with treatment; $ETCO_2$ levels above 45 mmHg and rising, despite treatment; or a clinical assessment that the patient is tiring and not keeping up with the work of breathing.

Signs of respiratory insufficiency and failure must be recognized in order to treat the patient in a timely manner before a deteriorating level of consciousness puts the patient past the point CPAP can help. There are many interventions besides bronchodilators to try including intubation, positive pressure noninvasive bag-mask supplementation of the patient's ventilation, CPAP, or BiPAP. Recent evidence-based reviews of the literature for pulmonary edema demonstrate improved outcomes with **noninvasive positive pressure ventilation (NIPPV)** compared with invasive ventilation. Rates of intubation were decreased in the CPAP group.[10] Fewer hospital and intensive care unit (ICU) days were utilized by the patient treated with NIPPV compared with the patient who was intubated.

DOT 5-1.9

Besides albuterol, other sympathomimetic medications that can be used to reverse bronchospasm include metaproterenol, terbutaline, epinephrine, and racemic epinephrine. Another class of drugs that can reverse bronchospasm is the methylxanthine derivatives, or xanthines as they are sometimes called. Xanthines include theophylline, aminophylline, and theobromine. The use of these drugs for the treatment at an acute asthma attack, however, has fallen out of favor. DOT 5-1.7

Another treatment strategy for asthma includes blocking the effects of the vagus nerve. Administration of inhaled ipratropium bromide (Atrovent™) targets specific receptors in the lungs to block the adverse effects of parasympathetic stimulation. Ipratropium bromide is an anticholinergic (muscarinic) antagonist.

DOT 5-1.7

Working in the Gray Zone

Bronchodilators and Cardiac Patients

Some prehospital protocols advise caution in administering beta$_2$ agonists to cardiac patients. At higher doses, there is more beta$_1$ stimulation and less beta$_2$ receptor specificity, which means that the heart (beta$_1$ receptors) may be stimulated following numerous treatments with drugs such as albuterol. Common side effects include palpitations, tremor, and tachycardia. Albuterol should not be withheld for concerns about tachycardia; the cause for the tachycardia is almost always the respiratory distress, and usually the tachycardia improves once the respiratory distress gets better with albuterol treatment. Less common, but more severe, adverse effects include hypokalemia, not usually clinically significant unless the patient has a low potassium level initially (potentially occurring with diuretic use).

CONNECTIONS To learn more about anticholinergic medications review Chapter 15: Pharmacology.

Corticosteroids

The third of three principal goals for treating an acute exacerbation of asthma is not typically performed in the prehospital setting. It is the administration of systemic corticosteroids, which act to reduce the inflammatory stimulus for bronchial hyperreactivity. These steroids (prednisone administered orally or methylprednisolone given intravenously) are very effective at reversing an acute asthma attack and are also effective when inhaled quick-relief medications are minimally to mildly effective. It is important to remember, however, that steroids typically take six to eight hours before improvement in the patient's condition is noted. DOT 5-1.7

Chronic Obstructive Pulmonary Disease (COPD)

Chronic obstructive pulmonary disease (COPD) includes multiple respiratory diseases (emphysema and chronic bronchitis are the two primarily thought of as COPD) and may share, in much smaller part, the feature of airflow obstruction with asthma. Some definitions of COPD include asthma within their definition; however, the more common definitions exclude asthma as a component. Therefore, COPD is usually defined as

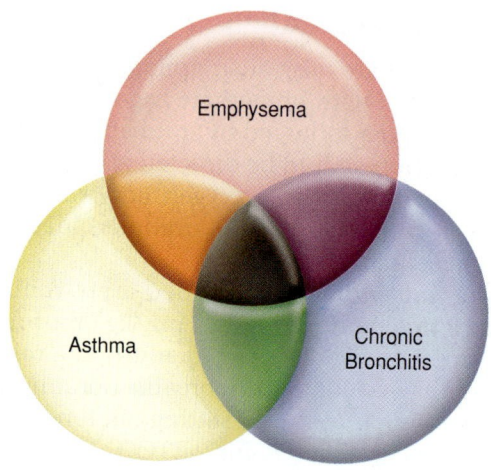

Figure 28-10 Patients can fall into any one of seven zones based upon their signs, symptoms, and disease patterns.

conditions *other than asthma* characterized by dyspnea, cough, sputum production, airflow limitation, and impaired gas exchange.[12] While asthma is characterized by hyperreactiveness of the airway, it is considered more reversible than COPD.

Chronic **bronchitis** is described as chronic sputum production that leads to airway inflammation in the bronchioles. Emphysema has a different pathology than bronchitis. Emphysema results in airway collapse and destruction of lung tissue, starting in the smallest airways and involving the alveoli. Comparing these diseases, asthma is the most reversible while COPD, with a variable component of bronchospasm, is more a chronic, progressive disease, which is less reversible. Of these two diseases, emphysema and chronic bronchitis, patients rarely have just one but commonly demonstrate features of both diseases. COPD and asthma should be thought of as overlapping zones (Figure 28-10). The patient can fall into one of seven zones with this configuration. DOT 5-1.10c

Chronic bronchitis begins as a morning cough, progresses to recurrent episodes of acute bronchitis, and finally is characterized by a chronic productive cough due to excessive bronchial mucus production and airway inflammation.[10]

By definition, the productive cough must be present for at least three months per year for at least two years in order to diagnose the patient as having chronic bronchitis.

Patients with chronic bronchitis are chronically short of breath and then have a decreased capacity to exchange oxygen and carbon dioxide secondary to a ventilation perfusion mismatch. When these patients have acute episodes of dyspnea, they often appear cyanotic or ashen.

CONNECTIONS Chapter 12: Airway Management, Ventilation, and Oxygenation describes ventilation perfusion (V/Q) mismatch.

Emphysema is characterized by destruction of the alveolar walls and enlargement of the alveolar air spaces. Following this destruction, collapse of the smallest airways (the terminal bronchioles) leads to further damage of the alveolar spaces, which leads to obstruction to airflow. Because the destruction is permanent and not reversible, the natural course of COPD, and more specifically emphysema, is one of progressive clinical worsening. The destruction of alveoli is the dominant component of the disease, with reversible bronchospasm a much smaller component. When damaged alveoli heal, they form into misshapen globules, called **blebs,** that are less elastic and less able to inflate and deflate compared to healthy alveoli. DOT 5-1i

With emphysema, gas exchange worsens secondary to a loss of surface area between the alveolar-capillary interface. When the patient becomes chronically hypoxic, the body attempts to compensate for a lack of oxygenation by increasing the production of red blood cells (called polycythemia) and hyperventilating. The increase in red blood cells increases the patient's ability to carry oxygen and also gives them a pink skin tone. DOT 5-1.5

Epidemiology of COPD

COPD affects approximately 14 million patients in the United States.[13] It is the fourth leading cause of death with a mortality rate of more than 50% in the 10 years following diagnosis.[12] The primary cause of COPD is tobacco use although up to 10% of COPD patient have never smoked. For nonsmokers, there are other environmental and occupational causes for COPD. Though mortality for men with COPD is leveling off, the mortality for women is increasing.[10]

Pathophysiology of COPD

The abnormal physiology in COPD occurs both at a cellular and at a clinical level. The cellular and tissue pathophysiology is helpful in understanding the clinical picture that you will encounter in the field. Though it is uncommon for either emphysema or chronic bronchitis to be present in isolation, description of the pure form of each will assist identification of the unique clinical presentations.

The pathophysiologic changes of chronic bronchitis occur in both small and large bronchi. Two predominant changes cause obstruction of the airway: Inflammation of the lining of the bronchi causes smooth muscle constriction and secretion of mucus. The combination of these two effects causes obstruction of the bronchi, worsened by frequent bouts of acute viral and bacterial infections.

As the disease progresses, the patient develops dyspnea on exertion (DOE), hypoxia, and hypercarbia. During this period, the bone marrow responds to the hypoxia by producing more red blood cells to the point that an abnormal number of red blood cells exists (polycythemia). Because the small bronchioles are plugged with mucus, the patient remains hypoxic. The combination of hypoxia and polycythemia causes cyanosis. In some patients, further progression results in pulmonary hypertension and eventually right heart failure (cor pulmonale).[10] The clinical signs of right heart failure are peripheral edema and jugular venous distension (JVD).

These changes combine to create the clinical picture of the chronic bronchitis patient.[12] The patient is generally overweight and cyanotic without significant dyspnea. These findings have led to the description of these patients as **"blue bloaters."** The chronically elevated carbon dioxide results in the abolishment of normal chemoreceptor sensitivity to CO_2, and the primary drive for respiration comes from the concentration of oxygen (the hypoxic drive takes over from the hypercarbic drive).

The patient with chronic bronchitis has a minor risk for medically applied oxygen therapy to suppress the internal drive to breathe.

Despite this, oxygen should never be withheld from COPD patients who are symptomatic for hypoxia.

Paramedics should be aware of the risk of respiratory suppression from oxygen and should be prepared to support ventilation as necessary.

At the other end of the spectrum is the patient with pure emphysema. The pathophysiologic changes in emphysema involve destruction of healthy alveoli which are replaced by blebs. On a cellular and tissue level, there is destruction of the septi between the air sacs as well as destruction of the capillary beds near the alveoli. Eventually, this destruction causes the loss of elastic recoil, which leads to the collapse of bronchi and significant obstruction to airflow.[10]

Clinically the patient responds by increasing minute ventilation. This increase in respiratory rate or tidal volume is directed at maintaining a normal or close to normal PO_2. Because the patient maintains a fairly normal PO_2, unlike chronic bronchitis, pulmonary

Nice to Know

Imagine the normal alveoli to be a bushel of grapes. During emphysema, these grapes are destroyed and are replaced by a blob of tissue that looks more like a nebulous cloud. There is much less surface area for blood cells to pass through and exchange oxygen and carbon dioxide.

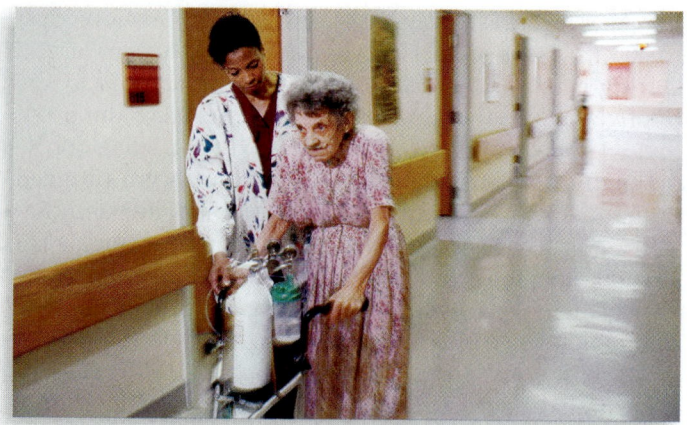

Figure 28-11   A patient with emphysema.

hypertension and right heart failure do not occur, and the patient usually has normal oxygen saturation. Rather, due to the increased work required to maintain the PO_2, the patient develops muscular wasting.

The classical emphysema patient is thin, tachypneic, and short of breath with a notably long expiratory phase in the respiratory cycle. The amount of effort required to maintain the PO_2 results in accessory muscle use and purse-lipped breathing. By pursing the lips, the patient is providing their own **positive end expiratory pressure (PEEP),** which keeps airways open, reducing the work of breathing. The clinical description of this emphysema patient is the **"pink puffer"** (Figure 28-11). Though most COPD patients have a combination of chronic bronchitis and emphysema (refer back to Figure 28-10), enough patients have a relative predominant clinical picture that these descriptions can be helpful to providers.

Primary Survey

As is the case with asthma, patients with COPD typically have acute exacerbations of their disease, manifested by complaints of shortness of breath. Physical examination may reveal wheezes, rhonchi, rales, or very little apparent air movement in the lungs. Also similar to asthma, complications of COPD that prompt immediate intervention include apnea, tension pneumothorax, altered mentation compromising airway patency, and decreased respiratory effort.

Treatment of COPD

There are a number of challenges faced by paramedics treating patients with COPD. Unlike patients with asthma, the baseline pulmonary function of patients with COPD is frequently abnormal. The problem is made worse because the daily baseline oxygen saturation, or normal $ETCO_2$, of these patients is not available to you. Goals for treatment then are for improvement of the initial presentation or to meet a minimally acceptable threshold for values such as oxygen saturation.

Oxygen

Due to the chronic, progressive nature of COPD, many patients are on home O_2 therapy, one of the only treatments (besides smoking cessation) shown to reduce mortality and improve quality of life for COPD patients.[13] In order for patients to qualify for home O_2 therapy and to obtain the mortality benefit, patients must have severe COPD with chronic hypoxemia (PO_2 less than 55 mmHg). Therefore, when encountering a patient on home O_2 therapy, it is safe to assume that the patient's baseline O_2 saturation on room air would be less than 90% (roughly correlating with a PO_2 of 60 mmHg).

Patients with COPD usually have abnormal baseline oxygen saturation and may have abnormal baseline noninvasive $ETCO_2$. Despite the variability between patients, some general guidance can be given. Oxygen saturations less than 90% should be interpreted to represent severe hypoxia in all patients.[10] The goals of therapy can be described in both absolute and relative terms. The absolute goal of oxygen therapy for an acute exacerbation of COPD should be to maintain PaO_2 greater than 60 mmHg, corresponding to an SpO_2 greater than 90%.[12] (See Table 28-3 for more information.) Relative goals would include an improvement in oxygen saturation from baseline or from initial assessment following treatment. In this way, even the chronic bronchitis patient, the "blue bloater" with the hypoxic drive to breathe, should be treated with oxygen for dyspnea. Providers should monitor the patient's mental status closely and be prepared to support breathing.

Beta$_2$ Agonist Medications

The quick-relief medication, albuterol, and its dosage for treating respiratory distress in patients with COPD are the same as they are in asthma. The difference compared with asthma is that the response to therapy is much less. Bronchodilators cause only a small, less than 10%, improvement in pulmonary function in COPD patients.[13] Despite this small improvement, nebulizations improve the patient's subjective dyspnea and should be used. As the patient experiences a decrease in anxiety, their minute ventilation volume will decrease, which can cause a decrease in the sensation of dyspnea. DOT 5-1.8

TABLE 28-3   **The 30-60-90 Rule for Oxygen Saturation**

Oxygen saturation (%) (SpO$_2$)	Oxygen pressure (mmHg) (PaO$_2$)
90	60
60	30

Parenteral Beta Agonist Medications

COPD patients who are in severe distress may be unable to self-administer nebulized medication. There are nebulizer units that connect directly to the nonrebreather face mask. There is also a nebulizer that attaches to the bag-mask unit. It is placed between the bag-mask unit and the face mask or the connector that allows for attachment to the ET tube.

Some patients are also candidates for parenteral beta agonist medications. The side effects seen with parenteral administration are relatively more than with nebulized medications. COPD patients tend to have cardiac disease more frequently than asthma patients, and COPD patients are generally old enough that they are at risk for undiagnosed cardiac disease. Both situations increase the risk of treatment with beta agonists. In some cases, terbutaline is a slightly better alternative compared to epinephrine. Refer to your protocols and medical direction for guidance on which patients are appropriate candidates for parenteral beta agonist treatment. DOT 5-1.8

Anticholinergic Medications

Anticholinergic medications are more effective at treating chronic COPD than beta agonists. This is different from treating asthma, which responds better to beta agonists.[13] However, the onset of action for anticholinergics (such as ipratropium) is slower than that of beta agonists, so they should be secondary to beta agonists in treatment priority or be used in combination with beta agonists.[12] Unlike albuterol and beta agonists, ipratropium is typically only administered one time in the prehospital setting. DOT 5-1.8

Treatment Measures

Patients with mild to moderate exacerbations of COPD should have pulse oximetry, ECG monitoring, peak flow reading measurement, rating of dyspnea on a one-to-ten numerical scale (see Figure 28-8), and noninvasive $ETCO_2$ monitoring. Severity of the COPD exacerbation can be evaluated with the same severity tool developed

for asthma (Table 28-2); the clinical classifications are the most accurate, but paramedics should realize that the numbers for pulse oximetry, PFR, and $ETCO_2$ are not "normal" at the baseline for the COPD patient. In fact, cardiorespiratory disease increases the difference between the arterial PCO_2 and the $ETCO_2$ to greater than the usual difference of less than 6 mmHg.[14] Goals should be as stated previously in the text: improvement in pretreatment measurements or attaining a minimally acceptable threshold. Patients should be given supplemental oxygen with a goal of improving oxygen saturation to above 90% or improved compared with pretreatment levels. Peak flow readings should be measured and repeated after each treatment. Serial albuterol nebulizations (up to one every twenty minutes to a total of three) can be combined with ipratropium one time.

COPD patients in acute ventilatory failure display an alteration in mental status; usually confusion or somnolence; cyanosis; and ineffective respirations. If patients are unable to follow commands or breathe effectively, they should receive positive pressure ventilation. Bag-mask ventilation should be performed initially with the Sellick maneuver, followed by intubation (Figure 28-12). Once intubation is successful by primary and secondary confirmation, institute the technique of permissive hypoventilation discussed previously.

COPD patients that are tiring may allow other ventilatory support options. These patients have already been treated aggressively with oxygen and nebulization treatments. Following treatment, their O_2 saturation may fall, specifically below 90% despite maximal therapy. Alternatively, if following treatment, the noninvasive $ETCO_2$ is rising, specifically above 45 mmHg, this may define respiratory insufficiency. When coupled with a tiring patient, ventilatory support is indicated. If the patient can follow commands, noninvasive ventilation with mask CPAP may be tried. Consult with your

Nice to Know

Albuterol and ipratoprium bromide can be purchased as a combination drug under the trade name Duoneb™. No additional fluid needs to be added to the drug; it simply needs to be opened and poured into the nebulizer unit. If a second nebulizer treatment is required, only albuterol is given for the next dose.

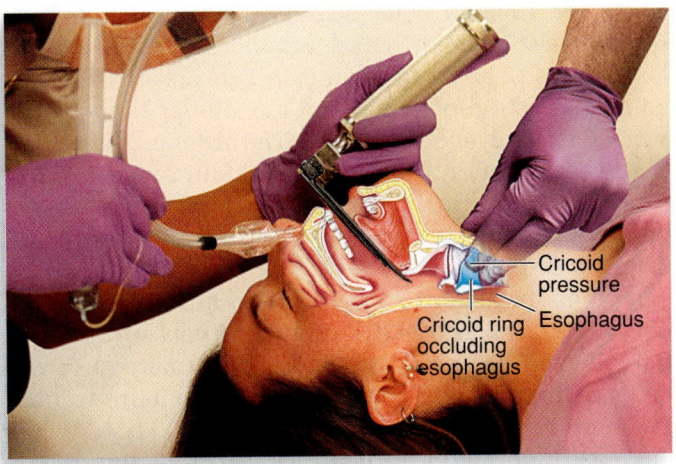

Figure 28-12 The Sellick maneuver can limit aspiration and assist in visualization of the trachea.

medical director to determine whether this COPD patient population qualifies for the CPAP protocol in your EMS system.

Summary of COPD

COPD patients are more difficult to treat and demonstrate less response to treatment compared with asthma patients. Despite this difference in responsiveness to therapy, these patients should be treated with oxygen, beta$_2$ agonist nebulizations, or injection, and ipratropium nebulization, along with transportation to the ED for further evaluation and initiation of corticosteroid therapy. DOT 5-1.10c, d

CONNECTIONS   The differentiation between acute pulmonary edema/congestive heart failure (APE/CHF) and COPD can be challenging. Chapter 29: Cardiology, Section II, discusses CHF and pulmonary edema in association with heart failure. That chapter has a discussion on differentiating between CHF, pulmonary edema, and COPD beginning on page 713.

Physician-Prescribed Medications for Respiratory Illnesses

Medications prescribed by physicians for asthma and COPD are long-term control medicines. The long-term control medicines are divided into different categories: long-term inhaled beta$_2$ agonist medications, antiinflammatory medicines, and leukotriene modifiers (Figure 28-13).[8] In addition, theophylline will be discussed briefly.

Long-term beta$_2$ agonist medications are a mainstay of therapy for bronchospasm. When the goal is long-term control of the symptoms, compliance with therapy is improved when medications are taken less frequently. There are inhaled beta$_2$ agonist medications such as salmeterol (Serevent™) and formoterol (Foradil™) that last at least 12 hours following a single dose. The mechanisms of action of salmeterol are similar to those described for beta$_2$ agonists above. The difference is in both the onset of action (longer) and the duration of action (longer). One critical point for paramedics: If a patient becomes acutely short of breath and uses either of these drugs, it is unlikely there will be improvement of the symptoms in a short time frame because the onset of action for each is 15–30 minutes. If you encounter a patient who has used salmeterol or formoterol for an acute asthma attack, you should use albuterol to treat the continuing symptoms. DOT 5-1.8

Antiinflammatory medicines are the most important therapy for long-term control of asthma. There are many different types of these medications and different

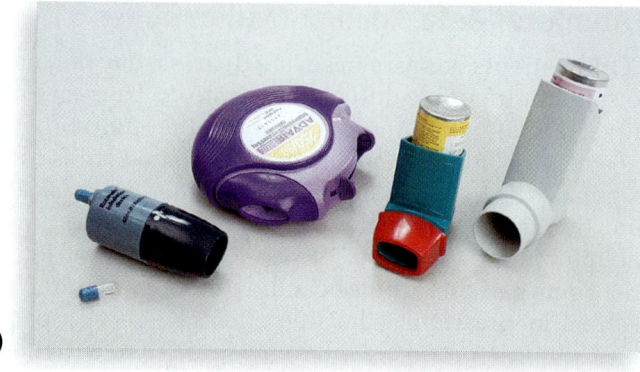
(a)

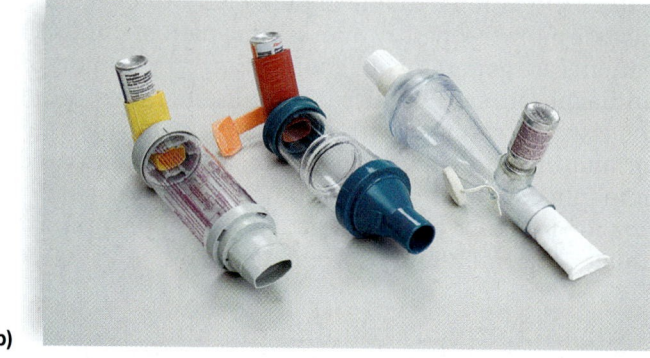
(b)

Figure 28-13   Examples of commonly used inhalers.

delivery methods. Steroid medications (corticosteroids) are physician-prescribed medications used to combat inflammation. Inhaled steroids target the lung, the specific organ affected by the disease, while minimizing systemic side effects. There are many steroid inhalers. A few examples are triamcinolone (Azmacort™), fluticasone (Flovent™), and budesonide (Pulmicort™).

Though inhaled steroids are very effective at controlling asthma long-term, they are not effective for quick relief.

Patients are also prescribed systemic oral steroids either for acute exacerbations of asthma or for chronic maintenance. Examples of oral steroids include prednisone and methylprednisolone. Patients who have recently run out of oral steroids are at higher risk of recurrence of symptoms. DOT 5-1.8

Other inhaled medications prevent inflammation through different mechanisms than steroids. They stabilize mast cells, an important component of the inflammatory reaction that causes symptoms. One example of this type of medicine is cromolyn sodium (Intal™), which comes in an inhaler or as a solution for nebulization. Another example of a medication that works through a similar mechanism is nedocromil (Tilade™). DOT 5-1.8

When allergy or infection stimulates inflammation in the patient, the expression of that inflammation at the cellular level occurs via several different pathways.

The pathway that stimulates bronchospasm involves leukotrienes. Recently, medications that can modify the leukotriene response have been developed. You may encounter patients on montelukast (Singulair™), zafirlukast (Accolate™) tablets, or zileuton (Zyflo™). These are long-term control medications that patients with moderate asthma may use prior to, or in addition to, inhaled steroids.

Theophylline is used much less frequently than previously prescribed. Theophylline is a **methylxanthine** that provides mild to moderate bronchodilation in asthma. The difference between therapeutic levels and toxic levels (called the therapeutic index) of the drug is very narrow, so patients can easily become toxic. Some patients may take more of their theophylline pills when they have an acute episode in an attempt to improve their breathing and instead ingest a toxic amount of medication.

Signs of methylxanthine toxicity include the following:

- Tachycardia
- Muscle tremors
- Narrow complex tachydysrhythmia
- Nausea
- Vomiting

If the patient with a methylxanthine overdose is symptomatically toxic but also significantly short of breath, wheezing should still be treated with nebulized beta$_2$ agonist medications. DOT 5-1.8

Pulmonary Embolism

A life-threatening **pulmonary embolism (PE)** occurs in 1 to 2 persons per 1,000 annually in the United States.[15] It can cause death or disability in a high percentage of patients that have the disease, but if treated promptly, mortality is reduced. Patients typically present with shortness of breath, chest pain, tachycardia, and tachypnea. Depending on the size and location of the embolism, oxygen saturations may be low. The diagnosis of pulmonary embolism can be difficult to make and is more commonly missed than other diseases causing respiratory complaints. For prehospital providers, identifying this condition depends upon a thorough history and physical exam. Having an associated condition, such as **deep venous thrombosis (DVT)**, predisposes patients to and increases the risk of PE. Patients most at risk for developing a PE are patients with a history of cancer, recurrent pregnancies with loss of the fetus, or a history of previous DVT or PE. Definitive testing for diagnosis of PE is available in the hospital (spiral CT scan, V/Q scan, pulmonary angiogram). DOT 5-1.5, 5-1.10l

Pathophysiology of PE

There are three basic mechanisms underlying DVT and PE that help to explain the different risk factors associated with an increased probability of developing the diseases. These three mechanisms include the following:

1. Pooling (stasis) of blood.
2. An increased likelihood of clotting (hypercoagulability).
3. An injury to the inner lining of a blood vessel (intimal injury).

Risk factors associated with pooling of blood include immobilization in a hospital or nursing home, lower extremity fracture (immobilized in a cast), or lower extremity paralysis. Risk factors for hypercoagulability include cancer and other inflammatory conditions. Risk factors for blood vessel injury include trauma, fracture and surgery.

The basic mechanisms and risk factors for DVT are the same as those for PE, and the presence of swelling of one leg with pain on palpation of the deep veins of the calf are clinical signs of DVT. The presence of a DVT increases the likelihood of PE in a patient with dyspnea or chest pain. Increasing age also increases the risk for DVT or PE: An age greater than 50 identifies increased risk in one clinical decision rule while in another, ages 60–79 are more likely to have greater risk, but ages greater than 80 have even higher risk.[15] DOT 5-1.101

Primary Survey

After evaluating the patient's risk factors, assessment can also identify patients with the potential for DVT or PE. Patients with PE commonly complain of acute onset of chest pain or breathlessness. Vital signs often reveal tachypnea and tachycardia (P greater than 100). If hypoxia (SpO$_2$ less than 95%) exists, the diagnosis is more likely. Prehospital lung and heart exam are not likely to provide any specific signs that would confirm the suspicion. A unilateral swollen, tender leg increases the risk for DVT and the likelihood that the patient's shortness of breath or chest pain is from a PE.

Treatment of PE

Prehospital treatment for PE is supportive care and rapid transport. Apply supplemental oxygen, and attempt to improve oxygen saturation to 95% or above. An IV should be established and IV hydration provided if the patient is hypotensive. Maintenance of vital signs is the primary goal. Infrequently, the embolus is very large and lodges in the main branch between the two pulmonary arteries (termed a saddle embolus). This embolus could obstruct blood flow to both lungs and thus prevent any oxygenation of blood in the lungs. In this setting, the patient can develop severe hypotension and hypoxia.

The standard of hospital treatment for a massive saddle embolus is fibrinolytic therapy such as tPA. This would only be considered after the diagnosis is made by imaging, so would be not possible in the field. DOT 5-1.10g

Pneumonia

Pneumonia, an infection of the lower airway, affects 4 million people per year in the United States and results in 15% of these patients (400,000) being admitted to the hospital annually.[16] Pneumonia is the primary cause of death in patients with the flu virus. Patients with pneumonia may call 9-1-1 and present complaining of shortness of breath and chest pain, making it challenging at times to differentiate from other respiratory complaints. For certain populations, pneumonia causes significant illness and can cause death, ranking as the sixth leading cause of death. Diagnosis is usually made after physician evaluation of the history and physical examination and chest x-ray. DOT 5-1.5, 5-1.10j

Pathophysiology of Pneumonia

Pneumonia is caused by infection of the lung by pathogens. Pathogens include viruses, bacteria, fungi, and parasites. Typical host defense mechanisms prevent pneumonia in healthy people. If bacteria are introduced into the lung of a healthy person, the lung defense mechanisms of mucus secretion and ciliary action work to eliminate the pathogen from the lung. The typical source for infection with these pathogens is aspiration from the oropharynx.

Any patient with impaired lung defenses or other chronic illnesses is at risk for pneumonia. Pneumonia can occur in young or healthy people; it causes severe illness and death in the elderly and patients with chronic medical illnesses (alcoholism, cancer, CHF, liver disease, renal disease, cerebrovascular disease, AIDS).

Once the pathogen establishes itself in the lung, the patient's immune system mounts a response to control and fight the infection. The inflammation causes a systemic fever. In the example of a bacterial pneumonia, if the body is successful in fighting the infection, then the pneumonia is surrounded and limited to a local area of the lung. In the area involved, there is fluid in the lung tissue and in the alveoli. When listening with a stethoscope, the paramedic would hear crackles (rales) over the anatomic area of consolidation (infection). If the body is not successful, then toxins or eventually bacteria spread to the bloodstream, and the infection spreads, which may lead to septic shock, hypotension, or death.

Primary Survey

Patients generally complain of cough and production of sputum, usually yellow-green in color that is often streaked with blood, for a period of days to weeks before they seek care. They usually experience fever and chills. For patients complaining of shortness of breath, the presence of productive cough and fever make pneumonia more likely than other diagnoses. On exam, tachycardia and tachypnea are frequently present. Signs of a more serious infection include respiratory rate greater than or equal to 30 breaths/minute, pulse greater than or equal to 125, temperature less than 95 or greater than or equal to 104°F, and oxygen saturation less than 90%. If the infection spreads to the bloodstream (bacteremia), the patient is more ill and may experience septic shock with a systolic BP less than 90 mmHg and altered mental status. Examination with the stethoscope will identify crackles or consolidation over the lobe of the lung that is infected.

Street Secrets

The classic presentation of pneumococcal pneumonia is a sudden onset of **rigors** (uncontrolled shaking chills) followed by a high fever and a cough productive of purulent or rust-colored sputum.

All patients should be evaluated with vital signs, pulse oximetry, and noninvasive $ETCO_2$. Patients that exhibit hypoxia (SpO_2 less than 90%) or hypercarbia (noninvasive $ETCO_2$ greater than 45 mmHg) initially have respiratory insufficiency and should be treated aggressively.

Treatment of Pneumonia

Apply oxygen either by nasal cannula or face mask to increase the oxygen saturation to greater than 90% and with a goal of greater than 94%, unless of course the patient has coexistent COPD. Some patients have associated wheezing; treat them with albuterol nebulization to attempt to improve their oxygenation. Follow vital signs, pulse oximetry, and noninvasive $ETCO_2$ after treatment. If the trends are worsening and the patient is tiring, be prepared to intubate the patient. Patients who are hypotensive due to systemic illness from pneumonia require fluid resuscitation with crystalloid IV fluids. Definitive treatment involves antibiotics or other agents directed at the specific pathogens. Patients with other associated illnesses, hypoxia, or respiratory distress are admitted to the hospital. DOT 5-1.10e

Spontaneous Pneumothorax

Spontaneous pneumothorax occurs without an obvious immediate precipitating cause such as trauma or a medical procedure attempt. Spontaneous pneumothorax is divided into two categories: (1) primary spontaneous pneumothorax with no apparent underlying lung disease and (2) secondary spontaneous pneumothorax caused by an underlying disease, usually lung disease.[10] It occurs more commonly in men compared to women and in smokers. Patients with connective tissue disease such as Marfan's syndrome are more likely to develop a spontaneous pneumothorax. DOT 5-1.5, 5-1.10o

Pathophysiology of Spontaneous Pneumothorax

Patients at higher risk for primary spontaneous pneumothorax typically have weak connective tissue in the lung, which results in blebs (air-filled sacs) on the surface of the lung. When breathing normally, the pressure in the lung during inspiration causes rupture of the bleb, resulting in a leak of air between the lung and the inside of the chest cavity. Secondary spontaneous pneumothorax is characterized by the same surface blebs; however, the cause of the weakness is underlying lung disease. Diseases associated with secondary spontaneous pneumothorax include COPD, pneumocystis carinii pneumonia in AIDS patients, tuberculosis, and lung cancer. There is a minimal association between asthma and the development of spontaneous pneumothorax.

The leak of air between the lung and the pleura lining the inside of the chest disrupts the negative pressure in the pleural space, which normally is the driving force for inspiration. Due to the leak of air, the lung collapses away from the chest wall.

Primary Survey

Patients with a spontaneous pneumothorax usually experience a sudden onset of a one-sided chest pain. The pain is sharp in nature, pleuritic, and made worse by deep breathing or coughing. Following the initial onset, there may be a dull, persistent, aching pain. Patients may delay seeking care for days to a week.[10] In addition to the pain, patients usually demonstrate tachypnea and may have associated tachycardia. If the pneumothorax is small, these may be the only signs encountered by the paramedic. Conversely, if the pneumothorax is large, then decreased breath sounds and resonance with percussion may be present.

Treatment of Spontaneous Pneumothorax

Supportive care will treat the majority of spontaneous pneumothoraces. Patients should be placed on supplemental oxygen and have an IV established. If the patient develops signs of tension pneumothorax (hyperresonance on percussion, hemodynamic compromise [systemic hypotension], and tachycardia) and jugular venous distention (venous hypertension), then needle decompression should be performed. **See Skill Sheet 77: Management of Chest Trauma (also see Step-by-Step 77).**

Any intubated patient, especially a COPD patient, treated with positive pressure ventilation that develops hemodynamic compromise should be suspected of having a tension pneumothorax and should undergo chest decompression. The application of positive pressure ventilation can easily convert a spontaneous pneumothorax into a tension pneumothorax; paramedics must be aware of this possibility and must frequently reassess patients for signs of this condition. Volume resuscitation, with 20 mL/kg boluses, may help reverse tachycardia and decreased blood pressure. DOT 5-1.10j

Adult Respiratory Distress Syndrome (ARDS)

A syndrome is a group of symptoms and signs that occur together lacking a single pathophysiologic cause. **Acute respiratory distress syndrome** is a form of noncardiogenic pulmonary edema caused by damage to the lung from a variety of illnesses and injuries. Common features include hypoxemic respiratory failure (PO_2 less than 60 mmHg) in the presence of one of the risk factors but the absence of congestive heart failure, fluid overload, or chronic lung disease.[10] DOT 5-1.10a

Cardiogenic pulmonary edema occurs because vascular preload and afterload increase, the heart cannot compensate for the pressure, and fluid backs up into the pulmonary capillaries causing a pressure gradient, leading to leakage of fluid into the alveoli. In ARDS, pulmonary pressures are not high, but instead, direct injury to the lung or circulating inflammatory mediators cause inflammation of the alveolar membrane. Once damaged, the alveolar membrane becomes leaky, and fluid and protein enter the alveoli. Findings on examination include signs of respiratory failure, wet rales on auscultation of the lungs, and absence of signs of CHF. Some common causes of ARDS include direct injury, pulmonary aspiration, severe viral infections, near drowning, and toxic gas or smoke inhalation. Circulating inflammatory mediators come from sepsis, shock, pneumonia or other infection, opiate overdose, trauma, burns, and pancreatitis. DOT 5-1.10k

Treatment of ARDS is primarily supportive. If patients develop respiratory failure not responding to supplemental oxygen, they may require intubation and positive pressure ventilation. In this setting, administering adequate oxygen to maintain oxygen saturations above 90% is recommended. Ventilation pressures are high, so "controlled hypoventilation" can be used to minimize barotrauma and the risk of pneumothorax. Diagnosis in the hospital requires chest x-ray. Once identified, treatment of the underlying cause is instituted.

Most cases of ARDS take hours to days to become clinically severe and are unlikely to occur during the phase of prehospital care from the time of the insult until transfer of care to the ED. One possible exception would be opiate overdose. Following IV injection of opiate, patients may develop respiratory distress more rapidly. Rapid assessment, evaluation for signs of respiratory failure, and supportive care are essential. DOT 5-1.5

Upper Respiratory Infections

Upper respiratory infections (URI) are common occurrences, but rarely represent a true life-threatening emergency. While not directly life-threatening, upper respiratory infections can exacerbate or worsen asthma or COPD. These infections occur in the upper respiratory tract, defined in the anatomy section above. Common historical and assessment findings can help distinguish life-threatening respiratory infections from more common viral colds. DOT 5-1.5, 5-1.10n

Pathophysiology of URIs

Upper respiratory infections are caused predominantly by viruses. Exposure occurs from virus particles sneezed or coughed into the air. Once the virus establishes itself on the mucus membranes of the nose and mouth, infection begins. Inflammation ensues with secretion of mucus, runny nose (rhinorrhea), coughing, and hoarseness. The patient may report a fever. These symptoms produce discomfort and, at times, pain.

Bacterial upper respiratory infections occur less frequently. Bacteria can cause specific infections in the upper airway. Pharyngitis or tonsillitis can be caused by Streptococcus or other bacteria. In this setting, the patient develops an infection specific to the tonsils or pharynx; there is usually an absence of the viral symptoms (runny nose, cough). The infection on the tonsils causes white blood cells to respond, and pus forms on the surface of the infected tonsil.

Hyperventilation

Hyperventilation can refer to a rapid respiratory rate (which more correctly should be called hyperpnea) or a condition resulting from the lowering of $PaCO_2$ levels, resulting in mild respiratory alkalosis. **Hyperventilation syndrome** is a respiratory problem with a combination of both: a faster than normal respiratory rate that results in the loss of excessive amounts of CO_2. There are many possible causes for hyperventilation, including both physical illness and anxiety. Some of the diseases causing hyperventilation are life-threatening including pulmonary embolism, CHF, acidosis (for example diabetic ketoacidosis), emphysema, asthma, and COPD. Other physical causes include fever, pain, and pregnancy. DOT 5-1.10p

When encountering a hyperventilating patient, you should realize that there are many medical causes that cannot be identified easily. The patient should be assessed and evaluated for medical causes of hyperventilation. Because the various medical causes often cannot be excluded, providers should be very careful to evaluate for the medical causes first and not assume the cause to be anxiety. If the patient has perioral (mouth) or digital numbness or tingling associated with hyperventilation, it is possible the patient has raised the pH enough to even affect consciousness. DOT 5-1.10k, 5-1.5

Neoplasms of the Lung

Cancer is the second leading cause of death in the United States, second only to vascular disease (cardiac and cerebral). Among the different types of cancer, lung cancer is the leading cause of cancer death in many developed countries. Patients with neoplasms of the lung can develop many complications. Tumors may partially or completely obstruct a bronchus, causing trouble breathing. Also, cancer can erode into a blood vessel and cause bleeding, which will, in most cases, present as a patient who is coughing up blood (hemoptysis). DOT 5-1.10m

Lung cancer patients are frequently assigned to receive chemotherapy, which weakens their immune systems and makes them more at risk to develop an infection in the days to weeks following the chemotherapy. These patients, with minimal white blood cells to protect against infection, are at higher risk for an overwhelming bacterial infection (pneumonia, UTI, or others). Cancer patients, as well, are hypercoagulable and at higher risk for clotting (DVT or PE).

One additional complexity in the management of lung cancer patients is that they may have advance directives, a prehospital DNR order requesting no CPR or no intubation. In these patients, supportive care fills a critical role to humanely reduce suffering. You should, however, remember that patients can revoke their advanced directives at any time and request ALS treatment for their symptoms. DOT 5-1.5

CONNECTIONS Review Chapter 4: Legal Issues for more information on advance directives.

Symptomatic treatment should be provided to lung cancer patients. Support initiatives including oxygenation, ventilation, and blood pressure maintenance are critically important goals. Supplemental oxygen, position of comfort, and narcotics for pain relief are essential. If the local prehospital DNR protocol differentiates between ALS and BLS supportive care, some patients electing BLS care are candidates for ALS medicines directed at relieving symptoms.

Special Procedures Used for Pulmonary Conditions

Chapter 12: Airway Management, Ventilation, and Oxygenation provides information on BLS and ALS airway management skills. Please refer to the end of Chapter 12 (page 234) to review this material. The following information was not discussed in detail in Chapter 12. This information serves as additional techniques to include with the basic airway management techniques discussed previously.

Controlled Hypoventilation (Permissive Hypercapnia)

When treating a critically ill asthmatic or COPD patient with respiratory insufficiency, the goal is for aggressive treatment to provide a significant clinical improvement as rapidly as possible. When this turn-around does not happen, these patients generally require intubation and positive pressure ventilation. Positive pressure ventilation (PPV) has many detrimental effects. The barotrauma from PPV combined with increased pulmonary pressures due to the intrinsic disease increases the risk of pneumothorax or tension pneumothorax. The risk of pneumothorax is made more likely by either increasing the ventilation rate or increasing the tidal volume. Additionally, both asthma and COPD are characterized by obstruction to airflow and incomplete emptying of lung capacity. Overzealous ventilation, both in rate and tidal volume, results in the development of "auto-PEEP."[12] Auto-PEEP keeps the alveoli open, but it also increases intrathoracic pressures, which can lead to decreased venous return and decreased cardiac output, which leads to clinical hypotension.

Controlled hypoventilation is directed at maintaining acceptable oxygen saturation while also tolerating the higher CO_2 concentrations and minor respiratory acidosis. It allows respiration to continue because oxygen continues to be delivered. Although hypercarbia is not ideal, it is necessary to allow it to occur because the complete correction of the imbalance is not possible without worsening the patient through creating a positive pressure in the thorax.

The actual technique involves administering as high a concentration (high FiO_2) of inspired oxygen as needed to obtain adequate oxygenation, at minimum above 90%, while tolerating hypercarbia by utilizing small tidal volumes (8–10 mL/kg) and slow ventilatory rates (less than or equal to 10 breaths/minute).[8,10] This ventilation strategy, once intubation is necessary in asthma or COPD, minimizes the risks of barotrauma and hypotension resulting from stacking of breaths and diminished venous return. DOT 5-1.6

Noninvasive Capnography

CONNECTIONS See additional information on invasive (attached to the endotracheal tube) and noninvasive capnography in Chapter 12: Airway Management, Ventilation, and Oxygenation.

Clinical use of the capnograph for noninvasive monitoring involves placing a nasal cannula in the patient's nares, which is then connected to the capnograph. Once connected, verify that there is a characteristic waveform indicating a tracheal or alveolar sample. Evaluate the shape of the wave: A shark fin configuration is diagnostic for asthma and obstruction to airflow. After confirming an adequate waveform, analyze the $ETCO_2$ value. If $ETCO_2$ is used to monitor an asthma patient, for example, note the $ETCO_2$ reading. This reading will usually fall within a range of 6 mmHg of the $PaCO_2$. Initially, make note of the value; if it is above 45 mmHg, this suggests failure to compensate for the CO_2 produced by the cells.

This is especially important because the typical compensating asthmatic will have increased respiratory rate and minute ventilation and should have an $ETCO_2$ value below 35 mmHg (lower limit of normal). In this setting, if the patient is still breathing adequately and not tiring, treat the patient aggressively with beta$_2$ agonists and ipratropium and monitor the response of the $ETCO_2$ following treatment. If the $ETCO_2$ value is decreasing, then therapy is working and should be continued. If the $ETCO_2$ value is rising, check to see if the patient is tiring and breathing ineffectively. If so, you will need to prepare for intubation.

When monitoring the COPD patient, you may note the initial $ETCO_2$ reading to be 48 mmHg. Since you will not know where this patient's $ETCO_2$ baseline is, you should make your assessment on the patient's clinical condition. Treat the patient with oxygen with a goal of increasing oxygen saturation greater than 90%. Give serial albuterol nebulizations and ipratropium, and reevaluate the $ETCO_2$. If the patient is responding positively, the $ETCO_2$ will decrease. DOT 5-1.6

Continuous Positive Airway Pressure (CPAP)

CPAP is a procedure used for patients in respiratory insufficiency or failure in order to support ventilations, improve their cardiac and respiratory parameters, and potentially avoid the need to intubate the patient (Figure 28-14). Mask CPAP can be applied to various causes of respiratory failure including congestive heart failure or pulmonary edema, COPD, and asthma. In order to apply CPAP, the patient must be awake and alert enough to follow commands, have adequate

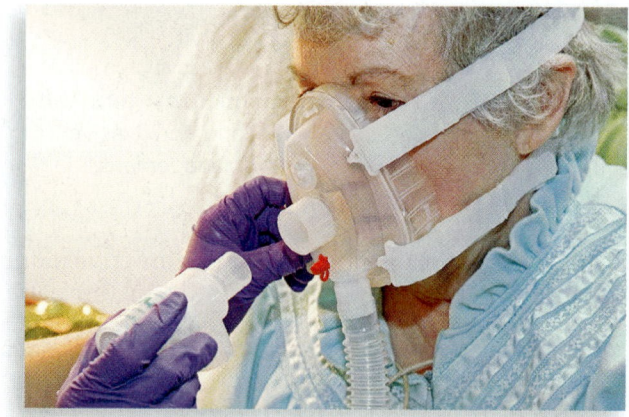

(a)

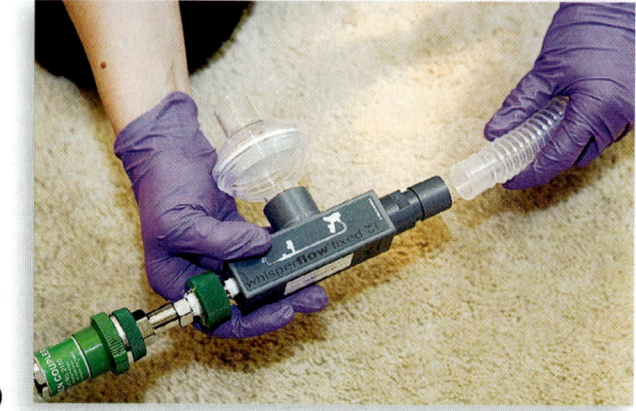

(b)

Figure 28-14 Using CPAP on patients in respiratory failure may prevent them from needing to be intubated.

respiratory effort, and have the ability to protect their own airway.[17] The application of the CPAP device may be difficult if the patient has a high level of anxiety. DOT 5-1.6, 5-1.9

Physiology

CPAP delivered by a mask snugly applied to the face has multiple beneficial effects in respiratory failure. The intended effect is to deliver air with an adequate concentration of oxygen (to improve the oxygen saturation to greater than 90%) via a tightly fitting, closed system at a pressure higher than air pressure. The effect of this increased pressure is to inflate collapsed alveoli, resulting in an increase in the volume of gas in the lung at the end of expiration (increase the functional reserve capacity). The result of this inflation of collapsed alveoli is to improve oxygenation.

Patients in respiratory failure are unable to keep up with the oxygenation and ventilation demands of their body. At this critical point of failure, the **work of breathing (WOB)** exceeds the patient's energy production. Because the alveoli are maintained open, it takes less energy for the patient to take the next breath, thus decreasing the work of breathing. This allows the patient to conserve some energy and rest, improving their ability to handle the WOB on their own at a later time.

In pulmonary edema specifically, alveoli are not functioning because there is fluid in the air sacs due to the heart not pumping adequately. The increased pressure in the alveoli produced by CPAP at end-expiration serves as a force to prevent further leakage of fluid due to the pressure gradient from the capillary to the alveoli (due to the failed pumping of the heart). The CPAP also serves to reverse the pressure gradient and encourage fluid to move back toward the interstitial space near the capillaries. Finally, CPAP serves to reduce afterload, improving cardiovascular hemodynamics in heart failure. Following application of CPAP in pulmonary edema, both heart rate and blood pressure are reduced as well as decreasing sympathetic tone.[10]

Indications and Contraindications

The indications for application of CPAP include respiratory insufficiency or failure combined with the clinical findings of an awake, alert patient who is able to follow commands and has continued respiratory effort. In addition, CPAP is better utilized for conditions that are reversible in a time frame of minutes to hours (such as pulmonary edema and acute respiratory failure) rather than chronic respiratory failure. The benefits in pulmonary edema are fairly clear. The benefit when applied to an asthmatic or COPD patient in respiratory failure is tempered by slightly more risk. There are many studies in which application of CPAP to patients in obstructive respiratory failure avoided intubation and its complications. Contraindications include apnea, unconsciousness, and full cardiopulmonary arrest. Relative contraindications include trauma with suspicion for elevated intracranial pressure and abdominal distension with risk for vomiting or hypotension.

CPAP applied to a patient in respiratory failure can be a frightening experience for the patient, worsening pulmonary function. The key to success with CPAP application is to educate the patient about the procedure, apply it in a gradual way, and complete the mask seal once the patient is comfortable with the application. Properly educating the patient and applying the facemask allows the paramedic to initiate therapy and titrate it to the desired clinical effect.

Initially, have the patient hold the mask loosely to their face. Explain to the patient that the oxygen will feel cool and will help them breathe. After the patient gets used to the mask, apply it more firmly to the face. When the patient appears comfortable, apply the mask snugly to the face with the face straps so that any air leak is minimized. Once the patient is connected to the CPAP device, monitor vital signs and the patient's condition. CPAP will often show a clinical effect within a short time period, five to ten minutes.

Bi-Level Positive Airway Pressure (BiPAP)

BiPAP is a variation of CPAP. CPAP provides a single level of positive pressure during both inspiration and expiration. Patients in respiratory insufficiency need an adequate level of pressure support during inspiration but a lesser level of pressure to 'stent' the alveoli open on expiration. BiPAP allows the provider to set a separate level of inspiratory positive airway pressure (IPAP) and expiratory positive airway pressure (EPAP). BiPAP machines are more expensive, and there have not been adequate prehospital studies to demonstrate effectiveness. DOT 5-1.9

Summary

Respiratory distress is one of the most common reasons EMS is called. In many situations, the primary survey may reveal life-threatening breathing problems that require rapid intervention before you have a thorough understanding of the disease or illness that is affecting the patient. Determining the actual cause of the breathing problem is not as important as quickly performing an appropriate patient assessment and history. From this, treatment decisions can be made that will enable you to properly care for the patient.

Respiration involves the delivery of oxygen to the tissues; ventilation involves the removal of carbon dioxide from the body. Some chronic respiratory diseases may cause an above normal CO_2 level (by $ETCO_2$ reading), which may not require treatment, provided the O_2 reading (by pulse oximetry) indicates hypoxemia is not present. A patient with chronic lung disease switches the trigger to breathe from high CO_2 levels and acidic pH levels to low oxygen levels. Maintaining the patient in a well-oxygenated but also slightly hypercarbic state may be necessary in order to minimize the disruption to cardiac output.

Notes

1. R. Maio, "Emergency Medical Services Outcomes Evaluation," "DOT HS 809 603" (National Highway Traffic Safety Administration, July 2003), http://www.nhtsa.dot.gov/people/injury/ems/emsoutcomes03/EMSOPfinal.pdf (accessed March 10, 2005).
2. R. B. Gerein, M. H. Osmond, I. G. Stiell, L. P. Nesbitt, and S. Burns (OPALS Study Group), "What Are the Etiology and Epidemiology of Out-of-Hospital Pediatric Cardiopulmonary Arrest in Ontario, Canada?" *Academic Emergency Medicine* 13(6)(June 2006):653–658.
3. V. N. Mossesso, J. Dunford, T. Blackwell, J. K. Griswell, "Prehospital Therapy for Acute Congestive Heart Failure: State of the Art," Presented at the Turtle Creek Conference IV. *Prehospital Emergency Care* 7(2003): 13–23.
4. P. Kleinschmidt, "Chronic Obstructive Pulmonary Disease and Emphysema," http://www.emedicine.com/emerg/topic99.htm (accessed February 9, 2006).
5. *Dorland's Medical Dictionary* 30th ed. (Philadelphia, PA, WB Saunders, 2003).
6. J. B. West, *Pulmonary Pathophysiology: The Essentials* 6th ed. (Baltimore, MD: Lippincott, Williams & Wilkins, 2003), p. 20.
7. American Heart Association, 2005 Guidelines, Part 7.1: Adjuncts for Airway Control and Ventilation; *Circulation* 112(2005):51 (Greenville, Texas: American Heart Association, 2005).
8. "Guidelines for the Diagnosis and Management of Asthma, July 1997," NIH Publication Number 97-4051. http://nhlbli.nih.gov/nhlbi/nhlbi.htm (accessed June 3, 2005).
9. W. Busse, "Clinical Crossroads: A 47-Year-Old Woman with Severe Asthma," *Journal of the American Medical Association* 284(17)(November 1, 2000):2225–2233.
10. J. A. Marx, ed., *Rosen's Emergency Medicine Concepts and Clinical Practice,* 5th ed. (St. Louis, MO: Elsevier Mosby, 2002).
11. National Institutes of Health, National Heart, Lung and Blood Institute, "Clinical Practice Guideline. Expert Panel 2 Report: Guidelines for the Diagnosis and Management of Asthma. July 1997," NIH Publication Number 97-4051. http://nhlbli.nih.gov/nhlbi/nhlbi.htm (accessed June 3, 2005).
12. A. Harwood-Nuss, *The Clinical Practice of Emergency Medicine,* 3rd ed. (Baltimore, MD: Lippincott, Williams & Wilkens, 2001), p. 661.
13. P. J. Barnes, "Chronic Obstructive Pulmonary Disease," *The New England Journal of Medicine* 27 343 (4)(July 2000): pp. 269–275.
14. R. W. N. Wahba and M. J. Tessler, "Misleading End-Tidal CO_2 Tensions," *Canadian Journal of Anaesthesia* 43(6)(1996): 862–866.
15. S. D. Chunilal, J. W. Eikelboom, J. Attia, M. Miniati, A. A. Panju, D. L. Simel, and J. S. Ginsberg "Does This Patient Have Pulmonary Embolism?" *Journal of the American Medical Association* 290(21)(December 3, 2003): 2849–2858.
16. American College of Emergency Physicians, "Clinical Policy for the Management and Risk Stratification of Community-Acquired Pneumonia in Adults in the Emergency Department," *Annals of Emergency Medicine* 38(1)(July 2001): 107–113, http://mdconsult.com (accessed June 1, 2005).
17. J. Roberts, *Clinical Procedures in Emergency Medicine,* 4th ed. (St. Louis, MO: Elsevier, Mosby 2004), http://www.mdconsult.com (accessed August 19, 2005).

chapter

29

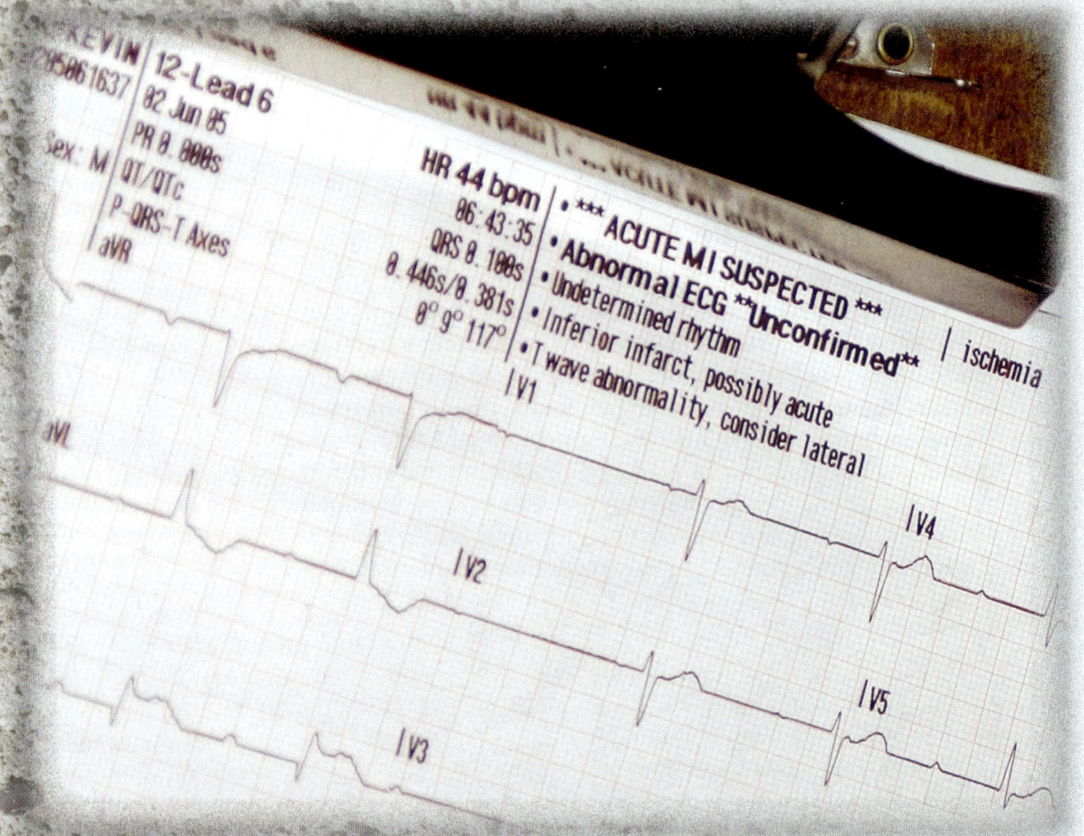
12-Lead 6
02 Jun 05
Sex: M
PR 0.000s
QT/QTc
P-QRS-T Axes
aVR
HR 44 bpm
06:43:35
QRS 0.100s
0.446s/0.381s
0° 9° 117°
• *** ACUTE MI SUSPECTED ***
• Abnormal ECG **Unconfirmed**
• Undetermined rhythm
• Inferior infarct, possibly acute
• T wave abnormality, consider lateral ischemia
aVL
V1
V2
V3
V4
V5

Cardiology

Section I: Physiology and ECG Interpretation

"We must emphasize the importance of feeling the pulse and teach that an intermittent pulse carries a poor prognosis and might be a harbinger of sudden death."

—Galen (AD 132–201)

Need to Know

► There are three critical components for perfusion to take place: the pump (heart), the pipes (vascular system), and the fluid (blood). The ECG only shows a piece of the picture of what is happening with the heart; it shows nothing about the pipes and fluid.

► ECG monitoring is an important tool in managing patients, but it should never replace a thorough history and physical examination.

► The ECG shows electrical activity in the heart—it does not show mechanical activity. Pulse assessment is an appropriate adjunct to ECG assessment to get a total picture of the heart.

► Proper rhythm interpretation requires a consistent approach that utilizes an analysis of the waves associated with the conduction of electricity through the heart's electrical conduction system.

► A normal ECG does not mean the patient is not sick. If signs and symptoms suggesting shock or an altered mental status are present, the patient is sick. Conversely, an "abnormal" ECG for a patient with stable vital signs and a normal mental status may be a normal finding.

► Remember that the ECG is a powerful tool, but it only provides some information for management. The whole clinical picture, including vital signs, physical examination, and history, must be used to determine the treatment regimen.

Introduction

If you ask any practicing paramedic what type of emergency they routinely respond to, they most likely will tell you cardiac or respiratory. These emergencies represent both routine and unique situations. They are often routine in their frequency, but each one can present with unique signs and symptoms.

The signs and symptoms of cardiac disease may follow some patterns, but at the same time, a lack of obvious (or patterned) signs or symptoms does not rule out serious illness. Subjective information from the patient interview must be combined with objective data from the physical exam. Assessment tools such as the electrocardiogram (ECG), pulse oximeter, glucometer, and the like add information needed to form a complete picture of what is going on with the patient.

Seldom will one piece of information fully explain your patient's illness. For example, a patient may be exhibiting signs and symptoms of a myocardial infarction, but the 12-lead ECG appears normal. Conversely, a patient's 12-lead ECG may show changes indicating ischemia (a low oxygen state) or infarction (with actual heart damage); however, the patient may not even be having a cardiac event. To be able to put all the pieces together, one must have a good understanding of the cardiovascular system, how each component works and relates to the others, and how to interpret information gathered from assessment tools such as the ECG. DOT 5-2.30

This chapter will review the anatomy and physiology of the cardiovascular system. It begins with the cellular level and progresses to the complex interrelationship between each of the components of the system. You will learn how electricity is produced and propagated (spread) throughout the heart and how that electrical flow is recorded on the ECG (Figure 29-1). Once the workings of the system are explored, Section II of this chapter will discuss what happens when the system fails and cardiovascular disease results. **This section of the chapter is supported by Skill Sheet 37: ECG Acquisition (also see Step-by-Step 37).**

The Roots of Good Patient Care

The study of the human body goes back centuries. Galen, an ancient Roman physician, taught the value of a good assessment and how to look to the patient for answers. Etienne Marey, a French physiologist, is credited with inventing the first sphygmograph (Figure 29-2). This device gave physicians and physiologists a way to record the pulse patterns. It led to the development of the modern-day equivalent of the

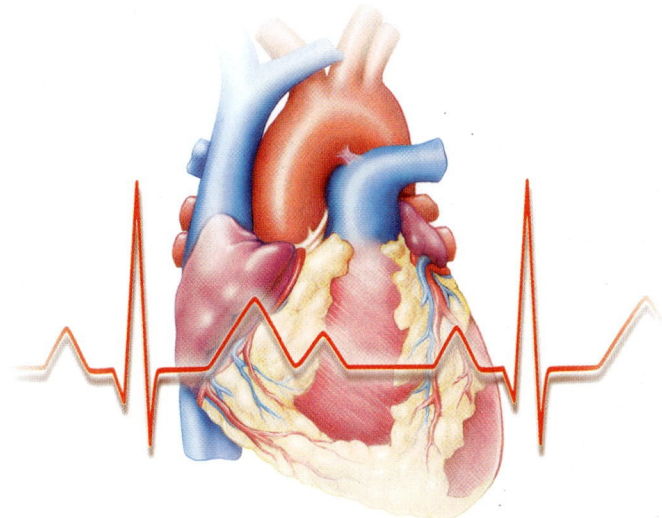

Figure 29-1 The flow of electricity throughout the heart is recorded on ECGs.

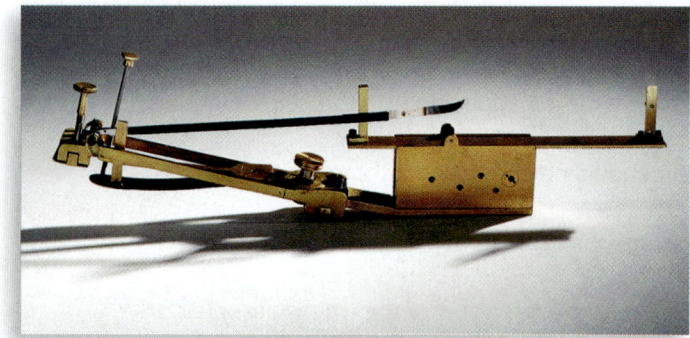

Figure 29-2 The first sphygmograph.

blood pressure cuff (called a sphygmomanometer). In 1903, a Dutch physician named Karel Wenckebach wrote, "The facts which we have obtained from physiology towards an explanation of the irregularities of the heart will form the groundwork on which the future study of these irregularities must be based."[1] Dr. Wenckebach went on to make many significant contributions to the study of electrophysiology, most notably with his work on heart blocks. Today, one specific type of second degree block still bears his name.

While the concept of a thorough patient assessment remains the backbone of modern cardiology, the invention of the **electrocardiograph (ECG)** around 1903 heralded a new era in cardiac care. The ECG allowed clinicians to trace the electrical patterns resulting from the flow of electricity throughout the heart. A Dutch physiologist named Willem Einthoven developed a device capable of recording the electrical activity of the heart. In 1906, Einthoven published the first electrocardiographic tracing depicting a heart block in a dog.[2] His work earned him the title of "the father of modern electrocardiography." Other physiologists were quick to realize the potential of this device and utilized it in their research.

Countless other physicians and electrophysiologists have contributed much to what is now known and understood regarding the workings of the heart. Knowledge continues to advance, and it is common for physiology coursework for the paramedic to incorporate information on the genetic and molecular level of function. Even in light of all these new advancements, never forget the lessons taught by those early physicians—never underestimate the value of good patient assessment and remember to treat the patient, not the monitor.

The Cardiovascular System

The cardiovascular system is a complex network of three primary components:

1. The pump (heart).
2. Circulating blood and all its components (oxygen, wastes, glucose and electrolytes, among others).

3. The vascular structures such as arteries, veins, and capillaries that make up the "pipes" of the system. DOT 5-2.7

The purpose of this three-component system is to circulate blood containing oxygen and nutrients to the cells while providing a means for waste removal at the same time (Figure 29-3). The metabolic reactions taking place in the cells occur under relatively narrow parameters of temperature and pH and require a continuous supply of raw materials for energy. Failure of the system will eventually result in cellular death and ultimately death of the patient.

The circulatory system is closely tied to the pulmonary system. This relationship is so interdependant that changes in one will quickly result in changes in the other. For example, a decreasing respiratory rate will trigger a physiologic response that results in the heart increasing its pumping rate and being forced to compensate for the reduced intake of oxygen by circulating blood more efficiently. Although this process is helpful, the muscular heart, which is now working very hard, has an increased demand and need for oxygen, and this workload cannot be sustained permanently. If the respiratory compromise is not corrected, the cardiac

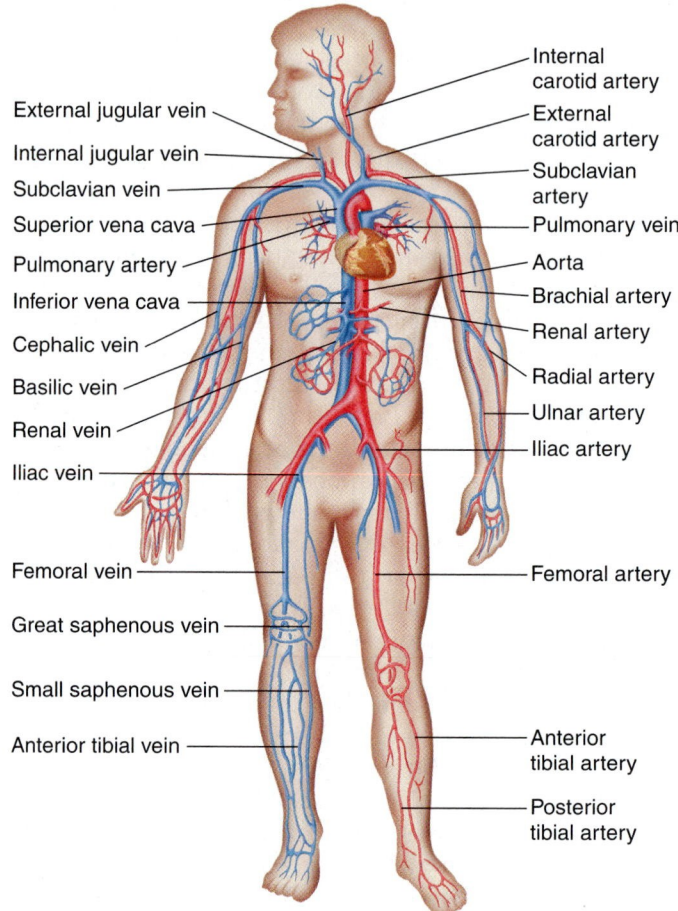

Figure 29-3 The cardiovascular system.

corrective action will soon begin to deteriorate. The result is a slower rhythm known as bradycardia. Again, if not corrected, it will ultimately result in complete cessation of the activity of the heart, causing asystole.

Street Secrets

The pump (heart), blood volume, and pipes (vascular structures) make up the three components of the cardiovascular system. Problems with any of the three components lead to inadequate tissue perfusion and, at the extreme, death. You should always remember that the primary energy source moved around within the body—oxygen—comes from the respiratory system. It is critical that both the cardiac and respiratory systems function together for the individual to remain healthy.

Blood Vessels

At an average rate of 70 heartbeats (cardiac cycles) per minute, the heart beats about 100,800 times per day. With an average volume of approximately 70 mL

pumped with each heartbeat, the heart pumps approximately 1800 gallons of blood daily through the complex system of blood vessels (arteries, veins, and capillaries) that total about 60,000 miles in length. This almost unbelievable feat is accomplished every day throughout a lifetime. This incredible network of vessels extends to almost every region of the body, and, in fact, almost every cell in the body lies adjacent to a capillary. DOT 5-2.5

The Systemic Circulation

Starting with the left side of the heart, the blood leaves the left ventricle and is propelled though a large artery called the aorta. This vessel branches out into smaller arteries, then ultimately becomes arterioles and terminates in the capillary beds (Figure 29-4). The blood carried by the arteries, with the exception of the pulmonary arteries discussed later, is oxygen-rich. Within the capillary bed, oxygen is exchanged with carbon dioxide (Figure 29-5). Much of this process occurs through diffusion and between pressure gradients found on each side of the membranes making up the blood cells and capillaries.

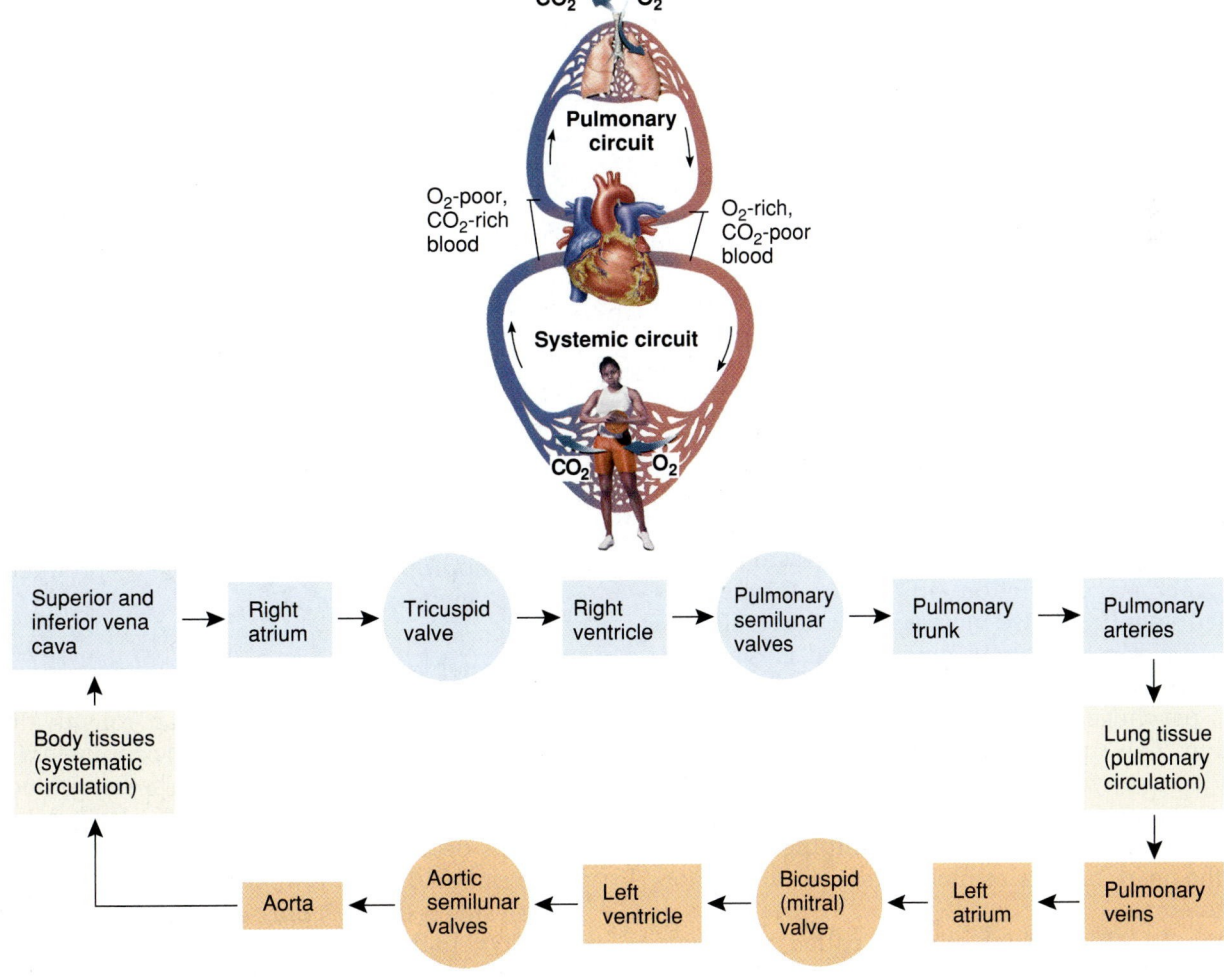

Figure 29-4 Blood flow through the heart.

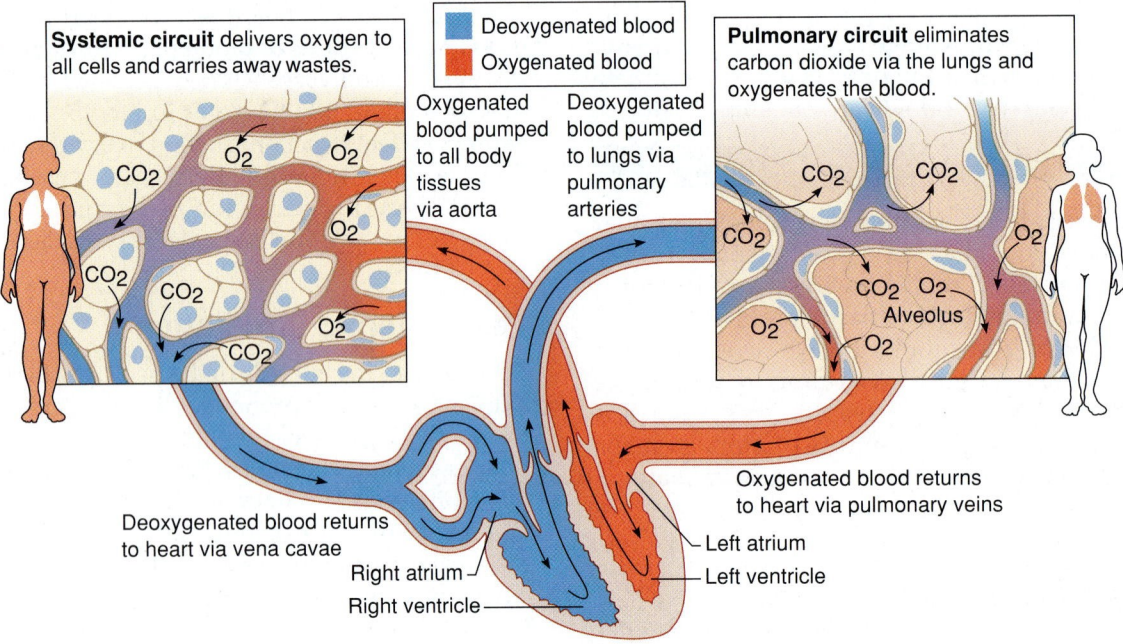

Figure 29-5   The cardiovascular system transports blood to the body cells and organs in order to deliver oxygen and remove carbon dioxide.

Nutrients and waste products are also exchanged at this point. The capillaries are so tiny that they will only allow blood cells to pass through in a single file line.

At the beginning of the capillary bed, the red blood cell is oxygenated, and once gasses are exchanged, the red cell now carries deoxygenated blood. The "ends" of the capillary beds come back together to form the beginning of the venous side of the circulatory system. At this point, the tiny veins are called venules. The net pressure within the capillary beds and initial venules is very low, almost zero. Deoxygenated blood collects into progressively larger vessels that ultimately empty into the ascending (or inferior) and descending (or superior) vena cava. The inferior and superior vena cava end by dumping their blood into the right atrium of the heart.

The venous system provides an important function, serving as a reservoir for blood not currently needed by the body.[3] It does this by increasing or decreasing its size through venous constriction or dilation (sometimes also called **"pooling"**). By increasing or decreasing its capacity, it can control how much blood is being returned to the heart. This system is influenced by blood pressure, psychogenic (emotion controlled) factors, or medication. This mechanism allows the body to adjust to blood loss, dehydration, and overhydration by altering the container size to accommodate the fluid volume. This, along with adjustments in the pumping speed and force of the heart, maintains blood pressure within normal parameters.

Simple fainting, which is also called vasovagal syncope, may be the result of increased **capacitance** (or size change) of the vascular system, which decreases blood flow to the heart and ultimately to the brain. As

with all compensatory mechanisms, vascular system constriction or dilation has its limitations.

To summarize the role of the vascular system in maintaining adequate circulation, the cardiovascular system is dependent on the following:

- An intact system of properly functioning blood vessels.
- Appropriate capacitance of the venous system.

The remaining two components, the heart and blood, will be discussed next. They supply the following components:

- A functioning myocardium to serve as a pump.
- Blood of the appropriate viscosity (thickness) providing an adequate supply of oxygen and nutrients and appropriately removing the by-products of cellular metabolism.

The Heart

The heart is a hollow muscular organ, roughly the size of an adult fist, and it averages about 14 centimeters long and 9 centimeters wide (Figure 29-6). The heart functions as a two-stage pump. The right side is the low pressure side. It pumps deoxygenated blood to the pulmonary system where carbon dioxide is off-loaded and oxygen is loaded. The left side is the high pressure side. It provides oxygenated blood to the rest of the body. DOT 5-2.4

The heart sits in the middle of the chest between the lungs, backed by the vertebral column and covered anteriorly by the sternum. This area of the chest is called

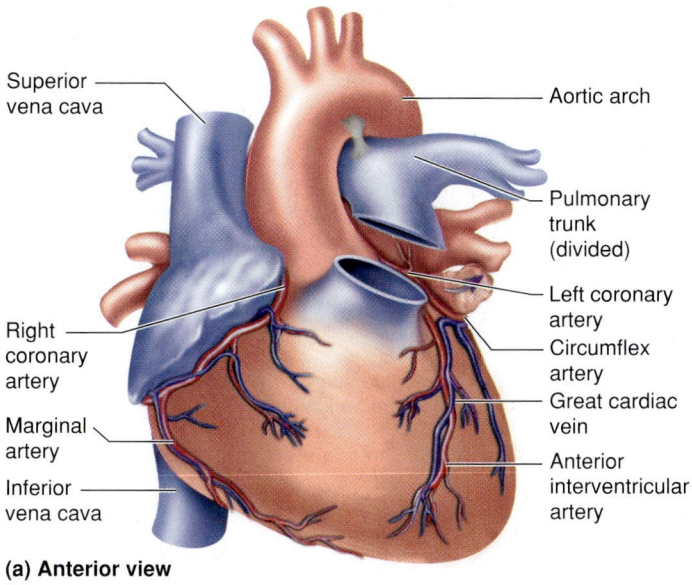

Superior vena cava
Aortic arch
Pulmonary trunk (divided)
Left coronary artery
Right coronary artery
Circumflex artery
Marginal artery
Great cardiac vein
Inferior vena cava
Anterior interventricular artery

(a) Anterior view

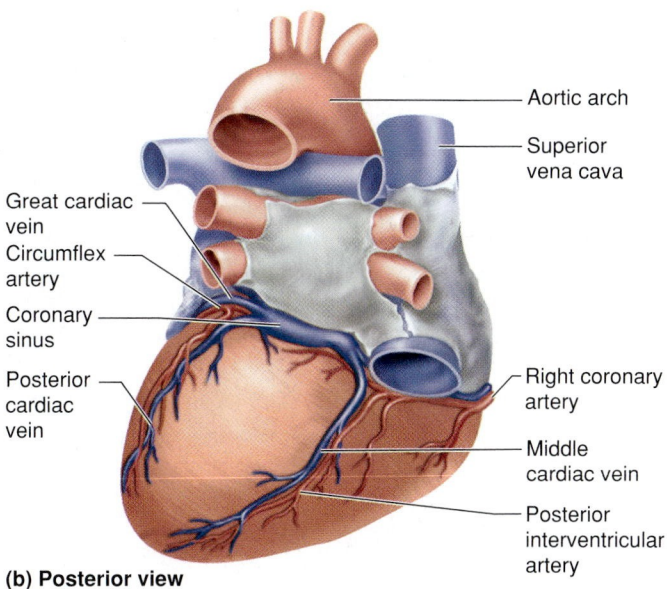

Aortic arch
Superior vena cava
Great cardiac vein
Circumflex artery
Coronary sinus
Posterior cardiac vein
Right coronary artery
Middle cardiac vein
Posterior interventricular artery

(b) Posterior view

Figure 29-6   Anatomy of the heart and major blood vessels.

the mediastinum (Figure 29-7). In most people, the heart extends from just beneath the second rib downward and ends around the fifth rib.[4] In a few individuals, the heart actually is tipped to the right, instead of to the left. This condition is referred to as **dextrocardia.**

If you were to cut out a valentine shape and place it in the very center of your chest, you would not be accurate in the shape, placement, or orientation of the actual heart. The actual heart is more cone-shaped than "heart-shaped," with a somewhat flattened top portion, and it actually lies on its side. The bottom, or pointed portion of the heart, is called the apex. It is the closest part of the heart to the chest wall. The apex is located

just left of the sternum at the fifth rib. This location is the optimal position to listen with a stethoscope to the closure of the valves that are found between both the left and right atria and ventricles. This auscultatory site is called the **point of maximal impulse,** or **PMI.** DOT 5-2.25

The superior aspect of the heart is referred to as the base. It is flattened somewhat and is where all the major blood vessels enter and exit the heart. If you were to peel off the layers of skin, muscle, and bone covering the chest to expose the heart, you would note that the portion of the heart that is the most visible is the left ventricle. The lower portions of the right ventricle rest directly on the diaphragm. The heart moves a little within the chest as the diaphragm rises and falls with breathing.

The heart is covered and protected by fibrous tissue called the pericardium (Figure 29-8). The pericardium covers the entire heart and the proximal ends of the major blood vessels, which connect to the base of the heart. The pericardium is one continuous tissue that forms two layers of covering over the heart. The tough, outer layer, called the **parietal pericardium,** actually turns on itself, covering over the beginning of the major blood vessels, and then forms a layer directly adhered to the epicardium of the heart. The more delicate, inner layer attached to the heart is called the **visceral pericardium.**

Both layers are separated by a very thin layer of fluid. The fluid keeps the layers separated and provides lubrication. The fluid-filled space between the layers is so thin that it is classified as a "potential space" and is called the **pericardial space.** The pericardial membrane secretes a small amount of serous fluid, which serves to lubricate the layers so there is no friction as the heart beats within the sac. The parietal pericardium has little stretching ability while the visceral pericardium can stretch a lot more. Neither membrane will provide an excessive amount of stretch, and any collection of fluid

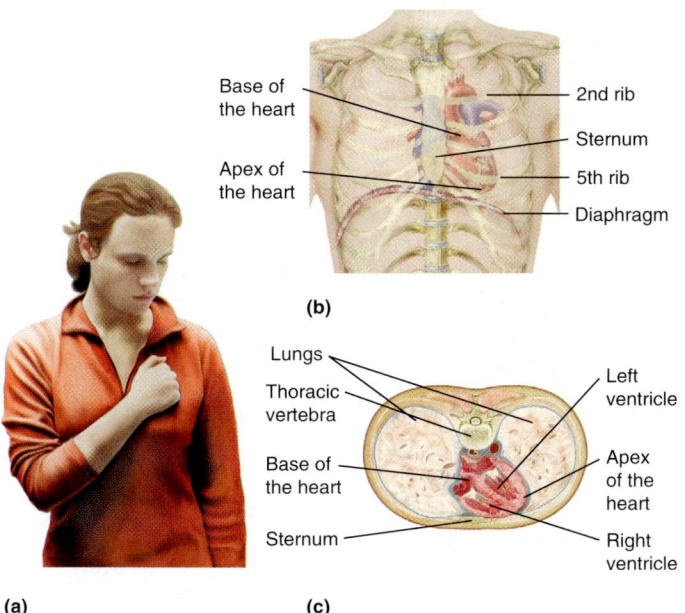

Base of the heart
2nd rib
Sternum
Apex of the heart
5th rib
Diaphragm

(b)

Lungs
Left ventricle
Thoracic vertebra
Base of the heart
Apex of the heart
Sternum
Right ventricle

(a)   **(c)**

Figure 29-7   Position of the heart.

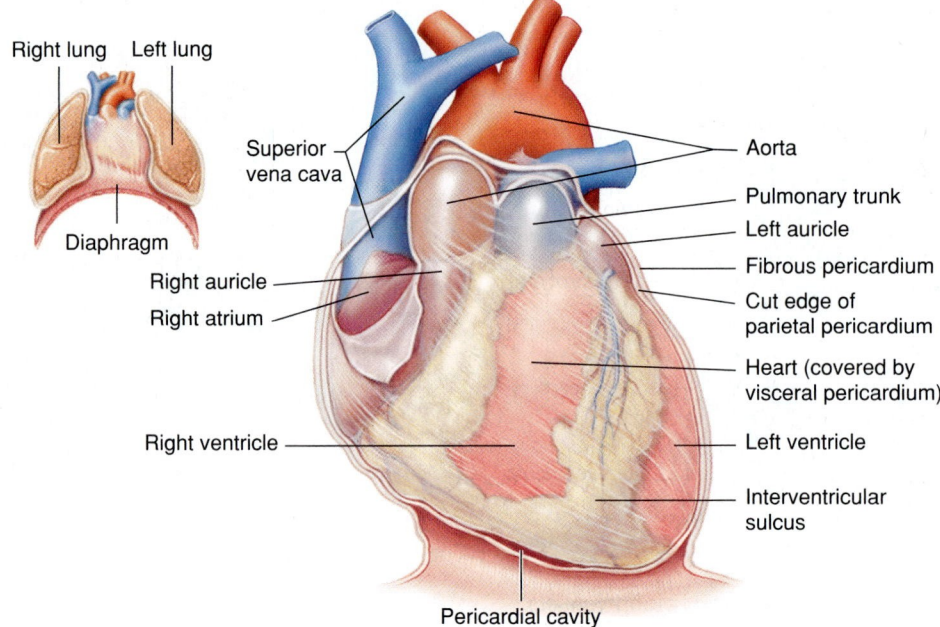

Figure 29-8   The heart within the pericardium.

between the membranes can cause problems for the patient. On occasion, bacteria or viruses find their way between the layers of the heart, causing an infection known as **pericarditis.** The resulting inflammation can cause chest pain, which in many ways mimics that of a myocardial infarction.

The heart itself is comprised of three distinct layers (Figure 29-9):

1. The epicardium
2. The myocardium
3. The endocardium

Nice to Know

Potential Spaces Within the Body

The body has numerous places where different tissue types come together within organs or between structures. These areas are so thin or so similar in form and function that they may not be visible with the naked eye. Although they may produce or contain fluid that serves to lubricate the layers, they are not meant to contain air or allow for the formation of pockets of blood or infection. These areas are called **potential spaces** for this reason. Although they are not actual spaces, there is the potential to form a space in this location if fluid or air were to accumulate. Another very important potential space paramedics should be aware of is found between the visceral and parietal plural lining covering the lung and inner rib cage. This potential space also contains a small amount of fluid for lubricating purposes. When air collects between these layers, the result is a pneumothorax, and when blood collects between the layers, it is a hemothorax.

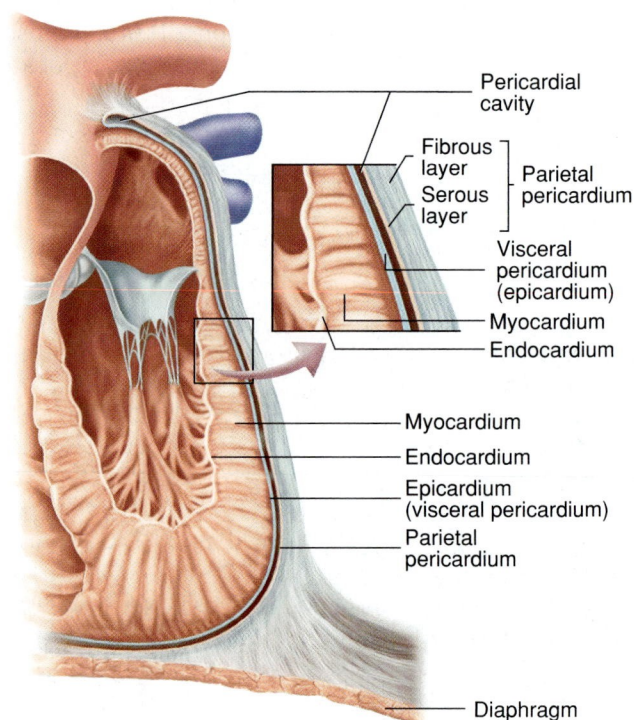

Figure 29-9   Cross section of the heart.

The outermost layer, the **epicardium,** serves as the "skin" of the heart and is a protective layer that contains most of the heart's blood vessels, lymph vessels, and nerve fibers. The **myocardium** makes up the bulk of cardiac muscle tissue and also contains a rich blood supply of capillaries. The innermost layer is the **endocardium** and is comprised of mostly connective tissue, a few blood vessels, and the system of nerve fibers known as the purkinje fibers. The endocardium serves as the inner lining of the four chambers of the heart.

The heart muscle is an organ, and it receives its blood supply in the same manner that all organs in the body do: Arteries supply oxygenated blood to the capillaries, capillaries exchange products, and the veins take the deoxygenated blood back to the heart and then the lungs for reoxygenation. Even though blood comes into direct contact with the endocardium lining within the chambers, the heart does not actually receive oxygen directly from the chambers. This will be discussed in more detail.

To summarize the role of the heart in maintaining adequate circulation, the cardiovascular system is dependant upon the following:

■ A properly functioning myocardium.

The Blood Supply to the Heart

Although the heart is filled with blood as it performs its function, it is not able to directly utilize this blood for its own oxygen and nutrient supply. The supply of oxygen to the heart is instead provided by a system of coronary arteries and veins that surround the heart and reach deep into the muscle through a network of capillary beds. Because of the pressure generated within the heart muscle, this blood flows freely into the vessels only when the heart is "resting" or during the final portion of the diastolic phase of the cardiac cycle. DOT 5-2.6, 5-2.8

Systole describes the period of the cardiac cycle when the high pressure ventricles of the heart are contracting. During contraction, they squeeze and push the blood within them out of the heart into either the aorta or the pulmonary artery. **Diastole** is the relaxation phase of the cardiac cycle when the ventricles are done squeezing and are then passively refilling with blood that comes from the atria. At the end of this process, just before they begin squeezing again, the pressure within the heart is at its lowest point, and the coronary arteries are perfused.

Blood flow through the coronary system is dependent on the backpressure in the arterial system from systole and occurs at the end of diastole. This pressure is referred to as **afterload.** Afterload is also described as the pressure found throughout the body that is created by the combined pressure within each of the arteries and veins. Remember that the capillaries measure almost no pressure, and the veins have little pressure. Most of the

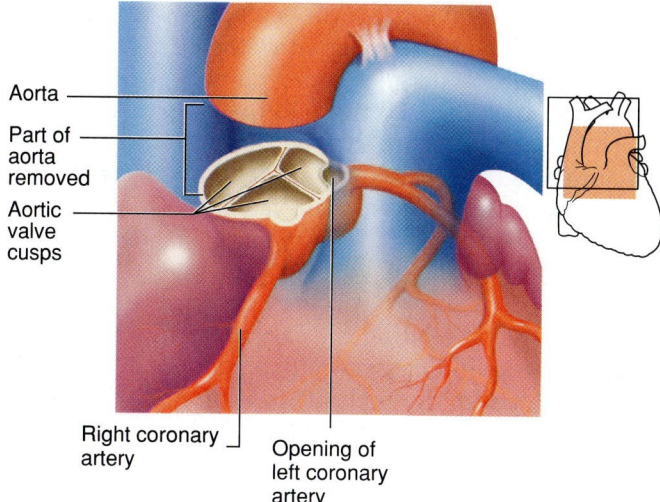

Aorta

Part of aorta removed

Aortic valve cusps

Right coronary artery

Opening of left coronary artery

Figure 29-10 Coronary arteries above the aortic valve cusps are fed by backpressure in the arterial system.

pressure of afterload, which is also called **vascular resistance,** comes from the arteries.

As the heart beats during systole, blood is pushed out of the heart, engorging the arterial system. The aortic valve, which is located between the left ventricle and aorta, is forced closed as the engorged arteries pressurize the arterial system. The coronary arteries branch off the aortic arch just superior to the aortic valve (Figure 29-10). Some of the blood that was pushed out into the aorta during systole is "sucked" back toward the heart as the muscle begins to relax and refill during diastole. At this time, the coronary arteries are opened and blood quickly flows into them, perfusing the heart and supplying the cardiac muscle with needed oxygen and nutrients.

CONNECTIONS Chapter 28: Pulmonary describes the refilling of the heart during diastole in relationship with intrathoracic pressure. A review of this section will help reinforce the interrelationship between the cardiovascular and respiratory systems.

The pressure generated within the heart is transmitted throughout the arterial system to the capillary beds. Since the capillary beds allow only a small amount of blood to pass at a time, this pressure is expended over a longer period of time, supplying a constant flow of blood through the capillary system.

Korotkoff Sounds in Blood Pressure

The pressure in the arterial system over time is reflected by the Korotkoff sounds heard during auscultation of the blood pressure. When you record a patient's blood pressure, you listen for the first sounds as blood is pushed through an artificially constricted artery covered by the BP cuff. This reading is the highest pressure point or the systolic pressure. You continue to listen to the point where the sounds disappear altogether. This is the diastolic pressure and reflects the point at which blood flow is no longer forced through the constricted artery, thus it is equalized with the pressure distal to the blood pressure cuff. This reading represents the lowest point of pressure within the arterial system.

The Role of Blood Pressure

A blood pressure reading is a very important diagnostic sign and can be indicative of any number of problems or conditions within the body. This section looks at some correlations between blood pressure and the cardiovascular system. Having an adequate supply of blood passing through an organ is vital to its survival. This flow is called perfusion. For example, if the brain is not adequately perfused, it cannot function properly. If blood flow to an organ such as the brain is compromised, a message is sent to the heart to increase the heart rate and contraction strength. Simultaneously, the arterial system is stimulated to constrict, enhancing blood flow to target areas and diminishing it to others considered less vital. The end result of the combined action is an increased blood pressure in vital areas. Hopefully, this increased blood pressure will be adequate to push blood through the compromised organ, keeping it functioning until conditions can be normalized. On the other hand, an excessive blood pressure over an extended period of time can overwork the system, putting increased strain on the heart as well as the arterial system. This strain could result in cardiovascular failure later in life.

> The shorter the length of the diastolic period, the less the amount of time available for coronary blood flow.

Excessively rapid heart rates can be very stressful to the heart. The heart is one of three vital organs that require a constant flow of blood to meet their metabolic demand. The other organs are the brain and the kidneys. Because these organs function continuously, even in times of stress, they have a limited ability to store oxygen for later needs.

These organs extract a maximum amount of oxygen from the passing blood. In fact, cardiac cells contain the highest concentration of **mitochondria** of any part of the body. Mitochondria are the organelles (cell components) that use oxygen to create ATP energy for use by the cell. Mitochondria make up an estimated 20% of the number of structures within heart cells and 5% in other body tissue. Even a short period of reduced or interrupted blood flow (hypoxia) will cause ischemia and eventually cellular death. Since the heart normally has already extracted as much oxygen from the blood as it can, the only other way to increase its oxygen supply is to either increase blood flow or increase the oxygen concentration of the blood. The use of supplemental oxygen for patients with suspected or actual heart disease is of benefit in either circumstance.

Afterload and Opening Doors

Another way of thinking of afterload is to draw a parallel with opening a door. The act of pushing open a closed door is usually not a problem. However, think of a bunch of people on the other side of that door holding it closed. How much more force will it take to push that door open, and how long are you going to be able to push against such a force? That force you are working against is afterload. While you may be able to open the door a few times in the face of that force, eventually either you will have to get stronger or you will wear yourself out in the process. This is similar to how blood pressure can affect the heart. The heart muscle can become stronger for a while, but eventually it won't be able to maintain its working ability against the pressure, and it will fail.

The Coronary Circulation

The coronary artery system of the heart consists of two major vessels coming off of the aorta: the **left main coronary artery** and the **right coronary artery (RCA)** (Figure 29-11). The left main coronary artery further branches into two other major arteries called the **circumflex** and the **left anterior descending (LAD)** arteries. The circumflex artery supplies the walls of the left atrium and left ventricle with blood. In about 10% of the population, it also branches off into the **nodal artery,** supplying the atrioventricular and sinus nodes with blood. Cardiologists refer to these people as left dominant. DOT 5-2.9, 5-2.10

The left anterior descending coronary artery supplies the septum and ventricular walls. If the left main coronary artery is blocked, a majority of the left ventricle will become ischemic, and if uncorrected, this may result in sudden death (Figure 29-12). It is for this reason that the left main coronary artery has earned the nickname "the widowmaker."

The right coronary artery (RCA) supplies a majority of the right atrium and right ventricle. The RCA continues around the posterior side of the heart, taking a downturn at a region known as the crux. The artery is thereafter referred to as the **posterior descending artery.** In 90% of the population, the nodal artery branches off the RCA around the crux and provides blood to the sinus node and atrioventricular node. The significance of these nodes will be discussed in detail later in the chapter, but for now, understand that they are the primary and secondary pacemakers for the heart.

Coronary veins are found in close proximity to the coronary arteries and serve the function of collecting blood from the capillary beds, moving it through progressively larger veins to the **coronary sinus.** The coronary sinus terminates in the wall of the heart very near

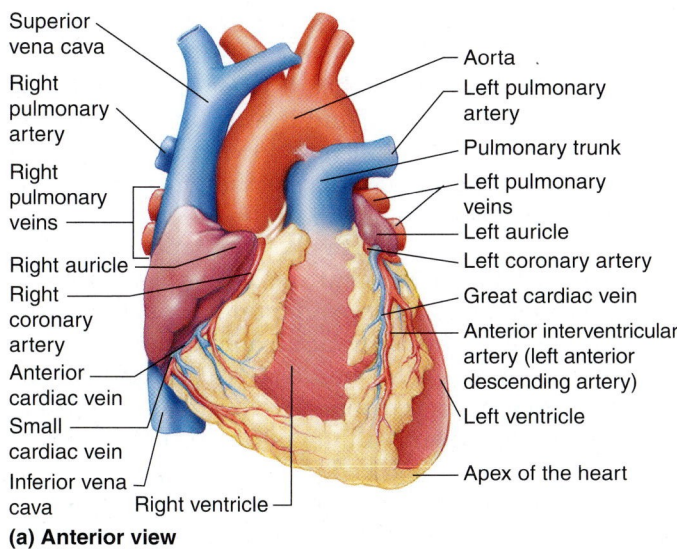

(a) Anterior view

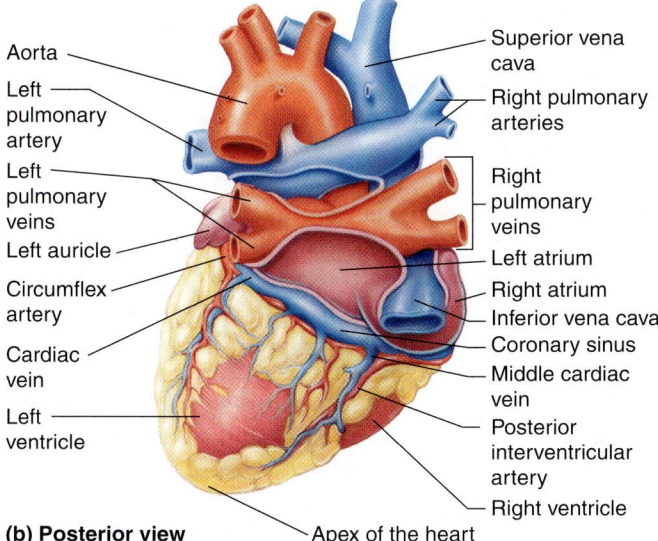

(b) Posterior view

Figure 29-11   Coronary artery system.

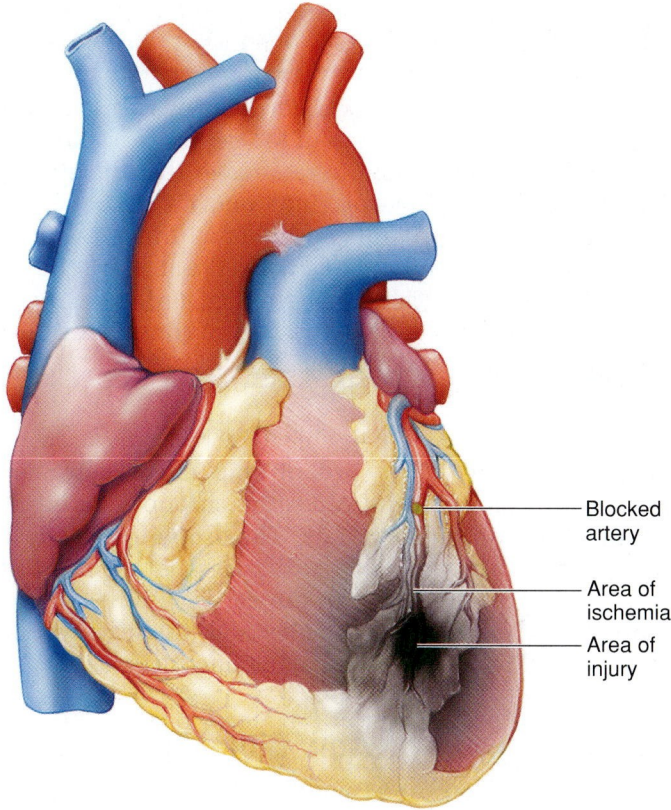

Figure 29-12   The "widowmaker"—left coronary artery.

where the inferior vena cava is found and deposits its blood directly into the right atria.

Interruption of blood flow in any of the coronary arteries can result in hypoxia, ischemia, necrosis, and death of myocardial tissue. The vessels can spasm or become blocked with debris from a blood clot or a broken-off piece of atherosclerotic plaque. Stable or unstable angina pectoris conditions (which will be discussed later) are reversible conditions with intermittent coronary arterial block, while a myocardial infarction is an actual block.

Cardiac Properties and Effects

The heart is made up of specialized muscle tissue found nowhere else in the body. It has the normal properties of muscle tissue in that it will contract and relax when stimulated by electrolytes such as calcium and magnesium. These specialized cells express the additional unique properties of **automaticity,** the ability to initiate an electrical impulse without outside nervous system stimulation, and **excitability,** the ability to readily receive and respond to an electrical impulse. These properties both involve the nervous system. **Contractility** is the ability to contract when stimulated. This property deals with the muscular pumping action of the heart. Both types of properties, those targeting electrical responses and those targeting mechanical responses, are required for the heart to pump effectively. DOT 5-2.14

While every cardiac cell possesses these properties, certain cells have specialized further to function primarily as pacemakers, conduction fibers, or muscle fibers. When each is doing its job correctly, the pacemaker initiates the impulse at the appropriate time, the conduction fibers propagate (spread) this impulse for maximum advantage in pumping, and the contractile cells perform an orchestrated contraction, which moves blood through the heart.

Inotropy, Chronotropy, and Dromotropy

Other terms associated with cardiac function and properties include inotropy, chronotropy, and dromotropy. The **inotropic effect** refers to the strength of the cardiac contraction. For example, a drug with a positive inotropic

Nice to Know

The contraction of the ventricle of the heart is called systole, and the relaxation of the ventricle is called diastole. It is important to remember that the atria and ventricles are performing opposite tasks (constriction or dilation) timed together within the same cardiac cycle. Simply stated, when the atria are contracting, both ventricles are relaxing, and when the atria are relaxing, both ventricles are contracting.

effect on the heart would be able to increase the strength of a contraction. The **chronotropic effect** describes influence on the heart rate. A positive chronotropic effect would speed up the heart rate. The **dromotropic effect** describes the excitability, or willingness, of the heart to conduct an impulse through the cardiac cells. A drug with a negative dromotropic effect on the heart would slow down the rate of electrical conduction. DOT 5-2.21

Coronary and Systemic Blood Flow

Blood flow is continuous and cyclic in nature. It can be examined from virtually any starting point and traced around the body to return to that point. A common means to follow this path is to begin this process where deoxygenated blood enters into the heart, at the right atria, or where oxygenated blood enters into the left atria (Figure 29-13).

We start our discussion with blood returning from the body via the superior and inferior vena cava and depositing in the right atria. At about this same time, oxygenated blood is flowing into the left atria from the lungs via the pulmonary veins. To be most accurate in this discussion, you need to know that the timing of blood moving through the left side of the heart is milliseconds faster than the right side of the heart be-

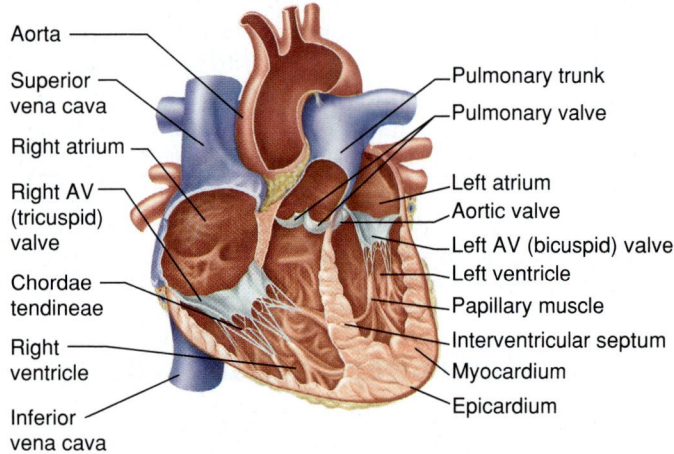

Aorta
Superior vena cava
Right atrium
Right AV (tricuspid) valve
Chordae tendineae
Right ventricle
Inferior vena cava

Pulmonary trunk
Pulmonary valve
Left atrium
Aortic valve
Left AV (bicuspid) valve
Left ventricle
Papillary muscle
Interventricular septum
Myocardium
Epicardium

Figure 29-13   Interior of the heart.

cause the left ventricle begins its contraction sooner. This results in the valves closing at different times (resulting in the two sounds heard when listening to the heart with a stethoscope), and it results in a directionally improved flow as it pushes blood through the heart in the direction it should go. For the purposes of this portion of the discussion, think of the left heart and right heart activity occurring virtually simultaneously.

There are no valves controlling the flow of blood into the atria, and it is dependant upon pushing from behind caused by the continuous venous flow of blood. The flow of blood into the atria is continuous. The pressure from this process is called **preload.** The higher the preload, the more volume of blood that is moved into the right atria. Reduced preload means that not as much blood will flow into the heart. Although preload is occurring within both atria, in our discussion of the impact of it upon the overall pumping force, we focus on the preload of the right side of the heart.

Another feature of cardiac muscle is called the **Frank-Starling mechanism** of the heart. Frank-Starling mechanism (also sometimes described as a "law") states that the force of blood ejected by the heart is determined primarily by the length of the fibers of its muscular wall.[5] Simply stated, the more a cardiac muscle is stretched, the harder it will contract.[6] Reexamining the principal of preload with respect to Frank-Starling mechanism, the more blood that flows into the atria, the harder they will contract, pushing the blood more forcefully into the ventricles. The atria are relatively thin muscles, lacking significant pumping strength; however, since their job is basically to fill the ventricles, they are adequate for the task. DOT 5-2.18

This movement of blood into the ventricles associated with the atrial contraction is referred to as the **atrial kick** and is responsible for providing a little extra blood to the ventricles beyond what would flow passively once the valves opened. (Remember, the atria do not have much pumping force.) It occurs just at the conclusion of the blood transfer between the atria and ventricles. Without this atrial kick, the heart may lose as much as 25% of its output capability.

Once the atria contract, they push blood through the tricuspid and bicuspid valves into the right and left ventricles, respectively (Box 29-1). The Frank-Starling mechanism described earlier also applies to the ventricles; the more blood that is pushed into them (thus stretching them more), the harder they will contract, increasing cardiac output. At a normal heart rate of around 80 beats/minute, approximately 80 milliseconds after the cardiac cycle starts, the ventricles themselves contract, pushing blood through the pulmonic and aortic valves into the pulmonary system and systemic circulation, respectively. This 80 millisecond delay allows adequate time for the ventricles to fill with blood. If this time interval is shortened, cardiac

BOX 29-1 The Group Names of the Heart Valves

The tricuspid and bicuspid are also referred to as the AV valves because they separate the atria from the ventricles. The pulmonic and aortic valves are called semilunar valves because of the appearance of their shape when viewed from the inside of the heart; they look like moons. The opening and closing of each set of valves is opposite; when the semilunar valves are open, the AV are closed, and when the AV valves are open the semilunar are closed.

output will be decreased. This may happen during episodes of extremely rapid heart beats or during atrioventricular conduction abnormalities, which will be discussed later.

Attached to the ventricular walls are specialized tissue called **papillary muscles.** Attached to them are tough cords called **chordae tendinae** and the various pieces, called leaflets, of the tricuspid and bicuspid (mitral) valves. These muscles contract, along with the ventricular wall, and pull the valve shut, sealing the ventricle and preventing backflow of blood into the atria.

As previously discussed, the heart is actually a two-stage pump, with the right side pumping blood under relatively low pressure into the pulmonary system and the left side pumping blood at a higher force throughout the body via the arterial system. Because of the difference in workload between the two ventricles, the left ventricle is much thicker than the right. Due to its increased size and heavier workload, the left ventricle is often the first to fail from increased stress or reduced oxygen or nutrient supply.

Cardiac output is the measure of how much blood is pumped out of the heart per minute. It is defined as the stroke volume (amount of blood pumped out of the heart with each beat) times the heart rate per minute. Applying the principles discussed in the last section, the amount of blood pumped out of the heart, or cardiac output, is dependent upon the following:

- Blood supply available to flow into the heart or *preload.*
- Ability of the atria to push blood into the ventricles or *atrial kick.*
- Ability of the ventricles to pump blood efficiently against the *afterload.*
- An adequate heart rate, which allows for optimal filling times for the chambers.

If any one of these factors is compromised, the others must somehow compensate to maintain adequate cardiac output. For example, should the blood supply be reduced because of hemorrhage, preload is reduced; therefore, atrial kick is reduced, limiting the pumping ability of the ventricles. In this scenario, the only way the appropriate level of cardiac output can be maintained would be to increase the heart rate. This happens during hemorrhagic shock.

Another example of this mechanism is a patient who has taken the medication nitroglycerin for angina pain. Nitroglycerin has the ability to relax or dilate blood vessels. Earlier in this chapter, the venous system was described as a type of holding tank for blood. Nitroglycerin will increase the capacity of the venous system by dilating key vessels resulting in **vascular pooling.** With more blood being retained in the venous system, less blood will flow into the atria, thus reducing cardiac output by reducing preload. Instead of an actual blood loss as seen in the hemorrhage example, nitroglycerin creates the same effect called **relative hypovolemia** (Box 29-2). If the heart rate cannot compensate adequately for this, systemic blood flow and organ perfusion will be reduced. This will be reflected through a falling blood pressure reading. It may also be appreciated by noting a difference in strength or an absence of the radial pulse when the carotid and radial pulses are palpated simultaneously. Should the brain become affected by this reduced cardiac output, unconsciousness may result.

BOX 29-2 Absolute Versus Relative Hypovolemia

Relative hypovolemia is a condition that results from a discrepancy between the size of the container (blood vessels) and the volume of blood that is available to fill it. By contrast, absolute hypovolemia is due to an actual loss of blood volume, either through bleeding, dehydration, or other causes. Both situations are potentially life-threatening. The treatment for each condition will vary as the paramedic must consider the impact to each part of the cardiovascular system as treatments are rendered. For example the problem may be primarily due to relative hypovolemia caused perhaps by anaphylaxis induced from a bee sting. The paramedic "treats" the low blood pressure by administering a large amount of isotonic crystalloid IV fluid into the patient while also giving the patient injections of medication to counteract the anaphylaxis. Once the medicine begins to work, vasoconstriction begins, and now the patient may appear to be overhydrated. Pulmonary edema may develop as more fluid leaves the capillaries than returns back to the bloodstream, and the increase of preload and afterload may lead to a rise in blood pressure as well.

Electrophysiology of the Myocardium

To understand how the conduction system works and to later understand the ECG pattern, the basic electrophysiology of a single cardiac cell must first be understood. A functioning heart is dependent on the interaction of cardiac muscle fibers, conduction fibers, and specialized clumps of cells known as pacemaker sites. The properties of each will be discussed, but to start, the workings of a single cardiac cell will be examined. Cells are comprised of a bilipid (double fat-composed) membrane, embedded with proteins specifically constructed to act as selective gates or pores. These gates provide semipermeability to the cell wall, giving it the ability to control fluid and electrolyte particles entering into and exiting from the cell.

To better understand this interaction, remember that specific rules govern cellular function throughout the entire body. First, the body always wants all electrical forces to be neutral, meaning the number of positive forces must equal the number of negative forces. Second, the body will always attempt to maintain the numbers of particles in balance by diluting an area with higher concentrations of particles by water crossing a semipermeable membrane from an area with lower concentrations of particles. If these balanced conditions do not exist, a pressure difference develops, and this pressure difference is known as a gradient (Box 29-3).

For example, if a greater concentration of sodium (Na^+) exists outside of a cell, and the influx of Na^+ into the cell is limited by the protein gates within the cell membrane, there will be a force trying to push the Na^+ into the cell's interior as the body tries to equalize the concentration. The same principal applies to an excess of charged particles outside the cell wall. This pressure gradient creates a "potential" to do something. One may draw a parallel between this electrostatic and concentration gradient to that of cocking the hammer of a gun. Keeping all the Na^+ outside the cell would be like cocking the hammer (Figure 29-14). The gun would now have the potential of firing, should the right conditions occur, like someone pulling the trigger. So it is with the cell. Sodium is building up outside the cell, until a force opens the protein gates of the cell, allowing Na^+ to rush into the interior of the cell. This initiates a series of events known as the action potential of the myocardial cell. DOT 5-2.16

While the complete function of the cardiac cells requires the interaction between a host of electrolytes and other substances, we will concentrate now on the three chief ions that make the cells function. The main ions are Sodium (Na^+), Potassium (K^+), and Calcium (Ca^{++}). At rest, a higher concentration of Na^+ is found outside the cell and K^+ is found in higher concentration inside the cell while Ca^{++} exists mainly outside the cell and within invaginations (channels) deep in the cell.

BOX 29-3 Demystifying Particle Movement (Osmosis, Diffusion, and Facilitated Diffusion)

The concept of particle movement between gradients is often a difficult concept for paramedics to grasp. However, it follows concrete laws, and a simplified description may help. Remember, equilibrium is achieved when an equal amount of particles on each side of a membrane results in equal pressure. It is important to focus on not having a one-to-one ratio of particles but having an overall equality of pressures. When there is not an equality of pressures, substances are forced to move to reach the equilibrium state. (Ironically, when true equilibrium is achieved, movement pretty much stops—and that would be a bad thing!)

Think of a semipermeable membrane as a slice of Swiss cheese. Place this slice of cheese into a glass of water so that it divides the container exactly in half. Now let us add some beads of various sizes (some of which are larger than the holes) to one side of the glass and watch what happens. Over time, the water will flow back and forth freely through the holes. The small molecules of water freely move through the holes. Water movement is from **simple diffusion** and is called osmosis.

The movement of the beads will be another story. Any beads that are smaller than the hole will move around freely, eventually obtaining equilibrium through simple diffusion. Any that are too large to pass will remain where they are. Machinery imbedded in the cheese could allow any bead to be grabbed and forced through the cheese. In the cell, these structures are membrane-bound proteins, and they move particles through **active transport**, or **facilitated diffusion.**

Every particle present within the glass container is contributing pressure to the whole system, including the cheese, water molecules, and the beads. If the pores are too small to allow larger beads to pass and there are no membrane-bound proteins, the only components capable of moving between the two sides are the water and smaller particles. In order to achieve equality of pressures, when particles cannot freely move, water is forced to migrate (in other words, be drawn) into the area to change the concentration balance to bring the pressures together. Water's movement is seldom inhibited by the membrane until the pressures reach a point where movement is prevented due to the pressure from the other side of the membrane.

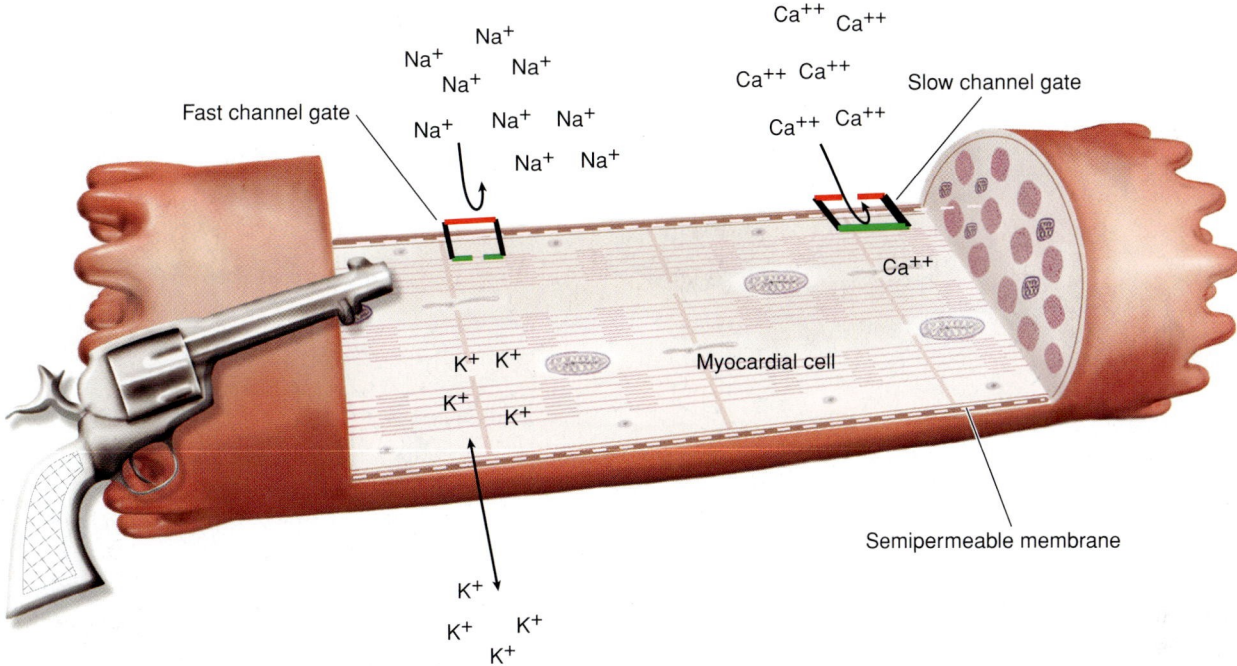

Figure 29-14 The body tries to equalize the concentration.

This sets up the interplay between electrostatic and concentration gradients.

Let us examine this cellular environment closer (Figure 29-15). Sodium is found in its highest concentration outside the cell. It remains there as long as the protein gates, called the sodium channel gates, are closed. These gates are very specialized and remain closed until activated by an electrical impulse. Once activated, they open and allow Na^+ to flow freely into the cell. Sodium carries a positive charge and due to its abundance is a major contributor to the high positive charge outside the cell.

Meanwhile, potassium is allowed into the cell, balancing the concentration gradient of potassium inside and outside the cell. Inside the cell, potassium, which also

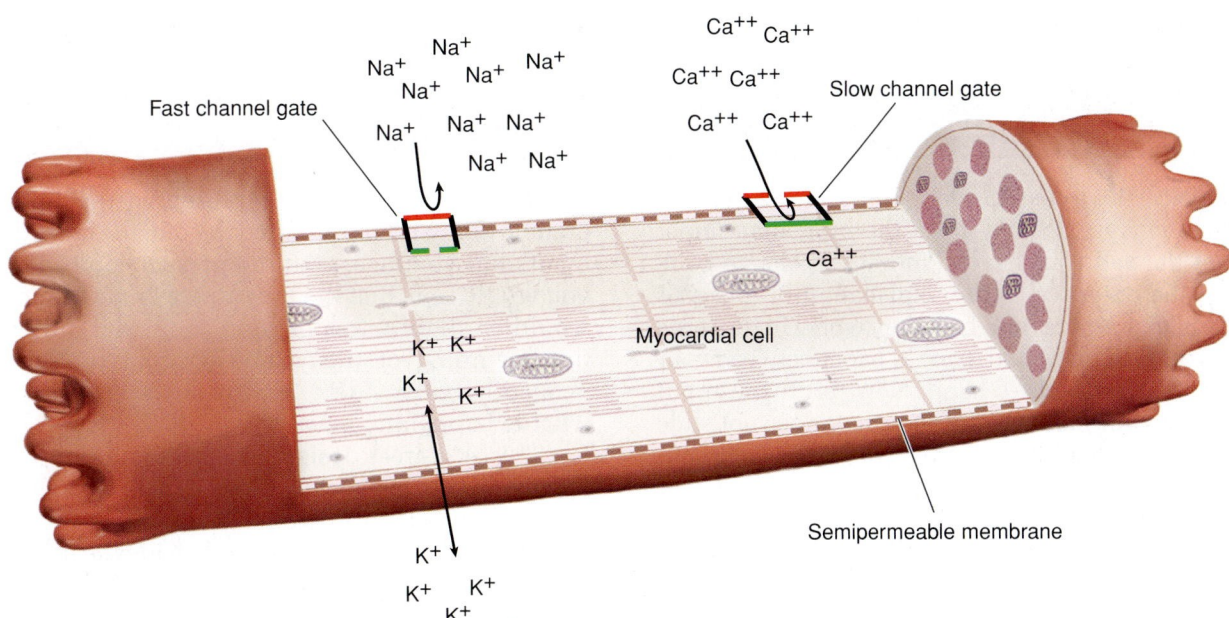

Figure 29-15 Resting membrane potential. Na^+ can't enter the cell. Ca^{++} can't enter the cell. K^+ can pass freely. This creates pressure that has the potential to make something happen. Cells will remain in this phase until a stimulus from another cell opens the gates.

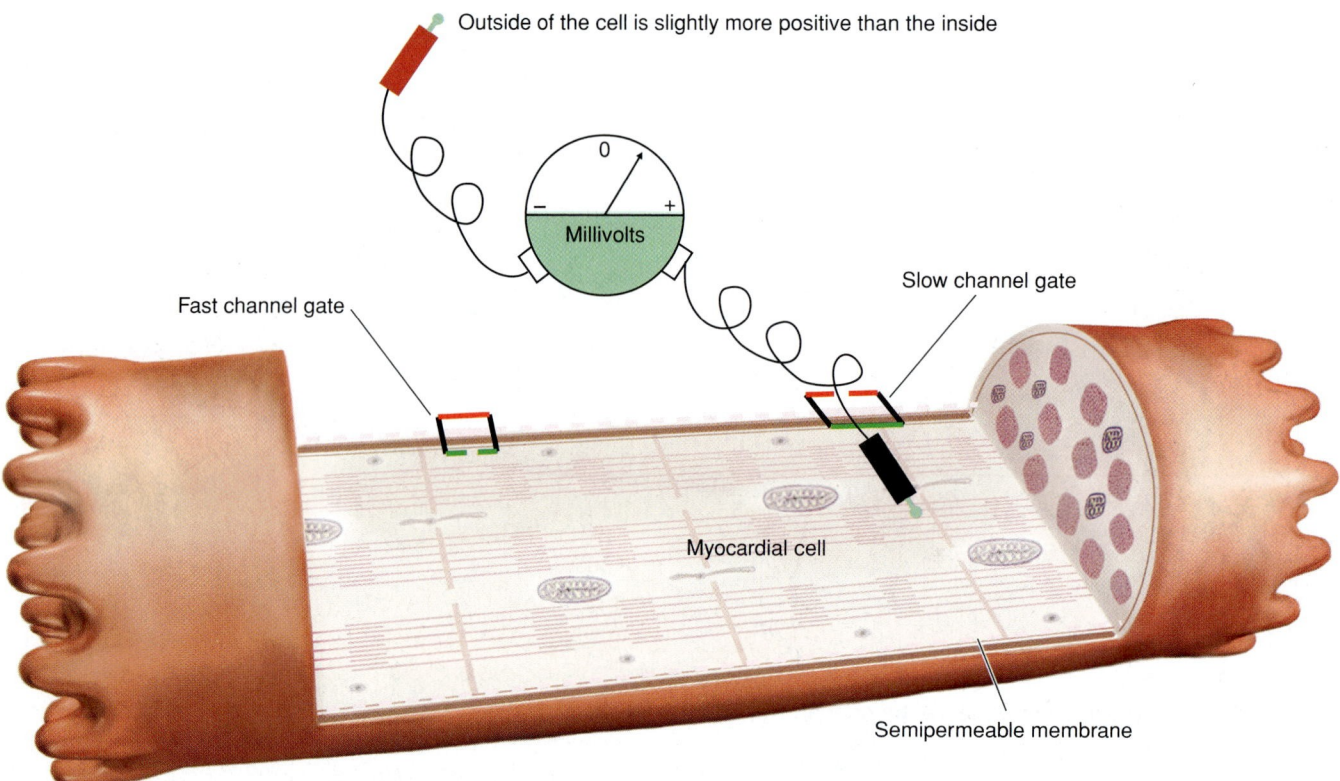

Outside of the cell is slightly more positive than the inside

Millivolts

Fast channel gate

Slow channel gate

Myocardial cell

Semipermeable membrane

Therefore, an electrical pressure exists, because the body tries to neutralize all forces!

Figure 29-16 Electric potential. When the inside of the cell has a different chemical charge than the outside, a potential difference exists. However, some ions can't easily cross the cell wall.

carries a positive charge, contributes to the resulting interior electrical charge, along with many other substances. If the electrostatic charges were measured on both sides of the cell wall of a cell at rest, it would be found that, due to the high concentration of Na^+ outside the cell, it would be slightly more positive than the inside

(Figure 29-16). Therefore, two pressure gradients exist: electrostatic pressure as the inside and outside try to neutralize and concentration pressure as Na^+ tries to balance between the outside and inside of the cell (Box 29-4).

This resting phase, when nothing is flowing in or out of the cell, is referred to as the **resting membrane**

BOX 29-4 How Do Two Positive Charges Make a Negative?

Potassium carries a positive charge. Sodium also carries a positive charge. So why does the immediate inner lining of the cell wall have a "negative" charge compared to the outer wall? The explanation of this goes back again to pressures and how they work. To illustrate this for yourself, place one piece of paper between your hand and someone else's hand. Now tell them to put pressure on your hand so that the paper does not slide out. Note that when they do this, you will have to put some pressure back toward them or your hand will move. Try to keep the paper from moving and try to keep your hands from moving while still applying pressure. Note that if pressure on one side is increased slightly, pressure on the other side must also increase to prevent movement.

If your friend's hand represented the cell membrane, your hand represented the outside cell environment, and you measured the pressures on each side, you would note that the pressure on your friend's side would be slightly less than on your side. But wait, in the beginning of this exercise equal pressure was needed on each side of the paper to keep it still, so what is happening now?

This is a great design because if suddenly a hole opened up in the paper to allow something to flow into the cell, the slightly higher pressure on the outside would prevent the contents from inside the cell leaking out and would also encourage material on the other side to flow in. Allowing an influx of material, in the case of the cell sodium ions, starts the electrical exchange.

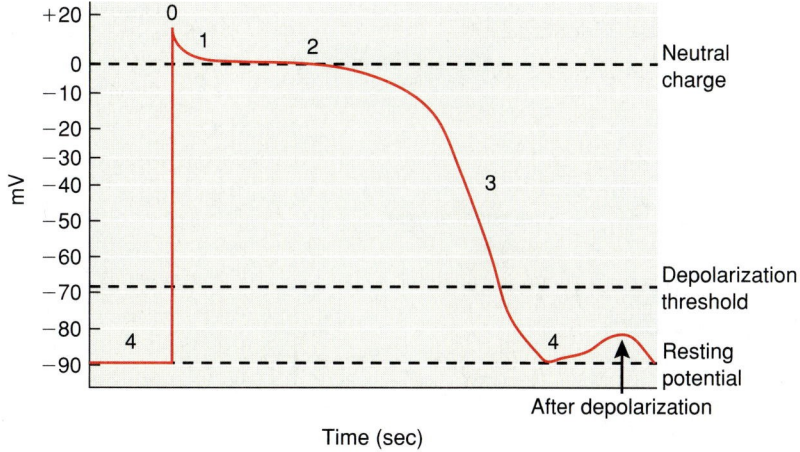

Figure 29-17 Action potential graph showing the phases of the action potential.

potential. At this point, the importance of the proper balance of electrolytes within the system can be appreciated. The amount of pressure trying to push Na^+ into the cell is offset by the amount of K^+ inside the cell. The action potential that results in cardiac activity is divided into phases. The resting membrane potential is phase four (Figure 29-17). DOT 5-2.15, 5-2.17)

Action Potential

Phase 4: Resting

The cardiac cell is at rest, and Na^+ is under a great deal of pressure to enter the cell to balance electrostatic and concentration gradients while potassium concentration has balanced itself with the exterior of the cell, effectively setting the electric potential inside the cell. Calcium is waiting outside the cell, also trying to balance its concentration with the inside of the cell. The "hammer" is now cocked, waiting for something to pull the trigger.

Phase 0: Sodium Moves Inside the Cell

The "trigger" in the case of the cardiac cell is an electric impulse passed on from specialized pacemaker cells or from the adjacent cell. This electrical impulse activates the sodium channels by binding with specific receptor sites, effectively opening them up to allow sodium to cross the membrane at will. Remember that Na^+ is under a great deal of pressure and rushes into the cell very rapidly. This begins phase 0 of the action potential (Figure 29-18).

As sodium rushes in, the rapid change in electrostatic pressure begins to force K^+ out of the cell. In fact, Na^+ rushes in so fast that it overshoots the desired balance in electrostatic forces, causing the interior to become more positive than the exterior of the cell. This reversing of electrostatic gradients is called **depolarization,** a term which has become synonymous with the beginning of a heartbeat. Sodium moves into the cell until the electrical charge inside that cell reaches a certain level. Once this

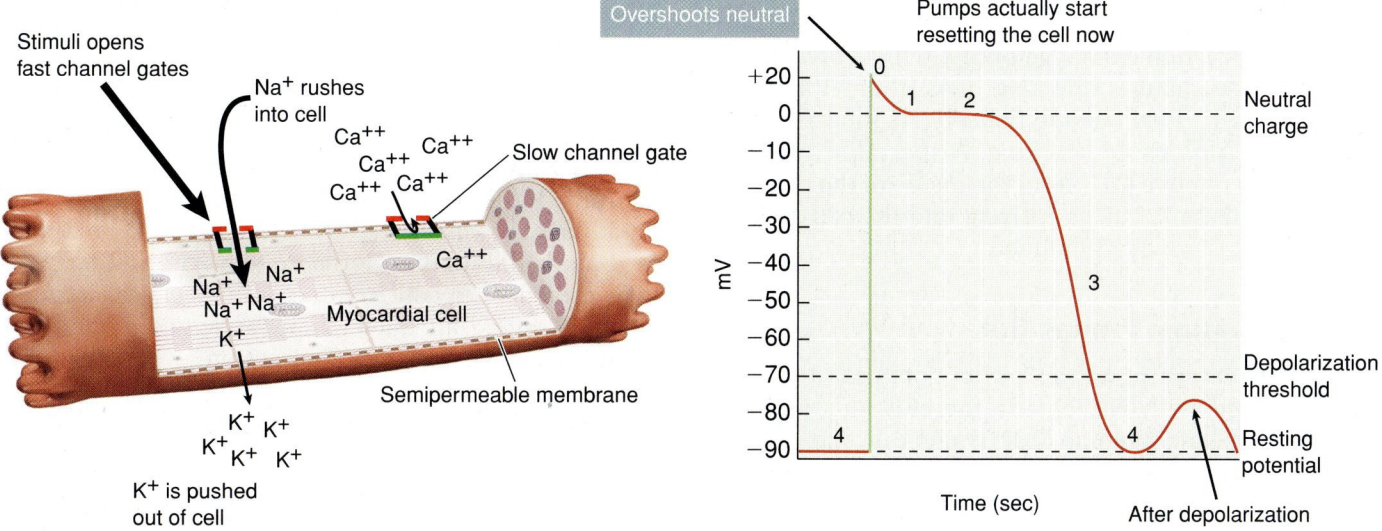

Figure 29-18 Phase 0: Depolarization—sodium moves inside the cell.

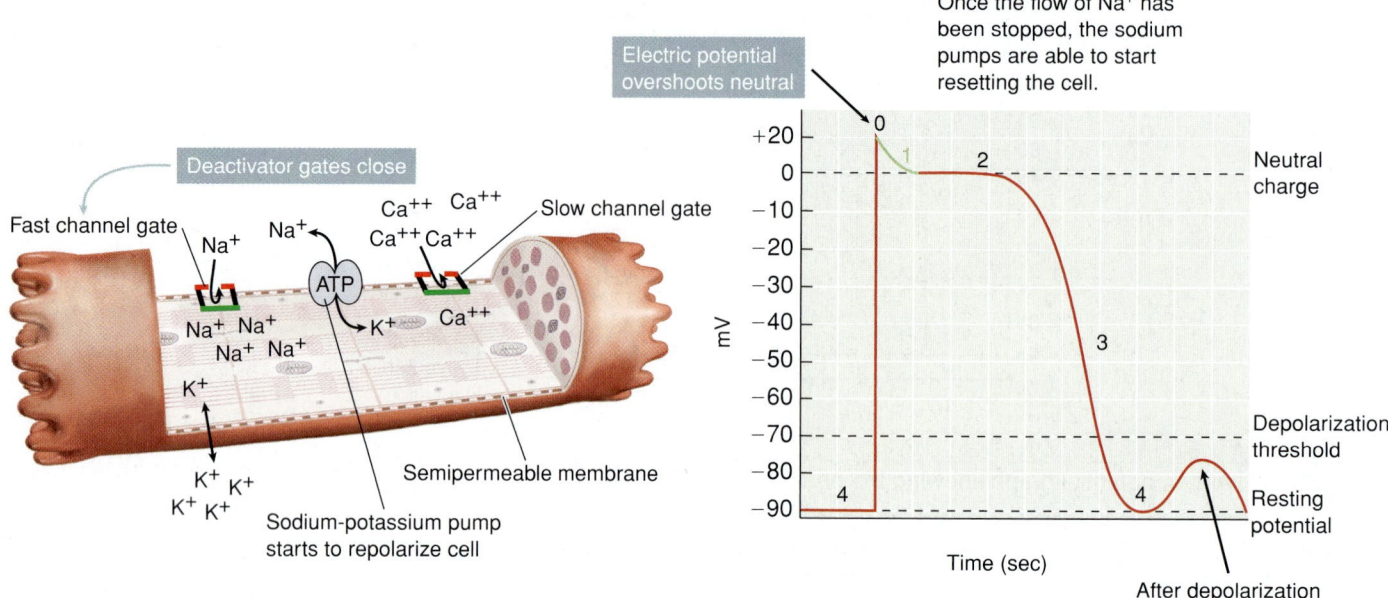

Figure 29-19   Phase 1: ATP grabs sodium inside the cell and pushes it back out.

level is achieved, the sodium channel gates are once again closed, and the influx of Na⁺ is halted.

At this point another important feature of the cell wall is introduced. Many specialized protein gates exist in the cell wall. As previously discussed, some gates control sodium influx in the cell while other gates allow potassium and calcium into the cell. There is another type of protein channel that acts as a biochemical pump. These channels require the use of adenosine triphosphate (ATP) as a fuel for the active transport mechanism, which grabs sodium inside the cell and pushes it back out (Figure 29-19).

Because this pump is required to push Na⁺ outside the cell in spite of how much Na⁺ is already out there, fuel is required. (This is an example of facilitated diffusion.) This is how Na⁺ is built up outside the cell against a concentration gradient. This pump is actually a sodium/potassium exchange pump, which, on activation by ATP, exchanges three Na⁺ ions from within the cell with two K⁺ ions outside the cell. As long as there is fuel, these pumps are working. A specialized pump also exists to remove Ca⁺⁺ from the inside of the cell. At the time of phase 0, Na⁺ is rushing into the cell so fast that the pumps are overwhelmed.

Phase 1: Sodium Pumps Out

Once again, returning to the action potential, the cell is depolarized with Na⁺ inside the cell, the sodium channel gates have become deactivated due to the electrostatic changes inside the cell, and the sodium/potassium exchange pumps are trying to move the Na⁺ back out of the cells again. This begins phase 1 of the action potential.

Remember, at the end of phase 0, Na⁺ overshoots the balance of electrical forces across the cell membrane. As the sodium channels shut down, the ion exchange pump starts to lower the Na⁺ level within the cell. The electrical charge inside the cell is now able to activate the calcium channel gates, allowing calcium to begin moving inside the cell. This now begins phase 2 of the action potential.

Phase 2: Calcium Moves In

In phase 2, we have Na⁺ still being pushed out of the cell, K⁺ being pulled in, and now Ca⁺⁺ flowing into the cell (Figure 29-20). At this phase, the electric charges remain relatively constant, creating a period of little change in electric gradient across the cell membrane. This is also called the **plateau phase.** This is important for two reasons. It protects the cell from being influenced by any other electrical impulses that may come along and, perhaps more importantly, it allows calcium to perform its primary function. Once inside the cell, calcium binds with receptors, causing fibers of actin and myosin to pull together, effectively causing the cell to contract. Millions of these cells, contracting in a coordinated fashion, cause the heart to contract and squeeze the blood out into the arterial system. The plateau phase thus protects the cell from ectopic electrical impulses while allowing adequate time for enough calcium to enter the cell to initiate a contraction.

Phase 3: Calcium Moves Out

Phase 3 of the action potential begins when enough calcium has entered the cell to change the normal balance of electrical charges to a point which deactivates the Ca⁺⁺ channel gates (Figure 29-21). When the

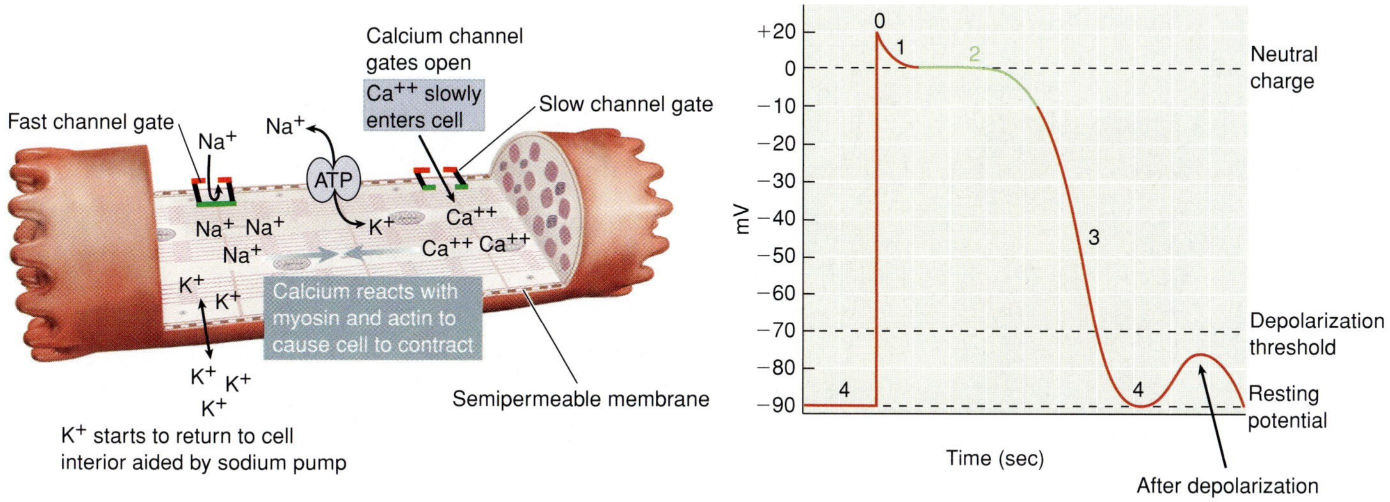

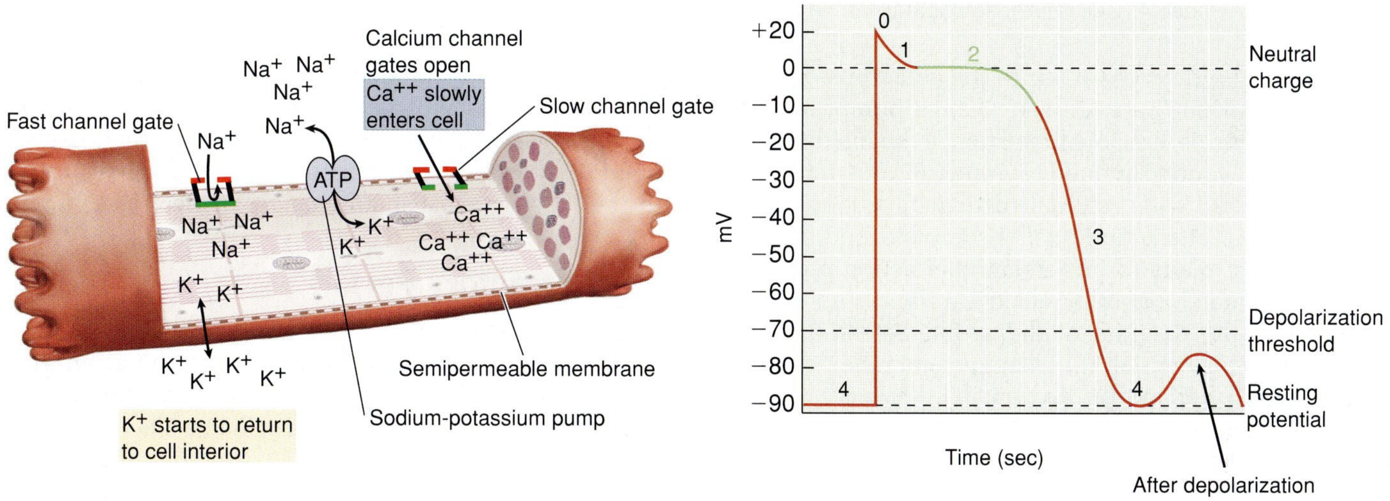

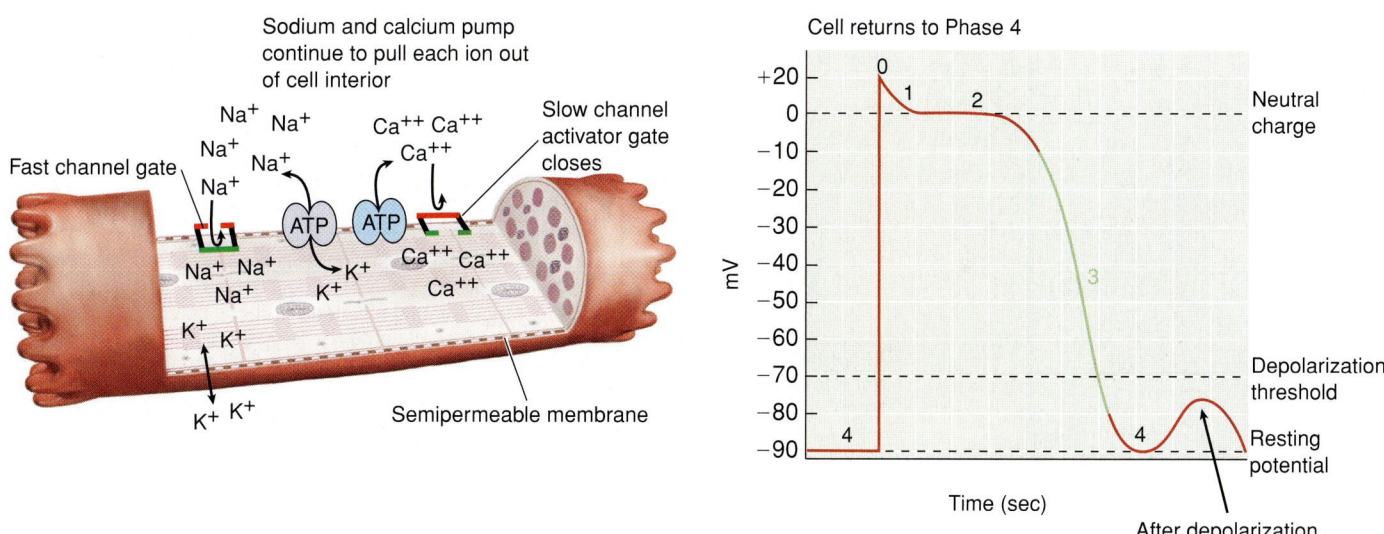

Figure 29-20   Phase 2: Plateau phase—calcium moves in.

Figure 29-21   Phase 3: Repolarization—calcium moves out.

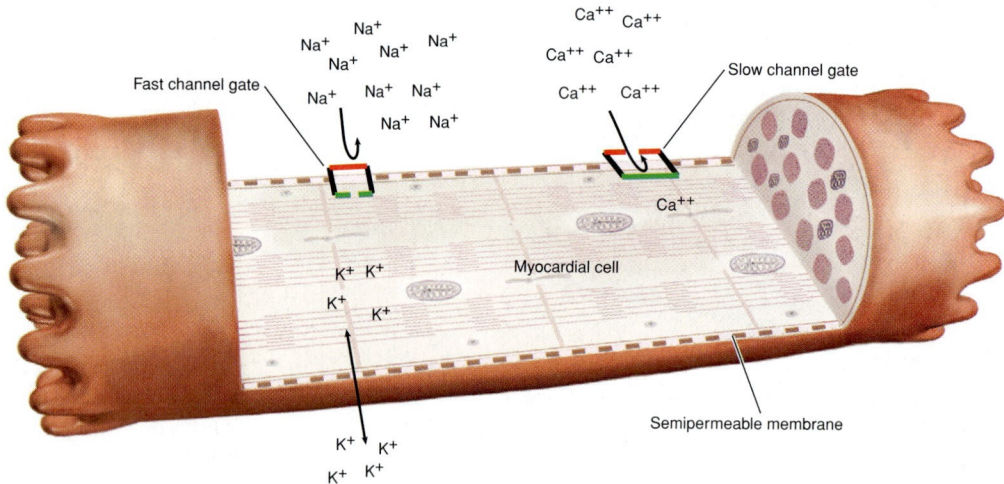

Figure 29-22   Phase 4: Cell returns to original resting state.

gates close, the flow of Ca^{++} into the cell stops. At this point, the sodium/potassium exchange pump, as well as the Ca^{++} pumps, are able to influence the inside of the cell fully. They move enough Na^+ and Ca^{++} out of the cell to reset the cell to its original resting state, or phase 4 (Figure 29-22). The action is now complete, and the cell is repolarized, ready to initiate another action potential when stimulated by another electrical impulse.

Refer to the diagram of the action potential graph (Figure 29-17). Note that the resting membrane potential occurs around −90 mV (millivolts) in the average cardiac cell. This is assuming that all electrolyte levels are correct and no problems with the cell membrane exist. It is estimated that a single myocardial cell membrane contains around a million sodium channel gates. The point at which enough sodium gates have opened to start the massive influx of sodium into the cell is called the **membrane threshold.** It is then reasonable to assume

that the stronger the electrical impulse, the greater the number of gates will be opened. Conversely, a weaker impulse will not be able to stimulate enough gates to open to cause a depolarization to occur. This protects the cell against most small changes in electrical flow.

The Refractory Period

Once the cell is in the depolarized state, the electrical gradient is such that no matter how strong an impulse comes along, the cell is not capable of responding to it (Figure 29-23). This part of the cardiac cycle is known as the **absolute refractory period.** As stated, during the absolute refractory period, the cell is incapable of receiving, responding to, and passing along an electrical impulse.

During repolarization, in phase 3, electrical gradients are moved back to the original resting membrane potential. This can be thought of as "resetting" back to

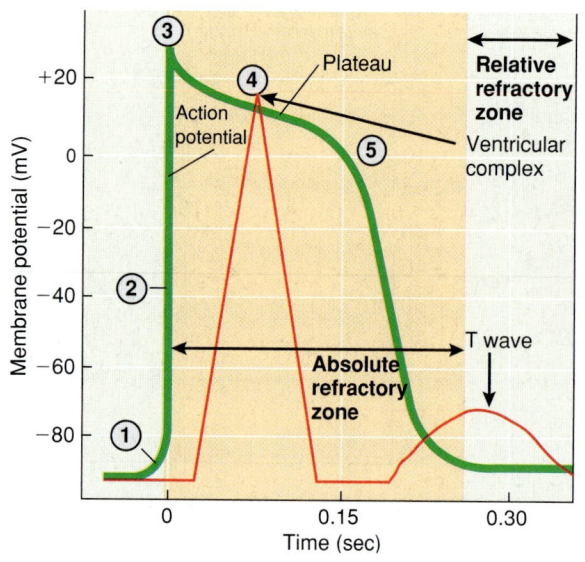

1. Voltage-gated sodium channels open.

2. Na^+ inflow depolarizes the membrane and triggers the opening of still more Na^+ channels, creating a positive feedback cycle and a rapidly rising membrane voltage.

3. Na^+ channels close when the cell depolarizes, and the voltage peaks at nearly +30 mV.

4. Ca^{2+} entering through slow calcium channels prolongs depolarization of membrane, creating a plateau. Plateau falls slightly because of some K^+ leakage, but most K^+ channels remain closed until end of plateau.

5. Ca^{2+} channels close and Ca^{2+} is transported out of cell. K^+ channels open, and rapid K^+ outflow returns membrane to its resting potential.

Figure 29-23   The refractory period.

the original state. There is, however, a small period of time during phase 3 when enough of an electrical gradient has been achieved to theoretically respond to a new electrical impulse if it is of sufficient size. This is called the **relative refractory period.** Should a strong enough impulse reach the cell at this time, a depolarization could possibly be initiated. However, since the cell is not fully reset to its resting membrane potential, the depolarization would not be as strong, resulting in a weaker than normal contraction that is not properly coordinated with the rest of the cardiac cells. A strong enough impulse hitting at this time may be sufficient to interfere with the coordinated activity of the conduction system, effectively destabilizing the entire heart. This destabilization could result in chaotic electrical activity known as ventricular fibrillation or ventricular tachycardia, and it could be life-threatening.

Of the two states, absolute and relative refractory periods, the absolute refractory period is stable, and any impulse coming along at that point in time will not cause a disruption to the cardiac cycle. The relative refractory period occurs when the cardiac cycle is not finished and is unstable, and an impulse coming along may or may not result in depolarization of cells. If it does not result in disruption, the impulse is not transmitted and it is harmless. If it is transmitted, it could result in the occurrence of a relatively harmless single impulse, or it could result in the development of a lethal cardiac rhythm. Because of the potential for causing a life-threatening situation, always be on the lookout for this, and, if observed on the ECG tracing, take steps to try to correct it. Treatment for this situation will be explored in detail later.

Pacemaker Cells

As mentioned, each cardiac cell possesses the properties of automaticity, excitability, and contractility. Therefore, any cardiac cell in the right circumstances is capable of initiating an impulse that could start a chain reaction of depolarization throughout the entire heart. The task of initiating depolarization waves at the appropriate time is usually performed by a group of specialized cells called **pacemaker cells.** DOT 5-2.12

Electrophysiological studies have identified several potential pacemaker sites within heart tissues, but three are clearly defined as the primary sites: the sinus or sinoatrial (SA) node, the atrioventricular (AV) node, and the purkinje fibers. These three groups of specialized cells function together as the primary pacemaker site (sinus node) and two backup systems (AV and purkinje), creating a fairly reliable system to initiate depolarization at the appropriate time in a coordinated manner. Physiologically, pacemaker cells differ from ordinary cardiac cells in that they have far fewer sodium channel gates (the fast response gates), which initiate phase 0. The reduced number of gates results in a shorter plateau phase as well as slower repolarization. The cellular membrane of pacemaker cells is designed to allow a programmed "leakage" of sodium into the cell, thus reaching depolarization threshold after a prescribed period of time. Pacemaker action potential time may be influenced by the activity of the autonomic nervous system or by the administration of cardioactive medications such as calcium channel blockers (Figure 29-24).

The **primary pacemaker,** or **sinus node,** is able to initiate depolarization at a rate of 60–100 times per minute. Should the sinus node fail to initiate an impulse, the AV will then fire. Should both fail, the purkinje fibers take over at an intrinsic rate of 20–40 times per minute. When "lower" positioned pacemaker sites fire because a higher site has failed, the term **escape** is used to describe the rhythm that results.

While not adequate in most cases to effectively perfuse the patient, impulses generated from the lower sites (the AV or purkinje fibers) are usually rhythmic and fast enough to keep the patient alive until corrective actions can be initiated.

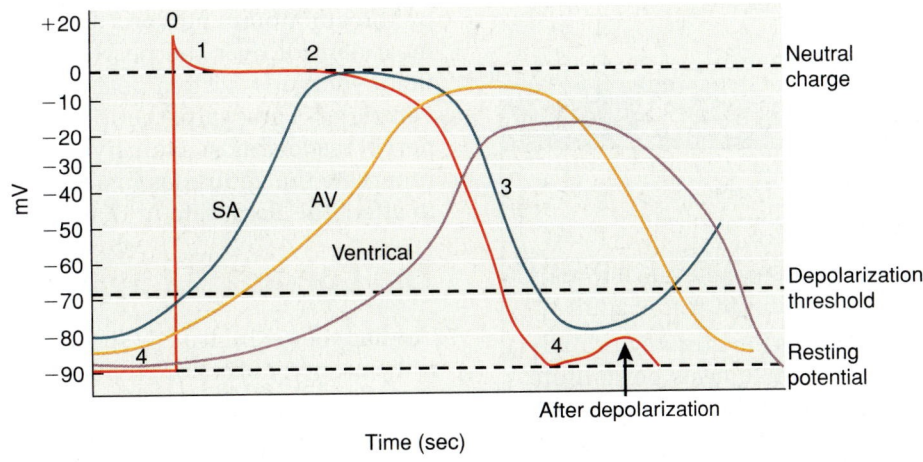

Figure 29-24 Leakage of various pacemaker groups.

1. Baroreceptors are responsible for detecting changes in pressure, usually within the heart or the main arteries. Chemoreceptors sense changes in the chemical composition of the blood. This information is transmitted to the cardioregulatory center in the medulla oblongata.

2. When the blood pressure is elevated, the cardiorespiratory center may activate the parasympathetic nervous system, which acts to slow the heart rate and lower the blood pressure.

3. If the blood pressure is low the cardiorespiratory center will activate the sympathetic nervous system, which acts to increase the heart rate and contractility. This increases cardiac output and raises the blood pressure.

4. The cardioregulatory center causes the release of epinephrine and some norepinephrine from the adrenal medulla into the general circulation. Epinephrine and norepinephrine increase the heart rate and stroke volume.

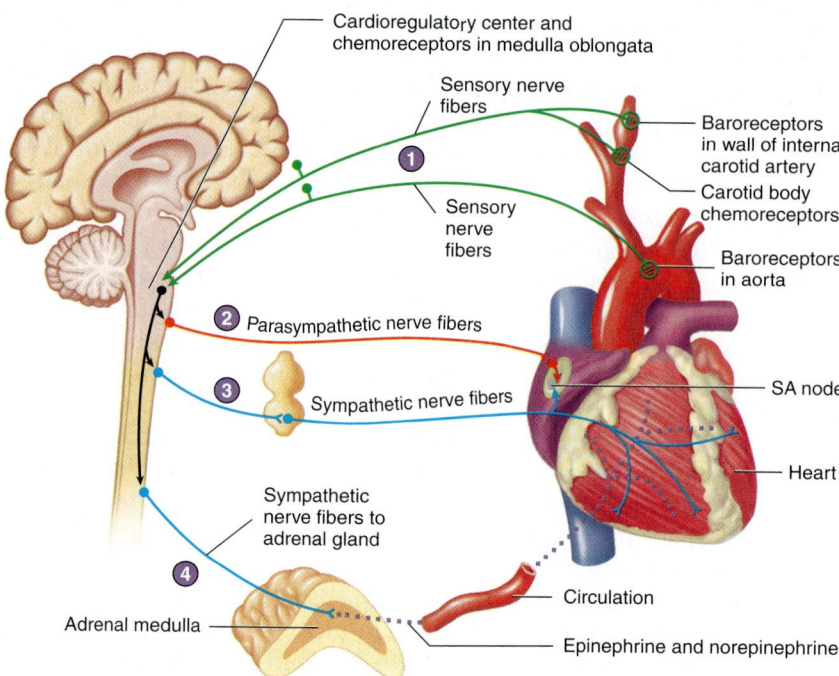

Figure 29-25   Innervation of the heart.

To keep the pacemaker sites from interfering with each other, secondary pacemaker sites are kept in check by a phenomenon known as **overdrive suppression.** Overdrive suppression occurs when a cell is driven to depolarization by a higher or stronger pacemaker. That cell becomes hyperpolarized, or reset to a lower resting membrane potential than would normally occur. It is believed that the overdriving of pacemaker cells increases the activity of the sodium ion pumps, hyperpolarizing the interior of the cell. Consider now the way pacemaker cells reach threshold through a controlled leakage. If they start from a lower level, it will take them longer to reach that threshold level thus effectively suppressing their pacemaker potential until needed.

Nice to Know

Inherent Automaticity Rates for Each Pacemaker Site

SA node = 60–100 impulses per minute normally with a top rate of 160 per minute in the adult

AV node = 40–60 impulses per minute normally with the top rate of about 220 beats per minute

Purkinje rate = 20–40 impulses per minute with a top rate close to 300 beats per minute

Control of the Heart Rate

The actual heart rate is influenced by the sympathetic and parasympathetic branches of the autonomic nervous system (Figure 29-25). It can also be influenced by drugs and hormones such as insulin or glucagon. All of these influences give the heart the ability to adjust its output based on the needs of the rest of the body. For example, increasing blood pressure, which is sensed by **baroreceptors** (pressure receptors) found in the carotid arteries, aorta, and in other sites, can trigger the brain to tell the heart to slow down. The parasympathetic nervous system then exerts its influence via the tenth cranial nerve (the vagus nerve) to slow the heart rate down. DOT 5-2.19, 5-2.20

The SA nodes and AV nodes are innervated directly by the autonomic nervous system and thus exhibit the most control over the heart rate. Fibers of the sympathetic nervous system reach into both the atria and ventricles. Parasympathetic fibers (primarily the vagus nerve) reach almost exclusively into the atria and do not innervate the ventricles in a significant enough manner to affect the heart rate in that area directly.

The Conduction System of the Heart

Cardiac cells exhibit a few special properties; among these is the property of conductivity. Cardiac cells are interconnected end-to-end, progressively branching out throughout the entire heart (Figure 29-26). Each cell is coupled to the next through an intercalated disk. Inside these intercalated disks are specialized plasma membrane channels

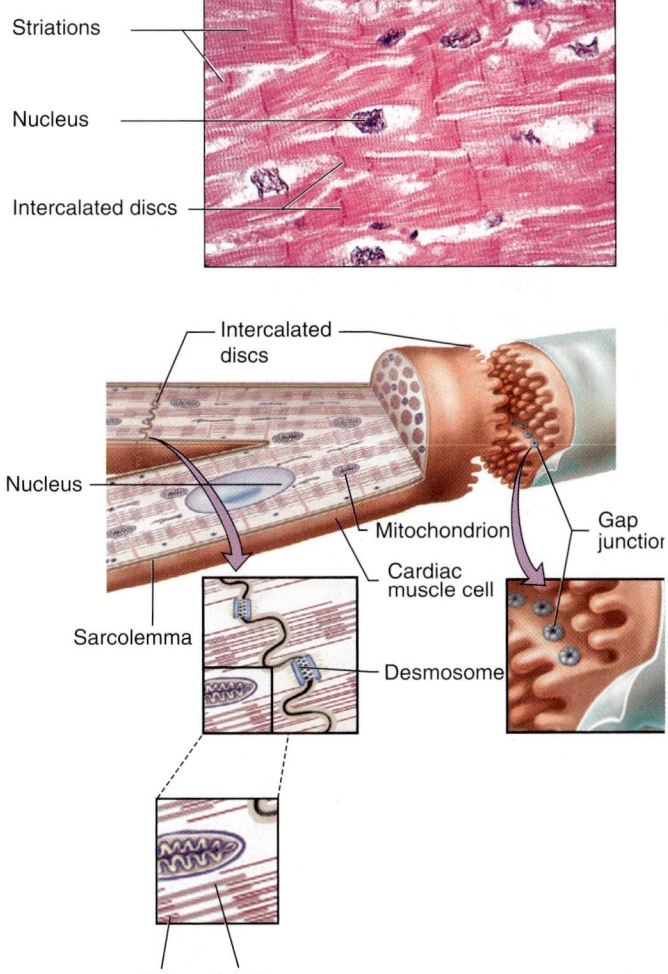

Figure 29-26 Myocardial cell.

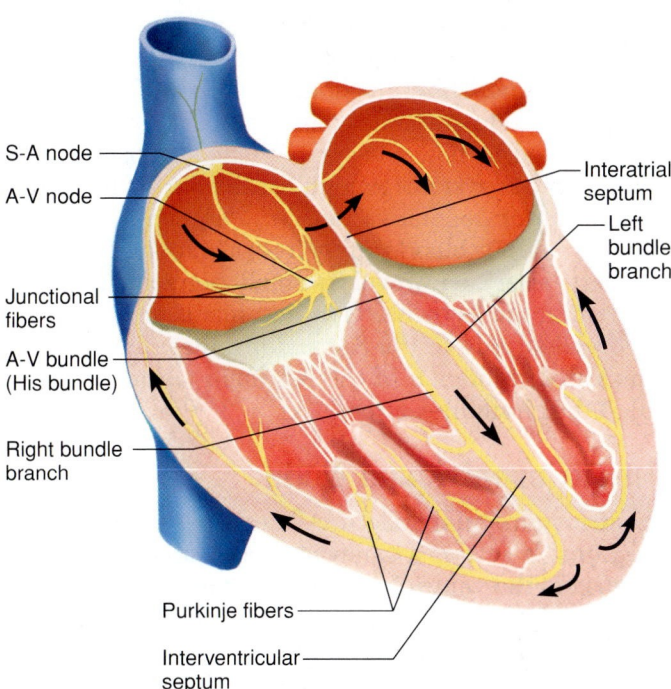

Figure 29-27 The cardiac conduction system.

called gap junctions. These **gap junctions** allow ions and small molecules to pass between cells. They also facilitate conduction between cells and keep the heart beating in a synchronized manner. DOT 5-2.11

There are specialized conduction fibers identified in the heart that are capable of conducting impulses at a much faster rate than the average cardiac cell. These are called **conduction fibers.** The conduction fiber system allows the impulse to travel all the way down to the apex of the heart (the ventricles) to cause them to begin their contraction from the apex moving towards the base. This action results in the chambers squeezing themselves from the "bottom" up with the squeeze ending at the valve. The result is effective emptying of nearly all the blood contained within the chamber.

Components of the Conduction System

It is important to understand that the chambers of the heart are electrically isolated from each other by a cartilaginous structure known as the cardiac skeleton. This structure primarily supports the valves and gives

shape and structure to the heart. The cardiac skeleton also separates the chambers electrically, so the impulses typically must travel through the conduction pathway to reach each chamber. Conduction of an impulse from one chamber to the next is then usually dependent upon a functioning and stable conduction system.

The conduction system of the heart consists of several specialized structures (Figure 29-27). The impulses usually originate within the dominant pacemaker: the **sinus node.** As the impulses leave the node, they begin to travel throughout the atria. The impulses are picked up through a system of **internodal pathways** and dispersed quickly throughout both atria. Conduction to the left atria is facilitated by a conduction fiber called the **Bachmann's bundle,** and this branch is often called the **interatrial pathway.** Three pathways have been identified that move between the SA and AV node. Both atria depolarize at virtually the same time.

At the base of the left atria is the secondary pacemaker called the **atrioventricular node** or **AV node.** Immediately after this is the **AV junction.** This structure connects to the **bundle of His,** which further branches into the **left** and **right bundle branches.** The left and right bundle branches terminate in a network of conduction fibers called the **purkinje network.** The purkinje network is the location of the third pacemaker.

The Sinus Node

The sinus node, or SA node, is a group of round, cardiac cells arranged in a crescent-shaped mass. It is located in the posterior aspect of the heart, where the superior vena cava meets the right atrium. The sinus node acts as the primary pacemaker, controlling the heart rate under normal conditions. The sinus node usually initiates an impulse from 60 to 100 times per minute. The sinus node is innervated by both the sympathetic and parasympathetic nervous systems, which exhibit strong influence on the rate of depolarization. In most people, the SA node receives its blood supply from a branch of the right coronary artery. However, a small percentage of the population are known as left dominant, meaning that the blood supply to the SA node in these individuals comes from a branch of the left main coronary artery called the circumflex artery.

The Atrioventricular Node

The atrioventricular node, or AV node, has three primary functions. It acts as a gateway, electrically connecting the atria to the ventricles. But almost as importantly, it slows down the conduction on the average of 0.08 milliseconds. This delay allows the atria a little extra time to fill the ventricles with blood (the **atrial kick**) before the ventricles themselves begin to contract.

The third function of the AV node is to act as the secondary pacemaker for the heart. In the event that the sinus node or the conduction system of the atria fails, the AV node would begin to fire at a rate of 40–60 beats per minutes. Since these impulses would essentially "escape" from overdrive suppression, the resulting rhythm would be called an escape rhythm.

The atrioventricular node is a very complex structure in itself, accepted to be comprised of three functional areas. These areas are referred to as the AN (antinodal), N (nodal), and NH (nodal His) regions. It is believed that the conduction delay occurs within the N region. The accepted location of the secondary pacemaker is within the NH region, or the junction between the AV node and the bundle of His. Hence, it is called the AV junction, or junction for short. Any rhythm that originates from within this area is then referred to as a junctional rhythm. While the NH region is the accepted location of the pacemaker, studies have also shown that the AN region is also capable of producing pacemaker-like activity under certain conditions. Pacemaker activity from within this region could account for some beats out of sequence, or dysrhythmias. DOT 5-2.13

The AV node communicates with the bundle of His to allow the impulse to pass into the ventricles. The bundle itself functions as only a conduction fiber; however, if damaged, it may be the location of a conduction block.

The Bundle Branches

Once the impulses have traveled through the bundle of His, they bifurcate (or split) into the left and right bundle branches. These serve the purpose of quickly transmitting the impulse to the apex of the ventricles, insuring that the ventricles depolarize from the apex up, effectively "milking" the blood from the apex into the pulmonary artery and the aorta. Both bundle branches terminate in a network of small conduction fibers known as the purkinje network.

The right bundle branch transmits the electrical impulse into the right ventricle. Since this ventricle is relatively smaller than the left, the right bundle branch is also simpler. The left bundle branch actually bifurcates further into the **anterior and posterior fascicles.** The posterior fascicle is a broad and flat series of conduction fibers, not unlike a horse's tail. Because of the area it covers, it is only damaged in cases of extensive muscle damage.

The anterior fascicle runs anteriorly around the bicuspid valve and is more susceptible to damage during ischemic episodes. The left bundle branch is responsible for the depolarization of the **myocardial septum,** which is the wall between the chambers.

The Purkinje Network

The bundle branches terminate in a network of conduction fibers called the purkinje network. These fibers have the responsibility of dispersing the impulse through the remainder of the myocardium and up the outer walls. The purkinje fibers are also capable of acting as the third and final primary pacemaker site. These cells depolarize at an intrinsic rate of 20–40 beats per minute. Since this is the third pacemaker site, the other two pacemaker sites must have failed before it activates, or the conduction between the atria and ventricles must have been interrupted. This may either be at the level of the AV node or the bundle branches.

The Electrocardiogram

We have described how the heart relies upon an orderly depolarization to work properly. Unfortunately this does not always happen. In the 1800s, Dr. Wilhem Einthoven captured the electrical activity of the heart. For the first time, physicians were able to visualize the electrical impulse as it traveled through the heart. Equipment has improved since then, but the principles he developed are still important to this day.

Early electrocardiography was based upon three points of connections or electrodes. The ECG monitor measures the relationship between these electrodes two at a time. The combination of a negative and positive electrode is called a lead. The remaining electrode serves as a ground to help improve the appearance of the tracing. The ECG monitor measures the flow of electricity that is occurring between a negative and positive electrode over time, giving a graphic portrayal of the movement of electricity through the heart. DOT 5-2.31, 5-2.32, 5-2.33, 5-2.34, 5-2.36

Early studies used a series of three limb leads, called leads I, II, and III. Einthoven discovered a relationship between these leads, which became known as **Einthoven's triangle** (Figure 29-28). The relationship can be expressed

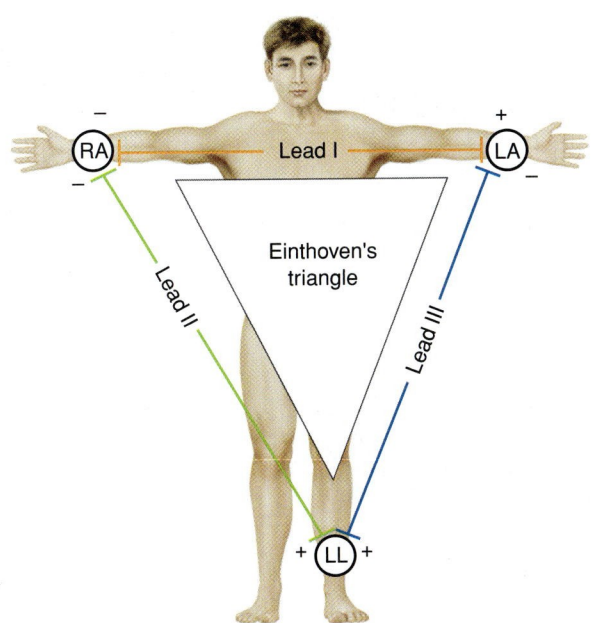

Figure 29-28   Einthoven's triangle.

several principals that dictate the most reliable location for lead placement. First, the farther away one gets from the heart, the more attenuated (dispersed) the electrical signal becomes, resulting in a smaller ECG size. Second, all muscles create electrical impulses. So, the farther away from the heart the leads are placed, the more other muscle tissue's electrical activity creates interference (called artifact) with the accuracy of the ECG tracing. Since each lead records electrical activity between a negative and positive pole, placing the leads in different locations will cause them to look slightly different. To minimize the effect of all these factors, standardized lead placement has been developed. There are almost endless possibilities for these leads, each with its own specific purpose, but the discussion will begin with six limb leads and six precordial, or chest, leads. Together these result in 12 distinct views of the heart from different angles and directions.

Looking closer at an ECG lead, there are three rules that dictate an ECG's appearance (Figure 29-29):

1. All electrical impulses traveling toward a positive lead will result in an upright deflection (or waveform) on the ECG pattern.
2. All electrical impulses traveling away from the positive lead will result in a negative deflection of the ECG pattern.
3. Electrical impulses traveling perpendicular to the lead will result in a biphasic pattern with equal

mathematically as the electrical summation of current in lead I plus lead III is equal to the sum of the current measured in lead II. This relationship will be discussed a little later. However, these three leads are still used today.

Electrical energy is conducted throughout the body. Therefore, the electrical activity of the heart could theoretically be picked up anywhere on the body. There are

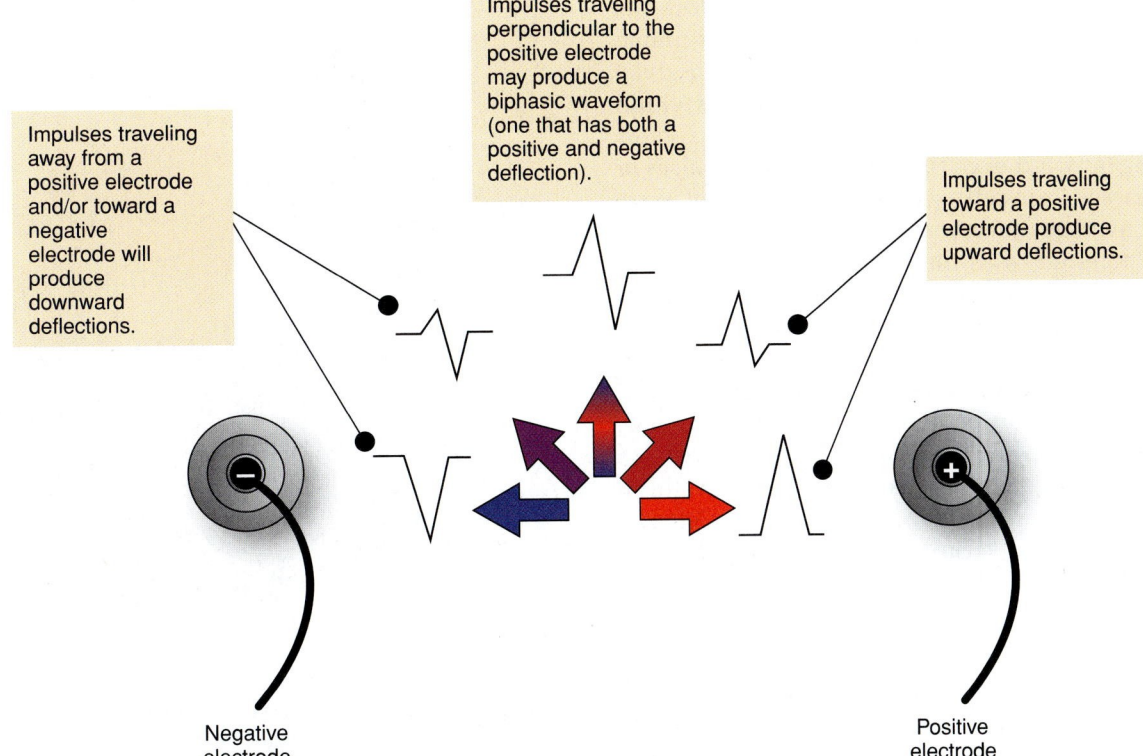

Figure 29-29   ECG pattern resulting from different vectors.

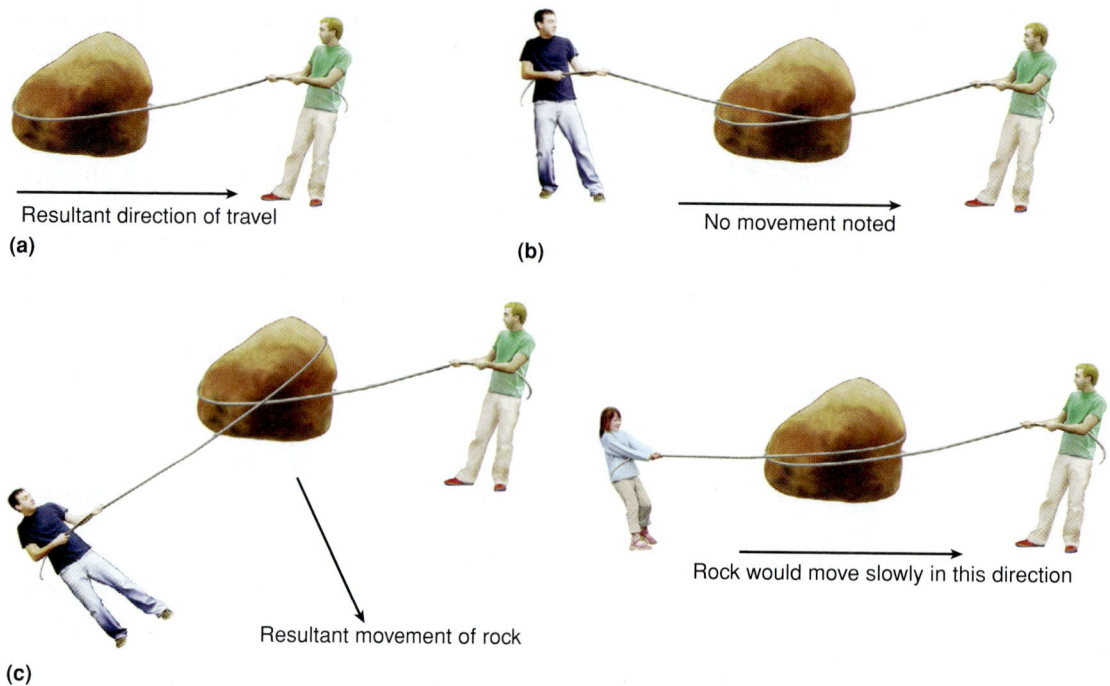

Resultant direction of travel
(a)

No movement noted
(b)

Resultant movement of rock
(c)

Rock would move slowly in this direction

Figure 29-30 (a) Force applied to the rock in one direction will move it in that direction. (b) Two equal and opposing forces will cancel each other. No resultant directional flow is measured. (c) Unequal opposing forces will cancel each other to some extent but will result in movement toward the larger force.

deflection both positive and negative. This may also appear as a flat line on the ECG. The flatline on the ECG is also called the **isoelectric line.**

As the current travels through the heart, it moves in many different directions. Some impulses are stronger than others while some go toward the positive electrode and some go away (Figure 29-30). The ECG is the summation of all these impulses, referred to as **vectors,** at a given period of time. Since the impulse usually originates within the SA node in the upper portion of the right atria, vectors begin moving outward from there. While the impulses or vectors are passed from cell to cell in every direction, there is a mean or average movement of the electrical impulse. This is also referred to as the resultant force or axis of electrical flow (Figure 29-31). Simply stated, the electrical impulse generally starts at the base of the heart and propagates to the apex then back up the outer walls. The greatest amount of current would be flowing toward the apex. The **electrical axis** of the heart may be influenced by size, position, and pathophysiology of the heart (Figure 29-32). Knowing the electrical axis of the heart can be useful in identifying anterior or posterior hemiblocks. The electrical axis of the heart is determined by examining the limb leads. It will be covered in more detail later.

The Limb Leads

Limb leads get their name because of the standard placement of the lead on each of the limbs (Figure 29-33). The limbs afford a very standard placement for the leads because they are always attached at the same place, no matter who places the electrodes. On any part of the limb, it will always appear electrically as if the electrodes are located on the hips or shoulders. Remember that the farther you get from the heart, the

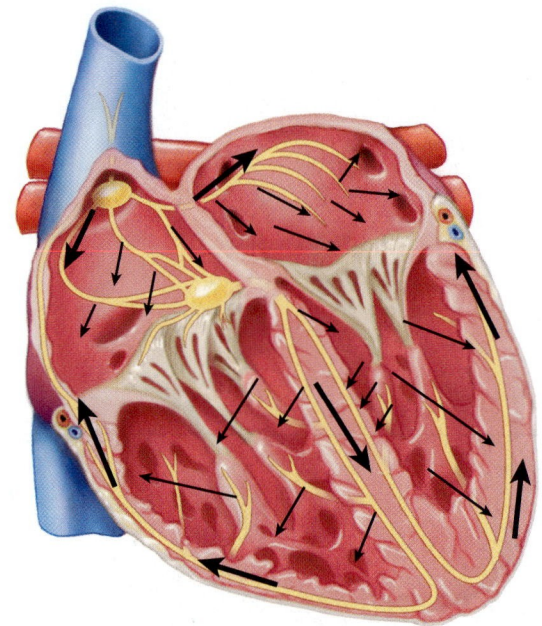

Figure 29-31 Impulses travel through the heart in many directions. The summation of all these impulses results in a mean directional flow of electricity. This resultant flow is called the electrical axis of the heart.

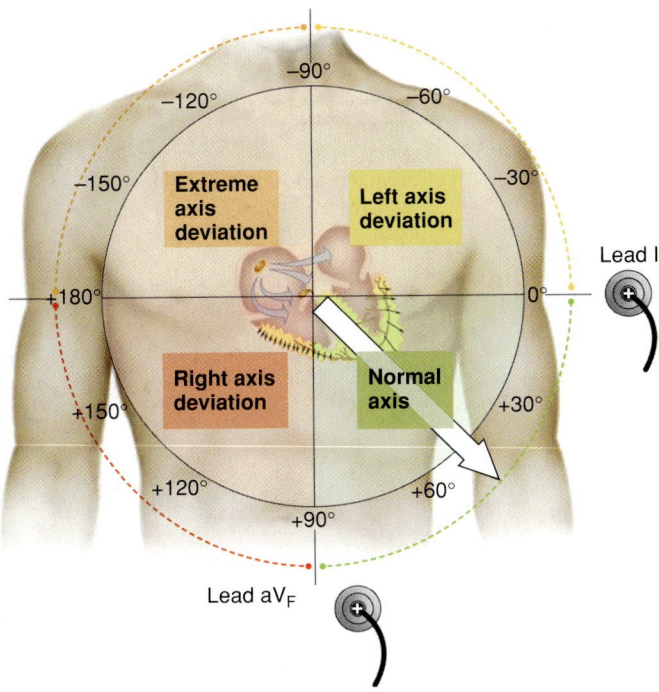

Figure 29-32 Diagram of heart axis.

smaller the signal and higher the risk of muscle artifact. Therefore, placements on the upper arms and thigh are beneficial. To minimize artifact even further, and to eliminate artifact from arm or leg movement, electrodes can be placed on the upper chest and anterior lower thorax. When placed in this location, they are still referred to as limb leads even though they are now on the

trunk of the body. The most important rule in electrode placement is consistent placement. Bony prominences may make good landmarks, but they often result in increased muscle artifact.

There are six limb leads commonly used today: leads, I, II, and III, the traditional leads, and aV_L, aV_R, and aV_F. The latter three are called augmented leads because their signal is so small; they must be amplified or augmented by the monitor in order to be visualized. Leads I, II, and III are called bipolar leads because they require at least two electrodes, one reading negative and one reading positive to obtain their reading. Lead I is created by placing the negative electrode (typically white in color) on the right arm and the positive electrode (red) on the left arm. There is a ground wire (black) usually located on the left leg. Lead II is created by keeping the negative electrode on the right shoulder but putting the positive lead on the left leg, and the ground moves up to the left shoulder. Lead III is then created by placing the negative lead on the left shoulder and keeping the positive lead on the left leg while the ground moves up to the right shoulder.

This all seems kind of confusing, so ECG monitors are designed to move the electrodes around internally, based upon a switch or lead selection button. All that is necessary is to correctly place the electrodes as they are labeled. RA for right arm, LA for left arm, and LL for left leg. Lead II is the most commonly used lead for general rhythm monitoring because it usually gives the tallest ECG complex and also because it observes the impulse traveling "down" through the conduction pathway.

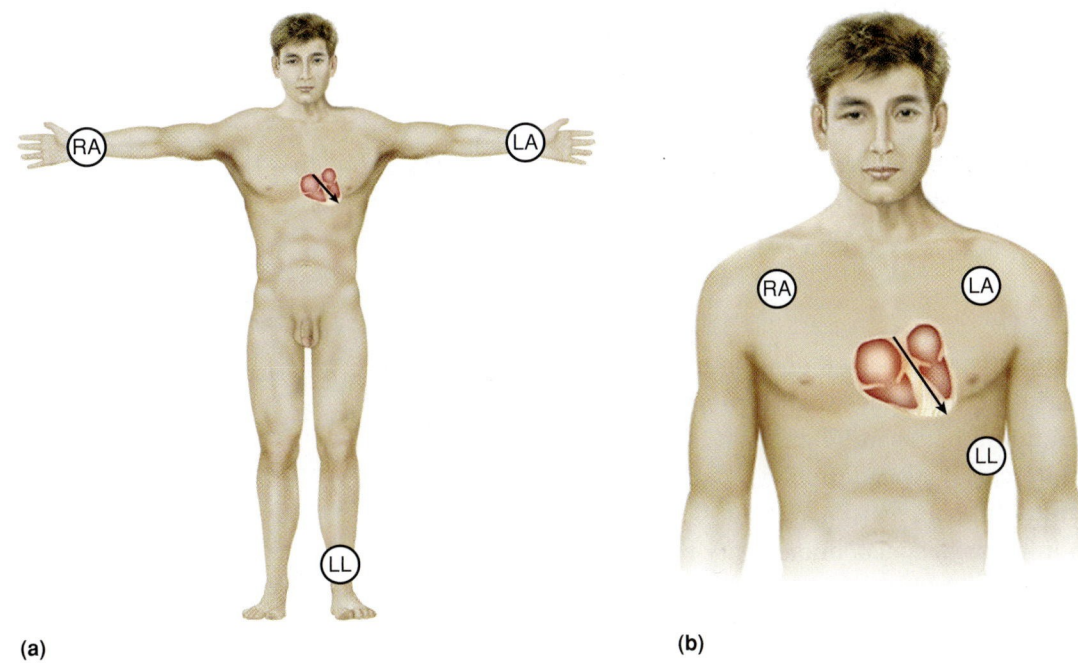

(a)   (b)

Figure 29-33 Limb leads.

To be able to monitor the augmented leads, a fourth electrode is required. This electrode is placed on the right leg, is labeled RL, and is typically green in color. As mentioned earlier, the augmented leads have a very tiny electrical signal on their own, so they are amplified. Primarily, this is because they are calculated leads (Figure 29-34). The ECG monitor uses three electrodes to calculate the center or average in the leads to create the ground electrode. By using the average of the electrical potential, the negative electrode is placed approximately in the middle of the heart. Once again, by internal switching in the monitor, three more views electrically of the heart can be obtained.

The limb leads are useful for looking at specific areas of the heart and determining electrical axis. But they assume that the heart is a one-dimensional organ, thin as paper. Since the heart is a three-dimensional organ, other leads are needed to create a full picture of the heart.

The Precordial Leads

To get a better view of the heart as a three-dimensional object, six more leads are added to the standard ECG analysis. These, in conjunction with the six limb leads, create the standard 12-lead ECG. The precordial leads get their name because of their placement around the heart on the chest. The precordial leads are also known as unipolar leads because, just as in the augmented leads, the negative component is calculated using three limb leads. Once again, this puts the negative electrode roughly in the middle of the heart.

These leads must be properly placed to achieve consistency and to be able to compare one 12-lead ECG to the next. Poorly placed leads will render the tracing worthless when compared to another ECG taken with proper lead placement. The precordial leads are labeled as V1, V2, V3, V4, V5, and V6. Figure 29-35 shows proper lead placement on the chest.

V Lead Placement

- V1 = fourth intercostal space R of sternum
- V2 = fourth intercostal space L of sternum
- V3 = the midpoint between V2 and V4
- V4 = fifth intercostal space, midclavicular line
- V5 = the midpoint between V4 and V6
- V6 = sixth intercostal space, midaxillary line

To properly place the leads on the chest, utilize landmarks on the chest. V1 should be placed to the right of the sternum at the fourth intercostal space

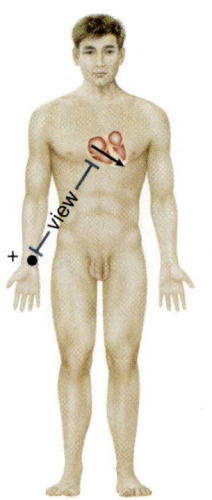

Impulses moving away from the positive lead.

(a) Lead aV_R

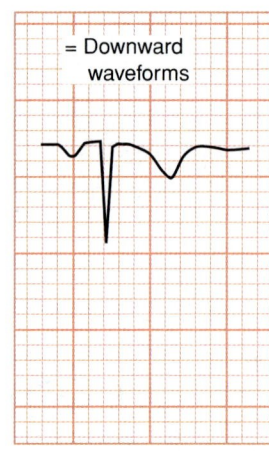

= Downward waveforms

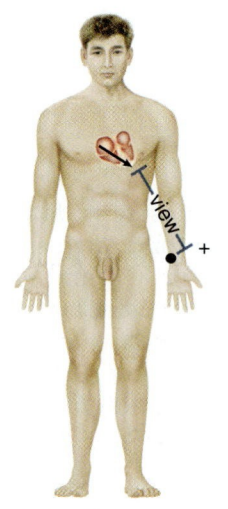

Impulses moving toward the positive lead.

(b) Lead aV_L

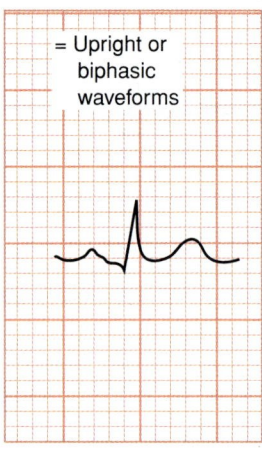

= Upright or biphasic waveforms

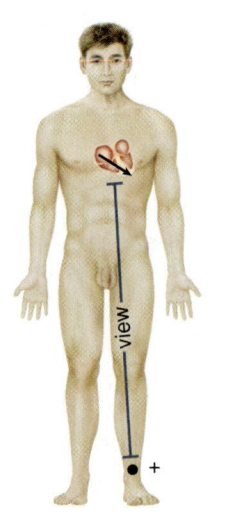

Impulses moving toward the positive lead.

(c) Lead aV_F

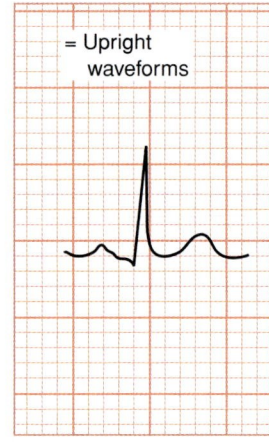

= Upright waveforms

Figure 29-34 Augmented leads.

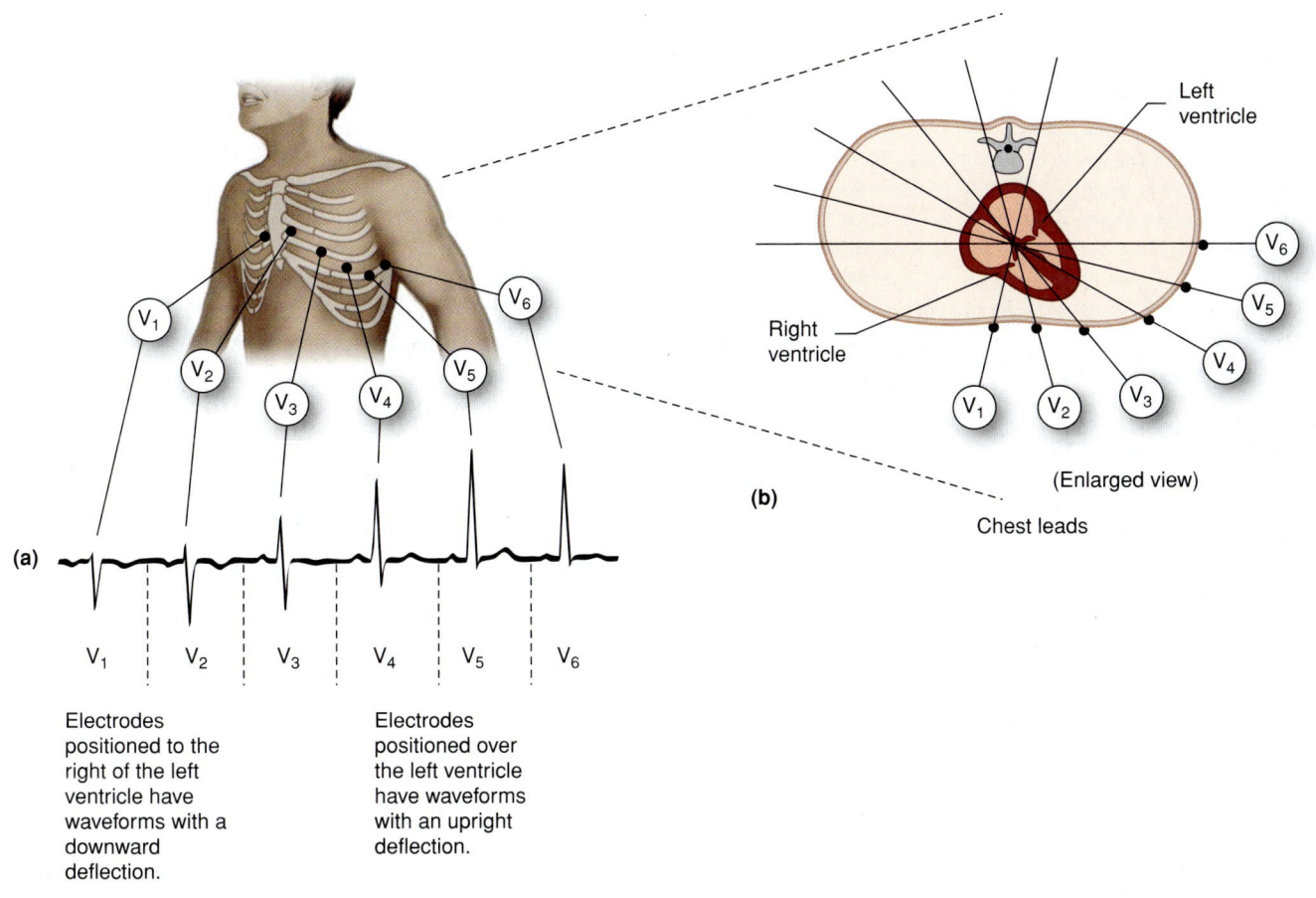

(a)

V₁ ┊ V₂ ┊ V₃ ┊ V₄ ┊ V₅ ┊ V₆

Electrodes positioned to the right of the left ventricle have waveforms with a downward deflection.

Electrodes positioned over the left ventricle have waveforms with an upright deflection.

Figure 29-35   Precordial lead placement.

(Figure 29-36). You may find the fourth intercostal space by locating the angle of Louis or sternal angle where the manubrium meets the sternal body. At this point, the second rib is attached to the sternum. Once you find the second rib, the second intercostal space is right below it. Count down two more spaces to the fourth space. The fourth intercostal space is also closely associated with the average nipple line. V2 is located directly across from V1, just to the left of the sternum. V4 is located in the fifth intercostal space, midclavicular line. You then locate V3 at the midpoint between V2 and V4. V6 is placed in the sixth intercostal space, midaxillary line, and V5 is placed at the midpoint between V6 and V4.

If your patient is female, leads should be placed as close as possible to the correct position beneath the breast. If placed over the breast, the fatty tissues can shift, resulting in inaccurate placement, and the tracing will not be as strong as the impulse will have to travel through too much tissue.

For general cardiac monitoring, often only the limb leads are used with either three or four electrodes. The optional electrode in this case is the right leg. The limb leads configured properly for lead II are all that is required for rhythm identification. However, limb leads

are notorious for rounding off electrical patterns, often making them difficult to read. By examining the precordial leads (V1 through V6) along with the limb leads, the accuracy of interpretation is improved.

The ECG Monitor

The ECG monitor is a device designed to measure and graphically display the movement of electricity through the body. It is capable of monitoring several leads simultaneously and displaying the pattern on a screen.

The ECG monitor does not display any mechanical activity. This is determined through assessment of the level of consciousness, pulse, and blood pressure.

When no electrical activity is detected, the monitor screen and any paper tracing will show a flat, isoelectric line. As mentioned earlier, when a specific lead is monitored, any electric activity moving toward the positive electrode will cause the line to be deflected positively, or upward. Conversely, any current measured moving away from the positive electrode causes the line to be deflected negatively, or downward. Essentially, the ECG

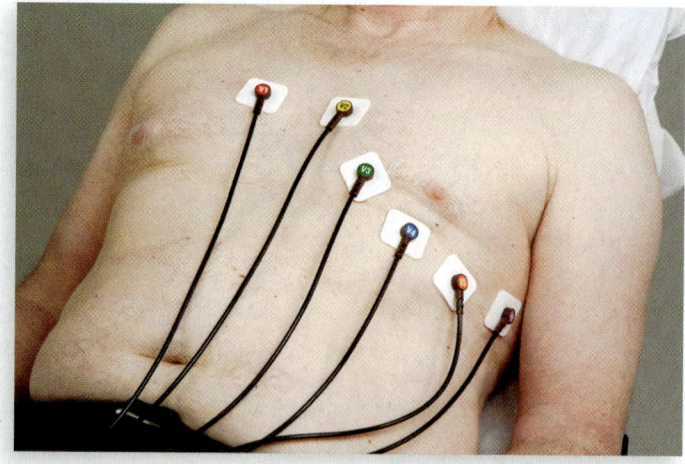

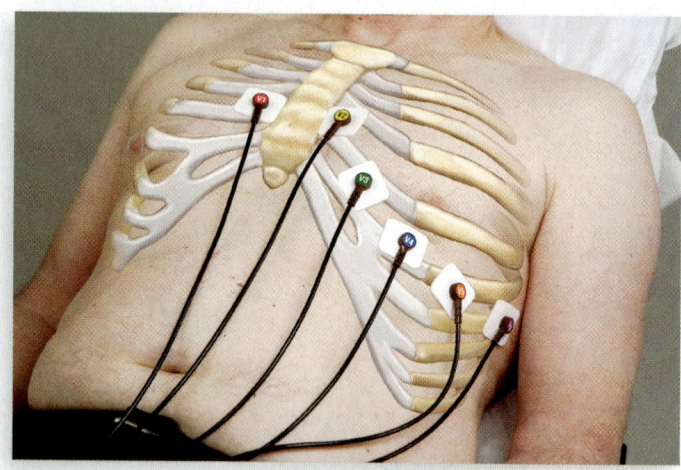

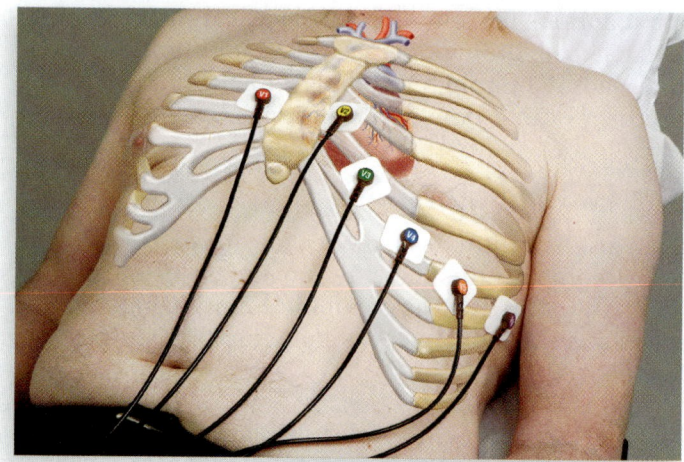

Figure 29-36   Proper placement of leads on the chest.

pattern is simply electrical current measured over a given time frame.

This activity is printed out on paper specifically designed for that purpose. ECG paper is graph paper with 1 millimeter markings (Figure 29-37). The paper is fed out of the ECG at exactly 25 millimeters per second. The horizontal axis of the paper measures time in

milliseconds while the vertical axis measures electrical amplitude in mVolts. The paper is further marked every 5 millimeters in both directions, with darker or thicker lines. Five small boxes equals the length of one big box.

These standardized markings are used to measure both timing and amplitude of the wave patterns. At 25 mm/sec, each 1 mm (one small box long) represents 0.04 seconds of time, and each larger box, or 5 mm, represents 0.20 seconds. Therefore, a waveform lasting the length of three little boxes would have lasted for 0.12 seconds.

The vertical axis is the amplitude of the electrical current. In the standard ECG, one small box (1 mm tall) equals 0.1 mV of current. One big box or 5 mm equals 0.5 mV of current. A standardized ECG monitor must deflect two large boxes or 10 mm when a current of 1 mV is introduced into the system. All modern ECG monitors automatically set this during the start-up procedures. Older models can be tested by depressing a button that marks the ECG tracing, which can then be counted to determine if it is calibrated accurately.

Through the use of these standardized markings on the ECG tracing, heart rate is determined as well as how long it takes for current to travel through a given area of the heart, and how much current is actually being measured.

Always remember that the ECG is not perfect. It measures all electrical activity in the body although this is minimized by a series of filters (Figure 29-38). **Muscle artifact** was discussed earlier, but there are other kinds of interference as well (Figure 29-39). Two other common types of artifact include **loose leads** and **60 cycle-interference.** Sixty cycle-interference is caused by proximity to other electrical devices.

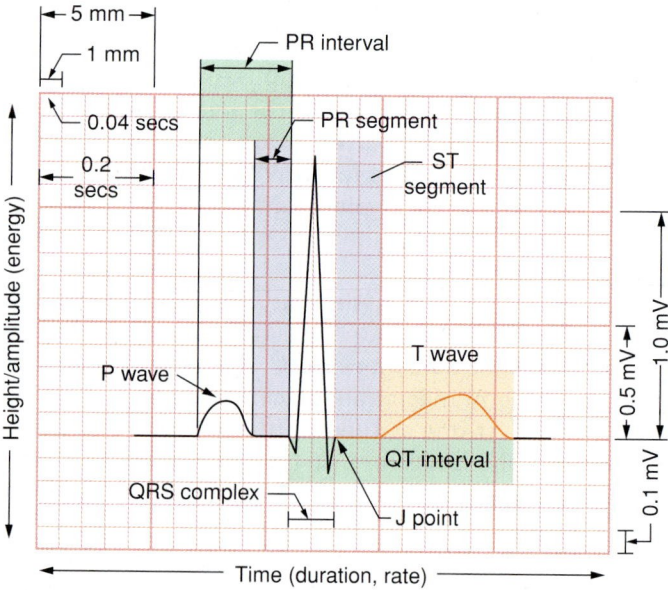

Figure 29-37   ECG complex.

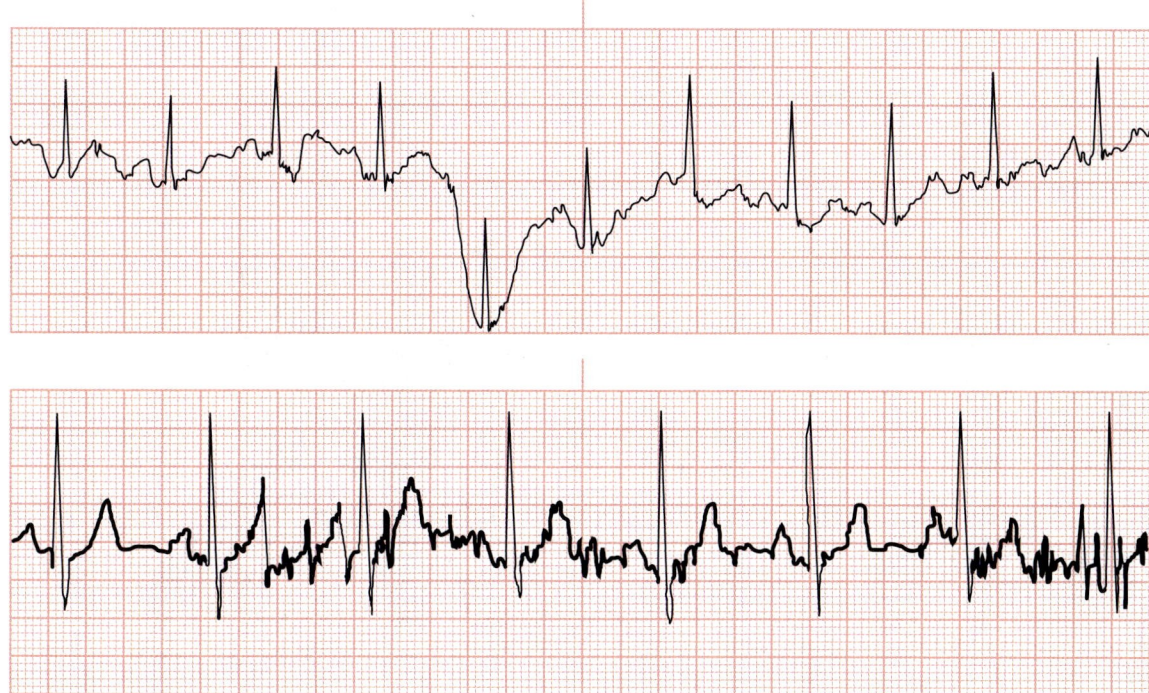

Figure 29-38   Muscle artifact.

Practical Points for Recording an ECG[7]

- Ensure effective contact between the electrode and skin
  - Electrodes should not be outdated
  - Electrolyte gel or paste should be fresh
  - Skin should be dry
  - The site of lead placement should be free of excessive amounts of hair and dead skin cells (Consider shaving hair and abrading the skin lightly to ensure good contact with living tissue)
- Recording techniques and placement should be consistent
- The position of the patient is important; the patient should be lying flat or in a 30-degree, head up position called semi-Fowler's and should remain motionless while the 12-lead tracing is being acquired

The ECG Wave Pattern

For simplicity in this introduction to the ECG waveform, lead II will be used as the primary lead, which is the standard lead used in ECG interpretation. Remember that in lead II, the negative electrode is on the right arm while the positive electrode is on the left leg. Given the position of the heart within the chest, this placement looks "down" the conduction pathway.

Also remember that any impulse traveling toward the positive electrode will result in a positive deflection of the wave above the isoelectric line, and any impulse traveling towards the negative electrode will result in a negative waveform below the isoelectric line. All waves return to the isoelectric line when they are finished.

The P Wave

The first deflection noted with the start of the cardiac cycle is called the **P wave** (Figure 29-40). It identifies atrial depolarization and shows the impulse originating in the sinus node. As the impulse begins to spread out

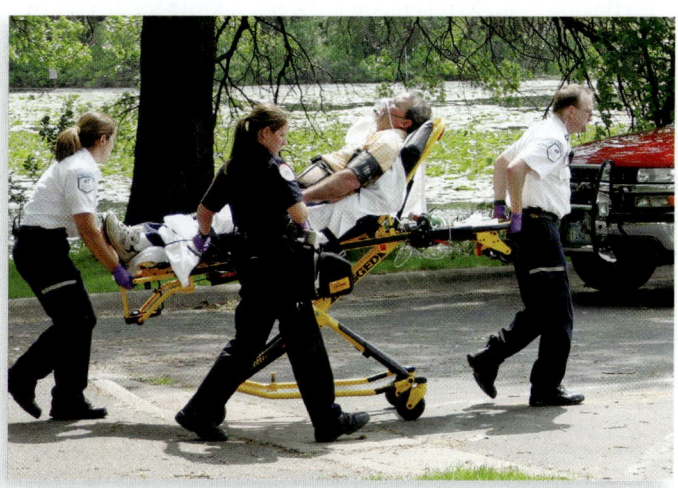

Figure 29-39   Moving patients interferes with an ECG.

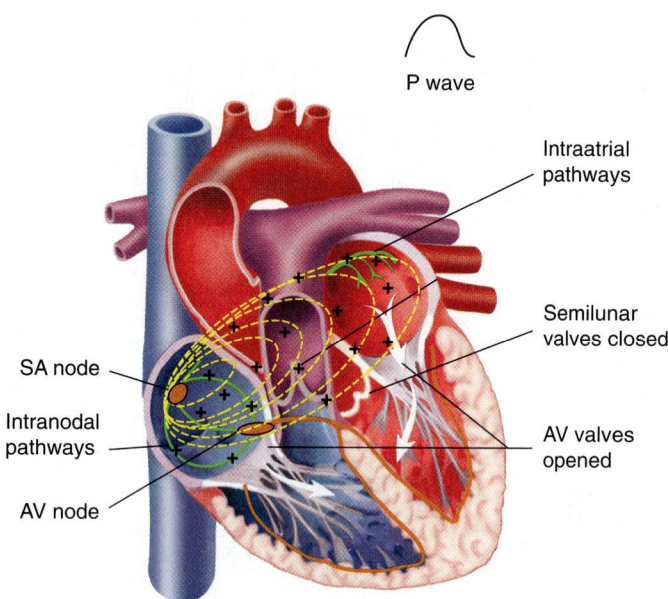

Figure 29-40   Formation of the P wave during atrial depolarizaiton.

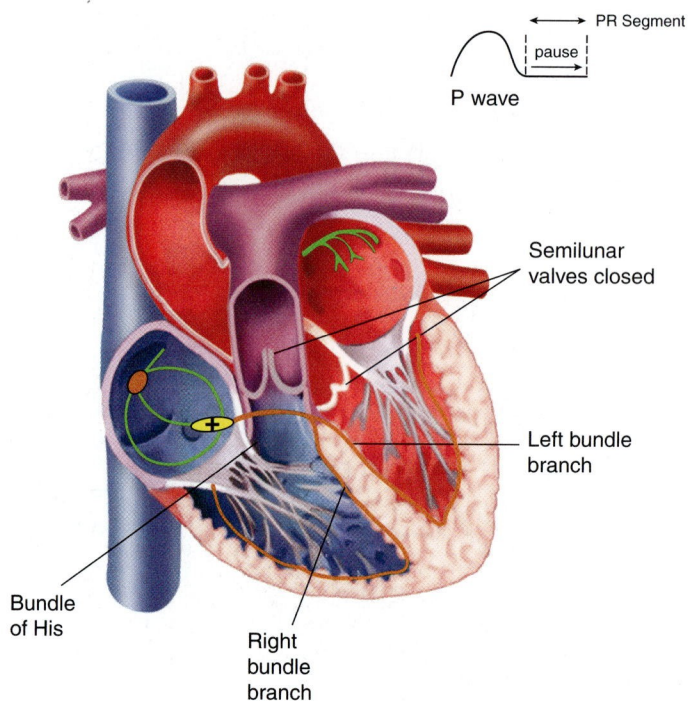

Figure 29-42   PR segment occurs on the egg as impulse is delayed in the AV node.

to depolarize the atria, electrical movement is detected traveling towards the positive electrode. The electrical current travels down the internodal pathway from the SA node to the AV node. This results in a positive deflection beginning on the ECG. As the atrial depolarization is completed, the electrical impulse subsides, and the ECG pattern is returned to the isoelectric line.

The P wave is usually upright and rounded in lead II, but in other leads it may be inverted or biphasic. The duration is 0.10 seconds or less and is rarely over 2 mm high (Figure 29-41). Abnormal P waves are over 2.5 mm in amplitude, in which case it is called P-pulmonale and may be associated with respiratory problems. This P wave is usually peaked instead of rounded. In cases where the left and right atria are depolarizing at slightly different times, or one is larger than the other, the P wave may take on a notched appearance.[8]

A "normal" P wave is generally assumed to originate from the sinus node. In some cases, it may come from another location within the atria. This would be called an ectopic P wave. Ectopic beats originate away from the normal conduction pathway, or they occur out of sequence of the normal process. This P wave may have an unusual appearance, such as be longer in duration, peaked, or notched, and may be slightly closer to the QRS complex.

P to R Segment

The impulse has now reached the AV node, and, as you recall, one of the duties of the AV node is to slow down the impulse to allow the ventricles to finish filling. This slow down is represented by an isoelectric line approximately 0.08 seconds long (2 small boxes). Since no electrical impulses are detected during this time, the line should be straight. This line is called the **PR segment** (Figure 29-42). The PR segment may be shorter if the P wave comes from an ectopic site.

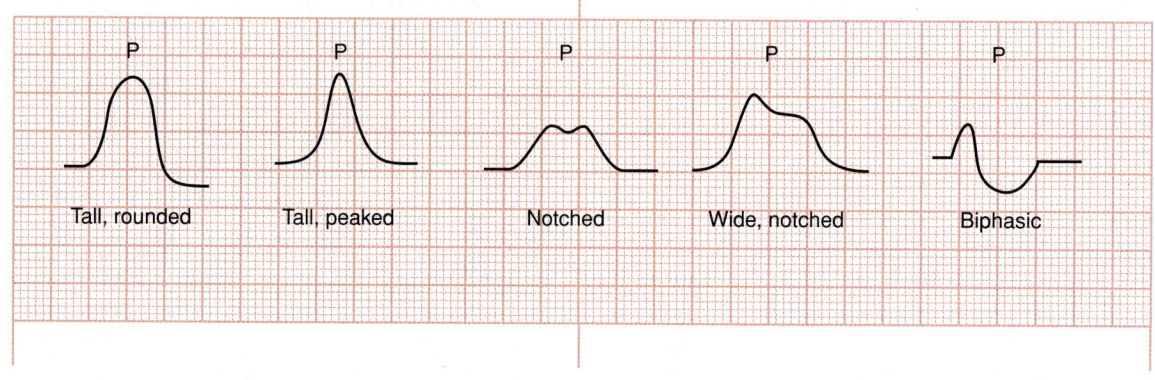

Figure 29-41   Different shapes of P waves.

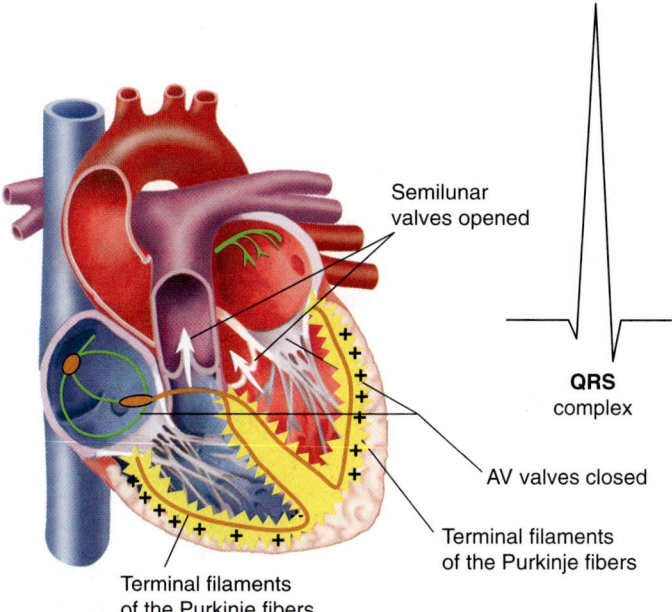

Semilunar
valves opened

QRS
complex

AV valves closed

Terminal filaments
of the Purkinje fibers

Terminal filaments
of the Purkinje fibers

Figure 29-43   Formation of the QRS complex.

The PR Interval

The **PR interval (PRI)** is calculated by adding the time from the beginning of the P wave to the end of the PR segment. This interval normally measures between 0.12 and 0.2 seconds in duration. This interval is very important and will serve as one of the measurements used to name rhythms captured by the ECG tracing. Usually, any PRI of less than 0.2 seconds (one large box) with an upright P wave is considered "normal."

The QRS Complex

The **QRS complex** represents depolarization of the right and left ventricles (Figure 29-43). The electrical waveform usually travels very quickly down the pathway though the ventricles to the apex of the heart, finishing within 0.12 seconds (three small boxes).

The components of the QRS complex are the Q wave, R wave, and S wave. The Q wave is the first negative deflection from the isoelectric line. It is not necessarily seen with every person or in every lead. The R wave is the first positive deflection from the isoelectric line. The S wave is the first negative deflection after the R wave, and it terminates when it returns to the isoelectric line.

Not all waves need be present in the QRS complex. A wave form called the QS wave consists entirely of a single negative deflection; however, it is still usually referred to as a QRS complex. A QRS complex may also contain extra waves such as a second upright wave after the original R wave. This wave is referred to as the R prime wave and is usually designated by r′. QRS complexes may also exhibit a notching in the waveform, usually caused by a conduction defect or off timing

between the left and right ventricles. More of the abnormalities associated with QRS complexes will be discussed later.

Examining the QRS formation in greater detail, the impulse originating in the SA node has reached the AV node, where it paused. Now continue to trace the impulse as it travels through the AV node, reaching the bundle of His and the bundle branches. As the impulse hits the left bundle branch, the septum begins to depolarize, and once again, some electrical movement is detected by the monitor. Since the left bundle branch depolarizes the ventricular septum, the impulses travel across the septum to the right bundle branch. The result is a very tiny deflection away from the positive electrode called a Q wave. This wave is usually so small it often is not seen at all. Other forms of the Q wave will be discussed when the 12-lead ECG is examined.

The impulse rapidly spreads down the bundle branches, and the largest part of the heart begins to depolarize. As this impulse spreads downward through the heart, the electrodes detect a large current traveling towards the positive electrode, resulting in a positive deflection of the isoelectric line called the R wave. Now the impulse has depolarized most of the heart, but the purkinje network is still spreading the impulse to the outer wall of the heart from the apex. Because the current is traveling away from the positive lead, it results in a negative deflection of the isoelectric line.

In review, the P wave reflects atrial depolarization, the PR segment relates to the slowdown in the AV node for ventricular filling, and Q, R, and S waves result from ventricular depolarization.

Each waveform identifies a distinct event occurring in the cardiac cycle: The P equals atrial depolarization, and the QRS equals ventricular depolarization. During depolarization of the QRS, the atria are undergoing repolarization. Due to the magnitude of the forces during ventricular depolarization, the atrial repolarization is seen only under rare conditions. Remember that what you see in an ECG complex is the result of millions of tiny vectors occurring at a specific point in time, adding up to a resultant flow of current. For example, an impulse that would deflect the ECG positive at least 5 mm may occur at the same instant a negative impulse with amplitude of −2 mm formed. The result would be waveform with a positive deflection of no more than 3 mm.

The T Wave

The normal **T wave** represents the repolarization of the ventricles (Figure 29-44). Normally, we are only concerned about the height, shape, and direction of the T wave. The ventricles repolarize from the epicardium inward, the reverse of the depolarization process.[8] This phenomenon is believed to be caused by the pressure

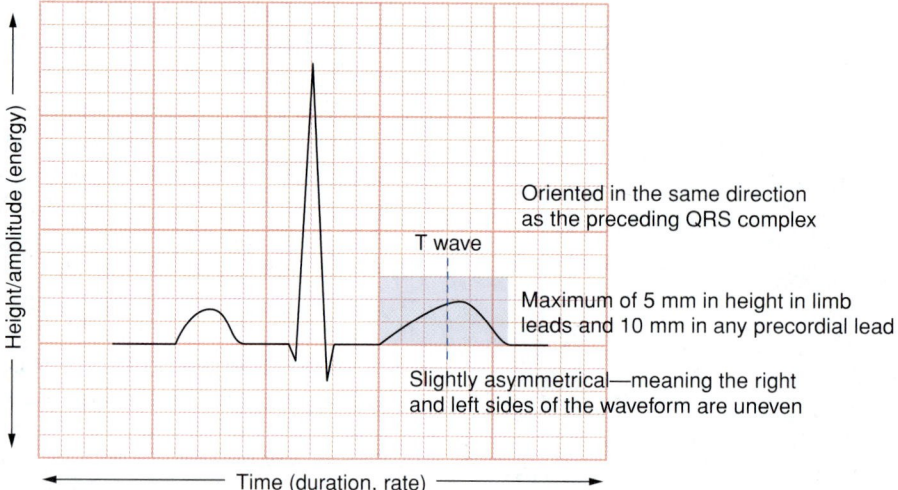

Figure 29-44 T wave following ST segment.

in the heart during contraction, inhibiting the repolarization from the endocardial layer. The normal direction of the T wave is upright and 0.10 to 0.25 seconds in duration.[8] The normal T wave is also asymmetrical and slightly rounded (Figure 29-45).

An abnormal T wave is usually associated with abnormal ventricular depolarization and usually is the result of myocardial ischemia, infarction, myocarditis, pericarditis, ventricular hypertrophy, or electrolyte imbalance.[8] The appearance of an abnormal T wave may be inverted, tall and peaked, or biphasic. DOT 5-2.46 and 5-2.48

The segment between the S wave and the T wave is known as the **ST segment** (Figure 29-46). The point at which the S wave ends is called the **J point.** This area will be very important when reading the 12-lead ECG.

The J point can be difficult to determine in some leads, especially lead II. For now, its position relative to the baseline and its general shape are the main concerns.

The QT Interval

The **QT interval** is the time represented from the start of the QRS complex to the end of the T wave (Figure 29-47). In other words, it represents complete ventricular activity. The QT interval is rate dependant; it gets longer as a rate gets slower. For that reason, it is not significant in initial rhythm interpretation. It is discussed here only to provide a more complete picture of the ECG's cardiac cycle, and once basic rhythm interpretation is attained, this information should be added to your understanding of the waveforms.

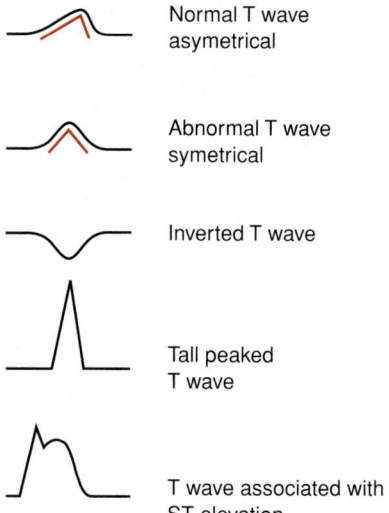

Figure 29-45 Common shapes seen in the T wave. Remember that abnormal depolarization results in abnormal repolarization. Tall, peaked T waves may be the result of early infarction or hyperkalemia.

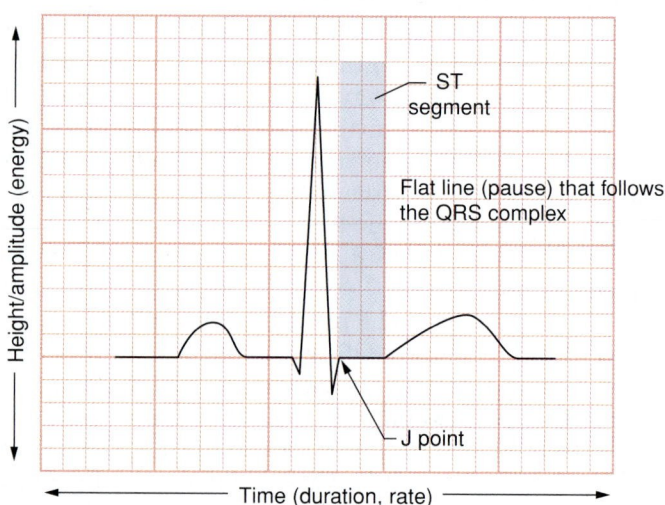

Figure 29-46 ST segment at the J point.

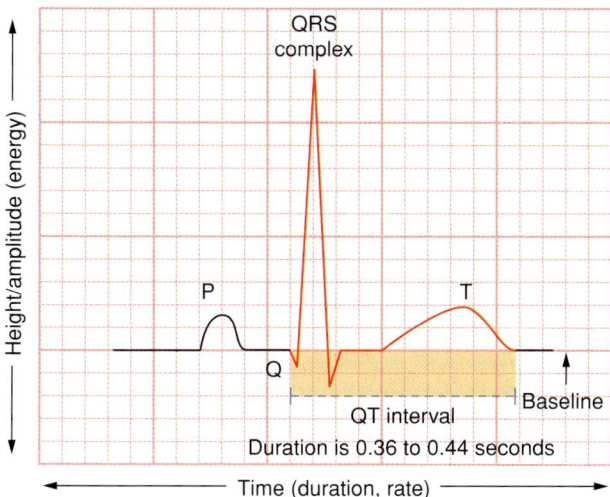

Figure 29-47   QT interval.

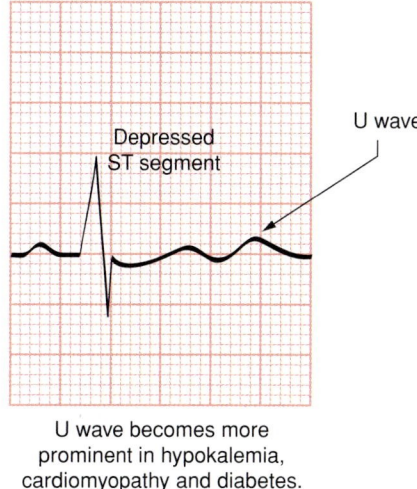

Figure 29-48   U wave.

The QT interval length will be an important measurement due to its prolongation from the use of antidysrhythmic drugs such as quinidine, procainamide, and disopyramide. Lengthening of the QT interval may indicate the heart is at risk to develop a malignant polymorphic ventricular tachycardia called Torsade de Pointes. (This will be discussed later in the chapter.)

You may see a corrected QT interval listed on 12-lead ECG tracings. This is calculated by the computer within the monitor and is reported for interpretation purposes. Because the interval is rate dependant, researchers have noted that the QT interval varies with the square root of the cycle length (Bazett's formula).[11] The actual normal measurement remains under investigation.

As a general rule, the QT interval should not be more than one-half of the R to R interval. To check this, measure out a QT interval with your calipers. Then, without moving the point on the right, rotate the calipers over; the next point of contact should fall before the next QRS starts. If it goes beyond the start of the next QRS, the QT interval is probably prolonged and warrants further investigation by a cardiologist.

The U Wave

It is believed that the **U wave** represents the final stage of ventricular repolarization although it is not commonly seen (Figure 29-48).[8] Some have thought that it signifies the repolarization of the papillary muscles attached to the cordae tendinae or the purkinje system.[7] The U wave is usually upright and immediately follows the T wave. The amplitude is normally under 2 mm and of little importance, but abnormally tall U waves may be present in hypokalemia, cardiomyopathy, and diabetes and on some occasions may be associated with administration of certain antidysrhythmic medications.[8,9]

Reading the Electrocardiogram

When beginning to read ECGs, it is vital that you remember what an ECG will tell you and what it will not tell you. DOT 5-2.36

An ECG can tell you

- How long it takes an impulse to travel through each part of the heart
- The electrical heart rate
- The regularity of the rhythm

An ECG cannot tell you

- If the heart is responding to the electrical impulse (in other words, actually contracting)
- How strong the heart is pumping

It is, therefore, extremely important to remember to verify anything you see on the ECG monitor with your patient's condition. Remember the old saying, "Treat your patient, not the monitor."

There are a few ECG patterns you will learn to identify by sight, such as the life-threatening dysrhythmias. This will come after you learn a systematic approach to rhythm interpretation. Some rhythms can be difficult, and not every rhythm you will encounter falls into a defined pattern. For every ECG, you should train yourself to identify the rhythms by following this five-step process:

1. Rate
2. Rhythm (including the presence of ectopic beats)
3. Presence and shape of the P wave and its relationship to the QRS
4. PR interval
5. QRS complex

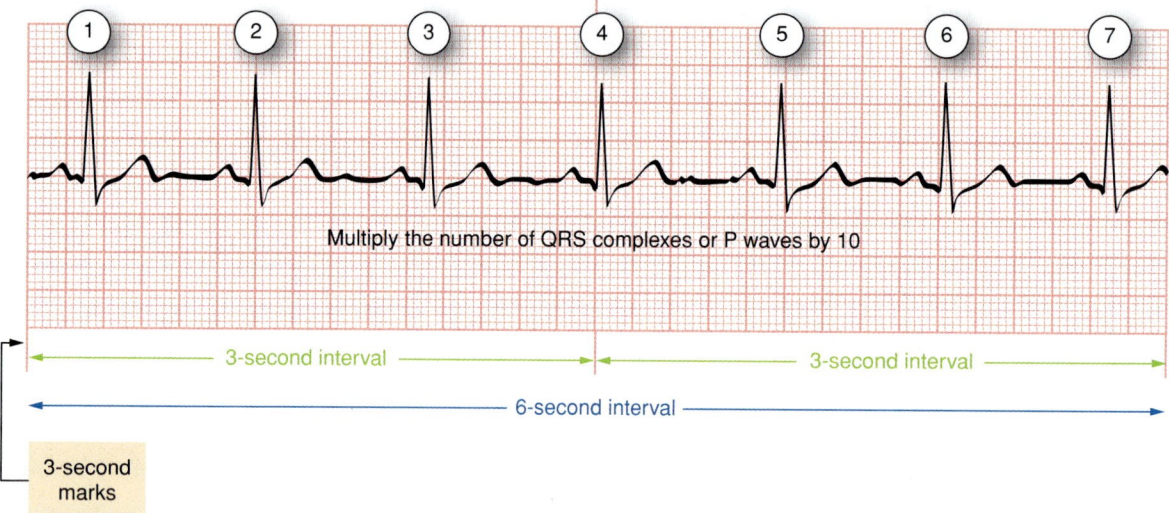

Multiply the number of QRS complexes or P waves by 10

3-second interval

3-second interval

6-second interval

3-second marks

Figure 29-49 Six second method.

Following these five steps will ensure that you don't miss anything and make an incorrect reading.

Rate

Most modern ECG monitors will give you a fairly accurate reading regarding the heart rate. They will even print it out on the paper. However, there can be problems with this. The heart rate displayed by your monitor is a calculated rate with at least a three-second delay. It counts only the QRS complexes since these are the ones that indicate ventricular depolarization, which correlate to mechanical contractions and pulse beats when everything is functioning normally. But because the machine reads electrical impulses that look like QRS complexes, it often can add artifact into the count. In some instances, not every beat that shows up on the ECG is actually perfusing (resulting in a heart beat) through the body.

> You must learn to check your patient's pulse rate and then compare that to the ECG rate from the tracing.

There are four acceptable methods to calculate heart rate from the ECG tracing: the six-second strip method, two counting methods, the triplicate method, and using rate meters.

The Six-Second Strip Method

ECG paper, as we already learned, is marked off in 1-mm (small) boxes and 5-mm (large) boxes. ECG paper is also marked off in three-second and six-second intervals. These markings are typically noted at the top or bottom of the ECG paper. Fifteen large boxes equals three seconds of time, and 30 large boxes equals six seconds (Figure 29-49).

The easiest method to estimate heart rate is to count the number of complexes contained within a six second strip and multiply that number by 10.[7] This method only really works for regular or very slightly irregular rhythms.

The 300 and 1500 Counting Methods

For regular or slightly irregular rhythms, and when the three- or six-second markings may not be visible, you can estimate the heart rate by identifying the R waves of two consecutive complexes, counting the number of large (5-mm) boxes between them, and dividing that number into 300. For even more accuracy, count the number of small (1-mm) boxes between the R waves, and divide that number into 1500 (Figure 29-50). You don't have to count all the little boxes, as you know, each larger box has five smaller boxes. Simply count the number of little boxes in the last partial bigger box and add the rest. Neither of these counting methods work very well with irregular rhythms.

The Triplicate Method

The triplicate method requires a regular rhythm (Figure 29-51). It works the best when an R wave falls directly on a heavy, vertical line in a large box. Once mastered, this method can be used going either forward or backwards on the ECG tracing. To learn it initially, go from left to right. Move one large box to the right of your starting point, and label this line "300." Continue jumping one large box at a time, and mark the next boxes with "150," "100," "75," "60," and "50." The heart rate is indicated by association of the next R wave with the number closest to it. You will usually have to do some estimating for an exact heart rate, but this method is a quick way to estimate the approximate rate, either fast or slow.

Heart Rate Meters

Many ECG books contain heart rate meters. These devices are small paper or plastic gauges with heart rates

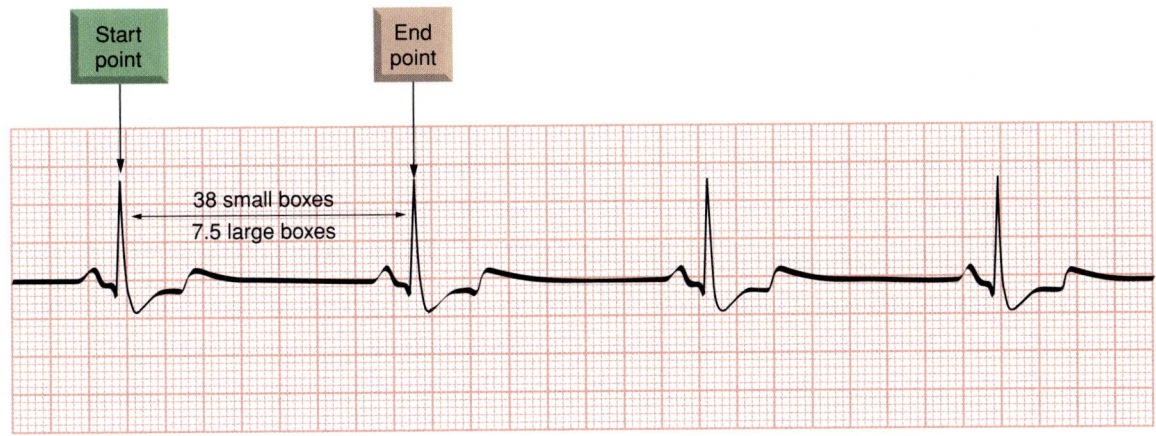

Figure 29-50   The 1500 counting method: 1500 divided by 38 small boxes = 40 beats per minute. The 300 counting method: 300 divided by 7.5 large boxes = 40 beats per minute.

listed along the meter. They are used by aligning an arrow or point on the gauge with the peak of a QRS complex (usually an R wave) and measuring over to the right of the next QRS complex. The number of the line on the meter corresponds with the heart rate. This device is only accurate for regular rhythms.

Rhythm

The rhythm refers to how regular or irregular the cardiac cycles are occurring (Figure 29-52). To be considered regular, the timing intervals (measured as the distance between each RR interval) should march across the ECG strip from R to R without major changes. The faster the rhythm, the more exact it should be. Slower rhythms may be up to two small boxes off either way and may still be considered essentially regular.[8]

A rhythm may be classified in one of many ways. The choices are regular, essentially regular, regularly irregular, and irregularly irregular. The presence of ectopic beats will influence how you classify regularity and irregularity.

If the distance between the shortest RR interval and the longest RR interval is greater than 0.16 sec (four small boxes), the rhythm is considered **irregular.**[8] Any time an irregular rhythm is encountered, determine if there is a definite pattern to the rhythm. This could occur as a result of grouped or paired beats, with certain heart blocks occurring rhythmically, or with a beat being dropped consistently as you look across the ECG strip. When this occurs, the rhythm is classified as **regularly irregular.** It is irregular, but a predictable pattern is present. **Irregularly irregular rhythms** have no predictable pattern to their irregularity.

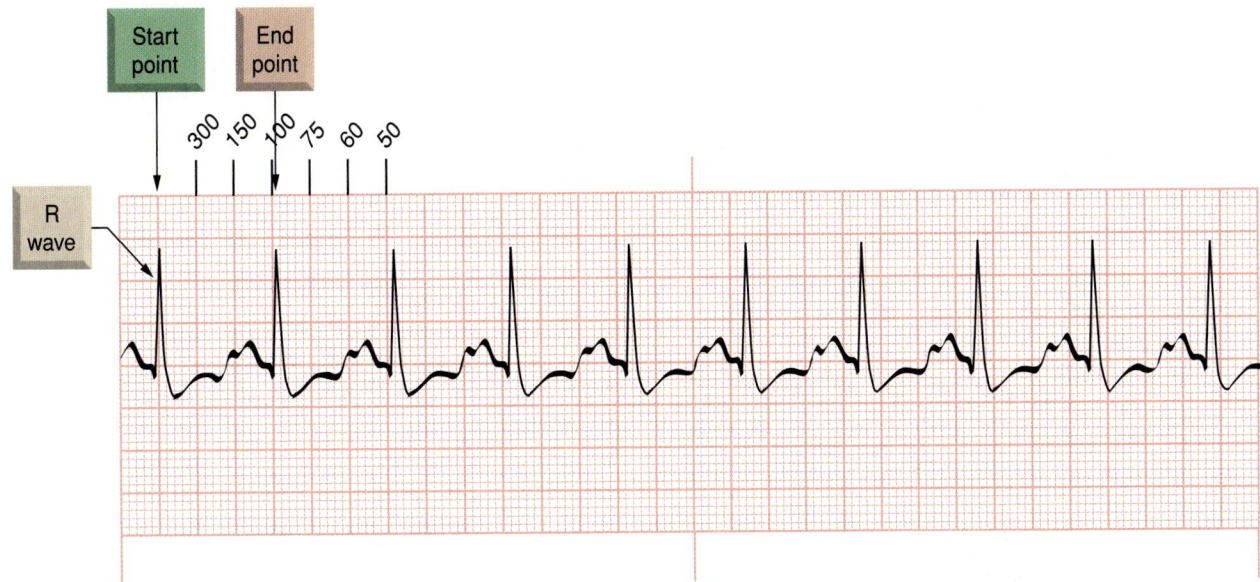

Figure 29-51   Triplicate method of rate determination.

In this rhythm, each R-R and P-P interval is 21 small boxes apart. For this reason it is classified regular.

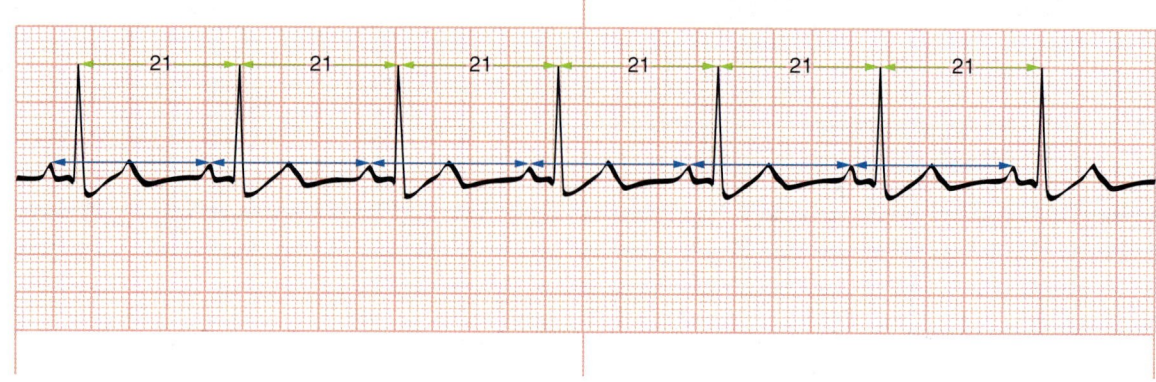

In this rhythm, the number of small boxes differs between some of the R-R and P-P intervals. For this reason it is considered irregular.

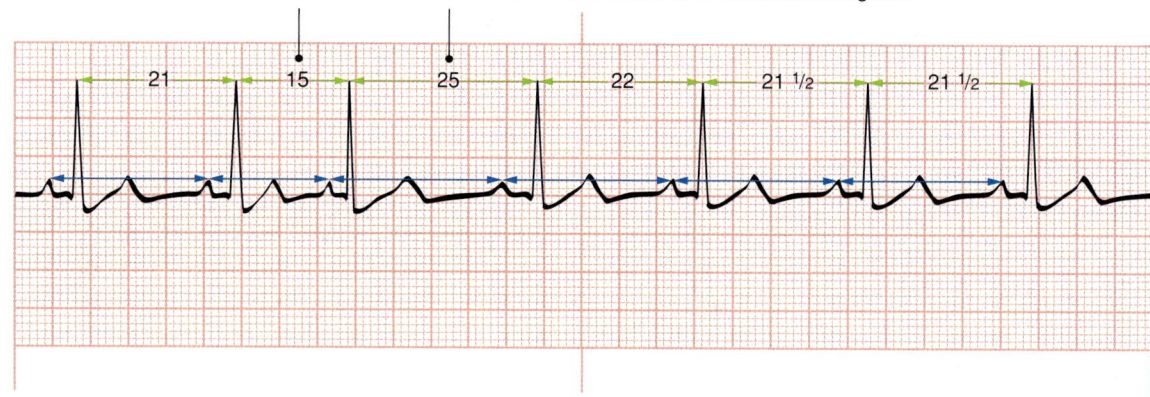

Figure 29-52 Regular versus irregular rhythms.

It is also very important to identify the **underlying rhythm** if there is ectopy. For example, a rhythm may look irregular, but closer inspection shows that you have a very slow regular pattern showing up, and every so often, an ectopic beat such as an escape beat appears.

When this occurs, there are essentially two rhythms to interpret. First interpret the underlying rhythm, and then interpret the ectopy. Report and record the name of this rhythm, first with the name of the underlying rhythm, then include the name of the ectopic beats. For example, "The ECG showed normal sinus rhythm with frequent PVCs." These rhythms are often classified as *essentially regular with ectopy* since the underlying rhythm would be regular if the ectopic beats were not present. You will learn more precise terminology as you get into the specific rhythms.

Nice to Know

The Use of Calipers to Interpret ECG Rhythms

Calipers are special tools used to measure the length between the waves for ECG tracings. They provide a high level of accuracy and are very useful. They are very sharp pointed instruments that resemble a compass. To maintain their shape and accuracy, and because they are pointed, they require special handling and storage. They are not always available for use in the ambulance, so you should learn to interpret rhythms without them.

P Wave

P waves represent the depolarization of the atria and typically precede every QRS complex in a sinus rhythm. A word of caution: Do not assume every small bump you see on the ECG is a P wave. If you see something that looks like a P wave, then prove it; there should be more of them, and they should march out with your calipers or upon visual inspection. If not, then what you are looking at may not be a P wave. Often artifact or malformed complexes may mimic P waves (Box 29-5).

The P wave is normally upright in leads I and II but may be inverted or biphasic in lead III and the left

BOX 29-5 Getting Over the Hump in Rhythm Interpretation

Early on in the process of learning how to interpret ECGs, you will encounter frustration, and unfortunately it will stick with you until you "get it." You learn a lot of rules and then quickly learn that not all rhythms follow all the rules, and now you don't know which rules to disregard and which matter most. You learn how to measure intervals and waves because you are told that it is important, and then an instructor or senior medic looks over your shoulder at that same rhythm and says, "It's close enough." Sometimes, once the regularity of the rhythm is determined (step two of the five-step process), you need to revisit step one: rate, and calculate it over again. What is really frustrating is when you have narrowed your interpretation down to one of two rhythms, and the one you pick is based more upon how "sick" the patient is than on what the actual rhythm really is. Finally, when you match up the names of the rhythms with the treatment algorithm for rhythms, you find out that many rhythms are actually treated in the same manner because of where they came from (their origin) in the heart or how potentially deadly they are; and for many rhythms the treatment ends up being "IV, oxygen, monitor, and transport," immediately making you question why you had to learn all this in the first place. All we can tell you is, "Hang in there, apply the rules of the five-step process religiously, and soon you will see the big picture and the frustration will be over." It happened to us as providers, and it happens to nearly every student we teach.

precordial leads (V_1–V_4). Its amplitude should not exceed 2 or 3 mm of height in any lead.[7] The P wave should be gently rounded and is considered abnormal if peaked, inverted, or notched. In cases of a biphasic P wave, where the second half of a P wave is grossly more negative in V_1, it could indicate enlargement of the left atria.[7]

While examining the P waves, pay close attention to their association with the QRS complex. There should be a one-to-one relationship between the Ps and QRSs. This relationship should translate both directions, meaning there should be one P with every QRS, and every QRS should have a P. Also, if the distance between the P wave and the QRS far exceeds 0.20 seconds, it may not be associated. This means that although the P wave precedes the QRS, it is possible that the impulse represented by that P wave did not transmit through the AV junction, causing ventricular depolarization.

PR Interval

The PR interval (PRI) marks the time it takes for the atria to depolarize and pass the impulse into the ventricles (Figure 29-53). It is measured from the beginning of the P wave to the beginning of the QRS complex, including the PR segment and is normally between 0.12 and 0.20 seconds.[7] This interval varies slightly with heart rate, with slower rhythms often approaching or exceeding 0.20 sec. If this interval is prolonged beyond 0.20 seconds, a block within the AV node or junction exists. In cases where the PR interval is very prolonged, you may notice a shallow inversion behind the P wave. This inversion is called the T_p wave and actually shows that the atria have repolarized.[7] Since this wave is usually merged (or buried) within the QRS, it is only seen in these circumstances. A PRI of less than 0.12 seconds is also considered abnormal and indicates that the impulse originated either very low in the atria or right in the AV node or used an accessory bypass pathway.

QRS Complex

Because it reflects the electrical conduction within the ventricle, the QRS complex is often considered the most important part of ECG interpretation (Figure 29-54). While inspecting the QRS, you must look at the following:

- The duration (width) of the complex
- Amplitude (height) of the complex
- The presence of Q waves and their length and size
- The general configuration of the complex, noting any notching or slurring of the waves and how the QRS flows into the T wave

The duration or width of the QRS should be from 0.05 to 0.10 seconds, measured from the beginning of the QRS to the J point (which was discussed earlier). In some cases, an incomplete block in one of the bundle branches may widen this slightly, so one can say that any QRS complex less than 0.12 seconds (three small boxes) is most likely originating from above the

Nice to Know

Origination of Electrical Impulses Causing the QRS Wave

The fastest pathway for electricity to take through the ventricles is if it comes through the AV node and junction and zips down the bundle branches to the Purkinje fibers. For this reason, any QRS that is less than 0.12 seconds in duration is believed to have followed this pathway and is classified as "narrow" and "normal."

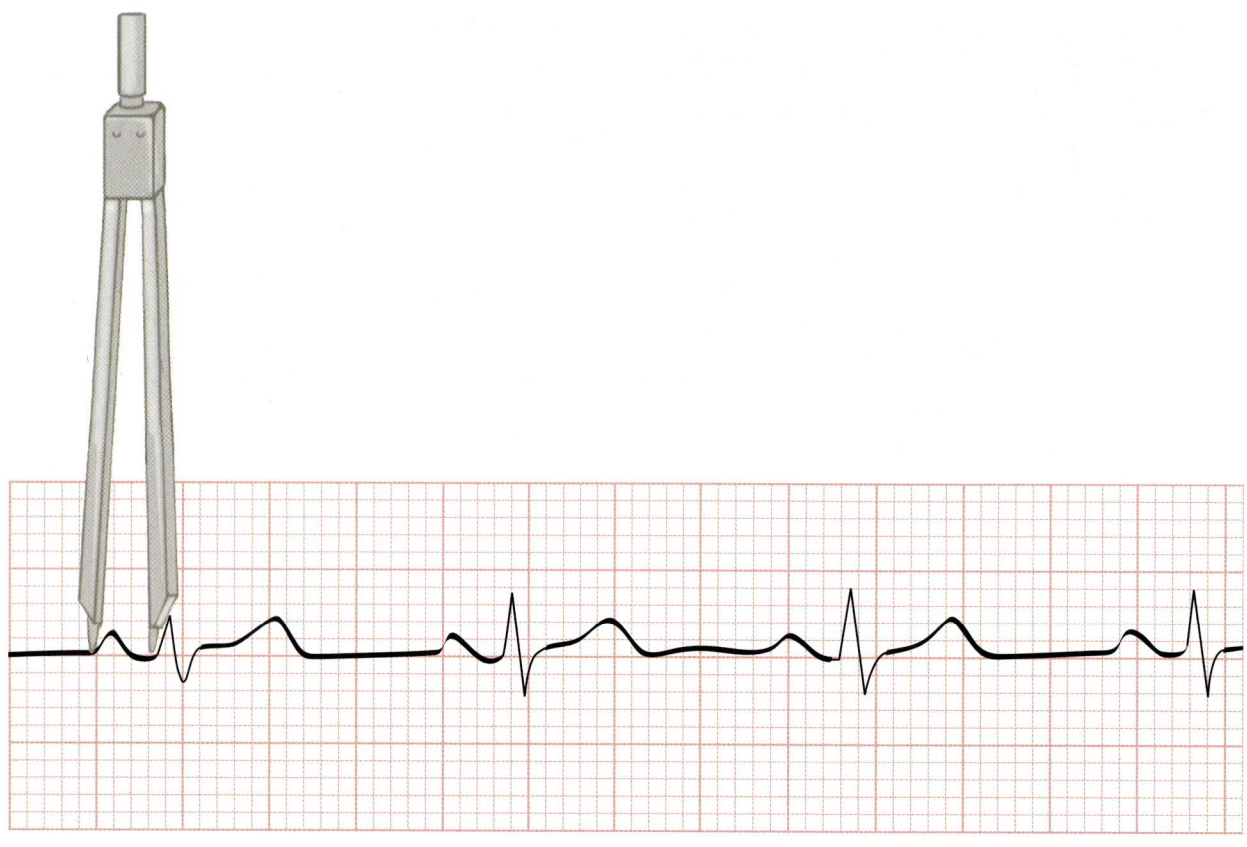

Figure 29-53 Measuring the PR interval with calipers.

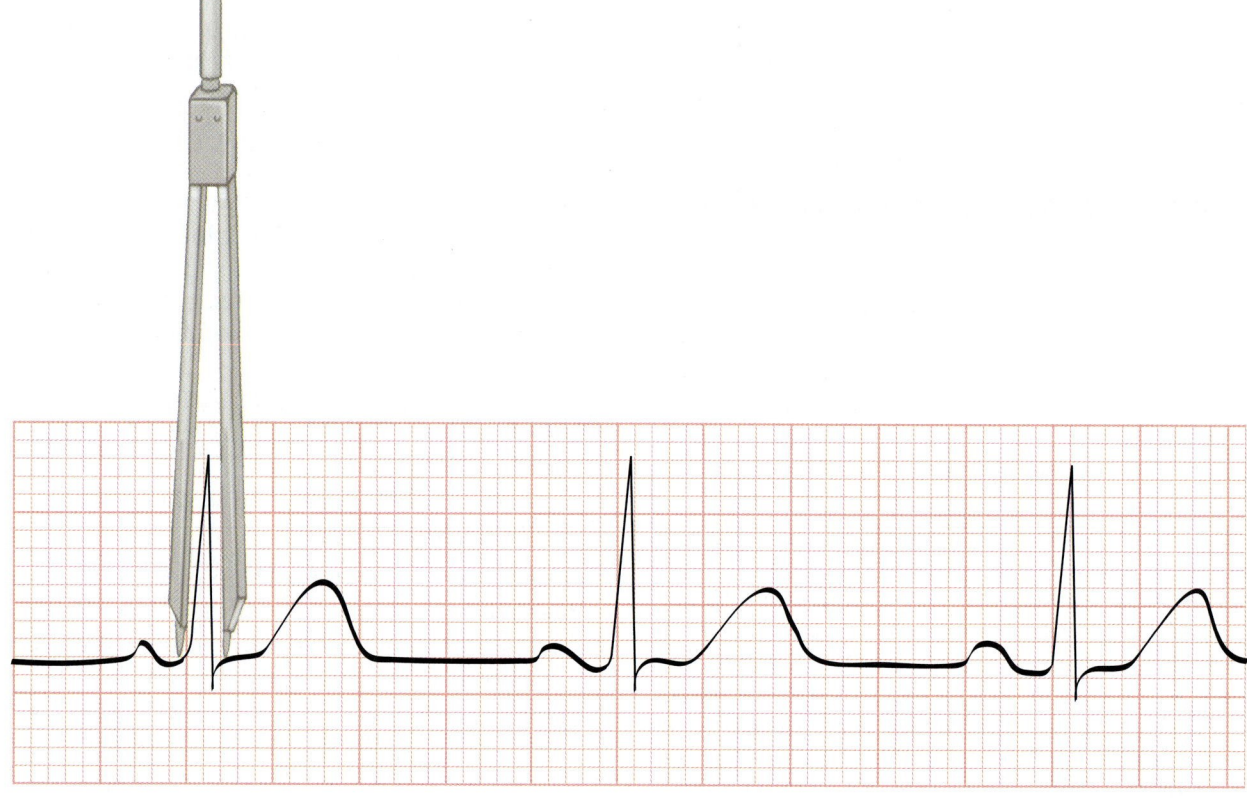

Figure 29-54 Measuring the QRS interval with calipers.

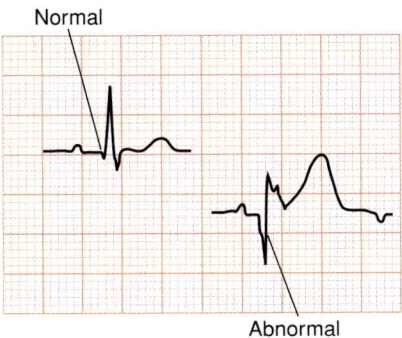

Figure 29-55   Abnormal Q wave accompanied by ST segment elevation indicates both infarct and injury stages are present.

ventricles or following the normal ventricular conduction pathways.[8]

The size or amplitude of the QRS wave may vary widely from very tiny to very tall. Generally, if the total amplitude (sum of positive and negative forces) for the QRS in each of leads I, II, and III is 5 mm or less, it is considered abnormal, possibly due to coronary disease, pericardial effusion (fluid in the pericardium), myxedema (a severe form of hypothyroidism discussed in detail in Chapter 31), emphysema, generalized edema, or obesity. Before jumping to any conclusion about heart health, remember that the amplitude of the QRS can vary due to many reasons, such as thickness of the chest wall, size of the chest, and distance the electrodes are placed from the heart.[7] All of these things must be taken into consideration before reaching a conclusion regarding the presence of heart disease.

The presence of a Q wave may also mean several different things. Our main concern is if they are normal Q waves reflecting septal depolarization or if they are pathologic Q waves. Pathologic Q waves often develop on the ECG after a myocardial infarction (Figure 29-55). Generally, Q waves smaller that 1 mm wide are not considered significant while Q waves greater than 0.03 seconds are consider pathologic. One must always consider the clinical appearance of the patient when making this decision. Do not confuse the Q wave with a QS wave as discussed earlier.

QRS patterns which are slurred, notched, or otherwise bizarre looking must be examined closely (Figure 29-56). If all the QRS complexes in a rhythm have the same abnormality present, it may mean that there is a conduction defect or a bundle branch block. However, occasional bizarre looking complexes may indicate a ventricular or ectopic origin for those impulses such as those noted with a premature ventricular contraction (PVC).

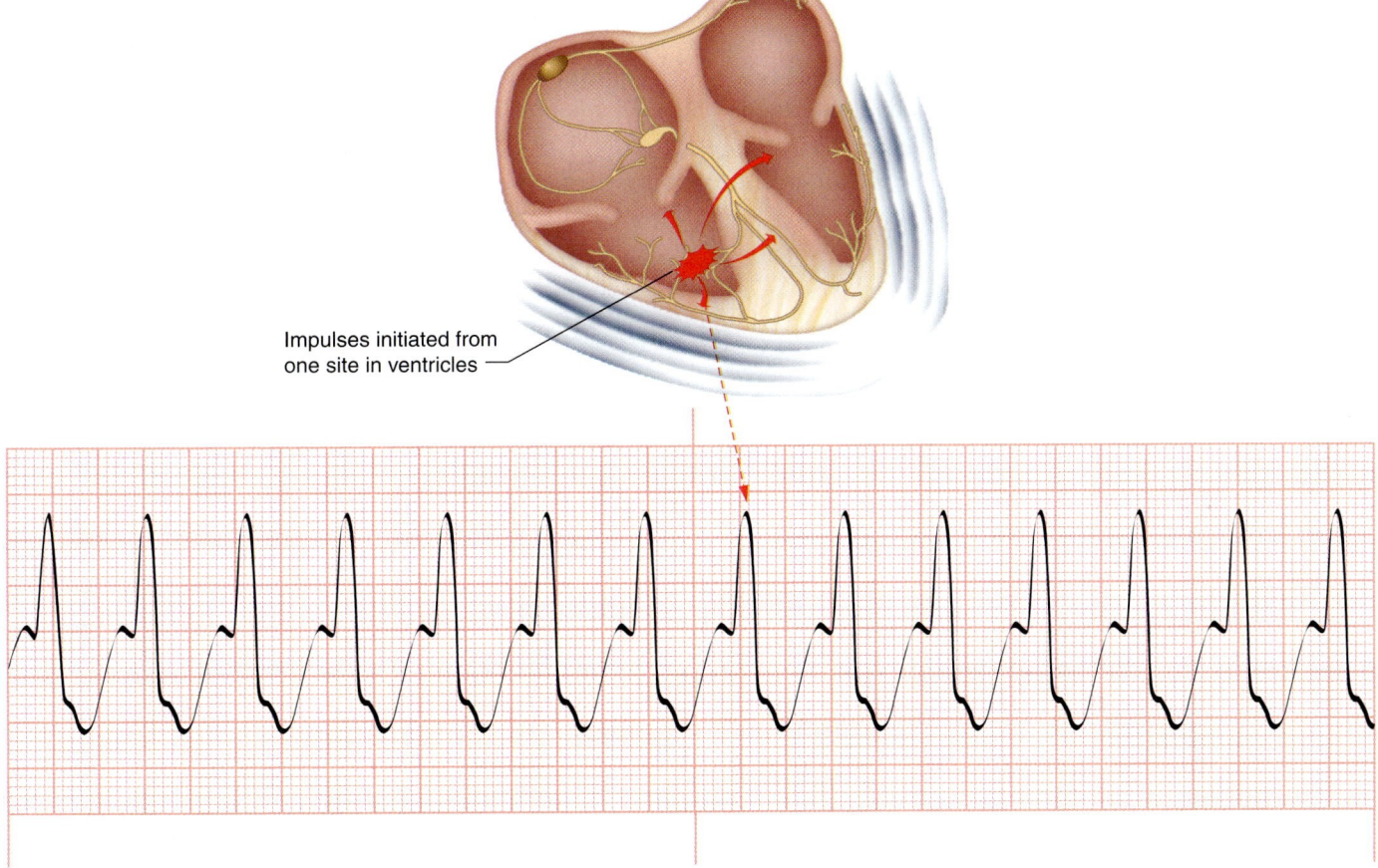

Figure 29-56   Wide bizarre-looking complexes.

Once you have obtained all the information you can from the rhythm, you should have enough information to identify this rhythm. Compare the findings from the five-step analysis process to the ECG rhythm definitions to derive a name for the rhythm. The next section will classify rhythms based on their origin. In other words, they are grouped together by which portion of the conduction pathway and which chamber of the heart they come from.

Dysrhythmias through Dr. Marriott's Eyes

Dysrhythmias are any rhythm outside the parameters of a normal sinus rhythm. Many of these look similar and may be hard to distinguish from one another without good investigative techniques. Dr. Henry Marriott described some principles to help identify and classify dysrhythmias. They are as follows[7]: DOT 5-2.27, 5-2.28

- *Use a lead containing maximum information*
  - One lead is usually not enough to fully appreciate a rhythm, so use limb leads and V leads and compare the results in several leads.
- *Learn all you can about what causes each dysrhythmia*
  - Know the rules for each rhythm and use the five-step process every time until it is routine.
- *Milk the QRS*
  - Get as much information as you can out of the QRS complex; remember that lead II may be a

good monitoring lead, but it is not the best lead to diagnose bundle branch or other blocks, so use several leads.

- *Cherchez le P (look for the P)*
  - If the information you need is not in the QRS, then closely examine the P wave.
  - Make sure you note the relationship of the Ps and the QRSs. Is it a 1:1 relationship? Are there more Ps than QRSs? Are there more QRSs than Ps?
- *Mind your Ps*
  - Be wary of things that look like P waves but are not.
  - T waves often look like P waves.
- *Dig the break*
  - If you find a break in the underlying rhythm, that is where you are likely to find the solution to the rhythm.
- *Who's married to whom?*
  - Is that P wave really associated with the QRS complex, or is its appearance at that position on the ECG tracing a coincidence (i.e., as what occurs with a complete heart block)?
- *Pinpoint the primary rhythm*
  - Make sure you identify the underlying rhythm. Usually the rhythm coming from the highest part of the conduction pathway (like the SA node) is the underlying rhythm and the other complexes represent the ectopy.

Normal sinus rhythm arises from the SA node. Each impulse travels down through the conduction system in a normal manner.

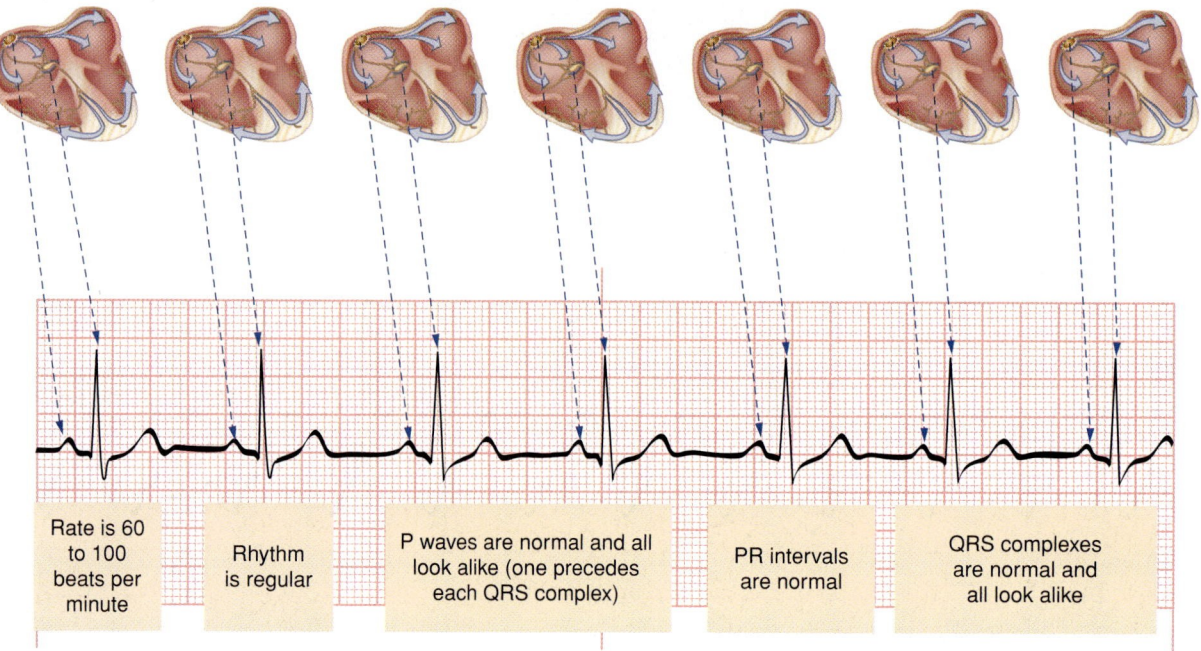

Rate is 60 to 100 beats per minute

Rhythm is regular

P waves are normal and all look alike (one precedes each QRS complex)

PR intervals are normal

QRS complexes are normal and all look alike

Figure 29-57 Normal sinus rhythm.

Rhythms Originating within the Sinus Node

Normal Sinus Rhythm (NSR)

The most common rhythm is the **normal sinus rhythm** (Figure 29-57). In this rhythm, the electrical impulse originates within the sinus node and follows normal conduction pathways to the AV node and then the ventricles. To qualify to be called the normal sinus rhythm, the following rules must apply:

- The heart rate must be between 60 and 100 beats/minute.
- The rhythm must be regular.
- The P wave should be present and precede every QRS complex, every QRS must have a P, and the overall relationship should be 1:1.
- The PRI must be between 0.12 and 0.20 seconds (one large box or less) and relatively constant.
- The QRS complex follows each P wave and measures 0.12 seconds (three small boxes) or less.

This rhythm is normal, and typically only supportive treatment is indicated: Administer IV and oxygen, monitor ECG and vital signs, and transport as necessary. The term "normal" implies that all the above criteria are met without exception.

Diagnostic Criteria for NSR

Rate: 60–100
Rhythm: regular without any ectopy
P waves: present and precedes each QRS, 1:1 relationship
PRI: 0.12–0.20 seconds
QRS: < 0.12 seconds, uniform in shape

Arrhythmias

The term **arrhythmia** literally translates into "an ECG that is without a rhythm." This term has historically meant an abnormal rhythm instead of no rhythm at all. The term is most often used synonymously with **dysrhythmia,** which literally translates as a difficult, painful, or bad rhythm. Some linguistic purists would argue that if properly used, the only true arrhythmia would be **asystole,** or complete lack of a rhythm. The current terminology standard is to favor the use of the term "dysrhythmia" over "arrhythmia" when identifying rhythms just like the use of the term "ECG" is now favored over "EKG."

Although either term—arrhythmia or dysrhythmia—may be used to describe a rhythm that is not normal, the preference in this text is for dysrhythmia.

Sinus Arrhythmia

This specific rhythm, **sinus arrhythmia,** is a title with historical significance and is universally recognized within the medical community, so for this instance "arrhythmia" will be used instead.

With sinus arrhythmia, although the rhythm originates from the sinus node, it is not normal. The distinguishing factor between this rhythm and normal sinus is the rhythm, or timing intervals between cardiac cycles, making it regularly irregular. In sinus arrhythmia, the heart rate increases during inspiration and decreases during expiration (Figure 29-58). All other criteria are identical to the normal sinus rhythm.

Sinus arrhythmia is a normal variant in children, young adults, and elderly individuals and is usually of no clinical significance. It is also often noted in world-class athletes with highly conditioned cardiovascular systems with a high level of vagal tone. Even the normal sinus impulse will vary due to exercise, stress, blood pressure, and thermoregulation.

The most common cause of sinus arrhythmia is a mild parasympathetic vagal influence associated with intrathoracic pressure changes during breathing.[10] Remember that the vagus nerve stimulates the heart to slow its rate, and in the case of excessive amounts of vagal stimulation (also called vagal tone), the tendency is for the heart rate to slow down. A very pronounced sinus arrhythmia could conceivably cause dizziness or syncope should the rate slow too much.

To qualify as a true sinus arrhythmia, the distance between the shortest P to P interval and longest P to P interval must be greater than 0.12 seconds in duration.[11] Unless other signs or symptoms exist, treatment for this arrhythmia is generally unnecessary.

Diagnostic Criteria for Sinus Arrhythmia

Rate: 60–100
Rhythm: regularly irregular with respiration and without any ectopy
P waves: present and precedes each QRS with a 1:1 relationship
PRI: 0.12–0.20 seconds
QRS: < 0.12 seconds, uniform in shape

Sinus Tachycardia

Sinus tachycardia identifies a regular rhythm originating from the sinus node but beating at a rate greater than 100 (Figure 29-59). The rate is the result of increased

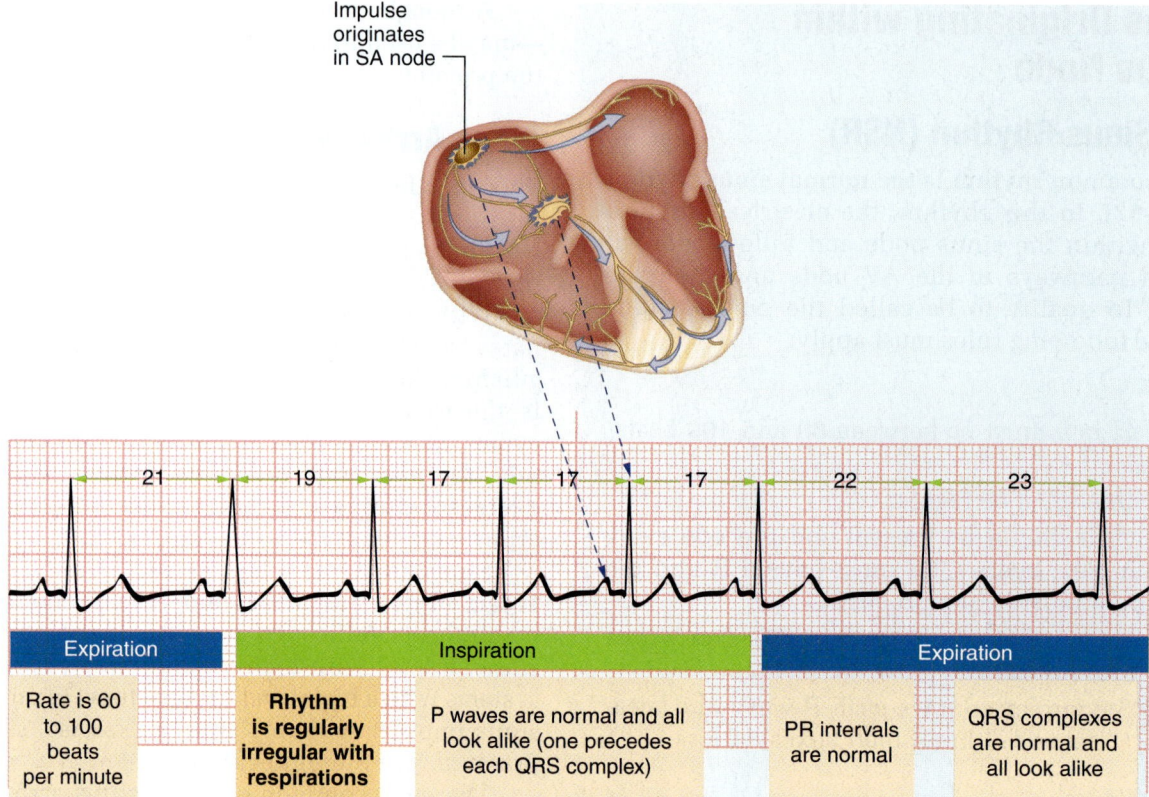

Figure 29-58 Sinus arrhythmia.

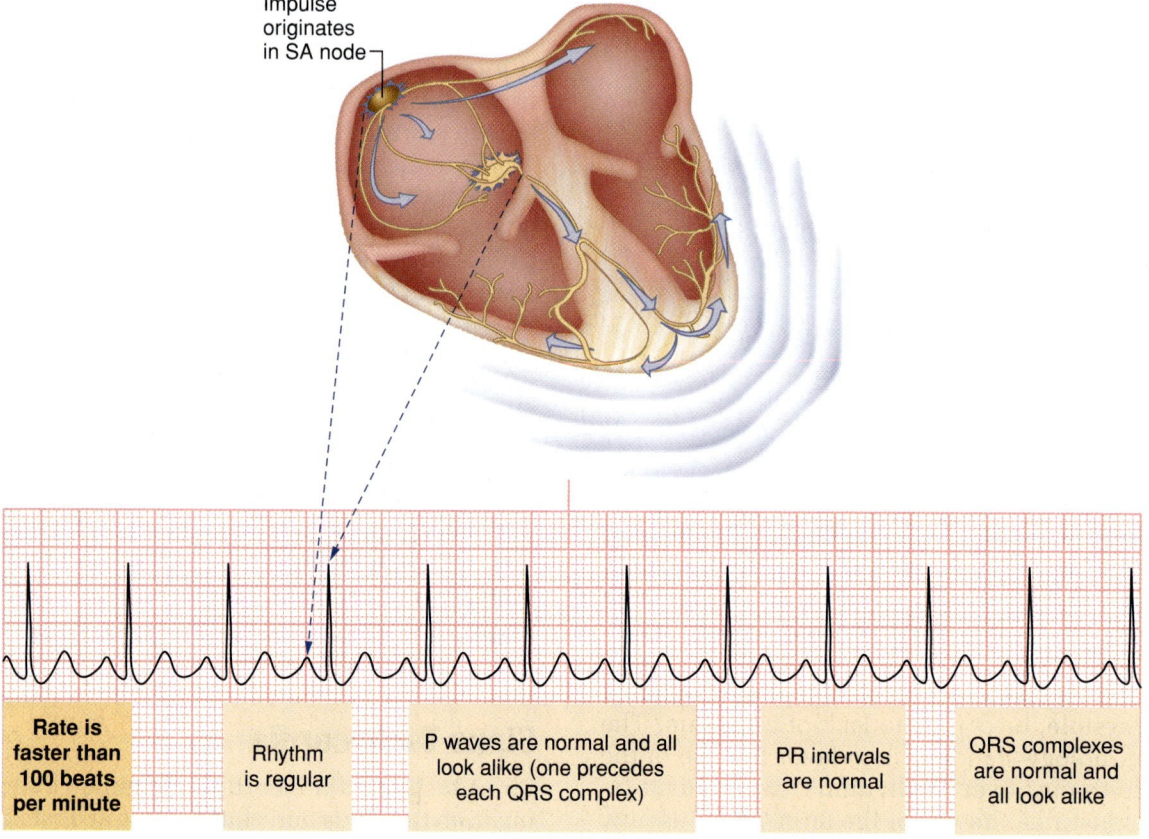

Figure 29-59 Sinus tachycardia.

Sinus bradycardia arises from the SA node. Each impulse travels down through the conduction system in a normal manner.

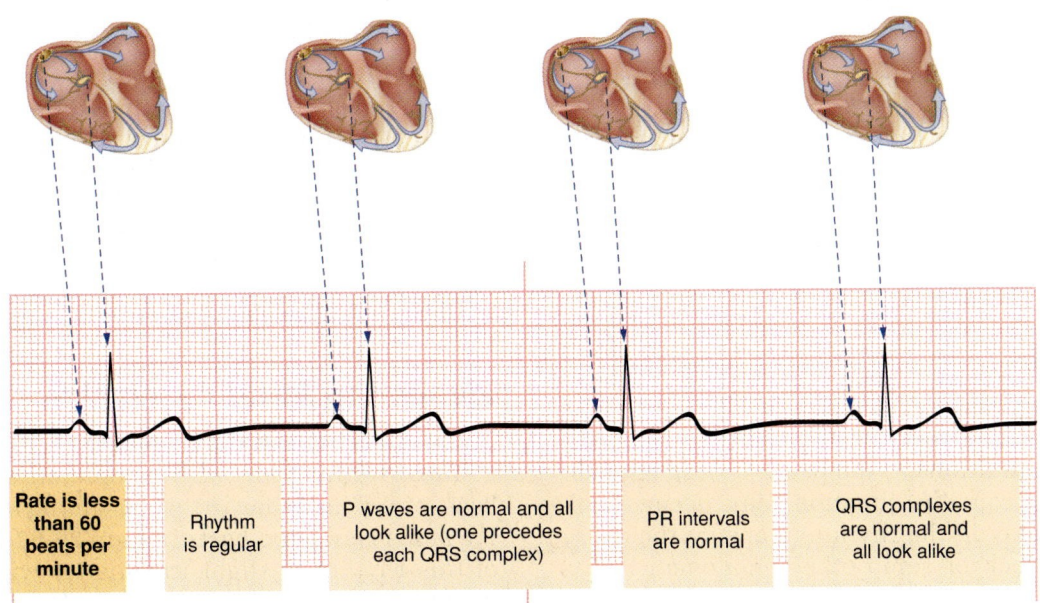

| Rate is less than 60 beats per minute | Rhythm is regular | P waves are normal and all look alike (one precedes each QRS complex) | PR intervals are normal | QRS complexes are normal and all look alike |

Figure 29-60 Sinus bradycardia.

automaticity of the sinus node, which speeds up the heart rate to anything between 100 and 150 beats/minute. On rare occasions, the sinus node will reach rates approaching 180 beats/minute, but 160 is generally the fastest it fires.[7] In a pediatric patient, sinus-generated heart rates may exceed 200 beats/minute.

Increased automaticity is the result of any number of causes such as sympathetic stimulation, emotional stress, exercise, pain, drug abuse, myocardial infarction, and many more.[10] The important thing to remember is that sinus tachycardia exists as the result of some other stimulus or problem and is not a primary dysrhythmia in itself. It is most likely compensation for something else and presents as an attempt to maintain adequate cardiac output and blood pressure. Therefore, the treatment lies in finding and correcting the underlying cause. The question to answer here is, "Is the rhythm causing the problem, or is the problem causing the rhythm?" In most cases of sinus tachycardia, the problem is causing the rhythm, so the treatment lies in correcting the problem.

Diagnostic Criteria for Sinus Tachycardia

Rate: 100–160

Rhythm: regular without any ectopy

P waves: present and precedes each QRS with a 1:1 relationship

PRI: 0.12–0.20 seconds

QRS: < 0.12 seconds, uniform in shape

Sinus Bradycardia

Sinus bradycardia occurs when the sinus node fires at a rate less than 60 beats/minute (Figure 29-60). Some possible causes include excessive parasympathetic stimulation (increased vagal tone), myocardial infarction, and drugs such as digitalis, beta blockers, and others.[10]

The only abnormality with sinus bradycardia is the rate. Some adults normally are bradycardic, especially well-trained athletes. Sinus bradycardia is very rare in children. Clinical implications of this rhythm range from a very benign condition, such as vagal stimulation, to more serious conditions, such as inferior wall myocardial infarctions.[11] This emphasizes the need to very carefully assess each patient clinically. In the presence of an infarction, a slow heartbeat can be beneficial by reducing the workload and demand on the heart. However, decreased cardiac output can also lead to serious symptoms such as dizziness, hypotension (especially orthostatic hypotension) mental confusion, and fainting.

Treatment for sinus bradycardia must then be based on the clinical presentation of symptoms and not on the actual heart rate. A patient mentating properly (who is awake, alert, and oriented to person, place, time, and situation), with no serious symptoms such as hypotension, chest pain, or difficulty breathing, may simply be observed until a cause is determined. The presence of serious signs or symptoms may require drug therapy or electrical intervention such as cardiac pacing to increase the heart rate and maintain the blood pressure.

Diagnostic Criteria for Sinus Bradycardia

Rate: < 60

Rhythm: regular to essentially regular without any ectopy

P waves: present and precedes each QRS with a 1:1 relationship

PRI: 0.12−0.20 seconds

QRS: < 0.12 seconds, uniform in shape

Diagnostic Criteria for Sinus Arrest

Rate: depends upon the frequency of the arrest

Rhythm: regular to essentially regular with obviously dropped beats; ectopic beats may be present if the AV node or purkinji fibers tried to pace the heart during the sinus arrest beat

P waves: present and precedes each QRS with a 1:1 relationship

PRI: 0.12−0.20 seconds

QRS: < 0.12 seconds, uniform in shape

Sinus Arrest

A **sinus arrest** or **pause** occurs when the sinus node fails to initiate an impulse at the expected time (Figure 29-61). Under normal conditions, if the pause is long enough, an escape beat from the junction may occur. Look closely at the break in the rhythm to ensure the cause is not an AV block or some other phenomena. ECG recognition of sinus arrest begins with the observation of a long pause in the rhythm when the sinus node failed to fire. The rhythm may be normal before and after this pause.

If the missed beat situation is infrequent, there will be no treatment required. If the missed beats are occurring frequently, the patient may require supportive care to maintain blood pressure.

Wandering Atrial Pacemaker (WAP)

The **wandering atrial pacemaker (WAP)** is essentially a sinus dysrhythmia with ectopic atrial or junctional beats occurring in fairly regular timing intervals replacing sinus-generated beats (Figure 29-62). The hallmark of this rhythm is slight irregularity with at least two variations in the appearance of the P wave. The P wave morphology will change as the origin of the beat occurs in various locations in the atria.

What typically occurs prior to the onset of WAP is that the sinus-generated rhythm starts to slow down, permitting an opportunity for an ectopic impulse to escape and initiate the next complex. On a few occasions, the normal sinus beat and the ectopic impulse may

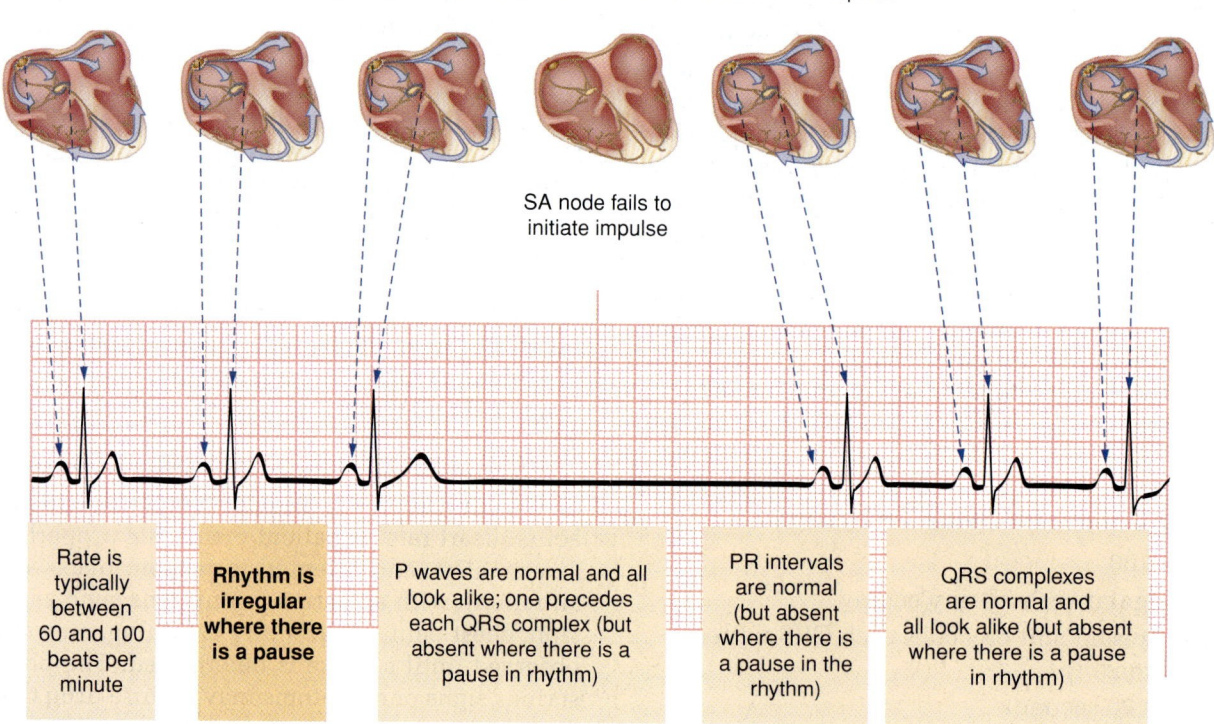

Sinus arrest occurs when the SA node fails to initiate an impulse.

SA node fails to initiate impulse

Rate is typically between 60 and 100 beats per minute

Rhythm is irregular where there is a pause

P waves are normal and all look alike; one precedes each QRS complex (but absent where there is a pause in rhythm)

PR intervals are normal (but absent where there is a pause in the rhythm)

QRS complexes are normal and all look alike (but absent where there is a pause in rhythm)

Figure 29-61   Sinus arrest.

Wandering atrial pacemaker arises from different sites in the atria.

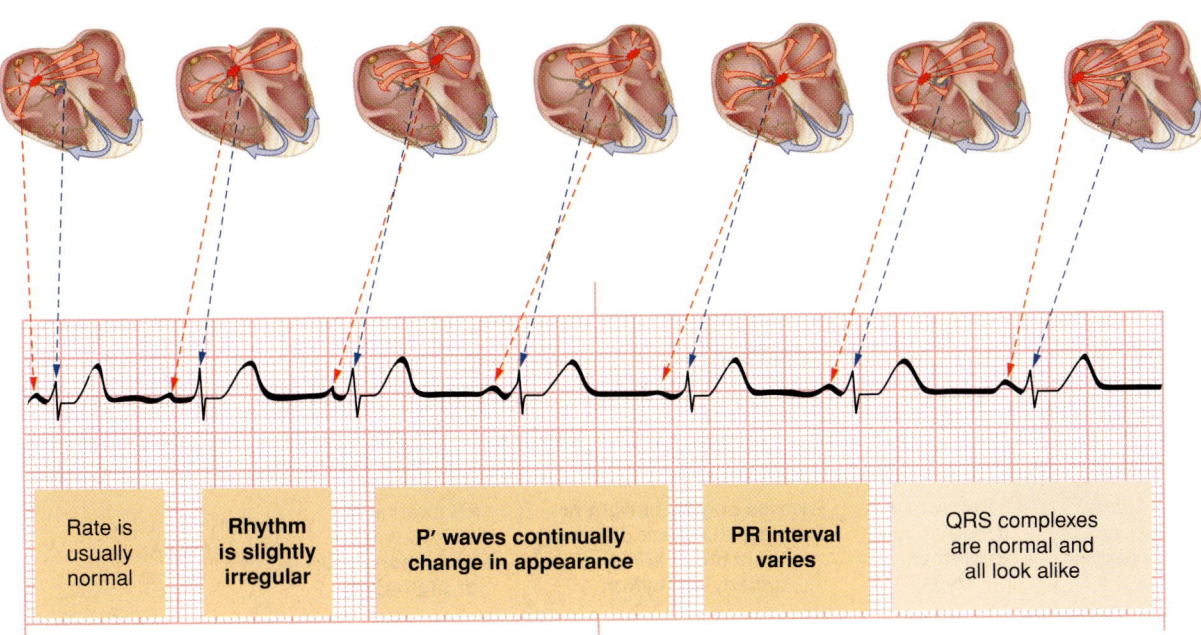

| Rate is usually normal | **Rhythm is slightly irregular** | **P′ waves continually change in appearance** | **PR interval varies** | QRS complexes are normal and all look alike |

Figure 29-62 Wandering atrial pacemaker (note the different shapes of P waves).

occur near the same time, resulting in an atrial fusion beat. A fusion beat results when two or more impulses occur simultaneously and meet at a central location. They tend to produce a complex with a much different appearance than other normal sinus impulses.

In most cases, the prehospital treatment of the wandering atrial pacemaker consists of supportive care. If the heart rate is too slow to support adequate cardiac output, the bradycardic WAP rhythm may require treatment. In that case, the ACLS algorithm for bradycardia would be followed.

Diagnostic Criteria for WAP

Rate: 60–100, but frequently < 60

Rhythm: regular to essentially regular, usually no additional ectopic beats other than the wandering pacer site

P waves: vary in morphology but a 1:1 relationship generally exists

PRI: varied

QRS: < 0.12 seconds, uniform in shape

Dysrhythmias Originating within the Atria

Certain dysrhythmias that originate in the atria are not from the sinus node. Under most conditions, automaticity in cells outside of the conduction pathway is usually prevented by overdrive suppression from one of the pacemakers. However, under certain conditions, heart disease, sympathetic stimulation, influence of stimulant drugs like caffeine, cocaine or others, or in times of stress, any cardiac cell can become "irritable" and initiate an impulse earlier than expected, which may result in a takeover as the primary pacemaker site. DOT 5-2.39

Premature Atrial Contractions (PAC)

The **premature atrial contraction (PAC)** is a beat originating from somewhere in the atria other than the sinus node (Figure 29-63). The beat is named "premature" because it occurs earlier than expected with respect to the underlying rhythm. The PAC is not dysrhythmia in itself but rather an irregularity in an underlying rhythm. This premature beat occurring in an otherwise healthy heart is common and is not clinically significant. However, if it occurs in the presence of existing heart disease, it may indicate irritability due to congestive heart failure or an acute myocardial infarction.[8] The most common causes of PAC include enhanced automaticity due to emotion, stimulant use (e.g., alcohol, caffeine, and tobacco), or even the use of cardioactive drugs such as epinephrine, digitalis, or others.[8] When PACs are seen in the presence of congestive heart failure, it is most likely due to increased atrial pressure.

Another important key in identifying the PAC is to examine the P wave closely. Since the ectopic beat is probably not originating from the SA node, it is following a different electrical pathway, and it should have a slightly different P wave morphology. However, all PAC beats will have a P wave and a fairly normal PRI and QRS. If the premature complex is occurring very close

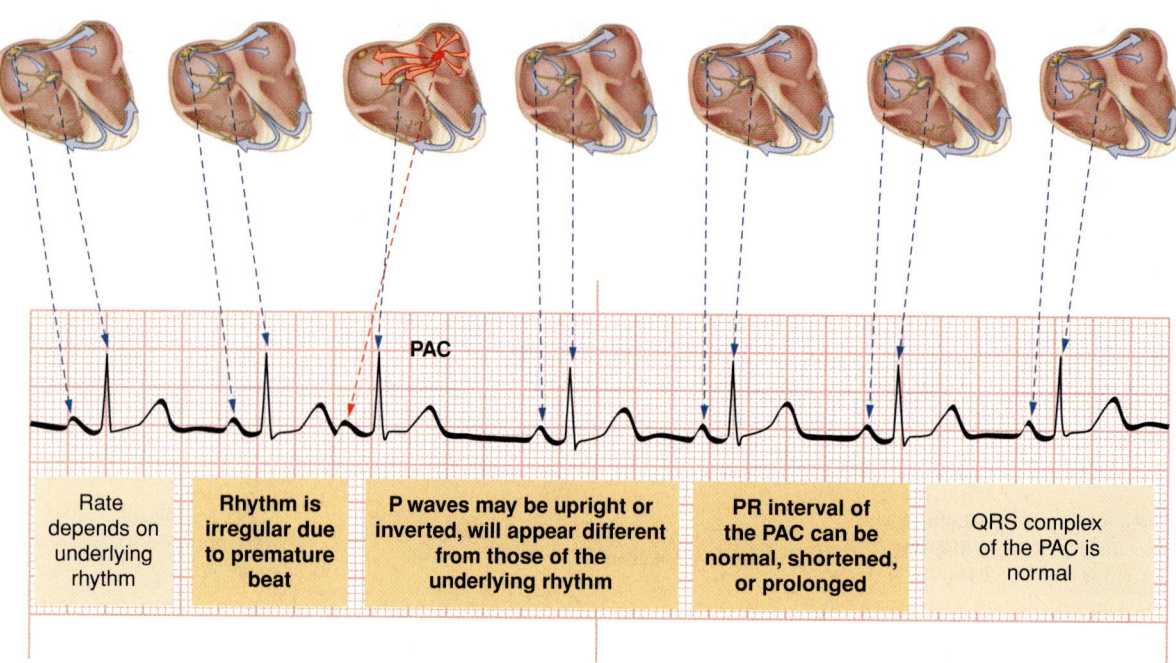

Premature atrial complexes arise from somewhere in the atrium.

| Rate depends on underlying rhythm | Rhythm is irregular due to premature beat | P waves may be upright or inverted, will appear different from those of the underlying rhythm | PR interval of the PAC can be normal, shortened, or prolonged | QRS complex of the PAC is normal |

Figure 29-63 Premature atrial complex (note the absence of compensatory pause).

to the preceding normal complex, the P wave may be on top of or closely associated with (or buried within) the T wave of the preceding complex (Box 29-6).

An additional factor in recognizing a PAC is the absence of a **compensatory pause** after the premature contraction. When a PAC occurs, it depolarizes the atria and "re-sets" the SA node. Therefore the sinus beat after the PAC occurs sooner than expected. In contrast, a premature ventricular contraction usually does not re-set the SA node, which will fire normally but not result in a conducted beat. The next sinus beat after the PVC occurs two (or slightly more) cycles after the sinus beat that preceded the premature beat. This results in what appears to be a long compensatory pause after the premature beat (see Figure 29-80, page 652, PVCs).

Although the majority of PACs are relatively benign, they could be associated with an underlying problem that needs to be evaluated. Any abnormality should be investigated until a reasonable explanation can be found. For example, a very fast rhythm called reentrant atrial tachycardia almost always begins from a single PAC.

Diagnostic Criteria for PAC

Rate: matches that of the underlying rhythm

Rhythm: slightly irregular due to extra complex

P waves: present and precedes each QRS in a 1:1 relationship, slightly different morphology

PRI: 0.12–0.20 seconds (less on premature complex)

QRS: < 0.12 seconds, uniform in shape

BOX 29-6 Comparing Premature Beat Morphology to NSR Beats

Of the three types of premature beats, the PAC looks the most similar to the normal SA node-generated beats. The other two premature complexes: premature junctional complex (PJC) and premature ventricular complex (PVC) look different because they are originating lower down on the conduction pathway.

Nice to Know

Complex versus Contraction

Ectopic beats are commonly referred to by their initials: PAC, PVC, PJC. The 'C' can refer to the word complex or contraction. The 'C' stands for 'complex' when one is referring to the ECG and stands for 'contraction' if the complex was conducted resulting in a palpable beat.

Atrial tachycardia arises from a single focus in the atria.

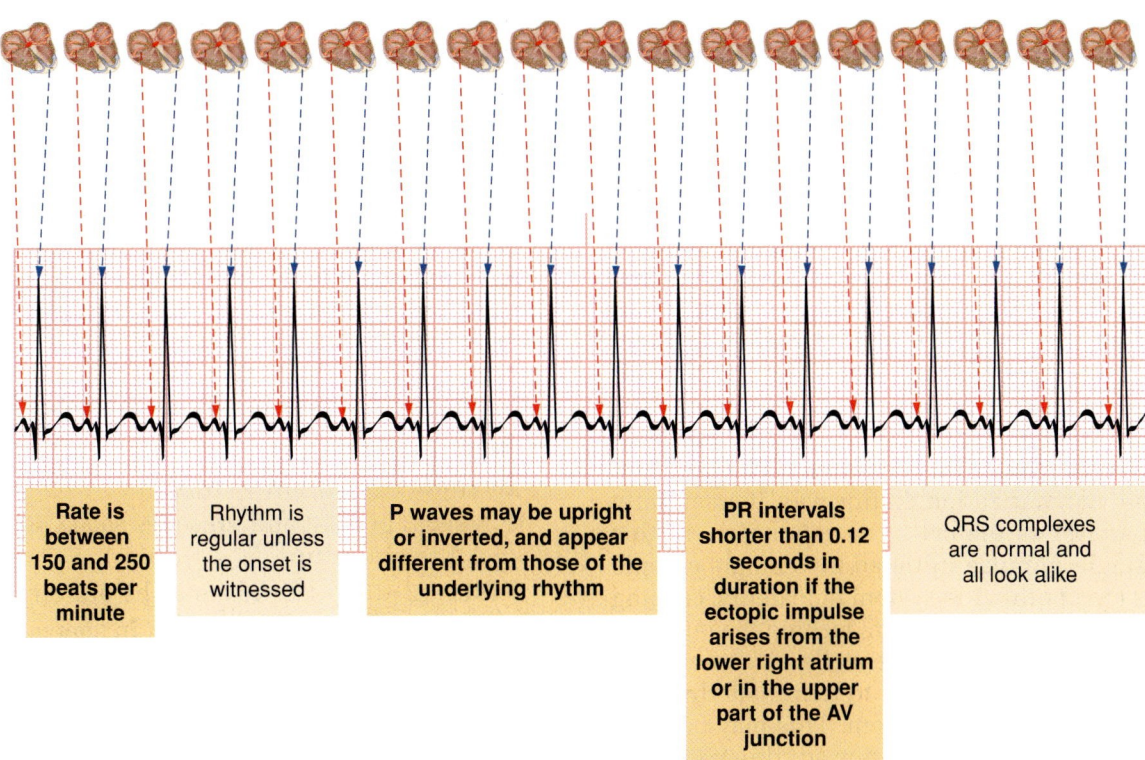

| Rate is between 150 and 250 beats per minute | Rhythm is regular unless the onset is witnessed | P waves may be upright or inverted, and appear different from those of the underlying rhythm | PR intervals shorter than 0.12 seconds in duration if the ectopic impulse arises from the lower right atrium or in the upper part of the AV junction | QRS complexes are normal and all look alike |

Figure 29-64   Atrial tachycardia.

Atrial Tachycardia

Atrial tachycardia describes a dysrhythmia originating from an ectopic site somewhere within the atria (Figure 29-64). It typically occurs at a rate between 160 and 240 beats/minute.[8] The cause of atrial tachycardia is essentially identical to that of a PAC, but it keeps firing at an accelerated rate and it eventually becomes the primary pacemaker for the heart. The impulse may continue to form at that ectopic site for one of two reasons. First, the ectopic site keeps firing due to enhanced automaticity or structural damage, or second, the rhythm may actually replicate itself in a phenomenon known as a reentry mechanism (Figure 29-65).

The reentry mechanism is responsible for several different dysrhythmias, such as SVT or PVCs. To understand how it works, the conduction system of the heart within the atria must be revisited. Recall that the sinus node is located in the upper right portion of the right atria and is connected to the rest of the atria through a system of specialized conduction fibers called the internodal pathways. By nature, some of those pathways conduct at different rates of speed. Researchers have identified fast fibers and slow fibers connecting the SA node to the AV node. Normally, the impulses entering the slow fibers reach depolarized tissue at the AV node because the fast fibers have already passed the impulse through them, and they are in the refractory period of

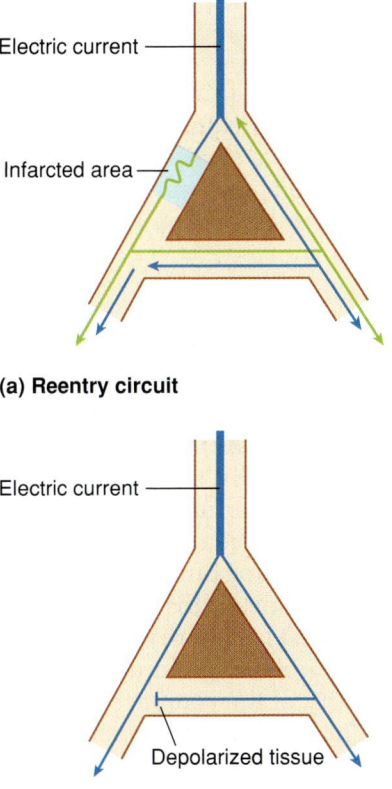

Electric current

Infarcted area

(a) Reentry circuit

Electric current

Depolarized tissue

(b) Normal circuit

Figure 29-65   (a) Current is delayed in damaged region and reenters the system after repolarization. (b) Current is blocked by depolarized tissue.

the action potential. The slow fiber impulses basically terminate within the tissue.

This can be different in the case of reentry. For this example, assume an ectopic site is located very near the slow fibers in the atria. This site may fire out of sequence before the SA node can do its job. When this occurs, the impulse travels through the atria and the slow fibers before it can reach the fast fibers. The impulse is then free to travel to the AV node and depolarize the ventricles. When this occurs, the ECG tracing image will show a PAC. At this time, the impulse has also started up the fast fibers in a retrograde fashion. Most of the time, it too will run into the impulse initiated by the next sinus beat and simply dissipate in the tissue. But on some occasions, it escapes the fast fiber and is allowed to reenter the conduction pathway and cause another depolarization. In this way, it essentially feeds itself as fast as the cells can repolarize. In this manner, a single impulse initiated by a single ectopic site reenters the conduction system repeatedly, causing a run of a very high-speed rhythm, lacking the rate control inherent within the pacemaker cells. It is essentially a rhythm out of control. In order to terminate this dysrhythmia, the cycle must be broken. This may be done through vagal maneuvers, medication administration, or synchronized cardioversion.

Street Secrets

When the heart is beating too fast there is not enough time to allow for adequate ventricular filling, which eventually leads to a significant drop in cardiac output and a drop in blood pressure. Symptomatic tachycardias need aggressive intervention with either drugs or electrical therapy.

The term **paroxysm** refers to something that starts or ends abruptly. Atrial tachycardia initiated by reentry does just that, so it is often referred to as **paroxysmal atrial tachycardia (PAT).** An irritable focus or ectopic site that fires repeatedly, usurping the duties of the pacemaker, is called either nonparoxysmal or simply atria tachycardia. In the event that there are three or more irritable sites, all firing out of control, the result may be an irregular high-speed rhythm called **multifocal atrial tachycardia (MAT).** This rhythm can be irregularly irregular and completely void of any pattern due to the unpredictability of the ectopic sites. However, one important diagnostic clue to remember is to identify a P wave associated with the QRS complex in order to say it has an atrial origin.

Clinically, atrial tachycardia is significant for the workload it places on the heart. On top of this, the ventricles are unable to fill completely because of the fast rate. When the ventricles cannot fill properly, the re-

sult is reduced cardiac output and decreased perfusion of the brain. The patient may become confused and light-headed and may complain of palpitations. **Palpitations** are fluttering or odd beating sensations that the patient feels in the chest when the heart is beating erratically. In the case of preexisting heart disease, the workload increase during the tachycardia could trigger or exacerbate (worsen) an infarction or congestive heart failure. Symptomatic atrial tachycardia must be treated promptly to limit the consequences of reduced cardiac output and reduce the risk of life-threatening dysrhythmias.

Diagnostic Criteria for Atrial Tachycardia

Rate: 160–240
Rhythm: regular unless MAT
P waves: present and precedes each QRS, 1:1 relationship
PRI: 0.12–0.20 seconds, may be prolonged
QRS: < 0.12 seconds, uniform in shape

At times, it may be impossible to identify P waves, due to the inherent fast rate of the rhythm: The cardiac cycles are occurring so quickly that the waves are appearing to merge together and there is not enough distance between them to clearly see the Ps and PRIs. In these cases, it may also be impossible to differentiate atrial tachycardia from junctional tachycardia. For these cases, the term **paroxysmal supraventricular tachycardia** (PSVT) was coined. The term supraventricular means "from above the ventricles," so basically, this term describes any tachycardic rhythm originating from somewhere above the ventricles.

Street Secrets

The classification of "SVT" is an umbrella term that is used to cover all tachycardia rhythms that originate from any site above the ventricles: the SA node, the atria, and the AV node or junction. All of these rhythms are firing too fast for a view of the isoelectric line, P wave, and PRI. Because of this, the rhythm is virtually unidentifiable. Fortunately, the treatment is focused on signs and symptoms instead of rhythm identification. However, every attempt should be made to try to identify the rhythm, and looking at the rate of the rhythm can help. For example, if the tachycardia is around 150 beats per minute, it could be sinus tach, atrial tach, junctional tach, or atrial flutter, but when the rate is around 220, it cannot be sinus tach or junctional tach as both of those pacemaker sites are unable to fire that quickly.

In prehospital emergency care, it is usually not important to decide where an SVT rhythm is actually

Atrial flutter arises from rapid depolarization of a single focus in the atria.

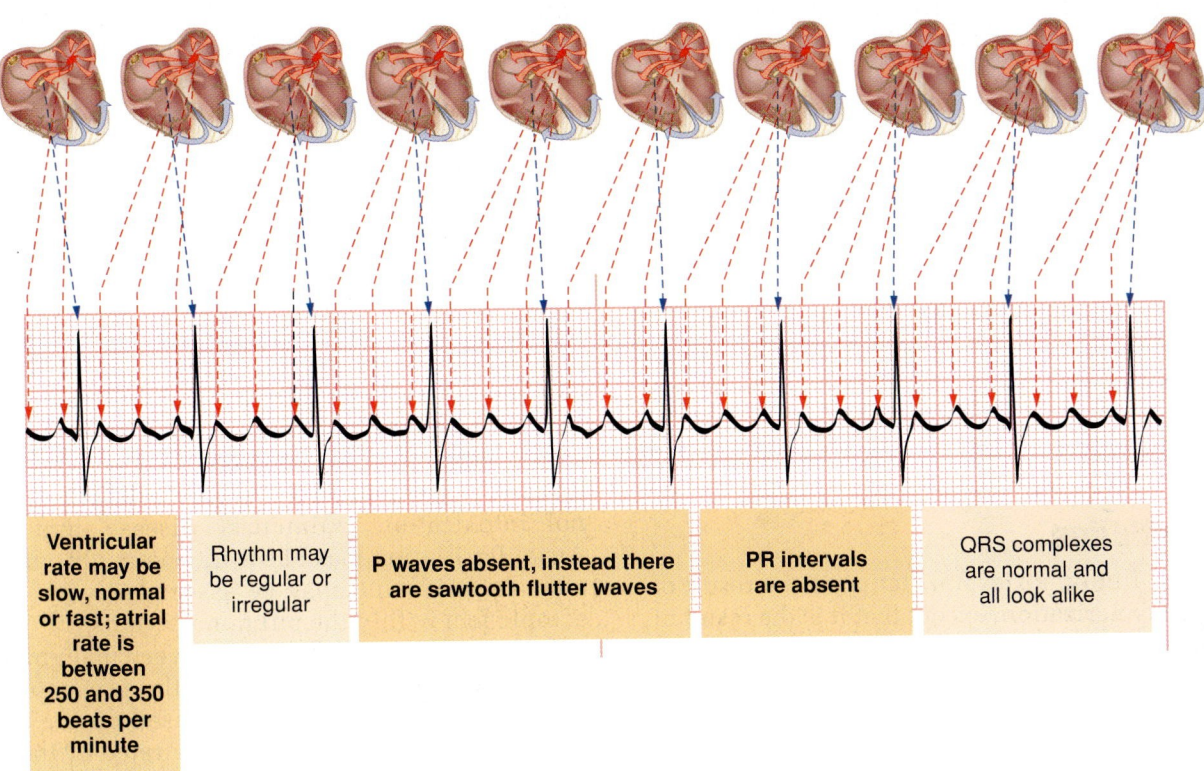

| Ventricular rate may be slow, normal or fast; atrial rate is between 250 and 350 beats per minute | Rhythm may be regular or irregular | P waves absent, instead there are sawtooth flutter waves | PR intervals are absent | QRS complexes are normal and all look alike |

Figure 29-66   Atrial flutter.

coming from as the treatment in most cases will be virtually identical and is focused on the signs and presenting symptoms. The primary goal is to recognize the rhythm, assess the patient for stability, and take prompt steps to terminate this arrhythmia.

Atrial Flutter

Atrial flutter appears to be the result of a well-defined ectopic pacemaker within the atria, firing at a rate of 250–350 times a minute (Figure 29-66).[10] The ectopic site depolarizes the atria so fast that the sinus node is overdriven and the AV node can't keep up. The atria depolarize and repolarize so quickly that the result is a very characteristic sawtooth wave called the F wave or flutter waves. These are not to be confused with multiple P waves. The ventricular response is often within normal limits (60–100 beats/minute) due to the AV node doing its job and controlling the entry into the ventricles. However, the ventricular rate can often reach rates as high as 150 or more. There are often several F waves for every QRS complex, and they can often be buried within the QRS itself.

Do not assume that the P wave immediately before the QRS complex is the one that resulted in the formation of the QRS. Any impulse could get through and generate the QRS, or the AV node could generate the QRS. Atrial flutter is most commonly a very regular rhythm, but under certain circumstances displays varied conduction into the ventricles. This is called **atrial flutter with variable block.**[10]

Signs and symptoms related to atrial flutter are directly related to the ventricular response rate. The faster the ventricles depolarize, the less time they have to fill, thus reducing cardiac output. Another factor involves the atria's ability to pump blood into the ventricles, or as discussed earlier in this chapter, atrial kick. Since the atria are not functioning properly, they lose effective pumping action. Recall that although blood is always flowing into the ventricle when the valves are open, the atrial contraction right at the end of the ventricular stretch "kicks" in the last of the blood in the atria.

Loss of this atrial kick can reduce cardiac output as much as 25%.[8]

Atrial flutter may be associated with thromboembolisms that may precipitate a stroke.[12] When the atria are not contracting normally, blood can collect in the chamber. Blood cells have a lifespan of about 120 days. When they die in the atria and are not removed, they begin to break down. As several dead cells clump together, they form microemboli. These small clots can move out of the atria, especially if they are "kicked" out with an atrial contraction, and then this could lead to blood clots compromising circulation in the lungs or arteries.

At times of rapid ventricular response, a brief vagal maneuver may be useful to verify the interpretation of atrial flutter with the appearance of distinct F waves. In cases of hemodynamic instability, synchronized cardioversion may be required to terminate this dysrhythmia.

Diagnostic Criteria for Atrial Flutter

Rate: atrial 250–350 ventricular; varied dependant upon AV conduction

Rhythm: regular, may be irregular

P waves: replaced by F waves

PRI: replaced by FR intervals, and the PRI is not reliable or determinable

QRS: < 0.12 seconds, uniform in shape

Atrial Fibrillation

As with atrial flutter, **atrial fibrillation** is the result of rapid atrial depolarization, except that it is the result of multiple ectopic sites within the atria, resulting in an atrial depolarization rate of 350–600 (Figure 29-67). Atrial fibrillation may be paroxysmal or chronic in nature with no apparent cause. It is believed to be the result of multiple coexisting reentry circuits or multiple rapidly discharging ectopic foci.[13] The hallmark of this rhythm is the gross irregularity of the ventricular response. Due to the shear volume of atrial impulses, it is impossible to predict which impulse will be conducted to the ventricles and when.

There are two main concerns with this rhythm: the rate of ventricular response and the chaotic dysrhythmic action capable of releasing blood clots into the general circulation, resulting in embolisms. It is very likely that one of them might lodge in the brain and cause a stroke.

Atrial fibrillation is a very common dysrhythmia, occurring in either diseased or healthy hearts, with a higher incidence occurring in the elderly. Research has shown a high correlation between atrial fibrillation and congestive heart failure.[13] Other disorders associated with atrial fibrillation include arterial hypertension, coronary artery disease (CAD), valvular heart disease, cardiac surgery, electrolyte disturbances, ethanol intoxication, pulmonary disease, and sepsis.[13] Atrial fibrillation may show up about 30% of the time after surgery[11] and may be associated with reentrant ectopic foci within the pulmonary veins.[11,14] Whatever the cause, atrial fibrillation is a very malignant, difficult to control dysrhythmia. In the prehospital environment, treatment should be based on the degree of hemodynamic instability demonstrated by the patient. Hemodynamic instability is most commonly the result of a very fast ventricular response rate and quite often

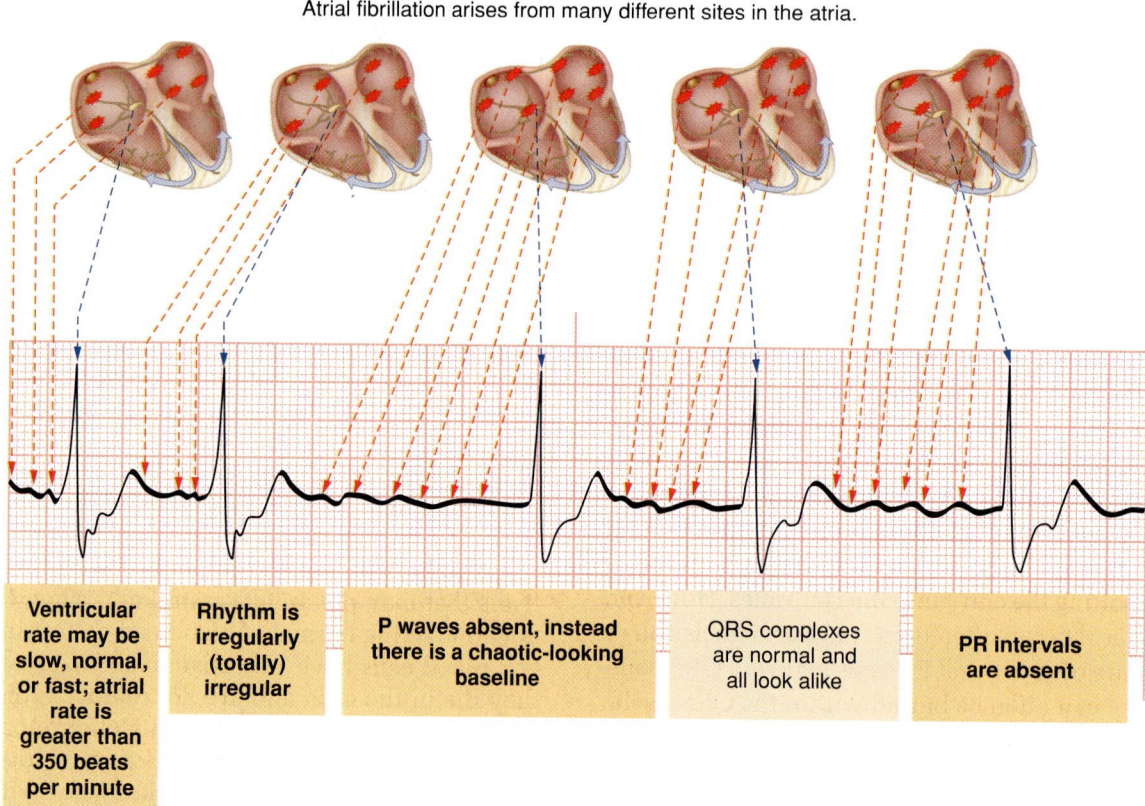

Atrial fibrillation arises from many different sites in the atria.

> **Ventricular rate may be slow, normal, or fast; atrial rate is greater than 350 beats per minute**
>
> **Rhythm is irregularly (totally) irregular**
>
> **P waves absent, instead there is a chaotic-looking baseline**
>
> **QRS complexes are normal and all look alike**
>
> **PR intervals are absent**

Figure 29-67 Atrial fibrillation.

requires synchronized cardioversion. Hospital treatment will focus on evaluating how long the rhythm has been occurring with an emphasis on treating the patient with heparin or other medication designed to reduce the formation of blood clots before the rhythm is corrected.

A diagnosis of this dysrhythmia is usually based upon its irregularly irregular ventricular response. Characteristically, no P waves are identifiable due to a very chaotic baseline produced by multiple incomplete depolarizations from many groups of cells. As in atrial flutter, atrial kick is lost, resulting in loss of cardiac output. This, along with a rapid ventricular response, produces most of the clinical symptoms, such as light-headedness and dizziness similar to atrial flutter. Atrial fibrillation is said to be controlled if, by natural or pharmacological means, the ventricular response is maintained at a rate that will afford good cardiac output to the patient. This is often produced by a relatively rhythmic ventricular response of less than 100. However, a ventricular response at a rate of greater than 150 is often present and causes treatable symptoms in the prehospital environment.

Diagnostic Criteria for Atrial Fibrillation

Rate: variable in ventricles
Rhythm: irregularly irregular
P waves: undetectable
PRI: none
QRS: < 0.12 seconds, uniform in shape

Dysrhythmias Originating from the Junction

Junctional rhythm describes any electrical rhythm that originates from within the junction. As discussed previously, the accepted location of the junction is in the nodal HIS (NH) region of the AV node. Junctional rhythms are relatively rare compared to other dysrhythmias and can be grouped into four types: primary abnormalities, those that appear after surgery, those that are secondary to drug effects, and escape rhythms due to bradycardia.[13] DOT 5-2.40

Premature Junctional Contractions (PJC)

The **premature junctional contraction (PJC)** is a complex that originates from within the AV junction (Figure 29-68). By definition, it is an ectopic beat that occurs earlier than the next expected normal beat. There are many causes, and they can occur in a healthy heart from no apparent cause. Most of the time, they are the result of drug toxicity, especially digitalis. Other less common causes include congestive heart failure and hypoxia.

As in the PAC, this dysrhythmia is not a primary rhythm but an irregularity in the underlying rhythm. Therefore, the heart rate would be that of the underlying rhythm. The rhythm would then be irregular at the time of the PJC, the degree of irregularity dependant upon how many PJCs are occurring. The most significant identifying feature would be the P wave that is associated with the PJC. Considering that this beat originates from

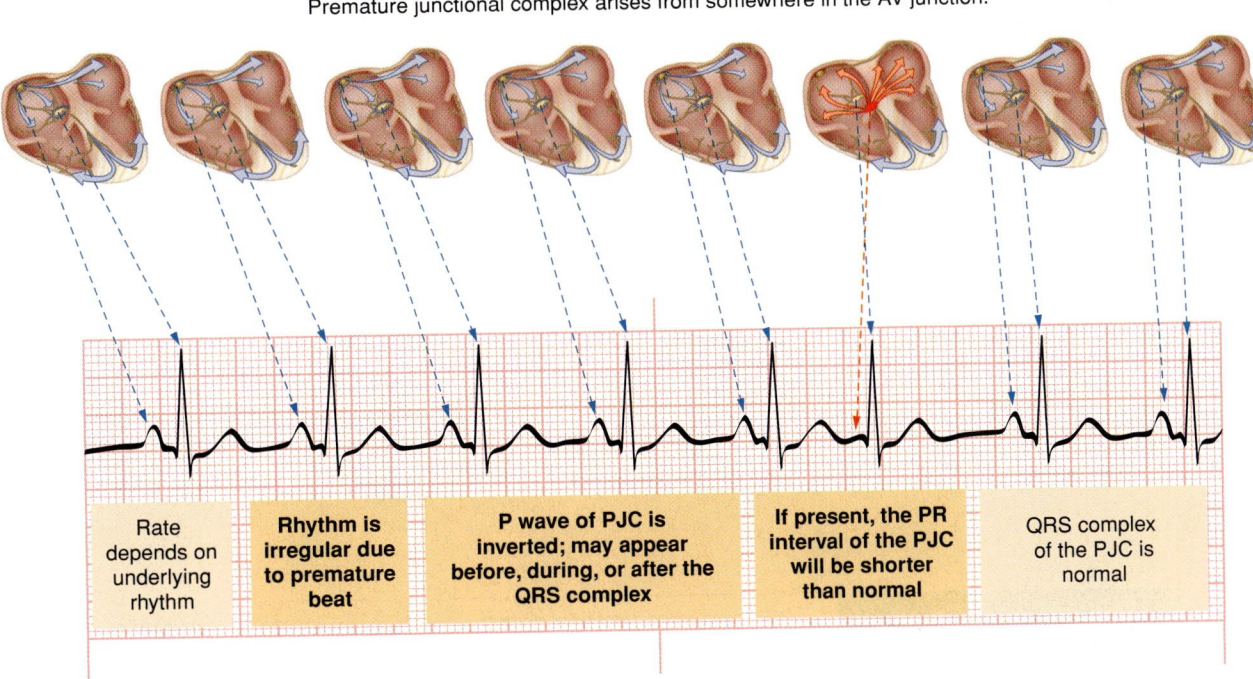

Premature junctional complex arises from somewhere in the AV junction.

| Rate depends on underlying rhythm | Rhythm is irregular due to premature beat | P wave of PJC is inverted; may appear before, during, or after the QRS complex | If present, the PR interval of the PJC will be shorter than normal | QRS complex of the PJC is normal |

Figure 29-68   Premature junctional complex.

within the AV junction, it may or may not propagate to the atria. In fact, it may collide with a sinus impulse coming down from the sinus node or be buried in the T wave of the preceding beat. An impulse originating in the proximal portion of the junction could make it to the atria and possibly depolarize them in a retrograde fashion, resulting in an inverted P wave in lead II. Impulses arising from the distal end of the junction may also depolarize the atria in a retrograde fashion. However, the P wave will most likely be buried within the QRS complex or actually occur following the QRS complex. Therefore, the identifying feature of the junctional complex in lead II is the appearance of an inverted P wave that occurs immediately before, during, or after the QRS complex.

The PR interval in a PJC usually becomes shorter than normal or less than 0.12 seconds. It could conceivably be normal or even prolonged in the presence of delayed AV conduction. The QRS complex is usually normal, unless other conduction defects exist within the ventricles.

Isolated PJCs are not usually clinically significant and do not warrant specific treatment. It is a good policy to investigate their appearance in patients taking drugs designed to regulate AV conduction such as the cardiac glycoside drug digoxin. Frequent PJCs may herald the onset of a more serious junctional dysrhythmia and also merit close monitoring.

Diagnostic Criteria for PJC

Rate: dependant upon underlying rhythm
Rhythm: occasionally irregular
P waves: inverted, prior, during or after QRS
PRI: usually < 0.12 sec (if visible)
QRS: < 0.12 seconds, uniform in shape

Junctional Escape Rhythm

The **junctional escape rhythm** is the AV junction doing its job as the secondary pacemaker in the event of failure of the SA node to function properly (Figure 29-69). Recall that the inherent firing rate of the AV junction is 40–60 beats per minute. Junctional escape occurs at a rate of 40–60 beats/minute when the sinus node fails or slows down too much. When the junction is allowed to reach threshold, a beat "escapes" and causes a depolarization, hence the name, escape rhythm.

The diagnostic characteristics of the junctional rhythm are essentially the same as the PJC, with the exception that they continue until they are suppressed by a higher pacemaker. By definition, three or more junctional complexes in a row may be called a junctional rhythm.

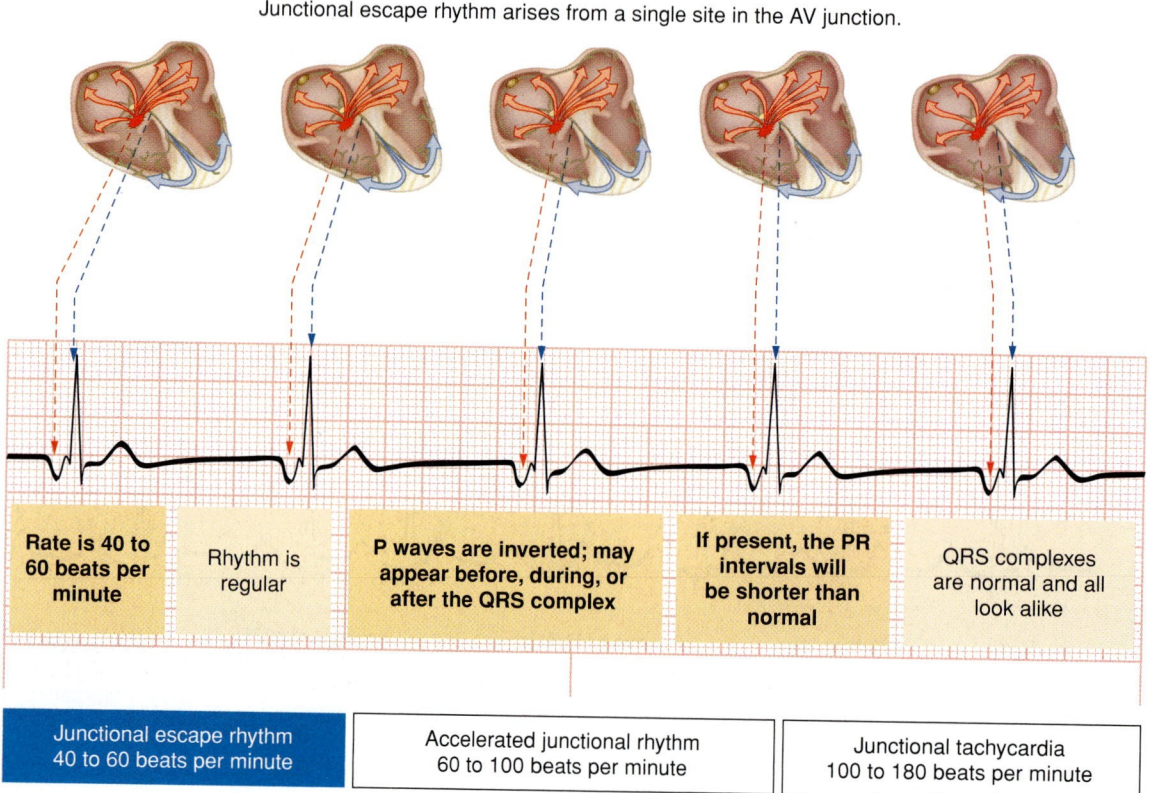

Junctional escape rhythm arises from a single site in the AV junction.

| Rate is 40 to 60 beats per minute | Rhythm is regular | P waves are inverted; may appear before, during, or after the QRS complex | If present, the PR intervals will be shorter than normal | QRS complexes are normal and all look alike |

| Junctional escape rhythm 40 to 60 beats per minute | Accelerated junctional rhythm 60 to 100 beats per minute | Junctional tachycardia 100 to 180 beats per minute |

Figure 29-69   Junctional escape rhythm.

Clinically, the signs and symptoms are the same as sinus bradycardia, in that the heart is beating too slow and may be unable to adequately perfuse the body. At the higher end of the rate, approximately 60 beats, the patient may be entirely asymptomatic and warrant only close observation and standard care, such as IV, oxygen, and so on. Always be alert for signs of deterioration of the rhythm to something more serious. Should the patient be symptomatic due to this rhythm, treatment should be promptly initiated. This rhythm would be treated as a bradycardic rhythm.

Diagnostic Criteria for Junctional Escape

Rate: 40–60
Rhythm: regular
P waves: prior, during, or after QRS complex
PRI: < 0.12 seconds
QRS: < 0.12 seconds, uniform in shape

Accelerated Junctional Rhythm

The **accelerated junctional rhythm** resembles the junctional escape rhythm with the exception of the rate (Figure 29-70). This rhythm fires at a rate of greater than 60 but still less than 100. The rules of ECG rhythm naming define tachycardia as a rhythm greater than 100 beats per minute and bradycardia as less than

60 beats per minute. In the case of junctional escape, the inherent firing rate of the junction is 40–60. Junctional tachycardia, by definition would be a heart rate greater than 100. The term accelerated junctional rhythm is very descriptive: It is firing faster than the inherent rate top rate of 60, but not fast enough to be called tachycardia.

The patient is usually asymptomatic unless other conditions exist. Seldom does this dysrhythmia warrant specific treatment in the prehospital environment. Monitor the patient closely for any changes in condition or rhythm. Enhanced automaticity of the junction and digoxin toxicity remain the primary causes.

Diagnostic Criteria of Accelerated Junctional

Rate: 60–100
Rhythm: regular
P waves: prior, during, or after the QRS
PRI: < 0.12 seconds if visible
QRS: < 0.12 seconds, uniform in shape

Junctional Tachycardia

Junctional tachycardia identifies any rhythm originating from the junction at a rate greater than 100 (Figure 29-71). It is usually between 100 and 180 beats per minute. The

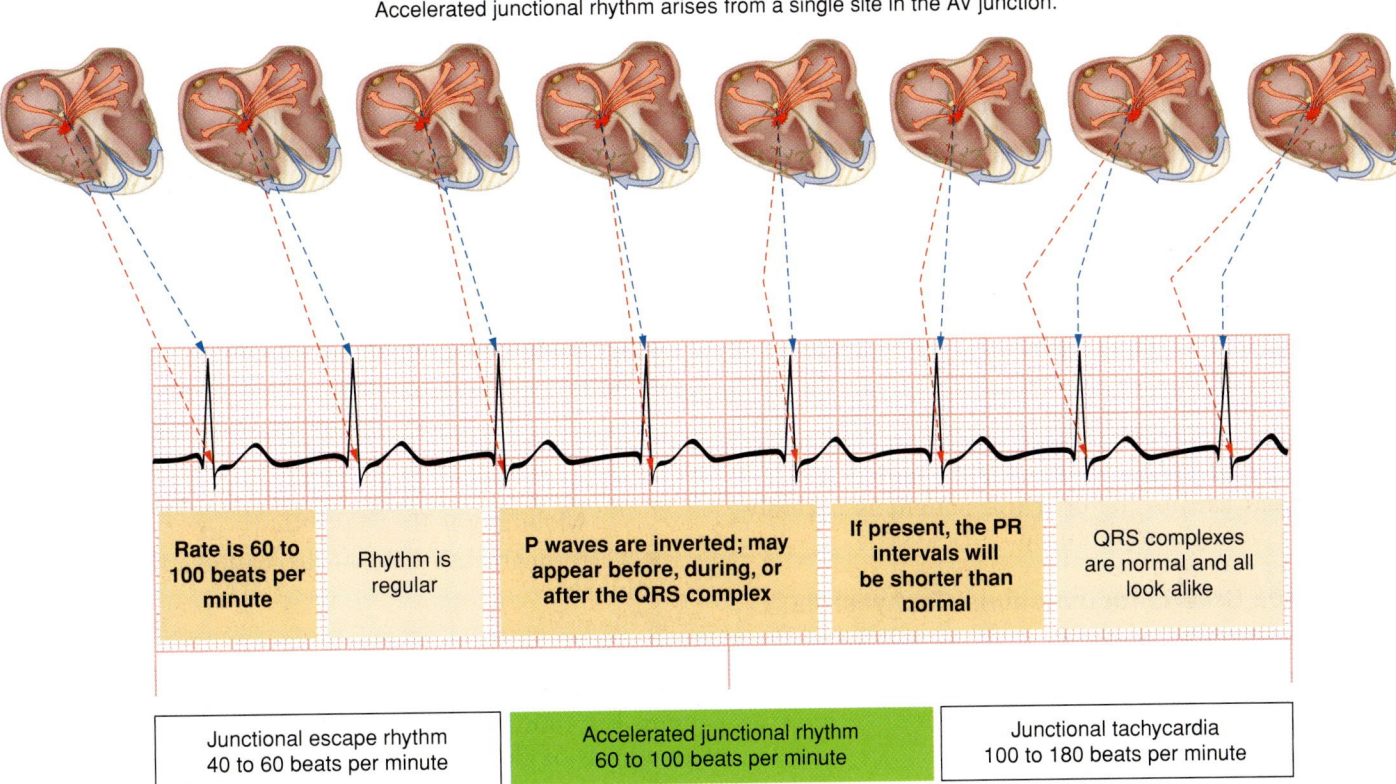

Accelerated junctional rhythm arises from a single site in the AV junction.

| Rate is 60 to 100 beats per minute | Rhythm is regular | P waves are inverted; may appear before, during, or after the QRS complex | If present, the PR intervals will be shorter than normal | QRS complexes are normal and all look alike |

| Junctional escape rhythm 40 to 60 beats per minute | Accelerated junctional rhythm 60 to 100 beats per minute | Junctional tachycardia 100 to 180 beats per minute |

Figure 29-70 Accelerated junctional rhythm.

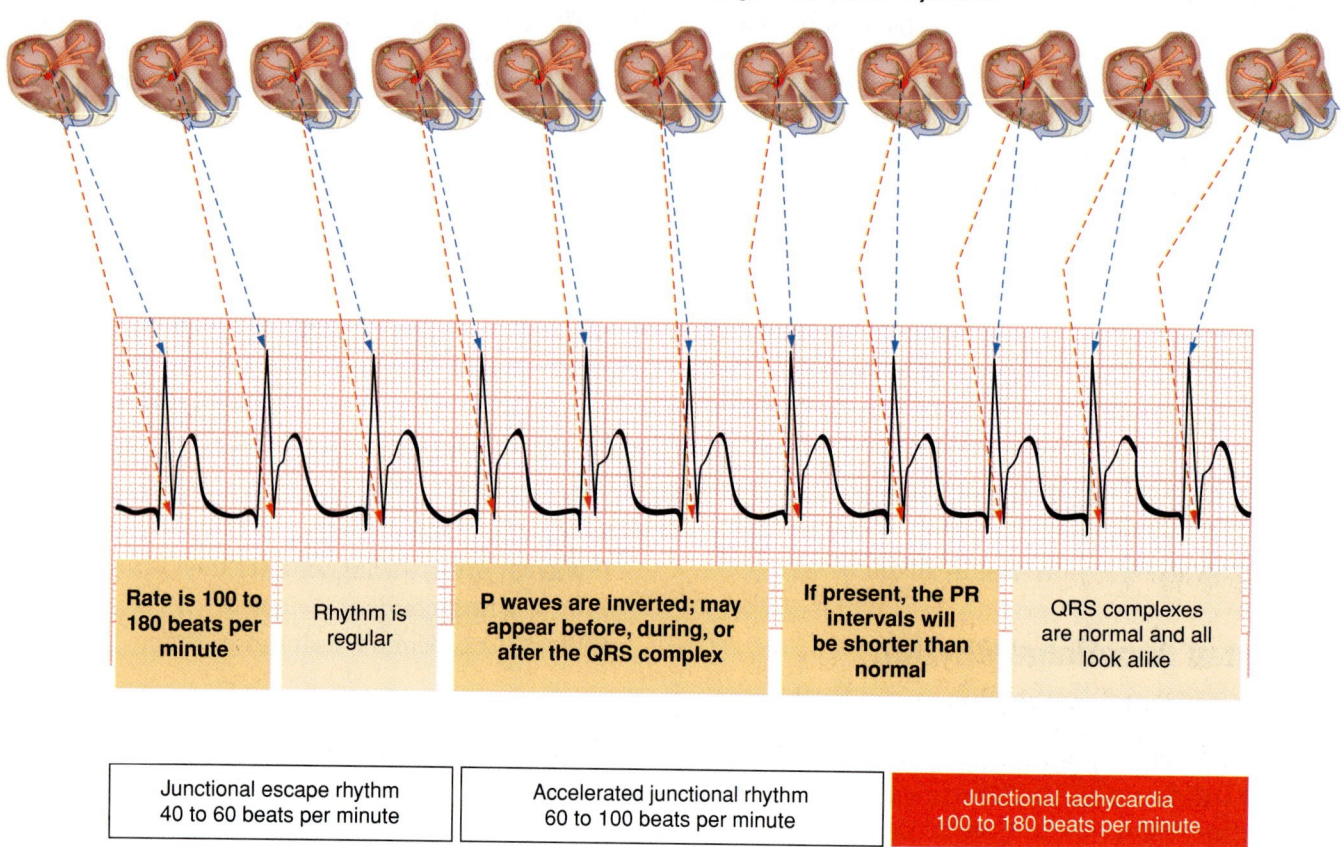

Junctional tachycardia arises from a single focus in the AV junction.

| Rate is 100 to 180 beats per minute | Rhythm is regular | P waves are inverted; may appear before, during, or after the QRS complex | If present, the PR intervals will be shorter than normal | QRS complexes are normal and all look alike |

| Junctional escape rhythm 40 to 60 beats per minute | Accelerated junctional rhythm 60 to 100 beats per minute | Junctional tachycardia 100 to 180 beats per minute |

Figure 29-71   Junctional tachycardia.

cause is usually related to digoxin toxicity or a reentry mechanism around the AV node. Since at high rates this rhythm may be difficult to differentiate from atrial tachycardia, it falls into the same category as a supraventricular tachycardia and is treated as such. You may observe a retrograde P wave behind the QRS complex, or you may see none at all.

At the slower end of the spectrum, the patient may appear asymptomatic, but as the rate approaches or exceeds 150, serious symptoms of hemodynamic compromise may develop. Because the atria are not regularly depolarized, atrial kick is lost. Couple this with decreased ventricular filling time, and cardiac output will fall.[8] Management of this rhythm centers on eliminating the cause but may require direct intervention such as synchronized cardioversion if the patient is severely hemodynamically compromised.

Diagnostic Criteria for Junctional Tachycardia

Rate: > 100 (100–180)
Rhythm: regular
P waves: prior, during, or after the QRS
PRI: < 0.12 seconds if visible
QRS: < 0.12 seconds, uniform in shape

Atrioventricular Blocks

The term *block* implies an interruption or termination of normal cardiac conduction along normal pathways. Quite often, the impulse is not completely blocked but forced to take a different route.[10] **Atrioventricular blocks** occur when the pathway is blocked within the AV node, bundle of His, or the bundle branches. They are usually categorized into three groups:

- First-degree AV block
- Second-degree AV block
  - AV block type I—also called Wenckebach or Mobitz type I
  - AV block type II—also called Classic block or Mobitz type II
- Third-degree AV block—also called complete heart block

It is important to understand that the degree of block doesn't always denote the severity of the dysrhythmia, but rather it is a simplified classification. Several methods of classification have arisen in the past in an attempt to make the terminology more descriptive, but these names have prevailed and continue to be widely

In 1st-degree AV heart block impulses arise from the SA node but their passage through the AV node is delayed

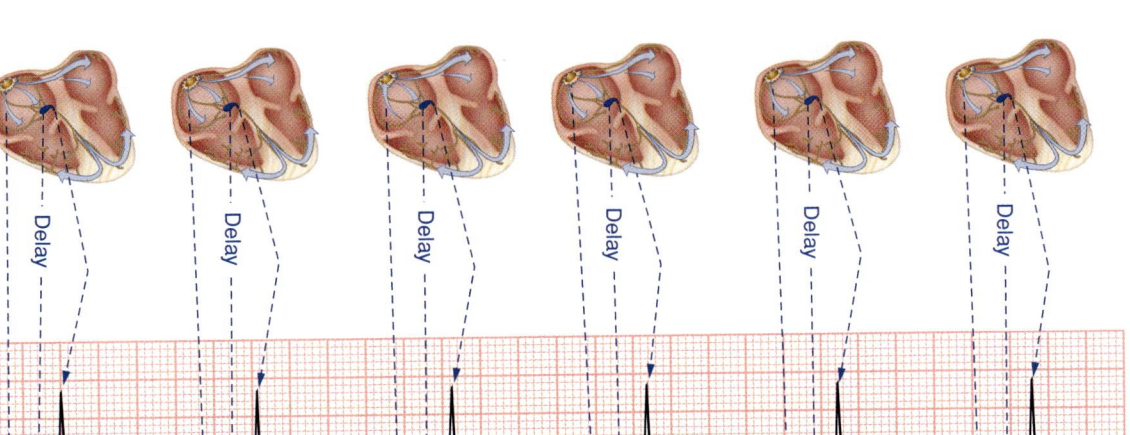

| Underlying rate may be slow, normal, or fast | Underlying rhythm is usually regular | Present and normal and all are followed by a QRS complex | PR interval is longer than 0.20 seconds and is constant | QRS complexes are normal |

Figure 29-72   First-degree heart block.

accepted. All AV blocks share the feature that communication between the atria and ventricles is delayed, occasionally blocked, or permanently blocked. With the exception of the first-degree AV block, all of the other blocks will have more P waves than QRS complexes. This feature makes AV block relatively easy to identify.

First-Degree AV Block

The term **first-degree AV block** can be a little misleading due to the fact that there is a delay rather than a block occurring within the AV node (Figure 29-72). The PR interval is prolonged to longer than 0.20 seconds, but every P wave results in the formation of a QRS. First-degree AV block is typically considered to be a nonmalignant rhythm because it doesn't produce any real symptoms unless the rhythm is accompanied by bradycardia significant enough to cause symptoms.[10] Approximately 13% of patients with acute myocardial infarction present with prolonged PR intervals.[11] This is usually associated with inferior infarctions due to involvement of the RCA, which provides blood to the AV and SA node in 90% of the population. Treatment of the first-degree AV block by itself is not indicated, but it must be monitored in the event of progression to a more lethal dysrhythmia.

Diagnostic Criteria for First-Degree Block

Rate: that of underlying rhythm
Rhythm: regular
P waves: present and precede each QRS
PRI: > 0.20 seconds
QRS: < 0.12 seconds, uniform in shape

Second-Degree AV Block Type I

Second-degree AV block is an actual block resulting from a progressive delay in conduction through the AV node until an impulse is blocked entirely (Figure 29-73). This is noted through the progressive increasing of the PR interval until a QRS fails to appear. This is often described as a "dropped beat." The progressive delay is described by the Wenckebach phenomenon (which describes the progressive PRI until a beat is dropped); therefore, it is commonly referred to as the **Wenckebach rhythm.**[5]

The pathology causing the second-degree AV block type I is almost always in the AV node and very rarely within the bundle of His. This dysrhythmia is commonly seen during an inferior wall myocardial infarction but may appear due to acute infections, myocarditis, and drug toxicity and occasionally in well-trained athletes due to enhanced vagal tone.[8,11] Identification is

In 2nd-degree AV heart block, Type I (Wenckebach), impulses arise from the SA node but their passage through the AV node is progressively delayed until the impulse is blocked.

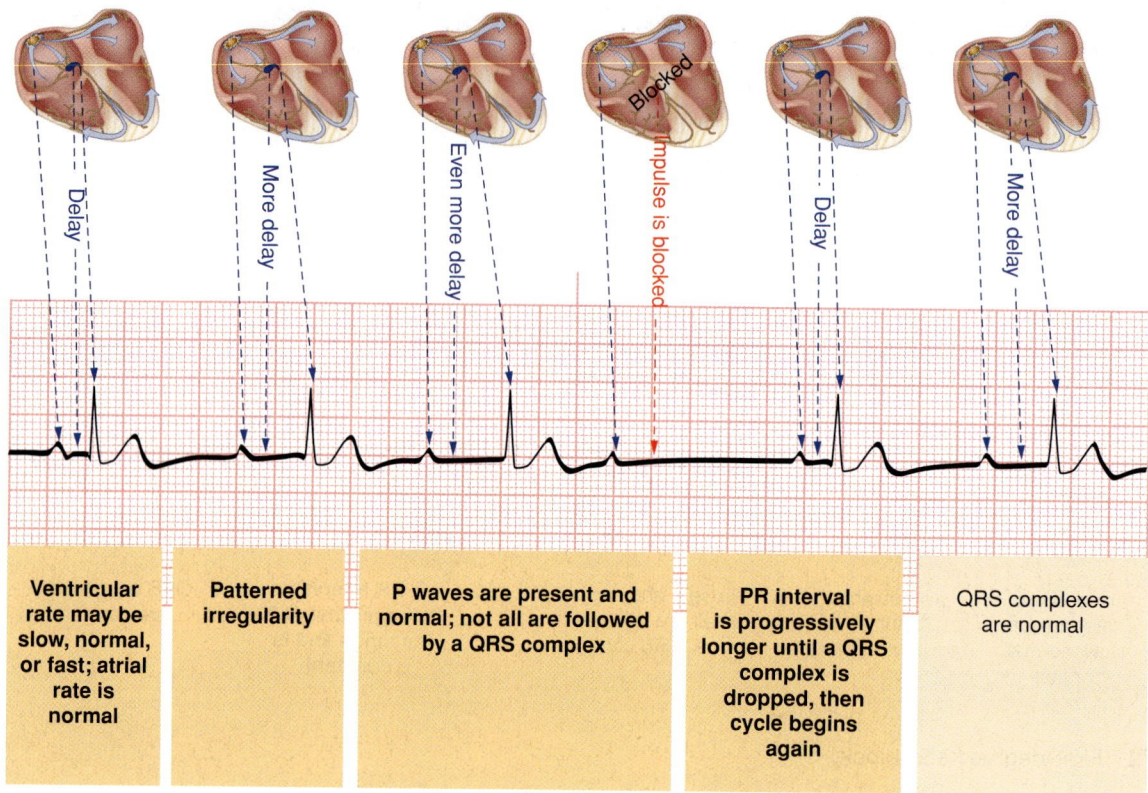

| Ventricular rate may be slow, normal, or fast; atrial rate is normal | Patterned irregularity | P waves are present and normal; not all are followed by a QRS complex | PR interval is progressively longer until a QRS complex is dropped, then cycle begins again | QRS complexes are normal |

Figure 29-73 Second-degree heart block, type I.

usually based upon the appearance of the Wenckebach phenomenon but is also characterized by periods of grouped beats. Because the PP and RR are getting shorter until a beat is actually dropped, the complexes appear in clusters.

The second-degree AV type I block is usually transient and reversible when the cause is resolved. Treatment of signs and symptoms remains the focus of prehospital treatment. In the event this rhythm is producing serious signs and symptoms due to bradycardia, direct treatment may be required involving the administration of atropine, a catecholamine drug by IV drip, or external cardiac pacing.

Diagnostic Criteria for Second-Degree Type I

Rate: that of underlying atrial rhythm

Rhythm: regularly irregular

P waves: present and precede QRS when it occurs because of the unconducted beat there are more Ps than QRSs

PRI: gradually lengthens

QRS: < 0.12 seconds, uniform in shape

Second-Degree AV Block Type II

While the second-degree type I AV block tends to have a more normal rate, the second-degree AV block type II is usually somewhat slower (Figure 29-74). It is essentially regular with consistent PP and PR intervals until a QRS complex is dropped. This rhythm tends to have a consistent ratio of conducted to nonconducted P waves, (for example, 2 conducted, 1 nonconducted, or 3 to 1). The location of this block may be in the bundle of His but is usually found infranodal, with an intermittent block of one bundle branch and a complete block of the other. In this case, the QRS pattern tends to be wide because the impulse is forced to take an alternate route through the ventricles. This block is more serious than the type I and could progress to a complete heart block.

The **second-degree type II AV block** is commonly the result of extensive damage to the bundle branches caused by an anteroseptal infarction. This block tends to be very unpredictable in the presence of heart disease and represents a very serious condition for the patient. The patient may show signs of hemodynamic compromise due to heart rate, myocardial infarction, or any combination of either. The patient may complain of an odd sensation from the skipped beats.

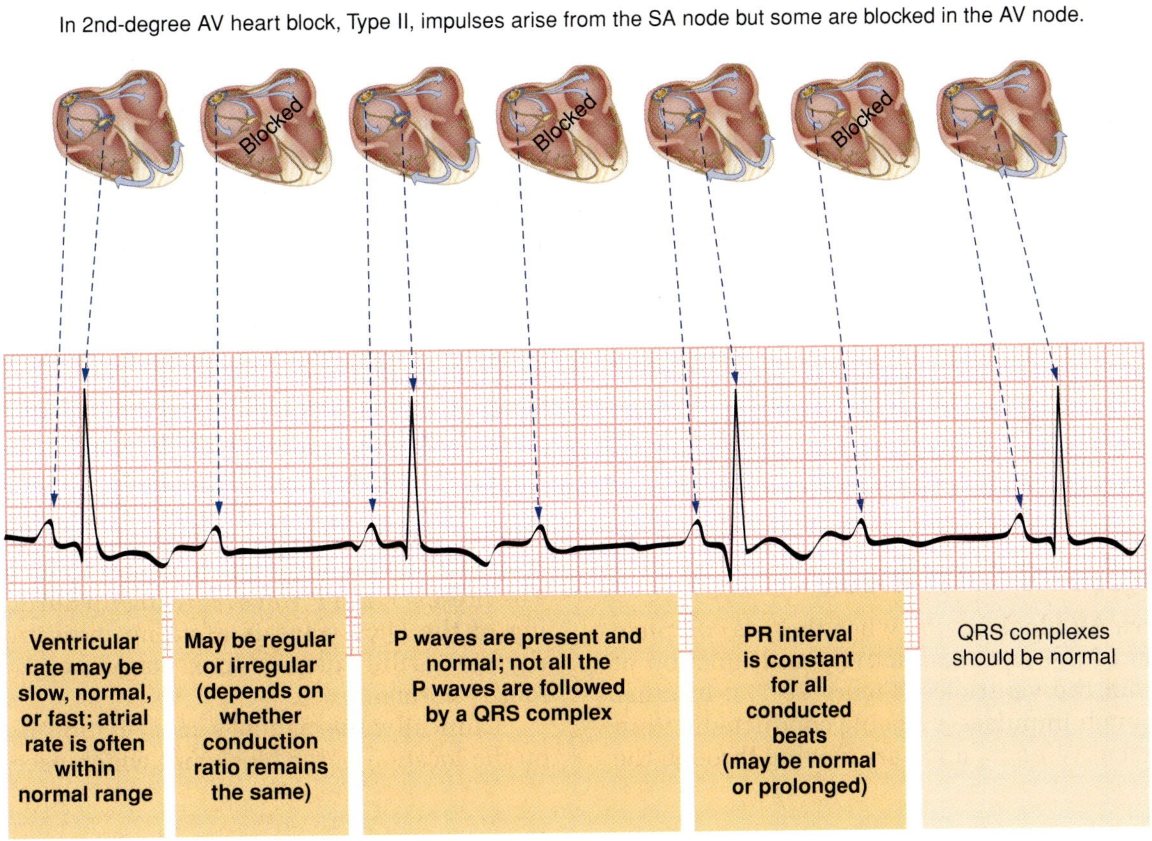

In 2nd-degree AV heart block, Type II, impulses arise from the SA node but some are blocked in the AV node.

| Ventricular rate may be slow, normal, or fast; atrial rate is often within normal range | May be regular or irregular (depends on whether conduction ratio remains the same) | P waves are present and normal; not all the P waves are followed by a QRS complex | PR interval is constant for all conducted beats (may be normal or prolonged) | QRS complexes should be normal |

Figure 29-74   Second-degree heart block, type II.

Treatment for this rhythm revolves around treatment of the underlying condition and supporting the heart rate so that it improves cardiac output. This is accomplished usually through external cardiac pacing. The parasympathetic blocker atropine is not recommended with this rhythm because of a risk in creating a higher grade block. The use of atropine can also increase myocardial oxygen demand, which could worsen an already weakened myocardium if an AMI is present.

Diagnostic Criteria for Second-Degree Type II

Rate: atrial rate due to underlying rhythm, ventricular rate is lower

Rhythm: irregular
P waves: regular and precede conducted QRS
PRI: consistent until QRS is dropped
QRS: typically > 0.12 seconds

2:1 AV Block

A **2:1 AV block** is a term that applies to a rhythm with a conduction ratio of two P waves to every QRS complex (Figure 29-75). Since the hallmark of distinguishing between type I and type II AV blocks is the PR interval, it is very difficult to conclusively identify this rhythm as either one. One clue may be that the width of the QRS

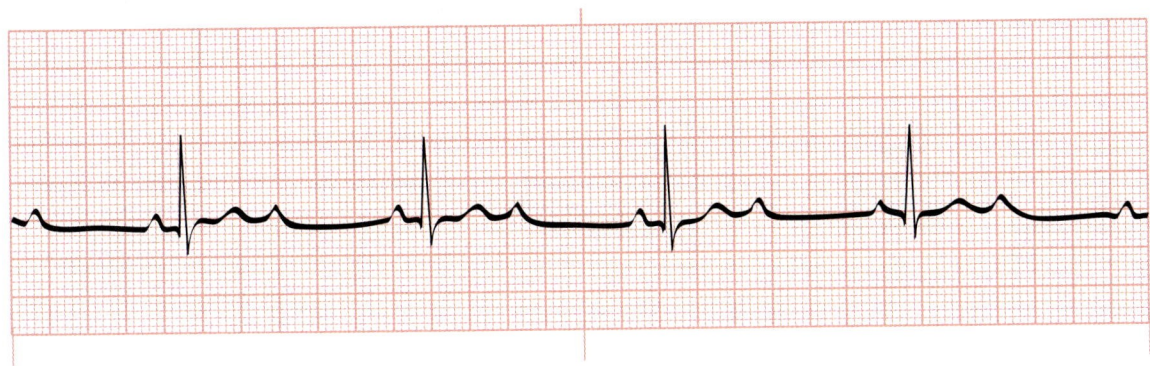

Figure 29-75   ECG of a 2:1 AV block.

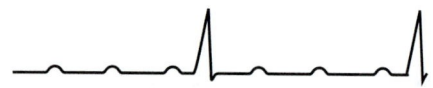

At least three P waves for every QRS complex

Figure 29-76   High grade second-degree AV block.

complex is usually wider in the type II. All other treatment and assessment remains the same.

High-Grade Second-Degree AV Block

A **high-grade second-degree AV block** occurs when two or more consecutive atrial beats fail to reach the QRS complexes due to the block itself (Figure 29-76).[11]

Third-Degree AV Heart Block

Third-degree AV block occurs when there is complete dissociation of the electrical activity and function of the atria from the ventricles (Figure 29-77). In other words, although impulses are being conducted within the atria to the AV node, none are moving through the

AV junction into the ventricles, and the ventricles pace themselves. This block may be located at the AV node, in the bundle of His, or within the bundle branches. When the ventricular complexes are generated from the atria, they follow the inherent rates for automaticity in that area of the heart. Since there is dissociation at or near the AV junction or node, the ventricular rate matches either the node inherent rate (40–60) or the purkinje fibers rate (20–40).

The hallmark of identification of third-degree block is a regular atrial rate and a regular ventricular rate, but one is different from the other, and the relationship between them (as noted in the PRI) is nonexistent. The sinus node may be firing at 80 beats/minute, but the ventricles may be running on the ventricular pacemaker at a rate of 40. As you look across the ECG strip, you will see that the P waves appear to "march" across the strip. The QRS complexes have a similar appearance. The presence of a P wave showing up during the drawing of the QRS wave is a strong indication that the rhythm is a third degree block, particularly if the P wave looks "normal."

Clinically, the patient's presentation is dependant on the location of the block and which pacemaker is in

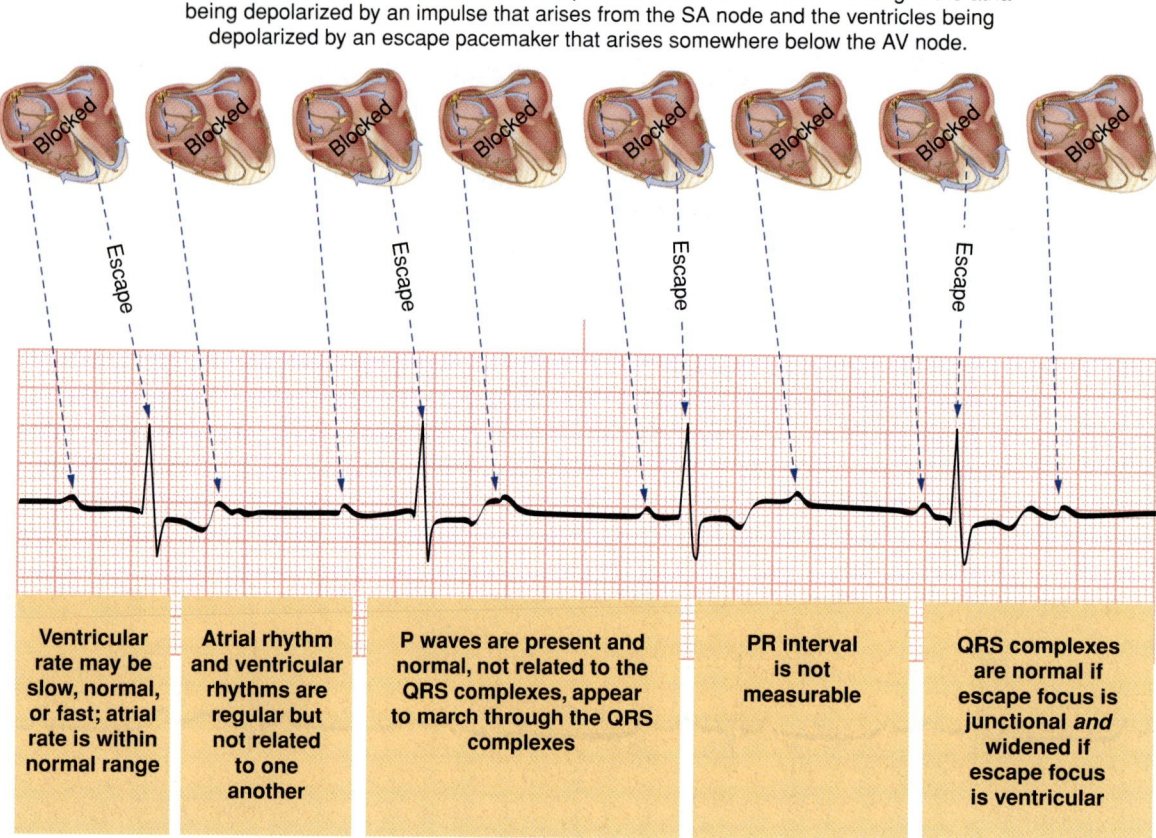

In 3rd-degree AV heart block there is a complete block at the AV node resulting in the atria being depolarized by an impulse that arises from the SA node and the ventricles being depolarized by an escape pacemaker that arises somewhere below the AV node.

| Ventricular rate may be slow, normal, or fast; atrial rate is within normal range | Atrial rhythm and ventricular rhythms are regular but not related to one another | P waves are present and normal, not related to the QRS complexes, appear to march through the QRS complexes | PR interval is not measurable | QRS complexes are normal if escape focus is junctional *and* widened if escape focus is ventricular |

Figure 29-77   Complete heart block.

control. A block within the AV node may result in a ventricular rate of 60, and although without appreciable atrial kick, the patient may still appear quite normal. On the other hand, a block located in the bundle branches will result in the ventricular pacemaker driving the ventricular rate, and the patient may present with signs of profound bradycardia due to reduced cardiac output.

In rare cases, the ventricles will begin to depolarize at a more rapid rate than the atria, creating a condition very similar to the complete heart block. This is called **atrioventricular dissociation.**[10] Again, this is rare and is often confused with traditional third-degree block but has a different etiology.

Diagnostic Criteria for Third-Degree Block

Rate: atrial rate that of underlying rhythm
  ventricular rate typically 20–60
Rhythm: regular
P waves: not associated with QRS
PRI: vary widely
QRS: narrow or wide dependant upon location of
  block and origin of the QRS

AV blocks are significant because they can reflect serious heart disease or myocardial infarction. Signs and symptoms associated with the blocks are almost always due to reduced cardiac output as the result of the bradycardic rhythm. The decision to treat must be weighed carefully against the risk of exacerbating the underlying condition and hemodynamic compromise. In the emergency setting, treatment is only recommended in the presence of signs of hemodynamic compromise. Signs of significant hemodynamic compromise include an altered level of consciousness, presence of shock, diaphoresis (sweating), dyspnea, and signs of cardiac insufficiency such as chest pain.

Ventricular Dysrhythmias

Ventricular dysrhythmias are probably the most significant of all dysrhythmias (Figure 29-78). These dysrhythmias often degrade into life-threatening conditions leading to cardiopulmonary arrest. This is due to the fact that if the ventricles are not working rhythmically, there is no cardiac output at all. While there are several types of ventricular dysrhythmias, and some more dangerous than others, they all represent some degree of irritability within the ventricles and warrant investigation.

Ventricular dysrhythmias all have several characteristics in common that will help you identify them. First, the width of the QRS complex is greater than 0.12 seconds. This is explained by the fact that most ectopic beats originate outside of the normal conduction fibers, so they will propagate slowly until the fibers are reached. This also explains the bizarre shape. The complex may be biphasic, monophasic, notched, or slurred (Figure 29-79). Ventricular beats typically have larger amplitude than normal beats. To understand how this is possible, look at how the ventricles are normally depolarized. First, the septum is depolarized; then the right and left ventricles depolarize almost simultaneously. The left ventricle is much larger than the right, so it becomes the dominant force of energy picked up by the ECG electrodes. As the impulse spreads, the currents from the left ventricle cancel out the currents moving through the right ventricle.[11] In the case of the ventricular beat, the ventricles don't simultaneously depolarize, so there is no cancellation of the currents, resulting in a larger perceived amplitude by the monitor.

Another feature of ventricular dysrhythmias is that the T wave tends to have opposite polarity from the QRS. This means that if the ventricular-generated beat has a positively deflected QRS, there is a good chance the T wave will be negatively deflected. During abnormal depolarization, the repolarization pattern is also abnormal, resulting in a secondary T wave change.[11]

When discussing atrial contractions, the compensatory and noncompensatory pause were mentioned. Recall that this basically means that the ectopic impulse either depolarized the sinus node or it did not. In the case of ventricular beats, the SA node is seldom affected, allowing the basic rhythm to go on unaffected after the ectopic beat. This is another very common identifying feature of ventricular beats; they are usually associated with full compensatory pauses.

Premature Ventricular Contractions

Most people experience **premature ventricular contractions (PVCs)** at some point in their life; in fact, daily occurrence of a few PVCs is the norm rather than the exception. However, in the presence of other symptoms or conditions, they must be carefully assessed and occasionally suppressed to protect the patient from life-threatening dysrhythmias. Historically, it was suspected that certain types of PVCs were more likely to initiate dangerous dysrhythmias, but recent studies have shown this to be untrue.[9] Consider, instead, the presentation of the patient and the patients history to decide whether to simply monitor the PVC or be more aggressive with treatment. While it is true that most patients experiencing an AMI with ventricular ectopy will respond to antidysrhythmic therapy, the therapy itself is not without risks.[9] Antidysrhythmic drugs all have the potential to suppress automaticity, and there is always a risk of allergic reaction or adverse effect with the administration of any medication.

Also, some dysrhythmias may be serving a protective function for the patient. Consider what may happen if an antidysrhythmic drug were administered to a patient whose heart rate was 60 beats per minute with

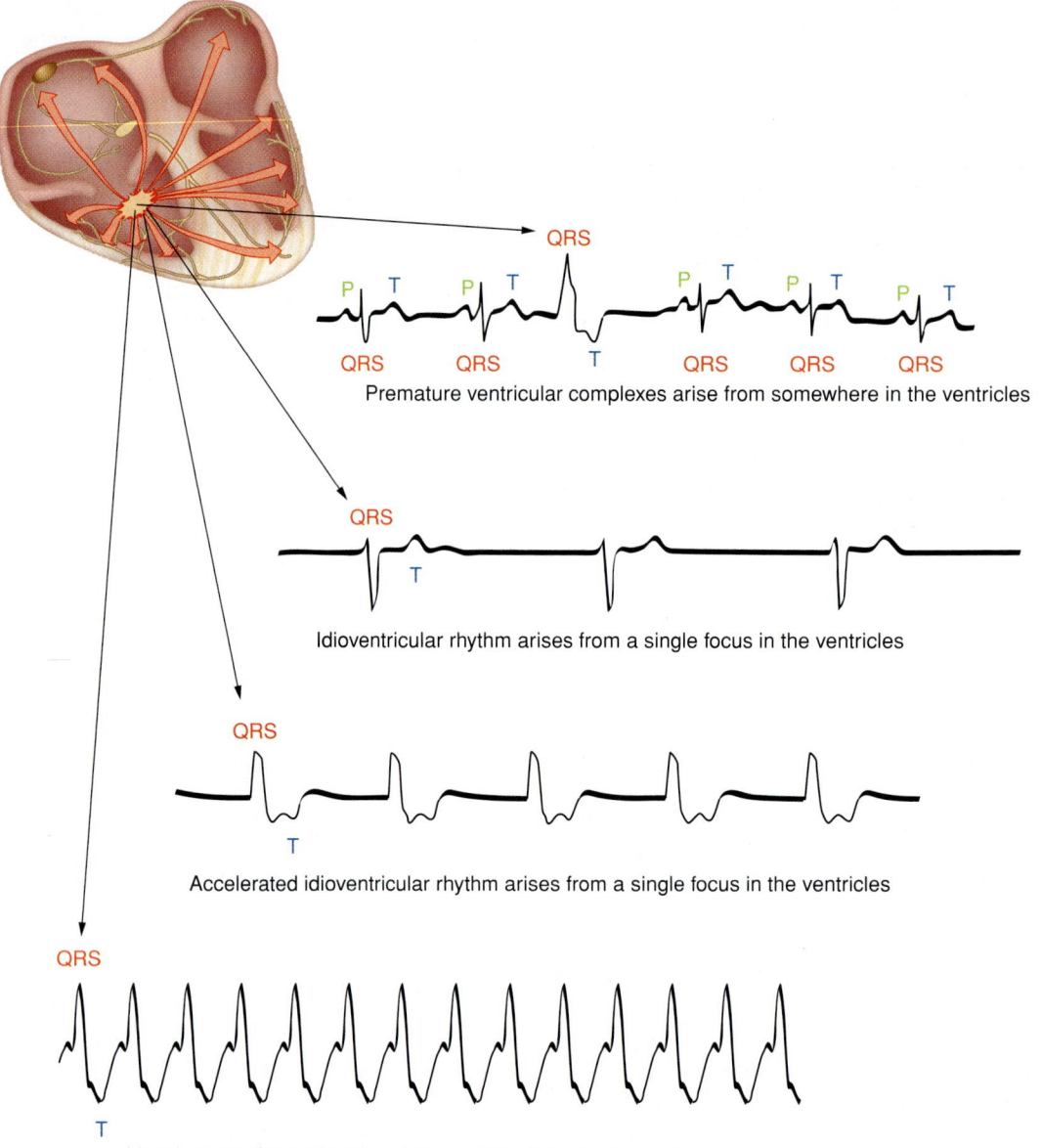

Premature ventricular complexes arise from somewhere in the ventricles

Idioventricular rhythm arises from a single focus in the ventricles

Accelerated idioventricular rhythm arises from a single focus in the ventricles

Ventricular tachycardia arises from a single focus in the ventricles

Figure 29-78   Ventricular dysrhythmias.

every one of those "abnormal beats" actually a perfusing ventricular escape beat. Once the ectopy is suppressed, the patient now has a rhythm of 30 and a corresponding drop in cardiac output to a dangerous level. It is necessary always to assess the patient for signs and symptoms and try to get all of the pieces of the clinical picture before treating a dysrhythmia just because it exists.

A PVC is a ventricular complex or pair of complexes that occur early, before the next normal beat is expected. Because it originates from within the ventricles and is not following traditional pathways, its appearance is usually wide and bizarre. Remember that the fastest route through the ventricle is from the atria through the AV junction. Any other pathway takes longer, thus in the case of PVCs, the QRS complex will be wider than 0.12 seconds.

Some of the characteristics of the PVC follow:

- They are all premature, wide complexes.
- They are not associated with a P wave and most do not affect the sinus node.
- The ST segment and T wave of the PVC are often deflected in opposite directions.
- Some may be directed into the atria, causing retrograde conduction.

PVCs result from several causes, but most are the result of enhanced automaticity, trigger activity, and re-entry mechanisms. Enhanced automaticity could result from stimulation from drugs or stress or may be the result of damaged cellular membranes, causing irritability

Premature ventricular complexes arise from somewhere in the venticle(s)

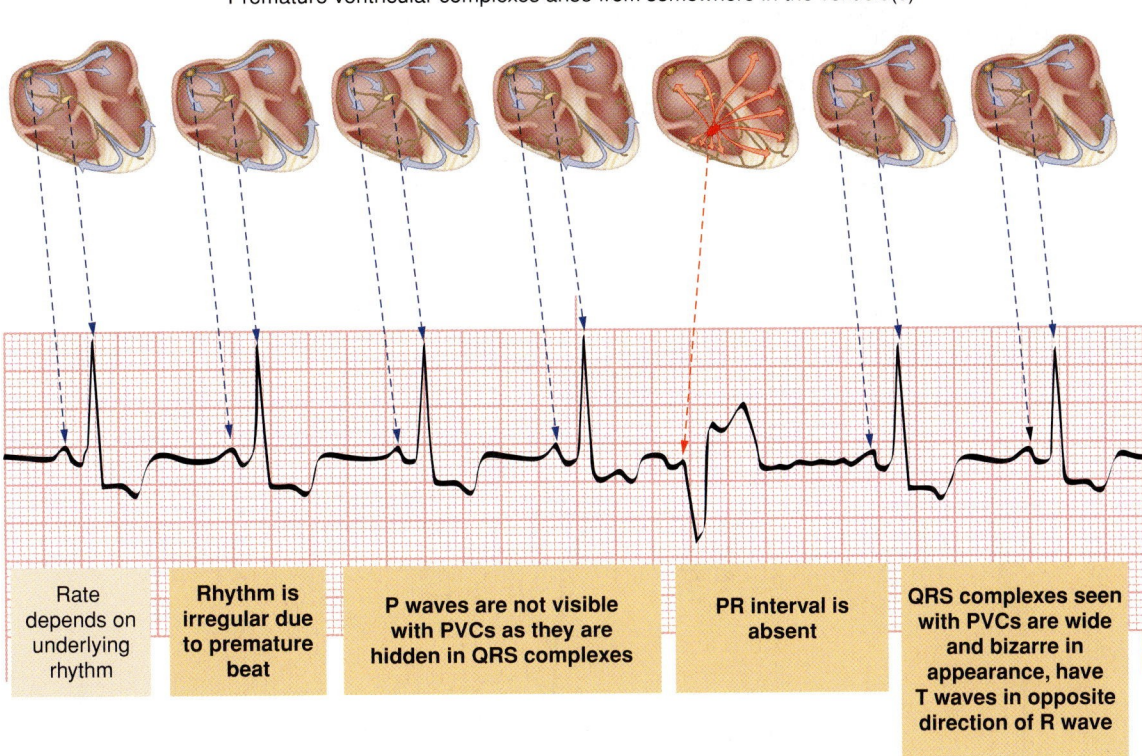

| Rate depends on underlying rhythm | Rhythm is irregular due to premature beat | P waves are not visible with PVCs as they are hidden in QRS complexes | PR interval is absent | QRS complexes seen with PVCs are wide and bizarre in appearance, have T waves in opposite direction of R wave |

Figure 29-79   Premature ventricular complexes.

or cellular dysfunction. Reentry mechanisms were discussed earlier in atrial dysrhythmias. The same principle applies to ventricular conduction. Delayed conduction in damaged tissue may reenter the conduction system and generate an ectopic impulse.

To understand triggered activity, we must revisit the action potential once again. If you recall, phase 3 is the repolarization of the cell, terminating in phase 4 or the return to the resting membrane potential (RMP). As the RMP is reached, there is a small depolarization rebound that normally goes unnoticed.[7] If this after-potential is of sufficient height to reach threshold, a depolarization may be initiated, thus a premature beat is formed. In order to reach threshold, the RMP must be nearer the threshold than normal or the threshold is lower. This may occur through the effects of medication, electrolyte imbalance, or ischemic or injured tissue. In this manner, affected cells in the ventricles may produce PVCs through triggered activity, which is often called irritability.

PVCs are typically named for their timing and association with other beats. These names are important in describing the frequency and, in some cases, the severity of the rhythm. A basic PVC originating from one focus (tissue site) is referred to as a unifocal PVC. It describes a PCV originating from one spot and following the same conduction pathway every time it occurs, so each ectopic beat is identical in morphology (Figure 29-80).

Contrast this to the multiformed PVC that may arise from the same location, but the conduction follows a different pathway through the ventricles, making them appear slightly different. A third type of PVC is referred to as the multifocal PVC, where the complexes are obviously originating from different locations within the ventricles. Multiformed and multifocal PVCs are difficult to distinguish from one another. Multifocal PVCs are more ominous because there are numerous irritable foci.

PVCs are also known to occur in patterns such as when they follow every other beat, every third beat, or every fourth beat. Respectively, they are named bigeminal, trigeminal, and quadrigeminal rhythms. Therefore, a rhythm in which every other beat is a PVC would be called ventricular bigeminy. Occasionally, PVCs will occur in groups or pairs known as couplets. A group of three or more PVCs are either referred to as a salvo, burst, or run of ventricular tachycardia (Figure 29-81).

If the sinus node remains intact and is firing normally and the patient is also experiencing PVCs, every so often the timing of a PVC impulse is going to occur right at the same instance as the sinus beat. The two impulses would then meet somewhere in the middle of the conduction system. The complex that results from this collision is a funny looking beat known as a fusion beat. It has a bizarre appearance not resembling any other complex either sinus or ventricular in

Measure first R-R interval that precedes the early beat

Rotate or slide the calipers over until the left leg is lined up with the second R wave— mark the point where the tip of the right leg falls

Rotate or slide the calipers over until the left leg is lined up with your first mark

When the tip of the right caliper leg lines up with the next R wave it is considered a compensatory pause

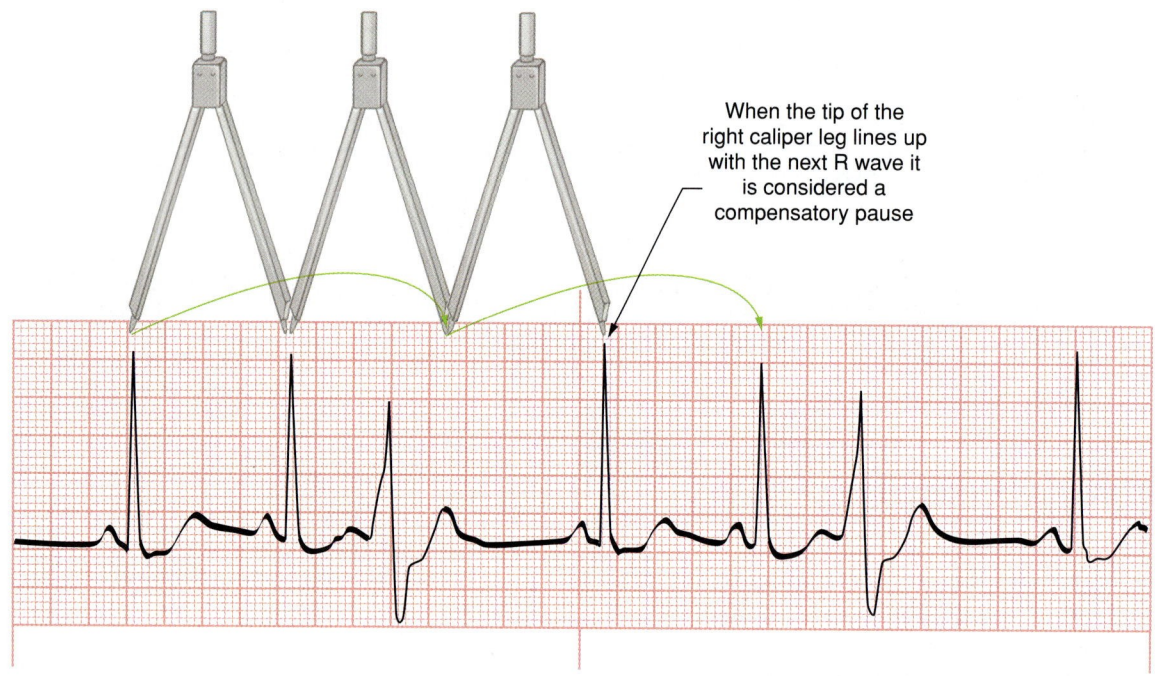

(a)

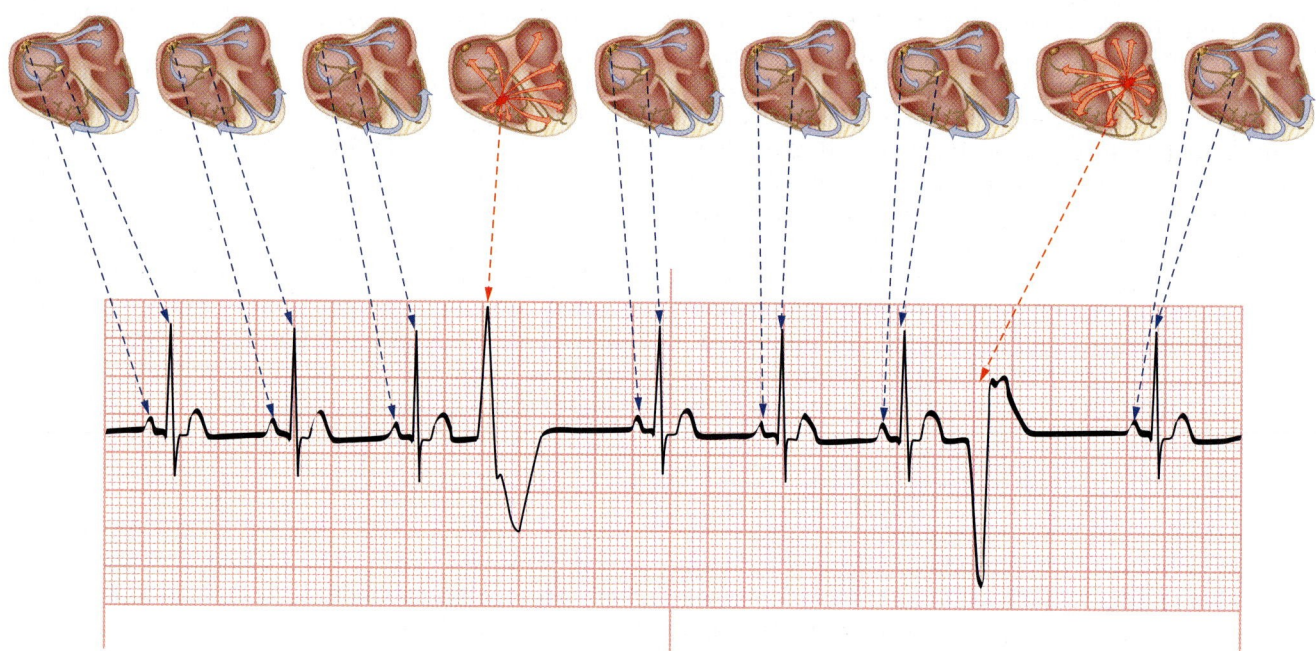

(b)

Figure 29-80 Unifocal (a) and multifocal (b) PVCs.

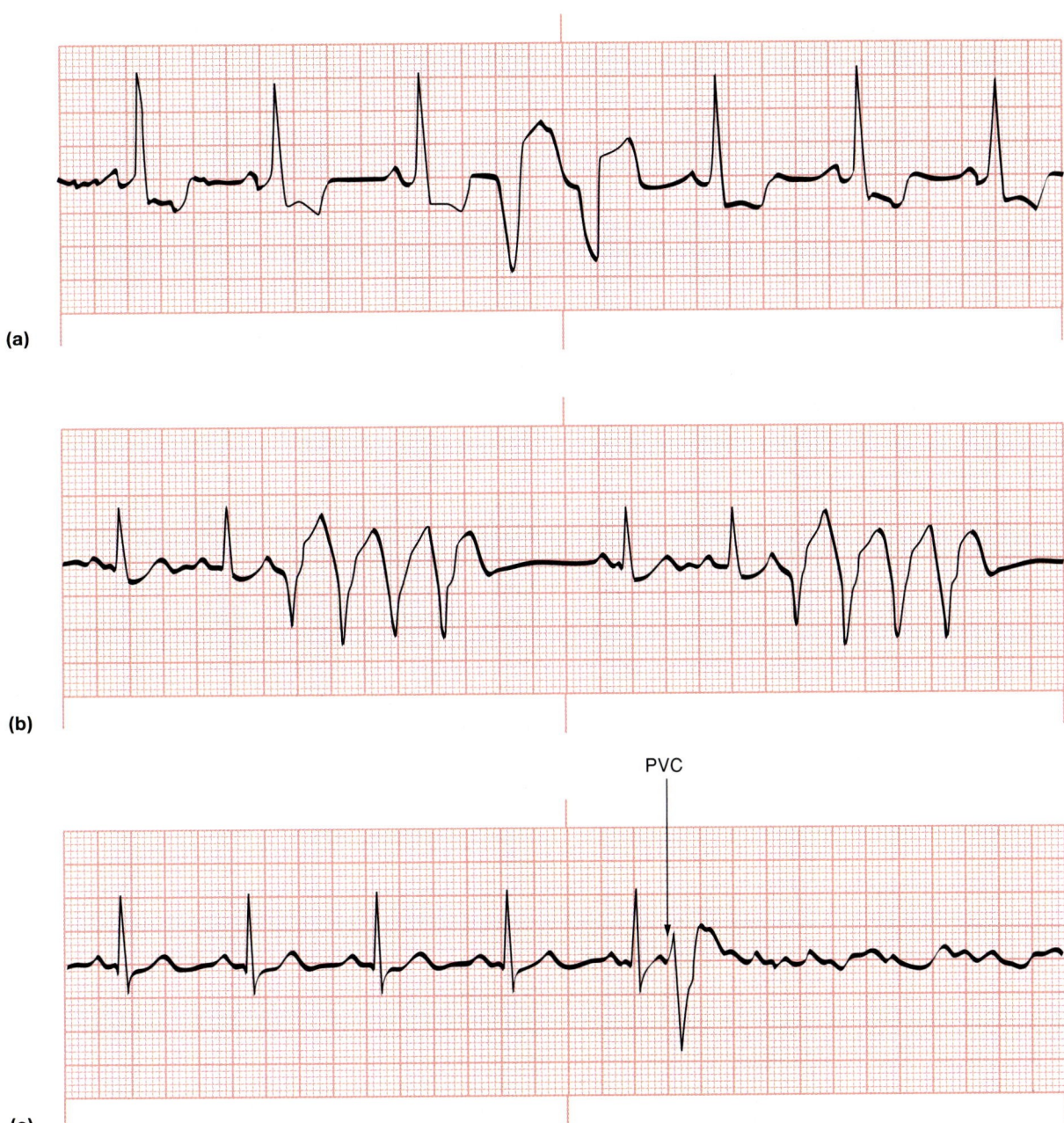

(a)

(b)

PVC

(c)

Figure 29-81   Pairs and groups of PVCs. (a) Two PVCs in succession are a couplet. (b) Three or more in a row are called a run. (c) A PVC on or near a T wave can precipitate ventricular tachycardia or fibrillation.

origin. In the case of sustained ventricular activity, fusion beats may be an encouraging sign that there is still atrial activity occurring in spite of ventricular dominance.

The **R on T phenomenon** has been used to describe a PVC beat that occurs within a T wave of the preceding complex (Figure 29-81(c)). It was believed that because this is depolarizing a cell at a very vulnerable period (the relative refractory zone), it could destabilize the entire heart and result in ventricular fibrillation or ventricular tachycardia. Recent analysis has downplayed this effect,

but it is still a noteworthy occurrence and should be monitored closely.

Diagnostic Criteria For PVCs

Rate: that of underlying rhythm

Rhythm: irregular when PVC is present

P waves: may or may not be associated with PVC

PRI: none associated with PVC

QRS: > 0.12 and premature

Life-Threatening Dysrhythmias

The life-threatening dysrhythmias are ventricular fibrillation, ventricular tachycardia without a pulse, asystole, and pulseless electrical activity (PEA).

In each of these conditions, the patient has absolutely no cardiac output and cannot survive unless definitive treatment is initiated immediately. Often, these patients die even when appropriate treatment is rendered. DOT 5-2.42, 5-2.43

Ventricular Fibrillation (VF)

Ventricular fibrillation, or **VF,** is the leading cause of sudden cardiac death in the United States.[13] VF is a disordered electrical activity resulting in unsynchronized depolarization within the ventricles (Figure 29-82). The result of the chaotic discharge of electrical energy removes the possibility of an organized mechanical contraction. Since no blood is pumped, there is no cardiac output.

The ECG tracing consists of disorganized, chaotic waves of varied amplitude and frequency, resulting in either a coarse or fine appearance. It appears that coarse VF starts early and will progress to fine VF if not successfully treated. In hearts with extensive disease, coarse VF may not be seen.

The most effective method of terminating VF is electrical defibrillation. To be effective, this needs to occur quickly, optimally within the four- to six-minute window before cellular death begins to occur within the brain and other vital organs.

Several studies have demonstrated the value of public access to defibrillators by showing a higher rate of return of spontaneous circulation in areas with publicly available defibrillators.[15] Defibrillation is a single dose of energy delivered at one time that forces depolarization of all of the muscle fibers. If successful, an organized rhythm will start up again.

Recent research has indicated that VF is not as disorganized as originally thought. It actually moves through the heart muscle in waves, resulting in thousands of depolarizations as it passes through.[13] The VF rhythm can result from many things, but most commonly it is caused by advanced heart disease. Electrocution, drug toxicity, hypoxia, metabolic disorders, or electrolyte imbalances can also cause VF.

Although the most effective method of terminating VF is prompt defibrillation, it can also cause VF. Defibrillation should only be used when the patient is pulseless and in the presence of only two rhythms: VF or pulseless ventricular tachycardia.

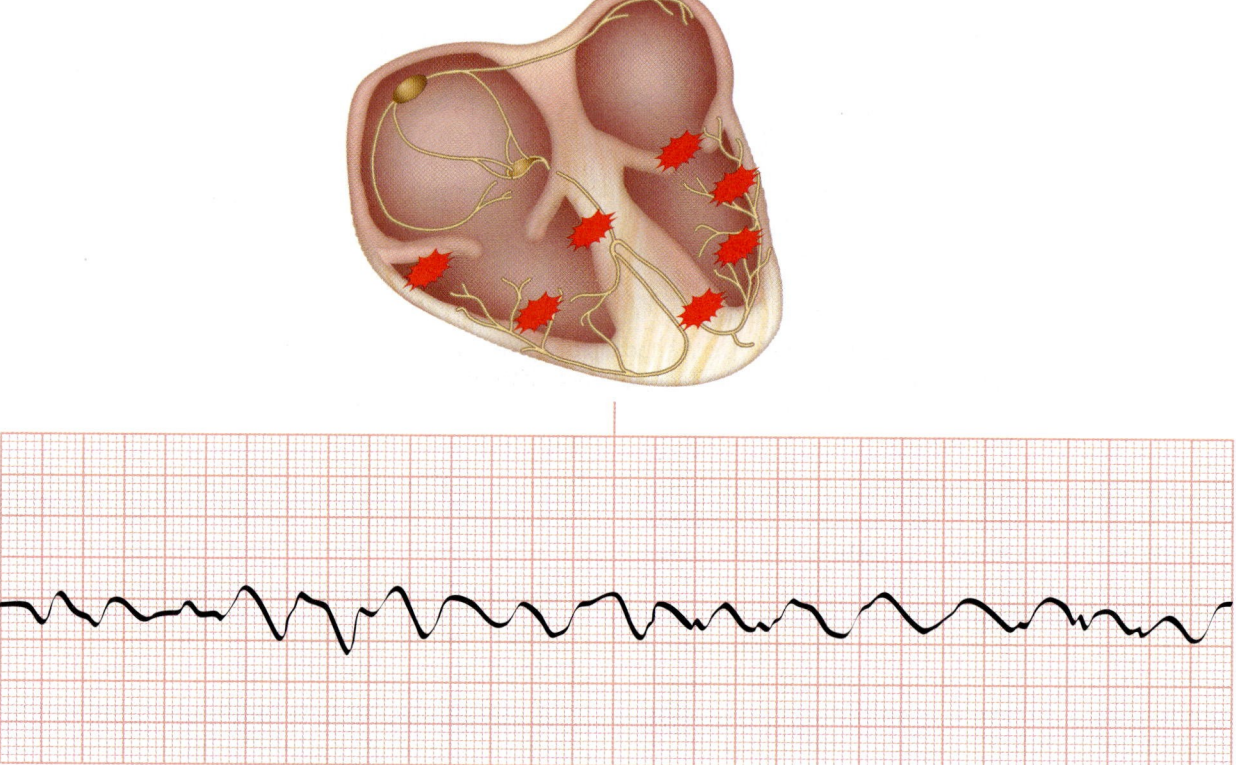

Figure 29-82   Ventricular fibrillation.

On May 4, 2006, Brian Burba was working at a job site when his life was changed forever. His job as a renovation specialist was physically demanding, and he always got enough sleep. But at 42 years of age, he was not in the best of health because of a recent return to smoking (after quitting for two years). He had hypertension (which was controlled with medication) and a steady diet of fast food. He had recently gained thirty pounds, bringing him to his heaviest weight of 230 pounds on a 6'2" frame.

That day, he began experiencing severe chest pain that he said felt like "somebody pulling a cinder block out of my chest." Co-workers called 9-1-1, and he was transported. At the hospital, he recalls saying, "The pain is gone." Noting the sudden occurrence of VF, the doctor administered a precordial thump while requesting the nurse to charge the paddles for defibrillation. Never losing consciousness, Brian looked at the doctor and immediately asked him why he punched him in the chest. Brian received two stents in the cardiac catheterization laboratory. His LAD

(the "widowmaker") was 95% occluded, and his circumflex was 90% occluded. He is no longer smoking and is now eating a healthy, low-fat diet and exercising regularly. He shows no interest in returning to his previous lifestyle.

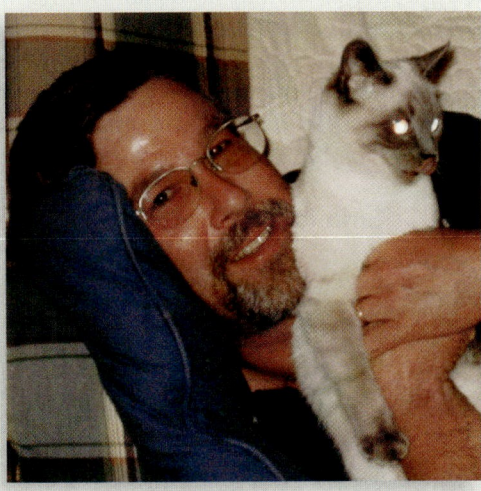

In the last few years, another type of defibrillation, called biphasic defibrillation, has been studied, and it appears promising.[13] Biphasic defibrillation utilizes a split phase depolarization in which the first phase appears to defibrillate similar to that of monophasic defibrillation (the original form of defibrillation), and then the second phase seems to lower the fibrillatory threshold, terminating the event.[13] Studies are ongoing in this respect. The fact remains that early defibrillation, whether biphasic or monophasic, is still the best method to terminate VF.

The Fibrillatory Threshold

The **fibrillatory threshold** is the point at which fibrillation is likely to occur. When you speak in terms of the fibrillatory threshold, to raise it means the possibility of the heart moving from one state to the other is less likely. In the case of fibrillation, a low threshold is not a good thing because a low threshold means fibrillation is likely to reoccur. If the threshold is higher, it is less likely to reoccur.

The Precordial Thump

Treatment of VF must be immediate, with no delays in performing defibrillation. For the patient on an ECG who suddenly goes into VF, you may try a **precordial thump** while charging the defibrillator to deliver a shock. The precordial thump is thought to produce an electrical depolarization of between two and five Joules.

This extremely small shock may disrupt a reentrant pathway dysrhythmia if delivered at the right moment. The likelihood of this procedure being successful is very small, so performing it should not take precedence over defibrillation (Box 29-7).

Diagnostic Criteria For Ventricular Fibrillation

Rate: none
Rhythm: none
P waves: none
PRI: none
QRS: none; isoelectric line is chaotic

Asystole

Asystole is the complete lack of any electrical activity within the heart. Once it occurs, it is very difficult to restore any meaningful electrical activity. Remember that any impulse traveling perpendicular to a given lead may either show up as a biphasic or isoelectric deflection on the monitor. For this reason, it is mandatory that the patient is checked in multiple leads, preferably perpendicular leads, to ensure the patient is actually in asystole. Once this is determined, CPR should be initiated at once, followed by pharmacologic intervention with further assessment to try to determine the causes. Some of the causes include hypoxia, hypovolemia, AMI, hypothermia, acidosis, drug overdose, tension pneumothorax, or cardiac tamponade. DOT 5-2.126

Previously, treatment for asystole focused on correcting the cause, as well as using a combination of drug therapy and electricity to bring the patient out of asystole. Initially, defibrillation was the recommended therapy, and then a few years later, pacing was recommended. Research into this over the past few years has led to the belief that applying electricity is usually of no value in treating asystole, so defibrillation and pacing are not recommended. The only exception to this recommendation is for an immediate attempt at pacing when the monitored patient enters into asystole. More research into this will help clarify whether this will be of any benefit.

Diagnostic Criteria for Asystole

Rate: none
Rhythm: none
P waves: none
PRI: none
QRS: none; isoelectric line is flat and "silent"

Pulseless Electrical Activity (PEA)

Pulseless electrical activity (PEA) is not so much a rhythm in itself, but a life-threatening condition that can look like any normal or abnormal rhythm. Basically, there is electrical activity visible on the cardiac monitor, but no perceivable pulse is felt. There is no cardiac output and no perfusion. Typically, the term PEA is descriptive of any rhythm that would normally be expected to have a pulse, for example, normal sinus rhythm, which for some reason is pulseless. Ventricular fibrillation, which by its nature is pulseless, should not be classified as PEA. DOT 5-2.44

With PEA, it is difficult to determine if there is no myocardial activity (pumping action) or simply no blood volume to generate a pulse. Either way, steps must be taken immediately to rule out possible causes. All of the possible causes listed above for asystole should also be considered for PEA as well. While this is being done, CPR must be started, and pharmacologic intervention may be initiated. Continuous cardiac monitoring and frequent pulse assessments should also be performed.

Street Secrets

Earlier in the chapter, there was discussion about the three components required for perfusion: the pump (heart), pipes (vascular vessels), and a well-oxygenated, adequate blood volume. When trying to determine the problem causing PEA, be sure to investigate each of these three components. The focus should be on the volume and pipes as the pump is the least likely suspect.

Diagnostic Criteria For PEA

Rate: depends upon rhythm
Rhythm: depends
P waves: depends
PRI: depends
QRS: present and depends upon rhythm, the problem is there is no pulse to accompany the rhythm, which means there is electrical activity but no mechanical response or perfusion

Ventricular Tachycardia (VT or V Tach)

Ventricular tachycardia is a problematic rhythm for many reasons. Primarily, it represents an extreme workload on the heart and must be terminated as soon as possible (Figure 29-83). How that is accomplished is entirely dependant upon the presentation of the patient. A patient in this rhythm may present either with or without a pulse. They may initially be relatively stable or may be experiencing severe hemodynamic compromise. Whatever the presentation, aggressive action should be taken to restore this dysrhythmia to a normally perfusing rhythm.

Ventricular tachycardia without a pulse is a rhythm that is perfusing so poorly that no pulse can be perceived. There should be no delay in treatment to try to determine the cause; it should be treated just as VF, using the same protocol. The acute lack of perfusion will cause this rhythm to progress to VF or asystole very quickly if immediate steps are not taken to correct the problem.

Ventricular tachycardia, by definition, is an ectopic rhythm, originating from one of the ventricles, beating anywhere from 100 to 250 beats per minute or in a run of three or more beats during another rhythm. As with any rhythm, rates in the lower 100s may be slow enough to allow adequate ventricular filling and perfuse the patient well enough to be relatively asymptomatic. However, at rates exceeding 150, ventricular filling time decreases to the point where hemodynamic compromise starts becoming a problem. If the patient is perfusing well, blood pressure is adequate, and there are no signs of impending cardiac failure or arrest, a pharmacologic approach may be considered first to break the rhythm. If medication fails to slow the rhythm, cardioversion may be needed.

If any signs of hemodynamic compromise exist, such as frank hypotension, chest pain, altered level of consciousness, or shortness of breath attempt to resolve this rhythm immediately through the electrical therapy of synchronized cardioversion. Pharmacologic support can be used to sedate the patient prior to the procedure. The overall guide should not be so much the

Ventricular tachycardia arises from a single site in the ventricles.

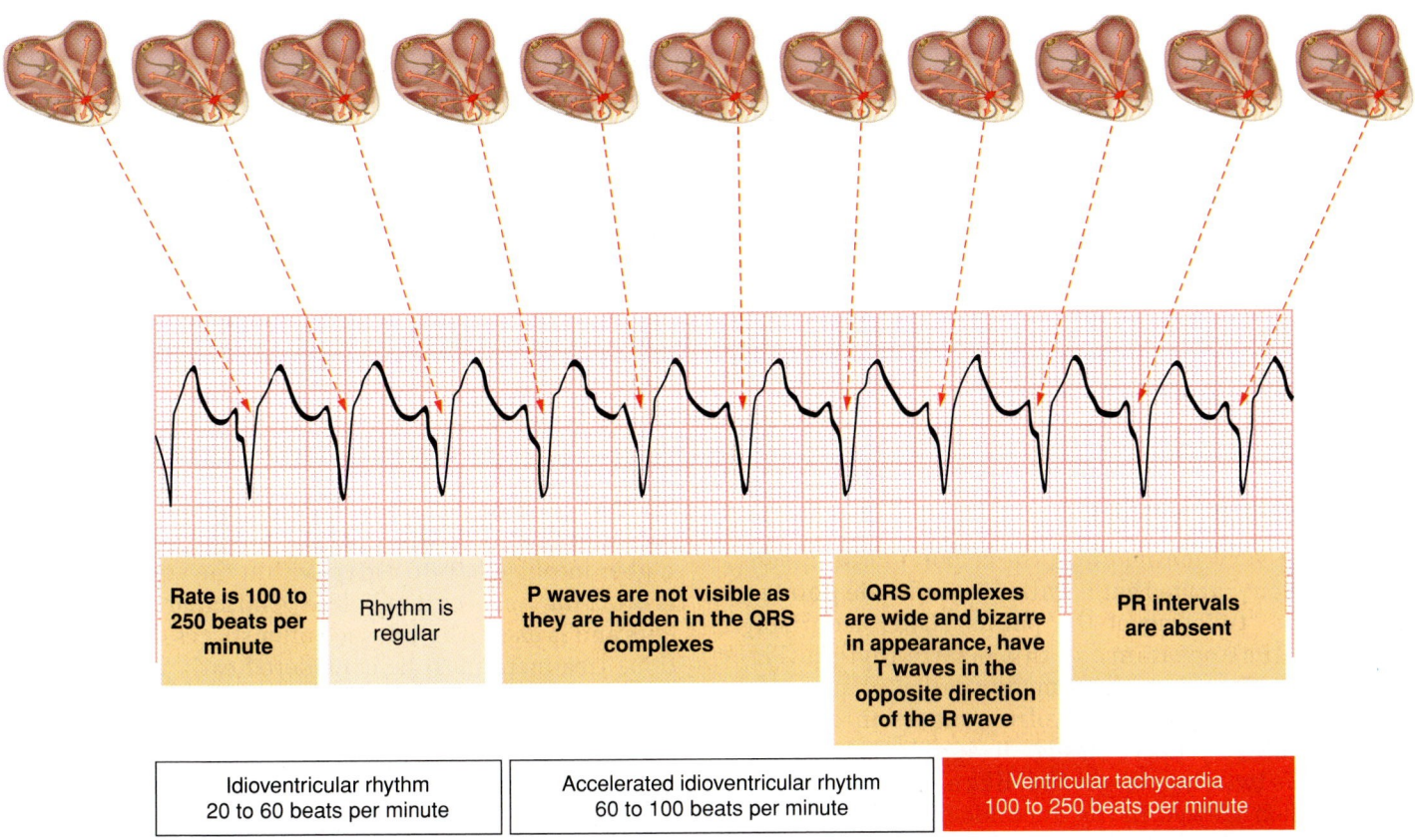

| Rate is 100 to 250 beats per minute | Rhythm is regular | P waves are not visible as they are hidden in the QRS complexes | QRS complexes are wide and bizarre in appearance, have T waves in the opposite direction of the R wave | PR intervals are absent |

| Idioventricular rhythm 20 to 60 beats per minute | Accelerated idioventricular rhythm 60 to 100 beats per minute | Ventricular tachycardia 100 to 250 beats per minute |

Figure 29-83   Ventricular tachycardia.

actual rate but how the patient is presenting: stable or unstable.

The mechanisms for ventricular tachycardia are the same as for the PVC, but the rhythm is sustained, not just an isolated impulse. The evidence strongly suggests that reentry is the causative mechanism for V Tach in the postmyocardial infarction period.[13] VT usually occurs in runs of three or more beats or short bursts for a period of time. Occasionally, it can go on for a long period of time, and then it is called **sustained ventricular tachycardia.** It is not however abbreviated as SVT.

Differentiating between ventricular tachycardia and supraventricular tachycardia may be confounded by the presence of a conduction defect within the ventricles, such as a bundle branch block that will make a supraventricular-generated beat appear widened. It is best to assume any tachycardic rhythm with a wide QRS complex is ventricular tachycardia until proven otherwise. Looking for features, such as the presence of fusion beats or AV dissociation, may help confirm the final diagnosis. A 12-lead may also be helpful at this point. First, focus on stabilizing the patient before diagnosing the rhythm further.

Ventricular tachycardia occurs most often in the presence of cardiac disease. The main cause is a myocardial infarction. Some other causes are cardiomyopathy, mitral valve prolapse, and CHF. It may also be seen it as a result of digoxin toxicity.

The appearance of ventricular tachycardia may either be monomorphic or polymorphic. Most VT is monomorphic where all the complexes look relatively identical because they are arising from a single site within the ventricle and are traveling a consistent route during conduction. There may be slight variations in appearance due to the multiformed effect in damaged heart tissue, and some slight irregularities in the rate may be seen. For the most part, the complexes look the same.

Diagnostic Criteria for Ventricular Tachycardia

Rate: 100–250

Rhythm: depends, usually regular

P waves: none

PRI: none

QRS: wider than 0.12 seconds, often the QRS wave is deflected in the opposite direction from the T wave

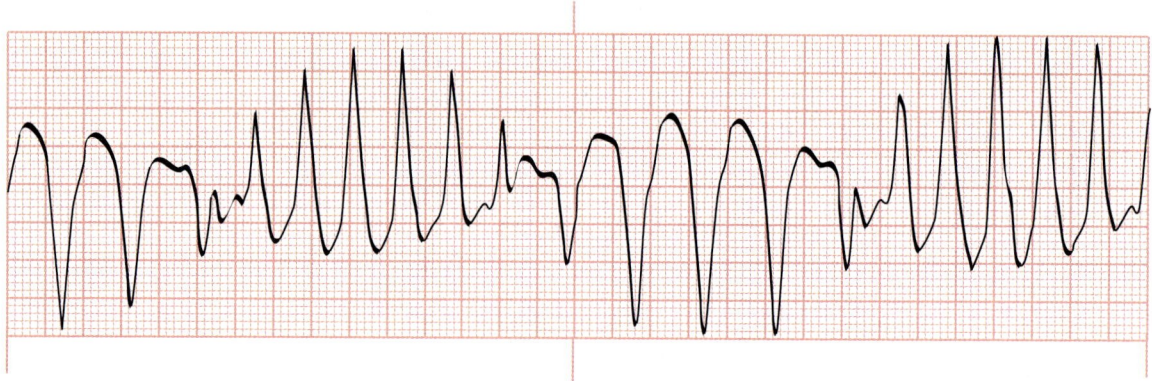

Figure 29-84   Torsades de pointes.

Torsades De Pointes

There is a very malignant form of polymorphic ventricular tachycardia that is called **torsades de pointes,** French for "twisting of the points." This accurately describes the appearance of this bizarre rhythm (Figure 29-84). There is a phenomenon called phase shifting as the polymorphic wavefront moves throughout the destabilized heart tissue. It appears as though someone is twisting the rhythm like a spring, hence its name. When viewed in the dynamic mode on the ECG monitor, torsades appears to spiral on itself.

Torsades de pointes (TdP) usually occurs in patients with serious heart disease who have prolonged ventricular repolarization evident by a prolonged QT interval. Drugs such as quinidine, given as an antidysrhythmic, may exacerbate this dysrhythmia. This dysrhythmia tends to be very malignant and difficult to resolve. Special treatment for this dysrhythmia may be either overdrive pacing electrically or chemically with isoproterenol.[9] Recent evidence has shown that magnesium sulfate may also be effective in terminating this rhythm and to date remains the standard in the prehospital environment.

Diagnostic Criteria for Torsades De Pointes

Rate: 100–250
Rhythm: regular
P waves: not associated with ectopic complex if any are seen
PRI: if P waves are seen they are disassociated with the complex
QRS: > 0.12 seconds, wide and bizarre appearance

Ventricular Escape Rhythm—Idioventricular Rhythm

This rhythm, as the name implies, is the result of the third and final pacemaker site within the purkinje network doing its job (Figure 29-85). The purkinje fibers have an inherent pacemaker rate of 20–40 beats/minute. This rhythm can appear within about 1.5–2.0 seconds after a higher impulse fails to arrive within the ventricles. This is often the final rhythm before ventricular standstill occurs and is also a rhythm seen after successful defibrillation. Treatment must be considered early as the patient is almost always compromised by the bradycardic rate. The treatment goal is to increase the rate through external cardiac pacing or pharmacological intervention.

Diagnostic Criteria for Idioventricular Rhythm

Rate: 20-40 (or slower)
Rhythm: regular
P waves: none
PRI: none
QRS: > 0.12 bizarre appearance

Accelerated Idioventricular Rhythm (AIVR)

There is a faster version of ventricular escape rhythm, which occurs when the ventricular pacemakers experience abnormal automaticity and is commonly seen in reperfusion dysrhythmias and inferior or anterior infarctions. This dysrhythmia is known as **accelerated idioventricular rhythm** or **AIVR.** This dysrhythmia occurs as a rate of 60–110 beats per minute and may be well tolerated by the patient.[11] It is usually transient in nature and seldom requires specific treatment unless signs of hemodynamic compromise exist. In that case, external cardiac pacing would be considered.

Diagnostic Criteria for AIVR

Rate: 60–110
Rhythm: regular
P waves: none
PRI: none
QRS: > 0.12 seconds, bizarre shape, uniform

Idioventricular rhythm arises from a single site in the ventricles.

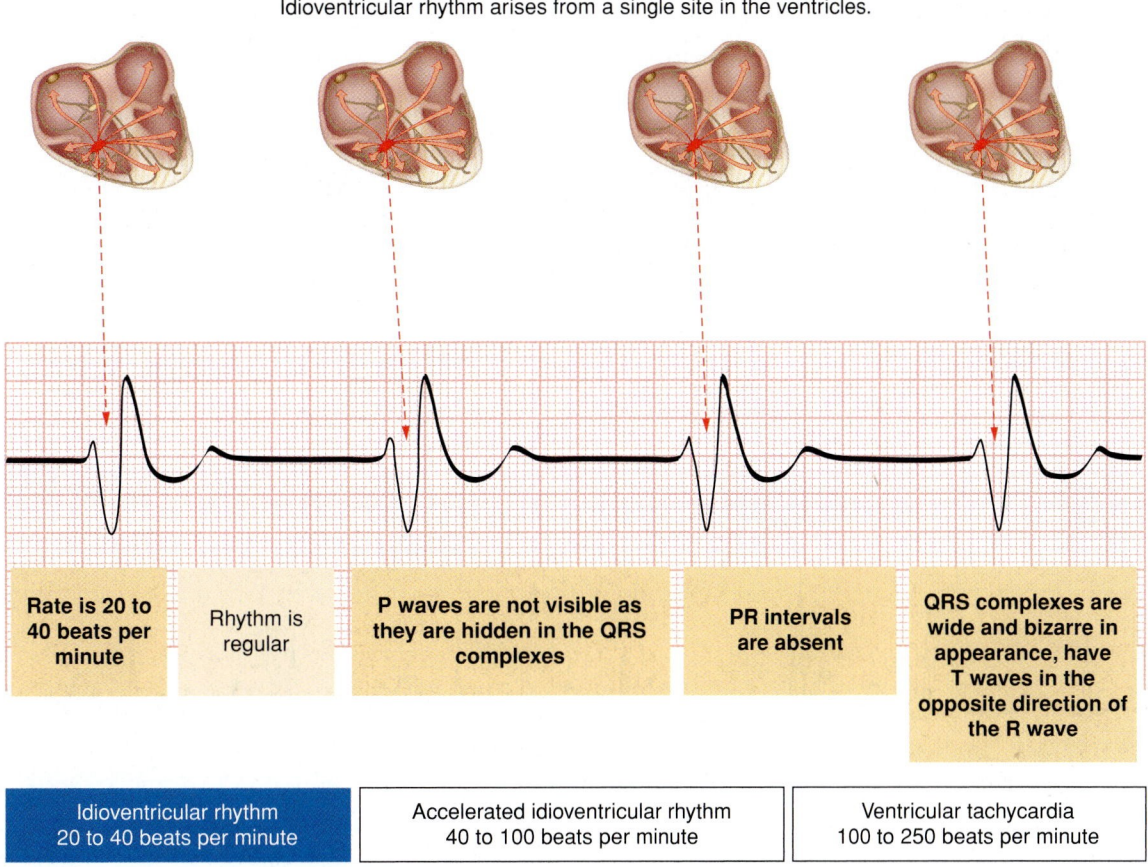

| Rate is 20 to 40 beats per minute | Rhythm is regular | P waves are not visible as they are hidden in the QRS complexes | PR intervals are absent | QRS complexes are wide and bizarre in appearance, have T waves in the opposite direction of the R wave |

| Idioventricular rhythm 20 to 40 beats per minute | Accelerated idioventricular rhythm 40 to 100 beats per minute | Ventricular tachycardia 100 to 250 beats per minute |

Figure 29-85   Idioventricular rhythm.

Aberrant Ventricular Conduction

Aberrant ventricular conduction is not as much a rhythm as it is a conduction problem, which can confound the correct identification of dysrhythmias such as SVT versus VT. During aberrant conduction, there appears to be a delay in the repolarization of one of the bundle branches (Figure 29-86). This appears usually in the right bundle branch since the left begins to depolarize first. Should an impulse appear in one bundle branch earlier than expected, before the bundle branch is fully repolarized, the conduction may be abnormal, resulting in a very different looking complex.

This situation is seen frequently with the presence of PACs. In this case, when you examine the strange looking complex, you will see it is associated with a P wave and should be normal, but the delayed conduction in the bundle branch gives it a wide appearance, making it look like a PVC. Treatment for aberrant conduction is usually not indicated in the emergency setting unless the patient also has significant symptoms.

Bundle Branch and Fascicular Blocks

The left and right bundle branches run down along the wall between the ventricles called the ventricular septum. They facilitate the movement of the electrical impulses to the ventricles and begin the depolarization contraction at the apex of the heart. The right ventricle is smaller, so it depolarizes much quicker and with less current than the left ventricle. On the ECG tracing, the current of the left ventricle overshadows the smaller current from the right, so the QRS complex seen in lead II is primarily showing the electricity of the left bundle branch. DOT 5-2.41, 5-2.45

The time it takes for an impulse to depolarize the septum, right ventricle, and most of the left ventricle is called the **ventricular activation time (VAT)** and is normally less than 0.05 seconds.[8] Because of the conduction delay with a bundle branch block, the VAT is delayed in the left bundle branch, changing the appearance of the complex. The right bundle branch block will produce similar delays, but since the right ventricle is usually a smaller component in the ECG, it has a slightly different effect on the complex.

The right bundle branch is a very thin fiber, easily damaged from ischemia or infarction. Blood for the right bundle branch is supplied by the left anterior descending artery. The left bundle branch actually splits into two branches or fascicles. The posterior branch is wide and thick, receiving a blood supply from two coronary arteries, creating a condition of collateral (or backup) circulation to the branch. The posterior branch is seldom damaged because of the collateral circulation unless the patient has extreme heart disease.

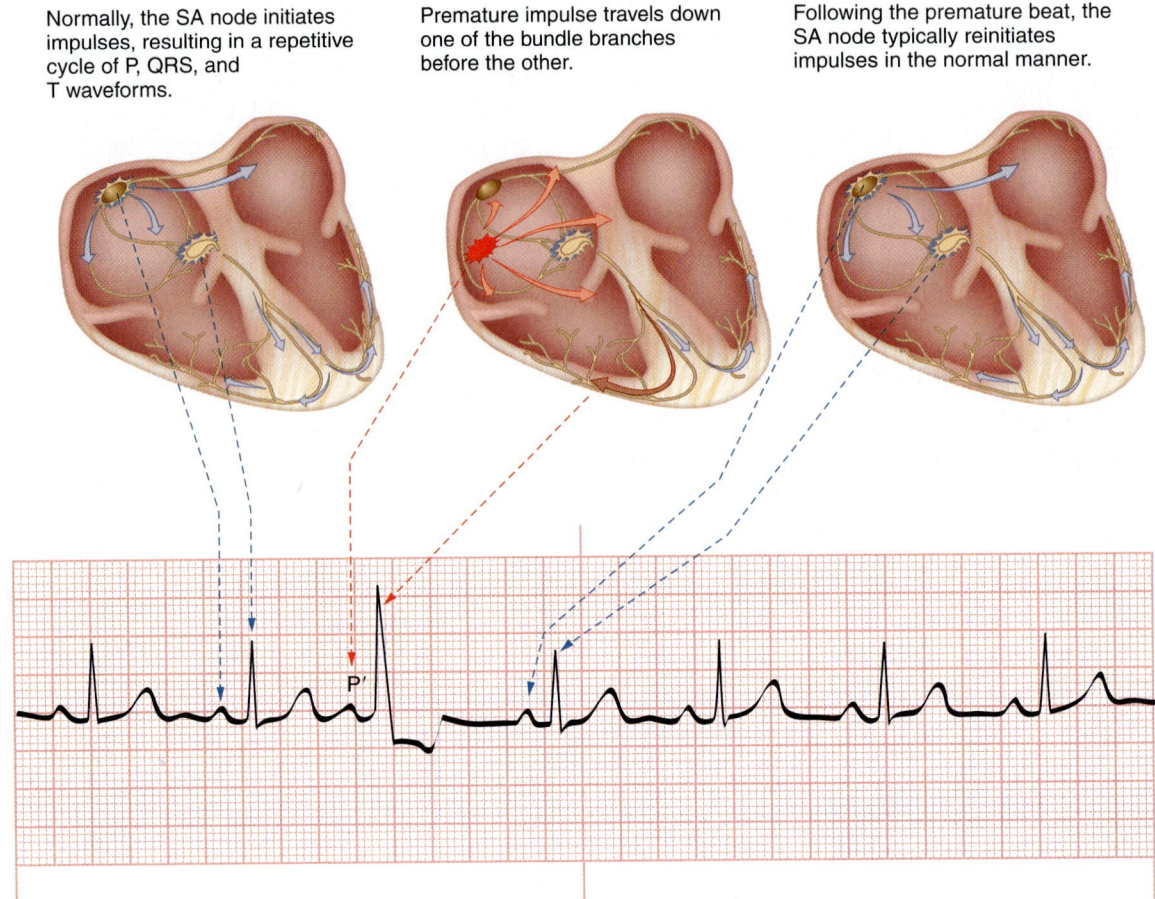

Normally, the SA node initiates impulses, resulting in a repetitive cycle of P, QRS, and T waveforms.

Premature impulse travels down one of the bundle branches before the other.

Following the premature beat, the SA node typically reinitiates impulses in the normal manner.

P'

Figure 29-86   Aberrant conduction.

The left anterior branch resembles the right bundle branch in that it is thin and prone to damage. It receives its blood supply via the left anterior descending coronary artery. Understanding where the blood supply comes from will help to understand the benefits of recognizing bundle branch and fascicular blocks and learn when to anticipate potential problems.

Bundle branch and **fascicular blocks** may appear in normal hearts, but they are usually associated with heart disease. Some of the causes are ischemia, degeneration of the conduction system, cardiomyopathy, and left ventricular hypertrophy.[8] In myocardial infarction, you may see damage to both the right and left bundle branches during anteroseptal infarctions. The left bundle branch may also be affected by inferior infarctions, while the right is rarely damaged by them. The left anterior fascicle is susceptible to damage during an anteroseptal infarction.[8]

Specific treatment is usually not indicated for bundle branch blocks in the prehospital setting, but some physicians will decide to install a pacemaker in certain cases. One of the most important features of bundle branch blocks is their ability to produce ST elevation similar to that of an acute myocardial infarction. Therefore, ST elevation becomes an unreliable sign when assessing a 12-lead for infarction when a bundle branch block is also suspected. You must rely heavily on your clinical assessment of the patient and treat accordingly.

In describing the electrophysiology of the bundle branch blocks, use V_1 and V_2 leads. These are the best leads to identify a bundle branch block and distinguish between the origins of the various sites.

During right bundle branch block, the impulse traveling down the bundle of His is not allowed to propagate normally down that branch (Figure 29-87). The ventricle must then be depolarized from impulses traveling across the ventricular septum from the left bundle branch. Electrically, you will see a small R wave signifying septal depolarization, and a deep S wave will appear as the left ventricle depolarizes normally. Finally, a wide, slurred R wave will appear as the left ventricle finishes depolarization and the right ventricle is depolarized. This gives a classic triphasic, "M" or "rabbit ear" appearance to the right bundle branch pattern.

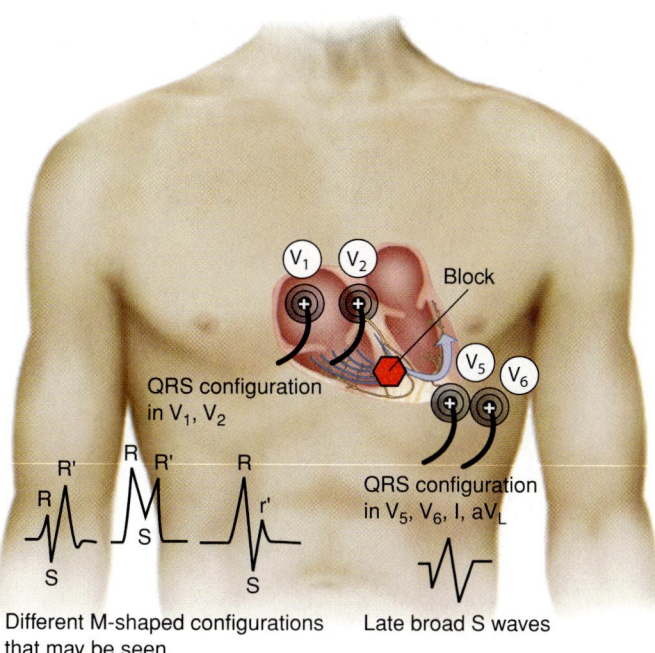

Figure 29-87   Right bundle branch block.

abnormally from the right to left pattern. The early depolarization of the right ventricle may produce a tiny R wave but is usually small as current is moving the opposite direction to the larger left ventricle. Since the impulse arrives late to the left ventricle, the VAT is delayed past 0.05 seconds, resulting in a widened complex with a classic QS appearance with ST elevation very common.

Hemiblocks are seldom problematic unless in the presence of a RBBB or acute myocardial infarction. In those cases, recognition of these blocks can help to rapidly identify high-risk cardiac patients.

The left anterior hemiblock (LAH) occurs with blockage of the LAD coronary artery and, in some cases, the nodal artery branching off the posterior descending artery (Figure 29-89). Since most of the left ventricle can depolarize normally, the prolonged (wide) QRS does not appear. Instead, there are other forces in play as the impulses travel upward to the left through the area and are usually depolarized by the LAF. These extra forces cause the appearance of left axis deviation to appear on the ECG. This is the classic sign of a left anterior hemiblock: normal QRS width with left axis deviation. When in combination with a RBBB, the LAH will produce a classic RBBB pattern with left axis deviation. In this patient, a complete heart block is very possible. This situation is called the **bifascicular block.**

The left posterior hemiblock (LPH) is relatively rare due to its sturdy design and backup blood supply

The typical ECG pattern seen in the left bundle branch block usually consists of a deep QS or RQS wave (Figure 29-88). Again, looking at V_1, we see the impulse traveling down the bundle of His normally, reaching the right and left bundle branches. It travels down the right bundle branch normally, but the septum is depolarized

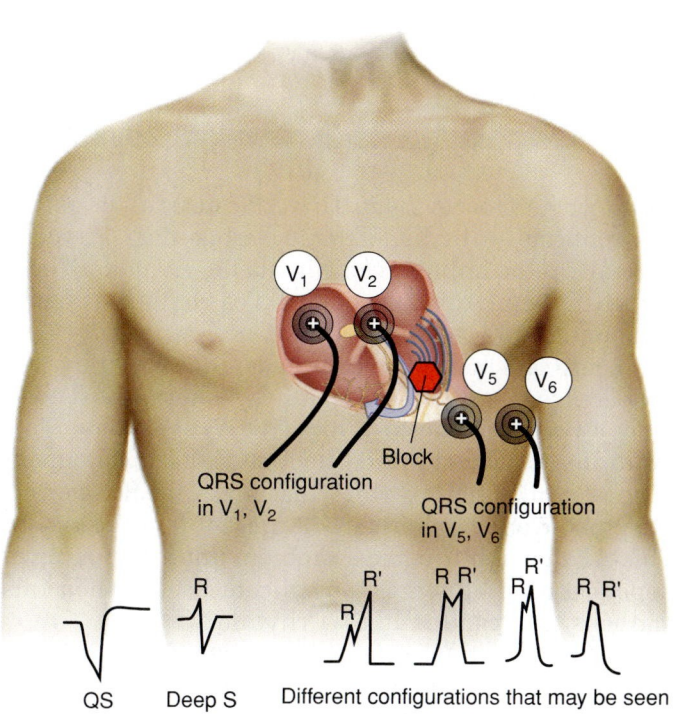

Figure 29-88   Left bundle branch block.

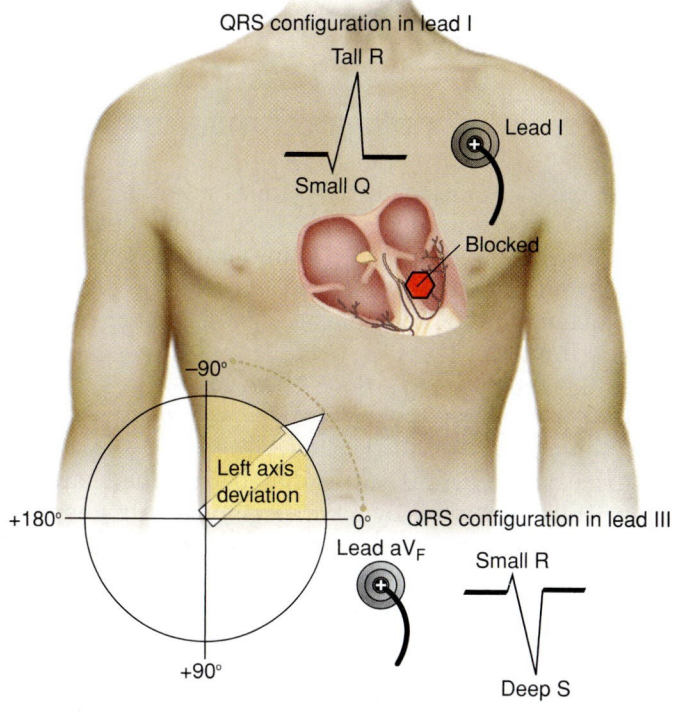

Figure 29-89   Left anterior hemiblock.

Nice to Know

Axis Determination

The electrical axis of the heart is the mean or resultant direction of current through the heart. If the lead vectors are superimposed on a circle, all crossing through the center point, a very distinctive pattern emerges with the lead vectors falling about 30 degrees apart on a circle. This is known as the hexaxial diagram (Figure 29-90). Degrees are assigned at each point, beginning at 0 degrees on the far right side or the 3 o'clock position. They progress positively in the clockwise direction to 180 degrees in the 9 o'clock position, running negative from the 0-degree location again. A normal heart will have an axis of 0 degrees to +90 degrees. Any axis that falls from 0 degrees to −90 is called left axis deviation, and any that fall between +90 and 180 degrees is then right axis deviation. The remainder fall into an area called extreme right axis deviation.

There are several methods to calculate the exact degree of axis deviation, and the calculation is actually written on the 12-lead printout. For quick analysis, you can get a good estimate of axis deviation by looking at leads I and II. The rules are as follows:

- If the complexes in both leads I and II are predominantly upright, the axis is normal.
- If lead I is upright and lead II is negative, there is left axis deviation.
- If lead I is negative and lead II is upright, there is right axis deviation.
- If both leads are predominantly negative, the axis is extreme right.

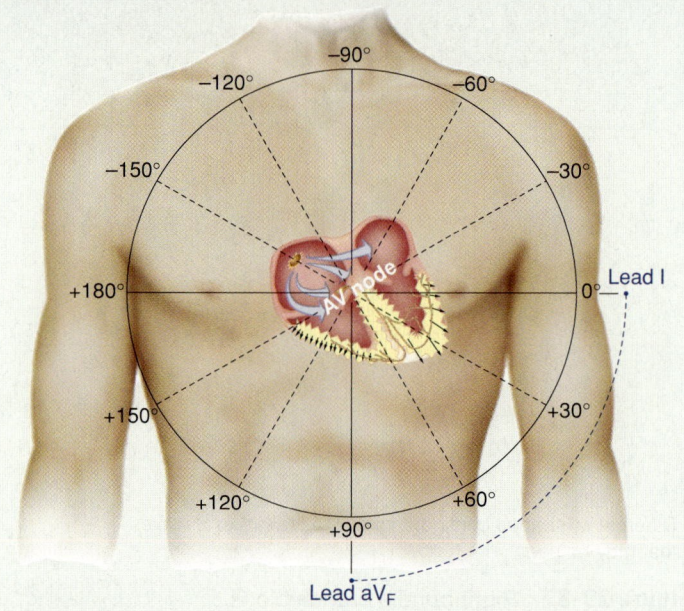

Figure 29-90 Use an imaginary circle to envision the heart's axis divided into equal 30-degree segments.

Left axis deviation is commonly associated with left ventricular hypertrophy, inferior wall myocardial infarction, and block in the left anterior portion of the left bundle branch.

Right axis deviation is commonly associated with right ventricular overload, such as might occur with a large pulmonary embolus, lateral wall myocardial infarction, and block in the posterior portion of the left bundle branch.

(Figure 29-91). Usually, it only appears in the case of a massive infarction, involving several parts of the heart. ECG recognition of the LPH is similar to the LAH, with the exception that it produces right axis deviation instead of left. The QRS complexes in both cases are within normal limits.

Preexcitation Syndromes

As discussed previously, the chambers of the heart are electrically separated by a cartilaginous cardiac skeleton. This tissue supports the heart valves and helps the heart maintain its shape. It prevents electrical impulses from crossing from the atria to the ventricles at just any location. In some individuals, an **accessory pathway** (AP) shows up, creating another pathway into the ventricles from the atria. There are many identified locations for these AP, but it takes very special cardiac

monitoring to locate them. This AP causes all or part of the ventricle to be depolarized earlier than it would normally if the impulse came in via the AV node. These AP are the source of many of the PSVT rhythms you will encounter.

There are several syndromes identified by the appearance of an accessory pathway, but the most common is **Wolff-Parkinson-White (WPW) syndrome.** This syndrome is characterized by a flaw in the development of the annular fibrous rings that make up the cardiac skeleton, leaving a short circuit present in the skeleton. This AP may not become a problem until the timing of depolarization allows it to replicate itself. When this happens, the result is a PSVT rhythm.

To examine the cause, start by reviewing the depolarization of the atria through normal channels. As the impulse reaches the AV node and the AP, they both start to depolarize the ventricles. However, in normal cases,

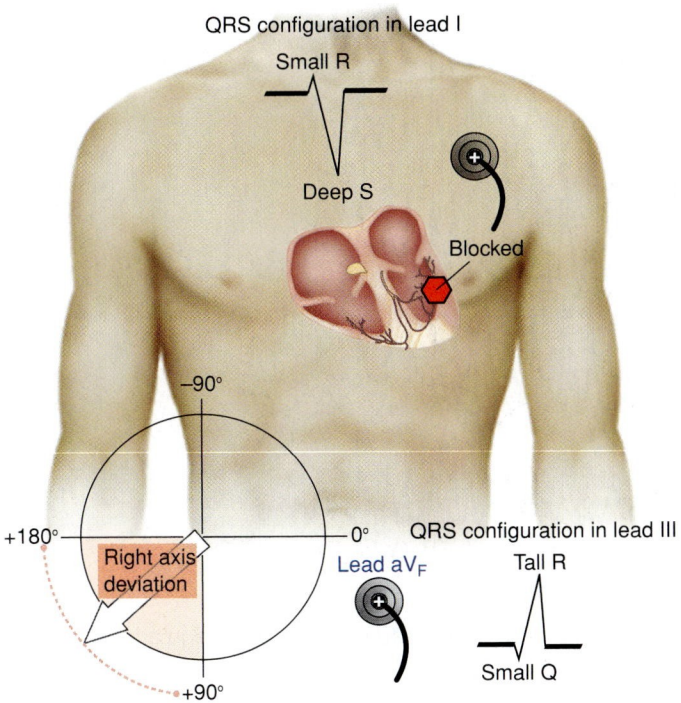

Figure 29-91   Left posterior hemiblock.

the normal conduction fibers of the ventricles depolarize the majority of the ventricles, and the AP-conducted impulse just dissipates in the depolarized tissue.

However, should the impulse be delayed in the AV node slightly longer than normal, the AP impulse may actually reach the conduction system first and affect the depolarization. This could go one step further and travel back through the AV node and atria and depolarize them also, with the impulse once again heading down the AP. This starts a circuitous movement without any controls that is also referred to as retrograde conduction. This is what initiates the PSVT dysrhythmia. To terminate the event, the circuit must be broken. This usually happens spontaneously or requires pharmacologic intervention or synchronized cardioversion.

The ECG of a patient with Wolff-Parkinson-White has a classic characteristic called the delta wave (Figure 29-92). The delta wave is a slurring of the initial

Nice to Know

Excitation Syndrome: Lown-Ganong-Levine

Another less common cause of preexcitiation is a condition known as Lown-Ganong-Levine syndrome. This condition produces shortened PR intervals and is also capable of producing PSVT although the slurred QRS (delta wave) is usually not seen.

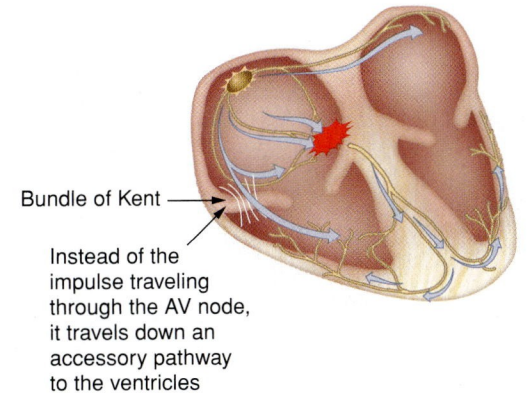

Bundle of Kent

Instead of the impulse traveling through the AV node, it travels down an accessory pathway to the ventricles

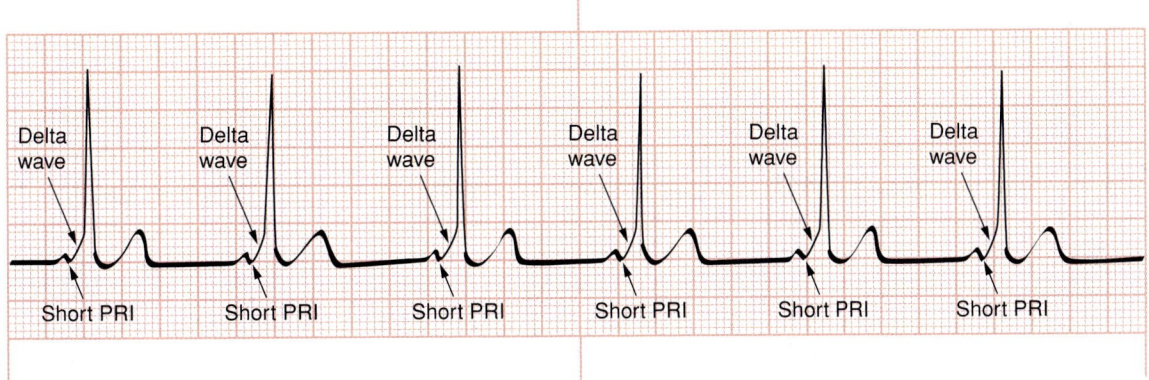

Figure 29-92   WPW.

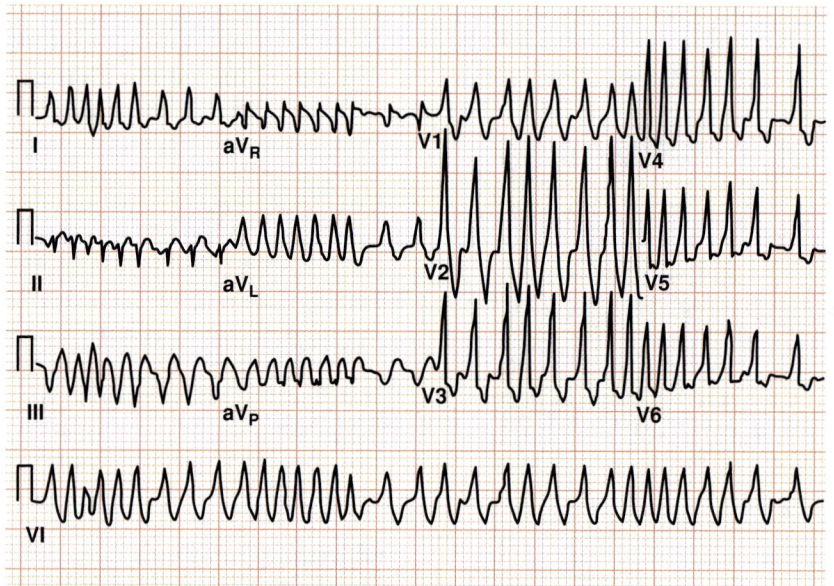

Figure 29-93 When WPW occurs with atrial fibrillation, it can be a lethal rhythm. The key is to discover the irregularity in the rhythm. The ECG can be easily misinterpreted to be ventricular tachycardia.

deflection of the QRS complex, created as the AP allows a tiny portion of the ventricles to begin depolarization before the normal conduction catches up. The early depolarization also results in a shorter than normal PR interval. Patients with WPW can remain perfectly normal for extended periods of time, until conditions are just right for the AP to take over.

While most patients with WPW can lead normal lives, and episodes of SVT may be managed through traditional methods, surgical ablation (correction

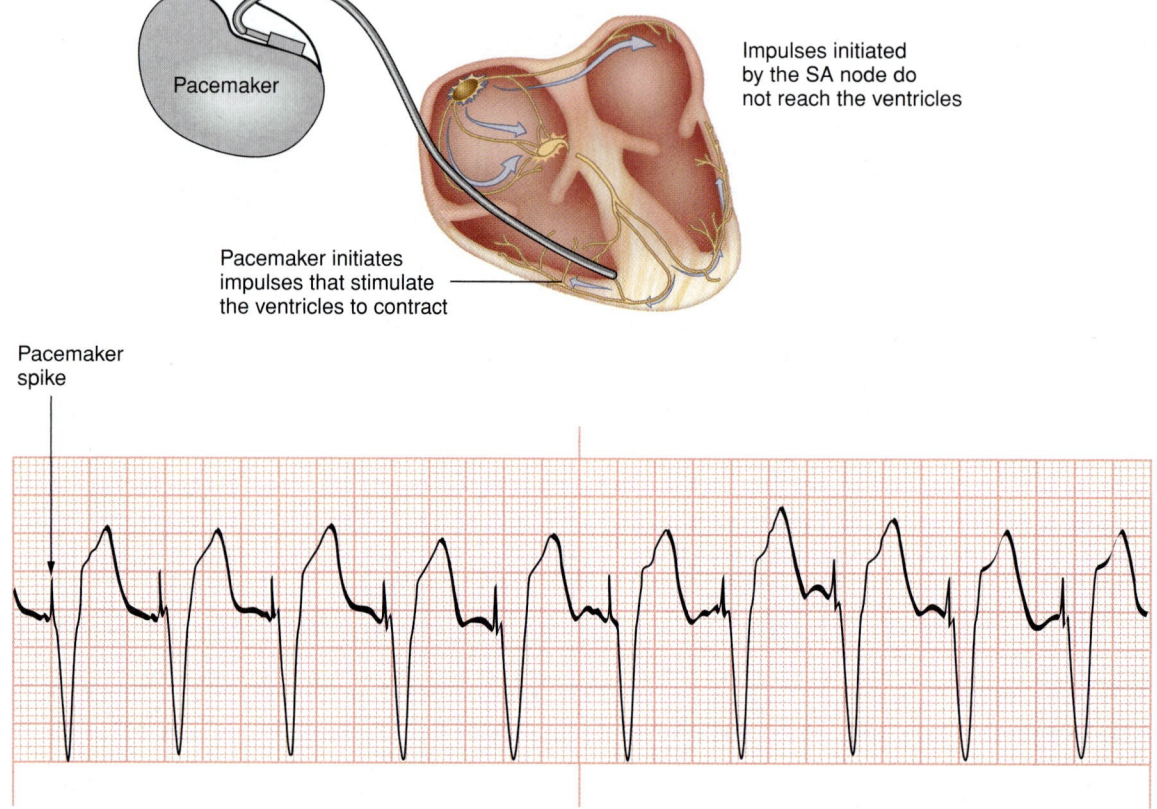

Figure 29-94 Cardiac pacemaker (note the small pacemaker spike before each QRS complex).

through destruction of the affected cells) of the APs may be necessary if the WPW gets to be problematic for the patients. In some cases, if it occurs along with atrial fibrillation, the first sign of WPW may be sudden death. This combination results in an extremely fast rhythm due to the rapid atrial rate and relatively short refractory period of the AP.[16] This rhythm can deteriorate into ventricular fibrillation very quickly, so it must be recognized and treated aggressively (Figure 29-93). Recognition of this rhythm is focused on the very fast, regularly irregular rhythm, with a QRS wider than 0.12 seconds due to the preexcitation through the AP and retrograde impulse transmission. At first glance, this rhythm may be misinterpreted as ventricular tachycardia. A careful review of clinical signs and past medical history will help with the interpretation.

Pacemaker Rhythms

Patients with a cardiac history may have an internal pacemaker in place. The internal pacemaker is a device that monitors the patient's heartbeat, compares it with its internal program, and either initiates or inhibits a pacemaker-generated impulse (Figure 29-94). Pacemaker are often placed in patients with an unreliable sinus node or complete AV dissociation. They have allowed countless people who have experienced significant cardiac illnesses to lead a near-normal life. DOT 5-2.156, 5-2.158, 5-2.167

A pacemaker is a small electronic device connected to a wire and electrodes (Figure 29-95). The wires usually run into the subclavian vein and into the right ventricle via the right atria and tricuspid valve (Figure 29-96). The device is able to sense an electrical impulse and, according to its programming, initiate a small impulse, which causes the heart to depolarize. The device is capable of sensing or triggering an impulse and can be programmed many ways. For example, in the case of a patient with a third-degree AV block, the pacemaker may sense an impulse within the atria and then trigger an impulse in the ventricles. In contrast, the pacemaker may be set to sense a true impulse in the atria and then decide not to trigger an impulse in the atria or ventricles. It is programmed to trigger only if an impulse is not sensed. As you can see, they are very sophisticated devices capable of managing a wide range of cardiac problems. DOT 5-2.55, 5-2.60

Most patients will tell you if they have pacemakers, but not many will be able to tell you how they are programmed or what they are doing other than "helping the heart beat better." Some people will carry cards with that information on it. If the patient is unable to assist with needed information, rely on the assessment for information. Most often, the pacemaker unit is implanted just beneath the skin on the upper left or right chest (Figure 29-97). You should notice or feel a small bump under the skin.

The presence of an actively firing pacemaker is noted by small vertical lines, or spikes on the ECG. These can be seen immediately before the P wave or QRS complex, depending upon the programming of the pacemaker (Figure 29-98). There can also be two spikes if the pacemaker is firing two times during the same

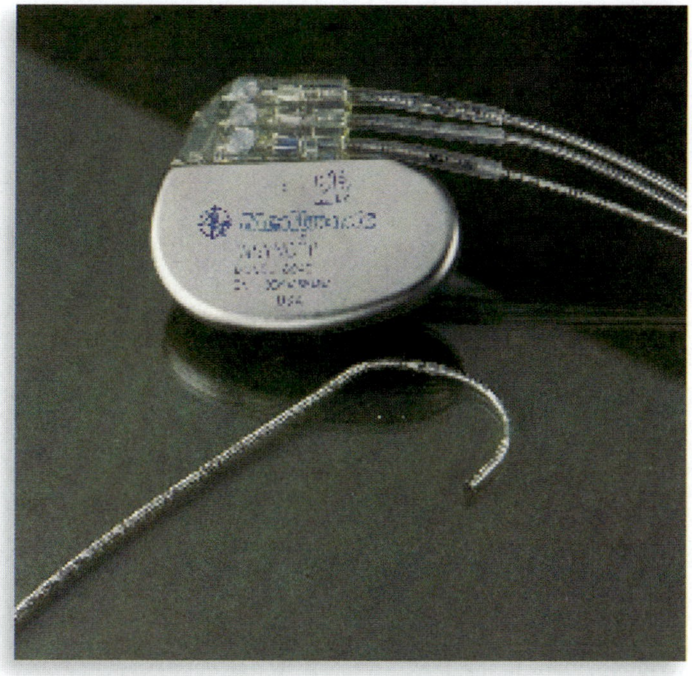

Figure 29-95   An implantable cardiac pacemaker.

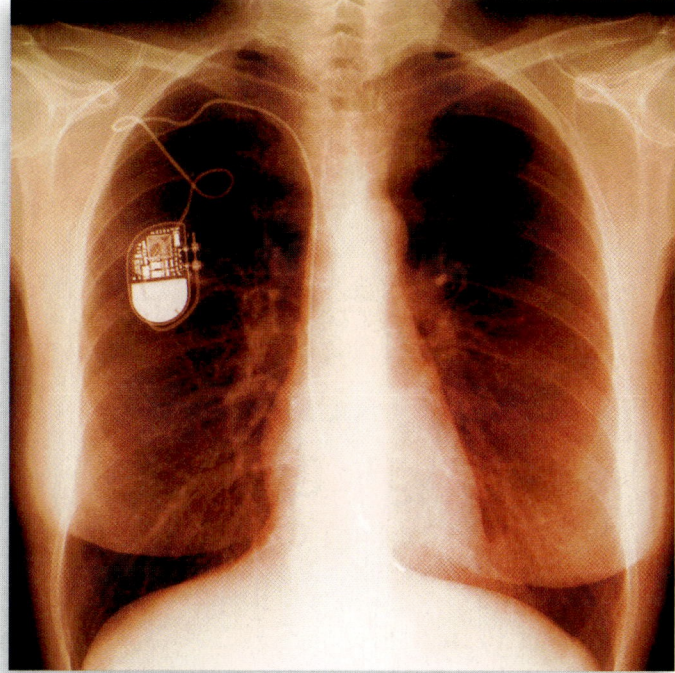

Figure 29-96   X-ray of implanted pacemaker.

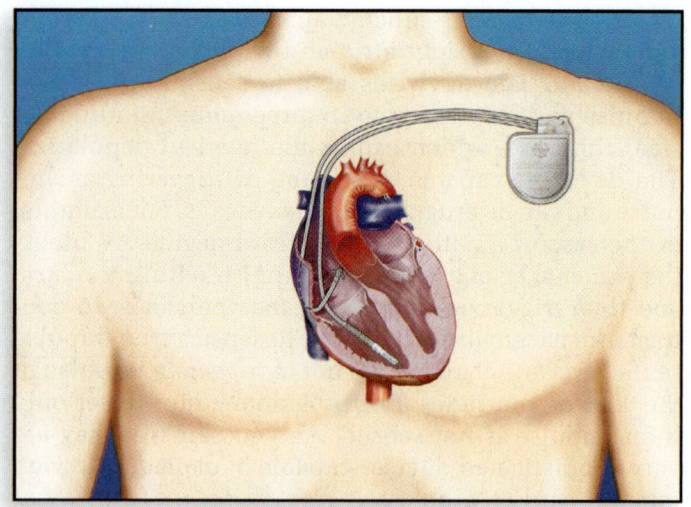

Figure 29-97   Chest wall with pacemaker implanted.

cardiac cycle. Again, depending upon the programming of the pacemaker, it may fire occasionally, frequently, or continuously. A word of caution, however, you may not always see a pacemaker spike; it may be too small or perpendicular to the monitoring lead. DOT 5-2.60, 5-2.61

You should always question the presence of a pacemaker when you see a wide regular complex occurring at a normal or near-normal rate. The wide complex is very characteristic of a ventricular paced rhythm since the electrode is located against the ventricular wall and that is the point of origin of the impulse. DOT 5-2.63

As good as pacemakers are, at times they do malfunction or run low on electrical power. When this occurs, they may be programmed to gradually increase the rate of fire, which alerts the patient to have it checked. Pacemakers do have other potential complications beyond battery power. The wires may corrode or become misplaced, the pacemaker wires may actually perforate the ventricular wall, or they may come loose from their anchor point. Should this happen, the loose wire could initiate an ectopic beat anywhere it strikes the wall of the ventricle, resembling ventricular ectopy. DOT 5-2.60, 5-2.64

Other Implanted Cardiac Devices

Other implanted cardiac devices include the **automatic internal cardiac defibrillator (AICD),** implanted Holter monitors, and ventricular access devices (VAD). There are three types of VADs: left ventricular devices (LVAD), right ventricular devices (RVAD), and devices placed in both ventricles, called BiVADs. A brief description of each of these devices is included, so that you can

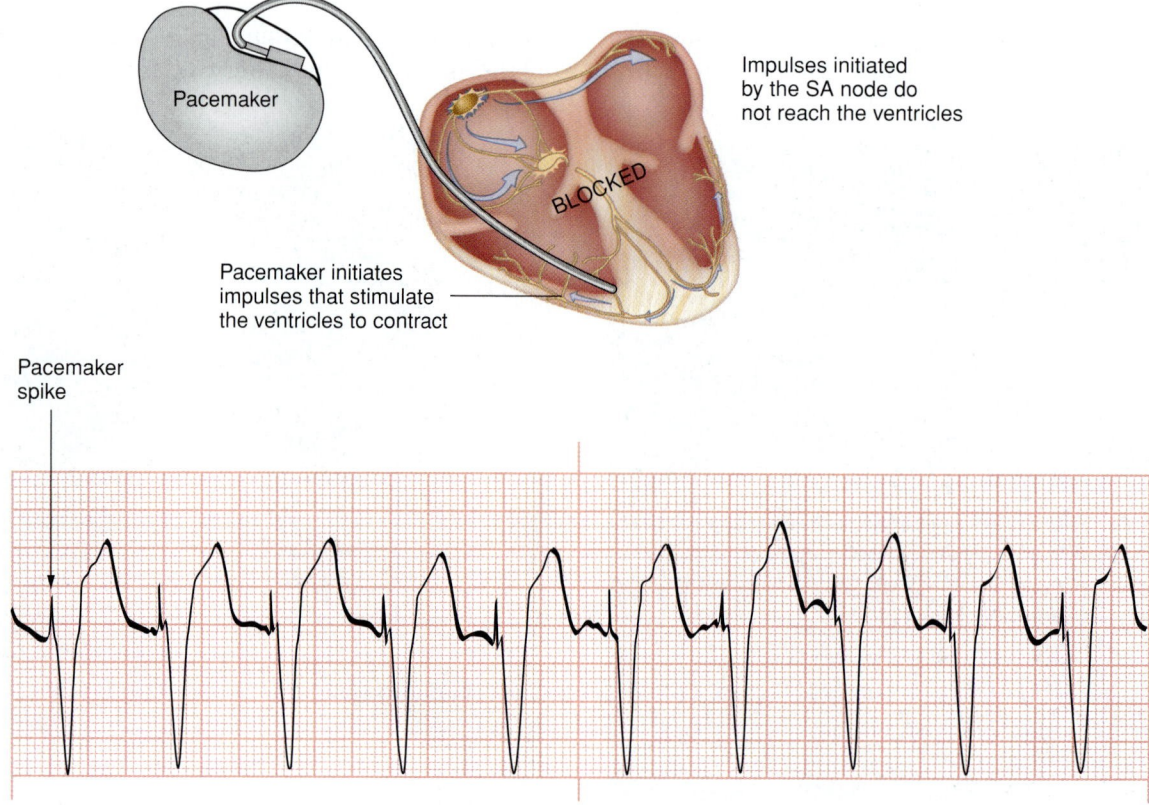

Figure 29-98   Ventricular pacemaker initiating a QRS complex.

become familiar with them. Actual training on managing patients with these devices is beyond the scope of the entry-level paramedic curricula.

Automatic Internal Cardiac Defibrillator

An AICD works in a similar fashion to a pacemaker. It is a small computer and cardiac monitor that is programmed to defibrillate a patient when it senses the onset of ventricular fibrillation or ventricular tachycardia. These devices are implanted in patients who continue to have these rhythms after other treatments have failed. It allows them to resume a normal life. The device occasionally causes a little pain when it fires, and it may cause muscle twitching. You may sense a slight amount of current if you are touching the patient when the AICD fires, particularly if you are performing CPR, but there has not been a reported case of injury to anyone from this.

Holter Monitor

Holter monitors are portable ECG machines that have been used for years to record the heart rhythm of a patient undergoing a cardiac study. It may be worn for a few hours or for months at a time. There are leads attached to the patient's chest, and the monitor is worn on the hip of the patient. If the device is to be used for a long period of time, the entire device can now be implanted into the patient's chest wall to allow the greatest amount of mobility for the patient. Implanted Holter monitors will not interfere with the appearance of the ECG tracing.

Ventricular Access Devices

Ventricular assist devices (LVADs, RVADs, and **BiVADs)** are artificial heart devices that are implanted internally or externally, which take the functional place of the diseased ventricle. They are used for a variety of purposes, including to act as a bridge to buy more time for patients who are waiting for heart transplants, to allow the heart time to heal following myocardial damage, and to provide an alternative to patients who are not candidates for heart transplants (because of social habits, age, insurance denial, or other sources) who are not responding to other therapy.

All VADs require power sources, and most have hand or foot pumps to use as back-up in the event that the electrical pump fails. The systems have both electrical and battery back-up, and many have car adaptors that plug into the cigarette lighter. Patients are sent home with power source back-up systems, and they must have a support system of individuals who know how to troubleshoot problems as well.

At the time this chapter was written, there were only 25 centers across the United States implanting these devices, and because there is not currently a national registry of the number of patients with these devices, it is unknown exactly how many people have them. It is estimated that the number is somewhere around 250 patients as many centers average around 10 patients with the device at any time. The largest center, which is located in Utah, currently has an average of 25 patients at any time with a VAD discharged into the community.

These devices allow an otherwise critically ill person the opportunity to leave the hospital and return to a fairly normal life. However, their life is highly regimented. These patients travel, resume work, and resume normal intimate relationships, and it is reported that at least one patient opted to keep the LVAD device when a heart transplant became available. Patients are not allowed to leave the hospital until they have proven their ability to troubleshoot their device and manage it if problems arise.

LVAD devices typically last 18 months before the pumps require surgical replacement, but they can last longer. Currently, a device is under investigation that is believed to be able to remain in place for up to five years.

LVAD patients are on aspirin or coumadin to prevent the formation of blood clots, but they do not require immunosuppression, steroids, or any of the other medication that heart transplant patients require.

These devices may or may not generate enough pressure to allow for a palpable pulse, even when the VAD is functioning properly. This is because some of the devices have continuous flow, and some have a "pumping" action similar to the ventricle. The ones that "pump" can generate a pulse, but not all of them do. Also, mechanical blood pressure cuffs cannot be used to assess blood pressure, only manual cuffs can. Again, this is due to the lack of the pulsatile flow of blood into the extremities that is required for the BP cuff to obtain a reading.

Heart sounds will be mostly unaffected with the VAD device in place, but the hum of the motor (which sounds like an airplane engine from a long way off) or the clicking of the diaphragm on the pump may be heard in addition to the patient's heart valves.

The ECG of the patient will not be affected by the VAD because it is a mechanical assistant device, not an electrical device such as a pacemaker. Tachydysrhythmias in these patients pose a problem. Most VADs rely on good right heart function (even when a RVAD is in place), and in the presence of right heart failure (which tachycardia can quickly cause), cardiac output can be disrupted significantly.

CPR is not recommended for these patients as it will tear the device from its attachment to the heart muscle, but certain electrical therapy such as defibrillation and cardioversion can be performed when the electrical pump and computer are disconnected first.

Chest trauma of any type, including airbag deployment, is potentially dangerous to the attachment points of the device to the myocardium, and the patient should be transported immediately.

Typically, the hospital that implanted the device will provide education to the local ambulance service that is likely to respond to the patient. Also, they are the ones to call in the event that an emergency occurs.

Infarctions and 12-Lead Acquisition

The 12-lead ECG tracing is a helpful tool to use in identifying possible myocardial infarctions or AMI (heart attack). The 12-lead ECG is one piece of a total assessment package that includes a comprehensive physical examination and history. An abnormal ECG gives strong evidence for a heart attack, but the lack of ECG findings does not rule out the possibility of a heart attack. This next section will discuss the 12-lead ECG and also provide an overview of the types of infarctions based upon their location within the heart.

The 12-Lead ECG

To appreciate the value of the 12-lead ECG, it is necessary to revisit some principles of how impulses move through the heart and how they are perceived by the ECG monitor. The primary purpose of the 12-lead ECG is to assess for the presence of heart disease. In several studies on the accuracy of computer-interpreted electrocardiography in the presence of heart disease, the computer performed quite well in identifying patients with acute MI.[17,18] Always remember that no matter what the 12-lead ECG shows, it should not supercede your patient assessment and clinical judgment but should augment it. Not every cardiac event shows up on the ECG, so you must always be prepared to treat patients based on their presentation.

The 12-lead ECG uses a combination of limb leads and precordial leads to give a three dimensional view of the heart (Figure 29-99). Typically, all six limb leads are used, and the six mostly left-sided precordial leads make up the standard 12-lead ECG. There are times when between one and three additional right side precordial leads are used to provide further evaluation for

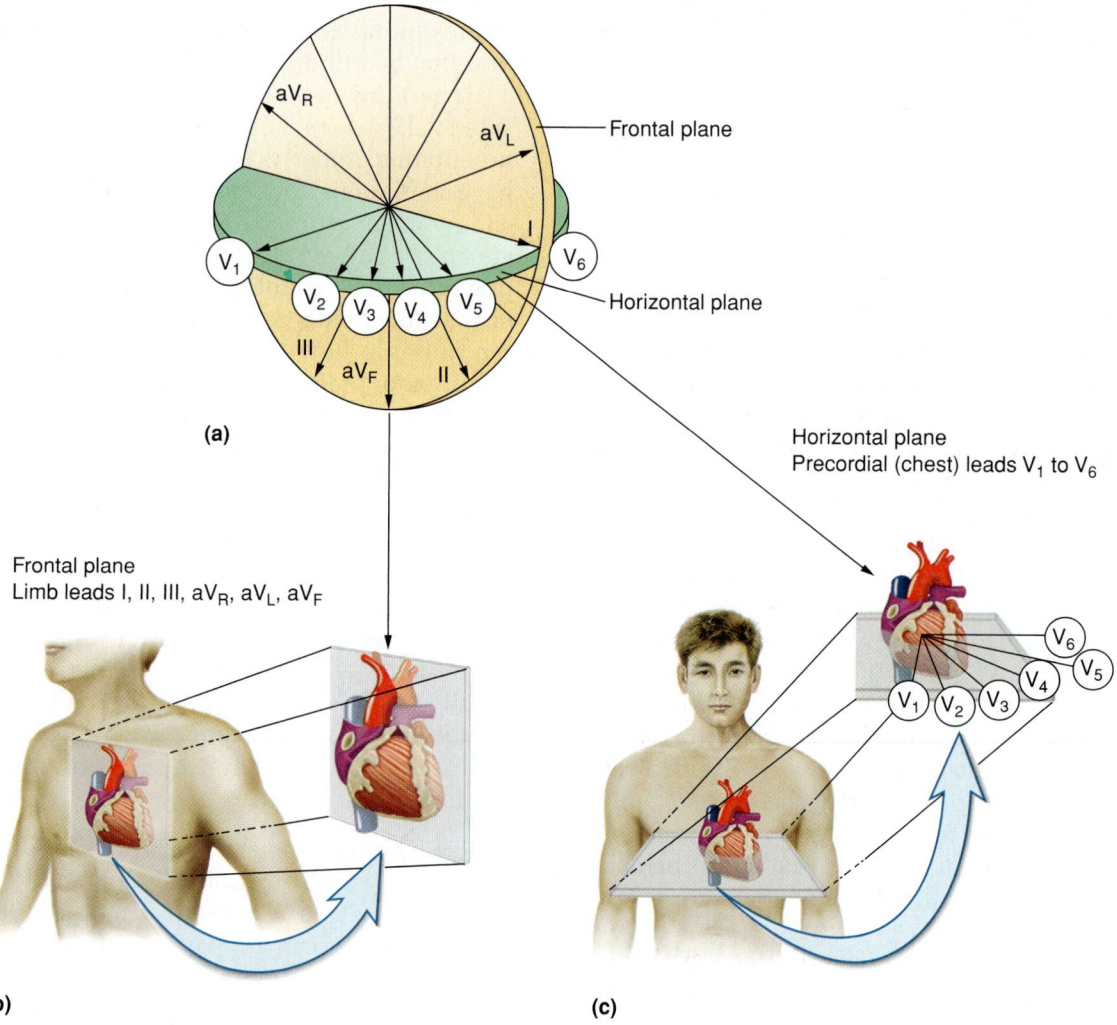

(a)

Frontal plane
Limb leads I, II, III, aV_R, aV_L, aV_F

Horizontal plane
Precordial (chest) leads V_1 to V_6

(b)

(c)

Figure 29-99   The 12-lead ECG components.

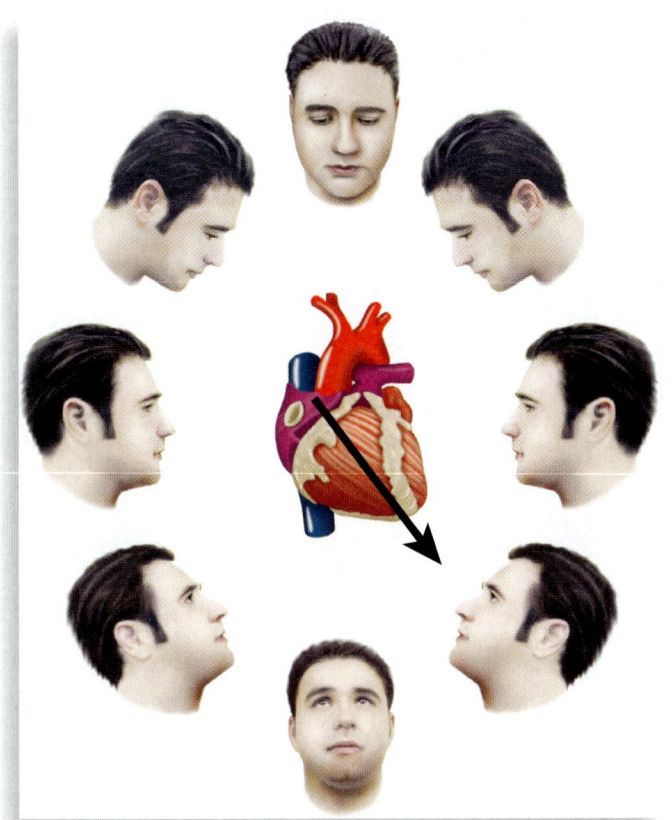

Figure 29-100   Each ECG lead provides a different view of the heart.

an inferior myocardial wall infarction. This will be discussed later.

The precordial leads are unipolar leads. This means that the negative lead is a calculated negative, theoretically located in the center of the heart. Lead placement is extremely important for consistency in the 12-lead ECG. Think of each electrode as an "eye" looking toward the heart (Figure 29-100). Each "eye" looks at a very specific portion of the heart. Since the electrical conduction travels many different directions in different areas of the heart, the ECG pattern will appear slightly different in all leads. Keep in mind that the measurements of waves and intervals shouldn't change. This also means that a change involving only one portion of the heart will only be seen in the leads that look to that area. For example, an infarction involving the inferior aspect of the heart will only be evident in the leads that look at that area, specifically leads II, III, and avF.

When examining a 12-lead ECG, you should already have identified the rhythm, or significantly narrowed it down, using the five-step process. Occasionally, the 12-lead ECG is needed to confirm the suspected diagnosis, but that is not a common reason to run the 12-lead ECG. The 12-lead ECG is typically used to look for some indication of ischemia or infarction. It is important to use a well-defined procedure to ensure something is not missed. A recommendation would be to use the 5 + 3

method, where you look at the rate, rhythm, P waves, PR interval, and the QRS pattern to make your judgment on the rhythm as described earlier. Then look for ST depression, ST elevation, and Q waves, all of which will be discussed here. By using this disciplined approach, fewer important items will be missed.

The 12-lead ECG is a very good tool, yielding a wealth of information. As you become comfortable with these items, you will want to learn more about the 12-lead in the future. An important thing to remember is that the 12-lead ECG tracing is no more important a tool than a comprehensive patient assessment and history. Continue to treat the signs and symptoms, not the ECG monitor. Also, the absence of the clinical findings listed above does not mean the patient is not having a heart attack. There can be a heart attack and a "normal" ECG.

Research has shown that the ECG displays very characteristic patterns as a myocardial event takes place (Figure 29-101). For this information early in the timeline of the event (as determined by the onset of symptoms), look primarily at the ST segment and T wave. As an area of the heart becomes ischemic, the T wave often will become inverted (Figure 29-102). This is followed by the appearance of ST segment deviation. When looking for the ST segment deviation, remember that changes should be at least 1 mm above or below the baseline in the limb leads and at least 2 mm above or below the baseline in the V leads to be considered a significant finding. As the ischemic area starts to experience actual injury (infarction), the ST segment begins to show signs of elevation above the baseline; early signs may also include the T wave as it becomes tall and peaked in an upright formation. This is known as the hyperacute phase of an infarction.

A word about the T wave is appropriate here. As a rule, when depolarization is abnormal, so too will be repolarization. So ST changes will also include changes in the appearance of the T wave. As a general rule, the T wave should be asymmetric in appearance and will often become symmetrical during an infarction. Also remember that there are a lot of flowing electrical forces present during depolarization and repolarization; abnormal conduction confounds this further. As a result, you won't always see each of the changes described above.

As the injury pattern extends through the heart, the ST segment continues to elevate, creating a classic appearance commonly called the "tombstone" or "screaming T wave" (Figure 29-103).

If intervention to restore blood flow doesn't occur, the injured region will begin to die, which is evident by the appearance of pathologic Q waves. Small Q waves are often seen as a normal component of the ECG complex signifying septal depolarization. If the Q waves are at least 1 mm in width and greater than one-third the size of the R wave in the same lead, they can be considered abnormal and pathologic in origin. To understand why this occurs, think of an infarcted area like an open

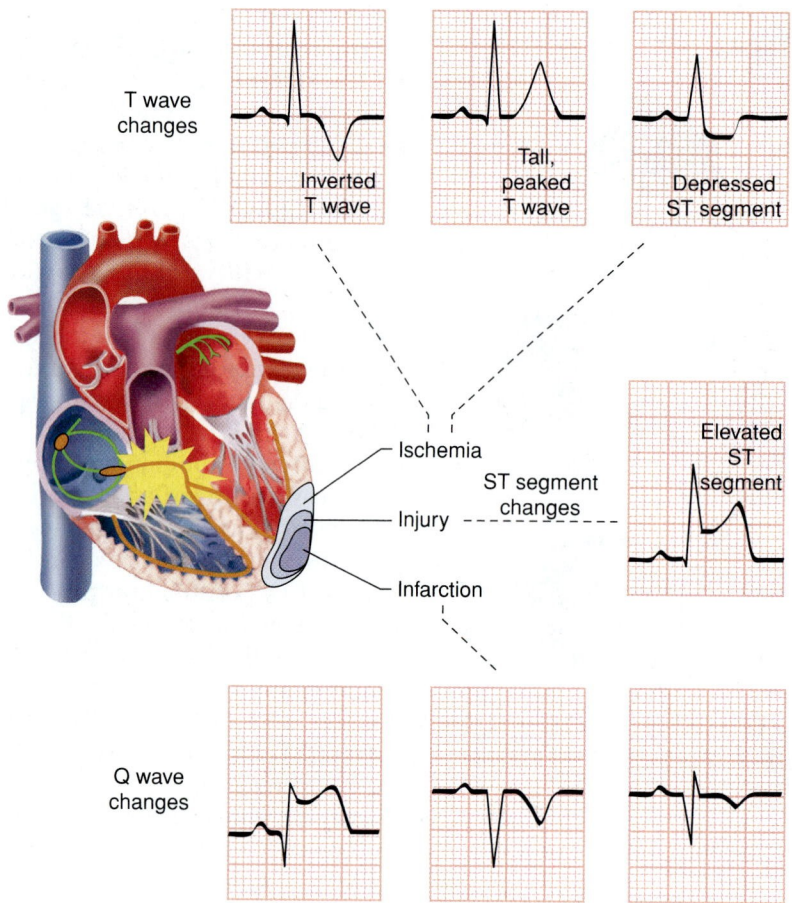

Figure 29-101   ECG changes with ischemia, injury, or infarction.

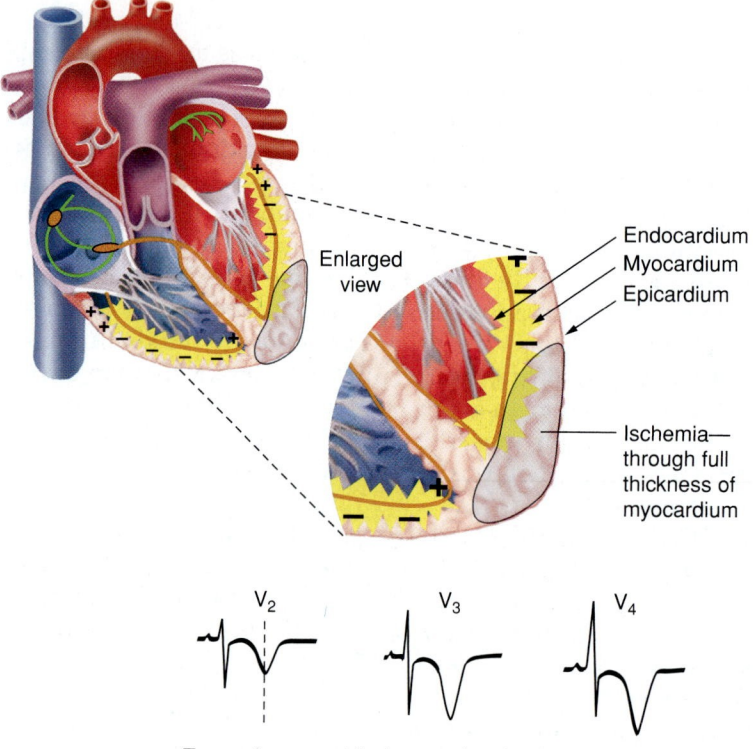

T wave is symmetrical—meaning the right and left sides of the waveform are the same size and inverted.

Figure 29-102   ECG pattern of ischemia.

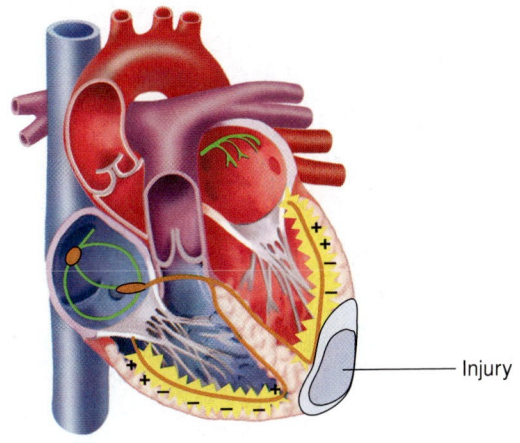

Injury

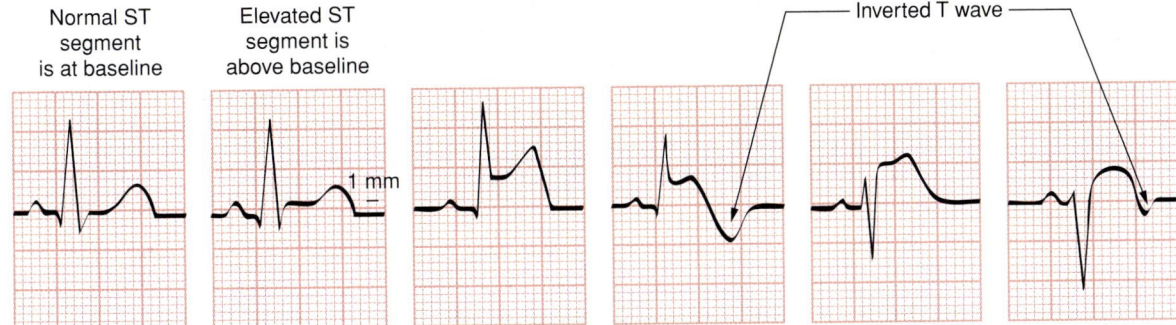

Normal ST
segment
is at baseline

Elevated ST
segment is
above baseline

1 mm

Inverted T wave

Examples of ST segment elevation

Figure 29-103   ST segment signs of myocardial infarction.

window. Since no electrical current is occurring within the necrotic tissue, the electrode is actually picking up the electrical impulse from the opposite wall of the ventricle, which is obviously reversed in polarity. Q waves usually become a permanent fixture in the complex from then on, indicating necrotic or electrically inert tissue.

The next important step in reading the 12-lead ECG is to correlate which lead is associated with which area of the heart. Refer to Figure 29-99 (on page 668). Examine the hexaxial diagram of leads, with the precordial leads superimposed over the heart, to understand this better. Think of the heart as two types of structures—the left and right ventricles—each with its own geometric shape with the septum separating them. The right ventricle, has septal, anterior, and inferior aspects. The left ventricle, has septal, anterior, lateral, and posterior aspects. Remember that the left ventricle is much larger than the right and commands much more electrical current (Figure 29-104).

Using this as a guide, notice that leads II, III, and avF are looking at the heart's inferior aspect; they are referred to as the inferior leads. Leads V1 and V2 look at the septal region. Leads V3 and V4 look at the anterior aspect while V5, V6, and leads I and avL look at the lateral wall. There is some crossover between the leads; for example, changes affecting the septum and anterior

wall are diagnosed with an anteroseptal infarct. This is observed in leads V1 through V4. There may also be involvement of more than one wall of the heart such as the inferolateral or anterolateral areas. In each case, changes should be present in all the leads that normally look at those areas.

One exception to the ST elevation rule is the case of the posterior infarction. In the standard 12-lead ECG, no leads look directly at the posterior portion of the heart. Therefore, the identification of a posterior aspect of the heart is evident by looking for something called reciprocal changes. **Reciprocal changes** are a reversal of ST changes seen in a lead or leads opposite of the actual location. For example, during an inferior infarction, ST elevation should be present in the inferior leads: leads II, III, and avF. On the opposite side of the heart, the anteroseptal leads V1 through V4 may be showing ST depression. This emphasizes why it is so important to use a methodical approach to 12-lead ECG interpretation. What may appear to be anterior ischemia may in fact be an inferior infarction with reciprocal changes.

Another word of caution during interpretation of a 12-lead ECG is to be wary of the interpretation provided by the monitor itself. Most modern 12-lead ECG-capable monitors will provide an interpretation based upon a database of known measurements and changes. While

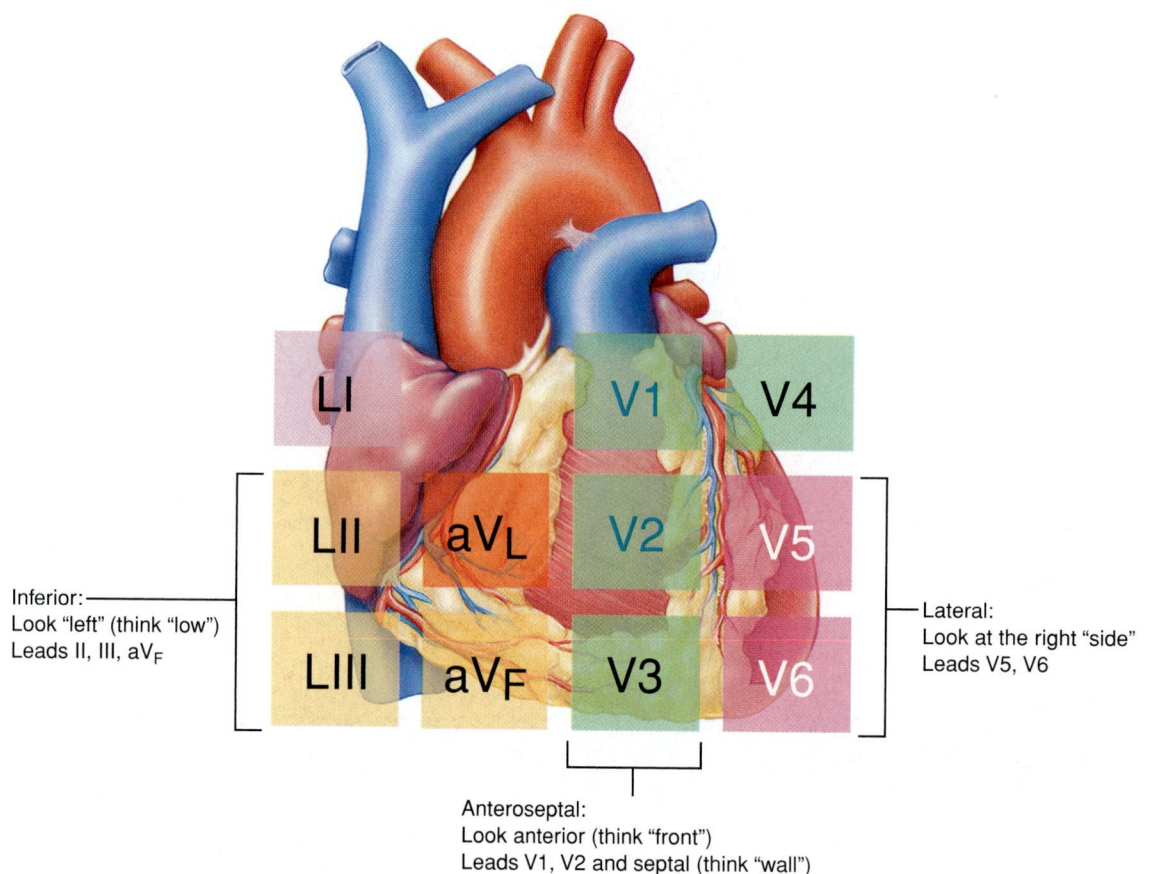

Inferior:
Look "left" (think "low")
Leads II, III, aV$_F$

Lateral:
Look at the right "side"
Leads V5, V6

Anteroseptal:
Look anterior (think "front")
Leads V1, V2 and septal (think "wall")

Figure 29-104   The concept of "contiguous leads" on an ECG can be difficult to understand at first. Think of this figure as a roadmap to understanding 12-lead ECGs. The contiguous leads are looking at sections of the heart.

- Look "left" (think "low") leads II, III, and aV$_F$ = inferior.
- Look anterior (think "front"): leads V1, V2, and septal (think "wall") = anteroseptal.
- Look at the "right" side: leads V5 and V6 = lateral.

studies have shown them to be reliable at identifying infarctions, they do make mistakes. It is always advisable to make your own determination first, then verify with the interpretation provided by the monitor for a second opinion. Do not assume the monitor is always right. Any confusion should be discussed with a physician or medical control.

Inferior Infarction

An **inferior infarction** is the result of blockage of the right coronary artery involving the right ventricle. But possibly as important, in 90% of the population, the RCA supplies blood to the nodal artery, which in turn supplies blood to the sinus and AV nodes. Disruption of this blood supply could result in sinus node dysfunction or AV block. For this reason, it is helpful to know if the obstruction is in the proximal or distal end of the RCA. To determine this, you should perform a right precordial 12-lead ECG with attention to the V4r

lead. The right precordial electrodes are placed in the same location as the left, just on the opposite side of the chest. Remember to label the 12-lead as right precordial, as the monitor will not know the difference and anybody reading the report at a later date will not know it was a right-sided tracing.

Since damage to the right ventricle can lead to hypotensive problems, it is valuable to assess the extent of right ventricular involvement. You can estimate this by examining leads II and III. If the degree of ST elevation in lead III exceeds that of lead II, the right ventricle is involved (Figure 29-105).

Another clue may be the presence of ST elevation in V1 along with leads II, III, and aV$_F$. Right ventricular failure may precipitate hypotension in approximately 50% of patients and may prevent the use of standard medications (nitrates and morphine) normally used with an acute coronary syndrome. Careful fluid boluses may be required along with medications to treat the problem. This infarct may also involve the inferior wall of the left ventricle (see Box 29-8).

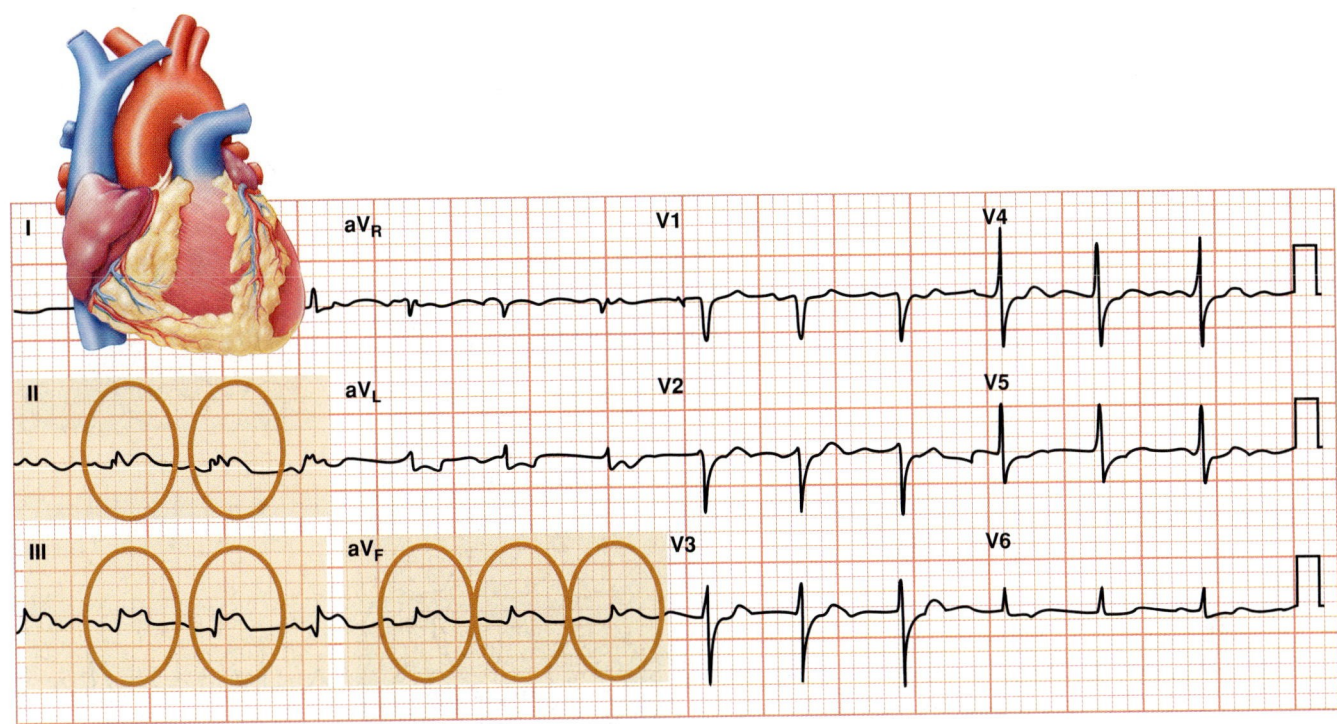

Figure 29-105 Inferior myocardial infarction. Note the elevated ST segment in leads II, III, and aVF.

BOX 29-8 Usual ECG Leads Affected—Inferior MI

I	aV$_R$	V1	V4
II	aV$_L$	V2	V5
III	aV$_F$	V3	V6

BOX 29-9 Usual ECG Leads Affected—Septal MI

I	aV$_R$	V1	V4
II	aV$_L$	V2	V5
III	aV$_F$	V3	V6

Septal Infarction

Isolated **septal infarctions** are, by themselves, rare as most also involve the left ventricle. Blockage high in the left anterior descending coronary artery may result in a conduction defect along the bundle branches within the septum. Isolated septal infarctions are evidenced by ST elevation in V1 and V2 and usually result in a QS wave in V1 (see Box 29-9). Complications such as second-degree type II AV block, complete heart block, and bundle branch block are common.

Anterior Infarction

Anterior infarctions represent problems with the left ventricle. Whenever the left ventricle is involved in an infarction, it not only compromises systemic circulation but could also engorge the pulmonary vasculature, resulting in pulmonary edema and breathing difficulty.

The combination of decreased cardiac output and respiratory compromise results in very serious signs and symptoms (see Box 29-10). Not only is a significant area of muscle involved, but the appearance of critical conduction abnormalities such as second-degree type II AV block and complete heart block are also more common.

BOX 29-10 Usual ECG Leads Affected—Anterior MI

I	aV$_R$	V1	V4
II	aV$_L$	V2	V5
III	aV$_F$	V3	V6

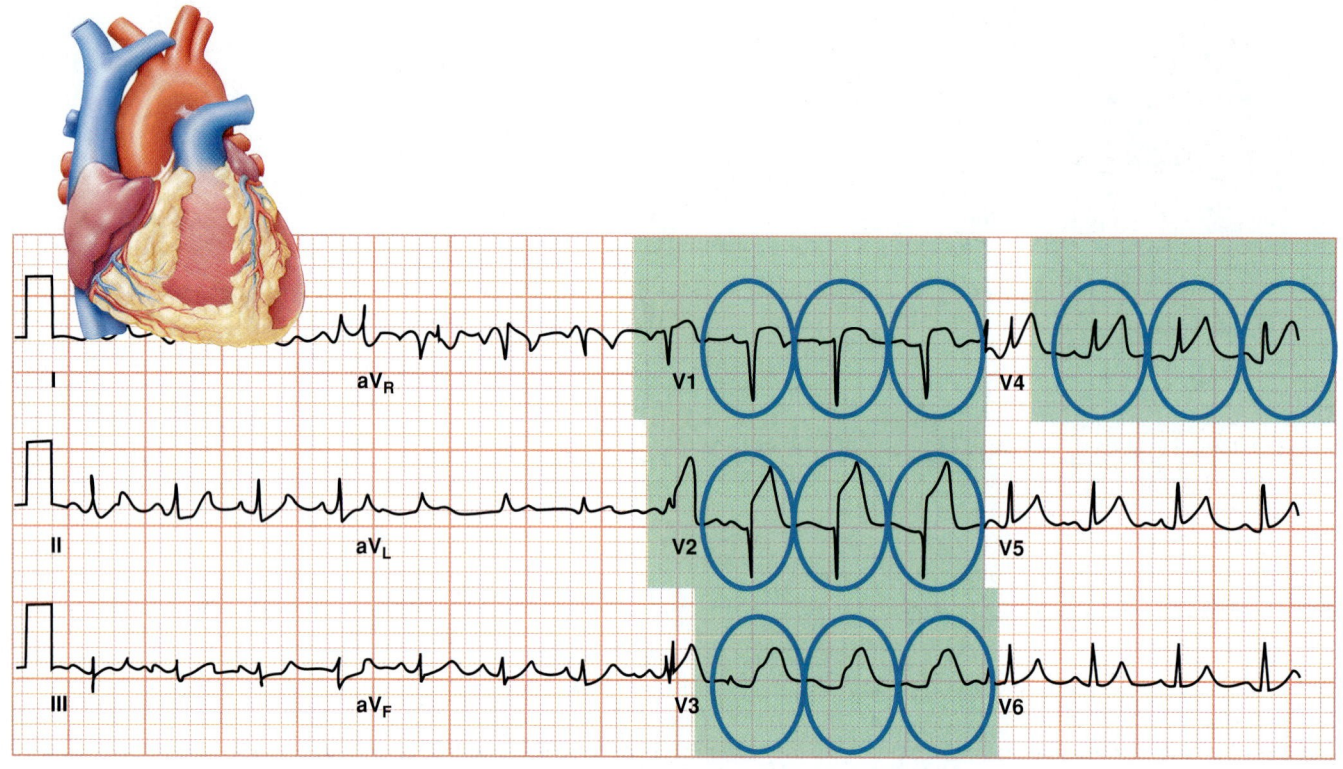

Figure 29-106   Anteroseptal myocardial infarction. Note the elevated ST segment in leads V1, V2, V3, and V4.

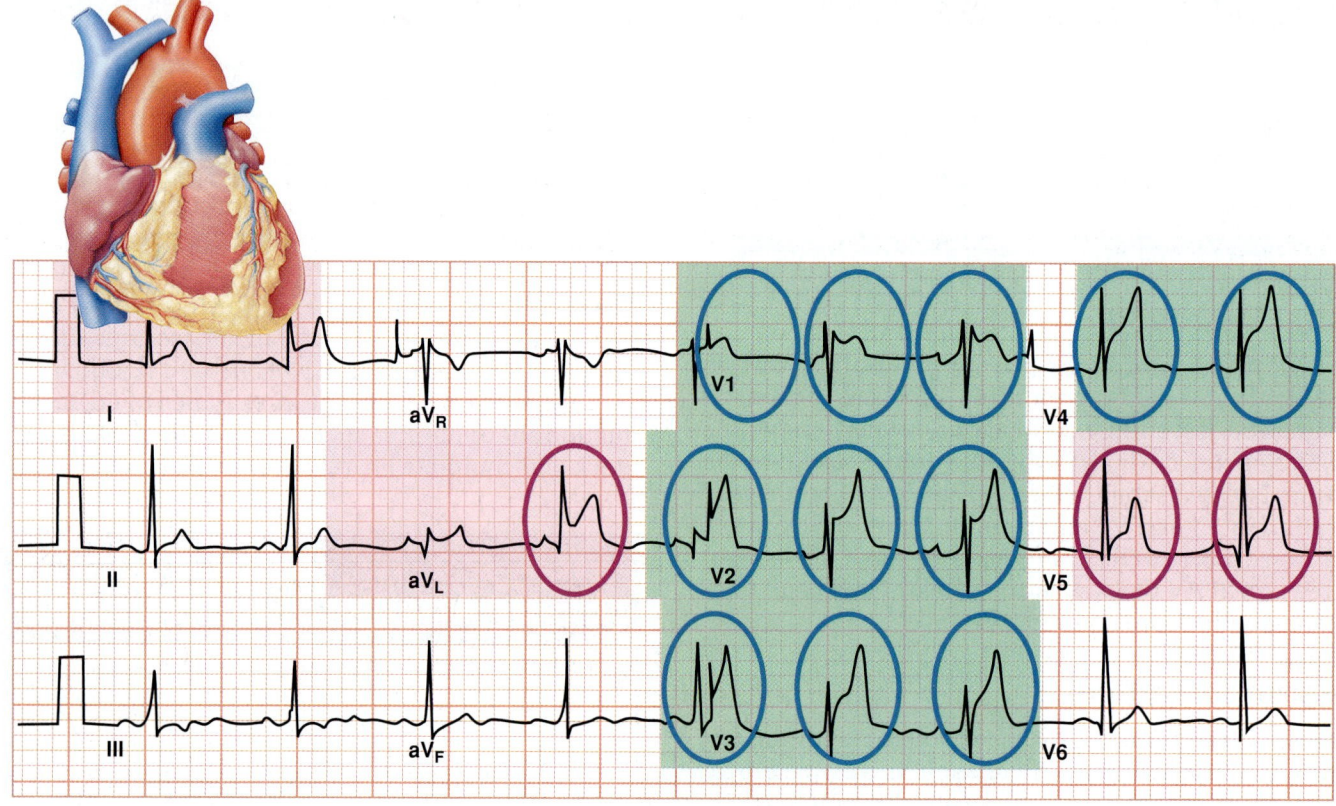

Figure 29-107   Anterolateral myocardial infarction. Note the elevated ST segment in leads V1, V2, V3, and V4 and lateral leads V5, lead I, and aVL.

BOX 29-11 Usual ECG Leads Affected— Anteroseptal MI			
I	aV$_R$	V1	V4
II	aV$_L$	V2	V5
III	aV$_F$	V3	V6

BOX 29-12 Usual ECG Leads Affected— Anterolateral MI			
I	aV$_R$	V1	V4
II	aV$_L$	V2	V5
III	aV$_F$	V3	V6

There is a high risk of the development of lethal dysrhythmia for several days postinfarct associated with anterior involvement.

The primary leads associated with the anterior AMI are V3 and V4 (Box 29-11). It is also common to see either septal or lateral involvement. These are respectively referred to as anteroseptal and anterolateral infarcts. The anteroseptal infarct would include ST changes in V1, V2, V3, and V4 (see Box 29-11 and Figure 29-106). Risks would include all of those associated with the anterior infarction, along with the potential conduction problems associated with septal involvement.

Anterolateral changes would be evident by ST changes in V3 to V6 plus lead I and avL (see Figure 29-107 and Box 29-12).

Lateral Infarction

Lateral wall ischemia or **infarctions** involve the circumflex coronary artery, and like the septal wall infarction, isolated lateral wall infarction is rare. It is most commonly associated with anterior wall or posterior wall involvement. In about 10% of people, the circumflex coronary artery also supplies the nodal artery on the posterior aspect of the heart. Since this artery supplies the AV and SA nodes, conduction problems associated with those areas are not unusual.

Lateral wall changes are observed in leads I and avL, along with precordial leads V5 and V6 (see Figure 29-108 and Box 29-13).

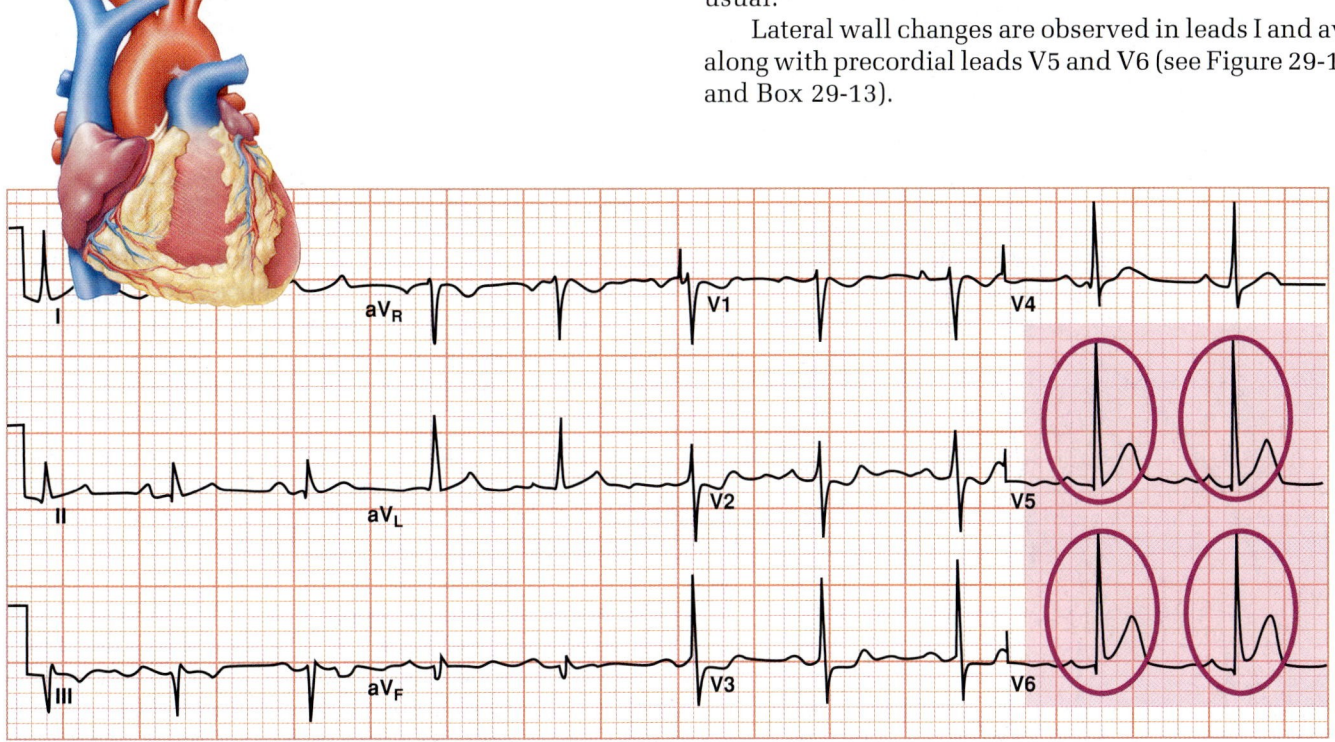

Figure 29-108   Lateral myocardial infarction. Note the elevated ST segment in leads V5 and V6. Also note reciprocal changes (ST depression in leads V1, V2, and V3.) ST depression alone is not a reliable indicator of infarction, but when it is accompanying ST elevation, it helps confirm the interpretation.

BOX 29-13 Usual ECG Leads Affected—Lateral MI			
I	aV$_R$	V1	V4
II	aV$_L$	V2	V5
III	aV$_F$	V3	V6

BOX 29-14 Usual ECG Leads Affected—Posterior MI			
I	aV$_R$	V1	V4
II	aV$_L$	V2	V5
III	aV$_F$	V3	V6

Posterior Wall Infarction

Because the posterior wall in a significant part of the population is supplied with blood through the RCA, it is not unusual to see a posterior wall infarction associated with inferior infarctions (Figure 29-109). In the standard 12-lead configuration, there are no leads that look directly at the posterior wall. Occasionally for diagnostic purposes, leads may be changed slightly to include V7, V8, and V9 running around the back with V9 attached just left of the spine at the fifth intercostal space, V8 at the midscapular line in the fifth intercostal space, and V7 on the postaxillary line in the fifth intercostal space. Remember that the monitor will not perceive this change, so if you use it, all the altered leads must be properly labeled.

Instead of changing the lead configuration, suspect posterior wall infarctions based upon ST depression in leads V1, V2, and V3 (Box 29-14). Another clue is a tall R wave in V1. Consider using the standard configuration to suspect posterior involvement; then change the leads for verification. Posterior wall involvement is commonly associated with either inferior or anterolateral involvement; therefore, expect serious conduction problems to appear, dependant upon the time and extent of the problem.

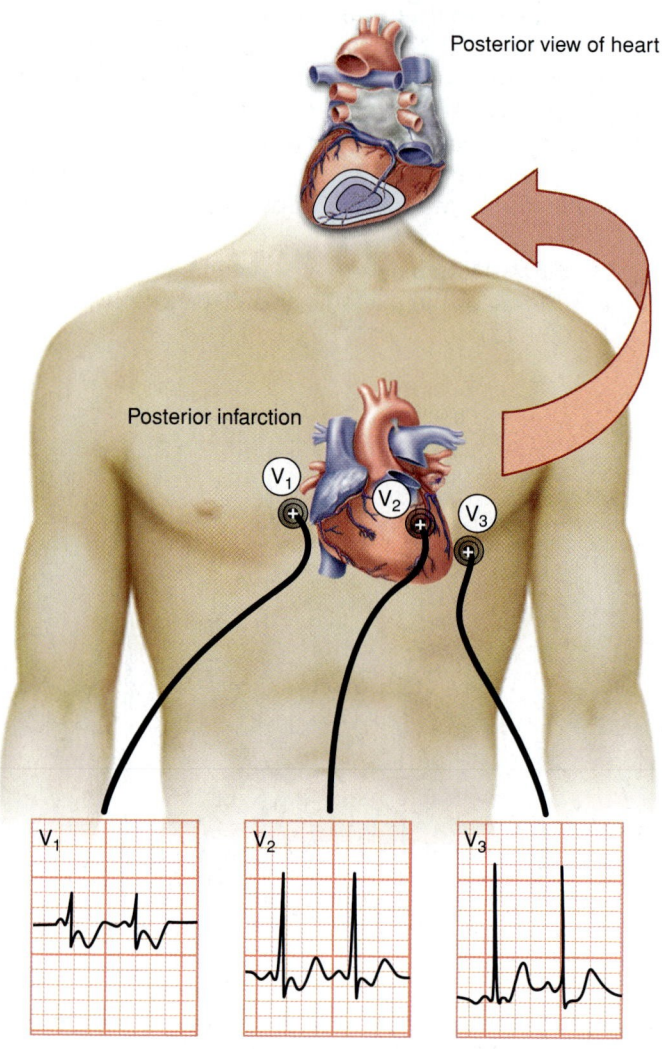

Posterior view of heart

Posterior infarction

Figure 29-109   Posterior myocardial infarction.

Summary

This section introduced the process for ECG interpretation. It started with a review of the anatomy and physiology of the cardiovascular system. The heart was explored from the cellular level and progressed to the complex interrelationship between each of the components of the electrical conduction system. An examination of the conduction system showed how electricity was produced and propagated throughout the heart and how that electrical flow was recorded on the ECG.

A five-step process for evaluating the ECG was introduced. It was applied to all the ECG rhythms, including those from the atria, junction, and ventricle. Interpretation of the 12-lead ECG was also discussed.

The next section of this chapter will discuss the diseases associated with the cardiovascular system. It will take the information learned in this section and use it in discussions of the management of these patients.

Section I Notes

1. K. F. Wenckebach, *Arrhythmia of the Heart: A Physiological and Clinical Study,* trans. T. Snowball (Edinburgh, Scotland: William Green, 1904).

2. W. Einthoven, "Le Telecardiogramme," *Archives International de Physiologie* 4(1906):132–164.

3. C. C. Pang, "Measurement of Body Venous Tone," *Journal of Pharmacological and Toxicological Methods* 44(2) (September–October 2000):341–360.

4. Shier, Butler, and Lewis, *Hole's Human Anatomy & Physiology,* 10th ed. (New York, NY: McGraw-Hill, 2003).

5. *Taber's Cyclopedic Medical Dictionary,* 20th ed. (Philadelphia, PA: FA Davis, 2005).

6. N. Fukuda and H. Granzier, "Role of the Giant Elastic Protein Titin in the Frank-Starling Mechanism of the Heart," *Current Vascular Pharmacology* 2(2) (April 2004):135–139.

7. H. J. L. Marriott, *Practical Electrocardiography,* 8th ed. (Baltimore, MD: Lippincott Williams & Wilkins, 1988).

8. R. J. Huszar, *Basic Dysrhythmias,* 2nd ed. (St. Louis, MO: Mosby-Year Book, 1994).

9. J. E. Tintinalli, G. D. Kelen, J. S. Stapczynski, O. J. Ma, and D. M. Cline, *Tintinalli's Emergency Medicine: A Comprehensive Study Guide,* 6th ed., McGraw-Hill's AccessMedicine (accessed September 18, 2006).

10. R. Wiederhold, *Electrocardiography: The Monitoring and Diagnostic Leads,* 2nd ed. (Philadelphia, PA: Elsevier Saunders, 1999).

11. M. B. Conover, *Understanding Electrocardiography,* 7th ed. (St. Louis: MO: Elsevier Mosby, 1996).

12. W. A. Ghali, B. I. Wasil, R. Brant, D. V. Exner, and J. Cornuz, "Atrial Flutter and the Risk of Thromboembolism: A Systematic Review and Meta-Analysis," *The American Journal of Medicine* 118(2) (February 2005):101–107.

13. D. P. Zipes and J. Jalife, *Cardiac Electrophysiology: From Cell to Bedside,* 4th ed. (Philadelphia, PA: Elsevier Saunders, 2004).

14. "Spontaneous Initiation of Atrial Fibrillation by Ectopic Beats Originating in the Pulmonary Veins," The *New England Journal of Medicine* 339(10) (September 3, 1998):659–666.

15. Allison Gandey, "Evidence Supports Bystander CPR and Rapid Defibrillation," http://www.theheart.org/viewArticle. do?primaryKey=122127 (accessed May 29, 2005).

16. H. J. Wellens, L. M. Rodriguez, C. Timmermans, and J. P. Smeets, "The Asymptomatic Patient with the Wolff-Parkinson-White Electrocardiogram," *Pacing and Clinical Electrophysiology* 20(8) part 20 (August 1997):2082–2086.

17. P. J. Kudenchuk, "Accuracy of Computer-Interpreted Electrocardiography in Selecting Patients for Thrombolytic Therapy," *Journal of the American College of Cardiology* 17(7) (June 1, 1991):1486–1491.

18. M. F. O'Rourke, "Accuracy of a Portable Interpretive ECG Machine in Diagnosis of Acute Evolving Myocardial Infarction," *Australian and New Zealand Journal of Medicine* 22(1) (February 1, 1992):9–13.

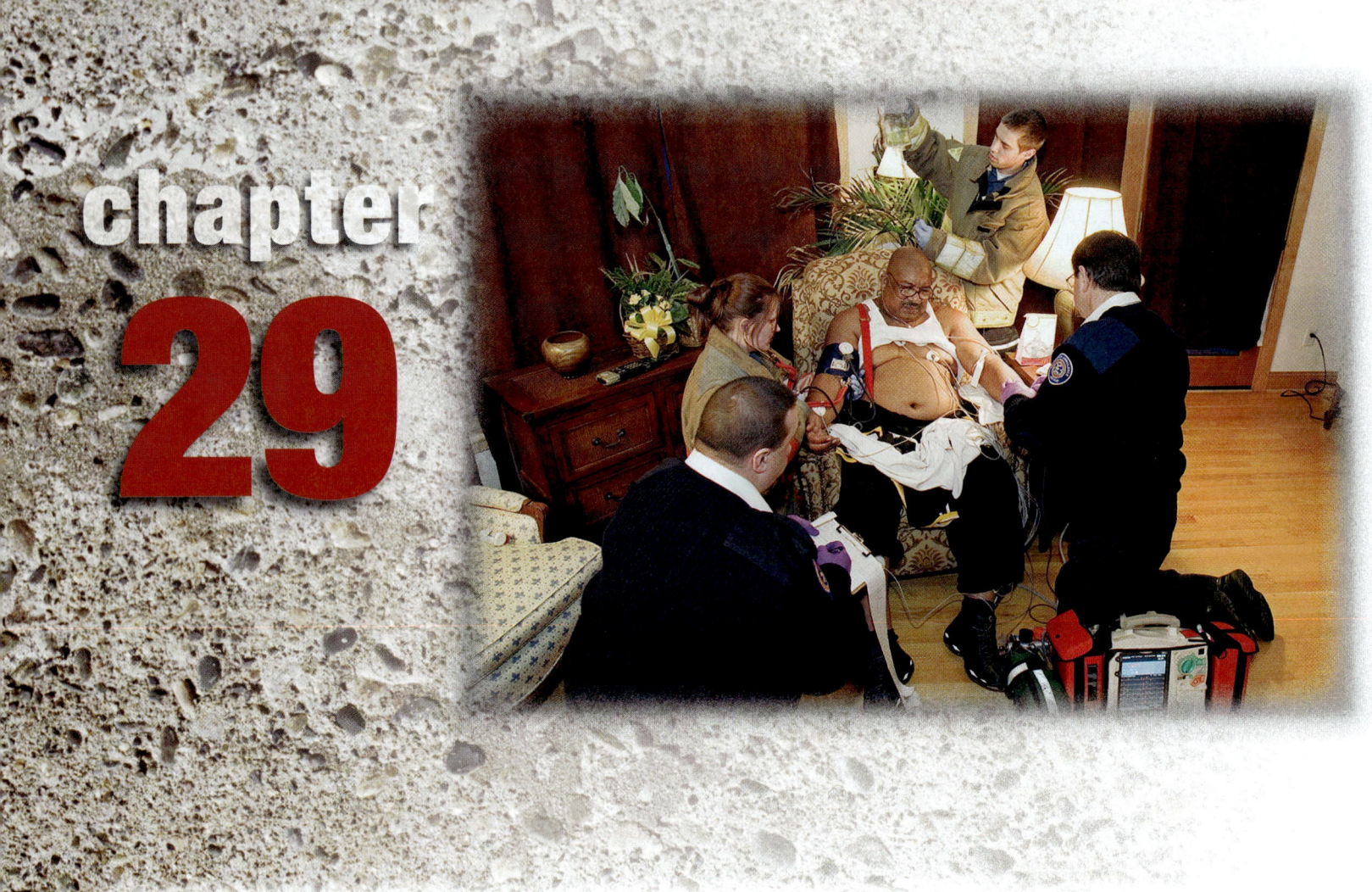

Cardiology

Section II: Cardiovascular Diseases

"*If I can stop one heart from breaking I shall not live in vain; if I can stop one life the aching or cool one pain, or help one fainting robin unto its nest again, I shall not live in vain.*"

—Emily Dickinson

Need to Know

▶ Cardiovascular emergencies are commonly encountered by paramedics, so it is important to understand the pathophysiology of sudden cardiac death, myocardial infarction, heart failure, hypertensive emergencies, and vascular diseases.

▶ Dysrhythmias may be treated conservatively by monitoring or by rapid transport with minimal interventions or more aggressively with electricity or medications.

▶ Accurate rhythm interpretation is required in order to treat dysrhythmias.

▶ An acute myocardial infarction can lead to other cardiovascular diseases such as left or right heart failure, chronic dysrhythmias, or vascular disease.

▶ Sick	▶ Not yet sick
• Any cardiac patient with signs of shock should be transported promptly to a medical facility capable of managing cardiovascular emergencies. • Diagnosis of AMI requires three components: history suggestive of an AMI, ECG changes, and the presence of elevated cardiac enzymes. Not all of these are recognizable or obtainable in the prehospital setting (and some may never show up despite the presence of an AMI), so it is important that the paramedic maintain a high index of suspicion for cardiac disease based on the history, physical examination, and chief complaint. • Treat chest pain with MONA drugs (morphine, oxygen, nitroglycerin, and aspirin) as the vital signs and circumstances permit. The goal is to reduce chest pain as much as possible toward a "0" on the one-to-ten scale.	• Patients have compensatory mechanisms that preserve blood pressure and cardiac output and may not appear sick on first assessment. It is important to remember that these patients may not be able to compensate for a long period of time, and prompt recognition of the severity of their condition is important. • Ask about cardiovascular risk factors, particularly about the history of cardiac problems in a first-degree relative (father, mother, or siblings).

Introduction

The previous section of this chapter discussed cardiovascular physiology and introduced ECG rhythm interpretation. This section continues the discussion of cardiovascular disease, including signs, symptoms, patient presentation, and prehospital treatment plans. The cardiovascular disorders discussed include sudden cardiac death, cardiac arrest resuscitation, myocardial infarction (heart attack), heart failure, hypertensive emergencies, and vascular diseases.

A related condition, pulmonary embolism, is covered in detail in Chapter 28: Pulmonary. It will be discussed briefly here.

CONNECTIONS A full discussion of pulmonary embolus can be found in Chapter 28: Pulmonary (page 583).

This section of the chapter is supported by Skill Sheet 34: Chest Pain Assessment, Skill Sheet 35: Dyspnea Assessment, Skill Sheet 37: ECG Acquisition (also see Step-by-Step 37), Skill Sheet 38: Synchronized Cardioversion and Defibrillation (also see Step-by-Step 38), Skill Sheet 39: Transcutaneous Cardiac Pacing (also see Step-by-Step 39), Skill Sheet 40: Vagal Maneuvers, Skill Sheet 86: NREMT Dynamic Cardiology, and Skill Sheet 87: NREMT Static Cardiology.

The Incidence of Cardiovascular Disease

Cardiovascular disease (CVD) includes coronary artery disease (CAD), stroke, and peripheral vascular disease (PVD). CVD is the leading cause of death in the United States. Each year, more than 900,000 CVD deaths occur in the United States. CVD is the major cause of mortality in most developed countries and is becoming a major cause in developing countries as well. It is difficult to assess the true extent of cardiovascular disease morbidity, but over thirteen million Americans have CAD, and nearly seven million have active chest pain in the form of angina. DOT 5-2.1

The cost of CAD in the United States for 2003 was estimated to be $133.2 billion.[1] As the American population ages, there is no doubt that these diseases will affect more and more people.

Over 13 million Americans have CAD alone, and nearly 7 million have active chest pain (angina).

The incidence of cardiovascular disease can be reduced. The majority of known risk factors for CVD are modifiable. A large study published in *The New England Journal of Medicine* suggests that, with appropriate exercise, diet, and lifestyle modifications, the risk for heart disease can be reduced by 84%.[2] There are many modifiable cardiovascular risk factors including abnormal cholesterol levels (dyslipidemia), hypertension (high blood pressure), smoking, improper diet, physical inactivity, obesity, and diabetes mellitus. Additional ways to prevent heart disease (called **primary prevention** strategies) include having regular physician check-ups, making healthy lifestyle changes, and taking aspirin and other medication when indicated. DOT 5-2.2, 5-2.3

Cardiac Risk Factors

There are multiple risk factors that predispose patients to coronary artery disease (CAD). Certainly, paramedics do not have a grasp on all of these factors, but they can recognize someone at higher risk based on the risk factors in Box 29-15. DOT 5-2.22

Dyslipidemia

Hyperlipidemia or an increased cholesterol level is a significant risk for CAD. Cholesterol levels clearly play a role in the buildup of atherosclerosis, which is the vascular change that leads to a heart attack. There are two types of lipids: **low-density lipoprotein (LDL),** which is also referred to as "bad cholesterol," and **high-density lipoprotein (HDL),** which is called "good cholesterol." Having a high LDL and low HDL are each independent risk factors for CAD. The ratio of total cholesterol to HDL cholesterol should be less than 5.0 in order to be categorized as low risk. Additional protein

BOX 29-15 Coronary Artery Disease Risk Factors

- Abnormal cholesterol levels (dyslipidemia)
- High blood pressure (hypertension)
- Diabetes mellitus
- Tobacco abuse
- Male gender
- Family history
- Obesity/Metabolic syndrome
- Kidney disease

and lipid factors in the bloodstream may contribute to (or are at least markers of) CAD, including homocysteine and high-sensitivity C-reactive protein. Medications are available to assist patients in lowering their cholesterol levels. Diet and exercise have also been shown to help control cholesterol.

Hypertension (HTN)

High blood pressure has a direct relationship to CAD as it predisposes patients to vascular injury. It increases stress on the heart by increasing the work and size of the left ventricle and causes increased oxygen delivery needs. HTN decreases blood delivery in patients with preexisting coronary artery atherosclerosis. Medications are available to assist patients in controlling hypertension. Diet and exercise have also been shown to help control HTN.

Cigarette Smoking

Smoking is one of the highest risks for CAD and is also potentially the most modifiable. The effects of smoking on CAD and atherosclerosis are multiple and not well-delineated at the pathophysiologic level. These likely include direct vascular toxicity of smoke, decreased oxygen delivery, decreased effectiveness of medicines, and enhanced vascular stress by drugs such as epinephrine. Patients with previously documented CAD who smoke have significantly higher risks of sudden death, AMI, and mortality. Most importantly, smoking cessation clearly reduces cardiac risk.

Family History

A patient is at particularly high risk for CAD if a primary relative (parent, sibling, or child) has had early onset coronary disease. For males, early onset is considered the development of CAD prior to age 55. For females, the early onset age is prior to 65. One of the largest cardiovascular databases ever compiled, the Framingham database, showed that after correcting for all other risks, a strong family history of heart disease increases the likelihood of heart attack by twofold in men and 1.7 times in women.[3] Obviously, this is a risk factor that cannot be modified, but it certainly allows a better understanding of risk and should stress the importance of gathering a thorough history from the patient.

Diabetes Mellitus

Diabetes is another very important modifiable risk factor with major implications for CAD as well as vascular disease in general. The increased cardiovascular risk in diabetes is correlated with the severity of glucose intolerance. In an analysis of over 13,000 participants in the Copenhagen Heart Study, the relative risk of incidence of MI or stroke was increased two- to threefold in those with type 2 diabetes (noninsulin dependant), and the risk of death was increased twofold, independent of other CAD risk factors.[4] Obesity makes diabetes more prevalent and severe. Proper diet and exercise both have a positive impact on diabetes.

Kidney Disease

This is a relative newcomer to the CAD risk category. It has long been known that patients with end-stage renal failure (requiring dialysis) have increased risk of heart disease, but more recent research is suggesting that any level of renal impairment can be considered a CAD equivalent. Practice guidelines from the National Kidney Foundation in 2002 and the American College of Cardiology/American Heart Association task force in 2004 recommended that chronic kidney disease be considered a CAD risk equivalent.[5,6]

Obesity and the Metabolic Syndrome

Patients with all of the following—abdominal obesity, hypertension, diabetes, and dyslipidemia—have **metabolic syndrome.** These are important CAD risks because they affect all of the above risk factors, and also indicate lack of cardioprotective activities such as regular exercise, healthy diet, appropriate lifestyle, and so on.

Additional Emerging Risks

New risk factors are not yet well understood in mechanism or severity. These are under active study and include C-reactive protein (an inflammatory protein), microalbuminuria, collagen vascular diseases, coronary artery calcification, and plasma fibrinogen levels. As research uncovers more information on each of these, they may or may not be included as future CAD risk factors.

The Cardiac History and Physical Examination

History

The initial history in the patient with known or suspected cardiovascular disease should include a description of the patient's symptoms such as onset, duration, character and intensity of symptoms, and any interventions that have improved or worsened the condition. The OPQRST mnemonic is a helpful tool to use when assessing chest pain because it contains all of the elements just described. DOT 5-2.67

CONNECTIONS Chapter 11: The Normal Physical Examination and Chapter 14: Patient Assessment discuss the OPQRST mnemonic.

A frequent complaint in patients with cardiovascular disease is chest pain. Chest pain can have many characteristics and can take many forms. It should always be thoroughly investigated to avoid missing life-threatening cardiac events. Chest pain is discussed extensively in the next section.

Other symptoms may accompany the pain including dyspnea, palpitations, lightheadedness, diaphoresis, edema, cyanosis or pallor, cool and clammy skin, and nausea and vomiting. Dyspnea should be evaluated to determine whether it occurs at rest or with exertion (**dyspnea on exertion** is abbreviated DOE). It may occur when lying supine, as in **orthopnea,** or may happen as the patient tries to sleep, as in **paroxysmal nocturnal dyspnea** (PND) (Box 29-16). In fact, patients may mention needing more pillows to sleep on at night to improve breathing.

Prior history of heart disease or heart surgery is especially important and may identify recurrence of a chronic problem or a complication of a recent treatment. A thorough review of the cardiac risk factors listed previously is key to assessing the probability of cardiac disease. Remember to inquire if a first-degree family member (parent or sibling) has a cardiac history, and determine at what age this problem occurred. A childhood history of congenital heart defects is also important as these problems may lie dormant for many years before expressing themselves.

The social and dietary history may also help establish the diagnosis. Tobacco use should be quantified to assess risk of heart disease. The use of alcohol and illicit drugs should also be ascertained. Stimulant drugs such as cocaine or methamphetamine can cause vasospasm, resulting in cardiac ischemia and chest pain. DOT 5-2.151

BOX 29-16   Paroxysmal Nocturnal Dyspnea (PND)

PND occurs when sleeping patients are awakened at night experiencing severe difficulty breathing. Patients often report they can no longer breathe while lying flat, and they must resort to propping up in bed or sleeping in a chair. This condition may accompany severe upper respiratory infections, or it may indicate an ongoing disease process such as heart failure or chronic obstructive pulmonary disease. DOT 5-2.92

Physical Exam

Inspection

The initial part of the cardiovascular exam should begin by thoroughly observing the patient's general appearance, which can be done simultaneously with history taking. Note whether the patient is obese or frail. A pronounced barrel-shaped chest usually indicates chronic obstructive pulmonary disease (COPD) is present. Patients with COPD often have heart disease as well. DOT 5-2.23

Skin color can help indicate the condition of the patient; the presence of pallor, cyanosis, or flushing can imply poor oxygenation status. Breathing patterns should be noted as well as the posture and position of the patient as they try to breathe.

The presence of edema, whether localized to the legs or diffuse, gives clues that heart failure may be present. Jugular venous distension can also indicate fluid overload. Endocarditis, which is an infection of the inner lining and valves of the heart, often presents with splinter hemorrhages, subcutaneous nodules at the fingertips, and petechiae. Splinter hemorrhages are small areas of bleeding or hemorrhage under fingernails or toenails and may represent vessel damage from inflammation of the blood vessels or microscopic clots. Petechiae are tiny red spots on the skin.

Street Secrets

For patients who are chronically bedridden, edema will most likely not develop in the legs and feet. Instead, these patients should have their posterior surfaces, particularly the sacral area, inspected for evidence of edema. DOT 5-2.93

Pulses

Assess the carotid and radial pulses, and compare them for intensity and equality. Note if pulse deficit, pulsus paradoxus, or pulsus alternans is present as these all indicate there is a problem.

Pulse deficit is a notable difference between the apical and peripheral pulse rates. The apical pulse is the rate captured while listening with a stethoscope to the "lub-dub" sound of the heart beating as the valves close. Peripheral pulses are assessed by palpation of the extremities. Pulse deficit occurs when heartbeats are not conducted to the peripheral artery, potentially signifying a dysrhythmia or perfusion problem. DOT 5-2.24, 5-2.100

Pulsus paradoxus refers to a 10 mmHg or greater drop in the systolic blood pressure that occurs during inspiration. It is classically noted in cardiac tamponade, constrictive pericarditis, and restrictive cardiomyopathy. Pulsus paradoxus is explained further in the description of cardiac tamponade. DOT 5-2.24, 5-2.100

Pulsus alternans describes a pulse intensity that alternates between weak and strong. The changing intensity of the pulse indicates that the ventricle is alternating between stronger and weaker contraction forces. These pulses generally differ by at least 20 mmHg and signify severely depressed cardiac function. DOT 5-2.24, 5-2.100

Auscultation

Heart tones can be difficult to auscultate in the prehospital environment; however, proper assessment may provide clues to certain heart problems. The best way to develop the ability to discern normal and abnormal heart tones is to listen to these sounds often and in all patients, whether they have a cardiac complaint or not.

Normal heart sounds are single, distinct sounds. The names S_1 and S_2 are given to the normal first and second heart sounds, respectively, and are used as the guideposts for the heart exam (Figure 29-110). S_1 is produced by closure of the mitral and tricuspid valves, which are the AV valves, and marks the beginning of ventricular systole. These valves are located between the atria and ventricles. S_2 is produced by closure of the aortic and pulmonic valves, which are located between the ventricles and the vessels found immediately after the ventricles: the aorta and pulmonary artery. The S_2 sound marks the beginning of ventricular diastole and can be split into the aortic and pulmonic components. Additional sounds, like S_3, S_4, murmurs, or other sounds represent abnormal findings. DOT 5-2.26

Abnormal Heart Sounds

Early systolic sounds are most commonly ejection "clicks" and may represent a calcified (sclerotic) or

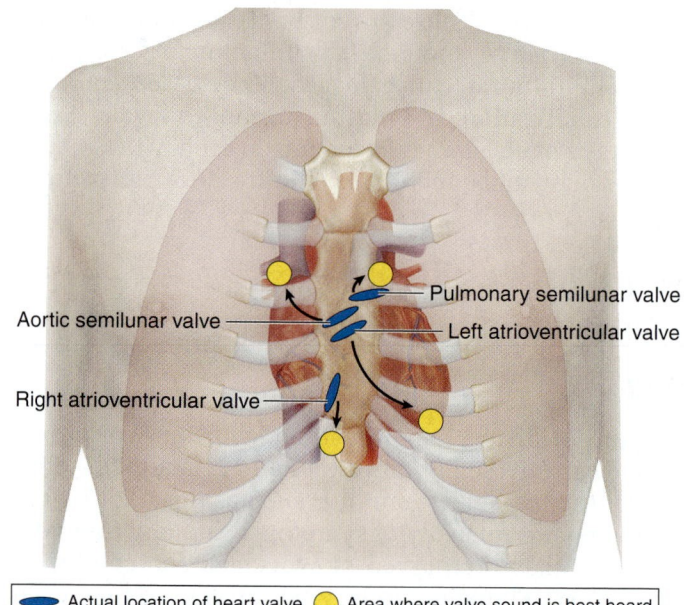

Aortic semilunar valve

Pulmonary semilunar valve

Left atrioventricular valve

Right atrioventricular valve

━━ Actual location of heart valve   ◯ Area where valve sound is best heard

Figure 29-110   Guideposts for the heart examination.

prosthetic aortic valve. Midsystolic sounds are most commonly the "click" from mitral valve prolapse. The best-known early diastolic sound is the opening snap heard in rheumatic mitral stenosis, which produces the S_3 sound. S_3 sounds are produced by stiffening and distension of ventricular walls and are often heard with congestive heart failure. Late diastolic sounds are almost always S_4 sounds and are produced by blood hitting a stiffened ventricular wall. S_4 sounds are often heard in patients with hypertension and ischemic heart disease. DOT 5-2.27, 5-2.28

A **pericardial friction rub** is a scratchy sound that can be heard at any point within the cardiac cycle. It is heard as the exterior surface of the heart rubs against the inner lining of the pericardium as the heart moves within the chest as it beats. It indicates the presence of inflammation from fluid, blood, pus, or other substances. As the layers move over each other, friction produces the sound that is heard during auscultation. It may also produce discomfort or pain. It is best heard with the patient upright and leaning forward, and may be exaggerated with inspiration.

Murmurs

Murmurs are sounds produced by turbulent blood flow within the heart and vessels. They are described by their timing within the cardiac cycle, intensity, pitch, shape (or configuration), quality, duration, and direction of radiation. It is not within the scope of your paramedic practice to name the various types of murmurs. As previously discussed, hearing murmurs and most abnormal heart sounds is a skill that takes practice to acquire. It is important for you to listen to heart sounds often, even when the complaint is not cardiac in nature. Over time, you will begin to appreciate what normal sounds like and will be able to quickly identify "abnormal," even if you do not actually name the murmur you hear.

Chief Complaint: Chest Pain

One of the most frequent calls to emergency medical personnel is for chest pain. The history and physical examination are key elements in sifting through the multitude of chest pain etiologies. Chest pain can be caused by myocardial ischemia (angina) or infarction (heart attack) (Box 29-17). Clearly, not all chest pain is due to cardiac problems. In fact, chest pain as a complaint carries one of the largest differential diagnosis lists in all of medicine. Atypical symptoms or unusual presentations of pain are more common in diabetics, women, and elderly patients. DOT 5-2.29, 5-2.159, 5-2.160, 5-2.161, 5-2.162

It is often easiest to think of the possible causes of chest pain in a system-based manner, with the most

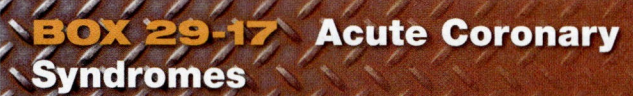

BOX 29-17 Acute Coronary Syndromes

Acute myocardial infarction (AMI) and **unstable angina (UA)** are part of a spectrum of disease identified as **acute coronary syndrome (ACS)**. Stable angina can become UA, which can lead to an AMI. The cause of each of these diseases is a ruptured or eroded arthrosclerotic plaque in one or more of the coronary arteries. ACS is the most common cause of sudden cardiac death.

common systems affected being cardiac, pulmonary, vascular, gastrointestinal, musculoskeletal, and psychological. Other systems almost never lead to chest pain. A brief discussion of the differential diagnosis of chest pain will be presented here, and more detailed presentation of the specific etiologies of chest pain follows later in this chapter. DOT 5-2.68

Each of the systems and syndromes are included in Table 29-1, with typical clinical descriptions and some important distinguishing features. **Skill Sheet 34: Chest Pain Assessment provides a format for obtaining a history of chest pain.** DOT 5-2.149, 5-2.150

Table 29-1 covers the basics of chest pain etiologies. In the real world, patients may have more than one of these disorders, and their symptoms are seldom "classic" in appearance. Therefore, the paramedic must have all the disorders in mind when evaluating patients with chest pain. Also, an understanding of the life-threatening potential is important. The most life-threatening of the disorders in Table 29-1 are acute myocardial infarction, aortic dissection, and pulmonary embolism (PE). Others certainly have life-threatening potential, including peptic ulcer disease (if ruptured ulcer or severe bleeding), pneumothorax, or esophageal rupture. However, the initial work-up and concern should be aimed at ruling out MI, PE, and aortic dissection. DOT 5-2.82

Life-Threatening Causes of Chest Pain

- Heart attack (acute myocardial infarction)
- Pulmonary embolism
- Aortic dissection

The paramedic needs to be adept at distinguishing characteristics of these disorders. This is done by using clinical judgment and evaluating the patient for the risk factors previously described as well as current signs and symptoms.

TABLE 29-1 Causes of Chest Pain and Typical Features DOT 5-2.68

System	Diagnosis	Clinical Features	Distinguishing Features
Cardiac	Angina	Retrosternal chest pain, pressure, burning, heaviness; can radiate to jaw, neck, epigastrum, shoulders, or arms	Worse with exertion, distress, cold; often lasts 2–10 minutes and relieved by rest
	Unstable angina	Similar to angina symptoms	Any change to typical angina pattern, new angina, angina at rest, or "accelerated" angina
	Acute myocardial infarction	Same as angina; may be more severe, longer lasting	More likely to be sudden onset, lasting more than 30 minutes, and more likely to be associated with shortness of breath, nausea, and vomiting
Vascular	Pericarditis	Sharp, pleuritic chest pain (worse with breathing), worse with position changes or swallowing, better with leaning forward, variable duration	Exam reveals a loud "rub"—a constant sound heard throughout the cardiac cycle
	Aortic dissection	"Ripping," excruciating pain that typically starts suddenly and anteriorly but radiates to the back	Severe pain, usually in the setting of hypertension or a patient with known connective tissue disorder such as Marfan's syndrome
	Pulmonary embolism (PE)	Sudden onset of pain and shortness of breath; typically pleuritic pain	Risks include history of clotting disorder, inactivity (long car/plane ride); typically patients have tachycardia, shortness of breath, rapid breathing, and signs of right heart failure (elevated neck veins, peripheral edema); common cause of sudden hemodynamic collapse
Pulmonary	Pneumonia	Less commonly painful, but is generally a pleuritic type pain	Usually pain lateralizes to the side of pneumonia if present; often with cough, producing sputum, fevers, chills
	Pneumothorax	Sudden onset of unilateral pain and shortness of breath	Abrupt onset, patients may have a history of pneumothorax or chest tube; often thin people or women during menses (*catamenial* pneumothorax)
Gastrointestinal	Esophageal reflux	Burning pain, often epigastric but can be as high as into throat	Typically worse after meals, especially if large and fatty meal; relieved by antacid
	Esophageal spasm	Similar to reflux but more periodic and severe	May be relieved by nitroglycerin
	Peptic ulcer disease	Prolonged burning, epigastric pain	Often improved with antacids; patients may have a history of ulcers or be on acid blocker

TABLE 29-1   *(Continued)*

System	Diagnosis	Clinical Features	Distinguishing Features
Gastrointestinal	Gallbladder disease	Epigastric pain, usually persistent and localized to the right upper quadrant of abdomen, sometimes radiates to the right shoulder	Also often associated with meals; typically patients are obese and younger (30–40); female more common Remember the "4Fs": Fat, Female, Forty, Fertile (usually several children)
	Pancreatitis	Epigastric or back pain	Alcohol and gallstone disease are biggest risks
Musculoskeletal	Costochondritis	Often a sharp pain	Reproducible with pressure on affected joint, worse with arm movements
Psychological	Panic disorder or anxiety	Chest tightness, aching, short of breath, tingling or numbness of extremities. Usually no association with movement or exertion	May have history of anxiety or evidence of emotional disorder
Infectious	Herpes zoster (shingles)	Prolonged burning pain in dermatomal distribution	May not yet have characteristic vesicular rash

Source: Adapted from D. P. Zipes, P. Libby, R. O. Bonow, and E. Braunwald, *Braunwald's Heart Disease: A Textbook of Cardiovascular Medicine,* 7th ed., Vol. 2, 2004 (Philadelphia, PA: Elsevier Saunders) p. 1130.

Assessing and Treating Acute Coronary Syndromes

Describing the pain is an essential first step. The quality of the pain can be helpful although myocardial ischemia is rarely described as "pain." Ischemic pain is more typically described as pressure, tightness, constriction, burning, or a squeezing band-like sensation of compression around the chest. The pain location is less helpful as ischemic pain is usually felt diffusely throughout the chest. Patients with cardiac ischemia or infarction may demonstrate a clenched fist over their chest when asked to describe what they are feeling. This classic gesture is called the **Levine sign.** However, a pain localized to a very small area of the chest is more likely to be musculoskeletal in nature. DOT 5-2.163, 5-2.164, 5.2-165

CONNECTIONS Use the OPQRST mnemonic to ask about cardiac pain. This tool, which is found in Chapters 11 and 14, covers the full spectrum of issues related to cardiac pain and will help focus history taking.

Reproducible pain is pain that can be caused following a stimulus such as pressing and releasing the chest wall. Reproducible pain, which was once thought to be noncardiac in origin, has been shown to occasionally be cardiac. The pain of myocardial ischemia can radiate into the neck, jaw, teeth, arm, or shoulder. Although classical myocardial ischemia pain is described

Nice to Know

Acute cholecystitis (inflammation or infection of the gallbladder) can also present with pain in the right shoulder, but this is more commonly associated with epigastric or right upper quadrant pain. Additionally, pain that radiates to the back may be due to aortic dissection.

as radiating to the left arm, radiation to the right arm or both arms has been shown to be a strong predictor of myocardial ischemia as well.[7,8] DOT 5-2.163, 5-2.164, 5.2-165

The trajectory of the pain is also an important factor. Pain having an abrupt onset, with greatest intensity of pain initially, is typically associated with pneumothorax, pulmonary embolism, or aortic dissection. In contrast, the pain of myocardial ischemia is often gradual with increasing intensity over time. This type of pain is also associated with esophageal disorders. The duration of the pain is helpful in that ischemic myocardial pain generally lasts at least several minutes while musculoskeletal pain may have been going on for hours or days.

Provoking factors can also be helpful in differentiating the types of chest pain. Pain provoked with eating or swallowing tends to correlate with esophageal disease. Pain worsening with exertion highly suggests cardiac origin. In addition, pain that is worsened by respiration or lying down is highly suggestive of pleuritic chest pain, the causes of which include pulmonary embolism, pneumonia, and pneumothorax. Alleviating factors can also be helpful. Pain reliably relieved by antacids is likely gastroesophageal in origin although occasionally patients with ACS have reported improvement of their cardiac symptoms with antacids. Pain that is **palliated** (relieved) with rest is suggestive of a cardiac cause. Although nitroglycerin relieves myocardial ischemia pain, it can also relieve esophageal pain.

Symptoms associated with chest pain can also help determine the origin of the chest pain. Pain associated with belching, difficulty swallowing, or a bad taste in the mouth is likely to be gastroesophageal in origin. Dyspnea, palpitations, and diaphoresis are more likely to be associated with myocardial ischemia. Chest pain associated with cough or fever is commonly seen with pneumonia. A patient presenting with syncope and chest pain should be carefully monitored for a catastrophic event such as a ruptured aortic aneurysm, acute aortic dissection, or a large pulmonary embolus.

Assessing the patient's past medical history and risk factors for cardiac disease can aid in determining the cause of the pain. Risk factors for coronary artery disease, including previous myocardial infarctions, should be elicited. The patient's medical history may also provide clues to the cause of the pain, particularly if the patient's symptoms closely resemble a previous event.

The physical examination provides an assessment for severity. The patient's general appearance suggests the severity and possibly the seriousness of the symptoms. An attempt should be made to establish a baseline of the severity of pain using a zero-to-ten scale, with zero being pain free and ten the worst pain the patient can imagine. By itself, it may be an indication of the patient's level of anxiety or fears, but a comparison of pain level after treatment could indicate effectiveness of the treatment.

A full set of vital signs can provide valuable clues to the clinical significance of the pain and may in some cases aid in establishing its origin. For example, a marked difference in blood pressure between the two arms suggests the possibility of an aortic dissection. Physical examination should include palpation of the chest wall to assess for tenderness and auscultation of the heart and lungs. In addition, the abdomen should be palpated to assess for tenderness, paying particular attention to the right upper quadrant, epigastrium, and the abdominal aorta. DOT 5-2.142

A 12-lead electrocardiogram (ECG) should be obtained on every patient with suspected cardiac symptoms.

As discussed in the previous section, the absence of findings such as ST elevation, ST depression, and reciprocal changes does not rule out a possible cardiac event, but the presence of these findings is strongly suggestive of one.

The 12-lead ECG can expedite treatment by allowing you to alert the receiving hospital of an incoming cardiac event. This can reduce the time it takes to initiate therapy in the hospital. Remember, when the history sounds like a cardiac process, a normal electrocardiogram should not divert the course of therapy. DOT 5-2.47

Normal Cardiac Physiology

To briefly review normal cardiac physiology: The heart provides sufficient blood flow to the body in its normal state. This process is dependent on three principles: **preload, afterload,** and **contractility.** You will recall these principles from Section I of this chapter. The various cardiovascular diseases and their treatments are related to each of these in different ways.

The Three Pillars of Cardiac Function
- Preload
- Afterload
- Contractility

Preload is how tightly stretched the ventricular myocardium is just prior to contraction and is measured by the ventricular pressure just before each heart contraction. It is assessed by left ventricular end-diastolic pressure, or LVEDP, and measured in the hospital using a direct left ventricle (LV) catheter in the cardiac catheterization lab or by Swan-Ganz balloon catheter wedged in the smaller pulmonary arteries. How preload affects cardiac function is analogous to a balloon blown up with two breaths and then released. It exhausts the air out with low pressure, making minimal noise. If the same balloon is blown up with 10 breaths and then released, air is expelled with much greater pressure. Cardiac ventricular distention just prior to contraction (end-diastolic volume) is directly correlated to the volume of blood ejected with systole (stroke volume). This is known as the **Frank-Starling relationship** (Figure 29-111). DOT 5-2.18

As ventricular end-diastolic volume increases, its pressure also increases. As end-diastolic volume and pressure increase (i.e., preload) within normal physiologic ranges, stroke volume also increases. After a certain limit, myocardial contractile elements are stretched too far, they generate less contractile force, and the once beneficial mechanism of more stretch yielding stronger contractions becomes compromised (see Figure 29-112). The Frank-Starling curve flattens at this point, and additional preload leads to worsening pulmonary and venous congestion.

Afterload is the pressure against which the ventricle must pump. Afterload is clinically measured as systolic blood pressure. This is an indirect measure of the pressure inside the left ventricle when the aortic valve is open and blood is ejected, barring any obstruction between the

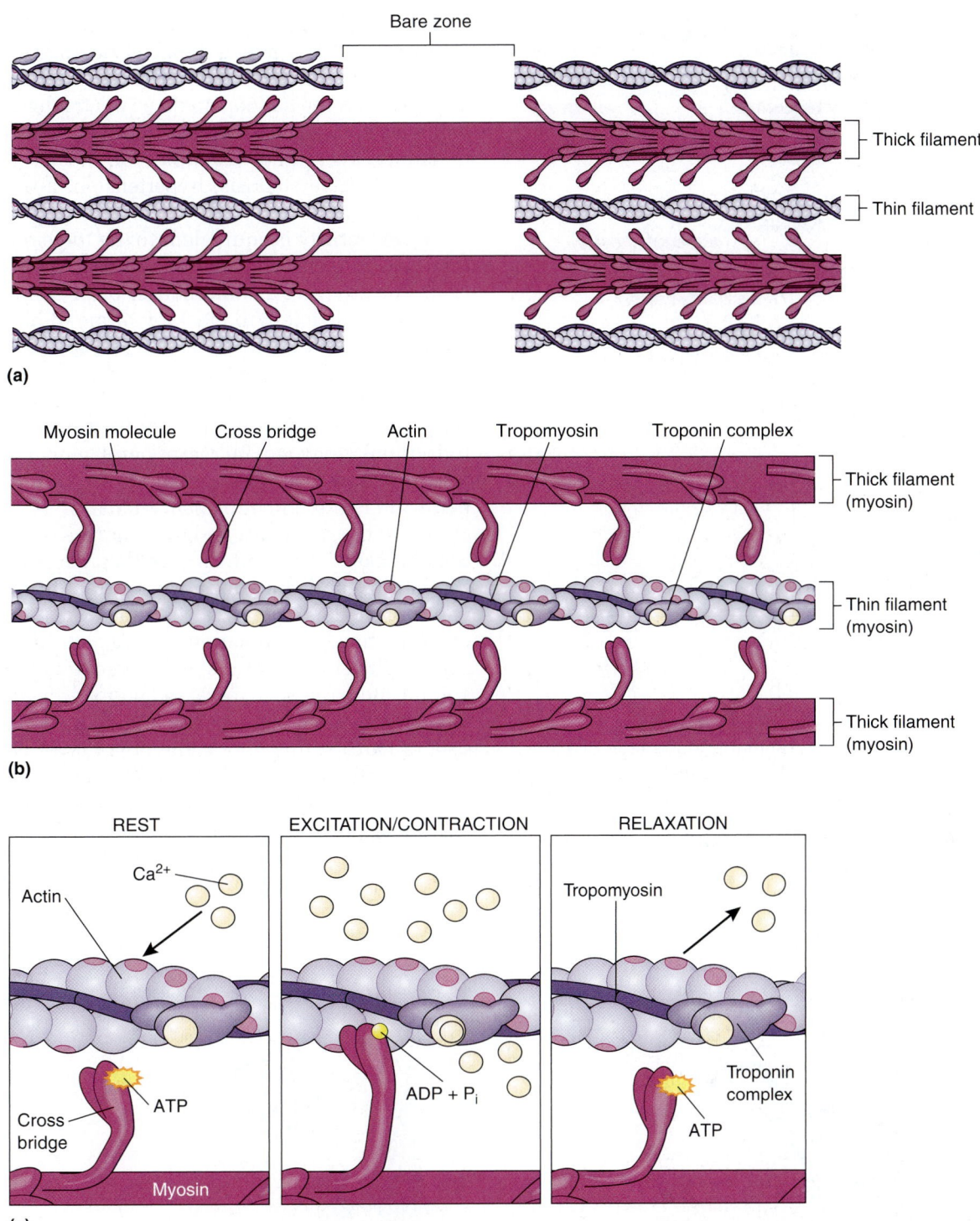

Figure 29-111   (a) Longitudinal section of filaments within one sarcomere of a myofibril. The further the fibers stretch, the more actin-myosin cross bridges can be made and the greater the force of the contraction. (b and c) Excitation-contraction coupling and the interaction between actin and myosin. Depolarization of the muscle cell membrane allows entry of calcium into the cell and release of calcium stored in the sarcoplasmic reticulum. (b) The structure of the actin-myosin complex. (c) Calcium binds troponin, allowing interaction between actin and myosin.

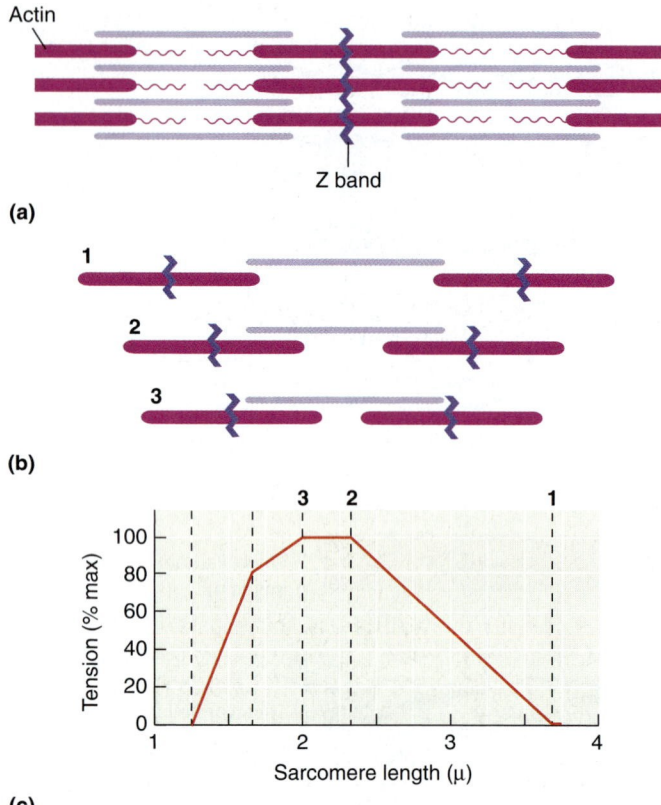

Actin

Z band

(a)

1

2

3

(b)

100
80
60
40
20
0

3 2   1

Tension (% max)

1   2   3   4

Sarcomere length (μ)

(c)

Figure 29-112 The relationship between myocardial sarcomere length and tension. (a) In this illustration of a sarcomere, the thin filaments (actin) are attached at the Z band. (b) Point 1 shows extreme sarcomere stretch with zero tension development. Points 2 and 3 show maximum actin-myosin overlap with maximal tension. (c) Graph of points 1, 2, and 3 from (b).

ventricle and the artery from which blood pressure is being measured. The greater the afterload, the more pressure the ventricle must produce to empty its volume, or in keeping with the balloon analogy, the tighter the inflated balloon's neck, the more pressure it takes for the balloon to empty over time. Examples of increased afterload are aortic valve stenosis, hypertension, and peripheral vasoconstriction.

Contractility is equivalent to the force each **cardiac myocyte** (muscle cell) generates during systolic contraction. For any given combination of preload and afterload, the ventricle will eject a volume of blood **(stroke volume).** Individual myoctes can increase their contraction force independent of preload and afterload, depending on the concentration of calcium within them. As calcium is increased, the contraction force from an individual myocyte increases, and global contractile force increases with increased stroke volume. Norepinephrine is a medication that increases calcium availability to the myocytes and thus increases contractility. Beta-blockers are medications that decrease calcium availability and thus decrease contractility and stroke volume, weakening cardiac contraction.

Any fixed combination of preload, afterload, and contractility results in a specific stroke volume. Stroke volume increases with increased preload, decreased afterload, or increased contractility (Figure 29-113). The measure of cardiac function at the organ level is not based solely on stroke volume but instead on cardiac output.

Cardiac output is stroke volume multiplied by heart rate (HR × SV) and is thus the number of liters per minute of blood a heart pumps.

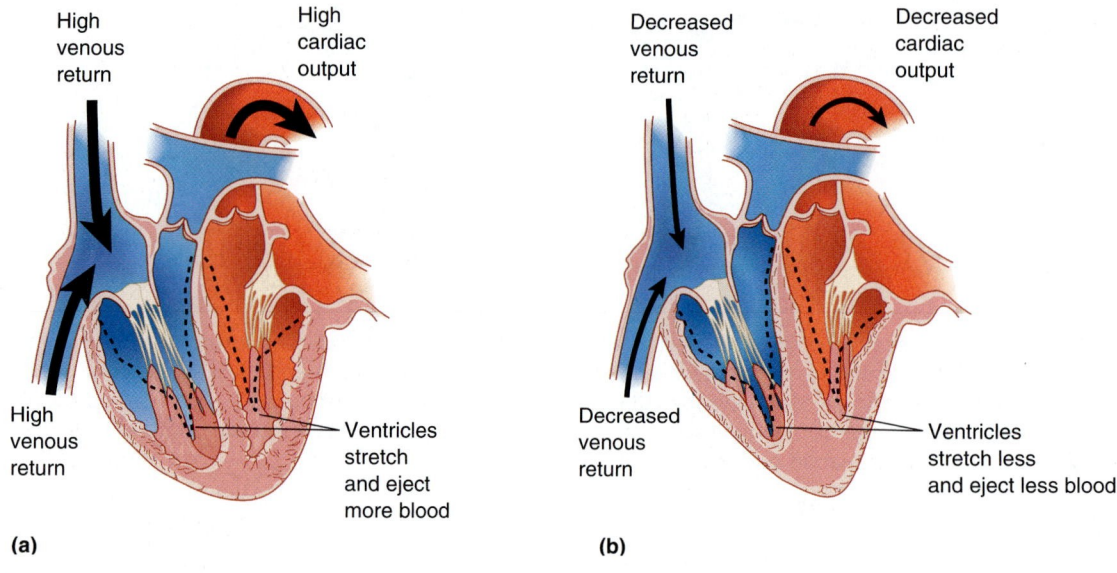

High venous return

High cardiac output

High venous return

Ventricles stretch and eject more blood

(a)

Decreased venous return

Decreased cardiac output

Decreased venous return

Ventricles stretch less and eject less blood

(b)

Figure 29-113 The Frank-Starling relationship. Cardiac ventricular distention just prior to contraction (end-diastolic volume) is directly correlated to the volume of blood ejected with systole (stroke volume). (a) Large venous return. (b) Smaller venous return.

At the organ level, a low stroke volume can be accommodated by an increasing heart rate, and vice versa, to meet metabolic demands and explains why heart failure patients have rapid heart rates: It is because of an attempt to increase (or maintain) cardiac output. DOT 5-2.7

Cardiac Ischemia and Infarction

Many episodes of chest pain are not of cardiac origin. However, when chest pain is thought to be cardiac ischemia or infarction, this sets into motion a series of standardized events in an effort to "preserve the myocardium."

The American Heart Association algorithm for managing patients with an acute coronary syndrome recommends the use of the following medications to treat an acute coronary syndrome (Figure 29-114). They can be summarized by the acronym MONA:

MONA

M morphine

O oxygen

N nitroglycerin

A aspirin

This acronym is meant to be a memory aid only; it is not meant to imply the order of administration of these drugs. The order for administration will be discussed further. DOT 5-2.84

Myocardial Ischemia

Angina pectoris is a chest discomfort caused by myocardial ischemia, where coronary artery plaque restricts blood flow and needed oxygen into the heart during activity. As previously mentioned, more than 7 million Americans experience angina regularly. From a pathophysiologic perspective, angina is caused either by increased myocardial oxygen needs or by decreased oxygen supply. DOT 5-2.65, 5-2.66

Stable angina is brought on with exertional activity, and is similar to previous episodes of cardiac-related chest pain. Often, patients will report having a diagnosis of CAD, and they may have a prescription for nitroglycerin or take aspirin or other cardiac, antilipid, or HTN drugs. Their reported episodes of angina should be fairly similar in character and duration. It is important to evaluate patients with a history of stable angina to determine whether or not the character of the current episode is different from prior episodes as this could indicate a transition into unstable angina.

Unstable angina is accelerated angina, meaning angina that is either new, occurring at rest, changing from its previous state (pain lasts longer, is more severe, comes on with less exertion, new location, etc.), or is more frequent.

Typical patient descriptions of cardiac-related chest pain include comments like "an elephant is sitting on my chest," "vice-like," "a belt around my chest," or "pressure." It may have unusual presentations such as a heartburn sensation or neck, jaw, shoulder or arm pain. It is rarely sharp. It lasts minutes to hours (it is not fleeting) and usually disappears after physical activity is ceased. In other patients, the quality of the sensation is vague and is described as a "mild pressure-like discomfort," an "uncomfortable numb sensation," or a "burning sensation." The site of the discomfort is usually retrosternal (behind the sternum), but radiation to other locations is common and usually occurs down the ulnar surface of the left arm; the right arm and the outer surfaces of both arms may also be involved (Figure 29-115). Epigastric discomfort alone or in association with chest pressure is not uncommon. Anginal discomfort above the mandible or below the epigastrium is rare, leading some medical facilities to adopt a protocol that any pain between the epigastrum and sternal notch is considered to be cardiac until proven otherwise.

Coronary ischemia can produce other symptoms either with or without myocardial ischemia. These include dyspnea, faintness, fatigue, and nausea, all of which are more common in the elderly. Importantly, diabetic patients may be less likely to feel chest pain with coronary ischemia.

Another form of angina pain is called **variant** or **angiospastic angina.** Angiospastic angina is capable of producing symptoms identical to unstable angina but is related to a spasm of a coronary artery rather than blockage. Typically, the spasm will occur at rest as in **Prinzmetal's variant angina** but may also be triggered by exertion or periods of high stress. During an attack, ST segment elevation may be evident on the ECG, and the symptoms will respond to the administration of nitroglycerin. The ST segment changes will resolve once the vasospasm subsides and oxygenation is restored. Variant anginal attacks may appear in clusters over a short period of time or may subside for weeks or months. DOT 5-2.69

The typical anginal episode begins gradually and reaches its maximum intensity over a period of minutes before resolving. It is unusual for angina pectoris to reach its maximum severity within seconds, and patients with angina usually prefer to rest, sit, or stop walking during episodes.

Symptoms that are less likely to be anginal include pleuritic pain (respiratory variation of pain), pain localized to the tip of one finger, pain reproduced by movement or palpation of the chest wall or arms, and constant pain lasting many hours or, alternatively, very brief episodes of pain only lasting seconds. Pain radiating into the lower extremities is also a highly unusual manifestation of angina pectoris.

Acute Coronary Syndromes Algorithm

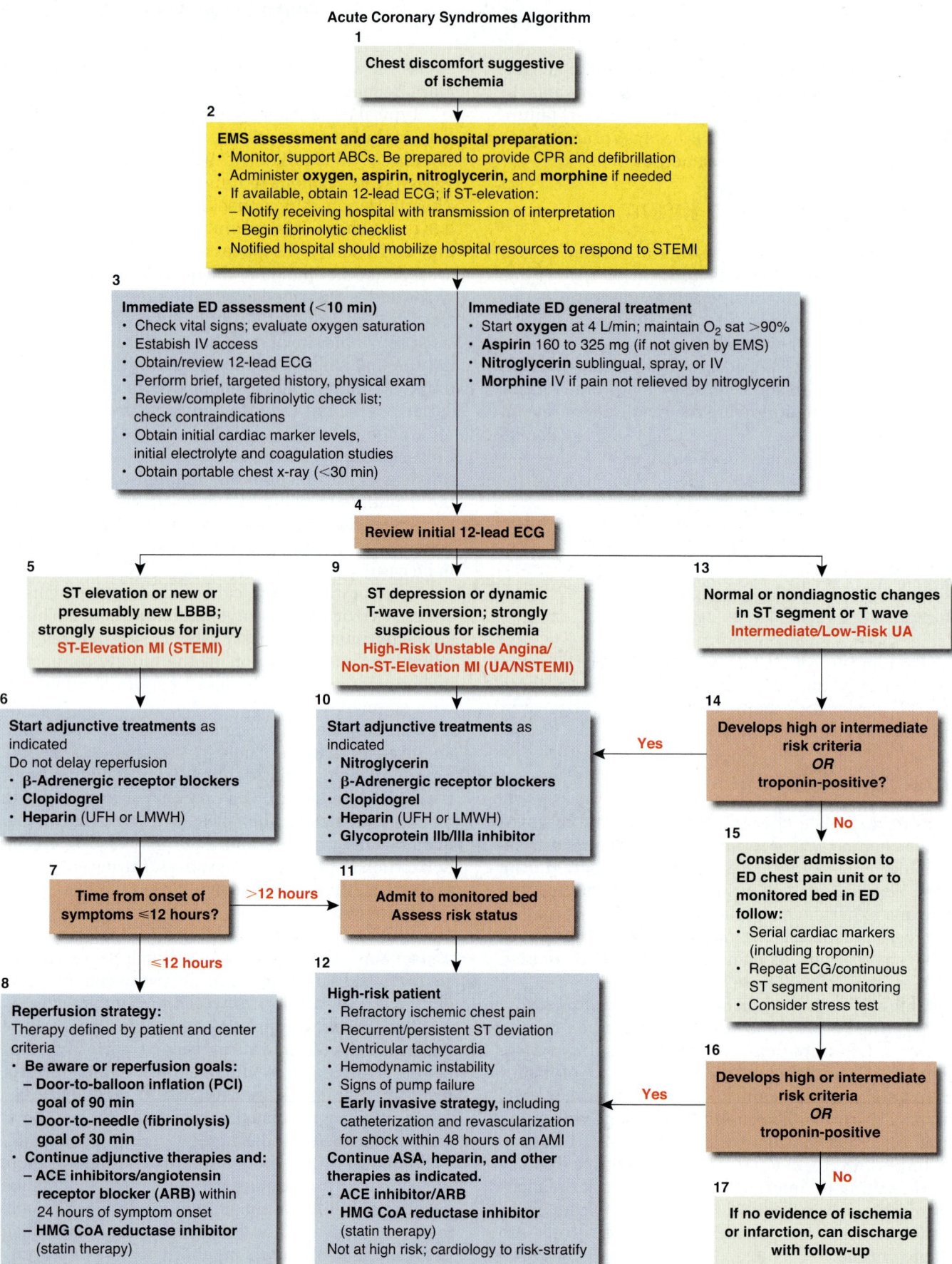

Figure 29-114 AHA algorithm for the treatment of acute coronary syndrome. Reproduced with permission 2005 American Heart Association *Guidelines for Cardiopulmonary Resuscitation and Emergency Cardiovascular Care* © 2005, American Heart Association.

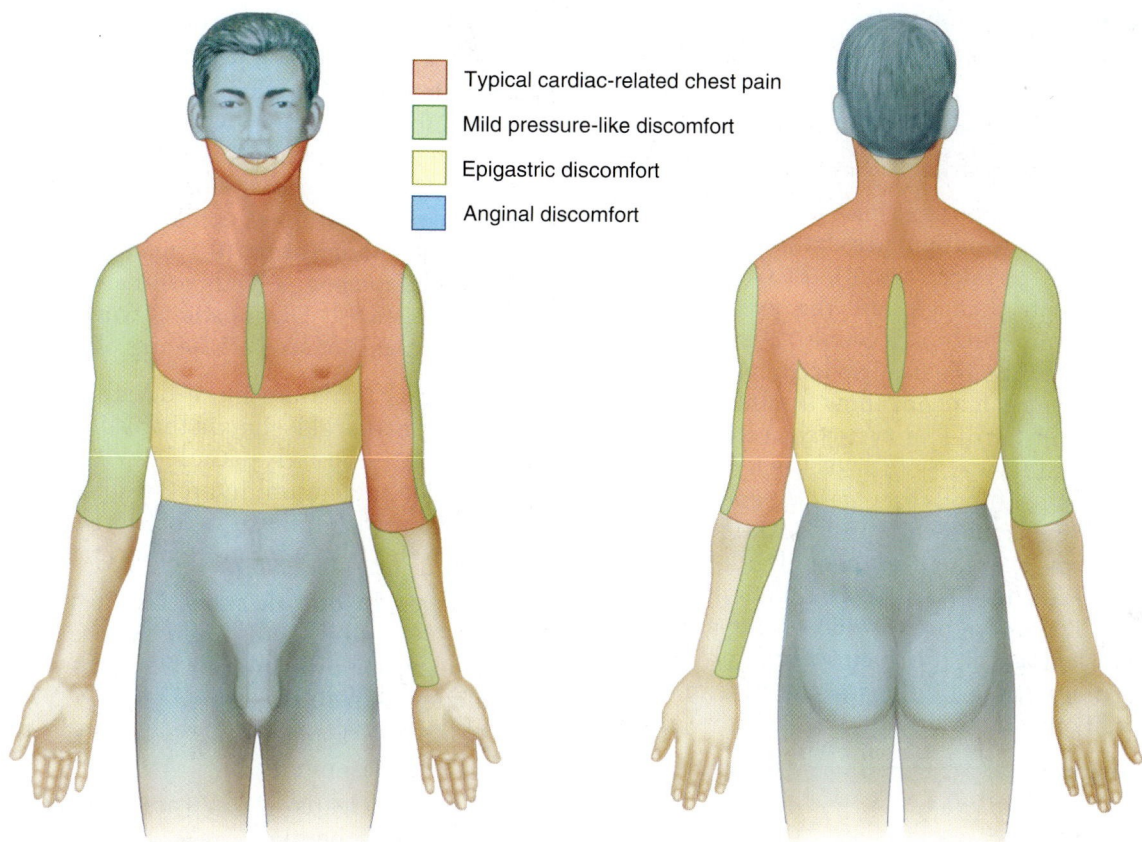

Figure 29-115   Cardiac-related chest pain and referred pain.

Typical angina pectoris is relieved within minutes by rest or by the use of nitroglycerin. The response to the latter is a useful diagnostic tool, but as previously mentioned, other noncardiac syndromes such as esophageal spasm and pain may also respond to nitroglycerin. A delay of more than five to ten minutes before relief is obtained by rest and nitroglycerin suggests that the symptoms are either not due to ischemia or, alternatively, are due to severe ischemia as with acute myocardial infarction or unstable angina.[9] DOT 5-2.77

The ECG is a valuable tool for distinguishing acute myocardial infarction from angina. The ECG will show characteristic changes during the acute myocardial infarction that would not be present in typical angina. These will be discussed further when AMI is discussed.

Chest Pain Characteristics Consistent with Angina (Coronary Artery Disease)

- Related to exertion
- "Pressure" or "vice-like;" rarely sharp
- Associated with nausea, sweating, or shortness of breath
- Radiates to either arm, the neck, or jaw

A good history is the most important and useful way to diagnose angina. The history in the paramedic setting may be brief by necessity but is nonetheless vital to guide what management steps will follow. The OPQRST mnemonic is essential to remember when taking a history. Answers to these questions alone will often provide a sufficient history to trigger a decision to treat for a possible cardiac event.

Acute Myocardial Infarction (AMI)

Chest pain unrelieved by rest, oxygen, or nitroglycerin and lasting longer than a few minutes must be assumed to be an acute myocardial infarction until proven otherwise. Symptoms may be similar to anginal pain but often persist regardless of treatment. Be suspicious of any changes in anginal history such as increased level of pain and duration, accompanied with shortness of breath or anything that would indicate the progression of angina from stable to unstable.

The clinical diagnosis of AMI requires an integrated assessment of the history with some combination of evidence of myocardial necrosis using biochemical, electrocardiographic, and imaging modalities (Box 29-18). Each of these will be discussed later in this chapter.

BOX 29-18 The Three Elements of Diagnosing an AMI

The three elements important for a physician diagnosis of an AMI are the **patient presentation** (including history and physical exam), **ECG changes** suggestive of acute damage, and the **presence of cardiac enzymes** in the blood. Some 12-lead ECGs do not change, despite the occurrence of a heart attack. Q wave changes may not show up until weeks after the infarction. Cardiac enzymes can be assessed in the prehospital setting, but this is not a common practice. Also, most blood tests lack the specificity to identify these enzymes early in the AMI process as there may not be enough of them circulating in the blood to result in a positive test. Patients suspected of an AMI in the prehospital setting should be treated based upon the history and physical exam, regardless of the findings of the ECG or the availability of enzyme tests.

There are four major types of acute coronary artery syndromes in which myocardial ischemia leads to different ECG manifestations. DOT 5-2.49, 5-2.50, 5-2.78

The Acute Coronary Syndromes Include the following:

- Classic angina (subendocardial ischemia)
- Unstable angina
- Non-ST elevation myocardial infarction (Non-Q wave MI)
- ST-elevation myocardial infarction (Q wave MI)

- **Subendocardial ischemia** (classic angina) without infarction is manifested by transient ST segment depression.

Remember: ST elevation usually means injury; ST depression is ischemia.

- **Noninfarction transmural ischemia** (Prinzmetal's variant angina, from coronary artery spasm) is manifested by transient ST segment elevations or paradoxical T wave normalization.
- **Non-ST elevation (Non-Q wave) MI** is manifested by ST depressions or T wave inversions without pathologic Q waves. Remember: the circumflex coronary artery is typically 'silent' by ECG criteria.

That is, an infarct due to circumflex artery occlusion may occur without visible surface ECG changes.

- **ST elevation (Q wave) MI** is manifested in most patients by pathologic Q waves that are usually preceded by hyperacute T waves and ST elevation, followed by T wave inversion. Clinically significant ST segment elevation is considered to be present if it is greater than 1 mm (0.1 mV) in at least two contiguous precordial leads or in at least two adjacent limb leads.[10,11] Diagnostic Q waves are wider than 0.04 seconds or are half the size of the QRS complex.

The ECG leads are more helpful in localizing regions of transmural ischemia than subendocardial ischemia.[10,11] Based on early pathologic studies, the anatomic location of a transmural infarct is determined by which ECG lead shows ST elevation or increased T wave positivity. See Box 29-19 for more information.

1. Changes in one or more of the precordial leads (V1–V6) and in leads I and aV$_L$ are consistent with acute transmural anterior wall ischemia, often with lateral extension.
2. Changes in leads V1 to V3 are consistent with anteroseptal ischemia.
3. Changes in leads V4 to V6 are consistent with apical or lateral ischemia.
4. Changes in leads II, III, and aV$_F$ are consistent with inferior wall ischemia.

Medications to Think of in Acute Coronary Syndromes

- Aspirin
- Beta-blocker (usually not prehospital)
- Heparin or other anticoagulant (usually not prehospital)
- Pain medication (morphine)
- Clopidogrel (Plavix) (usually not prehospital)
- Oxygen
- ACE inhibitors and statins in the first 24 hours (usually not prehospital)

It is very important to note that an initially normal ECG does not exclude ischemia or even acute infarction. As a result, if the initial ECG is not diagnostic yet the patient remains symptomatic with high clinical suspicion for AMI, the ECG should be repeated at five to ten minute intervals.[12] Clinical suspicion and intuition are very important in guiding patient care; if the history is classic for AMI or unstable angina but ECG changes are not yet consistent with ST elevation AMI, the patient should be treated aggressively for an acute coronary syndrome.

Patients treated for ACS require medication delivered early, including aspirin, beta-blockers, heparin or other anticoagulant, morphine or other IV pain

BOX 29-19 ECG Lead Tracing with Corresponding Ventricular Wall Views

Lead I lateral wall	Lead aV_R quality control	Lead V1 septal wall	Lead V4 anterior wall
Lead II inferior wall	Lead aV_L lateral wall	Lead V2 septal wall	Lead V5 high lateral wall
Lead III inferior wall	Lead aV_F inferior wall	Lead V3 anterior wall	Lead V6 high lateral wall

medication, oxygen, and more recently recommended medicine such as clopidogrel (Plavix). The decision to use lipid-lowering agents (called statins) and ACE inhibitors is beneficial in ACS and AMI patients but not a priority for paramedics.

Regarding the ECG diagnosis of AMI: Not all ST elevation is from myocardial infarction.

Pericarditis typically induces diffuse ST segment elevation, in contrast to acute myocardial infarction in which the ST segment elevation is localized. With pericarditis, ST elevation occurs in the chest leads and also in leads I, aV_L, II, and aV_F. Reciprocal ST depression is often seen in lead aV_R. An important clue to pericarditis in addition to the diffuse nature of the ST elevation is PR segment elevation in aV_R and PR depression in other leads (usually II, III or aV_F) due to a concomitant energy current flow through the atria. Abnormal Q waves do not occur, and ST elevation is followed by T wave inversion after a variable time period.[13]

Also, ST segment elevation, which occurs in some normal patients, is known as early repolarization. In some healthy subjects, particularly young men (especially African Americans), the ECG shows a normal variant ST segment elevation (an early repolarization pattern is typically seen in the mid to lateral chest leads [V3–V6]). Comparison with an old ECG is ideal, although it is often difficult in the prehospital setting. Clinical suspicion and an overall assessment of the situation remain the best guide for the need for treatment. Figure 29-116 shows an ECG as it transitions through several changes during an AMI. The first two figures show early and late changes in the 12-lead ECG, and the last figure shows a "normal" ECG for comparison.

The Cardiac Enzyme Evolution of ST-Elevation Myocardial Infarction

The biochemical evaluation for myocardial infarction includes assessing for the presence of specific enzymes that are found with cardiac tissue damage. This includes obtaining cardiac troponin levels, occasionally creatine kinase (CK), and specifically creatine kinase—MB isoenzyme (CK-MB) fractions. The CK-MB typically elevates early (about four hours after the event) and lasts 24 to 48 hours. Cardiac troponin, a more specific and sensitive test for AMI, typically rises six to eight hours after the event, and can remain present in the blood for one week although levels usually peak in 24 to 48 hours.

Cardiac enzyme studies may be important tests for which to draw blood, but from a paramedic's perspective, the

Working in the Gray Zone

ST Elevation—To Treat or Not to Treat

Although the text discusses some possible causes of ST elevation that are not from an AMI, it is important to remember to treat all symptoms and signs as they present, including persistent chest discomfort or pain. ST elevation is a possible sign of AMI, so it is appropriate to treat each patient with ST elevation for a possible AMI, observing each treatment for improvement. The hospital will work on obtaining an actual diagnosis of the problem, ruling out whether or not the actual cause is a heart attack or something else.

Nice to Know

Cardiac Enzymes

Cardiac enzymes (cardiac troponin, creatine kinase [CK], and creatine kinase MB isoenzyme [CK-MB]) are chemicals that are released by dying cardiac cells. They circulate in the blood and can be detected by blood studies. Their presence generally indicates damage has occurred and is a reliable indicator for AMI. Currently, there is no technology to allow testing of cardiac enzymes in the prehospital setting.

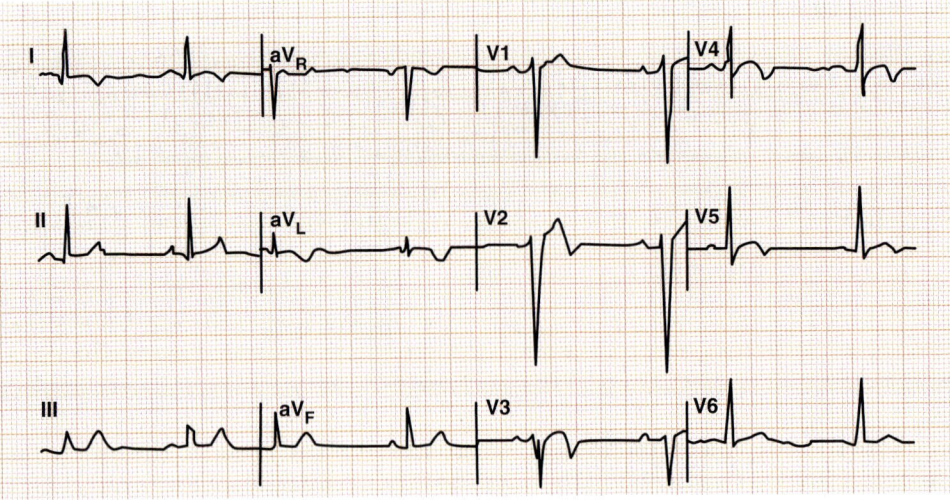

(a)

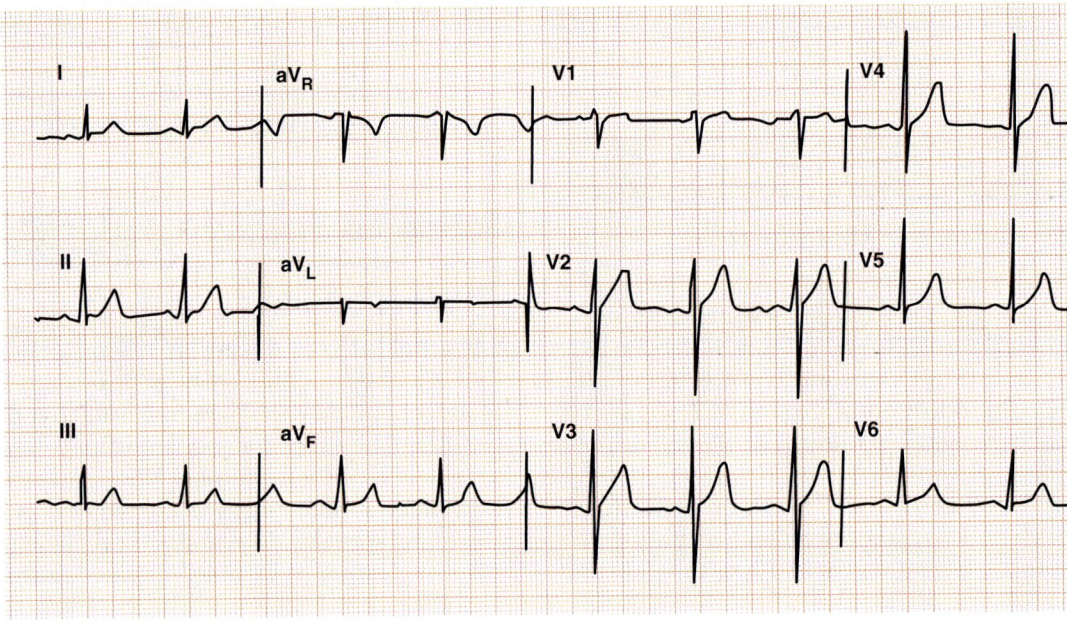

(b)

(c)

Figure 29-116 (a) Evolving anterior myocardial infarction. (b) Late evolution of anterior MI. (c) Normal ECG.

management of an AMI lies in the history, physical exam, and the ECG.

The ECG remains the gold standard for diagnosis of AMI in the first four to six hours after the event. Reeder and Kennedy suggest the four most important goals of early management of ST elevation myocardial infarction are as follows: DOT 5-2.70

1. Confirmation of the diagnosis by electrocardiogram (ECG) and laboratory tests.
2. Relief of ischemic pain.
3. Assessment of the hemodynamic state and correction of abnormalities that are present.
4. Initiation of reperfusion therapy (discussed in next section).[14]

Acute chest trauma can lead to cardiac contusion and direct physical cardiac muscle injury. Trauma is an unlikely cause of myocardial infarction although a ventricular wall rupture may occur. Also, biochemical markers can be elevated in chest trauma patients if the heart tissue has been injured by contusion or rupture. DOT 5-2.73

Complications and Hemodynamic Changes Associated with Myocardial Infarction

Mortality from myocardial infarction has steadily declined since the 1950s with the advent of different treatment modalities including medications (beta-blockers, aspirin), reperfusion strategies (thrombolytics and percutaneous coronary intervention, PCI), and better diagnostic tools. However, the most recent publications about ST elevation myocardial infarction still report mortality rates in the 5–10% range at one month following the event. The cause of death is most often a complication of the myocardial infarction such as cardiogenic shock or ventricular failure, rather than the initial event itself. DOT 5-2.71, 5-2.72, 5-2.76, 5-2.79

As with any critically ill patient, the initial assessment and workup should include an assessment of the ABCs. The history, electrocardiogram, and other diagnostic steps must take a back seat to airway protection and preserving breathing and circulation. Careful hemodynamic monitoring of the patient with suspected ACS is vital. DOT 5-4.75

The primary hemodynamic complications during acute myocardial infarction include hypotension, poor perfusion, pulmonary edema, and cardiogenic shock, all from myocardial stunning or necrosis and sometimes from dysrhythmia. Each of these bears further discussion. DOT 5-2.74

Myocardial Stunning

Myocardial stunning is not well-defined from an epidemiological perspective but clearly occurs in many patients with acute myocardial infarction, even after reperfusion therapy. It frequently results in postischemic contractile dysfunction, where cardiac myocytes (muscle cells) that are not technically dead are unable to contract normally. Stunning plays a major role in the development of acute pulmonary edema following an AMI.

Acute Pulmonary Edema (APE)

This syndrome is also known as **flash pulmonary edema.** It can be caused by other problems aside from myocardial infarction, and not all pulmonary edema is due to myocardial infarction or ischemia. However, AMI must be the primary consideration in any patient presenting with APE (with or without chest pain or "classic" symptoms). Pulmonary edema is discussed in detail in Chapter 28: Pulmonary.

Cardiogenic Shock

A severe and deadly complication of AMI is shock due to low cardiac output. **Cardiogenic shock** is defined as inadequate tissue perfusion due to cardiac dysfunction. Two large clinical trials (the GUSTO-I and SHOCK trials) showed this complication occurs within the first 24 hours and often after hospital admission (5.3% of patients). In the SHOCK trial, the median time from AMI to onset of cardiogenic shock was 5.5 hours, and 75% of the patients who developed cardiogenic shock did so within 24 hours.[15,16] DOT 5-2.112

Cardiogenic shock is accompanied by pulmonary edema more than two-thirds of the time. Management consists of fluid resuscitation, vasopressor support, airway management, and mechanical devices including an intra-aortic balloon pump. Hypotension is a frequent manifestation of right ventricular infarction, which can produce cardiogenic shock despite a normal left ventricle. In this syndrome, the left ventricle cannot fill adequately and thus cannot produce adequate blood pressure. A more thorough examination of cardiogenic shock can be found later in the chapter. DOT 5-2.113

Dysrhythmias

The most lethal acute complication of AMI is **cardiac dysrhythmia.**

Both atrial and ventricular dysrhythmias can occur during and after the initial phase of an acute AMI. These include atrial fibrillation or flutter, which can cause symptomatic hypotension or hypoperfusion due to rapid heart rate, and life-threatening ventricular tachycardia (VT) or ventricular fibrillation (VF). Atrial fibrillation and flutter are also the leading cause of strokes. DOT 5-2.124

The most data on MI-related VT and VF comes from the GUSTO-I trial. This study included nearly 41,000 patients, and found the incidence of VT or VF was 10.2%: 3.5% developed VT, 4.1% VF, and 2.7% both VT and VF. Approximately 80–85% of these dysrhythmias occurred in the first 48 hours.[16] Prophylactic measures against these dysrhythmias include early administration of an intravenous beta-blocker and treatment of hypokalemia and hypomagnesemia, if present. Once VF or VT occurs, the treatment is defibrillation or cardioversion as per AHA ACLS guidelines. VF remains the most common cause of sudden cardiac death. DOT 5-2.37, 5-2.48, 5-2.54

Treatment Goals and Options in Acute Myocardial Infarction

The goal for acute AMI therapy is to prevent early complications and provide definitive treatment as rapidly as possible. "Time is muscle" is a commonly used phrase in the cardiology community, indicating that the sooner an occluded artery is opened, the faster blood and oxygen will be provided, the more heart muscle will be saved, and thus the patient prognosis will be better. DOT 5-2.51, 5-2.52, 5-2.53

As recently as 15 years ago, acute AMI was treated only with medications and supportive measures. The advent of emergent coronary intervention has changed the decision tree for managing acute MI. This tree has three branches. The first is conservative medical management and supportive treatment as was done previously. This option is rarely used today, principally in situations of non-ST elevation MI, especially in the elderly. The other two options seek to reopen the infarct-related artery as rapidly as possible, which is the definitive treatment. One option is by mechanical reperfusion using balloon angioplasty and coronary artery stenting. The other option for reperfusion is intravenous thrombolytic medication (tPA, uPA, streptokinase, etc.).

The paramedic's role is vital in caring for patients with acute myocardial infarction. Many barriers exist to the performance "in a timely manner" for PCI and include delayed patient recognition of the symptoms, transport delays, inaccessibility to catheterization labs, or delays in starting fibrinolysis. Each of these steps can be made more efficient, so more lives can be saved. The paramedic can prevent complications and initiate treatment for acute myocardial infarction before hospital arrival, resulting in a reduction of time between the AMI event and reperfusion therapy. Managing pain, maintaining cardiac output, performing serial 12-lead ECGs, and transporting to a facility capable of managing patients with an AMI is critical. As time permits during transport, initiating additional IVs and completing a fibrinolytic checklist will help facilities that utilize this therapy be able to provide the medication sooner upon arrival at the hospital (Box 29-20). DOT 5-2.80, 5-2.81

Fibrinolysis Versus Percutaneous Coronary Intervention (PCI)

In recent years, the advantages of fibrinolysis versus angioplasty have stirred vigorous debate. This question

---

BOX 29-20   Fibrinolytic Inclusion Criteria

- 18 years or older
- Ischemic discomfort lasting 30 minutes or more
- ST segment elevation greater than 1 mm in two or more than two contiguous limb leads *or* 2 or more mm in two or more than two contiguous chest leads *or* new (or presumably new) left bundle branch block
- Ability to administer the first bolus of thrombolytic within 12 hours of onset of pain

Exclusion Criteria

- History of stroke or transient ischemic attack (TIA)
- Known cranial neoplasm, AV malformation, or aneurysm
- Major surgery, trauma, or internal bleeding within four weeks
  - Ask about bloody or tarry stools
- A blood pressure reading greater than 180 SBP or 110 DBP
- Cardiogenic shock or pulmonary edema resulting in intubation
- Known bleeding disorder
- Known oral anticoagulation within past three days, including Coumadin
- Symptoms consistent with aortic dissection
  - Unequal pulses or BPs
- Cocaine or amphetamine use within past three days
- Pregnancy

---

has been resolved through multiple comparative clinical trials, randomizing patients to fibrinolysis or stenting. **Percutaneous coronary intervention (PCI)** is clearly now the preferred method if performed in a timely manner. An important advantage of primary PCI is that it restores normal cardiac blood flow in more than 90% of cases compared to only 50–60% with fibrinolysis.[17,18,19,20,21] If PCI is available at a center with skilled, high-volume operators, mutiple randomized trials have shown this intervention enhances survival compared to fibrinolysis and has lower rates of intracranial hemorrhage and recurrent MI (Figure 29-117).[22] Situations still exist where PCI cannot be performed in a timely manner, and thrombolytics are appropriate in these situations.

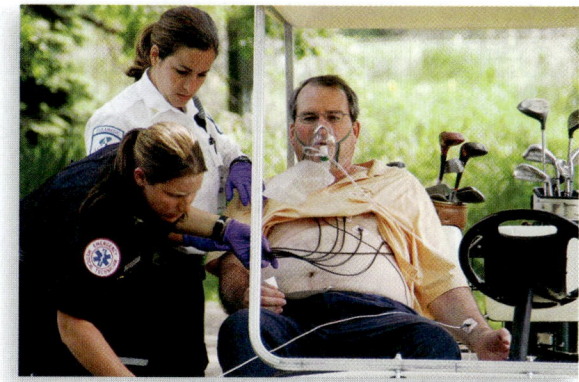

(a)

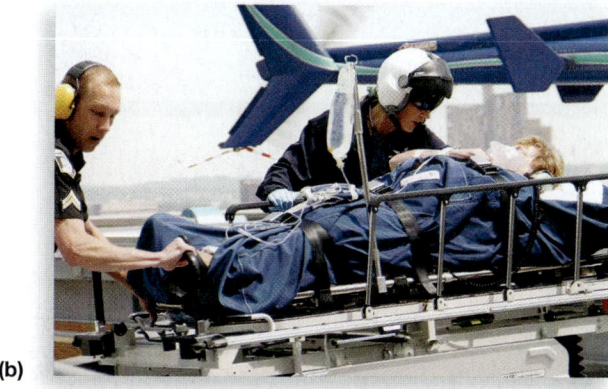

(b)

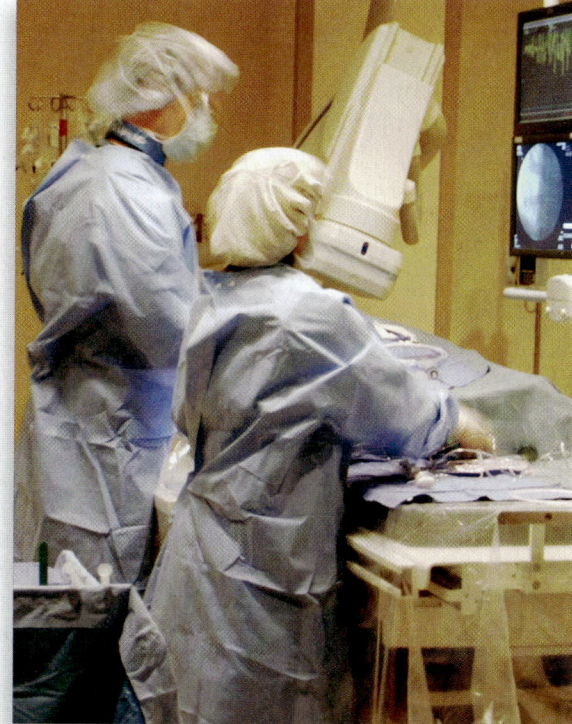

(c)

Figure 29-117 Paramedics can play a large role in getting the patient to a specialized cardiac care center where PCI is available. Rapid identification with a scene 12-lead ECG, (a) alerting the receiving hospital to have a catheterization lab team ready, and rapid transfer to a specialized hospital (b) are some of the ways EMS can reduce the time it takes to get the occluded artery open (c).

Thrombolytic medications improve outcomes in MI compared to no intervention at all but have associated complications, and therefore multiple contraindications. A generally accepted way to approach the MI patient who may be a candidate for lysis follows:

1. Has the patient experienced chest pain for greater than 15 minutes and less than 12 hours? If yes, then . . .
2. If any of the questions listed in Box 29-21 are answered "yes," thrombolytics are probably contraindicated.
3. Does the patient have cardiogenic shock or severe heart failure, making PCI preferable? These are typically clinically evident based on the evaluation, including the absence of hypotension or hypertension, cold and clammy extremities, and lung crackles or pulmonary edema.[9,12]

If the patient meets these criteria and is unable to have PCI in a timely manner, thrombolytics are the preferred method of treatment.

What is "a timely manner" for PCI? This is a complicated question without a clear answer. According to recent guidelines from the American College of Cardiology/American Heart Association (ACC/AHA), a "timely manner" is the infarct-related artery opened by PCI within 90 minutes of first contact with a hospital.[12] The time from presentation to a hospital to the opening of the artery is called "door-to-balloon" time. Studies suggest a door-to-balloon time ranging up to 120 or 150 minutes as still providing benefit over fibrinolysis.[21] Regardless of the final door-to-balloon time goal, time is muscle.

The main goal of rapid and effective AMI management is preventing morbidity and mortality. Preserving cardiac tissue prevents abnormal cardiac remodeling (enlarging of the heart) and shortens the time for acute complications, therefore decreasing short- and long-term cardiac dysrhythmias, heart failure, and other major contributors to cardiovascular morbidity and mortality. Two of the frequent complications of myocardial infarction are cardiac arrest and cardiogenic shock. These will now be examined in greater detail.

DOT 5-2.83

Cardiac Arrest

Sudden cardiac death (SCD) is used to describe cardiac arrest with cessation of cardiac function, whether resuscitation or spontaneous reversion of the dysrhythmia occurs. Despite the term "death" in SCD, not all patients who have cardiac arrest die as some are resuscitated. There is a clear connection between the time interval to initiate resuscitation and patient

BOX 29-21	Fibrinolytic Exclusion Criteria		
Systolic blood pressure greater than 180 mmHg		YES	NO
Diastolic blood pressure greater than 110 mmHg		YES	NO
Right versus left arm systolic blood pressure difference greater than 15 mmHg		YES	NO
History of structural central nervous system disease		YES	NO
Significant closed head or facial trauma within the previous three months		YES	NO
Recent (within six weeks) major trauma, surgery (including laser eye surgery), gastrointestinal or genitourinary bleed		YES	NO
Bleeding or clotting problem or on blood thinners		YES	NO
Pregnant female		YES	NO
Serious systemic disease (e.g., advanced or terminal cancer, severe liver or kidney disease)		YES	NO

survival in cardiac arrest. The global medical community has improved outcomes with better CPR training and AED (automatic external defibrillator) use through public access defibrillator (PAD) programs. A recent series from Seattle shows that bystander CPR performance has increased from 27% to 50%.[23] Paramedics see cardiac arrest as often as any other members in the healthcare community. DOT 5-2.121, 5-2.122, 5-2.123, 5-2.124, 5-2.125

The initial assessment taught in ACLS and BCLS remains the preferred approach to the patient with cardiac arrest. For example, resuscitating a cardiac dysrhythmia that originated as a result of airway blockage is not helpful for patient survival if the airway blockage is not corrected.

Defibrillation

Defibrillation is the administration of unsynchronized electrical therapy with the intent of depolarizing a critical mass of vulnerable cardiac cells to terminate ventricular fibrillation. Once this wavefront is terminated, there exists an opportunity for the heart to regain normal electrical activity. For successful defibrillation to occur, the shock must affect a critical mass of cardiac tissue, estimated to be 80–90% of the total mass of the heart. The amount of current actually reaching the heart may be influenced by such things as electrode contact pressure, transthoracic impedance, and the amount of applied current. Effective defibrillation requires the optimization of these variables to insure a maximal current reaches and travels through the heart. DOT 5-2.178, 5-2.179, 5-2.180

Electrode placement plays a critical role in ensuring the current travels through the heart. If electrodes are too close together, current will travel just below the skin from electrode to electrode without reaching the heart. With electrodes that are too far apart or placed without proper electrolyte conduction medium, the current will be attenuated to the extent that the critical mass cannot be depolarized. There are two options for placement of paddles or multifunction pads on the chest wall (Figure 29-118). First is the anterolateral position in which a single paddle or pad is placed on the left fourth or fifth intercostal space on the midaxillary line; the other paddle or pad is placed just to the right of the sternal edge on the second or third intercostal space.

The second option is the anteroposterior position. A single paddle or pad is placed to the left of the sternum, over the apex of the heart and the other paddle or pad is placed between the tip of the right scapula and the spine. Since the skin can conduct away a significant portion of the current, electrolyte-rich conductive gel or pre-gelled pads are commonly used to ensure good contact. Under ideal circumstances, only 10–30% of the total current reaches the heart.

Transthoracic impedance may be affected by poor electrode contact or an excessive amount of subcutaneous tissue. The level of current applied is recorded in watts/sec or Joules (J). Studies have shown that shocks as low as 50 Joules may be effective, and those in excess of 400 Joules have no clear benefit and may indeed inflict substantial myocardial damage. It is therefore recommended to defibrillate at 360 J with monophasic defibrillators and 150 J to 200 J for biphasic defibrillators.

Traditional defibrillation utilizes a monophasic waveform. Many modern defibrillators now use a biphasic waveform. Studies have shown that biphasic waveforms appear to be more effective and operate at lower joules than a monophasic waveform.[24] The actual shape of the biphasic waveform remains controversial, and defibrillator manufacturers have designed equipment that varies in waveform type and applied Joules. The paramedic must become familiar with the equipment

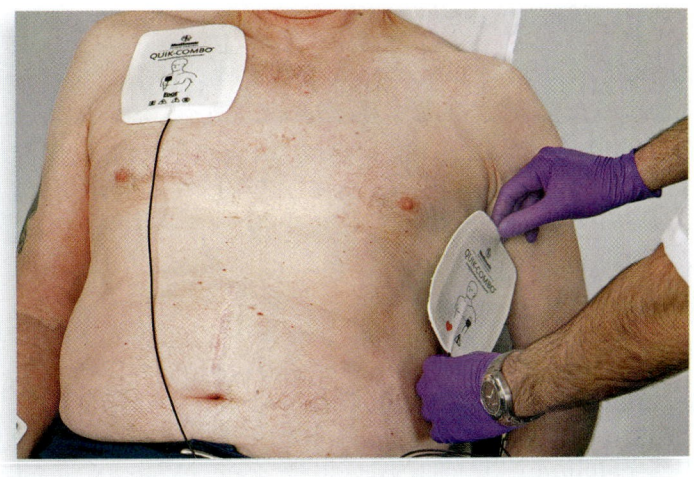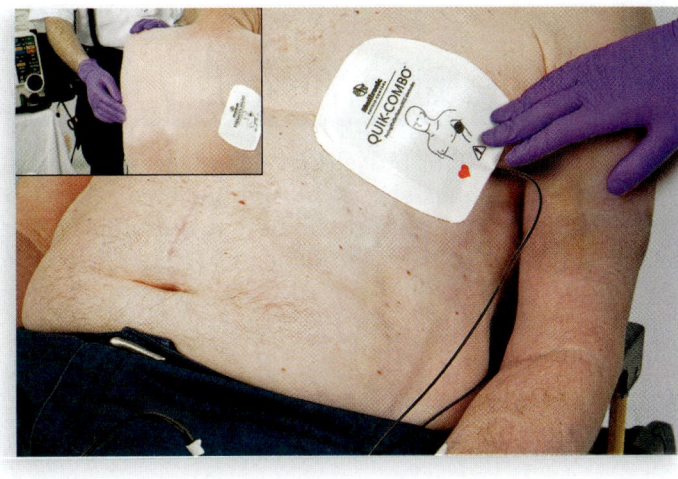

(a)   (b)

Figure 29-118   Two choices for multifunction pad placement. (a) Anterolateral. (b) Anteroposterior.

used in his or her service. The basic idea behind biphasic defibrillation is that the first wave will depolarize the critical mass as in the monophasic waveform, but then the second waveform (occurring milliseconds later during the same defibrillation) reduces the fibrillatory threshold to prevent reinitiating the fibrillatory wavefront. Another theory suggests that the first wave hyperpolarizes cellular membranes to increase the chances of successful defibrillation by the second wave.[22,25] Whatever the exact mechanism, it appears that biphasic defibrillation is more effective and has lower energy requirements than monophasic defibrillation.

Synchronized cardioversion is similar to defibrillation in that an electrical current is applied to the patient with the intent of terminating potentially lethal dysrhythmias and restoring a normal rhythm (Box 29-22). If you recall the discussion about the absolute and relative refractory periods in the action potential, then you will understand that the application of an electrical current to a group of cells in the relative refractory period may have the effect of destabilizing the cells and inducing

ventricular fibrillation. By "synchronizing" the defibrillator to the existing ECG complex and instituting a precisely timed delivery, the vulnerable period may be avoided, lessening the chances of inducing VF. The ECG monitor senses and marks the underlying rhythm of the heart by examining the R wave of the QRS complex. The shock is then timed and delivered to avoid the relative refractory period.

During cardioversion, should the QRS complex be too small to be reliably identified, you should increase the size of the QRS through the controls on the monitor itself. The effective current for cardioversion varies with the type of dysrhythmia but is usually begun at 50–100 joules and is increased up to 360 J (100 J–200 J–300 J–360 J) if the rhythm is refractory to lower levels of energy. The monitor has a button that turns on the synchronization mode, which must be reset on each successive cardioversion. Failure to do this will result in the delivery of a nonsynchronized shock, which can cause VF.

If you see *ventricular fibrillation* or *ventricular tachycardia,* with no pulse . . . DEFIBRILLATE!

Ventricular dysrhythmias are often lethal. Placing the patient on a cardiac monitor or obtaining an ECG rhythm strip is of utmost importance after CPR initiation and airway control (Box 29-23). The most common fatal dysrhythmias are ventricular fibrillation (VF) and ventricular tachycardia (VT) (see Figure 29-119 page 701, the AHA Pulseless Arrest Algorithm). VF will rarely convert to a normal rhythm without intervention, and the treatment is to defibrillate at 360 J with monophasic defibrillators and 150 J to 200 J for biphasic defibrillators. Based on how quickly one is able to defibrillate, success in terminating VF can be high. If VF persists without definitive intervention for longer than four minutes, neurologic brain damage is often irreversible.[26] DOT 5-2.124

BOX 29-22   What Is the Difference between Cardioversion and Defibrillation?

Cardioversion delivers energy synchronized with the cardiac cycle (with the QRS complex), while defibrillation is an unsynchronized delivery of energy, meaning the shock is delivered randomly during the cardiac cycle without any regard for the relative refractory period. DOT 5-2.127

BOX 29-23   CPR Versus Defibrillation: Which Is First?

If the onset of VF or pulseless VT is witnessed, one defibrillatory shock should be administered immediately followed by approximately two minutes of CPR. If the patient is found to be in VF or pulseless VT when you begin your ABC assessment, then perform two minutes of CPR prior to a single defibrillation attempt.

BOX 29-24   Causes and Treatment of PEA

In addition to CPR, intubation, oxygen, IV, epinephrine, ECG, and rapid transport, consider adding the following treatments:

Hypovolemia: Give 20mL/kg boluses crystalloid IV

Hypoxia: Ensure 100% oxygen is being delivered

Acidosis: Ensure 100% oxygen is being delivered and give bicarbonate if necessary

Hyperkalemia: Give sodium bicarbonate or calcium

Hypokalemia: No additional treatment available in the prehospital setting; rapid transport

Hypothermia: Passive rewarming, warmed IV fluids, remove wet clothing

Overdose: Provide antidote (atropine, bicarbonate, naloxone, flumazenil, 2 PAM (pralidoxime) chloride, among others)

Cardiac tamponade: Rapid transport for pericardiocentesis

Tension pneumothorax: Needle decompression **(see Skill Sheet 77: Management of Chest Trauma)**

AMI: Rapid transport, most MONA drugs are not indicated if the patient is pulseless

Pulmonary embolus: Rapid transport

While defibrillation remains the primary and most efficacious treatment of VF and pulseless VT, pharmacologic intervention may be of some benefit also. Such pharmacologic intervention includes epinephrine or vasopressin, or use of an antidysrhythmic such as lidocaine, amiodarone, or magnesium sulfate.[27]

Asystole is the term used for no visible electrical activity in the heart. This marks the cessation of cardiac function and cardiac electrical activity. Asystole and fine ventricular fibrillation are so similar in appearance that the rhythm should be confirmed by checking it in at least two leads. If any leads show more than a completely flat line, consider that the rhythm could be fine VF and treat following that algorithm (see Figure 29-119, AHA Pulseless Arrest Algorithm). Other acute treatments include CPR, an attempt at transcutaneous pacing (if the onset of asystole was witnessed), and using epinephrine, vasopressin, or atropine. DOT 5-2.84

Street Secrets

Confirming Asystole: When a three- or four-lead system is used to monitor the patient, switch the view from lead II to lead I or III to confirm asystole, or place the paddles (which reads lead II) on the chest to confirm the lead. If the paddles are placed on the chest, lift the (+) paddle (the one on the apex) and move it up toward the right shoulder, directly across from the other paddle near the left shoulder; this changes the view from lead II to lead I. If the multifunction pads are on the chest, attach the limb leads to verify asystole in another lead. You cannot switch leads with the multifunction pads as they read lead II only. DOT 5-2.126

Another common cardiac rhythm seen in arrest settings is **pulseless electrical activity (PEA)** (Box 29-24). This is defined as electrical activity seen on the cardiac monitor when the patient is without a pulse. Using this description, PEA is reserved for pulseless electrical rhythms that are normally expected to have a pulse (see

Figure 29-119, AHA Pulseless Arrest Algorithm). For example, ventricular fibrillation and asystole are always pulseless, so they would not be classified as PEA, but sinus tachycardia without a pulse is a PEA rhythm.

Every patient in PEA needs CPR and regular pulse checks. Drugs used to treat PEA include epinephrine, vasopressin, and atropine. Atropine is only indicated if the PEA rate is slow. If a pulse returns and a recognizable rhythm comes on the monitor, change algorithms accordingly. It is important to consider the possible causes of PEA in order to treat it effectively. Causes to consider include hypovolemia, hypoxia, acidosis, hyperkalemia, hypokalemia, hypothermia, overdose, cardiac tamponade, tension pneumothorax, AMI, and pulmonary emboli. DOT 5-2.84

Symptomatic bradycardia can cause cardiac arrest. Medical management usually starts with the drug atropine, and if this is ineffective, transcutaneous pacing is indicated until more definitive cardiovascular therapy is available (see Figure 29-120, the AHA Algorithm for Bradycardia). Caution must be used when using atropine if the bradycardia is accompanied by a second-degree type II AV block or a third-degree AV block.

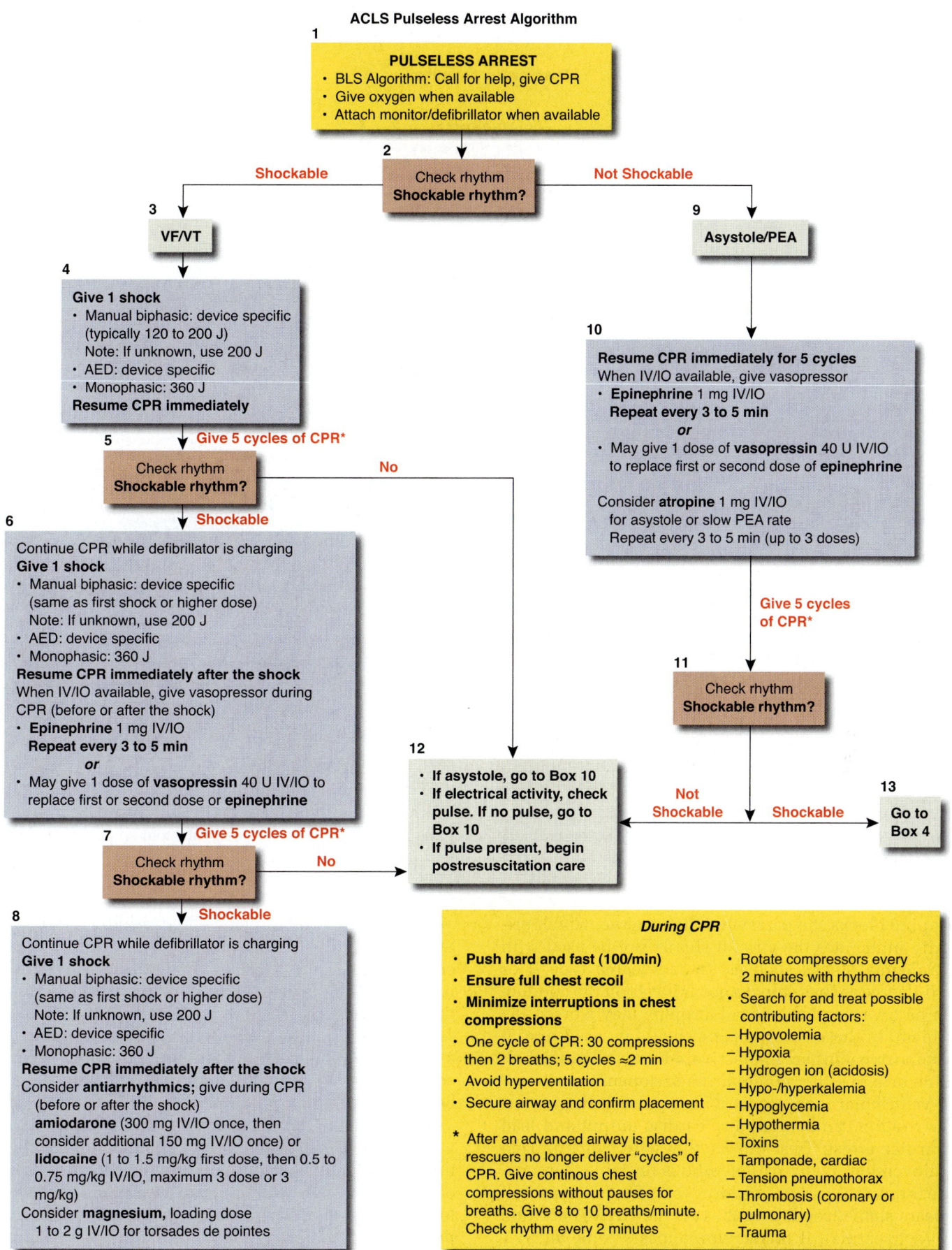

Figure 29-119 AHA Algorithm for Pulseless Arrest. Reproduced with permission 2005 American Heart Association *Guidelines for Cardiopulmonary Resuscitation and Emergency Cardiovascular Care* © 2005, American Heart Association.

Bradycardia Algorithm

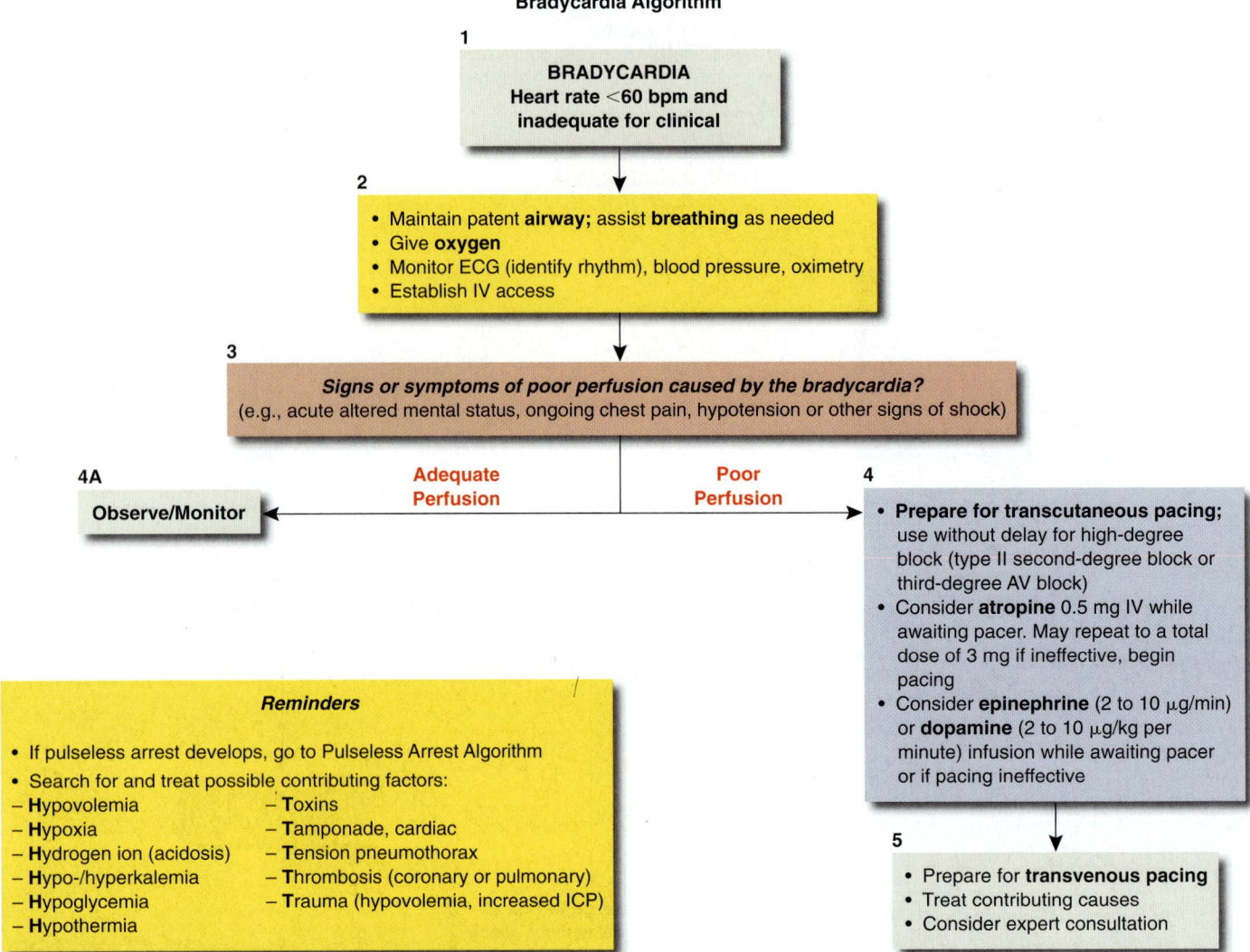

1

BRADYCARDIA
Heart rate <60 bpm and
inadequate for clinical

2
- Maintain patent **airway;** assist **breathing** as needed
- Give **oxygen**
- Monitor ECG (identify rhythm), blood pressure, oximetry
- Establish IV access

3
Signs or symptoms of poor perfusion caused by the bradycardia?
(e.g., acute altered mental status, ongoing chest pain, hypotension or other signs of shock)

4A
Observe/Monitor

Adequate
Perfusion

Poor
Perfusion

4
- **Prepare for transcutaneous pacing;** use without delay for high-degree block (type II second-degree block or third-degree AV block)
- Consider **atropine** 0.5 mg IV while awaiting pacer. May repeat to a total dose of 3 mg if ineffective, begin pacing
- Consider **epinephrine** (2 to 10 μg/min) or **dopamine** (2 to 10 μg/kg per minute) infusion while awaiting pacer or if pacing ineffective

5
- Prepare for **transvenous pacing**
- Treat contributing causes
- Consider expert consultation

Reminders

- If pulseless arrest develops, go to Pulseless Arrest Algorithm
- Search for and treat possible contributing factors:
  - **H**ypovolemia
  - **H**ypoxia
  - **H**ydrogen ion (acidosis)
  - **H**ypo-/hyperkalemia
  - **H**ypoglycemia
  - **H**ypothermia
  - **T**oxins
  - **T**amponade, cardiac
  - **T**ension pneumothorax
  - **T**hrombosis (coronary or pulmonary)
  - **T**rauma (hypovolemia, increased ICP)

Figure 29-120 AHA Algorithm for Bradycardia. Reproduced with permission 2005 American Heart Association *Guidelines for Cardiopulmonary Resuscitation and Emergency Cardiovascular Care* © 2005, American Heart Association.

Atropine blocks the parasympathetic nerve, which primarily innervates the atria. It should not be used with high-degree blocks such as second-degree type II or third-degree as these blocks occur lower on the conduction pathway, and the use of atropine may worsen the problem. In these cases, pacing should be used first. If atropine or pacing are ineffective, administer a catecholamine drip of either epinephrine or dopamine.

Ventricular tachycardia with a pulse is dangerous. This rhythm can compromise cardiac output and lead to cardiac arrest. Treat this rhythm with synchronized cardioversion in any patient who is unstable. Amiodarone is the antidysrhythmic drug to try first if the patient appears stable (see Figure 29-121, the AHA Algorithm for Tachycardia). If the rhythm appears to be an SVT rhythm with aberrancy that is causing the QRS to appear wide (mimicking VT), a trial of adenosine can be attempted. Magnesium sulfate is the recommended antidysrhythmic drug if the rhythm is torsades de pointes.

Most narrow-complex tachydysrhythmias do not typically lead to cardiac arrest; however, under some circumstances they can, usually by causing myocardial ischemia. Rapid, narrow, complex dysrhythmias sometime respond to vagal maneuvers such as carotid massage (make sure there is no carotid bruit present first) or the Valsalva maneuver. Additional therapies include adenosine, the calcium channel blocker diltiazem, or beta-blockers.

The Valsalva maneuver causes vagal stimulation, which may cause the heart rate to slow, thus breaking the cycle of tachycardia. While there are several methods to accomplish this, the most common method is to instruct patients to take a deep breath and hold it, putting pressure on a closed glottic opening. The patient can also be instructed to bear down as if having a bowel movement while holding their breath. An ECG recording should be running during this maneuver so you can watch for changes in the heart rate.

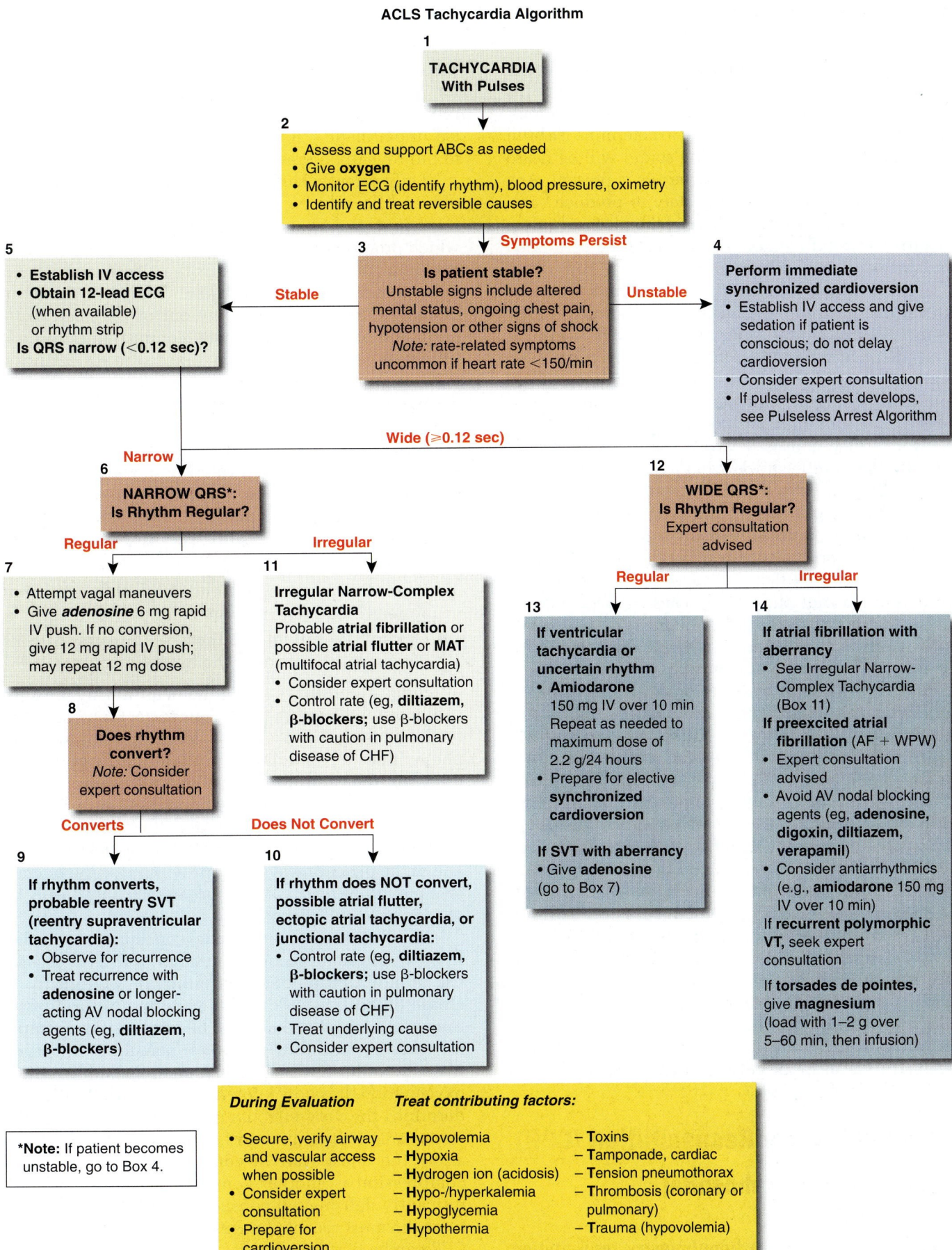

Figure 29-121 AHA Algorithm for Tachycardia. Reproduced with permission 2005 American Heart Association *Guidelines for Cardiopulmonary Resuscitation and Emergency Cardiovascular Care* © 2005, American Heart Association.

Massage of the carotid artery may also be an effective method of slowing the heart rate but is seldom used in the prehospital environment due to potential complications. The neck should first be auscultated to determine if a bruit is present. If present, a whooshing sound will be heard that indicates significant atherosclerosis is present. Any pressure applied to the carotid artery to produce vagal stimulation may result in breakage of the plaque, leading to a stroke. Carotid massage should never be performed simultaneously on both sides of the neck.

Cardiac arrest has many causes and includes both cardiac and noncardiac features. Cardiac etiologies include myocardial infarction, prolongation of the QT segment, cardiac tamponade, cardiogenic shock, congestive heart failure (low ejection fraction and left ventricular changes), and cardiac medications (beta-blockers, calcium channel blockers, digoxin, and others.) Noncardiac causes of arrest that lead to cardiac dysrhythmia include shock (from hypovolemia or sepsis), hypoxia, acidosis, tension pneumothorax, pulmonary embolus, hypothermia, and drug overdose.

A **respiratory arrest** (the heart is beating but there are no, or few, spontaneous respirations) often leads to cardiac arrest if the offending cause is not reversed or respirations are not supported. These causes include overmedication with respiratory depressants (examples include narcotics), large mucous plugs, or endotracheal tube plugging in mechanically ventilated patients.

Patients who have had prior episodes of VF or VT may have had an implantable automatic defibrillator placed. Under normal circumstances, the implantable defibrillation device will activate if it senses either ventricular tachycardia (VT) or ventricular fibrillation (VF). However, these devices may be ineffective at times, either due to inaccurate rhythm determination or an inadequate energy to defibrillate. This is evident in cases of VT or VF appearing on the monitor, yet no shocks are apparent from the implanted defibrillator. In this case, the algorithm for pulseless VT and VF should be followed, which includes prompt CPR and external defibrillation. Do not place the multifunction pads or paddles directly over the implanted defibrillator or for that matter directly over any device implanted into the chest. Place pads and paddles at least two inches away from these devices, and make sure the electrolyte paste or gel is not smeared over these devices. DOT 5-2.128

Cardiopulmonary Resuscitation (CPR)

Latest Trends in Prehospital Resuscitation

Despite the practice of **cardiopulmonary resuscitation (CPR)** for over 40 years, survival rates after out-of-hospital cardiac arrest have remained around 5%

nationwide for decades. Statistics are not much better for in-hospital arrest survivors; on average, about 20% return home, and many of those have severe neurological impairment.[28] As such, there is ample opportunity to improve upon these dismal outcomes. DOT 5-2.129, 5-2-130

Only recently have new insights into the physiology of blood flow during CPR resulted in radical new treatment strategies, some of which are counterintuitive, but which promise to increase survival rates after cardiac arrest. It has been known for years that chest compressions raise intrathoracic pressure and compress the heart, thereby increasing blood flow out of the heart to the brain and other vital organs. By contrast, until recently, little or no attention has been paid to the importance of refilling the heart after each compression.

No pump is effective unless the pump reservoir is filled after each cycle. In other words, how does blood get back into the heart for the subsequent compressions? Recent research has discovered new ways to enhance venous blood flow back to the heart (preload).

Venous return is dependent upon small but critical pressure changes within the thorax itself. As a general rule,

- Increased (positive) intrathoracic pressure *prevents* venous blood return to the heart.
- Lowered (negative) intrathoracic pressure *increases* venous blood return to the heart.

Since blood flows out of the heart during the chest compression phase, the only time to get blood back into the heart is during the chest decompression or recoil phase. Indeed, blood flow to both the main reservoirs in the heart, the ventricles, as well as the coronary arteries that provide blood to the heart muscle occurs only during the decompression phase of CPR. Without preload or blood flow back to the heart, CPR is ineffective. Thus, one of the primary ways to improve CPR's effectiveness is to maximize negative pressure in the chest during the recoil phase of CPR. DOT 5-2.6

Based upon this fundamental concept, some changes in the traditional practice of manual CPR, as well as the use of new CPR adjuncts, provide ways to greatly increase blood flow to the heart and brain during CPR, thus increasing the likelihood of survival. For example, for years healthcare workers were taught to hyperventilate patients in cardiac arrest to maximize tissue oxygenation. It is now known that hyperventilation undermines the very effectiveness of CPR by increasing intrathoracic pressure and is deadly.[29] Also, failing to allow the chest wall to completely recoil following compression is another common CPR error with significantly detrimental consequences.[30] Box 29-25 outlines the most recent changes in the way conventional CPR can be performed to maximize venous blood flow back and fill the heart for the next compression. Remember, it doesn't do any good to administer numerous

BOX 29-25   Points to Remember When Performing Adult CPR

1. Compress the chest 100 times/minute to a depth of 1.5–2 inches.

2. Assure that the chest wall recoils *completely* after each compression. An alternative hand position, which brings the palm of the compressing hand slightly but completely off the chest during the recoil phase, may facilitate this (Figure 29-122).

3. Every positive pressure ventilation diminishes blood return to the heart! Avoid hyperventilation and ventilations of long duration. For an unsecured airway (e.g., facemask), ventilate over 1.5–2 seconds until the chest rises. For a secured airway (e.g., endotracheal tube), ventilate over 1–1.5 seconds until the chest rises.

4. Avoid prolonged interruptions in compressions. During facemask ventilation, stop only for delivering ventilations. Except for intubation and defibrillation use, chest compressions should never be stopped for more than a few seconds while the patient remains pulseless.

5. Proper CPR is tiring! Rotate duties frequently (every two minutes) to avoid fatigue and the poor CPR quality that results.

6. Consider use of an impedance threshold device to enhance circulation and provide guidance on proper ventilation rate. Remember to maintain a tight face seal with the facemask during chest compressions. A two-person ventilation technique facilitates this.

7. Provide resuscitative efforts for at least 30 minutes. Blood flow is much lower during CPR, even if properly performed. It takes longer to get vital nutrients and oxygen to the heart and brain, especially after prolonged down times. Give good CPR a chance to work.

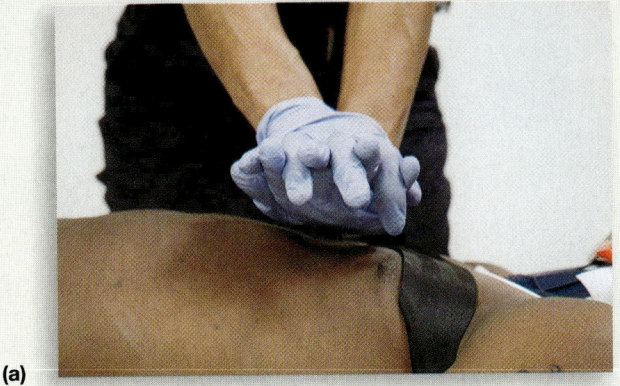
(a)

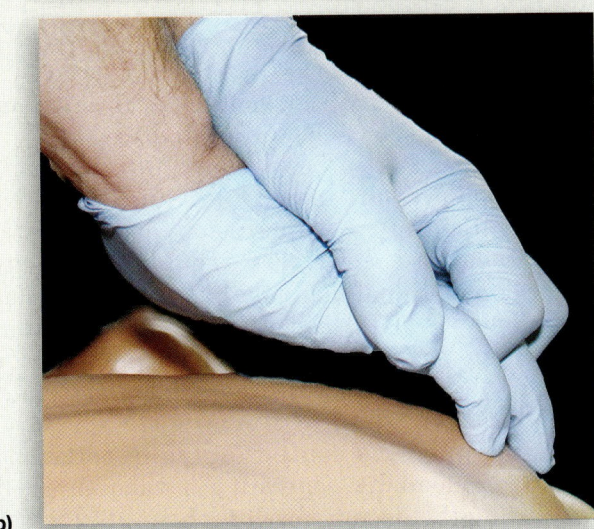
(b)

Figure 29-122   (a) Full recoil of the chest involves taking all pressure off the chest in the upstroke of the compression. In this example, the rescuer has interlocked her fingers and is completely off the chest. (b) In this alternate technique, the rescuer leaves the tips of his fingers on the chest to make sure he does not lose his landmark and curls his palms off the chest. He must take care not to rest his hands and fingers too heavily on the chest.

medications during resuscitation if good basic life support is not performed to circulate them.

Circulation-Enhancing Devices

In addition to changes in conventional manual CPR technique, several devices have been evaluated and shown to increase circulation during CPR. One device, the ResQPOD®, also known as an impedance threshold device (ITD), works by selectively preventing airflow into the lungs when the chest wall recoils back to its natural position after each compression (Figure 29-123). This results in an enhanced vacuum (negative pressure) within the thorax, which increases venous blood return to the heart during the decompression or chest wall recoil phase. Improved preload results in enhanced cardiac output on the subsequent compression.

In animals and patients, use of the ResQPOD doubles blood flow to the heart, increases cerebral perfusion, doubles the systolic blood pressure in humans, and doubles 24-hour survival rates in patients with any

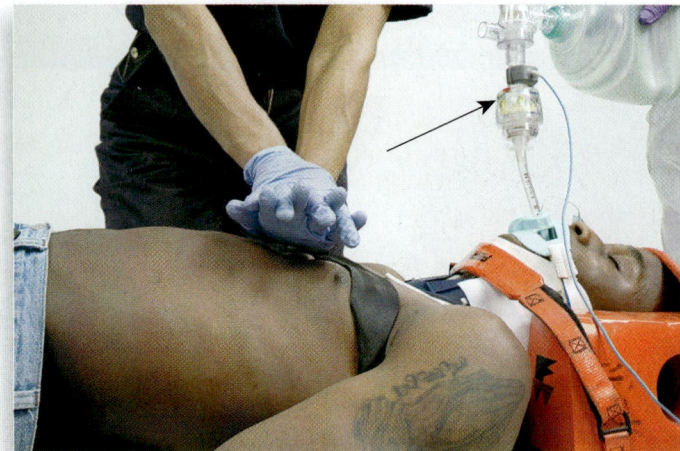

Figure 29-123 ResQPOD®.

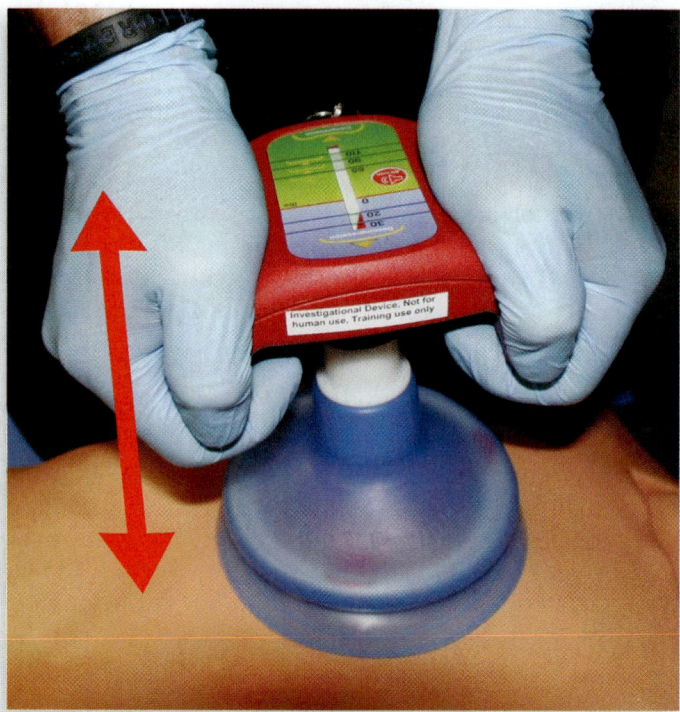

Figure 29-124 ResQPump®. The rescuer pushes down, observing a gauge to measure the force of the compression, and pulls up, manually creating an enhanced negative pressure in the chest. This may increase blood return to the heart.

initial electrical activity (e.g., ventricular fibrillation or tachycardia or pulseless electrical activity).[31,32,33,34,35,36] The ResQPOD has also been shown to significantly increase blood pressure in patients with asystole who are undergoing active compression decompression CPR and to increase survival rates in patients in asystole after conventional manual or active compression decompression CPR. Based upon extensive clinical trials in humans, the ResQPOD was highly recommended by the American Heart Association's Guidelines in 2005.[37,38,39,40]

Building upon the concept of the importance of enhancing preload by generating a vacuum in the thorax during the decompression phase of CPR, both manual (ResQPump®) and automated (LUCAS™) active compression decompression devices have been developed (Figures 29-124 and 29-125). These devices attach to the chest wall, transforming the chest into an active bellows. The addition of the ResQPOD to active compression decompression CPR results in a fourfold increase in blood flow to the heart and brain compared with conventional manual CPR.[41] The clinical trial results with this device combination are striking, especially in patients with the greatest chance for survival, those with a witnessed arrest and an initial rhythm of ventricular fibrillation. This group of patients fails to respond to initial defibrillation about 75% of the time, but after receiving treatment with the ResQPOD and active compression decompression CPR, they have a greater than 65% 24-hour survival rate.[37] A second clinical trial showed that adding the ResQPOD to active compression decompression CPR resulted in a 50% improvement in survival to 24 hours compared with active compression decompression CPR alone.[40]

The automated version of the active compression decompression device (LUCAS) is more expensive than the manual version but offers the advantages of any mechanical device. Moreover, it is easier to perform continuous CPR with the automated version, and continuous (asynchronous) CPR during ventilation with a secured airway has been shown to provide enhanced circulation compared with results when chest compressions are interrupted to provide ventilations.[42]

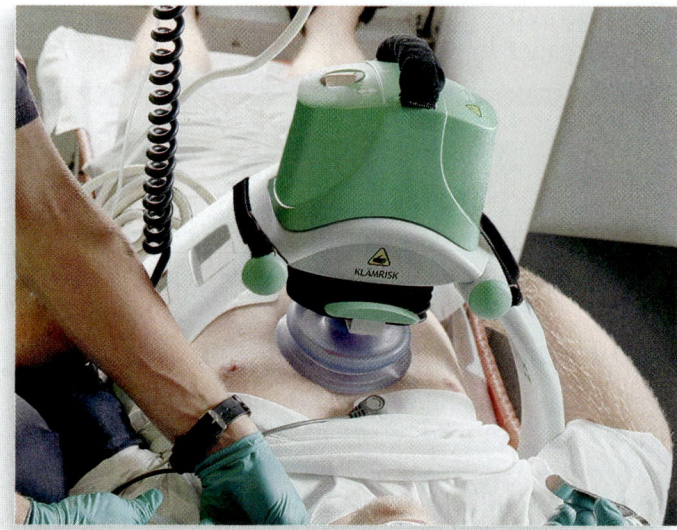

Figure 29-125 LUCAS™ (Jolife).

After an invasive airway device, such as an endotracheal tube, Combitube, laryngeal mask airway, or other similar devices, is in place and placement is confirmed, CPR should be performed continuously with ventilations delivered at a rate of eight to ten per minute. Of course, the rhythm should be checked every two minutes while CPR is being performed.

Finally, another automated device, called the Auto-Pulse™, applies compression with a band, thereby increasing intrathoracic pressure more by squeezing the entire anterior section of the thorax than by compressing only the sternum (Figure 29-126). This device has been shown to increase hemodynamics in animals and patients and to increase the return of spontaneous circulation in one small, non-randomized, historical control study.[43,44,45] At the time of this writing, there are no published clinical trials demonstrating longer-term benefit.

Automated CPR devices (e.g., LUCAS and Auto-Pulse™) have some advantages over manually performed conventional CPR; they

1. Provide continuous CPR, thus reducing interruptions.
2. Eliminate the fatigue factor which results in errors that compromise CPR effectiveness.
3. Potentially reduce the number of personnel needed at the scene of the cardiac arrest.

Regardless of whether manual or automated CPR is performed, the key to survival is maintaining optimal circulation and blood flow to vital organs until a spontaneous pulse can be restored. Attention to performing good

CPR and the use of promising new technology will offer patients the greatest opportunity for survival.

Cardiogenic Shock

Cardiogenic shock occurs when enough damage to heart muscle has occurred to interfere with its ability to pump, causing low blood pressure and significantly reduced tissue perfusion and decreased oxygen delivery. This hypoxic effect may be reversible if treated early but if left untreated quickly becomes irreversible and causes cell death with end-organ damage and failure, which can be fatal. DOT 5-2.114

Cardiogenic shock refers to failure of the heart to adequately pump and distribute oxygen. Cardiac output and systolic function are reduced. It is most commonly caused by acute myocardial infarction but may also be the result of cardiomyopathies, chronic congestive heart failure (CHF), dysrhythmias, valvular or septal defects, or obstructive disorders such as pulmonary embolus, tension pneumothorax, or pericardial tamponade. Proper treatment of cardiogenic shock requires addressing and potentially correcting the underlying defect, most commonly the treatment of acute myocardial infarction (Box 29-26). DOT 5-2.115, 5-2.117

In contrast to the pump failure of cardiogenic shock, hypovolemic shock is a result of profound hemorrhage or fluid loss. Stroke volume is decreased as well, and tachycardia is the normal physiologic response. It can be corrected with replacement of the lost fluids. Vasodilatory shock—seen in sepsis, anaphylaxis, or toxin reactions—is a result of a severe drop in systemic vascular resistance, often with increased cardiac output and tachycardia. In addition to potential dehydration or actual fluid loss, the leaky vascular system allows blood

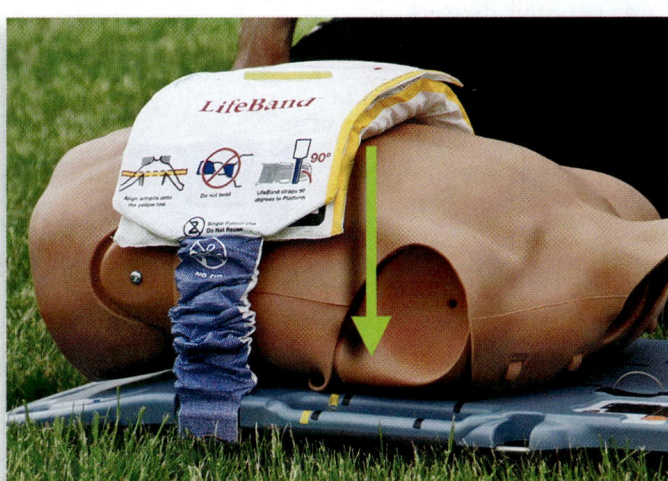

Figure 29-126 AutoPulse™ (Revivant Corporation). The AutoPulse applies pressure over a wide area. Compression and release happen rapidly and evenly. This is a mechanical device and does not involve a rescuer doing compressions.

BOX 29-26 Types of Shock and Treatment

Cardiogenic (pump failure)

Treat by correcting underlying problem

Reverse ischemia, if present

Relieve pulmonary congestion

Support cardiac function

Hypovolemic (massive fluid or blood loss)

Replace lost fluid or blood

Vasodilatory (sepsis, anaphylaxis, toxins)

Treat underlying cause

Supportive care

plasma to leave the vascular space. This fluid enters the interstitial tissues, causing edema, and creates a relative hypovolemia state. Effective treatment involves replenishing any fluid losses, appropriate antibiotics, and, if needed, vasopressive agents to keep the vascular system from leaking fluids and maintaining the blood pressure. DOT 5-2.116

Stages of Cardiogenic Shock

Once the cardiogenic event has occurred and circulation becomes disrupted, shock progresses through three stages. Initially, the homeostatic mechanisms will compensate for the diminished perfusion; this is known as preshock. In this stage, the patient may be asymptomatic or may have only modest tachycardia or hypotension. There is little change in mental status during this state, but the patient may report they feel something is wrong. This can lead to anxiety or restlessness.

As preshock develops into the true shock stage, the homeostatic mechanisms are no longer sufficient to maintain adequate tissue perfusion, resulting in end-organ impairment. This impairment is clinically recognized by tachycardia, tachypnea, metabolic acidosis, decreased urine output, and cool and clammy skin. Tachycardia and tachypnea result from homeostatic attempts to correct the problem. Metabolic acidosis occurs as wastes build up in the tissues. Urine output drops off due to the drop in blood pressure and homeostatic controls to preserve perfusion to more vital organs. Cool, clammy skin occurs because blood is shunted from the extremities.

Finally, the persistent hypoperfusion leads to irreversible end-organ damage, specifically a significant or total loss of urine output, increasing restlessness and confusion, and a worsening of acidosis. Ultimately, multiple organ system failure leads to the death of the patient. DOT 5-2.115

Compensation

In shock, cardiac output is significantly diminished, so other organ systems in the body must compensate if death is to be prevented. To accomplish this, systemic vascular resistance (SVR) increases in the microcirculation to maintain perfusion to the heart and brain, sacrificing other tissues such as kidneys, muscles, skin, and the gastrointestinal tract. The kidneys produce an enzyme called angiotensin, which contributes to the constriction of peripheral arteries, and it also increases reabsorption of water and salt in an attempt to halt the progression of shock. Additional water retention results from the release of vasopressin by the posterior pituitary

gland. The lungs respond by decreasing tidal volume and increasing minute ventilation, resulting in a respiratory alkalosis to compensate for the metabolic acidosis present in the shock state.

Pathophysiology of Cardiogenic Shock

As mentioned earlier, cardiogenic shock results from cardiac pump failure, which can be due to direct damage to the heart itself (intrinsic) or restriction of the output of the heart (compressive).

Intrinsic cardiogenic shock is most commonly seen as a complication following AMI but can also be seen in CHF, severe dysrhythmias, or valvular heart disease. Cardiac output is decreased, and SVR is increased. This drop in peripheral perfusion can result in hypoxia to the affected organ systems, resulting in the clinical features described below. Elevated pulmonary vascular pressures also lead to pulmonary congestion.

Compressive cardiogenic shock is the result of a mechanical impairment of cardiac output. Accumulation of blood or fluid in the pericardial sac can compress the heart and prevent it from filling, a condition known as cardiac tamponade. A pulmonary embolus can impede right-sided blood flow and result in right heart failure as well. Tension pneumothorax or overaggressive positive pressure ventilation can also lead to compressive cardiogenic shock.

Causes of Cardiogenic Shock

Intrinsic
- MI
- CHF
- Severe dysrhythmia
- Valvular disease

Compressive
- Pericardial tamponade
- Pulmonary embolus
- Tension pneumothorax

Clinical Features of Cardiogenic Shock

The patient may not be able to provide adequate historical information, so the patient's family may be helpful in this regard. A review of the patient's prior medical and medication history may indicate existing ischemic heart disease, CHF, or cardiomyopathy.

Physical exam may reveal severe hypotension with a systolic blood pressure less than 90 mmHg or a mean arterial pressure 30 mmHg less than the patient's usual blood pressure. In approximately two-thirds of patients, respiratory distress due to pulmonary congestion will be present.[46] Other signs of decreased perfusion of the skin, kidneys, and brain will likely be seen, including cool extremities, decreased urine output, or altered mental status, respectively. DOT 5-2.175, 5-2.176

Clinical Features of Cardiogenic Shock

- Severe hypotension
- Tachycardia
- Tachypnea
- Metabolic acidosis
- Low urine output
- Cool, clammy skin
- Decreased mental status

Specific to compressive cardiogenic shock, cardiac tamponade may demonstrate the triad of hypotension, jugular venous distension (JVD), and muffled heart sounds. Pulsus paradoxus may also be noted. Tension pneumothorax should be suspected when decreased breath sounds on one side, tracheal deviation, and JVD are noted.

Diagnosis in the field relies chiefly on the history and physical examination, specifically noting signs and symptoms of AMI, pulmonary congestion, or any other of the above conditions. An ECG and a chest radiograph will assist further in making the diagnosis, but these are not always available outside of the hospital.

Treatment of Cardiogenic Shock

Initial treatment should be focused on stabilizing the patient for immediate transport to the hospital. Because AMI is the most common cause for cardiogenic shock, it would be prudent to give 160–325 mg of aspirin (either by mouth, rectally, or by crushing and placing it in the buccal space), as well as to initiate intravenous heparin if allowed and no contraindications are present.[12,47] Heparin doses of a 5000-unit bolus, followed by a drip at 1000 units/hr have shown no increase in hemorrhagic complications.[48] DOT 5-2.118, 5-2.119, 5-2.120

Nice to Know

Beck's Triad

Beck's triad is the three classic, clinical manifestations of cardiac tamponade:

- JVD
- Muffled heart tones
- Hypotension

In patients without evidence of pulmonary congestion or respiratory distress, a 250 mL bolus of normal saline may improve systemic perfusion. However, overly aggressive fluid support may result in significant pulmonary edema, especially in left ventricular infarction and in the elderly. If there is evidence for pulmonary congestion, the drug furosemide or another potent diuretic can be given.[49]

Treatment of Cardiogenic Shock

- Aspirin
- Heparin (if available prehospital)
- Fluids, if dehydrated
- Furosemide, if pulmonary congestion
- Oxygen
- Vasopressors, if necessary

Supplemental oxygen should be given with the goal of maintaining oxygen saturation above 90%. Ventilator support may be required in order to protect the airway and ensure adequate oxygenation. End tidal CO_2 should also be monitored. DOT 5-2.177

Intravenous vasopressors such as dopamine, norepinephrine, dobutamine, epinephrine, or isoproterenol may be necessary to maintain adequate blood pressure.[49,50] DOT 5-2.84

- **Dopamine** is the most frequently used vasopressors both in the hospital and on the ambulance, and it is started at a dose of around 15 mcg/kg/min or higher, and titrated to a maximum of 50 mcg/kg/min. Dopamine increases cardiac contractility but leads to vasoconstriction of peripheral vessels and tachycardia and also raises the pulmonary capillary wedge pressure (which can adversely affect cardiac output), so it should be given at the lowest effective dose (Box 29-27).

- **Norepinephrine** is also commonly used in the hospital: An appropriate starting dose is 2–4 mcg/min, and it has similar effects on cardiac contractility, vasoconstriction, and heart rate. Caution should be used as norepinephrine may lead to tissue necrosis if the intravenous line infiltrates.

- **Dobutamine** is sometimes used for severe or refractory cardiogenic shock. It is not considered first-line, single therapy, so it is often used in conjunction with dopamine.[50] It increases cardiac contractility with minimal effect on vasoconstriction or heart rate and is started at 2.5 mcg/kg/min and titrated to a maximum of 25 mcg/kg/min.

- **Epinephrine** and **isoproterenol** infusions are infrequently used. They are potent catecholamine drugs that increase myocardial contractility, but they have systemic side effects that may be undesirable.

Drugs that cause significant vasoconstriction (called positive inotropic agents) must be used with caution. Although they can maintain perfusion by causing vasoconstriction or can improve the pumping force of the heart, they can "overcorrect," which leads to compromised blood flow in tissues when blood flow is reduced because of excessive vasoconstriction. These drugs should be **titrated to effect.** This means the amount of drug used should be just enough to provide the desired therapeutic effect without further compromising tissues. These drugs are given as IV drips, and the use of pumps improves the delivery of the drug to precisely calculated doses. Using several of these drugs together allows for the combined desired effect with the use of less total amount of each drug.

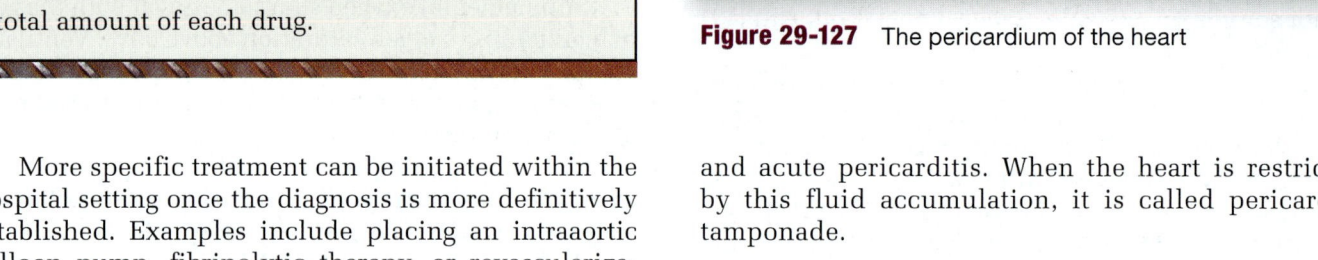

Pericardium overlying the heart

Figure 29-127 The pericardium of the heart

More specific treatment can be initiated within the hospital setting once the diagnosis is more definitively established. Examples include placing an intraaortic balloon pump, fibrinolytic therapy, or revascularization. Compressive etiologies can also be treated, including needle thoracostomy for tension pneumothorax or pericardiocentesis for cardiac tamponade.

Cardiac Tamponade

The pericardium is normally an elastic, double-layered, fibrous sac that encases the heart (Figure 29-127). One layer is attached to the surface of the heart (the visceral pericardium) and is separated from the other layer (the parietal pericardium) by a thin film of pericardial fluid. The pericardium has some elasticity, so when cardiac volumes change, it can expand a little with the heart. There are many conditions in which the pericardium is no longer elastic and capable of accepting changing intracardiac volumes. This can occur in patients with pericarditis, fibrosis, or infiltrative processes that form a thickened and scarred pericardium. The inelastic sac becomes a restrictive force around the heart that can prevent chamber expansion during diastole. DOT 5-2.96, 5-2.97, 5-2.98, 5-2.99

The pericardium can also constrict the heart when excess fluid accumulates between its two layers. The fluid present is called a **pericardial effusion** and may or may not be symptomatic. Pericardial effusions occur in patients with cancer, infections, renal failure, liver failure, congestive heart failure, severe hypothyroidism,

and acute pericarditis. When the heart is restricted by this fluid accumulation, it is called pericardial tamponade.

The volume of fluid, the rate at which it accumulates, and the compliance of the pericardium all determine whether a pericardial effusion causes hemodynamic changes and symptoms of tamponade.

The normal pericardium holds between 15 and 50 mL of fluid. An acute injection of as little as 20 mL can cause tamponade while chronically 500 mL or more can slowly accumulate without hemodynamic compromise. Typically, 100–120 mL of fluid can be added to the pericardial sac without increase in cardiac pressures, provided it accumulates gradually and the patient is not placing high demand upon the cardiovascular system.

When pericardial fluid accumulates at volumes or rates high enough to outweigh the compliance of the pericardial sac, cardiac tamponade occurs. The pericardial fluid acts in similar fashion to a PASG that has been placed around the heart, inhibiting diastolic filling of all chambers. This results in decreased stroke volume and thus decreased cardiac output, hypotension, and reflex tachycardia. Besides impairing forward cardiac output, it increases intracardiac pressures, so systemic venous congestion occurs from increased right heart pressure causing peripheral edema, and pulmonary venous congestion occurs from increased left-sided pressure resulting in pulmonary crackles or rales and hypoxia. Cardiac tamponade can be mildly symptomatic with hypoxia and shortness of breath or may present as cardiogenic shock, leading to death. DOT 5-2.93

The causes of cardiac tamponade overlap with those of pericardial effusion. However, some etiologies are more likely to progress to tamponade physiology. The most common causes of cardiac tamponade are malignant (cancer-induced) effusions, bacteria (including tuberculosis or mycobacteria), fungus, human immunodeficiency virus-associated infections, and bleeding into the pericardial sac known as hemopericardium. Hemopericardium most commonly occurs with trauma and malignancy.[51,52,53]

Common Causes of Pericardial Tamponade

- Malignant (cancer-induced) effusions
- Bacterial (including mycobacteria) or fungal infections
- Human immunodeficiency virus-associated infections
- Bleeding into the pericardial sac (hemopericardium)

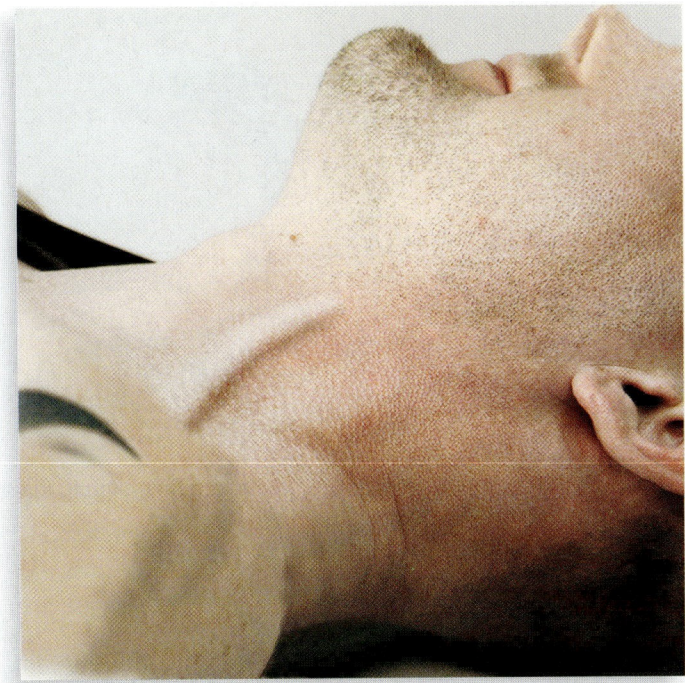

Figure 29-128 To properly assess jugular vein distention, the patient must be in a semi-sitting position.

When a patient presents with pericardial tamponade, they may have mild or severe signs and symptoms, ranging from mild shortness of breath to hypotension and cardiogenic shock. The basis for signs and symptoms associated with tamponade is the physiology of decreased cardiac output and secondarily increased pulmonary and systemic venous congestion.

There are several typical, clinical signs of cardiac tamponade that are important to recognize. Beck's triad is the classic occurrence of jugular venous distension (Figure 29-128), reflecting increased venous pressures from the right heart; hypotension, resulting from decreased cardiac output; and muffled heart tones, secondary to the effect of the excess pericardial fluid. Patients are usually tachycardic as the heart tries to maintain output in the setting of decreased stroke volume. They may have altered mentation levels due to hypotension or hypoxia. These patients frequently have chest pain, and their conditions can be mistaken for acute myocardial infarction.

In the chronic or subacute etiologies of tamponade, presenting symptoms may be subtle: fatigue (reflecting decreased cardiac output), orthopnea or paroxysmal nocturnal dyspnea (reflecting pulmonary venous congestion), and peripheral edema (reflecting venous congestion from right heart failure). The pain from pericarditis is sometimes positional, relieved by leaning forward and worsened with swallowing or breathing deeply, both of which mechanically tug on the pericardium.

In general, the jugular veins are evaluated for distension with patients sitting up at at least a 45° angle (see Figure 29-128). Patients with signs of shock, however, should not be elevated in order to check for JVD but rather should be kept in the supine position.

In addition to the basic history and physical exam findings in patients with cardiac tamponade, there are some stereotypical clinical findings often associated with the process. **Pulsus paradoxus** is a cyclic decrease in systolic blood pressure during the inspiratory phase of respiration. When normal patients inspire, intrathoracic pressure is negative, so air may easily enter the lungs. This negative pressure also increases venous return to the right heart. When the right heart fills with blood during inspiration, the intraventricular septum shifts slightly into the left ventricle, making room for the increased right heart volume. The flexible myocardium and surrounding pericardium allow the left ventricle to expand slightly away from the septum to maintain normal left ventricular volume and pressure. Even in this normal situation, there is a slight decrease in left ventricular filling in diastole during inspiration. Stroke volume is diminished, as is blood pressure. This normal physiologic process is exaggerated in cardiac tamponade because the left ventricle cannot expand outward due to pericardial restriction when the right heart fills with its increased volume during inspiration. As a result, the filling volume of the left ventricle is even less than in the normal setting, leading to an even lower stroke volume and systolic blood pressure during inspiration. DOT 5-2.100, 5-2.169, 5-2.170

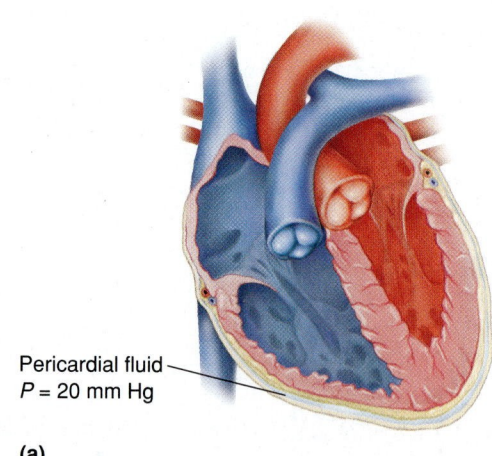

(a)

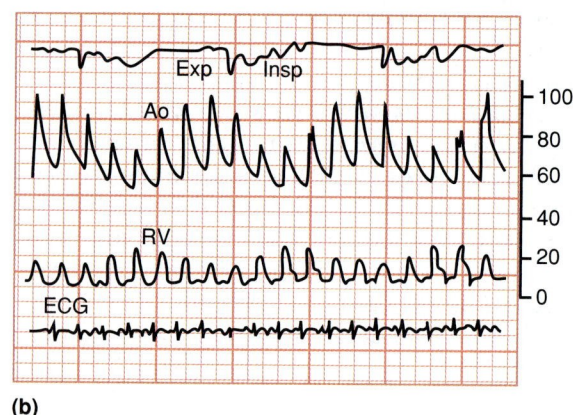

(b)

Figure 29-129 Pulsus paradoxus. (a) Fluid accumulating in the pericardial space. (b) Graph showing the drop in blood pressure during inspiration.

Pulsus Paradoxus

Criteria: difference of *10 mmHg* in systolic blood pressures between inspiration and expiration

Pulsus paradoxus is measured using a sphygmomanometer on the arm, but the cuff needs to be deflated more slowly than usual. During deflation, the first Korotkoff sounds are audible only during expiration (when left ventricular stroke volume is higher). With further deflation, Korotkoff sounds are heard throughout the respiratory cycle.

The difference between the systolic pressure at which the first Korotkoff sounds are heard during expiration and the pressure at which they are heard throughout the respiratory cycle quantifies pulsus paradoxus (Figure 29-129). A difference of more than 10 mmHg is the typical cutoff for defining pulsus paradoxus. It should be noted that pulsus paradoxus can also occur in severe asthma, COPD flare-ups, and pulmonary embolism.

Pulsus alternans is an alternating peripheral pulse amplitude occasionally seen in patients with cardiac tamponade. However, it usually signifies a failing left ventricle, and the mechanism behind pulsus alternans is not fully understood. DOT 5-2.100

The ECG can be helpful in diagnosing cardiac effusion and tamponade. **Electrical alternans** is a very specific finding but is not sensitive for pericardial effusion with tamponade. It is caused by an anterior-posterior swinging motion of the heart with each heartbeat inside the fluid-filled pericardial sac, another mechanism that is not well-understood.[54] A low-amplitude ECG is also frequently present in pericardial effusion and tamponade but can be present in any condition that increases the distance between the ECG leads and the myocardium (e.g., COPD, obesity, etc). Cardiac tamponade causing pulseless electrical activity (PEA) is usually associated with a narrow complex tachycardia on the ECG. Echocardiography, not available to most EMS providers, can clearly show a pericardial effusion and the diastolic collapse of the right atrium and ventricle in cardiac tamponade.

For patients *in pulseless electrical activity*, think of *tamponade* as the cause.

The only therapy for reversal of cardiac tamponade is drainage of the excess pericardial fluid. This is usually done in the cardiac catheterization lab; however, it rarely needs to be done emergently in the field, depending on patient condition and local protocols (Figure 29-130). It is frequently a final maneuver prior to discontinuing resuscitation efforts in patients with traumatic cardiac arrest. DOT 5-2.101, 5-2.171

The responsibility of EMS providers to patients with suspected pericardial tamponade is primarily rapid transportation to a facility where pericardiocentesis can

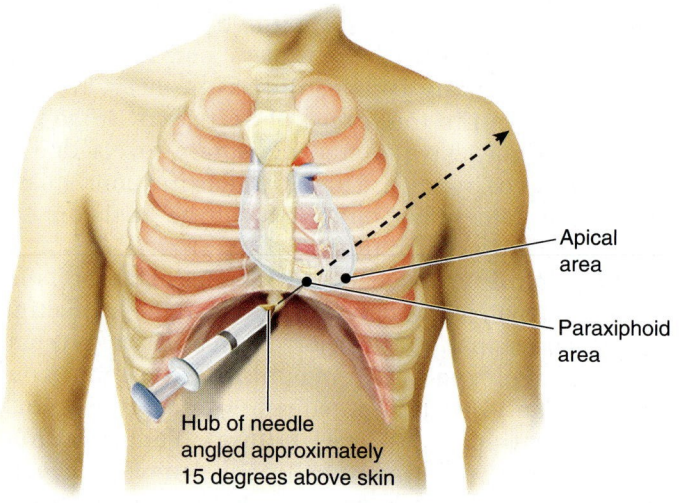

Figure 29-130 Pericardiocentesis drains excess pericardial fluid.

be performed. Intravenous fluids should be given to support the low filling volumes of the heart in patients who are hypovolemic. Inotropic support is controversial in this patient population, though dobutamine is theoretically the ideal agent in hypotensive patients. Mechanical ventilation (for example, with a bag-mask) should be avoided, if possible, in known cases of cardiac tamponade because it can further decrease stroke volume and can worsen hypotension. External cardiac compression is usually of minimal help in patients with cardiac arrest secondary to cardiac tamponade because there is very little additional room for ventricular filling.[54] DOT 5-2.101

Pacemakers

When the heart's intrinsic, automatic, electrical mechanism is compromised or ineffective, a cardiac pacemaker is required. Pacemakers can be either temporary or permanent, depending on the situation. Temporary pacemakers can be placed externally on the chest wall (transcutaneous) or placed internally through a vein (transvenous). In transcutaneous pacing, electrical current is passed from an external pulse generator through large pacing electrodes applied to the patient's chest. These electrodes are placed in the same location as for defibrillation, in the anterior/posterior position or the RA/LL (apex/sternum) configuration. Actual placement may be dictated through convenience and patient position. DOT 5-2.55

Transcutaneous pacing is based on the principle that an electrical current applied to a myocardial muscle cell during a susceptible period will result in the activation or stimulation of that cell, and rhythmic depolarization will ensue. Studies of pacing have shown that in the human heart, the ventricles depolarize, with atrial depolarization occurring in a retrograde pattern. Since "atrial kick" is lost in this case, cardiac output will suffer by a factor of around 20% during pacing. The heart rate for pacing should be set at a rate consistent with normal ranges for the patient's age group. The current should be started lower, around 10–20 milliamps, and increased until capture is obtained. Capture occurs when the ECG tracing rate matches the heart rate as palpated in the carotid or radial artery (Box 29-28).

BOX 29-28   Pacing and Asystole

In the case of asystole, it is recommended to move quickly to maximal energy to prevent delays in definitive care. Current AHA ACLS guidelines recommend pacing for asystole only when the onset of asystole is witnessed.

Guidelines for implantation of cardiac pacemakers have been established by a task force formed jointly by the American College of Cardiology, the American Heart Association, and the North American Society for Pacing and Electrophysiology (ACC/AHA/NASPE).[55,56] These guidelines are based on current evidence for the benefit of placement of cardiac pacemakers. Although these guidelines apply to permanent pacemakers, the conditions for which they are indicated are applicable to a patient in the field in need of transcutaneous pacing.

The conditions for which a pacemaker is definitely indicated are:

- Third-degree or advanced second-degree atrioventricular (AV) block. There is controversy over pacemaker placement in asymptomatic patients Second- or third-degree blocks can arise from many disorders.
- Following AMI when there is persistent second-degree AV block in the His-Purkinje system with bilateral bundle branch block or third-degree AV block within or below the His-Purkinje system, transient advanced infranodal AV block and associated bundle branch block, and persistent and symptomatic second- or third-degree AV block.
- Symptomatic Mobitz II AV block.
- Symptomatic Mobitz I AV block.
- Symptomatic sinus bradycardia in which the symptoms are clearly related to the bradycardia. The most significant symptoms include syncope, seizures, congestive heart failure, dizziness, or confusion in patients with a heart rate below 40 beats/minute.

In addition, there are multiple other conditions for which a pacemaker may be indicated, but the supporting evidence is either lacking or shows a less clear benefit. Thus, in general, a patient is in need of a pacemaker when a faulty electrical system in the heart causes ineffective mechanical functioning, leading to a decreased cardiac output. This can manifest itself in a patient as subjective lightheadedness, confusion, weakness, or even syncope. In addition to these symptoms, the signs that a patient may need a pacemaker may include bradycardia, hypotension, or congestive heart failure. When these symptoms are found in association with the above ECG indications, placement of a cardiac pacemaker may be the essential component of a treatment plan.

Heart Failure

Congestive heart failure (CHF) is the common clinical syndrome for many cardiac diseases that result in inadequate cardiac output. There are many causes, including ischemic coronary artery disease (heart attack, necrosis, scarring), valvular heart disease, hypertension, congenital cardiac malformations, and the various cardiomyopathies (infiltrative, restrictive, and dilated). Because heart failure is a common endpoint for so many cardiac diseases, nearly 5 million Americans have this diagnosis today, and it accounts for at least 20% of hospital admissions in patients older than 65.[57,58] These numbers are increasing due to the aging population and the ability to prolong survival of cardiac patients. Nearly 75% of patients with heart failure are older than 65 to 70 years of age, and 8% of patients between 75 and 86 years old have heart failure. Heart failure is thus the leading cause of hospitalization in the geriatric age group.[59,60] In addition to its high prevalence, congestive heart failure is quite lethal. Mortality rates for patients with congestive heart failure are about 18% and 55% at one and five years, respectively, from time of diagnosis.[58,61,62] DOT 5-2.85, 5-2.86, 5-2.87, 5-2.88

The American College of Cardiology/American Heart Association Guidelines (ACC/AHA) define heart failure as a "complex clinical syndrome that can result from any structural or functional cardiac disorder that impairs the ability of the ventricle to fill with or eject blood."[63] The clinical effects of heart failure are manifest when the heart cannot pump sufficient blood to the organs to meet their metabolic demands or when abnormally high filling pressures are needed to do so. Emergency medical personnel see many clinical presentations of heart failure, demonstrating how complex the disease truly has become. Signs and symptoms are commonly a result of intravascular and interstitial volume overload and include shortness of breath, lung crackles or rales, and peripheral edema. Other clinical presentations result from tissue underperfusion and include renal insufficiency, dyspnea, easy fatigability, angina, and poor exercise tolerance.

Pathophysiology of Heart Failure

Heart failure has multiple pathophysiologic mechanisms (Figure 29-131). As described previously, cardiac output is the end product of several individual components, and heart failure results when cardiac output is insufficient to meet the body's metabolic demands. Therefore, preload impairment, poor contractility, or high afterload can all decrease stroke volume and cause heart failure. Failure can occur in the left, right, or both ventricles. Left heart failure is more common. Most principles associated with left-sided heart failure also pertain to right-sided failure.

Heart failure is grouped into two categories: systolic and diastolic dysfunction. Decreased contractility or increased afterload results in the inability of the left ventricle to eject its normal stroke volume and is known as *systolic dysfunction*. By contrast, if the left ventricle does not fill properly, if, for example, it is too stiff, *diastolic dysfunction* and shortness of breath result.

Systolic Failure

Two-thirds of patients with heart failure have systolic failure.[64] A major contributor to systolic heart failure is impaired contractility (Figure 29-132). Decreased contractility frequently results from either myocyte loss or decreased function of remaining myocytes, as occurs in myocardial infarction and ischemia. Other causes of myocyte death and dysfunction include myocarditis (inflammation of the heart) and toxins affecting the myocardium. Decreased contractility also occurs with chronic volume overload in conditions such as aortic and mitral valve insufficiency or valve leakage. In these cases, the forward blood flow for each stroke is decreased. Subsequently, the blood volume that did not go "forward" to the body returns to the ventricle (aortic insufficiency) or left atrium (mitral insufficiency) and causes a larger volume than normal in the respective chambers. This results in a chronically elevated end diastolic volume and pressure in the ventricle, which further decreases contractility.

Systolic failure also results from increases in afterload. A balloon can be used to illustrate the concept. If the balloon neck is pinched off, significantly more

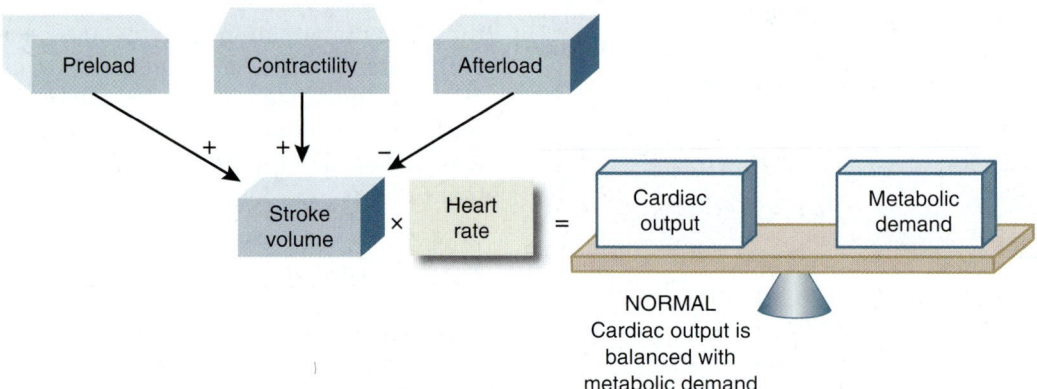

Figure 29-131   Contributors to cardiac output. Increased preload and contractility increase stroke volume; increased afterload decreases stroke volume. Cardiac output is the product of stroke volume and heart rate.

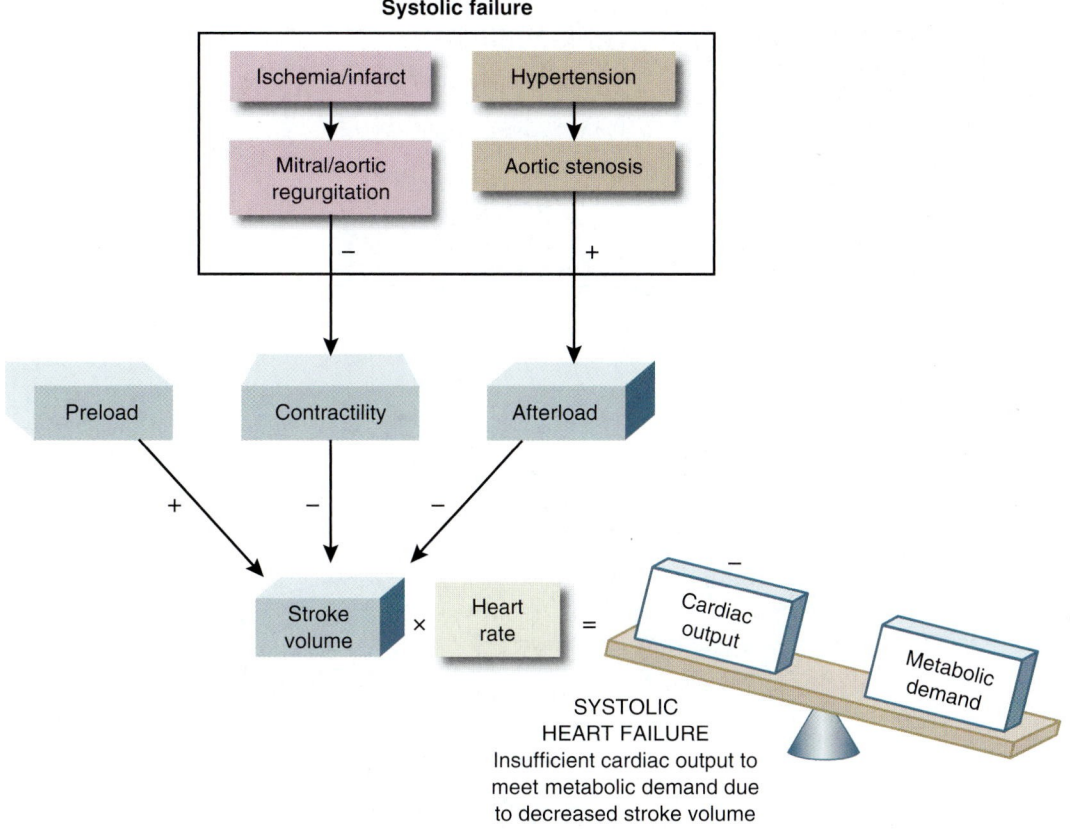

Systolic failure

Figure 29-132 Contributors to systolic heart failure. By decreasing contractility and increasing afterload, these mechanisms decrease stroke volume.

pressure is needed to expel the air. Similarly, if the left ventricle is pumping against a narrowed or stenotic aortic valve, it must generate higher pressures to eject the same amount of blood. If the balloon neck is taped with a narrow, noncompliant drinking straw as its exit, increased pressure is also needed to eject blood. Similarly, hypertension causes stiff and noncompliant arteries that also act to increase afterload.

Diastolic Failure

The less common (and less intuitive) heart failure is *diastolic dysfunction,* which occurs due to either impaired ventricular relaxation or a stiffened left ventricle (Figure 29-133). In either case, there is insufficient ventricular volume to accept blood at the end of diastole, either because it is slow to relax or because it is stiff and cannot fully relax. Diastolic dysfunction occurs both acutely as in an ischemic ventricle and in cases of pericardial tamponade. Diastolic dysfunction also occurs chronically in hypertrophied ventricles, from chronic hypertension, and in hypertrophic cardiomyopathy. Stiff ventricles also result with infiltrative cardiomyopathies such as amyloidosis or sarcoidosis or in a ventricle restricted from expanding by pericarditis.[64]

Each of these conditions increases the end diastolic pressure of the ventricle, which is transferred back into the left atrium and eventually into the venous beds of the lungs, causing symptoms of diastolic heart failure.

Right-Sided Heart Failure

The most common cause of right-sided heart failure is left-sided heart failure.

Right-sided heart failure has similar pathophysiologic mechanisms to left-sided failure but with some differences. Differences typically result from the thin muscular wall of the right ventricle compared with that of the left. The RV has a thinner wall than the LV because it pumps against a pulmonary system with significantly lower pressure than that of the systemic circulation. As a result, mild increases in pulmonary pressures cause right ventricular strain. The most common cause of increased pulmonary pressures, and subsequently the most common cause of right heart failure, is left-sided heart failure. The pressure backup from the left side of the heart is transmitted through the pulmonary system and ultimately into the right ventricle.

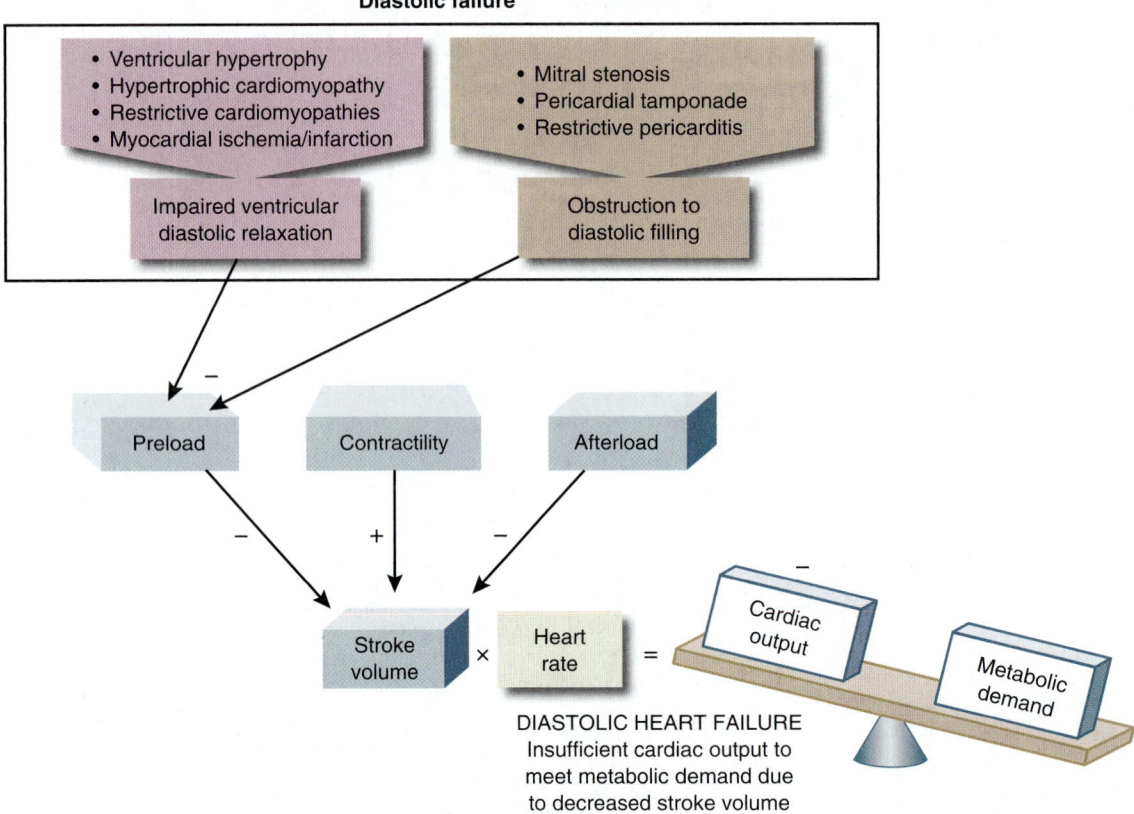

Figure 29-133 Contributors to diastolic heart failure. When on the physiologic portion of the Frank-Starling curve, preload is beneficial to stroke volume. Therefore, impaired ventricular relaxation during diastole, or obstructed blood flow into the ventricle, results in decreased preload and subsequently decreased stroke volume.

Right-sided heart failure can also occur with normally functioning left ventricles. In these cases, there is usually an intrinsic pulmonary disease such as pulmonary fibrosis, primary pulmonary hypertension, pulmonary embolism, interstitial lung diseases, COPD, or acute respiratory distress syndrome (ARDS) that increases afterload on the right ventricle.

Right-sided failure secondary to an intrinsic pulmonary etiology is referred to as cor pulmonale. Right-sided valvular abnormalities (e.g., pulmonary valve stenosis, tricuspid regurgitation) can cause right heart failure similar to the effect of their left-sided counterparts.

In the failing left ventricle, the left atrium and subsequently the pulmonary vasculature receive increased pressures. On the right side of the heart, a failing right ventricle transmits its increased pressure and volume to the right atrium and to the systemic venous return through the superior and inferior vena cavae. Just as left-sided failure results in pulmonary edema, right-sided failure results in peripheral edema.

While the right ventricle suffers from a failing left ventricle, the opposite is also true. The preload of the left ventricle relies heavily on the volume of blood pumped through the pulmonary system by the right ventricle (right ventricular stroke volume). As right ventricular stroke volume decreases, left-sided preload and subsequently cardiac output also decrease. In the case of a massive pulmonary embolism, the right ventricle is unable to pump a sufficient amount of blood into the new high-pressure pulmonary system, or in a large right ventricular infarct, where contractility is significantly impaired, left ventricular preload can be severely depressed, resulting in decreased stroke volume and hypotension. DOT 5-2.90

The Body's Response to Heart Failure

Systolic and diastolic dysfunction can remain silent for many years before the patient presents with clinical heart failure. This is due to the body's multiple complex compensatory mechanisms to accommodate systolic and diastolic dysfunction. The first mechanism results from the Frank-Starling relationship (see again Figure 29-113). As ventricular volumes and pressures rise because the ventricle cannot fully eject its blood volume, preload increases, and so does stroke volume. However, this relationship has a limit, occurring when the positive effects of increasing end diastolic pressure do not improve stroke volume and in fact become detrimental, with excess blood backing up into the pulmonary and systemic venous systems, with left and right heart failure respectively. DOT 5-2.166, 5-2.167

The second adaptation in heart failure is ventricular hypertrophy. This adaptation is helpful early on as it provides additional contractility and increases stroke volume. However, one reason for diastolic dysfunction is a thick, hypertrophied ventricle. Eventually, the detrimental effect that hypertrophy has on diastolic function outweighs the benefit it has on contractility, further adding to the pathophysiology of congestive heart failure. DOT 5-2.91

The third heart failure adaptation mechanism of the body is also the most complex. It is an orchestra of hormonal signals, each playing different roles, but each also unaware of the detriment they cause. The first major hormonal response to heart failure is sympathetic nervous outflow that results when carotid artery baroreceptors do not sense sufficient blood pressure from the failing heart. They, in turn, rapidly increase sympathetic tone via release of the hormone norepinephrine, resulting in increased contractility, increased heart rate, and increased vasoconstriction (returning more blood to the heart and increasing preload). Sympathetic activation also increases arterial constriction, which elevates blood pressure.

The next compensatory mechanism is from the kidneys. They are activated by the sensing of inadequate blood pressure from the failing heart and are stimulated by sympathetic hormones. They are also activated when they do not sense enough blood chloride. This mechanism is called the **renin-angiotensin system** and it involves the conversion of angiotensin I to angiotensin II via angiotensin converting enzyme (ACE). Angiotensin II is a potent vasoconstrictor that also increases sodium absorption and triggers thirst. These mechanisms all increase preload and thus improve stroke volume for a period of time. The third major hormonal adaptive mechanism is the release of antidiuretic hormone (ADH). ADH increases the amount of water the kidney retains and thus also increases preload.

These compensatory mechanisms are helpful early on in heart failure, but as heart failure severity outweighs compensation, the mechanisms actually worsen heart failure and its associated symptoms. The effects of increased sympathetic tone via norepinephrine on heart rate causes increased metabolic demands on an already fatigued heart. The vasoconstrictive effect of norepinephrine returns more blood to the heart than it can adequately move forward through the circulation, resulting in backup into the lungs and congestion. Arterial vasoconstriction provides more afterload for the already weakened heart to pump

against. Angiotensin II and ADH result in similar problems.

Acute Pulmonary Edema

A common life-threatening heart failure presentation is flash or acute pulmonary edema. This is a rapid fluid increase within the pulmonary interstitium and alveoli, resulting in rapid onset of shortness of breath, hypoxia, pulmonary rales, a "frothy" cough, and usually tachycardia with hypertension. Hypotension in this setting may be a sign of profound cardiac failure. DOT 5-2.89, 5-2.94

The causes of flash pulmonary edema are many; however, the most frequent cause is myocardial ischemia that leads to a stiff left ventricle (diastolic dysfunction) that has poor contractility as well (systolic dysfunction). This results in increased intracardiac pressure that is transmitted back to the lungs, causing pulmonary edema. The acute onset of aortic insufficiency or mitral insufficiency can also lead to an acute increase in left ventricular and left atrial pressures that transmit to the pulmonary system as well cause pulmonary edema. Acute valvular insufficiency can be caused by ischemia, valve chordae tendineae rupture, or trauma such as an aortic dissection.[65] Treatment of acute pulmonary edema in the field involves placing the patient in an upright position to decrease venous return to the already overloaded heart; supplemental oxygen with noninvasive positive pressure ventilation, if needed (CPAP); intravenous diuretics, if available; nitrates to reduce venous return to the heart by way of vasodilation; occasionally inotropic agents (such as dopamine or dobutamine) in cases of cardiogenic shock with hypotension; and lastly intravenous morphine sulfate to decrease venous return, dilate coronary blood supply, decrease anxiety, and decrease the work of breathing. Ultimately, treatment is aimed at the underlying cause of the acute increase in intracardiac pressures that leads to the flash pulmonary edema.[65,66] DOT 5-2.95

Treatment for Acute Pulmonary Edema

- Patient in upright position
- Oxygen
- Diuretics
- Nitrates
- Morphine
- Inotropic agents

While many patients live comfortably with "compensated" heart failure, there are several triggers for other exacerbations of heart failure. These are shown in Figure 29-134.

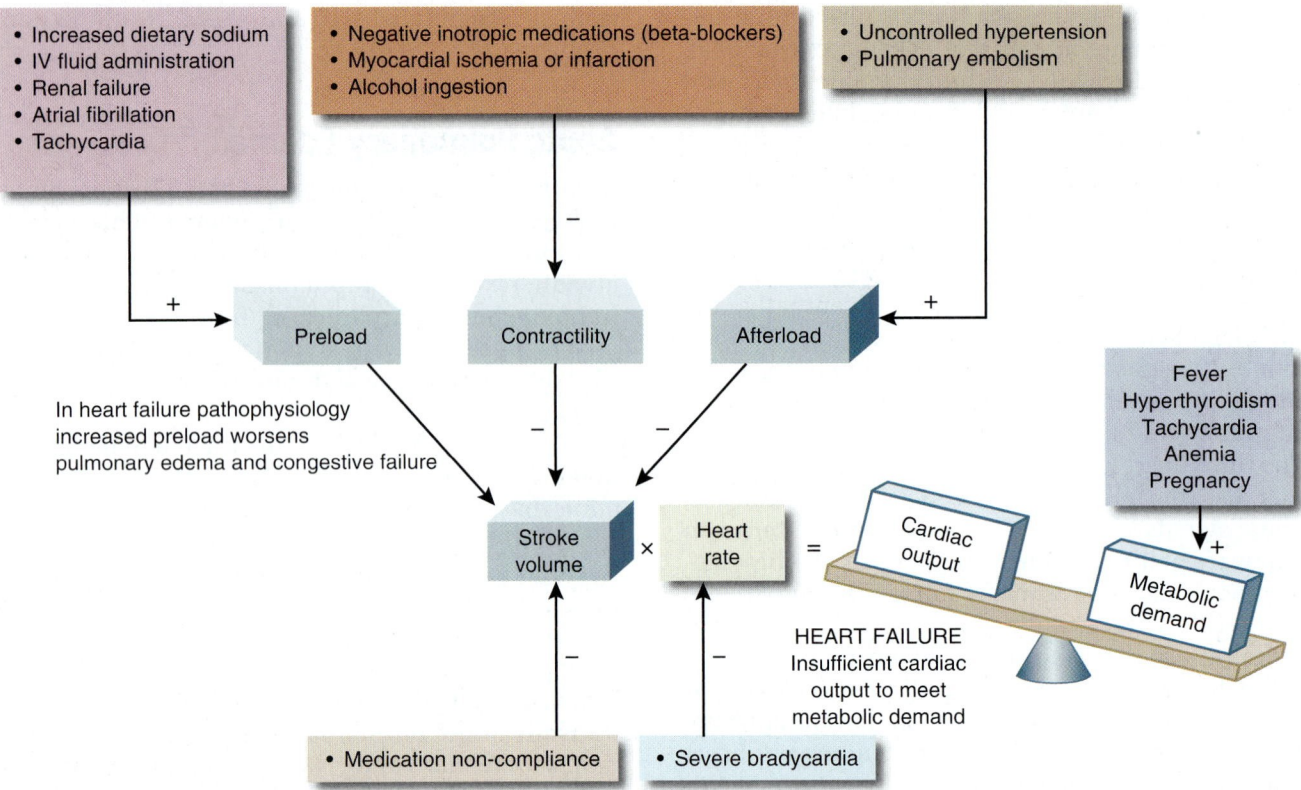

Figure 29-134   Contributors to exacerbations of congestive heart failure. Note that once a patient is in congestive heart failure, the goal is to decrease preload to a level that returns him or her to the physiologic portion of the Frank-Starling curve. Increased preload in the failing heart worsens symptoms of heart failure and does not provide any additional contractile stimulus.

Other Signs and Symptoms of Heart Failure

The common symptoms of heart failure are shown in Table 29-2. The mechanism for most signs and symptoms is intuitive from the pathophysiology discussed above. Shortness of breath is a common chief complaint. There are two frequently asked questions to patients presenting with possible congestive heart failure that can help confirm a cardiac etiology for their shortness of breath:

- "Do you wake up at night gasping for air and have to sit up in bed to catch your breath?" (This indicates paroxysmal nocturnal dyspnea.) DOT 5-2.92
- "Do you have to sleep on multiple pillows or put phonebooks under the head of your bed to avoid being short of breath?" (This indicates orthopnea.)

TABLE 29-2   Signs and Symptoms of Left- and Right-Sided Heart Failure

	Signs	Symptoms
Left-sided failure	Lung crackles/rales Extra heart sounds: S_3 (dilated cardiomyopathy), S_4 (diastolic failure) Diaphoresis Tachypnea Tachycardia	Dyspnea Orthopnea Paroxysmal nocturnal dyspnea Fatigue Palpitations (in patients with dysrhythmias)
Right-sided failure	Bowel distention Hepatomegaly Peripheral edema Elevated jugular venous pressure	Anorexia Right upper quadrant pain

These are two common presenting symptoms in patients who have excess venous return (preload), which the heart cannot handle when they are supine. This results in a backup of blood into the pulmonary system, in turn causing shortness of breath that is typically relieved by sitting up and subsequently decreasing venous return (preload) to the heart.

Treatment of Heart Failure

The goal of heart failure therapy is to improve survival, alleviate symptoms, and slow progression of the disease process. Targets for systolic heart failure therapy are aimed at the neurohormonal compensatory mechanisms discussed above. The hospital treatment of heart failure is first and foremost to correct the underlying etiology, if possible, which includes angioplasty and coronary artery bypass for ischemic failure, replacement of stenotic or insufficient valves, or decreasing blood pressure in hypertensive patients. While some therapy overlaps between systolic and diastolic heart failure, this section will focus on treatment of systolic failure.

Common prehospital treatment for systolic heart failure therapy includes oxygen, ECG monitoring, rapid transport, and cardiovascular support. Drugs may include diuretics, vasodilators, cardiac glycosides, beta-adrenergic agonists, and beta-adrenergic antagonists (beta-blockers). DOT 5-2.84

When the renin-angiotensin system and ADH are activated in heart failure, it leads to the retention of sodium and water. Loop diuretics such as furosemide and bumetanide are the primary drugs of choice for counteracting this detrimental compensatory mechanism because eventually, the heart cannot handle the increase in intravascular volume and preload that results from increased water and sodium retention.

Intracardiac pressures increase to the point where pulmonary edema occurs from the backup of fluid into the lungs. Diuretics act by inhibiting sodium and water reabsorption at the kidney, thus decreasing the volume overload and intracardiac pressures. Thiazide diuretics are also used with a similar effect; however, they are not primary diuretics. A major concern with loop diuretics is the risk for hypokalemia; therefore, patients are typically on potassium replacement in combination with their diuretic. Aldosterone antagonists such as spironolactone offer an alternative medication that specifically blocks the mechanism of ADH at the kidneys and promotes diuresis *without* the loss of potassium. This diuretic class is called potassium sparing diuretics. DOT 5-2.95, 5-2.168

Treatment of Congestive Heart Failure

- Diuretics
- Vasodilators
- Cardiac glycosides
- Beta-adrenergic agonists
- Beta-adrenergic antagonists (beta-blockers)

Another group of medications, the vasodilators, decrease preload on the overloaded ventricle but also have other effects. When the venous bed is vasodilated, less blood is returned to the heart, preload is decreased, and intracardiac pressures are also decreased, resulting in less pulmonary congestion from the overloaded heart. The most common example of vasodilators that act primarily on the venous system are the nitrates such as nitroglycerin. There are also vasodilators that act primarily on the arterial system (e.g., hydralazine). Their beneficial effect in heart failure comes through a decrease in afterload on the struggling left ventricle, allowing improved cardiac output. Additionally, angiotensin-converting enzyme inhibitors (ACE inhibitors) and angiotensin receptor blockers (ARBs) act as vasodilators on both the arterial and venous systems. These medications also play a beneficial role in the inhibition of sodium and water retention due to angiotensin. DOT 5-2.95, 5-2.168

Loss of contractile function in systolic CHF is a major contributor to worsening symptoms and progression of the disease. Therefore, the next logical target for pharmacotherapy is to increase ventricular contractile force. This type of medication is referred to as an inotropic agent (an agent that increases contractile force) in contrast to a chronotropic agent (an agent that increases heart rate). Digoxin, a cardiac glycoside, is the classic inotropic agent. It increases cardiac output and shifts the Frank-Starling curve upwards (Figure 29-113).

Digoxin toxicity can occur; therefore, serum digoxin concentrations are typically monitored, especially in patients with renal insufficiency. Common signs of toxicity include ectopic junctional and ventricular beats or escape rhythms, bradycardia, an excessively slow ventricular rate response to atrial fibrillation, and atrioventricular conduction blocks. The bradycardic effects of digoxin toxicity usually respond to atropine, but temporary pacing is also a treatment for refractory cases.[67]

Other examples of medications that increase contractility are beta adrenergic agonists. These medications act to stimulate the beta receptors similar to activation of the heart and vasculature by the sympathetic nervous system.[68] They are typically used over the short term for acute decompensated CHF, are given intravenously, and do not only increase inotropy, but are chronotropic agents as well. Common examples include dobutamine, dopamine, epinephrine, and norepinephrine.

Juxtaposed to the beta adrenergic *agonists* that are used in *acute* decompensated heart failure to increase inotropy and chronotropy, the beta adrenergic *antagonists* (also known as beta-blockers) are a mainstay of therapy in *chronic* heart failure. It may seem counterintuitive to decrease the sympathetic stimulation of norepinephrine on the heart in CHF; however, similar to the other compensatory mechanisms the body has to deal with in heart failure, too much sympathetic stimulation of the heart with norepinephrine can be toxic to the myocardium. In addition, the oxygen requirement of the myocardium increases as sympathetic stimulation rises.[69] When used in patients with heart failure, beta-blockers have been shown to increase cardiac function, decrease progression of cardiac dysfunction, and increase survival.[70,71,72,73] The main beta-blockers are metoprolol, atenolol, bisoprolol, and carvedilol. Side effects of beta-blockers include bradycardia and worsening of AV nodal blocks. They may also increase depressive symptoms, fatigue, and sexual dysfunction.[74] Beta-blockers have been shown to decrease bronchodilation and potentially worsen reactive airway disease, as well as worsen hypoglycemia in patients with diabetes.[75,76,77] However, recent studies have shown these side effects are much less likely with the current selective beta$_1$-blockers such as metoprolol, atenolol, bisoprolol, and carvedilol than in the nonselective beta-blockers such as propranolol.[78,79,80,81] Do note that while treatment with beta-blockers may result in side effects, abrupt discontinuation of beta-blockers may cause serious complications such as worsening ischemia, infarction, and even death.[82,83,84,85]

Hypertensive Emergencies

A frequent precipitant of acute congestive heart failure and pulmonary edema is acute hypertension. Hypertensive emergency is an acute, marked elevation in blood pressure that results in damage to vital organs, and is therefore life-threatening. By contrast, hypertensive urgency refers to a marked elevation in blood pressure without the end-organ damage. These end-organ effects will be discussed below. DOT 5-2.102, 5-2.103

Those at risk include patients with long-standing uncontrolled hypertension, especially those who may have abruptly discontinued treatment. Patients with renal artery stenosis may be at-risk for this, as are pregnant patients with preeclampsia. DOT 5-2.104, 5-2.107

Hypertensive Emergencies: Risk Factors

- Long-standing HTN
- Uncontrolled HTN
- Abrupt discontinuation of treatment
- Renal artery stenosis
- Pregnant patients with preeclampsia

Even with effective treatment of hypertension, its effects on blood vessels, kidney function, and survival are still significant. Blood vessel damage puts patients at higher risk for future coronary, cerebrovascular, and renal disease. Survival rates are significantly reduced, especially in those with renal insufficiency.

Pathophysiology of Hypertensive Conditions

With mild to moderate increases in blood pressure an autoregulatory response is activated, resulting in arterial and arteriolar vasoconstriction. This process maintains consistent tissue perfusion and prevents the higher pressures from damaging the smaller distal blood vessels.

However, as blood pressure increases, this regulatory mechanism is overwhelmed, and the rise in pressure results in endothelial injury in the arterioles and capillaries. This injury allows vascular contents to infiltrate the endothelium, eventually narrowing and occluding the blood vessel. Following failure of the vasoconstrictive regulation, dilation of these arterioles and capillaries within the brain leads to cerebral edema and the clinical signs of hypertensive encephalopathy. DOT 5-2.106, 5-2.109

Sustained hypertension results in chronic hypertrophy of vascular endothelium, effectively narrowing the lumen. In settings of sudden, acute changes in blood pressure, these already narrowed vessels are then predisposed to complete occlusion.

Clincal Features of Hypertensive Conditions

Malignant hypertension is severely elevated blood pressure (diastolic blood pressure greater than 100 mmHg) with retinal hemorrhages, retinal exudates, and papilledema. Malignant nephrosclerosis (hardening of kidney tissues) can lead to acute renal failure, hematuria (blood in the urine), and proteinuria (protein in the urine). Continued damage to the kidney can potentially result in worsening of the hypertension. DOT 5-2.105, 5-2.108, 5-2.111

Hypertensive Emergencies: Clinical Features

- Marked blood pressure elevation
- Retinal hemorrhage, retinal exudates, and papilledema
- Renal failure, low urine output
- Encephalopathy: headache, confusion, restlessness

Uncontrolled malignant hypertension can result in intracerebral or subarachnoid bleeding as well as cerebral infarcts. Hypertensive encephalopathy can occur from cerebral edema. It is characterized by gradual onset of headache, nausea, vomiting, confusion, and restlessness. If left untreated, this can lead to seizures and coma. In contrast to the gradual onset and nonlocalizing signs of hypertensive encephalopathy, cerebral hemorrhages or strokes typically have an abrupt onset of focal neurologic findings.

Treatment of Hypertensive Conditions

The treatment goal in hypertensive emergency is to reduce the diastolic blood pressure (DBP) to about 100–105 mmHg over the first two to six hours. The initial drop in blood pressure should not exceed 25% in order to prevent too low pressures to vital organs, leading to ischemia or infarct. Once initially controlled, oral anti-hypertensive therapy should be directed to gradually reduce DBP to around 85–90 mmHg over the next two to three months. DOT 5-2.172, 5-2.173, 5-2.174

Nitroprusside is perhaps the most effective medication for treatment of hypertensive emergencies, dilating both arterioles and veins, but is difficult to prepare and is not commonly used in the field. The onset of action is very rapid (within seconds), and its duration of action lasts for approximately two to five minutes. Blood pressure must be closely monitored, but because of its short duration of action, the risk of hypotension is much less than with longer acting medications (see Drug Box 29-1).

The most significant drawback to nitroprusside use is its metabolism to cyanide. Cyanide toxicity can result in clinical deterioration, altered mental status, and lactic acidosis and is potentially fatal. It can, however, be prevented by limiting the use of nitroprusside to the lowest necessary dose for short periods of time. The recommended starting dose for nitroprusside is 0.25–0.5 mcg/kg/min, with a maximal dose of 10 mcg/kg/min. High or maximal doses should be used for less than 10 minutes to prevent cyanide toxicity, and nitroprusside should not be used in pregnant women. DOT 5-2.110

Nitroglycerin acts in a manner similar to nitroprusside, except that it preferentially dilates veins over arterioles and does not carry the risk of cyanide toxicity (Drug Box 29-1). It is most useful in hypertensive patients with coronary artery disease and in those who have had coronary artery bypass surgery. The most common adverse effects are headache (a product of vasodilation) and reflex tachycardia. Onset of action is two to five minutes, and its effects last five to ten minutes. The initial IV drip dose is usually 5 mcg/min, with a maximal dose of 10 mcg/min. DOT 5-2.110

Labetalol blocks both alpha and beta adrenergic receptors (Drug Box 29-1). It acts rapidly—within five minutes—and is therefore the only beta-blocker useful in this setting. Labetalol can be given as bolus doses or as an infusion. Typically, an initial 10–20 mg bolus is given, then an additional 10–80 mg every 10 minutes as needed for adequate blood pressure control, to a maximum total of 300 mg. Alternatively, an infusion can be maintained between 0.5–2 mg/min. Labetalol should be avoided in patients with congestive heart failure, bradycardia, heart block, or asthma or chronic obstructive lung disease. DOT 5-2.110

Other medications can be used in hypertensive emergencies but are either less commonly used or fall outside of the scope of this text. These include nicardipine, fenoldopam, esmolol, enalaprilat, and phentolamine.

Vascular Disease

The heart plays the central role in the cardiovascular system; however, the vascular portion of this system's name is just as important. Vascular disease encompasses diseases of large arteries and veins of the thorax, abdomen, and vessels in the extremities. This section discusses disorders of the aorta and the peripheral arterial system, with a brief discussion of venous disorders that often present similarly to arterial disease.

Diseases of the Aorta

The aorta is the largest artery in the human body, carrying blood from the heart to the vital organs and the peripheral circulation. It is a strong and dynamic artery that is able to withstand the demands of carrying some 200 million liters of blood over the course of an entire lifetime.

CONNECTIONS Refer to Chapter 7: Anatomy Overview for more on the aorta.

The aorta is composed of three layers of tissue (Figure 29-135). The innermost layer is the tunica intima, a thin layer of tissue encased by a thicker layer of muscle and connective tissue called the tunica media. The media is further encased by a fibrous tissue layer called the tunica adventitia. Aortic strength is attributed largely to

Drug Box 29-1   Treatment for Hypertensive Emergencies

Medication	Mechanism of Action	Dosing	Limitations
Nitroprusside	Dilates arterioles and veins	0.25–0.5 mcg/kg/min	Causes cyanide toxicity
Nitroglycerin	Dilates veins	5 mcg/min	Headache, reflex tachycardia
Labetalol	Alpha- and beta-blocker	10–20 mg bolus, then 10–80 mg every 10 min or 0.5–2 mg/min infusion	Patients with CHF, bradycardia, Heart block, COPD

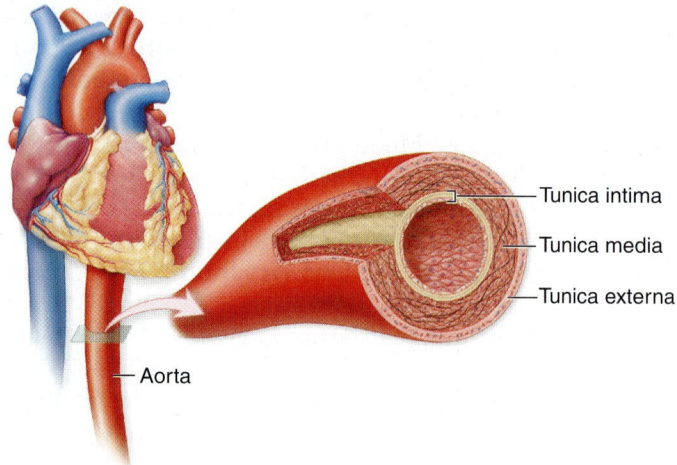

Figure 29-135 The three layers of the aorta.

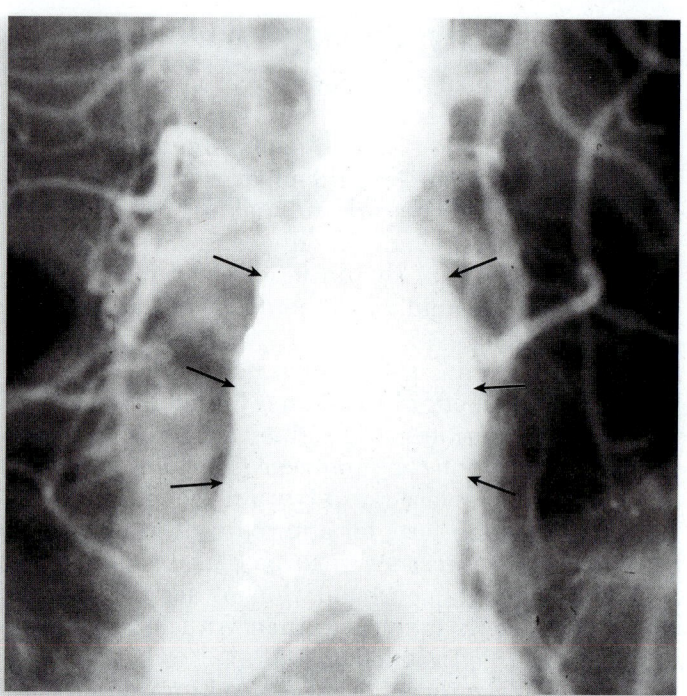

Figure 29-136 Angiogram image of an abdominal aortic aneurysm (AAA), indicated by the arrows.

its middle layer, the media, which is composed of laminated and intertwined layers of smooth muscle and connective tissue. The arrangement of connective tissue within the media aids the left ventricle in pumping blood to the periphery. The aorta is divided into two parts, the thoracic and abdominal segments. Disorders of the aorta involve breakdown or weakness of one or all of the anatomic layers. DOT 5-2.135

Aneurysm

An **aneurysm** is a focal dilation or expansion of an artery compared to an adjacent arterial segment. In general, aneurysms are defined as segments that are permanently dilated to 1.5 times the diameter of the adjacent artery. Aneurysms can occur anywhere along the aorta but generally are characterized as involving either the thoracic or abdominal aortic segments. This is because the incidence, risk factors, and pathophysiology differ somewhat between the two types. DOT 5-2.135

Abdominal Aortic Aneurysm (AAA)

Abdominal aortic aneurysms are much more common than thoracic aortic aneurysms. The incidence of abdominal aortic aneurysms rises rapidly for men ages 55 and older and for women 70 years and older. Men have five to ten times more abdominal aneurysms than women. Screening studies show that abdominal aortic aneurysm occurs in 2–13% of men and 6% of women over the age of 65 (Figure 29-136). Besides age and gender, cigarette smoking is a very important risk factor for AAA. One survey of 73,000 veterans determined smoking was the most significant risk, with an odds ratio of 5:6.[86] Atherosclerosis, hypertension, and family history are also factors that increase abdominal aortic aneurysm risk. DOT 5-2.134, 5-2.137

Risk Factors for AAA

- Tobacco use
- Hypertension
- Atherosclerosis
- Family history

The pathogenesis of abdominal aortic aneurysms is not completely understood at present, but it is likely due to the combination of a variety of factors. Atherosclerosis may be either the cause or an effect of aneurysmal dilation.[87] Genetics are also important. A study of 36 families with abdominal aortic aneurysm led to an identification of a gene locus on chromosome 19.[88] In addition, animal models suggest that increased protease activity (enzymes that degrade connective tissue) promote aneurysms. It is theorized that the durable structure of the aorta is weakened by increased activity of these enzymes.[89] Inflammation may play a role in aneurysm formation, as evidenced by elevated markers of inflammation in those patients with abdominal aortic aneurysm.[90] DOT 5-2.136

The major concern of abdominal aortic aneurysms is the risk of rupture. It is well-established that rupture risk increases with aneurysm diameter. A patient with a ruptured abdominal aortic aneurysm typically describes an acute onset of abdominal or back pain, often described as "gnawing" and constant. A pulsatile mass can often be felt in the abdomen, and the abdomen is tender to palpation. The pain can mimic many other entities such as renal colic, mesenteric ischemia, biliary colic, inferior myocardial infarction, or pancreatitis. Because the pain is not specific to this problem, it is not surprising that aneurysms are initially misdiagnosed in up to 30% of all cases.[9] Acute rupture can lead to retroperitoneal bleeding and, if severe, can be associated with profound and unstable hypotension. Prompt identification and treatment are crucial, as the mortality of a ruptured abdominal aortic aneurysm is over 50%. Elective surgical repair of aneurysms is very successful and is usually suggested for aneurysms that reach 5 cm in diameter.

Field treatment is supportive with fluid administration targeted to maintain the systolic blood pressure at 90–100 mmHg.

Thoracic Aortic Aneurysm

Thoracic aortic aneurysms are much less common than abdominal aortic aneurysms. They occur in 6 per 100,000 patients. Men are affected two to four times more often than women.[91] Risk factors for a thoracic aortic aneurysm are similar to those of AAA, such as association with atherosclerosis and smoking.

The major difference in thoracic aneurysms is their strong association with genetic disorders, most importantly Marfan's syndrome and Ehlers-Danlos syndrome. These are inherited defects of collagen and elastin production, two major structural elements of the aorta. There are other less well-defined familial disorders that are associated with thoracic aortic aneurysms.[92] In addition, certain infections, classically syphilis, and other inflammatory conditions can cause a breakdown in the structure of the aorta, leading to aneurysm formation.

Thoracic aortic aneurysms are often asymptomatic but can present in many ways, depending on their location along the aorta and the surrounding structures involved. If the aneurysm occurs at the aortic root, near the aortic valve, congestive heart failure may result from the damaged aortic valve. This occurs because the root dilation causes the valve leaflets to no longer close properly.

Dilatation near the aortic root may also compromise a coronary artery, which can lead to myocardial infarction. Thoracic aneurysms may also move into adjacent structures such as the mediastinum. This can cause many symptoms, such as hoarseness if the vagus nerve is involved, wheezing and hemoptysis (spitting up blood) if the bronchi or alveoli are involved, or back and chest pain if the aneurysm erodes into bone. Thrombus formation can also occur within the aneurysm, which can cause embolism to any of the major branch vessels of the aorta. This causes ischemic injury to the brain, mesentery, or the extremities. Just as in AAA, rupture is the

major concern and requires prompt identification and surgical treatment. Chest pain is severe, abrupt in onset, and associated with profound hypotension or shock.

Complications of Thoracic Aortic Aneurysms

- *Congestive heart failure* secondary to valvular dysfunction.
- *Myocardial infarction* due to compromise of coronary arteries by aneurysm.
- *Ischemia of brain, mesentery, and extremities* due to thrombus formation within the aneurysm, and distant embolization.
- *Hypotension and shock* due to aneurysmal rupture.

Aortic Dissection

An **aortic dissection** creates a second "false lumen" within the walls of the aorta (Figure 29-137). The inciting event for an aortic dissection is a tear in the intimal layer. This tear allows pulsatile blood to enter the media, separating the intima from the media or adventitia. This causes a false lumen within the wall of the aorta, which can spread both proximally and distally, causing a variety of symptoms. DOT 5-2.143

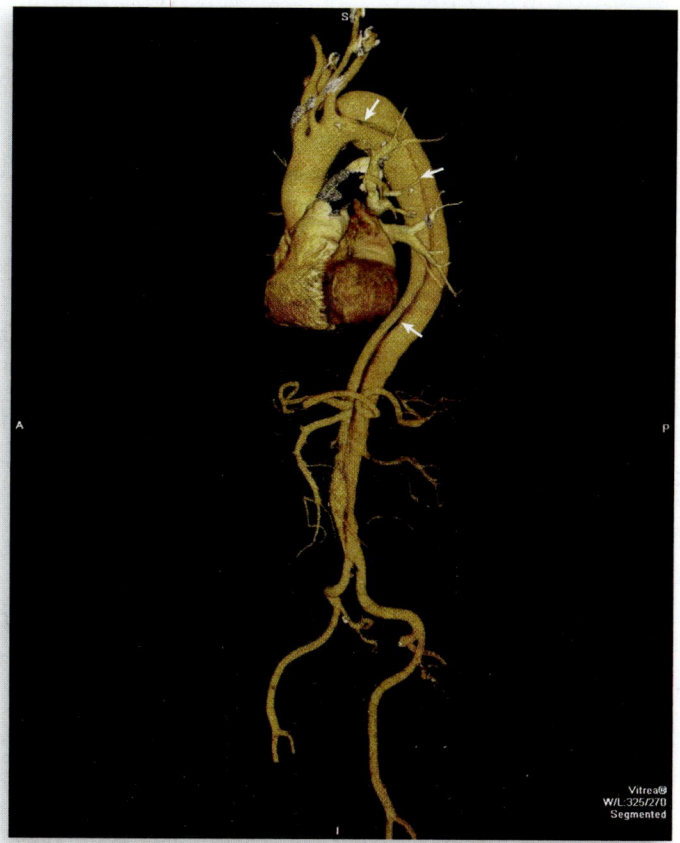

Figure 29-137 Spiral aortic dissection down the length of the aorta (arrows) is visualized in three dimensions by multislice CT.

Although the primary event is an intimal tear, aortic medial degeneration is the main cause. Thus, the same conditions associated with aneurysm formation are also associated with aortic dissection, namely inherited conditions, Marfan's and Ehlers-Danlos syndrome, in addition to infections and inflammatory vascular conditions. In fact, preexisting aortic aneurysm is a risk factor for aortic dissection.[93] However, the major risk factor associated with aortic dissection is hypertension, particularly in older patients.[94] DOT 5-2.139

The most common symptom of aortic dissection is pain, often sharp or tearing. The pain location depends on the affected aortic segment. Chest pain is more common in dissections involving the ascending aorta while back and abdominal pain are more common in dissections of the descending aorta. A classic sign of dissection is a "pulse deficit," which is a weak or absent carotid, brachial, or femoral pulse in relation to the contralateral side. This occurs as a result of the involvement of a branch vessel by the intimal flap or a resulting hematoma.[94] However, this sign has been described in only 9–30% of cases.[93,94,95] The other symptoms manifest as a result of involvement of the dissection with major branch vessels of the aorta, resulting in ischemia of the coronary, cerebral, spinal, or visceral circulations. Ascending aortic dissection deserves special note, as this can cause several life-threatening complications. Myocardial infarction can occur if the dissection involves the coronary arteries. Acute aortic valve insufficiency can occur if the aortic root is involved, leading to congestive heart failure. Tamponade or hemothorax can also arise if the aorta ruptures into the pericardial or intrapleural spaces. In addition, neurological deficits can develop if the dissection involves the carotid arteries. DOT 5-2.143, 5-2.144, 5-2.145

Initial management of a dissection involves lowering the blood pressure, which is elevated in approximately 70% of cases.[94] Additional management involves supportive care as well as treating the sequelae of dissection, such as stroke, congestive heart failure, or other ischemic events. Differentiation of aortic dissection from MI in the field is often extremely difficult. In most cases, treatment will be initiated as for an MI; however, heparin should not be given. DOT 5-2.146, 5-2.147

Peripheral Arterial Disease

The term **peripheral arterial disease (PAD)** refers to atherosclerosis obstructing the blood supply to the extremities (Figure 29-138). The prevalence of PAD varies with the selected population, the definition used, and the method of measurement but generally ranges between 4.6% and 29%. The prevalence of PAD increases with age as PAD is detected in about 20% of those aged greater than 75 years compared with 3% in those younger than 60 years.[9] Some studies have shown an equal

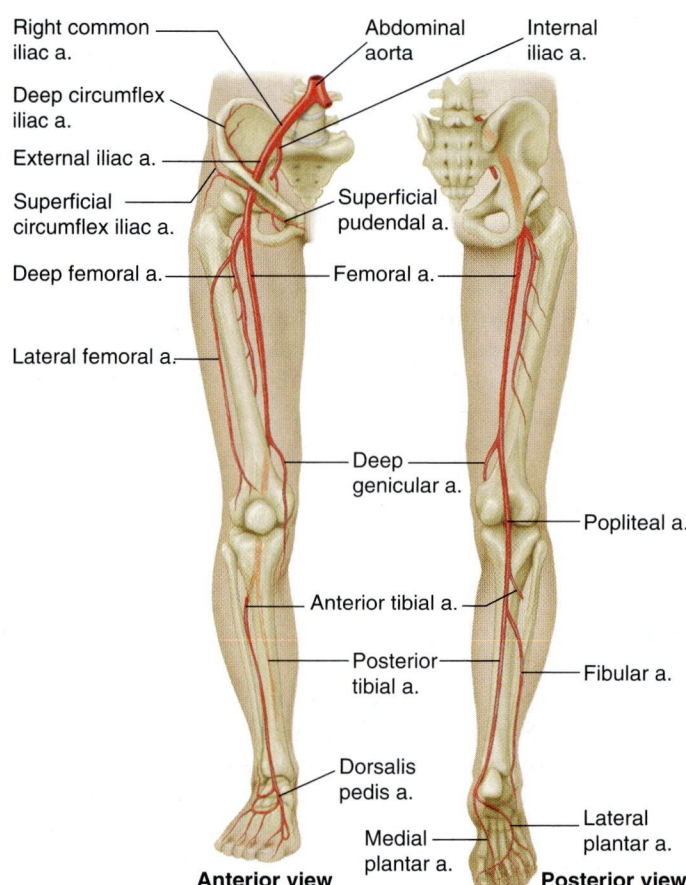

Figure 29-138   Anatomy of the peripheral (i.e., lower extremity) arterial system.

prevalence between men and women while others have shown a slight male predominance. DOT 5-2.140, 5-2.141

The major risk factors for PAD include cigarette smoking, diabetes mellitus, hypertension, dyslipidemia, and hyperhomocysteinemia. Cigarette smoking and diabetes mellitus appear to be the most significant, with a relative risk between 2.0 and 5.0 for both conditions.[9] Studies show that PAD risk increases progressively with the number of contributing risk factors in any patient. DOT 5-2.134

Risk Factors for Peripheral Arterial Disease

- Cigarette smoking
- Diabetes mellitus
- Hypertension
- Dyslipidemia
- Hyperhomocytseinemia

PAD narrows arteries, compromising blood flow to an extremity. This causes a spectrum of symptoms, ranging from mild pain to life-threatening limb ischemia. The primary process of PAD is atheromatous plaques forming in an artery, most often occurring at branch points. These plaques progressively enlarge over time, further narrowing the lumen of the artery. This narrowing increases the potential for complete or partial arterial occlusion. Arterial occlusion can occur by a variety of mechanisms, generally divided between thrombotic and embolic mechanisms. Thrombosis occurs when a previously stable plaque ruptures, causing a local inflammatory reaction and clot formation at the plaque rupture site. This results in compromise of blood flow downstream from the blockage. Thrombosis can also occur in the setting of a hypercoagulable state where either an acquired or inherited defect in the coagulation process leads to a propensity for thrombus formation. Arterial occlusion can occur from an embolus that has traveled from a distant source, most often the heart.[96] Thrombi from aneurysms can travel distally and cause arterial occlusion. PAD can occur in any vessel, but it is common in the legs. DOT 5-2.138, 5-2.148

PAD symptoms are pain during rest and intermittent claudication. Intermittent claudication (derived from the Latin word for limp) is a reproducible discomfort of a defined muscle group brought on by exercise and relieved with rest. The discomfort is usually described as an ache, fatigue, or cramping in the affected muscle group. This disorder results from an imbalance between blood supply and oxygen demand that fails to satisfy ongoing metabolic requirements. It is analogous to angina, except it is occurring in the legs. Persons with chronic arterial disease often give a history of intermittent claudication, which over time may progress to rest pain, indicating that the narrowed artery can no longer supply the basic metabolic needs of the extremity. This can lead to skin ulcer formation, typically involving the distal digits and pressure points such as the metatarsal heads (bones of the foot) and lateral malleolus (ankle bone). Skin of the affected limb is often thinned, and hair loss may occur. DOT 5-2.137

Depending on the severity of disease, peripheral pulses may be faintly palpable or absent. Distal pulses such as dorsalis pedis, posterior tibial, and radial pulses are more likely to be absent before more proximal pulses disappear. Auscultation of the arteries, such as the femoral, subclavian, and popliteal, may reveal bruits as a result of turbulent and rapid blood flow through the narrowed artery.

Acute arterial occlusion presents with new symptoms that represent acute worsening of chronic symptoms (as in the case of thrombosis of an atherosclerotic plaque) or an acute onset of new symptoms. Determining the onset and trajectory of pain is essential in determining the nature of the ischemia. An acute worsening of chronic ischemic pain is more likely to be thrombosis; whereas, acute pain where there was none previously is more likely embolic.

The Symptoms and Signs of Acute Limb Ischemia

- Pain
- Pallor
- Paresthesias
- Paralysis

The pain usually starts distally, then progresses proximally as the ischemia persists. Eventually the pain wanes as the sensory nerves deteriorate from ischemia. Comparison of pulses between an affected and asymptomatic limb is also important as a diminished pulse in an asymptomatic limb most likely represents diffuse arterial disease and thus is more likely to be thrombotic.

The skin of an affected limb typically displays pallor and, when compared to an asymptomatic limb, is often cool to the touch, displaying delayed capillary refill in the nail beds. Further inspection of the skin may reveal signs of chronic ischemia, such as skin thinning and hair loss. Finally, as the ischemia persists, sensory nerves are affected and sensation is often diminished in the ischemic limb, leading to paresthesia. As motor nerves are affected, paralysis sets in, which indicates advanced ischemia is taking place.

A slightly different acute ischemic process deserves mention due to its unusual presentation. The "blue toe syndrome" is the showering of atheromatous debris such as platelets, fibrin, and cholesterol fragments from the aorta to the small digital arteries in the lower extremities. Although the ischemia is localized, it often is a sentinel marker for more extensive disease or an unstable plaque. It differs from the usual presentation of acute ischemia in that it is localized to one or a few toes, and thus dorsalis pedis and posterior tibial pulses are often present.

The management of acute arterial occlusion includes analgesia for pain and keeping the affected limb below the level of the heart so that gravity can assist perfusion. Care must also be taken to minimize trauma to the affected limb, including removing compressive stockings or restrictive clothing that may impair circulation. Prompt management of acute arterial occlusion is imperative, as urgent revascularization, either by thrombolytics, anticoagulation, surgery, or intraarterial intervention, will increase the chances that the limb may be salvaged.

Diseases of the Venous System

Diseases of the venous system fall into two broad categories: chronic venous insufficiency and thrombosis.

Chronic Venous Insufficiency

Chronic venous insufficiency is very common. Although specific numbers are not known regarding incidence and prevalence, the morbidity involved with chronic venous insufficiency and its complications are significant for the 6 to 7 million Americans who are affected with this condition.[97] The main risk factors are a history of venous thrombosis, age, obesity, and a history of leg injury.[98] The final common pathway for chronic venous insufficiency is increased venous pressure. There are many causes of this increased pressure: obstruction in venous outflow, deterioration of venous valves in the extremities, and defects in the normal pumping physiology of the venous system.

The clinical presentation of chronic venous insufficiency spans a spectrum from asymptomatic (but cosmetically troublesome) small surface veins and varicosities, to severe and chronic skin inflammation, edema, and ulceration. Symptomatic patients may complain of leg fullness, aching discomfort, heaviness, nocturnal leg cramps, or bursting pain upon standing. Pain may be severe enough to make walking difficult or even impossible. Ulcer formation is common and when present is often chronic, recurrent, and resistant to treatment. Cellulitis, which is tissue inflammation, occurs commonly with chronic venous insufficiency.

The physical findings in venous insufficiency are characteristic and can help distinguish venous disease from other disorders. The skin characteristically has a bronze discoloration starting near the ankles or feet. The edema in chronic venous insufficiency differs from other causes of edema based on its improvement with elevation of the extremity, its poor response to diuresis, and its asymmetric distribution.

Chronic venous insufficiency ulcers can be distinguished from those resulting from arterial disease (Table 29-3). Venous ulcers tend to be shallow, tender, red-based, and located along the medial malleolus (inner ankle bone). This is in contrast to arterial ulcers, which tend to form along the lateral malleolus (outer ankle bone) and other pressure points and are often dry. Venous ulcers are generally not painful compared to arterial ulcers, which tend to be painful.

Venous Thrombosis

Venous thrombosis is the formation of a blood clot within a vein. This can occur within superficial veins or within the larger, deeper veins (Figure 29-139). The distinction between superficial and deep venous thrombosis is important as the clinical consequences of the two disorders differ greatly. When thrombosis occurs in superficial veins, it produces inflammatory reactions called *phlebitis*. There is local warmth, tenderness, and occasionally induration (a hardening of tissues) over the area of the thrombosed vein. The vein can also occasionally be palpated as a firm cord beneath the skin. This condition, although very bothersome for the

TABLE 29-3 **Distinguishing Arterial from Venous Ulcers**

Venous	Arterial
Relatively painless	Painful
Irregular margins	Sharply demarcated
Superficial	Deep
Exudative	Dry
Located medially and along veins	Located at pressure points and at distal extremities

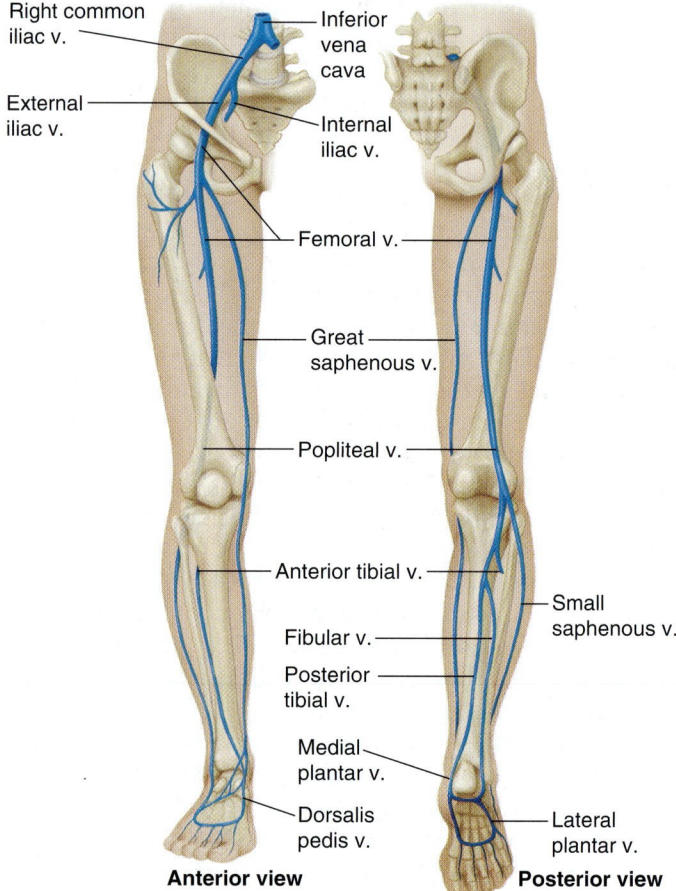

Figure 29-139 Illustration of the lower extremity venous system.

patient, typically is benign and is treated conservatively with ice, compression stockings, and nonsteroidal antiinflammatory medications. However, occasionally thrombosis of a superficial vein may be a sentinel marker for thrombosis of a deeper vein and thus may warrant further investigation. DOT 5-2.137

Thrombosis of larger veins, or **deep venous thrombosis (DVT),** is a more serious condition due to the risk of embolism to the pulmonary arteries. DVTs occur commonly.[99] Risk factors for DVT are numerous, but the major risk factors include the following:

- History of immobilization or prolonged hospitalization or bed rest or long airline flights
- Recent surgery
- Obesity
- Prior episode(s) of venous thromboembolism
- Lower extremity trauma
- Malignancy
- Use of oral contraceptives or hormone replacement therapy, particularly in smokers
- Pregnancy or postpartum status
- Stroke

The classic DVT symptoms include swelling, redness, and pain in the affected limb. The area of swelling does not necessarily correlate with the actual location of the thrombosis. In addition, there are many conditions that mimic the presentation of DVT, some of which include venous insufficiency, muscle sprain or strain, lymph outflow obstruction, cellulitis, and knee disorders. Thus DVT identification begins with suspicion based on the above risk factors. The initial DVT management includes immobilizing the affected limb and avoiding walking if possible. Treatment of DVT in the field includes transport to the hospital for diagnosis and treatment with anticoagulation to prevent extension of the clot and embolization to the lungs. This is particularly true with large, proximal clots, as 50% of these clots eventually embolize to the lung if left untreated.[100]

Resuscitation Issues

When the complex cardiovascular system and all of its compensatory mechanisms described throughout this chapter fail, emergency medical personnel are frequently confronted by the need for resuscitation. The basic foundation for resuscitation lies on the restoration of the ABCs. Specifically, loss of airway, impaired ability to breath, or inadequate circulation all demand immediate attention. Resuscitation, therefore, is the restoration of any or all ABCs. DOT 5-2.122, 5-2.131, 5-2.133

Upon arrival at a scene, the most important question is "can and should this patient be resuscitated?" The typical answer in emergency medicine is usually yes, as time is too precious to gather enough information to assess potential causes underlying medical conditions. In the field, EMS personnel should err on the side of initiating resuscitation. There are, however, some instances where the answer to the question is no.

One of the frequently encountered issues upon arrival at a resuscitation scene is the presence of do not resuscitate orders (DNR), do not intubate orders (DNI), living wills, advanced directives, and durable power(s) of attorney. With the modern move toward hospice care, do not hospitalize orders, and comfort care, many patients have their wishes already established. In crises, family members still call EMS personnel even when patients have documented end-of-life orders for DNR, DNI, or no-transport to the hospital. EMS personnel face difficult, timely interpretations in the field in these cases, so individual states have guidelines for EMS-DNR programs. These programs describe what documents in certain situations dictate action or lack thereof. The goal is to have all concerned parties educated on policy, to provide efficient resuscitation when warranted, and to respect a patient's wishes when resuscitation is not wanted.

When advanced directive documents are not available, some situations still occur where resuscitation is not recommended. The National Association of EMS Physicians published two position papers on the issue to help guide cessation of resuscitative efforts in the prehospital setting. They divide their recommendations into guidelines for patients with traumatic and non-traumatic cardiopulmonary arrest. The recommendations shown in Boxes 29-29 and 29-30 are taken directly from their position papers and are used to guide local practice. DOT 5-1.132

Summary

Cardiac diseases account for a significant number of patient encounters for paramedics. Many cardiovascular diseases have similar signs and symptoms, but some have presentations unique to that particular disease. Sudden cardiac death and myocardial infarction require aggressive management. Conditions such as heart failure, hypertensive emergencies, and vascular disease may require aggressive management or simply require monitoring of the patient during transport. A thorough history and physical examination will help guide the decision-making process for treatment of each of these conditions.

BOX 29-29 Termination of Resuscitation in Prehospital Traumatic Cardiopulmonary Arrest[102]

1. Resuscitation efforts may be withheld in any *blunt* trauma patient who, based on out-of-hospital personnel's thorough primary patient assessment, is found apneic, pulseless, and without organized electrocardiographic (ECG) activity upon the arrival of emergency medical services (EMS) at the scene.

2. Victims of *penetrating* trauma found apneic and pulseless by EMS, based on their patient assessment, should be rapidly assessed for the presence of other signs of life, such as pupillary reflexes, spontaneous movement, or organized ECG activity. If any of these signs are present, the patient should have resuscitation performed and be transported to the nearest emergency department (ED) or trauma center. If these signs of life are absent, resuscitation efforts may be withheld.

3. Resuscitation efforts should be withheld in victims of penetrating or blunt trauma with injuries obviously incompatible with life, such as decapitation or hemicorporectomy.

4. Resuscitation efforts should be withheld in victims of penetrating or blunt trauma with evidence of a significant time lapse since pulselessness, including dependent lividity, rigor mortis, and decomposition.

5. Cardiopulmonary arrest patients in whom the mechanism of injury does not correlate with clinical condition, suggesting a nontraumatic cause of the arrest, should have standard resuscitation initiated.

6. Termination of resuscitation efforts should be considered in trauma patients with EMS-witnessed cardiopulmonary arrest and 15 minutes of unsuccessful resuscitation and cardiopulmonary resuscitation (CPR).

7. Traumatic cardiopulmonary arrest (TCPA) patients with a transport time to an ED or trauma center of more than 15 minutes after the arrest is identified may be considered nonsalvageable, and termination of resuscitation should be considered.

8. Guidelines and protocols for TCPA patients who should be transported must be individualized for each EMS system. Consideration should be given to factors such as the average transport time within the system, the scope of practice of the various EMS providers within the system, and the definitive care capabilities (that is, trauma centers) within the system. Airway management and intravenous (IV) line placement should be accomplished during transport when possible.

9. Special consideration must be given to victims of drowning and lightning strike and in situations where significant hypothermia may alter the prognosis.

10. EMS providers should be thoroughly familiar with the guidelines and protocols affecting the decision to withhold or terminate resuscitative efforts.

11. All termination protocols should be developed and implemented under the guidance of the system EMS medical director. On-line medical control may be necessary to determine the appropriateness of termination of resuscitation.

12. Policies and protocols for termination of resuscitation efforts must include notification of the appropriate law enforcement agencies and notification of the medical examiner or coroner for final disposition of the body.

13. Families of the deceased should have access to resources, including clergy, social workers, and other counseling personnel, as needed. EMS providers should have access to resources for debriefing and counseling as needed.

14. Adherence to policies and protocols governing termination of resuscitation should be monitored through a quality review system.

Exceptions

Situations in which trauma is complicated by significant hypothermia should not be included in these recommendations. Profound hypothermia below 32°C will cause progressive bradycardia, decreased cardiac output, loss of consciousness, and, ultimately, loss of brainstem reflexes—effectively mimicking death but with the potential for successful resuscitation with appropriate medical treatment and rewarming. Examples of hypothermia complicating trauma may include cold water submersion (particularly in children), avalanche burial, and minor trauma with subsequent environmental exposures. In these situations, patients should be aggressively resuscitated and transported to a center capable of rewarming the victim.

BOX 29-30 Termination of Resuscitation in the Prehospital Setting for Adult Patients Suffering Nontraumatic Cardiac Arrest[101]

1. **Patient Population:** Termination of resuscitation may be considered for any patient who suffers sudden cardiac death that is likely to be medical. Patients who are likely suffering from hypothermia or cold water drowning should generally not be considered candidates for field termination of resuscitation.

2. **Collapse-to-Treatment Interval:** Important intervals include the time from collapse to the times the patient is found, CPR is started, defibrillation is administered, and ACLS is initiated. Unwitnessed cardiac arrests with unknown downtimes, delayed initiation of CPR beyond six minutes, and delay to defibrillation of more than eight minutes carry a poor prognosis. These intervals are often hard to define and although they are associated with poor outcomes, should be used as considerations but not as criteria for termination of resuscitation.

3. **Treatment Requirements:** A full resuscitative effort is required prior to consideration for termination of resuscitation in the out-of-hospital setting. This includes definitive airway management, intravenous access, defibrillation or cardioversion if necessary, CPR, and 20 to 30 minutes of treatment following Advanced Cardiac Life Support guidelines or local protocols.

4. **Response to Therapy:** Patients without return of spontaneous circulation (ROSC) are candidates for termination of resuscitation. Those patients whose rhythm changes to, or remains in, VF or VT should have continued resuscitative efforts. Patients in asystole or PEA are considered to be in terminal rhythms, and termination of resuscitation should be considered.

5. **Logistic Factors:** Consideration should be given to family wishes. If the family wishes efforts be continued, or if the family's wishes remain unclear, particularly if there is a communication barrier, it may be preferable to continue resuscitative efforts. Other logistic factors may be considered, including collapse in a public place, weather, and safety of the crew and public.

6. **Education of EMS Personnel:** Emergency medical services providers should be educated regarding the ramifications of termination protocols. This includes education regarding the natural history and pathophysiology of cardiac arrest and the inherently poor prognosis it carries.

7. **Medical Oversight:** All termination protocols need to be developed and implemented under the guidance of the system medical director, with input from physicians responsible for providing on-line direction. On-line medical direction should be established prior to termination of resuscitation in the field. The final decision to terminate resuscitative efforts should be a consensus between the paramedic and on-line physician.

8. **Care of the Deceased:** After the decision to terminate resuscitative efforts has occurred, many important steps need to occur. These include notification of local law enforcement, involvement of the medical examiner or coroner, and completion of the patient call report and on-line direction documentation. Policies and protocols for termination of resuscitative efforts in the field should outline the steps that are needed based on local practices and must be in place before programs terminating resuscitation in the field are implemented.

Section II Notes

1. American Heart Association, *Heart Disease and Stroke Statistics-2004 Update* (Dallas, TX: American Heart Association, 2004).

2. M. J. Stampfer, F. B. Hu, J. E. Manson, E. B. Rimm, and W. C. Willett, "Primary Prevention of Coronary Heart Disease in Women Through Diet and Lifestyle," *The New England Journal of Medicine* 343(1)(2000): 16–22.

3. D. M. Lloyd-Jones, B. H. Nam, R. B. D'Agostino, Sr., D. Levy, J. M. Murabito, T. J. Wang, et al., "Parental Cardiovascular Disease as a Risk Factor for Cardiovascular Disease in Middle-Aged Adults: A Prospective Study of Parents and Offspring," *Journal of the American Medical Association* 291(18)(2004): 2204–2211.

4. T. Almdal, H. Scharling, J. S. Jensen, and H. Vestergaard, "The Independent Effect of Type 2 Diabetes Mellitus on Ischemic Heart Disease, Stroke, and Death: A Population-Based Study of 13,000 Men and Women with 20 Years of Follow-Up," *Archives of Internal Medicine* 164(13)(2004): 1422–1426.

5. S. Yusuf, S. Hawken, S. Ounpuu, T. Dans, A. Avezum, F. Lanas, et al., "Effect of Potentially Modifiable Risk Factors Associated with Myocardial Infarction in 52 Countries (The INTERHEART Study): Case-Control Study," *Lancet* 364(9438)(2004): 937–952.

6. P. W. Wilson, "Established Risk Factors and Coronary Artery Disease: The Framingham Study," *American Journal of Hypertension* 7(7 Pt 2)(1994): 7S–12S.

7. J. P. Berger, T. Buclin, E. Haller, G. Van Melle, and B. Yersin, "Right Arm Involvement and Pain Extension can Help to Differentiate Coronary Diseases from Chest Pain of Other

Origin: A Prospective Emergency Ward Study of 278 Consecutive Patients Admitted for Chest Pain," *Journal of Internal Medicine* 227(3)(1990): 165–172.

8. A. A. Panju, B. R. Hemmelgarn, G. H. Guyatt, and D. L. Simel, "The Rational Clinical Examination. Is This Patient Having a Myocardial Infarction?" *Journal of the American Medical Association* 280(14)(1998): 1256–1263.

9. D. P. Zipes, P. Libby, R. O. Bonow, and E. Braunwald, ed., *Braunwald's Heart Disease E-dition* (Philadelphia PA: Elsevier Saunders, 2005).

10. A. L. Goldberger and E. Goldberger, *Clinical Electrocardiography: A Simplified Approach*, 5th ed. (St. Louis, MO: Mosby, 1994).

11. A. L. Goldberger, *Myocardial Infarction: Electrocardiographic Differential Diagnosis*, 4th ed. (St. Louis, MO: Mosby Year Book, 1991).

12. E. M. Antman, D. T. Anbe, P. W. Armstrong, E. R. Bates, L. A. Green, M. Hand, et al., "ACC/AHA guidelines for the Management of Patients with ST-Elevation Myocardial Infarction—Executive Summary. A Report of the American College of Cardiology/American Heart Association Task Force on Practice Guidelines (Writing Committee to Revise the 1999 Guidelines for the Management of Patients with Acute Myocardial Infarction)," *Journal of the American College of Cardiology* 44(3)(2004): 671–719.

13. A. M. Goldberger, "Electrocardiogram in the Diagnosis of Myocardial Ischemia and Infarction," *Up To Date* (2005), www.uptodate.com (accessed January 2005).

14. G. S. Reeder, K. Ma, and L. Harold, "Diagnosis of an Acute Myocardial Infarction," *Up To Date* (January 2005), www.uptodate.com (accessed June 1, 2005).

15. J. G. Ebb, L. A. Sleeper, C. E. Buller, J. Boland, A. Palazzo, E. Buller, et al., "Implications of the Timing of Onset of Cardiogenic Shock After Acute Myocardial Infarction: A Report from the SHOCK Trial Registry. Should We Emergently Revascularize Occluded Coronaries for Cardiogenic Shock?" *Journal of the American College of Cardiology* 36(3 Suppl A)(2000): 1084–1090.

16. D. R. Holmes, Jr., E. R. Bates, N. S. Kleiman, Z. Sadowski, J. H. Horgan, D. C. Morris, et al., "Contemporary Reperfusion Therapy for Cardiogenic Shock: The GUSTO-I Trial Experience. The GUSTO-I Investigators. Global Utilization of Streptokinase and Tissue Plasminogen Activator for Occluded Coronary Arteries," *Journal of the American College of Cardiology* 26(3)(1995): 668–674.

17. R. H. Mehta, K. J. Harjai, D. Cox, G. W. Stone, B. Brodie, J. Boura, et al., "Clinical and Angiographic Correlates and Outcomes of Suboptimal Coronary Flow Inpatients with Acute Myocardial Infarction Undergoing Primary Percutaneous Coronary Intervention," *Journal of the American College of Cardiology* 42(10)(2003): 1739–1746.

18. G. W. Stone, C. L. Grines, D. A. Cox, E. Garcia, J. E. Tcheng, J. J. Griffin, et al., "Comparison of Angioplasty with Stenting, with or Without Abciximab, in Acute Myocardial Infarction," *The New England Journal of Medicine* 346(13)(2002): 957–966.

19. J. L. Anderson, L. A. Karagounis, and R. M. Califf, "Metaanalysis of Five Reported Studies on the Relation of Early Coronary Patency Grades with Mortality and Outcomes After Acute Myocardial Infarction," *American Journal of Cardiology* 78(1)(1996): 1–8.

20. Anonymous, "An International Randomized Trial Comparing Four Thrombolytic Strategies for Acute Myocardial Infarction: The GUSTO Investigators," *The New England Journal of Medicine* 329(10)(1993): 673–682.

21. Anonymous, "The Effects of Tissue Plasminogen Activator, Streptokinase, or Both on Coronary-Artery Patency, Ventricular Function, and Survival After Acute Myocardial Infarction, The GUSTO Angiographic Investigators," *The New England Journal of Medicine* 329(22)(1993): 1615–1622.

22. E. C. Keeley, J. A. Boura, and C. L. Grines, "Primary Angioplasty Versus Intravenous Thrombolytic Therapy for Acute Myocardial Infarction: A Quantitative Review of 23 Randomised Trials," *Lancet* 361(9351)(2003): 13–20.

23. T. D. Rea, M. S. Eisenberg, L. J. Becker, J. A. Murray, and T. Hearne, "Temporal Trends in Sudden Cardiac Arrest: A 25-Year Emergency Medical Services Perspective," *Circulation* 107(22)(2003): 2780–2785.

24. "The Effects of Biphasic and Conventional Monophasic Defibrillation on Postresuscitation Myocardial Function," *Journal of the American College of Cardiology* 34(3)(September 1999): 815–822.

25. P. P. Zipes and J. J. Zalife, *Cardiac Electrophysiology: From Cell to Bedside*, 4th ed. (Philadelphia, PA: Elsevier Saunders 2004).

26. R. S. Baum, H. Alvarez, III, and L. A. Cobb, "Survival After Resuscitation From Out-of-Hospital Ventricular Fibrillation," *Circulation* 50(6)(1974): 1231–1235.

27. "American College of Emergency Physicians, "Use of Pressors in the Treatment of Cardiac Arrest," *Annals of Emergency Medicine* 37(4) (April 2001).

28. J. P. Ornato and M. A. Peberdy, *Cardiopulmonary Resuscitation* (Totowa, NJ: Humana Press, 2005).

29. T. P. Aufderheide and K. G. Lurie, "Death by Hyperventilation: A Common and Life-Threatening Problem During Cardiopulmonary Resuscitation," *Critical Care Medicine* 32(9)(2004): S345–351.

30. D. Yannopoulos, S. McKnite, et al., "Effects of Incomplete Chest Wall Decompression During Cardiopulmonary Resuscitation on Coronary and Cerebral Perfusion Pressures in a Porcine Model of Cardiac Arrest," *Resuscitation* 64(2005): 363–372.

31. K. G. Lurie, K. A. Mulligan, et al., "Optimizing Standard Cardiopulmonary Resuscitation with an Inspiratory Impedance Threshold Valve," *Chest* 113(4) (1998): 1084–1090.

32. K. G. Lurie, W. G. Voelckel, et al., "Improving Standard Cardiopulmonary Resuscitation with an Inspiratory Impedance Threshold Valve in a Porcine Model of Cardiac Arrest," *Anesthesia and Analgesia* 93(3)(2001): 649–655.

33. K. G. Lurie, T. Zielinski, et al., "Use of an Inspiratory Impedance Threshold Valve Improves Neurologically Intact Survival in a Porcine Model of Ventricular Fibrillation," *Circulation* 105(1)(2002): 124–129.

34. T. P. Aufderheide, R. G. Pirrallo, et al., "Clinical Evaluation of an Inspiratory Impedance Threshold Device During Standard Cardiopulmonary Resuscitation in Patients with Out-of-Hospital Cardiac Arrest," *Critical Care Medicine* 33(4)(2005): 734–740.

35. R. G. Pirrallo, T. P. Aufderheide, et al., "Effect of an Inspiratory Impedance Threshold Device on Hemodynamics During Conventional Manual Cardiopulmonary Resuscitation," *Resuscitation* 66(2005): 13–20.

36. R. C. Thayne, D. C. Thomas, et al., "Use of an Impedance Threshold Device Improves Short-Term Outcomes Following Out-of-Hospital Cardiac Arrest," *Resuscitation* 67(2005): 103–108.

37. B. B. Wolcke, D. K. Mauer, et al., "Comparison of Standard Cardiopulmonary Resuscitation Versus the Combination of Active Compression-Decompression Cardiopulmonary Resuscitation and an Inspiratory Impedance Threshold Device for Out-of-Hospital Cardiac Arrest," *Circulation* 108(18)(2003): 2201–2205.

38. P. Plaisance, K. G. Lurie, and D. Payen, "Inspiratory Impedance During Active Compression-Decompression Cardiopulmonary Resuscitation: A Randomized Evaluation in Patients in Cardiac Arrest," *Circulation* 101(9)(2000): 989–994.

39. P. Plaisance, C. Soleil, et al., "Use of an Inspiratory Impedance Threshold Device on a Facemask and Endotracheal Tube to

Reduce Intrathoracic Pressures During the Decompression Phase of Active Compression-Decompression Cardiopulmonary Resuscitation," *Critical Care Medicine* 33(5)(2005): 990–994.

40. P. Plaisance, K. G. Lurie, et al., "Evaluation of an Impedance Threshold Device in Patients Receiving Active Compression-Decompression Cardiopulmonary Resuscitation for Out-of-Hospital Cardiac Arrest," *Resuscitation* 61(3)(2004): 265–271.

41. K. G. Lurie, W. Voelckel, et al., "Use of an Inspiratory Impedance Threshold Valve During Cardiopulmonary Resuscitation: A Progress Report," *Resuscitation* 44(2000): 219–230.

42. K. B. Kern, R. W. Hilwig, et al., "Importance of Continuous Chest Compressions During CPR," *Circulation* 105(2002): 645.

43. H. R. Halperin, N. Paradis, et al., "Cardiopulmonary Resuscitation with a Novel Chest Compression Device in a Porcine Model of Cardiac Arrest: Improved Hemodynamics and Mechanisms," *Journal of the American College of Cardiology* 44(11)(2004): 2214–2220.

44. S. Timerman, L. F. Cardoso, et al., "Improved Hemodynamic Performance with a Novel Chest Compression Device During Treatment of In-Hospital Cardiac Arrest," *Resuscitation* 61(3)(2004): 273–280.

45. M. Casner, D. Andersen, and S. M. Isaacs, "The Impact of a New CPR Device on Rate of Return of Spontaneous Circulation in Out-of-Hospital Cardiac Arrest," *Prehospital Emergency Care* 9(1)(2005): 61–67.

46. V. Menon, H. White, T. LeJemtel, J. G. Webb, L. A. Sleeper, and J. S. Hochman, "The Clinical Profile of Patients with Suspected Cardiogenic Shock Due to Predominant Left Ventricular Failure: A Report from the SHOCK Trial Registry. Should We Emergently Revascularize Occluded Coronaries in Cardiogenic Shock?" *Journal of the American College of Cardiology* 36(3 Suppl A)(2000): 1071–1076.

47. T. J. Ryan, E. M. Antman, N. H. Brooks, R. M. Califf, L. D. Hillis, L. F. Hiratzka, et al., "1999 Update: ACC/AHA Guidelines for the Management of Patients With Acute Myocardial Infarction: Executive Summary and Recommendations: A Report of the American College of Cardiology/American Heart Association Task Force on Practice Guidelines (Committee on Management of Acute Myocardial Infarction)," *Circulation* 100(9)(1999): 1016–1030.

48. A. Lincoff, "Heparin in Acute ST Elevation (Q Wave) Myocardial Infarction," *Up To Date* (2004), www.uptodate.com (accessed June 1, 2005).

49. D. L Kasper, E. Braunwald, A. S. Fauci, S. L. Hauser, D. L. Longo, and J. L. Jameson, eds., *Harrison's Principles of Internal Medicine,* 16th ed. (New York, NY: McGraw-Hill, 2006).

50. V. Menon and J. S. Hochman, "Treatment of Cardiogenic Shock Complication Acute Myocardial Infarction," *Up To Date* (December 15, 2004), www.uptodate.com (accessed June 1, 2005).

51. T. G. Roberts and L. S. Lilly, "Diseases of the Pericardium," In *Pathophysiology of Heart Failure,* 2nd ed., L. S. Lilly, ed. (Baltimore, MD: Lippincott Williams & Wilkins, 1998).

52. M. M. LeWinter and S. Kabbani, "Pericardial Diseases," In *Braunwald's Heart Disease E-dition,* D. P. Zipes, P. Libby, R. O. Bonow, and E. Braunwald, ed., 7th ed. (Philadelphia, PA: Elsevier Saunders, 2005).

53. R. Shabetai, "Pericardial Compressive Syndromes," *Up To Date* (December 8, 2004), www.utdol.com/application/topic. asp?file=hrt_fail/2458&type=A&selectedTitle=1~7 (accessed May 13, 2005).

54. D. H. Spodick, "Acute Cardiac Tamponade," *The New England Journal of Medicine* 349(7)(2003): 684–690.

55. G. Gregoratos, J. Abrams, A. E. Epstein, R. A. Freedman, D. L. Hayes, M. A. Hlatky, et al., "ACC/AHA/NASPE 2002 Guideline Update for Implantation of Cardiac Pacemakers and Antidysrhythmia Devices: Summary Article: A Report of the American College of Cardiology/American Heart Association Task Force on Practice Guidelines (ACC/AHA/NASPE Committee to Update the 1998 Pacemaker Guidelines)," *Circulation* 106(16)(2002): 2145–2161.

56. G. Gregoratos, M. D. Cheitlin, A. Conill, A. E. Epstein, C. Fellows, T. B. Ferguson, Jr., et al., "ACC/AHA Guidelines for Implantation of Cardiac Pacemakers and Antidysrhythmia Devices: Executive Summary: A Report of the American College of Cardiology/American Heart Association Task Force on Practice Guidelines (Committee on Pacemaker Implantation)," *Circulation* 97(13)(1998): 1325–1335.

57. M. Jessup and S. Brozena, "Heart Failure," *The New England Journal of Medicine* 348(20)(2003): 2007–2018.

58. B. M. Massie and N. B. Shah, "Evolving Trends in the Epidemiologic Factors of Heart Failure: Rationale for Preventive Strategies and Comprehensive Disease Management," *American Heart Journal* 133(6)(1997): 703–712.

59. M. Kupari, M. Lindroos, A. M. Iivanainen, R. Heikkila, and J. Tilvis, "Congestive Heart Failure in Old Age: Prevalence, Mechanisms and 4-Year Prognosis in the Helsinki Ageing Study," *Journal of Internal Medicine* 241(5)(1997): 387–394.

60. K. A. Schulman, D. B. Mark, and R. M. Califf, "Outcomes and Costs Within a Disease Management Program for Advanced Congestive Heart Failure," *American Heart Journal* 135(6 Pt 2 Su)(1998): S285–292.

61. K. K. Ho, K. M. Anderson, W. B. Kannel, W. Grossman, and D. Levy, "Survival After the Onset of Congestive Heart Failure in Framingham Heart Study Subjects," *Circulation* 88(1)(1993): 107–115.

62. R. J. Rodeheffer, S. J. Jacobsen, B. J. Gersh, T. E. Kottke, H. A. McCann, K. R. Bailey, et al., "The Incidence and Prevalence of Congestive Heart Failure in Rochester, Minnesota," *Mayo Clinic Proceedings* 68(12)(1993): 1143–1150.

63. S. A. Hunt, D. W. Baker, M. H. Chin, M. P. Cinquegrani, A. M. Feldmanmd, G. S. Francis, et al., "ACC/AHA Guidelines for the Evaluation and Management of Chronic Heart Failure in the Adult: Executive Summary A Report of the American College of Cardiology/American Heart Association Task Force on Practice Guidelines (Committee to Revise the 1995 Guidelines for the Evaluation and Management of Heart Failure)," *Circulation* 104(24)(2001): 2996–3007.

64. M. R. Zile and D. L. Brutsaert, "New Concepts in Diastolic Dysfunction and Diastolic Heart Failure: Part I: Diagnosis, Prognosis, and Measurements of Diastolic Function," *Circulation* 105(11)(2002): 1387–1393.

65. G. Gardner, D. S. Pinto, and S. Lewis, "Flash Pulmonary Edema," *Up To Date* (October 22, 2004), www.utdol.com/application/ topic.asp?file=hrt_fail/2458&type=A&selectedTitle=1~7 (accessed May 12, 2005).

66. S. K. Frankel and M. A. Fifer, "Heart Failure," In *Pathophysiology of Heart Failure,* 2nd ed., L. S. Lilly, ed. (Baltimore, MD: Lippincott Williams & Wilkins, 1998).

67. M. R. Bristow, S. Linas, and J. D. Port, "Drugs in the Treatment of Heart Failure." In *Braunwald's Heart Disease E-dition,* D. P. Zipes, P. Libby, R. O. Bonow, and E. Braunwald, ed., 7th ed. (Philadelphia, PA: Elsevier Saunders, 2005).

68. R. I. Shorr, W. A. Ray, J. R. Daugherty, and M. R. Griffin, "Antihypertensives and the Risk of Serious Hypoglycemia in Older Persons Using Insulin or Sulfonylureas," *Journal of the American Medical Association* 278(1)(1997): 40–43.

69. W. S. Colucci and E. Braunwald, "Pathophysiology of Heart Failure." In *Braunwald's Heart Disease E-dition,* 7th ed., D. P. Zipes, P. Libby, R. O. Bonow and E. Braunwald, eds. (Philadelphia, PA: Elsevier Saunders 2005).

70. J. M. Brophy, L. Joseph, and J. L. Rouleau, "Beta-Blockers in Congestive Heart Failure. A Bayesian Meta-Analysis," *Annals of Internal Medicine* 134(7)(2001): 550–560.

71. S. Bonet, A. Agusti, J. M. Arnau, X. Vidal, E. Diogene, E. Galve, et al., "Beta-Adrenergic Blocking Agents in Heart Failure: Benefits of Vasodilating and Non-Vasodilating Agents According to Patients' Characteristics: A Meta-Analysis of Clinical Trials," *Archives of Internal Medicine* 160(5)(2000): 621–627.

72. M. L. Fisher, S. S. Gottlieb, G. D. Plotnick, N. L. Greenberg, R. D. Patten, S. K. Bennett, et al., "Beneficial Effects of Metoprolol in Heart Failure Associated with Coronary Artery Disease: A Randomized Trial," *Journal of the American College of Cardiology* 23(4)(1994): 943–550.

73. M. Packer, M. R. Bristow, J. N. Cohn, W. S. Colucci, M. B. Fowler, E. M. Gilbert, et al., "The Effect of Carvedilol on Morbidity and Mortality in Patients with Chronic Heart Failure," U.S. Carvedilol Heart Failure Study Group, *The New England Journal of Medicine* 334(21)(1996): 1349–1355.

74. D. T. Ko, P. R. Hebert, C. S. Coffey, A. Sedrakyan, J. P. Curtis, and H. M. Krumholz, "Beta-Blocker Therapy and Symptoms of Depression, Fatigue, and Sexual Dysfunction," *Journal of the American Medical Association* 288(3)(2002): 351–357.

75. D. Dunlop and R. G. Shanks, "Selective Blockade of Adrenoceptive Beta Receptors in the Heart," *British Journal of Pharmacology* 32(1)(1968): 201–218.

76. E. A. Abramson, R. A. Arky, and K. A. Woeber, "Effects of Propranolol on the Hormonal and Metabolic Responses to Insulin-Induced Hypoglycaemia," *Lancet* 2(7478)(1996): 1386–1388.

77. W. S. Reveno and H. Rosenbaum, "Propranolol and Hypoglycaemia," *Lancet* 1(7548)(1968): 920.

78. B. N. Singh, R. M. Whitlock, R. H. Comber, F. H. Williams, and E. A. Harris, "Effects of Cardioselective Beta Adrenoceptor Blockade on Specific Airways Resistance in Normal Subjects and in Patients with Bronchial Asthma," *Clinical Pharmacology & Therapeutics* 19(5 Pt 1)(1976): 493–501.

79. C. Skinner, J. Gaddie, and K. N. Palmer, "Comparison of Effects of Metoprolol and Propranolol on Asthmatic Airway Obstruction," *British Medical Journal* 1(6008)(1976): 504.

80. T. E. Sirak, S. Jelic, and T. H. Le Jemtel, "Therapeutic Update: Non-Selective Beta- and Alpha-Adrenergic Blockade in Patients with Coexistent Chronic Obstructive Pulmonary Disease and Chronic Heart Failure," *Journal of the American College of Cardiology* 44(3)(2004): 497–502.

81. S. P. Deacon and D. Barnett, "Comparison of Atenolol and Propranolol During Insulin-induced Hypoglycaemia," *British Medical Journal* 2(6030)(1976): 272–273.

82. M. C. Houston, "Abrupt Cessation of Treatment in Hypertension: Consideration of Clinical Features, Mechanisms, Prevention and Management of the Discontinuation Syndrome," *American Heart Journal* 102(3 Pt 1)(1981):415–430.

83. R. R. Miller, H. G. Olson, E. A. Amsterdam, and D. T. Mason, "Propranolol-Withdrawal Rebound Phenomenon. Exacerbation of Coronary Events After Abrupt Cessation of Antianginal Therapy," *The New England Journal of Medicine* 293(9)(1975):416–418.

84. B. M. Psaty, T. D. Koepsell, E. H. Wagner, J. P. LoGerfo, and T. S. Inui, "The Relative Risk of Incident Coronary Heart Disease Associated with Recently Stopping the Use of Beta-Blockers," *Journal of the American Medical Association* 263(12)(1990): 1653–1657.

85. P. J. Podrid, "Major Side Effects of Beta Blockers," *Up To Date* (September 20, 2004); http://www.utdol.com/application/topic.asp?file=carrhyth/31775 (accessed May 11, 2005).

86. F. A. Lederle, G. R. Johnson, S. E. Wilson, E. P. Chute, F. N. Littooy, D. Bandk, et al., "Prevalence and Associations of Abdominal Aortic Aneurysm Detected through Screening," Aneurysm Detection and Management (ADAM) Veterans Affairs Cooperative Study Group, *Annals of Internal Medicine* 126(6)(1997): 441–449.

87. D. Reed, C. Reed, G. Stemmermann, and T. Hayashi, "Are Aortic Aneurysms Caused by Atherosclerosis?" *Circulation* 85(1)(1992): 205–211.

88. H. Shibamura, J. M. Olson, C. van Vlijmen-Van Keulen, S. G. Buxbaum, D. M. Dudek, G. Tromp, et al., "Genome Scan for Familial Abdominal Aortic Aneurysm Using Sex and Family History as Covariates Suggests Genetic Heterogeneity and Identifies Linkage to Chromosome 19q13," *Circulation* 109(17)(2004): 2103–2108.

89. K. M. Newman, J. Jean-Claude, H. Li, W. G. Ramey, and M. D. Tilson, "Cytokines That Activate Proteolysis Are Increased in Abdominal Aortic Aneurysms," *Circulation* 90(5 Pt 2)(1994): II224–227.

90. G. K. Sukhova, G. P. Shi, D. I. Simon, H. A. Chapman, and P. Libby, "Expression of the Elastolytic Cathepsins S and K in Human Atheroma and Regulation of their Production in Smooth Muscle Cells," *Journal of Clinical Investigation* 102(3)(1998): 576–583.

91. L. K. Bickerstaff, P. C. Pairolero, L. H. Hollier, L. J. Melton, H. J. Van Peenen, K. J. Cherry, et al., "Thoracic Aortic Aneurysms: A Population-Based Study." *Surgery* 92(6)(1982): 1103–1108.

92. D. M. Milewicz, H. Chen, E. S. Park, E. M. Petty, H. Zaghi, G. Shashidhar, et al., "Reduced Penetrance and Variable Expressivity of Familial Thoracic Aortic Aneurysms/Dissections," *American Journal of Cardiology* 82(4)(1998): 474–479.

93. E. W. Larson and W. D. Edward, "Risk Factors for Aortic Dissection: A Necropsy Study of 161 Cases," *American Journal of Cardiology* 53(6)(1984): 849–855.

94. P. G. Hagan, C. A. Nienaber, E. M. Isselbacher, D. Bruckman, D. J. Karavite, P. L. Russman, et al., "The International Registry of Acute Aortic Dissection (IRAD): New Insights Into an Old Disease," *Journal of the American Medical Association* 283(7)(2000): 897–903.

95. E. Bossone, V. Rampoldi, C. A. Nienaber, S. Trimarchi, A. Ballotta, J. V. Cooper, et al., "Usefulness of Pulse Deficit to Predict In-Hospital Complications and Mortality in Patients with Acute Type A Aortic Dissection," *American Journal of Cardiology* 89(7)(2002): 851–855.

96. W. Quinones-Baldrich, "Acute Arterial and Graft Occlusion." In *Vascular Surgery: A Comprehensive Review*, W. Moore, ed. (Philadelphia, PA: W.B. Saunders, 1993).

97. W. W. Coon, P. W. Willis, 3rd, and J. B. Keller, "Venous Thromboembolism and Other Venous Disease in the Tecumseh Community Health Study," *Circulation* 48(4)(1973): 839–846.

98. T. E. Scott, W. W. LaMorte, D. R. Gorin, and J. O. Menzoian, "Risk Factors for Chronic Venous Insufficiency: A Dual Case-Control Study," *Journal of Vascular Surgery* 22(5)(1995): 622–628.

99. M. Cushman, A. W. Tsai, R. H. White, S. R. Heckbert, W. D. Rosamond, P. Enright, et al., "Deep Vein Thrombosis and Pulmonary Embolism in Two Cohorts: The Longitudinal Investigation of Thromboembolism Etiology," *The American Journal of Medicine* 117(1)(2004): 19–25.

100. S. Landaw, "Approach to the Diagnosis and Therapy of Suspected Deep Vein Thrombosis," *Up To Date* (2004), www.uptodate.com (accessed April 15, 2005).

101. L. R. Hopson, E. Hirsh, J. Delgado, R. M. Domeier, J. Krohmer, N. E. McSwain, Jr., et al., "Guidelines for Withholding or Termination of Resuscitation in Prehospital Traumatic Cardiopulmonary Arrest," *Journal of the American College of Surgeons* 196(3)(2003): 475–481.

102. E. D. Bailey, G. C. Wydro, and D. C. Cone, "Termination of Resuscitation in the Prehospital Setting for Adult Patients Suffering Nontraumatic Cardiac Arrest," National Association of EMS Physicians Standards and Clinical Practice Committee, *Prehospital Emergency Care* 4(2)(2000): 190–195.

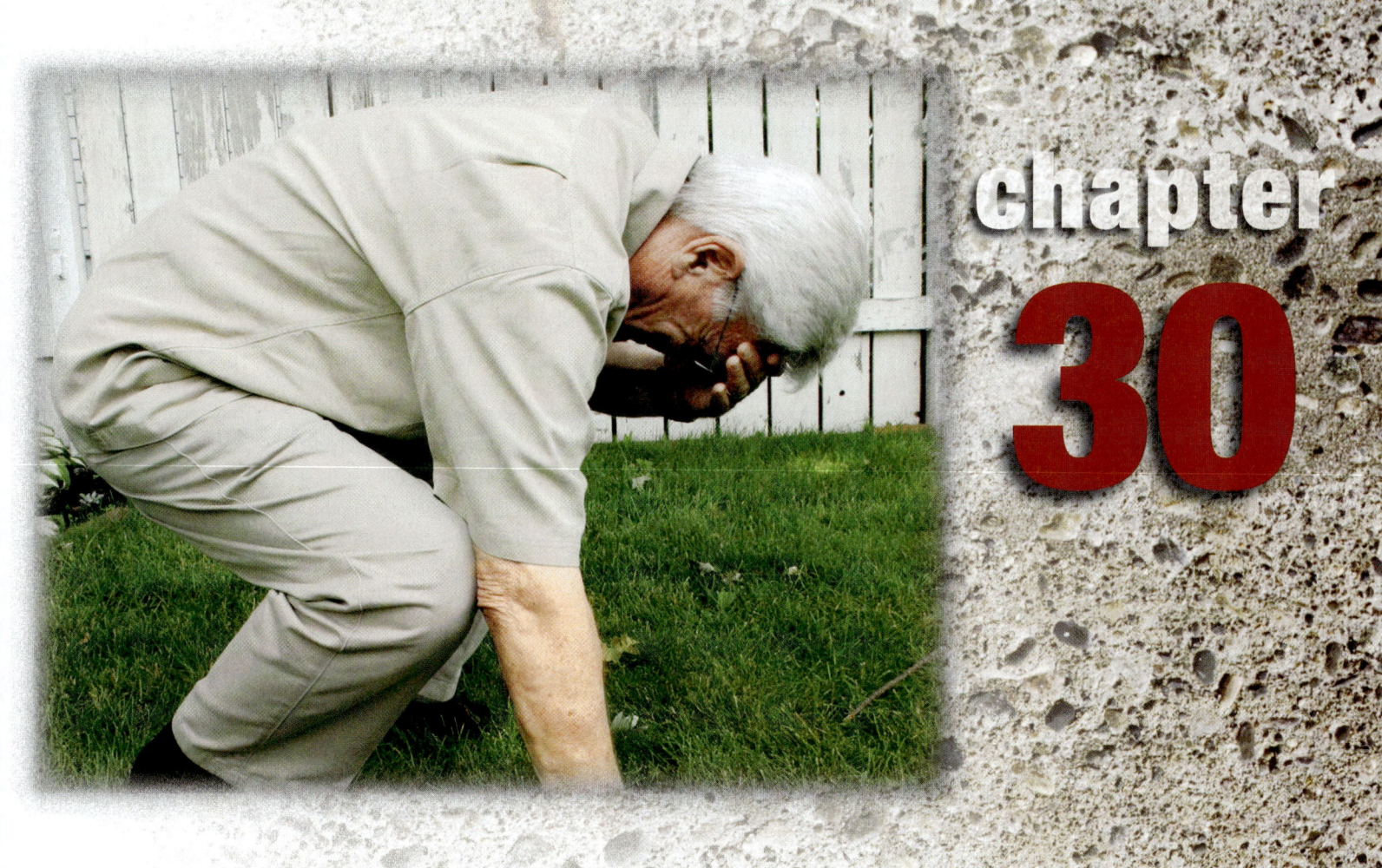

Neurology

"Somewhere, something incredible is waiting to be known."

—Carl Sagan

Need to Know

▶ The cause of altered mental status (AMS) is hypoxia until proven otherwise.

▶ Always provide oxygen; don't wait for cyanosis to develop as this is a very late sign.

▶ Use basic adjuncts to control the airway. Attempt BLS techniques before ALS.

▶ Assist ventilations if the patient is hypoventilating or there are signs of hypoxia (despite a normal respiratory rate) that persist after initial interventions with supplemental oxygen.

▶ Never hyperventilate a patient unless there are obvious signs of herniation present.

▶ Rule out immediately treatable causes for AMS such as hypoglycemia or narcotic overdose before performing advanced airway procedures.

▶ Sick	▶ Not Yet Sick
• Status epilepticus and stroke are true life-threatening situations that require prompt action. • Altered mental status and unconsciousness require further assessment in an attempt to discover the root cause; however, stabilization of the ABCs is still the first priority. • Use the Cincinnati Prehospital Stroke Scale (CPSS) or the Los Angeles Prehospital Stroke Screen (LAPSS) to assess suspected stroke victims. • Perform a rapid neurologic examination for the unconscious patient, including looking at pupils, assessing for any eye movements, and checking motor response (grimacing or posturing) to painful stimuli.	• Consider the possible causes listed in the AEIOU-TIPS memory aid to guide your assessment.

Introduction

The nervous system is a complex and intricate network of neurons and neural connections that regulates senses, controls motor functions, and houses human intelligence and emotion.

A clear understanding of basic neuroanatomy and physiology will help you determine the appropriate treatment of the patient with altered mental status or evidence of neurological impairment. The elements of the neurological exam are based on this understanding of the structure and function of the nervous system. **This chapter is supported by Skill Sheet 30: Prehospital Stroke Evaluation (also see Step-by-Step 30).**

Basic Function of the Nervous System

The nervous system is divided into two main systems: the **central nervous system (CNS),** which consists of the brain and spinal cord, and the **peripheral nervous system (PNS),** which includes the cranial and spinal nerves. There are two divisions of the peripheral nervous system: the **somatic** or "voluntary" and the **autonomic** or "involuntary." The autonomic nervous system consists of two divisions: the **sympathetic** and **parasympathetic** nervous systems (Figure 30-1). DOT 5-3.3

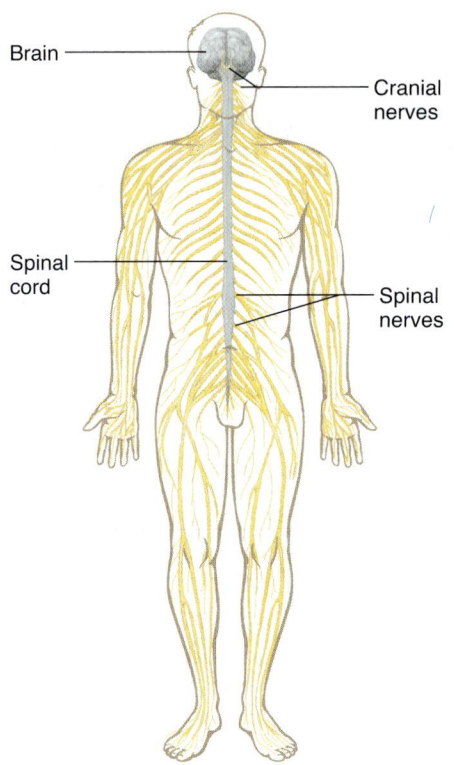

Figure 30-1 The central (gray) and peripheral (yellow) nervous systems.

Cells of the Nervous System

There are several types of cells found in the nervous system, including neurons and glial cells.

The neuron or nerve cell is the functional unit of the nervous system.

There are three main types of neurons. **Sensory** (or **afferent**) neurons detect stimuli and changes in the environment and carry electrical signals into the CNS. **Motor** (or **efferent**) neurons carry electrical signals to the effector cell such as a muscle or gland. Most nerves include both sensory and motor fibers, and they are called **mixed nerves. Interneurons** carry electrical signals from one neuron to another. Other important cell types include glial cells; astrocytes, which form the blood brain barrier; oligodendrocytes, the myelin-producing cells of the CNS; and ependymal cells, which line the ventricles of the brain (Figure 30-2). **Myelin** forms a sheath or covering around some nerve cells and allows for faster transmission of the nerve impulse down the length of the neuron. DOT 5-3.3

Nerve Fiber Classification

Nerves that originate from the brain and communicate with other parts of the body are called cranial nerves. Those that originate from the spinal cord and communicate with other parts of the body are called spinal nerves. The nerve fibers within these structures are further subdivided into four groups:

1. General somatic efferent fibers: carry motor impulses outward from the brain or spinal cord to skeletal muscles and stimulate them to contract.
2. General visceral efferent fibers: carry motor impulses outward from the brain or spinal cord to various smooth muscles and glands associated with internal organs, causing certain muscles to contract or glands to secrete.
3. General somatic afferent fibers: carry sensory impulses inward to the brain or spinal cord from receptors in the skin and skeletal muscles.
4. General visceral afferent fibers: carry sensory impulses to the CNS from blood vessels and internal organs.

The Cranial Nerves

There are 12 pairs of cranial nerves that arise directly from the underside of the brain and connect to parts of the head, neck, and trunk. The first two pair arise from the cerebrum, and the remaining 10 pairs arise from the brainstem. The names of the cranial nerves indicate their primary functions or the general distribution of their fibers. Table 30-1 lists the names of the nerves, their classification, and where they innervate.

Most cranial nerves are mixed (both sensory and motor), but some are pure sensory or pure motor. Some cranial nerves are somatic, and others are autonomic. In addition to the four subdivisions of nerve fibers just described, cranial nerves have three other specialized groups of fibers because of their direct connection to the brain:

1. Special somatic efferent fibers carry motor impulses outward from the brain to the muscles used in chewing, swallowing, speaking, and forming facial expressions.

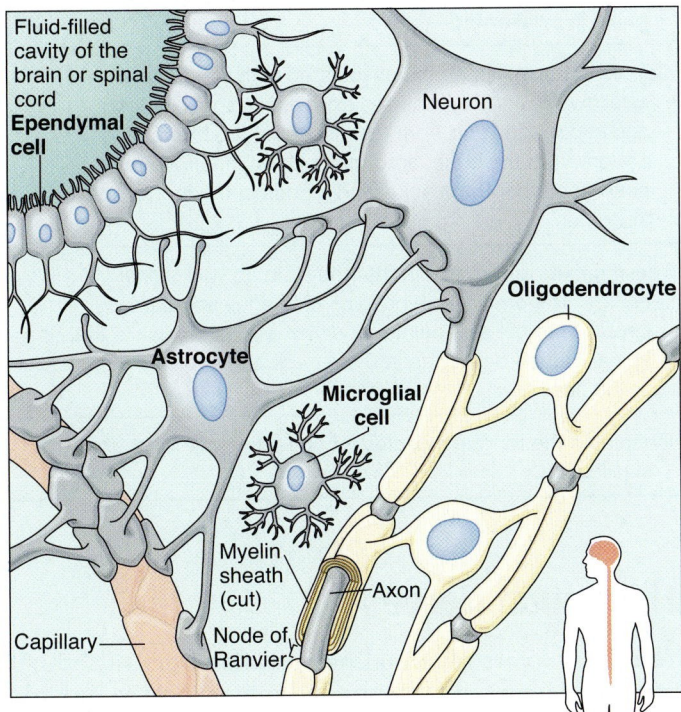

Figure 30-2 The cellular structure of the peripheral nervous system.

Nice to Know

A disorder of the trigeminal nerve (CN-V) causes severe recurrent pain in the face and forehead on the affected side. If drugs cannot control the pain, the nerve can be severed surgically. If this occurs, the patient loses sensation to all the areas of the head this nerve serves, so they must be careful when eating and drinking hot foods and beverages, and they must carefully inspect their mouth for the development of sores. DOT 5-3.66e

TABLE 30-1   The Twelve Pairs of Cranial Nerves

Number and Name	Classification Type	Innervation Site
I Olfactory	Sensory	Nose—receptor sites for the sense of smell
II Optic	Sensory	Connects the eyes to the brain
III Oculomotor	Motor	Controls involuntary muscles in the eyes, constrict and dilate pupil and help focus the eye
IV Trochlear	Motor (mainly)	Supplies the superior oblique muscle of the eye (which is not innervated by CN-III)
V Trigeminal (so named because it has three divisions: ophthalmic, maxillary, and mandibular)	Mixed	Brings impulses from the eye, tear gland, some of the scalp, forehead, and upper eyelid; carries impulses from the upper teeth, lip, and gum and palate. The third division is mixed and it transmits impulses from behind the ear, skin of jaw, lower teeth, gum, and lip; it also allows for mastication (chewing) and moves muscles in the floor of the jaw.
VI Abducens	Motor (mainly)	Supplies motor function to the lateral rectus muscle of the eye
VII Facial	Mixed	Sensation of taste on the anterior two-thirds of the tongue and motor response for facial expressions, and stimulates secretions from tear ducts and salivary glands
VIII Vestibulocochlear (also called acoustic or auditory nerve)	Sensory	Each nerve has two parts, vestibular and cochlear, that sense positional changes in the head, help maintain equilibrium, and provide for hearing
IX Glossopharyngeal	Mixed (predominately sensory)	Carries impulses from the pharynx, tonsils, and posterior third of the tongue to the brain; they innervate some salivary glands and constrict muscles in the pharynx to aid in swallowing
X Vagus	Mixed with somatic and autonomic fibers (autonomic predominate)	Carries impulses to larynx, associated with speech and swallowing, carries impulses from the pharynx, larynx, and esophagus and from the viscera of the thorax and abdomen to the brain; autonomic fibers innervate the heart and smooth muscles and glands in the thorax and abdomen
XI Accessory (spinal accessory)	Motor with some sensory	These nerves are unique in that they join up with spinal nerves. The cranial branch joins the vagus and carries impulses to the soft palate, pharynx, and larynx while the spinal branch descends into the neck and supplies muscles of the neck
XII Hypoglossal	Motor with some sensory	Innervates the tongue muscles for speaking, chewing, and swallowing

2. Special visceral afferent fibers carry sensory impulses inward to the brain from the olfactory and taste receptors.

3. Special somatic afferent fibers carry sensory impulses inward to the brain from the receptors of sight, hearing, and equilibrium.

The Spinal Nerves

Thirty-one pairs of spinal nerves arise from the spinal cord. These mixed (sensory and motor) nerves provide two-way communication between the spinal cord and the neck, trunk, and upper and lower limbs. Spinal nerves are not named individually, but they are grouped according to the spinal level from which they arise and are numbered sequentially. The intervertebral foramen is associated with the inferior portion of each vertebra, so each spinal nerve that passes through the foramen is associated with the vertebra above it. The exception is the cervical spine in which each spinal nerve root passes superior to the vertebra. There are eight pairs of cervical nerves (numbered C1 to C8), 12 pairs of thoracic nerves (numbered T1 to T12), five pairs of lumbar nerves (numbered L1 to L5), five pairs of sacral nerves (numbered S1 to S5), and one pair of coccygeal nerves labeled C0.

Each nerve emerges by a dorsal and ventral nerve root. The dorsal root contains sensory fibers and has a dorsal root ganglion. The ventral root contains motor fibers. Just beyond its foramen, each spinal nerve divides into several branches. Most spinal nerves combine to form plexuses that direct nerve fibers to a particular body part.

The Anatomy and Function of the Neuron

The **neuron** has a distinct cell body (or **soma**) where metabolic processes take place. The cell body contains the nucleus and organelles for producing structural proteins, enzymes, and other substances for neuron cell function (Figure 30-3). **Dendrites** are the projections of the nerve cell that contain receptors for specific substances and carry electrical signals toward the cell body of the neuron. The electrical signal is carried away from the cell body via the **axon**, which then branches into axon terminals.[1]

Action Potential

The neuron generates electrical impulses called **action potentials** that travel along the axon to the synaptic terminals. The neuron cell membrane, at its resting membrane potential, is **polarized** with a relative negative charge on the inside of the cell membrane. The resting membrane potential is caused by a build-up of potassium ions on the inside of the cell and an excess of sodium ions on the outside of the cell. A transmembrane protein, known as the sodium-potassium ATPase (or the sodium-potassium "pump"), removes or "pumps" out three sodium ions from the cell for every two potassium ions it pumps into the cell. These events and conditions create an electrochemical gradient across the cell membrane, and the electrical impulse travels along the axon to the next structure (another nerve or perhaps the brain) along the way (Figure 30-4).

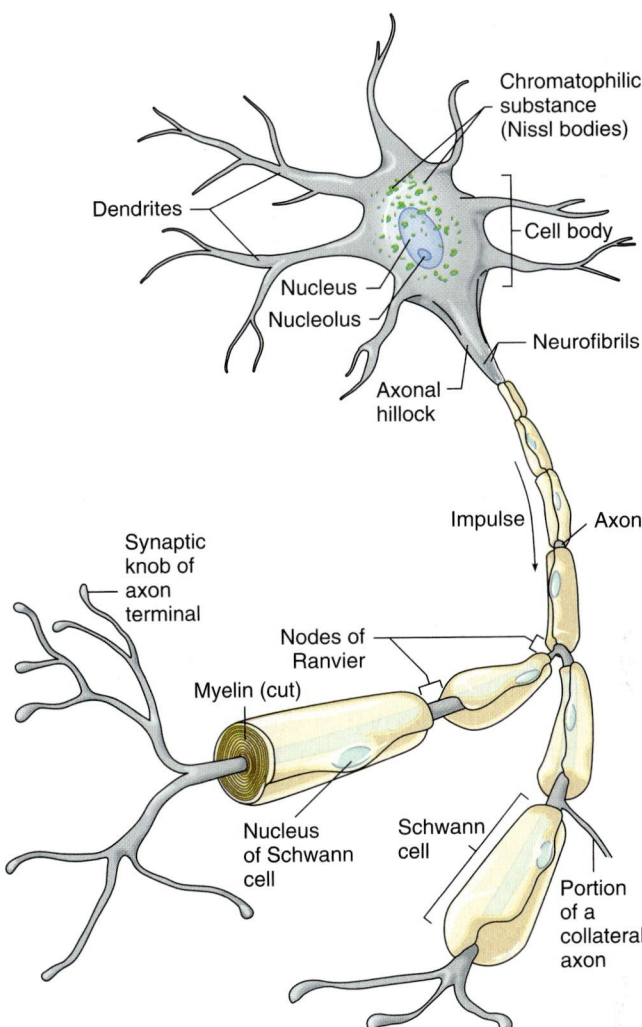

Figure 30-3 The relationship of neurons, dendrites, and axons in the peripheral system.

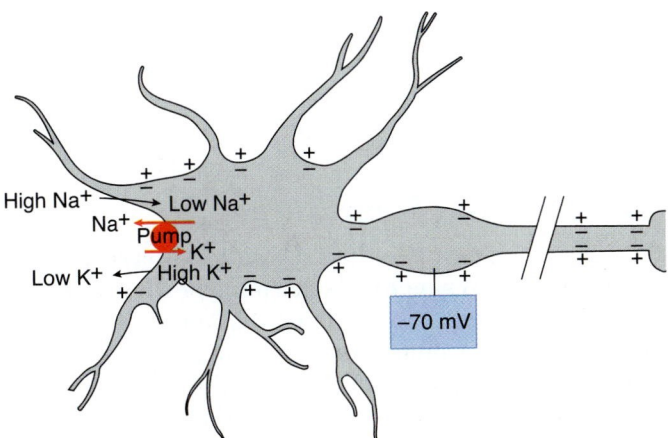

Figure 30-4 In the neuron cell membrane, an electromechanical gradient is created by the movement of sodium ions out of the cell and potassium ions into the cell.

Threshold Potential: Depolarization and Repolarization

Once the neuron reaches its **threshold potential,** voltage-gated sodium channels open, and sodium rapidly enters the cell, causing **depolarization** across the membrane. Slower potassium channels open, and potassium ions rush out of the cell, causing repolarization of the membrane. The sodium-potassium ATPase then restores the membrane to the **resting membrane potential,** and the cycle begins again. **Repolarization** is occurring at this time. This cycle of depolarization and repolarization is known as an action potential.[2]

CONNECTIONS This process is similar to that which occurs in the pacemaker cells of the heart and is described in more detail in Chapter 29: Cardiology.

The Response to the Action Potential

At the axon terminal (the presynaptic membrane), vesicles contain stored **neurotransmitters** that are released upon the arrival of the action potential. The neurotransmitter is released into the synapse. The **synapse** is the small space between the presynaptic membrane and the postsynaptic membrane of another cell (e.g., another neuron, a muscle cell, glands, etc.) (Figure 30-5).

At the synapse, the signal changes from electrical (as the action potential) to chemical (as the released neurotransmitter).

This process of electrochemical signaling is the basis of neurologic function. Some common neurotransmitters include acetylcholine, norepinephrine, dopamine, and serotonin; there are many others, and many still are yet to be discovered.

Mapping the Brain: Neuroanatomy Review

Regions of the Brain

The brain consists of distinct regions: the **cerebrum** (including the **basal ganglia** and **cortex**), the **diencephalon** (including the **thalamus** and **hypothalamus**), the **limbic system,** the **brainstem** (including the **midbrain, pons, medulla,** and **reticular formation**) and the **cerebellum** (Figure 30-6). The **cerebral hemispheres** are responsible for most of what are considered human abilities, including senses, memory, and personality. The **cerebral cortex** is the thin layer of gray matter (neuron cell bodies) that makes up the outer portion of the cerebrum.

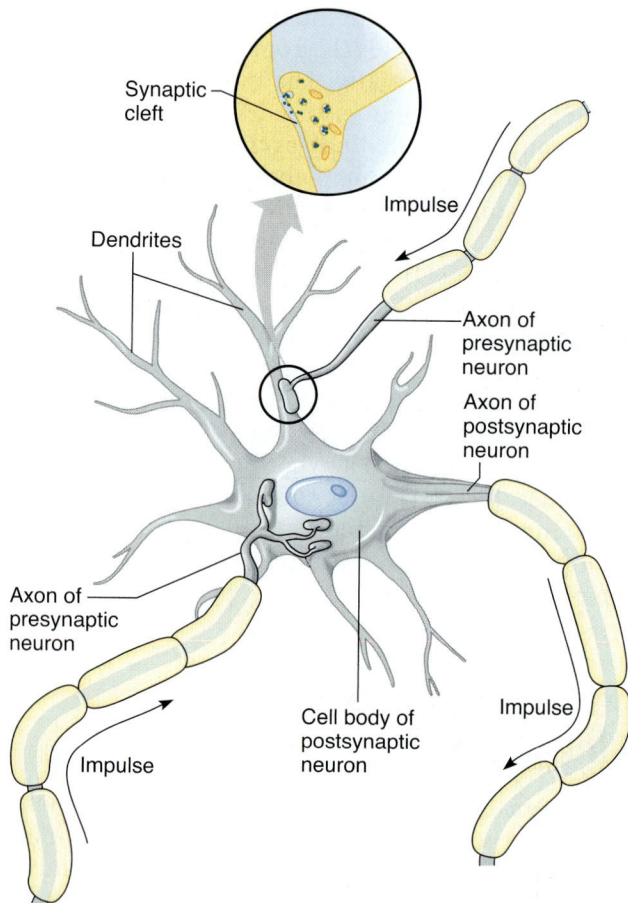

Figure 30-5 The synapse is the small space between the presynaptic membrane and the postsynaptic membrane of another cell (e.g., another neuron, a muscle cell, glands, etc.).

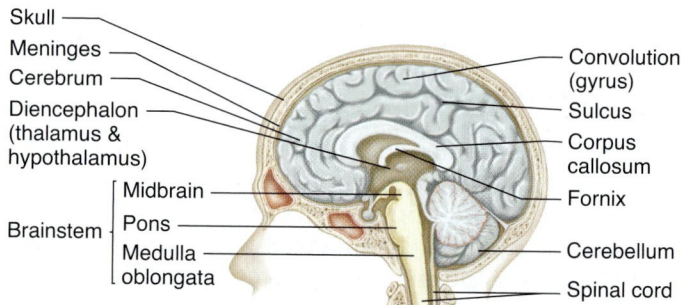

Figure 30-6 The regions of the brain include the cerebrum, the diencephalon, the midbrain, the brainstem, and the cerebellum.

Hemispheres of the Cerebrum

Each hemisphere is divided into paired **frontal, parietal, temporal,** and **occipital** lobes (Figure 30-7). Each hemisphere has a **lateral ventricle,** and **cerebrospinal fluid** (CSF) is produced in the ventricular system of the brain and circulates throughout the subarachnoid space.

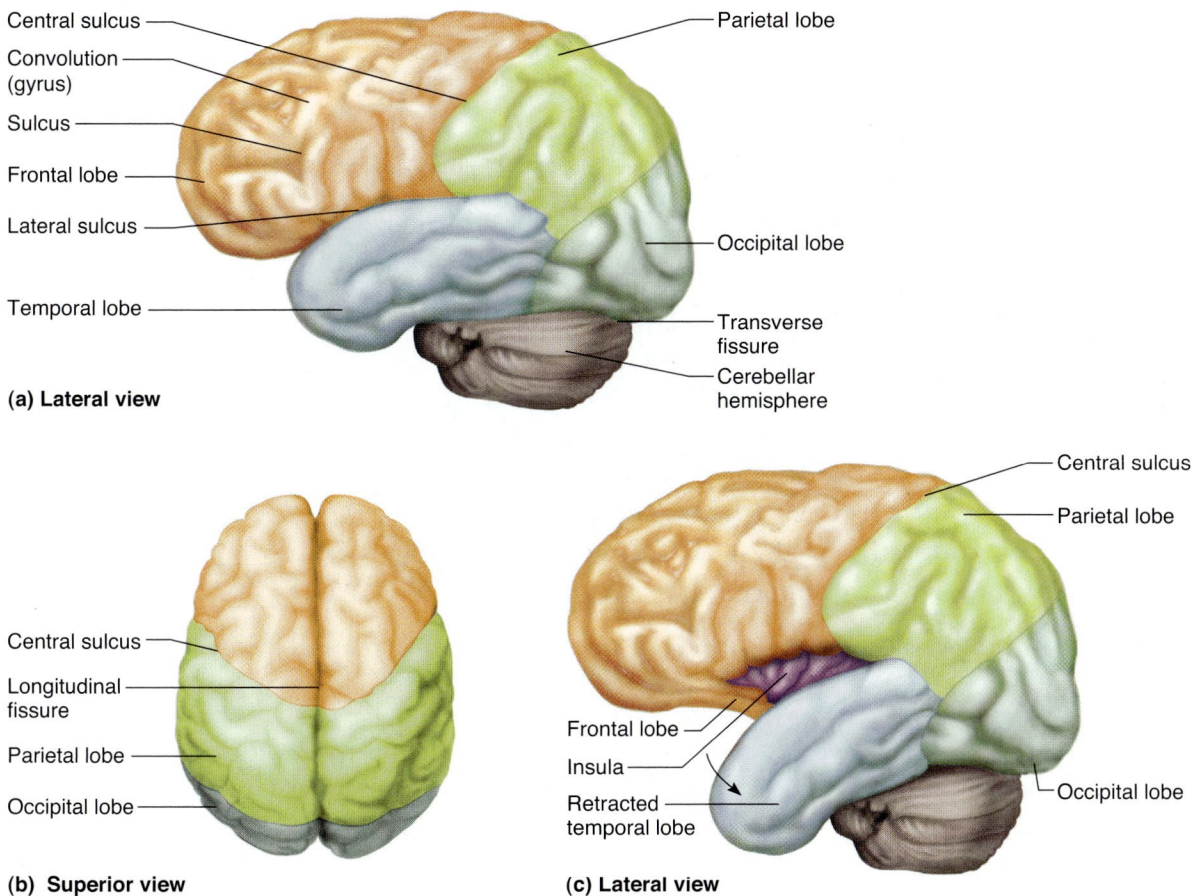

Figure 30-7   Each hemisphere of the brain is divided into frontal, parietal, temporal, and occipital lobes.

Two smaller ventricles, which bring the total number of ventricles to four, are located within the brain, close to the brain stem. The brain secretes approximately 500 mL of CSF daily, with 140 mL continuously found within the nervous system. CSF is continuously being reabsorbed into the blood.

The cerebral hemispheres contain some shared functions, found in both the right and left hemispheres, such as motor control, sensation, vision, hearing, and memory. **Motorsensory function** is located around the area of the central sulcus, which divides the frontal and parietal lobes. **Motor function** is located in the precentral gyrus of the frontal lobe, and **sensory function** is located in the postcentral gyrus of the parietal lobe. The frontal lobe is also responsible for higher thought and emotional behavior (Figure 30-8).

Specialized functions of the cerebral hemispheres include language and understanding spacial relationships. The ability to understand and convey language is most commonly located in the left hemisphere, the "dominant" hemisphere, in the frontal and parietal lobes. The right, or "nondominant," parietal lobe controls the sensory input for understanding spacial relationships. A basic understanding of these areas of the brain is critical to your ability to recognize the signs of focal damage to the brain as seen, for example, in stroke victims.

Basal Ganglia

Basal nuclei are masses of gray matter, called **basal ganglia,** located deep within the cerebral hemispheres. The neurons of the basal nuclei interact with other brain areas to facilitate voluntary movement, such as swinging your arms when you walk.

Nice to Know

Some older anatomy reference texts describe five ventricles instead of just four. The fifth one, when listed, is described as a continuation of a portion of the longitudinal fissure, which was shut off from the two hemispheres when the corpus callosum formed. It is typically no longer described as a ventricle since it does not secrete or contain cerebrospinal fluid as do the other four ventricles.

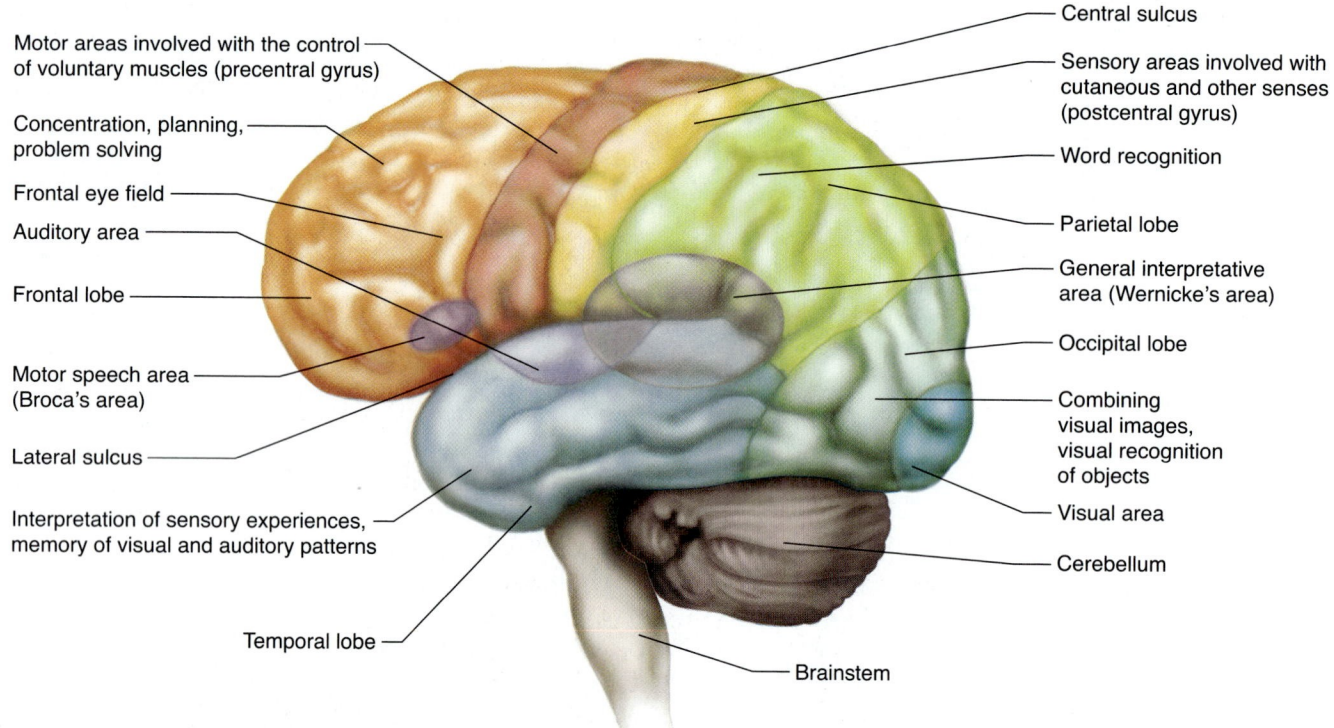

Figure 30-8   A basic understanding of the brain is critical to your ability to recognize signs of focal damage to the brain.

The Cerebral Cortex

The cortex covers the convolutions of the brain and dips into the sulci and fissures. The cortex contains nearly 75% of all neuron cell bodies in the nervous system. The cortex is responsible for motor and sensory functions. The occipital cortex is responsible for vision. The left occipital cortex is responsible for what you see in your right visual field of both eyes and the right occipital cortex is responsible for what you see in your left visual field of both eyes. The **auditory cortex** is located in the temporal lobe.

Street Secrets

Are we only skin deep? One way to think of the relationship between the cortex and the cerebrum is to think of the cortex as the skin covering the body of the cerebrum. In this case, because most every nerve (75%) is located in the cortex on the surface or "skin," all of our sensing abilities really are only "skin deep."

Diencephalon

The diencephalon consists of the thalamus and hypothalamus (Figure 30-9). The **thalamus** receives all incoming sensory messages (except those associated with the sense of smell) and relays them to the cortex. The thalamus not only receives and passes on messages, but it also has the ability to modify messages.

The **hypothalamus** regulates autonomic functions and homeostasis by linking the nervous and endocrine

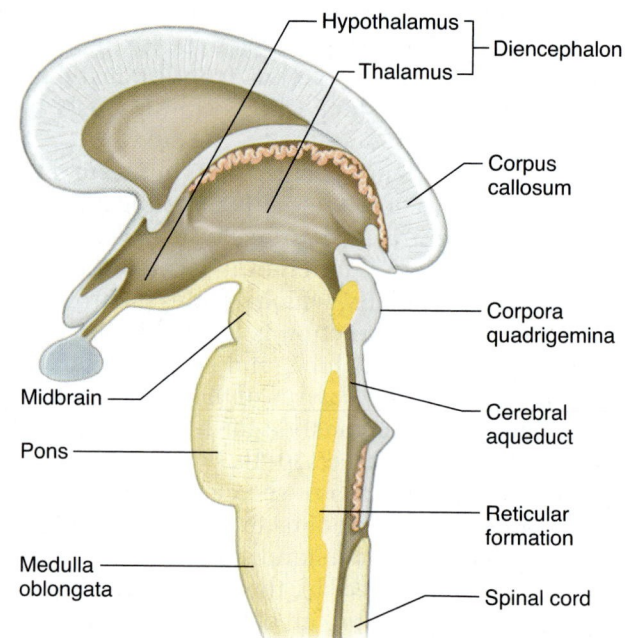

Figure 30-9   The diencephalon consists of the thalamus and hypothalamus.

systems. Specifically the hypothalamus regulates the following:

- Heart rate and arterial blood pressure
- Body temperature
- Water and electrolyte balance
- Control of hunger and body weight
- Control of movements of glandular secretions of the stomach and intestines
- Production of neurosecretory substances that stimulate the pituitary gland to release hormones that help regulate growth, control various glands, and influence reproductive physiological responses
- Sleep and wakefulness

Limbic System

The limbic system is a specialized portion of the brain that is located near the diencephalon. The **limbic system** controls emotional responses. It is comprised of portions of the cerebral cortex, and it connects to the hypothamalus, thalamus, basal nuclei, and other deep nuclei. In addition to controlling emotional experiences and expressions, it also modifies the way a person acts and produces fear, anger, pleasure, and sorrow. The

Nice to Know

Have you ever wondered why a certain smell triggers a feeling or emotion? Some pleasant examples may include a specific perfume that reminds you of your grandmother or the smell of turkey cooking reminding you of Thanksgiving dinners from years past. Because the olfactory receptors are located within the limbic system, triggering them may also cause a triggering of emotions that are tied to the memory of a certain smell.

limbic system is thought to guide a person by creating emotional responses that increase the chance of survival. The limbic system also interprets olfactory receptor impulses connected to the sense of smell.

Brainstem

The **brainstem** extends from the base of the brain to the spinal cord. It consists of the **midbrain, pons, and the medulla oblongata** (Figure 30-10). Axons from the neurons in the cerebral cortex extend down

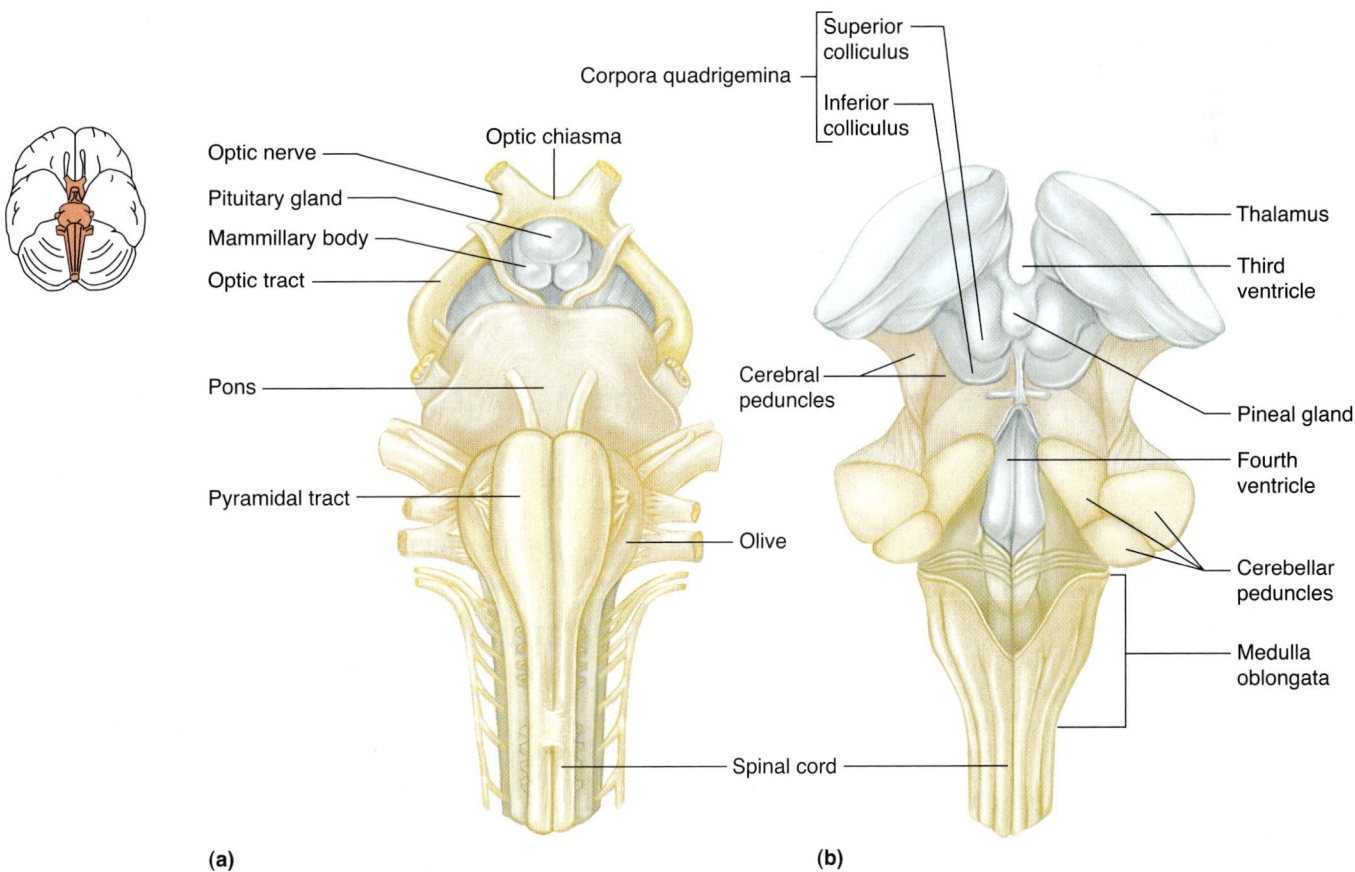

(a) **(b)**

Figure 30-10 Ventral (a) and dorsal (b) views of the brainstem.

through the brain and cross over in the brainstem to the opposite side of the body. For example, the right side of the brain controls motorsensory function of the left side of the body, and vice versa. Within the brain stem are areas that control autonomic functions such as cardiovascular and respiratory regulation. Nerves that control eye movements are located within the midbrain and pons.

Midbrain

The mesencephalon, or **midbrain,** is a short section of the brainstem between the diencephalon and pons. It joins lower parts of the brainstem and spinal cord with the higher parts of the brain. Reflex centers are located within the midbrain.

Pons

The **pons** separates the midbrain from the medulla oblongata. It relays messages between the cerebrum and medulla and between the cerebrum and cerebellum. Several nuclei relay impulses from peripheral nerves to higher brain centers. Other nuclei function with centers of the medulla to regulate the rate and depth of breathing.

Medulla Oblongata

The **medulla oblongata** is a continuation of the spinal cord. It extends from the foramen magnum of the skull up to the pons. Because of its location, all of the nerve fibers connecting the brain and spinal cord pass through it. Centers of control found within the medulla include the following:

- Cardiac center: Peripheral nerves transmit impulses to the heart to increase or decrease heart rate.
- Vasomotor center: Impulses travel to certain smooth muscles in blood vessel walls and stimulate contraction (vasoconstriction), which increases blood pressure. A decrease in the activity of these cells leads to vasodilation, which drops blood pressure.
- Respiratory center: The primary respiratory control center is located in the medulla. It regulates rate, rhythm, and depth of breathing. In the event of damage to this center, others can take over.
- Other centers: The medulla contains the control centers for some nonvital functions including coughing, sneezing, swallowing, and vomiting.

Reticular Formation

The **reticular formation** (or the reticular activating system or RAS) is responsible for arousal and alertness. The RAS is a complex network of nerve fibers scattered throughout the medulla, pons, and midbrain. A sensory impulse passes through this area to the cerebral cortex and "awakens" it to the incoming impulse. The RAS has the ability to filter impulses, and it may opt not to send them on. Decreased activity in the RAS results in sleep. Lesions of this area will cause a loss of consciousness.

What is consciousness? A patient who is comatose or unconscious has lost awareness, arousal, and the ability to meaningfully interact with the environment. Consciousness depends on the normal function of two main brain regions, the reticular formation (or RAS) and the cerebral cortex of the bilateral cerebral hemispheres. A collection of thousands of neurons dispersed throughout the brain stem, the RAS is the "light switch" that turns on the signal to the cerebral processes of thought and emotion. Damage or insult to the RAS or to both hemispheres of the cerebral cortex results in a loss of consciousness (coma).[3] **DOT 5-3.8**

Cerebellum

The **cerebellum** is responsible for unconscious control of somatic motor activity. It is composed of white matter with a thin layer of gray matter, just like the cerebrum. The gray matter is also called a cortex. The cerebellum communicates with other parts of the CNS through one of three pairs of nerve tracks called cerebellar peduncles. Sensory information from the body passes through this area and is filtered and transmitted to appropriate parts of the brain. Motor responses are then passed downward toward the pons, medulla, and down the spinal cord. The cerebellum integrates sensory information concerning body position and coordinates skeletal muscle responses. Dysfunction of the cerebellum will result in a staggered gait. It also receives and interprets sensory information from the eyes and ears.

The Meninges

Membranous protective layers, called the **meninges,** surround the brain and spinal cord and include the outer **dura mater,** the **arachnoid mater**, and the innermost layer, the **pia mater** (Figure 30-11).

The Peripheral Nervous System

The peripheral nervous system (PNS) consists of the 12 pairs of cranial nerves (that arise directly from the brain) and the 31 pairs of spinal nerves.

Sensory nerve tracts carry electrical impulses into the CNS, and motor nerve tracts carry impulses away from the CNS.

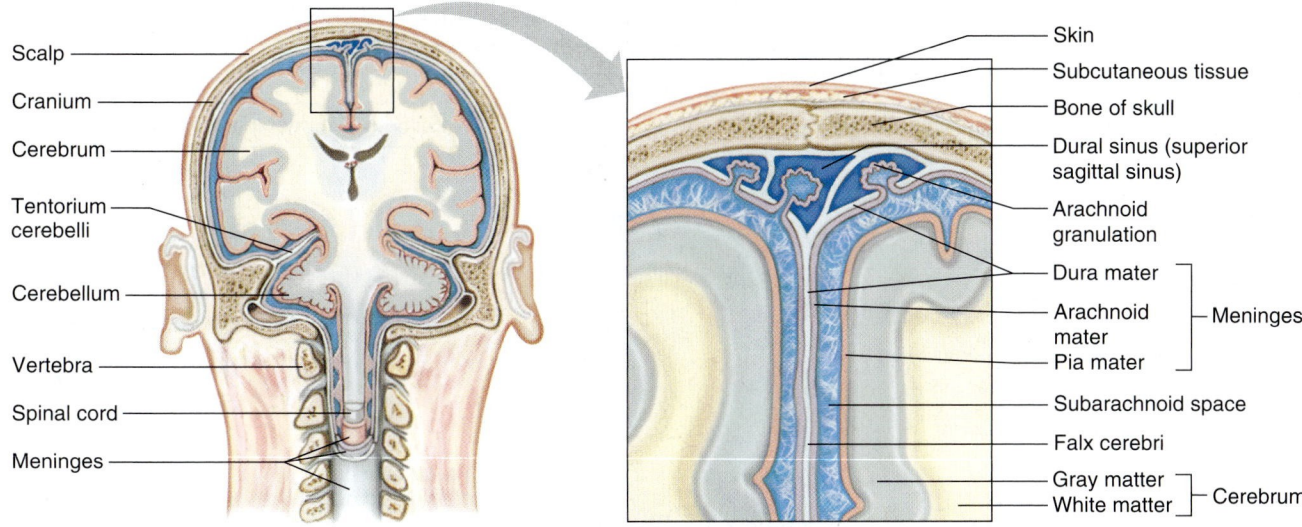

Scalp
Cranium
Cerebrum
Tentorium cerebelli
Cerebellum
Vertebra
Spinal cord
Meninges

Skin
Subcutaneous tissue
Bone of skull
Dural sinus (superior sagittal sinus)
Arachnoid granulation
Dura mater
Arachnoid mater — Meninges
Pia mater
Subarachnoid space
Falx cerebri
Gray matter
White matter — Cerebrum

Figure 30-11   The brain is protected by the skull and layers of meningeal tissue.

The PNS is divided into the somatic and autonomic systems. The somatic system controls voluntary movement of skeletal muscle while the autonomic nervous system (ANS) controls involuntary functions such as respiration, circulation, and digestion.

The **ANS** has two divisions: the **sympathetic** and **parasympathetic** nervous systems (Figure 30-12).

Sympathetic Nervous System

The sympathetic nervous system controls the "fight or flight" response. Sympathetic stimulation causes pupil dilation, increases in heart rate and the force of cardiac contraction, dilation of the bronchioles, and shunting of blood away from the skin and digestive organs, with increased blood flow to the skeletal muscles and the vital organs (heart, lungs, and brain). Sympathetic nervous system stimulation also causes an increase in blood glucose through the breakdown of glycogen in the liver.

Parasympathetic Nervous System

The parasympathetic nervous system controls the "rest and digest" response. Parasympathetic stimulation causes pupil constriction, an increase in gastric and digestive secretions, a reduction in heart rate, and constriction of the bronchioles.[4]

CONNECTIONS   Chapters 8: Physiology Overview, 15: Pharmacology, and 29: Cardiology discuss the nervous system from the perspective of the unique controls of the sympathetic and parasympathetic divisions of the ANS.

Cerebral Circulation

The brain receives its blood supply through anterior and posterior circulations. The internal carotid arteries branch into the left and right middle cerebral arteries (MCA) and the anterior cerebral arteries (ACA) (Figures 30-13 and 30-14). The MCAs provide most of the cerebral blood flow to the hemispheres, and interruption of blood flow within these arteries causes dramatic neurologic deficits. The ACAs supply oxygenated blood to areas of the brain that include motor and sensory functions of the lower extremities. The posterior circulation to the brain is provided by the paired vertebral arteries, which enter the base of the skull and then join at the brainstem to form the large basilar artery. At the top of the midbrain, the basilar artery branches to form the posterior cerebral arteries (PCA), which supply blood to the occipital lobes.

Some important areas of the brain are perfused by small blood vessels. Disruption in blood flow of even one of these small vessels can cause dramatic neurologic symptoms. Some of these small vessels arise from the middle cerebral artery (MCA) to supply a region known as the internal capsule. The internal capsule carries the axons from neurons that extend from the cerebral cortex to the spinal cord. Other small vessels branch from the basilar artery and feed the thalamus and brain stem.[5]

Blood flow to the brain is constant despite changes in blood pressure and metabolic activity. The cerebral perfusion pressure (CPP) is equal to the mean arterial pressure (MAP) minus the intracranial pressure (ICP). If the intracranial pressure rises, the cerebral perfusion pressure will fall, and cerebral ischemia will result. Examples of conditions that can increase intracranial

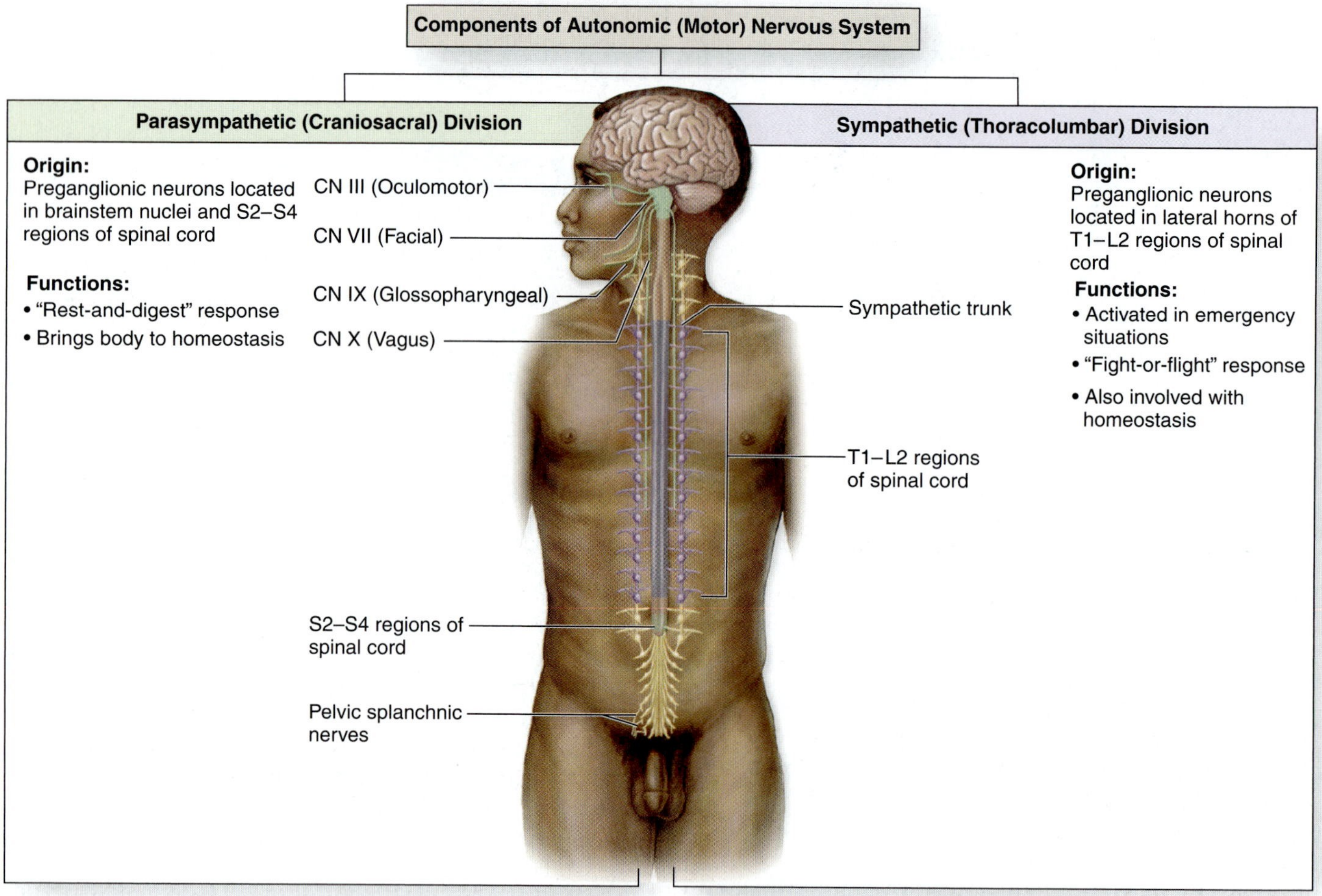

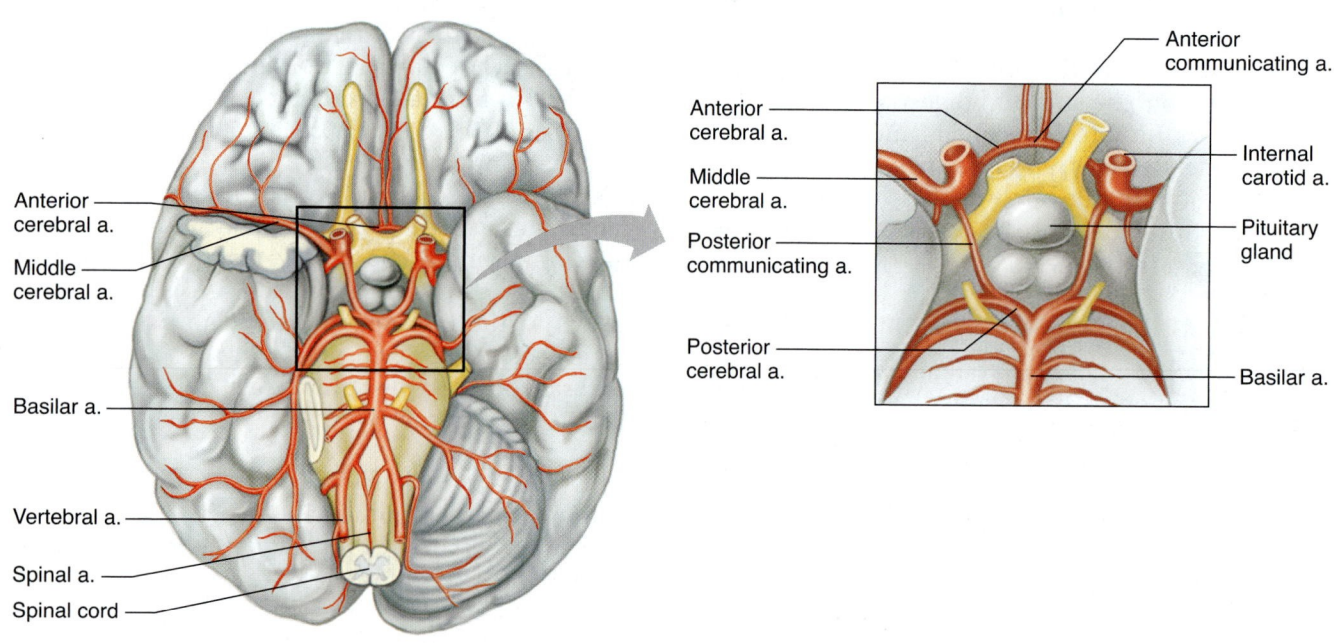

Components of Autonomic (Motor) Nervous System

Parasympathetic (Craniosacral) Division

Origin:
Preganglionic neurons located in brainstem nuclei and S2–S4 regions of spinal cord

Functions:
• "Rest-and-digest" response
• Brings body to homeostasis

CN III (Oculomotor)
CN VII (Facial)
CN IX (Glossopharyngeal)
CN X (Vagus)

S2–S4 regions of spinal cord

Pelvic splanchnic nerves

Sympathetic (Thoracolumbar) Division

Origin:
Preganglionic neurons located in lateral horns of T1–L2 regions of spinal cord

Functions:
• Activated in emergency situations
• "Fight-or-flight" response
• Also involved with homeostasis

Sympathetic trunk

T1–L2 regions of spinal cord

Figure 30-12   The autonomic nervous system is made up of the parasympathetic and sympathetic divisions.

Anterior cerebral a.
Middle cerebral a.
Basilar a.
Vertebral a.
Spinal a.
Spinal cord

Anterior cerebral a.
Middle cerebral a.
Posterior communicating a.
Posterior cerebral a.

Anterior communicating a.
Internal carotid a.
Pituitary gland
Basilar a.

Figure 30-13   Cerebral circulation.

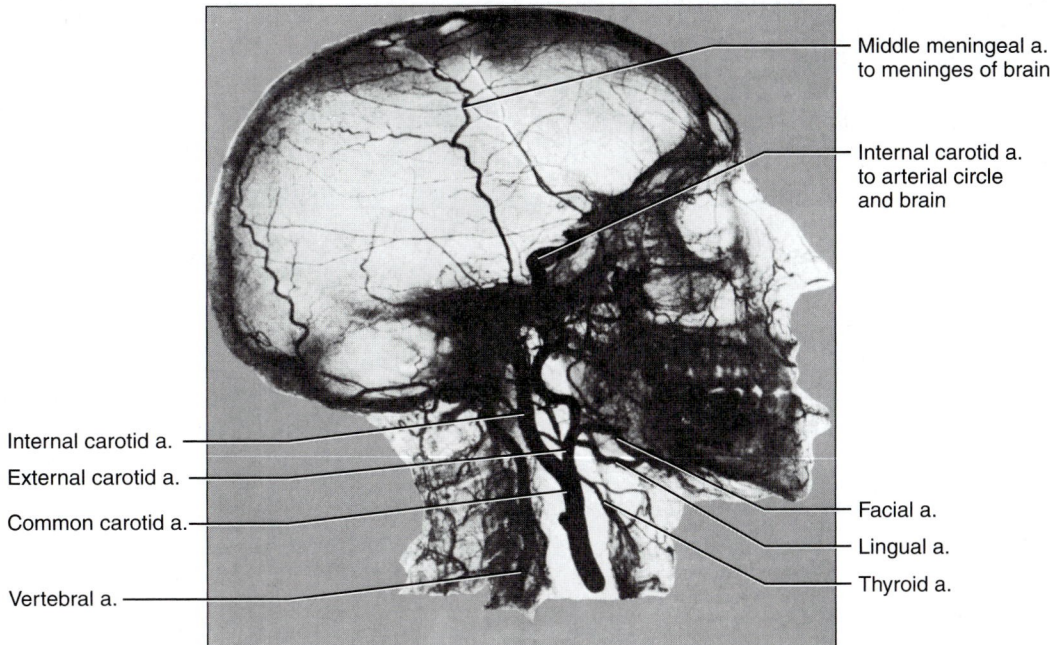

Internal carotid a.
External carotid a.
Common carotid a.
Vertebral a.

Middle meningeal a.
to meninges of brain

Internal carotid a.
to arterial circle
and brain

Facial a.
Lingual a.
Thyroid a.

Figure 30-14   Arteries that deliver blood to the head.

pressure include traumatic brain injury, intracranial hemorrhage, cerebral edema, and certain metabolic conditions such as hypoxia (low oxygen) and hypercapnea (high carbon dioxide). DOT 5-3.4

Cerebral Perfusion Pressure

Cerebral perfusion pressure (CPP) = Mean arterial pressure (MAP) − Intracranial pressure (ICP)

MAP = Diastolic pressure + 1/3 of Pulse pressure

Pulse pressure = Systolic pressure − Diastolic pressure

ICP is typically 0–15 mmHg and CPP is typically around 70 mmHg (60–90 mmHg)

The Neurologic Exam

Components of the neurologic examination cross over both the primary and secondary surveys. A general level of consciousness baseline assessment is performed during the initial assessment by using the AVPU assessment. If the patient appears to have a traumatic brain injury (TBI), the Glasgow Coma Scale (GCS) may be calculated as a part of the initial assessment as well. If the patient is severely injured, has a significant mechanism of injury, or is unconscious, the appropriate initial assessment may include the "D" element (which stands for disability) and "E" (expose) component added to the standard ABC assessment for serious trauma situations. If this is the case, the disability assessment will include a quick palpation of

the extremities and a pulse, motor, and sensory check of both feet and both hands. DOT 5-3.6

The secondary survey components of the neurologic examination include such elements as the cranial nerve assessment, blood glucose monitoring, and notation of areas of the body that have alterations in sensation or motor. It may also include using stroke assessment tools such as the Cincinnati Prehospital Stroke Scale or the Los Angeles Prehospital Stroke Screen. Each of the tools will be explored in more detail. DOT 5-3.5

Elements of the Neurological Exam

The following procedures, evaluations, and tests are included in the neurological assessment of a patient. Not every item is used on each patient encounter, even when the source of the emergency is a neurologic system problem. Experience and protocols will help guide which assessment tools are appropriate. The following are elements of the neurologic assessment to consider during your assessment:

- Assess the level of consciousness (LOC) with the AVPU or GCS
- Pupil evaluation for reactivity to light and speed of reaction
- Facial muscle and symmetry evaluation
- Motor ability and grip strength
- Sensation evaluation
- Language ability assessment
- Cranial nerve assessment

BOX 30-1   The Glasgow Coma Scale

Eye Opening

4 = spontaneous
3 = to voice
2 = to pain
1 = no response

Verbal Response

5 = oriented (aware of surroundings, knows person, place, time, and event)
4 = confused
3 = inappropriate words
2 = incomprehensible words
1 = no response

Motor Response

6 = obeys commands
5 = localizes pain (purposefully attempts to stop a painful stimuli)
4 = withdraws from pain (moves away from painful stimuli)
3 = abnormal flexion to pain (decorticate posturing) (Figure 30-15[a])
2 = abnormal extension to pain (decerebrate posturing) (Figure 30-15[b])
1 = no response

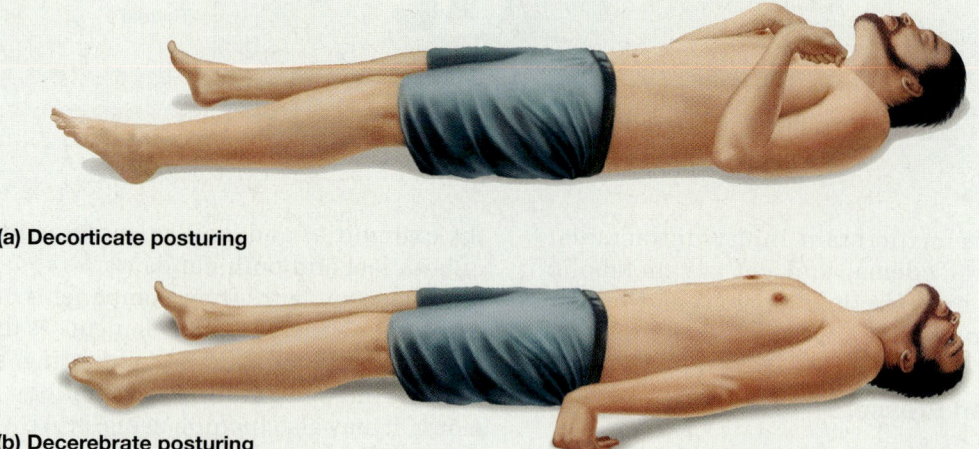

(a) Decorticate posturing

(b) Decerebrate posturing

Figure 30-15   Decorticate and decerebrate posturing.

- The Cincinnati Prehospital Stroke Scale or Los Angeles Prehospital Stroke Screen assessment
- SAMPLE history focusing on AEIOU-TIPS criteria
DOT 5-3.2

Assessing the Level of Consciousness

The neurologic exam is an important assessment tool that you will use to determine whether or not the patient is suffering from an insult to the nervous system, and it begins with evaluating the level of consciousness. Patients may be fully conscious at one end of the spectrum or comatose at the other end. Alterations of consciousness can occur anywhere between these two endpoints. DOT 5-3.8

Assessing level of consciousness in the prehospital setting involves an initial evaluation of the basic responsiveness of the patient using the simple AVPU scale. Is the patient awake, responsive to verbal stimuli, responsive to painful stimuli, or unresponsive?

AVPU

A = Awake
V = Verbal stimuli, responsive to
P = Painful stimuli, responsive to
U = Unresponsive

Once the basic level of responsiveness has been established, perform the primary assessment evaluating the airway, breathing, and circulation, and correct any immediate life threats. After treatment of any identified life threats, the Glasgow Coma Scale (GCS) will give you a more detailed evaluation of the level of consciousness. The pupils may be assessed during the initial assessment, but most often they will be checked during the secondary survey. DOT 5-3.9

Use the GCS to evaluate the patient's state of consciousness at regular intervals (Box 30-1). One of the first signs of hypoxia is a deterioration of the patient's mental status, which may present initially as combativeness, irritability, confusion, or agitation. If this condition is untreated, it will progress to obtundation (insensitivity to stimuli) and eventually coma. If the airway, breathing, and circulation are stabilized and the patient has a persistent altered mental status, consider other metabolic abnormalities (e.g., hypoglycemia, sepsis, hypothermia, overdose) or structural abnormalities (e.g., stroke, traumatic injury, tumor, abscess), and treat according to protocol.

Street Secrets

Another way to learn the GCS score is to think of it as the "EVM-456" scale. The eyes, verbal, and motor (or EVM) score has four points, five points, and six points, respectively, which may make it easier to learn as each letter is now a clue to what is assessed and not a random name. The EVM-456 scale should be performed routinely on all patients, time permitting, on each ambulance transport until the scale becomes second nature and is memorized.

Evaluating the level of consciousness is the most important element of the neurological exam. Other important components collectively evaluate for evidence of focal (specific) or global neurologic deficits. Structural abnormalities most often present with focal (asymmetric) signs such as unequal pupils, hemiparesis, or hemiplegia. Metabolic or toxicologic abnormalities most often present with global neurologic deficits such as altered mental status, bilaterally dilated or pinpoint pupils, or coma.

Pupil Evaluation

Evaluate pupils for size, equality, and reactivity to light. Evaluate eye movements in the awake patient by asking the patient to follow horizontal and vertical movements. In the unconscious patient, evaluate eye movements by using the oculocephalic or "doll's eyes" maneuver.

This maneuver, however, should not be performed in the patient with suspected cervical spine or head injury.

In a conscious patient, the eyes will move in the same direction as the head is turned; whereas, in the unconscious patient, the eyes appear to move to the opposite side as the head is turned. Evaluate visual fields in the conscious patient by facing the patient and extending your arms on either side of the patient's visual field. Instruct the patient to look at your nose, and then alternately wiggle the right, the left, and then both index fingers while instructing the patient to point to the side of their visual field where they see movement.

Facial Muscle and Symmetry Evaluation

Observe the face for signs of asymmetry (one-sided facial droop). Ask the patient to show his teeth. Facial droop will appear as a flattening of the nasolabial fold and the inability to raise the corner of the mouth in a smile. If there is asymmetry, determine if this is a new event, an ongoing situation, or perhaps their normal, baseline appearance. Note if there is a progressive worsening to the droop, and document the times you noted changes in the patient care report.

Motor Ability and Grip Strength

Does the patient move all extremities equally? Ask patients to extend their arms with palms facing up in front of them. Look for signs of weakness in one or both arms. **Arm drift** occurs as patients are unable to hold one or both arms straight out in front for longer than a few seconds or if they are unable to hold them at the same height. Ask patients to squeeze your hands or two fingers, and note if their grip is equal on each side of the body. You can also ask patients to push or pull against your hands to test their strength.

Evaluate for evidence of weakness in the lower extremities. To perform this test, ask patients to push down on your hands placed on the soles of their feet (like a gas pedal), and ask patients to lift up their foot with your hands placed on the top of the foot.

If patients are ambulatory, evaluate the gait by observing patients walk a short distance. Be sure to support patients while doing this if there is any question of their stability.

Street Secrets

Avoid knuckle smashing grips by presenting patients with two fingers to squeeze instead of your whole hand. If you cross your two extended fingers first, patients will not grind your knuckles into each other as they squeeze your hands. Place your middle finger fingertip directly over your first finger nailbed, and ask patients to grasp your fingers.

Sensation Evaluation

Note if the patient complains of pain, numbness, loss of feeling, heat or cold sensation, or a tingling sensation anywhere. Evaluate the patient's ability to sense touch in all extremities by lightly stroking your fingers along the side, top, and bottom of the foot, and sides and back of the hand. Never use a sharp instrument or anything capable of penetrating the skin to perform this test.

Street Secrets

When you grasp a toe or finger, do so out of the patient's line of vision, and then ask which one you grasped. Pick either the great or small toe for the foot and either the thumb or smallest finger for the hand. Picking a digit from somewhere in the middle just confuses the examination and may confuse the patient trying to cooperate and respond to you. The neurologist will perform detailed intricate assessments of sensatory or motor deficit if it is appropriate to do so. You are simply performing a gross assessment to establish a baseline for your own treatment of the patient.

Language Ability Assessment

As you speak to the patient, note any difficulties in language such as halting speech (expressive aphasia) or difficulty understanding (receptive aphasia). Ask the patient to name a few simple objects that you hold up (such as a pen, watch, or flashlight) and to repeat a simple phrase to test for language deficits. The Cincinnati Prehospital Stroke Scale asks the patient to say "You can't teach an old dog new tricks."

Cranial Nerve Assessment

The cranial nerve assessment is presented in Box 30-2. This evaluation takes approximately one minute to perform, and it allows for the evaluation of all 12 cranial nerves. DOT 3-2.57, 3-2.58

Cincinnati Prehospital Stroke Scale or Los Angeles Prehospital Stroke Screen Assessment

The CPSS and LAPSS are two stroke screening tools. The CPSS tool is based on a physical examination only. It assesses three physical findings: facial droop, arm weakness or drift, and speech abnormalities. The presence of a single abnormality on the CPSS has a sensitivity for stroke of 59% and a specificity of 89%.[6] The LAPSS tool requires the paramedic to rule out other causes of altered mental status (such as hypoglycemia or seizures) as a part of the evaluation process and then identify asymmetry in any of three examination categories: facial smile or grimace, grip strength, and arm strength. The LAPSS has a specificity of 97% and sensitivity of 93%.[7] Tables 30-2 and 30-3 have additional information on each tool.

BOX 30-2   The One-Minute Cranial Nerve Exam

Evaluate all 12 cranial nerves with this series of simple tests:

1. Ask the patient to close their eyes and smell a common thing (alcohol prep) and identify the odor.
2. Light penlight, ask the patient to hold their head still, and to track the light with their eyes as you move the light around the head in an "H" pattern.
3. Ask the patient to clench teeth. You palpate the masseter and temporal muscles for tone.
4. Test sensation at forehead, chin, and each cheek.
5. Ask the patient to smile and show clenched teeth.
6. Ask the patient to open their mouth and say "Ahhhh," and watch uvula move.
7. Test gag reflex with tongue blade.
8. Test balance with Romberg test. Ask the patient to stand up straight with feet together and close their eyes and observe for sway. The patient should not move if normal.
9. Test hearing by leaning in close and whispering a simple sentence like, "Can you hear me?"
10. Ask the patient to shrug their shoulders upward while you push downward and to rotate their head to left and right while you put gentle counterpressure on each side of the face.

SAMPLE History and AEIOU-TIPS

Ask the SAMPLE history questions to look for clues that may help identify the cause of the problem. For example, a diabetic patient may be having a hypoglycemic emergency instead of a stroke. A memory aid to use when assessing a patient for causes of altered mental status or unconsciousness follows:

AEIOU-TIPS

A = Acidosis or alcohol
E = Epilepsy
I = Infection
O = Overdose
U = Uremia (kidney failure)
T = Trauma, tumor, or toxins
I = Insulin (hypoglycemia or hyperglycemia)
P = Psychosis or poisoning
S = Stroke, seizure, or sepsis

TABLE 30-2   Los Angeles Prehospital Stroke Screen

Criteria	Yes	Unknown	No
Age >45 years	[ ]	[ ]	[ ]
History of epilepsy or seizures absent	[ ]	[ ]	[ ]
Symptom duration <24 hours	[ ]	[ ]	[ ]
Patient not bedridden or wheelchair bound at baseline	[ ]	[ ]	[ ]
Blood glucose between 60 and 400 mg/dl	[ ]	[ ]	[ ]
Obvious asymmetry in any of the following three exam categories:	[ ]	[ ]	[ ]
	Equal	**Right weak**	**Left weak**
Facial smile/grimace	[ ]	[ ] Droop	[ ] Droop
Grip	[ ]	[ ] Weak grip	[ ] Weak grip
		[ ] No grip	[ ] No grip
Arm strength	[ ]	[ ] Drifts down	[ ] Drifts down
		[ ] Falls rapidly	[ ] Falls rapidly

This memory aid prompts you to consider common causes associated with AMS or unconsciousness. It is not an exhaustive list, but it is a good place to start. The list of causes is not by order of frequency of occurrence, it is simply arranged into an easily recallable list.

Differential Diagnosis of Neurologic Disorders

One of the most difficult EMS calls is for a patient with a neurologic disorder or a patient with an altered mental status of an unknown or uncertain etiology. Begin looking for clues to the cause of the patient's condition from the moment you arrive on scene when you begin the scene size-up. As you approach the patient, form a general impression based upon the patient's age, appearance, and the position in which they are found. Be sure to look for evidence for a possible traumatic mechanism. If one is suspected, order or take spinal precautions by manual stabilization of the head in a neutral alignment as you assess the level of consciousness. DOT 5-3.71, 5-3.72, 5-3.73, 5-3.74

During the initial assessment, pay particular attention to performing a careful assessment, and ensure control of the airway. A patient who is obtunded may suffer from a partially obstructed airway when in the supine position as the relaxed tongue blocks the posterior pharynx. If the patient has suffered a brain injury, the patient may not be able to cough or gag and thereby at risk for aspiration of gastric contents. DOT 5-3.7

Open the airway, position the patient to maintain airway patency, and attempt to place an oropharyngeal airway to displace the tongue from the oropharynx. If the patient has a gag reflex and cannot tolerate an oral airway, use a nasopharyngeal airway. Remember to keep

TABLE 30-3   Cincinnati Prehospital Stroke Scale

Test Item	Procedure	Normal Exam	Abnormal Exam
Facial Droop	Have patient show teeth and smile	Both sides of face move equally	One side of face does not move as well
Arm Drift	Close eyes and hold both arms straight out for 10 seconds	Both arms move the same or not at all	One arm stays stationary and one drifts down
Abnormal Speech	Ask patient to say "You can't teach an old dog new tricks."	Uses correct words and no slurring	Patient slurs words, uses wrong words, or is unable to speak

a working suction device and advanced airway kit nearby.

Rule out immediately treatable causes for the altered mental status (opiate overdose, hypoglycemia) before performing invasive advanced airway procedures such as endotracheal intubation. This is particularly true if you know the patient may quickly regain consciousness following therapeutic interventions such as the administration of naloxone or glucose. DOT 5-3.10

Assess the patient's work of breathing and tidal volume. Provide immediate ventilatory support using a bag-mask unit if the patient who accepts an oral adjunct shows signs of inadequate ventilations. Remember that altered mental status means hypoxia until proven otherwise, so complete a thorough assessment of the patient's breathing, and provide the appropriate level of support and oxygenation before continuing your examination. Complete the initial assessment by evaluating the patient's circulation by examining skin signs, pulse rate and quality, and signs of external bleeding.

Working in the Gray Zone

Assess Respiration and Ventilation

Remember that when assessing a patient for adequacy of breathing, it is important to assess for both respiration and ventilation. Just observing for chest rise and fall is not enough. Tools such as the pulse oximeter and end-tidal CO_2 detector (capnography) provide valuable information about the adequacy of each. The pulse oximeter measures oxygenation, and capnography measures ventilation. If a nonrebreather mask is applied, observe how much air the patient inhales from the nonrebreather reservoir with each ventilatory effort. Count the rate and depth of respirations and watch for signs of inadequate breathing such as retractions, shoulder shrugging, purse-lipped breathing, nasal flaring, cyanosis, or pallor.

Obtain a thorough history of the present illness and past medical history from the patient or any bystanders, witnesses, or family members; evaluate blood pressure, pulse oximetry, and blood glucose; and perform a head-to-toe examination of the patient to assist in your differential diagnosis of the patient's condition. Evaluate the ECG for cardiac dysrhythmias. Continuously re-evaluate the patient's level of consciousness, ABCs, vital signs, and neurologic function for changes and responses to treatments rendered. The mnemonic AEIOU-TIPS contains reminders of possible causes to consider

Working in the Gray Zone

Flumazenil has been shown to cause seizures in some patients with overdoses of multiple drug combinations.[8] It is not recommended for use in many adult overdose situations for this reason as often several drugs are involved in the overdose. Flumazenil may also precipitate immediate drug withdrawal, so the dose should be given in small increments and patient response monitored closely.

when assessing a patient who is unconscious or has an altered mental status.

Rule out treatable causes of the neurologic disorder. Assess blood glucose, and treat suspected hypoglycemia with intravenous administration of 25 grams of 50% Dextrose, 10–15 grams of oral glucose if the patient is awake and can swallow, or 1 mg of intramuscular glucagon if an IV cannot be established. If opiate overdose or illicit narcotic drug use is suspected, administer 0.4–2 mg naloxone via the intramuscular or intravenous route. Flumazenil (Romazicon) may be used to treat overdoses of benzodiazepines such as diazepam and midazolam.

Street Secrets

Ensure the IV remains patent by performing frequent aspiration during the injection procedure whenever administering dextrose since infiltration may cause soft tissue necrosis.

When taking the history and vital signs and performing the physical exam, look for signs of increasing intracranial pressure. Increased intracranial pressure causes compression of cranial nerves, ischemic damage to neurons, and eventually herniation of the brain. Signs of herniation include altered mental status (persistent unconsciousness) and decerebrate posturing or flaccid paralysis and one or both pupils become dilated and unresponsive to light. Rising blood pressure, slowing pulse, and an irregular respiratory pattern are collectively referred to as Cushing's triad, which is a clear but late sign of increasing intracranial pressure (Box 30-3).

CONNECTIONS Chapter 20: Head, Face, and Neck Trauma has more information on ICP and herniation.

High levels of arterial carbon dioxide cause cerebral vasodilation and increase intracranial pressure. This occurs because capillary beds dilate in an attempt to draw in oxygenated blood. One way to rapidly treat increasing

BOX 30-3 Cushing's Triad

Rising ICP results when the brain is injured and is swelling. Primary brain injury occurs at the time of injury, but secondary injury, which is a preventable complication, results from hypotension and hypoxia, both of which lead to additional swelling.[9] As the body tries to compensate for the increasing intracranial pressure, tachycardia develops and blood pressure must also rise, or the brain will not be perfused. As pressure continues to rise, the heart rate will begin to decline. Respiratory patterns change as various parts of the damaged brain attempt to compensate for the damaged respiratory control center.

intracranial pressure with signs of herniation is to moderately hyperventilate the patient using 100% oxygen at a rate of approximately 20 breaths per minute for adults (Box 30-4). Hyperventilation will reduce the arterial CO_2 levels and cause cerebral vasoconstriction, which reduces intracranial pressure, but the trade-off is that it also reduces cerebral perfusion. Only hyperventilate a patient who has the three distinct signs that herniation is imminent. These signs include abnormal pupil reactivity and symmetry, persistent unconsciousness, and flaccid paralysis or extensor posturing. Prophylactic hyperventilation for suspected brain injury is not recommended in the absence of signs of herniation as the reduction in cerebral perfusion may further compromise an already damaged brain. Maintain oxygen

BOX 30-4 Signs of Cerebral Herniation

The Brain Trauma Foundation guidelines for management of traumatic brain injury (TBI) identify the following three criteria that must be present prior to initiating hyperventilation as the treatment for herniation:[9]

- Persistent coma or unconsciousness
- Decorticate posturing (see Figure 30-15[a]) or flaccid paralysis
- One or both pupils fixed and dilated (unresponsive to light)

When herniation is noted, hyperventilation with a bag-mask unit and 100% oxygen, at a rate of 10 breaths per minute more than the normal respiratory rate, should be performed.

saturation levels above 90% and systolic blood pressure above 90 mmHg.[9]

Stroke

A **stroke** is a disruption in the blood supply to the brain and can be caused by either a hemorrhage or a clot (from embolus or thrombus) of one or more of the cerebral arteries. A few cases of stroke each year are caused by systemic hypoperfusion resulting from cardiac failure.[10]

Stroke is the third leading cause of death and the leading cause of adult disability in the United States. The risk of stroke increases with age. Early treatment for certain types of stroke holds the promise of reducing the impact of stroke on victims and their families. Proper and prompt treatment requires accurate identification of the stroke in the prehospital setting. This involves taking an accurate history and performing a focused neurological exam. It also requires the prehospital personnel to suspect stroke in the first place (Box 30-5). This clinical judgment comes with specific education and experience. DOT 5-3.1, 5-3.2, 5-3.43

Over 500,000 people will suffer a new stroke each year in this country. Between 15% and 30% of strokes are fatal. Over 150,000 will die, and half will survive with a permanent disability. Recurrent stroke is frequent; about 25% of people who recover from their first stroke will have another stroke within five years.[11]

There are over 3 million stroke survivors in the United States, many of whom are severely disabled and dependent on others for their care. The direct cost of care is estimated at over 30 billion dollars per year, including the direct cost of hospital care and lost productivity.[12] DOT 5-3.44

Hypertension and diabetes are the most common risk factors associated with stroke.[13] Both conditions lead to atherosclerosis. The most important risk factor for atherosclerosis is systolic or diastolic hypertension. In one study of more than 5,000 symptom-free men and women from 30 to 60 years of age followed prospectively for 18 years, the likelihood of hypertensive subjects developing stroke was seven times that of the nonhypertensive subjects. A blood pressure of 160 mmHg systolic or 95 mmHg diastolic observed during any clinic visit tripled the risk of stroke, suggesting that such patients should receive antihypertensive treatment.[10]

Smokers have a significantly higher risk of large vessel stroke. Carotid artery disease is a significant risk factor for embolic stroke, and atrial fibrillation is a well-known risk factor for cardio-embolic stroke.

Modification of only two risk factors reduced stroke risk in controlled trials. Advances in the treatment for hypertension have drastically reduced the incidence of stroke in this group of patients over the past 30 years.

BOX 30-5   An Atypical Stroke Patient

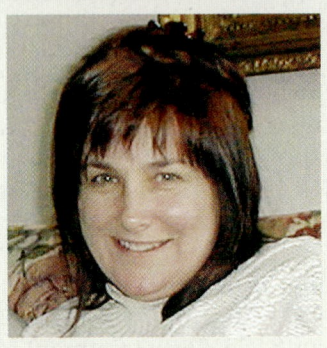

In November 2005, Grace was out doing errands. As reported by other drivers, Grace was driving well—obeying traffic rules, using turn signals, and so on. Suddenly, she had what felt like a "panic attack" and then lost consciousness. Her car crossed the center line and hit another vehicle head-on. The driver of the second car had minor injuries. Grace was unconscious. She had to be cut out of her car.

She regained consciousness briefly, and she panicked again when the paramedics were putting a cervical collar on her. She felt like it was choking her, and she couldn't breathe. The paramedics sedated her for the trip to the hospital. The EMS team and the emergency department assumed that she had had a seizure. Grace was 46 years old and of average weight. She was not hypertensive, diabetic, or a smoker.

Two days later, it was discovered from an MRI that Grace had had a significant stroke. It was in the language processing area of her brain. It was then determined that she has a clotting disorder, and Grace is now on Coumadin. She has no residual effects from the stroke.

Because Grace did not fit the profile of a typical stroke victim, no one suspected stroke as the cause of her crash and the diagnosis was delayed for two days.

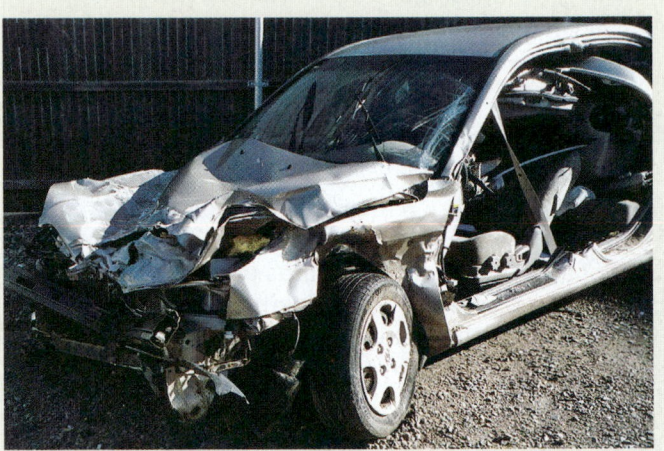

Treatment with anticoagulants, antidysrhythmics, and in some cases a pacemaker, controls atrial fibrillation, which reduces the risk of stroke. Since the leading cause of death following a stroke is heart disease, stroke survivors also must learn to modify these risks. DOT 5-3.43

Between 66% and 80% of all strokes are ischemic (due to a clot), and the rest are hemorrhagic.[10] Rupture of a cerebral blood vessel causes hemorrhagic stroke. These strokes are classified by the location of the hemorrhage. Ischemic strokes can be classified both structurally (by location) and mechanistically (by actual causative agent). DOT 5-3.44, 5-3.45

Hemorrhagic Strokes

Intraparenchymal hemorrhage (or intracerebral bleeding) is bleeding within the brain itself and appears on a CT scan as a dense, white area. Neurologic signs of intraparenchymal hemorrhage depend on the location of the bleeding site within the brain. Many of these hemorrhages are not treatable due to their location, and intraparenchymal hemorrhage has a high mortality rate.

Hemorrhagic stroke in young patients is commonly due to drug use (typically cocaine) or a ruptured vascular malformation such as an aneurysm or arteriovenous malformation (AVM). Patients with significant hypertension are at higher risk than the general population for hemorrhagic stroke.

Ischemic Strokes

Ischemic strokes can be classified by the size of the artery affected and divided into two groups: large vessel or small vessel. Large vessel strokes are typically embolic (caused by debris or emboli) but may be thrombotic (from a blood clot). The large vessels involved and the associated stroke symptoms that are seen when blood flow is disrupted in these vessels are described in Table 30-4.

Large Vessel Strokes. The middle cerebral artery (MCA) is the major blood vessel of the brain and supplies blood to the majority of the cerebral cortex (see Figure 30-13, page 744). When the MCA is occluded, the patient can show a range of neurologic deficits, depending upon

TABLE 30-4   Large Vessel Strokes

Cerebral blood vessel	Stroke signs
Middle cerebral artery (MCA)	Aphasia (dominant hemisphere—left) Neglect (nondominant hemisphere—right) Hemiparesis Gaze deviation toward affected side May have visual field deficit
Anterior cerebral artery (ACA)	Hemiparesis of leg
Posterior cerebral artery (PCA)	Visual field deficit
Basilar artery	Coma Dysconjugate gaze Vertigo Respiratory changes

how much of the brain is affected. MCA stroke of the dominant (left) hemisphere produces aphasia and hemiparesis of the right side of the body and face (facial droop). **MCA stroke** of the nondominant (right) hemisphere produces hemiparesis of the left side and face and may produce a syndrome known as "neglect," in which the patient is unaware of their own body and body space in one-half of their field of vision (usually the left). A patient with **neglect** may only pay attention to people who stand in their right field of vision and may ignore their own symptoms and claim to be normal. MCA strokes may also produce visual field deficits and gaze deviation toward the side of the stroke.

Anterior cerebral artery (ACA) strokes produce deficits of one of the legs, which the patient usually describes as a feeling of heaviness, numbness, or weakness. **Posterior cerebral artery (PCA) strokes** result in a visual field deficit on the opposite side of the stroke (a right PCA stroke will result in a left visual field deficit).

Strokes of the basilar artery can produce dramatic symptoms depending upon how much of the brain stem area is affected. Strokes affecting the brain stem may affect all descending commands from the cerebral hemispheres and cause a patient to be "locked in," which means that the patient is conscious but unable to move from the eyes down. The patient may be able to move his eyes upward to command and may have a sympathetic response (increased heart rate and pupil dilation) to a painful stimulus.

Small Vessel Strokes. Small vessel strokes, also known as **lacunar infarcts,** affect the tiny blood vessels that branch from the MCAs and the basilar artery and provide blood to the internal capsule, the thalamus, and the brain stem. Hypertension, diabetes, and ad-

vanced age all increase the risk of small vessel stroke. Occlusion of the small vessels of the internal capsule will produce "pure motor" symptoms described as a loss of motor function of the face and arm and leg of one side of the body. Small vessel occlusion of the blood vessels leading to the thalamus will cause a "pure sensory" or hemisensory loss. If the brain stem is affected, the patient may experience a wide variety of signs and symptoms from vertigo and nausea to dysconjugate gaze and respiratory dysfunction, depending upon the severity of the insult.

Ischemic Strokes Classified by Mechanism. Ischemic strokes can also be classified by the mechanism and are either embolic or thrombotic. **Embolic strokes** account for the majority of ischemic strokes and arise from a clot that travels from another location in the body (usually the heart) to the brain where it lodges in one of the cerebral arteries blocking blood flow beyond. **Thrombotic strokes** occur because of a thrombus (blood clot) that develops within a cerebral artery or one of the smaller branches. Thrombosis occurs as a result of long-term arteriosclerosis and progressive narrowing of the cerebral arteries.

Transient Ischemia Attack

A **transient ischemic attack (TIA)** occurs when a patient exhibits the neurologic signs and symptoms of stroke that last less than 24 hours and resolve without any intervention. TIAs typically last less than 30 minutes, and frequently, the symptoms resolve prior to the arrival of EMS. These patients should still be transported to a hospital and evaluated to ensure that the risk of future stroke is recognized and appropriate preventive therapy with antiplatelet or anticoagulant agents is initiated. Because it is impossible to differentiate between stroke and TIA, these patients should be treated the same as patients with suspected strokes. DOT 5-3.53, 5-3.54, 5-3.55, 5-3.57, 5-3.58, 5-3.61

Stroke Patient Management

Field assessment of the stroke patient emphasizes accurate identification of stroke symptoms and early notification to the hospital during transport.[14]

Stroke is a clinical diagnosis. That is, the diagnosis is based upon the clinical examination of the patient. A CT or MRI scan is used to evaluate for the presence of a hemorrhage or other structural abnormality such as a tumor, abscess, or edema that may account for the neurologic deficits. If the patient presents with the neurologic signs and symptoms and medical history suggestive of stroke and the absence of hemorrhage on CT scan, then the patient may be eligible to receive thrombolytic treatment. DOT 5-3.46, 5-3.47

In 1995, the FDA approved **tissue plasminogen activator (tPA)** for use in acute ischemic stroke within three hours of the onset of symptoms in patients who meet a specific set of criteria. Criteria for receiving tPA are based on the risk of causing potentially fatal bleeding into the brain from the drug treatment itself versus the benefit of restoring blood flow to the injured area of the brain. Since its approval, many hospitals have instituted a stroke protocol for treating acute ischemic stroke patients and to measure the outcome of patients who receive such treatment. Unfortunately, most patients are not eligible for treatment simply because they are beyond the three-hour window at the time they present to the hospital emergency department. DOT 5-3.51

Some academic medical centers are evaluating other treatments for acute ischemic stroke that may extend the time window. Mechanical Embolus Removal for Cerebral Ischemia (the MERCI trial) is a multicenter trial designed to evaluate the efficacy of using a specialized catheter threaded into the brain to the site of the embolus and mechanically removing the embolic material.

As the care for stroke victims becomes more specialized, the need for specialty destinations or "stroke centers" must be addressed. Some regions have already determined specialty care centers for stroke based upon the American Heart Association guidelines that state that suspected stroke victims should be transported to a hospital capable of providing thrombolytic therapy within the three-hour window. DOT 5-3.52

Prehospital personnel must be proficient at the accurate identification of stroke signs and symptoms and performing a focused neurologic exam. Two focused stroke-specific examinations (the Cincinnati Prehospital Stroke Scale and the Los Angeles Prehospital Stroke Screen) have been validated for use in the prehospital setting and have been shown to improve the sensitivity and specificity of prehospital identification of stroke victims. DOT 5-3.50, 5-3.56

As previously discussed, the CPSS and LAPSS are tools used by prehospital personnel to evaluate patients with suspected stroke symptoms. The CPSS evaluates three elements (see Table 30-3): language, motor function, and facial droop. The LAPSS (see Table 30-2) is a screening tool used on noncomatose, atraumatic patients who present with neurologic symptoms. Although the LAPSS does not evaluate for aphasia, in clinical studies it had 93% sensitivity and 97% specificity for identifying stroke in patients evaluated using this screening tool. The likely explanation for this is that most stroke victims who experience aphasia also have other obvious asymmetry such as facial droop or motor deficit.

Note that neither scale evaluates for visual field abnormalities (PCA occlusion). Prehospital personnel should consider evaluating for visual field deficits since these may indicate a category of stroke not commonly identified in the emergency setting.

Stroke scales and screening tools should be used to *enhance* the accuracy of stroke identification based on the initial physical examination. The information obtained from such tools must be used together with the information obtained from the medical history and history of the present illness to make an accurate diagnosis of stroke.

Prehospital stroke treatment is focused on accurate identification and early hospital notification. Assess the airway, breathing, and circulation, and provide oxygen and ventilatory support, as needed. Pay particular attention to airway management since the patient with acute stroke may not be able to maintain airway patency due to impaired gag and swallowing reflexes or excess secretions. Correct hypoxia, test blood glucose, and treat hypoglycemia if present. Sometimes a metabolic abnormality (such as hypoglycemia or infection) can produce the same signs as a stroke, particularly in patients with prior history of stroke. Monitor the patient's heart rhythm, and start an IV of crystalloid solution. DOT 5-3.48, 5-3.49, 5-3.58

Transport the patient to a hospital capable of administering thrombolytic therapy within the three-hour window. Stroke treatment facilities have a list of questions that must be answered before thrombolytic agents can be administered. The EMS crew can begin asking the patient these questions while transporting to the hospital to help expedite the time to treatment.[15] DOT 5-3.59, 5-3.60, 5-3.61

Intracranial Hemorrhages

Patients who sustain intracranial, epidural, subdural hemorrhages may present with a wide variety of complaints and symptoms, depending upon the location and size of the hemorrhage. Most commonly, these hemorrhages occur as a result of trauma to the head. The symptoms may develop slowly over days to weeks or may occur suddenly and progress within minutes to coma. In addition, the symptoms may vary significantly in intensity and severity and range from persistent headache to focal neurologic findings to unresponsiveness and posturing. DOT 5-3.50, 5-3.51

CONNECTIONS Chapter 20: Head, Face, and Neck Trauma discusses epidural, subdural, and intracerebral hemorrhages in detail. Please consult that chapter for additional information on managing these trauma-related injuries.

Seizures

A **seizure,** or **ictus,** is a temporary disruption in normal neuronal activity, resulting in abnormal repetitive and synchronous firing (action potentials) of neurons in the brain. The physical features seen during a seizure depend on the location of the seizure activity within the brain. There are two main classifications of seizures based upon their clinical features: generalized and partial. Generalized seizures involve simultaneous, ictal activity in both cerebral hemispheres. Partial seizures originate in one or more localized regions or "foci" of the brain. Partial seizures may spread to other areas of the brain and become generalized. This is known as secondary generalization. There are many subtypes of generalized seizures (Table 30-5). **Epilepsy** is an umbrella term for a variety of disorders that cause electrical disturbances within the central nervous system, and are characterized by convulsing motor activity. DOT 5-3.11, 5-3.12

TABLE 30-5   **Classification of Seizures**

Generalized	Generalized tonic-clonic (grand mal)
	Absence (petit mal)
	Tonic
	Atonic
	Clonic and myoclonic
	Infantile spasms (a specific epileptic syndrome)
Partial	Simple partial
	Complex partial
	Partial with secondary generalization

Absence Seizures

Absence seizures are commonly seen in childhood epilepsy and are characterized by a loss of interaction, staring off into space, and returning to normal with no memory of the event. Patient may smack their lips, blink their eyes, or perform another repetitive action. Absence seizures are thought to be caused by ictal activity between the thalamus and cerebral cortex. DOT 5-3.14, 5-3.16

Grand Mal Seizures

Generalized **tonic-clonic** or **grand mal seizures** are the most common type of generalized seizure in the adult patient with a history of seizures. This type of seizure is characterized by several distinct phases. Prior to the muscular convulsions, the patient may or may not experience an **aura** (which is a smell or visual disturbance or other sensation signaling a seizure is coming). The seizure has a tonic phase, which generally lasts from 15 to 30 seconds. During this time, the patient loses consciousness, is typically apneic, and has muscle rigidity. When the tonic-clonic phase begins, the skeletal muscles have rhythmic contraction and relaxation, and the patient appears to shake. This movement can be violent and dramatic or look like shivering or shuddering. This phase may last up to two minutes. During this time, the patient may become incontinent of urine or sometimes even feces. The patient may injure soft tissues, bones, or spine while flailing about and may bite the tongue or lip. DOT 5-3.13, 5-3.14

When the tonic-clonic period ends, the **postictal** phase begins. At this time, the seizure and convulsive activity ceases, and the patient gradually regains consciousness. Confusion or amnesia of the event is common. As the patient's mind clears, embarrassment often sets in, and the patient is typically exhausted and requires rest. The post-ictal phase may last 20–30 minutes or longer. During this period, the patient is vulnerable to airway obstruction by the tongue, secretions, vomitus, or blood. Airway management using basic maneuvers, adjuncts, suction, and proper patient positioning is the highest priority. DOT 5-3.17

Partial Seizures

Partial seizures begin in a specific region or *focus* of the brain. **Simple partial** seizures occur in the motor area of the frontal lobe or the sensory area of the parietal lobe and produce focal motor or focal sensory seizures. Simple partial seizures will not impair normal consciousness. **Complex partial seizures** occur in the frontal or temporal lobe and can produce bizarre behavior that may mimic a psychiatric disorder. Patients who experience complex partial seizures may display repetitive behaviors such as lip smacking, chewing, or picking at clothing or may wander aimlessly. Complex partial seizures disrupt normal consciousness but do not cause unconsciousness unless the focus spreads to a generalized seizure.[16] DOT 5-3.14, 5-3.15

Status Epilepticus

Status epilepticus is a major medical emergency that is associated with significant morbidity and mortality. There are approximately 102,000–152,000 cases of adult status epilepticus and 55,000 deaths each year in the United States. Status epilepticus in the adult patient is defined as a continuous seizure that lasts longer than five minutes or when two or more seizures occur with no intervening period of consciousness. DOT 5-3.1

Although status epilepticus can occur with any of the seizure types listed in Table 30-5, the most dangerous type is **generalized convulsive status epilepticus** (GCSE). Complications of prolonged GCSE include severe physiologic disturbances such as hypoxia, airway compromise, hypoventilation, metabolic acidosis, hyperthermia, rhabdomyolysis (skeletal muscle breakdown), electrolyte abnormalities, and cardiovascular collapse.

Status epilepticus lasting over 30 minutes can cause cerebral injury due to continuous firing of the neurons, even in the absence of overt convulsive activity. As GCSE progresses, the clinical manifestations may become subtle, and the diagnosis of ongoing status epilepticus will take careful clinical observation. Patients may only show repetitive twitching of the face or extremities, nystagmus (rapid oscillations of the eyes), and persistent unconsciousness. Some patients may have no observable convulsive activity, overt or subtle, and may require in-hospital electroencephalographic (EEG) confirmation of seizure activity.[17] Remember that the use of paralytic agents to facilitate intubation will mask clinical signs of seizure activity due to neuromuscular blockade.

Paralytic drugs will not terminate the seizure.

These patients are still at-risk for cerebral injury and require prompt treatment for the seizure, which will continue in their brain.

Status epilepticus is caused by acute or chronic disease processes. Acute causes of status epilepticus include intracranial hemorrhage, infection, drug toxicity, hypoxia, and metabolic disturbances (i.e., hypoglycemia, sepsis, electrolyte abnormalities). Chronic processes include preexisting epilepsy with subtherapeutic blood levels of antiseizure medications, breakthrough seizures, chronic alcoholism, and remote processes such as a CNS tumor or stroke that lead to status epilepticus after a latent period of many weeks to years.

Outcomes of adult patients with status epilepticus are dependant upon two main factors: underlying etiology and duration of the status epilepticus event. Patients with acute etiologies such as head trauma and hypoxia have poorer outcomes than those with chronic etiologies such as preexisting epilepsy. The duration of status epilepticus is independently associated with outcome, so the longer the seizure activity continues, the more likely it is that cerebral injury and systemic complications will occur, which will worsen patient outcome.

There is some evidence that indicates that the longer the seizure event lasts, the more difficult it is to terminate it with traditional pharmacologic agents such as benzodiazepines, barbiturates, and other anti-seizure medications. Prehospital treatment should focus on the proper assessment and control of the airway and ventilation, treatment of any reversible etiology that may exist (i.e., hypoglycemia, opiate overdose, or hypoxia), and prompt termination of continuous seizure activity through use of antiepileptic medications such as diazepam (Valium™).[18]

Treating Uncomplicated Seizures

Treatment of the patient who has experienced an isolated, uncomplicated seizure is directed toward avoiding traumatic injury and maintaining a patent airway and normal ventilation.

If the patient is actively seizing, protect the patient from injury without restraint by placing padding between the patient and the surface the patient is lying on.

Once the seizure activity has subsided, place the patient on the patient's side and assure patency of the airway, and adequacy of ventilations. Evaluate the blood oxygen saturation level, and provide oxygen as appropriate. Continuously assess the patient's level of consciousness during the postictal period. Assess the patient's blood glucose level, and treat hypoglycemia if it exists. Monitor the patient for changes in level of consciousness, and continuously assess the ABCs. Obtain a thorough medical history from bystanders or family members who are familiar with the patient's medical condition. If the patient has a preexisting seizure history, obtain information about the current episode, medications the patient is prescribed (see Table 30-6 for common epilepsy medications), and recent changes in the patient's healthcare and health status. Be prepared to treat status epilepticus.

Despite the periods of apnea and cyanosis that occur during the tonic phase of a seizure, most patients breathe sufficiently during the clonic phase as

TABLE 30-6   Common Medications Used to Treat Chronic Epilepsy

Type of seizure	Medications
Partial and grand mal (or generalized tonic-clonic)	Phenytoin (Dilantin) Carbamazepine (Tegretol) Phenobarbital (Luminal)— *less common* Vigabatrin Lamotrigine Gabapentin
Generalized absence	Ethosuximide Valproic acid

long as the airway remains clear. Administer 100% oxygen, and maintain airway patency using an oral or nasopharyngeal airway. If there is clinical evidence of hypoventilation, assist ventilations with a bag-mask, and consider nasal or oral intubation if basic airway maneuvers are insufficient.

Acute Pharmacologic Therapy

Benzodiazepines are the first-line pharmacologic therapy used to terminate active seizures during status epilepticus. Intravenous administration of lorazepam (Ativan™) 2–4 mg is the most effective initial pharmacological agent for the treatment of status epilepticus.[19] Since lorazepam is heat sensitive, it may not be practical for storage on the ambulance and for prehospital use; therefore, intravenous diazepam (Valium™) in 5–10 mg increments may be used instead.[20] Both agents are fast acting, potent, antiseizure drugs and are preferred as initial therapy. Another benzodiazepine, midazolam (Versed™) has been used in the prehospital setting as a first-line agent in the treatment of both adult and pediatric status epilepticus, despite a lack of clinical trials to evaluate efficacy and safety of use in this manner and setting. Midazolam is a water-soluble benzodiazepine and may be administered via the intramuscular route. In the hospital setting, the use of midazolam for status epilepticus has been limited to cases of refractory status epilepticus and is only administered as a continuous infusion in the intensive care unit where the patient can be closely monitored.

Administer intravenous benzodiazepines slowly, and monitor for side effects, which include respiratory depression and hypotension.

Benzodiazepines depress consciousness and respiratory drive in a dose-dependant manner, meaning that the higher the dose, the more respiratory depression that occurs.

Repeat doses will increase the likelihood of these adverse events. Also, since the benzodiazepines depress consciousness, evaluation of the patient's mental status after apparent termination of the status epilepticus is difficult. The patient may remain in a postictal state for a longer period than for a typical isolated seizure, due to prolonged seizure activity or adverse effects of the medications that are used to terminate status epilepticus.

Suppresive Pharamacologic Therapy

Phenytoin (20 mg/kg administered IV at 50 mg/min) and fosphenytoin (a water-soluble prodrug of phenytoin) are effective for maintaining prolonged antiseizure effects once the termination of active seizures in status epilepticus has been accomplished with a benzodiazepine. These pharmacologic agents are commonly administered in the emergency department setting.[21]

Syncope

Syncope is a temporary loss of consciousness and postural tone, usually due to a brief, sudden drop in cerebral perfusion. It may be caused by a cardiac dysrhythmia or by an alteration in blood volume or distribution. Vasovagal syncope is a condition during which an increase in parasympathetic tone causes a sudden and brief drop in cardiac output and cerebral perfusion. Often a patient will become dizzy or light-headed (called presyncope) prior to losing consciousness. Noncardiac syncope usually does not require treatment and often resolves by positioning the patient supine with the legs elevated. Ensure the patient has not injured themself while falling. DOT 5-3.18, 5-3.19, 5-3.20

CONNECTIONS Cardiac syncope is different from the type of syncope described in this section. Refer to Chapter 29: Cardiology for a discussion on cardiac syncope.

Sometimes a person with syncope can have **myoclonus** (muscle twitching) that a bystander may misinterpret as seizure activity. There are some distinctions between syncope and seizure that are important to be aware of when obtaining a history of the event from a witness. Syncope is sudden, and it causes a temporary loss of consciousness with an immediate return to consciousness once the patient is lying flat. By contrast, an isolated generalized tonic-clonic (GTC) seizure typically lasts from one to two minutes and is followed by a postictal phase, as previously described.

Twitching noted during a syncopal episode is brief and not as symmetrical or repetitive as seen in a GTC seizure although some seizure patients may have atypical convulsive features. The syncope patient will

TABLE 30-7 Comparison between Seizure and Syncope

Syncope	Seizures
• Cause: increased parasympathetic tone	• Cause: epilepsy, hypoxia, trauma, etc.
• May be light-headed or dizzy prior to event	• May have aura prior to event
• Sudden onset of LOC with immediate return to consciousness when prone or supine	• Sudden onset of LOC that persists for several minutes
• Skin: cool, moist, pale	• Tonic-clonic activity, or other repetitive muscular activity noted
• Some muscle twitching may be noted but nothing organized or resembling tonic-clonic activity	• Patient may urinate or defecate
• The patient may sustain an injury during the fall (uncommon event)	• Soft tissue, bone, or spinal injury may occur
• Treatment: none required, but positioning with legs elevated may result in faster recovery	• Gradual return to consciousness
	• Treatment: varies from supportive care to resuscitation of ABCs

typically have cool, pale, and moist skin; a patient with GTC seizures may appear cyanotic or flushed or may have normal skin signs. As with any medical emergency, direct your patient care based upon the information obtained through taking a thorough history and performing a complete physical exam.

Table 30-7 is a comparison between the signs and symptoms of a seizure with syncope.

Headache

There are four main types of headaches:

1. Vascular
2. Tension
3. Traction
4. Inflammatory

The most common type of **vascular headache** is the migraine headache, which is described as a severe pain on one or both sides of the head often accompanied by nausea and visual disturbances. Migraine headaches are more common in women than men. Cluster headaches (more common in men) are repeated episodes of severe pain thought to be caused by high blood pressure. **Tension headaches** involve muscle tension in the muscles of the face and neck. **Traction** and **inflammatory headaches** are symptoms of other disorders such as stroke, sinus infection, or inflammatory disorders. Headache may also be a warning sign of a serious neurological disorder such as tumor, hemorrhagic stroke, or meningitis. DOT 5-3.21, 5-3.22, 5-3.23

The following signs indicate the need for prompt medical attention:

- Sudden severe headache
- Sudden headache associated with a stiff neck, fever, seizures, confusion, or loss of consciousness or following a blow to the head.

Infection

Bacterial or viral infections may lead to inflammatory disease of the membranes that surround the brain and spinal cord (the meninges) and cause **meningitis** or may affect the brain itself causing **encephalitis.** Symptoms of this type of inflammation include sudden fever, headache, stiff neck, vomiting, increased sensitivity to light, confusion, irritability, seizures, and loss of consciousness. **Viral meningitis** typically resolves within 10 days, but other, more aggressive types of **bacterial meningitis** may be deadly if not treated promptly. Field treatment of these patients is primarily supportive. Treat symptoms such as seizures with anti-seizure medications, maintain an adequate airway and ventilation, and provide circulatory support, as needed.

Street Secrets

Take appropriate infection control precautions, including respiratory isolation protection with an N95 or high efficiency particulate air (HEPA) mask, if meningitis is suspected.

Some patients with a history of recent intracranial surgery (i.e., craniotomy) or oral surgery may develop an intracranial abscess, which is a collection of pus that develops in the cranial vault. The signs and symptoms will depend upon the location of the abscess and the region of the brain displaced and most commonly present as other structural abnormalities such as stroke or tumor. DOT 5-3.34, 5-3.35, 5-3.36, 5-3.37, 5-3.38

Neoplasms

Brain and spinal tumors are abnormal growths of cells that are found within the brain or around the spinal cord. Malignant tumors are cancerous and benign tumors are noncancerous growths. Primary brain tumors originate from the neuroglial cells. These cells are non-neuron cells found in the brain. As the tumor develops and becomes larger, it places pressure on the brain. DOT 5-3.24, 5-3.25, 5-3.26

Signs and symptoms of a brain tumor will depend upon the region of the brain displaced by the tumor and will commonly present as headache, personality change, seizure, or stroke. Patients with a prior history of brain tumor may be prescribed steroid anti-inflammatory agents to prevent swelling and increase in intracranial pressure. DOT 5-3.27, 5-3.28

Other Neurologic Disorders

Detailed Anatomy and Pathophysiology of Myelin Sheaths

Normal function of the nervous system is based on elec-trochemical signals. The dendrites and axons of neurons are surrounded by a myelin sheath that promotes smooth and rapid conduction of electrical impulses. Schwann cells form the myelin sheath around neurons of the pe-ripheral nervous system, and oligodendrocytes form the myelin sheath around the neurons of the central nervous system. Spaces between the cells that form the myelin sheath are small nodes known as the nodes of Ranvier (see Figure 30.3, page 737). As the action potential trav-els down the myelinated axon, electrical conduction "jumps" from one node to the next; therefore, the trans-mission of electrical impulses is very rapid. Without a myelin sheath, the neuron transmission is slowed and eventually halted. Normal neurons are capable of trans-mitting impulses at velocities of up to many meters per second. DOT 5-3.63

Detailed Pathophysiology of Neurotransmitter Binding

When the electrical impulse arrives at the axon termi-nals, the chemical neurotransmitter that is stored in the vesicle is released into the synapse (the small space between the presynaptic membrane and the postsyn-aptic membrane). The neurotransmitter diffuses across the synapse and binds to a receptor site on the postsyn-aptic membrane.

Not all the neurotransmitter binds to the receptor sites. Unbound neurotransmitter is taken up by the pre-synaptic membrane by reuptake mechanisms or broken down by a specific enzyme that acts as a chemical inac-tivator. For example, acetylcholine is the neurotransmit-ter released at the presynaptic membrane of a motor neuron. Acetylcholine receptor sites are found on the membrane of skeletal muscle. This synaptic region is known as the neuromuscular junction.

Once released into the synapse, acetylcholine binds to its receptor sites on the skeletal muscle cell and causes depolarization of the skeletal muscle cell membrane. This initiates a cascade of events, leading to muscle contraction. Unbound acetylcholine is either taken up by the presynaptic membrane through reuptake mecha-

nisms or inactivated by acetylcholinesterase. This enzyme breaks down acetylcholine into its chemical constituents, acetyl and choline, which are then taken up by the neuron for the manufacturing of more acetyl-choline. This electrochemical signal can be disrupted if the amount of acetylcholine released or maintained in the synapse is altered from normal or if there is a change in the number of available acetylcholine receptor sites. DOT 5-3.67, 5-3.68

Many chronic neurologic diseases disrupt electrical conduction along axons and dendrites or interfere with the electrochemical communication at the level of the synapse. DOT 5-3.63, 5-3.64

Multiple Sclerosis (MS)

Multiple sclerosis (MS) is a "demyelinating" disease caused by the destruction of the myelin sheath in the CNS. MS is thought to be an autoimmune disease or the result of a viral infection. This disease usually affects young adults in their most productive years, and disease progression varies greatly. Symptom onset may begin with numbness and paresthesias, double vision, ataxia, and bladder control problems as selective axons of the CNS are progressively demyelinated. Once the diagno-sis is made, treatment includes corticosteroids to reduce the inflammatory process and interferon to control dis-ease progression and prolong periods of remission. Finding medications to remyelinate these neurons is the focus of research efforts. There is currently no cure for multiple sclerosis. Field management of these patients is based upon the patient's presenting complaint and, in most cases, is supportive. DOT 5-3.62, 5-3.65, 5-3.66b

Movement Disorders

Movement disorders are characterized by abnormal movements and result from neurologic impairment in the central or peripheral nervous system. There are sev-eral different types of movement disorders. **Tremors** are rhythmic oscillatory movements around a joint and may be more prominent at rest (as in Parkinson's disease), during sustained posture (postural tremor), or during movement (intention tremor).

Chorea is an abnormal movement characterized by irregular, unpredictable, involuntary, muscle jerks that impair voluntary activity. Other abnormal movements include slow writhing movements known as **athetosis** or sustained abnormal postures known as dystonia.

Dystonia can appear as a contorted posture with arms or legs flexed in various rigid positions and the head turned to the side. Dystonia may occur with cere-bral lesions, as an acute complication of specific drugs (i.e., neuroleptic agents such as phenothiazines), or as an idiopathic (meaning an unknown cause) neurologic disorder. A dystonic reaction to neuroleptic agents may be reversible with administration of an antimuscarinic agent such as diphenhydramine (Benadryl®). The pathophysiologic basis of chronic dystonia is unclear. DOT 5-3.62, 5-3.65, 5-3.66c

Muscular Dystrophies

Muscular dystrophies (MD) are inherited disorders characterized by progressive muscle weakness and wasting. The various diseases within the MD category are subdivided by mode of inheritance, age of onset, and clinical features.

Signs and symptoms primarily include muscle weakness. Some individuals, with a specific disease process called Duchenne dystrophy will have stiff muscles, skeletal deformities, muscle contractures, and often cardiac involvement and intellectual retardation. Field treatment is based on the presenting complaint and is usually supportive. DOT 5-3.62, 5-3.65, 5-3.66b

Miscellaneous Neurologic Disorders

Parkinson's Disease. **Parkinson's disease** is a condition that affects the dopamine-producing cells of the basal ganglia. The exact cause of the disease is unknown, and though it commonly appears after age 60, it can present in younger patients. The hallmark signs of Parkinson's disease are muscle rigidity, bradykinesia (extreme slowness of movement and reflexes), and tremor. The tremor is commonly noted as involuntary shaking of the hands that worsens at rest. Muscles remain partially contracted, so when the joint is bent, sudden catches known as "cogwheel rigidity" result. Facial muscles also stiffen, and the face takes on a mask-like appearance. Eventually, voluntary movements become slower and more difficult and balance may become impaired. DOT 5-3.66d

Treatment is directed toward increasing the amount of dopamine in the brain. Since dopamine does not cross the blood-brain barrier, it cannot be administered directly; therefore, drugs such as Sinemet®, which contain L-dopa, the immediate metabolic precursor to dopamine, are used to increase dopamine levels. Unfortunately, L-dopa loses its effectiveness over time and can also cause adverse effects such as dyskinesias and blood pressure changes. Recently, the drug deprenyl has been used to slow the progression of Parkinson's disease, and some believe that the drug may actually prevent the death of neurons in the basal ganglia. DOT 5-3.62, 5-3.65

Transplantation of stem cell tissue to replace the dying dopamine-producing cells is the focus of much research on Parkinson's disease. Field treatment of Parkinson's patients is primarily supportive and based on the presenting complaint.

Bell's Palsy. **Bell's palsy** is thought to be a viral immune-mediated disease that involves the segmental demyelination of the facial nerve (cranial nerve VII). After the primary infection, the virus becomes latent in the nervous system. Reactivation of the virus induces an inflammatory response along the nerve axons. Diabetics are four to five times more likely to develop Bell's palsy than the general population. The disease presents as unilateral facial numbness, paralysis, and decreased tearing. The facial droop can appear similar to that of stroke; however, Bell's palsy often involves the face from forehead to chin and does not involve hemiparesis of the limbs as is often seen in stroke. DOT 5-3.66f

Patients with Bell's palsy must pay particular attention to protecting the eye from drying and damage. Bell's palsy is treated with antiviral and antiinflammatory medications, and most patients make a complete recovery with this treatment. The inflammatory response and the signs and symptoms of Bell's palsy can reoccur. Field treatment is symptomatic. DOT 5-3.62, 5-3.65

Amyotrophic lateral sclerosis (ALS). **ALS,** also known as "Lou Gehrig's disease," is a degenerative disease caused by the selective destruction of motor neurons in the peripheral nervous system. The etiology of this disease is unknown. The disease begins with a slowly progressive muscle weakness and wasting, initially involving the muscles of the limbs. As the disease progresses, the weakness becomes more widespread and involves the respiratory muscles and those controlling speech and swallowing. Death occurs from pulmonary infection and insufficiency. Field treatment is based on the presenting complaint and is usually supportive. DOT 5-3.62, 5-3.65, 5-3.66g

Peripheral Neuropathy. **Peripheral neuropathy** means literally "peripheral nerve damage" and has many causes. The neuropathy may involve sensory function (numbness or loss of sensation), motor function (weakness or paralysis), or autonomic function. Some common causes of peripheral neuropathy include diabetes, alcoholism, bacterial or viral infection, and autoimmune disorders. Nearly 60% of all diabetic patients suffer symptoms of peripheral neuropathy. Common symptoms of peripheral neuropathy include sharp pain, weakness, tingling, or burning or the sensation of wearing a glove or sock. Patients can also have difficulty walking or moving their arms, a loss of balance or coordination, and abnormalities in blood pressure and pulse. Field treatment is based upon the presenting complaint and is usually supportive. DOT 5-3.62, 5-3.65, 5-3.66h

Myoclonus. **Myoclonus** refers to a sudden involuntary jerking movement that is caused by a sudden contraction of muscle or group of muscles followed by relaxation. "Sleep starts" refers to the myoclonic jerking that occurs in normal individuals as they are drifting off to sleep. Myoclonic jerking may occur repetitively and abnormally in patients with multiple sclerosis, Parkinson's disease, Alzheimer's disease, and Creutzfeldt-Jakob disease. Myoclonic activity in patients with epilepsy is described as convulsions that result from seizure activity in the brain. Field treatment is based upon the presenting complaint and is usually supportive. If myoclonic activity is concurrent with a seizure, benzodiazepine therapy may be used to stop the seizure, which may stop the myoclonus. DOT 5-3.62, 5-3.65, 5-3.66i

Spina Bifida. **Spina bifida** occurs as a result of incomplete development of the brain, spinal cord, or meninges in the first month of fetal development. Spina bifida results from an incomplete closure of the neural tube and may leave the infant with an opening of the spine to the outside of the body and significant neurologic impairment. There are three main types of spina bifida: myelomeningocele, the most severe form in which both spinal cord and meninges protrude from an opening in the spine; meningocele in which the spinal cord develops normally but the meninges protrude from the opening in the spine; and occulta in which one or more vertebrae are malformed and covered only by a layer of skin. The spinal opening is repaired surgically shortly after birth; however, the infant is often left with severe neurologic impairment such as nerve damage from missing vertebrae, various physical and mobility difficulties, and sometimes learning disabilities. Field treatment is based upon the presenting complaint and is usually supportive. DOT 5-3.62, 5-3.65, 5-3.66j

Poliomyelitis. **Poliomyelitis** is a highly infectious disease caused by the polio virus that invades the tissue of the nervous system and can cause rapid onset of paralysis. The virus enters through the mouth and multiplies in the intestine, causing the initial symptoms of fever, fatigue, headache, vomiting, stiffness in the neck, and pain in the extremities. One in 200 persons infected with the polio virus will become paralyzed, and 5–10% of those will die because of paralysis of the respiratory muscles. Because of a worldwide effort to eradicate polio, the number of new cases of polio has decreased by 99% since 1988. Most EMS calls relate to complications of polio in patients who previously had the disease. Field treatment is based on the presenting complaint and is usually supportive. DOT 5-3.62, 5-3.65, 5-3.66k

Summary

Although there are various causes for neurologic impairment, a paramedic must take a common and systematic approach to each patient, treating any life-threatening airway, ventilatory, and circulatory abnormalities during the initial assessment and paying particular attention to maintaining a patent airway in the patient who is obtunded or comatose. Rule out immediately treatable causes of the neurologic insult such as hypoglycemia, hypoxia, and opiate overdose. Perform a thorough physical exam, and take a complete history to assist in the differential diagnosis of the patient's condition.

Neurological diseases and conditions may present with a wide variety of symptoms and signs; however, treatment is consistent for many of these problems: Support the ABCs and transport for further evaluation. Some conditions such as active seizures or status epilepticus have specific therapies designed to prevent death or disability from continuous seizure. Strokes have treatment therapies in the hospital that branch into one of two pathways, depending on their cause, but in the prehospital setting, supportive care of the ABCs and rapid transport are the primary treatment. Altered mental status and unconsciousness may be difficult to treat due to the wide variety of possible causes. In addition to providing support to the ABCs, the paramedic must also search for a possible cause.

Notes

1. V. Scanlon and T. Sanders, *Essentials of Anatomy and Physiology* (Philadelphia, PA: FA Davis Company, 2002), p. 569.
2. E. Kandel, J. Schwartz and T. Jessell, *Essentials of Neural Science and Behavior* (Stamford, CT: Appleton and Lange, 1995), p. 717.
3. A. Dalton, D. Limmer, J. Mistoich, and H. Werman, *Advanced Medical Life Support* (Upper Saddle River, NJ: Brady/Prentice Hall Publishing, 1999), p. 476.
4. A. Guyton, *Textbook of Medical Physiology,* 11th ed. (Philadelphia, PA: W. B. Saunders, 2005).
5. S. G. Waxman, *Clinical Neuroanatomy,* 25th ed. (New York, NY: McGraw-Hill, 2003).
6. R. U. Kothari, A. Pancioli, T. Liu, T. Brott, and J. Broderick, "Cincinnati Prehospital Stroke Scale: Reproducibility and Validity," *Annals of Emergency Medicine* 33(1999):373–378.
7. C. S. Kidwell, J. L. Saver, G. B. Schubert, M. Eckstein, and D. Starkman, "Design and Retrospective Analysis of the Los Angeles Prehospital Stroke Screen (LAPSS)," *Stroke* 31(2000):71–76.
8. J. E. Tintinalli, G. D. Kelen, J. S. Stapczynski, O. J. Ma, and D. M. Cline, "Nonbenzodiazepine Hypnosedatives," *Tintinalli's Emergency Medicine: A Comprehensive Study Guide,* 6th ed., McGraw-Hill's AccessMedicine (accessed June 15, 2006).
9. Brain Trauma Foundation, *Guidelines for the Prehospital Management of Traumatic Brain Injury,* www2.braintrauma.org/guidelines (accessed September 28, 2006).
10. J. E. Tintinalli, G. D. Kelen, J. S. Stapczynski, O. J. Ma, and D. M. Cline, "Stroke, Transient Ischomic Attack, and Other Central Focal Conditions," *Tintinalli's Emergency Medicine: A Comprehensive Study Guide,* 6th ed., McGraw-Hill's AccessMedicine (accessed June 15, 2006).
11. National Institute of Neurological Disorders and Stroke, "What Is the Prognosis?" www.ninds.nih.gov/disorders/stroke/stroke.htm# (accessed June 23, 2006).

12. American Heart Association, *Advanced Cardiac Life Support Guidelines* (Dallas, TX: American Heart Association, 1999).

13. M. J. Aminoff, D. A. Greenberg, and R. P. Simon, "Stroke," *Clinical Neurology,* 6th ed., McGraw-Hill's AccessMedicine (accessed June 23, 2006).

14. W. Smith, *Recognition and Evaluation of Stroke: Training Program for Emergency Medical Technician-Paramedic* (San Francisco, CA: University of California at San Francisco Department of Neurology, 1996).

15. R. Sahni, "Acute Stroke: Implications for Prehospital Care," *Prehospital Emergency Care* 4 (3)(July/September 2000):270–272.

16. B. S. Chang and D. H. Lowenstein, "Epilepsy," *The New England Journal of Medicine* 349(13)(September 25, 2003): 1257–1266.

17. J. M. Murthy and T. J. Naryanan, "Continuous EEG monitoring in the Evaluation of Non-Convulsive Seizures and Status Epilepticus," *Neurology India* 52(4)(December 2004):430–435.

18. D. H. Lowenstein and B. K. Alldredge, "Status Epilepticus," *The New England Journal of Medicine* 338 (14)(April 2, 1998): 970–976.

19. B. K. Alldredge, A. M. Gelb, S. M. Isaacs, M. D. Corry, F. Allen, S. Ulrich, N. O'Neil, J. M. Neuhaus, M. R. Segal, and D. H. Lowenstein, "A Comparison of Lorazepam, Diazepam, and Placebo for the Treatment of Out-of-Hospital Status Epilepticus," *The New England Journal of Medicine* 345(9)(August 30, 2006):631–637.

20. M. D. Gottwald, L. C. Akers, P. K. Liu, P. J. Orselak, P. Bacchetti, M. D. Corry, S. M. Fields, D. H. Lowenstein, and B. K. Alldredge, "Prehospital Stability of Diazepam and Lorazepam," *The American Journal of Emergency Medicine* 17(4)(July 1999): 333–337.

21. D. H. Lowenstein, "Treatment Options for Status Epilepticus," *Current Opinions in Pharmacology* 3(1)(February 2003): 6–11.

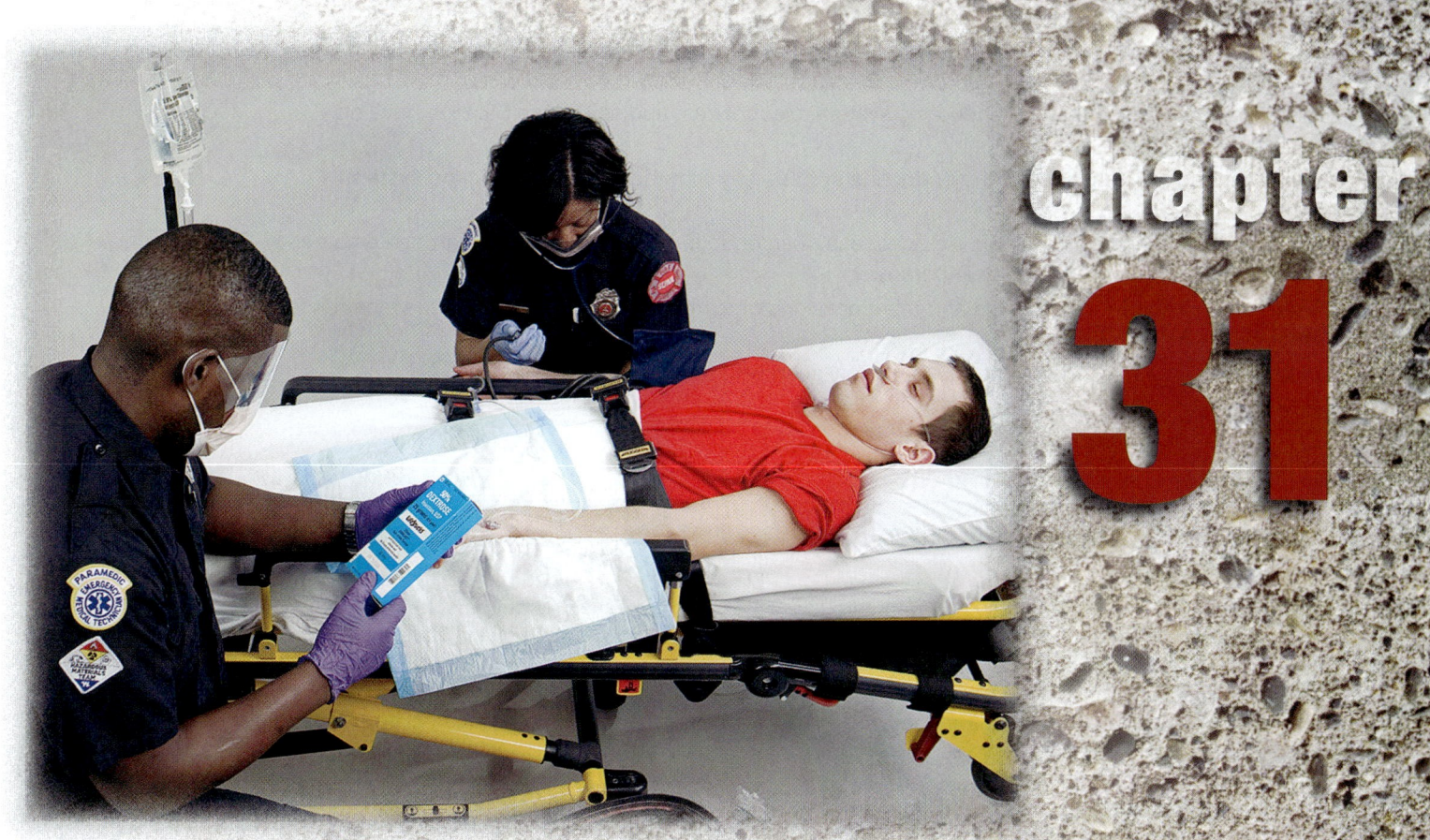

Endocrinology, Electrolytes, and Acid/Base

*"**W**hen health is absent, wisdom cannot reveal itself, art cannot manifest, strength cannot fight, wealth becomes useless, and intelligence cannot be applied."*

—Herophilus

Need to Know

▶ Recognize the importance that the endocrine system, electrolytes, and acid/base balance have on homeostasis.

▶ Be familiar with normal functions of the endocrine system and with the signs of endocrine system dysfunction.

▶ Be able to recognize when a patient is sick because of an endocrine, electrolyte, or acid/base emergency, and provide the appropriate supportive therapy.

▶ Understand the important electrolytes and the main signs or symptoms that occur when the electrolytes are out of balance.

▶ Be familiar with the signs and symptoms commonly seen with acid or base imbalances.

▶ Sick	▶ Not Yet Sick
• Use the AEIOU-TIPS memory aid to help you work through the possible causes for unconsciousness. • Test blood sugar on every unconscious patient, and treat with dextrose or glucagon, as appropriate. • Any patient with a significant number of the signs described for each problem should be considered sick, particularly if a potential life-threatening sign is present. • Patients with deteriorating mental status or vital signs are sick. • Suspect endocrine, electrolyte, or acid/base emergencies in any nonhead injured unconscious patient.	• Ask the patient about personal information such as last menstrual period, bowel habits, or urine output in a professional manner to minimize embarrassment for both of you. • Patients with minor symptoms and stable vital signs should be transported for hospital follow-up. • Avoid glucagon administration, if possible, as it can cause severe muscle pain.

Introduction

Healthcare providers are involved in a variety of patient care situations. In some cases, such as a myocardial infarction or a gunshot wound, the underlying illness or injury is often readily apparent. In other cases, such as altered mental status, the patient's chief complaint and symptoms may be more challenging to pinpoint. This chapter discusses conditions in which the prehospital assessment of the patient is often not specific.

The signs and symptoms associated with endocrine conditions cover a wide spectrum. In some cases, they are easily identified. In other cases, they may be very challenging to identify, requiring comprehensive assessments only available in tertiary care facilities. The intent of this chapter is that healthcare providers will gain additional confidence in their ability to understand and recognize these conditions.

The endocrine system consists of hormone-producing glands that control basic body functions. The hormones may affect one or several organs throughout the body;

depending on hormone type, they influence metabolism, growth, and sexual development. Many of the hormones produced by the endocrine glands interact with each other to maintain the homeostatic balance. The amount of hormones produced by each gland is regulated by complex feedback loops. Abnormal over- or underproduction of the hormones has numerous effects that can result in endocrine disorders. Table 31-1 provides an overview of the organs and their functions.

Medical conditions involving the endocrine system consume a variety of healthcare resources. For example, there are 10 million people in the United States diagnosed with diabetes and another estimated 5.4 million undiagnosed. There are approximately 80,000 cases of acute pancreatitis annually.[1] Hypothyroidism, the most common thyroid disorder, affects more than 6 million individuals.[1] Hyperparathyroidism, which involves an overactive parathyroid, affects about 250 out of every 100,000 individuals.[1] DOT 5-4.1, 5-4.2 **This chapter is supported by Skill Sheet 26: Blood Glucose Assessment (also see Step-by-Step 26).**

TABLE 31-1   **Overview of Endocrine Glands**

Gland	Function
Hypothalamus	Secretes hormones that stimulate or suppress the release of hormones in the pituitary gland. The hypothalamus is located in the brain. It influences water balance, sleep, temperature, appetite, and blood pressure.
Pituitary gland	Secretes hormones to stimulate the adrenals, thyroid, pigment-producing skin cells, and gonads (ovaries and testes). Also secretes growth hormone, an antidiuretic hormone, prolactin (a hormone that affects milk production after childbirth), and oxytocin (a hormone that plays a role in childbirth). The pituitary gland is located at the base of the brain. It controls many functions of the other endocrine glands earning it the name "Master Gland".
Thyroid gland	Secretes thyroxin, triiodothyronine, and calcitonin, which affect metabolism, body heat, and bone growth. The thyroid plays an important role in the body's metabolism.
Parathyroid glands	Secretes parathyroid hormone (PTH), which affects calcium levels in the blood. Both the thyroid and parathyroid glands have a role in the regulation of the body's calcium balance.
Adrenal cortex of the adrenal gland	Secretes hydrocortisone, which affects metabolism. Also secretes androgen hormone and aldosterone, which affect blood pressure and saline balance. It secretes epinephrine and norepinephrine. The adrenal glands are located on top of the kidneys. Adrenal glands work in conjunction with the hypothalamus and pituitary gland.
Pineal body	The pineal body is located in the brain. It produces melatonin and serotonin.
Gonads	The male and female reproductive glands (testes and ovaries) produce and secrete a variety of hormones related to sexual maturation and function.
Thymus	The thymus is located in the upper part of the chest and produces T-lymphocytes, which are white blood cells that fight infections and destroy abnormal cells.
Pancreas	Secretes insulin and glucagon, which affect the body's absorption of glucose. The pancreas is located across the back of the abdomen, behind the stomach. The pancreas plays a role in digestion as well as hormone production.

The Endocrine Glands

The major glands of the endocrine system include the hypothalamus, pituitary, thyroid, parathyroids, adrenals, pineal body, gonads, thymus, and the pancreas (Figure 31-1).

The endocrine system is regulated by a complex feedback system that is similar to a thermostat. When an individual sets a particular temperature on a thermostat, the device then measures the actual temperature. If the temperature exceeds the set point, the thermostat turns off the heating system, and when the temperature falls below the set point, it turns the system back on. The endocrine system works in much the same fashion.

For example, for the hormones that are regulated by the pituitary gland, a signal is sent from the hypothalamus to the pituitary gland in the form of a "releasing hormone." This causes the pituitary to secrete a "stimulating hormone" into the circulation. The stimulating hormone then signals the target gland to secrete its hormone. As the level of this hormone increases in the circulation, the hypothalamus and the pituitary gland recognize the increased level of the hormone and decrease secretion of the releasing hormone and the stimulating hormone, which in turn slows the secretion by the target gland. This feedback system results in stable blood concentrations of the hormones that are regulated by the pituitary gland.[1-4] Other systems function in a similar manner. DOT 5-4.4

Hypothalamus

The **hypothalamus** is located in the lower part of the brain. It is involved in the regulation of metabolism and body temperature. It secretes hormones that either stimulate or suppress the release of hormones in the pituitary gland. These hormones include thyrotropin-releasing hormone (TRH), corticotropin-releasing hormone (CRH), gonadotropin-releasing hormone (GnRH), prolactin releasing hormone (PRH), prolactin-inhibiting hormone (PIH), growth hormone-releasing hormone (GHRH), and somatostatin. Five of these hormones are

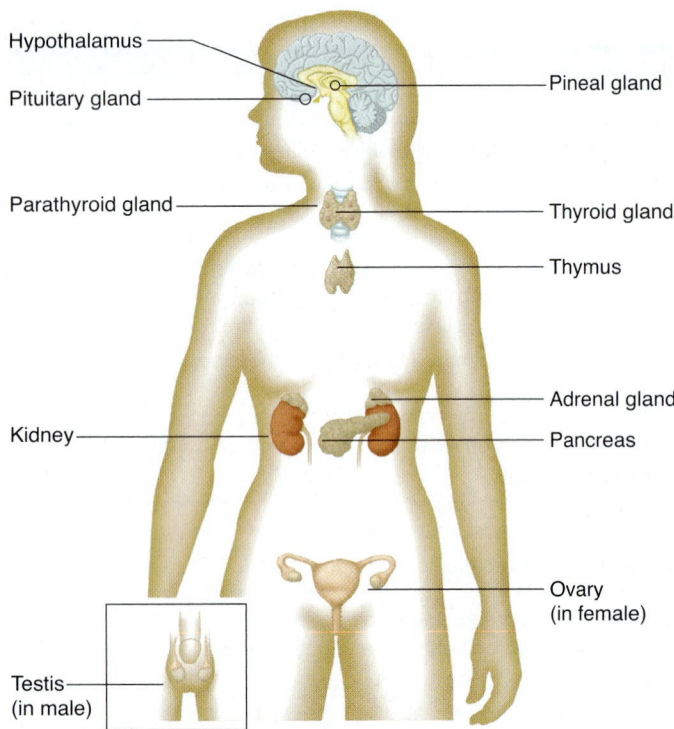

Figure 31-1   The locations of the endocrine glands.

releasing hormones, which are secreted into arteries, thereby allowing them to directly influence the pituitary gland. Once they reach the pituitary gland, the releasing hormones signal secretion of stimulating hormones.[1–5] Two of these hormones, PIH and somatostatin, are inhibitory hormones that suppress the release of other pituitary hormones. DOT 5-4.3

Pituitary Gland

The **pituitary gland,** referred to as the *master gland,* is located in the brain beneath the hypothalamus (see Figure 31-1). It is considered to be one of the most important parts of the endocrine system because it produces hormones that control many of the functions of other endocrine glands. The pituitary gland controls the release of thyroid hormones, which help to maintain blood pressure, heart rate, digestion, muscle tone, and reproductive functions.[1–4] Hypopituitarism occurs when the pituitary gland fails or does not produce adequate amounts of one or more of its hormones. Hyperpituitarism is just the opposite—when the pituitary produces too much of a hormone.

The pituitary gland has anterior and posterior lobes. The anterior lobe produces a variety of hormones including follicle-stimulating hormone (FSH), luteinizing hormone (LH), thyroid-stimulating hormone (TSH), adrenocorticotropic hormone (ACTH), prolactin (PRL), and somatotropin (also called growth hormone or GH). The posterior lobe secrets antidiuretic hormone (ADH,

which is also called vasopressin) and oxytocin (OT). ADH and OT are actually produced within the hypothalamus and are stored in the posterior lobes until their release is triggered. The secretion of hormones from the pituitary gland is controlled by the hypothalamus. Oxytocin stimulates contractions in pregnancy and is involved in the production of breast milk. ADH results in the renal system retaining water. TSH stimulates the thyroid gland to release its hormones. This results in an increased metabolic rate. ACTH stimulates the adrenal cortex to release its hormone. The pituitary gland also influences the production and release of follicle stimulating hormone (FSH) and luteinizing hormone (LH), which have roles in the maturation and release of eggs from the ovary.[1–4] DOT 5-4.3

Thyroid Gland

The **thyroid gland** is located in the lower portion of the anterior neck and is the largest endocrine gland. The follicular cells within the gland produce hormones including triiodothyronine (T3) and tetraiodothyronine (T4, which is also called thyroxine) which are collectively referred to as thyroid hormone. Thyroid hormones are secreted in response to TSH from the pituitary. These hormones regulate the body's metabolism, have a role in bone growth, and are involved in the development of the brain and nervous system. Calcitonin is also produced by the thyroid gland. It comes from parafollicular or C (for calcitonin) cells. Calcitonin antagonizes the action of parathyroid hormone.[1,2,6] DOT 5-4.3

Street Secrets

The thyroid gland receives one of the highest rates of blood flow per gram of any tissue in the body.[7] Therefore, great caution must be exercised when surgical airways are performed or when anterior lacerations are found on the neck.

Parathyroid Glands

The **parathyroid gland** consists of small pea-shaped glands that are located on the surface of the thyroid gland. Typically, there are four glands. They release parathyroid hormone, which plays a role in regulating calcium levels in the blood and bone metabolism. Removal or disruption of the parathyroid glands may lead to hypocalcemia.[1–5] DOT 5-4.3

Adrenal Glands

The **adrenal glands** are located on top of each kidney. They consist of the adrenal cortex and the adrenal medulla, the outer portion, and inner portion, respectively.

The cortex produces steroid hormones including glucocorticoids (cortisol and corticosterone), mineralocorticoids (aldosterone), and androgenic, or sex, hormones (like dihydroepiandrosterone (DHEA), testosterone, and small amounts of estrogen). They influence the body's metabolism, the balance of salt and water, the immune system, and sexual function. Glucocorticoids are produced by the adrenal cortex and account for the majority of the adrenal cortex hormone production. They are released in response to traumatic situations (e.g., stress, infections, or injury), and they increase blood glucose levels. They are also involved in antiinflammatory activities and immune suppression. Mineralocorticoids are involved in the regulation of potassium and sodium. If the adrenal cortex produces excessive amounts of hormones, Cushing's disease may develop.[8,9] The adrenal medulla produces hormones called catecholamines, including norepinephrine and epinephrine. These hormones help the body respond to physical and emotional stress via the fight or flight syndrome.[1-4] DOT 5-4.3

Pineal Gland

The **pineal gland,** or **pineal body,** is located in the middle of the brain. It secretes melatonin at night and serotonin during the day. These help regulate the sleep and wake cycles of the body and both hormones are believed to be connected to mood as well. It shrinks as a child grows and its volume of secretions peaks between the ages of one to five. The amount of secretion declines by 75% by the end of puberty.[1-4] DOT 5-4.3

Gonads

The **gonads** are both endocrine and exocrine glands. Their exocrine products are eggs and sperm. The endocrine products are gonadal hormones. Most of these hormones are steroids. The ovaries secrete estradiol, progesterone, and inhibin. The testes secrete testosterone, estrogen, inhibin, and weaker androgens. DOT 5-4.3

Thymus

The **thymus** is found in the mediastinum just above the heart. Like the pineal gland, it is large in infants and small children, and shrinks (or involutes) after puberty. It secretes thymopoietin, thymosin, and other hormones that regulate the development and activation of T lymphocytes (or T cells) that help fight infection.

Pancreas

The **pancreas** is located toward the posterior portion of the upper abdomen, behind the stomach. It has both exocrine and endocrine functions. The exocrine pancreas secretes digestive enzymes through ducts that empty into the duodenum to help with digestion of food and nutrients. The endocrine pancreas secretes insulin and glucagon. The alpha cells of the pancreas secrete glucagon, and the beta cells secrete insulin. Like all endocrine glands, the pancreas secretes these hormones directly into the bloodstream.[1-4] DOT 5-4.3

Diabetes, Glucose, and Insulin

One of the most common endocrine-related diseases encountered by prehospital care providers is **diabetes mellitus.** Glucose is a simple sugar that provides energy to the body.[3,10] Cells receive glucose, or dextrose, from the blood and break it down for energy. While many sources of energy—including carbohydrates, fats, and proteins—can be used by body cells, certain cells, such as brain cells and red blood cells, are primarily dependent on glucose as their main source for energy. When food is ingested, glucose is absorbed from the intestines and distributed throughout the body via the bloodstream. The body attempts to keep a constant supply of glucose for the cells by maintaining a consistent glucose concentration in the blood. Without this, the cells would have excessive glucose following a meal and would be glucose-depleted between meals and while a person sleeps.[1-4]

Insulin

Insulin is produced by the beta cells of the pancreas. It is required by almost all of the body's cells as a facilitator to allow the passage of glucose into the cells. Its major targets include the liver, fat cells, and muscle cells. Insulin has several key functions. It stimulates the liver and muscle cells to store glucose as glycogen and to create proteins. Insulin is also a key element for glucose to enter the cell. When glucose is present in the circulation, it interacts with insulin to allow glucose to enter the cell. Without insulin, the amount of glucose that enters the cell is insufficient to meet the body's demands.[9-17] Once inside the cell, the glucose is converted to energy. When there is excess glucose in the bloodstream, the body stores the excess in the liver and muscles in the form of glycogen. When glucose levels are low, the body mobilizes glucose from stored glycogen or it stimulates hunger. These activities are an attempt to maintain blood sugar levels.[10]

Glucagon

Glucagon is a protein hormone that is produced and secreted by the alpha cells of the pancreas. Glucagon acts on the same cells as insulin but has opposite effects. It stimulates the liver and muscles to break down stored glycogen (glycogenolysis) and release glucose. It also stimulates the liver and muscles to enhance gluconeogenesis (the formation of glucose).[10,11]

When there is a reduction in blood sugar levels, glucagon secretion is stimulated from the pancreatic alpha cells. This inhibits insulin secretion from the beta cells and results in an increase in blood glucagon levels. Glucagon then acts on liver, muscle, and kidney tissue to mobilize glucose from glycogen or to make glucose that gets released into the blood. These activities prevent blood glucose levels from drastically falling.[10-18]

Balancing Insulin and Glucagon Levels

The body must determine when to secrete glucagon versus insulin. In normal situations, the levels of insulin and glucagon are balanced in the bloodstream. For example, after food is ingested, the body prepares to receive the glucose, fatty acids, and amino acids that are contained within the food. The presence of these substances in the intestine stimulates the pancreatic beta cells to release insulin into the blood. This activity also inhibits the pancreatic alpha cells from secreting glucagon.[10-18] The levels of insulin in the blood begin to rise and act on cells. Liver, fat, and muscle absorb the incoming glucose, fatty acids, and amino acids. Through this mechanism, insulin prevents the blood glucose concentration from increasing excessively in the bloodstream. When these mechanisms function correctly, the blood glucose balance is maintained (Figure 31-2).[10-18]

When insulin is not effective or is lacking, the body's utilization of glucose is impaired. For example, when there is insufficient insulin, regardless of the reason, it causes high blood glucose levels to develop. Without insulin, cells cannot absorb glucose from the bloodstream.[11-14]

Because the cells are unable to receive glucose from the bloodstream, the body reacts as if it were actually glucose deficient. The alpha cells of the pancreas respond by secreting glucagon. The glucagon stimulates specific organs, such as the liver and muscles, to break down stored glycogen and to release glucose into the blood. This results in a further increase in blood glucose levels.[11-14]

As blood glucose levels continue to increase, the amount of glucose that is filtered by the kidneys increases. Eventually, the kidney's filtration rate is exceeded, and glucose spills into the urine. At the same time, the filtered glucose attracts water, which leads to increased urine production. The increased urine flow causes an increase in the frequency and rate of urination. With high blood glucose concentrations, increased osmotic pressures of the blood, lost sodium, and an increased urine output, thirst is triggered.[11-14] DOT 5-4.8, 5-4.15, 5-4.16, 5-4.17

A deficiency or lack of insulin has additional effects. Fats and proteins are broken down. This results in weight loss, even though the individual eats and drinks more. The metabolism of fatty acids leads to the production of acidic ketones, which leads to the development of **ketoacidosis.** This can result in a variety of

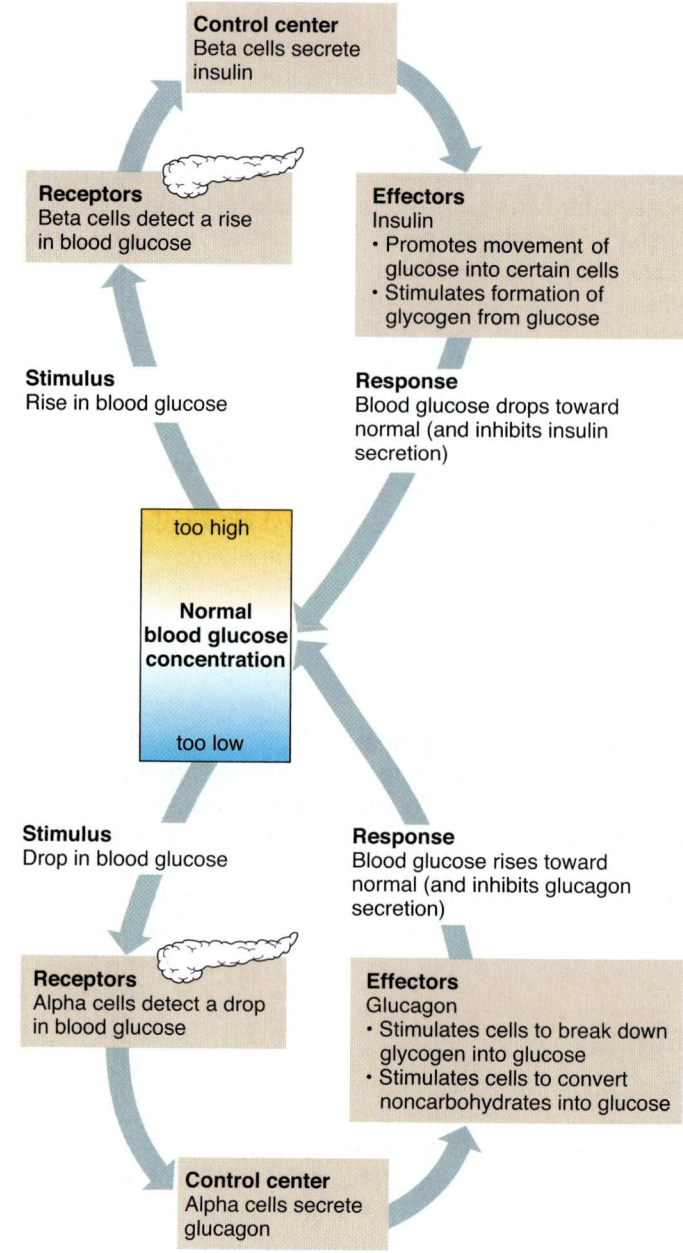

Figure 31-2 Insulin and glucagon work together to stabilize blood glucose levels.

complications, including dyspnea, cardiac dysrhythmias, and unconsciousness.[11-16] DOT 5-4.19

Street Secrets

Diabetics are often "poly" patients. Diabetics commonly have a triad of symptoms called the **Three Ps:**

- Polyuria (increased urine output)
- Polydipsia (increased thirst)
- Polyphagia (increased appetite)[5,13] DOT 5-4.18, 5-4.20

Diabetes Mellitus

In the United States, more than 10 million people have been diagnosed with diabetes.[18] It is estimated that an additional 5.4 million have undiagnosed diabetes.[18–22] The morbidity and mortality associated with diabetes is related to short- and long-term complications. Complications can include hypoglycemia, hyperglycemia, infections, microvascular complications (e.g., retinopathy, nephropathy), neuropathic complications, and macrovascular disease. Diabetes is the major cause of blindness in adults between the ages of 20 and 74 years of age. It is also the leading cause of nontraumatic lower extremity amputation and end-stage renal disease (ESRD).[18–20] Approximately 10% have type I diabetes, and the remaining 90% have type II.[17–21] DOT
5-4.11, 5-4.20

Diabetes—Type I

Type I diabetes, also referred to as insulin-dependent diabetes mellitus (IDDM), or juvenile onset diabetes (JODM), develops because of a lack of natural insulin. As a result, individuals with type I diabetes are required to administer exogenous (external) sources of insulin either by injection or continuous pump (Figure 31-3). In some cases, the exogenous insulin must be taken several times a day. Type I is typically diagnosed during childhood, adolescence, or early adulthood. It can also develop in older adults. It tends to peak during the adolescent years among individuals with a lean build.[10,14,18–22]

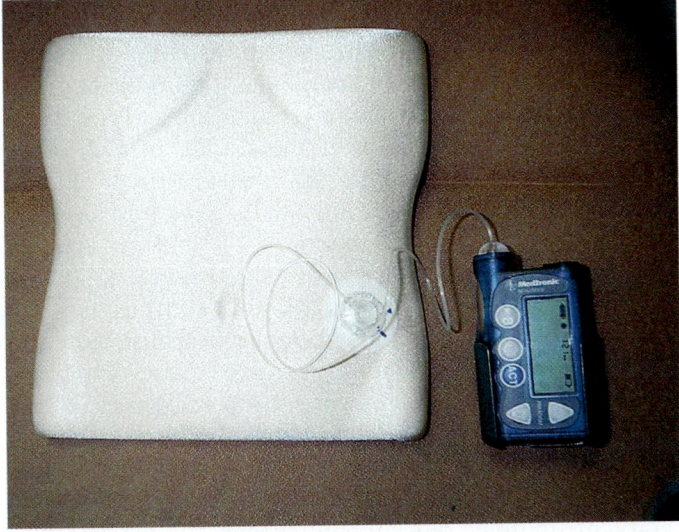

Figure 31-3   A typical insulin pump and the manner in which it is attached to the patient.

Type I diabetes is characterized by the inability of the pancreas to secrete insulin. This is most often due to autoimmune destruction of the pancreatic beta cells. Without insulin, glucose cannot enter cells. This leads to the situation in which the individual experiences a glucose-depleted state despite the actual presence of glucose in the blood stream. In order to correct this, type I diabetics are dependent on an external source (exogenous) of insulin to maintain homeostasis.[10,14,18–22]

The type, amount, and frequency of insulin injections vary among type I diabetics. The administration may be influenced by numerous factors, including meals and exercise. The intent of treatment is to provide optimal management of the glucose levels. Because of the need for injections, patients must monitor their blood glucose levels throughout the day, adjusting the injections accordingly. By monitoring blood sugar levels and adjusting the insulin injections, type I diabetics attempt to maintain their blood glucose concentration from fluctuating excessively. If the exogenous insulin administration is impaired or interrupted, ketosis and ketoacidosis can develop.[10,14,18–22] The following website provides detailed information regarding insulin: http://www.fda.gov/diabetes/insulin.html. **Skill Sheet 26: Blood Glucose Assessment (and Step-by-Step 26) outlines the use of a glucometer.** DOT 5-4.10

Diabetes—Type II

Type II diabetes, also referred to as adult onset diabetes (AODM) or noninsulin-dependent diabetes (NIDDM), differs from type I. Type II is more common in individuals who are older than 40 in which there is a family history of diabetes. In this form of diabetes, there is a resistance to insulin with an insulin-secretion defect. Maturity-onset diabetes of the young, MODY, is another form of type II diabetes. It tends to affect many generations in the same family with an onset in individuals who are younger than 25 years of age.[3,10,18,20,22]

In contrast to patients with type I diabetes, patients with type II diabetes have the ability to secrete endogenous (internal or natural) insulin. In type II, the amount of insulin that is released may be insufficient to allow for optimal glucose metabolism. However, it is sufficient enough to keep the development of diabetic ketoacidosis (which is explained in the next section) at bay. Type II patients who receive exogenous insulin do not tend to develop diabetic ketoacidosis if they stop taking the exogenous form. Because of this, they are not considered to be insulin "dependent."[12–14,18,21]

The number of cases of type II diabetes is increasing as people live longer. While type II diabetes occurs most often in those aged 40 years or older, its incidence is increasing rapidly in adolescents and young adults. Part of this is attributed to the increase in childhood obesity. There are several risk factors associated with type II diabetes. Examples include individuals who are over the age of 45; are obese; have a family history; are of Hispanic, Native American, African American, Asian American, or Pacific Islander descent; have a history of impaired glucose tolerance (IGT) or impaired fasting glucose (IFG); or have hypertension and/or dyslipidemia. The incidence is equal in females and males.[12–14,18,22]

Type II diabetes may be managed through several approaches, including monitoring body weight through diet and exercise and, in certain cases, the use of medications. Many of the medications used for type II diabetes are taken orally and have specific mechanisms of action. Examples include stimulating the pancreas to release more insulin to help reduce blood glucose, interfering with the absorption of glucose by the intestine (thereby preventing glucose from entering the bloodstream), improving insulin sensitivity, and reducing glucose production by the liver. Depending on the specific etiology of the diabetes, the diabetic type II patient may be using more than one type of medication to control their blood sugar levels.[3,10,18,20,22]

New Therapy for Type II Diabetes

A new therapy for type II diabetes was approved in early 2005. Exenatide (Byetta™) is a glucagon-like peptide-1 (GLP-1) that stimulates beta cells to secrete insulin, inhibits glucagon secretion, and slows gastric emptying.[23] Exenatide improves postprandial (after eating) and overall glycemic control in patients with type II diabetes without increasing the incidence of hypoglycemia or causing weight gain. Both of these are potential side effects from the use of antihyperglycemic therapies such as sulfonylurea drugs like glimepiride, glipizide, or glyburide. Byetta is administered by injection only, and it comes in a prefilled pen with multiple doses inside the unit. It is currently administered twice daily, but a long-acting formula that would allow a single weekly dose is under investigation.

Secondary Diabetes

In addition to type I and type II diabetes, other forms of diabetes are often caused by the presence of another illness or medication and are referred to as **secondary diabetes.** Depending on the primary process involved (e.g., destruction of pancreatic beta cells), these cases present in a manner similar to type I or type II diabetes. Common causes include diseases that destroy the pancreatic beta cells (e.g., pancreatitis, cystic fibrosis, pancreatic cancer), hormonal syndromes that interfere with

insulin secretion (e.g., pheochromocytoma), disease processes that cause peripheral insulin resistance (e.g., acromegaly, polycystic ovarian syndrome, Cushing syndrome), and drug-induced diabetes (e.g., phenytoin, glucocorticoids, estrogens).[18,22] DOT 5-4.9

Gestational Diabetes

Gestational diabetes mellitus (GDM) is related to pregnancy. GDM can be defined as any degree of glucose intolerance with an onset or first recognition during pregnancy. GDM complicates approximately 4% of all pregnancies in the United States although a range of 1–14% has been reported.[17,21] Untreated GDM can lead to fetal macrosomia (overly-large sized fetus), hypoglycemia, hypocalcemia, and hyperbilirubinemia. In addition, mothers with GDM have higher rates of cesarean delivery and chronic hypertension.[18,22]

Hypoglycemia

Hypoglycemia, or low blood sugar, involves a glucose level that is inadequate to effectively fuel the body's blood cells. Depending on the sources consulted, the "normal" range of blood glucose levels may vary somewhat. For this discussion, the normal range of blood sugar will be considered to be approximately 60 to 120 mg/dL (milligrams of glucose per deciliter of blood).[18–22] DOT 4-5.22

When hypoglycemia occurs, it is dangerous because glucose is the major source of energy for the brain. Hypoglycemia can have numerous effects, including brain damage or death, if the glucose deficit is prolonged. There are a variety of causes of hypoglycemia. Examples include a pancreatic tumor that produces insulin, a diabetic patient who missed a meal, strenuous exercise by the diabetic patient, the consumption of alcohol without eating, the ingestion of medications, and an overdose (either accidental or intentional) of insulin or other antidiabetic medications. Hypoglycemia may be a condition by itself, or it may be a complication of diabetes or other disorders. It is most often seen as a complication of diabetes and is often referred to as an insulin reaction.[12–14,18–22] DOT 4-5.23, 4-5.24

When an individual's blood sugar level falls, they begin to experience hypoglycemic symptoms. The symptoms are the result of poor cerebral function and autonomic nervous system responses. Since the brain relies on glucose as its main source of energy, hypoglycemia will result in impaired cerebral function. Autonomic nervous system responses will include skin that is often cool and clammy to touch and a tachycardic heart rate. In some cases, the patient may be mistakenly assessed to be intoxicated.[12–14,18–22]

DOT 5-4.21, 5-4.25

Signs and symptoms of hypoglycemia include

- Sweating
- Tremors
- Anxiety
- Hunger
- Dizziness
- Headache
- Impaired vision
- Confusion or altered mental status
- Abnormal behavior
- Seizures
- Loss of consciousness
- Slurred speech
- Pale skin
- Diaphoresis
- Tingling sensation around the mouth
- Nausea
- Sympathetic nervous system response: anxiety, sweating, vasoconstriction (pale, cool skin), tachycardia
- Parasympathetic nervous system response: hypotension, bradycardia, nausea, hunger

Hyperglycemia

The individual with **hyperglycemia** has a reduction in the ability of insulin to trigger cells to absorb glucose molecules from the blood. Whether this is due to a decreased amount of insulin produced or from an insensitivity of the cells to a normal amount of insulin, the results are the same—blood glucose levels become abnormally high. In some cases, blood sugar levels may exceed 300 mg/dL. If left uncorrected, hyperglycemia can subsequently lead to diabetic ketoacidosis.[4,5,10,14–16,18,22] DOT 5-4.31

The development of hyperglycemia may be influenced by a variety of factors. Examples include infection, the ingestion of certain medications (e.g., diuretics), a myocardial infarction, or cerebral vascular accident. If the signs and symptoms of hyperglycemia are noted, the healthcare provider should suspect the presence of high blood sugar levels. This should also be considered a precursor to the potential development of ketoacidosis.[4,5,10,14–16,18,22] DOT 5-4.33

The signs and symptoms of hyperglycemia differ from those of hypoglycemia.

The more common findings of hyperglycemia include

- Polyphagia (excessive hunger)
- Polyuria (excessive urination)

- Polydipsia (excessive thirst)
- Recurrent infections
- Visual difficulties
- Fatigue
- Weight loss
- Wounds that do not heal well
- Dry mouth
- Dry, itchy skin
- Impotence (males)

Polyphagia develops because the individual with diabetes is unable to metabolize the glucose as an energy source within cells. As a result, even though there is glucose in circulation, the body is unable to utilize it. The hunger mechanism **(polyphagia)** is triggered in an effort to compensate for the perceived cellular hypoglycemia. Also, because the cells are unable to use the sugar as fuel, as blood filters through the kidneys, some of the sugar is not reabsorbed. This excess blood sugar "spills" into the urine. The extra sugar that is now contained in the urine causes water molecules to follow. As a result, the individual experiences increased urination, or **polyuria,** which can produce dehydration. This leads to the development of **polydipsia,** or excessive thirst. The body can sense that excess water is being lost **(polyuria)** due to the frequent urination. In response, the brain is stimulated to trigger the thirst response.[4,5,10,14–16,18,22] DOT 5-4.35

The symptoms of hyperglycemia vary and are influenced by the individual's underlying health and age. For example, younger individuals may present with specific complaints, such as polyuria or polydipsia. Older patients, however, may experience severe hypovolemia, acute changes in mental status, and acute renal failure. It is also possible for the signs and symptoms to be masked by the presence of preexisting conditions. This may complicate the identification and subsequent treatment of the hyperglycemia.[4,5,10,14–16,18,22] DOT 5-4.12

Diabetic Ketoacidosis

Diabetic ketoacidosis (DKA) results from a lack of insulin and involves a change in metabolism. In DKA, normal glucose utilization does not occur; therefore, alternative energy sources, including lipids, are metabolized. In type I diabetics, DKA can be triggered by a variety of events, including a lapse in insulin treatment, an acute infection, trauma, or any condition that creates a situation in which the availability of insulin becomes inadequate. While DKA is rare in type II diabetes, type II patients may also experience the formation of ketones and subsequent acidosis.[3,5,11–26] DOT 5-4.43

DKA involves marked hyperglycemia that causes the osmotic diuresis discussed earlier in this chapter.

Diuresis involves fluid losses via urination, including water and electrolytes, such as sodium and potassium. The patient may experience fluid shifting and acidosis that results from increases in hepatic ketone body production and release. The presence of ketone bodies, or strong acids, results in hyperketonemia. This in turn leads to metabolic acidosis, which contributes to increases in the excretion of additional acids and electrolytes. The acetone that develops may initially be excreted through the respiratory system; however, this may be a short-term solution if the cycle continues.[5,11–26] DOT 5-4.8, 5-4.30, 5-4.44

The onset of DKA tends to be gradual and may evolve over 12–24 hours or longer.

Early symptoms of DKA include

- Increased thirst
- Excessive hunger
- Urination
- Malaise

General symptoms may include nausea, vomiting, and, in children, abdominal pain. Lethargy or somnolence may occur later. In untreated patients, DKA may progress to coma. In uncomplicated DKA, the patient's temperature is usually normal or low. Signs of dehydration are usually present, and some patients are hypotensive. Kussmaul's respirations, a distinctive pattern of deep sighing breaths that may be slow, rapid, or normal, may also be noted. The presence of acetone odor may be detected on the breath. [3–5,11–26] DOT 5-4.46

Street Secrets

Suspect diabetic ketoacidosis when the blood sugar level is over 300 mg/dL. When the patient is in DKA, they should not engage in strenuous activity as this will result in metabolism of additional muscle mass for fuel.

Hyperosmolar Hyperglycemic Nonketotic Syndrome

Hyperosmolar hyperglycemic nonketotic syndrome involves severe hyperglycemia in which the blood sugar often exceeds 600 mg/dL and electrolyte imbalances occur. This may be referred to as hyperosmolar hyperglycemic state (HHS) or hyperosmolar hyperglycemic nonketotic syndrome (HHNS). In either case, ketonemia and metabolic acidosis may also develop at some point.[3,4,27,28] DOT 5-4.36

HHNS is the result of cumulative events. There is decreased insulin utilization that results in an increase in hepatic glucogenesis and glycogenesis. These factors contribute to the development of hyperglycemic blood glucose levels, hypovolemia, the development of ketones, and subsequent acidosis.[27,28]

The symptoms and pathology of HHNS and DKA are very similar. Hyperglycemia, volume depletion, electrolyte imbalance, and acidosis are possible with both situations. In HHNS, the acidosis may be due to the hypoperfusion of tissues. HHNS occurs less frequently than DKA. The mortality rates with HHNS exceed DKA, at 15–30%, compared to 5%, respectively.[27,28] The metabolism of lipids that occurs in DKA is considered by some to be the differentiating factor between HHNS and DKA. [3,4,27,28] DOT 5-4.37

Cases of HHNS tend to be found in the elderly patient population. Early findings in the elderly may include mental status changes or fluctuations in vital signs. Because of the pathology involved in HHNS, a variety of symptoms can be seen. DOT 5-4.40

Symptoms of HHNS in the elderly

- Poor skin turgor
- Dry mucous membranes
- Sunken eyes
- Hypotension

The patient's central nervous system functions may be impaired, leading to complications such as altered mental status, seizures, unconsciousness, and possibly death. The patient may also experience weakness, anorexia, fatigue, cough, dyspnea, or abdominal pain. More than 25% of these cases involve the presence of pneumonia and urinary tract infection.[3,4,27–30]

Thyroid Disorders

In addition to being prepared to respond to a diabetic emergency, healthcare providers must also be ready to assist in a variety of other types of calls. The following section discusses thyroid disorders, focusing on hypothyroidism, hyperthyroidism, and myxedema coma.

Hypothyroidism

Hypothyroidism is an endocrine-mediated disease process that slows normal body functions. It results from the impairment or absent production of the thyroid hormone. The disease can progress slowly over a period of months or years, or it can have an acute onset. Normally thyroid hormone is secreted in response to stimulation of the thyroid gland by thyroid stimulating hormone (TSH). When this system does not function normally, hypothyroidism may develop. There are different forms of hypothyroidism. Primary hypothyroidism results from the inability of the thyroid gland to produce adequate amounts of thyroid hormone. Secondary hypothyroidism is the result of pituitary dysfunction causing impaired release of thyroid stimulating hormone. Tertiary hypothyroidism is caused by a hypothalamic abnormality.[3–5,31–34]

Two leading causes of hypothyroidism include treatment for Graves' disease as well as autoimmune destruction of the thyroid gland. **Graves' disease** is a severe form of hyperthyroidism where the thyroid is swollen (it forms a goiter on the anterior surface of the neck), exophthalmos occurs (bulging eyes), and toxic signs of hyperthyroidism are present (Figure 31-4). In Graves' disease, the thyroid gland is removed either surgically or radioactively. Autoimmune destruction of the thyroid gland may be seen in cases of Hashimoto's thyroiditis. This is a type of autoimmune thyroid disease in which the patient's own immune system attacks and destroys the thyroid gland.[3,4,31–34]

While the exact incidence of hypothyroidism is debated, reports suggest an approximate incidence of less than 6%.[31–34] Many patients are not aware that they have the condition. The signs and symptoms are largely dependent on the degree of hormone deficiency.[31–34]

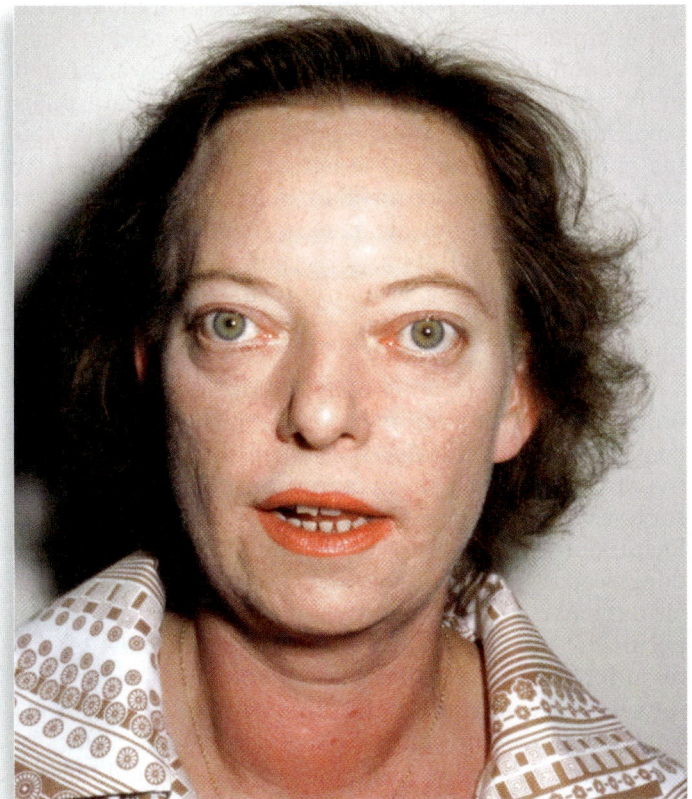

Figure 31-4   Graves' disease can cause protruding eyes. Treatment of Graves' disease can lead to hypothyroidism.

Signs and symptoms of hypothyroidism include:

- Weakness (99%)
- Skin changes (79%)
- Mononeuropathy
- Menstrual irregularity
- Menorrhagia
- Lethargy
- Loss of energy
- Deep, husky voice
- Cold intolerance
- Weight gain
- Muscle or joint pain or weakness
- Inability to concentrate
- Drowsiness
- Constipation
- Emotional lability
- Forgetfulness
- Headaches
- Blurred vision
- Fullness in throat
- Dry hair
- Depression
- Hypothermia
- Nonpitting, waxy, dry edema
- Dependent edema
- Loss of axillary and pubic hair
- Pallor
- Loss of scalp hair
- Abdominal distention
- Pseudomyotonic reflexes
- Goiter (Figure 31-5)
- Unsteady gait
- Pericardial effusion
- Dull facial expression
- Coarsening or huskiness of voice
- Periorbital puffiness
- Bradycardia
- Decreased systolic blood pressure and increased diastolic blood pressure

Myxedema Coma

Myxedema coma is a severe and potentially life-threatening condition that can occur during the progression of hypothyroidism. The term myxedema is sometimes used interchangeably with hypothyroidism, but this is not exactly correct as myxedema is on the far

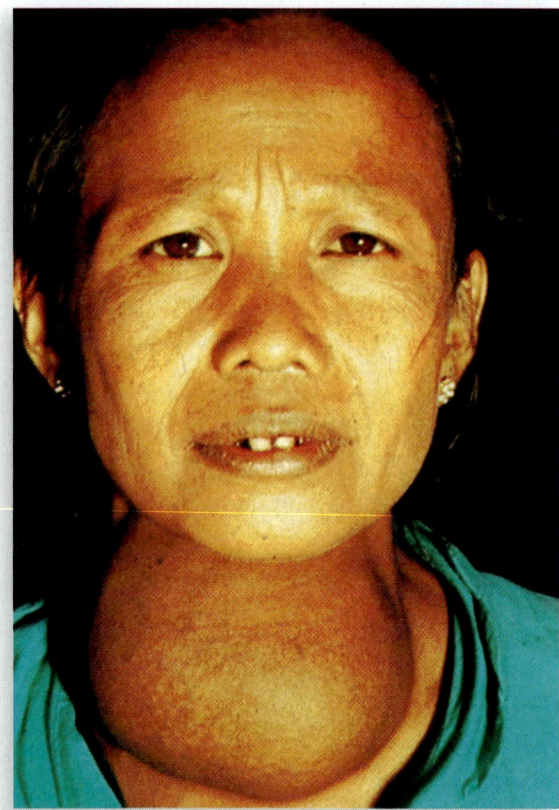

Figure 31-5 An example of physical changes that can be brought on by hypothyroidism is the goiter on this patient's neck.

precipitated by a secondary insult such as hypothermia, infection, other systemic diseases, or drug therapies.[35]

Potential causes of myxedema coma include:

- Burns
- Carbon dioxide retention
- Gastrointestinal hemorrhage
- Hypoglycemia
- Hypothermia
- Pneumonia
- Sepsis
- Surgery
- GI hemorrhage
- Stroke
- Trauma
- Influenza
- Urinary tract infection or urosepsis
- Medication ingestion: amiodarone (Cordarone), anesthesia, barbiturates, beta-blockers, diuretics, lithium, narcotics, phenothiazines, phenytoin (Dilantin), rifampin (Rifadin, Rimacta)

end of the continuum of the hypothyroidism state. It is reported in less than 0.1% of all cases of hypothyroidism.[35,36] In the United States, hypothyroidism is present in 8% of women and 2% of men who are older than 50 years.[35,36] The incidence of hypothyroidism increases with age, and myxedema coma is predominantly seen in elderly individuals, especially Caucasian women.[35,36]

A majority of the cases occur during the winter months. It is suspected that the increased winter rate is due to the older patient's age-related loss of the ability to sense temperature and the lower heat production secondary to hypothyroidism. The mortality rate for untreated or unrecognized myxedema can exceed 95%.[35,36]

The reports of the frequency of myxedema coma vary based upon the definition used. For example, if only comatose patients are considered, the rate of myxedema coma is low. Between 1953 and 1996, there were 200 cases reported. If the definition is widened to include more than just those cases in which the patient is in a coma, the number of cases increases considerably. Mortality rates range between 30% and 60% with numerous factors (e.g., core body temperature, cardiac function) influencing the patient's outcome.[35,36]

Myxedema coma is more common in patients with long-standing untreated hypothyroidism and is usually

There are a variety of signs and symptoms associated with myxedema coma. Hypoventilation may occur due to the decreased respiratory response to hypoxia and hypercapnia. Respiratory dysfunction may lead to sleep apnea, and respiratory difficulties may be exacerbated by myxedematous infiltration of the tongue and pharynx. Diaphragmatic weakness may develop. Mental status changes can include lethargy, stupor, delirium, or coma. While the exact mechanisms causing changes in mental status are not clear, it is suspected reductions in cerebral blood flow and oxygen delivery, reduced oxygen and glucose consumption, and the lack of thyroxine (T4) and triiodothyronine (T3) influence brain function.[35,36]

Additional symptoms of hypothyroidism are present including weight gain, cold intolerance, a deep voice, coarse hair, and dry, pale, cool skin. Elderly patients with hypothyroidism may have atypical initial presentations, such as decreased mobility as the primary finding. Respiratory muscle function may be compromised, and a depressed respiratory drive may develop. Fluid accumulation may cause pleural effusions, causing ventilation-perfusion mismatch. These factors contribute to the retention of an excessive amount of carbon dioxide in the blood (hypercapnia). Dysfunction of other organ systems may have profound effects. If present, obesity causes decreased lung volumes. This, in combination with reduced flow rates, may be the primary cause of the hypoventilation, hypoxia, hypercarbia, and depressed respiratory drive that is often noted in these patients.[3–5,35,36]

TABLE 31-2   Effects of Hypothyroid Myxedema Coma

Organ or System	Possible Effects
Cardiac	Normal systolic pressure, elevated diastolic pressure, bradycardia.
Thyroid	Enlarged, not palpable, scar suggesting previous thyroidectomy.
Respiratory	Slow respiration rate, congestion, pleural effusion.
Abdomen	Distension secondary to ileus or ascites, diminished or absent bowel sounds.
Extremities	Cold, nonpitting edema of hands and feet.
Skin and nails	Pale, dry, scaly, thickened skin; dry brittle nails; ecchymoses, purpura.
Neuromuscular	Confusion, stupor, obtunded, coma, slow speech, seizures.

Table 31-2 outlines the effects of hypothyroid myxedema coma. DOT 5-4.55, 5-4.56, 5-4.58 & 5-4.60

Hyperthyroidism

Hyperthyroidism occurs from an overactive thyroid gland. It is a subset of thyrotoxicosis, which is caused by excess synthesis and secretion of thyroid hormone by the thyroid. Although distinct disease processes, the terms hyperthyroidism and thyrotoxicosis are sometimes used interchangeably.[3–5,31,32,34]

Hyperthyroidism affects every organ and body system. Thyroid hormone is needed for normal growth, development, and the regulation of cellular metabolism. Excess thyroid hormone causes an increase in the body's metabolic rate. This is associated with increased total body heat and cardiovascular activity. This can result in increased heart contractility and vasodilation. Hyperthyroidism leads to an increase in sympathetic nervous system symptoms, including nervousness, stare, tremor, and tachycardia. The specific symptoms of hyperthyroidism vary and may be influenced by the patient's age.[3–5,31,32,34]

One of the most common causes of hyperthyroidism is **Graves' disease,** an organ-specific autoimmune disorder (see Figure 31-4). It accounts for more than 50% of these cases. In this situation, certain thyroid hormones bind to their receptors, triggering the release of thyroid hormone and growth of the thyroid (hypertrophy).[31,32,34]

Another cause of hyperthyroidism is **subacute thyroiditis.** This involves an increased release of thyroid hormones and accounts for approximately 20% of these cases. **Toxic multinodular goiter,** or **Plummer disease,**

occurs in 15–20% of patients with thyrotoxicosis. It is most common in elderly individuals, especially in patients with a chronic goiter. In this situation, the excess of thyroid hormone develops gradually over time.[31,32,34]

Hyperthyroidism can also be classified as "hyperthyroidism" or "apathetic hyperthyroidism." In hyperthyroidism, patients tend to be younger with symptoms that indicate multiorgan involvement. **Apathetic hyperthyroidism** is associated with older patients in which the signs and symptoms seen in younger patients are less obvious. Symptoms of cardiovascular compromise may be noted in the latter case.[31,32,34]

Thyroid conditions occur more frequently in women than in men. Thyroid disease occurs with the same frequency in whites and Asians; it occurs less frequently in the black population.[31,32,34]

Symptoms of hyperthyroidism include:

- Periorbital (tissues around the eyes) edema
- Chemosis (swollen eyelids) or conjunctival edema
- Proptosis (bulging eyes)
- Weakness
- Weight loss
- Heat intolerance
- Nervousness
- Palpitations

Hyperthyroidism may also be associated with other autoimmune diseases such as pernicious anemia, myasthenia gravis, adrenal insufficiency, and type I diabetes.[31,32,34]

Additional symptoms associated with hyperthyroidism:

- Anxiety
- Increased perspiration or diaphoresis
- Tremor
- Hyperactivity or hypermetabolic state
- Oligomenorrhea (abnormally light menses)
- Tachycardia
- Hypertension
- Warm skin
- Smooth skin
- Stare
- Tremor
- Muscle weakness
- Atrial fibrillation or high output failure (in elderly individuals)

(continued on next page)

- Sweating
- *Younger patients* tend to exhibit more sympathetic activation, such as anxiety, hyperactivity, and tremor
- *Older patients* have more cardiovascular symptoms, such as dyspnea and atrial fibrillation with unexplained weight loss

Thyrotoxicosis and Graves' Disease

As mentioned, the most common cause of thyrotoxicosis is Graves' disease (known as Basedow's disease in Europe). It is an autoimmune disorder affecting the thyroid gland, characterized by an increase in synthesis and release of thyroid hormones. The thyroid gland is typically enlarged, which is called a goiter, and the eyes typically protrude from the sockets (exophthalmos). Graves' disease should be suspected if any evidence of thyroid eye disease exists, including periorbital edema, diplopia (double vision), or proptosis (eyes protrude outward). DOT 5-4.49, 5-4.50, 5-4.52, 5-4.54

Signs of thyrotoxicosis:

- Exophthalmos
- Sinus tachycardia
- Atrial fibrillation
- Systolic hypertension
- Soft smooth skin
- Excessive perspiration
- Palmar erythema (red palms) and sweating
- Lid lag
- Extension tremor (when a limb is fully extended it trembles)
- Hyperkinesis (abnormal and sometimes uncontrolled muscle movements)
- Large-muscle weakness

Cushing's Syndrome

Cushing's syndrome is the result of excess cortisol levels. This can result from excessive cortisol production, excessive use of cortisol (topically, in pill form, or in injections), or other similar steroid (glucocorticoid) hormones. Cortisol is a hormone produced by the adrenal gland. It mobilizes nutrients, influences the body's response to inflammation, stimulates the liver to raise the blood sugar, helps control the amount of water in the body, and helps the body respond to stress. The production of cortisol is regulated by adrenocorticotrophic hormone (ACTH), which is produced in the pituitary gland. When an excess amount of cortisol is produced or when an excess amount is ingested in the

course of treating other diseases, the resulting changes are referred to as Cushing's syndrome.[8,9] DOT 5-4.61

Most cases of Cushing's syndrome are caused by the administration of *exogenous* glucocorticoids. Annual incidence of *endogenous* Cushing's syndrome has been estimated at 13 cases per 1 million individuals.[8,9] Of these cases, approximately 70% are caused by Cushing's disease (pituitary ACTH-producing tumor), 15% by ectopic ACTH, and 15% by a primary adrenal tumor.[8,9] Cushing's syndrome caused by an adrenal or pituitary tumor has a female-to-male incidence ratio of approximately 5:1.[8,9] The peak incidence of Cushing's syndrome is 25 to 40 years of age (Figure 31-6). The morbidity and mortality associated with Cushing's syndrome are primarily related to the effects of excess glucocorticoids.[8,9] DOT 5-4.62, 5-4.64, 5-4.66

Symptoms of Cushing's syndrome:

- Headache
- Visual disturbances
- Amenorrhea (cessation of menstruation)
- Thinning of skin
- Irregular menses
- Prolonged wound healing
- Increased rate of infections
- Fatigue
- Bruise easily
- Muscle weakness
- Depression
- Cognitive dysfunction
- Weight gain, especially in the face (moon face), supraclavicular region, upper back, and torso

Adrenal Crisis: Addison's Disease

Acute adrenal crisis is a life-threatening condition caused by insufficient levels of cortisol, a hormone that is produced in the adrenal gland. Cortisol assists in glucose regulation and influences the body's response to stress. Adrenal crisis can develop if the adrenal gland deteriorates (such as in the case of **Addison's disease,** or primary adrenal insufficiency), if the pituitary gland is injured (referred to as secondary adrenal insufficiency), or if preexisting adrenal insufficiency is not treated appropriately. In these situations, there is an insufficient amount of cortisol, leading to the development of acute adrenal crisis. The onset of the crisis can be acute or may develop over a period of days. DOT 5-4.67, 5-4.68

The presence of underlying disease processes can result in adrenal crisis. Bilateral massive adrenal

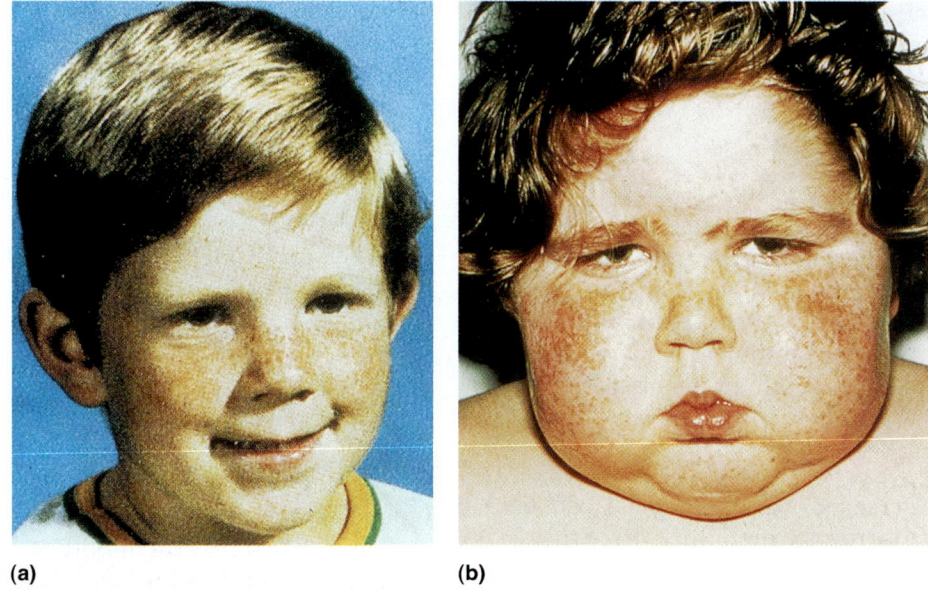

(a)   (b)

Figure 31-6   These photos, taken only four months apart, show the effects of Cushing's syndrome on a young boy.

Nice to Know

Adrenal insufficiency may be noted in patients with long-term steroid use. Any patient with a suspected electrolyte imbalance, endocrine disorder such as Addison's disease, or genitourinary complaint should have their history for urination and defecation explored. The patient should be asked if their toilet habits (frequency, volume, appearance, etc.) have been normal or abnormal.

hemorrhage (BMAH) may occur when there is a severe physiologic stress, such as myocardial infarction, septic shock, complicated pregnancy, or coagulopathy. If BMAH develops, the patient may have a poor outcome.[36–38] DOT 5-4.70, 5-4.72

Factors that lead to the development of adrenal crisis include physical stressors such as infection, trauma or surgery, adrenal gland or pituitary gland injury, and premature termination of steroid treatment. Steroid use, AIDS, and tuberculosis are also associated with the development of adrenal crisis. Symptoms associated with adrenal crisis cover a wide spectrum of findings.[37–39]

Signs and symptoms of adrenal crisis:

- Dizziness
- Weakness
- Sweating
- Abdominal pain
- Nausea
- Vomiting
- Altered level of consciousness
- Weight loss
- Fever
- Tachycardia
- Hypotension

Electrolytes

The prehospital care provider should be familiar with the various electrolytes of the body. Electrolytes have a key role in maintaining homeostasis (Figure 31-7). They assist in regulating water balance, assist in acid/base regulation, contribute to enzyme reactions, and support neuromuscular activity. Alterations in

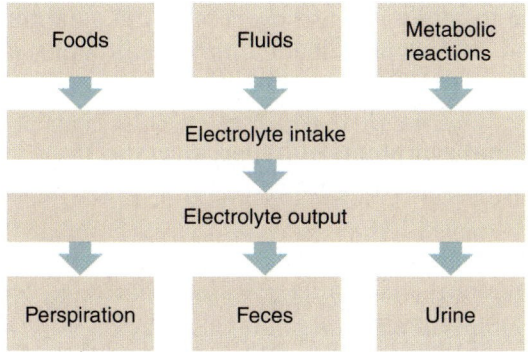

Figure 31-7   Electrolyte balance exists when the intake and output from all sources is equal.

electrolytes can affect any organ or system. It is also possible for the signs and symptoms of electrolyte imbalances to mimic symptoms of other potential disease pathology.[3–5,40]

Calcium

Calcium is needed for normal cell function, neural transmission, membrane stability, bone structure, and blood coagulation. Calcium balance is maintained through a variety of mechanisms, including the parathyroid hormone (PTH), vitamin D, calcitonin, and magnesium. More than 95% of calcium is found in the bone.[40–42]

Hypercalcemia

Hypercalcemia, or increased calcium levels, can be caused by several disorders, including hyperparathyroidism, malignancy, and certain medications. Hypercalcemia can be divided into PTH-mediated hypercalcemia and non–PTH-mediated hypercalcemia. PTH-mediated hypercalcemia is related to an increase in calcium absorption from the intestine. As a reminder, PTH is parathyroid hormone; it was discussed in the beginning of the chapter. In non–PTH-mediated hypercalcemia, the hypercalcemia is most commonly associated with malignancy and metastases which cause increased osteoclastic (resorption) activity within the bone.[3,4,42]

Primary hyperparathyroidism can lead to hypercalcemia. It occurs in 25 per 100,000 persons in the general population.[40,42] The rate of primary hyperparathyroidism increases with age.[40,42] There are more than 50,000 new cases that occur each year. Cancer patients are also prone to hypercalcemia. The prognosis of hypercalcemia associated with malignancy is poor.[40,42] The one-year survival rate is between 10% and 30%. The rate of hypercalcemia is higher in women, and the annual incidence in women older than 65 years of age is 250 per 100,000.[40,42]

The symptoms of hypercalcemia depend on the underlying cause of the disease, the time over which it develops, and the overall health of the patient.[3,4,40,42] Similar to many disease processes, the symptoms associated with hypercalcemia may mimic other disease pathology.

Signs and symptoms of hypercalcemia:

- Nausea
- Vomiting
- Altered mental status
- Abdominal or flank pain
- Constipation
- Lethargy
- Depression
- Weakness
- Polyuria
- Coma
- Hypertension
- Bradycardia
- ECG: shortened QT interval, various degree of heart blocks

Hypocalcemia

Hypocalcemia, or low calcium levels, can be caused by the impaired ability to mobilize calcium from bone stores, abnormal binding of calcium, abnormal losses from the kidneys, or the decreased absorption of calcium from the intestines. In most cases, hypocalcemia presents in a mild form and is usually the result of a chronic disease or illness. Chronic or subacute complaints (secondary to mild or moderate hypocalcemia) are more likely to be a chief complaint in the emergency department versus acute symptoms of hypocalcemia. When acute cases are encountered, they may involve cardiac dysrhythmias and cardiovascular collapse.[3,4,40,41]

Causes of hypocalcemia:

- Hypoalbuminemia (low blood albumin levels), most common cause
- Hypomagnesemia (low blood magnesium levels)
- Hyperphosphatemia (high blood phosphate levels)
- Medication effects
- Surgical effects
- PTH deficiency (parathyroid hormone)
- Vitamin D deficiency
- Acute pancreatitis
- Rhabdomyolysis (destruction of muscle tissues with resultant toxin release)
- Sepsis
- Toxic shock
- High calcitonin (excess amount of the hormone that lowers blood calcium levels)
- Renal insufficiency
- Sarcoidosis (formation of nodules in the lymph nodes of an unknown cause)
- Tuberculosis
- Hemochromatosis (an iron metabolism disorder)
- Toxicologic causes

Hypocalcemia occurs equally in males and females of all ages. Neurologic symptoms, including seizures, can develop. Deaths, although rare, have been reported. In some cases, the disease causing the hypocalcemia may have greater impact on morbidity than the hypocalcemia itself.[3,4,40,41]

Signs and symptoms of hypocalcemia:

- Muscle cramps
- Shortness of breath due to bronchoconstriction
- Seizures
- Distal extremity numbness
- Tingling sensations
- CHF
- Angina
- Cataracts
- Dry skin
- Coarse hair
- Brittle nails
- Psoriasis
- Syncope
- Laryngeal stridor
- Scars over the thyroid indicating removal or injury
- Dysphagia
- Intestinal colic
- Altered mental status
- Hypotension
- Wheezing
- Rales
- Bradycardia
- Focal numbness
- Muscle spasms
- Tetany

Potassium

Potassium is an important electrolyte that has several functions. It helps to regulate the activity of all muscle tissues, including smooth muscles, the myocardium, and skeletal muscles. It is involved in the enzyme reactions that occur during digestion and metabolism, and it influences homeostasis. More than 95% of the potassium is located inside cells, with the remainder being located extracellularly.[3,4,40]

Hyperkalemia

Hyperkalemia involves an excessive level of potassium. This can be the result of increased total body potassium or excessive release of potassium from the cells into the bloodstream. Factors include renal failure, adrenal insufficiency, metabolic acidosis, and excessive potassium release secondary to tissue trauma.[3,4,43]

In normal situations, the kidneys remove excess potassium from the body. A majority of the cases of hyperkalemia are caused by conditions that impair the kidneys' ability to remove excess potassium. Insufficient kidney function may result from a variety of conditions, including acute or chronic renal failure, lupus nephritis, or the rejection of a transplanted kidney.[3,4,43]

When potassium is released from cells, it may accumulate in the extracellular fluid and the bloodstream. Reasons why potassium moves into the extracellular fluids include traumatic injury, surgery, tumor, burns, or hemolytic conditions. Aldosterone, which is a hormone, regulates the kidney's excretion of sodium and potassium. Aldosterone deficiency can result in hyperkalemia. Similar to other disease processes, gradual increases in potassium may be better tolerated than acute increases. The symptoms associated with hyperkalemia can include a spectrum of findings.[3,4,43]

Signs of hyperkalemia:

- Nausea
- Bradycardia
- Heart blocks
- Ventricular fibrillation
- Weakness
- Muscle cramps
- Diarrhea
- Gastrointestinal distress
- ECG changes: peaked T waves, depressed ST segment, depressed P waves, widened QRS

Hypokalemia

Hypokalemia, or low potassium, can result from a variety of causes, including renal or GI losses, inadequate diet, transcellular shift (movement of potassium from serum into cells), and the ingestion of certain medications. Up to 20% of hospitalized patients are reported to experience hypokalemia.[43] Of this group, 5% of these patients are considered to be clinically significant.[43] Severe hypokalemia is relatively uncommon. For patients who are receiving diuretics, it is thought that almost 80% experience hypokalemia at least once. The rate is equal in males and females.[44]

Street Secrets

Certain diuretics, such as the thiazide drugs (hydrochlorothiazide is an example), can cause hypokalemia. Patients on these types of diuretic are often also prescribed potassium supplements. Potassium tablets, however, are extremely acidic and frequently cause stomach upset. Many of these tablets are enteric coated, so they do not begin to break down until they pass through the stomach. Unfortunately, many elderly patients with digestive problems pass the enteric coated pills right through their GI tract without absorbing the medication. If patients exhibit signs of hypokalemia, even when they tell you they take potassium supplements, assume that could be the root problem.

The patient with hypokalemia may present with a vague medical history or symptoms. The provider must consider the patient's overall state of health as well as their history when attempting to formulate a clinical impression.[3–5,44]

Common symptoms of hypokalemia:

- Palpitations
- Skeletal muscle weakness
- Paralysis
- Constipation
- Nausea, vomiting, and diarrhea (including severe and prolonged diarrhea or vomiting from eating disorders such as bulimia)
- Abdominal cramping
- Polyuria, nocturia (frequent voiding at night), or polydipsia
- Psychosis, delirium, or hallucinations
- Depression
- Lethargy
- Hypotension
- Cardiac dysrhythmias
- Bradycardia or tachycardia
- Hypoventilation, respiratory distress
- Respiratory failure
- Cardiac arrest
- Decreased muscle strength

Sodium

Sodium has a significant role in the regulation of water. In fact, it is often noted that "water follows sodium."[5] When sodium levels increase, it is referred to as hypernatremia. If there is a decrease, it is called hyponatremia. Sodium is the dominant electrolyte, and its balance is vital to normal cellular functions.[3–5,45–47]

Hypernatremia

Systemic sodium levels are controlled through the regulation of urine production and the thirst response. **Hypernatremia** can be caused by abnormal thirst responses or behavioral responses that lead to problems with the renal concentrating mechanism. These factors can be the result of kidney pathology, hormonal control complications, or from water losses secondary to other causes. In individuals with a functioning thirst response, hypernatremia is rare. When it does develop, it is associated with a mortality rate that exceeds 50%.[3–5,45–47]

In hypernatremia, cells become dehydrated and the body attempts to compensate for this through a variety of mechanisms. If, for example, the intracellular sodium concentration is excessive, the cells may respond by actively pumping sodium out of the cell. This can result in dehydration, and the cells shrink from the lost water and sodium.[3–5,45–47]

Cells respond to these structural changes and fluid losses by altering electrolyte balances. For example, after a period of hypernatremia, intracellular compounds are created in an effort to restore the cell's fluid volume and to avoid structural damage. These activities are intended to be protective and to assist in avoiding further cellular compromise. Once these mechanisms are initiated, and as fluid replacement begins, there needs to be adequate time for the excretion of the intracellular compounds that accumulated. If fluid replacement occurs too quickly (e.g., during fluid resuscitation) and the cellular compounds are not allowed to be removed, fluid overload and cerebral edema may occur.[3–5,45–47]

The effects of hypovolemia and cellular dehydration can be observed in the patient's CNS function. Due to the changes associated with dehydrated neurons, as well as the alteration of membrane potentials from electrolyte shifting, CNS functions become ineffective. If the cellular changes are severe, cerebral veins may be stretched and torn, leading to the development of subarachnoid hemorrhage.[3–5,45–47]

Hypernatremia occurs in approximately 1% of hospitalized patients. The mortality rate from hypernatremia varies, depending on the severity of the condition as well as the presence of other medical conditions. In acute hypernatremia the mortality rate ranges between 42% and 85%; for chronic hypernatremia, the rate is 10–60%.[40,45,47]

Mortality secondary to hypernatremia is more common among the elderly. If a patient with hypernatremia has other underlying diseases, it is difficult to precisely evaluate the degree of mortality that is directly the result of hypernatremia. Most deaths are due to the underlying

TABLE 31-3   **Summary of Hyponatremia and Hypernatremia**

Hyponatremia		Hypernatremia	
Causes	**Symptoms**	**Causes**	**Symptoms**
• Excessive sodium losses • Sweating • Diuresis • Gastrointestinal losses • Nausea, vomiting • Diarrhea	• Headache • Confusion, altered mental status • Lethargy • Seizures • Abdominal cramps • Impaired thirst mechanism	• Excessive sodium intake • Diuretic therapy • Watery diarrhea • Inability to swallow • Unconsciousness • Decreased blood pressure	• Skin dry and flushed • Decreased tendon reflexes • Seizures • Unconsciousness • Increased body temperature • Tachycardia

disease process and not the hypernatremia. For survivors, the effects of the morbidity are significant. Many patients experience permanent neurological deficits. Patients who arrive at the hospital in a hypernatremic state tend to be at the extremes of age, either very young or very old. There is no difference in rates between males and females. Examples of symptoms are listed in Table 31-3.[40,45,47]

Hyponatremia

Hyponatremia involves a low sodium level. It can occur by itself or as a complication of other conditions. Hyponatremia becomes clinically significant when it results in a reduction in serum osmolality, as in the case of hypotonic hyponatremia. Hypo-osmolality indicates that there is an excess of total body water relative to electrolytes. This imbalance can be due to electrolyte depletion, dilution of the electrolytes, or a combination of these factors.

Because hyponatremia influences cellular edema and central nervous system function, the treatment of hyponatremia will be guided by the onset of the condition. Acute hyponatremia (duration of less than 72 hours) can be safely corrected more quickly than chronic hyponatremia. Correction that occurs too rapidly can precipitate severe neurologic complications.[46,47]

Hyponatremia affects all races and has no gender difference. It is more common among the elderly because of the increased incidence of comorbid conditions, such as cardiac or renal failure. In these cases, the patient may seek medical attention as the result of symptoms that are attributed to hyponatremia, or they may seek medical attention due to their comorbid condition (e.g., CHF, liver failure), with the hyponatremia being identified coincidentally.[3,4,46,47]

The severity of neurologic symptoms is influenced by both the acuteness of the onset as well as the severity of the drop in the serum sodium. A more gradual drop of the serum sodium is often better tolerated versus an acute

change. The patient may also have vague complaints such as nausea, malaise, or flu-like symptoms. Neurological symptoms, such as headache, seizure, or coma, are often the result of a severe and acute drop of the serum sodium level that results in intracerebral fluid shifting and brain edema. Table 31-3 provides a summary of the causes and symptoms associated with hyponatremia.[3,4,46,47]

Magnesium

Magnesium is a mineral salt. It influences several processes, including the regulation of the absorption of calcium and myocardial function. It is helpful in relaxing the smooth muscle of the bronchioles and arterioles. It has been used to treat a variety of conditions, including asthma and hypertension.[3–5,48,49]

Hypermagnesemia

Hypermagnesemia (excessive magnesium) is less common than hypomagnesemia. It is more common in patients with chronic renal disease or rhabdomyolysis, which is the breakdown of muscle fibers resulting in the release of muscle cell contents into the circulation.

Signs and symptoms of hypermagnesemia include:

• Nervousness
• Decreased blood pressure
• Widened QRS
• T wave segment elevation
• Confusion
• Respiratory distress
• Flushing
• Nausea
• Vomiting

Hypomagnesemia

Hypomagnesemia (magnesium deficiency) may be caused by a variety of conditions that increase magnesium losses or shift the electrolyte balance. Examples include renal disease and diuretic therapy, including antihypertensive medications, as well as hyperthyroidism, pancreatitis, diabetes, parathyroid gland disorders, and diarrhea.[3–5,48,49]

The symptoms of hypomagnesemia can be difficult to attribute to only the hypomagnesemia itself. Examples include fatigue, irritability, weakness, muscle tightness or spasms, dysmenorrhea, high blood pressure, cardiomyopathy, nerve conduction problems, anorexia, insomnia, sugar cravings, poor nail growth, and anxiety. Specific cardiac findings can include the widening of the QRS complex and peaking of the T wave, as well as the prolongation of the PR interval and the flattening of the T wave.[3–5,48,49]

Acid/Base Balance

The following provides an overview of acid/base balance, including some of the more common complications that can be encountered.

Normally, the body maintains a specific pH (Figure 31-8). The pH is measured using the pH scale. The pH scale is inversely related to hydrogen ion concentration. For example, if the hydrogen ion level increases, the pH drops. If the hydrogen ion level decreases, the pH rises. The pH scale ranges from 1 to 14 with the blood ideal pH ranging between 7.35 and 7.45. When the pH is below 7.35, it is called acidosis; when it is greater than 7.45, it is referred to as alkalosis.[50–55]

Acid/Base Pathology

During normal metabolism, the body produces hydrogen ions, H^+ (acids). For normal body function to occur,

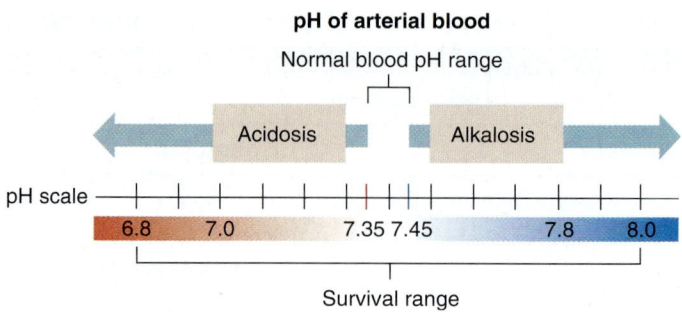

Figure 31-8   Normal pH ranges from 7.35 to 7.45. A pH as low as 6.8 or as high as 8.0 for any period of time is not compatible with life.

the acids must be removed from the body. There are three systems that can assist in this process:

1. The chemical buffer system
2. The respiratory system
3. The renal system

They work collaboratively in an effort to maintain an acid/base balance for optimal body functions.[3–5,50–55]

The chemical buffer system consists of carbonic acid (H_2CO_3) and bicarbonate (HCO_3^-). Under normal circumstances, the bases, or alkaloids, are in balance with the hydrogen ion concentration. Depending on the acid/base balance needed during metabolism, some of the carbonic acid will dissociate into bicarbonate and hydrogen, or hydrogen will combine with bicarbonate to form carbonic acid. In Box 31-1, the section referred to as "Balance" provides an illustrative overview of this process.[3–5,50–55]

Within the bicarbonate/carbonic acid system, complex interactions and chemical exchanges occur. These interactions are designed to maintain the body's normal pH range and optimal body function.[3–5,50–55] For example, when there is a change in hydrogen concentration, the body responds using several systems, such as the respiratory and renal systems (Figure 31-9). In response

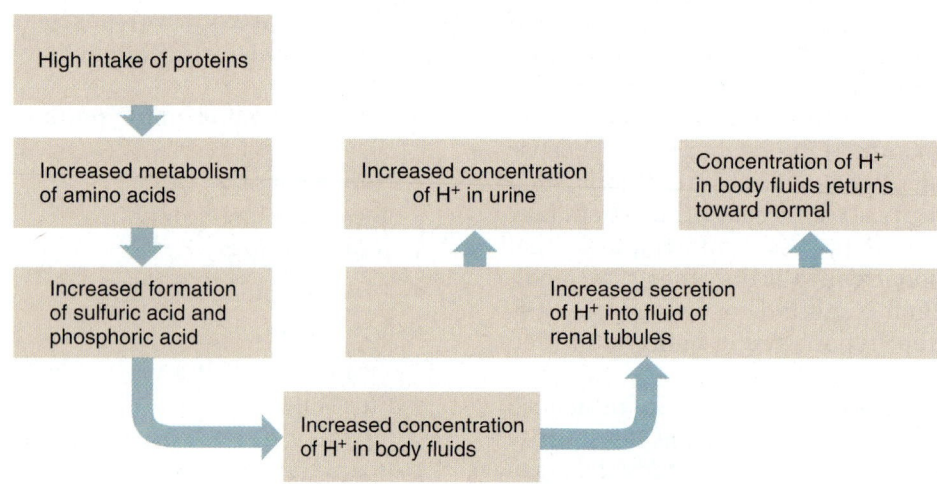

Figure 31-9   This flowchart illustrates the renal system compensating for increases in hydrogen.

BOX 31-1 An Overview of Acid/Base Balance

Balance:
$$H^+ + HCO_3^- \longleftrightarrow H_2CO_3$$
Hydrogen ion + Bicarbonate $\longleftrightarrow$ Carbonic acid

Increased acid:
$$\uparrow H^+ + HCO_3^- \rightarrow \uparrow H_2CO_3$$

Decreased acid:
$$\downarrow H^+ + HCO_3^- \rightarrow \downarrow H_2CO_3$$

Respiratory acidosis:
$$\downarrow \text{Respirations} = \uparrow CO_2 + H_2O \rightarrow \uparrow H_2CO_3 \rightarrow \uparrow H^+ + HCO_3^-$$

Respiratory alkalosis:
$$\uparrow \text{Respirations} = \downarrow CO_2 + H_2O \rightarrow \downarrow H_2CO_3 \rightarrow \downarrow H^+ + HCO_3^-$$

Metabolic acidosis:
$$\uparrow H^+ + HCO_3^- \rightarrow \uparrow H_2CO_3 \rightarrow H_2O + \uparrow CO_2$$

Metabolic alkalosis:
$$\downarrow H^+ + HCO_3^- \rightarrow \downarrow H_2CO_3 \rightarrow H_2O + \downarrow CO_2$$

to acidosis, the respiratory rate may increase. This type of change normally occurs within minutes or hours of acid/base fluctuations. The kidneys also have a role. They may adjust the renal excretion of acid or base in an effort to maintain homeostasis. Renal responses develop over a period of several days.[3–5,50–55]

The body's pH buffers also reduce significant fluctuations in hydrogen ion concentrations. Buffers are weak acids that are in balance with the bases (alkaloids). Buffers respond to changes in hydrogen ion concentrations by combining with excess hydrogen ion to minimize the impact of the change in pH. While the primary pH buffer in the blood is the bicarbonate/carbonic acid system, a variety of compounds, including phosphates, ammonia, proteins, and bone also provide pH buffering.[3–5,50–55]

Disturbances of acid/base metabolism can also influence carbon dioxide (CO_2) and bicarbonate (HCO_3^-) concentrations. Increases or decreases in HCO_3^- are referred to as **metabolic alkalosis** or **acidosis,** respectively. Increases or decreases in $PaCO_2$ are referred to as **respiratory acidosis** or **alkalosis** (Table 31-4).[3–5,50–55]

TABLE 31-4 Summary of Acid/Base Disorders

Condition	Summary
Metabolic acidosis	Results from production of acids—several of which may use bicarbonate ions. May be the result of vomiting, diarrhea, diabetes, and certain medication use. Develops when there is a build-up of acid. If the acid load overwhelms respiratory capacity, acidemia (arterial pH > 7.35) can develop. Can be due to increased acid production or acid administration.
Metabolic alkalosis	Results from net extracellular fluid acid loss or alkali gain. May be associated with the use of diuretics. If alkalosis overwhelms the pH buffering capacity, alkalemia (arterial pH > 7.45) results. Can develop through the loss of acid-containing gastric secretions via protracted vomiting or nasogastric suction or excessive losses of acid via the urine or stool. Can also develop from the movement of hydrogen ions into cells, resulting in a next loss of acid from loss of the extracellular fluid.
Respiratory acidosis	Results from the retention of CO_2. This may be caused by the depression of the central respiratory center, secondary to a variety of causes such as chest injuries, COPD, pneumonia, or pneumothorax. When there is a decrease in alveolar ventilation, this leads to pulmonary CO_2 retention and results in respiratory acidosis.
Respiratory alkalosis	Results from increased respirations and excessive removal of CO_2. Can result from a variety of causes, including hyperventilation, anxiety, over-ventilation of patients on assisted ventilation, CNS disorders, liver failure, coma, and fever. Increased respiratory rate and depth lead to hyperventilation, leading to excessive loss of CO_2 in expired air. As the PCO_2 and cerebral tissue PCO_2 fall, plasma and brain pH rise. Cerebral vasoconstriction results and may produce cerebral hypoxia.

TABLE 31-5   Comparison of Symptoms in Metabolic and Respiratory Acidosis and Alkalosis

Metabolic Acidosis	Metabolic Alkalosis	Respiratory Acidosis	Respiratory Alkalosis
• Nausea	• Confusion	• Headache	• Numbness of fingers or toes
• Kussmaul's respirations	• Hyperactive reflexes	• Respiratory distress	• Dizziness
• Vomiting	• Tetany	• Depression	• Panic
• Abdominal pain	• Seizures	• Paranoia	• Tetany
• Weakness and lethargy	• Decreased rate and depth of respirations	• Tremors	• Seizures
• Altered mental status	• Hypokalemia	• Paralysis or weakness	• Cardiac dysrhythmias
• Cardiac dysrhythmias	• Hypovolemia	• Warm, flushed skin	
• Hypotension, tachycardia	• Polyuria	• Coma	
• Warm, flushed skin		• Tachycardia	

It is possible for the acid/base balance to be influenced by a number of factors that result in "mixed acid/base" balances. In this case, the acid/base disturbance is more complex, and there are often two or more primary alterations occurring simultaneously. Mixed disturbances occur when the body reacts with either less than or greater than the expected level of compensation in response to changes in the acid/base balance. This is significant because the treatment that is provided must address each of the disturbance's causes. In the hospital setting, the measurement of pH, $PaCO_2$, and HCO_3^- in conjunction with the recognition of the underlying disease process, is usually sufficient to correctly solve most acid/base disturbances.[3–5,50–55]

Fluctuations in the acid/base balance can affect the delivery of oxygen and other compounds to tissues. This can result in both immediate and long-term complications for the patient. Table 31-4 provides examples of common acid/base conditions encountered by prehospital care providers. Table 31-5 provides an overview of the symptoms associated with acid/base imbalances.[3–5,50–55] Table 31-6 describes some of the ways the body compensates for acid/base abnormalities.

Patient Assessment

Primary Survey

Upon initial patient contact, rapidly determine the patient's level of consciousness and the status of their airway, breathing, and circulation. For their level of consciousness, consider using the AVPU system. If the patient has an altered level of consciousness or is unconscious, attempt to determine the cause. Life-threatening findings, such as respiratory or cardiac arrest, should be immediately managed.[5,55]

TABLE 31-6   Compensatory Mechanisms in Response to Acid/Base Imbalances

Respiratory system	Increased respirations assist with the removal of CO_2. Decreased respirations result in the retention of CO_2.
Bicarbonate system	Responds to changes in hydrogen concentration.
Renal system	Can regulate the pH by influencing concentration of bicarbonate in blood.

CONNECTIONS   Chapter 11: The Normal Physical Examination and Chapter 14: Patient Assessment discuss the AVPU assessment tool.

Note the condition of the patient's skin. Is it warm, pink, and dry, or is it cool, moist, and "clammy?" Are there any obvious signs of trauma? Compare proximal (e.g., carotid) and distal (e.g., radial) pulses for presence, quality, rate, strength, and regularity. Subtle dermal and cardiac findings may provide clues as to the cause and severity of the patient's condition.[5,55]

The initial patient assessment provides valuable information. For example, the provider can determine whether or not the patient is alert and oriented to person, place, and time as well as if there are any life-threatening conditions. Following the initial assessment, treatment plans can be formulated. Details regarding the patient's medical history and the events surrounding this episode can be obtained during the secondary assessment.[5,55]

Secondary Survey

The secondary assessment allows for a more comprehensive and detailed assessment of the patient. This includes conducting a head-to-toe survey as well as obtaining a complete set of vital signs. During the secondary survey, additional patient information may be obtained. The SAMPLE technique can be used to obtain this information.[5] This includes obtaining a detailed patient history, including symptoms, allergies, past medical history, medications being taken, last meal, and events that occurred prior to this episode.

Baseline vitals should be obtained as early as possible. At a minimum, vital signs should include heart rate, respiratory rate, blood pressure, and skin temperature. If available, pulse oximetry and capnometry may also be applied. Vital signs should be assessed every five to ten minutes. Depending on the patient's condition and provider's judgment, the frequency of taking vital signs may vary. For example, if volume depletion is suspected, providers may consider assessing for orthostatic vital signs changes. Reassessing the patient, including noting any changes in mental status and vital signs, should be part of any patient assessment.[5,55]

The physical exam may include an assessment of orthostatic vital signs. This can assist in the assessment of volume status. In addition, this determination (e.g., hypervolemic, euvolemic [normal volume], hypovolemic) often guides treatment decisions. Assessing for medical comorbidities (e.g., preexisting conditions) is also important.[4,5] DOT 5-4.6, 5-4.7, 5-4.27, 5-4.39

Treatment

Differentiating among endocrine conditions, electrolyte imbalances, and acid/base complications can be extremely difficult in the prehospital environment. Treatment should focus on improving circulatory volume, maintaining tissue perfusion, assessing and correcting blood glucose levels, reducing serum osmolality, clearing ketones from urine and serum, correcting electrolyte imbalances, and identifying precipitating factors. The severity of fluid and electrolyte imbalance is determined by the duration of the hyperglycemia, renal function, and fluid intake. This type of information is obtained once the patient has been evaluated in the emergency department.[4,5,55–57] DOT 5-4.5

The prehospital treatment of a patient experiencing a potential endocrine, acid/base, or electrolyte imbalance will be influenced by a variety of factors. This includes the patient's medical history and current presentation, local protocols, medical direction, provider skill level, provider judgment, and distance to an emergency department. While it may be possible to determine the patient's exact diagnosis in the prehospital setting, this is not always the case. In fact, many of the topics included in this chapter are impossible to "diagnose" in the field. Because of this, the prehospital care provider may need to treat the patient based on a rapid evaluation of the patient's signs and symptoms in combination

with information gathered on-scene. The following and Table 31-7 provide an overview of treatment options.[4,5,55–57]

Upon initial patient contact, determine if the patient is conscious. Any patient with an altered level of consciousness or acute complaint such as dyspnea, chest pain, or dizziness should receive supplemental oxygen. The status of the patient's airway, breathing, and circulation should be quickly assessed. If the patient's airway is at risk (e.g. snoring respirations), manual airway support, such as intubation, may be needed.[4,5,55–57]

Street Secrets

Consider using the AEIOU-TIPS mnemonic as a guide to critically think through the causes of unconsciousness. This memory aid can be found in Chapter 14: Patient Assessment.

Note the presence, rate, and quality of proximal and distal pulses. Although tachycardia can exist in any of the conditions discussed in this chapter, the patient may be bradycardic from beta-blockers or profound volume depletion. Blood pressure may vary and is influenced by infection, dehydration, and medication use. The combination of tachycardia, hypotension, dry mucous membranes, and febrile skin should indicate the potential for dehydration. Hypotension is considered a late finding and will require fluid therapy.[4,5,55–57]

If volume depletion is suspected, an intravenous line (IV) should be established. While starting the IV, blood samples may be obtained. Intravenous fluid administration will be influenced by factors including the patient's medical history and the patient's clinical

TABLE 31-7 Prehospital Treatment Considerations

Treatment	Summary
Oxygen	Acute complaints, altered mental status, unconsciousness
Intravenous line	Fluid administration, medication administration
Naloxone	Altered mental status or unresponsiveness, narcotic ingestion
Thiamine	Given in conjunction with Dextrose
Dextrose	Hypoglycemia, altered mental status or unresponsiveness
Sodium bicarbonate	Metabolic acidosis, select drug overdose
Anticonvulsants	Seizure activity

Nice to Know

How Many Calories are in an Amp of D50?

Carbohydrate contains 4 calories per gram. (Protein also contains 4 calories, and fat contains 9 calories.) An amp of D50 has 25 grams of dextrose, so each 50 mL ampule of 50% dextrose contains 100 calories. That is about one-half or one-third of the amount of sugar in a typical candy bar or sugar-containing soft drink. For patients who are severely hypoglycemic, a second bolus of D50 may be required. Reassess the blood sugar after about five minutes, and note the mental status to help guide this decision. Your protocols may require that you consult for the second bolus.

response. In cases of hypotension, tachycardia, or suspected hyponatremia (e.g., water intoxication), normal saline (0.9% sodium chloride) is recommended. Aggressive fluid replacement will assist in restoring intravascular volume. It will also reduce circulating blood glucose levels and will assist with the replacement of fluid and electrolyte loss.[4,5,55–57] DOT 5-4.65

Street Secrets

Patients with hyperglycemia are in danger of life-threatening cellular dehydration. These patients, with blood sugar levels above 300, often need several boluses of crystalloid IV solution. Begin with 20 mL/kg boluses, and consult with medical direction, if required, for additional fluid boluses. DOT 5-4.32, 5-4.45

When administering intravenous fluids, patient monitoring is important. Complications of over-aggressive fluid replacement, including cerebral edema, pulmonary edema, and acute respiratory distress syndrome (ARDS), have been reported.[4,5,55–57]

All patients with altered mentation or known diabetics, complaining of weakness, lightheadedness, sweating, or clamminess, should undergo blood glucose determination with a dextrostick and glucose meter.[4,5,55–57] DOT 5-4.8

In suspected or confirmed hypoglycemia, the blood sugar level should be restored to normal as quickly as possible. Early hypoglycemia can be managed through the oral intake of energy sources including cheese, crackers, sandwiches, and milk in awake patients who can protect their airway when swallowing. In acute hypoglycemia with altered mental status or unconsciousness, blood glucose levels can be restored with the administration of 25 gm of 50% dextrose intravenously.[55–57] DOT 5-4.73, 5-4.74

Recovery from an episode of hypoglycemia is influenced by the level of circulating insulin or oral antihyperglycemic agent. Higher levels of insulin may require more time for recovery. Restoring blood sugar levels in a patient who takes oral medications can be challenging as the half-life of certain hypoglycemic agents can exceed 24 hours. Diabetics who take oral medications, are over the age of 60, have kidney or liver disease, or do not regularly monitor their blood sugar are at-risk for experiencing prolonged hypoglycemia. In certain situations, a glucose infusion with repetitive blood glucose monitoring (e.g., once the patient has been admitted) may be required to correct the hypoglycemia.[4,5,55–57] DOT 5-4.26

If the patient is a child, pediatric doses of medications will need to be used. Adult dextrose is packaged as D50 (25 grams of dextrose in a 50 mL vial). In pediatric cases, it is suggested that the patient receive 2–4 mL/kg of D25 (e.g., diluted D50). Following the administration of the dextrose, the IV line should be flushed. Providers should consult with their local protocols regarding the use of medications for pediatric patients.[4,5,55–57]

Thiamine may be administered in conjunction with dextrose. It is a vitamin that promotes the metabolism of glucose and supports optimal energy production. Thiamine deficiencies tend to be associated with certain patient populations, such as those who regularly use or abuse alcohol. In these cases, the administration of dextrose without thiamine may contribute to the development of complications such as Wernicke's syndrome (encephalopathy with poor gait, eye muscle weakness, and mental derangement) and Korsakoff's psychosis (memory disorder). If indicated, 100 mg of Thiamine should be given either IV or IM in accordance with local protocols.[4,5,55–57] DOT 5-4.63, 5-4.75, 5-4.76

Naloxone, which is an opiate antagonist, may be considered if the patient has an altered mental status or is unconscious. The adult dose usually ranges between 0.4–2.0 mg. The route of administration, IV, IM, or ET, should be in accordance with local protocols.[4,5,55–57]

Street Secrets

The amount of naloxone to give should be driven by the patient's response to 0.2–0.4 mg divided doses. Give only enough naloxone to restore normal respirations. A return to full consciousness is not required if it is understood that the problem with the patient is limited to narcotic overdose. A 2-mg dose of naloxone given to a chronic drug user may precipitate withdrawal symptoms.

Glucagon may be needed in cases of hypoglycemia where an intravenous line cannot be established in the patient with AMS or unconsciousness. When the liver has an adequate supply of glucose, glucagon works by

Working in the Gray Zone

Administering glucagon can result in painful spasms in the abdomen or legs. Glucagon works by triggering the muscles to release the glycogen that is stored within the muscle tissue. When the body regulates this process, it is gradual and painless. When a single bolus is given IM, the process can be abrupt. Caution should be exercised with the use of glucagon. Its use should be limited to those circumstances when an IV truly cannot be established and oral glucose administration is not appropriate.

raising the patient's blood sugar by increasing the release of glucose from the liver. It can be administered intramuscularly (IM), intravenously (IV), or subcutaneously (SQ). The standard adult dose is 0.5–1 mg given IV, IM, or SC (pediatric dose is 0.3 mg/kg up to 1mg). It may take up to 20 minutes for glucagon's effects to occur.[4,5,55–57]

If the patient is experiencing a seizure, treatment may include airway management and medication administration (e.g., oxygen, dextrose, thiamine, naloxone). Anti-convulsants (e.g., benzodiazepine) may be indicated if the seizure activity continues.[4,5,55–57]

In the prehospital setting, the administration of sodium bicarbonate may be indicated in select cases, such as hyperkalemia or profound acidosis. An alkalinizing agent, sodium bicarbonate, is a salt that provides bicarbonate in an effort to buffer metabolic acidosis. It is usually administered as 1 meq/kg via IV. It may be repeated in ten minutes at a dose of 0.5 meq/kg. Calcium may also be administered in cases of hyperkalemia or hypocalcemia. The dosage is usually 2–4 mg/kg via IV.[4,5,55–57]

Cardiac monitoring (ECG) can be used to assess for myocardial involvement and potential electrolyte abnormalities. Peaked T waves suggest hyperkalemia; a prolonged QT interval suggests hypokalemia. Pulse oximetry and end-tidal CO_2 may also be used to monitor the patient's condition.[4,5,54,55,56]

Additional assessments (e.g., insulin or steroid administration), including laboratory testing in the hospital, are required in most cases to determine the specific etiology of the patient's condition. Prehospital care providers should document the initial patient findings as well as interventions provided and subsequent changes in the patient's status. These reports may guide the treatment that is provided in the hospital. In addition, providing the hospital staff with a thorough report will promote the continuum of care from the prehospital setting through discharge from the hospital.[4,5,55–57] DOT 5-4.7, 5-4.13, 5-4.14, 5-4.28, 5-4.29, 5-4.34, 5-4.35, 5-4.38, 5-4.41, 5-4.42, 5-4.47, 5-4.48, 5-4.51, 5-4.53, 5-4.57, 5-4.59, 5-4.69, 5-4.71

Summary

Endocrine emergencies account for a large percentage of hospital visits each year and a significant number of ambulance transports. For example, the most common cause of unconsciousness in nonhead injured patients is hypoglycemia in diabetes.

Hormones (secreted by endocrine organs) and electrolytes maintain the homeostatic balance. When any of these are out of balance, the life of the patient may be at stake. Most endocrine, acid/base, and electrolyte emergencies require supportive care of the ABCs. Once the patient arrives at the hospital, additional tests can pinpoint the root cause of the problem, and preventative measure or treatment can occur. Outcomes for endocrine, electrolyte, and acid/base emergencies will depend on the paramedic's understanding of the potential for life threats and rapid application of appropriate interventions.

Notes

1. University of Virginia, "Statistics related to the endocrine system" (2005), http://www.healthsystem.virginia.edu/UVAHealth/adult_endocrin/stats.cfm (accessed February 3, 2005).
2. "Anatomy of the Endocrine System," *Emedicine* (2004), http://www.emedicinehealth.com/articles/37539-1.asp (accessed September 28, 2006).
3. A. Spence and E. Mason, *Human Anatomy and Physiology*, 3rd ed. (Menlo Park, CA: Benjamin/Cummings, 1987).
4. C. Porth, *Pathophysiology: Concepts of Altered Health States*, 3rd ed. (Philadelpia, PA: J. B. Lippincott, 1990).
5. M. Londer, D. Hammer, and G. D. Lelen. Fluid and Electrolyte Problems in *Emergency Medicine: A Comprehensive Study Guide*, J. Tintinalli (ed.), 6th ed. (New York: McGraw-Hill, 2005), pp. 167–179.
6. D. Gardner, "Thyroid Disorders" (2002), http://www.muhealth.org/~daveg/thyroid/thy_dis.html (accessed February 5, 2005).
7. K. S. Saladin, *Anatomy & Physiology: The Unity of Form and Function*, 4th ed. (Dubuque, IA: McGraw-Hill, 2007), p. 647.
8. G. Adler, "Cushing Syndrome," *Emedicine* (2004), http://www.emedicine.com/emerg/topic117.htm (accessed February 3, 2005).
9. P. Margulies, "What Is Cushing's Syndrome?" (2005), http://www.medhelp.org/www/nadf4.htm (accessed February 3, 2005).
10. "Diabetes Overview," *Emedicine* (2004), http://www.emedicinehealth.com/articles/17044-1.asp (accessed February 3, 2005).
11. J. Koeslag, "Gluconeogenesis and Ketogenesis" (2005), http://academic.sun.ac.za/med_physbio/med_physiology/dept/footnote.htm (accessed February 3, 2005).
12. "Insulin's Mechanism of Action" (2005), http://www.medbio.info/Horn/PDF%20files/how_insulin_works.pdf (accessed February 5, 2005).
13. Becton, Dickinson and Company, "How Insulin Works," (2005), http://www.bddiabetes.com/us/yourinsulin/intro_how.asp (accessed February 5, 2005).
14. American Heart Association, "Hyperglycemia and Hypoglycemia" (2005), http://www.americanheart.org/presenter.jhtml?identifier=4593 (accessed February 5, 2005).
15. A. Hemphill, "Hyperglycemia," *Emedicine* (2005), http://www.emedicine.com/emerg/topic260.htm (accessed February 5, 2005).

16. Endocrine Web and the Norman Endocrine Surgery Clinic, "Symptoms of Hyperglycemia," http://www.endocrineweb.com/diabetes/hyperglycemia.html (accessed February 5, 2005).

17. C. Freudenrich, "Insulin, Glucagon and Blood Glucose," *Merck, How Stuff Works* (2005), http://health.howstuffworks.com/diabetes1.htm (accessed February 5, 2005).

18. R. Mathur, "Diabetes Mellitus," *MedicineNet.com* (2005), http://www.medicinenet.com/diabetes_mellitus/article.htm (accessed February 3, 2005).

19. S. Votey and A. Peters, "Diabetes Mellitus, Type 1—A Review," *Emedicine* (2005), http://www.emedicine.com/EMERG/topic133.htm (accessed February 3, 2005).

20. S. Votey, "Diabetes Mellitus, Type 2—A Review," *Emedicine* (2005), http://www.emedicine.com/emerg/topic134.htm (accessed February 3, 2005).

21. American Diabetes Association, "Type I Diabetes," http://www.diabetes.org/type-1-diabetes.jsp (accessed February 5, 2005).

22. American Diabetes Association, www.diabetes.org (accessed September 28, 2006).

23. L. Schmeltz, "Hot Topic: Approval of Exentide for Type 2 Diabetes," in: D. L. Kasper, E. Braunwald, A. S. Fauci, S. L. Hauser, D. L. Longo, J. L. Jameson, and K. J. Isselbacher, eds., *Harrison's Principles of Internal Medicine*, 16th ed., McGraw-Hill's AccessMedicine (accessed June 23, 2006).

24. Merck, "Diabetic Ketoacidosis," *HowStuffWorks* (2005), http://health.howstuffworks.com/framed.htm?parent=diabetes.htm&url=http://www.merck.com/pubs/mmanual/section2/chapter13/13b.htm (accessed February 5, 2005).

25. D. Rucker, "Diabetic Ketoacidosis," *Emedicine* (2004), http://www.emedicine.com/emerg/topic135.htm (accessed February 3, 2005).

26. W. Lamb, "Diabetic Ketoacidosis," *Emedicine* (2004), http://www.emedicine.com/ped/topic582.htm (accessed February 3, 2005).

27. J. Gonzalez-Campoy, "Hyperosmolar Coma," *Emedicine* (2003), http://www.emedicine.com/med/topic1091.htm (accessed February 5, 2005).

28. M. Sagarin and A. McAfee, "Hyperosmolar Hyperglycemic Nonketotic Coma," *Emedicine* (2005), http://www.emedicine.com/emerg/topic264.htm (accessed February 5, 2005).

29. Merck, "Nonketotic Hyperglycemic-Hyperosmolar Coma," *HowStuffWorks* (2005), http://health.howstuffworks.com/framed.htm?parent=diabetes.htm&url=http://www.merck.com/pubs/mmanual/section2/chapter13/13d.htm (accessed February 5, 2005).

30. M. Lipsky, "Management of Diabetic Ketoacidosis," *American Family Physician* Vol. 49(1) (Kansas City, MO: American Academy of Family Physicians, January 1994).

31. S. Lee, "Hyperthyroidism," *Emedicine* (2004), http://www.emedicine.com/med/topic1109.htm (accessed February 5, 2005).

32. C. Manifold, "Hypothyroidism and Myxedema Coma," *Emedicine* (2004), http://www.emedicine.com/emerg/topic280.htm (accessed February 5, 2005).

33. P. Orlander, "Hypothyroidism," *Emedicine* (2005), http://www.emedicine.com/med/topic1145.htm (accessed February 5, 2005).

34. D. Fitz-Patrick, "Thyroid Disorders," *Diabetes and Hormone Center of the Pacific* (1996), http://www.endocrinologist.com/thyroid.htm (accessed February 5, 2005).

35. C. Wall, "Myxedema Coma: Diagnosis and Treatment," *American Academy of Family Physicians* (2000), http://www.aafp.org/afp/20001201/2485.html (accessed February 5, 2005).

36. E. Citkowitz, "Myxedema Coma or Crisis," *Emedicine* (2004), http://www.emedicine.com/med/topic1581.htm (accessed September 28, 2006).

37. L. Kirland, "Adrenal Crisis," *Emedicine* (2003), http://www.emedicine.com/med/topic65.htm (accessed February 3, 2005).

38. N. Rennert, "911! Adrenal Crisis, Addison's/Adrenal Insufficiency" (2004), http://www.nlm.nih.gov/medlineplus/ency/article/000357.htm (accessed February 3, 2005).

39. K. Klauer, "Adrenal Insufficiency and Adrenal Crisis," *Emedicine* (2004), http://www.emedicine.com/emerg/topic16.htm (accessed February 3, 2005).

40. C. Weaver, "Electrolyte Imbalance," *Cancer Consultants* (2004), http://patient.cancerconsultants.com/supportive_treatment.aspx?id=23137 (accessed February 3, 2005).

41. C. Beach, "Hypocalcemia," *Emedicine* (2004), http://www.emedicine.com/EMERG/topic271.htm (accessed February 5, 2005).

42. R. Hemphill, "Hypercalcemia," *Emedicine* (2005), http://www.emedicine.com/emerg/topic260.htm (accessed February 5, 2005).

43. I. Agha, "Hyperkalemia," *Medline Plus* (2004), http://www.nlm.nih.gov/medlineplus/ency/article/001179.htm (accessed September 28, 2004).

44. D. Garth, "Hypokalemia," *Emedicine* (2004), http://www.emedicine.com/emerg/topic273.htm (accessed February 5, 2005).

45. S. Stephanides and M. Wilson, "Hypernatremia," *Emedicine* (2004), http://www.emedicine.com/emerg/topic263.htm (accessed February 5, 2005).

46. M. El-Twal and R. Crausman, "Hyponatremia," *Emedicine* (2004), http://www.emedicine.com/med/topic1130.htm (accessed February 5, 2005).

47. P. Fall, "Hyponatremia and hypernatremia: A systematic approach to causes and their correction," *Postgraduate Medicine* 107, http://www.postgradmed.com/issues/2000/05_00/fall.htm (accessed September 28, 2006).

48. Mineral Resources International, "*Magnesium*" (2003), http://www.2pmltd.com/Mineral%20Resources/magnesium.html (accessed February 5, 2005).

49. L. Dube and J. Granry, "The Therapeutic Use of Magnesium in Anesthesiology, Intensive Care and Emergency Medicine: A Review," *Canadian Journal of Anesthesia* (2003), http://www.cja-jca.org/cgi/content/full/50/7/732 (accessed February 5, 2005).

50. World Federation of Societies of Anaesthesiologists, "*Pharmacology: Acid Base Balance*" (2001), http://www.nda.ox.ac.uk/wfsa/html/u13/u1312_03.htm (accessed February 3, 2005).

51. "Acid-Base Balance" (2005), http://www.merck.com/mrkshared/mmanual/section2/chapter12/12g.jsp (accessed February 3, 2005).

52. K. Doerschug, K. Kline, J. Hornick, et al., "Basic Concepts: Acid-Base Disturbances," *Virtual Hospital* (1994), http://www.vh.org/adult/provider/internalmedicine/abg/BasicConcepts3.html (accessed February 3, 2005).

53. A. Edgren, "Metabolic Acidosis," *Health A to Z, Gale Encyclopedia of Medicine* (2002), http://www.healthatoz.com/healthatoz/Atoz/ency/metabolic_acidosis.jsp (accessed February 5, 2005).

54. A. Edgren, "Respiratory Alkalosis," *Health A to Z, Gale Encyclopedia of Medicine* (2002), http://www.healthatoz.com/healthatoz/Atoz/ency/respiratory_alkalosis.jsp (accessed February 5, 2005).

55. T. Kiriakopoulos, "Consciousness, Decreased," *Medline Plus* (2004), http://www.nlm.nih.gov/medlineplus/ency/article/003202.htm (accessed February 3, 2005).

56. V. Peragallo-Dittko, "Diabetes: Acute Complications," *RN* 58(8) (Montvale, NJ: Medical Economics, 1995).

57. A. Kitabchi and B. Wall, "Management of Diabetic Ketoacidosis," *American Family Physician* 60(2) (Kansas City, MO: American Family Physician, 1999).

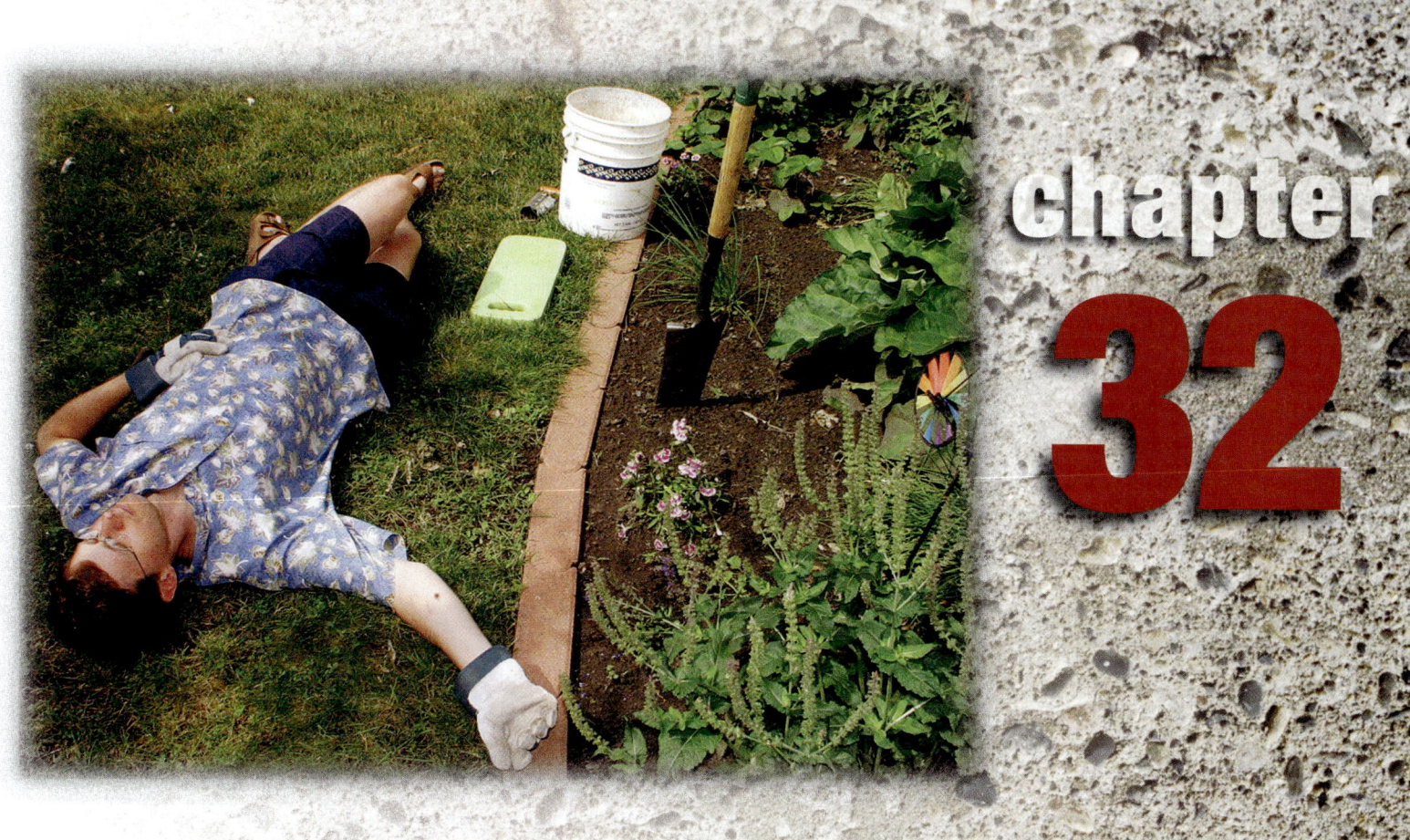

Allergies and Anaphylaxis

" 'Tis the maddest trick a man can ever play in his whole life, to let his breath sneak out of his body without any more ado, and without so much as a rap o'er the pate, or a kick of the guts; to go out like the snuff of a farthing candle, and die merely of the mulligrubs, or the sullens."

—Miguel De Cervantes (1547–1616)

Need to Know

▶ Allergic reactions have a wide range of severity and also a wide range in the speed with which the problem progresses.

▶ Patients can deteriorate very quickly and should be monitored closely even if symptoms appear mild when you arrive on the scene. Minor itching and skin rashes can rapidly progress to difficulty breathing and swelling of the airway.

▶ Any swelling of the upper airway structures should be considered life-threatening and should be treated immediately with either epinephrine or an antihistamine such as diphenhydramine.

▶ A person may be exposed to a substance once or many times before developing a sensitivity to it. The number of exposures is not as important as recognizing the signs and symptoms of a reaction and appropriately treating it.

▶ Exposure to commonly known allergens, such as insect bites and stings, certain foods, and medications are important clues that an allergic reaction may be occurring.

▶ Profound, life-threatening hypotension as a result of vasodilation can occur with anaphylaxis, with or without airway compromise.

▶ Sick	▶ Not Yet Sick
• The patient with a fast moving reaction to the exposure to an allergen that includes systemic (full body) involvement or has facial edema or dyspnea.	• Ask about exposure to known allergens such as medication, food, insect, and latex.
• If the patient faints and is hypotensive following the allergen exposure.	• Ask if the throat is tightening or there are symptoms of upper airway obstruction.
• Administer epinephrine 0.3 mg IM/SC or use an autoinjector.	• Patient has localized dermatologic reaction to allergens and has *no evidence* of systemic reactions like full body hives, dyspnea, lightheadedness, dizziness, or facial edema.
• Administer diphenhydramine 25–50 mg to prevent anaphylaxis or after use of epinephrine to help prevent recurrence of anaphylaxis.	• Look for signs of dyspnea, hypoxia, and hypotension.
• With facial and tongue swelling, ask about ACE inhibitor use because this can promote the formation of angioedema.	

Introduction

Allergic reactions are bothersome at a minimum and life-threatening at their worst. Allergic reactions are a hypersensitive immune response to exposure to a foreign substance.[1] The severity of the reaction can vary greatly from one person to the next and depends on the type of substance involved and the route, duration, and amount of exposure, as well as history of prior exposure to the inciting allergen. Antibiotics, latex, foods, and insect bites or stings are some of most common causes of allergic reactions.[2,3] DOT 5-5.1

The problem for the paramedic is that the transition between these two states (bothersome versus life-threatening) is not always predictable. For one thing, the transition does not always take place. For another, the speed with which it takes place varies from person to person. For example, three people are stung on the arm at the same time by the same type of bee. One patient experiences pain, localized swelling, and itching. A second patient experiences hives over his entire body,

and his skin is hot and itchy. A third patient appears to faint, and 30 seconds later her face and lips quickly swell and she cannot breathe. While all three are obviously allergic and reacting to the sting, patient number three is having an obvious anaphylactic reaction as well. Patient number two is the one who is difficult to assess; is he "on his way to anaphylaxis" or is he just having a "bad" allergic reaction? This makes determining the difference between a sick and not-yet-sick patient difficult. DOT 5-5.2

Few medical problems compare to anaphylaxis in the need for the paramedic to clearly differentiate between the sick anaphylactic patient and the not yet sick allergic patient. This medical illness could actually be said to have a category between the two called "quickly transitioning" from not yet sick to sick. Local protocol may even authorize administration of epinephrine or an antihistamine such as diphenhydramine to prevent the continued development of anaphylaxis in a patient with significant signs and symptoms of allergic reaction, even without signs of anaphylaxis.

This chapter will discuss the difference between allergies and anaphylaxis and will discuss assessment and management strategies for each group of patients. Skill Sheet 50: Intramuscular Drug Administration (and Step-by-Step 50), Skill Sheet 52: Nebulized Drug Administration (and Step-by-Step 52), Skill Sheet 53: Subcutaneous Drug Administration (and Step-by-Step 53), and Skill Sheet 59: Autoinjector Drug Administration Device support this chapter.

Pathophysiology of Allergy and Anaphylaxis

Under normal circumstances, the immune system functions as an automatic self-defense mechanism. It identifies and neutralizes harmful foreign substances that threaten the body. In the case of allergic reactions, however, a substance that is normally identified as harmless is instead identified as a potential threat by the body's immune system, and the reaction begins. When a person is exposed to a substance the body recognizes as a threat, the immune system can react vigorously and can set in motion a potentially deadly chain of events.[4,5]

The term *allergy* was first used in 1906 by the pediatrician Clemens von Pirquet, when he observed two patterns of reaction in his patients: immunity and allergy. **Immunity,** the older concept, resulted in protection for the patient from foreign invaders. **Allergy,** which he noted was an "altered reactivity," was deemed harmful to the patient.[6] The substance that caused the allergic reaction was later named the **allergen.** Traditionally, the terms **anaphylaxis** and **anaphylactic shock** have been reserved for immediate severe systemic reactions (Box 32-1).[3–7] DOT 5-5.1, 5-5.2

Allergies are categorized according to the anatomical location where the signs and symptoms of the reaction occur:

- Atopic dermatitis: itching and raised hives (urticaria), redness, and swelling of the skin.
- Atopic rhinitis: nasal passages are irritated, causing sneezing, itching, runny nose, and itchy, watery eyes.
- Atopic asthma: lungs are irritated, causing coughing, wheezing, or dyspnea.
- Food allergies: nausea, vomiting, diarrhea, or upset stomach in gastrointestinal system.
- Anaphylaxis: systemic reaction, causing airway swelling or massive vasodilation and hypotension.[6]

Working in the Gray Zone

Are the Terms *Anaphylaxis* and *Allergic Reaction* the Same?

Traditionally, the term *anaphylaxis* has been reserved for the most severe systemic and life-threatening reactions, which makes it different from *allergic reaction.* Some researchers differentiated anaphylaxis from a less severe reaction mediated by the antibody immunoglobulin E (IgE).[8] The term **anaphylactoid reaction** was, for a time, used by physicians and other hospital clinicians to describe the reaction that was IgE-mediated. Since these are clinically indistinguishable on gross examination, both terms, anaphylactic and anaphylactoid reaction, are used interchangeably.[2]

It may be helpful to think of allergic reactions and the term "anaphylaxis" as a continuum in degrees of severity.[3] Mild reactions are usually *localized* to a specific part of the body or organ. More severe reactions affecting more than one organ are considered **systemic.**[5] DOT 5-5.14

BOX 32-1 Do You React the *First* Time You Are Exposed?

One way to remember the pathophysiology of allergic reactions is to look back on how it was discovered. In 1902, Charles R. Ricket and Paul Jules Portier observed that fatal results would occur after the *second* administration of a particular protein to the dogs in the experiment. The dogs had no reaction to the first exposure of the protein; it was only after the second exposure that they reacted and died. They coined the term **anaphylaxis,** meaning *against or without protection.* One way to remember this, is by thinking of the opposite term **prophylaxis** which means *to protect.*[6,7,8]

Anaphylaxis is a true medical emergency that requires immediate recognition and intervention. Even the reaction appearing mild should be watched carefully. Patients can rapidly deteriorate into respiratory or cardiovascular compromise.[9] Primary treatment of the patient with anaphylaxis centers on maintenance of airway, breathing, and circulation. Epinephrine and diphenhydramine are indicated for patients showing signs and symptoms of airway and breathing compromise or signs of shock as the result of an allergic reaction.[10]

BOX 32-2   Common Causes of Anaphylaxis

Antibiotics

  Penicillin
  Cephalosporins
  Tetracyclines
  Nitrofurantoin
  Streptomycin
  Vancomycin

Foreign Proteins

  Latex
  Insulin
  Hymenoptera venom (honeybee, yellow jacket, wasp, hornet)
  Fire ant
  Kissing bug (triatoma) saliva
  Deerfly venom
  Rattlesnake venom

Modulators of Arachidonic Acid Metabolism

  Acetylsalicylic acid
  NSAIDs
  Benzoates (presumed)
  Tartrazine (possibly)

Therapeutic Agents

  Hydrocortisone
  Esters

  Amides
  Acetaminophen
  Egg-based vaccines: measles, mumps, rubella
  Whole blood
  Immunoglobulin
  Plasma
  Radiopaque contrast media
  Local anesthetics

Foods

  Milk
  Egg white
  Shellfish
  Nuts
  Bananas
  Chocolate
  Bisulfites
  Metabisulfites

Physical Factors

  Exercise
  Food-independent
  Food-dependent
  Food-specific

Epidemiology

Good statistics about the frequency and severity of allergic reactions are not available. While some report that allergic reactions are not commonly encountered in the prehospital setting, there is no consensus about the exact definition, classification, and reporting of allergic reactions.[2,3,9] Estimates of the numbers of anaphylactic cases presenting to North American emergency departments range from 10 to 20 per 100,000 people per year.[3] The most frequent causes triggering these events include exposure to antibiotics (specifically penicillin), hymenoptera stings (bees, hornets, wasps, and imported fire ants), and food.[2,5,11] Additionally, approximately 0.9% (or 9 in 1,000 persons) of patients who take aspirin will experience anaphylaxis.[5] DOT 5-5.3, 5-5.4, 5-5.11

  Severe reactions are more likely to be associated with older patients, insect venom, and medically induced (iatrogenic) causes.[9] Also, anaphylactic reactions after parenteral exposure (via injections or skin punctures such as bites or stings) are usually more immediate and severe than topical or oral exposures.[2]

  Patients in anaphylaxis who also have a history of asthma have a higher risk for poor outcome.[3]

Race, sex, and geography seem to have little impact on the rates or severity of anaphylaxis.[2] Exercise can also lead to anaphylaxis, but as many as half of these cases may have been related to food ingestion prior to exercise.[12,13] Box 32-2 lists some common causes of anaphylaxis.

Applied Anatomy and Physiology

The immune system is the body's security system against foreign agents. It may be helpful to think about immunity as a self-defense system, with various specialized defense teams, such as genetic and acquired immunity, in place to perform different protective functions. DOT 5-5.5

Genetic Immunity

Before birth the body takes an inventory of all the large molecules and proteins present. It then codes this information on the cells of the immune system, labeling these molecules as "self." The immune system is coded to consider these "friendly cells" and to "tolerate" and not harm them. This process is called **immunotolerance**. When the body encounters an unknown (not previously cataloged) substance, it mounts a defense against this "nonself" molecule that is presumed to be a hostile attacker. DOT 5-5.9

In addition to this cataloging, the body also inherits lists of known "enemies" and how to defend against them. This is called **genetic immunity.** For example, newborn babies develop antibodies against a number of common diseases as a result of their mother's prior exposure to disease.

> Just as height, eye, and hair color are inheritable traits, the tendency to develop allergic reactions is also an inherited characteristic.

Although you may have the genetic predisposition to develop allergies, you are not automatically allergic to specific allergens. Certain factors must be present for you to develop an allergic sensitivity:

- Inheritance of the necessary genes from your parents.
- Exposure to the enemy substance that you are genetically programmed to respond to.
- The extent and length of the exposure.

Acquired Immunity

In addition to genetically passing on immunity, the body can acquire immunity throughout its lifetime. It does so by being exposed to a disease or foreign substance naturally (such as contracting a disease or being exposed to an allergen) or by being artificially or deliberately exposed (such as vaccination). When the body is exposed for the first time to an unknown substance (an **antigen**), it will produce **antibodies** to attack it. During this defense, specialized memory cells have the job of recording and cataloging the method of defense used to rid the body of the invader. The next time the antigen invades the body, the immune system can respond more quickly.[1–7,14] It is when this response is overexaggerated that the person can have an anaphylactic reaction. DOT 5-5.10

Autoimmune Disorders

When the immune system malfunctions, it can overreact and turn against its own body's cells. It basically relabels "friendly" substances inside the organs as foreign, "nonself" cells and attacks them. This process is called **autoimmunity.** When this occurs, the patient may develop chronic diseases that have episodic flare-ups during times when the immune system is actively damaging body cells and tissues. Some examples of autoimmune disorders that are encountered in the prehospital setting include the following:

- Lupus
- Type I diabetes mellitus
- Graves disease
- Hemolytic anemia
- Multiple sclerosis

CONNECTIONS   Read more about these autoimmune disorders in Chapter 30: Neurology, Chapter 31: Endocrinology, Electrolytes and Acid/Base and Chapter 37: Hematology.

Immune System Activation

The First and Second Lines of Defense: Nonspecific Immunity

Our body's first and second lines of defense are through innate, nonspecific defensive measures called **species resistance.** These two lines of defense are in operation all of the time, independent of an allergic or anaphylactic situation. The first line of defense includes simple reflexes (such as coughing), mechanical barriers (such as the skin), and chemical barriers (such as tears or stomach acids). These barriers and secretions can help prevent or limit penetration and exposure or help the body shed the allergenic substance.

The second line of defense is an internal response that occurs once an allergen penetrates the body (Figure 32-1). Enemy antigenic molecules trigger the immune defense system for a nonspecific response during the second line of defense. The body recognizes these foreign cells and begins attacking back. Once it learns more about them, the third line of defense neutralizes any further threat they may pose.

Natural killer, or NK, cells are special lymphocytes that provide protection by secreting cytolytic (cell cutting) substances called perforins that lyse (cut) cell membranes. The NK cells destroy any infected body cells in an attempt to limit further spread of the antigen. NK cells also secrete chemicals that enhance the development of inflammation.

Increased circulation (via the inflammatory response) to the affected area helps bring more blood and phagocytic cells into the area to eat up and destroy the foreign substance.[1,15,16] The **phagocytes** are cells programmed to identify nonself cells, surround them, and eat them. Phagocytes operate as fluid is shifted from one body compartment to another. For example, they clean the lymph that is in the interstitial space before it passes into the blood stream. The white blood cells' neutrophils and monocytes are the most active phagocytic cells. They are attracted to the affected area (called **chemotaxis**) by the release of the chemicals from the cells killed by the NK cells. DOT 5-5.12

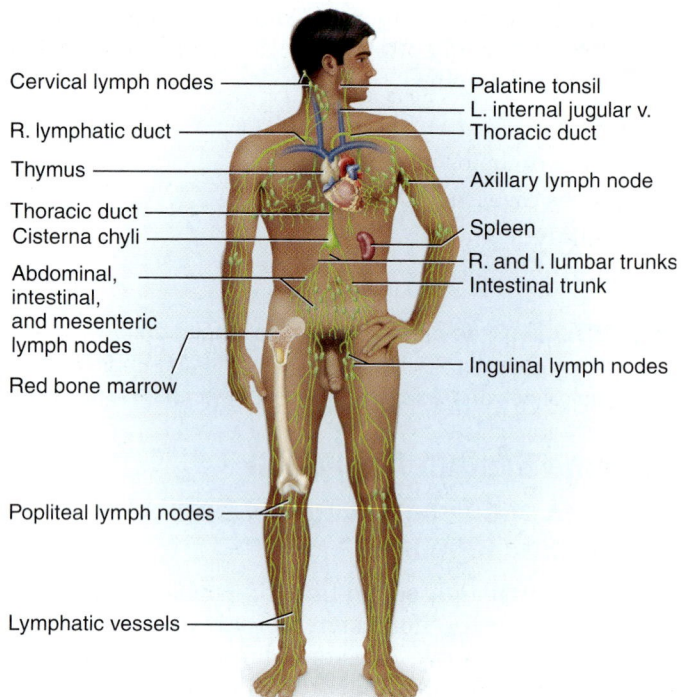

Cervical lymph nodes

R. lymphatic duct

Thymus

Thoracic duct

Cisterna chyli

Abdominal, intestinal, and mesenteric lymph nodes

Red bone marrow

Popliteal lymph nodes

Lymphatic vessels

Palatine tonsil

L. internal jugular v.

Thoracic duct

Axillary lymph node

Spleen

R. and l. lumbar trunks

Intestinal trunk

Inguinal lymph nodes

Figure 32-1 The lymphatic system and organs involved in the development of B cells and T cells.

CONNECTIONS Chapter 37: Hematology provides more detail on nonspecific immunity. Nonspecific immunity is always in operation, protecting the body.

The Third Line of Defense: Specific or Adaptive Immunity

Mild allergen exposures are ideally handled by our first or second lines of defense. If this fails, particular substances may require a third line of defense that is more specific to the substance (called **specific,** or **adaptive, immunity**). In response to an antigen entering the body, the immune system attempts to recognize the antigen from its list of known "hostiles" and dispatches specific **antibodies** (also called immunoglobulins), which mount the third line of defense.

In this third line of defense, the body calls up the Special Forces, which are specialized white blood cells

called **lymphocytes,** to fight the invader. This third line of defense is often at play during severe allergic reactions. Understanding it will improve the ability to recognize and treat allergic reactions.

Lymphocytes are created by **stem cells** in the bone marrow. Once formed, these special cells are sent off to circulate in the bloodstream throughout the body to mature. The lymphocytes that reach maturity in the thymus gland are called **T cells** (think of T for thymus). The others, thought to initially mature in the fetal liver and throughout the rest of life in the bone marrow, are called **B cells** (think of B for bone marrow) (see Figure 32-1).

T cells and B cells are the individual soldiers in the Special Forces third line of defense and play key roles in allergic reactions (see Table 32-1). T cells attack antigens one-on-one at the cellular level, so think of them as doing hand-to-hand combat against antigens in **cell-mediated immunity.** B cells are capable of organizing a massive, group response, using millions of antibodies (called **immunoglobulins**) in a **humoral immunity** response.

The immunoglobulins are manufactured by the B cells and are secreted into the blood. Within this category, there are five different classes of immunoglobulins—IgM, IgA, IgG, IgE, IgD—and each has a specific role in providing immunity (Table 32-2).

> Other than the brain, the immune system is the only other system that has a memory.

Once created in the marrow, B cells migrate to the lymph nodes, spleen, and other lymphoid structures where they complete development and are ready to respond to an antigen threat. The next stage of development occurs with activation. When an antigen enters the body, the B cell will bind to the antigen and undergo many cellular divisions (mitosis), producing both plasma cells and memory B cells. The many **plasma cells** produced from a single antigen-activated B cell can either be short- (a few days) or long-lived (months), producing and secreting 2,000 antibody molecules per second while they are alive.[17] The **memory B cells** do not secrete antibodies; their only job is to remember the antigen and the defensive measures required for future attacks. When stimulated a second time by a previously

TABLE 32-1 The Differences between T Cells and B Cells

T cells	B cells
Provides cell-mediated immunity	Provides humoral immunity
Mature in thymus gland	Mature possibly in bone marrow
Mount a cellular-mediated defense	Mount an antibody-mediated defense
Long-lived cells that split into new cells	New cells continuously created in bone marrow
Actually attack allergens, stimulate the development of more B cells, and trigger other T cells into action	Secrete immunoglobulin to fight allergen

TABLE 32-2 Immunoglobulins

Note: The letters for these immunoglobulins have been arranged in this table to spell the word "Imaged," which can be used as a memory aid for these antibodies: IgMAGED.

Antibody Name	Concentration and where it is most concentrated in the body	Role in Immunity
IgM	6% of all antibodies, found in plasma	Reacts with antigens occurring naturally on some RBC membranes following transfusions, activates compliment
IgA	13% of all antibodies, secreted by exocrine glands	Defends against bacteria and viruses
IgG	80% of all antibodies, found in plasma and tissue fluid	Defends against bacteria, viruses, and toxins, activates compliment
IgE	<1% of all antibodies, secreted by exocrine glands	Promotes inflammation and allergic reactions
IgD	<1% of all antibodies found on the surface of most B lymphocytes	Activates B cells to begin working

experienced antigen, these cells will respond by generating many new plasma cells, secreting large amounts of antibodies.

Pathophysiology

The previous section reviews what should normally happen when the immune system functions ideally. During an allergic reaction, the body labels an antigen as an enemy, but for some unknown reason, the reaction is overblown and excessive. Instead of simply destroying the allergen and returning the body to homeostatic balance, the body sets into motion a process that destroys normal cells as well. DOT 5-5.7, 5-5.17

Nice to Know

HIV and AIDS

When T cells are "activated for combat," they divide themselves into several subgroups. One of these subgroups is called a "helper T-cell." This helper T cell enhances the immune response by activating the creation of more B cells and the division of more T cells. Human immunodeficiency virus (HIV) attacks helper T cells. Without these helper T cells, the immune system is crippled and cannot defend itself. The disease syndrome that can result from the HIV virus is called acquired immunodeficiency syndrome or AIDS. To read more about AIDS, see Chapter 33: Infectious and Communicable Diseases.

More specifically, when the allergen is detected, B cells are dispatched and immediately activate millions of IgE antibodies. The IgE antibodies bind with **mast cells** (primarily in target organs) and **basophils** (primarily in the blood stream), resulting in the massive release of **histamine, prostaglandin D,** and **leukotrienes** (Figure 32-2). These substances cause dilation of blood vessels, increased vascular permeability (which causes edema), bronchospasm, increased mucus production, and contraction of the smooth muscle in the intestinal tract. This cascade of events can lead to devastating respiratory failure or cardiovascular collapse.

Specific Allergens

Aeroallergens

Aeroallergens are airborne proteins and glycoproteins from a variety of sources, including pollinating trees and grasses, mold spores, animal dander (cat, dog, and rodent), and particulates produced by dust mites and cockroaches. It has been shown that airborne mouse allergen concentrations in as many as a quarter of inner-city homes are sufficiently high to elicit symptoms in sensitized individuals.[11] Whereas indoor allergens are more closely associated with the development of asthma, outdoor allergens appear more important in the development of allergic rhinitis.[4] DOT5-5.8

Food Allergens

Food allergies can be life-threatening and result in a significant reduction of quality of life.[18] Even though thousands of different foods are available and consumed,

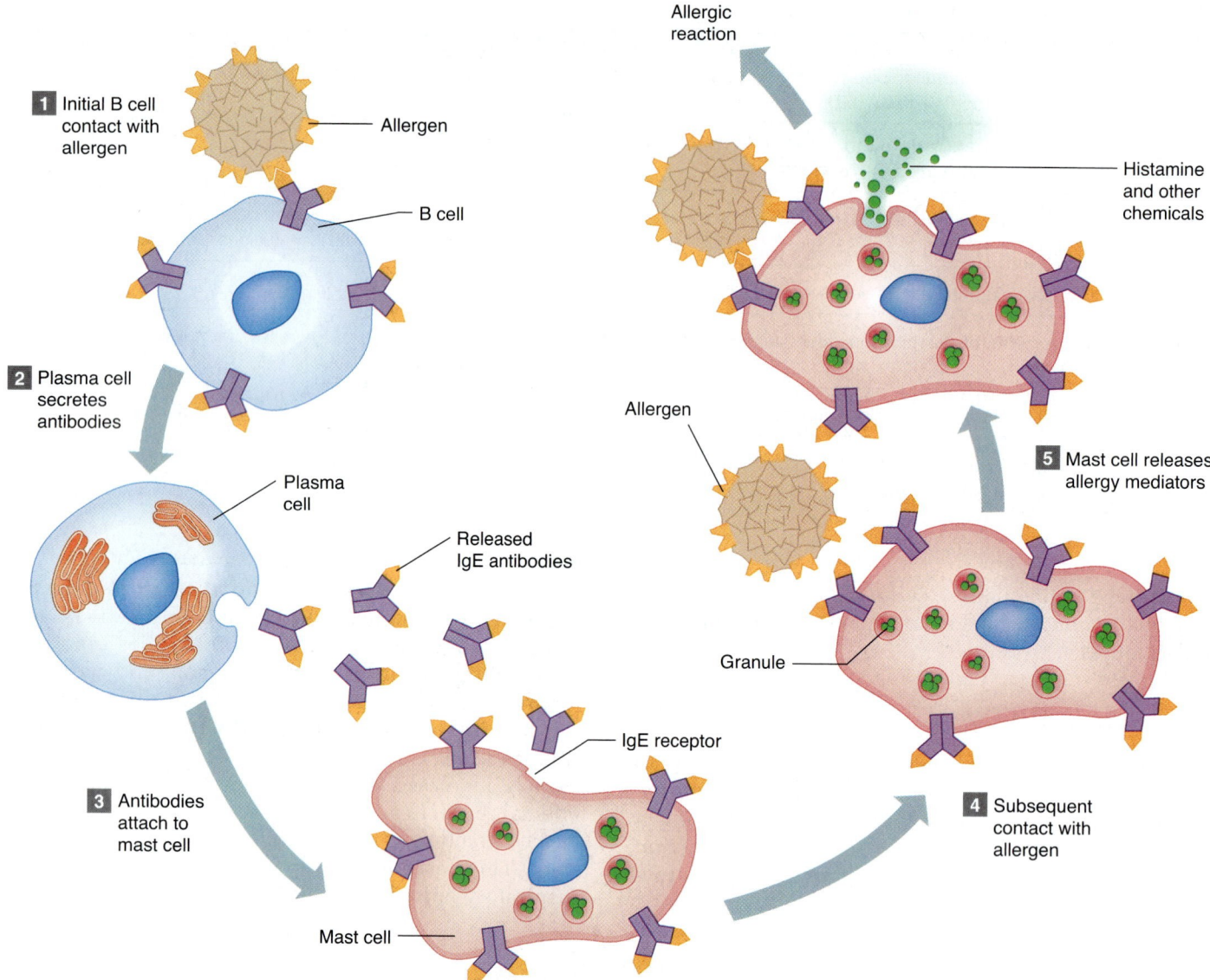

Figure 32-2   Immediate-reaction allergy. Part 1 shows B cells activated when they contact an allergen. Part 2 shows an activated B cell differentiating further into an antibody-secreting plasma cell. Part 3 shows antibodies attaching to mast cells. Part 4 shows that when allergens are encountered, they combine with the antibodies on the mast cells. Part 5 shows the mast cells releasing allergy mediators which cause the symptoms of the allergy attack.

only a very small number of these foods are responsible for food allergies. These allergies can be subdivided into childhood and adult allergies. The most common food allergies in childhood are the result of milk, eggs, peanuts, soy, and wheat. Food-related allergies are more common in children less than two years of age. As they grow older, these allergies sometimes resolve or go away without further problems. Adult food allergies usually involve peanuts, tree nuts, fish, and shellfish. Reactions to food allergies can be fatal. The most frequently observed severe food reactions are the result of peanut allergies.[6]

Latex Allergens

In the last few years, a new antigen has been identified that is linked to immediate hypersensitivity reactions to latex rubber. This allergy is most commonly seen in healthcare workers, rubber industry workers, and patients who underwent multiple surgical procedures in early infancy.[20,21] However, there have been documented cases of latex allergies in infants younger than one year with no physical abnormalities or previous operations.[22] Symptoms include contact urticaria, asthma, rhinoconjunctivitis (red, itchy, and watery nose and eyes), and mucosal swelling (Figure 32-3). Severe reactions and even death have occurred as the result of exposure of the rectal mucosa to latex, especially in children with spina bifida.[19]

Street Secrets

Watch Out for Peanut Allergies!

A recent case report identified a cross-reaction between persons allergic to peanuts and lupin flour. Lupin flour is used in Europe and other countries as a replacement for soy flour. Persons with known allergies to peanuts need to avoid foods containing lupin flour.[19] There is also concern for individuals with peanut or soy allergies for receiving the parasympatholytic blocking drug ipratoprium (Atrovent™), and its use is contraindicated for these patients. The combination of ipratoprium with albuterol (called a DuoNeb) is often used to try to reverse bronchoconstriction during an allergic reaction; however, it should not be used in these patients.

It has also been shown that persons with allergies to certain fruits, such as banana, avocado, kiwi, and chestnuts, develop clinical symptoms following contact with latex.[23] It is believed that this condition is the result of IgE being reactive to enzymes present in both the fruits and nuts.[9] Latex allergies had been increasing but appear to have stabilized, perhaps due to increased awareness and decreased use of latex in medical products.[24]

Medication Reactions

Allergic reactions to drugs are a common medical emergency. Most drugs are low-molecular weight compounds that attach to proteins. Once attached to the protein, the drugs generate an allergic response (penicillin is a classic example). The drug is often administered parenterally, which is twice as likely to produce a rapid and fatal reaction.[2] Cephalosporin antibiotic drugs are similar to penicillin in chemical structure and may also cause a reaction in penicillin-allergic individuals. It is estimated that 5–16% of patients that are allergic to penicillin will have a cross-reaction with cephalosporins.[5] Other agents, such as quaternary ammonium compounds (neuromuscular blocking agents) and sulfonamides (antibiotics) are also common stimuli for allergic reactions.[9]

Insect Venom Allergens

Insect stings that cause allergic reactions belong to the order *Hymenoptera*. This order includes three families of insects: Apidae (honeybees), Formicidae (fire ants), and Vespidae (wasps, yellow jackets, and hornets).[2] These stings can cause a wide range of reactions, from a simple rash to a severe anaphylactic reaction.[25]

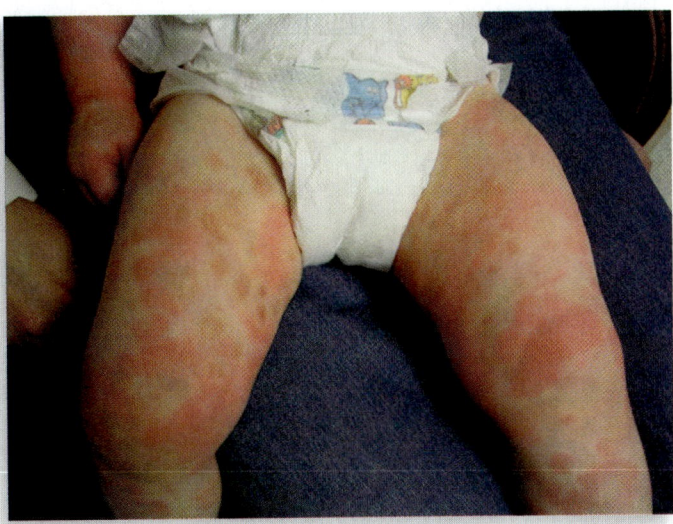

Figure 32-3 Urticaria.

The venom in each of these types of insects is made of similar proteins, but being allergic to one insect's sting does not necessarily mean that a person will have the same reaction to a different member of the order. For example, being allergic to honeybees may or may not mean that you are also allergic to yellow jackets. Being sensitive to fire ants, however, is likely to cause the same reaction (*cross-reaction*) as a yellow jacket.[9]

CONNECTIONS Chapter 38: Enviromental Conditions has more information on bites and stings.

Street Secrets

Maintain a high index of suspicion. Even though reactions are more likely to be severe in patients who have been previously stung, patients may develop a severe reaction any time they are exposed to the venom.[2,5]

The Onset of Allergic Reaction Symptoms

The patient with an allergic reaction will first notice a sensation of warmth or tingling of the face, mouth, or upper chest or at the site of the exposure. Pruritus (itching) is the most common symptom, along with generalized flushing and urticaria (Figure 32-4). This exposure can lead to respiratory distress, cough, tightness of the chest, dyspnea, and wheezing. Hypotension may be observed, with the patient complaining of light-headedness and syncope. Gastrointestinal manifestations will follow. The patient may complain of cramps and abdominal pain, nausea, vomiting, and diarrhea. The patient may also have a sense of impending doom. Table 32-3 describes a three-stage grading system for allergic reactions.[19]

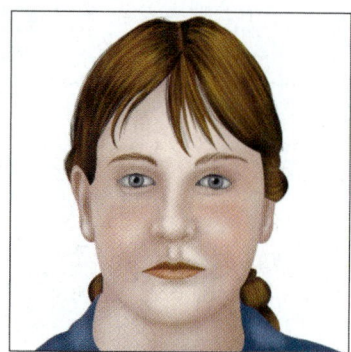

Figure 32-4 Flushed face from vasodilation.

Progressing from an Allergic Reaction to Anaphylaxis

One study reported the median time from exposure to cardiac arrest was five minutes for medications, 15 minutes for insect venom, and 30 minutes for food.[26] However, cases have been reported of delays of clinical signs and symptoms for several hours.

In general, the more rapid the onset of symptoms following exposure, the more severe the reaction.[3]

Biphasic or **multiphasic anaphylaxis** occurs when symptoms reoccur after a previously resolved allergic reaction.[25] This patient will be exposed to an antigen, will display some of the signs and symptoms of anaphylaxis, and, with proper treatment, all symptomatic conditions will resolve. However, within 1 to 72 hours

following complete resolution of symptoms, a small percentage of patients will develop a second anaphylactic reaction without being re-exposed to the offending antigen. **Recurrent** or **multiphasic anaphylaxis** has been estimated to affect 3–20% of patients with anaphylaxis.[27] The threat of biphasic or multiphasic reactions is a strong reason to perform transport to the hospital for every allergic reaction, even for patients with seemingly mild symptoms at the time. DOT 5-5.13

Angioedema

Angioedema is a rare and specific form of localized allergic reaction that is usually of short duration and frequently resolves itself.[2,5,28] Angioedema usually involves swelling of the lips, tongue, oral cavity, and upper

Nice to Know

Bee Stings

If anaphylaxis is the result of honeybee stings, remember that the stinger has a barb on the end that keeps the stinger in the patient even after the insect is gone. The poison sac will continue to pump bee venom into the patient until it is removed or the venom sac is empty. Remove the stinger and venom sac using the flat surface of a credit card or other similar object. Tweezers should be avoided because they will only inject more venom into the patient.

TABLE 32-3 Three-Stage Grading System for Allergic Reactions

Reaction	Description	Signs and symptoms
Mild reaction	The patient is **NOT YET SICK** but may progress **to that state.** Skin and subcutaneous tissues are the only parts involved.	Generalized erythema Urticaria Periorbital edema or angioedema
Moderate reaction	The patient is in transition between **NOT YET SICK and SICK.** Signs and symptoms suggest respiratory, cardiovascular, or gastrointestinal involvement	Dyspnea Stridor Wheezing Nausea Vomiting Dizziness (presyncope) Diaphoresis Chest or throat tightness Abdominal pain
Severe reaction (anaphylaxis)	The patient is **SICK.** Signs include hypoxia, airway compromise, hypotension, and neurologic compromise	Cyanosis $SpO_2 < 93\%$ at any stage (at sea level) Hypotension (SBP < 90 mmHg in adults) Confusion Collapse Loss of consciousness Incontinence

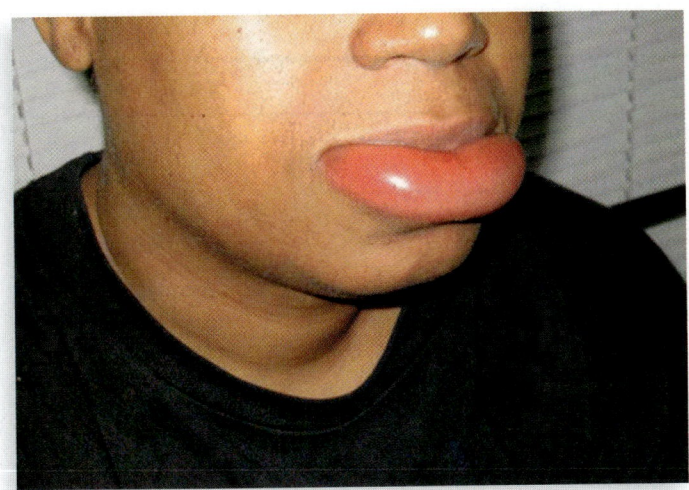

Figure 32-5   Angioedema as a result of a reaction to an ACE inhibitor medications.

airway (Figure 32-5). The swelling is nonpitting and has a tendency to manifest itself in areas where the skin is not taut (like the face). There are two main causes for the reaction. Typically, it is an allergic reaction to angiotensin converting enzyme (ACE) inhibitor medications. This occurs in 0.1–0.7% of people taking ACE inhibitor medications.[2] Nonsteroidal antiinflammatory (NSAID) medications may also cause angioedema.[28] Angioedema from this type of allergic reaction is not mediated by IgE and will usually not respond to standard treatments such as epinephrine and antihistamines.

The second main cause of angioedema is hereditary. In this second type, the body produces large amounts of tissue bradykinin.[28] Attacks can recur and can last a few hours to a few days.[2]

The main concern with angioedema is potential compromise of the airway. Fortunately, most cases resolve themselves before aggressive airway maneuvers are needed. Nevertheless, careful monitoring of the airway is the mainstay of treatment.[2]

Scene Size-Up

When responding to a call for a known allergic reaction, pay close attention to dispatch and prearrival information to determine potential hazards. The 9-1-1 operator and dispatcher may be able to give you valuable information about the cause of the reaction and the potential for dangerous conditions at the scene. Exposure to the source of the allergic reaction should be considered before entering the scene, if possible. DOT 5-5.8, 5-5.13, 5-5.15, 5-5.16

Once on the scene, be aware of changing conditions and recognize hazards. While ingestion or injection of antibiotics or other medication or a food allergy will have no effect on you and your crew, airborne chemicals (liquids or powders) and swarms of bees can be dangerous.

Minimizing scene time will shorten your exposure to danger and benefit a sick patient by providing a rapid transport to the hospital. Personal protective equipment (PPE) is another important step in protecting yourself. If a hazmat situation is anticipated, be sure the appropriate team is alerted to respond for patient decontamination. Ideally, the patient will be moved to a safe location away from the exposure.

CONNECTIONS   Review responses to incidents involving hazardous materials in Chapter 53: Hazardous materials incidents.

Primary Survey

In a severe anaphylactic reaction, the patient will present with labored breathing, bronchospasm, tachycardia, and hypotension or worse, be dead upon your arrival. If the patient is without vital signs, provide resuscitation following the standard algorithms for the management of cardiac arrest.

CONNECTIONS   Chapter 29: Cardiology discusses the various algorithms for cardiac arrest situations.

Labored breathing, bronchospasm, tachycardia, or hypotension indicate impending collapse of the circulatory system. Rapid intervention includes support for airway, breathing, and circulation.[2] The mainstay of prehospital care for severe anaphylaxis is epinephrine (See Drug Boxes 32-1 and 32-2).[2,3,5] Administer 0.3 mg epinephrine IM or SC as soon as possible, followed by the administration of diphenhydramine or other approved antihistamine. DOT5-5.18

Airway and Oxygenation

Examine the airway closely for signs of swelling. Early intervention is the key to assuring that the airway will remain open. Place the patient in a position of comfort, and protect the airway. High concentration oxygen via a non-rebreather mask should be started immediately. Early administration of epinephrine and diphenhydramine helps reverse swelling and may preempt the need for more aggressive airway maneuvers.[3] If swelling is impeding the airway, the patient may require airway support.

Oxygen saturation (SpO_2) should be maintained above 95%, with supplemental oxygen delivered by nasal cannula or mask as necessary.[2] The use of inhaled or nebulized bronchodilators is appropriate for the patient who does not initially respond well to first-line medications such as injectable epinephrine.

If the patient is apneic or the rate and quality of respiration are insufficient, initiate ventilatory support using a bag–mask with supplemental oxygen. Placement of oropharyngeal and nasopharyngeal airways should be avoided as they may generate laryngospasm.

If the above measures are not working, endotracheal intubation (ETI) may be needed. Have various sizes of endotracheal tubes are available since the glottic opening

Drug Box 32-1   Epinephrine[29]

Indications	Severe allergic reaction
Adult Dose	0.3–0.5 mg IM/SC (0.3–0.5 mL of a 1:1000 solution); may be repeated two times, every 5 to 10 minutes. DO NOT ADMINISTER 1:1000 VIA THE IV ROUTE.
Contraindications	There are no absolute contraindications to the use of epinephrine in a life-threatening situation.
Mechanism of Action	Sympathomimetic: Stimulates the sympathetic systems alpha and beta adrenergic receptors.
Precautions	Adverse effects include cardiac ischemia and dysrhythmias, but the benefits in anaphylaxis outweigh risks.

Drug Box 32-2   Diphenhydramine (Benadryl®)[29]

Indications	Allergic reactions, urticaria
Dose	25–50 mg PO/IM/IV
Contraindications	Nursing mothers, newborns, or premature infants
Mechanism of Action	Competitively binds with H1 histamine receptors, blocking their effects locally and systemically
Precautions	Asthma, elderly

may be smaller than expected because of swelling. If indicated, ETI should be performed early, before swelling completely obstructs the view of the larynx and passing the tube becomes more difficult.[2] A gum elastic bougie or Flex Guide™ may be helpful as a guide to insert the tube. Needle or surgical cricothyrotomy may become necessary if initial efforts to secure the airway fail.[30] These procedures are a last resort and are complicated considerably by the edema. Landmarks may be hard to identify and penetrate. The need to perform a cricothyrotomy correlates with poor outcomes for the patient.[31,32] DOT 5-5.18

Circulation

Keep a close watch on your patient for circulatory collapse. Due to the release of histamines, your patient may develop third-space fluid shift. When this occurs, the blood vessels have dilated, and fluid is leaking from the circulatory system into the interstitial tissues. The result is a state of low circulating blood volume (hypovolemia), even though the patient has not lost any fluid from internal or external bleeding. This will leave the patient hypovolemic and hypotensive. Initiate a large-bore IV as soon as possible with a crystalloid solution such as lactated Ringer's or normal saline. If there is time, placement of a second IV line will be appropriate. Maintain the blood pressure above 90–100 mmHg.[2,5] DOT 5-5.19

Commonly observed dysrhythmias include sinus tachycardia, premature atrial contractions, premature ventricular contractions, nodal dysrhythmias, and atrial fibrillation. Other ECG changes may include nonspecific and ischemic ST wave changes and intraventricular conduction changes.[5]

Working in the Gray Zone

Should First Responders and EMT-Basics Carry Epinephrine Auto-Injectors?

If a patient can carry and self-administer the medication, why shouldn't an EMT-basic? There are significant variations in state law or local protocol regarding the use of epinephrine by the basic life support providers: emergency medical responders and EMTs. There is no prehospital research to support the use of this drug by basic level providers.[3]

In 2002 the National Association of EMS Physicians published a position paper in support of this practice, provided adequate education is provided to the BLS provider and there are adequate medical control measures (specifically citing the need for strict indirect oversight) in place to guide the BLS provider.[33] This document, and their other position papers, may be accessed directly from the NAEMSP website at http://www.naemsp.org/.

Secondary Survey

Allergic reactions and anaphylaxis affect the cutaneous, respiratory, cardiovascular, and gastrointestinal systems. Signs and symptoms of these reactions are summarized in Table 32-4. Manifestations that may result in death are highlighted in yellow. DOT 5-5.13, 5-5.15, 5-5.16, 5-5.18

TABLE 32-4   **Clinical Manifestations of Allergic Reactions and Anaphylaxis**

Organ system	Reaction	Symptoms	Signs	Pathophysiology
Respiratory tract				
Upper	Rhinitis	Nasal congestion	Nasal mucosal edema	Increased vascular permeability
		Nasal itching	Rhinorrhea	Vasodilation
		Sneezing		Stimulation of nerve endings
	Laryngeal edema	Dyspnea	Laryngeal stridor	As above, plus increased exocrine gland secretions
		Hoarseness and tightness in the throat	Supraglottic and glottic edema	
		Hypersalivation		
Lower	Bronchospasm	Cough	Cough	As above, plus bronchiole smooth muscle contraction
		Wheezing	Wheeze, rhonchi	
		Dyspnea	Respiratory distress	
			Cyanosis	
Cardiovascular system	Circulatory collapse	Light-headedness	Tachycardia	Increased vascular permeability
		Generalized weakness	Hypotension	Vasodilation
				Loss of vasomotor tone
				Increased venous capacitance
		Syncope	Shock	
		Ischemic chest pain		
	Dysrhythmias	As above, plus palpitations	Tachycardia	Decreased cardiac output
			Nonspecific and ischemic ST-T wave changes	Decreased mediator-induced myocardial suppression
			Decreased vascular return affects R ventricle performance	Decreased effective plasma volume
			Premature atrial and ventricular contractions	Decreased preload
			Nodal rhythm	Decreased afterload
			Atrial fibrillation	Hypoxia and ischemia
				Dysrhythmias
				Iatrogenic effects of drugs used in treatment
				Preexisting heart disease
	Cardiac arrest		Pulseless	
			Ventricular fibrillation	
			Asystole	

(continued)

TABLE 32-4 (*continued*)

Organ system	Reaction	Symptoms	Signs	Pathophysiology
Skin	Urticaria	Pruritus	Urticaria	Increased vascular permeability
		Tingling and warmth	Diffuse erythema	Vasodilation
		Flushing		
		Hives		
	Angioedema (when it involves the airway)	Nonpruritic extremity, periorbital, and perioral swelling	Nonpitting edema, frequently asymmetrical	Increased vascular permeability
				Vasodilation
Eye	Conjunctivitis	Ocular itching	Conjunctival inflammation	Stimulation of nerve endings
		Increased lacrimation		
		Red eye		
Gastrointestinal tract		Dysphagia	Nonspecific	Increased mucus secretions
		Cramping, abdominal pain		Gastrointestinal smooth muscle contraction
		Nausea and vomiting		
		Diarrhea (rarely bloody)		
		Overwhelming urge to void urine or have a bowel movement		
Central nervous system		Apprehension	Anxiety	Secondary to cerebral hypoxia and hypoperfusion
		Sense of impending doom	Seizures (rarely)	Vasodilation
		Headache	Coma (late)	
		Confusion		
Hematologic	Fibrinolysis and disseminated intravascular coagulation	Abnormal bleeding and bruising	Mucous membrane bleeding, disseminated intravascular coagulation	Mediator recruitment and activation
Genitourinary		Pelvic pain	Increased uterine tone	Uterine smooth muscle contraction
		Vaginal bleeding	Vaginal bleeding	
		Urinary incontinence	Urinary incontinence	Bladder smooth muscle contraction

Pharmacological Intervention for Allergic Reactions

Common medications used to treat allergic reactions have already been discussed. This section will discuss a wider range of medications that may be useful in treating these patients. Patients with anaphylaxis are in need of immediate pharmacological intervention. The first drug to choose for patients with airway compromise is always oxygen. Administer high-concentration oxygen by an appropriate device.

DOT 5-5.16

Epinephrine

Epinephrine, with its combined alpha and beta adrenergic agonist actions, is the first drug to use for the treatment of severe anaphylaxis (see Drug Box 32-1 page 800). The alpha agonist effect increases peripheral vascular resistance. This will reverse peripheral vasodilation, vascular permeability, and systemic hypotension. The beta agonist effects will cause bronchodilation and increase cardiac contractile force. Keep in mind that this combined alpha and beta agonist effect can also result in elevated heart rates (chronotropy), stronger myocardial contractions (inotropy), and hypertension. All three can increase myocardial oxygen demand. Increased oxygen demand can result in tachycardia and myocardial ischemia or infarction. Caution should be used with administration of epinephrine in the elderly and in those patients with known coronary artery disease or pregnant patients.[5] The benefits of administering epinephrine in a severe allergic reaction typically outweigh the dangers.

When epinephrine is indicated for a severe reaction, the fastest route of medication administration should be chosen. Administer 0.3 mg epinephrine 1:1000 intramuscularly (IM) in the thigh.[34] Subcutaneous (SC) epinephrine is also effective and acceptable. Some studies have shown that SC rates of absorption are slower and less reliable than IM routes.[3,34] The standard dose for adults is 0.3 to 0.5 mg IM/SC; pediatric dose is 0.01 mg/kg IM/SC to a maximum of 0.5 ml of 1:1000 solution (0.5 mg).[35]

> Never administer the 1:1000 concentration via the IV route in an adult.

Epinephrine at a concentration of 1:10,000 may be administered intravenously (IV) for patients in severe shock.[36] The rationale behind this route is that, in extreme cases of shock, peripheral circulation may be so impaired that direct IV access is the only way to get the drug to the heart quickly for circulation throughout the body. The dose for this route of administration varies according to different sources, so you should check your local protocol and medical director preference. Intravenous administration of epinephrine is associated with significant complications including dysrhythmias, myocardial ischemia, and myocardial infarction. Continuous cardiac monitoring is recommended, so the administration may be stopped at the first sign of a cardiac dysrhythmia. There are no prehospital studies comparing IM or SC administration to IV administration.

Nebulized Beta Agonists

If bronchospasm is present during an allergic reaction, a beta selective bronchodilator should be administered to the patient.[5,39] Although numerous beta agonists can be used, albuterol (Proventil and Ventolin®) is the most common (see Drug Box 32-3).[39] In cases of severe bronchospasm, anticholinergic therapy may be used simultaneously with a bronchodialator. Ipratropium bromide (Atrovent) can be used for this purpose. In patients that are intubated, a nebulizer may be attached for ET administration.

Antihistamines

Antihistamines are especially helpful in counteracting allergic reactions. These medications act by competitively binding with either H_1 histamine receptors or H_2 histamine receptors and blocking their effects.[37] H_1 antagonists (such as diphenhydramine or Benadryl®) are especially useful for reversing capillary permeability (responsible for swelling), itching, and some smooth muscle contraction (see Drug Box 32-2, page 800). They are also central nervous system (CNS) depressants and cause sedation. In certain people and with certain doses, the CNS effects can be just the opposite and can cause excitation. H_1 blockers are not as effective as epinephrine or beta-agonists in reversing bronchospasm or systemic hypotension because these conditions are thought to be caused by other mediators, such as leukotrienes.[37]

Diphenhydramine and promethazine are both H_1 blockers and are used for several other conditions. Since they are effective in inhibiting muscarinic receptors, these medications have an anticholinergic effect. Over-the-counter and home uses include treatment of runny noses, coughs, insomnia, motion sickness, and parkinsonism. In the prehospital setting they are also used for motion sickness, nausea, and vomiting.

Drug Box 32-3   Albuterol

Indications	Bronchospasm
Adult Dose	2.5 mg diluted in 3 mL of normal saline nebulized; may be repeated every 15 minutes or given continuously as needed.
Contraindications	Hypersensitivity
Mechanism of Action	Stimulates Beta$_2$ adrenergic receptors
Precautions	Cardiac disease, elderly

CONNECTIONS See Chapter 34: Gastroenterology and Chapter 40: Behavioral and Psychiatric Disorders to read about dystonic reactions.

Diphenhydramine hydrochloride is the most commonly used H_1 antihistamine in the prehospital setting.[38] The standard dose is 25 to 50 mg IV or IM.[35] This medication needs to be administered slowly when given intravenously. The pediatric dose of diphenhydramine hydrochloride is 1 to 2 mg/kg up to a 50 mg maximum dose.

H_2 blockers (such as ranitidine and cimetidine) are effective in the reversal of shock when other first line treatments, epinephrine, fluids, and H_1 blockers, have not been sufficient, but are more commonly administered in the hospital setting. H_2 blockers are more commonly used to inhibit gastric acid secretion in gastrointestinal disorders.[37]

Corticosteroids

Corticosteroids (such as methylprednisolone or Solu-Medrol®) have a role in reversing bronchospasm and localized effects of allergic reactions.[5,39] They have an onset time of four to six hours following administration. Because of this, they have limited benefit in the field as an initial treatment consideration. Corticosteroids may also be effective in reducing the biphasic reaction of anaphylaxis.[39] One study showed that these are prescribed on discharge from the emergency department in 50% of the cases.[40] There is no evidence to suggest this treatment is effective or could be used in the prehospital setting.[3]

Vasopressors

Patients with persistent hypotension in spite of epinephrine and fluid resuscitation volumes may require vasopressors to maintain blood pressure. The intravenous use of dopamine, norepinephrine, and epinephrine can be used to support the severely hypotensive patient. Administration via infusion will support the blood pressure and cardiac output.[5]

Prevention

When it comes to prevention strategies, patient education is the key. If the situations that cause anaphylaxis can be avoided, then the consequences can be avoided. Simple things such as *not* going barefoot in the grass will eliminate the chance of stepping on a bee. Also, whenever spending time outdoors, avoid the use of aftershave, cologne, or perfume, and avoid wearing brightly colored clothing as both attract bees. Awareness of what is in foods being eaten and liquids being consumed is important. It is necessary for a susceptible individual to become an avid label reader. Knowing the ingredients in anything that is consumed will help prevent allergic reaction. DOT 5-5.6

Persons should wear or have in their possession information devices (such as a medical alert bracelet or wallet card) that indicate what they are allergic to. Items such as Medic-Alert® bracelets should be worn to alert others of their conditions if they are discovered unconscious. Patients can also begin their own care if they carry the epinephrine auto-injector called the EpiPen.® Parents and caregivers of children should also carry the EpiPen, Jr.® for younger susceptible patients.

Summary

Fortunately, the incidence of anaphylaxis and severe allergic reactions is low. However, when they do occur, action must be swift and direct because death can occur in minutes. Prehospital treatment of patients with anaphylaxis must begin as soon as the compromised airway and breathing are recognized.

The primary drug for treating anaphylaxis is epinephrine. Inhaled beta-agonists, such as albuterol or Proventil, can be used to treat bronchospasm and airway involvement. Antihistamines may also be useful in preventing a mild or moderate reaction from progressing to a more severe reaction if they can be used immediately after epinephrine in a severe reaction. In addition to respiratory compromise, circulatory compromise must be treated with intravenous fluids and vasopressors. Although the primary concern is airway protection, a patient can die from circulatory collapse as well, so both problems should be looked for and addressed promptly.

Notes

1. D. Shier, J. Butler, and R. Lewis, *Hole's Human Anatomy and Physiology,* 10th ed. (New York, NY: McGraw-Hill, 2004).
2. J. Tintinalli, *Emergency Medicine: A Comprehensive Study Guide,* 6th ed. (New York, NY: McGraw-Hill, 2004).
3. H. A. Sampson, "Symposium on the Definition and Management of Anaphylaxis: Summary Report," *The Journal of Allergy and Clinical Immunology* 115(3) (March 1, 2005):584–591.
4. T. Nowak and A. Handford, *Pathophysiology: Concepts and Applications for Health Care Professionals,* 3rd ed. (New York, NY: McGraw-Hill, 2004).
5. J. A. Marx, *Rosen's Emergency Medicine: Concepts and Clinical Practice,* 5th ed. (St. Louis, MO: Mosby, 2002).
6. William E. Paul (ed.), *Fundamentals of Immunology,* 5th ed., Chapter 46: Immunologic Mechanisms of Allergic Disease (Baltimore, MD: Lippincott Williams, & Wilkins, 2003).
7. K. N. Anderson, L. E. Anderson, and W. D. Glanze, eds., *Mosby's Medical Dictionary,* 5th ed. (St. Louis, MO: C. V. Mosby, 1997).
8. K. McCance and S. Huether, *Pathophysiology: The Biologic Basis for Disease in Adults and Children,* 3rd ed. (St. Louis, MO: Elsevier, 1998).

9. S. G. Brown, "Clinical Features and Severity Grading of Anaphylaxis," *The Journal of Allergy and Clinical Immunology* 114(2) (August 1, 2004):371–376.

10. K. E. Kane and D. C. Cone, "Anaphylaxis in the Prehospital Setting," *The Journal of Emergency Medicine* 27(2004):371.

11. D. L. Kasper, E. Braunwald, A. S. Fauci, S. L. Hauser, D. L. Longo, J. L. Jameson, and K. J. Isselbacher, eds., "Anaphylaxis," *Harrison's Principles of Internal Medicine,* 16th ed., McGraw-Hill's AccessMedicine (accessed August 23, 2006).

12. J. P. Dice, "Physical Urticaria," *Immunology and Allergy Clinics of North America* 24(2) (May 1, 2004):225–246.

13. R. Horan and A. Sheffer, "Food-Dependent Exercise-Induced Anaphylaxis," *Immunology and Allergy Clinics of North America* 11(1991): 757–766.

14. Joint Task Force on Practice Parameters, American Academy of Allergy, Asthma, and Immunology, American College of Allergy, Asthma, and Immunology, and the Joint Council of Allergy, Asthma, and Immunology, "The Diagnosis and Management of Anaphylaxis," *The Journal of Allergy and Clinical Immunology* 101 (6 pt 2): (1998): S465.

15. B. Herlihy, and N. Maebius, *The Human Body in Health and Illness* (Philadelphia, PA: WB Saunders, 2000).

16. D. Le Vay, *Teach Yourself Human Anatomy and Physiology,* 4th ed. (New York, NY: McGraw-Hill, 2001).

17. G. A. Thibodeau and K. T. Patton, *Anatomy & Physiology,* 5th ed. (St. Louis, MO: Mosby, 2003).

18. B. L. Cohen, "Development of a Questionnaire to Measure Quality of Life in Families with a Child with Food Allergy," *The Journal of Allergy and Clinical Immunology* 114(5) (November 1, 2004):1159–1163.

19. M. Radcliffe, G. Scadding, and H. M. Brown, "Lupin Flour Anaphylaxis," *Lancet,* 365(2005):593.

20. J. E. Slater, "Latex Allergy," *The Journal of Allergy and Clinical Immunology* 94(1994):139.

21. K. Turjanmaa, H. Alenius, and S. Makinen-Kiljunem, "Natural Rubber Latex Allergy," *Allergy* 51(1996):593.

22. H. Kimata, "Latex Allergy in Infants Younger Than 1 Year," *Clinical and Experimental Allergy* 34(2004):1910.

23. U. Theissen, J. L. Theissen, and N. Mertes, "IgE-Mediated Hypersensitivity to Latex in Childhood," *Allergy* 52(1997):665.

24. D. L. Hepner, and M. C. Castells "Latex Allergy: An Update," *Anesthesia and Analgesia* 96(2003):1219–1229.

25. D. B. Golden, "Insect Sting Allergy and Venom Immunotherapy: A Model and a Mystery," *The Journal of Allergy and Clinical Immunology* 115(3) (March 1, 2005):439–447.

26. R. S. Pumphrey, "Lessons for Management of Anaphylaxis from a Study of Fatal Reactions," *Clinical and Experimental Allergy* 30(2000):1144–1150.

27. W. J. Brady, Jr., S. Luber, and T. P. Joyce, "Multiphasic Anaphylaxis, Report of a Case with Pre-Hospital and Emergency Department Considerations," *The Journal of Emergency Medicine* 15(1997): 477.

28. A. P. Kaplan and M. W. Greaves, "Angioedema," *Journal of the American Academy of Dermatology* 53 (September 2005): 373–388.

29. T. P. Tran and R. L. Muelleman, "Allergy, Hypersensitivity, and Anaphylaxis," in *Rosen's Emergency Medicine: Concepts and Clinical Practice,* 6th ed., J. A. Marx, R. S. Hockberger, R. M. Walls, et al. (eds.) (Philadelphia, PA: Mosby-Elsevier, 2006), pp. 1818–1837.

30. P. Jabre, "Use of Gum Elastic Bougies for Prehospital Difficult Intubation," *The American Journal of Emergency Medicine* 23(4) (July 1, 2005):552–555.

31. G. N. Peterson, "Management of the Difficult Airway: A Closed Claims Analysis," *Anesthesiology* 103(1) (July 1, 2005):33–39.

32. P. Eisenburger, K. Laczika, M. List, A. Wilfing, H. Losert, R. Hofbauer, H. Burgmann, H. Bankl, B. Pilula, J. L. Benumof, and M. Frass, "Comparison of Conventional Surgical Versus Seldinger Techniques Emergency Cricothyrotomy Performed by Inexperienced Clinicians," *Anesthesiology* 92(2000):687–690.

33. D. C. Cone, "Position Paper for the National Association of EMS Physicians. Subcutaneous Epinephrine for the Out-of-Hospital Treatment of Anaphylaxis," *Prehospital Emergency Care* 6(1) (January/March 2002):67–68.

34. F. E. R. Simons, J. R. Roberts, X Gu, et al., "Epinephrine Absorption in Children with a History of Anaphylaxis," *The Journal of Allergy and Clinical Immunology* 10(1998a):33–37.

35. "Epinephrine," *DRUGDEX,* http://www.thomsonhc.com/hcs (accessed August 23, 2006).

36. M. Fisher, "Treating Anaphylaxis with Sympathomimetic Drugs," *British Medical Journal* 305 (1992):107–108.

37. L. L. Brunto et al., *Goodman & Gilman's The Pharmacological Basis of Therapeutics,* 11th ed., Chapter 24: Histamine (New York, NY: McGraw-Hill, 2006), http://www.accessmedicine.com (accessed October 15, 2005).

38. J. S. Lubin et al., "Evolution of Statewide EMS Drug Formularies and Regulations," *Prehospital Emergency Care* 9(2005):176–180.

39. R. S. Krause, "Allergy and Immunology Anaphylaxis," *Emergency Medicine Textbook* (April 29, 2005), http://www.emedicine.com (accessed October 14, 2005).

40. S. Clark, S. A. Bock, T. J. Gaeta, B. E. Brenner, R. K. Cydulka, and C. A. Camargo, "Multicenter Study of Emergency Department Visits for Food Allergies," *The Journal of Allergy and Clinical Immunology* 113(2004):347–352.

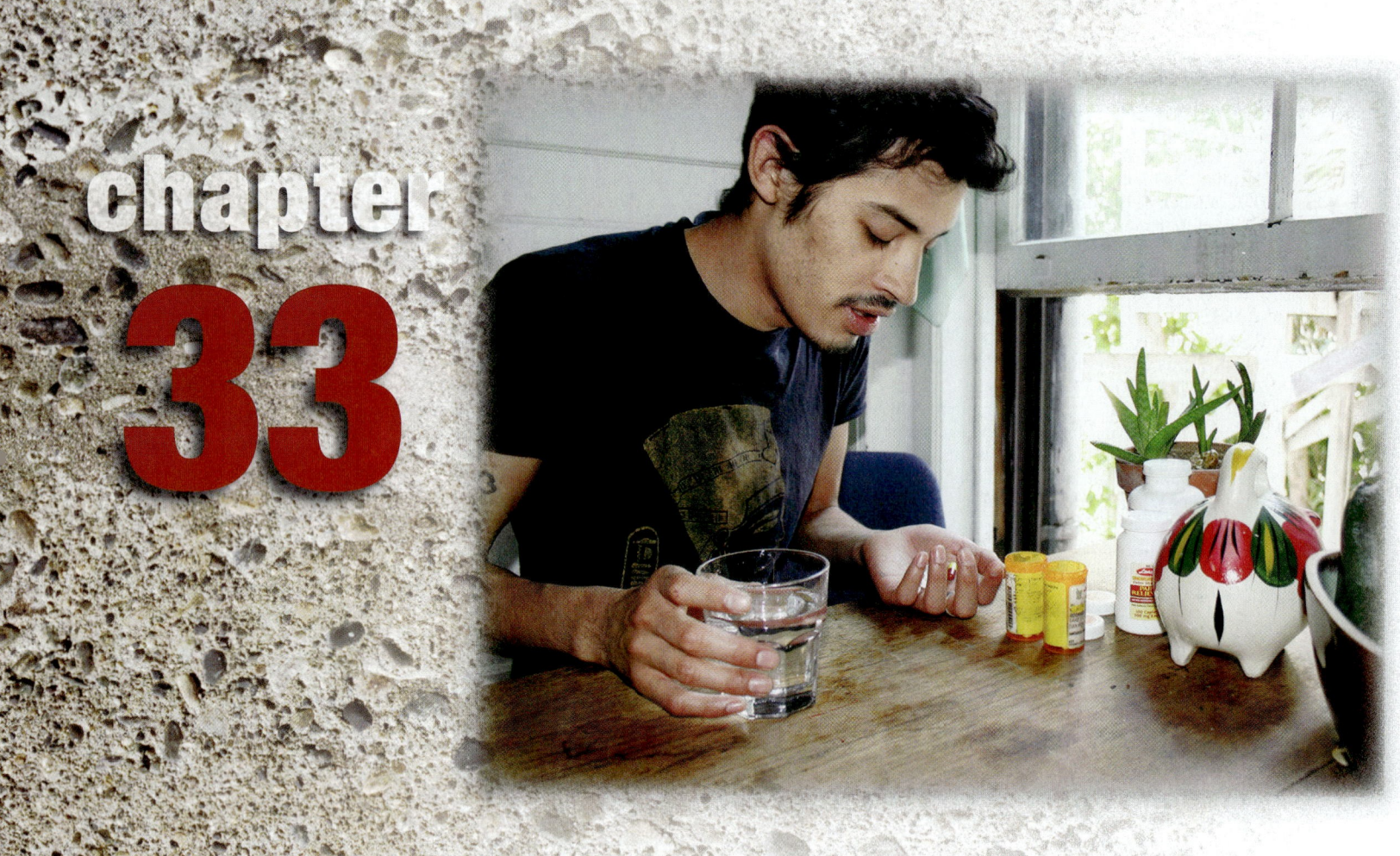

Infectious and Communicable Diseases

*"O*h, powerful bacillus,
With wonder how you fill us,
Every day!
While medical detectives,
With powerful objectives,
Watch your play."

—William Tod Helmuth, "Ode to the Bacillus"

Need to Know

▶ The variety of ways infectious agents are encountered and transmitted from one person to another.

▶ Paramedics need to know how to protect themselves, their patients, and their families from exposure to infectious disease.

▶ Paramedics need to be able to recognize infectious diseases based upon the presenting symptoms and signs.

▶ Sick	▶ Not Yet Sick
• During times of epidemic with airborne diseases, the use of respiratory protection (isolation level protection) is mandatory. • Patients with the following should be approached with caution: cough, high fever, headache, recent weight loss, stiff neck, and a history of recent antibiotic use.	• Ask what resources are available to you for infectious disease surveillance and prevention, and take advantage of any services available to you and your family. • Know which diseases must be reported and know the process to make an official notification or report to the appropriate agency. • Avoid work when you have signs of infection as described in this chapter. • Use the Ryan White Act to your advantage, and request testing when you believe you have been exposed to an infectious disease. • Do not be afraid to treat all patients, even those with infectious diseases, provided you have the appropriate BSI precautions and personal protective equipment.

Introduction

Infectious diseases (also known as **communicable diseases**) are those diseases that are caused by living organisms, such as bacteria and viruses. Those organisms that cause human disease are referred to as **agents** or **pathogens.** Paramedics must have an understanding of infectious diseases for both their patients' well-being and their own safety. DOT 5-11.2

Classification of Pathogens

Infectious agents include viruses, bacteria, fungi, and parasites such as protozoa and helminths. The agents infect the host, causing disease and, in some cases, death. Some of these agents also are transmissible, or pass from one individual to another, causing disease in that person as well. DOT 5-11.8

Viruses

Viruses are comprised of genetic material wrapped in a protein coat. When a virus infects a cell, it uses that cell's reproductive mechanisms to create new copies of itself. Therefore, viruses are unable to reproduce without the help of the host cell. Viruses are generally named for the disease they cause, such as mumps virus. A virus has only one function—to replicate itself.

Viruses are an enigma. They are not fully alive as are bacteria; they do not eat or burn oxygen for fuel, but they are not "nonliving" either. They do not engage in any

process that could be considered metabolic. They make no side products, whether by accident or design, nor do they produce waste. They do have sex, and in fact, they cannot reproduce independently. Several theories on their origins exist. Some suggest they were simple organisms that evolved into a higher state of being, and other theorists believe they de-evolved from a higher being to the simpler one they are today. It is possible that different viruses developed in different ways.[1]

Bacteria

Bacteria are single-celled organisms that are found in all environments on Earth. Bacteria are capable of reproducing without the aid of host cells and cause disease by direct infection of cells or by release of toxins that destroy cells. Standard terminology for bacteria includes the genus and species name, for example, *Escherichia coli.* The genus name is frequently abbreviated, giving the much more common *E. coli.* Some bacteria are referred to by their genus name alone (for example, "strep" for Streptococcus and "staph" for Staphylococcus).

Fungi

Fungi are multicelled organisms with capsules that protect them from the host's immune response. Life-threatening fungal infections are rare in a host with a normally functioning immune system. When fungal infections occur, symptoms are usually slow to develop. Because of the slowness with which fungi reproduce, treatment is usually necessary for weeks or months. The classification and naming of fungi is similar to that of bacteria. DOT 10.3

Parasites

Parasites are animals that infest a host. The most common are protozoa (amoeba), helminths (tapeworms), and insects (lice). Although parasites are given scientific names (*Pediculus humanis capitis)*, they are much more commonly referred to by their English names (head lice). DOT 5-11.2, 5-11.8

Medications Used to Treat Pathogens

Alexander Fleming discovered penicillin, the first antibiotic, in 1929. Since that time, dozens of **antimicrobials** (medications with actions against microorganisms) have been produced. **Antibiotics** are medications that treat bacterial infections, **antivirals** treat viral infections, and **antifungals** treat fungal infections.

All of these medications work by interfering with metabolic processes in the pathogen. For example, penicillin stops bacteria from building cell walls, which prevents the production of new bacteria. Stopping the formation of new bacteria gives the body's immune system a chance to fight the infection.

It is important to remember that antimicrobials only work when new organisms are being produced. Therefore, pathogens that reproduce slowly require prolonged treatment to ensure adequate treatment. A classic example is tuberculosis, which must be treated for six to twelve months.

Another medication used to treat infections is **immunoglobulin.** Immunoglobulin is a purified solution of antibodies from a person or animal that has been infected with a specific disease. It is used in situations in which the patient is unlikely to mount a sufficient immune response in sufficient time to prevent serious or life-threatening illness. For example, patients with signs of lockjaw (tetanus) may be given immunoglobulin, without which they would suffocate before their immune system could fight the infection.

Public Health Principles

Paramedics must understand that infectious diseases affect not only individuals but also larger populations. You are likely to encounter small outbreaks of non-fatal diseases, such as the common cold sweeping through a daycare center. However, you must be familiar with the potential for the rapid spread of a disease and the devastation that can occur. DOT 5-11.4

The bubonic plague spread through Europe between 1347 and 1352 AD, killing 25 million people, about one-third of the population. The winter of 1918–1919 saw an outbreak of influenza that killed between 25 and 40 million people worldwide, compared to 15 to 20 million killed in battle during World War I. In the last twenty-five years, nearly 40 million people worldwide have become infected with Human Immunodeficiency Virus, of whom more than 20 million have died.[2]

Knowledge of the transmission of an infection is necessary not only to understand the disease as it occurs in one patient but also to understand the consequences of transmitting that disease to others. As an example, the virus that causes hepatitis B is transmitted in bodily fluids, so there is no risk of infection with normal personal contact. However, getting stuck with a needle that was used in a patient with hepatitis B might spread the infection to you. On the other hand, tuberculosis is spread by respiratory droplets, so simply being in the back of an ambulance with a coughing patient with TB puts you at risk.

Public health agencies are involved in the monitoring, prevention, and management of outbreaks of disease. Municipal, city, and county health departments participate in disease surveillance and act as the first lines of defense in an outbreak. State agencies serve in a regulatory capacity and are responsible for overseeing the local health departments to ensure that federal guidelines are being followed and to allocate resources when necessary. Local and state health departments also enact and enforce regulations to protect the health of the people, such as mandatory reporting of infectious diseases. Once a disease has been reported, health departments will determine the appropriate steps to follow, such as finding and treating those at risk for infection or taking steps to contain the spread of a pathogen. DOT 5-11.3

The federal government integrates local, regional, and state health departments into a nationwide surveillance and management superstructure. The Occupational Health and Safety Administration (OSHA), a division of the Department of Labor, is responsible for assuring "the safety and health of America's workers by setting and enforcing standards; providing training, outreach, and education; establishing partnerships; and encouraging continual improvement in workplace safety and health."[3]

The Department of Health and Human Services includes the Centers for Disease Control and Prevention (CDC) and the National Institute for Occupational Safety and Health (NIOSH). The CDC, headquartered in Atlanta, is "the lead federal agency for protecting the health and safety of people—at home and abroad, providing credible information to enhance health decisions, and promoting health through strong partnerships . . . developing and applying disease prevention and control, environmental health, and health promotion and education activities designed to improve the health of the people of the United States."[4] NIOSH is "the federal agency responsible for conducting research and making recommendations for the prevention of work-related injury and illness."[5]

Other national agencies involved in public health include the Department of Defense, Federal Emergency Management Agency (FEMA), Department of Homeland Security, National Fire Protection Association (NFPA), and the U.S. Fire Protection Administration. DOT 5-11.4

Infection and Pathogenicity

Infection occurs when a pathogen invades a body and begins reproducing. Not every infection causes disease; many infections are cleared by the immune system before they ever cause symptoms. A **reservoir** is an animal, person, or environment in which an infectious agent reproduces without causing disease. You can think of a reservoir as the place a pathogen "hangs out" while waiting to infect a susceptible host. Infection occurs when an agent is transmitted from its reservoir to a susceptible individual.

The development of clinical disease depends on several factors. The **virulence** or **pathogenicity** of an agent is the ease with which it causes disease. The **dose** is the number of agents that make contact with the victim. The immune system confers **resistance** to infection. Finally, the agent must use the correct **mode of entry.** Infection can only occur if an adequate dose of an agent of sufficient virulence contacts the victim through the proper mode of entry when that victim's resistance is inadequate to ward off the infection. However, as stated above, infection does not necessarily mean that disease will occur. DOT 5-11.1, 5-11.5

Routes of Entry

Paramedics should be familiar with the different routes of entry of pathogens. The **oral** route involves ingestion of matter that has been contaminated with bacteria or their toxins. This can occur by drinking water or eating food that has been contaminated. It can also occur by eating food that was prepared under unsanitary conditions (i.e., prepared by someone who did not wash their hands after using the bathroom). **Respiratory droplets,** which are small globules of saliva that are expelled when the patient coughs, also spread infection. **Parenteral** infections require direct contact of infected bodily fluids with the bloodstream. This can occur through needle sticks or unprotected sexual contact. Contact with nonintact skin can lead to localized or systemic infections.

Stages of an Infection

An infection will progress through several phases. Any given infection may include some or all of these phases, and they may overlap. A **latent** period occurs when the

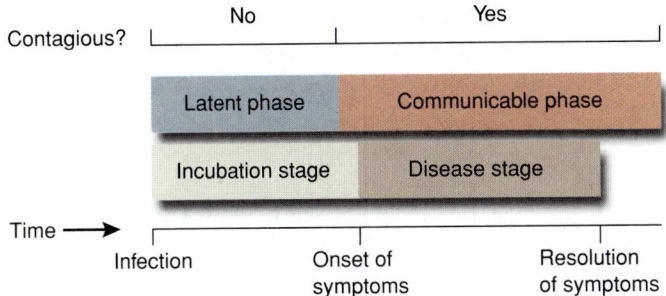

Figure 33-1 Stages of an infection.

infectious agent has entered the host and is present, reproducing, but causing no signs or symptoms. During the latent period, the agent generally cannot be transmitted to another host. The **communicable** phase is that period during which the infectious agent can be spread to another host. Note that not all diseases are communicable, and symptoms may or may not occur during this phase. The **incubation phase** is that time period between initial infection and the onset of symptoms. Finally, the **disease period** is when symptoms occur (Figure 33-1). DOT 5-11.5, 5-11.7

The Immune System

The human body is endowed with a remarkable and complex system for preventing and fighting infection. The immune system identifies infectious agents and isolates and destroys them. Persons with fully functional immune systems are said to be **immunocompetent.** Those whose immune systems are not fully functional are said to be **immunosupressed** or **immunodeficient** and are less able to fight off infection. Many treatments for cancer leave a patient immunosupressed; patients with AIDS are immunodeficient. DOT 5-11.6, 5-11.11, 5-11.12

The defenses of the immune system are categorized as nonspecific and specific.

Nonspecific Mechanisms

Nonspecific mechanisms block the entry into the body of any foreign substance. The body's first nonspecific defense is the skin, which is watertight and prevents entry of all but the most invasive organisms. Since most agents cannot enter the body through intact skin, they must either enter through defects in the skin (cuts, abrasions, or puncture wounds) or through other portals such as the respiratory and gastrointestinal tracts. DOT 5-11.9

Respiratory Tract

The respiratory tract is much more prone to allowing the entry of infectious agents than the skin. The environment within the respiratory tract is warm and moist, making it perfect for the incubation of pathogens. Furthermore, the membranes that line the respiratory tract are more permeable than the skin. Fortunately, the respiratory tract has several mechanisms for preventing the entry of infection.

Just inside the entry to the nose are many hairs that trap the largest particulate matter. Deeper in, the nose contains shelves of bone called **turbinates** that promote turbulent airflow, forcing particulate matter against the walls of the nasal cavity. These walls are covered with a thick mucus that traps foreign matter, preventing it from traveling deeper into the respiratory tract.

The mucous membrane covering of the nasal cavity extends down into the trachea and bronchi of the lungs. Tiny, hair-like projections on the surface of the trachea called cilia constantly beat the mucus upwards towards the mouth. This **mucociliary** "elevator" helps clear pathogens from the respiratory tract. The mucus from the trachea and nasal passages is either swallowed or coughed out as phlegm.

Gastrointestinal Tract

The **gastrointestinal tract** is another portal for the entry of pathogens but has its own protective mechanisms. The stomach acid destroys many ingested agents, while the digestive enzymes of the lower GI tract deal with other agents. Bacteria living in the colon **(normal intestinal flora)** compete with ingested pathogens for resources, helping to prevent infections. Finally, the GI tract can expel pathogens by making defecation more frequent, causing diarrhea.

Should a pathologic agent make its way into the body, a localized **inflammatory response** occurs in an effort to limit the spread of infection. This response is initiated by the body's recognition of foreign matter or the presence of tissue damage from trauma, heat, or chemical injury. Blood vessels dilate and become permeable to fluid. This leads to redness, warmth, and swelling. Increased blood flow into the area and decreased blood flow out of the area prevent spread of infection. The chemicals that initiate the inflammatory

response also attract white blood cells, which begin attacking the pathogen.

Specific Mechanisms

The specific immune response (also called the **adaptive immune response**) is designed to identify and attack pathogens. This system consists of white blood cells, the reticuloendothelial system, and the complement system.

White Blood Cells

White blood cells are formed in the bone marrow and differentiate into specialized cells with particular functions. Lymphocytes are the most important mediators of the specific immune response and are classified as **B cells** and **T cells**. DOT 5-11.10

Antigens are unique proteins on the surfaces of bacteria, viruses, and fungi. The body can use these to identify infectious agents. Proteins called **antibodies** that are produced by B cells recognize these antigens by fitting them in much the same way that a key fits a lock. Unless it is fighting an infection, the human body does not produce antibodies against a specific antigen; rather, it produces a wide range of random antigens in the hope that one of them will match a pathogenic organism (Figure 33-2).

When an antibody is successful at binding with an antigen, the specific immune response begins in earnest. First, the B cell responsible for the production of that particular antibody rapidly clones itself. Some of these cells will become **plasma cells,** producing large quantities of antibody. Antibodies help fight infection by identifying those organisms that need to be destroyed by white blood cells. The remainder of the newly produced B cells become **memory cells,** which present their specific antibody on the cell surface. These memory cells persist in the body for years and are responsible for a much more rapid immune response in the event of subsequent contact with the same pathogen.

Vaccines use the principle of antibodies and memory B cells to protect against disease. A person is

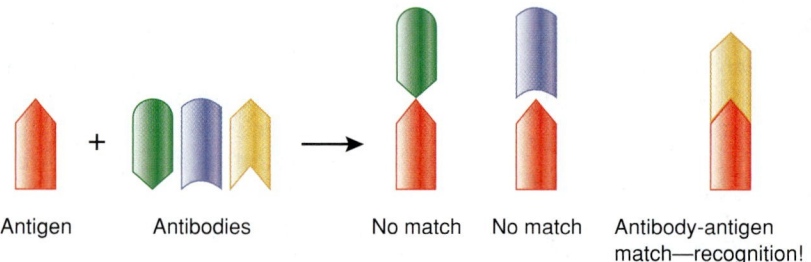

Figure 33-2 Antibody-antigen reactions.

administered a dose of a prepared antigen that produces an antibody response. If that person ever comes into contact with the agent that matches that antibody, the immune response is prepared to fight it off before it can cause disease. Vaccines have been successful in preventing numerous diseases. For example, due to the worldwide vaccination efforts of the United Nations, smallpox had been completely eradicated.

T cells are responsible for mediating the immune response. **T helper cells** (identified by a surface protein known as CD4) secrete substances called lymphokines that cause other white blood cells to migrate to the area. Other T cells, known as **T killer cells,** help to kill pathogens while **T suppressor cells** help to stop the immune response after the pathogen has been cleared. Both of these cells are identified by the CD8 protein on their surface.

Other white blood cells involved in the immune response include **monocytes** and **macrophages,** which engulf and destroy cells that have been coated with antibody. **Neutrophils** are also involved in destroying antibody-coated cells. **Eosinophils** and **basophils** release substances that assist in the immune response. DOT 5-11.11

Reticuloendothelial System

The **reticuloendothelial system** (RES) is the collection of white blood cells found outside the bloodstream, namely in the liver, spleen, lungs, lymph nodes, bone marrow, and intestines. These white blood cells help to clear the blood of any debris that results from fighting an infection. This system also stores T cells and B cells when they are not active in an immune response. Patients with liver disease or who have had their spleens removed are less capable of clearing an infection and are, therefore, more prone to prolonged infection. DOT 5-11.10

Complement System

The **complement system** is a collection of proteins in the blood that help to kill pathologic organisms. The proteins are activated by the binding of antibody to antigen or by the simple presence of a pathogen. Once activated, the complement system kills pathogenic cells, causes white blood cells to migrate to the area, and stimulates B cells to produce antibody. The complement system helps to activate the immune response before antibody is produced and helps intensify the immune response as antibody appears. DOT 5-11.9, 5-11.10

CONNECTIONS Chapter 37: Hematology and Chapter 32: Allergies and Anaphylaxis have more information on immunity.

Exposure to Infectious Disease

Every healthcare agency is responsible for protecting its employees by minimizing the risk of coming into contact with infectious agents. Each individual healthcare provider is responsible for understanding the roles of personal protective equipment and body substance isolation when caring for patients with known or suspected infectious disease. DOT 5-11.12

Universal Precautions

Universal precautions are a set of procedures to be used by every healthcare provider to prevent transmission of infectious disease. Universal precautions include the use of barriers to prevent direct contact with infected substances and the isolation of potentially infected bodily fluids.

It is important to realize that universal precautions must be used for *every* patient contact. You must get in the habit of treating all patients as if they had an infectious disease, so that you never put yourself at risk. DOT 5-11.13

CONNECTIONS See Chapter 2: The Well-Being of the Paramedic and Chapter 53: Hazardous Materials Incidents for more information on and illustrations of PPE.

Personal Protective Equipment (PPE)

A wide range of equipment is available to the healthcare provider to prevent the transmission of communicable diseases. This equipment includes but is not limited to gloves, masks, protective eyewear, gowns, and face shields. When properly used, these devices can prevent the spread of communicable disease from the patient to the healthcare provider or to other patients. The proper use of personal protective equipment (PPE) is critical in many public health emergencies. Proper training, fit testing, and storage of equipment such as N-95 masks, gloves, shoe covers, powered respirators, gowns, hoods, and eye protection are essential as these items will likely be utilized in cases of infectious outbreaks, chemical releases, bioterrorist attacks, or radiation releases. Protection for both the paramedic and the patient must be taken into consideration. Local protocols and guidelines will mandate which elements of PPE are to be utilized for a given situation.

Gloves must be worn whenever a paramedic is going to touch any body substance or when the paramedic is going to perform an invasive procedure such as venipuncture. Gloves should be removed after the contact with the patient has been concluded or after the procedure if the gloves have become contaminated.

The proper method of removing gloves involves using one gloved hand to grab the palm of the other glove, pulling it off the hand and turning it inside out at the same time. Then, the fingers of the bare hand are slid under the cuff of the glove still being worn, lifting it off the hand and turning it inside out. This method prevents contact with the external, contaminated surface of the gloves. Both gloves are immediately thrown into an appropriate container. **Skill Sheet 60: Putting On and Removing Gloves outlines how to don sterile gloves.**

Facemasks should be worn to prevent exposure to an airborne infection. As a rule, the paramedic should wear a mask whenever the patient is coughing. It is also sensible to place a mask on the patient to protect others. Masks are classified by the amount of protection they confer. Surgical masks will protect against direct contamination of the mouth but do not confer adequate protection against most airborne pathogens. Particulate filters such as the N-95 class of facemasks should be worn to protect against respiratory pathogens such as tuberculosis.

Face shields or protective eyewear must be worn whenever there is a risk of body fluids splashing or spattering, such as during intubation or childbirth. Gowns should also be worn in these situations to prevent contamination of work clothes.

Traumas are special situations in which the risk of exposure to bodily fluids is very high. In such cases, gloves, gowns, and protective eyewear must be used.

Finally, PPE must be properly disposed of after use. It is never appropriate to leave contaminated PPE at the scene or to throw it on the floor of the ambulance.

Hygiene Measures. A few simple hygiene measures can provide significant protection to patients and paramedics and should be followed regularly. DOT 5-11.15

- Frequent hand washing with antibacterial soap is the most important method of protection. When not able to wash, hands should be sanitized with alcohol-based hand cleansers. Paramedics should also avoid touching their faces with their hands. **See Skill Sheet 61: Hand washing.**

- Cover the mouth and nose when coughing or sneezing.

- Wear a surgical mask or N-95 mask when coughing or sneezing while working with patients, and consider covering patients' mouth and nose with a mask if they have respiratory symptoms. This becomes mandatory when epidemic illness is known to exist.

- Encourage additional airflow in the patient compartment of the ambulance by opening windows, if appropriate.

- Stay home from work when ill with respiratory illnesses to prevent the spread to others. This practice is called *social isolation.*

Protocols are necessary to address issues such as the transmission routes and incubation periods of various infectious agents; isolation and quarantine techniques and which types of exposures mandate either isolation or quarantine for paramedics and decontamination of vehicle equipment. In cases where decontamination procedures are complex and time-consuming, as in serious airborne diseases such as SARS, agencies frequently have protocols that allow for the transport of stable victims to the hospital by private car with a previously exposed driver after proper evaluation and initial treatment by EMS personnel. Patients transported by ambulance should only receive nebulizer treatments or other infectious aerosol-producing treatments if absolutely necessary, in an effort to minimize potential contamination of the passenger compartment environment. DOT 5-11.14

Body Substance Isolation (BSI)

Body substance isolation is the practice of treating all bodily fluids as if they were infected. Bodily substances should be contained, and PPE should be used before making direct contact with any bodily fluid.

Any sharp objects, such as needles or lancets, that were used on a patient must be placed in a rigid plastic container designed for the disposal of medical sharps. Never attempt to recap a needle or force a sharp into an overly full container, as a puncture wound can result. Sharps containers should be disposed of properly before they are full. DOT 5-11.16

Contaminated linens and trash should be placed in bags clearly marked "biohazard," and disposed of according to the regulations of your agency. Non-disposable equipment should be disinfected according to local regulations. Disinfection is usually classified as high-level or low-level. High-level disinfection involves heating to kill pathogens or soaking in sterilizing fluid. High-level disinfection is mandatory for equipment that will enter the patient's body (needles and scalpels) or come into contact with mucous membranes (laryngoscope blades). The best way to prevent the spread of disease is to use disposable equipment whenever possible.

Low-level disinfection is required for all other equipment. This can be achieved with Lysol™ spray or 10% bleach solution. DOT 5-11.17

Isolation and Quarantine. The need to quarantine or isolate potentially infected or ill paramedics may seriously decrease the number of EMS staff available to respond to calls for transport or transfer. During the Toronto SARS outbreak, 850 paramedics had 1,166 potential exposures to SARS, resulting in 436 medics being placed in 10-day home quarantine. During quarantine, paramedics had to wear N-95 respirators continuously. Sixty-two paramedics developed SARS-like illnesses. During the second phase of the outbreak, 200 more paramedics were quarantined.[6] Removing paramedics from duty obviously requires redeployment of available personnel and places stress on the remaining EMS staff.

It is generally better to err on the side of caution and suspicion when treating and transporting patients during times of public health emergencies, especially very early in the course of the incident. A high index of suspicion and vigilance on the part of the paramedic can prevent the spread of illness or contamination and prevent further trauma. DOT 5-11.15

CONNECTIONS Chapter 52: Teamwork and Operational Interface, Figure 52-1 (page 1263), and Figure 52-8 (page 1270), provide situation response guides for special pathogens.

Responsibility for Universal Precautions

Agency Responsibility

Infection control is the responsibility of every healthcare agency, including hospitals, clinics, and EMS providers. Each agency must identify the risk of communicable disease for its members and insure protection for its members by providing personal protective equipment.

An agency must have procedures for using PPE and disinfection of equipment and vehicles. The agency is responsible for providing containers for sharps and contaminated linens.

Personal Responsibility

It is the responsibility of paramedics to be proactive about infection control. Paramedics must be familiar with their agency's policies and procedures regarding infection control. They must utilize the appropriate PPE when necessary, and should always practice BSI. The important aspects of personal responsibility are outlined in Box 33-1.

Hand washing is the single most important aspect of personal responsibility and is recognized as the best protection from the spread of infection.

The Centers for Disease Control and Prevention have established the following guidelines for the washing of hands: Hands should be washed before direct patient contact or performing invasive procedures and after touching a patient's skin or any bodily fluids, after removing gloves, and before and after eating or using a restroom. Hands should be washed either with antimicrobial soap and warm water or with an alcohol-based hand cleanser.

When using soap and water, the soap should be applied to the skin and the hands rubbed together vigorously for 15 seconds prior to rinsing. A good rule of

BOX 33-1 Personal Responsibility in Infection Control

- Understand policies and procedures regarding infection control.
- Maintain a high level of wellness and ensure immunizations are current.
- Use personal protective equipment.
- Practice body substance isolation.
- Cover all open wounds with a watertight dressing.
- Wash hands after every patient contact.
- Remove work clothes when leaving work to avoid spreading contamination.
- Understand proper handling of work clothes that have been contaminated with bodily fluids.
- Do not prepare or eat food in patient care areas.
- Understand correct disposal of needles and sharps into appropriate containers.
- Understand correct disposal of linens and supplies contaminated with bodily fluids.
- Avoid rubbing face, nose, eyes, or mouth with gloved hands.

thumb is to sing "Happy Birthday" twice, "Row, Row, Row Your Boat" three times, or recite the alphabet twice to yourself to mark the time. Special attention should be paid to washing the web spaces between fingers. Hands should be dried with a disposable towel, which should then be used to turn off the faucet. The faucet should be considered contaminated and should not be touched with the bare hands after they have been washed.[7]

When using an alcohol-based hand rub, a sufficient amount should be used to cover both hands, and the hands should be rubbed together until dry. Studies have shown that alcohol-based hand rubs are as effective as bactericidal soap and water if there is no gross contamination of the hands.[8] DOT 5-11.13, 5-11.16

Street Secrets

Your best defense against infection is to maintain a healthy immune system. Eat a well-balanced diet, exercise regularly, get enough sleep, limit stress in your life, and keep up with routine health screening and immunizations. Chapter 2: The Well-Being of the Paramedic discusses wellness and provides tips on how to maintain a high level of wellness.

Bacteremia and Sepsis

Bacteremia is the presence of bacteria in the bloodstream. Bacteremia may be accompanied by fever, **malaise** (a generalized feeling of discomfort), and **myalgias** (muscle aches) but is frequently asymptomatic. Bacteremia can only be diagnosed with blood cultures.

Sepsis is a syndrome that is caused by the presence of bacteria or bacterial toxins in the blood.

Sepsis is characterized by the following:

- Fever *or* hypothermia
- Tachycardia greater than 90 beats per minute
- Tachypnea greater than 20 breaths per minute
- Evidence of decreased perfusion, such as altered mental status or hypoxia

Sepsis may progress to **septic shock**, in which blood is no longer adequately perfusing the body's tissues. Septic shock is usually accompanied by a blood pressure measurement below 90 mmHg. Untreated septic shock will lead to multisystem organ dysfunction, in which more than one organ shows signs of failure. Even with aggressive medical care, sepsis has a 30% mortality rate.[9]

Paramedics must be able to recognize sepsis due to its high mortality. Any patient with signs of an infection who is hypotensive or has altered mental status should be treated aggressively. Intubation is necessary in patients who cannot protect their own airways. Large-bore IV access and adequate fluid resuscitation to maintain perfusion is necessary. However, the most successful treatments for sepsis include administration of vasoactive medications and antibiotics that are beyond the scope of practice of most paramedics. Therefore, transportation to the closest appropriate facility should take priority over performing on scene interventions such as vascular access and fluid resuscitation.

The Approach to the Patient with a Suspected Infectious Disease

It is sometimes difficult to identify the patient with an infectious disease. Many patients will have a fever, but others (especially the elderly and those who are immunocompromised) may actually have a lower body temperature. Patients with pneumonia will almost always have a cough, but a cough could also indicate a noninfectious lung disease such as emphysema.

Although no single sign or symptom is guaranteed to diagnose an infection, the complete clinical picture is often clearer. For example, headaches are a common and nonspecific symptom, but the combination of headache, fever, and stiff neck suggests meningitis. Always take into account the constellation of complaints and physical findings when assessing for an infection.

After donning the appropriate personal protective equipment and reminding yourself to practice body substance isolation, you should begin your assessment of the patient. The history should focus on the onset of the chief complaint, the presence or absence of a fever, and the progression of symptoms over time. It is important to determine whether the patient used medicines that will decrease a fever, such as aspirin, acetaminophen, or ibuprofen. DOT 5-11.6

The past medical history should include questions regarding any history of chronic infections or inflammatory disorders. The use of steroids (such as prednisone) may prevent the patient from mounting an inflammatory response. The use of antibiotics indicates the presence of a preexisting infection.

Street Secrets

Always read the labels on the medication bottles. Patients sometimes stop taking antibiotics when they begin feeling better and they may reuse the remaining medication at another time. Make sure the medication is prescribed for the patient taking it.

Certain chronic diseases predispose patients to infection and impair the healing process. These diseases include diabetes and chronic lung disease. Finally, a history of organ transplant is important since most patients with a transplanted organ take drugs to suppress the immune system, thus decreasing organ rejection but increasing the infection risk.

Physical findings that should be assessed include skin color and temperature, flexibility of the neck (do not attempt to assess if there is any evidence of trauma), breath sounds, and abdominal tenderness. The skin should also be assessed for signs of localized infection such as redness, warmth, and swelling.

After disposition of the patient, the paramedic must ensure that all contaminated supplies are appropriately disposed of or disinfected. All sharps must be accounted for and placed in a sharps container. Linens should be bagged, and the ambulance cleaned and disinfected. Soiled uniform clothing should be removed and laundered separately from other clothes. Finally, hands must be washed. DOT 5-11.15, 5-11.52

Specific Infectious Diseases

Diseases Spread by Bodily Fluids

The following diseases are spread through the parenteral route, that is to say, by the exchange of bodily fluids. These diseases are of concern to the paramedic mainly for the risk posed by occupational exposure through needle sticks.

Human Immunodeficiency Virus (HIV) and the Acquired Immune Deficiency Syndrome (AIDS)

HIV-related disease was first described in the early 1980s in a group of homosexual men in Los Angeles who had a rare pneumonia usually seen only in patients with immune system failure.[10] The subsequent epidemic first spread amongst homosexuals, hemophiliacs, and IV drug users but now involves all populations.

HIV preferentially infects the T cells called T helper cells or CD4 cells that are responsible for mediating the immune response. Acute infection with the Human Immunodeficiency Virus is often accompanied by non-specific symptoms such as fever, malaise, and swollen lymph nodes that last for several days to weeks. Following this period, the infection lies dormant for a variable period (weeks to decades), during which time the infected individual is asymptomatic but contagious. When the infection is reactivated, possibly as a result of an immune response, HIV begins killing CD4 cells as well as cells of the central nervous system.

The clinical effects of HIV disease are primarily related to immunodeficiency. Numerous agents in the environment are rapidly and completely eradicated by a functioning immune system but cause disease in patients with immune deficiency. These are called **opportunistic infections.**

The Centers for Disease Control and Prevention defines Acquired Immune Deficiency Syndrome (AIDS) as a low CD4 cell count and the presence of opportunistic infections, signifying the defect in cell-mediated immunity. The list of opportunistic infections included in this definition is given in Box 33-2.[11]

It is estimated that, as of 2003, there are almost 1 million people in the United States living with HIV, of whom approximately 25% do not know they are infected. There

---

BOX 33-2 Opportunistic Infections Included in the Case Definition of AIDS

Candida in the esophagus, trachea, bronchi, or lungs

Invasive cervical cancer

Coccidioidomycosis

Cryptococcus outside the lungs

Cryptospiridiosis with diarrhea lasting for more than one month

Cytomegalovirus (CMV) retinitis

CMV disease outside the liver, spleen, or lymph nodes

Herpes simplex virus causing prolonged skin problems or involving the lungs or esophagus

HIV-related encephalopathy

Chronic intestinal isosporiasis lasting longer than one month

Kaposi's sarcoma (Figure 33-3)

Burkitt's, immunoblastic or primary brain lymphoma

Widespread *Mycobacterium avium intracellulare* (MAI) or *Mycobacterium kansasii*

Pneumocystis pneumonia

Recurrent bacterial pneumonia

Progressive multifocal leukoencephalopathy

Recurrent *Salmonella* septicemia

Toxoplasmosis of the brain

HIV wasting syndrome

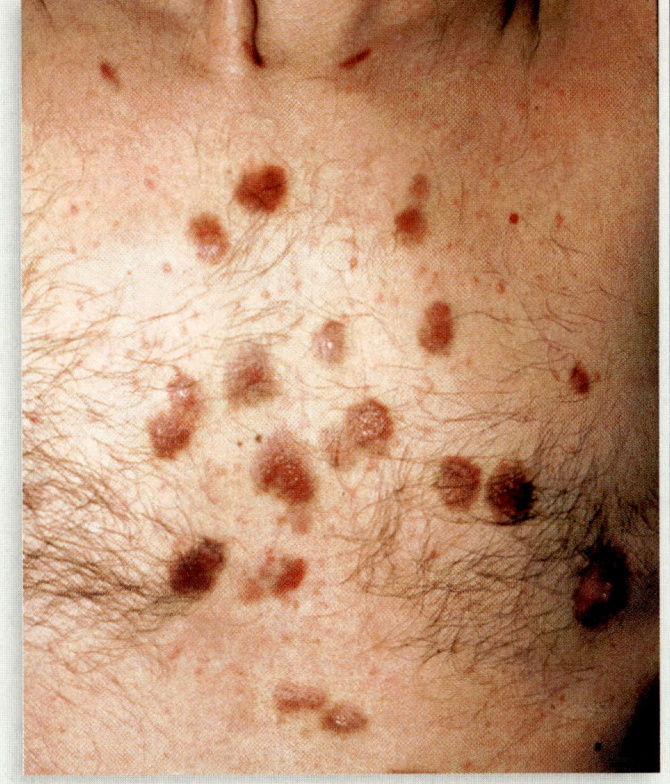

Figure 33-3 Kaposi's sarcoma lesions.

were over 40,000 new diagnoses of AIDS in the United States in 2003, bringing the cumulative total of American AIDS cases to a little over 900,000. In 2003, there were 18,000 deaths due to AIDS, bringing the cumulative total to more than half a million.[12] It is estimated that 40 million people have been infected with HIV worldwide, resulting in 20 million deaths over the last 25 years.

The clinical manifestations of AIDS are extremely variable and often difficult to diagnose without lab tests and X-rays. *Cryptococcus neoformans* (a fungus) or *Toxoplasmosis* (a parasite found in cats often spread through dirty litter boxes) can cause central nervous system infections such as meningitis. These will present like other forms of meningitis (headache, fever, stiff neck) but tend to develop slowly and have less intense symptoms. Progressive multifocal leukoencephalopathy (PML) presents with confusion and difficulty walking, paralysis, and blindness. The Human Immunodeficiency Virus can also cause direct damage to nerve cells, resulting in AIDS dementia, which causes cognitive impairment such as confusion and memory loss, progressing to coma. Infection with Cytomegalovirus (CMV) causes visual impairment and blindness.

Pulmonary opportunistic infections include tuberculosis, *Pneumocystis carinii* pneumonia (PCP), and community-acquired pneumonia. These will all present with cough, fever, and pleuritic chest pain. Gastrointestinal symptoms include thrush (growth of *Candida albicans* yeast in the oropharynx and mouth) and chronic diarrhea caused by the parasite *Cryptosporidium*. Dermatologic infections include Herpes simplex outbreaks and Kaposi's sarcoma (a purple lesion found on the skin and mucous membranes). Patients with AIDS are also more likely to develop cancer, particularly lymphoma.

HIV is transmitted through the exchange of bodily fluids and is found in large concentrations in blood, semen, vaginal fluid, and breast milk. The most common routes of infection include unprotected sexual intercourse and shared IV needles. Receptive anal intercourse and receptive vaginal intercourse are considered the riskiest behaviors. The risk of association with oral sex is unknown but is believed to be low. The transmission of HIV is reasonably guarded against with the use of *latex* condoms provided they remain intact and only a water-soluble lubricant is applied. Although nonoxynol-9, a spermicide, kills HIV, it is contraindicated because in some patients it may cause genital ulcers that could facilitate HIV transmission. Patients should be counseled that condoms are not 100% effective.[13]

Spread from mother to child can occur in 13–30% of pregnancies but can be largely prevented by giving the mother AZT at the time of delivery.[14] Although HIV has been detected in saliva, tears, urine, and bronchial secretion, there is no evidence of transmission of disease through contact with these fluids. There have been no reports of HIV transmission through insect bites.[15]

Healthcare workers must exercise caution when dealing with any bodily fluid because of the risk of HIV. The risk of transmission from a needle stick is low, occurring in 1 out of 300 needle sticks. Factors that increase the risk of seroconversion are depth of the needle stick, use of hollow bore needle (as opposed to solid, sewing-type needle), and the HIV viral load of the patient. To date, there have been twelve unconfirmed cases of occupational HIV transmission in paramedics.[16] There have been no cases of transmission after exposure of infected bodily fluids with intact skin or mucous membranes.

Although the risk of transmission to healthcare workers is low, the clinical implication is enormous. Since HIV tests will not become positive for four to six weeks after infection, it is important to treat the exposed healthcare worker with HIV medications at least until that time period has elapsed.

Treating occupational exposures is effective, and prompt use of postexposure prophylaxis has been shown to decrease seroconversion rates by 81%.[17] However, HIV medications have significant side effects, including nausea and vomiting and fatigue. Exposure also causes psychological stress for the affected healthcare workers and their families.

There is currently no immunization against HIV, although clinical trials are underway to investigate the possibility of a vaccine.

Prehospital treatment of the patient with AIDS is supportive, with particular attention to hydration and altered mental status. Paramedics must use personal protective equipment and must be sure to wash their hands after contact with any patient. Eye protection and facemasks should be used in situations in which exposure to large quantities of bodily fluids is possible (trauma, childbirth, or vomiting). Due to the high prevalence of tuberculosis in patients with AIDS, all patients with a cough should have a mask placed over their nose and mouth.

Infection with HIV is asymptomatic, and patients may be reluctant to disclose their HIV status to healthcare workers. Furthermore, one-quarter of all infected persons are unaware of their HIV status. For these reasons, it is important that paramedics practice body substance isolation on all patients.

It is imperative that paramedics familiarize themselves with the resources available to them after exposure. Early identification, testing, and treatment are necessary to minimize the risk of seroconversion.

Patients with HIV may or may not be treated with antiretroviral drugs, agents that slow the progression of disease. These patients may also be taking medications to prevent opportunistic infections. Hospital care of the patients with HIV or AIDS depends on the nature of problem but usually involves fluid resuscitation and antibiotics. Due to their inability to effectively fight infection, patients with HIV and AIDS are frequently admitted for IV antibiotics or observation. **DOT 5-11.18**

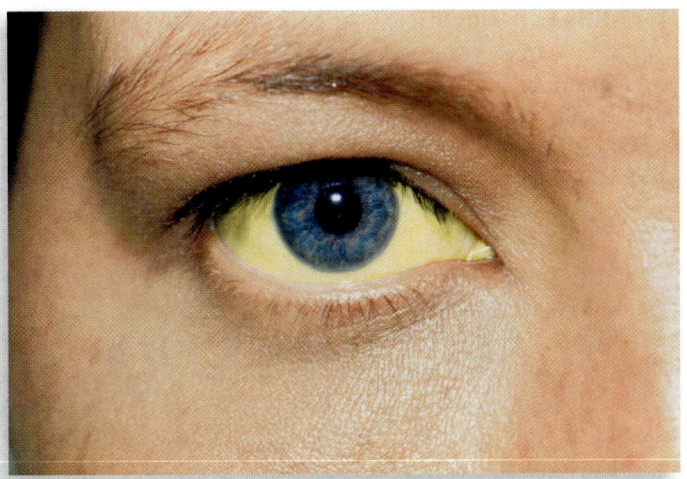

Figure 33-4 Yellow discoloration (jaundice) of the sclera of the eye.

Hepatitis

Hepatitis is a term used to describe any inflammation of the liver. Symptoms include abdominal pain and vomiting. Signs include abdominal tenderness and jaundice (yellow discoloration of the skin and eyes) (Figure 33-4). The most common causes of hepatitis are the hepatitis viruses but also medications or alcohol abuse.

Hepatitis A. Hepatitis A is the most common form of hepatitis in the United States, comprising almost half of all cases of hepatitis. The hepatitis A virus is transmitted by the fecal-oral route and has an incubation period of approximately 28 days. About one-quarter of all cases are asymptomatic, and there is evidence that one-third of the population of the United States has been exposed to the virus.

Hepatitis A is common in developing countries with poor sanitation, especially in Central and South America, Africa, the Middle East, and Southeast Asia. In the United States, hepatitis A is most common in the West and Southwest states, and the number of cases has been steadily dropping, from a high of 35,000 reported cases in 1989 to less than 8,000 in 2003.[18]

Acute infection with hepatitis A causes nausea, abdominal pain, diarrhea, and anorexia, followed in a few days by jaundice. Symptoms typically last for two to six weeks, although 15% of patients will have relapsing symptoms for up to nine months. There is no chronic infection, and exposure to the hepatitis A virus confers lifelong immunity. Children who become infected are usually less symptomatic than adults.[19]

Hepatitis A is spread most commonly through food prepared in unsanitary conditions. The virus can also be spread by close personal contact (most frequently in daycare centers), sexual contact, and occasionally through needle stick exposure. The hepatitis A virus can survive on unwashed surfaces for four hours.

A vaccine against hepatitis A has been available since 1995 and is extremely effective against the disease with few side effects. Since hepatitis A is relatively rare in the United States, routine immunization is only recommended for travelers to locations with high incidence of the disease, household contacts of persons with the disease, men who have sex with men, injection drug users, patients with hemophilia, and patients with chronic liver disease. Hepatitis A vaccine is not routinely recommended for healthcare workers.[18] The main complication of the hepatitis A vaccine is localized pain.[18]

Treatment of patients with hepatitis A is supportive, with fluid resuscitation as necessary. Personal protective equipment is required as is close attention to hand washing after patient contact. Most cases of hepatitis A are mild, and most patients are treated at home; those with severe nausea and vomiting will be admitted to the hospital for fluid resuscitation. DOT 5-11.19

Hepatitis B. Hepatitis B comprises one-third of all cases of hepatitis in the United States. Hepatitis B is transmitted through the parenteral route, with an incubation period of 12 weeks. Approximately 70% of infected persons will develop symptoms, although less than 10% of children under age five will develop symptoms. Approximately 5% of the American population has been exposed to the virus.[20]

Hepatitis B is endemic in Africa, Southeast Asia, and South America. The incidence of hepatitis B has been dropping in the United States from a high of 260,000 new cases reported in 1985 to 73,000 cases reported in 2003.[20]

The signs and symptoms of acute infection with hepatitis B are similar to hepatitis A with abdominal pain, nausea, anorexia, and jaundice. Thirty percent of infected persons will have no symptoms. Approximately 1% of all patients will die from liver failure in the acute stage.

Chronic infection occurs in 90% of children infected before one year of age, 30% of those infected between ages one and five, and 6% of patients infected after age five. Chronic infection can occur in symptomatic or asymptomatic patients. Chronic hepatitis B carries the risk of liver failure from cirrhosis and liver cancer. Of those people with chronic hepatitis B, 15–20% will die as a result of their disease. It is estimated that 1.25 million people in the United States have chronic hepatitis B, many of whom contracted the disease in infancy.

The hepatitis B virus is found in high concentrations in the blood, moderate concentrations in semen and vaginal fluids, and low concentrations in breast milk, urine, and tears. Transmission is through exchange of bodily fluids, including sexual intercourse, sharing IV needles, and transmission from an infected mother to her child during delivery. Transmission through blood transfusion is uncommon since donated blood has been tested for the presence of hepatitis B since 1971. Hepatitis B virus can survive on contaminated surfaces for seven days.

A vaccine against hepatitis B has been available since 1982. The vaccine is delivered in a series of three doses, with the second dose being given one month after the first, and the third dose being given five months later. Successful immunization occurs in 30–50% of people after the first dose, 75% of people after the second, and 96% of people after the third. Complications of the vaccine include localized pain at the injection site, fever, rash, and muscle pain.[21]

Since the mid-1990s, hepatitis B vaccine has been included in the routine childhood immunization schedule. Almost all states require hepatitis B vaccination before beginning first grade. Adolescents are also being vaccinated through a "catch-up" program to increase coverage of immunity. Hepatitis B vaccine is also recommended for IV drug users, people with multiple sex partners, hemodialysis patients, men who have sex with men, and inmates in correctional facilities.

Due to the risk of exposure to infected bodily fluids, it is recommended that *all* healthcare workers receive vaccinations to Hepatitis B and have immunoglobulin levels checked one to two months after the immunization series to verify immunity.[21]

The greatest risk to healthcare workers is from a needle stick. Percutaneous puncture with a hollow needle that has been used to draw blood from an infected individual carries a 6-30% risk of transmission of the disease.[22]

The treatment of patients with hepatitis B is supportive, with attention to fluid resuscitation. Personal protective equipment must be used, and special care must be taken when handling sharps or equipment that has been contaminated with bodily fluids. Disinfection of equipment is mandatory. Hospital care involves fluid resuscitation and arranging close follow-up to monitor liver function. DOT 5-11.21, 5-20.20

Street Secrets

Disinfectant solutions must be used exactly as recommended on the label. If they are supposed to be diluted before use, using a full strength solution may actually be less effective. If the solution needs to be used at a certain temperature (for example, with hot water) then that is what is required. If the solution is supposed to be in contact with the surface to be cleaned for five minutes, then it should be left in place for the full five minutes. Before any chemical is approved for use for disinfection, it undergoes a significant amount of testing for efficacy, and the proper method of use is very important to achieve the full benefit.

Hepatitis C. Hepatitis C accounts for 15% of cases of hepatitis each year. Its transmission is through the parenteral route, but it is far more virulent than hepatitis B. Only 20% of infected persons will develop symptoms, which are similar to those of hepatitis A and B, although jaundice is uncommon. Approximately 2% of people in the United States have been exposed to the virus.[23]

Chronic hepatitis occurs in 55–85% of persons infected with the virus, regardless of the presence of acute hepatitis. Of those patients with chronic hepatitis, 70% will develop chronic liver failure, and 1–5% will die as a result of their disease. Hepatitis C is associated with liver cancer and is the most common reason for liver transplant in the United States.[23]

Hepatitis C has been falling in incidence, from an estimated 300,000 new cases in 1989 to fewer than 30,000 new cases in 2003. The most common source of transmission of hepatitis C before 1990 was blood transfusions, but routine testing of donated blood has all but eliminated that source. Shared needles among IV drug users are currently the most common vectors. Sexual intercourse and transmission from an infected mother to her child are also common.[23]

There is no vaccine against hepatitis C. There are currently 2.7 million cases of chronic hepatitis C in the United States. Factors leading to more severe disease include alcohol consumption, age over 40 when first infected, concurrent chronic hepatitis B infection, and HIV coinfection.

The greatest risk to healthcare workers is through a needle stick. Percutaneous puncture with a hollow needle that was used to draw blood from an infected patient carries a 3–10% risk of transmission. Due to the lack of vaccine and the risk of development of chronic disease, healthcare workers should be especially wary of contracting this disease.[22]

Treatment of patients with hepatitis C is supportive. Hospital care of patients acutely infected with hepatitis C includes interferon and ribavirin, the combination of which significantly decreases the progression to chronic disease. Careful monitoring of liver function is also necessary. DOT 5-11.22

Hepatitis D. There are believed to be at least three other hepatitis viruses, which account for less than 3% of all cases in the United States. The first of these, the "delta virus," causes hepatitis D. The delta virus is an incomplete virus and cannot cause disease on its own. However, when coupled with hepatitis B infection, the delta virus can increase the severity of disease. Patients who are infected with hepatitis B and D at the same time are more likely to develop acute liver failure. Patients with chronic hepatitis B who become infected with the delta virus are more likely to develop cirrhosis.[24]

The symptoms of hepatitis D are similar to but more severe than symptoms of hepatitis B. There is no vaccine although vaccination against hepatitis B prior to infection with the delta virus will prevent disease. Treatment of patients with hepatitis D is supportive. DOT 5-11.23

Hepatitis E.   The hepatitis E virus causes hepatitis E. Signs and symptoms are similar to hepatitis A, and transmission is by the fecal-oral route. Hepatitis E is most commonly caused by drinking contaminated water, and disease tends to be more severe in women during the third trimester of pregnancy. Hepatitis E is endemic to Southeast Asia and North Africa and is rare in the United States. Treatment is supportive, and there is no vaccine.[25] DOT 5-11.24

Hepatitis G.   The hepatitis G virus has recently been identified. It is controversial whether infection is associated with clinical disease. Transmission is through the parenteral route, and there is no vaccine or treatment.[26]

Diseases Spread by Airborne Transmission

The following diseases are spread by airborne droplets. They are of chief concern to the paramedic for the risk of occupational exposure through close contact in an enclosed space (i.e., the back of an ambulance).

Tuberculosis

Tuberculosis is one of the greatest threats to public health in the United States. The incidence of tuberculosis has been steadily dropping since surveillance was started, from a high of 80,000 cases in 1953 to nearly 15,000 new cases in 2003. It is estimated that 10 to 15 million Americans have been infected with tuberculosis at one time or another. Worldwide, approximately 2 billion people are infected, with 3 million deaths a year attributable to active tuberculosis.[27]

Factors that contribute to an increased risk of tuberculosis include HIV infection, immigration from countries where TB is endemic, and living in cramped quarters with infected individuals (including homeless shelters). In recent years, immigrants have comprised over half of all new TB cases in the United States.

Tuberculosis is caused by the bacterium *Mycobacterium tuberculosis,* which is spread by respiratory droplets. Inhaled bacteria multiply in the lungs but are controlled by a T cell mediated response. Approximately 5% of all infected persons will develop clinical tuberculosis in the first weeks after infection while another 5% will develop active disease later in life.

Ninety percent of all infected patients will not develop any symptoms.[28]

Since T cells mediate the control of tuberculosis, persons with defective immune systems, particularly those with HIV disease, will be less likely to prevent active tuberculosis. In fact, the risk of developing active tuberculosis is 10% *per year* in HIV-infected patients.[29] Other conditions that increase the risk of developing active TB include substance abuse, diabetes, low body weight, and immunodeficiency from prolonged corticosteroid use, cancer, or end-stage renal disease.

Active tuberculosis disease most commonly occurs in the lungs and is called **pulmonary tuberculosis.** Untreated pulmonary tuberculosis carries a mortality of 50%. The use of antitubercular medications has decreased the mortality rate to 7%.[30] Tuberculosis can also spread to other body systems, causing meningitis, pericarditis, arthritis, bone infection (especially in the spine, called Pott's disease), lymph node infection (called scrofula in the neck), and disseminated or "miliary" tuberculosis. Infections outside the lungs are called **extrapulmonary tuberculosis.**

Symptoms of pulmonary tuberculosis include cough, fever, weight loss, and night sweats. **Hemoptysis** (blood in the sputum) is common. Tuberculosis should be suspected in at-risk patients with the above symptoms, especially if the symptoms have persisted for longer than three weeks. Symptoms of extrapulmonary tuberculosis are specific to the body systems affected and can include altered mental status, chest pain, bone pain, or localized swelling in the neck.

Patients who have been infected with *M. tuberculosis* will mount an immune response in the form of antibodies that can be detected by the Mantoux skin test. In this test, a small amount of tuberculosis antigen (purified protein derivative, or PPD) is injected into the skin. If antitubercular antibodies are present, redness and swelling will develop at the site of injection in 48 to 72 hours. A positive skin test indicates a history of infection but does not indicate active disease. Other tests used for diagnosing TB include chest x-ray and sputum culture.

Tuberculosis infection is classified as either active or latent. Active pulmonary tuberculosis is characterized by the presence of symptoms and indicates that the patient is capable of spreading disease. Latent infection means the bacteria are present in the body but are causing no symptoms. Patients with latent tuberculosis cannot spread the disease to others. It is generally believed that patients with extrapulmonary tuberculosis are not contagious.

Treatment regimens for tuberculosis last from six to twelve months due to the slow growth of the bacterium. Prophylactic treatment is often given to people after their skin test becomes positive to prevent development of active disease. Prophylaxis involves a six-month course of isoniazid (also known as INH). INH can cause paresthesias, seizures, nausea, vomiting, and hepatitis. INH also interferes with the metabolism of alcohol, resulting in violent nausea and vomiting.[31]

Due to the severity of side effects from prophylaxis and the mortality of untreated disease, it is imperative that healthcare workers protect themselves from infection. Infection control is as simple as wearing a NIOSH-approved N-95 particulate filter mask.[32] Since it is difficult to differentiate tuberculosis from other respiratory diseases in the prehospital setting, paramedics should place a mask on any patient with a cough and should wear masks when dealing with these patients.

Paramedics transporting suspected cases of tuberculosis must notify the receiving facility before arrival. This will give the emergency department staff time to prepare an isolation room for the protection of their other patients and themselves.

Patients with tuberculosis are frequently treated as outpatients although certain populations (patients who are institutionalized, jailed, or living in homeless shelters) are frequently admitted to the hospital to prevent spread of the disease to others in the community. If a patient is diagnosed with active tuberculosis, treatment involves multiple antibiotics to cover resistant organisms. The greatest risk of tuberculosis is multidrug resistance, in which the bacterium is not susceptible to most of the antibiotics used to treat TB. Close monitoring of patients for compliance with antibiotics is mandatory. DOT 5-11.25

Meningococcal Meningitis

Meningitis is an inflammation of the **meninges,** the linings of the brain and spinal cord. Viruses, tuberculosis, fungi, and multiple bacteria can cause meningitis. However, the most virulent and dangerous agent that causes meningitis is the bacterium *Neisseria meningitidis,* also known as meningococcus.

Meningococcus is spread by respiratory droplets and colonizes the mucosa of the nasopharynx. At any given time, 2–10% of the population is colonized with meningococcus, and there is evidence that almost all people have been exposed to the bacterium at some time during their lives.[33]

For reasons that are unclear, meningococcus occasionally invades the nasal mucosa, traveling to the meninges. This invasive behavior tends to occur in clusters of patients. Populations at risk include people living in close quarters, such as college students in dorms and military personnel in barracks.

Meningococcal meningitis develops quickly, with sudden onset of fever, headache, and neck stiffness. A petechial rash is common and is an ominous sign. Patients occasionally develop septic shock (known as Waterhouse-Friderichsen syndrome), characterized by adrenal insufficiency, disseminated intravascular coagulation, and coma. The disease can progress from onset of symptoms to death in as little as six hours.

The physical exam will often reveal fever, altered mental status, and a rash. The muscles of the back of the neck may be stiff (called **nuchal rigidity**). **Kernig's** sign is an inability to extend the knee when the hip is flexed to 90 degrees due to irritation of the meninges from the infection. **Brudzinski's** sign is involuntary flexion of the hips when the neck is flexed. The combination of these symptoms is referred to as **meningismus.**

Children from ages six months to two years are especially susceptible to infection but have less specific symptoms. Children with fever, vomiting, and signs of altered mental status (lethargy or irritability) should be considered to be at risk for having meningitis. Meningismus does not usually occur in children. If the cranial sutures have not yet closed, the fontanelles may be bulging.

Patients suspected of having meningitis must be immediately isolated. Facemasks and shields should be worn. Special care should be paid to body substance isolation. Paramedics should pay particular attention to patients' fluid status. Hospital treatment of meningitis involves aggressive fluid resuscitation and parenteral antibiotics.

Paramedics transporting suspected cases of meningitis must notify the receiving facility before arrival. This will give the emergency department staff time to prepare an isolation room for the protection of their other patients and themselves.

Paramedics who are exposed to cases of meningococcal meningitis should be treated with prophylactic antibiotics to prevent development of the disease.

A meningococcus vaccine exists and is effective in preventing the disease. However, due to the low incidence of disease in the population, routine immunization is not recommended.[34] DOT 5-11.26

Other Causes of Meningitis

Streptococcus pneumonia is the second most common cause of meningitis in adults and is also the most common cause of pneumonia in adults and the most common cause of inner ear infections in children. It is spread by respiratory droplets although contact with patients with streptococcal meningitis rarely results in disease in the caregiver. Universal precautions and body substance isolation should be initiated.

Haemophilus influenza type B used to be the most common cause of bacterial meningitis in children. However, the introduction of an *H. flu* vaccine in 1981 has all but eliminated the disease. *H. flu* meningitis in adults is relatively rare and presents similarly to other forms of meningitis.

Viruses, fungi, and tuberculosis can all cause meningitis. Signs and symptoms are similar to bacterial meningitis but are often less severe with a less rapid onset. These forms of meningitis are not considered to be communicable. However, since it is impossible to differentiate these forms of meningitis from bacterial meningitis in the field, universal precautions should always be taken for any patient suspected to have meningitis. DOT 5-11.27

Pneumonia

Pneumonia is an infection in the alveoli of the lungs. Pneumonia is frequently bacterial, and causative agents include *Streptococcus pneumoniae, Mycoplasma pneumoniae, Staphylococcus aureus, Haemophilus influenza, Klebsiella pneumoniae, Moraxella catarrhalis,* and the *Legionella* species. There are also numerous viruses and fungi that cause pneumonia. Tuberculosis is considered to be a special form of bacterial pneumonia and is described previously.

Pneumonia is generally spread from person to person through respiratory droplets. Susceptibility to disease is related to underlying health status and pulmonary function. Conditions that decrease the ability of the lungs to clear infection include chronic lung disease, smoking, influenza, and aspiration. Age and nutritional status also contribute to increased susceptibility. Other conditions that increase the risk of pneumonia are listed in Box 33-3.

Pneumonia may present with sudden onset of fever and chills or may develop slowly. Cough productive of yellow-green sputum and pleuritic chest pain are common symptoms. Treatment in the prehospital setting is supportive. Respiratory isolation precautions should be used to protect the paramedic. Hospital evaluation includes chest x-ray, and treatment usually involves antibiotic therapy.

There is a vaccine for streptococcal pneumonia, but immunization is generally reserved for patients with a risk for pneumonia, especially those without a spleen, young patients with chronic disease or immunosuppression, and the elderly. Routine vaccination of healthcare workers is not recommended.[35] DOT 5-11.28

Viral Diseases of Childhood

There are many viral diseases that typically affect children. Routine immunization against these diseases has made them uncommon, and it is unlikely that you will see them. However, the paramedic must be aware of the necessity of vaccination and the risk of disease in unimmunized populations.

Routine childhood immunizations have been performed since the 1960s and have resulted in the near eradication of many diseases. Most states have laws requiring immunization in children who are starting school. However, some populations are not routinely immunized for social, economic, or religious reasons. The paramedic must ask about immunization status when assessing any child. DOT 5-11.31

Varicella (Chickenpox)

A **pox** is any disease that causes **vesicles** (a rash characterized by small collections of fluid or pus). The most common form of pox is chickenpox and is still common in the United States. The name is believed to come from the fact that the pustules of chickenpox resemble chickpeas (and in fact has nothing to do with chickens) (Figure 33-5).

Chickenpox is caused by the varicella zoster virus, which is one of the herpes viruses. The virus is transmitted through airborne droplets and can also be transmitted by the fluid from the vesicles. After an

BOX 33-3 \ Conditions Leading to Increased Susceptibility to Pneumonia

Sickle cell anemia

Cardiovascular disease

Absence of a spleen (surgically removed or nonfunctional)

Diabetes mellitus

Chronic renal failure

HIV infection

Organ transplantation

Multiple myeloma

Lymphoma

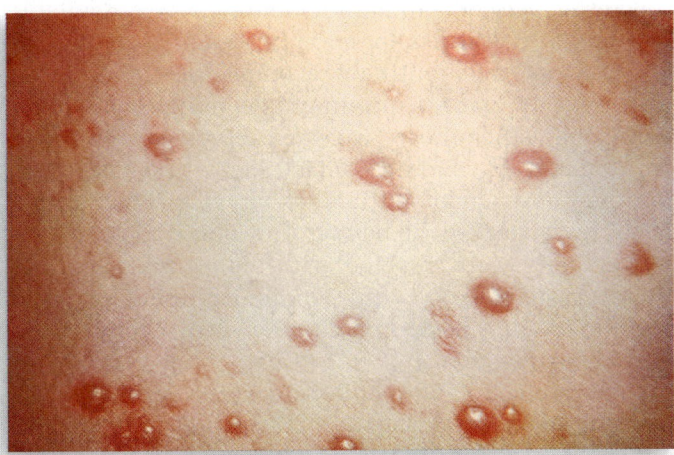

Figure 33-5 The most common form of pox is chickenpox, which is still common in the United States.

incubation period of one to three weeks, patients will begin to have nonspecific symptoms such as fever, malaise, and signs of an upper respiratory infection. The rash begins as red marks on the trunk that fill with fluid, rupture, and scab over. The vesicles are painful and then become intensely itchy as they heal. The entire course of symptoms typically lasts one week. Patients are contagious from one or two days before the rash appears until all pustules have scabbed over. Infection with chickenpox confers lifelong immunity.

Prior to 1996, there were 4 million cases of chickenpox in the United States every year, mostly in children under age 15. The vaccine that was introduced in 1996 is being added to the routine immunization schedule of most states and has reduced the rate of chickenpox by approximately one-half.[36]

Although the disease is painful, there are few sequelae in children. Adults who never had the disease in childhood are susceptible to infection. Chickenpox in adults is more complicated, occasionally causing pneumonia, encephalitis, and death. Pregnant women who have never been infected or immunized should be especially careful. Infection with chickenpox during the first six months of pregnancy can result in congenital varicella, causing limb deformities and neurologic deficits in the child.

Children with chickenpox require isolation from other children, unimmunized adults, and pregnant women. Since the complication rate is so low, transportation to the hospital is rarely necessary. If you are transporting a suspected chickenpox case, you must notify the emergency department, so proper isolation can be prepared. Paramedics should use BSI, including gloves and masks if the child is coughing.

Adults with chicken pox are usually much sicker than children and should be transported for further medical care. Similar precautions, including hospital notification, should be taken. Hospital care involves fluid resuscitation and treatment with the antiviral agent acyclovir. Varicella immunoglobulin is also available for populations at risk for complications.

Vaccination is routinely recommended for children under age 12 and for unimmunized adults who are at risk (such as healthcare workers). If you have not had chickenpox, you should contact your physician to test for the presence of antibodies. It is estimated that 70–90% of people who believe they never had chickenpox actually were infected with the virus but had no symptoms and do not require immunization. The risk of immunization is development of a rash or, occasionally, onset of active chickenpox.[36]

After infection with chickenpox, the varicella virus tends to survive in the nerves of the spinal cord but does not cause symptoms. Occasionally, this virus can reactivate, causing a disease called **zoster** or, more commonly, **shingles.** This name is derived from the Latin word "cingulus" meaning girdle, based on the belt-like rash caused by the disease. Shingles will occur in up to 20% of patients who have previously had chickenpox. Reactivation of varicella is more common with advanced age and immunodeficiency. The disease begins as nonspecific, burning pain, usually on the trunk, followed by outbreak of rash similar to chickenpox. The rash is limited to one dermatome of the skin (most commonly seen as a band on one side of the trunk). Patients with zoster are contagious until all pustules have scabbed over. Shingles is exquisitely painful, and symptoms occasionally persist for months or years. Shingles on the face is particularly dangerous due to the risk of damage to the eyes. The effect vaccination will have on shingles is unclear. DOT 5-11.32

Mumps

Mumps is caused by the mumps virus. The virus is spread by respiratory droplets and has an incubation period of two to four weeks. The disease typically causes swelling of the parotid glands in the cheeks, giving a chipmunk-like appearance (Figure 33-6). Complications are more common in adults and include meningitis, inflammation of the testicles with subsequent sterility, pancreatitis, and deafness.

Mumps vaccine has been available since 1945 and has been in routine use since the late 1960s. The incidence of disease has dropped from 212,000 cases in 1967 to 213 reported cases in 2003 although there was a surge in the spring and summer of 2006, mostly in the midwest. Vaccination is usually delivered as part of the **MMR** (measles, mumps, and rubella) shot.[37]

Paramedics should be immunized against mumps if they have not already been immunized in childhood. Paramedics treating a suspected case of mumps should wear gloves and facemasks and be scrupulous about washing their hands.[38] DOT 5-11.33

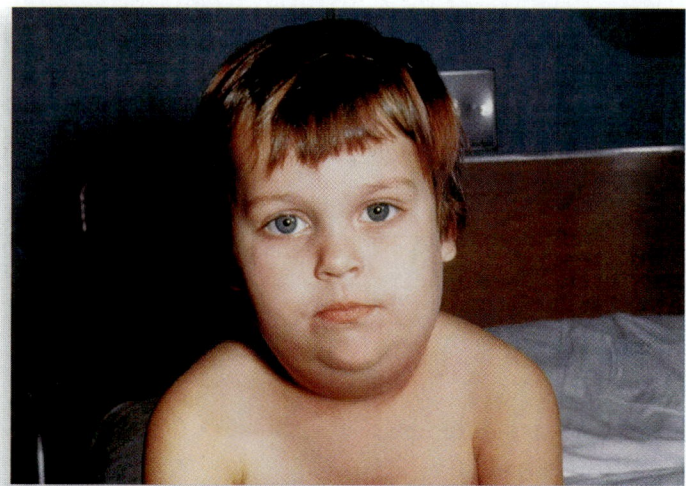

Figure 33-6 Mumps typically causes swelling of the parotid glands in the cheeks, giving a chipmunk-like appearance.

Rubella (German Measles)

Rubella is caused by the rubella virus and is also called German measles because it was first reported in Germany. The virus is spread through respiratory droplets and has an incubation period of two weeks. Symptoms include low-grade fever, swollen lymph nodes, and a generalized rash. Symptoms usually last three days, and the disease is without complications. Adults with rubella frequently experience arthritis that resolves with the disease. Patients are contagious from one week before the onset of rash to one week after the rash has resolved.

Rubella is passed through the placenta and causes congenital rubella syndrome. This syndrome can be devastating, causing deafness, blindness, mental retardation, and occasionally death. Infants with congenital rubella syndrome may be contagious for up to one year after birth.

The rubella vaccine was licensed in 1969 and is routinely given with measles and mumps vaccines as part of the MMR immunization. The incidence of rubella has fallen from 58,000 cases in 1969 to 18 cases reported in 2003.[39]

Patients should be treated symptomatically, with special attention to universal precautions, including facemasks.

Paramedics who are unaware of their immunization status should be screened for the presence of antibodies. Those who are found to be unprotected should receive the vaccine before beginning work.[38] DOT 5-11.34

Rubeola (Measles)

Measles is caused by the measles virus and is sometimes referred to as rubeola. The virus is spread by respiratory droplets and has an incubation period of two weeks. Symptoms begin with a fever that gradually increases over two days to a high of 103° to 105°. After the fever peaks, symptoms occur, including conjunctivitis, runny nose, and cough. A red, bumpy rash begins at the hairline, spreads downward to the trunk, and lasts for about a week (Figure 33-7). Small, white spots appear on the mucous membranes of the mouth and are called **Koplik's spots.** Complications of measles include diarrhea, otitis, pneumonia, and encephalitis. Death occurs in 0.1% of cases.

The measles vaccine was licensed in 1963 and decreased the incidence of measles from 500,000 cases with 500 deaths a year in the 1960s to a total of 44 cases and no deaths in 2002. Immunization is achieved as part of the MMR vaccine.[40]

Patients with measles are treated symptomatically, with special care towards universal precautions and facemask use.

Paramedics who are unsure of their immunization status should be tested for the presence of antibodies.

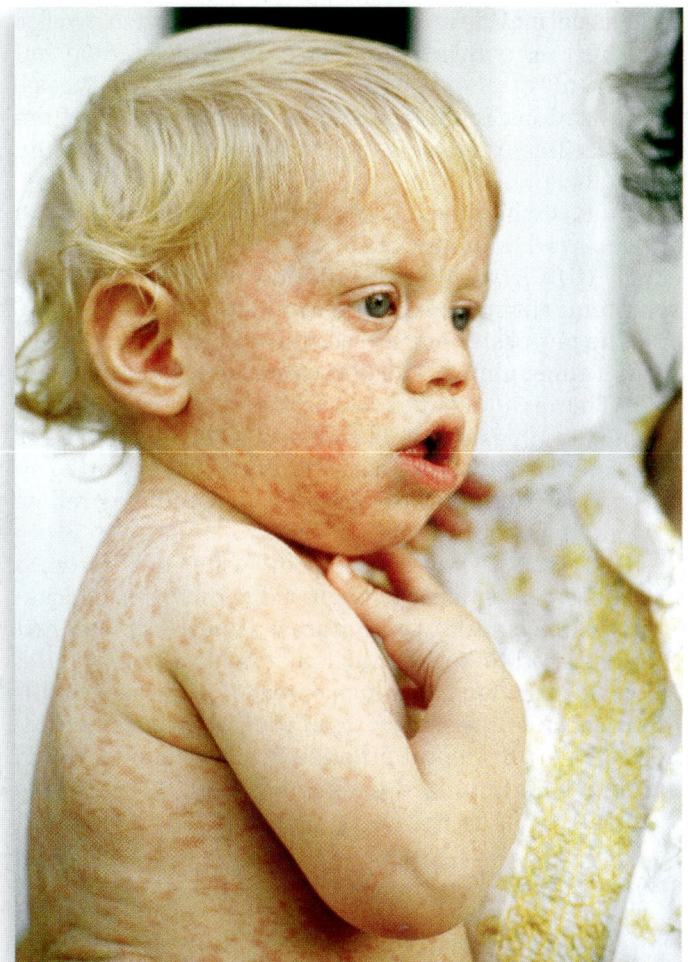

Figure 33-7 Measles is sometimes referred to as rubeola. Symptoms begin with a fever. After the fever peaks, other symptoms occur, including conjunctivitis, runny nose, and cough. A red, bumpy rash begins at the hairline, spreads downward to the trunk, and lasts for about a week.

Unimmunized paramedics should receive the vaccine prior to beginning work.[38] DOT 5-11.35, 5-11.36

Pertussis (Whooping Cough)

Although **pertussis** is not a viral disease, it is included in this section because it is a childhood disease that has been all but eliminated by routine immunization. It is caused by the bacterium *Bordetella pertussis* that is spread by respiratory droplets. Symptoms occur after an incubation period of one to two weeks.

The disease has three stages. The first, or catarrhal, stage, presents similar to the common cold, with runny nose, cough, and sneezing. This stage lasts one or two weeks, with the cough becoming more severe. The second, or paroxysmal, stage is characterized by bursts of coughing followed by a long inspiratory effort. The distinctive "whoop" sound made during this inspiration gives the disease its common name "whooping cough."

This stage may last anywhere from one to ten weeks. The third, or convalescent, stage, involves gradual improvement of the cough over two or three weeks. Complications include pneumonia and seizures from hypoxia. Twenty percent of all cases of pertussis require hospitalization.

Infants who develop pertussis are often too weak to create a "whoop" and will instead have a persistent cough with irritability. Adults have much less severe symptoms than children and rarely whoop.

The pertussis vaccine was introduced in the 1940s. At that time, almost 200,000 cases were reported each year. The incidence fell to a low of 3,000 cases a year during the 1980s. For unclear reasons, the incidence has been increasing, with nearly 12,000 cases reported in 2003. Many of these cases are in adults and may reflect a decrease in protection over time.[41]

Paramedics should be careful when dealing with patients with whooping cough, using universal precautions and facemasks. Unimmunized adults can contract the disease, but the clinical picture is usually mild. However, infected adults can spread the disease to children. Vaccination is performed routinely during childhood as part of the diphtheria-pertussis-tetanus (DPT) vaccine. Unimmunized paramedics should receive the vaccination.[42] DOT 5-11.37

Other Viral Diseases

The following diseases are caused by viruses and are prevalent in adults. Treatment is generally supportive, and few vaccines exist to prevent the diseases.

Influenza

Influenza is caused by the influenza virus, of which there are two main classes (influenza A and influenza B), with each class having several strains. A third class, influenza C, causes only mild disease and is generally not considered a health threat. Influenza is spread through respiratory droplets but can survive on environmental surfaces for several hours. Influenza has an incubation period of one to four days. Adults become contagious the day before symptoms occur and remain contagious for a week.

Symptoms of the flu include fever, runny nose, cough, body aches, and nausea. Symptoms typically last five to seven days and resolve with few complications in the healthy adult. Elderly patients and young children are at increased risk of complications, including pneumonia, sepsis, and death.

Influenza usually occurs during the winter months but can occur in late fall and early spring. Each season sees the spread of new strains of flu, and it is difficult to predict which strain will cause the majority of cases. Some strains are more virulent and cause more severe disease than others, resulting in years with more cases of serious influenza. Most cases of influenza are diagnosed clinically without laboratory confirmation, so it is impossible to determine exact prevalence. However, it is believed that there are 36,000 deaths a year due to influenza, mostly in the elderly population.[43]

Infection confers lifelong immunity to the particular strain that caused the disease. However, given the large number of strains and the frequent mutation of current strains, immunity is not considered protection against future disease.

Paramedics should be wary of influenza during the winter months and should practice universal precautions, including wearing facemasks, when contacting patients suspected of having the flu. Due to the survival of the virus on environmental surfaces, thorough disinfection of the ambulance is necessary after transportation. Care of the patient is symptomatic, with attention paid to hydration status.

Each year, the Centers for Disease Control and Prevention create a vaccine against two strains of influenza A and one strain of influenza B. This vaccine is produced before flu season begins, and the strains are chosen based on epidemiologic data from the last year's flu season. In essence, the CDC is making the best possible guess about which strains will be prevalent in the upcoming flu season.[44]

Immunization is recommended for persons at risk, particularly children, the elderly, and patients with chronic medical conditions. Healthcare workers should also be immunized, due to the risk of contacting patients with influenza, the risk of spreading influenza to patients at risk, and the large number of workdays missed due to illness.

Several antivirals exist to treat influenza. Amantadine (Symmetrel® or Symadine®) and rimantadine (Flumadine®) will shorten the duration of influenza A when given within two days of onset of symptoms. Zanamivir (Relenza®) and oseltamivir (Tamiflu®) will decrease the duration of symptoms of influenza A and influenza B. These medications are usually reserved for mitigating the effects of outbreaks in institutional settings such as nursing homes. DOT 5-11.38

Infectious Mononucleosis

Mononucleosis (or "mono") is caused by the Epstein-Barr virus (EBV), part of the herpes virus family. This virus was isolated from Burkitt's lymphoma tumors in 1964 by Drs. Michael Anthony Epstein and Yvonne Barr.

EBV is found in high concentrations in the saliva and is frequently transmitted by kissing (thus the common name "kissing disease"). Transmission through airborne droplets or close contact is not common. Children are infected with EBV by contact with infected care providers but rarely experience symptoms. Infection with EBV confers lifelong immunity, and there is evidence that 95% of adults have been infected at one time during their lives.[45]

Infectious mononucleosis in adults causes sore throat, swollen tonsils, fever, and swollen lymph nodes. Occasionally, swelling of the liver and spleen can lead to abdominal pain. Symptoms last up to two months but are rarely debilitating. EBV persists in cells of the immune system and has been implicated in the development of the cancers Burkitt's lymphoma and nasopharyngeal carcinoma. For reasons that are unclear, these cancers are rare in the United States.

Healthcare workers are generally not at risk for infection because of the high level of immunity in the adult population. Paramedics should, however, wear gloves and avoid direct contact with a patient's saliva.

There is currently no vaccine available for Epstein-Barr virus. DOT 5-11.39

Herpes Simplex Virus Type 1

Herpes simplex virus type 1 (HSV-1) causes painful blisters called cold sores on the lips, face, and oropharynx (Figure 33-8). HSV-1 is also implicated in infections of the hands, feet, and genitals. Conjunctival infection is also possible. HSV-1 can cause meningitis or encephalitis, manifesting with fever, headache, and altered mental status. The virus is spread by contact with saliva of carriers of the disease.

HSV-1 is common, affecting up to 90% of the adult population. HSV-1 remains in the body, causing sporadic outbreaks for the rest of the victim's life. Patients are contagious whether or not blisters are present.

Most infections with HSV-1 are self-limited and require no treatment. HSV-1 conjunctivitis carries the risk of permanent damage to the eye but is difficult to differentiate from other forms of conjunctivitis in the prehospital setting. Patients with frequent outbreaks may be treated with antiherpetic medications such as acyclovir (Zovirax), valcyclovir (Valtrex), or ganciclovir (Cytovene).

Paramedics should use universal precautions when dealing with patients with cold sores and should avoid contact with saliva in all patients. Proper hand washing is mandatory after patient contact. Paramedics with cold sores may continue to work, but should pay close attention to washing their hands, especially after eating or touching their mouths. DOT 5-11.40

Other Viral Diseases

There exist a large number of viruses that cause clinical disease. Many of these cause nonspecific illnesses of the upper respiratory tract, and are termed "upper respiratory infections" or URI. These diseases are spread through respiratory droplets, close contact, and contaminated surfaces. Symptoms include runny nose, congestion, cough, fever, and sore throat. The disease is self-limited and usually resolves without complications.

Paramedics should exercise judgment when dealing with patients with URI signs and symptoms. Gloves and hand washing are mandatory, and masks may be worn if the patient is coughing.

Viruses that are implicated in the nonspecific URI include the coronaviruses, rhinoviruses, myxoviruses, echoviruses, coxsackieviruses, adenoviruses, parainfluenza viruses, and respiratory syncitial virus. DOT 5-11.41

Sexually Transmitted Diseases

Sexually transmitted diseases (STDs) are transmitted through sexual contact. Human immunodeficiency virus and hepatitis B and C are often included in this category but are discussed in the section on bloodborne pathogens.

Syphilis

Syphilis is caused by the bacterium *Treponema pallidum*, which is found in high concentrations in the skin lesions of active syphilis, semen, blood, saliva, and vaginal secretions. Transmission is through contact with contaminated fluids or skin lesions. Transmission through needle stick is theoretically possible but has not been documented. It is estimated that only about 30% of exposures will result in infection.

Syphilis was once widespread in the United States, with over 500,000 cases reported per year in the 1940s. The introduction of antibiotics and public education about STDs has reduced that rate to less than 7,000 cases in 2003.[46]

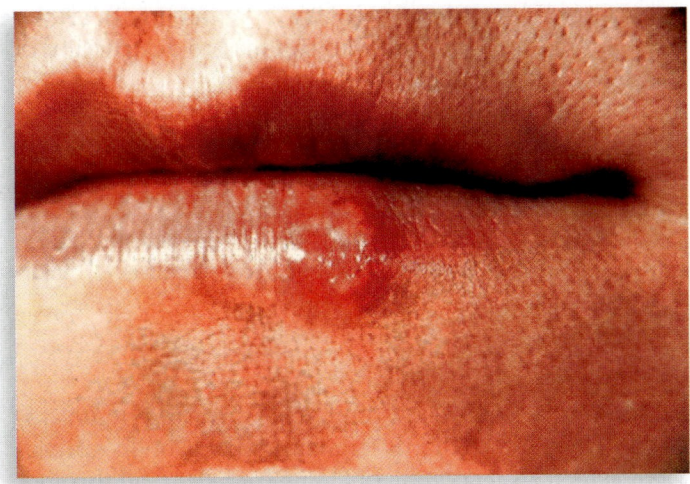

Figure 33-8 Herpes simplex virus type 1 (HSV1) causes painful blisters, commonly called cold sores, on the lips, face, and oropharynx.

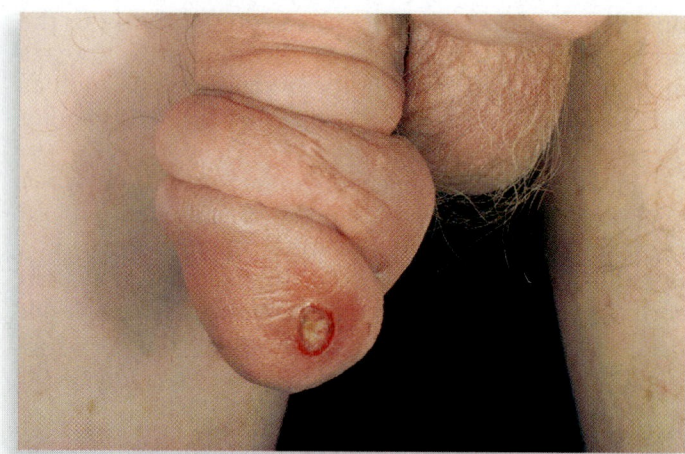

Figure 33-9 Primary syphilis occurs 3 to 6 weeks after initial contact and presents with a painless ulceration of the genitals called a chancre.

The clinical aspects of syphilis infection are divided into four stages. Primary syphilis occurs three to six weeks after initial contact and presents with a painless ulceration of the genitals called a **chancre** (Figure 33-9). This ulcer contains high concentrations of bacterium and is the main source of sexual transmission to others. The chancre will heal without treatment in three to six weeks.

Secondary syphilis begins approximately six weeks after the chancre has disappeared. The signs of secondary syphilis include a flat, red, raised rash on the palms of the hands and soles of the feet. Patients also develop **condyloma lata,** large, wart-like lesions in the inguinal area that are highly contagious. Rashes may occur in other parts of the body. Secondary syphilis lasts about six weeks and resolves spontaneously.

Latent syphilis is that period after secondary syphilis during which the patient has no symptoms. Two-thirds of all patients will remain asymptomatic for the rest of their lives. The other third will develop tertiary syphilis, which is characterized by skin lesions, cardiovascular complications, and neurologic disorders. The signs and symptoms of tertiary syphilis may present several decades after secondary syphilis.

The classic skin lesion of tertiary syphilis is called a **gumma.** These are large, painless ulcerations that occur on the skin. Gummas can also occur on bone, causing deep, gnawing pain. The cardiovascular effects of tertiary syphilis include destruction of the connective tissue in the aorta, leading to aortic dissection. Damage to blood vessels in the brain can lead to vascular obstruction and progressive deterioration of the mental status.

Neurosyphilis is characterized by high levels of *T. pallidum* in the cerebrospinal fluid. Symptoms include dementia, blindness, numbness, decreased coordination, and paralysis. Unrecognized neurosyphilis can be mistaken for senile dementia.

The treatment of syphilis is simple, with a single shot of penicillin. Patients allergic to penicillin can be given erythromycin or doxycycline. Treatment is only effective in killing the bacteria; the long-term effects of tertiary syphilis, once they have developed, are generally irreversible.

Paramedics should use universal precautions when dealing with suspected cases of syphilis. There is no immunization available. DOT 5-22.42

Gonorrhea

Gonorrhea is caused by the bacterium *Neisseria gonorrheae.* Gonorrhea typically affects the genital tract but can colonize the oropharynx or rectum or can result in disseminated disease. Transmission is through direct contact with the purulent exudates that form on infected mucous membranes. There are numerous strains of *N. gonorrheae,* meaning that the immunity conferred by infection will not prevent infection with a different strain.

It is estimated that 650,000 cases of gonorrhea occur in the United States each year.[47]

Symptoms in men include a burning sensation in the urethra, usually accompanied by a greenish discharge. Women may have vaginal burning or discharge, but the majority of women are asymptomatic. Women are less likely to be treated for gonorrhea since they do not experience symptoms, which contributes to the spread of the disease. In women, the bacteria may spread up from the cervix to the uterus and Fallopian tubes, causing a severe infection known as **pelvic inflammatory disease (PID).** PID carries the risk of abscess formation and disseminated infection and causes scarring in the Fallopian tubes that can lead to ectopic pregnancy or sterility.

Gonorrheal pharyngitis can occur after oral sex with an infected person and presents as a sore throat with fever. Gonorrhea infection is also associated with arthritis, usually of the knee, which can lead to destruction of the joint if left untreated.

Gonorrhea is treated with antibiotics, usually as an outpatient. Cases involving pelvic inflammatory disease and arthritis are frequently admitted for IV antibiotics.

Routine, universal precautions are necessary when treating patients with gonorrhea. No vaccine is available. DOT 5-11.43

Chlamydia

Chlamydia is caused by the bacterium *Chlamydia trachomatis.* Chlamydia is transmitted through unprotected sexual intercourse but can also be spread through clothing, towels, and hand-to-hand transfer.

The symptoms of infection with chlamydia are generally indistinguishable from gonorrhea. One-quarter of infected men and up to 95% of infected women will experience no symptoms. Chlamydia is also a cause of pelvic inflammatory disease, with complications similar to gonorrhea. Chlamydia can cause conjunctivitis in newborn babies by transmission from the mother during delivery. Chlamydia conjunctivitis is the leading cause of preventable blindness in the world.

There are an estimated 3 million new cases of chlamydia in the United States each year.[48]

Chlamydia is treated with antibiotics. Infection does not confer immunity, and no vaccine is available. Paramedics should use universal precautions when dealing with cases of suspected chlamydia. DOT 5-11.44

Herpes Simplex Virus Type 2

HSV-2 is genetically similar to HSV-1 and causes painful blisters. HSV-2 is less virulent than HSV-1 and generally causes genital lesions (Figure 33-10). Transmission is through close contact. Over one million new cases are diagnosed each year. Treatment is similar to HSV-1. DOT 5-11.45

Human Papillomavirus (Genital Warts)

Human papillomavirus (HPV) is spread by direct contact. More than 100 types of HPV have been identified and patients may or may not have symptoms associated with the infection. Types 6 and 11 cause visible genital warts. Other HPV types, such as 16 and 18, do not produce visible genital warts. These types, which may be found with a cervical exam (specifically a Pap test), are associated with precancerous cervical cell changes and cervical cancer. A vaccination now exists that can provide protection for some types of HPV that cause cervical cancer and should be considered for all sexually active women.

Parasitic Infestations

Parasites are animals that live in or on and feed off of another animal with no benefit to the host. The presence of a parasite is referred to as an **infestation** as opposed to an infection. Most parasitic infestations are rare in the United States and are beyond the scope of this discussion. However, two common infestations are mentioned due to the risk of transmission to the healthcare provider.

Scabies

Scabies is infestation of the skin with the insect *Sarcoptes scabei*. Scabies is generally transmitted through close contact with infested persons although they survive in bedding and clothes for up to 24 hours. Scabies can burrow into the skin in a matter of minutes.

The latent period of a person's first scabies infection is two to six weeks although subsequent infestations result in symptoms in a matter of hours. Symptoms are related to localized reactions to mites and eggs in the skin and include intense itching, with redness at the site of insect burrows. Scabies tend to live in the web spaces between fingers and toes and the lower abdomen or genital region (Figure 33-11). Infestation in infants may involve the head, the palms of the hands, and the soles of the feet.

Scabies is commonly treated with permethrin (Elemite) or lindane (Kwell), which are creams that are spread on the skin. Infestations may require multiple treatments.

Infestation with scabies does not provide any protective immunity. There is no vaccine available.

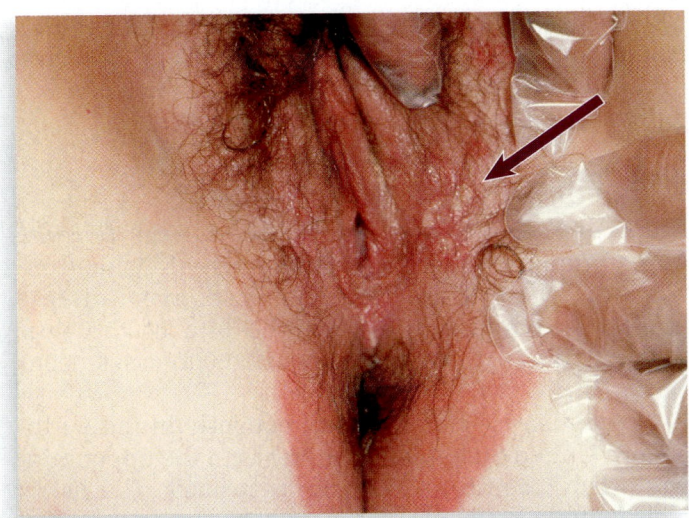

Figure 33-10   HSV2 is genetically similar to HSV1 and causes painful genital blisters.

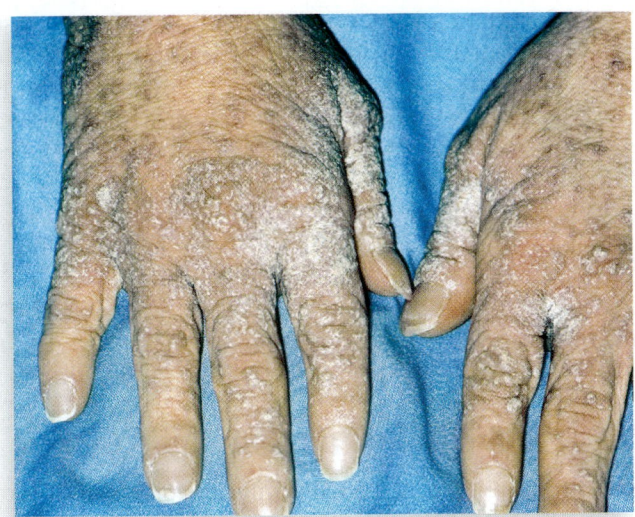

Figure 33-11   Scabies tend to live in the web spaces between fingers and toes.

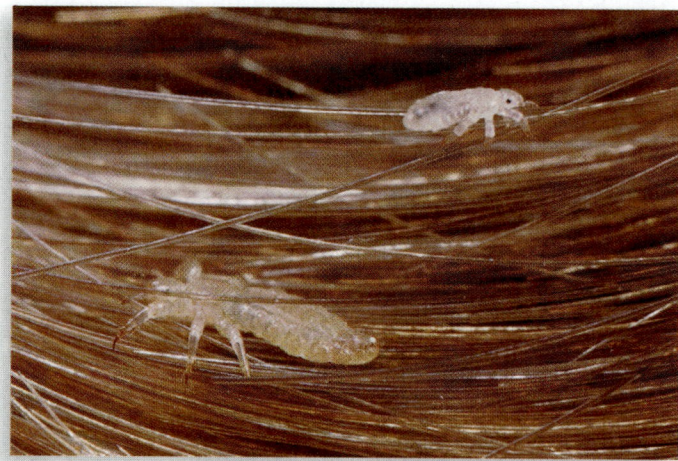

Figure 33-12 Lice are a collection of insects that infest human skin. *Pediculis humanus capitis* is commonly known as head lice and is found in the hair of the scalp.

Prehospital care involves wearing gloves and avoiding direct contact with bedding or clothing of infested patients. All linens should be bagged after use and disposed of appropriately. DOT 5-11.46

Lice

Lice are a collection of insects that infest human skin. *Pediculis humanus capitis* is also known as head lice and is found on the scalp (Figure 33-12). *Pediculis humanus corporis,* or body lice, are found anywhere on the body. *Phthirus pubis* are pubic lice that are usually found in the pubic hair and are often referred to as "crabs."

Lice feed off of human blood by making small bites in the skin. Intense itching is caused by these bites and the local reaction to them. Lice egg clusters, called nits, are tightly bound to hair follicles and are difficult to remove with even the finest tooth combs.

Lice are transmitted from person to person by close contact or contact with clothing or bedding. Body lice can transmit disease and are the major vectors for typhus and relapsing fever. Chronic infestation has also been associated with anemia, due to the constant, minute drainage of blood from each louse bite.

Treatment of lice is similar to scabies, with creams and shampoos and careful elimination of nits from hair. Clothing and bedding must also be properly disinfected. Paramedics should exercise universal precautions and bag all linens after use. No vaccine is available. DOT 5-11.47

Diseases Spread through Animal Vectors

The following diseases have animal reservoirs and are transmitted to humans through insect stings or animal bites. Prehospital care of patients with these diseases is supportive.

Rabies

Rabies is caused by the rabies virus. Rabies can survive in almost all mammals, and the natural reservoirs in the United States include skunks, raccoons, bats, foxes, wild dogs, jackals, wolves, mongooses, and coyotes. Routine vaccination has all but eliminated rabies in domestic animals. Fewer than 20 human cases have been reported in the United States in the last decade.[49]

Rabies virus is found in large concentrations in the saliva and is transmitted through biting. Airborne transmission is possible but is rare. Human-to-human transmission is theoretically possible but has never been documented. The disease has an incubation period of three to eight weeks although disease has been reported up to seven years after contact.

Rabies symptoms include anxiety, headache, fever, and altered mental status. The disease progresses to weakness, delirium, and convulsion. Paralysis of the muscles of the pharynx leads to an inability to swallow water, causing **hydrophobia** (fear of drinking water). Without treatment, the disease lasts two to six days. Although it was once thought to be universally fatal, a teenage girl in Wisconsin recently recovered from clinical rabies.[50]

Patients who sustain animal bites should be transported to the hospital for evaluation. If the animal is a domesticated pet, paramedics should attempt to ascertain its immunization status. Local animal control should be contacted immediately to find and capture the animal. ***Under no circumstances should paramedics attempt to capture the animal.*** Hospital care will include debridement of the wound, cleansing with soap and water, and administration of antibiotics, as needed. If exposure to rabies is suspected, rabies immune globulin and rabies vaccine will be administered.

Routine immunization is limited to people at high risk of exposure, such as animal care workers. Paramedics need not be routinely vaccinated against rabies.[51]
DOT 5-11.30

Lyme Disease

Lyme disease is caused by the bacteria *Borrelia burgdorferi* and is named for the town of Lyme, Connecticut, where it was first identified. Lyme disease is spread to humans through the bite of the deer tick, and it is estimated that over 20,000 cases occur each year.[52]

Lyme disease occurs most frequently in the northeastern United States, with outbreaks in the upper midwest, mid-Atlantic, and Pacific coast states. The risk is highest in those people who spend time in tick-infested woods, especially when camping, fishing, hiking, or hunting.

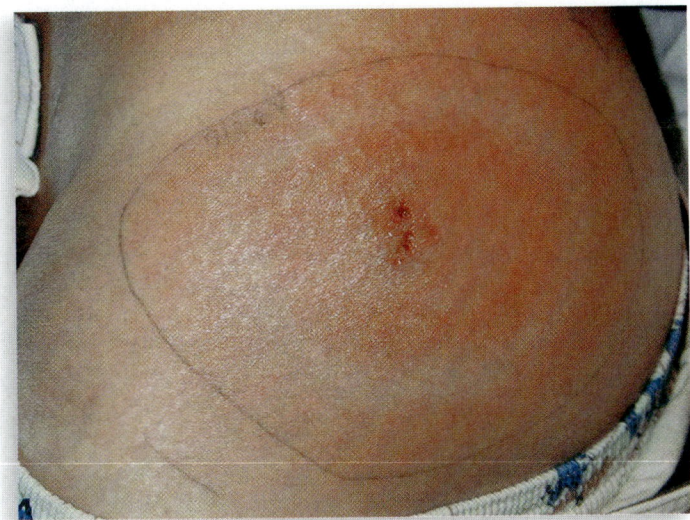

Figure 33-13 The classic sign of Lyme disease consists of a red, painless rash at the site of the tick bite called erythema migrans. As this rash gradually spreads outwards, the center clears or may turn blue, giving it a "bull's eye" appearance.

The earliest sign of Lyme disease occurs three to thirty days after exposure and consists of a red, painless rash at the site of the tick bite called **erythema migrans.** As this rash gradually spreads outwards, the center clears or may turn blue, giving it a "bull's eye" appearance (Figure 33-13). This rash is often associated with fever, muscle aches, and a stiff neck.

Several weeks after the initial erythema migrans occurs, multiple sites may erupt in a similar rash. Nervous system involvement is common at this time, with meningitis, weakness, and Bell's palsy (paralysis of the facial nerve on one side). Cardiovascular involvement also occurs, causing conduction abnormalities and dysrhythmias. Joint pain is also common.

Approximately 10% of untreated individuals will develop chronic arthritis, especially in the knees. Long-term neurologic deficits also occur, including insomnia, fatigue, and dementia.

Treatment with antibiotics is effective and reverses almost all symptoms. Paramedics who work in and around wooded environments must be vigilant for the presence of ticks. Universal precautions are recommended when dealing with patients with Lyme disease, but no evidence exists to suggest person-to-person transmission. There is no vaccine available for Lyme disease.

DOT 5-11.48

Rocky Mountain Spotted Fever

Rocky Mountain Spotted Fever (RMSF) is most frequently diagnosed, oddly enough, in the south central states (Oklahoma, Missouri, Arkansas, and the Carolinas have the largest number of cases).[53] The name comes from the fact that the first cases were identified in the Rocky Mountains.

The disease is caused by a bacterium, *Rickettsia rickettsii,* which is spread through the bite of infected wood ticks. Symptoms such as fever and malaise begin two to five days after the tick bite. The rash for which the disease is named begins about a week after the onset of fever and presents as red spots all over the body, including the palms of the hands and the soles of the feet (Figure 33-14). As many as 15% of patients will not develop a rash.

RMSF can be severe, spreading to the lungs, kidneys, or brain. Treatment includes antibiotics, and hospitalization is common. Long-term complications include paralysis, gangrene, and cognitive impairment.

There is currently no vaccine against RMSF. The best protection against the disease is to prevent tick bites by wearing long pants and long sleeved shirts when working in wooded areas.

Hantavirus

Hantavirus has a natural reservoir in mice and is shed in the mouse's feces, urine, and saliva. Transmission to humans occurs when the virus is dispersed into the air

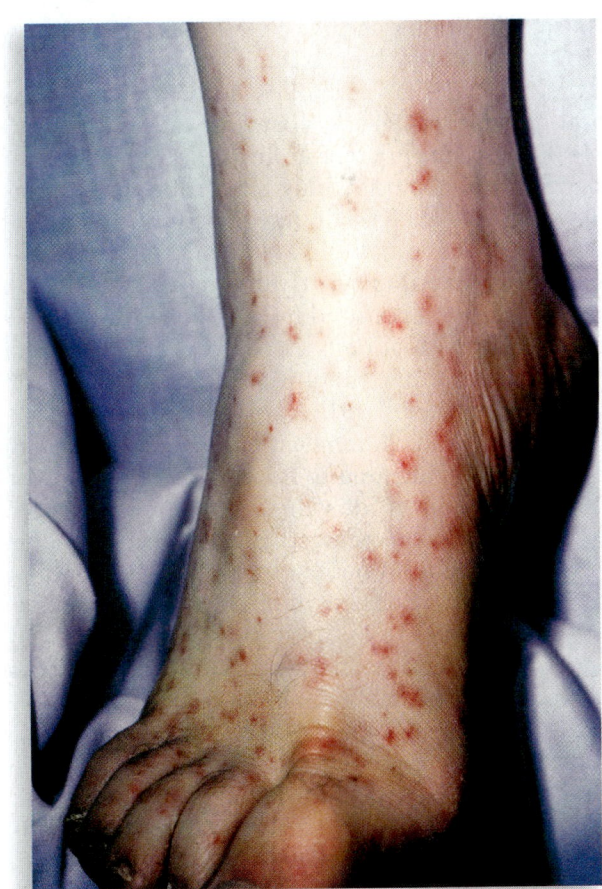

Figure 33-14 The rash of Rocky Mountain Spotted Fever begins about a week after the onset of fever and presents as red spots all over the body, including the palms of the hands and the soles of the feet.

by disturbing mouse droppings. The virus is inhaled and causes a severe pneumonia called hantavirus pulmonary syndrome. Hantavirus is not transmitted from person to person.

The mice that carry hantavirus are found in all environments although most cases in the United States have been in the Southwest "four corners" region in Colorado, New Mexico, Utah, and Arizona. There have been 387 documented cases in the last decade, of which 36 have died.[54] Risk factors include stirring up mouse droppings in basements or abandoned buildings.

Hantavirus pulmonary syndrome presents with fever, chills, myalgias, and cough. Abdominal pain, nausea, and vomiting are also common. Patients rapidly develop pulmonary pneumonia and hypotension that resembles septic shock.

Treatment of the patient with hantavirus pulmonary syndrome is supportive as there are no effective antivirals and no vaccine for this disease. DOT 5-11.29

H5N1 (Avian Flu)

The current epidemic of highly pathogenic H5N1 avian influenza within poultry populations in Southeast Asia raises serious concerns that genetic reassortment will result in a human influenza pandemic. Viruses can actually intensify their virulence as they pass through several generations in the host, but unless they jump species, for example cross from birds into swine and swine into humans, they may be harmless to humans. So far, the individuals who have come down with the virus seem to have had close contact with birds. For example, they handled poultry on a daily basis, and this disease could have resulted following another viral infection when the patient's immunity was weakened. In 2003 through 2006, there were 263 confirmed cases of human infection with H5N1 avian influenza in Vietnam, Thailand, Indonesia, China, and Cambodia, with a mortality rate greater than 50%.

Having first been identified in 1997, H5N1 (avian influenza A virus) reemerged in 2004 in eight Asian countries, infecting 44 people and killing 32, for a mortality rate of 73%. Because of a lack of comprehensive surveillance measures in these countries, the actual incidence of exposure and death is unknown and these numbers only represent estimates.

The greatest fear for H5N1 is that the virus will mutate and allow efficient person-to-person transmission. To date, no person-to-person infection has been definitively proven. One recent case may change that. An 11-year-old Vietnamese female was taken to the hospital with a severe febrile illness consistent with influenza. Within a few days, she died of progressive respiratory distress, hypoxemia, and shock. DOT 5-11.51

The patient's mother lived in a distant city and had no history of poultry exposure. The mother drove to the hospital the day she learned her daughter was sick, and she took over the girl's bedside care for sixteen to eighteen hours. She was in close contact with the child, kissing her daughter and coming into contact with her secretions. Nine days later, she was admitted to a hospital in her province; three days after admission, she died of pneumonia and progressive respiratory failure.[55,56]

There is also concern that if avian flu "jumps" to the human population, some deaths may not be attributed to H5N1 as the cause. A recent case appeared in patients without typical flu-like symptoms. In this case, two siblings presented to the hospital in their home country of Vietnam with diarrhea and encephalitis. Both quickly lapsed into coma and died. The male had throat and rectal swabs as well as cerebrospinal fluid and serum specimens obtained prior to his death. All of his specimens tested positive for H5N1. The female, who actually died the week before her brother, was cremated, so no specimens were available for testing. The doctors believe she died from the same virus because her symptoms were identical.[57]

To prevent and prepare for an increase in human cases, public health officials are working to improve detection methods and to stockpile effective antiviral medications. While vaccines are the mainstay of prophylaxis against influenza, there are technical and safety issues that must be overcome in the development of enough avian influenza vaccine for use in humans.[58]

Treatment of the patient with a virus like H5N1 is supportive. The use of respiratory protection by the EMS crew is paramount. The production of a vaccine is ongoing; however, most reports to date are that there is an insufficient amount of vaccine to immunize the general population.

Working in the Gray Zone

The flu epidemic of 1918 was the deadliest epidemic of flu ever in the world and is considered by many to be the deadliest epidemic of any disease. Many of the people who died during this time did not die from the flu but from either bacterial pneumonia or acute respiratory distress syndrome (ARDS). Both problems developed when the patient's immune systems went into overdrive to try to counteract the flu virus. Ironically, most of these deaths were in young and otherwise healthy individuals. The recent focus on the potential of a new pandemic has the concern that a mutation of the strain from 1918 may return or that H5N1 will cross over into humans. While many people underplay the importance of the flu, it has the potential to be deadly.[1]

Diseases Spread through the Environment

Agents that have environmental reservoirs and are contracted through contact with contaminated food or soil cause the following diseases.

Tetanus

Tetanus is caused by the bacterium *Clostridium tetani.* Tetanus spores exist in the environment and are frequently found in soil or animal feces. The spores enter the body through contaminated wounds. Mature bacteria produce a toxin that is released into the bloodstream. The toxin causes generalized **tetany,** which means painful, prolonged contraction of the muscles. Symptoms include inability to open the mouth **(trismus),** tightening of the neck muscles, and finally contraction of the muscles of the trunk. Death occurs by laryngospasm or paralysis of the diaphragm.

The incidence of tetanus in the United States has been declining since the introduction of tetanus immunization in the 1940s. There were only 25 reported cases in 2002, and effective treatment has reduced the mortality rate to 10%.[59]

Tetanus immunization typically begins in childhood and provides protection for up to a decade. It is recommended that all people receive booster shots at least every 10 years (more frequently if they experience a contaminated wound). Any patient with an open wound should be questioned regarding tetanus status, and that information should be passed on to the emergency department staff. Patients who have out-of-date or unknown immunization status should be encouraged to seek further medical care even if they only have minor scrapes. DOT 5-11.29

Gastroenteritis

Gastroenteritis is a collection of symptoms, including nausea, vomiting, abdominal pain, and diarrhea that are caused by a variety of infectious agents. Gastroenteritis is often caused by viruses such as rotaviruses, adenoviruses, caliciviruses, astroviruses, Norwalk virus, and a group of Noroviruses. These viruses can be spread by close personal contact but can also be spread by eating contaminated food or using contaminated utensils. Symptoms usually begin one to two days after infection and last for three to five days. Treatment is symptomatic, and care should be taken to wear gloves and wash your hands after patient contact. DOT 5-11.49

Parasites are also known to cause gastroenteritis. The most common are *Giardia lamblia, Cryptosporidium parvum,* and *Cyclospora cayetanensis.* These are contracted by the fecal-oral route and are often found in water that has been contaminated with sewage. Giardia is common amongst campers who drink unfiltered and unpurified water.

Bacterial gastroenteritis tends to be more severe than the viral or parasitic forms. Most cases of bacterial gastroenteritis involve virulent strains of normal intestinal flora. These include *Escherichia coli, Klebsiella pneumoniae, Enterobacter, Campylobacter jejuni, Vibrio cholerae, Shigella,* and *Salmonella.*

E. coli causes gastroenteritis either by direct infection of the intestines or by releasing toxins that cause cramping and diarrhea. A particularly virulent strain, *E. coli* O157:H7 has been implicated in fatal cases of gastroenteritis in otherwise healthy individuals. *E. coli* can be killed by thoroughly heating food.

Cholera is caused by *Vibrio cholerae* and is one of the leading causes of endemic gastroenteritis in developing nations. Cholera spreads through drinking water contaminated with feces and causes prolonged watery diarrhea.

Shigella and *Salmonella* both can cause gastroenteritis. *Shigella* is transmitted through food contaminated with feces and typically causes bloody diarrhea. *Salmonella* is typically found in chicken and eggs that have not been properly cooked and has the potential to spread from the intestines to other organ systems.

It is difficult to differentiate between viral, parasitic, or bacterial gastroenteritis based on the history and physical exam. All patients should be assessed for signs of dehydration and should be rehydrated, as necessary. Paramedics should wear gloves and wash their hands thoroughly after contact with infected patients. Furthermore, paramedics who are experiencing gastroenteritis should avoid work to prevent spread to susceptible patients.

There are no vaccines available for gastroenteritis. DOT 5-11.49

Botulism

Botulism is a particular case of food poisoning caused by the bacterium *Clostridium botulinum.* This organism lives in the soil and reproduces best in environments with low levels of oxygen. Botulism is typically found in home-canned foods. Botulism is also spread through sharing dirty needles. There are approximately 100 cases of botulism in the United States each year.[60]

C. botulinum releases a toxin that causes paralysis by preventing nerve signals from reaching muscles. Symptoms of botulism include double vision, drooping eyelids, slurred speech, difficulty swallowing, and muscle weakness. Untreated botulism can lead to loss of airway protection, respiratory failure, and death.

Botulinum toxin has recently been used in plastic surgery to reduce visible wrinkles on the face. "Botox" is also being investigated for use in migraines, managing neurological pain, and incontinence.

Paramedics who suspect botulism should be prepared to protect their patient's airway. Prehospital care is otherwise supportive and involves suctioning secretions and administering oxygen. Treatment in the

Nice to Know

Botulism is found in small amounts in honey. The amount is too small to cause symptoms in the adult but can be sufficient to cause clinical disease in infants. Small children who contract infant botulism will be limp with a weak cry and have difficulty feeding. Careful attention to the baby's airway is mandatory.

hospital involves administering antibiotics and antitoxin and frequently requires prolonged intubation. Botulism should be suspected in any patient with drooping eyelids, double vision, and slurred speech, especially if there is a history of eating home-canned foods or IV drug use.

Paramedics should utilize universal precautions when dealing with cases of botulism. No vaccine is available.

Bioterrorism

Increased attention has been paid to the risk of terrorism since the events of September 11, 2001. **Bioterrorism** is the use of infectious agents in terrorist activities. The spread of anthrax through the mail in the months following 9/11 confirmed that bioterrorism is a real threat.

Any infectious disease could potentially be used in a terrorist attack. The attributes that make an agent suitable for terrorist activity include the following:

- Terrorists must have easy access to the agent.
- The agent must be easy to grow in a lab or other controlled setting.
- The agent must be easy to spread.
- The agent must be sufficiently virulent to cause disease in a significant portion of those infected.
- The symptoms must appear quickly and with sufficient severity to disrupt medical facilities.

The scope of bioterrorism is far too broad to discuss in detail here. However, paramedics should be familiar with two pathogens thought to be most likely to be used in a terrorist attack.

CONNECTIONS Chapter 55: Responding to WMD Events discusses this topic in more detail.

Smallpox

Smallpox is caused by the variola virus and has a presentation similar to chickenpox (Figure 33-15). Transmission is through close contact with a patient or

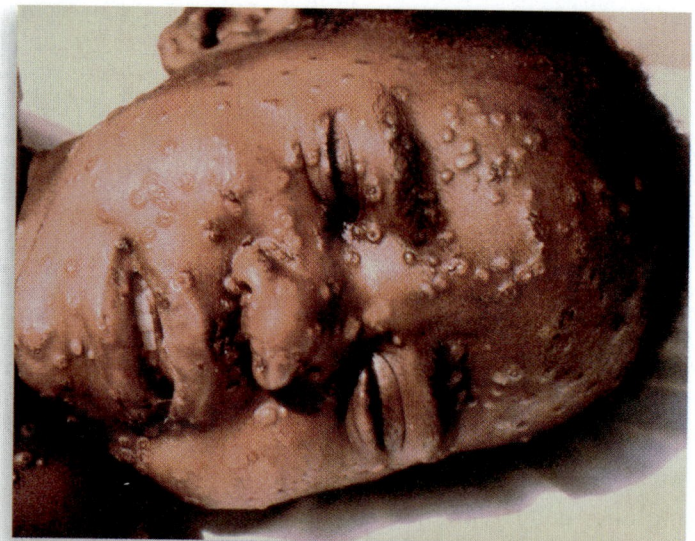

Figure 33-15 Smallpox is caused by the variola virus and has a presentation similar to chickenpox.

with the patient's clothing and bedding. Airborne transmission is also suspected. Smallpox disease is historically fatal in 30% of cases. It has been remarked that smallpox has killed more people than any other infectious disease in history, including over 500 million victims in the 20th century.[2]

Smallpox was the first disease for which a vaccine was created. In 1796, the British physician Edward Jenner realized that milkmaids who had been infected with cowpox (a mild disease that was transmitted to humans from infected cows and caused pustules on the hands) did not contract smallpox. As an experiment, Dr. Jenner injected the pus from a cowpox pustule into a young boy who was later exposed to smallpox. As expected, the boy did not contract the disease. Louis Pasteur would later coin the term vaccination from the Latin "vaca" meaning cow.

Smallpox is uniquely suited to immunization. The disease has no reservoir other than humans and cannot survive in the environment. Vaccination against the disease may confer lifelong immunity in almost all people. Finally, the disease is only spread through close contact, so cases can be easily quarantined.

Routine vaccination against smallpox began in the United States in the early 1900s. The last documented case of smallpox in the U.S. was in 1949. In 1967, the United Nations' World Health Organization (WHO) launched a program to eradicate smallpox on a global scale and declared the disease eradicated in 1980.

A decision was made to preserve two samples of variola virus, without which the virus would be entirely extinct. One of these samples is in the labs of the CDC in Atlanta. The other was kept at the Institute for Viral Studies in Moscow.

Before September 11, 2001, it was believed that smallpox was not a threat. Since that time, however, doubt has been cast on the security of the Russian sample. It is not known whether samples of the smallpox virus have been made available to terrorist groups.

Although the threat from smallpox is thought to be small, the disease is highly contagious and has a high mortality rate. Furthermore, immunization against smallpox was discontinued in the United States in the early 1970s, making a large percentage of the population susceptible to the disease. An outbreak of smallpox would be devastating.

Paramedics should be familiar with the differentiation of smallpox from chickenpox. First, smallpox lesions are found all over the body, while chickenpox tends to be concentrated on the trunk. Second, chickenpox pustules tend to be of various ages, with new red bumps, mature pustules, and crusted-over ulcers all seen at the same time. Smallpox lesions are all in the same stage of development at the same time.

Paramedics who suspect their patients have smallpox should take extreme caution to wear gloves, gowns, and facemasks. Notification to the receiving hospital is necessary to allow the emergency department staff to prepare an isolation room. All linens should be bagged and disposed of, and all surfaces should be disinfected.

Vaccination against smallpox is no longer routine, but doses were made available to healthcare workers wishing to prepare against terrorist attack.[61] Most healthcare workers have declined immunization since the threat of smallpox is still thought to be low and the vaccine has serious side effects. Paramedics should contact their physicians to discuss whether they should receive the vaccine.

Anthrax

Anthrax is caused by the bacterium *Bacillus anthracis*, which causes disease in livestock and can survive in soil for years. It is believed that several countries have experimented with weaponizing anthrax, but none have used it during wartime. In 1979, weaponized anthrax was inadvertently released from a military facility in Russia, causing up to 1,000 deaths. In late 2001, 22 people in the United States contracted anthrax from the mail attack, resulting in five deaths.

The majority of infections with *B. anthracis* are through direct contact, causing **cutaneous anthrax.** Symptoms include a raised bump at the site of inoculation that becomes necrotic (Figure 33-16). The mortality rate of untreated cutaneous anthrax is 20%, but death is rare with the use of antibiotics.

Gastrointestinal anthrax is caused by ingesting contaminated food and causes abdominal pain, vomiting blood, and diarrhea. Death occurs in 20–60% of cases, and the efficacy of antibiotics is not known.

Breathing in aerosolized *B. anthracis* causes **inhalation anthrax.** Symptoms are flu-like, with fever, chills, myalgias, and cough. Inhalation anthrax is fatal

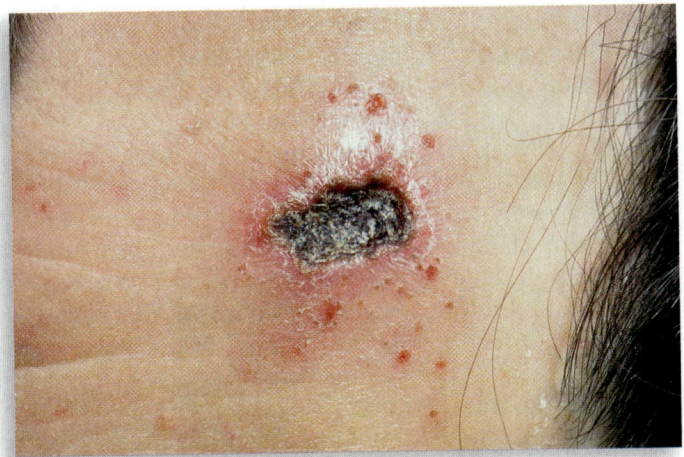

Figure 33-16 The majority of infections with *B. anthracis* occur through direct contact, causing cutaneous anthrax, which presents as a raised bump at the site of inoculation that becomes necrotic.

in 75% of cases regardless of antibiotic therapy using historical data; however, given advances in therapeutics and intensive care, the mortality rate in the 2001 attack was decreased to 40%.

Anthrax is difficult to differentiate from other forms of skin rash, gastroenteritis, or pneumonia. Fortunately, anthrax is not communicable from person to person. Paramedics should use universal precautions as appropriate.

A vaccine exists for anthrax, but its use is limited to military personnel traveling to areas with high rates of anthrax. Vaccination is unlikely to be available to prehospital care workers.

Reporting an Exposure to an Infectious Disease

Healthcare workers are constantly at risk of contracting disease through contact with their patients. A significant contact is defined as any blood or other bodily fluid coming into contact with the eyes, mouth, mucous membrane, or through puncture wounds in the skin. Any paramedic who experiences a significant contact should report it to the appropriate authorities. DOT 5-11.50

It is important to report exposure because many exposures will result in disease that can be prevented with appropriate prophylaxis. Reporting an exposure allows the paramedic to receive appropriate treatment and follow-up.

Each prehospital agency must designate an individual to investigate every significant exposure. Such investigations can determine how the exposure occurred and whether or not it was preventable. This can lead to procedural changes to avoid future exposures.

Finally, the United States Government passed the Ryan White Comprehensive AIDS Resources Emergency Act of 1990, which gives healthcare workers the right to request the infection status of the source patient.[62] However, the source always retains the right to refuse testing.

The agency that employs the healthcare worker is responsible for developing an Exposure Control Plan, and must tell the employee what to do in case of exposure. Paramedics must report exposure to their agency's designated infection control officer. That person will then determine whom to inform based on local, state, and federal requirements.[6,63]

Reportable diseases are listed in Box 33-4.

Healthcare agencies are also required to provide free medical evaluation and follow-up for workers who are exposed. This follow-up includes counseling about the risk of developing disease and appropriate prophylaxis, with discussion of side effects and contraindications to those medications. This follow-up exam may involve taking a blood sample to test for the presence of hepatitis or HIV. The employee retains the right to refuse this blood test. Finally, appropriate vaccinations will be offered as necessary.

The healthcare provider performing this examination must prepare a written statement for the employee's agency. This statement must include the results of the evaluation as well as a discussion of the treatment options recommended to the employee. This statement will also list those medical conditions caused by the exposure that will require further evaluation or treatment.

Both the agency and the employee should receive copies of this statement. All other parts of the medical record are confidential and cannot be disclosed without the written consent of the employee. **DOT 5-11.14, 5-11.50**

Preventing Transmission of Disease

It is your responsibility to prevent spreading infection to other healthcare workers or patients. This can be accomplished by following these rules:

1. *Avoid work when*
   - You have diarrhea.
   - You have a draining wound or any wet lesions (you may return to work when the lesions are crusted over).
   - You have jaundice.
   - You have infectious mononucleosis.
   - You are being treated for scabies or lice.
   - You have been diagnosed with strep throat (you may return to work when you have been treated with antibiotics for 24 hours).
   - You have a cold. If you must go to work when you have a cold, wear a mask.

2. *Stay up-to-date.* It is your responsibility to ensure that your immunizations are up-to-date. Check with your physician about your status in terms of:
   - Screening for tuberculosis (PPD or chest x-ray)
   - Measles, mumps, or rubella
   - Hepatitis B
   - Hepatitis A (if required by your agency)
   - Diphtheria-pertussis-tetanus
   - Polio
   - Chicken pox
   - Influenza (annual immunizations)
   - Rabies (if appropriate to your risk)

3. *Approach all patients with caution and the right attitude.* If you prepare for infectious disease and take the appropriate precautions as soon as possible, you will reduce your risk of contracting disease.

4. *Control the scene.* A chaotic scene increases the risk of making mistakes, including needle stick injuries.

5. *Observe body substance isolation.* Assume that all bodily fluids are infected, and avoid direct contact with them at all times. Do this by:
   - Always wearing gloves when in contact with your patient.
   - Wearing a face shield or protective eyewear when there is a risk of splashing.
   - Wearing a gown when large volumes of bodily fluids are expected.
   - Wearing a mask when your patient is coughing.

6. *Look out for dangerous signs and symptoms.* The following signs and symptoms should make you suspicious of serious infection:
   - Cough
   - Headache
   - Generalized weakness
   - Recent weight loss
   - Stiff neck
   - High fever
   - History of antibiotic use

7. *Recognize patients who may be immunocompromised.* Patients with AIDS have impaired immune systems, but so do patients with diabetes, chronic renal failure, and those who have received organ transplants. These patients will have difficulty fighting infection and may experience more severe symptoms than patients with fully functional immune systems.

8. *Don't treat your patients differently because you think they have an infection.* All patients deserve

BOX 33-4   **Infectious Diseases Designated as Notifiable at the National Level During 2006[64]**

Acquired Immunodeficiency Syndrome (AIDS)
Anthrax
Arboviral neuroinvasive and nonneuroinvasive
   diseases
      California serogroup virus disease
      Eastern equine encephalitis virus disease
      Powassan virus disease
      St. Louis encephalitis virus disease
      West Nile virus disease
      Western equine encephalitis virus disease
Botulism
      Botulism, foodborne
      Botulism, infant
      Botulism, other (wound and unspecified)
Brucellosis
Chancroid
Chlamydia trachomatis, genital infections
Cholera
Coccidioidomycosis
Cryptosporidiosis
Cyclosporiasis
Diphtheria
Ehrlichiosis
      Ehrlichiosis, human granulocytic
      Ehrlichiosis, human monocytic
      Ehrlichiosis, human, other or unspecified agent
Giardiasis
Gonorrhea
Haemophilus influenzae, invasive disease
Hansen disease (leprosy)
Hantavirus pulmonary syndrome
Hemolytic uremic syndrome, post-diarrheal
Hepatitis, viral, acute
      Hepatitis A, acute
      Hepatitis B, acute
      Hepatitis B virus, perinatal infection
      Hepatitis, C, acute
Hepatitis, viral, chronic
      Chronic Hepatitis B
      Hepatitis C Virus Infection (past or present)
HIV infection
      HIV infection, adult (> = 13 years)
      HIV infection, pediatric (< 13 years)
Influenza-associated pediatric mortality
Legionellosis
Listeriosis
Lyme disease
Malaria
Measles

Meningococcal disease
Mumps
Pertussis
Plague
Poliomyelitis, paralytic
Psittacosis
Q Fever
Rabies
      Rabies, animal
      Rabies, human
Rocky Mountain spotted fever
Rubella
Rubella, congenital syndrome
Salmonellosis
Severe Acute Respiratory Syndrome-associated
      Coronavirus (SARS-CoV) disease
Shiga toxin-producing *Escherichia coli* (STEC)
Shigellosis
Smallpox
Streptococcal disease, invasive, Group A
Streptococcal toxic-shock syndrome
Streptococcus pneumoniae, drug resistant, invasive disease
Streptococcus pneumoniae, invasive in children
      < 5 years
Syphilis
      Syphilis, primary
      Syphilis, secondary
      Syphilis, latent
      Syphilis, early latent
      Syphilis, late latent
      Syphilis, latent, unknown duration
      Neurosyphilis
      Syphilis, late, non-neurological
      Syphilitic stillbirth
      Syphilis, congenital
Tetanus
Toxic-shock syndrome (other than Streptococcal)
Trichinellosis (Trichinosis)
Tuberculosis
Tularemia
Typhoid fever
Vancomycin—intermediate *Staphylococcus*
      aureus (VISA)
Vancomycin—resistant *Staphylococcus*
      aureus (VRSA)
Varicella (morbidity)
Varicella (deaths only)
Yellow fever

to be treated with respect. Remember that you are not treating an infection, you are treating a patient with an infection.

9. ***Don't avoid treating your patients because of infections.*** Using universal precautions, personal protective equipment, and body substance isolation can protect you from infectious disease. Do not withhold care because you are afraid of contracting disease. However, do not put yourself at undue risk because of your duty to the patient. Remember that you cannot help others if you are sick.

10. ***Disinfect your equipment.*** After each call, wipe all equipment and each surface of the patient compartment of your ambulance with an approved disinfectant. Take the time to do this properly; do not put yourself or your patients at risk because you rushed or avoided disinfecting equipment.

11. ***Avoid lice and scabies.*** Although they are considered innocuous, infestations with lice and scabies are uncomfortable and difficult to treat. Wear gloves when treating a patient with scabies or lice. After transporting the patient with scabies or lice, bag all linens and dispose of appropriately.

12. ***Inspect your uniform for soil and damage.*** Change to clean clothing and launder the uniform separately or send it out for special cleaning by professionals as necessary.

13. ***Always wash your hands.*** Wash your hands before and after every patient contact, after removing gloves, and after each invasive procedure.

Summary

Infectious diseases are not easily diagnosed prehospital emergencies, which means that you will be less experienced identifying infectious disease than you will other, more common disorders such as trauma. However, infectious diseases have the potential to be spread to you and other caregivers. For these reasons, you must be vigilant when dealing with patients with potential infectious disease for your own protection.

As a paramedic, you are not responsible for definitively diagnosing infectious disease. You will, however, be responsible for suspecting those conditions that are highly contagious, such as tuberculosis, meningitis, and chickenpox. When you suspect a contagious disease, you must take the proper steps to protect yourself, such as wearing personal protective equipment. Always protect yourself by using the appropriate personal protective equipment and treat all bodily fluids as if they are infected. You must also effectively communicate your suspicions to receiving hospital staff to ensure their safety and the safety of their patients.

Notes

1. J. M. Barry, *The Great Influenza: The Epic Story of the Deadliest Plague in History* (New York, NY: Viking Press, 2004).
2. "Pandemic," http://en.wikipedia.org/wiki/Pandemic (accessed May 31, 2005).
3. "OSHA Mission Statement," http://www.osha.gov/oshinfo/mission.html (accessed May 31, 2005).
4. "Centers for Disease Control Mission Statement," retrieved http://www.cdc.gov/about/mission.htm (accessed May 31, 2005).
5. "National Institute of Occupational Safety and Health," http://www.cdc.gov/niosh/about.html (accessed May 31, 2005).
6. M. R. Loutify, A. Silverman, and A. Simor, "*Toronto Emergency Medical Services and SARS,*" Center for Disease Control, *Emerging Infectious Diseases* (September 2004), http://www.cdc.gov/ncidod/EID/vol110no9/04-0170.htm (accessed April 5, 2005).
7. Centers for Disease Control and Prevention, "Guideline for Hand Hygiene in Health-Care Settings: Recommendations of the Healthcare Infection Control Practices Advisory Committee and the HICPAC/SHEA/APIC/IDSA Hand Hygiene Task Force," *Morbidity and Mortality Weekly Report: Surveillance Summaries* 51(No. RR-16) (2002): 1–44.
8. J. M. Boyce et al., "Guideline for Hand Hygiene in Health-Care Settings: Recommendations of the Healthcare Infection Control Practices Advisory Committee and the HICPAC/SHEA/APIC/IDSA Hand Hygiene Task Force," *Infection Control and Hospital Epidemiology* 23(12 Suppl) (December 2002): S3-40.
9. E. Slade, P. S. Tamber, and J. Vincent, "The Surviving Sepsis Campaign: Raising Awareness to Reduce Mortality," *Critical Care* 7(1) (2003): 1–2.
10. Centers for Disease Control, "Pneumocystis Pneumonia—Los Angeles," *Morbidity and Mortality Weekly Report: Surveillance Summaries* 30 (1981): 250–252.
11. National Center for Infectious Diseases Division of HIV/AIDS, "1993 Revised Classification System for HIV Infection and Expanded Surveillance Case Definition for AIDS Among Adolescents and Adults," *Morbidity and Mortality Weekly Report: Surveillance Summaries* 41(RR-17) (1992).
12. http://www.cdc.gov/hiv/stats.htm#aidscases (accessed May 21, 2005).
13. M. H. Katz, A. R. Zolpa, and H. Hollander, *Current Medical Diagnosis and Treatment 2006. Infectious Diseases: HIV,* McGraw-Hill's AccessMedicine (accessed June 25, 2006).
14. P. Brocklehurst and J. Volmink, "Antiretrovirals for Reducing the Risk of Mother-to-Child Transmission of HIV Infection," *Cochrane Database Systemic Reviews* 1 (2002):CD003510.
15. Centers for Disease Control, "HIV and its Transmission," *HIV and Its Transmission* (1999) 1–4.
16. "HIV and the Health Care Worker," http://aidscentral.com/HIV_AND_THE_HEALTH_CARE_WORKER.html (accessed May 31, 2005).
17. D. M. Cardo, D. H. Culver, C. A. Ciesielski, et al., "A Case-Control Study of HIV Seroconversion in Health Care Workers After Percutaneous Exposure," *The New England Journal of Medicine* 337 (1997): 1485–1490.
18. Centers for Disease Control, "Prevention of Hepatitis A Through Active or Passive Immunization: Recommendations of the Advisory Committee on Immunization Practices (ACIP),"

Morbidity and Mortality Weekly Report: Surveillance Summaries 48(RR-12) (1999): 4–9.

19. Centers for Disease Control, "Hepatitis A Fact Sheet," http://www.cdc.gov/ncidod/diseases/hepatitis/a/fact.htm (accessed May 31, 2005).

20. "Hepatitis B Fact Sheet," http://www.cdc.gov/ncidod/diseases/hepatitis/b/fact.htm (accessed May 31, 2005).

21. Immunization Practices Advisory Committee, "Hepatitis B Virus: A Comprehensive Strategy for Eliminating Transmission in the United States Through Universal Childhood Vaccination: Recommendations of the Immunization Practices Advisory Committee (ACIP)," *Morbidity and Mortality Weekly Report: Surveillance Summaries* 40(RR-13) (1991): 1–19.

22. Centers for Disease Control, "Updated U.S. Public Health Service Guidelines for the Management of Occupational Exposures to HBV, HCV, and HIV and Recommendations for Postexposure Prophylaxis," *Morbidity and Mortality Weekly Report: Surveillance Summaries* 50(RR-11) (2001): 1–42.

23. "Hepatitis C Fact Sheet," http://www.cdc.gov/ncidod/diseases/hepatitis/c/fact.htm (accessed May 31, 2005).

24. "Hepatitis D Fact Sheet," http://www.cdc.gov/ncidod/diseases/hepatitis/d/fact.htm (accessed May 31, 2005).

25. "Hepatitis E Fact Sheet," http://www.cdc.gov/ncidod/diseases/hepatitis/e/fact.htm (accessed May 31, 2005).

26. M. C. Kew and C. Kassianides, "HGV: Hepatitis G Virus or Harmless G Virus?" *Lancet* 348 Suppl 2 (December 21–28, 1996): sII10.

27. Centers for Disease Control, "Trends in Tuberculosis-United States, 1998–2003," *Morbidity and Mortality Weekly Report: Surveillance Summaries* 53 (2004): 209–214.

28. Centers for Disease Control, "Core Curriculum on Tuberculosis: What the Clinician Should Know," 2000, www.cdc.gov (accessed September 28, 2006).

29. P. A. Selwyn et al., "A Prospective Study of the Risk of Tuberculosis Among Intravenous Drug Users with Human Immunodeficiency Virus Infection," *The New England Journal of Medicine* 320 (1989): 545–550.

30. C. Dye et al., "Consensus Statement: Global Burden of Tuberculosis: Estimated Incidence, Prevalence, and Mortality by Country. WHO Global Surveillance and Monitoring Project," *Journal of the American Medical Association* 282(7) (1999): 677–686.

31. American Thoracic Society, CDC, and Infectious Diseases Society of America, "Treatment of Tuberculosis," *Morbidity and Mortality Weekly Report: Surveillance Summaries* 53(RR-11) (2003): 1–77.

32. TB Infection-Control Guidelines Work Group, "Guidelines for Preventing the Transmission of *Mycobacterium Tuberculosis* in Healthcare Facilities, 1994," *Morbidity and Mortality Weekly Report: Surveillance Summaries* 43(RR-12) (1994): 1–132.

33. S. P. Yazdankhah and D. A. Caugant, "*Neisseria Meningitides:* An Overview of the Carriage State," *Journal of Medical Microbiology* 53(9) (2004): 821–832.

34. Centers for Disease Control, "Prevention and Control of Meningococcal Disease: Recommendations of the Advisory Committee on Immunization Practices," *Morbidity and Mortality Weekly Report: Surveillance Summaries* 49(RR-7) (2000): 3.

35. Centers for Disease Control, "Prevention of Pneumococcal Disease: Recommendations of the Advisory Committee on Immunization Practices (ACIP)," *Morbidity and Mortality Weekly Report: Surveillance Summaries* 46(RR-8) (1997): 1–31.

36. National Immunization Program, Centers for Disease Control, "Varicella" In *Epidemiology and Prevention of Vaccine-Preventable Diseases,* 8th ed. (Atlanta, GA: CDC, 2005), pp. 159–175.

37. National Immunization Program, Centers for Disease Control, "Mumps" In *Epidemiology and Prevention of Vaccine-Preventable Diseases,* 8th ed. (Atlanta GA: CDC, 2005), pp. 135–143.

38. Centers for Disease Control, "Measles, Mumps, and Rubella—Vaccine Use and Strategies for Elimination of Measles, Rubella, and Congenital Rubella Syndrome and Control of Mumps: Recommendations of the Advisory Committee on Immunization Practices (ACIP)," *Morbidity and Mortality Weekly Report: Surveillance Summaries* 47(RR-8) (1998): 1–57.

39. National Immunization Program, Centers for Disease Control, "Rubella" In *Epidemiology and Prevention of Vaccine-Preventable Diseases,* 8th ed. (Atlanta, GA: CDC, 2005), pp. 145–158.

40. National Immunization Program, Centers for Disease Control, "Measles" In *Epidemiology and Prevention of Vaccine-Preventable Diseases,* 8th ed. (Atlanta, GA: CDC, 2005), pp. 115–133.

41. National Immunization Program, Centers for Disease Control, "Pertussis" In *Epidemiology and Prevention of Vaccine-Preventable Diseases,* 8th ed. (Atlanta, GA: CDC, 2005), pp. 75–88.

42. Centers for Disease Control, "Diphtheria, Tetanus, and Pertussis: Recommendations for Vaccine Use and Other Preventive Measures Recommendations of the Immunization Practices Advisory Committee (ACIP)," *Morbidity and Mortality Weekly Report: Surveillance Summaries* 40(RR10) (1991): 1–28.

43. National Immunization Program, Centers for Disease Control, "Influenza" In *Epidemiology and Prevention of Vaccine-Preventable Diseases,* 8th ed. (Atlanta, GA: CDC, 2005), pp. 213–231.

44. "CDC—Influenza (Flu): Q & A Flu Vaccine" (November 2, 2004), http://www.cdc.gov/flu/about/qa/fluvaccine.htm (accessed May 31, 2005).

45. "Epstein-Barr Virus" (October 26, 2002), http://www.cdc.gov/ncidod/diseases/ebv.htm (accessed May 31, 2005).

46. Centers for Disease Control, "Primary and Secondary Syphilis—United States, 1999," *Morbidity and Mortality Weekly Report: Surveillance Summaries* 50 (2000): 113–117.

47. "Tracking the Hidden Epidemics 2000—Gonorrhea" (August 4, 2004), http://www.cdc.gov/nchstp/od/news/RevBrochure1pdfGonorrhea.htm (accessed May 31, 2005).

48. "Tracking the Hidden Epidemics 2000—Chlamydia" (August 4, 2004), http://www.cdc.gov/nchstp/od/news/RevBrochure1pdfChlamydia.htm (accessed May 31, 2005).

49. J. W. Krebs et al., "Rabies Surveillance in the United States During 2001," *JAVMA* 221(12) (2002): 1690–1701.

50. R. E. Willoughby, Jr., K. S. Tieves, G. M. Hoffman, et al., "Survival after Treatment of Rabies with Induction of Coma," *The New England Journal of Medicine* 352 (24) (2005): 2508–2514.

51. Centers for Disease Control, "Human Rabies Prevention—United States, 1999 Recommendations of the Advisory Committee on Immunization Practices (ACIP)," *Morbidity and Mortality Weekly Report: Surveillance Summaries* 48(RR-1) (1999): 1–21.

52. Centers for Disease Control, "Notice to Readers: Final 2002 Reports of Notifiable Diseases," *Morbidity and Mortality Weekly Report: Surveillance Summaries* 52(31) (2003): 741–750.

53. "Epidemiology—CDC Rocky Mountain Spotted Fever" (May 20, 2005), http://www.cdc.gov/ncidod/dvrd/rmsf/Epidemiology.htm (accessed May 31, 2005).

54. "Case Definition: CDC Hantaviruses" (May 4, 2005), http://www.cdc.gov/ncidod/diseases/hanta/hps/noframes/caseinfo.htm (accessed May 31, 2005).

55. K. Stöhr, "Avian Influenza and Pandemics—Research Needs and Opportunities (editorial)," *The New England Journal of Medicine* 352 (2005): 405.

56. K. Ungchusak et al., "Probable Person-to-Person Transmission of Avian Influenza A (H5N1)," *The New England Journal of Medicine* 352 (2005): 333.

57. M. D. de Jong et al., "Fatal Avian Influenza A (H5N1) in a Child Presenting with Diarrhea Followed by Coma," *The New England Journal of Medicine* 352 (2005): 686.

58. S. J. McPhee and M. Pignone, *Health Maintenance and Disease Prevention. Current Medical Diagnosis and Treatment 2006,* McGraw-Hill's AccessMedicine (accessed June 25, 2006).

59. National Immunization Program, Centers for Disease Control, "Tetanus" In *Epidemiology and Prevention of Vaccine-Preventable Diseases,* 8th ed. (Atlanta GA: CDC, 2005), pp. 65–73.

60. Centers for Disease Control, "Botulism in the United States 1899–1996," *CDC* (1998): 1–42.

61. Centers for Disease Control, "Vaccinia (Smallpox) Vaccine Recommendations of the Advisory Committee on Immunization Practices (ACIP), 2001," *Morbidity and Mortality Weekly Report: Surveillance Summaries* 50(RR10) (2001): 1–25.

62. Public Law. 101–381, Aug. 18, 1990, 104 Stat. 576.

63. John Hick, *Department of Health and EMS Regulatory Board. EMS Special Pathogen Guide* (St. Paul, MN: MDH, MN EMSRB, 2004).

64. Centers for Disease Control, "Nationally Notifiable Infectious Diseases—United States, 2006," www.cdc.gov/EPO/DPHSI/phs/infdis2006.htm (accessed September 24, 2006).

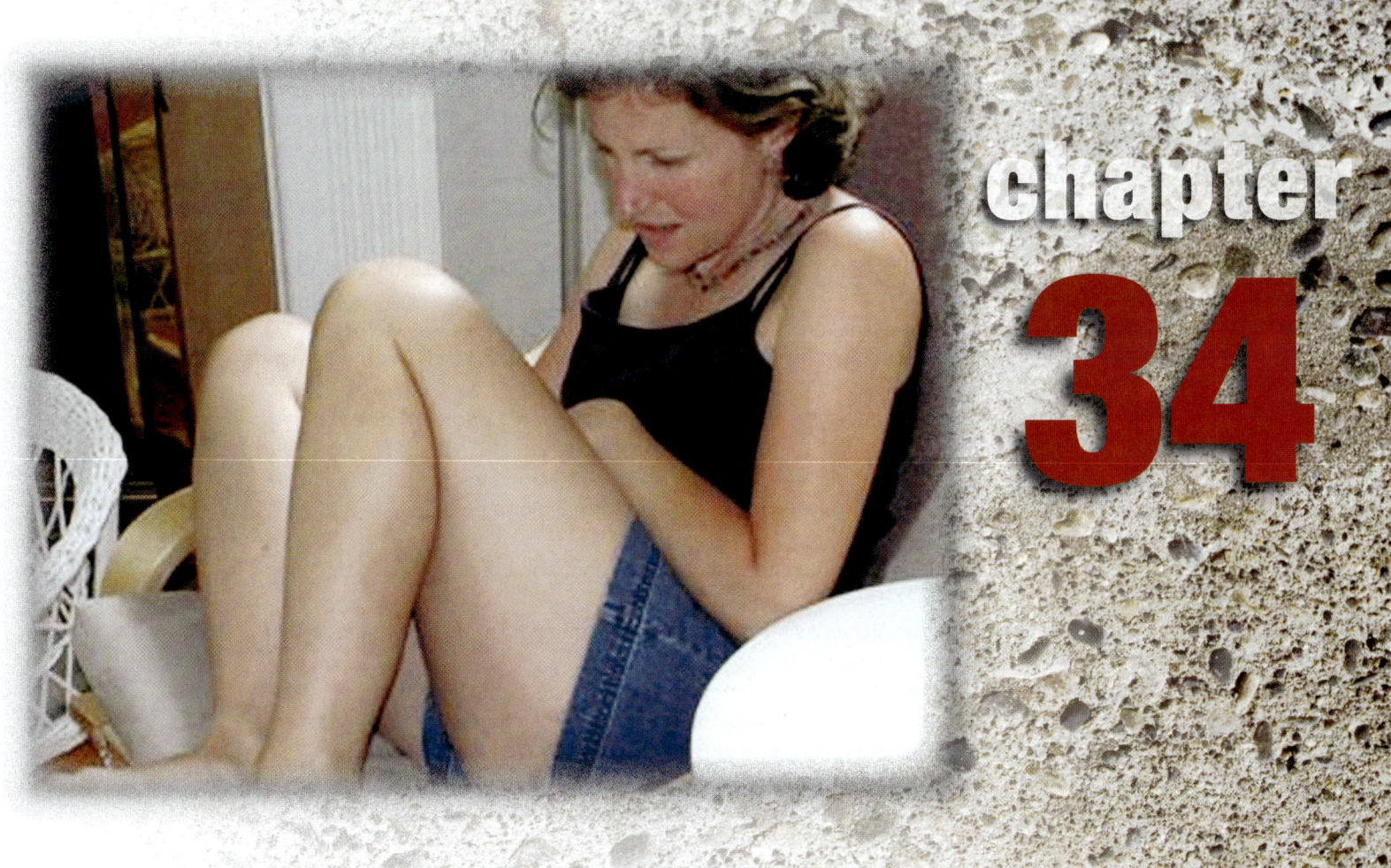

Gastroenterology

> "**I**n general, civilization affords chances of misuse of our digestive organs, and it is this difference between natural and civilized living that causes all ill health. In a word these diseases are primarily related to what we call Constipation, the Universal Malady of Modern Times."
>
> —Dr. Paul M. Koonin, D.D.Sc

Need to Know

▶ Consider abdominal pain as a potential sign for the following life-threatening conditions first: abdominal aortic aneurysm (AAA), acute myocardial infarction (AMI), pulmonary embolus (PE), bleeding from the spleen or liver, or a ruptured ectopic pregnancy.

▶ Keep an open mind and a high index of suspicion while treating abdominal pain. Do not try to make a rapid diagnosis. Abdominal pain is often misdiagnosed even by physicians.

▶ The GI tract can hold a large amount of blood, even the majority of the patient's blood volume, without any obvious external signs upon physical exam.

▶ Ectopic pregnancy should be considered in any female of childbearing age that is complaining of abdominal pain. You should ask the patient about her menstrual cycle and the date of her last menstrual period.

▶ Elderly patients and patients with diabetes mellitus may experience vague upper abdominal discomfort with nausea and sometimes vomiting when suffering from cardiac ischemia.

▶ An abdominal aortic aneurysm (AAA) should be an early consideration in patients over the age of 65 with the sudden onset of abdominal or low back pain, even if they have a normal blood pressure, no mass is detected, and the pain is no longer present.

▶ Acute appendicitis is caused by inflammation of the appendix and is a common condition that can develop at any age.

▶ The sympathetic nerves of the esophagus are very similar to that of the heart, which makes it hard to tell the difference between esophageal and cardiac pain.

▶ Esophageal varices are dilated veins in the esophagus that can bleed profusely. These are often a complication of alcoholic liver disease that raises venous blood pressure and increases venous return.

▶ **Cholecystitis** is the acute inflammation of the gallbladder and usually occurs when the neck of the gallbladder or cystic duct is obstructed, often by a gallstone. A classic presentation of cholecystitis is right upper quadrant pain when a patient has just finished a meal containing fatty foods. Other common findings are patients who are the "4 F's": female, fat, over forty, and fertile (still able to bear children).

▶ Patients with alcohol-related liver disease commonly complain of fatigue and poor appetite. Findings upon exam may include **spider angiomata** (small dilated blood vessels visible under the skin) or **ascites** (a distended abdomen with fluid wave, indicative of a build-up of ascitic fluid in the peritoneal cavity).

▶ Sick	▶ Not Yet Sick
• Obvious signs of shock, including hypotension or sustained tachycardia indicate the patient is very sick. • Significant pain may indicate the patient is sick, particularly if their position and appearance indicate the pain is severe. • Administer pain medication if indicated (consult MD if necessary) • Ask if the pain radiates. If it goes to the right shoulder, suspect the gallbladder. If it radiates to the left shoulder, suspect the spleen. If it is in the flank, suspect kidney stones.	• The abdomen is a difficult part of the body to evaluate and interpret. It is better to err on the side of caution and consider all abdominal complaints significant and needing transport. • Lights and siren or emergency transport may not be warranted unless obvious life threats are present. • Look for nausea, vomiting, and signs of dehydration (low BP, dry mucous membranes, positive orthostatic changes in VS). • Monitor the ECG and perform 12-lead ECG as appropriate. • Inspect the abdomen before palpating it. • Ask female patients about a history of previous ectopic pregnancy.

Introduction

Gastroenterology means, literally, the study of the gastrointestinal tract. A wide variety of disorders have their origins in the gastrointestinal tract, and while you may not be in a position to diagnose many of these problems, understanding the possible origins of a complaint and what might be causing certain symptoms can play a key role in proper prehospital management and disposition. In this chapter, the subject of gastroenterology is broken down into two sections: abdominal pain and gastrointestinal (GI) bleeding. Other symptoms and specific conditions discussed are nausea and vomiting, diarrhea, esophageal and gastric disease, bowel disease, appendicitis, pancreatitis, and liver disease.

Before considering the real subject of the chapter, gastrointestinal complaints, it is important to note that one of the most serious and life-threatening conditions that causes pain in the abdomen is actually not a gastrointestinal problem at all. In fact, the first thing you should consider when patients complain of abdominal pain is whether they could be having a heart attack. Myocardial infarctions may very well present with abdominal pain and can go undetected if your assessment is focused completely on gastrointestinal disorders. **Skill Sheet 42: Intravenous Access (and Step-by-Step 42) and Skill Sheet 47: Central Line Access for Fluids and Drug Administration support this chapter.**

Applied Anatomy and Physiology

The gastrointestinal tract **(alimentary tract)** is the system responsible for ingesting, processing, absorbing, digesting, and eliminating food (Figure 34-1). It starts with the mouth and ends at the anus. The digestion of food begins in the mouth. Mechanical digestion starts with the breaking up of food by the teeth (which is called **mastication**) and the forcing of the tongue against ridges of the hard palate to also break it down. Breakdown is necessary for the body to metabolize food as digestive enzymes will be more effective against a greater surface area. Some chemical digestion occurs within the mouth from salivary glands that secrete specific enzymes in the saliva. Fat and carbohydrate digestion begins here with lipase and amylase, respectively. Other glands secrete mucus that softens the food bolus.

As a food bolus is forced to the back of the mouth and into the posterior oropharynx, the soft palate moves to protect the posterior nasopharyngeal space, and the epiglottis drops down to cover the larynx and trachea and position food for movement into the esophagus. Up until now, the process has been completely voluntary. From this point on, it is an involuntary process. The esophagus is a tube approximately 10 inches long that passes through the diaphragm via the esophageal hiatus. The esophagus is where swallowing occurs, otherwise referred to as the deglutition reflex. Smooth muscle movement (peristalsis) propels food down the esophagus, through a ring-like band of fibers (gastroesophageal sphincter) that opens into the stomach. The sphincter also helps keep food from coming back up from the stomach.

CONNECTIONS During a cardiac arrest, when an overzealous caregiver is providing forceful ventilations (such as occurs with an oxygen resuscitator or two-handed forceful bag-mask ventilation) with a basic airway adjunct,

air may pass through the esophageal sphincter and distend the stomach. This often causes emesis and complicates airway management. For more information about the dangers of improper ventilation, turn to Chapter 12: Airway Management, Ventilation, and Oxygenation; and for more on cardiac arrest, turn to Chapter 29: Cardiology.

If the stomach pushes up through the esophageal hiatus, the condition is called a **hiatal hernia.** This type of hernia allows stomach acids to regurgitate into the esophagus, which is one of the principal causes of heartburn.

The stomach is responsible for storage of food until it can be accommodated in the lower GI tract. Mixing of this food with fluids, acids, and enzymes produced by the stomach occurs until it is a soft mixture called **chyme.** The stomach is also responsible for digestion of proteins and absorption of some water and alcohol. The food bolus, or chyme, leaves the stomach and heads into the small intestines by way of the pyloric sphincter.

The small intestines are approximately 21 feet long. The first 10 inches are the duodenum, and this is the area where a significant amount of the digestion of the food bolus occurs. There is a duct connecting to the duodenum that transports fluids, nutrients, and enzymes from the gallbladder, liver, and pancreas. The liver is responsible for producing bile that is stored in the gallbladder and necessary for the breakdown of fats in the duodenum. The pancreas produces glucagon, insulin, and enzymes necessary for digestion. From the duodenum, the bolus passes through the jejunum and then the ileum of the small intestines. Little digestion occurs here. Next, it passes through the ileocecal valve into the large intestine. The large intestine is made up of the cecum, transverse colon, descending colon, sigmoid colon, the rectum, and anus.

The appendix is a hollow, muscular, close-ended tube that arises from the posterior medial surface of the cecum, just a few centimeters beyond the ileocecal valve. Very little absorption occurs in the large intestine, except for some water and electrolytes. The large intestine is mostly responsible for the synthesis of vitamin K by bacteria and the synthesis of B-complex vitamins as well as the transport of waste products out of the body.

CONNECTIONS See the small and large intestines and the appendix on Plate B at the end of Chapter 7: Anatomy Overview, page 137.

The peritoneum is a large, essentially closed membrane sac that contains most of the GI tract distal to the esophagus (Figure 34-2). Inflammation or infection of organs within the peritoneal cavity can result in inflammation of the peritoneum **(peritonitis).** DOT 5-6.11

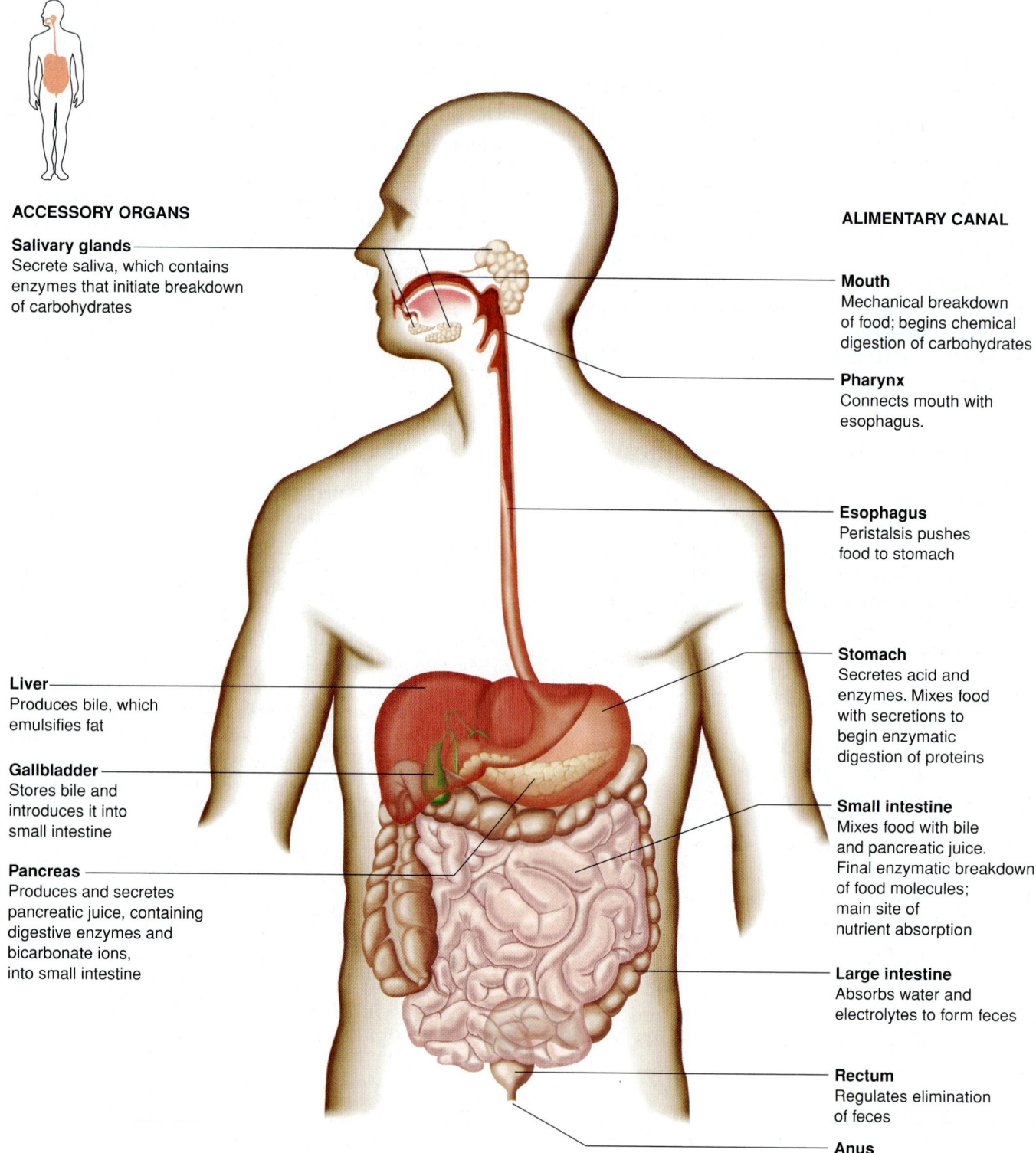

ACCESSORY ORGANS

Salivary glands
Secrete saliva, which contains
enzymes that initiate breakdown
of carbohydrates

Liver
Produces bile, which
emulsifies fat

Gallbladder
Stores bile and
introduces it into
small intestine

Pancreas
Produces and secretes
pancreatic juice, containing
digestive enzymes and
bicarbonate ions,
into small intestine

ALIMENTARY CANAL

Mouth
Mechanical breakdown
of food; begins chemical
digestion of carbohydrates

Pharynx
Connects mouth with
esophagus.

Esophagus
Peristalsis pushes
food to stomach

Stomach
Secretes acid and
enzymes. Mixes food
with secretions to
begin enzymatic
digestion of proteins

Small intestine
Mixes food with bile
and pancreatic juice.
Final enzymatic breakdown
of food molecules;
main site of
nutrient absorption

Large intestine
Absorbs water and
electrolytes to form feces

Rectum
Regulates elimination
of feces

Anus

Figure 34-1 The organs of the digestive system.

The liver has many functions, including storage and filtration of blood, metabolic functions, and processing much of what is eaten (Figure 34-3). The liver processes about 1500 milliliters of blood every minute. Kupffer cells protrude into the flowing blood and filter it of most debris, including almost all bacteria. The metabolic functions of the liver include carbohydrate metabolism (synthesis of glycogen for storage,

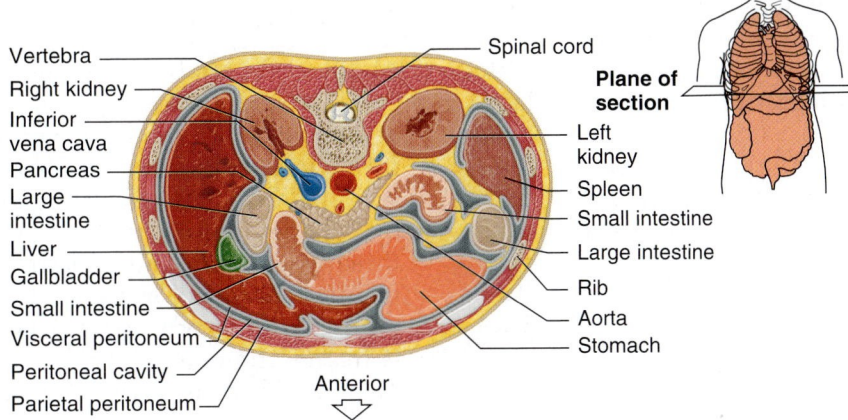

Figure 34-2   The peritoneum is a closed membrane that contains most of the GI tract. It is shown here in gray, with the peritoneal cavity in blue.

conversion of galactose and fructose to glucose, and gluconeogenesis), fat metabolism (beta oxidation of fatty acids, formation of lipoproteins, and synthesis of cholesterol and phospholipids), and protein metabolism (deamination of amino acids, formation of urea for removal of ammonia from body fluids, and formation of plasma proteins).

The liver is also involved in the storage of vitamins, formation of many of the blood substances utilized in the coagulation process, storage of iron, and removal and excretion of many drugs (such as penicillin), hormones, and other substances such as calcium. Finally, the liver forms bile from red blood cells that have reached the end of their life span and are too fragile to exist any longer in the circulatory system. The cell membranes are ruptured to release and process hemoglobin, which is broken down (phagocytized) into products the liver will ultimately use to form bile. After being manufactured by hepatic cells, this bile flows through the hepatic duct and common bile duct and empties into the gallbladder or directly into the

duodenum. Once in the duodenum, bile emulsifies (breaks down fat globules) and forms complexes with lipids to help in the absorption of fatty acids, cholesterol, and other lipids.

The biliary tract is made up of the hepatic (or liver) bile canaliculi, intrahepatic and extrahepatic bile ducts, the common bile duct, and the gallbladder. The pancreas serves multiple functions, including the synthesis of enzymes crucial to digestion and absorption. It is located in the retroperitoneal (behind the peritoneum) space. The main pancreatic duct goes from the tail of the pancreas, through the body, to the head of the pancreas, and enters the duodenum with the common bile duct. DOT 5-6.3

Primary Survey

As with any patient, the primary survey of the patient with a complaint related to the GI tract is really meant to determine if the patient is sick or not yet sick.

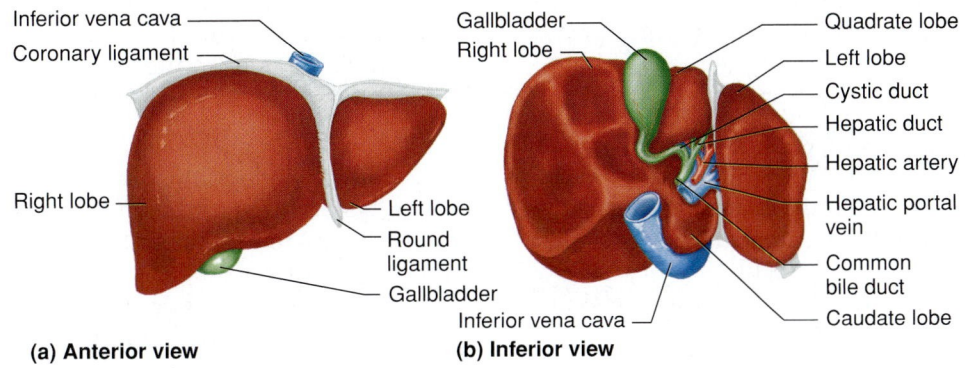

(a) Anterior view   **(b) Inferior view**

Figure 34-3   The anatomy of the liver.

The immediate life-threatening problems in patients with GI-related complaints need to be recognized quickly and treated aggressively. The primary life-threatening problem with gastrointestinal complaints is bleeding.

The four key life-threatening GI conditions associated with hemorrhage that your initial assessment should detect include:

1. Ruptured aortic aneurysm
2. Ruptured ectopic pregnancy
3. Ruptured spleen
4. Gastrointestinal bleeding

A patient with a ruptured abdominal aortic aneurysm may complain of abdominal as well as back pain. Although not often detected, a pulsating mass in the abdomen can be an important clue to this disease. Ectopic pregnancy is one of the rare diseases that kills otherwise healthy, young women and should be considered in all females of childbearing age with abdominal pain or syncope. A patient with a ruptured spleen may complain of abdominal pain and sometimes left shoulder pain. A patient who has recently suffered from mononucleosis and has resulting splenomegaly (enlarged spleen) is at particular risk for this, even with minimal trauma. Any bleeding of the upper or lower GI tract should be considered immediately life threatening. Even in the apparently stable patient, bleeding in the GI tract can be notoriously hard to control.

Finally, the healthcare provider should always keep in mind the potential for pathology outside of the GI tract that might be causing GI-related complaints. In particular, a patient with AMI may present with nausea or vomiting or a vague sense of discomfort in the upper abdominal region that could easily send the provider down the path of a GI tract evaluation. Keeping these issues in mind during the primary survey of the patient with GI complaints will be crucial to recognizing events that can be immediately life-threatening. Any patient who appears ill, such as one who is anxious, pale, diaphoretic, or has abnormal vital signs, should be considered sick until proven otherwise.

Street Secrets

A patient with knees drawn up is usually an indication of significant abdominal pain. A patient who has peritonitis or appendicitis usually will lie very still. A patient with colicky gallstones or ureteral stones may rock back and forth.

Abdominal Pain

Abdominal pain is a frequent complaint encountered by prehospital providers and accounts for up to 10% of patients presenting to the emergency department (ED).[1] In fact, one survey found abdominal pain was the single most frequently mentioned reason offered by patients for visiting the ED.[2] There are essentially three types of abdominal pain that most patients will manifest: visceral, somatic, and referred pain. Determining which category the patient's abdominal pain is in can often be helpful in generating a differential diagnosis and in determining appropriate treatment and disposition.

Visceral Pain

Visceral abdominal pain is caused by the stretching of visceral pain fibers, which are located in the walls of hollow organs (such as intestines or the gallbladder) and the capsules of solid organs (such as the liver, spleen, and kidneys). These nerve fibers become irritated by the stretching of these organs from distention or from vascular impairment, causing ischemia. Visceral pain is often felt at the midline of the abdomen but is generally difficult for the patient to specifically localize and is often ill-defined. Foregut organs in the upper GI tract, such as the stomach and biliary tract, will often produce pain in the mid-epigastric region while midgut organs such as the small bowel and appendix will cause periumbilical pain. The hindgut, or lower part of the GI tract such as the colon, genitourinary system, and pelvic organs, will typically cause pain in the area just above the pelvis (suprapubic) region. Patients with visceral pain will often appear in some distress, despite not being able to localize their pain very well. DOT 5-6.6, 5-6.16

Street Secrets

Patients with visceral pain generally are moving about while trying to find a comfortable position. For this reason, patients with visceral pain can sometimes be quite difficult to examine.

Visceral abdominal pain is often associated with other, systemic symptoms such as nausea and vomiting. Visceral pain tends to be intermittent, dull, or cramping and worsens over time. A small bowel obstruction in a patient who has had abdominal surgery in the past is an example of pathology that might cause visceral abdominal pain. DOT 5-6.9

Street Secrets

A mnemonic for assessing vomit is to think of the word "TACO." Ask about the following:

- **T**ype (for example, digested food, containing pill fragments, "coffee ground" appearance, etc.)
- **A**mount
- **C**olor (bloody, greenish, black, etc.)
- **O**dor

A greenish-yellow color might indicate a small bowel blockage. Vomit that is from a large bowel obstruction might have a fecal odor. Bleeding stomach or duodenal ulcers or esophageal varices may have a bright red blood or coffee ground appearance. Emesis might also be caused from increased intracranial pressure or myocardial infarction.

Somatic Pain

Somatic pain, also known as **parietal pain,** is caused by irritation of fibers that innervate the parietal peritoneum or abdominal wall. Because these nerve fibers return to the spinal cord on the same side as the origin of the pain, somatic abdominal pain is typically more localized than visceral pain is, and typically the pain localizes to an area very close to the site of the disease process causing the pain. As opposed to visceral pain, somatic abdominal pain is often described as constant, sharp, and aggravated by movement. While the patient with visceral pain will often be moving around trying to find a comfortable position, the patient with somatic pain often will be quite still and might even complain about the bumpy ride in the ambulance.

Street Secrets

A patient complaining about a rough ride in the ambulance, particularly when you did not notice an unusually bumpy ride, may have somatic pain as a possible etiology for their distress.

As the underlying disease process evolves, visceral pain may progress into somatic or parietal pain. Guarding of the abdomen may develop where the patient will tense the abdominal wall muscles when the abdomen is palpated. Appendicitis is an example of pathology that might cause visceral pain initially and then develop into somatic pain with guarding over the right lower quadrant. DOT 5-6.5, 5-6.10

Referred Pain

Referred pain is pain felt by the patient at a location distant from the site of the pathology causing the pain. Nerve segments that overlap and provide sensation to two or more areas can lead to pain originating in the abdomen but sensed at an extra-abdominal site. Referred pain is often intense and can sometimes be confusing for providers if they do not recognize the pattern of the pain. Pain resulting from pathology in the upper abdominal regions near the diaphragm can stimulate nerve fibers that instead suggest pain in the shoulder or neck. An abdominal abscess just under the diaphragm, such as one that might develop from an infection in the liver, gallbladder, or spleen, is an example of a process that might cause referred pain to the shoulder. Although this is not the only place referred pain can present, providers should consider an abdominal source as a cause in any patient complaining of nontraumatic shoulder pain. DOT 5-6.7

CONNECTIONS See Figure 14-10 (page 290) in Chapter 14: Patient Assessment for a diagram showing areas of referred pain.

Secondary Survey

History

The history can be very helpful in the focused assessment of patients with abdominal pain. As in most situations, open-ended questions should be used at the beginning of the history-taking process, allowing patients to describe in their own words what the pain feels like. Remember that the prehospital environment may be the best or only avenue to obtain important aspects of the history. Careful attention to your patients' responses could have an effect on patient outcome. Components of the history that can be particularly helpful include the following:

- Having patients describe the pain they are feeling. Do they describe it as cramping, sharp or dull, or do they use other words to describe their pain?
- How patients grade the pain on a scale of zero to ten, with ten being the worst pain they have ever experienced? This can be particularly helpful in tracking how the pain changes over time, whether you perform any interventions or not. Most hospitals will be tracking the pain in this same way, and consistency in this area can be helpful.
- Where, specifically, is the pain now, and where did it start? These may be in the same location, but when they are not, this can be particularly helpful information.

- When did the pain begin, and has it been constant or intermittent since that time?
- What are the other symptoms patients are experiencing that are associated with this pain? Nausea, vomiting, diarrhea, fevers, and shortness of breath are some of the potential associated symptoms that, when present, can help to direct the provider to what else to be concerned about (such as dehydration) and what the potential cause of the pain might be.

There are certain aspects of the history in patients with abdominal pain that should raise concern in the paramedic that a serious cause of the abdominal pain may exist. While these are in no way absolute, and the paramedic must always be ready for patients that do not follow these guidelines, they can be helpful points to keep in mind when assessing patients with abdominal pain.

- Which came first, the pain or the vomiting?
  - As a general rule, pain coming first is more concerning.
- How long have you had the pain?
  - Less than 48 hours tends to be more concerning.
- Is the pain constant or intermittent?
  - Constant pain is often a cause for greater concern.
- Have you ever had this pain before?
  - A history with no previous episodes of similar pain is often more concerning.[3]

Other important aspects of the history include whether they have had previous abdominal surgeries. Previous surgery in the abdomen raises the risk of bowel obstruction. Also, what medications patients are taking can be important as well. While this is usually part of the history paramedics seek from most patients encountered, pay particular attention to whether they are taking steroids or antibiotics. Both of these are known to sometimes mask infection and could be playing a role in masking the underlying etiology of the abdominal pain.

Street Secrets

All women of childbearing age should be asked about their menstrual cycle and when their last menstrual period was. Any irregularities should raise the concern for an ectopic pregnancy, a potentially life-threatening cause of abdominal pain and hemorrhage in women.

Always keep in mind that some patients, particularly the elderly and patients with diabetes mellitus, may experience vague upper abdominal discomfort with nausea and sometimes vomiting when suffering from cardiac ischemia.[4] In fact, up to 1–2% of elderly patients with abdominal pain will actually be having a myocardial infarction.

A good history taken from patients with abdominal pain will include questions regarding cardiac risk factors and symptoms. A history of human immunodeficiency virus (HIV) infection or cancer (particularly if patients have had recent chemotherapy) will be helpful as well. Immunodeficient states can mask underlying infection and can place the patient at risk for sepsis. DOT 5-6.13, 5-6.2

Physical Exam
General

A careful and skillful physical exam will be important in identifying patients with potentially serious causes of abdominal pain. The first aspect of this exam is, as with any patient, to note the general appearance of the patient and to assess the airway, breathing, and circulation. Is the patient sitting comfortably or is the patient obviously uncomfortable?

Street Secrets

The degree of pain a patient is experiencing does not necessarily correlate with the severity of the patient's illness.

Is the patient writhing around, unable to find a comfortable position or does the patient stay perfectly still, not wanting to move even slightly? The patient suffering from renal colic due to a kidney stone might be writhing around in pain (very similar to a patient suffering from a dissecting aortic aneurysm), while the patient with peritonitis (inflammation of the peritoneal lining surrounding the abdominal contents, generally as the result of inflammation of one of the abdominal organs such as the appendix) is more likely to want to remain still. Is the patient's skin pale, cool, and diaphoretic, signifying shock? Is there any alteration in the patient's mental status? In addition to a careful set of vital signs and the examination of the abdomen, a careful exam with particular attention to the heart, lungs, and pulses will be important. DOT 5-6.4, 5-6.14

Vital Signs

A careful, complete set of vital signs will be an early priority. Pulse and blood pressure should be followed for significant changes. A careful assessment of the respiratory rate for a full 15 seconds is important as well.

Respiratory rates can be elevated simply because of the pain a patient is experiencing, but following changes in the rate and pattern of respirations can give clues to other problems as well.

Street Secrets

Orthostatic changes can sometimes be helpful in detecting volume loss, with a 30-point difference in pulse correlating with the loss of approximately 1 liter of intravascular volume (blood).[5] It is important to remember, however, that an abnormal pulse or blood pressure on the initial set of vital signs should cause the provider to proceed with extreme caution when checking for orthostatic changes. Patients that already have abnormal vital signs while supine may respond with a worsening of those vital signs when asked to stand, and lightheadedness, syncope, or other undesirable effects can result. It is also important to remember that some patients, particularly the elderly, may not speed up their heart rate, as they normally should, to compensate for the drop in blood pressure when standing. This may be due to underlying heart disease or medications taken for preexisting diseases. The elderly are also more likely to have underlying hypertension, making interpretation of the initial blood pressure more difficult as what we might consider a normal blood pressure could be very low for that patient.

Abdominal Exam

The examination of the abdomen will include inspection, palpation, and, when possible, auscultation. The position of the patient during the physical examination is important; the patient should be supine, with head down and knees slightly flexed, if possible (Figure 34-4). However, the patient's position of comfort

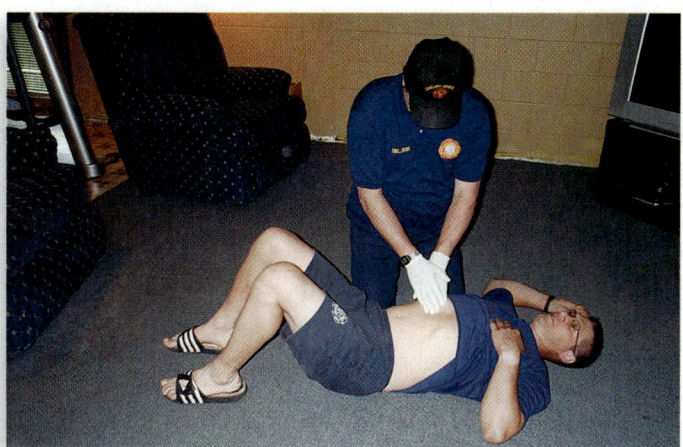

Figure 34-4   The best position for an abdominal examination is with the patient supine, head down, and knees slightly flexed.

will also have to be considered in choosing the best position in which to examine the abdomen. Explain to the patient what you are doing and why, not only to establish rapport, but also to increase cooperation and, therefore, the quality of the exam. Inspect the abdomen for obvious distention or masses. Also note any surgical scars, discoloration, or bruises that might be present.

Palpation of the abdomen should be gentle, using fingertip pressure, and should begin at the place furthest from the point of maximal pain identified by the patient. During your physical exam look for the following:

- ***Abdominal tenderness*** can generally be described as sensitivity or pain that is elicited by touch. It may be localized, generalized, or absent. Localized tenderness can provide clues as to an underlying cause. For example, pain that is localized on exam to the right lower quadrant area raises the concern for appendicitis. Generalized pain may raise the concern for peritonitis.

- **Guarding** occurs when the patient is contracting their abdominal muscles in response to or anticipation of your touch. It should be noted when present as it also raises the concern for peritonitis.

- **Rebound tenderness** is an increase in pain when pressure applied by the palpating hand is suddenly released. It can be a sign of peritoneal irritation and should be noted when found. You should not routinely check for rebound tenderness. This exam increases patient discomfort, can decrease patient cooperation with future examinations, and does not alter the prehospital treatment.[6]

- **Abdominal masses** felt on exam should be noted. A tender, pulsatile abdominal mass can indicate an abdominal aortic aneurysm, a potentially rapidly lethal cause of abdominal pain that should prompt the provider to seek a hospital such as a trauma center, when available, that can provide rapid access to a surgeon. DOT 5-6.14

Differential Diagnoses

The differential diagnosis of patients with abdominal pain is extensive, and many of these conditions cannot be definitively diagnosed in the field or even sometimes in the emergency department. Some of the more serious or common causes of abdominal pain will be briefly reviewed here, with a more extensive list noted in Box 34-1. As is always the case with emergency care, the more serious causes must be considered, and many times presumed, until proven otherwise.

Vascular causes of abdominal pain occur more commonly in the elderly and are nearly always serious, but patients suffering from these conditions do not always appear as sick as you might expect. **Abdominal aortic aneurysms,** which involve dilation of the abdominal aorta with resulting weakness of the aortic wall that can lead to leakage or frank rupture with massive intraabdominal hemorrhage, can cause pain in either the lower back or abdomen. Less than half of patients will have the well-described triad of hypotension, abdominal or back pain, and a pulsatile abdominal mass. More than three-quarters of patients

---

BOX 34-1   Differential Diagnoses of Abdominal Pain

Gastrointestinal
    Appendicitis
    Biliary tract disease
    Bowel obstruction
    Diverticulitis
    Esophageal perforation
      Boerhaave's syndrome
    Esophagitis
    Gastritis
    Gastroesophageal reflux disease
    Liver abscess
    Pancreatitis
    Peptic ulcer disease
    Splenic trauma
    Spontaneous bacterial peritonitis
    Tumor
    Volvulus
Vascular
    Abdominal aortic aneurysm
    Ischemic colitis
    Mesenteric ischemia
    Renal vein thrombosis
    Splenic rupture

Genitourinary
    Acute scrotum (infection or testicular torsion)
    Renal colic
      Kidney stones
      Pyelonephritis
    Urinary retention
Pelvic
    Ectopic pregnancy
    Ovarian torsion
    Pelvic inflammatory disease
    Ruptured ovarian cyst
    Tubo-ovarian abscess
Extra abdominal
    Abdominal wall hernias or hematomas
    Acute myocardial infarction
    Cardiac ischemia
    Hernias
    Metabolic derangements
    Pneumonia
    Pulmonary embolism
Neurogenic
    Herpes zoster

suffering from acute abdominal aortic aneurysms will have normal blood pressures. Pulsatile abdominal masses are notoriously difficult to detect, particularly in larger patients. Absent or decreased pulses cannot be relied upon. Therefore, an aortic aneurysm should be an early consideration in patients over the age of 65 with the recent onset of abdominal or low back pain, even if they are normotensive, no mass is detected, and the pain is no longer present.

Abdominal aortic aneurysms should be distinguished from aortic dissections, which are very uncommon causes of abdominal pain and generally begin in the chest or upper back and move lower as the dissection migrates downward.

Street Secrets

Abdominal pain, particularly above the umbilicus, should be considered to have a cardiac origin.

Splenic rupture is another cause of abdominal pain that must be considered. Although typically associated with victims of significant trauma, this is not always the case. A patient who has recently suffered from mononucleosis is at-risk for having an enlarged spleen (splenomegaly) that may rupture, even from minor trauma.

Bleeding into the peritoneal cavity often causes generalized abdominal pain. Any trauma can result in intra-abdominal hemorrhage, but nontraumatic causes, such as a ruptured abdominal aortic aneurysm or ruptured ectopic pregnancy, can result in bleeding and hemorrhagic abdominal pain as well. DOT 5-6.8

Mesenteric ischemia, where the vascular supply to the bowel provided by the mesenteric artery or vein is compromised, is a potentially life-threatening cause of abdominal pain seen more commonly in the elderly. The pain of mesenteric ischemia is classically described as out of proportion to the exam findings, so providers must consider this when caring for an elderly patient who appears to be in more pain than their physical examination seems to explain.

Although not part of the gastrointestinal system, **ectopic pregnancy** should always be considered in a female of childbearing age with abdominal pain as this can also be immediately life-threatening if it were to rupture and bleed. Care providers should always consider potentially life-threatening causes of abdominal pain from sources outside the abdomen.

In particular, **acute myocardial infarction, pulmonary embolism,** and **pneumonia** should be considered in the differential diagnosis of abdominal pain. Other causes of abdominal pain that are generally not immediately life-threatening include **inflammatory bowel disease** (ulcerative colitis or Crohn's disease) that will often have localized tenderness in the area of the inflamma-tion. Inflammatory bowel disease is often associated with diarrhea, and in the case of ulcerative colitis, it may be bloody. DOT 5-6.11, 12

Treatment

As the diagnosis in a patient with abdominal pain will rarely be made in the field, and although the cause of abdominal pain will rarely be immediately life-threatening, these patients should generally be transported to the emergency department for further evaluation. Responsibilities of the prehospital care provider include recognizing when a patient is seriously or critically ill, developing an appropriate differential diagnosis based on the patient's symptoms and presentation, selecting an appropriate destination based in part on that differential diagnosis, and providing appropriate pain control and transport based on the provider's assessment. Lights and siren use on the return to the hospital is generally not indicated unless the patient is hemodynamically unstable or otherwise appears ill (pale, diaphoretic, etc.).

Pain management in patients with abdominal pain has been a controversial issue for quite some time. Classic teaching has discouraged the use of narcotic analgesics in patients suffering from abdominal pain based on the concern that the diagnosis will be more difficult to make and a "surgical abdomen" may be masked by narcotics. Considerable research has shown, however, that judicious use of narcotic analgesia is safe, does not result in a delay in diagnosis, and may even aid in the management of some patients who will be easier to examine when more comfortable.[7] Local protocols will vary, but the idea that patients with abdominal pain should not be given reasonable doses of narcotic analgesia for fear of delaying the diagnosis is badly outdated. Fentanyl, which has a rapid onset and is short-acting (effects begin to decline after about 20 minutes), is an ideal drug to consider in these situations although longer acting medications may be appropriate as well. With the nearly immediate onset of fentanyl and the peak effect of morphine coming after about 20 minutes (just as fentanyl is beginning to wear off), this combination of medications might make sense for some situations. DOT 5-6.90, 5-6.91, 5-6.92, 5-6.93

Geriatric Patients with Abdominal Pain

Elderly patients (many consider elderly to be over the age of 65) with abdominal pain represent a particularly concerning population. The number of people over the age of 65 in the United States is rising, and it is very likely that paramedics will be called upon to care for elderly patients in the prehospital setting with increasing frequency. Up to one-third of patients over the age of

BOX 34-2   Causes of Abdominal Pain for Which the Elderly Are at Increased Risk

Abdominal aortic aneurysm

Mesenteric ischemia or infarction

Carcinoma

    Leading to bowel obstruction

Diverticulitis

    Although also seen in younger patients, the risk of diverticula increases with age

Volvulus

    From immobility

Myocardial infarction

Acute cholecystitis

    Also seen commonly in younger patients, but represents the most common surgical emergency in the elderly

65 who present to the emergency department with abdominal pain will require surgery. The mortality rate for the elderly presenting with abdominal pain is as high as 14%.[8,9] DOT 5-6.1

In addition to all the potential causes of abdominal pain that are seen in younger patients, the elderly are at increased risk for a number of very serious problems (Box 34-2). A good history and physical exam can be more difficult in the elderly as well, making these cases even more challenging. Ultimately, it is an appreciation for how complicated an elderly patient with abdominal pain can be, and the knowledge of the morbidity and mortality associated with abdominal pain in the elderly, that will direct paramedics to take appropriate caution and make appropriate management and destination decisions.

Pediatric Patients with Abdominal Pain

Like the elderly, pediatric patients with abdominal pain can present challenges that may differ from the adult population. The origin of abdominal pain in pediatric patients can be extra-abdominal and unrelated to the gastrointestinal tract, just as in the adult population, but with different sources in many cases.[10]

In the two- to six-year-old patients, tonsillitis has been a well-described source of abdominal pain. Lower lobe pneumonias can also result in a primary complaint of abdominal pain. Fussiness, lethargy, and altered level of consciousness may be the presenting complaint from the caregiver of children (particularly those less than two years of age) with abdominal pain. The child's gait may be affected and appear uncomfortable, or the child may prefer not to walk, but rather to lie still. Some healthcare providers will ask the child with evidence of abdominal pain to jump up and down for them, which the child is often reluctant to do if suffering from intraabdominal pathology.

As with the elderly, a good history and physical exam can be very challenging in pediatric patients and astute providers will look carefully for evidence of abdominal discomfort or other possible sources of abdominal pain in their pediatric patients. As with patients of all ages, causes of abdominal pain in pediatric patients can range from benign and self-limiting entities to life-threatening pathology, and it is sometimes only the meticulous and observant care provider that is able to tell the difference.

Causes of abdominal pain in pediatric patients are listed in Box 34-3. As with patients of all ages, it is not the role of the prehospital care provider to make the diagnosis of what is causing the abdominal pain in children. Instead, a good knowledge of potential causes and what types of things to be on the lookout for will help the prehospital care provider to appreciate subtle signs of serious pathology.

Women of Childbearing Age with Abdominal Pain

Women of childbearing age present particular challenges to the care provider, and knowledge of the unique aspects of this population is essential in order to appreciate potential life-threatening conditions. Childbearing age is the source of some debate, but to be on the conservative side, any female between nine and 60 years of age should be considered to be of childbearing age. In addition to nearly everything that can cause abdominal pain in males (with the exception of testicular pathology), females have a number of additional potential causes of abdominal pain. **Ectopic pregnancy** should be considered in any female of childbearing age with abdominal or pelvic pain, particularly if signs of hypovolemia are present. This should receive early and strong consideration as it is one of the few causes that can be immediately life-threatening in otherwise young, healthy patients.

CONNECTIONS See Chapter 41: Obstetrics and Gynecology for more information on ectopic pregnancy.

A careful history, preferably without parents present in the case of adolescents, is important, but keep in mind that even in the case of patients who reported normal menstrual periods and who denied any chance

BOX 34-3 Causes of Abdominal Pain in Pediatric Patients

Congenital anomalies
Usually in neonates
Colic
Generally in those under five months of age
Pyloric stenosis
Usually begins in the second or third week of life, presents with projectile vomiting after feeding, and an "olive"-sized mass may be noted in the right, mid-abdominal area.
Intussusception
Usually occurs in patients between three months and six years of age and is more common in males. Patients can appear ill, and caregivers may describe a "currant jelly"-like stool.
Volvulus
A complication of malrotation, it usually occurs in the first month of life.

Incarcerated hernias
Appendicitis
Meckel diverticulum
Toxins (lead, black widow spider bite)
Urinary tract infections
Gastroenteritis
Constipation
Pneumonia
Streptococcal pharyngitis
Generally in patients five to eleven years of age
Trauma
Torsion of the ovary or testicle
Usually over the age of five years
Diabetic ketoacidosis

of pregnancy, 7% were found to be pregnant.[11] Risk factors for ectopic pregnancy include previous ectopic pregnancy, pelvic inflammatory disease or sexually transmitted disease (STD), a history of tubal surgery (including tubal ligations), use of an intrauterine device, and assisted reproduction or fertilization techniques. Other causes of abdominal pain specific to women of childbearing age are listed in Box 34-4.

BOX 34-4 Causes of Abdominal Pain in Women of Childbearing Age

Ectopic pregnancy
Pelvic inflammatory disease
Usually associated with a vaginal discharge
Urinary tract infection
Ovarian torsion or abscess
Ruptured ovarian cyst
Endometriosis
Enlarging uterine fibroids
Trauma
Appendicitis
Incarcerated hernias

Gastrointestinal Bleeding

Gastrointestinal (GI) bleeding is a common and potentially life-threatening problem that prehospital care providers will be called on to manage, and it is potentially very serious, even when the patient looks well. Mortality from GI bleeding can be as high as 10%. There is an overall incidence of between 20 (lower GI) and 100 cases per 100,000 population (upper GI), with an increased incidence among males and in the elderly. Although GI bleeding can occur at any age, it most commonly affects those older than 50, and most deaths occur in those older than 60.[12] DOT 5-6.1, 5-6.23

GI hemorrhage can be very challenging, even for the experienced provider.[13] Any bleeding that occurs above the ligament of Treitz (suspensory ligament of the duodenum) is considered an upper GI bleed while anything distal to this ligament (including the lower quarter of the duodenum), is considered a lower GI bleed. One of the challenges in dealing with these patients is maintaining a sense of urgency in patients with acute GI hemorrhage as the large majority will be stable and remain so throughout their prehospital and emergency department care. The patients that become unstable, however, can do so very quickly and without warning. The astute provider will anticipate a deteriorating condition before it happens, even without any objective warning flags. DOT 5-6.15, 5-6.20

Patients suffering from GI hemorrhage, as with patients with most conditions, can be much more difficult to manage after they become unstable, and effective management sometimes depends on early, aggressive treatment even when faced with a "stable" patient. For this reason, GI bleeding should be considered life-threatening even when the patient does not appear seriously ill.

History

The history can be helpful in identifying the patient who may be experiencing GI bleeding and in differentiating upper from lower GI bleeding although this differentiation is neither absolute nor critical to managing these patients. A thorough history may reveal **hematemesis** (vomiting blood), coffee-ground emesis, **hematochezia** (bloody stools), or **melena** (black or tarry stools). Bloody or coffee ground emesis or melena suggest an upper GI source of the bleeding (esophagus, stomach, or upper or proximal duodenum) while hematochezia suggests a lower GI source (small intestines, colon, or rectum). Brisk upper GI bleeds can cause hematochezia, and lower GI bleeds have caused bloody emesis as well. Differentiation of upper from lower GI bleeds is not critical in the prehospital setting as treatment will be the same for both, but any history obtained by the prehospital provider may be of value to care providers at the hospital, particular if the patient deteriorates and is no longer able to give this information. Alcohol abuse is strongly associated with a number of causes of GI bleeding as is the use of certain medications, such as steroids, aspirin, nonsteroidal antiinflammatory medications (such as ibuprofen), and the anticoagulation medication warfarin, particularly in the elderly.

Physical Exam

A complete physical exam may not reveal any obvious external abnormalities even in a patient who is actively bleeding and seriously ill. Vital signs will often be normal, however even subtle abnormalities should raise concern. A decreased pulse pressure or mild tachypnea can be early signs of impending deterioration. Skin findings (cool or clammy) may suggest signs of shock or signs of chronic alcohol use (jaundice or spider angiomas). The abdominal exam may reveal tenderness.

> It is important to remember that the GI tract can hold a large amount of blood, even the majority of the patient's blood volume, without any external signs on physical exam.

Some patients can tolerate significant blood loss without changes in vital signs, and observed blood loss, either by the provider or the patient, may be minimal, even in the face of massive GI bleeding. It is safest

to assume GI bleeding is serious and manage it aggressively, even when physical evidence is lacking. DOT 5-6.17, 5-6.22

Causes of GI Bleeding

Although the cause will not often matter when managing a patient with GI bleeding, knowledge of the possible causes can sometimes lead to earlier suspicion that the patient is potentially suffering from acute blood loss.

- **Peptic ulcer disease** is a common cause of GI bleeding, accounting for up to 60% of upper GI bleeds.[14]
- **Gastritis** (seen more commonly in alcoholics and with certain medications such as aspirin or ibuprofen) is another common cause.
- **Esophageal varices,** which are strongly associated with alcohol abuse, are a less common cause of upper GI bleeding but are associated with higher morbidity and mortality.
- A patient who has had episodes of severe vomiting or retching and then notices blood in the emesis may be suffering from a **Mallory-Weiss** tear of the esophagus.
- Nose and throat sources of bleeding can result in large amounts of blood swallowed in the stomach and present as apparent upper GI hemorrhage.
- **Diverticulosis, carcinomas, inflammatory bowel disease, polyps,** and **hemorrhoids** are common causes of lower GI bleeding.
- Other causes include **anal fissures or varices, rectal foreign bodies, infectious diarrhea, mesenteric ischemia,** and **pseudomembranous colitis** (bloody diarrhea in patients who have been taking broad-spectrum antibiotics).

Treatment

Rapid resuscitative measures are a priority in any patient with suspected GI hemorrhage. Volume replacement should begin early with crystalloid administered through 2 large-bore intravenous (IV) lines. Early IV placement can be critical, as obtaining IV access in the stable patient will often be significantly easier than obtaining it in the unstable patient, and the only opportunity for relatively easy access may be in the prehospital setting. A critical patient in hypovolemic shock from GI blood loss can be one of the most challenging in which to gain IV access, and taking advantage of opportunities to start an IV early on in the management of such patients can prove invaluable.

Although the patient may not appear ill or short of breath, oxygen administration is important. Any significant blood loss will obviously limit the ability of the patient to deliver oxygen where it needs to go, and supplemental oxygen can be extremely valuable in reducing the effects of blood loss. It is also important to remember that your patient with GI bleeding may be in hypovolemic shock even if not yet hypotensive or tachycardic, and oxygen therapy is critical in any patient in shock. An appropriate appreciation for how serious gastrointestinal bleeding can be, even when faced with a normal-appearing patient with normal vital signs, will lead to appropriate priority being placed on rapid transport to the hospital. After initial resuscitative measures are performed, some of which will be initiated in the field, most patients with significant GI bleeding will be admitted to the hospital and will undergo endoscopy (either upper, lower, or both) to determine the actual source of the bleeding. Certain medications such as octreotide and vasopressin have been used in the emergency department and ICU with some success. DOT 5-6.18, 5-6.19, 5-6.23, 5-6.24, 5-6.73, 5-6.74

Nausea and Vomiting

Nausea and vomiting are among the most common complaints in patients seeking medical care, and are, therefore, a common problem faced by the prehospital provider. Most causes of nausea and vomiting are benign, but the provider will need to be aware of the potentially serious causes and be alert for signs of serious illness. Nausea and vomiting may be the primary complaint, or they may be a secondary problem related to the patient's illness. They may represent a GI illness (such as a small bowel obstruction) or a number of other systemic problems. Myocardial infarction, sepsis, medications, head injuries, and pregnancy are some examples of causes outside the GI system that may present as nausea and vomiting. Vomiting can also lead to potentially serious problems such as dehydration, aspiration, upper GI bleeding (Mallory-Weiss syndrome), and **esophageal rupture (Boerhaave's syndrome).** The most common causes of nausea and vomiting are acute gastroenteritis, febrile systemic illness, and drug effects.[15] DOT 5-6.25, 5-6.26, 5-6.27, 5-6.28, 5-6.29

History

There are several aspects of the history in a patient that is experiencing nausea and vomiting that may prove helpful. Other associated symptoms can help direct the provider as to what might be causing the symptoms. The timing of the symptoms can be helpful as well.

- Did the nausea or vomiting occur before or after other associated symptoms, such as abdominal pain?
- Do the symptoms occur primarily in the morning or after eating?

A past medical history may reveal previous abdominal surgery, which could raise the concern for bowel obstruction, as the most common cause of small bowel obstruction is adhesions from previous surgery. Medications the patient takes may reveal a potential cause for the symptoms the patient is experiencing.

Physical Examination

As with many presenting complaints, the physical exam in the patient who is experiencing nausea and vomiting may reveal significant findings that can help direct the care of the patient, or it may be entirely normal and reveal nothing even in the presence of serious pathology. Particular aspects of the exam to pay attention to in the patient with nausea and vomiting include vital signs and skin findings (orthostatic changes or poor turgor may be a sign of dehydration), the eye exam (nystagmus can indicate a neurologic cause of the symptoms), and the abdominal exam (significant tenderness raises the concern for intra-abdominal pathology, or distention could raise the concern for bowel obstruction). Checking for orthostatic changes in a patient who already has abnormal vital signs (tachycardia, hypotension, or both) can be dangerous and should be avoided.

Treatment

While the history and physical exam may raise the suspicion for certain potential etiologies, the definitive cause of the nausea and vomiting your patient is experiencing will rarely be identified in the field. This does not preclude use of treatment strategies aimed at improving the patient's symptoms. In general, IV access should be obtained, and fluid therapy with crystalloid therapy initiated. Aggressive fluid management may be appropriate in the severely dehydrated patient, with 2 liters or more given in the field. Antiemetics should not be routinely used in all patients with nausea as most of these medications will induce drowsiness, and the patient will be more difficult to get accurate information from (both on history and physical exam) upon arrival at the hospital.

There are a number of situations, however, where antiemetics are appropriate in the prehospital setting. Phenothiazines such as promethazine (Phenergan™) or prochlorperazine (Compazine™) have been used with success. Side effects such as dystonic reactions are not uncommon but can be treated successfully with diphenhydramine (Benadryl™), which can also be used by itself as an antiemetic. Metoclopromide (Reglan™) has also been used very effectively in the prehospital setting and is the only antiemetic that is a category B for pregnancy. It should be a first choice, if available, for the treatment of nausea and vomiting in women of childbearing age.

Gastroenteritis

Acute gastroenteritis is a syndrome that includes vomiting, diarrhea, and abdominal pain. It is usually caused by inflammation somewhere in the GI tract, which can result from a variety of causes, including foods, medications, and infections. Although viral gastroenteritis is a very common cause of nausea and vomiting, you should be very careful before deciding this is the cause of your patient's symptoms. Gastroenteritis has been called a "wastebasket" diagnosis as it seems to be the diagnosis providers turn to when they do not have a clear explanation for what their patient is experiencing. Appendicitis, acute myocardial infarctions, and even meningitis (particularly in children) have been labeled as gastroenteritis, often because of associated nausea and vomiting. It is often said it is not the role of the prehospital provider to diagnose. Whether you agree with this or not, the patient with nausea and vomiting is a particularly appropriate candidate for your immediate supportive care, not diagnosis. DOT 5-6.25, 5-6.26, 5-6.27, 5-6.28, 5-6.29

Once you assign a diagnosis, it is far too easy to let your guard down and not be alert to changing status or new developments. This "diagnosis" will often stick with the patient into the hospital or at follow-up, and it may decrease the chances of future providers keeping their minds open for other possibilities. You will hear the term gastroenteritis quite frequently, but it should not be a consideration in the field. If you assume a more serious entity and it turns out your patient had a viral gastroenteritis, no harm has been done; whereas, if you assume gastroenteritis is the cause of your patient's symptoms and you are wrong, there is the potential for harm. DOT 5-6.35, 5-6.36, 5-6,37, 5-6.38, 5-6.39

Diarrhea

Although not a frequent complaint encountered in the prehospital environment, diarrhea is a very common medical problem and can account for up to 5% of ED visits, particularly in children and in the fall and winter months. Diarrhea remains a significant worldwide problem, accounting for more than 4 million deaths per year, and it is estimated that in the United States, there are more than 200,000 hospitalizations annually due to problems related to diarrhea. The large majority of cases are caused by infections, and while most are self-limiting, serious complications can occur.[16] It is also estimated that up to 60% of persons infected with the human immunodeficiency virus (HIV) will suffer from significant diarrhea at some point in the course of their disease, and now that persons with HIV are living longer, there may be more opportunities to care for these individuals. Diarrhea in HIV patients can be

life-threatening and should be recognized as a potentially very serious complication.

Campylobacter is the most common cause of diarrhea in patients who seek medical attention. Other bacteria include Salmonella, Shigella, and *E. coli* (common cause of bloody diarrhea).

Field treatment is primarily directed at recognition of and treatment for dehydration. Intravenous access and crystalloid IV fluid administration are appropriate for patients with evidence of volume loss secondary to dehydration.

Esophageal Disease

The esophagus is a muscular tube located posterior and lateral to the trachea in the neck and mediastinum. It is slightly smaller in the upper (cervical) and lower (abdominal) aspects, which leads to some of the pathology related to this organ (see Figure 34-1). There are three anatomic constrictions within the esophagus: one at the top, at the level of the cricopharyngeus muscle; another at the level of the aortic notch; and a third at the gastroesophageal junction as the esophagus enters the stomach. These are common areas where food can get caught.

The sympathetic innervation of the esophagus is very similar to that of the heart, which explains why differentiating esophageal from cardiac etiology of a patient's pain can sometimes be very challenging. Although it would be unusual to make the diagnosis of an esophageal disorder in the field, a good understanding of the anatomy and types of symptoms esophageal disease can cause can help the paramedic in the evaluation of common problems they will manage. Complaints of **dysphagia** (difficulty swallowing), **odynophagia** (painful swallowing), ingested foreign body, chest pain, upper GI bleeding, and abdominal pain all can involve the esophagus.

Esophageal Varices

Esophageal varices are dilated veins in the esophagus, resulting from elevated venous pressure from a back-up of blood from the liver. They are often a complication of alcoholic liver disease (portal hypertension). The most concerning complication of the formation of esophageal varices is bleeding, which can be massive. Upper GI bleeding in patients with evidence of alcohol abuse and liver disease may be a result of esophageal varices. Management is discussed in the GI bleeding section of this chapter. DOT 5-6.70, 5-6.71, 5-6.72

Esophagitis

Defined as inflammation of the esophagus, **esophagitis** can be caused by gastroesophageal reflux disease (most common), infectious agents (particularly *Candida* *albicans* in HIV-positive patients), pills becoming lodged in the esophagus **(pill esophagitis),** or caustic ingestions (such as strongly acidic or alkaline substances). Treatment beyond appropriate pain control is generally initiated in the emergency department and will depend on the underlying cause.

Dysphagia

Dysphagia is defined as difficulty swallowing and is not a particularly common complaint seen in the prehospital setting. Causes vary and can include swallowed or impacted foreign bodies, esophageal cancer, strictures (often the result of scarring from gastroesophageal reflux disease [GERD]), motility disorders such as achalasia, esophageal spasm, or neuromuscular disorders such as cerebrovascular accidents (CVAs). Field treatment is primarily supportive with transport to the ED for evaluation.

Swallowed Foreign Bodies

Although the large majority of swallowed foreign bodies will pass spontaneously and cause no long-term problems, more than 1,500 people die every year in the United States as a result of ingesting foreign bodies.[17] Although much more common in the pediatric population, foreign body ingestion occurs in all age groups, with more common occurrences in prisoners, psychiatric patients, and those who wear dentures.

Most ingested foreign bodies in pediatric patients get caught in the proximal esophagus while those in the adult population are related to underlying esophageal disease (sometimes previously undiagnosed) and lodge in the distal esophagus. Most objects that get to the stomach will ultimately pass through the rectum without intervention, but exceptions may include irregularly shaped, sharp, or elongated objects and button batteries. A button battery lodged anywhere in the GI tract is a true emergency because the alkaline substance inside the battery can cause severe burns if the battery leaks. Objects lodged in the esophagus can result in airway obstruction, particularly in children, and is classically caused by coins getting lodged in the upper esophagus. Patients with foreign bodies stuck in the esophagus can be very accurate as to the location of the object (Figure 34-5). If they point to an area in their neck or chest where they are sensing the discomfort, it is very likely that either the foreign body is somewhere very near that location, or in the process of passing through the GI tract, the object caused an abrasion or other injury, leading to the discomfort the patient is experiencing in that location. Field care is primarily supportive. Patients with signs of airway obstruction should be allowed to assume a position of

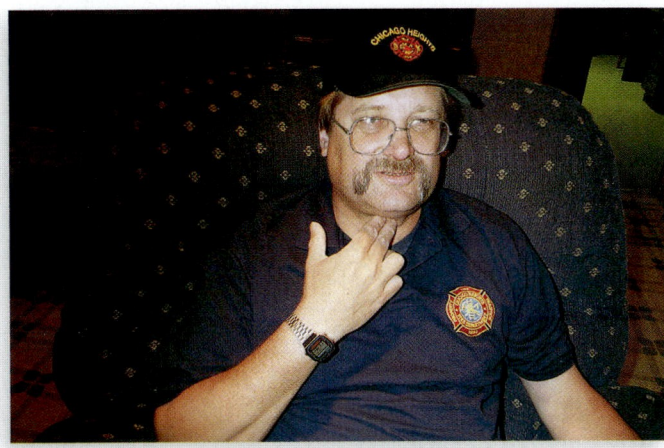

Figure 34-5 Patients are usually very accurate when describing the location of a foreign body.

comfort. On rare occasions, active airway management will be necessary to assure a patent airway.

Chest Pain

There are a number of esophageal disorders that can lead to the patient experiencing chest pain. This pain can be very similar to that experienced by patients who are suffering from cardiac ischemia. Since most pain caused by esophageal disorders is not immediately life-threatening while pain caused by cardiac ischemia obviously can be, it is prudent for the prehospital provider to assume a cardiac cause of a patient's complaints. Esophageal disorders that can cause the patient to experience chest pain include GERD (which affects up to 25% of the adult population and an even higher percentage in the elderly), esophageal spasm, esophagitis (more common in immunosuppressed individuals), and esophageal perforation (from trauma, foreign bodies, or severe retching) otherwise known as **Boerhaave's syndrome.**[18] Some of these entities, particularly GERD, may respond to treatments such as oxygen therapy or nitroglycerin, just as cardiac disease may respond to antacids or H_2 receptor blockers typically used to treat some esophageal or gastric disorders.

Gastric Disease

Gastroesophageal reflux disease (GERD) (sometimes referred to as **heartburn**) occurs when there is reflux of gastric contents into the esophagus. It occurs in up to 40% of adults in the United States each month.[19] The most common symptom is pain that is often described as a burning sensation beginning in the mid-epigastric area and moving toward the neck and mouth. There can be associated nausea, vomiting, and diaphoresis. As noted above, these symptoms can be very similar to angina, and cardiac causes should always be considered.

Peptic ulcer disease (PUD) and **gastritis** are common problems, with nearly 10% of the U.S. population over the age of 17 years suffering from PUD at some point in their lives, resulting in over 275,000 hospitalizations every year.[20] PUD is felt to arise when there is an imbalance between the production of acid within the stomach and the ability of the gastric mucosa lining the stomach to prevent itself from being damaged. While classically described as a burning pain that often occurs on an empty stomach and that may be relieved by certain foods, atypical presentations are common, particularly in the elderly.

Associated symptoms can include nausea, vomiting, and occasionally GI bleeding. Treatment is often symptomatic with a careful search for serious complications such as bleeding. H_2 blockers, such as ranitidine either orally or IV, have been used with some success, usually in patients who have been sent home from the hospital or doctor's office after the diagnosis has been confirmed. While a very common problem, the definitive diagnosis of PUD or gastritis will not be made in the field, and as with esophageal disease, it is most prudent for the paramedic to treat these symptoms as if they were caused by one of the more serious etiologies, such as cardiac, and not assume a gastric cause. DOT 5-6.50, 5-6.51, 5-6.52, 5-6.53, 5-6.54

Biliary Tract Disease

The biliary tract consists of hepatic bile canaliculi, which produce bile, the bile ducts, and the gallbladder. Gallbladder disease is primarily related to the formation of gallstones and is a common problem in patients seeking emergency medical care, with up to 25% of women and 15% of men older than age 50 having gallstones.[21] The gallbladder receives, concentrates, and secretes bile to assist in intestinal absorption of fats and fat-soluble nutrients. The presence of food in the stomach stimulates the gallbladder to contract, sending bile to the duodenum. Risk factors for gallbladder disease include advanced age, female gender, obesity, hyperlipidemia, and family history.

Cholecystitis is the acute inflammation of the gallbladder and usually occurs when the neck of the gallbladder or cystic duct is obstructed, often by a gallstone, and intraluminal pressure increases. The resulting inflammation leads to mucosal damage and ischemia. Pain is typically localized to the right upper quadrant (RUQ), nausea and vomiting are common, and a low-grade fever and tachycardia may be present. A **Murphy sign** (momentary inspiratory arrest during palpation of the RUQ) may be elicited. Infections can be associated with the obstruction, and a **Charcot triad** of RUQ pain, fever, and jaundice should raise the suspicion of **ascending cholangitis.** This will be more common in the elderly,

diabetics, and the debilitated, and mortality can approach 40%.[22] Treatment focuses on hydration, antiemetics, and analgesia, as appropriate. Antibiotics and emergency surgery will sometimes be required, particularly in the cases that don't respond to measures taken in the emergency department. DOT 5-6.1, 5-6.80, 5-6.81, 5-6.82, 5-6.83, 5-6.84

Pancreatitis

The pancreas is a retroperitoneal organ that lies across the posterior abdomen in the mid-epigastric area. The pancreatic duct enters into the duodenum with the common bile duct and produces digestive enzymes as well as bicarbonate (Figure 34-6). The pancreas also produces insulin and glucagon, and, therefore, has both exocrine (digestive enzymes) and endocrine (hormone) functions. DOT 5-6.68, 5-6.69

The two most common disorders associated with the pancreas are diabetes and acute pancreatitis. **Pancreatitis** is an inflammation of the pancreas, generally resulting in abdominal pain that is usually located in the mid-epigastric area or right upper quadrant. Most cases of pancreatitis are caused by either gallstones (45%) or alcoholism (35%).[23] It can also be caused by a number of medications, including many that are commonly taken by patients with HIV. Pancreatitis can range from mild to severe, and although mortality has significantly decreased in the past 30 years, it can still be life-threatening, particularly in HIV patients or the rare case of a child with pancreatitis.[24]

Treatment is generally supportive with IV fluid hydration and pain control, as appropriate. Although, as with many entities in gastroenterology, the diagnosis of pancreatitis will not be made definitively in the field, the prehospital care provider should be aware of this as a possible cause of abdominal pain. DOT 5-6.65, 5-6.66, 5-6.67

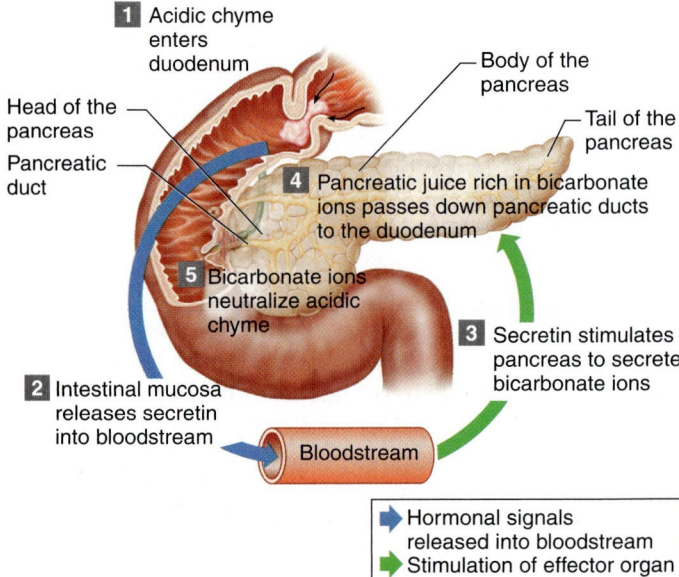

Figure 34-6   The anatomy and function of the pancreas.

Appendicitis

Acute appendicitis is caused by inflammation of the appendix, and it is a common condition that can develop at any age. About 7% of people will develop appendicitis at some point in their lifetimes, with most cases occurring in young adults and being slightly more common in men than in women.[25] The incidence of appendicitis in the United States appears to be decreasing although the reasons for this decrease are not entirely clear.[26]

Acute appendicitis is thought to begin with an obstruction of the lumen of the appendix from inflammation, adhesions, or even food. The appendix continues to secrete mucosal fluid, leading to a build-up of pressure within the appendix, resulting in the pain that a patient with appendicitis generally experiences. If medical attention is not sought or the diagnosis of appendicitis is not appreciated, this build-up of pressure can lead to perforation of the appendix and spilling of bowel contents into the peritoneal cavity. The initial inflammation triggers the visceral pain fibers supplying the appendix, resulting in vague, poorly localized pain (often in the periumbilical or epigastric area) that the patient often experiences early in the course of appendicitis. As inflammation continues, somatic pain fibers are inflamed, localizing the pain to the right lower quadrant area. DOT 5-6.64, 5-6.45

The history may reveal abdominal pain or discomfort, classically beginning in the periumbilical region and moving to the right lower quadrant (Figure 34-7). Patients may also describe a feeling similar to indigestion. This is often followed by anorexia, nausea, and sometimes vomiting. There may also be an associated low-grade fever although this often occurs later in the course of this disease. Upon physical exam, abdominal tenderness may be elicited, although early on there may not be any localized tenderness. As the pain becomes more localized, tenderness is classically elicited at McBurney point, which is below the middle of a line connecting the umbilicus and the anterosuperior iliac spine of the pelvis. Pain in the right lower quadrant with palpation of the left lower quadrant (Rovsing sign), is sometimes found. DOT 5-6.47

Although appendicitis may seem to be a relatively easy and straightforward diagnosis to make, this is often not the case.[21] Early in the course of appendicitis, the patient often experiences vague symptoms that might be consistent with many entities such as "food poisoning." If the appendix is lying in the retrocecal area, which may be more common than once thought, the patient may experience flank pain.[27] The pregnant uterus can displace the appendix up toward the right upper quadrant, resulting in pain higher in the abdomen than you think the appendix should be. Although diarrhea is not classically described as being associated with appendicitis, some patients may experience diarrhea as their appendix becomes inflamed, and the fact that a patient may have diarrhea does not in any way exclude the diagnosis of appendicitis.

As has been previously discussed, patients do not read a textbook of how signs and symptoms should present with illness and, therefore, may not have a "classic" presentation of a disease such as appendicitis. It is wise to keep appendicitis in the differential diagnosis of all patients with vague abdominal symptoms until the diagnosis has been ruled out (or unless the appendix has already been removed). Appreciation of how appendicitis can present and early consideration of the diagnosis in patients without classic symptoms may result in an earlier diagnosis and a better outcome in patients with this disease. DOT 5-6.49

Treatment of appendicitis in the field will be limited, but reasonable pain management is appropriate, and local protocols should allow prudent use of pain medications in the field for patients with abdominal pain. The diagnosis of appendicitis can be made by CT scan in the emergency department or by direct

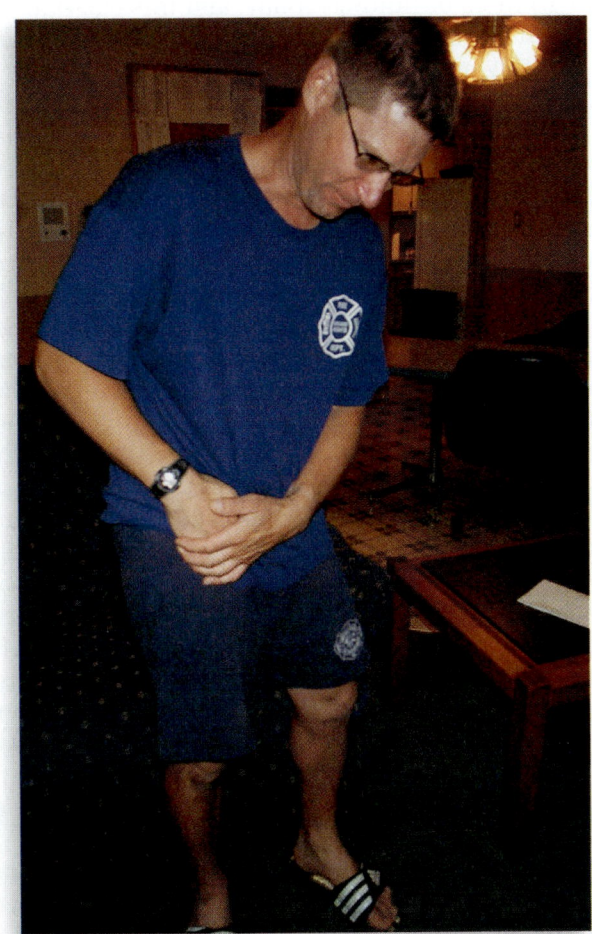

Figure 34-7 Pain from appendicitis is often felt in the periumbilical region and then moves to the right lower quadrant.

visualization in the operating room. The ultimate treatment for appendicitis is removal of the appendix in the operating room. DOT 5-6.48, 5-6.49

Intestinal Obstruction

Intestinal obstruction accounts for up to 20% of acute surgical admissions and has a mortality rate of approximately 5%.[28] The key to treatment is early recognition and surgical intervention, and that recognition can begin in the field. Knowing the likely presenting symptoms and findings, as well as who is at risk for bowel obstruction, will help direct the provider to consider this diagnosis and choose treatment and destination options that are appropriate.

Obstructions most commonly affect the small bowel, but up to 20% involve the colon. Up to 50% of small bowel obstructions are caused by adhesions from previous abdominal surgery.[29] Hernias, neoplasms, inflammatory bowel disease (Crohn's disease in particular), and intussusception (predominantly in children) are other considerations. The gastrointestinal tract produces up to 10 liters of fluid each day, and this can build up quickly when an obstruction occurs, even if the patient is not eating or drinking. DOT 5-6.1, 5-6.55, 5-6.56

Pain is generally the presenting complaint, and it is usually associated with nausea and vomiting. The pain is commonly described as intermittent and cramping, and the vomiting usually follows the onset of abdominal pain. The patient may describe decreased stool production, but some passage of stool and even diarrhea may be present. Patients also often complain of a distended abdomen. A history of previous abdominal surgeries, colon cancer, or previous similar episodes that have been obstructions can help raise the concern for bowel obstruction as a cause of the patient's complaints.

Vital signs will typically be normal or only minimally altered until late in the course of this disease. Abdominal tenderness is common, and distention may be appreciated. The remainder of the physical exam is often unremarkable.

The treatment for bowel obstruction is bowel rest (nothing by mouth), IV fluids, bowel decompression (by nasogastric tube), and symptomatic treatment (nausea and pain control). Surgery is sometimes needed to relieve the cause of the obstruction. DOT 5-6.57, 5-6.58, 5-6.59

Street Secrets

You should place a nasogastric tube into any patient who is in cardiac arrest, especially the pediatric patient, if protocols allow. Gastric distention secondary to forced ventilations can cause the stomach to push up on the diaphragm and impair ventilatory efforts.

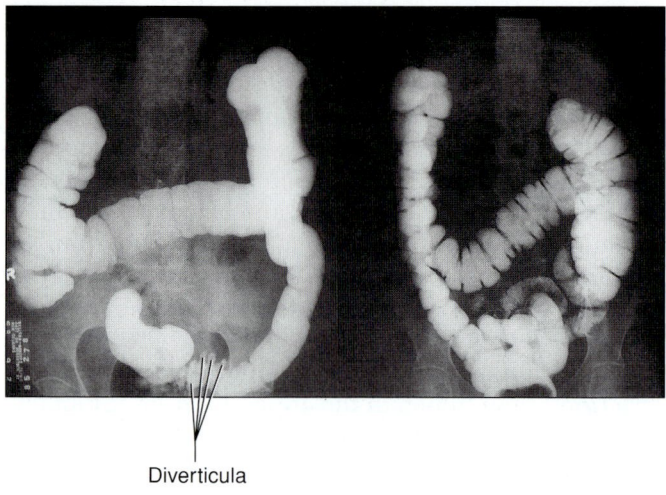

Diverticula

Figure 34-8   Diverticulosis. The large intestine on the left shows multiple diverticula. The one on the right is healthy.

Diverticulitis

Diverticulitis is inflammation of diverticula, which are sacs or pouches protruding out from the bowel. This inflammation can result in perforation of the diverticulum, abscess or fistula formation, or obstruction. Over 90% of diverticula are located in the sigmoid colon, with the rest located in the cecum, ascending colon, and transverse colon. **Diverticulosis** (the presence of diverticula) is equally common among men and women, and exists in over 50% of those older than age 70 (Figure 34-8).[30] DOT 5-6.40, 5-6.41

Clinical presentations related to diverticulitis are generally related to pain or bleeding. The pain of diverticulitis is often relatively sudden in onset and localized in the left lower quadrant area. It is sometimes associated with a fever. When diverticular disease results in bleeding, it is often sudden, severe, and painless rectal bleeding. The blood is usually bright or dark red. Treatment for diverticular disease and diverticulitis will focus on management of the bleeding, when present, and appropriate pain management. Antibiotics will be administered in the emergency department, and surgery is sometimes required to manage bleeding or cases that are unresponsive to antibiotics. DOT 5-6.42, 5-6.43, 5-6.44

Inflammatory Bowel Disease

Inflammatory bowel disease (IBD) consists of two chronic intestinal disorders: ulcerative colitis and Crohn's disease. The causes of both disorders are not completely understood. Onset of these diseases is most common in young adults (15 to 25 years old) and in patients 55 to 60 years of age. Ulcerative colitis is usually localized to the colon while Crohn's disease can be found anywhere in the intestinal tract and often in multiple locations, although it may not be continuous ("skip" lesions).

Patients tend to present with abdominal pain, chronic diarrhea, and anorexia and may have fever as well, but the presentation can be quite variable. Complications of IBD include bowel swelling and perforation, abscess formation, bowel obstruction, dehydration, and bleeding. These should be considered in all patients with an established diagnosis of IBD or in patients where the care provider has a high suspicion for IBD.

Treatment will include bowel rest and aggressive IV fluid management, when appropriate, and some patients will receive steroids and antibiotics in the emergency department. Surgery may be required for some of the complications related to IBD that do not respond to medical management. DOT 5-6.30, 5-6.31, 5-6.32, 5-6.33, 5-6.34, 5-6.60, 5-6.61, 5-6.62, 5-6.63, 5-6.64

Jaundice

Jaundice is defined as a yellowing of the skin, sclera of the eye, and other tissues due to excess circulating bilirubin (Figure 34-9). Bilirubin is a product of hemoglobin breakdown or metabolism, which is then conjugated in the liver and excreted from the body in urine or feces. Jaundice can affect patients of all ages, from neonates to the elderly, and will be seen in a variety of clinical settings. Jaundice can develop when there is excessive heme breakdown, failure of the liver to take up bilirubin, failure of the liver to conjugate and excrete bilirubin, or an obstruction of biliary excretion into the intestines. The principle causes of jaundice include liver disease, biliary obstruction, and hemolysis. Biliary disease leading to jaundice is often associated with pain.

Jaundice from underlying liver disease is often accompanied by other signs of that liver disease (such as ascites, evidence of malnutrition, spider angiomata, and palmar erythema). Jaundice without abdominal pain or other signs of liver disease should cause the provider to consider hemolysis or pancreatic cancer as a possible cause.

The actual diagnosis will not likely be made in the field, but awareness of what can lead to a patient presenting with jaundice can be helpful in predicting problems your patient may experience. For example, patients with liver (hepatic) failure are at risk for hypoglycemia, so any jaundice patient with altered mental status should have blood sugar checked. A careful exam for volume status should be performed, including listening to the patient's lungs and checking for peripheral edema as jaundice from hepatic congestion in the setting of congestive heart failure can occur. Mental status should be carefully assessed for early signs of hepatic encephalopathy, and signs of bleeding should be noted.

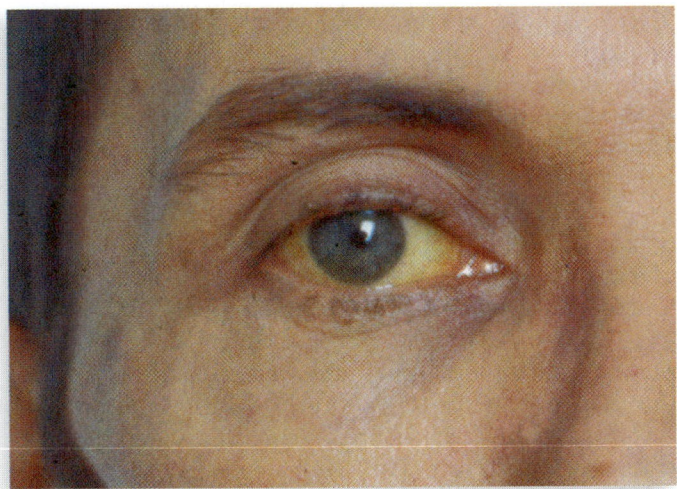

Figure 34-9 A patient with jaundice presents with yellowish skin and sclera.

Pregnant women presenting with jaundice can be very concerning. **HELLP syndrome** (**h**emolysis, **e**levated **l**iver enzymes, and **l**ow **p**latelets), which is often associated with nausea, vomiting, and right upper quadrant pain, as well as acute fatty liver of pregnancy generally accompanied by altered mental status, can lead to jaundice. Both will require emergency delivery.

Management of the jaundice patient in the field generally will include IV access and fluids if the patient is hypotensive without signs of fluid overload or if there is any evidence of bleeding. Naloxone and glucose should be considered if the patient has altered mental status.

Hepatitis

Hepatitis means an inflammation of the liver. It is most commonly the result of a viral infection but can also be due to bacterial and parasitic infections, prescribed medications, a toxic exposure (such as certain kinds of wild mushrooms), or an immunologic disorder. Most cases of viral hepatitis are caused by type A (infectious), type B (serum), and type C (classically described as posttransfusion, but also commonly associated with IV drug use or occupational exposure).

- Hepatitis A is caused by an RNA virus, and is generally spread by the fecal-oral route, either directly or through contaminated food or water. It is very unusual to contract hepatitis A from contact with blood.
- Hepatitis B is caused by a DNA virus and is generally contracted by exposure to blood or sexual contact.
- Hepatitis C is caused by an RNA virus as is hepatitis E, which is encountered most often in Asia, Africa, and the Soviet Union.

CONNECTIONS Hepatitis is discussed in more detail in Chapter 33: Infectious and Communicable Diseases, page 817.

Healthcare workers are most at-risk for contracting hepatitis B or C from needle sticks from equipment used on infected individuals. Widespread use of the hepatitis B vaccine, as well as increased awareness and safer sexual practices, have lead to the reduction in rates of hepatitis B.

Although there is no vaccine currently available for hepatitis C, a recent study showed some promising effects of treatment after contraction of hepatitis C from occupational exposure in healthcare workers. DOT 5-6.85, 5-6.86

The pathophysiology of viral hepatitis is not completely understood although it does appear that most of the liver injury occurs as a result of the immunologic response to the virus as opposed to damage to the liver from the virus itself. The clinical presentation is variable and can range from asymptomatic (the majority of cases) to fulminant hepatitis with liver failure and encephalopathy in 1% to 2% of cases.[30] Common complaints include malaise, fever, anorexia, nausea, vomiting, and abdominal pain. It is not unusual for the patient to seek medical care only when jaundice develops. Jaundice is sometimes best appreciated in the sclera, particularly in African Americans. On physical exam, jaundice may be evident as well as abdominal tenderness. An enlarged liver may be appreciated on exam.

Management

The management of patients with viral hepatitis is largely symptomatic. Fluid replacement and treatment of nausea are the most common interventions paramedics will be called upon to provide. Altered mental status can suggest liver failure with hepatic encephalopathy and should be managed as all altered mental status is treated in the prehospital setting, including dextrose stick and pulse oximetry. There is a risk of exposure to the disease for healthcare workers, and proper pre- and postexposure prophylaxis should be strongly considered. DOT 5-6.87, 5-6.88, 5-6.89

Alcohol-Related Liver Disease

Alcoholism is a major problem across the world, with an estimated 10 million chronic alcoholics in the United States alone.[31] While alcohol can affect all systems of the body, the liver is the most common site of injury from chronic alcohol use. Although the exact mechanism of injury is unclear, it is multifactorial, with accumulation of toxic metabolites, malnutrition, and alteration of immune function likely all playing a role.

Alcohol-related liver disease includes **alcoholic hepatitis,** which presents essentially the same way as does viral hepatitis, and **cirrhosis,** which is the end-stage of liver disease marked by the permanent destruction of hepatocytes. Patients with alcohol-related liver disease commonly complain of fatigue and poor appetite.

Findings on exam may include spider angiomata or ascites (a distended abdomen with a fluid wave, indicative of a build up of fluid in the peritoneal cavity). These patients are at-risk for developing other serious complications, including GI bleeding, **hepatic encephalopathy** (altered mental status from a build-up of ammonia in the blood), **ascites** (fluid accumulation in the abdomen), **spontaneous bacterial peritonitis** (infection of ascites fluid in the peritoneum), and **hepatorenal syndrome** (combined liver and renal failure of unclear cause). DOT 5-6.2

Summary

Abdominal pain is difficult to assess and manage. Many organs and systems are located in the abdominal cavity, including gastrointestinal, circulatory vessels, and genitourinary. Abdominal pain is a potential sign for several life-threatening conditions, including abdominal aortic aneurysm (AAA), acute myocardial infarction, pulmonary embolus (PE), bleeding from the spleen or liver, or a ruptured ectopic pregnancy.

It is not necessary to make a diagnosis. If the patient is not in need of immediate transport, perform a thorough history and physical examination and obtain as much information as possible. The GI tract can hold a large amount of blood, even the majority of the patient's blood volume, without any obvious signs on physical exam. An abdominal complaint may be minor or significant enough to cause loss of life. Keep an open mind and a high index of suspicion while treating abdominal pain.

Notes

1. J. A. Marx, ed., *Rosen's Emergency Medicine Concepts and Clinical Practice,* 5th ed. (St. Louis, MO: Elsevier Mosby, 2002), p. 185.
2. L. F. McCaig and L. Nghi, *National Hospital Ambulatory Medical Care Survey: 2000 Emergency Department Summary. Advance Data from Vital and Health Statistics: No. 326* (Hyattsville, MD: National Center for Health Statistics, 2002), p. 14.
3. S. A. Colucciello, T. W. Lukens, and D. L. Morgan, "Assessing Abdominal Pain in Adults: A Rational Cost-Effective, and Evidence-Based Strategy," *Emergency Medicine Practice* 1(1)(1999): 1–20.
4. J. L. Ponka, J. K. Welborn, and B. E. Brush, "Acute Abdominal Pain in Aged Patients: An Analysis of 200 Cases," *Journal of the American Geriatric Society* 11(1963): 993.
5. J. Koziol-McLain, S. Lowenstein, and B. Fuller, "Orthostatic Vital Signs in Emergency Department Patients," *Annals of Emergency Medicine* 20(1991): 606.
6. P. B. Fontanarosa, "Abdominal, Genitourinary, and Back Pain," In *Paramedic Field Care: A Complaint-Based Approach,* P. T. Pons and D. Cason, eds. (St Louis, MO: Mosby, 1997), 439–449.
7. G. S. Brewster, M. E. Herbert, and J. R. Hoffman, "Medical Myth: Analgesia Should Not be Given to Patients with an Acute Abdomen Because it Obscures the Diagnosis," *The Western Journal of Medicine* 172(2000): 209.

8. K. W. Kizer and M. J. Vassar, "Emergency Department Diagnosis of Abdominal Disorders in the Elderly," *The American Journal of Emergency Medicine* 16(1998): 357.

9. J. S. Bender, "Approach to the Acute Abdomen," *The Medical Clinics of North America* 73(1989): 1413.

10. J. D. Mason, "The Evaluation of Acute Abdominal Pain in Children," *Emergency Medical Clinics of North America* 14(1996): 629.

11. E. A. Ramosa, A. D. Sacchetti, and M. Nepp, "Reliability of Patient History in Determining the Possibility of Pregnancy," *Annals of Emergency Medicine* 18(1989): 48.

12. P. L. Henneman, "Gastrointestinal Bleeding," In *Rosen's Emergency Medicine: Concepts and Clinical Practice,* 5th ed., J. A. Marx, ed. (St. Louis, MO: Mosby, 2002), p. 194.

13. D. T. Overton, "Gastrointestinal Bleeding," In *Emergency Medicine: A Comprehensive Study Guide,* 6th ed., J. E. Tintinalli, G. D. Kelen, J. S. Stapczynski, eds. (New York, NY: McGraw-Hill, 2004), pp. 505–508.

14. G. F. Longstreth, "Epidemiology and Outcome of Patients Hospitalized with Acute Lower Gastrointestinal Hemorrhage: A Population-Based Study," *The American Journal of Gastroenterology* 92(1997): 419.

15. T. Heilenbach, "Nausea and Vomiting," In *Rosen's Emergency Medicine: Concepts and Clinical Practice,* 5th ed., J. A. Marx, ed. (St. Louis, MO: Mosby, 2002), p. 178.

16. J. E. Gough and P. A. Clement, "Diarrhea," In *Rosen's Emergency Medicine: Concepts and Clinical Practice,* 5th ed., J. A. Marx, ed. (St. Louis, MO: Mosby, 2002), p. 200.

17. G. F. Schwartz and H. S. Polsky, "Ingested Foreign Bodies of the Gastrointestinal Tract," *The American Surgeon* 42(1976): 236.

18. J. E. Richter, "Typical and Atypical Presentations of Gastroesophageal Reflux Disease: The Role of Esophageal Testing in Diagnosis and Management," *Gastroenterology Clinics of North America* 25(1996): 75.

19. O. T. Nebel, M. F. Frones, and D. O. Castell, "Symptomatic Gastroesophageal Reflux: Incidence and Precipitating Factors," *The American Journal of Digestive Disease* 21(1976): 953.

20. A. Sonnenberg and J. E. Everhart, "Health Impact of Peptic Ulcer in the United States," *The American Journal of Gastroenterology* 92(1997): 614.

21. J. D. Wilson, "Acute Diseases of the Biliary Tract," In *Harwood-Nuss' Clinical Practice of Emergency Medicine,* 4th ed., A. B. Wolfson, G. W. Hendey, P. L. Hendry, et al. (Philadelphia, PA: Lippincott Williams & Wilkins, 2005), pp. 361–5.

22. R. Elsakr, D. A. Johnson, Z. Younes, et al., "Antimicrobial Treatment of Intra-Abdominal Infections," *Digestive Diseases* 16(1998): 46.

23. W. M. Steinberg, "Diagnosis and Management of Acute Pancreatitis," *Cleveland Clinic Journal of Medicine* 64(1997): 182.

24. J. P. Neoptolemos et al., "Acute Pancreatitis: The Substantial Human and Financial Costs," *Gut* 42(1998): 888.

25. J. Wagner, P. Mckinnery, and J. Carpenter, "Does This Patient Have Appendicitis?" *Journal of the American Medical Association* 276(1996): 1589.

26. M. Feldman, *Sleisenger & Fordtran's Gastrointestinal and Liver Disease,* 6th ed. (Philadelphia, PA: WB Saunders, 1998).

27. D. C. Collins, "71,000 Human Appendix Specimens: A Final Report, Summarizing Forty Years' Study," *American Journal of Proctology* 14(1963): 365.

28. P. L. Henneman and S. P. Torrey, "Bowel Obstruction." In *Harwood-Nuss' Clincal Practice of Emergency Medicine,* 4th ed., A. B. Wolfson, G. W. Hendey, P. L. Hendry, et al. (Philadelphia, PA: Lippincott Williams & Wilkins, 2005), pp. 391–4.

29. K. N. Bass, B. Jones, and G. B. Bulkley, "Current Management of Small-Bowel Obstruction," *Advances in Surgery* 31(1997): 1.

30. R. C. Dickman and L. J. Checking, "Diverticular Disease in the Elderly," *Journal of the American Geriatric Society* 40(1993): 986–993.

31. W. Lee, "Acute Liver Failure," *The New England Journal of Medicine* 329(1993): 1862.

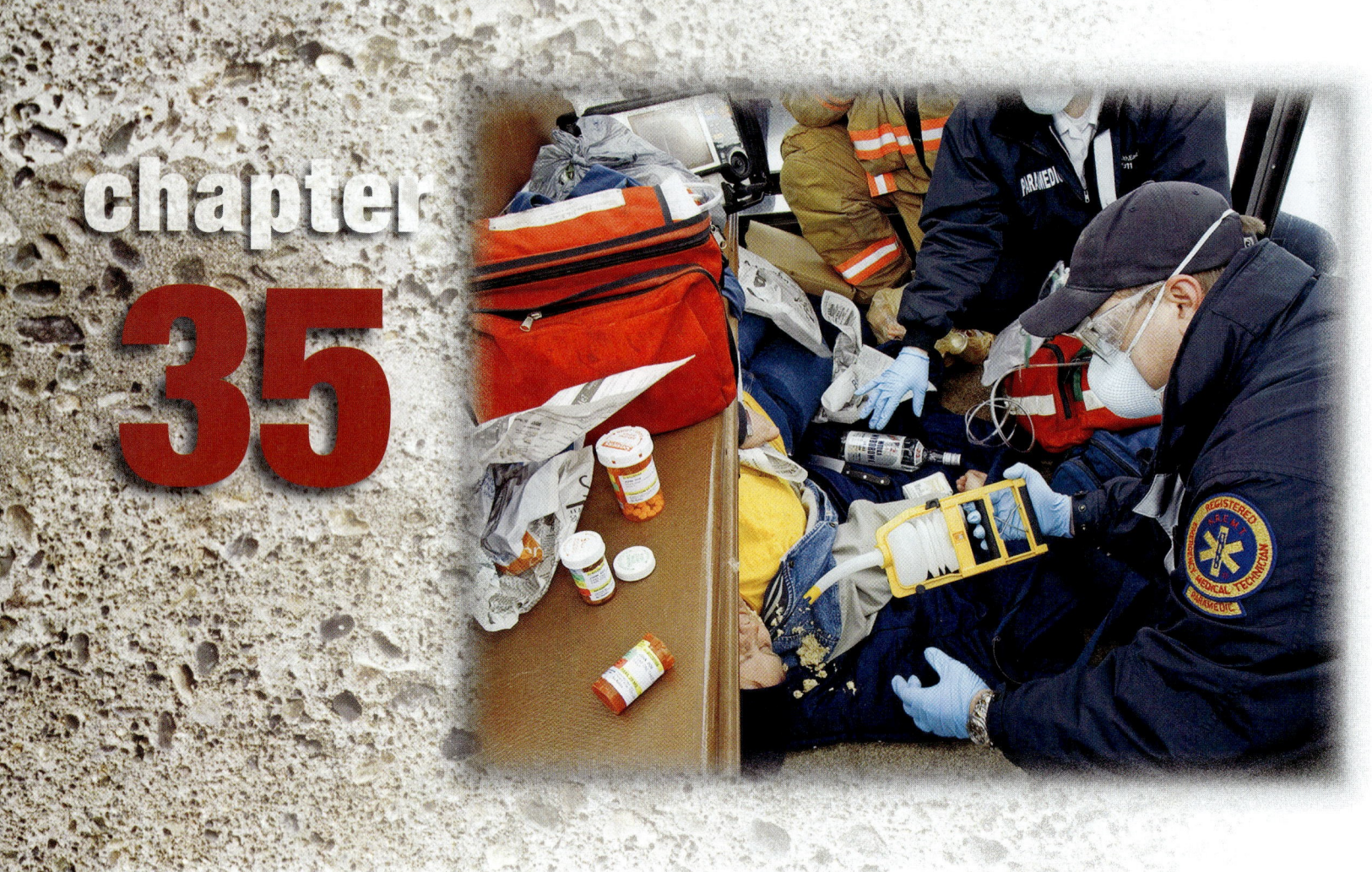

Toxicology

"**A**ll substances are poisons. . . . The right dose differentiates a poison from a remedy."

—Paracelsus

Need to Know

▶ Personal safety should be the initial consideration. Use appropriate protective equipment, and enlist help if the patient appears dangerous.

▶ Poisoning may result from exposure to medications, recreational drugs, environmental hazards, and natural toxins.

▶ Exposures may be intentional or accidental and may occur following skin (dermal) contact, inhalation, ingestion, or injection.

▶ Not all exposures cause toxicity. Consider the substance, duration, route, and clinical presentation when deciding if a patient is at-risk to develop toxicity.

▶ Consider a toxicological cause of symptoms if
  • There is no apparent reason for an alteration in vital signs or mental status.
  • Multiple patients have similar symptoms.

▶ The amount of poison absorbed is directly proportional to the duration of the exposure. Appropriate decontamination should be performed as soon as possible.

▶ Poisons often cause nonspecific symptoms; a diagnosis is often dependent on information gathered from witnesses or at the scene.

▶ Some poisonings cause a consistent set of symptoms (a toxidrome) that may help in diagnosis. Common drug overdoses you should recognize are narcotic overdoses, organophosphate (cholinergic) poisoning, anticholinergic poisoning, and sympathomimetic (stimulant) poisoning.

▶ Determining if the poisoning is accidental or intentional may also have scene safety implications, so exercise caution.

▶ Sick	▶ Not Yet Sick
• All of these patients should be treated as if they are sick. They should be monitored closely and transported. Those with obvious life threats are generally sicker than those with vital signs within the normal range, but all patients should be seen by a physician. • The nature of some toxic substances is that the patient can transition quickly from "stable" to "unstable," so observe all toxicology exposures closely.	• Look for hazardous conditions such as environmental poisons or dangerous patients. • Consider trauma. • Decontaminate for dermal and eye exposures. • Consider administration of antidotes. • Are there pill bottles, drug paraphernalia, product containers, or notes?

Introduction

Toxicology can be intimidating; there are literally thousands of poisons. Each year there are approximately 2 million exposures reported to poison centers in the United States. Fortunately, there are only approximately 1,000 deaths reported, suggesting that the overall mortality from poisoning is less than 1%. Most poisoned patients will develop no more than mild symptoms and do well without any treatment. Others will require supportive care such as airway management, treatment of seizures, or treatment of hypotension. Very few poisons have specific treatments, and these are almost always used after the patient has received supportive care. Table 35-1 lists the most common causes of poisoning death reported to U.S. poison centers in 2004. It is important to realize that even for the most deadly poisons,

less than 1% of exposures will be fatal. In this chapter, we will start with the initial evaluation and treatment of poisoning patients (with a focus on resuscitation), describe some basic pathophysiology and pharmacology that are relevant to poisoning, and finally, describe the manifestations and treatment of several common poisonings. DOT 5-8.1 **Skill Sheets 59: Autoinjector Drug Administration Device and 80: Eye Irrigation support this chapter.**

Reasons for Exposure to Poisons

There are several reasons that patients can be exposed to poisons. It is important that the exposure be appropriately classified for several reasons. The first reason is that there are important differences in prognosis. Another reason is that there may be social implications from mislabeling the reason for ingestion. The term "overdose" can imply

TABLE 35-1 The Most Lethal Poisons Reported to U.S. Poison Centers in 2004 DOT 5-8.12

Poison	Number of Deaths	Percent of Exposures to This Poison that are Fatal
Analgesics (acetaminophen and aspirin)	658	0.24%
Sedative/hypnotics/antipsychotics	371	0.29%
Antidepressants	299	0.47%
Cardiovascular drugs	162	0.22%
Alcohols (includes ethylene glycol and methanol)	114	0.15%

self-harming intent and may lead to insurance difficulties or other social stigmata if it is not appropriately qualified. The most common classification system divides exposures into deliberate and accidental. **Deliberate exposures** include abuse and misuse exposures, self-harming (suicidal) exposures, and malicious exposures, where a poison is used to harm another individual. In general, deliberate exposures result in larger doses of poisons and more serious effects than unintentional exposures. Intentional exposures are often harder to detect because the patient or others may want to conceal that a poisoning has occurred. DOT 5-8.40

There are specific criteria in the psychiatric literature that define substance abuse, but for our purposes, **drug abuse** involves taking a substance with a nontherapeutic, nonself-harming intent. The most common example is using a drug to get high. Most patients know how to use enough of the substance to obtain the desired high without causing serious toxicity. However, because the products are not prepared medications designed to deliver a specific amount, accidental toxicity is common. Patients will usually exceed the toxic dose by a small amount, so mild or moderate toxicity should be anticipated. **Drug misuse** occurs when a patient takes a substance with therapeutic intent but knowingly uses it in a nonstandard (usually excessive) dose. An example of misuse is taking excessive doses of acetaminophen to try to treat a toothache. While most patients will experience little or no effect from misuse, serious toxicity can occur. Patients frequently misuse pain medications, sleeping medications, and over-the-counter products. DOT 5-8.11, 5-8.41

Intentional exposures with self-harming (suicidal) intent often result in significant poisoning. Patients will take all of the poison that they can obtain, and ingestion of multiple products is common. The patients may deny the ingestion, and it may go unrecognized until symptoms develop. This will delay care, will limit the utility of some treatments, and may make it difficult to determine that a poisoning is the cause of a patient's symptoms. Patients with intentional exposures are at the greatest risk to develop serious effects, so it is important that these patients be carefully monitored. DOT 5-8.2, 5-8.13

Malicious poisonings are uncommon, but when they occur, the patients are often very ill. These poisonings usually involve exposure to high doses of dangerous poisons. There is rarely any history of exposure, and there may be multiple victims. On the other hand, threats of malicious poisoning without any exposure also may occur. This can result in mass panic and psychosomatic symptoms. Patients with nonspecific symptoms and a possible malicious poisoning should be monitored and transported without intervention unless symptoms develop. DOT 5-8.43

Accidental exposure to poisons is very common and includes accidental ingestions, therapeutic errors, environmental exposures, and adverse drug reactions. Most accidental ingestions are clinically insignificant: Either the substance is minimally toxic or the dose is insufficient to cause serious symptoms. It is critical to realize that most accidental pediatric exposures to medications fall into this category. The overall mortality for pediatric exposures reported to poison centers is 0.00003%. Given that the overall survival is excellent, it is probable that many well-intentioned interventions are more likely to cause harm than to help. With few exceptions, therapies with any potential for adverse effects should be withheld unless the patient has symptoms. DOT 5-8.44

A **therapeutic error** occurs when a medication is accidentally given in the wrong dose or by the wrong route. Common examples include taking an extra dose of a medication or giving an intramuscular dose of a medication as an intravenous dose. The severity of the effects ranges from minimal to life-threatening. Most extra dose errors cause minimal effects unless they are repeated several times. However, severe overdoses may occur (especially with children), and it is important to determine the dose administered.

Adverse drug reactions (ADR) are another cause of accidental poisoning. ADRs occur when a patient as an adverse event while using a medication appropriately. An ADR may occur from an allergic reaction, from a drug-drug interaction, from a change in drug metabolism, or because the patient is unusually sensitive to a medication. Allergic reactions are treated using standard protocols. The other types of ADRs are treated with supportive measures and antidotes, if appropriate. DOT 5-8.14, 5-8.15

CONNECTIONS Chapter 32: Allergies and Anaphylaxis discusses allergies and anaphylaxis in detail.

Applied Anatomy and Physiology

Pharmacokinetics is the study of how medications and poisons move into and out of the body. An understanding of pharmacokinetics is important to understand how to treat poisoned patients. It is also important to understand pharmacokinetics when deciding how to use many medications. Pharmacokinetic principles are commonly divided into absorption, distribution, metabolism, and excretion.

Absorption

For a poison to cause injury and for a medication to have a treatment effect, it must have contact with the cell. Poisons that cause injury to the skin or eye come in immediate, direct contact with the target cells. However, most poisons cause injury or dysfunction in organs that are not directly accessible. These poisons must be absorbed into the blood (systemic absorption), so they can be carried to the target organs. DOT 5-8.36

The most common ways for a poison to enter the body are ingestion, inhalation, injection, and transdermal absorption (Figure 35-1). Absorption can also occur through the ocular, vaginal, urethral, or rectal mucosa. These routes of exposure will not be discussed in detail, but it is critical to recognize that each of these exposures may lead to systemic poisoning. DOT 5-8.3, 5-8.33

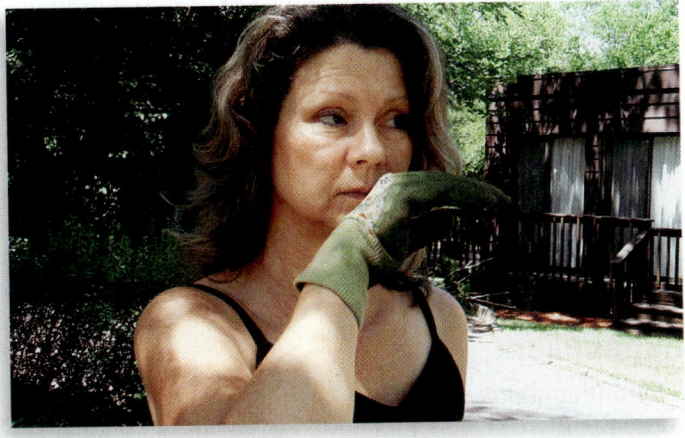

Figure 35-1   Poisons can be absorbed through many routes. Common garden products that are poisonous can be absorbed through the skin.

The extent of absorption is dependent on the following:

1. The properties of the poison
2. The route of exposure
3. The duration of contact DOT 5-8.4

The properties of several poisons will be discussed in detail later (see Common Poisonings section on page 871). Absorption varies greatly among the various exposure routes.

Intravenous exposure causes immediate absorption of all of the poison into the systemic circulation. The poison has immediate access to the target organs, and the onset of effects is usually rapid. When a poison is inhaled, it moves through the lung capillaries into the systemic circulation. Inhalation of poison results in a rate of absorption similar to intravenous exposure, but less of the poison may be absorbed because some may remain in the mouth and be exhaled before absorption occurs. Oral absorption occurs slowly compared to injection or inhalation. However, because the GI system is optimized to absorb nutrients rapidly, most ingested medications will have near complete absorption within 60 minutes. The rate of absorption can be altered significantly by recent meals, sustained release medications, or ingestion of massive amounts of poisons. The absorption of poisons following dermal exposure is very dependent on the properties of the poison. Most are not well-absorbed, and when absorption does occur, it is usually some time before symptoms develop. However, there are some poisons that have rapid systemic absorption following dermal exposure. DOT 5-8.6, 5-8.7, 5-8.20, 5-8.26, 5-8.27, 5-8.28, 5-8.29, 5-8.31, 5-8.32, 5-8.34, 5-8.35

Decontamination is the principle of limiting absorption by shortening the duration of exposure. Since absorption is immediate for injected poisons, decontamination is not useful. After inhalational exposures, patients should be placed on oxygen or moved to an area where ventilation will remove the poison from the environment. DOT 5-8.38, 5-8.45

Gastric decontamination is most commonly discussed for oral exposures. Systemic absorption can be limited by vomiting, trapping the poison in the intestinal lumen or moving the poison through the intestine so rapidly that it is never absorbed. Induced vomiting (mechanical or ipecac-induced) is no longer considered appropriate treatment for poisoned patients. Spontaneous vomiting should not be treated if there are pills in the vomitus, unless the patient is at risk for aspiration. DOT 5-8.39

Gastric lavage (stomach pumping) has fallen from favor over the past ten years, but it is occasionally useful for high-risk poisonings. Gastric lavage is performed by placing a large (40 French) orogastric tube and instilling 100–200 mL of water or saline; the fluid is then suctioned out or allowed to drain by gravity. This process is repeated until the fluid is clear. As placement of a large-bore orogastric tube dramatically increases the risk of aspiration, most patients should be intubated prior to gastric lavage.[1]

Activated charcoal (AC) is the most commonly used method of gastric decontamination. AC adsorbs many poisons and remains in the intestines, effectively trapping the poison and preventing systemic absorption. Charcoal aspiration into the lungs can be life-threatening; therefore, charcoal should not be used if the patient is at-risk to aspirate. The usual dose is 50 gm for adults and 1–2 gm/kg for children. There are some common poisons that are not bound by charcoal, including ethanol, methanol, ethylene glycol, iron, and lithium. Several studies have shown that prehospital administration of AC is safe and results in more rapid administration. However, a large recent study suggested that routine administration of AC to all poisoning patients is not necessary, so the role of prehospital AC administration is still unclear.[1]

In the past, **cathartics** (medications that increased intestinal movement) were used to try to move poisons through the intestines before systemic absorption can occur. Recently, **whole bowel irrigation** (WBI) (administration of a polyethylene glycol bowel preparation) has been used for the same purpose. The advantage of WBI is that there is less risk of fluid and electrolyte abnormalities than with cathartics. WBI has been used for treatment of sustained release medications, medications not bound by charcoal (iron and lithium), and body packers (see cocaine discussion on page 881 for a description of body packers).

Decontamination is also important for dermal and ocular exposures. When the poison causes direct injury to the skin (such as acids and alkali), the amount of injury is directly related to the duration of the exposure (Figure 35-2). All exposed surfaces should be copiously irrigated using the most readily available water source. Solid particles may need to be brushed off. In some cases, it may also be useful to use neutralizers or other agents to try to decrease the tissue injury, but irrigation should not be delayed while these adjuncts are prepared. Eye irrigation is best achieved by running the water source onto the patient's forehead and letting the water run into their eyes. Irrigation should be continued until symptoms resolve or for a minimum of 15 to 20 minutes.

Dermal decontamination may also be used to prevent the systemic absorption of poisons. Systemic poisoning from dermal absorption can occur after exposure to nerve agents and pesticides, paraquat (an herbicide), phenol, and hydrofluoric acid. Dermal absorption is also used for the administration of some medications, including nitroglycerin, fentanyl, clonidine, nicotine, and hormones. Prompt irrigation is the best way to limit systemic absorption. In some cases, adjuncts may be used such as dilute sodium hypochlorite (bleach) for organophosphate and nerve agents, polyethylene glycol for phenol, and calcium solution for hydrofluoric acid. However, it is never appropriate to delay decontamination while preparing these solutions.

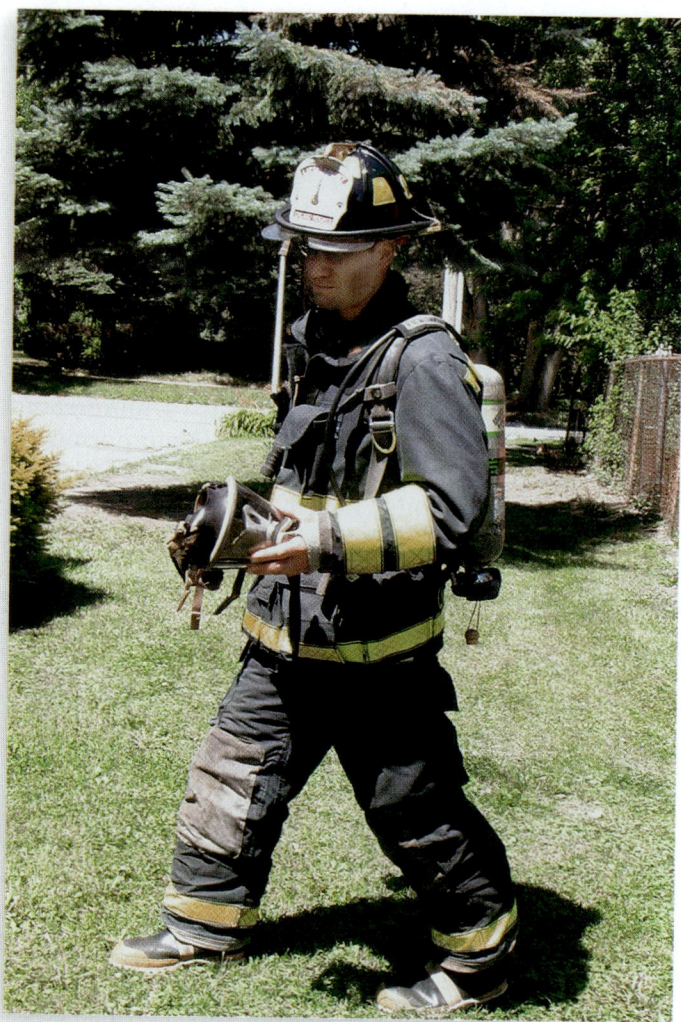

Figure 35-2 Be sure to wear the appropriate PPE when treating patients who have been poisoned.

Distribution

After the poison is absorbed into the blood, it is carried throughout the body and to the organs where it can produce effects. As the poison moves from the blood to the peripheral organs, the blood level of the poison will fall while the organ levels will increase. Organs with high blood flow, such as the liver, brain, kidneys, and heart, will quickly become saturated with the poison. Organs with lower blood flow, such as fat and skeletal muscle, will take longer to become saturated. Since the effects of the poison on the organ are related to the level of poison in that organ, high-flow organs usually show the effects of a poison before low-flow organs.

Metabolism

The human body has several systems to metabolize and remove poisons. The major site of poison metabolism is the liver, but poisons are also metabolized in the intestine and kidney and even by enzymes in the blood. In general, metabolism detoxifies the poison and increases the body's ability to clear the poison from the blood. However, some poisons are only toxic after they have been metabolized. In these cases, the patient may be treated by administering a medication to prevent the metabolism. One example of this is the use of ethanol to prevent the metabolism of methanol or ethylene glycol to their toxic metabolites. (See Common Poisonings section on page 874).

Poisons (and medications) that are ingested must pass through the liver before moving to the rest of the body. If the poison (or medication) is cleared effectively by the liver, much of the oral dose may be cleared before it reaches the rest of the body. This is known as a **first-pass effect.** When a drug has a large first pass effect, the oral dose is often many times the intravenous dose. For example, it takes a 15-mg tablet of morphine to provide the same effect as a 5-mg dose given IV. DOT 5-8.7

Excretion

Most poisons are eliminated from the body in the urine or the bile; some gases may be eliminated via the lungs. Other routes of elimination, such as the sweat, tears, and lactation, contribute little to the elimination of poisons but may be important for other reasons (e.g., transmission of medications during breastfeeding). Elimination of a poison may be dramatically impaired when a patient has renal or hepatic failure. Dosing adjustment is often required for patients with impaired renal or hepatic function. While these changes are not usually relevant for a single dose of medication used to treat an acute condition, impaired elimination can lead to chronic poisoning from many drugs, including lithium, digoxin, and aspirin.

Effects of Poisons

Pharmacodynamics is the study of how medications and poisons cause their effects. Most medications work by binding to specific receptors. This concept is well-demonstrated by the beta adrenergic receptor and the medication propranolol. Propranolol binds to the beta adrenergic receptor sites to slow the heart rate and lower blood pressure. Medications that bind to receptors usually adhere to the dose-response principle. This means that at low doses there is a small response while at higher doses there is a larger response. The difference between the dose of a medication that causes the desired effects and the dose that causes toxic effects is known as the **therapeutic window.** Dose-response relationships are important because they allow us to predict what the effects of an overdose will be. High doses of propranolol may cause severe bradycardia and hypotension. At very high doses, the medication may start binding to receptors other than the target receptor. These effects may be very different from the therapeutic effects. At very high doses, propranolol will bind to cardiac sodium channels and cause ventricular dysrhythmias. It is important to remember this concept when treating patients with large overdoses; they may not have the symptoms you would expect. DOT 5-8.51, 5-8.52, 5-8.53, 5-8.54, 5-8.55

There are several other common mechanisms of action for poisons and medications besides binding to receptors. Poisons may bind to specific enzymes and block cell metabolism or signaling; they may bind to DNA and alter cell reproduction; or they may bind to other cellular proteins and cause cell death. Each of these mechanisms is responsible for the effects of one or more poisons. The clinical effects of a poison will depend on the organs that are most affected by the poison.

There are several presentations that are very suggestive of poisoning.

Some life-threatening symptoms that are often caused by poisoning include the following:

- Decreased level of consciousness
- Seizures
- Dysrhythmias
- Shock

It is important to consider poisoning when patients present with these symptoms. Some poisons produce a characteristic combination of symptoms that can be used to identify the poison. These are called **toxidromes.** Table 35-2 shows the toxidromes of several important poisons. DOT 5-8.8, 5-8.9, 5-8.10

Information about Poisons

One of the most difficult aspects of caring for poisoned patients is knowing what effects are expected following a particular exposure. It is impossible to remember the therapeutic effects of all medications, let alone the toxic effects. There are many useful resources that may help in the care of poisoning patients. Poison centers are the most readily accessible source.

A regional poison center can be reached by calling 1-800-222-1222 anywhere in the United States.

Poison centers can provide assistance with the identification of poisons using descriptions of symptoms or pills provided by responders. They can also offer advice on assessment and treatment of poisoning patients. It is helpful to contact a poison center for all but the most trivial exposures. DOT 5-8.5

Other sources of useful information include packaging and **m**aterial **s**afety **d**ata **s**heets (MSDS) (Figure 35-3).

TABLE 35-2 The Signs and Causes of Several Common Toxidromes

Toxidrome	Symptoms	Common poisons that cause the toxidrome
Anticholinergic (parasympatholytic)	Dry skin, mouth, and eyes, delirium, dilated pupils, tachycardia, decreased bowel sounds	Atropine, jimson weed, sedating antihistamines
Cholinergic (parasympathomimetic)	Salivation, vomiting, wheezing, pulmonary edema, diarrhea, small pupils, seizures, fasciculations, muscle weakness	Organophosphate and carbamate pesticides, nerve agent chemical weapons
Opioids	Respiratory depression, small pupils, coma	Heroin, morphine, other opioid analgesics
Sympathomimetic	Tachycardia, agitation, seizures, diaphoresis, dilated pupils	Cocaine, amphetamines, other stimulants

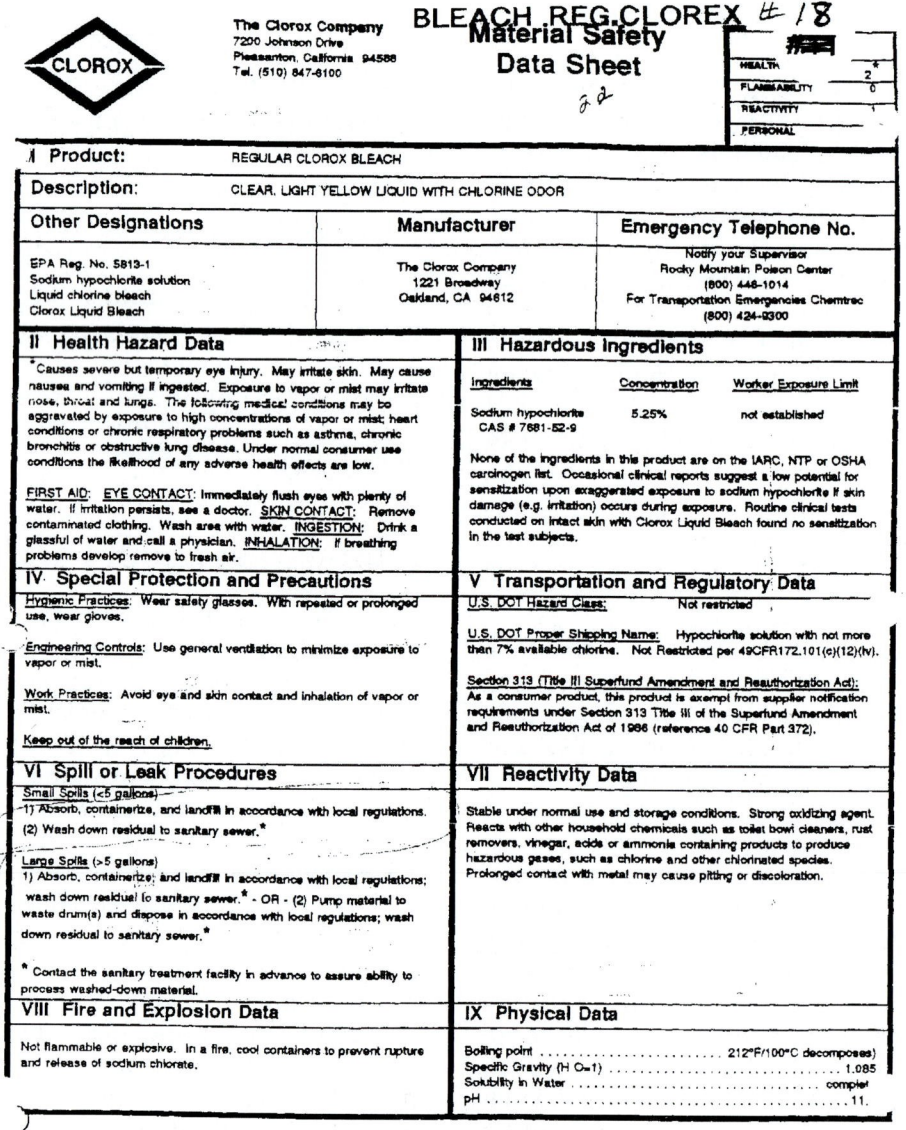

Figure 35-3 Manufacturer's Safety Data Sheets are a wealth of information, but you should also call a poison control center to verify the information.

Whenever possible, it is helpful to obtain product packaging. Many products have similar names, and misidentification may have serious consequences. Product data sheets will also have the exact concentration of each ingredient, which may help treatment decisions. Some packages will even have useful treatment information. The MSDS is a standard sheet that is produced by the manufacturer of common products. Employers are required to maintain copies of the MSDS for products used in the workplace. These sheets will have ingredient information and may have some initial treatment suggestions. However, the MSDS often contain outdated information, and it is often best to contact a poison center to ensure the accuracy of any recommendations beyond initial treatment.

Scene Safety and Decontamination

Personal protection must be the first priority at any scene. This is obvious when there is a mass exposure; many of the patients treated after the Tokyo sarin attack in 1995 were prehospital providers who were exposed to the sarin while caring for other victims. If environmental exposure is possible, the scene should be evaluated by a trained hazmat team and the victims should be removed and decontaminated *before* treatment is initiated.

CONNECTIONS Refer to Chapter 53: Hazardous Materials Incidents and Chapter 55: Responding to WMD Events for more information on decontamination.

Patients who have dermal exposures should have their clothing removed and skin decontaminated (personal decontamination). If the patients are ambulatory, they should be directed to do the following:

1. Remove their clothing. The clothing should be double-bagged and discarded.
2. Wash their entire body with any available water source. Ideally, they should wash for a minimum of 15 minutes.
3. Patients with eye symptoms should have their eyes irrigated for a minimum of 15 minutes, in addition to the dermal decontamination.

Obviously, it is important to avoid hypothermia during the decontamination process. Patients who are unable to decontaminate themselves should not be treated until they have been decontaminated by trained technicians with appropriate protective equipment.

While safety is an obvious concern with environmental exposures, it may be an issue in other situations. Patients poisoned by recreational drugs will often be violent. Suicidal patients are often irrational and desperate while family members may be anxious

and frightened. Any of these circumstances may result in violence directed at the paramedic. Law enforcement should be called to assist any time violence or altered behavior is a possibility.

CONNECTIONS Chapter 52: Teamwork and Operational Interface describes the importance of interfacing with law enforcement at the scene of a toxicological emergency.

Airway Assessment and Treatment

There are several causes of inadequate ventilation and oxygenation in poisoning patients. Airway obstruction can occur from loss of the gag reflex (as seen with sedative poisoning), airway swelling (as seen with acid or alkali ingestion), or secretions (as seen with organophosphate pesticide poisoning). Ventilatory failure most commonly occurs from opiate poisoning but may occur if the poison causes muscle weakness (as seen with some snake venoms). Inadequate oxygenation can occur from decreased environmental oxygen, bronchospasm, pulmonary edema (most commonly noncardiogenic), or abnormalities of hemoglobin. DOT 5-8.16

Poisoning is a dynamic process, so patients that appear stable may rapidly deteriorate. Monitor all patients for impending airway complications. Patients with an inadequate airway due to decreased consciousness will occasionally respond to stimulation, repositioning, or supplemental airway devices (nasal or oral airways). However, since vomiting is common in many poisonings, there should be a low threshold to intubate poisoned patients who have a decreased level of consciousness. Patients with airway swelling or secretions should be intubated as soon as possible as they will likely deteriorate with time. DOT 5-8.17, 5-8.18

Breathing Assessment and Treatment

Hypoventilation is treated with assisted ventilation. Many poisons cause a metabolic acidosis, so in general, it is better to overventilate patients in order to increase the loss of CO_2. Hypoventilation-induced hypoxia should improve rapidly with assisted ventilation. Inadequate oxygenation from decreased environment oxygen usually responds promptly to supplemental oxygen. Pulse oximetry is a valuable aid to help monitor the patient's level of oxygenation. DOT 5-8.46

A patient with bronchospasm should be treated with beta agonists, but steroids are not usually used unless the patient has a history of asthma. Pulmonary edema is treated initially with high-flow oxygen. If the patient does not improve, intubation with positive pressure ventilation is indicated. As most cases of pulmonary edema are noncardiogenic, diuretics, nitrates, and morphine are of little value. While pulse oximetry is a valuable tool for the assessment of oxygenation in most poisoning patients, it can be misleading in patients with carboxy-hemoglobin or methemoglobin. Patients with carbon monoxide poisoning require high-flow oxygen even if the pulse oximetry measurement is normal, while patients with even mildly elevated methemoglobin levels will appear cyanotic and have a low pulse oximetry measurement. Please refer to the specific discussions of these poisons on pages 874 and 879.

In general, standard airway management techniques should be used to intubate patients. Many patients will not require additional sedation to allow intubation. Succinylcholine carries a theoretical risk of hyperkalemia in digoxin and hydrofluoric acid poisoning or prolonged paralysis following organophosphate poisoning. However, the clinical significance of these complications is questionable, and if succinylcholine is needed to facilitate intubation, it should be used.[2]

Circulation Assessment and Treatment

Poisoning may cause abnormalities of blood pressure or heart rate and rhythm. As with airway and breathing, constant monitoring of cardiac function is essential.

The most common cardiac abnormalities are sinus tachycardia or bradycardia. If the heart rate is abnormal but the patient has adequate perfusion, there is no indication for immediate treatment. The patient should be monitored for deterioration. Treatment of the patient with symptomatic bradycardia or heart block should follow standard ACLS guidelines: atropine followed by external pacing.

Antidotes are available and may be required for some poisons that cause bradycardia or heart block (see beta-blockers, calcium channel blockers, and digoxin sections on page 875), but other poisonings require only supportive care. Sinus tachycardia most often occurs from CNS excitation. Therefore, the treatment is sedation. Benzodiazepines are an excellent first-line choice. Supraventricular (SVT) tachycardia may be treated with adenosine or cardioversion, but because these treatments do not reverse the poison, it is common for the SVT to recur. If this happens, it may be necessary to use a calcium channel blocker for rate control. Poison-induced, wide complex tachycardia is frequently due to sodium channel blockade.

Cardioversion will not effectively treat a wide complex dysrhythmia due to sodium channel blockade. The treatment of choice is hypertonic sodium bicarbonate (see antidote section on this page). Patients with wide complex tachycardia from other poisons may be treated with lidocaine and cardioversion although their utility is unproven, and recurrence should be anticipated.

Supportive Care of the Poisoning Patient

Poisoning patients may present with symptoms that respond to standard treatments. However, as the physiology of poisoning patients is abnormal, they may not respond to standard doses. For example, patients with hypotension from beta-blocker poisoning may only respond to high doses of epinephrine since many of their adrenergic receptors are occupied. This is true for most poisons that cause hypotension, so the standard "maximum doses" should not be considered ceiling doses for poisoned patients and medical direction should be sought early in the course of treatment.[3]

Seizures are another common symptom from poisoning. Most toxicological causes of seizures respond to standard doses of benzodiazepines (such as 5–10 mg of diazepam). The common antiseizure medication, phenytoin, is not considered useful for toxicological causes of seizures. Other sedatives, such as barbiturates and propofol, are generally considered useful for toxicological causes of seizures.[4]

The role of standard antidysrhythmics such as lidocaine and amiodarone is of unknown utility for poisoning-induced dysrhythmias. There is no evidence that suggests that they are harmful in the setting of cocaine poisoning (a common cause of ventricular dysrhythmias). Amiodarone may be useful for cardiac glycoside-induced ventricular dysrhythmias. Sodium bicarbonate is used to treat poisoning caused by sodium channel antagonism (see Table 35-3). Type 1A antidysrhythmics (such as procainamide) should be avoided when treating poisoning patients.[5] DOT 5-8.60, 5-8.61, 5-8.62

Working in the Gray Zone

Poison Control versus Medical Control: Who Is in Charge?
In some states, field providers are permitted to consult with poison control centers directly from the field. Make sure you know if you are allowed to accept orders from poison control centers directly or only upon approval of on-line medical direction.

Antidotes

Antidotes are treatments that specifically reverse the effects of a poison. There are very few antidotes relative to the number of poisons that are encountered. Table 35-3 lists several commonly used antidotes, the poisons they are used to treat, and the doses of the antidotes.

TABLE 35-3   Common Antidotes and the Standard Adult Doses

Antidote	Poison	Dose	Notes
Acetylcysteine	Acetaminophen	140 mg/kg PO	Loading dose followed by two infusions
Atropine	Cholinergic poisons	1–5 mg every five minutes until pulmonary symptoms improved	Severely poisoned patients may require more than 100 mg
Calcium chloride or gluconate	Calcium channel antagonists, hydrofluoric acid	1–3 gm IV bolus	Hydrofluoric acid poisoning may require several grams
Cyanide antidote			
Amyl nitrite	Cyanide	One ampoule inhaled 30 seconds on, 30 seconds off	Used until an IV established; each ampule lasts two to three minutes
Sodium nitrite	Cyanide	300 mg IV	
Sodium thiosulfate	Cyanide	12.5 gm IV	
Hydroxocobalamin	Cyanide	4 gm	Used as alternative to nitrites and thiosulfate
Glucagon	Calcium channel antagonists, beta-blocker	5–10 mg bolus	Most patients will require an infusion of 5–10 mg/hr
Glucose	Insulin, sulfonylurea oral hypoglycemic drugs	25–50 gm	Deliberate overdoses may require multiple doses
Methylene blue	Methemoglobinemia	1 mg/kg	
Naloxone	Opioids	0.4–2 mg IV or IM	
Pralidoxime	Organophosphate	1–2 gm IV	Used with atropine
Pyridoxine	Isoniazid	5–10 gm IV	
Sodium bicarbonate	Sodium channel antagonism	1–2 meq/kg	Administer for widened QRS

Common Poisonings

The remainder of this chapter will describe the clinical effects and the treatment for common poisonings. The chapter is divided into several medication classes, and includes some examples of drugs within each class. However, since new drugs are continually introduced, it is not possible to provide an exhaustive list of drugs that are in each medication class.

Environmental, Household, and Occupational Exposures

Acidic and Alkaline (Basic) Substances

Acids are substances with a low pH, and alkalis (or bases) are substances with a high pH. Exposure to substances that are strong acids (pH less than 3) or bases (pH greater than 11) may cause chemical burns. Patients will have pain and may have visible tissue necrosis. If the substances are ingested, airway swelling may be life-threatening. Inhalation will cause severe pulmonary irritation and bronchospasm and may cause pulmonary edema. Skin and corneal burns may be severe. The extent of injury is directly related to the duration of exposure, so decontamination should be started as soon as possible. Patients with ingestion should rinse their mouth, and if they can easily swallow, it is reasonable to have them swallow one to two ounces of water. There is no role for large volume dilution or forcing patients to take any fluids if they are having too much pain. Dermal and eye exposures should be treated with irrigation until the symptoms have resolved and for a minimum of 15 to 20 minutes.[6]

Hydrofluoric acid (HF) deserves special mention because it can cause severe systemic toxicity with minimal visible dermal or mucous membrane injury. Fluoride binds calcium with such affinity that less than one ounce of 5% HF will bind all of the free calcium in a human. Asymptomatic patients that have deliberately ingested HF should be treated with prophylactic calcium gluconate (1–3 grams IV over 20 minutes). Repeat dosing is required if the patient develops hypocalcemia. Patients who have cardiac arrest following HF poisoning should be treated with multiple doses of calcium.[7] DOT 5-8.56

Food Poisoning

Food poisoning is a nonspecific term. Although the term is frequently used to describe patients with self-limited vomiting, abdominal pain, and diarrhea, the actual etiology is rarely determined. The classic cause of food poisoning is bacterial toxins from bacteria such as *Staphylococcus aureus, Bacillus cereus,* and *Clostridium perefringens.* Patients will present with the abrupt onset of nausea, vomiting, and diarrhea. There is no specific treatment beyond supportive care. DOT 5-8.56

Plants

Plant exposures are commonly reported to poison centers. Fortunately, they rarely result in significant toxicity. Most plant ingestions will produce no symptoms or nausea and vomiting. Even ingestion of plants that contain poisons (such as oleander, which contains a compound similar to digoxin) rarely produces serious symptoms (Figure 35-4). DOT 5-8.56

Metals (Iron, Lead, Mercury)

Ingestion of iron-containing vitamins used to be a major cause of pediatric poisoning deaths. However, advances in treatment and new packaging restrictions have dramatically decreased the risk of death from iron poisoning. Large ingestions of iron (greater than 60 mg/kg of elemental iron) will cause gastrointestinal symptoms (including GI bleeding) and can progress to coma and shock.[8] Treatment is primarily supportive, but deferoxamine is occasionally administered in the hospital to bind and detoxify the iron. There is no significant toxicity from acute ingestion of lead, but chronic exposure may cause slowed learning and headaches and can eventually progress to cerebral edema.[9] Dimercaptosuccinic acid (DMSA) is an antidote that binds and inactivates the lead. Metallic mercury (quicksilver, liquid silver mercury found in thermometers) exposure rarely causes acute toxicity unless the mercury is heated and the vapors are inhaled. Ingestion of mercury salts, such as mercuric chloride, will produce severe gastroenteritis, GI bleeding, and shock. Patients with shock will require fluid resuscitation and may need vasopressor support. DMSA will also bind mercury and can be used to treat patients.[10] DOT 5-8.56

Cyanide and Hydrogen Sulfide

Cyanide and hydrogen sulfide bind to proteins in the mitochondria and prevent the formation of ATP. Cyanide is produced when many plastics are incinerated and is used in industry. Many burn patients suffer from cyanide poisoning. Hydrogen sulfide (HS) is formed by bacteria that are present in sewers and swamps. At low concentrations, it has a strong sulfur odor, but at toxic concentrations the smell goes away, and victims may not realize that they are in danger. Cyanide and HS both cause a rapid onset of headache, nausea, seizures, hypotension, and coma. HS is rapidly reversed by stopping the exposure; patients usually improve when moved to fresh air.

Cyanide poisoning requires specific treatment. Patients should be placed on oxygen and may require intubation, they should have an IV established, and they should be placed on a cardiac monitor. Hypotension is treated with fluids and vasopressors. The cyanide antidote kit includes amyl and sodium nitrite and sodium thiosulfate (Figure 35-5). The nitrites are used to induce

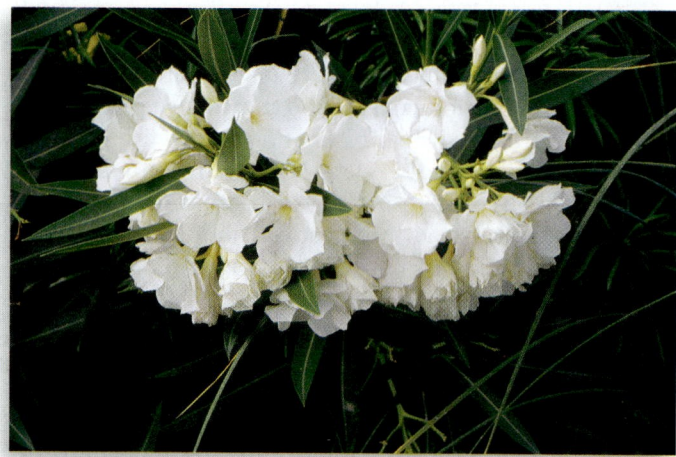

Figure 35-4 Oleander is a common plant that contains a poisonous compound. It rarely produces serious symptoms.

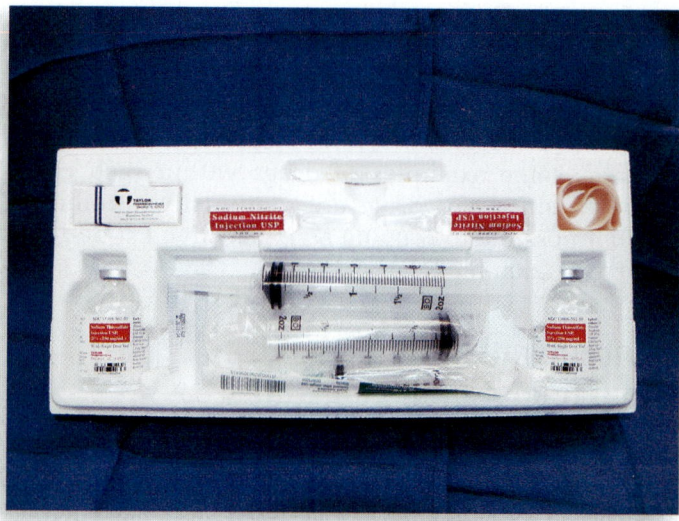

Figure 35-5 Cyanide poisoning antidote kit.

methemoglobinemia, which binds the cyanide and removes it from the mitochondrial proteins. Amyl nitrate is administered by breaking open the ampules and having the patient inhale the vapors. Sodium nitrite is administered by intravenous infusion. The adult dose is one ampule; administration of an adult dose to a child can cause life-threatening methemoglobinemia.[11] After the nitrite is given, sodium thiosulfate is administrated, which creates thiocyanate, which is then excreted in urine. DOT 5-8.56

Cholinergic Agents

Cholineric poisons include carbamate and organophosphate pesticides and nerve agent chemical weapons (such as sarin, tabun, and VX). These poisons all inhibit acetylcholinesterase, the enzyme that breaks down acetylcholine. Inhibition of this enzyme causes excess cholinergic activity. Common symptoms make up the SLUDGE syndrome:

SLUDGE

S = Salivation
L = Lacrimation
U = Urination
D = Defecation
G = Gastrointestinal upset
E = Emesis

Other symptoms include miosis (constricted pupils), bronchospasm, and pulmonary edema. Fasciculations (twitching muscles) and muscle weakness occur from acetylcholine excess at the neuromuscular junction. Because these substances are all readily absorbed through the skin, it is important that providers protect themselves and decontaminate all patients. The severity of these exposures may range from mild gastrointestinal symptoms to seizures, coma, and cardiovascular collapse. The cholinergic symptoms may require high doses (up to 1 gm) of atropine. In severe poisonings, atropine doses should be repeated until the patient's pulmonary symptoms improve. Seizures are treated with standard doses of benzodiazepines. Weakness may progress to loss of airway protection and respiratory failure, so patients with severe poisoning will require intubation and mechanical ventilation.[12] DOT 5-8.56

Pulmonary and Mucous Membrane Irritants

Many substances will cause irritation of the respiratory system and eyes. Common examples include ammonia, chlorine, acids, bases, and capsaicin. The main symptoms are upper airway burning, eye and nose irritation, and cough. Patients with prolonged exposure may develop more severe symptoms, including pulmonary edema and bronchospasm. Patients with asthma may be at high risk for severe symptoms. Treatment involves moving the patient to fresh air and irrigation of the mucous membranes. Most patients will recover within a few minutes. However, delayed symptoms may occur, so patients with any symptoms should be observed, and all patients should be instructed for return to care if symptoms recur.[13] DOT 5-8.56

Pepper Spray

EMS may be called to manage a patient with eye or skin irritation from pepper spray. There are several manufacturers of various chemical sprays, so exact concentrations and ingredients may be unknown, but all of the products are designed to provide enough irritation to the individual that they are incapacitated from continuing aggressive or threatening behavior. Signs and symptoms include intense lacrimation (tearing); intense burning sensation to the eyes, mucous membranes, and skin that come into contact with the chemical; chest tightness; sore throat; coughing; shortness of breath; and vomiting. Some patients have lost corneal epithelium following exposure. Permanent eye injury is unlikely, particularly with the pepper plant derivatives used in most preparations available today. The signs typically subside within 15–30 minutes after the exposure ends. Painful contact dermatitis may persist for hours following exposure to capsaicin (pepper).

Be very careful of overspray or walking into a closed or confined space with the chemical still in the air. Clothing from the patient may contain chemicals, and moving around the clothes may result in additional exposure, called off-gassing. Clothing should be removed and placed into plastic bags.

Additional treatments include moving the patient away from the chemical and into fresh air. Irrigate the eyes, mucous membranes, and skin with copious amounts of plain water, sterile water, or normal saline solution for 15 minutes. If irritation continues, repeat the irrigation process. Monitor the patient for respiratory distress, and suspect it if a cough develops. The patient may develop bronchitis or pneumonia, so the patient should be seen by a physician if a cough develops. Administer oxygen and assist ventilation, if required. Treat bronchospasm with beta$_2$ agonists such as albuterol. The patient should be encouraged to see a physician in the ED, but if the patient refuses further care or transport, the patient should be advised to shower immediately to remove any residual chemical.[14] DOT 5-8.56

Methanol and Ethylene Glycol

Methanol is commonly found in windshield wiper fluid and is also found in some fuel products used to heat food trays. Ethylene glycol is the major ingredient of automotive radiator antifreeze. Methanol and ethylene glycol both produce some degree of intoxication when ingested. However, their major toxic effects occur several hours after the exposure as they are metabolized to formic acid and oxalic acid, respectively. Both of these acids cause a life-threatening metabolic acidosis with serum pH often below 7.2 (normal pH is 7.35 to 7.45). Ultimately, formic acid will cause blindness, and oxalic acid will cause renal failure. Treatment of methanol and ethylene glycol includes administration of ethanol or fomepizole to prevent the formation of the toxic metabolites and hemodialysis to increase the elimination of methanol or ethylene glycol. There are no specific prehospital interventions beyond supportive care.[15,16] DOT 5-8.56

Carbon Monoxide (CO)

Carbon monoxide is an odorless, colorless gas that is produced by combustion. It is a common cause of deaths in fires, but it is also produced by heaters, gas stoves, and internal combustion engines. This poisoning often occurs during the first cold snap of a season when faulty furnaces and heaters are turned on. Carbon monoxide binds to proteins and blocks binding of oxygen. This is most readily recognized when carbon monoxide binds to hemoglobin and forms carboxyhemoglobin, but the major toxic effects of carbon monoxide occur when it binds to proteins in the brain and heart. The early symptoms of carbon monoxide poisoning are headache, nausea, and dizziness. More severe exposures cause confusion, seizures, coma, and hypotension.

High-flow oxygen and cardiac monitoring are the main prehospital interventions. The prehospital provider should determine, if possible, duration of exposure, identify if the exposure was in a closed space, and note when the patient was removed from the carbon monoxide. Pulse oximetry does not detect carboxyhemoglobin and will give a "normal" reading in the setting of carbon monoxide poisoning, although transcutaneous carbon monoxide detectors may soon become available. If transport time is prolonged, it is helpful to obtain a heparinized blood sample to determine baseline carboxyhemoglobin levels. Hyperbaric oxygen is used to treat severe carbon monoxide poisoning (Figure 35-6).[17] DOT 5-8.56

Hydrocarbons

The hydrocarbons are a diverse class of substances that have a carbon chain. Hydrocarbon poisoning occurs in two scenarios. The first is deliberate inhalation to produce intoxication. This is known as **huffing** or glue

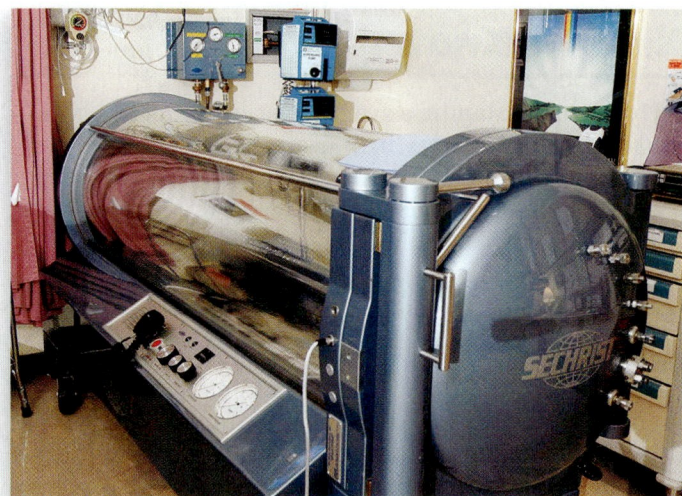

Figure 35-6 Hyperbaric oxygen chamber used to treat victims of carbon monoxide poisoning.

sniffing. Patients will present with CNS effects including somnolence, ataxia, slurred speech, and euphoria, and they will often smell like petroleum products. Pulmonary effects almost never occur from huffing unless the patient vomits and aspirates. The effects are usually short-lived, and treatment is removal of the patient from the exposure. It is important to identify the exact product that the patient is abusing because there may be other toxic ingredients that require specific treatment. DOT 5-8.19, 5-8.20, 5-8.21

Direct aspiration of hydrocarbon liquids is the second type of hydrocarbon poisoning. Lamp oil, kerosene, and paint thinner are hydrocarbons that are frequently aspirated. Gasoline is often ingested, but aspiration is uncommon. Aspiration should be suspected whenever a patient has choking, vomiting, or a cough after ingesting a hydrocarbon liquid. Hydrocarbon aspiration is the most common cause of pediatric poisoning death reported to poison centers. Initially, patients may have minimal symptoms. However, over several minutes to hours they go on to develop severe lung injury and often require prolonged intubation and respiratory support. Any patient with symptoms should be placed on oxygen and should be transported for monitoring. It is also important that any patient with vomiting be placed on their side to help minimize the risk of aspiration.[18] DOT 5-8.22, 5-8.23, 5-8.24, 5-8.25

Street Secrets

Huffing Gasoline: Avoid using beta agonistic bronchodilators (such as albuterol) to treat patients with intentional inhalation of gasoline. The bronchodilator will dilate the airways and allow for more absorption of the toxin, which can make the patient even sicker.

Cardiovascular Medications

Calcium Channel Blockers. Calcium channel blockers (CCB) are used principally to treat hypertension and occasionally for refractory migraine headaches. Verapamil and diltiazem primarily slow both sinus node (SA) firing and atrioventricular (AV) nodal conduction and cause mild peripheral vasodilatation. Nifedipine causes prominent vasodilatation with little inhibition of the SA and AV nodes. Other calcium channel blockers include amlodipine, felodipine, and isradipine. These have effects similar to nifedipine. All calcium channel blockers act by inhibiting voltage-gated calcium channels. The resultant effect is vasodilatation via contraction of vascular smooth muscle and slowing of cardiac conduction by inhibition of the SA and AV nodes.

Expect hypotension, bradycardia, and myocardial conduction delays with an acute CCB intoxication. Verapamil and diltiazem are more likely to cause bradycardia and conduction delays than the other agents. The cardiac effects can be severe and can occur abruptly. Patients may also develop drowsiness (with hypotension), vomiting, mild hyperglycemia, and acidosis.

Initiate gastrointestinal decontamination in all patients, even hours after ingestion, since CCB slows gastrointestinal motility and is very toxic. For controlled release preparations, decontamination may be performed up to 12 hours later, and whole bowel irrigation should be considered. Immediately perform endotracheal intubation if any significant cardiovascular compromise is apparent. Treatment for hypotension includes isotonic crystalloid fluid and vasopressors. Atropine can be used for bradycardia. Intravenous calcium and glucagon are also adjunct therapies for hypotension. Occasionally, cardiac pacing is needed. High-dose insulin with dextrose infusion is also used for patients that are refractory to standard therapy.[19] DOT 5-8.56

Beta Adrenergic Blockers. Beta receptor blockers competitively block the beta adrenergic receptor. These agents are used to treat hypertension, acute coronary syndrome, and occasionally migraine headaches. Beta$_1$ and Beta$_2$ receptors are the two primary receptors affected by these agents. Beta$_1$ receptors affect heart contraction and heart rate and are the most relevant to cardiac function. Beta$_2$ receptor agonists increase bronchodilatation, arterial vasodilatation, insulin release, and influx of potassium into cells. Common agents that affect both receptors (i.e., nonselective beta-blockers) are propanolol, labetalol, and timolol. Beta$_1$ selective drugs are more commonly prescribed and are used for their cardioselective effects. Examples are metoprolol, atenolol, and esmolol.

Beta-blocker (BB) intoxication usually manifests with hypotension and bradycardia. Heart block and myocardial conduction delay are also seen. Although generally beta-blockers are not as toxic as calcium channel blockers, a large beta-blocker overdose, or one in combination with another cardioactive medication, can be lethal. Some beta-blockers such as labetalol and carvedilol also inhibit alpha receptors, which can worsen hypotension. Propanolol is considered the most toxic BB. It inhibits myocardial sodium channels and can cause wide complex dysrhythmias. In addition, seizures have been reported after propanolol intoxication. Carvedilol, a newer BB, has similar characteristics to propanolol; however, significant toxicity has not been commonly reported.

Early, aggressive prehospital supportive care is important. Perform endotracheal intubation in the somnolent patient. Treat bradycardia with atropine. Treat hypotension with intravenous fluids and vasopressors. Intravenous glucagon and calcium are adjunct treatments (see Table 35-3 on antidotes). Occasionally, cardiac pacing is needed. Remedy seizures with benzodiazepines, and administer sodium bicarbonate bolus for widened QRS.[19] DOT 5-8.56

Cardioactive Steroids (Digoxin and Related Substances). Cardioactive steroids are derived from plants. Digoxin is the most commonly prescribed cardioactive steroid. Digoxin was originally produced from the foxglove plant. Other plants have cardioactive steroids, including red squill, yew berry, and oleander. Digoxin increases contractility of the heart by increasing intracellular calcium while simultaneously slowing the rate of ventricular contraction by slowing conduction through the AV node. Digoxin is used to treat congestive heart failure by increasing cardiac contractility. It is also used for patients with atrial fibrillation to slow the rate of ventricular contraction.

Clinical effects occur from both acute intoxication and chronic use. After acute overdosage, patients develop vomiting, bradycardia, heart block, dysrhythmias, and hyperkalemia. Adverse effects with chronic use are similar, and toxicity is usually from increased dose, a drug interaction, or decreased elimination from new or worsened renal insufficiency.

Place the patient on a cardiac monitor and perform a 12 lead electrocardiogram, if available, to assess for a dysrhythmia. Laboratory testing for serum potassium, digoxin level, and renal function are important to assess for toxicity. Consider atropine for symptomatic bradycardia. In the unstable patient with a ventricular dysrhythmia, use parenteral calcium with caution. Supplemental calcium with digoxin toxicity could lead to cardiac tetany and asystole. Because digoxin also causes myocardial irritability, electrical cardioversion could induce ventricular fibrillation; therefore, cardioversion should start at low levels, if needed urgently, or otherwise delayed until after antidotal therapy.

Administration of digoxin immune antibody fragments is the in-hospital treatment foundation of digoxin toxicity. Larger doses (approximately 10 vials) are given for acute toxicity and lower doses (approximately two vials) for chronic toxicity.[20] DOT 5-8.56

Type I Antidysrhythmic Medications. Class I antidysrhythmic agents block fast myocardial sodium channels and include a number of medications. They are used to treat ventricular dysrhythmias and are divided into three categories, based on additional mechanisms of action. Examples of Class IA agents are disopyramide, procainamide, and quinidine. Class IB agents are the most common and include lidocaine and its oral analog, mexiletine. Two common Class IC medications are flecainide and propafenone.

Dysrhythmias may occur after ingestion of any of these agents, particularly IA and IC. Symptoms of intoxication also include hypotension, somnolence, and generalized seizures. Upon initial evaluation, administer supplemental oxygen and place the patient on a cardiac monitor. Monitor for QRS widening and QT prolongation. Perform endotracheal intubation or bag-mask ventilation for respiratory failure. Treat seizures with parenteral benzodiazepines. Initially, treat hypotension with crystalloid infusion. Recalcitrant hypotension requires a vasopressor such as dopamine or norepinephrine. Treat wide complex dysrhythmias with sodium bicarbonate bolus (see Table 35-3 on antidotes).[21] DOT 5-8.56

ACE Inhibitors and Angiotensin Receptor Blockers. Angiotensin converting enzyme (ACE) inhibitors are commonly prescribed for hypertension. These medications are particularly beneficial for patients with concomitant diabetic nephropathy, congestive heart failure, or post-myocardial infarction. ACE inhibitors work by inhibiting ACE, which prevents the conversion of angiotensin I to angiotensin II. Angiotensin II is a potent vasoconstrictor. Commonly prescribed ACE inhibitors are captopril, lisinopril, enalapril, and ramipril.

Angiotensin receptor blockers (ARBs) also impede the effect of angiotensin II but act by directly blocking the angiotensin receptor. Examples of these medications are losartan, valsartan, irbesartan, and candesartan. ARBs are usually prescribed for similar indications as ACE inhibitors but are considered when ACE inhibitors are not tolerated by the patient. Future research will likely expand their therapeutic role.

Both categories of drugs are well tolerated with overdose. The most common effect of acute intoxication is mild hypotension. Occasionally, mild tachycardia and hyperkalemia can occur. Adverse effects of ACE inhibitors include a nonproductive cough, hyperkalemia, mild renal insufficiency, and, rarely, angioedema. Angioedema is characterized by facial and upper airway swelling and is usually insidious in onset. Symptoms may occur at any time after initiating the medication. ARBs may also produce mild hypotension and tachycardia. Cough and angioedema are much less common.

Because hypotension is usually mild, patients usually only need crystalloid infusion for treatment. Angioedema can cause airway obstruction and can be life-threatening. Early intubation may be needed. Antihistamine and antiallergic medications, such as diphenhydramine and prednisone, are not effective. Intramuscular epinephrine may be helpful to decrease severe edema. Patients should be monitored closely for progression of upper airway edema.[22,23] DOT 5-8.56

Clonidine and Alpha₂ Adrenergic Agonists

Clonidine is the most common alpha₂ adrenergic agonist. It is most commonly prescribed for attention deficient and hyperactivity disorder but is also used to control hypertension. Other uses are to treat Tourette's syndrome and to mitigate alcohol or opioid withdrawal.

Alpha₂ receptor agonists work by decreasing sympathetic flow, resulting in hypotension, sedation, and bradycardia. However, patients may develop transient hypertension before the sympathetic flow is inhibited. Lessened sympathetic stimulation of the pupillary muscles also produces miosis. Hypothermia is also common.

Symptomatic patients often present with miosis and sedation. Therefore, administer naloxone for possible opioid intoxication. Determine the blood glucose level, or administer glucose empirically to exclude hypoglycemia. Treatment is entirely supportive. Endotracheal intubation may be required if the patient is profoundly sedated. Administer atropine for bradycardia and crystalloid fluid and vasopressors for hypotension. No proven antidote exists.[24] DOT 5-8.56

Alpha₁ Adrenergic Antagonists

Alpha₁ receptors predominantly decrease vascular tone and bladder sphincter tone. Prazosin and terazosin are selective alpha₁ receptor antagonists and are routinely prescribed for urinary retention associated with benign prostatic hypertrophy. Phentolamine inhibits both alpha₁ and alpha₂ receptors and is administered subcutaneously for accidental epinephrine injections into a digit. It is occasionally given parenterally for severe hypertension from cocaine or other sympathomimetic agents.

The toxic effects are limited to orthostatic hypotension, mild tachycardia, dizziness, and occasionally syncope. Mild sedation and nasal congestion may also occur. Treatment is supportive. Crystalloid infusion is usually the only treatment needed for hypotension.[25] DOT 5-8.56

Over-the-Counter Medications

Acetaminophen. Acetaminophen is a common, mild analgesic and antipyretic. It is often combined with opioids such as codeine, hydrocodone, or oxycodone to treat moderate pain. Acetaminophen overdose causes no symptoms initially, but liver injury occurs 24 to 72 hours after the ingestion. The antidote for acetaminophen poisoning is N-acetylcysteine. There are no specific prehospital interventions beyond supporting the vital signs.[26] DOT 5-8.56

Nonsteroidal Anti-inflammatory Drugs (NSAIDs). NSAIDS are used to treat inflammation, pain, and fever. Common NSAIDs include ibuprofen, naproxen, ketoprofen, piroxicam, diclofenac, indomethacin, and ketorolac. Adverse effects during therapeutic use (such as GI bleeding and kidney failure) are relatively common. Acute NSAID ingestion can cause coma and metabolic acidosis, but these effects are only seen following massive ingestion. There are no specific prehospital interventions beyond supportive care.[27] DOT 5-8.56

Aspirin. Acetylsalicylic acid (aspirin) is commonly used for analgesia and antipyresis. It has also secured prominence as an antiplatelet agent in the treatment of acute coronary syndrome and cerebrovascular disease. Salicylates are available over-the-counter and are in several combination cold products. It is one of the most common poisonings reported to poison centers and is perennially one of the most lethal (see Table 35-1, page 864).

Nausea, vomiting, and abdominal pain are frequent symptoms after ingestion. Muffled hearing and tinnitus are also common. Moderate toxicity will induce hyperpnea, tachypnea, somnolence, and mild acidosis. Severe toxicity will produce cerebral and pulmonary edema, coma, and seizures.

Transport patients promptly to the emergency department. Initiate intravenous fluids for mild dehydration. Endotracheally intubate the comatose patient, and hyperventilate to prevent worsening acidosis. Most moderately intoxicated patients will require a sodium bicarbonate infusion; severely ill patients will need hemodialysis.[28] DOT 5-8.56

Antihistamines and Anticholinergics. Antihistamines are both prescribed and obtained over-the-counter. Histamine 2 (H2) blockers, such as ranitidine, cimetidine, famotidine, and nizatidine, decrease acid efflux into the stomach and are used for gastric and duodenal ulcers and gastroesophageal reflux disease. After overdose, H2 blockers are well tolerated with minimal adverse effects. Sedating histamine 1 (H1) blockers include diphenhydramine, doxylamine, brompheniramine, and hydroxyzine. These medications are used to treat allergic reactions. However, because they are sedating, they are also used as a treatment for motion sickness, vertigo, pruritus, and as a sleeping aide. Less-sedating H1 blockers include cetirizine, loratadine, desloratadine, and fexofenadine. These agents are used primarily for allergic reactions.

Sedating H1 blockers produce significant sedation, tachycardia, and anticholinergic effects. The anticholinergic toxidrome is described in Table 35-2. Occasionally, seizures occur after large ingestions. Ventricular dysrhythmias have rarely occurred after large diphenhydramine ingestions. Less-sedating H1 antagonists cause mild sedation and tachycardia.

In transport to the hospital, provide supplemental oxygen and cardiac monitoring. Administer benzodiazepines to agitated or delirious patients for sedation. Manually ventilate or endotracheally intubate somnolent patients. Treat seizures with parenteral benzodiazepines.[29,30] DOT 5-8.56

Herbal Remedies and Dietary Supplements. Herbal remedies and dietary supplements consist of an array of medications and products. Although many have been thought to have clinical benefit, the Food and Drug Administration has recognized few for clinical use. In general, few supplements and remedies have adverse effects beyond gastrointestinal upset.

Selected herbs can cause significant toxicity. Aconite from the *Aconitum* plants can cause hypotension, dysrhythmias, and heart blocks. Treatment is supportive. Jimsonweed seeds contain anticholinergic alkaloids and can produce toxicity, including prolonged delirium, tachycardia, dry skin, mydriasis, and urinary retention. Parenteral benzodiazepines for delirium and supportive care are sufficient prehospital treatment.

Cardiac glycosides from foxglove, oleander, lily of the valley, and squill can produce ventricular dysrhythmias and death. Treatment is the same as for cardiac glycoside poisoning from digoxin (see Cardioactive Steroids section). Kava can cause sedation and, rarely, liver injury. Pennyroyal oil is used as an abortifacient and can induce hepatotoxicity. N-acetylcysteine may be beneficial for the hepatoxicity. Ginseng and ginkgo biloba may cause problems with bleeding. Vomiting, sedation, and nystagmus are common symptoms of nutmeg toxicity. DOT 5-8.56

Psychiatric Medications

Benzodiazepines. The benzodiazepines are used to treat anxiety, seizures, insomnia, and ethanol withdrawal. Common benzodiazepines include diazepam, lorazepam, alprazolam, clonazepam, chlordiazepoxide, clorazepate, and many others. Benzodiazepine overdose causes CNS depression, but isolated benzodiazepine overdoses are rarely fatal, even without treatment.

Mixed ingestions, such as benzodiazepines and ethanol, can be fatal. Patients should be monitored for CNS depression and should be intubated if they have airway compromise.[31] DOT 5-8.56

Tricyclic Antidepressants (TCAs). The tricyclic antidepressants are a second-line therapy for depression but are commonly used to treat chronic pain, bedwetting, and insomnia. Common tricyclic antidepressants include amitriptyline, imipramine, desipramine, doxepin, and nortriptyline. Tricyclic antidepressant poisoning causes coma, seizures, hypotension, and wide complex cardiac dysrhythmias. These effects may develop very abruptly, and patients may progress rapidly from asymptomatic to life-threatening toxicity. All patients require constant cardiac monitoring, and paramedics must be prepared to treat any complications. Treatment of coma includes intubation and ventilation. Seizures usually respond to standard doses of benzodiazepines. Hypotension is treated with crystalloid infusion and dopamine or epinephrine infusions. Cardiac dysrhythmias are due to antagonism of cardiac sodium channels. Patients should be treated with hypertonic sodium bicarbonate boluses (see Table 35-3). These boluses are repeated, as needed. Hyperventilation may also be useful for preventing and treating dysrhythmias.[32] DOT 5-8.56

Street Secrets

Alkalinizing the urine occurs when sodium bicarbonate is administered. It alters the pH of the blood by raising it so that it is alkaline. This, in effect, inactivates much of the TCA drug, which prefers a more acidic pH level.

Selective Serotonin Reuptake Inhibitors (SSRIs). The selective serotonin reuptake inhibitors (SSRIs) are commonly used to treat depression and other psychiatric disorders. Common SSRIs include fluoxetine, paroxetine, sertraline, citalopram, escitalopram, and fluvoxamine. Other medications such as venlefaxine, trazodone, and mirtazepine also alter serotonergic neurotransmitters and are used for depression. Sedation is the most common effect of overdose. Other effects include agitation, seizures, and tachycardia, but the effects are usually self-limited. Serotonin syndrome is a collection of symptoms that may occur after overdose but is more commonly an adverse reaction that occurs when multiple serotonergic medications are taken simultaneously. The effects include CNS depression, fever, muscle rigidity, and tremor. Patients require aggressive sedation and cooling measures to prevent severe hyperthermia.[33] DOT 5-8.56

Monoamine Oxidase Inhibitors (MAOI). MAOIs, such as phenelzine (Nardil®) and tranylcypromine, are older antidepressants that are rarely used today. In overdose, they can cause hyper- or hypotension, seizures, coma, rigidity, and hyperthermia. The symptoms of MAOI toxicity may be delayed for more than a day after overdose. MAOIs may also cause a syndrome of flushing and severe hypertension when patients ingest tyramine-containing food such as wine, cheese, and smoked meats.[34] DOT 5-8.56

Lithium. Lithium carbonate is used to treat bipolar mood disorder. Most preparations are sustained release. The initial symptoms of acute ingestion are severe abdominal pain, vomiting, and diarrhea. Most patients will recover with supportive care and hydration to increase the renal clearance of lithium. However, some patients will develop confusion, seizures, and coma. Chronic lithium toxicity occurs when patients taking lithium become dehydrated. These patients present with confusion, somnolence, tremors, and muscle rigidity. While life-threatening effects are uncommon, patients may take several weeks to recover.[35] DOT 5-8.56

Antipsychotic Medications. Antipsychotic medications are used to treat schizophrenia and related psychiatric disorders. Common antipsychotic medications include haloperidol, fluphenazine, risperidol, olanzapine, ziprasidone, aripiprazole, and quetiapine. In overdose, these medications cause CNS depression that may be life-threatening and occasionally cause hypotension. No specific treatment beyond supportive care is indicated. Older antipsychotic medications such as haloperidol or fluphenazine also frequently cause dystonic reactions. These are involuntary muscle contractions that most commonly involve the neck but can involve any muscle group. These reactions usually respond to diphenhydramine 50 mg IV or IM.[36] DOT 5-8.56

Other Medications

Opioids (Narcotics). Common medicinal opiates include codeine, morphine, fentanyl, meperidine, oxycodone, hydrocodone, hydromorphone, buprenorphine, and methadone. Heroin is a morphine derivative that is commonly abused. Many of these products are combined with over-the-counter analgesics such as acetaminophen, ibuprofen, and aspirin. It is important to evaluate opioid-poisoned patients for co-ingestion of these products. The opioids are most commonly used to treat pain. They are also used to treat cough, diarrhea, and addiction.

The clinical effects of opioids include analgesia, CNS depression, cough suppression, decreased intestinal mobility, and miosis. Opioid overdose causes respiratory depression, which can lead to apnea and death.

Because of the high rate of opiate abuse and narrow therapeutic index, opioids are one of the most common causes of poisoning death. Patients that use opiates chronically will become tolerant to the effects, so very high doses of opiates may be required to provide analgesia. Chronic opiate users will also become dependent on opiates. This means they will develop withdrawal symptoms if their treatment is discontinued (or reversed with an antagonist). Opioid withdrawal causes nausea, diarrhea, abdominal cramping, piloerection, and anxiety. While withdrawal from opioids is not life-threatening, patients can develop severe symptoms and may benefit from supportive care such as antiemetics and IV fluids.

Opiate-poisoned patients require monitoring for CNS and respiratory depression. Their responsiveness and respiratory rate should be assessed. Patients may have apnea and may be severely hypoxic. Oxygenation should be assessed with pulse oximetry and the patient examined for cyanosis. Cardiovascular effects are almost always due to hypoxia, but mild hypotension may occur from histamine release.

The primary treatment for opioid-induced respiratory depression is support of ventilation and oxygenation. Naloxone is a specific antidote for opioid poisoning. It is most commonly administered intravenously or by intramuscular injection but can also be administered with an intranasal atomizer. Naloxone quickly reverses opioid effects (including analgesia) and will restore normal mental status within one to two minutes of administration. Naloxone has a short duration of action, and patients may have recurrence of symptoms after 30 to 60 minutes. While this is uncommon after heroin overdose, it is very common with longer-acting opioids. Nalmefene is a longer-acting antidote for opioid poisoning, but it is not commonly used.[37] DOT 5-8.56

Working in the Gray Zone

Naloxone is very effective in treating opiate overdoses. However, its use can also precipitate withdrawal symptoms in some individuals who are addicted to the drug. Opiate withdrawal is seldom life-threatening although it can be very unpleasant for patients; however, it can cause seizures in some patients. Generally naloxone should be given in small, divided doses to the point where respirations are restored. Patients who is monitored closely can remain asleep as long as the vital signs, including the respiratory rate, are within a normal range. It may be appropriate to check the blood sugar on these patients as well.

Barbiturates. Barbiturates are used as anesthetics and for the treatment of seizures and headaches. Common barbiturates include phenobarbital, pentobarbital, butalbital, and thiopental. Barbiturates cause intoxication, ataxia, confusion, slurred speech, and coma. Respiratory depression may be life-threatening, and intubation and respiratory support is the mainstay of treatment. DOT 5-8.56

Hypoglycemic Drugs. Insulin and sulfonylurea oral hypoglycemics are used to treat diabetes. Other diabetes medications, such as metformin, pioglitazone and rosiglitazone, do not cause hypoglycemia. The main toxic effects of insulin and the sulfonylurea medications are hypoglycemia and hypokalemia. There are several types of insulin; each type has a different onset and duration of action. Regular insulin has an onset of action within 60 minutes and duration of action of between two to five hours. Lispro and Aspart insulin have a more rapid onset and shorter duration of action. Most other insulin types (NPH, Lente, etc.) have a slower onset and longer durations of action. The treatment of hypoglycemia from insulin toxicity is dextrose. Insulin poisoning is often due to the patient missing a meal rather than from overdose. In these cases, patients will frequently respond to oral glucose or a single 25 gm of IV dose followed by a meal.

Although the sulfonylureas have the same major effect as insulin, there are substantial differences in the onset and duration of hypoglycemia. Sulfonylurea poisoning often causes profound, prolonged hypoglycemia that requires large doses of glucose. As the symptoms are delayed, nondiabetic patients that ingest these products or diabetics that ingest more than therapeutic amounts should be transported to the hospital and admitted for an observation period with serial glucose monitoring. Patients who develop hypoglycemia should be treated with a dextrose bolus and placed on a dextrose infusion.[38,39] DOT 5-8.56

Methemoglobinemia. Methemoglobinemia is a condition rather than a specific poison. Methemoglobin is formed when the iron in hemoglobin is oxidized and can no longer transport oxygen. Methemoglobinemia is usually an adverse reaction to a therapeutic dose of a medication in a sensitive patient. It has been reported after doses of benzocaine, nitrates, dapsone, and sulfonamides. Patients usually present with cyanosis and abnormal oxygen saturations on pulse oximetry. More severe cases may have symptoms of hypoxia such as headache, confusion, shortness of breath, and hypotension. Methylene blue is administered to patients with symptoms to convert methemoglobin back to hemoglobin.[40] DOT 5-8.56

Ethanol (EtOH). Ethanol is undoubtedly the most common drug of abuse and is the leading cause of drug abuse death. Although ethanol is sold as a beverage, it is also in a variety of medicinal and cosmetic preparations, including cough suppressants, mouthwash, perfumes, colognes, and industrial solvents.

Expected effects at low doses include euphoria, disinhibition, dysarthria, and impaired judgment. Symptoms of moderate toxicity are ataxia, disorientation, amnesia, uncoordination, and sedation. Severe toxicity manifests as respiratory depression, hypotension, hypothermia, and coma.

Monitor the patient for respiratory depression and hypoxia. Perform endotracheal intubation in the comatose patient. Monitor for hypotension and mild hypothermia. Administer crystalloid for hypotension. Determine if another process is causing the somnolence and altered mental status, such as intracranial hemorrhage, hypoglycemia, head trauma, or psychosis.[16] DOT 5-8.56

Marijuana and Cannabis. Marijuana is the most commonly used illicit drug. It is smoked or put into food. Hashish is the dried resin collected from the flowers of the marijuana plant.

Acute intoxication results in mild tachycardia, ataxia, and conjunctival injection. Euphoria, increased appetite, anxiety, impaired cognition, and, occasionally, dysphoria occur. Psychosis is unusual. Toxicity is not life-threatening, and the intoxicant effects are mild and transient. Place the patient in a quiet environment and offer reassurance. Treat agitation and anxiety with benzodiazepines. Assess for concomitant drugs of abuse. Treat mild hypotension with crystalloid infusion.[41] DOT 5-8.56

Gamma-Hydroxybutrate (GHB). Gamma hydroxybutyrate (GHB) is used for narcolepsy but is also abused for its mild euphoric effects. GHB has also been fallaciously associated with increasing muscle mass and is abused by body builders. Other GHB congeners are gamma-butyrolactone and 1,4 butanediol.

Hallmark features of intoxication are profound coma, myoclonus, and mild bradycardia. Somnolence occurs after an overdose and usually lasts less than six hours. During direct laryngoscopy without additional sedation or paralytic therapy, the patient retains airway reflexes waking quickly but transiently.

Upon initial evaluation, provide supplemental oxygen and cardiac monitoring. Most patients can be monitored without endotracheal intubation. Occasionally, intubation is needed for respiratory failure. Because of the patient's intact airway reflexes, pharmacologic paralysis is usually needed. Treat symptomatic bradycardia with atropine. Myoclonus is common and does not need to be treated; however, seizures may also occur and should be treated with benzodiazepines. In addition, chronic users of GHB develop a withdrawal state similar to alcohol and benzodiazepine withdrawal. GHB withdrawal can be treated similarly with benzodiazepines and supportive care.[42] DOT 5-8.56

Hallucinogens. There are several drugs classified as hallucinogens. The most common are lysergic acid diethylamide (LSD), tryptamines (e.g., "foxymethoxy"), and psilocybin in the *Psilocybe* mushrooms. LSD produces synesthesias, such as "feeling color" and "seeing sound." Patients have altered visual perception, are sensitive to sound, and may have mild depression. LSD also produces mild sympathomimetic effects such as tachycardia, diaphoresis, and mydriasis. Tryptamines and hallucinogenic mushrooms produce visual hallucinations and mild sympathomimetic symptoms.

Treatment entails providing reassurance in a calm, supportive environment. Treat agitation and anxiety with parenteral benzodiazepines. Monitor for mild tachycardia and hypertension.[43] DOT 5-8.56

Inhalant Abuse. Inhalant abuse is use of a volatile substance for the purpose of achieving euphoria. Examples of inhaled agents are toluene in paint, methanol in carburetor cleaner, and inhaled nitrites ("poppers"). Other volatile substances that are abused include gasoline, paint thinner, nail polish, and shoe polish. **Huffing** is when an individual holds a piece of cloth soaked in a volatile substance and breathes through it. **Bagging** is when the substance is sprayed into a bag, and the bag is placed over one's head. DOT 5-8.20

Inhalant abuse can produce sedation, mild euphoria, ataxia, and impaired cognition. Contact of the fluid with the skin may cause irritation. Aspiration of the inhalant can cause bronchospasm, hypoxia, and pneumonitis. Rarely, lethal dysrhythmias can occur if the inhalant sensitizes the myocardium and the individual is startled, also known as "sudden sniffing death." Abuse of nitrites can cause methemoglobinemia, which manifests as mildly low pulse oximetry, central cyanosis, and tachypnea. DOT 5-8.21, 5-8.22

The patient's airway should be monitored and supplemental oxygen administered. Assess the patient's pulse oximetry. Exclude other causes of altered mentation such as hypoglycemia and opioid intoxication. Sedation with benzodiazepines is occasionally needed for agitation. Administer intravenous fluids for dehydration. Treat methemoglobemia with supplemental oxygen. Methylene blue is the antidote and can be administered in the emergency department.[44] DOT 5-8.56

Stimulants: Amphetamines, Methamphetamines, and Cocaine. Cocaine, amphetamines, and methamphetamines are stimulants that are commonly abused. Some amphetamine derivatives such as methylphenidate and fenfluramine are used medically to treat attention deficient disorder and obesity. Methylene-dioxymeth-amphetamine (MDMA, Ectasy) is an amphetamine derivative abused for its euphoric and stimulant effects.

Tachycardia, diaphoresis, agitation, and mild hypertension are common. Pyrexia, seizures, and rhabdomyolysis occur with severe toxicity. Complications of stimulant use are myocardial infarction, intracerebral hemorrhage, intestinal ischemia, and ventricular dysrhythmias. Occasionally, bradycardia occurs with some amphetamine derivatives such as ephedrine.

The prehospital provider should place the patient on a cardiac monitor to assess for dysrhythmia, tachycardia, and hypertension. Administer supplemental oxygen. The mainstay of treatment is sedation with benzodiazepines and hydration for rhabdomyolysis. Treat chest pain after stimulant use with benzodiazepines and nitroglycerin. Hypertension is usually controlled with benzodiazepines, but occasionally, nitroglycerin or phentolamine are used for refractory hypertension. Lower the temperature of hyperthermic patients by administering benzodiazepines, removing the patient's clothing, and exposing the patient's skin to tepid water and fans. Treat ventricular dysrhythmias after cocaine use with sodium bicarbonate bolus to counteract cocaine's myocardial sodium channel blocking effects.[45,46]

Two other types of exposure to drugs of abuse are "body packing" and "body stuffing." The drugs that are most commonly "packed" or "stuffed" are cocaine, heroin, and methamphetamine. **Body packers** ingest a large amount of well-packaged drugs to smuggle the drug into a secured area (Figure 35-7). The most common scenario is the transport of cocaine into the U.S. from South America. It is rare for these packages to open, but when they do, the patient will have a massive exposure that is frequently lethal. Body packers are usually admitted to the ICU for observation, and whole bowel irrigation is used to clear the packets from the GI tract. Patients that develop symptoms must be treated aggressively and may need emergency surgery to remove the packets.

Body stuffers ingest drugs (or insert them in another body cavity such as the rectum or vagina) to avoid arrest. The amount of drug is much less than the amount involved in body packing, but the packaging of the drugs is much poorer. These patients usually develop mild to moderate symptoms within a few hours of the exposure. However, serious toxicity and even death may occur. These patients should be closely monitored and treated using the recommendations described in the specific drug sections above. If they remain asymptomatic for several hours, they can be discharged. DOT 5-8.56

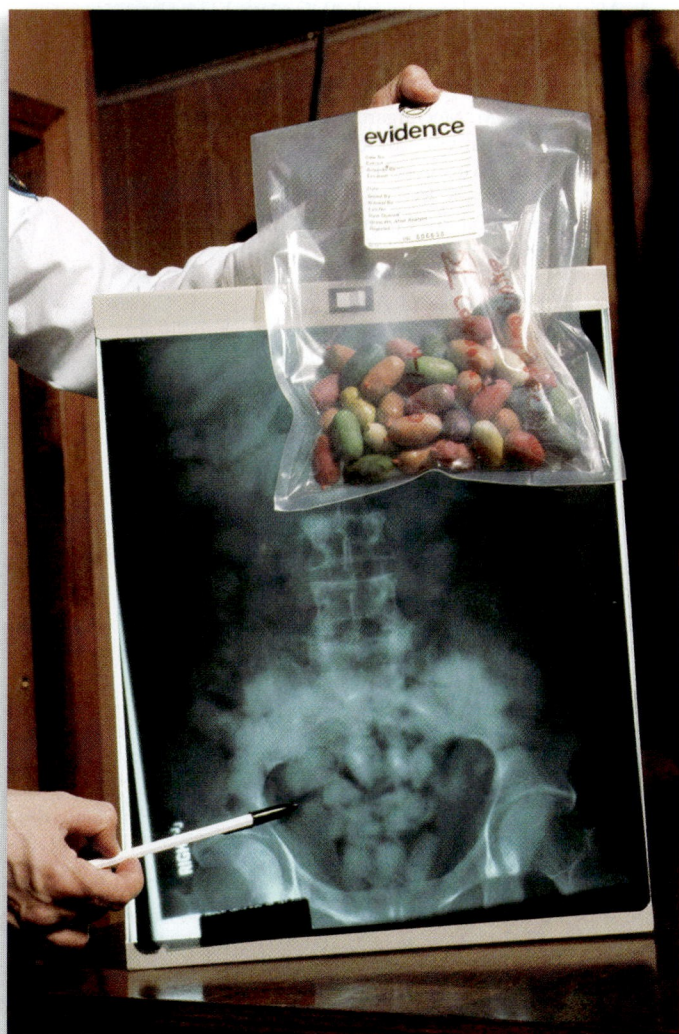

Figure 35-7 Abdomen X-ray of a "body packer" showing multiple drug packages inside the abdomen. The plastic bag holds the same balloons after they were expelled.

Summary

Poisonings can result from a wide variety of causes, both intentional and unintentional. The first priority of all responders is personal safety to prevent any responder from being injured. Careful evaluation of the presenting symptoms may allow for recognition of toxidromes, suggesting poisoning with certain classes of drugs.

In most cases, prehospital care is primarily supportive. Specific antidotes are available in cases of poisoning with certain drugs and may be administered in the prehospital setting.

Notes

1. K. Heard, "Gastrointestinal Decontamination," *The Medical Clinics of North America* 89(6) (2005): 1067–1078.
2. C. R. DeWitt and R. C. Dart, "Airway and Ventilatory Management," In *Medical Toxicology*, 3rd ed., R. C. Dart, E. M. Caravati, M. McGuigan, et al., eds. (Philadelphia, PA: Lippincott Williams & Wilkins, 2004), pp. 143–146.

3. R. C. Dart, "Hypotension and Shock," In *Medical Toxicology,* 3rd ed., R. C. Dart, E. M. Caravati, M. McGuigan, et al., eds. (Philadelphia, PA: Lippincott Williams & Wilkins, 2004), pp. 151–152.

4. G. Braitberg, "Treatment of Convulsions," In *Medical Toxicology,* 3rd ed., R. C. Dart, E. M. Caravati, M. McGuigan, et al., eds. (Philadelphia, PA: Lippincott Williams & Wilkins, 2004), pp. 156–159.

5. Part 10.2, "Toxicology in ECC," *Circulation* 112(24_suppl) (2005): IV126–IV132.

6. R. B. Rao and R. S. Hoffman, "Caustics and Batteries," In *Goldfrank's Toxicologic Emergencies,* 7th ed., L. R. Goldfrank, N. E. Flomenbaum, N. A. Lewin, M. A. Howland, R. S. Hoffman, and L. S. Nelson, eds. (New York, NY: McGraw-Hill, 2002), pp. 1323–1345.

7. K. Heard, "Hydroflouric Acid," In *Critical Care Toxicology,* J. Brent, K. L. Wallace, K. K. Burkhart, S. D. Phillips, and J. W. Donovan, eds. (St. Lous, MO: Mosby, 2005), pp. 1045–1050.

8. P. A. Chyka and W. Banner, "Hematopoietic Agents," In *Medical Toxicology,* 3rd ed., R. C. Dart, E. M. Caravati, M. McGuigan, et al., eds. (Philadelphia, PA: Lippincott Williams & Wilkins, 2004), pp. 605–614.

9. R. C. Dart, K. M. Hurlbut, and L. V. Boyer-Hansen, "Lead," In *Medical Toxicology,* 3rd ed., R. C. Dart, E. M. Caravati, M. McGuigan, et al., eds. (Philadelphia, PA: Lippincott Williams & Wilkins, 2004), pp. 1423–1431.

10. R. C. Dart and J. B. Sullivan, "Mercury," In *Medical Toxicology,* 3rd ed., R. C. Dart, E. M. Caravati, M. McGuigan, et al., eds. (Philadelphia, PA: Lippincott Williams & Wilkins, 2004), p. 1437.

11. A. R. Erdman, "Cyanide," In *Medical Toxicology,* 3rd ed., R. C. Dart, E. M. Caravati, M. McGuigan, et al., eds. (Philadelphia, PA: Lippincott Williams & Wilkins, 2004), pp. 1155–1168.

12. A. R. Erdman, "Insecticides," In *Medical Toxicology,* 3rd ed., R. C. Dart, E. M. Caravati, M. McGuigan, et al., eds. (Philadelphia, PA: Lippincott Williams & Wilkins, 2004), pp. 1475–1498.

13. R. C. Dart and K. M. Hurlbut, "Respiratory Irritants," In *Medical Toxicology,* 3rd ed., R. C. Dart, E. M. Caravati, M. McGuigan, et al., eds. (Philadelphia, PA: Lippincott Williams & Wilkins, 2004), pp. 1143–1145.

14. USP DI (r) and Advice for the Patients. Thomson MOCROMEDIX Healthcare Series, Vol. 128, June 2006.

15. H. A. Jollif and M. L. A. Sivilotti, "Ethylene Glycol," In *Medical Toxicology,* 3rd ed., R. C. Dart, E. M. Caravati, M. McGuigan, et al., eds. (Philadelphia, PA: Lippincott Williams & Wilkins, 2004), pp. 1223–1229.

16. M. L. A. Sivilotti, "Ethanol, Isopropyl and Methanol," In *Medical Toxicology,* 3rd ed., R. C. Dart, E. M. Caravati, M. McGuigan, et al., eds. (Philadelphia, PA: Lippincott Williams & Wilkins, 2004), pp. 1211–1222.

17. L. K. Weaver, "Carbon Monoxide," In *Medical Toxicology,* 3rd ed., R. C. Dart, E. M. Caravati, M. McGuigan, et al., eds. (Philadelphia, PA: Lippincott Williams & Wilkins, 2004), pp. 1146–1154.

18. R. C. Wang, "Hydrocarbon Products," In *Medical Toxicology,* 3rd ed., R. C. Dart, E. M. Caravati, M. McGuigan, et al., eds. (Philadelphia, PA: Lippincott Williams & Wilkins, 2004), pp. 1328–1351.

19. C. R. DeWitt and J. C. Waksman, "Pharmacology, Pathophysiology and Management of Calcium Channel Blocker and Beta-Blocker Toxicity," *Toxicological Reviews* 23(4) (2004): 223–238.

20. K. Heard, "Digoxin and Theraputic Cardiac Glycosides," In *Medical Toxicology,* 3rd ed., R. C. Dart, E. M. Caravati, M. McGuigan, et al., eds. (Philadelphia, PA: Lippincott Williams & Wilkins, 2004), pp. 700–705.

21. E. M. Caravati, "Type 1A Antidysrhythmic Agents," In *Medical Toxicology,* 3rd ed., R. C. Dart, E. M. Caravati, M. McGuigan, et al., eds. (Philadelphia, PA: Lippincott Williams & Wilkins, 2004), pp. 655–678.

22. S. Banerji, "Angiotensin-Converting Enzyme inhibitors," In *Medical Toxicology,* 3rd ed., R. C. Dart, E. M. Caravati, M. McGuigan, et al., eds. (Philadelphia, PA: Lippincott Williams & Wilkins, 2004), pp. 647–651.

23. S. Banerji, "Angiotensin Receptor Blockers," In *Medical Toxicology,* 3rd ed., R. C. Dart, E. M. Caravati, M. McGuigan, et al., eds. (Philadelphia, PA: Lippincott Williams & Wilkins, 2004), pp. 651–653.

24. R. C. Dart and D. L. Seeger, "Clonidine," In *Medical Toxicology,* 3rd ed., R. C. Dart, E. M. Caravati, M. McGuigan, et al., eds. (Philadelphia, PA: Lippincott Williams & Wilkins, 2004), p. 653.

25. K. M. Hurlbut, "Vasodilators," In *Medical Toxicology,* 3rd ed., R. C. Dart, E. M. Caravati, M. McGuigan, et al., eds. (Philadelphia, PA: Lippincott Williams & Wilkins, 2004), pp. 714–722.

26. R. C. Dart and B. H. Rumack, "Acetaminophen," In *Medical Toxicology,* 3rd ed., R. C. Dart, E. M. Caravati, M. McGuigan, et al., eds. (Philadelphia, PA: Lippincott Williams & Wilkins, 2004), p. 723.

27. A. C. Bronstein, "Non-Steroidal Anti-Inflamatory Drugs," In *Medical Toxicology,* 3rd ed., R. C. Dart, E. M. Caravati, M. McGuigan, et al., eds. (Philadelphia, PA: Lippincott Williams & Wilkins, 2004), p. 750.

28. L. Yip, "Salicylate," In *Medical Toxicology,* 3rd ed., R. C. Dart, E. M. Caravati, M. McGuigan, et al., eds. (Philadelphia, PA: Lippincott Williams & Wilkins, 2004), p. 739.

29. A. H. Dawson, "Antimuscarinic Drugs," In *Medical Toxicology,* 3rd ed., R. C. Dart, E. M. Caravati, M. McGuigan, et al., eds. (Philadelphia, PA: Lippincott Williams & Wilkins, 2004), p. 560.

30. I. MacGregor Whyte, "Sedating Antihistamines (H1 antagonists)," In *Medical Toxicology,* 3rd ed., R. C. Dart, E. M. Caravati, M. McGuigan, et al., eds. (Philadelphia, PA: Lippincott Williams & Wilkins, 2004), p. 396.

31. I. MacGregor Whyte, "Benzodiazepines," In *Medical Toxicology,* 3rd ed., R. C. Dart, E. M. Caravati, M. McGuigan, et al., eds. (Philadelphia, PA: Lippincott Williams & Wilkins, 2004), p. 811.

32. A. H. Dawson, "Cyclic Antidepressants," In *Medical Toxicology,* 3rd ed., R. C. Dart, E. M. Caravati, M. McGuigan, et al., eds. (Philadelphia, PA: Lippincott Williams & Wilkins, 2004), p. 834.

33. I. MacGregor Whyte, "Serotonin Reuptake Inhibitors," In *Medical Toxicology,* 3rd ed., R. C. Dart, E. M. Caravati, M. McGuigan, et al., eds. (Philadelphia, PA: Lippincott Williams & Wilkins, 2004), p. 843.

34. I. MacGregor Whyte, "Monoamine Oxidase Inhibitors," In *Medical Toxicology,* 3rd ed., R. C. Dart, E. M. Caravati, M. McGuigan, et al., eds. (Philadelphia, PA: Lippincott Williams & Wilkins, 2004), p. 823.

35. M. A. Miller and K. R. Olson, "Lithium," In *Medical Toxicology,* 3rd ed., R. C. Dart, E. M. Caravati, M. McGuigan, et al., eds. (Philadelphia, PA: Lippincott Williams & Wilkins, 2004), pp. 805–810.

36. N. A. Buckley, "Antipsychotic Medications (Neuroleptics)," In *Medical Toxicology,* 3rd ed., R. C. Dart, E. M. Caravati, M. McGuigan, et al., eds. (Philadelphia, PA: Lippincott Williams & Wilkins, 2004), p. 861.

37. S. A. Siefert, "Opioid Medications," In *Medical Toxicology,* 3rd ed., R. C. Dart, E. M. Caravati, M. McGuigan, et al., eds. (Philadelphia, PA: Lippincott Williams & Wilkins, 2004), p. 756.

38. K. M. Hurlbut, "Insulin," In *Medical Toxicology,* 3rd ed., R. C. Dart, E. M. Caravati, M. McGuigan, et al., eds. (Philadelphia, PA: Lippincott Williams & Wilkins, 2004), p. 953.

39. P. E. McKinney and S. A. McLaughlin, "Sulfonlyurea and Antihyperglycemic Drugs," In *Medical Toxicology,* 3rd ed., R. C. Dart, E. M. Caravati, M. McGuigan, et al., eds. (Philadelphia, PA: Lippincott Williams & Wilkins, 2004), p. 956.

40. A. B. Woolf and R. O. Wright, "Methemoglobinemia," In *Medical Toxicology,* 3rd ed., R. C. Dart, E. M. Caravati, M. McGuigan, et al., eds. (Philadelphia, PA: Lippincott Williams & Wilkins, 2004), p. 90.

41. E. M. Caravati, "Marijuana and Other Canabinoids," In *Medical Toxicology,* 3rd ed., R. C. Dart, E. M. Caravati, M. McGuigan, et al., eds. (Philadelphia, PA: Lippincott Williams & Wilkins, 2004), p. 1112.

42. J. E. Dyer and C. Haller, "Gamma Hydroxybutyrate, Gamma Butyrolactone and 1,4 Butanediol," In *Medical Toxicology,* 3rd ed., R. C. Dart, E. M. Caravati, M. McGuigan, et al., eds. (Philadelphia, PA: Lippincott Williams & Wilkins, 2004), p. 1096.

43. E. M. Caravati, "Hallucinogenic Drugs," In *Medical Toxicology,* 3rd ed., R. C. Dart, E. M. Caravati, M. McGuigan, et al., eds. (Philadelphia, PA: Lippincott Williams & Wilkins, 2004), p. 1103.

44. G. F. O'Malley, "Inhalent Abse," In *Medical Toxicology,* 3rd ed., R. C. Dart, E. M. Caravati, M. McGuigan, et al., eds. (Philadelphia, PA: Lippincott Williams & Wilkins, 2004), p. 1117.

45. J. E. Hollander, "Cocaine," In *Medical Toxicology,* 3rd ed., R. C. Dart, E. M. Caravati, M. McGuigan, et al., eds. (Philadelphia, PA: Lippincott Williams & Wilkins, 2004), p. 1083.

46. R. C. Lynton and T. E. Albertson, "Amphetamine and Designer Drugs," In *Medical Toxicology,* 3rd ed., R. C. Dart, E. M. Caravati, M. McGuigan, et al., eds. (Philadelphia, PA: Lippincott Williams & Wilkins, 2004), p. 1071.

36

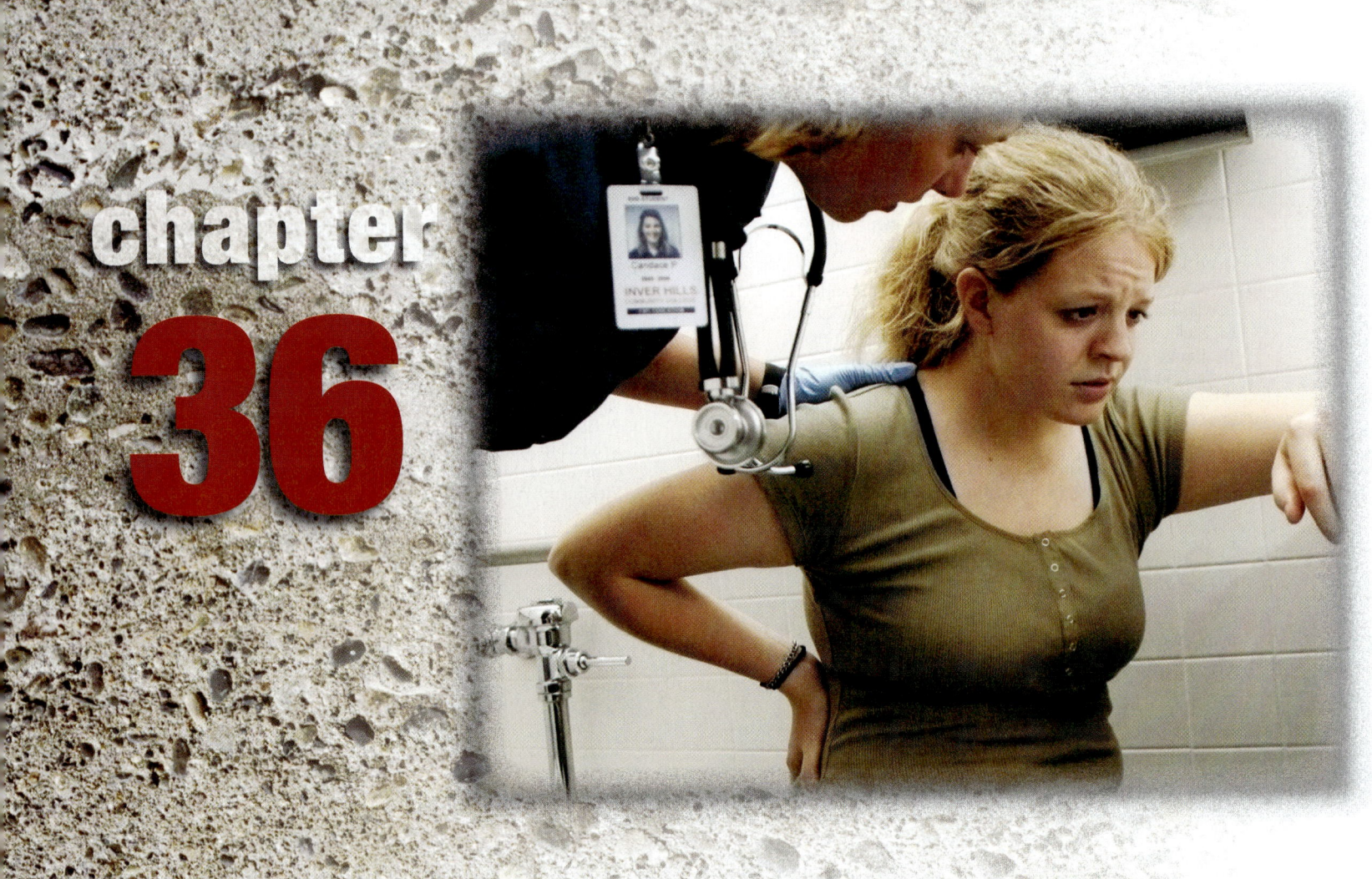

Nephrology and Urology

"*M*acduff: What three things does drink especially provoke? Porter: Marry, sir, nose-painting, sleep, and urine."

—William Shakespeare

Need to Know

▶ Kidney stones are extremely common, affecting one in ten people at some time during their lives.

▶ Acute renal failure (ARF) is the deterioration of renal function over a period of hours or days, which results in the accumulation of metabolic waste products, primarily nitrogenous compounds, in the blood.

▶ Fluid volume emergencies are common in acute renal failure (ARF).

- Too much fluid:
  - The most common fluid-related complications are due to fluid overload and include pulmonary edema, hypertension, and congestive heart failure.
  - Patients may present in pulmonary edema with symptoms of shortness of breath and dyspnea. The physical examination may show rales or rhonchi on lung auscultation, jugular venous distention, and peripheral edema.
  - Continuous positive airway pressure (CPAP) or biphasic positive airway pressure (BiPAP) devices may be used in severely compromised patients who are alert and not vomiting.
- Too little fluid:
  - Hypovolemia can occur due to vomiting, diarrhea, or inadequate intake of fluids. Hypotension, poor skin turgor, and dry mucous membranes may be noted on physical examination.

▶ Chronic renal failure (CRF) is a disease characterized by the gradual permanent and irreversible loss of kidney function due to destruction of the nephrons.

▶ Hyperkalemia should be considered in every CRF or end-stage renal disease (ESRD) patient encountered by the paramedic.

▶ Obtain the date of the patient's last dialysis treatment as part of your assessment. An AV shunt should only be used for IV access as a last resort in life-threatening situations.

▶ Sick	▶ Not Yet Sick
• Listen to lung sounds, look for pedal edema and fluid overload. Consider CPAP for respiratory distress.	• Determine: History of renal failure? Last dialysis? Or how far into current dialysis treatment?
• Patients passing kidney stones are frequently found writhing in pain, unable to remain still, and unable to find a comfortable position.	• Monitor fluid administration carefully; limit fluids if the patient is fluid overloaded.
• The most common causes of death in patients with ARF are sepsis, heart failure, and pulmonary failure. Therefore patients suspected of ARF and complications should be considered true medical emergencies and should be transported rapidly to a hospital. Hyperkalemia is the most common cause of metabolic death in ARF patients.	• Consider sepsis. What is the patient's temperature? • Treat suspected kidney stones with aggressive pain management.

Introduction

The genitourinary tract consists of several organs, including the kidneys, ureters, bladder, urethra, prostate, and testicles. The system organs occupy several different parts of the human body, including the abdomen, pelvis, and external genitalia. Most of the organs of the urinary tract cannot be directly visualized in the prehospital setting, and their function most often cannot be assessed without laboratory tests. Many other organ systems are adversely affected when the urinary tract is not functioning properly. Numerous problems, both medical and traumatic, can affect these organs primarily and other organs secondarily, causing a wide variety of signs, symptoms, and syndromes. Because of these factors, the paramedic must be aware of the interrelationships between the urinary tract and other organ systems as well as the individual disease entities that can affect the kidneys and related structures.

The urinary system helps maintain homeostasis by removing waste products from blood and by managing the volume of fluid in the body. **Nephrology** is the study and treatment of disorders of the kidney, primarily from a medical rather than surgical point of view. It is a complex discipline because kidney dysfunction negatively affects nearly every other organ system in the body. **Urology** is the study and treatment of diseases that affect the entire urinary tract from the kidneys to the genitalia. Nephrologists diagnose and treat medical conditions involving the kidneys; whereas, urologists primarily concentrate on surgical conditions affecting the kidneys as well as medical and surgical disorders of the collecting system, bladder, prostate, and genitalia. The EMS system may be activated for patients suffering from a wide variety of diseases and injuries to the organs of the urinary tract, many of which constitute true medical and surgical emergencies.

Applied Anatomy and Physiology

The paired, bean-shaped kidneys are roughly the size of a patient's fist and lie against the posterior wall of the abdomen in the retroperitoneal space (Figure 36-1). The renal arteries bring blood to the kidney directly from the aorta, and the renal veins drain blood from the kidneys to the inferior vena cava.[1] DOT 5-7.1

The glomerulus is the filtering unit of the kidney. Each kidney contains over one million glomeruli, which filter over 400 liters of blood daily to produce about two liters of urine per day in the average adult.[2,3] Each glomerulus is paired with a small, fluid-collecting tubule, forming a unit called a nephron

(Figure 36-2). The tubule collects wastes and water filtered from the blood.

Urine is collected first into the tubules, which then join larger tubes called calyces, which in turn join together to form the renal pelvis. The pelvis narrows to form a small diameter tube called the ureter, which connects the kidney to the bladder. The ureter drains urine by peristaltic contractions of its muscular walls toward the urinary bladder, which lies in the low anterior pelvis just behind the pubic symphysis. The bladder drains through the urethra, which passes directly to the outside of the body at the urinary meatus (Figure 36-3). In the male, the urethra passes through the prostate gland, which lies at the base of the bladder, and then through the penis. The testicles, each paired with an epididymus, are suspended by their vascular, ductal, and lymphatic structures in the scrotum, which hangs inferior to the base of the penis.

In females, the difference in the urinary system anatomy is that the urethra is significantly shorter. Physiologically, all structures function in a similar manner except that the mechanism for maintaining urine inside the bladder, called continence, is different between women and men. There is no internal sphincter in women to control continence. Instead, continence is maintained by the urethral mucosa and the external striated sphincter surrounding the distal two-thirds of the urethra.[4]

CONNECTIONS The organs of the female reproductive system are discussed in detail in Chapter 41: Obstetrics and Gynecology.

Pain

Pain in the abdomen and pelvis can be visceral or somatic. **Visceral pain** originates in the organs of the abdomen and pelvis. Visceral pain receptors (nociceptors) in the organs produce a vague, aching, difficult-to-localize pain as opposed to the **somatic pain** receptors of the skin, bones, tendons, or blood vessels, which produce a sharp, well-defined pain. For this reason, patients with infections or other disorders of the intra-abdominal urinary tract may experience a slowly developing, vague, nonlocalized pain that does not become localized until the infection reaches somatic receptors of the peritoneum, at which time the pain becomes sharper and more localized.

Referred pain may be present, causing discomfort that is perceived by the patient to be in an area completely unrelated to the injury or disease. Visceral pain may be referred to an area served by somatic receptors. Arm, neck, or jaw pain occurring with myocardial ischemia is an example of referred pain as is testicular or inguinal pain associated with ureteral stones, upper abdominal pain

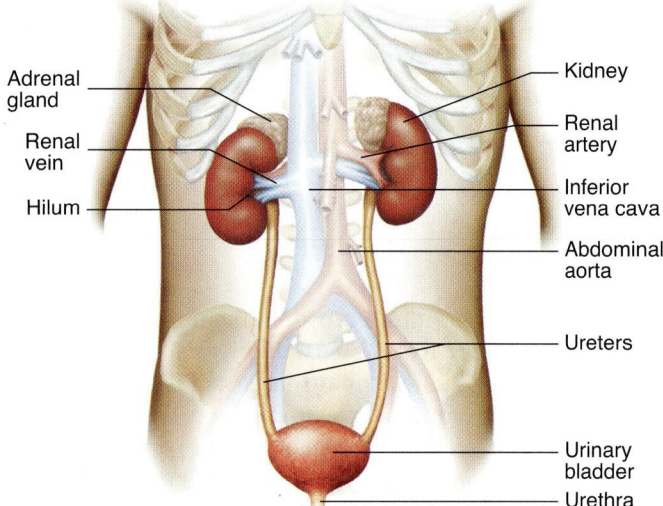

Figure 36-1   Anatomy of the urinary system.

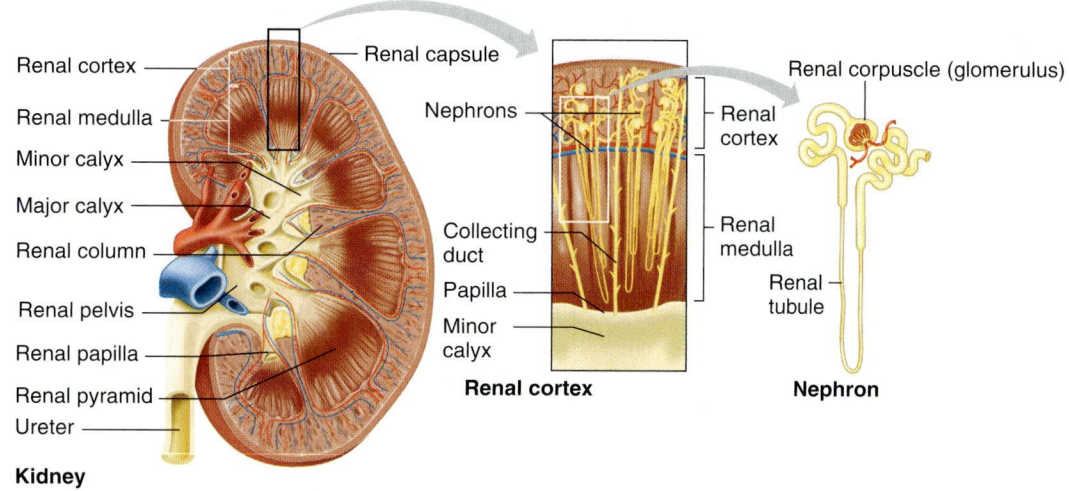

Figure 36-2   Anatomy of the kidney.

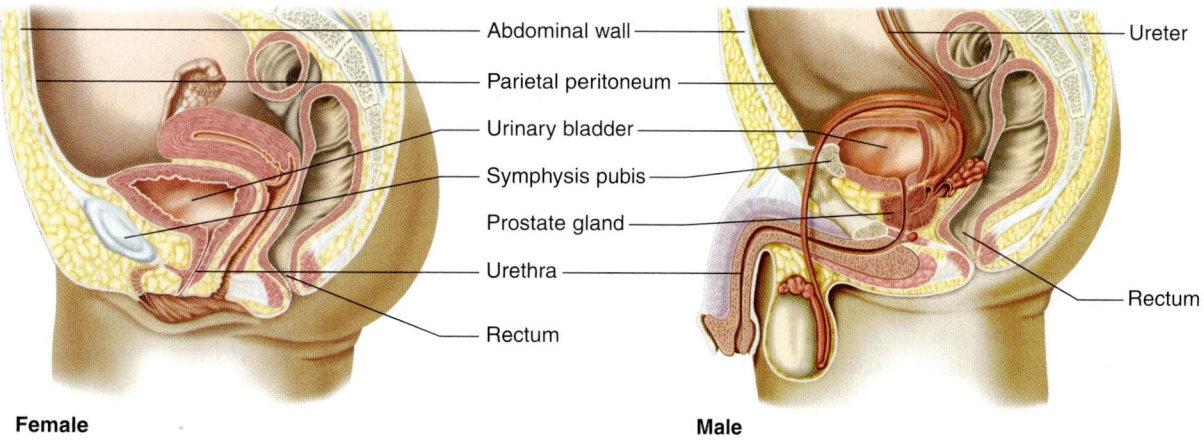

Figure 36-3   Female and male genitalia.

associated with certain pneumonias, or shoulder pain caused by biliary colic. These factors make the immediate and accurate diagnosis of intra-abdominal pathology very difficult in the prehospital setting based on examination and history alone. DOT 5-7.3, 5-7.29

CONNECTIONS   Chapter 34: Gastroenterology has more details about assessing abdominal pain.

Acute and Chronic Renal Failure

Acute renal failure (ARF) is the deterioration of renal function over a period of hours or days that results in the accumulation of metabolic waste products,

primarily nitrogenous compounds, in the blood.[5] The etiologies of acute renal failure can be classified into prerenal, intrinsic renal, and postrenal causes. **Chronic renal failure (CRF)** is a gradual and slowly progressive loss of renal function that may be mild or severe. CRF can lead to **end-stage renal disease (ESRD),** which is the irreversible loss of renal function. Without intervention in the form of dialysis therapy or renal transplantation, ESRD is a universally terminal condition. DOT 5-7.6

Prerenal Failure

Prerenal failure is the most common cause of ARF, accounting for 40–80% of all cases.[5] As its name suggests, prerenal describes any condition that decreases

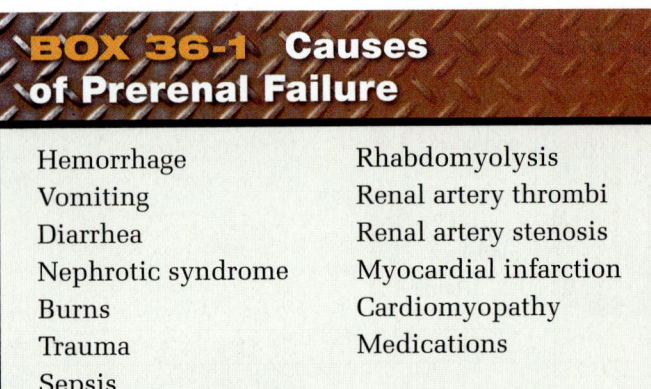

BOX 36-1   Causes of Prerenal Failure

Hemorrhage	Rhabdomyolysis
Vomiting	Renal artery thrombi
Diarrhea	Renal artery stenosis
Nephrotic syndrome	Myocardial infarction
Burns	Cardiomyopathy
Trauma	Medications
Sepsis	

perfusion before blood reaches the kidneys. This is mostly due to poor systemic perfusion (such as shock) or narrowing and blockage of vessels. The list of possible causes (differential diagnosis) of prerenal failure is long and complicated; the most frequent are listed in Box 36-1. Decreased renal perfusion can be caused by external or internal causes. For example, perfusion to the kidneys can be compromised if there is a lack of fluid volume. This can be the result of many problems, including hemorrhage, vomiting, or diarrhea. Fluid can also be lost if it is pooling in confined spaces (called **third spacing**) where it is not available for circulation. Burns, trauma, rhabdomyolysis, or sepsis are some of the conditions that can cause third spacing. DOT 5-7.7

High levels of protein in the urine **(proteinuria),** low levels of protein in the blood, and swelling can also result in third spacing of fluid and decreased perfusion of the kidneys. The combination of these symptoms is called the **nephrotic syndrome.** Clots in the renal arteries (thrombi) or diseases of the renal arteries such as atherosclerosis, resulting in narrowing (stenosis), can block blood flow to the kidneys. Over time, this is one of the causes of high blood pressure (hypertension) in patients with renal failure. When the cardiovascular system adjusts to ensure blood flow to the kidney, it must force the heart to beat stronger and the rest of the blood vessels to constrict, to force blood through the narrow opening into the kidney.

Any disease state that causes decreased cardiac output, such as myocardial infarction or cardiomyopathy, as well as certain medications, can result in low flow states and prerenal failure.

Intrinsic Renal Failure

Diseases of the kidneys themselves, involving the vasculature or glomeruli, may lead to intrinsic renal failure. There are many renal tubular diseases. They may be caused by acute tubular necrosis due to shock, sepsis, toxins, rhabdomyolysis, severe hemolysis or the intravascular destruction of red blood cells, which also results in clogged tubules. Certain antibiotics and radiographic contrast agents may also damage the tubules. DOT 5-7.7

Glomeruli may be damaged by several different mechanisms: diabetes mellitus, bacterial infections such as endocarditis or strep throat, systemic diseases like Goodpasture's syndrome, systemic lupus erythematosis, vasculitis or Wegener's granulomatosis, and primary kidney diseases including glomerulonephritis (Box 36-2). The signs and symptoms of glomerular disease include proteinuria (the presence of protein in the urine), hypoproteinemia (a decrease in blood protein levels due to excess excretion), hematuria (the presence of blood in the urine), edema (fluid which is third spaced into the extra-vascular spaces), and a reduced glomerular filtration rate.[2] DOT 5-7.7

Diseases and disorders of the renal blood vessels can also result in intrinsic renal failure. Occlusions of very small renal arteries or veins can cause renal cell death. Long-standing hypertension, malignant hypertension, or scleroderma, a disorder characterized by the deposition of hard, fibrous connective tissue in skin, joints, and blood vessels, may damage small vessels. Hemolytic uremic syndrome, thrombotic thrombocytopenic purpura, and polyarteritis nodosa are other causes of renal vascular damage that can lead to intrinsic renal failure.

Nice to Know

What Is Rhabdomyolysis?

When a muscle is injured, it can break down and release myoglobin into the bloodstream. Myoglobin has a devastating effect on the kidney and may cause renal failure. The disintegration of the muscle is called **rhabdomyolysis.**

Postrenal Failure

Postrenal failure is often called obstructive renal failure and is caused by obstruction of the urinary tract at any level (Box 36-3). The rapid recognition of an obstructive condition is very important, as this type of renal failure can be reversed by correcting the cause of obstruction. Renal function returns to normal if the obstruction is reversed before permanent damage is caused.

BOX 36-2 Causes of Intrinsic Renal Failure

Endocarditis
Streptococcal infections
HIV
Diabetes mellitus
Goodpasture's syndrome
Systemic lupus erythematosis
Vasculitis
Wegener's granulomatosis
Membranous nephropathy
Membranoproliferative glomerulonephritis
Renal artery or vein occlusion
Long-standing hypertension
Malignant hypertension
Scleroderma
Hemolytic uremic syndrome
Thrombotic thrombocytopenic purpura
Polyarteritis nodosa

The urinary tract may be obstructed at the level of the kidney or ureter by kidney stones, retroperitoneal tumors, blood clots, aortic aneurysms, or retroperitoneal

BOX 36-3 Causes of Postrenal Failure

Kidney stones (Calculi)
Retroperitoneal tumors
Blood clots
Aortic aneurysms
Retroperitoneal fibrosis
Medications
Bladder cancer
Bladder polyps
Neurogenic bladder
Benign prostatic hypertrophy
Prostate cancer
Phimosis
Trauma
Urethral strictures

fibrosis. Medications such as acyclovir or methotrexate can deposit in the kidney or ureter, causing obstruction.

Obstruction in the bladder can be caused by large kidney stones, blood clots, bladder cancers or polyps, neurogenic bladder due to diabetes or spinal cord injuries, medications, and, most commonly, by benign prostatic hypertrophy.

Outflow from the urethra can be obstructed by prostatic cancer, phimosis (constricted foreskin), calculi, trauma, and urethral strictures.

The most common problems arising in acute renal failure are electrolyte imbalances, acid/base imbalances, and fluid volume. When the kidneys are not able to excrete enough fluid, potassium may accumulate in the body. Too much potassium (hyperkalemia) is one of the most commonly encountered and most serious electrolyte complication. Metabolic acidosis can also occur.

CONNECTIONS Metabolic acidosis is covered in more depth in Chapter 31: Endocrinology, Electrolytes and Acid/Base.

The most common fluid-related complications are due to fluid overload, resulting in pulmonary edema, hypertension, and congestive heart failure. DOT 5-7.8

In the prehospital setting, the patient should be assessed for edema, jugular venous distension, and the presence of rales on lung auscultation. All patients with suspected complications of acute renal failure should receive oxygen therapy, intravenous access, cardiac monitoring, and blood glucose monitoring. Vitals signs must be monitored at regular intervals. DOT 5-7.9

Street Secrets

Renal failure affects the metabolism and action of many medications in unpredictable ways. On-line medical control is a very valuable resource that should be consulted at any time you feel unsure of treatment.

Hyperkalemia

Hyperkalemia is the most common metabolic cause of death in ARF patients.[3] The accumulation of potassium in the body with the resulting elevated serum potassium levels can result in skeletal muscle weakness and cardiac arrest. The ECG in hyperkalemia changes as the serum concentration rises and initially may show peaking of the T wave as well as shortening of the QT interval and ST depression. As the serum level rises, these changes may be followed by bundle branch block, flattening of the P wave, and increases in the PR interval (Figure 36-4).

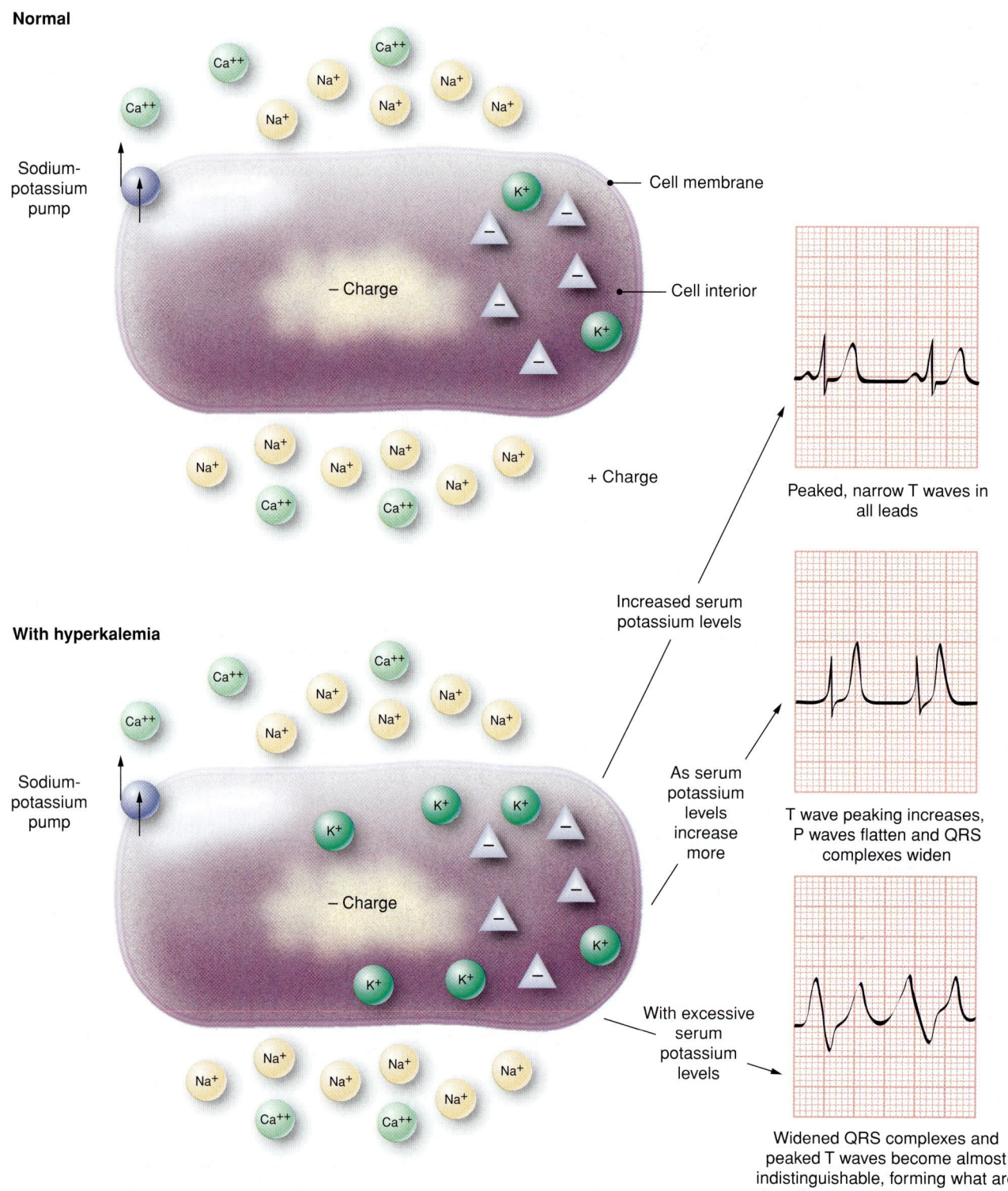

Normal

Sodium-potassium pump

Ca++ Ca++ Na+ Na+ Ca++ Na+ Na+ Na+

Cell membrane

K+ −

− Charge

Cell interior

− − K+

+ Charge

Na+ Na+ Na+ Na+ Na+ Ca++ Ca++ Na+

Peaked, narrow T waves in all leads

Increased serum potassium levels

With hyperkalemia

Sodium-potassium pump

Ca++ Ca++ Na+ Na+ Ca++ Na+ Na+ Na+

K+ K+ −

− Charge

− K+

K+ K+ −

As serum potassium levels increase more

T wave peaking increases, P waves flatten and QRS complexes widen

Na+ Na+ Na+ Na+ Na+ Ca++ Ca++ Na+

With excessive serum potassium levels

Widened QRS complexes and peaked T waves become almost indistinguishable, forming what are described as a "sine-wave pattern"

Figure 36-4 ECG changes seen in hyperkalemia.

CONNECTIONS To review a definition of the elements of the ECG, see Chapter 29: Cardiology, Section I.

Without treatment, the P wave disappears, and ventricular fibrillation and asystole can occur.[6] These ECG changes may correlate only roughly with the level of the serum potassium, and serious hyperkalemia may exist with no changes in the ECG.

The patient or the person giving the patient's medical history may not relate the presence of ARF or hyperkalemia, even if they are known. Your care should focus on ensuring adequate ABCs and treating respiratory

Street Secrets

In the prehospital setting, neither the patient nor you may be aware of the presence of acute renal failure. The patient may have suddenly developed ARF and its complications, and frequently, the conditions are undiagnosed when the ambulance is called.

distress (pulmonary edema) and hypotension. Patients who are unable to maintain an adequate oxygen saturation with supplemental oxygen are candidates for CPAP or BiPAP application, if available, or endotracheal intubation and positive pressure ventilation.

If hypotension or signs of cardiotoxicity such as QRS widening exist, 10% calcium carbonate or calcium gluconate may be given intravenously over two minutes. NOTE: Calcium should be avoided if digoxin toxicity is suspected, and it should not be used when the ECG shows only peaked T waves.[6]

EMS care for these patients is supportive. In the prehospital setting, bicarbonate and insulin given together with 50% dextrose may be appropriate. Bicarbonate is given with caution, however, as it could lead to fluid overload or seizures. Other metabolic disorders, such as hyperphosphatemia or metabolic acidosis, are generally not diagnosable in the prehospital setting; thus, specific treatments, other than supportive measures, are not possible.

Fluid Volume Emergencies

Fluid volume emergencies are common in acute renal failure. Nonoliguric patients, those who are still able to excrete some salt and water, may present with hypotension and signs and symptoms of hypovolemia. Patients with vomiting and diarrhea may also be hypovolemic. Physical examination of these patients may reveal poor skin turgor, dry mucous membranes, and hypotension. Treatment of these patients in the prehospital setting involves stabilizing life-threatening conditions. Reversal of hypovolemia by rapid fluid infusion often is sufficient to treat many forms of ARF. However, rapid fluid infusion can result in life-threatening fluid overload in patients with ARF, so it must be done with extreme care.[7] Bolus therapy using 200–500 mL boluses and rechecking vital signs can be used and repeated in an effort to prevent over-hydration. DOT 5-7.8

Hypervolemia

Hypervolemia may be present as a result of excessive fluid intake or the excessive excretion of protein from the body. Normally the molecule concentration in our blood exerts a pressure (called **oncotic pressure**) that keeps fluid from leaking out in the tissues. Decreased protein levels in the blood may result in a decreased oncotic pressure; this in turn causes fluid to leak and

accumulate in the lungs and periphery. Patients may present in pulmonary edema with symptoms of shortness of breath and dyspnea. The physical examination may show rales or rhonchi on lung auscultation, jugular venous distention, and peripheral edema. The usual approach to patients with such signs and symptoms in the absence of renal disease would normally involve diuretics (such as furosemide), nitroglycerin, and perhaps morphine. However, in ARF patients, a different approach is needed as nitrate administration may cause a significant blood pressure drop, and the use of morphine has been associated with increased morbidity in patients with ARF. DOT 5-7.8

Street Secrets

A memory aid for the medications for treating most causes of pulmonary edema is "give them L-M-N-O to make them Pee."

L = lasix
M = morphine
N = nitro
O = oxygen

This memory aid does not imply the order these medications should be given, but it does help you remember them.

The prehospital treatment of hypervolemic patients is difficult in the absence of lab studies and hemodynamic monitoring. Diuretics and vasodilators have been used in the past to treat ARF, but large, randomized studies have failed to show efficacy of either modality. In a person with normal kidney function, diuretics such as furosemide (Lasix) prevent the reabsorption of sodium in the nephron, resulting in the excretion of sodium and accompanying water into the urine. However, in the presence of renal failure, this mechanism does not function properly. Studies have shown that diuretics are usually ineffective in the treatment of ARF complications, but they may have some use in the fluid-overloaded patient with chronic renal failure.[8]

Likewise, most studies have shown that dopamine, which has been used in low doses as a vasodilator in ARF, does not improve morbidity or mortality in these patients.[9] A recent meta-analysis of studies looking at the use of dopamine in the setting of renal failure showed that low-dose (the so-called renal dose) dopamine had no significant effect on clinical outcomes in patients with, or at risk of, renal failure.[10] Continuous positive airway pressure (CPAP) or biphasic positive airway pressure (BiPAP) devices may be used in patients with severe respiratory compromise who are alert and not vomiting. Unstable patient suffering from complications of acute renal failure should be rapidly transported to a hospital where laboratory testing and hemodynamic monitoring are available. DOT 5-7.9, 5-7.10

Urinary Outlet Obstruction

Urinary outlet obstruction is a frequent cause of ARF. These patients will usually complain that they have not been able to urinate, and on physical examination, the bladder is often palpable above the pubic symphysis. They may present with lower abdominal pain and the urge to void. They may be able to pass small amounts of urine, but they are not able to fully drain the bladder. Catheterization to drain the bladder may be performed in patients with signs and symptoms of bladder outlet obstruction due to blood clots, prostatic hypertrophy, tumors, or swelling due to urologic procedures. Catheterization is indicated in situations involving prolonged transport times but is not warranted in most settings where EMS transport times are short.

The mortality rates of patients with acute renal failure remain high, ranging from 50–70%, despite advances in diagnosis, treatment, and dialysis. Since ARF is most frequently seen in conjunction with other severe illnesses, the causes of death are varied. The most common causes of death in patients with ARF are sepsis, heart failure, and pulmonary failure. Because of this, patients suspected of ARF and its complications should be considered true medical emergencies and should be transported rapidly to a hospital. DOT 5-7.1

Street Secrets

Although only a handful of EMS systems perform urinary catheterization, most paramedics will encounter catheterized patients. Many patients transported from long-term care facilities such as nursing homes have a catheter. Remember to note the volume of fluid in the drainage bag along with the color and consistency. If possible, ask if the bag can be drained prior to assuming care of the patient. If the bag becomes full en route, it will need draining, which can result in an accidental spill in a moving ambulance or create a disposal dilemma. Record the volume of fluid removed from the bag in your patient care report. Maintain the position of the bag below the level of the patient's hips at all times. If held above the level of the bladder, urine can backflow from the catheter tube and reenter the bladder, resulting in infection and perhaps even sepsis.

Chronic Renal Failure and End-Stage Renal Disease

Chronic renal insufficiency (CRI) is a condition in which the glomerular filtration rate is moderately reduced on a chronic basis but not to a degree sufficient to cause clinical symptoms.[3] The kidneys have a limited ability to function, reducing waste products and regulating the body's fluid status. **Chronic renal failure (CRF)** is a disease characterized by the gradual, permanent, and irreversible loss of kidney function due to destruction of the nephrons. CRF may exist for 10 to 20 years or more before ultimately progressing to **end-stage renal disease (ESRD)** at which point, kidney function is less than 10% of baseline. ESRD is universally fatal unless treated with either dialysis or renal transplantation. In the United States, nearly 300,000 people are on long-term dialysis, and more than 20,000 have a functioning transplanted kidney.[11] DOT 5-7.11, 5-7.12

The causes of chronic renal failure and ESRD are similar to those of acute renal failure and can be similarly classified as prerenal, intrinsic, and postrenal. The most common cause of ESRD in the United States is diabetes. Glomerular disease accounts for about 30–50% of all cases of ESRD, diabetic nephropathy being the single greatest cause.[3] Hypertension is another significant cause of ESRD in the United State, especially in the African-American population. HIV and ureteral reflux are common causes of ESRD in younger populations. DOT 5-7.13

Uremia

The clinical syndrome associated with ESRD is **uremia.** This term originally referred to the accumulation of urea in the blood due to loss of kidney function. Urea is a by-product of the breakdown of nitrogen containing molecules such as proteins and amino acids. It is a major component of urine and cannot be excreted in any other fashion. However, a multitude of other bodily functions are negatively impacted by the loss of renal function, and the entire constellation of signs and symptoms associated with chronic renal failure is termed uremia.[12]

Volume overload can occur due to the loss of ability to excrete ingested fluids into the urine. Electrolyte, acid/base, and hormone metabolism can be disrupted, leading to myriad signs and symptoms associated with uremia. In the cardiovascular system, anemia, hyperlipidemia, heart failure, hypertension, pericarditis, and pericardial tamponade can occur. Ventricular hypertrophy secondary to hypertension is seen. In the lung, pleural effusions, pleuritis, and pulmonary edema may develop. There are a host of neurologic abnormalities that result from uremia. The progression of neurologic signs and symptoms is the most common reason for starting kidney dialysis. Lethargy, difficulty concentrating, memory loss, seizures, and coma may occur. Fatigue, muscle cramps, and headache may be present. Patients can experience muscle twitching, hiccups, or restless legs syndrome. DOT 5-7.13

BOX 36-4 Clinical Abnormalities Present in Uremia

Fluid and Electrolyte Disturbances

Volume expansion or contraction
High or low levels of sodium and potassium
Metabolic acidosis

Endocrine and Metabolic Disturbances

High levels of uric acid
Hypothermia
High triglyceride levels
Impaired growth and development
Amenorrhea

Skin Disorders

Itching
Ecchymoses

Heart and Lung Disorders

Hypertension
CHF or pulmonary edema
Pericarditis
Pericardial tamponade
Cardiomyopathy
Hypotension
Dysrhythmias

Gastrointestinal Disturbances

Nausea and vomiting
Gastroenteritis
Peptic ulcer

Blood and Immune System Disorders

Anemia
Low white blood cell counts
Bleeding disorders
Splenomegaly

Neuromuscular Disorders

Fatigue
Sleep disorders
Headache
Impaired thinking
Lethargy
Peripheral neuropathy
Restless legs syndrome
Hiccups
Paralysis
Myoclonus
Seizures
Coma

Nearly every sign and symptom of uremia will resolve with renal transplantation. Many of these clinical abnormalities will improve with dialysis, though not all. A more complete listing of the signs and symptoms of uremia is in Box 36-4.[12]

Treatment of CRF Complications

Whereas patients with acute renal failure are prone to rapidly developing complications as a result of the acute nature of their disease, patients with CRF have a slowly progressive disease with relatively stable signs and symptoms. Acute problems in CRF patients are often caused by the sudden onset of acute concurrent illness or trauma.[3] Unlike ARF patients, the long-term history of CRF patients makes it unlikely that the paramedic will be able to intervene to treat the actual cause of the renal failure.

Many of the same complications associated with ARF are also found in CRF and ESRD. These patients may access the EMS system complaining of signs and symptoms of hyperkalemia and resulting ECG changes;

hypovolemia with hypotension and poor skin turgor; or hypervolemia, manifested by pulmonary edema or congestive heart failure. Neurologic complications tend to develop slowly and are not usually life-threatening. These patients have a compromised immune system and often present with infections. Hypothermia can also occur due to the accumulation of nitrogenous waste products.

As with ARF, patients with suspected complications of chronic renal failure should receive oxygen therapy, intravenous access, cardiac monitoring, and blood glucose monitoring in the prehospital setting. Vital signs should be monitored at regular intervals. These patients should be assessed for edema, jugular venous distension, and the presence of rales on lung auscultation. On-line medical control should be consulted at any time during patient encounters if the paramedic is unsure of treatment or management. DOT 5-7.14

Hyperkalemia should be considered in every CRF or ESRD patient encountered by the paramedic. Just as in hyperkalemia due to ARF, decompensation of the ECG due to elevated serum levels of potassium should be treated with calcium. Administration of inhaled albuterol by either metered dose inhaler or nebulizer promotes the movement of potassium across the cell membranes, thus temporarily reducing the serum levels in CRF patients, and may be used in patients with ECG evidence of hyperkalemia.[13]

Street Secrets

The administration of succinylcholine, sometimes used in rapid sequence intubation procedures, can produce life-threatening hyperkalemia and should be avoided in these patients in the prehospital setting. Succinylcholine allows potassium to leak out of cells into the extracellular space and into the serum, thus further raising the potassium level and increasing the potential risk of cardiac dysrhythmias or cardiac arrest.

Hypovolemia can occur due to vomiting, diarrhea, or inadequate intake of fluids. Hypotension, poor skin turgor, and dry mucous membranes may be noted on physical examination. Careful administration of intravenous normal saline can rapidly alleviate hypotension, but the patient must be carefully monitored for signs of fluid overload.

Hypervolemia with resulting pulmonary edema is one of the most common complications seen in CRF patients and is usually due to fluid overload. Patient should be questioned about recent weight gains and changes in fluid intake or output. Biphasic positive airway pressure (BiPAP) or continuous positive airway pressure (CPAP) may be applied to conscious, alert pulmonary edema patients who are not vomiting. Patients in profound respiratory distress will require endotracheal intubation and positive pressure ventilation. Sublingual nitroglycerin may be used with caution while monitoring patients carefully for hypotension. Unlike the ARF patient, diuretics such as furosemide can be used cautiously in patients with pulmonary edema associated with CRF. Furosemide, though ineffective as a diuretic in patients with only a few functioning nephrons, has potent vasodilatory effects in the lung. No matter what the treatment, the volume of fluid given, including IV medications, must be carefully monitored. Large doses of furosemide itself can lead to further fluid overload. DOT 5-7.13, 5-7.14

Other comorbid conditions should be treated appropriately, according to protocol. It should always be remembered that CRF patients are very susceptible to infections. Appropriate infection control precautions should be utilized. Patients suffering from acute complications of CRF should be rapidly transported to the hospital.

Treatment of End-Stage Renal Disease

Uremia caused by ESRD ultimately leads to death unless a patient receives a new functioning kidney via transplantation or receives dialysis. Uremic patients may eventually succumb to the illness that originally caused the renal dysfunction but may also die of infections, bleeding, or the other complications of ESRD already mentioned. They are also susceptible to iatrogenic causes of death due to mismanagement of fluid problems or their inability to excrete prescribed medications. Even over-the-counter medications such as supplements or antacids can lead to death.

In 2002, 91,049 patients began treatment for ESRD therapy with hemodialysis; 6,648 began peritoneal dialysis while 2,046 patients received a renal transplant.[14] Each modality is associated with complications that may be encountered in the prehospital setting. It is important to be familiar with the different modes of dialysis in order to be able to appropriately handle the problems that may arise in these patients. The paramedic must also be familiar with the complications of renal transplantation.

Renal Transplantation

The main causes of morbidity after renal transplant are hypertension (75–85% of patients), hyperlipidemia (60%), cardiovascular disease (15–23%), and diabetes (17–20%).[15] The main cause of mortality in the first year after a kidney transplant is infection.[15] Transplant patients may also experience acute renal failure, chronic renal failure, or end-stage renal disease for many of the same reasons as other nontransplant patients. They also have a significantly higher rate of cardiovascular disease than age-matched controls.[15] DOT 5-7.1

When the paramedic is summoned to care for an ill renal transplant patient, a thorough history of the transplant should be obtained:

- The patient should be asked whether the kidney was taken from a living donor or a cadaver.
- The date of the surgery and current medications, including immunosuppressants, should be noted as should any history of rejection or multiple previous transplants.
- A prior history of infection or recent exposures to infection should be determined.

A focused review of systems is crucial as is determining the presence of current or recent fever. A physical examination should be done, looking for the presence or absence of fever, signs of hypervolemia, and wound redness or drainage, if the transplant surgery was recent. Appropriate precautions to prevent the spread of infection to the immunocompromised transplant patient should be instituted. Treatment of complications such as pulmonary edema or hyperkalemia should be instituted as previously described in this chapter. Unstable patients should be rapidly transported to the ED, and on-line medical control should be utilized, as needed.

Dialysis

The urinary system is responsible for maintaining the body's homeostasis. When the kidneys fail, this mechanism fails, and if untreated, patients will become sicker and sicker until they die of septic shock, pulmonary edema, cardiac dysrhythmia, or a combination of these problems. **Dialysis** is the process of filtering blood to maintain homeostasis. It reestablishes the proper electrolyte balance and rids the body of wastes normally filtered out by the kidneys. There are two types of dialysis: hemodialysis and peritoneal dialysis.

Hemodialysis

In **hemodialysis,** an external filter replaces the diseased or absent kidney nephrons. The technology of removing toxins associated with uremia from the blood was developed in the 1940s, but human dialysis was not made practical until the development of the arteriovenous (AV) shunt in the 1960s. The pore size of the dialysis filter determines which solutes can pass through the filter and are removed from the blood. The pressure of the dialysis system determines how much fluid is removed from the body. Other factors, such as the duration of the dialysis run, also determine the amount of fluid and electrolytes removed from the blood. DOT 5-7.16

Before hemodialysis can begin, access to the vascular system must be obtained by creating a surgical fistula in which an artery and a vein are directly connected to each other in the patient's arm (Figure 36-5). In some cases, a synthetic graft is placed between the artery and vein (Figure 36-6). Both types of AV connections are called shunts. During the shunt healing process, a large-bore, double-lumen, central venous catheter is often placed in the subclavian vein and is used to access the vascular system for hemodialysis until the shunt is ready for use. Prior to the actual dialysis run, small doses of heparin are administered to prevent clotting of the patient's blood in the dialysis lines. Blood is drawn from the AV shunt or the dialysis catheter and circulated through the dialysis machine at a rate of 300 to 500 mL per minute. A dialysate fluid runs at a similar rate through the other side of the dialysis filter, and wastes from the patient diffuse across the filter from the blood into the dialysate due to differing osmotic gradients. The filtered blood is returned to the body through the shunt, minus urea, excess fluid, certain dialyzable drugs, and other waste products. Different filters may be utilized to withdraw larger amounts of fluid or specific medications or toxins, if needed, such as in the case of an overdose.

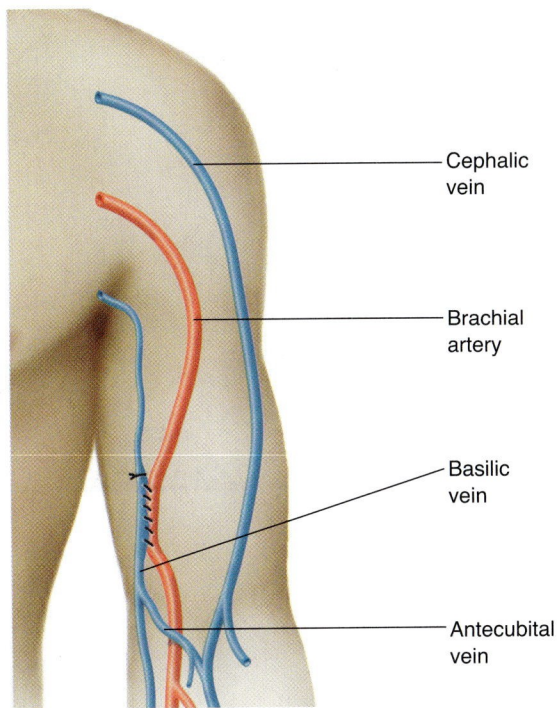

Figure 36-5   Arteriovenous dialysis shunt.

Cephalic vein

Brachial artery

Basilic vein

Antecubital vein

Patients are usually dialyzed three times a week, and the process can take up to eight hours. Approximately 65% of ESRD patients receive hemodialysis.[14]

Peritoneal Dialysis

The concept of peritoneal dialysis was actually developed in the 1920s, 20 years before hemodialysis, but **continuous ambulatory peritoneal dialysis (CAPD)** did not become practical until 1976.[5] In peritoneal dialysis, a silicone rubber catheter is inserted into the peritoneal cavity through a hole made in the abdominal wall. Dialysate fluid is circulated through the catheter into the cavity. Wastes and fluids diffuse across the peritoneum, which acts as the dialysis filter, into the dialysate, which is then drained from the abdomen by gravity after a prescribed time interval. The process can be done continuously during the day as a patient goes about his usual activities, or it can be done at night while the patient sleeps. The amount of waste and fluid filtered from the blood is determined by the glucose concentration of the dialysate. The osmotic pressure gradient between the blood and the dialysate determines how much fluid and waste is removed. A typical regimen involves the instillation of a total of eight liters of dialysate and removal of approximately ten liters of fluid per day in four cycles. Because this process occurs on an ambulatory basis during the day or during sleep at night, time-consuming trips to the dialysis unit are avoided. Due to

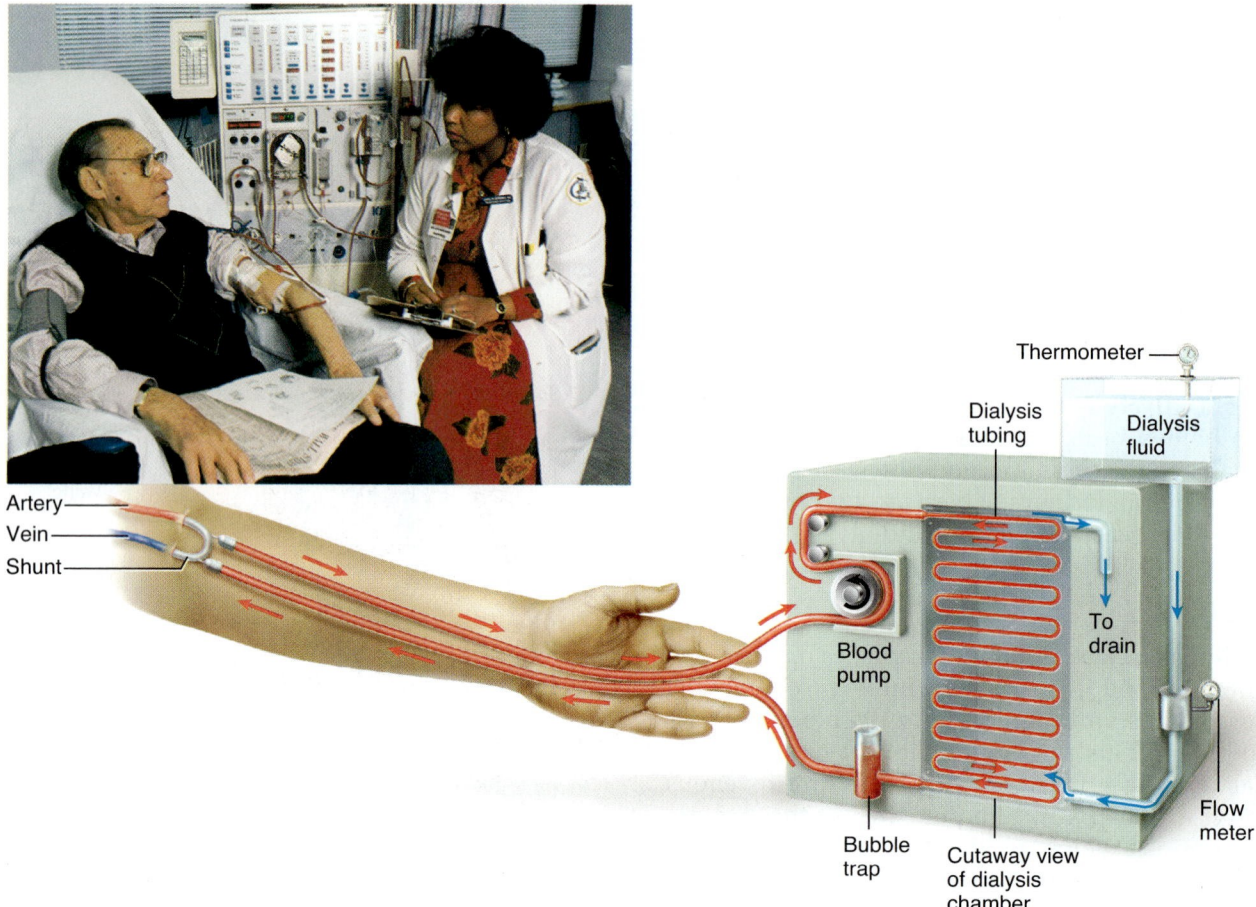

Figure 36-6   Arteriovenous dialysis graft.

Nice to Know

Because of their medical background, paramedics sometimes work for companies that perform at-home peritoneal dialysis. If you are interested in this area, you may find another opportunity to utilize your skills. You will need some additional training to perform this skill.

the lower cost and relative ease of peritoneal dialysis, it is the most common type of dialysis used in the world outside of the United States and Canada.[5]

Complications of Dialysis

Both hemodialysis and, to a lesser degree, peritoneal dialysis are associated with numerous complications, including those that occur from the underlying diseases that caused renal failure in the first place. The general, prehospital approach to patients who are receiving dialysis is similar to those with CRF or ESRD and includes the application of oxygen and the cardiac

monitor as well as obtaining vital signs and a blood glucose determination. A complete history should be obtained, and the date of the last dialysis treatment should be noted. The patient should be questioned about a history of prior problems caused by dialysis.

In cases of life-threatening illness or injury, the patient's AV shunt may be used for intravenous access. Ensure you communicate with medical direction prior to performing the procedure. However, in all other situations, an alternative IV site is preferred.

In general, IV fluids should not be administered unless severe hypotension is present. Most medications used in the prehospital setting can be used at the usual dose in dialysis patients.[16] Rapid transport to the hospital should be considered in any patient with unstable vital signs, and on-line medical control should be consulted, as needed. DOT 5-7.17

Infections of the dialysis vascular access shunt or the peritoneal catheter site are common. Local infection of a peritoneal catheter site can lead to peritonitis with symptoms of fever, abdominal pain, and a cloudy dialysate return. The incidence of peritonitis in peritoneal dialysis patients is one episode every

15 patient-months.[17] The peritoneal dialysis catheters may become kinked or occluded by fibrinous material. Hemodialysis shunt grafts tend to become infected more often than directly connected fistulae. Sepsis may develop, and septic emboli, frequently due to *Staph aureus*, can occur in the shunt. Often, the usual signs of localized infection like redness, swelling, induration, and tenderness are not present at the shunt site. Patients may present only with signs of systemic infection or sepsis, such as fever and hypotension.

Shunts may become occluded by thrombosis or stenosis. The usual bruit or thrill (vibration) under the shunt will be absent to palpation or auscultation when blood flow through the shunt ceases. The shunts may also bleed, either in the postoperative period after the surgical procedure to establish the access or after dialysis needle removal. As with other forms of hemorrhage from an extremity, treatment of such bleeding consists of the application of pressure to the bleeding site. In most cases, pressure alone is enough to control the hemorrhage. In rare cases, if bleeding persists or is life-threatening, it may be necessary to place a tourniquet proximally on the arm to stop the hemorrhage. This, however, will usually result in clotting of the shunt, necessitating placement of a new shunt. Tourniquets should never be placed above a dialysis shunt site without base station medical control contact. Though aneurysms of the vascular access site may occur due to repeated punctures by needles, they are rare, and they rarely cause serious hemorrhage. DOT 5-7.17

Complication During Dialysis

Occasionally, the EMS system may be activated for a patient experiencing hypotension during or immediately after a dialysis run. The cause is usually excessive removal of intravascular fluids without an adequate compensatory shift of intracellular fluid into the vascular space. Treatment consists of placing the hypotensive patient in the Trendelenburg position and carefully administering 100–200 mL boluses of normal saline until the blood pressure rises to acceptable levels. The paramedic must use extreme care to avoid inducing fluid overload.

Neurologic dysfunction during or immediately after dialysis is most frequently due to the **disequilibrium syndrome.** Affected patients may present with nausea, vomiting, and hypertension as well as seizures and loss of consciousness. The cause is thought to be cerebral edema due to osmolar differences between the newly filtered blood and brain tissue. If called for a dialysis patient with neurologic symptoms, the paramedic should also evaluate the patient for signs of hyperglycemia or hypoglycemia. Seizures should be treated in the usual manner and the airway protected in an obtunded or comatose patient.[18]

The assessment and prehospital management of patients with ARF, CRF, and ESRD can be difficult, especially if you are unable to obtain a good history from the patient or caregivers. You must approach renal failure and dialysis patients with a high index of suspicion, keeping in mind that very often, these patients will not exhibit the expected or usual signs and symptoms of many disease states. If the proper care of patients with renal disease is in doubt, or if signs and symptoms do not lead to a confident diagnosis or assessment, the paramedic should always provide supportive treatments, contact medical control, and transport unstable patients rapidly.

Urinary Tract Disorders

Urinary tract infection (UTI) is one of the most common infections in adults, resulting in over 6 million physician visits per year. Approximately 20% of all women will experience a UTI sometime in life.[19] In infancy, UTI is seen more often in males, but after infancy, it becomes more common in females. After age 50, the incidence of UTI goes up in males due to prostatic obstruction caused by benign prostatic hypertrophy or cancer.[20]

Urine is normally sterile, but bacterial infection of the organs of the urinary tract may develop due to the migration of fecal bacteria up the urethra into the bladder and urine. This occurs more often in females than in males due to the short urethra. Abnormalities in the urinary tract anatomy, such as obstruction or duplicate ureters or when the sphincter between the end of the ureter and the bladder does not close adequately can cause reflux of urine into the ureter and subsequent infection. Incomplete bladder emptying due to neurologic disorders, injuries, or diabetes can lead to the development of UTI. Bacteria can also travel from distant locations via the lymphatics or blood vessels, seeding the organs of the urinary tract. Obstruction of urine outflow, often seen in prostatic enlargement, can cause urine stasis and incomplete emptying, which in turn may lead to infection. *E. coli* is the most common bacterial pathogen in UTI.[19] DOT 5-7.23, 5-7.24

Symptoms of UTI depend on the genitourinary organ infected. Lower UTI, also known as bladder infection or **cystitis,** is often associated with burning on urination, frequency, urgency, and lower abdominal pain in the suprapubic area. Patients may also experience low back pain, nausea, and malaise. Referred pain to the flank may be present. Physical examination often reveals suprapubic tenderness and occasionally low back tenderness. Kidney infection (**pyelonephritis**) is associated with flank pain, fatigue, chills, malaise, nausea, fever, and in some cases, concurrent symptoms of bladder infection. Vomiting and diarrhea may be seen. Percussion or tapping over the flank or costovertebral angle may cause pain as can deep palpation of the

Nice to Know

Urinary Tract Fistulas

The urinary tract can be damaged in such a manner that a hole develops in the soft tissues between the ureter and vagina. When this occurs, urine leaks into the vagina. Urinary tract fistulas to the vagina are of three kinds: vesicovaginal (most common), uretero-vaginal, and urethrovaginal. They occur most often as a result of accidental injury to the urinary tract at the time of pelvic surgery or because of ischemic necrosis resulting from an impaired blood supply. The urethrovaginal fistula can occur either following radiation therapy for carcinoma of the reproductive organs (especially the cervix) or following prolonged impaction of the fetal head during labor. Fistulas may also occur as a result of tumor invasion of the vesicovaginal septum. In developing countries, urethrovaginal fistulas commonly occur in women who become pregnant when they are very young and their still-developing bodies are damaged during pregnancy. In some societies, these women become outcasts and end up living away from their families.

Constant urinary leakage is the cardinal symptom. Urine can usually be seen coming through an opening in the vagina. A strong urine odor becomes apparent, making the patient socially isolated. The presence of urine on the skin and soft tissues of the vagina can result in irritation and infections as well. Urinary tract fistulas rarely close spontaneously. Fistulas caused by urinary tract injury can be corrected surgically.[21]

kidney. Some patients, particularly the elderly, may show signs and symptoms of septic shock, with hypotension, tachycardia, fever, skin mottling, and low oxygen saturations. Urinary tract infections are among the most common causes of sepsis in the elderly or immunocompromised patients. DOT 5-7.25

The differential diagnosis of lower UTI includes urethritis, vaginitis, or pain due to irritants. Endometriosis, ovarian cysts, ovarian torsion, or pelvic inflammatory disease can mimic the symptoms of lower UTI.[22] Differential considerations in pyelonephritis include kidney stones, muscular back pain, gallbladder disease, or influenza syndromes.

Most patients with UTI present to a physician's office or emergency department on an ambulatory basis. Immunocompromised patients or those with signs and symptoms of sepsis due to UTI may access the EMS system for transport to the ED. Where appropriate,

intravenous or intramuscular analgesics such as fentanyl or morphine may be given for severe pain. Oxygen should be considered in patients with decreased mental status, hypotension, or other systemic symptoms. Patients showing signs of shock such as tachycardia or hypotension may require IV fluid administration.[19] Rapid transport should be accomplished in unstable patients. DOT 5-7.26, 7.27

Other GI Complications

Fournier's Gangrene

Fournier's gangrene is an uncommon polymicrobial necrotizing fasciitis of the perineal, perianal, or genital areas that can occur in males or females, although males are affected ten times more frequently (Figure 36-7). Signs and symptoms include edema, tenderness, induration, fever, blistering, purulent or foul-smelling drainage, cyanosis of the genitalia, and frank gangrene.[23] The infection spreads rapidly through tissues following the fascial planes, infiltrating deeply into the genital and pelvic areas. Fournier's gangrene is a life-threatening disorder with a mortality rate reported to be anywhere from 4–75% but typically running around 20%.[24] Prehospital care should include a careful examination and assessment for other coexisting conditions, oxygen administration, analgesics, and rapid transport to the hospital. Appropriate infection control measures must be taken. Other associated serious conditions like shock or respiratory failure should be treated aggressively.

Hernias

The protrusion of an organ or other bodily structure through the wall that normally contains it is called a **hernia.** Hernias can protrude through the abdominal wall due to congenital weakness or defects in the muscle. A pouch of peritoneum called a hernia sac may form

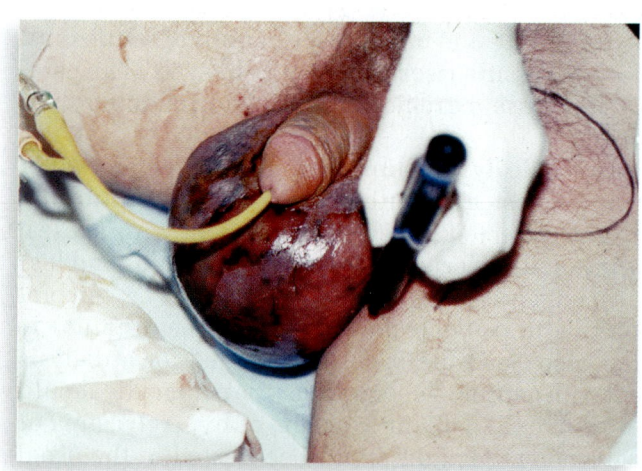

Figure 36-7   Fournier's gangrene.

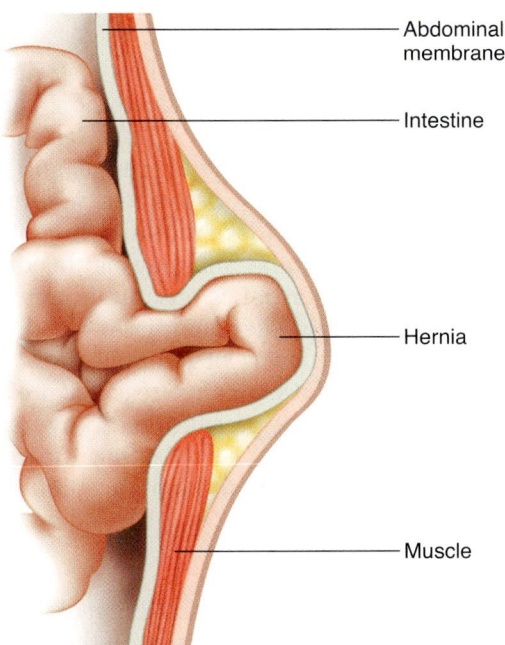

Figure 36-8   Abdominal hernia and sac.

Labels for Figure 36-8:
- Abdominal membrane
- Intestine
- Hernia
- Muscle

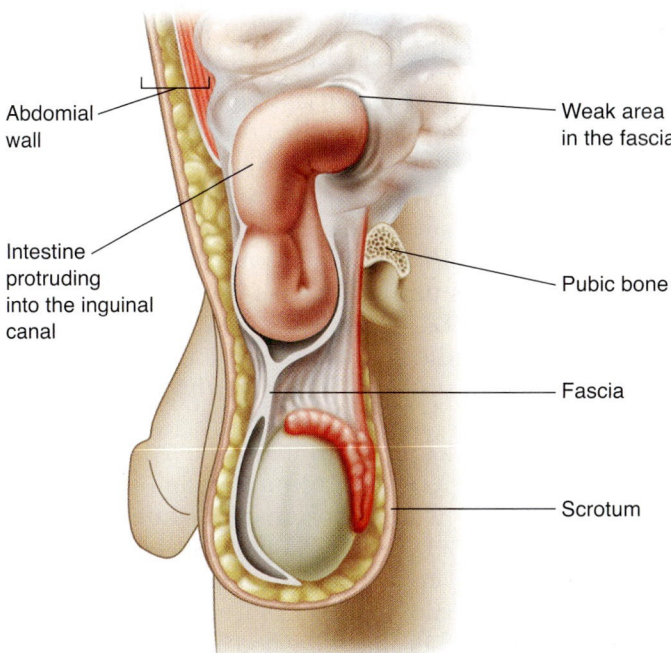

Figure 36-9   Inguinal hernia.

Labels for Figure 36-9:
- Abdomial wall
- Intestine protruding into the inguinal canal
- Weak area in the fascia
- Pubic bone
- Fascia
- Scrotum

outside of the body cavity. Areas of scarring or defects caused by surgery can lead to the protrusion of bowel through the abdomen wall (Figure 36-8). Structurally weak points in the abdominal wall occur naturally where blood vessels, nerves, and ducts enter or leave a body cavity and may be found in the lower abdomen, in the diaphragm where the esophagus passes from the chest to the abdominal cavity, or in the region around the navel. Obesity, pregnancy, chronic coughing, heavy lifting, and straining can cause intestine loops to push against the abdominal wall and eventually protrude through over time. Severe trauma can occasionally result in an acute hernia.

An **inguinal hernia** occurs in the inguinal or groin region (Figure 36-9). Because of increased intra-abdominal pressure, intestinal loops can push through a weak spot into the inguinal canal, which is a triangular opening between layers of abdominal muscle just superior to the attachment of the leg at the hip, through which vascular and ductal structures pass in and out of the abdomen. Untreated, any hernia may become incarcerated, meaning that a loop of intestine or piece of intra-abdominal fat becomes stuck and can no longer be reduced or pushed back to where it belongs in the abdominal cavity. The structures become trapped outside the abdomen. Swelling can ensue, resulting in the intestine becoming even more tightly trapped in the hernia sac. In some cases of severe swelling, the blood supply to the intestinal loop or fat mass may be cut off or strangulated, resulting in the death of the incarcerated mass if the hernia is not quickly reduced or surgically corrected.

In the prehospital setting, a patient may complain of a new or recurrent lump in the abdomen or inguinal region. The presence of pain in the area can indicate incarceration or strangulation, both of which are medical emergencies. If the hernia is not reduced, the intestinal loop, which has lost its blood supply, can die and become infected.

Street Secrets

Left untreated, the patient with a hernia can become septic and ultimately die. When assessing a patient complaining of a painful lump in the abdominal inguinal region, the paramedic should examine the area gently.

The entire abdomen should be palpated for diffuse tenderness, guarding, and rebound, which can indicate the presence of peritoneal irritation. Auscultation of the "lump" may reveal the presence of bowel sounds, indicating herniated intestine. Depending on the stage of incarceration, bowel sounds may be high-pitched and hyperactive, normal, or absent. Pain should be treated with intravenous or intramuscular narcotics.

The patient should be kept NPO, which means allowing nothing to be taken by mouth, and should be transported without delay to the hospital.

In the hospital, an attempt will be made to reduce the incarcerated structure manually. If this cannot be accomplished, the patient will be brought to the operating room where the incarceration may be relieved

Working in the Gray Zone

Nearly every study in the past five years has shown that administering appropriate doses of narcotic analgesics has no adverse effect on subsequent assessment of the pain in the Emergency Department (ED); however, many surgeons still maintain an attitude that patients with abdominal pain should not be given analgesics until they have been formally examined in the ED. Follow your local protocol, and consult your medical director to be sure you are following the wishes of the physician who is receiving the patient.

Recent studies of pain management strategies in the ED show a reluctance to provide pain relief in that setting as well. Unfortunately, acute pain accompanies 50–60% of all ED patient visits in the United States. The studies cite that resistance to treating acute pain in the ED is diminishing as physicians have become educated and comfortable with the benefits of treating pain in this patient population.

The route of administration of analgesics is less important than the need for adequate dosing and rapid onset. In selected patients, oral or intramuscular injection of analgesics is adequate, but most patients with severe pain are best served by titrated doses of intravenous analgesics, anxiolytics (antianxiety medication), and comfort measures.

Guidelines and standards for acute pain management have been published by the Agency for Health Care Policy and Research and the Joint Commission on Accreditation of Healthcare Organizations.[25,26] These documents are a useful guide for ED and hospital use, and they may serve as a helpful guide for the development of protocols for EMS.[27]

manually or surgically under general anesthesia. At the same time, the hernia of the abdominal wall will be closed. In some cases, a piece of mesh may be placed over the defect to provide additional strength to the repair or to close a defect too large to be closed by drawing the surrounding tissues together.

Disorders of the Male Genital Tract

There are many disorders that can affect the male genital tract, including infections, trauma, loss of blood supply, or tumor. Though ambulance calls for these problems are not common, the paramedic should be familiar with the various conditions that can develop as well as management techniques, where applicable.

Genital Lesions

Sores or lesions on the male genitalia may result from many causes. Among the most common causes are sexually transmitted diseases (STDs). Genital herpes, syphilis, chancroid, granuloma inguinale, and lymphogranuloma venereum are all associated with ulcers on the genitals.[28] Venereal warts or molluscum contagiosum can develop on the genitalia, and they may become ulcerated, causing genital sores. Lesions on the genitalia may be painless or painful. They may itch, bleed, or drain fluid or pus. Upon discovery of genital lesions, the paramedic should carefully cover any areas that are bleeding or oozing, taking proper precautions to avoid contact with, or dissemination of, the fluids. Specific treatments are generally not necessary in the prehospital setting.

Epididymitis and Orchitis

Epididymitis is inflammation or infection of the epididymis, a convoluted, worm-like structure that lies against the posterior surface of the testicle. If the infection extends into the adjacent testicle, the condition is called **epididymo-orchitis.** The testicle alone may be infected, a condition called **orchitis.** The most common cause of intrascrotal inflammation and infection is epididymitis.[29] In prepubertal males and after age 35, fecal coliform bacteria are the most commonly isolated pathogens. In the group from puberty to age 35, *Chlamydia trachomatis* is responsible for nearly 50–60% of cases while *Neisseria gonorrhoeae* is the second most common pathogen.[29]

Patients with epididymitis or orchitis may experience swelling and severe pain of the scrotal contents; urinary tract infection symptoms such as urinary frequency, urgency, or burning; urethral discharge; nausea; fever; and low abdominal or flank pain. The differential diagnosis includes urinary tract infection, hydrocele, and torsion of the testicle. Infection of the epididymis or testicle is not usually a medical emergency, but because it may not be possible to differentiate other emergent conditions such as torsion of the testicle from epididymitis in the prehospital setting, these patients should either be transported quickly to the hospital or encouraged to see a physician immediately in the case of a no-transport situation. Prehospital care consists of treating severe pain with analgesics, applying ice packs to the scrotum, and elevating the testicle and epididymis by placing a towel across the thighs and under the scrotum of the supine patient.

Prostatitis

The term **prostatitis** actually refers to four different entities involving the prostate.

1. **Acute bacterial prostatitis** is characterized by chills; fever; pain in the lower back, perineum, base of the

penis, or genital area; urinary frequency or urgency; dysuria; and white blood cells and bacteria in the urine. The treatment is antibiotic therapy and frequent ejaculations to help clear bacteria and cellular debris from the prostate and its ducts.

2. **Chronic bacterial prostatitis** occurs when an acute infection persists, whether treated or not, due to a defect in the prostate itself, which allows the continued existence of bacteria in the urinary tract.

3. **Chronic prostatitis** is a poorly understood syndrome of symptoms and signs of bacterial prostatitis, including at times the presence of white cells in the semen or urine but with no evidence of a bacterial causative agent. Symptoms may persist or may come and go, but antibiotic therapy is ineffective in treating this form of prostatitis.

4. **Asymptomatic inflammatory prostatitis** is defined as the presence of white blood cells in the semen in the absence of symptoms or a causative agent.[30] Other disorders, such as benign prostatic hypertrophy, lower UTI, prostate stones, ureteral stones, and prostate tumors, may present with similar symptoms. A patient may relate a past history of prostatitis to the paramedic, but in most cases in the prehospital setting, the diagnosis will likely not be known. Treatment is supportive and nonspecific and includes transport in a comfortable position and analgesics if the patient is extremely uncomfortable or if the transport time is very long.

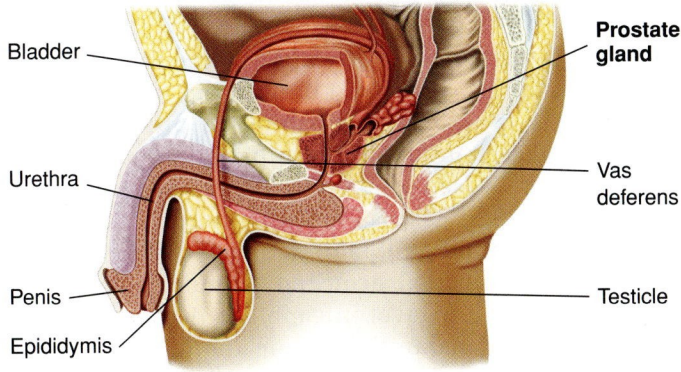

Figure 36-10 Anatomy of the prostate gland.

Prostatic Hypertrophy

The prostate gland, present only in the male, is a walnut-sized gland that produces the fluid that carries sperm during ejaculation. The prostate is composed of two lobes encased by a capsule. It lies at the base of the urinary bladder and completely surrounds the urethra as it leaves the bladder (Figure 36-10). As men age, the prostate gland enlarges for unknown reasons, causing a condition known as **benign prostatic hypertrophy.** This growth appears to require the presence of normally functioning testicles that produce testosterone. Men who have had their testicles removed in youth, such as those suffering from certain forms of testicular cancer, do not develop prostatic hypertrophy.[36]

While the prostate grows in physical size, the smooth muscle of the prostate that surrounds the urethra also contracts more. This combination of increased prostate mass and increased smooth muscle tone results in an overall decrease in the diameter of the lumen of the urethra. As the urethral diameter decreases, the flow rate of urine passing out of the bladder decreases. The symptoms of benign prostatic hypertrophy include difficulty starting urine flow, a weak or slow urine stream, persistent dribbling after

voiding, incomplete emptying of the bladder, increasing nocturia, and urinary retention. Urinary tract infections may develop due to stagnant urine accumulation in the bladder, and obstruction of the bladder outflow tract can result in acute renal failure if not relieved promptly. Bladder stones may form, and hematuria may be present.

Treatment of prostatic hypertrophy consists of giving medication to decrease smooth muscle tone at the bladder outlet and surgery to debulk the prostate gland where it surrounds the urethra. In the prehospital setting, there are no specific treatments for prostatic hypertrophy; however, it is important to recognize possible complications such as urine outflow obstruction and urinary tract infection. In these cases, prompt transport to the hospital is in order.

Urethritis

The tube that leads from the urinary bladder to the outside of the body is called the urethra. Urine drains from the bladder through the urethra in males and females, as do semen and sperm in males. **Urethritis** is inflammation of the urethra due either to trauma or infection. Traumatic causes of urethritis include frequent bladder catheterization and surgical instrumentation. Infections of the urethra occur primarily in adult males and are usually caused by sexually transmitted bacteria such as *Neisseria gonorrhoeae, Chlamydia trachomatis, Ureaplasma urealyticum, Mycoplasma hominis,* or *Trichomonas vaginalis.*[31] The signs and symptoms of urethritis primarily include dysuria and urethral discharge. Prehospital care includes the use of appropriate infection control methods. Long-term complications of urethritis include urethral stenosis or abscess formation.

Paraphimosis and Phimosis

The foreskin of the penis in young, prepubertal males is frequently too tight to retract or pull back over the head of the penis, the **glans**. This natural condition is sometimes called **congenital phimosis.** As males age, the foreskin usually loosens, and retraction over the glans becomes possible. Occasionally, the foreskin tightens, and it becomes impossible to pull back over the glans. This condition, called **acquired phimosis,** can result from a chronic low-level infection or inflammation of the glans called **balanitis** or from trauma such as repeated efforts by parents to retract the foreskin of a young male for cleaning.

Paraphimosis results when a tight foreskin is retracted over the glans penis and becomes entrapped. The glans usually swells, making it even more difficult to slide the foreskin back to its normal position over the glans. Paraphimosis usually occurs in elderly men although occasionally, it occurs after piercings or penile rings are inserted through the glans.[32] Phimosis is usually not considered an emergency condition while paraphimosis is definitely a urologic emergency. Failure to promptly reduce the paraphimosis can result in necrosis or gangrene of the glans.[33] There is no specific treatment in the prehospital setting, but it is important for the paramedic to transport the patient or to advise prompt evaluation and treatment, if necessary, when the problems are encountered.

Priapism

Priapism is a persistent erection of the penis. It is sometimes associated with systemic conditions such as sickle cell disease, leukemia, or tumors.[34] Other causes include blunt perineal injury; spinal cord injury; abuse of cocaine, ecstasy, or other drugs; and injections or popular oral medications used to treat erectile dysfunc-

tion. This persistent erection may be painless in some cases, but it usually becomes quite painful after time. A patient who complains of an erection lasting longer than four hours, especially in the presence of these predisposing conditions, should receive treatment. If evaluated and treated early in the course of the disorder, most cases respond to conservative measures.[35] In the prehospital setting, the paramedic may apply ice packs to the penis or perineum. Patients suspected of having a spinal cord injury should be appropriately immobilized. There is evidence to suggest that having a nontrauma patient walk up a flight or two of stairs may relieve the erection through an arterial steal phenomenon that pulls blood away from the engorged penis to supply the exerting muscles. Prompt transport to the hospital is recommended.

Testicular Torsion

Pain and swelling of the scrotal contents may be caused by torsion of the testicle in young to middle-aged men. Torsion is the twisting of the spermatic cord and testicle upon itself, initially resulting in venous occlusion and engorgement of the testicle and ultimately leading to obstruction of the artery supplying the testis and epididymis (Figure 36-11). Experimental evidence indicates that 720 degrees of torsion is required to compromise flow through the testicular artery and result in ischemia.[37] If the testicle is not quickly detorsed and untwisted, the lack of blood and oxygen can lead to ischemia and ultimately infarction of the testicle, with loss of its function. Salvage of the testicle is usually successful if the detorsion occurs within six hours of onset. After twelve hours, the salvage rate is nearly 0%.[37]

In addition to unilateral testicle swelling and pain, symptoms of torsion include fever, urinary frequency,

Normal Anatomy   Testicular Torsion

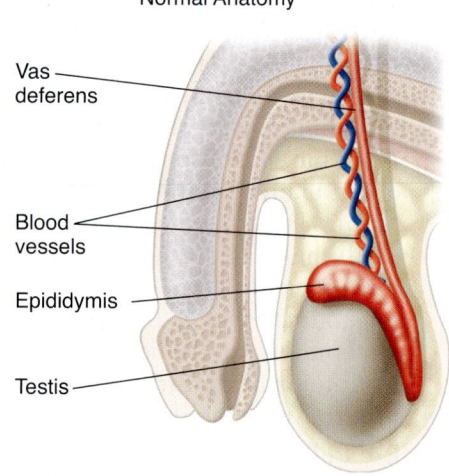
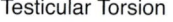
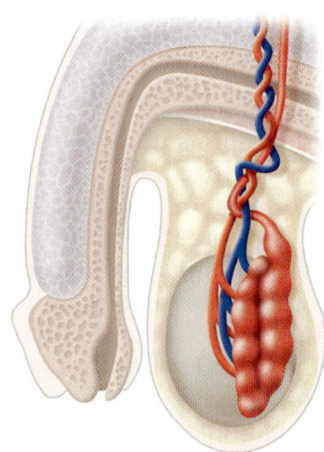

Vas deferens

Blood vessels

Epididymis

Testis

Figure 36-11 Testicular torsion.

nausea, and abdominal pain, much like epididymitis. The testicle may ride high in the scrotal sac compared to the contralateral testicle. The diagnosis in the emergency department is made by physical examination aided by color Doppler ultrasonography. Whereas epididymitis patients show normal or increased testicular blood flow, torsion patients show markedly decreased or absent flow on Doppler. As with epididymitis, prehospital care involves pain management, elevation of the scrotum, and prompt transport to the emergency department.

Testicular and Scrotal Masses

While the EMS system is not frequently activated for patients with isolated testicular or scrotal masses, knowledge of the causes of such masses is appropriate. While epididymitis, orchitis, and testicular torsion usually cause pain, other masses in the testicle or scrotum may be painful or painless. The pain may radiate up the scrotum into the spermatic cord and into the low abdomen, or it may be localized to a specific point on the testicle or scrotum. An inguinal hernia sac may extend down into the scrotum and may be tender to palpation. A small BB-like mass in the scrotum may be an appendix testis, which is a small, benign appendage attached to the testicle. Testicular cancer usually presents as a painless, solid lump of varying size on the testicle. A fluid-filled sac in the scrotum may be a spermatocele or a hydrocele. Both are benign cystic masses requiring no emergent treatment. A varicocele is a painless mass of dilated veins lying posterior to the testicle, frequently on the left side. Often described as feeling like a "bag of worms," varicoceles require no treatment unless they become very large or interfere with fertility.

Kidney Stones and Urinary Tract Calculi

Stones, or calculi, may form in the kidney, in the collecting system, or in the bladder. **Kidney stones** are extremely common, affecting one in ten people at some time during their life. In the year 2000 in the United States, patients made 2.7 million visits to healthcare providers and more than 600,000 patients went to emergency rooms for kidney stones.[38] Stones occur more often in men than women, and the prevalence is higher in industrialized countries. There also appears to be a genetic predisposition to form urinary tract stones. DOT 5-7.18

A kidney stone forms when crystals precipitate out from urine and build up on the inner surfaces of the kidney or its collecting system. The exact reason that some people form kidney stones and others do not is not completely understood. Certain factors make a person more likely to form kidney stones, including inadequate hydration (which causes concentration of the urine) and the lack of certain inhibitors in the urine, which normally prevent stone formation. Infections in the kidney can also lead to the formation of stones. The stones, which range in size from microscopic crystals to large casts of the entire collecting system, can be composed of calcium salts, struvite, cystine, uric acid, and even drugs taken by the patient. DOT 5-7.19

When stones break loose from their point of origin and travel from the kidney through the ureter to the bladder, they can cause excruciating pain as they scrape, scuff, and occlude the ureter. Once a stone breaks loose from its point of formation and travels through the ureter, it encounters three particularly narrow areas: the ureteropelvic junction (the junction of the kidney collecting system and the ureter), the pelvic brim (the point where the ureter passes from the abdomen into the pelvis), and ureterovesical junction (the junction of the ureter and the bladder). While the stone causes severe pain as it travels the entire distance of the ureter, the pain becomes especially severe as the stones negotiate these narrow areas, primarily due to ureteral obstruction and dilatation. Once the stone reaches the bladder, the pain usually disappears quickly. While some stones become permanently lodged in the trabeculae of the bladder, most pass undetected and without pain in the urine stream. DOT 5-7.19

The symptoms of **ureterolithiasis** (the presence of a kidney stone in the ureter) vary depending on where the stone is on its trip from the kidney to the bladder. The pain is caused by both ureteral spasm and obstruction. Patients passing kidney stones are frequently found writhing in pain, unable to remain still, and unable to find a comfortable position. The patients may complain of pain, which waxes and wanes, in the flank, abdomen or groin, and they may complain of radiation to the vulva or testicles. Other symptoms include nausea, diaphoresis, dysuria, urinary urgency or frequency, and the urge to defecate. Examination of these patients may reveal little or no tenderness in the abdomen and no peritoneal signs. They may have costovertebral angle or flank tenderness to palpation. Bowel sounds may be normal or hypoactive due to a mild ileus caused by the severe pain. DOT 5-7.20

The differential diagnosis is extensive and includes almost any cause of abdominal pain. Depending on which side of the abdomen is affected, the paramedic must consider the possibility of appendicitis, abdominal aortic aneurysm, gallbladder stones, testicular torsion, bowel obstruction, kidney infection, or diverticulitis, to name only a few entities. Prehospital evaluation includes assessment of vital signs and palpation of the abdomen, flanks, and possibly the genitalia. Because the pain of ureteral stones is one of the most excruciating pains a person can experience, intravenous access should be obtained, and the patients should be treated with appropriate analgesics, which include both nonsteroidal antiinflammatory agents and opiates.

Ketorolac, in particular, has been shown to be effective in treating the pain of ureterolithiasis.[39] Antiemetics may be necessary to treat severe nausea. Intravenous fluid bolus therapy is controversial. DOT 5-7.21

Eighty to eight-five percent of patients with kidney stones eventually pass the stones without invasive medical interventions. In addition to analgesics and antiemetics, patients may receive steroids and smooth muscle relaxing agents in the hospital. In cases where stones become impacted in the ureter and cannot pass, there are several methods of removing the stones. Extracorporeal shock wave lithotripsy utilizes underwater shock waves aimed at an anesthetized patient to pulverize the stone into small passable fragments. Endoscopy of the ureter from the urethra and bladder may be utilized to retrieve the stone with a basket or to fragment the stone directly with subsequent removal. Occasionally, it is necessary to approach the stone surgically through the skin of the flank with wires, endoscopes, or other instruments.

Recurrence rates after an initial episode of kidney stones are 14%, 35%, and 52% at one, five, and ten years, respectively.[40] Patients are encouraged to strain their urine with a fine mesh strainer for several days after an episode to capture the stone for lab analysis. The composition of the stone can be determined, and in some cases, dietary or medical interventions can be instituted to decrease the likelihood of recurrence. In most cases, the patients are advised to increase their consumption of water.

Primary Survey

As you can see from the discussion of the various genitourinary problems, immediate threats to life from urinary and renal emergencies fall into three categories:

1. Breathing problems (due to fluid overload resulting in pulmonary edema).
2. Septic shock (due to a urinary tract or shunt infection becoming severe).
3. Low blood pressure (due to fluid loss or possibly blood loss).

Airway compromise should always be a concern with any patient. In this case, it is unlikely that the airway will be compromised because of a urinary or renal problem. If it is present, it is likely to be secondary to a different condition such as an altered level of consciousness.

Breathing difficulty may occur in patients with chronic renal failure if they fail to get their dialysis, and they accumulate excess fluid.

The general status of the patient should be evaluated, looking for signs of fever, diaphoresis, shortness of breath, anxiety, inability to remain still or find a comfortable position, weakness, dehydration, confusion, or other changes in mental status. Supportive measures should be instituted as indicated by the history and clinical appearance of the patient.

Infections and other disorders can develop in every organ of the urinary tract, including the kidneys, urinary bladder, prostate, gonads, urethra, and external genitalia. Because most of these organs lie within the abdomen or pelvis, abdominal or pelvic pain may be the first symptom of infection, obstruction, or loss of blood supply.

Secondary Survey

When faced with a patient complaining of abdominal or pelvic pain, the paramedic should obtain a focused history of the pain, including the location, duration, and character of the discomfort:

- Has the pain moved, e.g., from the flank to the groin or from the periumbilical region to the right lower quadrant?
- Has the character of the pain changed, e.g., from dull and aching to sharp and localized?
- Are there other associated symptoms such as burning on urination, the urge to void or defecate, blood in the urine, frequent urination, nausea, vomiting, or diarrhea?
- Has the patient experienced chills, diaphoresis, fever, or headache?
- Is there a history of recent surgery, illness, or trauma?
- Has the patient experienced this type of pain before?
- Are there precipitating factors that either cause the pain or make it better or worse?

The patient should be asked about past medical history, surgeries, medications, and allergies. A brief review of the patient's family history may be helpful. Is there a history of kidney disease, ureteral stones, frequent infections, or bleeding disorders in family members? DOT 5-7.4, 5-7.5

Examination of the Abdomen

The abdomen should be palpated for signs of tenderness, rigidity, or guarding. Tenderness is pain that results when the abdomen is compressed by the examining hand. Guarding is the voluntary or involuntary tightening of the abdominal muscles to prevent deeper palpation. Rebound tenderness is the increase in pain felt when the examining hand exerting pressure on the abdomen is suddenly released. It is an indicator of peritoneal inflammation. Increased pain with coughing or when walking or going over bumps in a car may also indicate peritoneal inflammation. The anatomic locations of these findings should be noted. Does palpation of one region of the abdomen cause pain in another area? Can you palpate deeply, or does the patient push the examining hand away? The abdomen should be palpated for masses.

Examine the abdomen for signs of trauma, bruising, or unusual bulging, which may indicate a hernia. Does the umbilicus appear normal? Does the skin appear normal in color and temperature?

The examination of the abdomen traditionally includes auscultation for the presence or absence of bowel sounds and assessment of their character; however, this is extremely difficult in the usually noisy environment of the prehospital setting and provides little additional information that will change the treatment plan.

Physical Examination of the Flank and Groin

The flanks should be gently palpated or tapped looking for pain and tenderness. Discomfort in the flank after trauma suggests possible kidney injury and in the nontrauma patient may indicate infection or other problems. If full of urine, the bladder may be palpable as a round, frequently tender mass superior to the pubic symphysis. In a thin patient, a full bladder may actually be visible in the lower abdomen. In patients with pain in the external genitalia, the areas should be carefully examined. Are there signs of infection, purulence, or discoloration? Is swelling or tenderness present? Do the testicles appear to be of normal size and in the normal position? Is the foreskin retracted or swollen? Are there signs of trauma, bruising, or lacerations?

DOT 5-7.4, 5-7.5

Summary

Genitourinary (GU) complaints can cause intense pain or discomfort to the patient. The genitourinary system is critical for maintaining homeostasis. Patients with GU complaints may present with mild or life-threatening symptoms, so care must be taken to perform a thorough assessment of the patient. GI complaints are not encountered as often as respiratory or cardiovascular emergencies, but they have the potential to be just as dangerous for the patient.

Notes

1. J. Anderson, *Grant's Atlas of Anatomy,* 7th ed. (Baltimore, MD: Williams and Wilkins, 1978), pp. 2-99 to 2-114.
2. National Kidney and Urologic Diseases Information Clearinghouse, "Glomerular Diseases," National Institute of Diabetes and Digestive and Kidney Diseases (December 2003), http://kidney.niddk.nih.gov/kudiseases/pubs/glomerular/ (accessed August 10, 2005).
3. A. B. Wolfson and R. L. Maenza, *Rosen's Emergency Medicine: Concepts and Clinical Practice,* 5th ed., vol. 2, J. A. Marx, ed. (St. Louis, MO: Mosby, 2002), p. 1360.
4. F. C. Brunicardi, D. K. Andersen, T. R. Billiar, D. L. Dunn, J. G. Hunter, J. B. Matthews, R. E. Pollock, and S. I. Schwartz, "Urology," *Schwartz's Principles of Surgery,* 8th ed., McGraw-Hill's AccessMedicine (accessed June 30, 2006).
5. R. Sinert, *Emergency Medicine: A Comprehensive Study Guide,* 5th ed. (New York, NY: McGraw-Hill, 2000), p. 611.
6. D. Garth, "Hyperkalemia," Department of Emergency Medicine, Mary Washington Hospital (January 5, 2005), http://www.emedicine.com/emerg/topic261.htm (accessed August 18, 2005).
7. R. Sinert and P. R. Peacock, Jr. "Acute Renal Failure," State University of New York College of Medicine (January 11, 2005), http://www.emedicine.com/emerg/topic500.htm (accessed August 19, 2005).
8. I. R. Shilliday, K. J. Quinn, and M. E. Allison, "Loop Diuretics in the Management of Acute Renal Failure: A Prospective, Double-Blind, Placebo-Controlled, Randomized Study," *Nephrology, Dialysis, Transplantation* 12(12) (December 1997): 2592–2596.
9. M. Denton, G. M. Chertow, and H. R. Brady, "'Renal-Dose' Dopamine for the Treatment of Acute Renal Failure: Scientific Rationale, Experimental Studies and Clinical Trials," *Kidney International* 50 (1996).
10. J. O. Friedrich, "Meta-Analysis: Low-Dose Dopamine Increases Urine Output But Does Not Prevent Renal Dysfunction or Death," *Annals of Internal Medicine* 142 (7) (April 5, 2005): 510.
11. I. A. Agha, "End-Stage Kidney Disease," *Medline Plus,* Renal Division, St. Louis University (October 17, 2003), http://www.nlm.nih.gov/medlineplus/ency/article/000500.htm#Causes, %20incidence,%20and%20risk%20factors (accessed August 11, 2005).
12. B. M. Brenner and J. M. Lazarus, *Harrison's Principles of Internal Medicine,* 13th ed. (New York, NY: McGraw-Hill, 1994), pp. 1274–1275.
13. M. Allon, R. Dunlay, and C. Copkney, "Nebulized Albuterol for Acute Hyperkalemia in Patients on Hemodialysis," *Annals of Internal Medicine* 110 (1989): 426, 1.
14. U.S. Renal Data System, *USRDS 2004 Annual Data Report: Atlas of End-Stage Renal Disease in the United States* (Bethesda, MD: National Institutes of Health, National Institute of Diabetes and Digestive and Kidney Diseases, 2004).
15. R. Sinert and M. Erogul, "Renal Transplants," State University of New York College of Medicine, State University of New York Health Sciences Center, Brooklyn (September 2, 2004), http://www.emedicine.com/emerg/topic607.htm (accessed August 25, 2005).
16. R. S. Krause, "Chronic Renal Failure and Dialysis Complications," http://www.emedicine.com/emerg/topic501.htm (accessed August 23, 2005).

17. G. R. Bailie, R. Rasmussen, A. Hollister, and G. Eisele, "Incidence of CAPD Peritonitis in Patients Using UVXD or O-Set Systems," *Clinical Nephrology* 33 (1990): 252.

18. A. H. Ropper and R. H. Brown, "The Acquired Disorders of the Nervous System," *Adams and Victor's Principles of Neurology*, 8th ed., McGraw-Hill's AccessMedicine (accessed June 30, 2006).

19. D. S. Howes, "Urinary Tract Infection, Female," University of Chicago/Pritzker School of Medicine (April 25, 2005), http://www.emedicine.com/EMERG/topic626.htm (accessed August 24, 2005).

20. D. S. Howes and W. F. Young, "Urinary Tract Infections," *Tintinalli's Emergency Medicine: A Comprehensive Study Guide*, 5th ed. (New York, NY: McGraw-Hill, 2000), p. 625.

21. H. H. Woo et al., "The Treatment of Vesicovaginal Fistulae," *European Urology* 29 (1996):1.

22. J. I. Escobar II, E. R. Eastman, and A. L. Harwood-Nuss, "Selected Urologic Problems," *Rosen's Emergency Medicine: Concepts and Clinical Practice* (St. Louis, MO: Mosby, 2002), pp. 1406–1407.

23. R. Vick and C. C. Carson, "Fournier's Disease" *The Urologic Clinics of North America* 26(4) (November 1999): 841–849.

24. T. W. Thomsen and E. Legome, "Fournier's Gangrene," Department of Emergency Medicine, Mount Auburn Hospital (September 14, 2005), http://www.emedicine.com/emerg/topic929.htm (accessed September 21, 2005).

25. Acute Pain Management Guideline Panel, *Acute Pain Management: Operative or Medical Procedures and Trauma. Guideline Report.* Agency for Health Care Policy and Research Publication No. 92-002 (Rockville, MD: Agency for Health Care Policy and Research, Public Health Service, U.S. Department of Health and Human Services, 1993).

26. Joint Commission on Accreditation of Healthcare, *Pain Management Standards*, http://www.jcaho.org (accessed October 2, 2006).

27. J. E. Tintinalli, G. D. Kelen, J. S. Stapczynski, O. J. Ma, and D. M. Cline, "Acute Pain Management in the Adult Patient," *Tintinalli's Emergency Medicine: A Comprehensive Study Guide*, 6th ed., McGraw-Hill's AccessMedicine (accessed June 30, 2006).

28. D. Levy, "Genital Sores—Male," Greater Baltimore Medical Center (January 16, 2004), http://www.nlm.nih.gov/medlineplus/ency/article/003221.htm (accessed August 25, 2005).

29. M. B. Brooks, "Epididymitis" (2005), http://www.emedicine.com/emerg/topic166.htm (accessed September 21, 2005).

30. National Kidney and Urologic Diseases Information Clearinghouse, "Prostatitis: Disorders of the Prostate," National Institute of Diabetes and Digestive and Kidney Diseases, National Institutes of Health (December 2003), http://kidney.niddk.nih.gov/kudiseases/pubs/prostatitis/ (accessed September 22, 2005).

31. E. Walter and M. C. Plewa, "Urethritis, Male," Medical College of Ohio and Saint Vincent Mercy Medical Center (April 4, 2005), http://www.emedicine.com/emerg/topic623.htm (accessed September 22, 2005).

32. S. A. Jones and R. J. Flynn, "An Unusual (and Somewhat Piercing) Cause of Paraphimosis," *British Journal of Urology* 78(5) (November 1996): 803–804.

33. J. C. Williams, P. M. Morrison, and J. R. Richardson, "Paraphimosis in Elderly Men," *The American Journal of Emergency Medicine* 13(3) (May 1995): 351–353.

34. S. T. Miller, S. P. Rao, E. K. Dunn, and K. I. Glassberg, "Priapism in Children with Sickle Cell Disease," *The Journal of Urology* 154 (2 Pt 2) (August 1995): 844–847.

35. M. J. Carey, "Priapism," Department of Emergency Medicine, University of Arkansas for Medical Sciences (September 6, 2005), http://www.emedicine.com/emerg/topic486.htm (accessed September 22, 2005).

36. "Enlarged Prostate," *Encyclopedia*, MEDLINE PLUS (October 28, 2004), http://www.nlm.nih.gov/medlineplus/ency/article/000381.htm (accessed September 22, 2005).

37. T. J. Rupp and M. Zwanger, "Testicular Torsion," Emergency Medicine, Methodist Health Systems, Dallas, Texas (August 25, 2005), http://www.emedicine.com/EMERG/topic573.htm (accessed September 21, 2005).

38. F. L. Coe, "Kidney Stones in Adults," The National Kidney and Urologic Diseases Information Clearinghouse, The University of Chicago (December 2004), http://kidney.niddk.nih.gov/kudiseases/pubs/stonesadults/index.htm (accessed September 22, 2005).

39. G. L. Larkin, W. F. Peacock, S. M. Pearl, et al., "Efficacy of Ketorolac Tromethamine Versus Meperidine in the ED Treatment of Acute Renal Colic," *The American Journal of Emergency Medicine* 17(1) (January 1999): 6–10.

40. S. Craig, "Renal Calculi," Department of Emergency Medicine, University of North Carolina at Chapel Hill, Carolinas Medical Center (January 12, 2005), http://www.emedicine.com/EMERG/topic499.htm (accessed September 22, 2005).

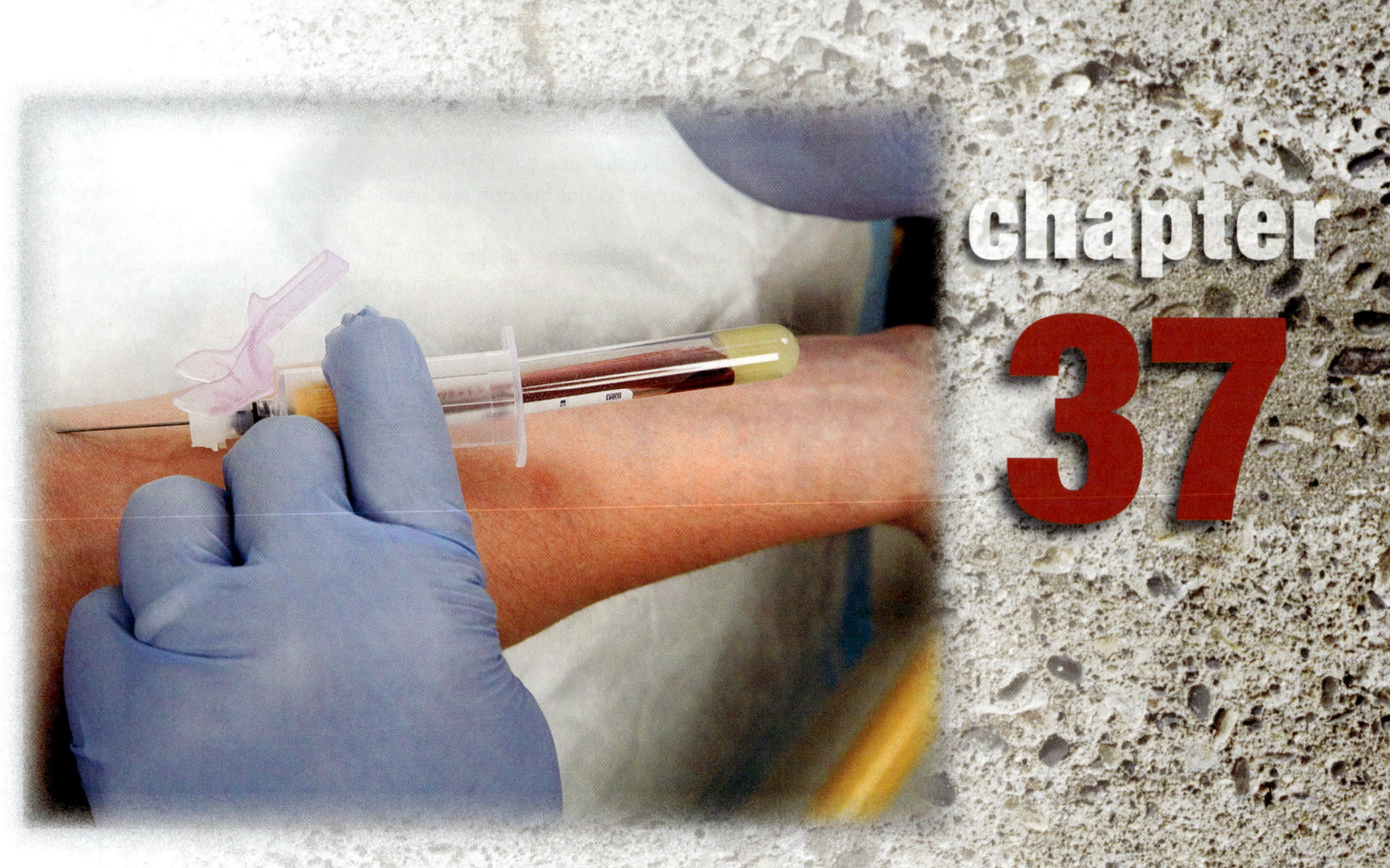

Hematology

*"**B**lood is inherited and virtue is acquired."*

—Venezuelan proverb

Need to Know

▶ The presence of hematologic disease compounds other medical conditions and diseases.
 • Typically, a hematologic disease becomes a chronic condition and is not the primary reason EMS is called—unless the patient is in a crisis.

▶ The basic management principles for patients with hematologic disorders are similar to most medical patients: support the ABCs in a manner consistent with the severity of the signs and symptoms presented.

▶ Understand that although most hematologic diseases do not present a true life-threatening emergency, when one does occur, time is critical and the patient should be transported immediately for management in the emergency department.
 • Many medications and treatments designed to counteract a hematologic emergency are not available in the prehospital setting.

▶ Sick	▶ Not Yet Sick
• If a patient has called EMS, they have exhausted their coping mechanisms or are in a crisis they cannot manage on their own.	• These patients are usually chronically ill and in most cases understand their disease and how to manage it.
• If the patient has not yet received a diagnosis of their condition, they will likely present as a sick medical patient. A thorough history and physical exam focused on the body system in question is important, but you should also consider performing a general physical exam, gathering additional clues for the hospital staff.	• Obtain a thorough history and be on the lookout for patients with hematologic disease as their conditions compound other medical conditions.
• Supportive care of the airway, breathing, and circulation is often the best treatment to render to these patients.	

Introduction

Hematology is the study of blood and blood-forming tissues and the disorders associated with them.[1] The **hematopoietic system** is made up of all the organs and tissues responsible for the formation of blood cells, including lymphoid organs and lymphatic tissues, spleen, liver, kidney, and bone marrow.

Hematological disorders such as leukemia, lymphoma, and anemia, are common, but they are rarely the sole reason EMS is called. Rather, these disorders complicate other health problems due to the immunosuppression that accompanies many of the hematologic disorders. Because there are often other health problems present, a thorough patient assessment needs to be performed to treat patients appropriately. Understanding the physiology behind hematologic disorders will allow the paramedic to perform a more complete patient assessment and prepare for possible complications. **Skill Sheet 42: Intravenous Access (and Step-by-Step 42) and Skill Sheet 47: Central Line Access for Fluids and Drug Administration support this chapter.**

Applied Anatomy and Physiology

Blood consists of both formed elements and plasma. The formed elements are red blood cells, white blood cells, and platelets, all of which arise from a single cell type called a pluripotent hematopoietic stem cell. Stem cells are capable of producing red blood cells (erythrocytes), white blood cells (granulocytes and agranulocytes), platelets (thrombocytes), and the cells of the immune system (Figure 37-1).[2] The process of blood cell formation occurs in the bone marrow in an adult. In the developing fetus, it occurs in the liver, spleen, thymus, and lymph nodes.

The pluripotent stem cell differentiates into either a lymphoid progenitor cell or a myeloid progenitor cell. The lymphoid progenitor cell further differentiates into T cells and B cells, both of which are types of white blood cells. The myeloid progenitor cell further differentiates into red blood cells, platelets, and other types of white blood cells: eosinophils, neutrophils, basophils, mast cells, and monocytes.

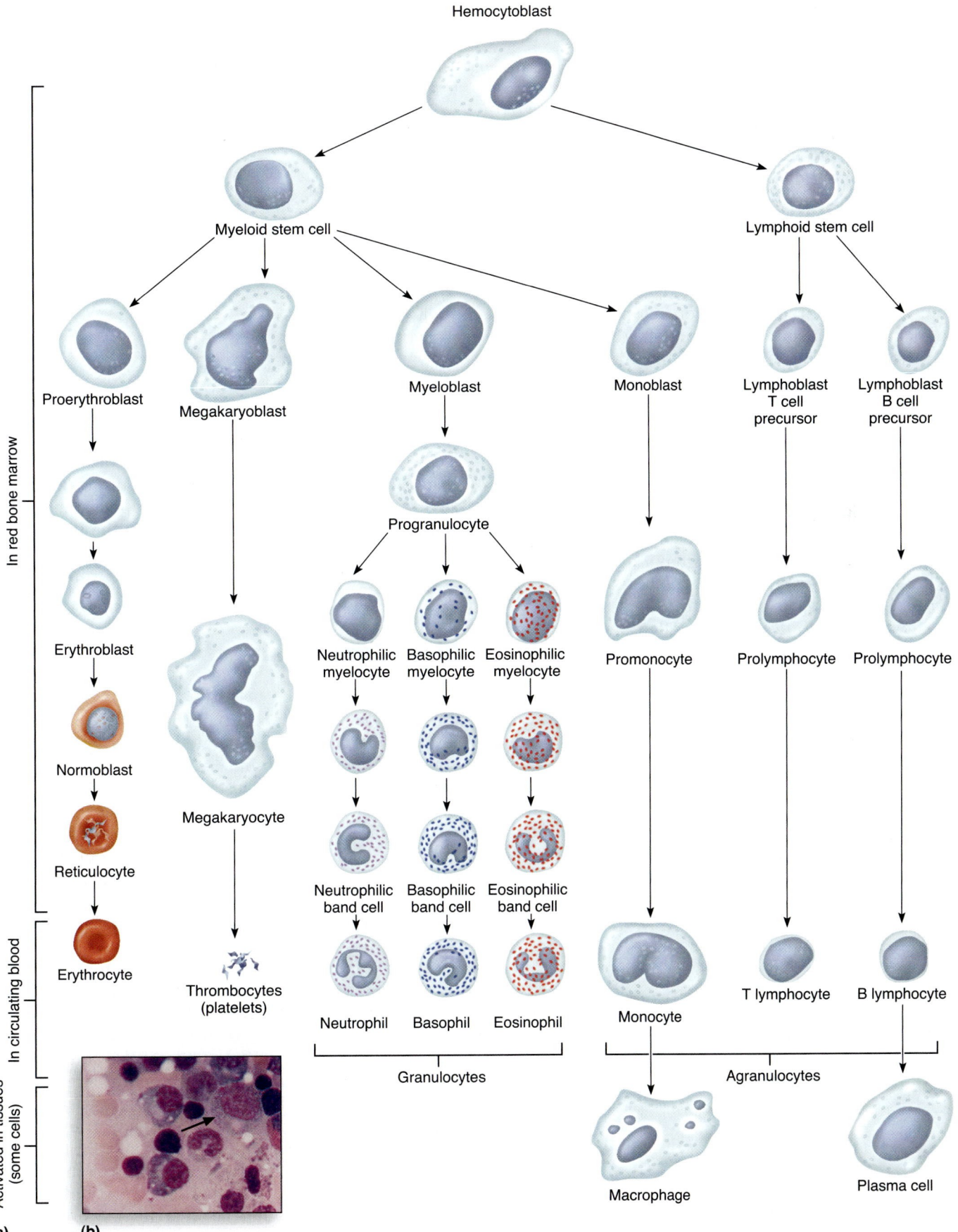

Hemocytoblast

Myeloid stem cell

Lymphoid stem cell

Proerythroblast

Megakaryoblast

Myeloblast

Monoblast

Lymphoblast T cell precursor

Lymphoblast B cell precursor

Erythroblast

Progranulocyte

Normoblast

Megakaryocyte

Neutrophilic myelocyte

Basophilic myelocyte

Eosinophilic myelocyte

Promonocyte

Prolymphocyte

Prolymphocyte

Reticulocyte

Neutrophilic band cell

Basophilic band cell

Eosinophilic band cell

Erythrocyte

Thrombocytes (platelets)

Neutrophil

Basophil

Eosinophil

Monocyte

T lymphocyte

B lymphocyte

Granulocytes

Agranulocytes

Macrophage

Plasma cell

In red bone marrow

In circulating blood

Activated in tissues (some cells)

(a)

(b)

Figure 37-1 (a) Blood cells start developing in the bone marrow, where hemocytoblasts differentiate into stem cells, which then produce red blood cells, white blood cells, platelets, and the cells of the immune system. (b) Light micrograph of a hemocytoblast (arrow) in red bone marrow (500x).

Other organs such as the kidneys and liver play a critical role in the hematopoietic system. **Erythropoietin** is an important hormone that is produced primarily by specialized cells in the kidneys and can also be produced in the liver. The specialized kidney cells are capable of sensing the oxygen level of the blood. When there is a low oxygen level, these cells secrete erythropoietin, which in turn stimulates bone marrow stem cells to produce more red blood cells. The liver is responsible for detoxifying the blood as well as producing six of the thirteen clotting factors. Clotting factors are the chemicals required for the blood clotting process to take place. The spleen is an important immune organ that filters blood and disposes of invading pathogens and dead or dying red blood cells. The spleen is also an important storage area for platelets.

Blood volume accounts for approximately 7–8% of total body weight and is made up of roughly 55% plasma and 45% formed elements (red blood cells, white blood cells, and platelets) (Figure 37-2). A healthy individual is capable of compensating for a 25–30% blood loss before progressing to decompensated shock.[3] Thus, an average person who weighs 75 kg (165 pounds) will have 5.625 liters of blood (see Table 37–1) and can potentially lose approximately 1.7 liters of blood before showing signs of decompensated shock. DOT 5-9.1, 5-9.2, 5-9.3

CONNECTIONS The various stages of shock are discussed in Chapter 13: Shock Overview. Hemorrhagic shock is covered in Chapter 19: Trauma and Hemorrhagic Shock.

Compensated shock occurs with early blood loss. As long as the bleeding is minimal and the patient is otherwise healthy, the body can maintain blood pressure and cellular perfusion by shunting blood from

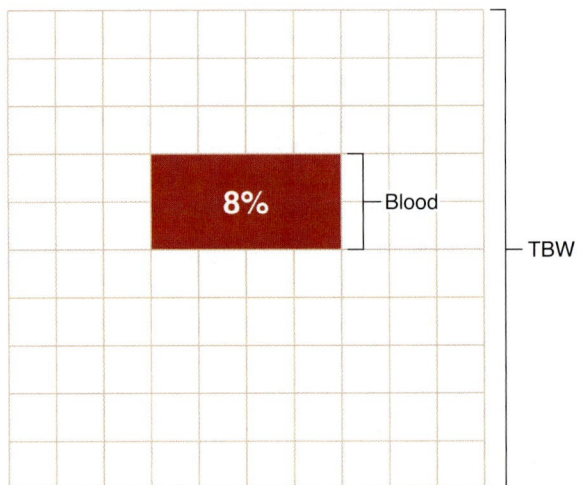

Figure 37-2   Blood volume accounts for approximately 8% of total body weight (TBW).

TABLE 37-1   **Average Blood Volumes**

Age	Blood Volume
Neonates	
Premature	95 mL/kg
Full-term	85 mL/kg
Infants	80 mL/kg
Adults	
Men	75 mL/kg
Women	65 mL/kg

Source: G. E. Morgan, Jr., M. S. Mikhail, and M. J. Murray, *Clinical Anesthesiology, 4th ed.* (McGraw-Hill Online, 2006). Copyright © 2006 The McGraw-Hill Companies, Inc. Reprinted with permission.

less critical areas such as the skin and organs of the GI tract, increasing the heart rate, force of contraction, respiratory rate, and vasoconstriction of the blood vessels. As the ability to compensate is lost, the patient slips into a decompensated state, and the blood pressure drops. If not corrected, irreversible shock develops, and the patient eventually dies from cellular hypoxia.

Blood Components

Plasma

Plasma is the liquid portion of the blood. It is pale yellow in color when it is separate from the blood cells. It consists of 90% water and 6–7% proteins, and the remainder is made up of waste products, nutrients (such as lipids [fats] and carbohydrates), gasses, and regulatory substances (such as electrolytes, hormones, and antibodies). Plasma is responsible for transporting blood cells and nourishment to the cells for metabolism and transporting waste products from the cells. The waste products in plasma are eliminated from the body through the lung, kidney, or liver.

Many of the components dissolved in plasma have the capability to diffuse across the capillary membrane in order to transport nutrients to the cells. This means they can leave the blood stream (the intravascular space) and pass into cells or other areas of the body such as the interstitial space. One exceptionally large protein molecule, albumin, is too large to diffuse easily out of the vascular space. This is actually a good thing because if it could leave the vascular space, most of the water in the plasma would follow it, leaving little fluid in the vascular compartment. Thus, plasma not only carries nutrients to the cells but also carries the proteins responsible for maintaining the fluid integrity of the vascular space. Other plasma proteins are responsible for blood clotting, dismantling of clots, and acid/base balance buffering.

Red Blood Cells

Red blood cells **(erythrocytes)** are formed through a process called **erythropoiesis.** In adults, erythrocytes are formed in the bone marrow from a pluripotent stem cell.

It takes about seven days to produce an erythrocyte. In healthy adults, RBCs live for about 120 days. After that, they are destroyed by macrophages (a special type of WBC) found in the spleen. A normal red blood cell count ranges from 4 million per microliter (abbreviated million/μL) of blood for an adult female to 6 million/μL of blood for an adult male. Erythrocytes are biconcave anucleated cells, meaning they resemble a donut and they have no nucleus (Figure 37-3). Their primary purpose is to carry oxygen (O_2) molecules to the cells and tissues for metabolism and pick up the waste product

carbon dioxide (CO_2). They then transport CO_2 to the lungs where it is exhaled. DOT 5-9.4

To accomplish this feat, each red blood cell contains about 270 million hemoglobin molecules, and each hemoglobin molecule is capable of carrying four oxygen molecules at a time (Figure 37-4). That is over one *billion* oxygen molecules carried per single red blood cell. A normal hemoglobin level in males is 13.5–18 grams per 100 milliliters (abbreviated g/100 mL) and 12–16 g/100 mL in females. The **hematocrit** measures the amount of space in the blood that is taken up by the red blood cells and is expressed as a percentage of red blood cells in whole blood. The hematocrit of healthy males is 40–54% and 38–47% in females.[4] A decrease in the number or the size of the red blood cell will result in a decrease in the hematocrit level. **Anemia** is a condition where a lower than normal level of red blood cells is found in the blood. There are several different causes of anemia, and they will be discussed later in the chapter. DOT 5-9.5, 5-9.6

The Oxyhemoglobin Dissociation Curve

The ability for two chemical substances to bind together is called **affinity.** Hemoglobin and oxygen are naturally supposed to bond together, so they have a high affinity for each other. Low affinity would describe two chemicals that do not readily bond together. Oxygen and carbon dioxide do not bond together, so there is low affinity between these two chemicals.

Hemoglobin's high affinity for oxygen is how it acquires and releases the oxygen molecule to the surrounding tissues. The oxyhemoglobin dissociation curve expresses how readily hemoglobin releases oxygen (Figure 37-5). The curve can be divided into an upper oxygen association curve, which represents what is happening in the alveolar-capillary environment (in the lung where oxygen is attached), and the lower portion of the curve describes what is happening in the tissue-capillary environment (where oxygen is released).[5] The curve of the graph is said to shift to the left or the right in response to the ability of oxygen to bind or unbind, depending upon the direction of shift, because of various factors. Shifts of the curve have their greatest impact at the steep portion because they affect oxygen delivery.

This graph relates oxygen saturation, which is abbreviated as SaO_2, to the partial pressure of oxygen, which is abbreviated as PaO_2. Oxygen saturation (SaO_2) is a ratio of the amount of oxygen bound to hemoglobin, compared to the oxygen-carrying capacity of hemoglobin. It measures the total amount of oxygen currently bound and compares it to the amount that could be bound if all the available hemoglobin was used. The amount of oxygen actually bound to hemoglobin is expressed as the partial pressure of oxygen (PaO_2). This

Top view

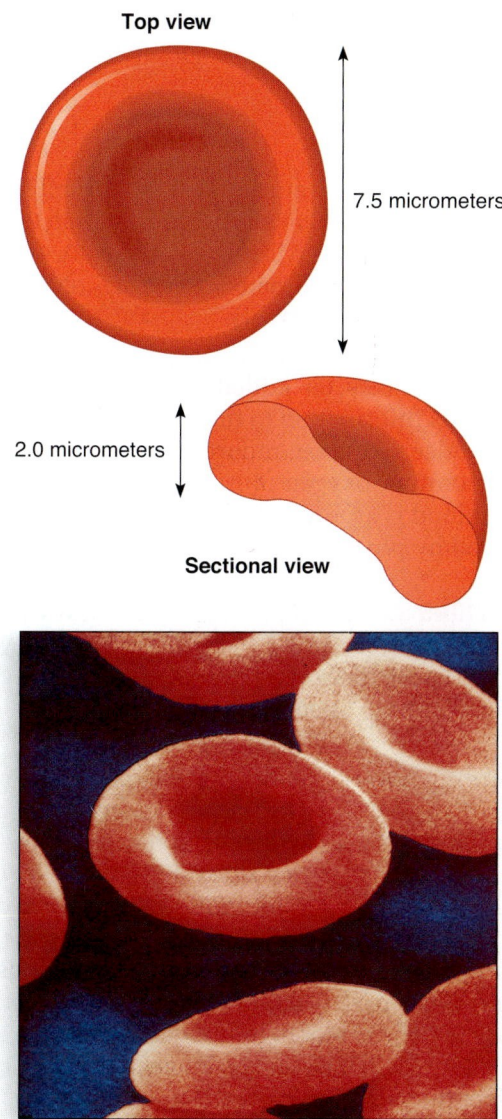

7.5 micrometers

2.0 micrometers

Sectional view

Figure 37-3   Size and shape of red blood cells.

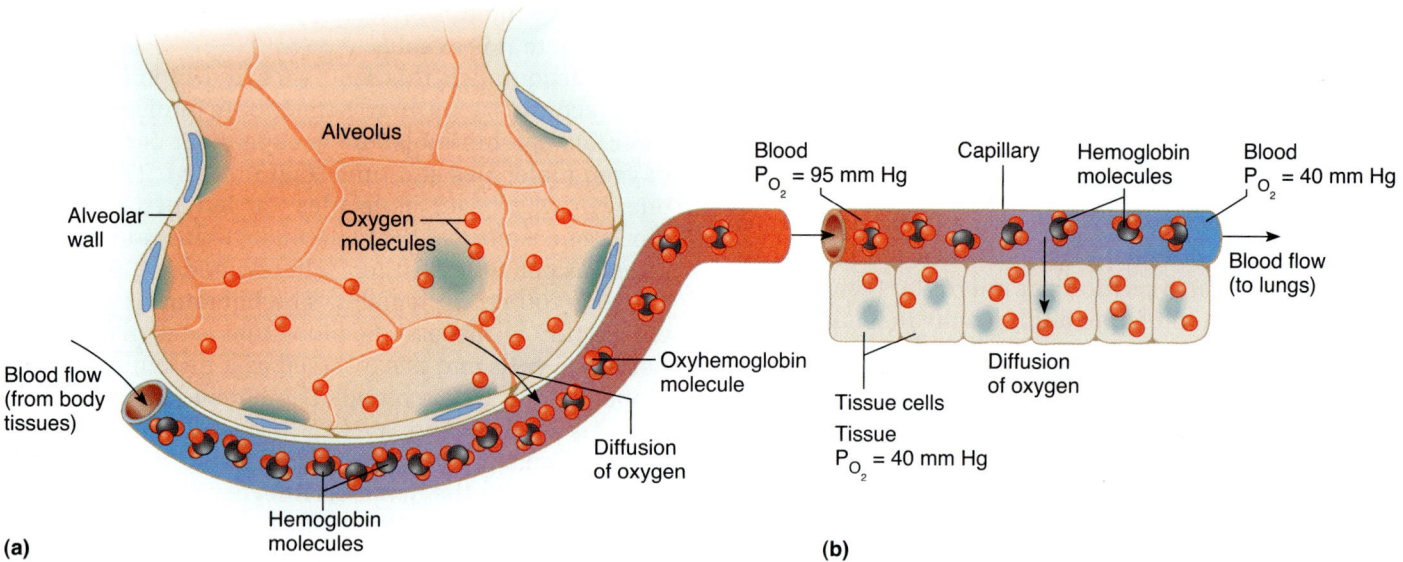

(a)

(b)

Figure 37-4   Oxygen molecules enter the bloodstream and bond to hemoglobin molecules, which carry four oxygen molecules at a time. Each erythrocyte contains millions of hemoglobin molecules. The oxyhemoglobin molecules are carried throughout the body where some of the oxygen molecules are diffused into the body's cells.

percentage does not consider the amount that could be bound if all of the hemoglobin was used; it simply states the amount that currently is bound. The partial pressure of oxygen in the lungs is relatively high, and this causes oxygen to readily bind to hemoglobin; whereas, the partial pressure of oxygen in the tissues is relatively low, forcing oxygen to disassociate (unbind) from hemoglobin and diffuse into the tissues.

A normal PaO_2 level at sea level is 95 mmHg, which relates to a 97% SaO_2 level. A simplification to remember for clinical practice is that a PaO_2 of 30, 40, 50, and 60 correspond approximately to a SaO_2 of 60%, 70%, 80%, and 90%, respectively.[6]

This concept takes on added significance when you compare this information to the use of a pulse oximeter. When a pulse oximeter reports the SaO_2 at 90%, the actual amount of oxygen present (PaO_2) within the circulating blood is around 60 mmHg, which is commonly considered by physicians to be hypoxemia![6]

CONNECTIONS   Chapter 28: Pulmonary discusses the oxyhemoglobin dissociation curve, hypoxemia, and hypoxia. Chapter 31: Endocrinology, electrolytes and acid/base discusses acid/base balance.

There are several factors that can influence a left or right shift in the standard dissociation curve. A right shift of the standard curve means that a greater partial pressure of oxygen is necessary for oxygen to bind to hemoglobin, whereas a left shift of the standard curve means that a lesser partial pressure of oxygen is necessary for oxygen to bind to hemoglobin. The most common and best known factors that affect the standard curve are pH of the blood, temperature, and 2,3 diphosphoglycerate (2,3-DPG) levels. Exercise and PCO_2 levels also affect the curve.[6]

A decrease in pH (causing the blood to be acidic) causes a right shift of the standard curve, meaning oxygen is released more readily. An increase in pH (causing

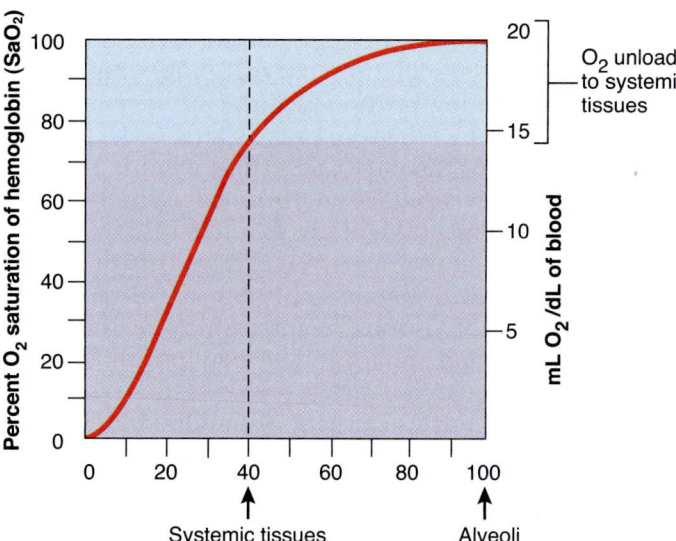

Figure 37-5   The oxyhemoglobin dissociation curve shows the relative amount of hemoglobin that is saturated with oxygen (SaO_2) as a function of ambient oxygen concentration (PaO_2).

the blood to be alkaline) causes a left shift of the standard curve, and hemoglobin holds onto oxygen more readily. Since pCO_2 is a waste gas that is directly related to pH, a decrease in pH will cause a right shift (releasing oxygen) while an increase will cause a left shift (retaining oxygen).

2,3-DPG is a compound produced by red blood cells during glycolysis. (Glycolysis is the breakdown of the carbohydrate glycogen into smaller sized sugar molecules for metabolism.) High levels of 2,3-DPG are seen with hypoxemia (low blood oxygen states), chronic lung disease, congestive heart failure, and anemia. All of these conditions cause a right shift of the standard curve to more easily release oxygen. Low levels of 2,3-DPG found in patients in septic shock result in a left shift of the standard curve.

Temperature does not have as dramatic an effect on the oxyhemoglobin dissociation curve as the other factors, but, nevertheless, it has an effect. Hyperthermia causes a right shift of the curve while hypothermia causes a left shift. Thus, oxygen is supplied to the tissues and organs at a greater capacity during periods of fever because of this right shift. This helps the body in its healing process because more oxygen is available for metabolism.

Carbon monoxide and methemoglobinemia both cause a left shift of the standard curve. Methemoglobinemia is a disorder of the RBC that prevents the hemoglobin from binding in a reversible fashion with oxygen. Carbon monoxide occurs as a by-product of combustion (from burning) and quickly reaches toxic levels in confined spaces. CO has a 240 to 260 times greater affinity for hemoglobin than does oxygen. This means CO binds much more readily to hemoglobin than does oxygen. Also, when carbon monoxide binds to hemoglobin (which results in a condition called **carboxyhemoglobin),** it alters all the binding sites, so any oxygen that is bound to a receptor is bound so tightly it may not be released to the tissues.

A pulse oximetry reading for a patient with CO poisoning may still show a reading of 100% because all the receptor sites on the hemoglobin molecule are bound with oxygen-containing molecules (CO and O_2), but the patient is hypoxic because little oxygen is actually being released to the tissues. DOT 5-9.4, 5-9.5, 5-9.6, 5-9.7

White Blood Cells

Leukocytes, also called **white blood cells (WBC)** travel throughout the blood stream and provide protection from foreign invaders such as bacteria and viruses. These extremely versatile cells are capable of responding to an infection very quickly. When a WBC encounters a foreign invader **(antigen),** it recognizes that it is not a normal part of the body. The WBC signals other white blood cells (through a process termed **chemotaxis**) that an antigenic

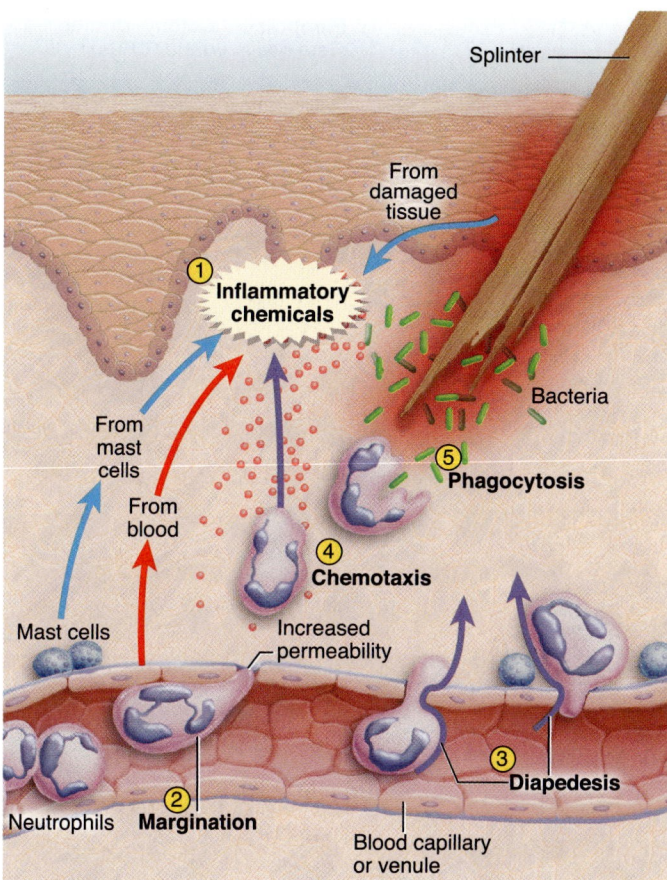

Figure 37-6 The response of white blood cells to invaders.

material has been recognized. The signaling process alerts other WBCs to respond and aide in the destruction of the invaders (Figure 37-6).

Some leukocytes do not travel in the blood stream, rather they remain in a certain area of the body and perform a function on blood that is circulating through their specific tissue. For example, splenic macrophages are found only in the spleen and are responsible for destroying dead and dying red blood cells.

Leukocytes are produced in the bone marrow by a process called leukopoiesis and differentiate from the same pluripotent stem cell from which red blood cells are derived. Under the influence of specific growth factors, the pluripotent stem cell differentiates into three forms, called **blasts,** which are the immature forms of white blood cells. The various blast forms are myeloblasts, monoblasts, and lymphoblasts. The myeloblasts further differentiate into granulocytes, which become neutrophils, basophils, and eosinophils. The monoblasts differentiate into monocytes, which are then called macrophages when they leave the blood stream and move into the tissues. Lymphoblasts differentiate

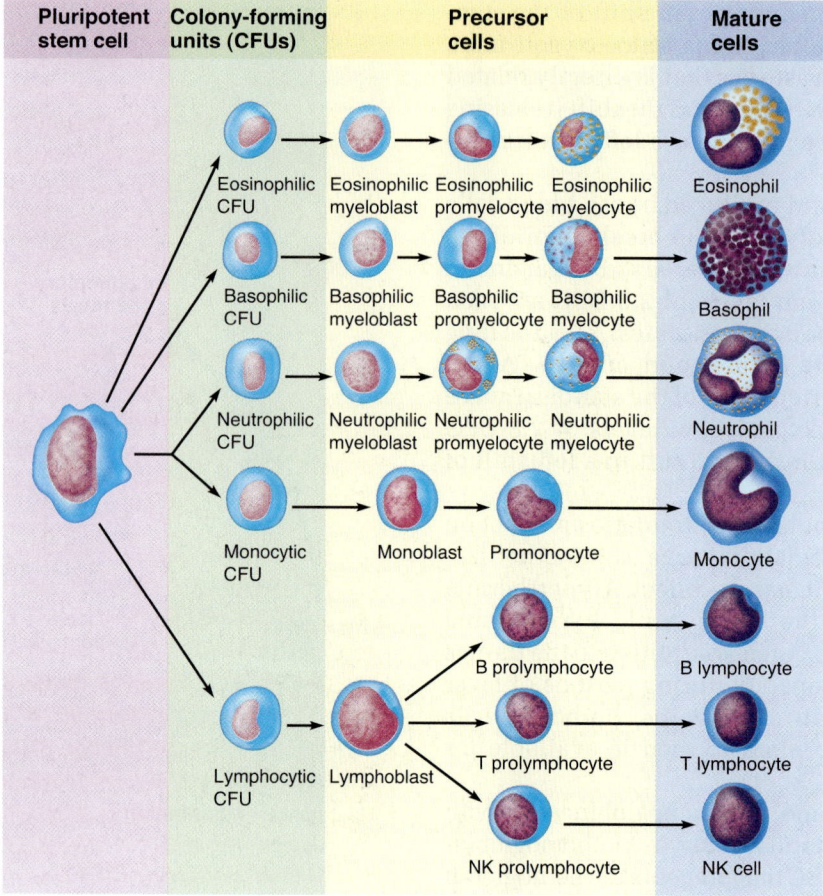

Figure 37-7 The formation of mature cells from pluripotent stem cells.

into lymphocytes, which become either T cells or B cells (Figure 37-7). DOT 5-9.8

Granulocytes

Granulocytes have a lobed, irregularly shaped nucleus and contain many granules that contain substances such as acid hydrolases, lysozyme, histamine, heparin, and slow reactive substance of anaphylaxis. These cells do not have any specificity for antigens, which means they are not coded or designed to recognize specific foreign invaders. They are capable of phagocytizing (meaning consuming or eating) antigen and fusing with the granules to break down the foreign invader.

Neutrophils

Neutrophils make up about 95% of the circulating granulocytes. They are also called **polymorphonuclear lymphocytes,** or PMNs or *polys* for short. They respond to chemotactic signals from platelets, other leukocytes, and the products of some bacteria. These are short-lived cells that have a life span of two to three days and are released from the bone marrow at a rate of about 700 million per minute. Since neutrophils comprise the

majority of granulocytes in the blood, if their level is low (called **neutropenia**), the body is incapable of mounting an appropriate defense against infectious particles. This may result in the death of the individual. The normal range for a neutrophil count is 38–80% of all white blood cells or an absolute count of between 1,650 and 8,000 cells per milliliter of blood.

Basophils

Basophils only make up about 0.2% of the circulating leukocytes. These cells play a dominant role in the inflammatory process and have a role in anaphylaxis as well. Basophilic granules contain substances such as histamine, serotonin, prostaglandins, and leukotrienes. When stimulated, basophils will degranulate, meaning they will spill their insides and release the contents of their granules into the extracellular space. These granulocytic substances cause increased vascular permeability, vasodilation, and chemotaxis of other leukocytes. Increased vascular permeability results in increased loss of fluid from the blood stream while vasodilation results in an increased blood flow into the affected area. The result of both processes is tissue edema. Chemotaxis results in more WBCs being called into the area to help fight the invader. The normal range for a basophil count is 0–2% or an absolute value of 0–125 cells/mL.

Eosinophils

Eosinophils make up about 2–5% of the circulating granulocytes. These cells are important in parasitic infections. When parasites are detected, the eosinophil will degranulate, releasing the contents of its granules onto the parasitic worm, which kills it. The toxic substances released by eosinophils are major basic protein and eosinophil cationic protein. Eosinophils also release histaminase, which inactivates histamine and another chemical, called slow reactive substance of anaphylaxis, which was released by the basophil. Histaminase helps slow or regulate the inflammatory process and granulocyte migration to the site of infection. This provides a helpful balance to the whole inflammation process and hopefully prevents an overaggressive response, which could result in anaphylaxis. A normal range for an eosinophil count is 0–8% of WBCs or an absolute value of 30–600 cells/mL.

Monocytes

Monocytes may live for months to years. These are the most important of the long-lived phagocytic cells. They are capable of engulfing foreign particles and internalizing and destroying them. These cells, when found in the liver, are known as Kupffer cells and when found in the synovial (joint) cavity, are known as synovial A cells. They are responsible for filtering the blood for foreign particles. When theses cells migrate out of the bloodstream into the tissues, they are then called macrophages. The normal range for a monocyte count is 0–13% of WBCs or an absolute value of 40–900 cells/mL.

Lymphocytes

There are two subpopulations of lymphocytes: T cells and B cells. B cells mature in the bone marrow and are then released directly into the bloodstream. T cells mature in the thymus gland, which is located in the mediastinum in the chest, after they are released from the bone marrow. These two types of lymphocytes are responsible for orchestrating two types of immunity: cellular and humoral.

In **cellular immunity,** pathogens are first attacked by a phagocyte cell, such as a macrophage. The phagocyte may be joined by a specific type of T cell (a helper T) which in turn aides the phagocyte in destroying the pathogen. DOT 5-9.10

In **humoral immunity,** B cells produce antibodies following their exposure to an antigenic stimulus. This results in the creation of future B cells capable of

"remembering" an infectious particle. Because of this, the body is capable of responding to the pathogen much quicker the next time it enters the body. DOT 5-9.10, 5-9.12

Autoimmune diseases, immunodeficiency, and hypersensitivity all cause alterations in the immune response. Autoimmunity is when immune processes within the body turn on its own cells, resulting in tissue destruction. A disease such as systemic lupus erythematosus (SLE) is a type of autoimmune disease in which the body's own antibodies are directed against nuclear components of their own cells. Immunodeficiency occurs when an element of the immune system does not work appropriately. Some immunodeficiencies are hereditary while others, such as the disease AIDS, are acquired. Hypersensitivity occurs when the immune system overreacts to an antigen with an exaggerated response, which may cause more damage than the offending antigen. An anaphylactic reaction is a type of exaggerated hypersensitivity reaction. DOT 5-9.11

Some leukocyte disorders consist of leukemia, lymphomas, and multiple myeloma. These disorders will be discussed later in the chapter. DOT 5-9.13

Platelets

Platelets (thrombocytes) have the primary function of providing hemostasis by forming blood clots. Platelets are derived from the pluripotent stem cells located in bone marrow. The stem cell first differentiates into a megakaryocyte, which then disassociates (breaks up) into platelets (Figure 37-8). One-third of all platelets stay in the spleen while the remaining two-thirds circulate in the blood.[2] Platelets are not really complete cells but are fragments, or parts of cells. The normal life span for a platelet is seven to ten days, after which it is removed by a phagocytic cell. DOT 5-9.14

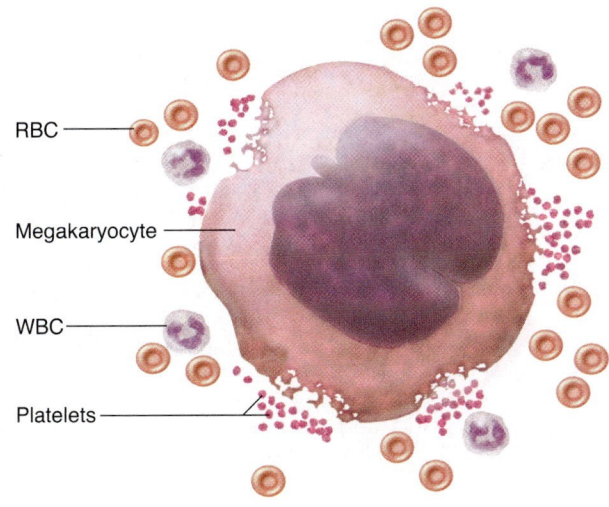

Figure 37-8   The formation of platelets from megakaryocytes.

Nice to Know

Hemostasis is not the same as homeostasis. Hemostasis is arrested bleeding, or the process of controlling bleeding. Homeostasis is the maintenance of a relatively stable internal environment in the body. Hemostasis contributes to homeostasis.

When the platelet count is too low, thrombopoietin, a hormone produced by the liver, signals the bone marrow to produce more platelets. A normal platelet count is 150,000–400,000/μL of blood. If the level drops below 50,000/μL of blood, the person is in danger of uncontrollable bleeding. The condition of too few platelets is called **thrombocytopenia.** Thrombocytopenia may lead to life-threatening bleeding due to the inability to form a clot when needed. The condition of too many platelets is called **thrombocytosis.** Thrombocytosis may lead to unnecessary clot formation, which can cause a stroke, heart attack, or blood clot in the arteries of the bowel or extremity.

Platelets are activated (triggered to clump together and form a clot) by several different mechanisms. Only a few are mentioned here. One means of activation occurs when platelets come into contact with collagen. Collagen is a fibrous protein, and it is exposed to the circulating blood when the endothelial lining of the blood vessel is damaged. Other ways to activate platelets include coming into contact with fibrin or the receptors on a leukocyte. Once activated, platelets release many different coagulation factors, which start or continue the

blood clotting process. The step-by-step process of blood clotting is called the **coagulation cascade.** During coagulation, platelets adhere to each other by attaching to adhesion receptors, known as integrins, found on their outer lining. They then attach to the underside of the endothelial cells that are lining the damaged wall of the blood vessel. When many platelets aggregate together in a given area, they are called a platelet plug. As the clot formation continues, the protein fibrin is deposited, forming a mesh-like structure, and the platelet plug becomes a stable clot (Figure 37-9). DOT 5-9.14

The Inflammatory Process

The body responds to infection and trauma through a process called **inflammation.** The cells that are involved in the inflammatory process are distributed throughout the body, and when an infection or trauma occurs, those cells are "called" to the infection or injured site so that the area can be walled off from the rest of the body and healing can begin. In order for these cells to migrate to the area, three processes must occur. DOT 5-9.9

- First, the blood supply to the affected area is increased.

- Then, permeability in the capillary bed, small arterioles, and venules is increased, so WBCs can leave the bloodstream through the small openings forming in the membranes.

- Finally, leukocytes migrate through the blood vessel wall (by diapedesis) to the site of infection. As previously described, this process is called chemotaxis. The leukocytes that show up early in the process of fighting an infection are the neutrophils

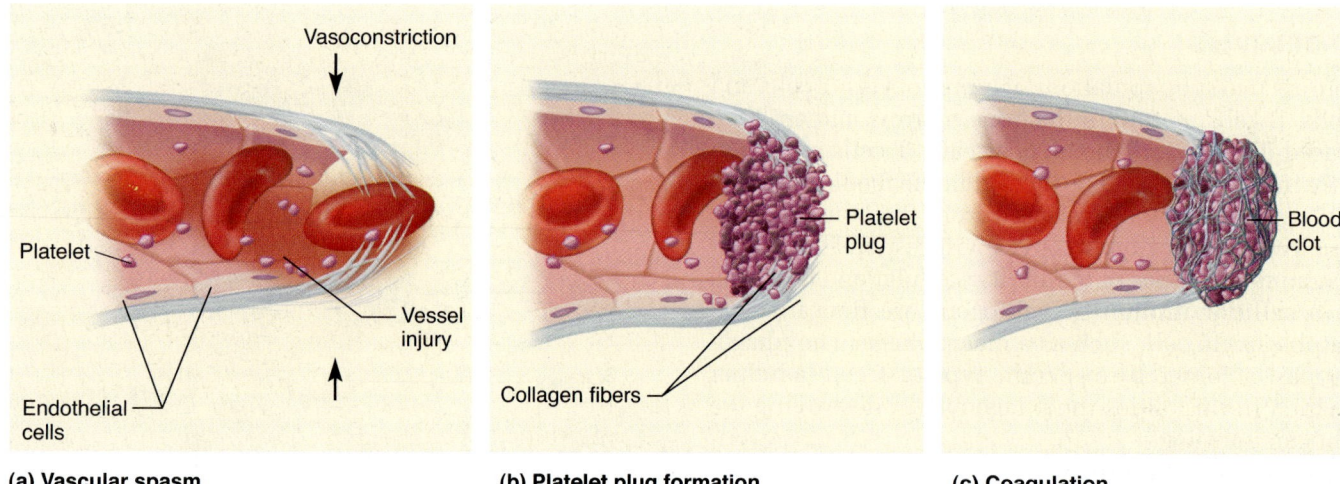

(a) Vascular spasm　　　　**(b) Platelet plug formation**　　　　**(c) Coagulation**

Figure 37-9　The process of clot formation.

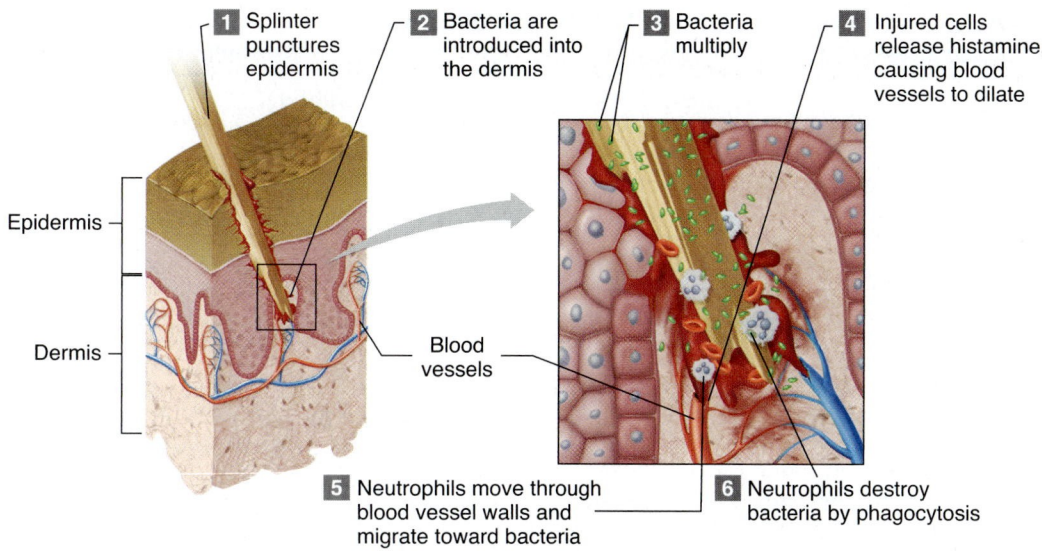

1 Splinter punctures epidermis

2 Bacteria are introduced into the dermis

3 Bacteria multiply

4 Injured cells release histamine, causing blood vessels to dilate

Epidermis

Dermis

Blood vessels

5 Neutrophils move through blood vessel walls and migrate toward bacteria

6 Neutrophils destroy bacteria by phagocytosis

Figure 37-10 Neutrophils are the first cells to start the fight against an infection.

(Figure 37-10). Monocytes and lymphocytes arrive later. DOT 5-9.9

Hemostatic Mechanisms

Hemostasis is restored when bleeding from an injured vessel is stopped. The process requires three mechanisms to work together in a coordinated effort to be successful.

1. When a blood vessel is damaged, the vessel first spasms and constricts, slowing the flow of blood into the damaged area.

2. Platelets will not adhere to normal vessel endothelial cells; however, they will adhere to the subendothelial cells that are exposed in the damaged vessel. The platelets become "sticky" and adhere to the damaged area, beginning to form a platelet plug.

3. The last mechanism is the deposition of fibrin on the platelet plug to form a stable fibrin clot. **Thrombosis** is clot formation while **fibrinolysis** (lysis means destruction) is the process that occurs to break down the clot. DOT 5-9.15, 5-9.20

These mechanisms are regulated by several factors. Platelets release two chemicals, serotonin and thromboxane A_2, which aide in vasoconstriction and initiate vessel repair. Thromboxane A_2 also causes platelet aggregation. Endothelial cells secrete von Willebrand's factor, which is needed for proper platelet adhesion. As long as these factors and others in this process work appropriately, bleeding will be stopped by clot formation, the injury will heal, and the clot will be dismantled. However, as will be seen later in the chapter, these processes do not always work appropriately. DOT 5-9.15

The Coagulation Cascade

The coagulation cascade can be stimulated by one of two pathways: the extrinsic or intrinsic pathway. The extrinsic pathway is activated by a damaged blood vessel, and the intrinsic pathway is activated by platelets damaged in turbulent blood flow through a damaged vessel. Eventually, both pathways converge into a common pathway. It is important to realize that once a clot is formed, the coagulation cascade does not stop, rather fibrinolysis begins to occur almost as soon as the clot finishes forming. Fibrinolysis begins as plasminogen is released from the clot. Plasminogen is converted to plasmin, which is a serine protease that is capable of lysing (breaking up) the clot. DOT 5-9.16, 5-9.17

Because there are so many steps in the clotting process, diseases can cause a breakdown of the process at any step along the pathways. The diseases hemophilia A and hemophilia B are both inherited disorders. In each, a key coagulation factor is deficient, resulting in a longer time frame for clotting to occur. Hemophilia will be discussed in more detail later in the chapter. Von Willebrand's disease is the most common inherited blood disorder and causes a deficiency in the von Willebrand's factor.[7]

Medications can also have an effect on the factors involved in the coagulation cascade. Heparin activates antithrombin III, which prevents thrombin formation. Warfarin sodium (Coumadin) prevents the vitamin K-dependent reactions that are necessary for thrombin and clotting factors VII, IV, and X to function properly. Aspirin blocks platelet aggregation by reducing the production of thromboxane A_2. All three of these drugs interfere with the normal blood clotting cascade, which could lead to difficult-to-control bleeding situations. DOT 5-9.16, 5-9.17

TABLE 37-2   Antigens and Antibodies of the ABO Blood Groups

Blood type	Antigen	Antibody
A	A	Anti-B
B	B	Anti-A
AB (universal recipient)	A and B	Neither anti-A nor anti-B
O (universal donor)	Neither A nor B	Both anti-A and anti-B

ABO Blood Types

Medically, the most important advance for blood transfusions was recognition of the ABO blood types discovered in 1900.[2] There are four types of blood in this blood group: A, B, AB, and O (Table 37-2). These types are based on the surface antigen or lack of surface antigen, on the red blood cell and the antibody or lack of antibody, that is produced. DOT 5-9.18

- Type A blood has surface antigen A but does not have surface antigen B. In addition, type A blood has anti-B antibody present but does not have anti-A antibody present.
- Type B blood contains surface antigen B but not surface antigen A, and anti-A antibody but not anti-B antibody.
- Type AB blood has both surface antigen A and surface antigen B, but does not have either antibody present.
- Type O blood has neither surface antigen present but has both antibodies present.

Rh Blood Types

Many other surface antigens are also present on the surface of the red blood cells. The second most important blood type for transfusion purposes is the Rh factor, also known as surface antigen D.[2] When this surface antigen is present, the person is Rh^+, and if it is absent, the person is Rh^-. Rh^- people make antibodies against the Rh^+ surface antigen, but Rh^+ people do not make antibodies against Rh^- blood. It is important to match the Rh factor of the recipient's blood with that of the donor's blood as a mismatch in this surface antigen can lead to a hemolytic reaction. Approximately 15% of the population lacks the Rh antigen. DOT 5-9.19

Erythroblastosis fetalis is a rare but sometimes fatal hemolytic disease seen in Rh^+ newborns in which an Rh^- mother has been sensitized to the Rh^+ surface antigen. The mother's exposure could be from a previous pregnancy in which the fetus was Rh^+ or from a blood transfusion of Rh^+ blood. The previous exposure causes the mother to make antibodies against the Rh^+ surface antigen. As with any antibody-antigen situation, any future encounter with the Rh^+ surface antigen will bring about an attack by that antibody on the red blood cell, that has that antigen, leading to its subsequent destruction. However, today it is common for Rh^- mothers to receive a RhoGAM immunization, which inhibits the formation of anti-Rh antibodies. All pregnant women should be checked for their Rh status in the third trimester of pregnancy prior to delivery.[7] The incidence of this disease has dropped dramatically in the United States since the introduction of ABO and Rh compatibility testing. Few infants manifest any signs of incompatibility, even though the rate of incompatibility with Rh in the United States is 20–25%.[8]

Because type O Rh^- blood has none of the three major surface antigens present, it is considered the universal donor. On the other hand, type AB blood has neither antibody present, so it is the universal recipient.

Transfusion Reactions

Acute intravascular hemolysis (a transfusion reaction) is usually due to ABO incompatibility. The reported frequency is approximately one in 38,000 transfusions. The most common cause of the reaction is human error by misidentification of a patient, blood specimen, or transfusion unit. These reactions are often severe. The risk of a fatal hemolytic reaction is about one in 100,000 transfusions or one to four per one million units of blood product transfused. The fatality rate from a transfusion reaction is 50%.[9,10] In awake patients, symptoms include chills, fever, nausea, and chest and flank pain.[9]

Cross matching blood prior to administering it reduces the likelihood of a transfusion reaction. When cross matching is performed for the ABO and Rh types, the incidence of a transfusion reaction is less than 1%.[9] The process involves taking blood from the donor and the recipient and mixing it together to see if the blood clumps, or agglutinates. If the blood does not agglutinate, then the two blood types are compatible; however, if agglutination occurs, then they are not compatible. DOT 5-9.18, 5-9.19

Although cross matching is the standard of care in the hospital setting, it is not practical for EMS to perform the procedure. It takes time to perform the test (five minutes for ABO and Rh and 45 minutes for other antibody tests), and the materials to conduct the test are sensitive to temperature changes.

There are many other surface antigens on red blood cells that can lead to nonhemolytic reactions. Nonhemolytic reactions do not involve the actual destruction of blood cells, but the patient is still reacting to the blood transfusion. Signs and symptoms of a nonhemolytic reaction are fever, chills, diaphoresis, hypertension, and tachycardia.

Blood and blood products are not used very often in the prehospital setting. They require specific storage temperature ranges (some products must be kept frozen until used), do not have a long shelf life (requiring frequent replacement), and are dangerous if given without proper cross checking of blood type. Some parts of the country with transport times longer than a few hours may need to use blood products. Some interfacility or critical care transports may have patients with infusions of blood or blood products. It is possible that such a patient could have a transfusion reaction while the ambulance service is transporting the patient. Depending on your treatment protocol or guideline, these types of transports may require other health professionals (nurses, physician assistants, or transfusionists) to accompany the patient in the ambulance.

It is also possible for a patient to receive a transfusion of blood or blood products and be discharged within hours or days of the procedure. Some transfusion reactions may be delayed for up to 10 days before the patient develops any signs or symptoms.[10] Although the incidence of transfusion reactions is low, it may happen, and because there is such a high mortality rate, it is important for the paramedic to be aware of the signs and symptoms and appropriate treatment.

Hemolytic reactions involve the destruction of red blood cells because the antibodies present in the recipient's blood attack the donor's blood. Destruction of the red blood cells leads to the release of toxins, which results in organ failure and death.

Signs and symptoms of a hemolytic reaction can include any of the following: hyperventilation, tachycardia, facial flushing, hives, fever, chills, chest pain, and wheezing. If the signs and symptoms are seen early in the reaction, it is possible to prevent end organ failure and death if treatment is begun immediately.

Prehospital guidelines will vary, depending on the availability of some of the medications or the ability to perform some of the procedures such as urinary catheterization. If a transfusion reaction is suspected, immediately stop the transfusion, and change out all blood and IV tubing. Start two large bore IVs of normal saline or lactated Ringer's, and administer enough fluid to maintain good perfusion. This means titrate the volume infused to obtain the blood pressure target established per your protocol. If no guideline exists, ensure the patient has peripheral pulses in the extremities. Of course on-line direction via consultation is always appropriate if you do not have a clear guideline or standing order to follow or if you are unsure as to how to proceed. Be sure to monitor the patient closely for signs of overhydration.[9]

Medications such as diphenhydramine (Benadryl™), epinephrine, or steroids may be indicated if signs and symptoms of an allergic reaction appear. Since hypotension can lead to renal failure and further build-up of toxic by-products, consider administering furosemide (Lasix) or other diuretic to promote excretion of the toxins from the body. Rapid transport is critical for these patients. Monitor vital signs, and use the cardiac monitor. Administer oxygen as well. Select the appropriate adjunct and delivery device based upon the patient's signs and symptoms, level of consciousness, and vital signs.

Overview of the Assessment and Management of the Hematologic System

Because the hematologic and immune systems are closely related, when there is a problem with one system, it often affects the other. Although hematological disorders are fairly common, they are rarely an emergency with the exception of a transfusion reaction. Using good aseptic technique and protecting these patients from infections is highly important as most of these patients will have alterations in their immune systems.

Primary Survey

The patient with a hematologic complaint should receive a standard ABC primary survey. Any life-threatening problems noted should be addressed before proceeding to the secondary survey. Since few hematologic complaints are life-threatening, the secondary survey may be started prior to initiating transport.

Upon questioning a patient with a hematological disorder about the chief complaint, the symptoms may seem vague or unrelated. Sometimes a patient may have an acute problem, such as trauma, that is impacted by the hematologic disorder. The classic example is the patient who has hemophilia and has a laceration with heavy bleeding. It may require administering the patient's own prescribed clotting factors along with standard bleeding control measures to effectively manage the emergency.[11] Oxygen support will be necessary for many of these patients to prevent hypoxia, and fluid replacement may be necessary to support perfusion.

Secondary Survey

Patients with hematological disorders often have crossover complications with other body systems. A thorough and complete assessment is crucial to uncover all of the signs and symptoms that are present. The following provides focus for your assessment of patients with known or suspected hematologic disorders. DOT 5-9.21, 5-9.23

Skin

Excessive paleness, also called **pallor,** often indicates loss of circulating blood volume, but it may indicate the patient has anemia. Anemia is a lack of the proper number of RBCs, a lack of the proper blood volume, or a deficiency in hemoglobin. Yellowing of the skin (called jaundice) may indicate the patient has liver failure or a significant amount of hemolysis of red blood cells. Facial flushing can be a sign of polycythemia, which is an overabundance of red blood cells. Thrombocytopenia may present with petechiae, which appear as a rash-like discoloration made up of small, pinpoint sized hemorrhages just under the skin. Deep hematomas (large, dark bruises), hemarthroses (hemorrhage found within joints), and purpura (purplish patches of discoloration from bleeding into skin or mucous membranes) may indicate a coagulation disorder. Leg and ankle ulcers may be present in patients with sickle cell anemia. Each of these conditions will be discussed in more detail. DOT 5-9.7, 5-9.22d

Street Secrets

Assess the conjunctiva of the eyes when looking for signs of anemia. This is one of the most sensitive areas to check. A normal conjunctiva should appear pink, if it is pale and colorless, that is a good indication the patient may be anemic.

Cardiorespiratory

Tachycardia (fast heart rate) and tachypnea (fast respiratory rate) are commonly present in patients with anemia. Anemic patients also may exhibit dyspnea upon exertion (DOE), which is trouble breathing or becoming out of breath with mild to moderate exertion because they don't have enough red blood cells to carry an adequate supply of oxygen. Orthostatic changes in blood pressure can also occur. Orthostatic changes are noted as a drop in the blood pressure of 20 mmHg or greater with the positional change from sitting to standing or from lying down to sitting.[10] Tachycardia may accompany the orthostatic drop in blood pressure change as the body attempts to compensate for the drop. Patients

with polycythemia often have angina and hypertension as a result of the blood thickening from the extra cells. Microemboli (extremely small clots of just a few blood cells that lodge in or near capillary beds) often form in their blood, resulting in tiny areas of ischemia (lack of oxygen) or infarction (tissue death) in organs or tissues. If the area is small enough, it may cause only minor tissue or organ dysfunction, but if it is large enough, it could cause death.

Gastrointestinal and Genitourinary

Inflammation in the spleen, lymphatic ducts, and liver is often seen in patients with hematological disorders. Collected debris from dead cells can result in damage to the liver or kidneys. Pallor of the mucous membranes may indicate anemia. Frequent bleeding from the nose and gums may indicate a coagulation abnormality.

Neurological

Headaches and dizziness are common with anemia or polycythemia. Thrombotic thrombocytopenic purpura (bleeding into the skin and mucous membranes) may be present along with altered mental status, dysphasia (problems with speaking or understanding language), coma, seizures, paresis (slight or partial paralysis), and visual disturbances. Patients with coagulation disruptions may suffer hemorrhages in the brain, which can result in a stroke with or without increased intracranial pressure. DOT 5-9.21

Red Blood Cell Disorders

Anemia

Anemia is classified into one of three groups centered on the cause:

1. Marrow production deficit or hypoproliferation anemia
2. Ineffective erythropoiesis, resulting in red cell maturation deficit anemia
3. Anemia caused by decreased red cell survival due to blood loss or hemolysis[2]

Anemia is suspected with a hematocrit level less than 37% in women or less than 40% in men. Most people with anemia are often not symptomatic until the hematocrit levels drop below 30%.[12] DOT 5-9.22a

Anemias from marrow production deficit include aplastic, iron-deficiency, megaloblastic (pernicious), and sickle cell anemia. At least 75% of all cases of anemia are the result of absolute or relative failure of the bone marrow.[2] The majority of hypoproliferative anemias are due to mild to moderate iron deficiency or inflammation. Cell maturation anemias occur in some chronic disease states such as renal failure, infection, and cancer. Decreased cell survival anemias include hemolytic anemia, thalassemia (also called Cooley's anemia), and blood loss that is either acute or chronic.

Marrow Production and Hypoproliferation Anemias

Aplastic anemia is seen when the bone marrow is incapable of producing sufficient numbers of red blood cells due to a decrease in the number of pluripotent stem cells. Causes may include viral infections, exposure to toxic chemicals, antibiotic therapy, antiseizure medications, and cancer medications. Treatments may include blood transfusions, medications, or bone marrow transplants.

The most common form of anemia is iron deficiency anemia, which occurs with excessive bleeding or a lack of iron intake or absorption. Treatment includes addressing the underlying cause of the bleeding and treating with oral iron supplements. IM or IV iron supplements may be needed in patients with poor intake or absorption of iron.[3]

Megaloblastic anemia is caused by a deficiency in vitamin B_{12}, folate, or both. It is caused by a decrease in the ability of the GI tract to absorb these elements. Vitamin B_{12} is necessary for the body to process carbohydrates and produce red blood cells. Megaloblastic anemia is mostly inherited but may be caused by surgery of the stomach or small intestine, abnormal bacterial growth in the small intestine, Crohn's disease, or celiac disease. However, it is rarely caused by a diet lacking in vitamin B_{12}.[13] Treatment includes IM or SQ injections of B_{12} for patients deficient in vitamin B_{12} absorption and oral folate supplements for patients with a folate deficiency. DOT 5-9.22a

Sickle cell anemia will be discussed in a section by itself. Although it is not the most common type of anemia, it is frequently encountered by EMS providers.

Cell Maturation Anemias

Anemia seen in chronic diseases is caused by several factors. One is the inability of the phagocytes to recycle iron, which leads to a decrease in the amount of iron available for new red blood cell formation. Second is an increase in the number of macrophages produced, which leads to cytokine release and suppression of red blood cell production. Other causes are a reduction in the life span of the red blood cell and a decrease in erythropoietin levels. Treatment may include any of the following: correcting the underlying cause, transfusion, or recombinant erythropoietin therapy.[14]

Blood Loss and Hemolytic Anemias

Thalassemia is marked by abnormal and short-lived red blood cells. Thalassemia major, also known as **Cooley's anemia,** is a severe form of anemia that causes rapid red blood cell destruction and deposition of iron in the skin and vital organs. Thalassemia minor involves only mild anemia and minimal red blood cell changes. Treatment for thalassemia major is a blood transfusion every two to three weeks.

Hemolytic anemia is characterized by destruction of red blood cells. This condition can be either congenital or acquired and can vary in severity. Hemolytic anemia is the rarest form of anemia.[2] About 90% of congenital hemolytic anemia is due to a deficiency in glucose-6-phosphate dehydrogenase and pyruvate kinase. A deficiency in these enzymes causes the cells to lyse when exposed to certain kinds of stressors such as oxidative stress, drugs, pregnancy, and infections. Treatment for patients with a glucose-6-phosphate dehydrogenase deficiency is hydration and avoidance of oxidative medications while treatment for patients with pyruvate kinase deficiency may include transfusion and splenectomy.[3] Many different factors may be the cause of an acquired hemolytic anemia, such as abnormal microvasculature, thrombotic thrombocytopenic purpura, and disseminated intravascular coagulation.[3] Treatment focuses on treating the underlying condition.

Prehospital Treatment For Anemia

Prehospital treatment of anemia will require a thorough patient assessment. The ABCs should be supported, as necessary. Vital signs should be monitored frequently. Monitor for occult bleeding. Oxygen should be given to these patients as the total number of red blood cells available to transport oxygen to the cells is diminished and the patient is often hypoxic. Transport in a position of comfort.

Sickle Cell Disease

Sickle cell disease is possibly the most common form of anemia encountered by prehospital care providers; thus, it is important to understand the physiology of this disease process. Sickle cell anemia is an autosomal recessive disease, meaning a sickle cell gene must be obtained from each parent in order to actually develop the disease. Sickle cell disease is most common in dark skinned individuals such as Africans. The gene is carried by 8% of African Americans, and one birth out of every four hundred in American blacks will produce a child with sickle cell anemia.[10] The condition sickle cell trait results when only one recessive gene is inherited. Patients with sickle cell trait rarely experience any symptoms of the disease except in low-oxygen environments such as a high altitude.[15,16] Patients with sickle cell disease typically die from organ failure after a long history of multiple system problems. Although there is no specific preventative treatment for the disease, patients who take folic acid supplements and who also receive prompt care in a crisis have an average life expectancy between forty and fifty years of age.[10]

Pathophysiology of Sickle Cell Anemia

Normal hemoglobin is called hemoglobin A. Hemoglobin in sickle cell anemia is hemoglobin S. Hemoglobin S is an abnormal, sickle-shaped hemoglobin molecule that has inferior oxygen-carrying capacity. Hemoglobin S is formed when the amino acid valine is substituted for glutamic acid in the sixth amino acid position of the beta globulin chain of hemoglobin from both parents.[17] Hemoglobin S crystallizes when it is exposed to low oxygen states, causing the red blood cells to sickle in shape. These sickle-shaped cells are destroyed easily, and their life span is reduced to 10 to 20 days (Figure 37-11).

Sickle cell crisis can be triggered by dehydration, low oxygen states, low pH, infection, trauma, extremes in temperature, and strenuous physical activity. Sickle cell crisis occurs when the rigid, sickle cells become lodged in the microvasculature of the body, causing vaso-occlusion. Patients suffer extreme and intense pain with occlusion of the microvasculature due to the lack of oxygen being supplied to that area. Infarction of the tissue or organ can occur if oxygen supply is not returned quickly. People with sickle cell crisis are at an increased risk of CVA, kidney failure, retinal damage,

and infarction of the tissues of the fingers and toes that may result in the need for amputation. Splenic infarction is common as well due to the occlusion of vessels in the spleen. As the spleen is damaged from the recurrent infarctions, scarring develops and the organ shrinks in size. This condition is known as autosplenectomy. Acute chest syndrome results if the vaso-occlusion occurs in the lungs. This decreases the flow of blood through the lungs and can be life-threatening.

Street Secrets

Both strenuous exercise and dehydration can cause a right shift of the oxyhemoglobin dissociation curve. For the sickle cell patient, the loss of oxygen can lead to a sickle cell crisis event.

Treatment of Sickle Cell Disease

Treatment of sickle cell disease involves hydration of the patient to decrease blood viscosity and to maintain perfusion of the kidneys. High-flow oxygen via nonrebreather mask should be administered since red blood cells are more likely to sickle in the low oxygen state. Pain is normally severe, so pain medications such as meperidine (Demerol ™) or morphine should be administered to patients in sickle cell crisis. Infection control measures should be instituted since these patients are normally immunocompromised. Hospital care may include a blood transfusion. DOT 5-9.22g

Street Secrets

The level of pain a patient experiences during a sickle cell crisis is excruciating. It is appropriate to provide pain medication to these patients. If medical direction is needed, perform the consult as soon as possible.

Polycythemia

Polycythemia is an increase in the number of red blood cells, which results in an increase in the hematocrit level. Hematocrit levels greater than 50% in men or 45% in women are slightly abnormal, but hematocrits over 60% in men and 55% in women are almost always associated with increased red cell numbers. Patients with polycythemia often have one of the following in their history: smoking, living at a high altitude, congenital heart disease, peptic ulcer disease, sleep apnea, chronic lung disease, or renal disease.[2] DOT 5-9.22d

Neurologic symptoms such as vertigo, tinnitus, headache, and visual disturbances may occur. Hypertension is often present. Patients may have easy bruising, epistaxis (nose bleed), or bleeding from the

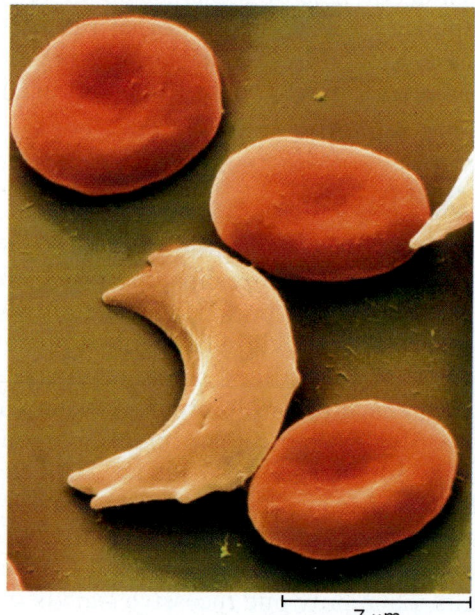

7 μm

Figure 37-11   Sickle-shaped cells found in sickle cell anemia.

gastrointestinal tract. Patients with hypoxemia may develop cyanosis on minimal exertion or have a headache, impaired mental acuity, and fatigue.[2]

Polycythemia causes an increase in the viscosity of the blood, vascular insufficiency and decreased tissue oxygenation and leads to an increased risk of thrombosis (clot formation). Thrombosis formation may lead to a heart attack, stroke, occlusion of the large veins (called deep vein thrombosis), or a pulmonary embolus (blood clot in the circulatory system of the lung). It can also cause bleeding complications due to the relative dilution of platelets.[14]

Treatment for patients with emergencies from polycythemia includes the administration of supplemental oxygen, initiation of IV therapy with an isotonic crystalloid solution, ECG monitoring, and support of the ABCs, as necessary. Long-term therapy in the hospital may include phlebotomy (removal of the excess blood volume) and bone marrow suppression to slow the formation of new RBCs. DOT 5-9.22d

White Blood Cell Disorders

Introduction to Lymphoma and Leukemia

Malignancies of lymphoid cells range from extremely aggressive and life-threatening to those causing little pain and growing slowly. All of these cancers arise from cells of the immune system at different stages of growth and development, resulting in a wide range of immunological, morphological (varying shapes), and clinical findings. Some malignancies of the lymphoid cells almost always result in leukemia, especially those primarily involving bone marrow and blood. Other malignancies present as solid tumors of the immune system. These are called lymphoma. There are other malignancies that can begin as either leukemia or lymphoma and can change over the course of the illness. In other words, the patient begins with one condition, for example lymphoma, and later leukemia develops. The frequency with which the disease progresses from one form to the other is about 1% of all cases.[2]

Leukemia

Leukemia is a cancer of the blood-forming stem cells located in the bone marrow. There are two major types of leukemia, myelogenous or lymphocytic, and each of these has acute and chronic forms.[10] Acute forms of leukemia have cells that proliferate quickly and do not develop properly while the chronic forms of leukemia have cells that do not die normally. Acute leukemias develop rapidly and affect immature cells while chronic leukemias have a slower progression and affect mature cells. DOT 5-9.22b

The overall survival rate for all types of leukemia combined is about 50%.[7] Adults with leukemia are more likely to have **acute myelogenous leukemia (AML)** or **chronic lymphocytic leukemia (CLL).** Another form of acute leukemia, **lymphoblastic leukemia (ALL),** makes up 20% of all cases of leukemia in adults, and it is the most common form found in children. AML is found mainly in adults. The average age when a patient first notices the signs of the disease is around 60. The incidence of AML increases with age.[7]

Children are more likely to have one of the acute forms of leukemia than a chronic form. Eighty percent of the type of acute leukemia found in children is acute lymphoblastic leukemia. The peak age of the disease in childhood is between three and seven. Survival rates are higher for children than adults.[7]

Leukemia Pathophysiology

Most cases of acute leukemia arise with no obvious cause although radiation, chemotherapy, and some toxins have been shown to cause it.[7] These cancerous cells may have an exaggerated proliferation (meaning too many develop) or a development problem where immature cells are released from the bone marrow. This leads to functional immaturity with an inappropriate response when stimulated to protect the body from invaders. Other problems that arise for leukemia cells are that some do not die when they should, which again causes an increase in the number of white blood cells. These cells are also functionally immature and, therefore, not as effective in providing immunity.

Signs and symptoms of leukemia include frequent infections, poor healing of minor wounds, anemia, bleeding or easy bruising, fatigue, fevers, night sweats, and weight loss. Other symptoms may include headache; confusion; balance problems; blurry vision; abdominal pain or swelling; pain in other areas including the neck, underarms, groin, bones, joints, and testicles; loss of muscle control; and seizures. Some patients are at risk for developing a life-threatening condition called disseminated intravascular coagulation, or DIC. DIC is extremely difficult to treat outside of the hospital.

Prehospital Treatment for Leukemia

Prehospital treatment of patients with leukemia should be targeted to support the ABCs and provide relief of any symptoms presented.[7] Use appropriate aseptic technique when managing these patients as their immune system is weakened, putting them at risk for infection.[7] Many of these patients may be complaining of the nausea, vomiting, and weakness that follow chemotherapy or radiation treatments. They may also report having a great deal of fatigue. Perform a thorough patient assessment, and look for signs of dehydration or altered mental status. Supplemental oxygen should be given if patients have any sign of hypoxia. If patients are dehydrated, provide fluid therapy and transport to the hospital. Some patients may present with an altered mental status (AMS). The standard protocol for treating patients with AMS is appropriate for the person with leukemia. This includes performing glucose monitoring. If patients are stable, transport them in a position of comfort to the hospital for evaluation of the chief complaint. Analgesics should be considered for patients in significant pain. DOT 5-9.22b

Lymphoma

Lymphoma is a cancer of the lymphocytes and consists of about 35 different subtypes. All lymphomas are characterized into one of two categories. The first category is **Hodgkin's lymphoma,** also known as Hodgkin's disease, and the other category is **non-Hodgkin's lymphoma.** Hodgkin's lymphoma and non-Hodgkin's lymphoma have very similar symptoms, and they are also hard to distinguish upon physical exam. Laboratory evaluation is needed to find the exact cell type that is being affected to differentiate the two types of lymphoma. Hodgkin's lymphoma affects a specific subtype of B lymphocytes while non-Hodgkin's lymphoma affects other B lymphocytes or T lymphocytes. There are five subtypes of Hodgkin's lymphoma and thirty subtypes of non-Hodgkin's lymphoma, and while they may appear the same, their therapies and cure rates are different.[18] DOT 5-9.22c

Other conditions present with the same signs and symptoms as lymphoma, which makes the diagnosis more difficult. Drug reactions, particularly to phenytoin or carbamezepine (both are antiseizure medications) can mimic the signs of lymphoma. Other immune system disorders such as rheumatoid arthritis and lupus or certain viral infections (cytomegalovirus and Epstein-Barr virus) or bacterial infections such as cat scratch fever can have similar signs and symptoms to those of lymphoma.[2] About 10% of lymphomas present in the head and neck. The frequency of lymphoma arising in AIDS patients is an increasing concern due to the difficulty in managing these patients because of complications from their disease.[18] The cure rate for lymphoma in children is around 85%, and around 50% of adults are long-term survivors.[2]

Signs and symptoms of lymphoma include swollen lymph nodes, enlargement of the spleen, pain from swollen lymph nodes pressing on nerves and vessels, fever, chills, unexplained weight loss, night sweats, lack of energy, and itching.[18] Prehospital management of patients with lymphoma is the same as the leukemia patient; support the ABCs, and perform a thorough history for the hospital to use in guiding further treatment.

DOT 5-9.22c

Multiple Myeloma

Multiple myeloma is a disorder affecting plasma cells characterized by replacement of healthy bone marrow with cancerous cells, bone destruction, and paraprotein formation. Paraproteins are abnormal serum globulins with unique physical characteristics that prevent them from functioning normally. Myeloma is a disease found primarily in older adults with a median age at the time of diagnosis of 65 years of age.[2] DOT 5-9.22h

Multiple Myeloma Pathophysiology

Plasma cells differentiate from B cells and are the cells responsible for producing immunoglobulins (antibodies). Cancerous plasma cells accumulate in the bone marrow and overproduce immunoglobulins. The excess paraproteins are known as M proteins.[14]

The pathophysiology of myeloma includes a decrease in the production of red blood cells, white blood cells, and platelets due to overcrowding in the bone marrow of cancerous plasma cells. Increased blood viscosity and electrolyte imbalances are seen due to the increase in the circulating immunoglobulins. Renal dysfunction is common as a result of the decrease in perfusion to the kidneys. Bone destruction, pain, fractures, and hypercalcemia occur from cytokines produced by the M proteins. Immunosuppression will ensue from the lack of normal immunoglobulins being produced.[14]

Prehospital Treatment for Myeloma

Many patients with multiple myeloma are asymptomatic, meaning they may be unaware they even have the disease because they have no signs or symptoms of the problem.[10] Patients with myeloma often seek treatment because of signs or symptoms associated with renal failure or spinal cord compression or because they are experiencing problems stemming from the **hyperviscosity** (thickening) of the blood. Renal failure often occurs without any obvious signs or symptoms in patients. However, as the condition worsens, patients may note a decrease in the volume of urine produced or the frequency of urination. They may also note the presence of blood in the urine as the number of cells present reaches a quantity sufficient enough for them to see a change in color. Spinal cord compression can result in intense pain, numbness, tingling, sensations of heat or cold, or any other common indication that nerves are irritated. Hyperviscous blood can present as mucosal bleeding, vertigo, nausea, visual disturbances, or altered mental status.[2]

Examination may reveal pallor, bone tenderness, and masses in the soft tissues. Patients may have an enlarged tongue, neuropathy, hepatomegaly (enlarged liver), or congestive heart failure. If they also have an infection present, fever is likely.[10] The most common presenting complaints are those related to anemia, bone pain, and infection. Bone pain is by far the most common complaint for these patients. It is generally localized to the back or ribs. Lumbar pain is the primary symptom in over 70% of all patients with myeloma.[7,10]

The patient may also have pathologic fractures.[7] A **pathologic fracture** is a fracture that results from the bone being porous and brittle or weakened from tumor cells. It does not take much force for a patient with this condition to experience a pathologic fracture. It can occur without any history of trauma. They can even occur spontaneously as the patient rolls over in bed while sleeping. The patient is frequently in a lot of pain, and gentle movements are critical.

Treatment may include chemotherapy, radiation, and glucocorticoid therapy. Prehospital treatment will include supporting the ABCs as appropriate. As previously mentioned, handle these patients gently, and if they are not in a life-threatening state, allow them to progress through positional changes and treatments at their own pace. This will help them maintain some control and dignity and may minimize pain. Administer oxygen as tolerated and indicated by the vital signs and clinical findings. IV fluid therapy should be instituted for any patient experiencing dehydration from the nausea and vomiting that is common with chemotherapy and radiation treatments. Patients experiencing significant pain should be given analgesics. Fractures should be splinted as appropriate, making sure that pulse, motor function, and sensation are consistent both before and after splinting. Special attention should be paid to using aseptic techniques to protect the patient from infection. Transport in a position of comfort with lots of padding to support the patient and minimize movements once they are settled on the ambulance cot. DOT 5-9.22h

Coagulation Disorders

Coagulation disorders can be acquired, congenital, or inherited (genetic). Acquired coagulation diseases occur as a result of other primary problems such as liver disease or sepsis. A congenital disease is a form of the acquired disease process that comes about during fetal development. The developing baby is exposed to a disease. Congenital problems are not due to genetics or heredity but are the result of something in the environment or an event (such as infection) that occurs during pregnancy.[2] For example, exposure of the mother to the cytomegalovirus or rubella may result in the infant acquiring many complications, including thrombocytopenia coagulation disorder.[6]

Patients with congenital coagulation defects typically bleed into muscles, joints, and body cavities for hours or days after an injury occurs. Most inherited coagulation disorders are due to defects in a single protein line factor such as factor VIII or IX deficiency, which account for the majority of inherited disorders. These patients may have severe bleeding and chronic disability. Most of these disorders prolong clotting time once bleeding occurs.[2]

Acquired coagulation diseases are more frequent and complex. They may arise from deficiencies in multiple coagulation proteins, which can affect multiple parts of the coagulation cascade. The most common acquired disorders are, in order, disseminated intravascular coagulation (DIC), hemorrhagic problems in liver disease, and vitamin K deficiency.[2] Occasionally, patients receiving medications to prevent coagulation may bleed as well.

The incidence of congenital and acquired bleeding disorders is relatively rare. For example, the incidence of factor VII deficiency is predominant in males and occurs at a rate of one per five thousand male births.[19]

Disseminated Intravascular Coagulation

Disseminated intravascular coagulation (DIC) is a systemic triggering of the coagulation cascade, resulting in the body becoming depleted of coagulation factors as many clots are formed and broken down.[6] In the normal clot formation response of hemostasis, the process is confined to a local area in response to injury, and the clotting factors are replaced as they are used. DIC, however, results in widespread thrombus formation in the microvasculature with depletion of platelets and other coagulation factors, which are not quickly replaceable. During the DIC process, bleeding and thrombosis are occurring simultaneously. DOT 5-9.22e

DIC is associated with a variety of disorders, including infection (mainly bacterial and leading to sepsis), surgery (from fat embolism), burns, liver disease, obstetrical complications, malignant tumors (adenocarcinoma, acute leukemia, and lymphoma), and environmental disorders (for example, hyperthermia or animal or insect envenomation).[7] DIC can occur acutely or become a chronic condition that can be managed as episodes occur.

Pathophysiology of DIC

Activation of the coagulation cascade system also activates the fibrinolytic system, which utilizes the hormone plasmin to degrade clots. However, the breakdown of fibrin by plasminogen results in the production of toxic by-products that cause platelet dysfunction, which prevents the formation of more fibrin clots necessary to maintain hemostasis. Plasmin can also activate substances that lead to increased vascular permeability, which increases bleeding and fluid loss from the vascular system, leading to hypotension and shock.[7]

Prehospital Treatment of DIC

Clinical presentations of DIC will vary, depending on the underlying precipitating medical problem. A patient may have bleeding, thrombosis, purplish rashes looking like petechia or large, deep purple bruises, and signs of multiple organ failure. The most common presentation is unexplained bleeding. Bleeding can come from the gastrointestinal tract, genitourinary tract, a surgical wound, mucous membranes, or any incision or puncture such as an IV site.[2]

Signs may include altered mental status, the presence of gangrene, oliguria (low urine output), kidney failure, and adult respiratory distress syndrome. The rash is seen most commonly when large amounts of bacteria are present in the blood. This condition is called bacteremia. Patients who develop DIC acutely have a poor prognosis. They are difficult to manage because they are extremely difficult to stabilize. They are high-priority patients. Support their ABCs aggressively; give oxygen, provide fluid resuscitation to maintain blood pressure, and transport quickly.

Some patients develop a chronic DIC state. The prognosis for patients with chronic DIC is closely related to the prognosis for the disease that caused them to have the DIC episodes. These patients are often able to compensate for the loss of clotting factors because the bone marrow is able to keep up with the production of new platelets.[2]

Hospital treatment for DIC involves treatment of whatever is causing DIC in addition to supporting the patient and resuscitating them while they are in crisis. It may include the use of drugs to cause vasodilation or improve cardiac output or the infusion of blood or blood products, including fresh frozen plasma and platelets. Heparin remains a controversial treatment, but it may be administered in low doses to prevent clot formation and the continued consumption of clotting factors. Heparin has not been shown to be helpful in managing acute forms of DIC.[3,7] DOT 5-9.22e

Hemophilia

Hemophilia is a sex-linked, inherited bleeding disorder that is the result of low levels or the absence of certain proteins necessary for clot formation. There are two types of hemophilia (hemophilia A and hemophilia B) that account for 99% of all hemophilia disorders. Hemophilia A is characterized by low clotting factor VIII availability. Hemophilia B (also called Christmas disease) involves low levels of clotting factor IX. In the United States, hemophilia A is the most common, affecting one in 10,000 males, and hemophilia B affects approximately one in 25,000 to 35,000 patients.[7] DOT 5-9.22f

The severity of the disease is proportionate to the amount of clotting factor available in the blood. When less than 1% of the normal amount of clotting factor is available, patients have severe hemophilia. About 70% of patients with hemophilia A have a severe form. When the clotting factor level rises to 5% or more of normal, patients are considered to have a mild form of the disease.[7]

Patients with near normal levels of clotting factors may not experience any problems clotting after minor wounds or injuries and may have no problem with abrasions. Patients with levels between 25% and 50% of normal may never even be aware they have the disease. Patients with 5–25% of normal levels are classified as having mild disease and usually only bleed following trauma. Patients with factor levels of 1–5% of normal have moderate disease and may bleed spontaneously, but they too typically only bleed in response to trauma. Patients with clotting factor levels below 1% have severe disease. These people will experience severe spontaneous bleeding episodes that are difficult to control.[19]

Treatment of Hemophilia Emergencies

Signs and symptoms of hemophilia consist of bleeding in the joints **(hemarthrosis)**, bleeding of the gums, nose bleeds, and blood in the urine or stool. Intracranial bleeds can also occur and result in the same signs and symptoms seen with increasing intracranial pressure or stroke. Intracranial bleeding is the leading disease-related cause of death for hemophilia patients. Up to 80% of these intracranial hemorrhages are not trauma-related.[19]

Treatment for hemophilia consists of providing the clotting factors that are in low supply in the blood. Patients with severe hemophilia may have injectable clotting factors in their possession. Paramedics can administer these factors when directed by protocol, by standing order, or after base station contact. Infusion of the clotting factor is as important as bleeding control measures, so its use should not be delayed.[3] Focus treatment on stopping any bleeding that is occurring by using standard techniques. Treat any ABC problems, as needed. Oxygen therapy is warranted due to blood loss. If bleeding is not controllable, expedite the transport of these patients to the hospital. DOT 5-9.22f

Summary

Hematology is the study of blood and the organs involved in blood cell production and maturation. Blood consists of plasma and formed elements. Plasma consists of about 90% water, and the rest is made up of proteins, carbohydrates, lipids, electrolytes, hormones, and gases. Plasma is essential to the acid/base balance of the body as well as to maintaining a consistent vascular pressure. The formed elements consist of red blood cells, white blood cells, and platelets. Red blood cells' primary responsibility is to transport oxygen to the tissues and carbon dioxide back to the lungs. Red blood cells transport oxygen and carbon dioxide on a molecule called hemoglobin. White blood cells' responsibility is to fight off foreign invaders. White blood cells, through the use of many chemical mediators, orchestrate cellular and humoral immunity. Platelets are instrumental in the clotting process. The coagulation cascade encompasses not only the formation of the clot but also the dismantling of the clot.

Due to the complexity of the hematopoietic system, there are many areas in which disorders can occur. In this chapter, several disorders of the red blood cell, white blood cell, and platelets were discussed. Although hematological disorders are rarely an emergency, they often complicate other health problems. Thus, a complete and thorough patient assessment is needed to identify all that is wrong with patients so that they may be treated appropriately.

Notes

1. "A Dictionary of Nursing," *Oxford Reference Online* (2003), http://www.oxfordreference.com/views/ENTRY.html?subview=Main&entry=t62.e3785 (accessed September 24, 2005).
2. D. L. Kasper, E. Braunwald, A. S. Fauci, S. L. Hauser, D. L. Longo, J. L. Jameson, and K. J. Isselbacher, eds. *Harrison's Principles of Internal Medicine,* 16th ed., McGraw-Hill's AccessMedicine (accessed October 3, 2006).
3. F. C. Brunicardi, D. K. Andersen, T. R. Billiar, D. L. Dunn, J. G. Hunter, J. B. Matthews, R. E. Pollock, and S. I. Schwartz, *Schwartz's Principles of Surgery,* 8th ed., McGraw-Hill's AccessMedicine (accessed October 3, 2006).
4. E. Nester, D. Anderson, C. Robert, Jr., N. Pearsall, and M. Nester, *Microbiology: A Human Perspective,* 4th ed. (New York, NY: McGraw-Hill, 2004).
5. F. G. Cunningham, K. L. Leveno, S. L. Bloom, J. C. Hauth, L. C. Gilstrap, and K. D. Wenstrom, *Williams Obstetrics,* 22nd ed., McGraw-Hill's AccessMedicine (accessed October 3, 2006).
6. J. E. Tintinalli, G. D. Kelen, J. S. Stapczynski, O. J. Ma, and D. M. Cline, *Tintinalli's Emergency Medicine: A Comprehensive Study Guide,* 6th ed., Mcgraw-Hill's AccessMedicine (accessed October 3, 2006).
7. L. M. Tierney, S. J. McPhee, M. A. Papadakis, eds., and R. Gonzles, and R. Ziegler, online eds., *Current Medical Diagnosis and Treatment 2006,* McGraw-Hill's AccessMedicine (accessed October 3, 2006).
8. A. H. DeCherney and L. Nathan, *Current Obstetric and Gynecologic Diagnosis and Treatment,* 9th ed., McGraw-Hill's AccessMedicine (accessed October 3, 2006).
9. G. E. Morgan, M. S. Mikhail, and M. J. Murray, *Clinical Anesthesiology,* 4th ed., McGraw-Hill's AccessMedicine (accessed October 3, 2006).
10. R. L. Humphries and K. Stone, *Current Emergency Diagnosis and Treatment,* McGraw-Hill's AccessMedicine (accessed October 3, 2006).
11. Maryland Institute for Emergency Medical Systems, *The Maryland Medical Protocols for Emergency Medical Providers.* http://miemss.umaryland.edu/MdMedProtocols2006.pdf (accessed October 3, 2006).
12. J. E. South-Paul, S. C. Matheny, and E. L. Lewis, *Current Diagnosis and Treatment in Family Medicine,* McGraw-Hill's AccessMedicine (accessed October 3, 2006).
13. "Vitamin B Complex," Mama'sHealth.com http://www.mamashealth.com/blood/peranemia.asp (accessed October 3, 2006).
14. P. Morton, D. Fontaine, C. Hudak, and B. Gallo, *Critical Care Nursing: A Holistic Approach,* 8th ed. (Philadelphia, PA: Lippincott Williams & Wilkins, 2005).
15. E. Mayfield, "New Hope for People with Sickle Cell Anemia," *FDA Consumer* (May 1996), 9 May 2005, http://www.fda.gov/fdac/features/496_sick.html (accessed May 9, 2005).
16. A. Taher, "Sickle Cell Anemia" (January 2005), http://www.emedicine.com/emerg/topic26.htm (accessed May 13, 2005).
17. "The Sickle Cell Information Center," The Georgia Comprehensive Sickle Cell Center at Grady Health System, The Sickle Cell Foundation of Georgia, Inc., Emory University School of Medicine Department of Pediatrics, Atlanta, Georgia Morehouse School of Medicine (October 16, 1997), http://www.scinfo.org/prod05.htm (accessed May 5, 2005).
18. "Lymphoma Overview," http://www.emedicinehealth.com/Articles/25799-1.asp (accessed May 5, 2005).
19. W. W. Hay, M. J. Levin, J. M. Sondheimer, and R. R. Deterding, *Current Pediatric Diagnosis and Treatment,* 17th ed., McGraw-Hill's AccessMedicine (accessed October 3, 2006).

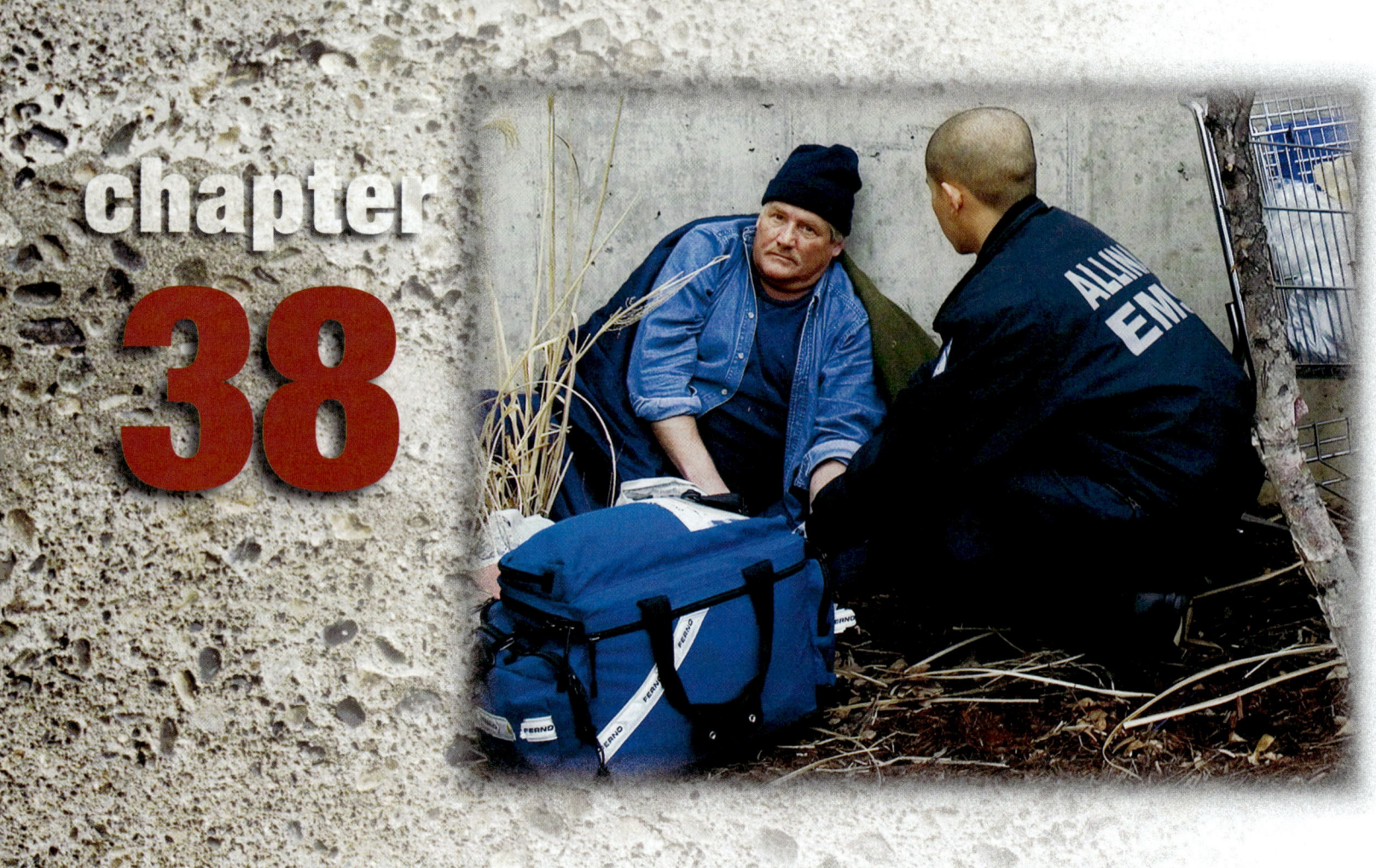

Environmental Conditions

"In wildness is the preservation of the world."

—Henry David Thoreau

Need to Know

▶ The body's response to changes in temperature.

▶ The way the body conserves and loses heat.

▶ The signs and symptoms associated with exposure to extremes of temperature.

▶ The effects of submersion, immersion, and diving-related illness.

▶ The effects of exposure to high altitudes and related signs and symptoms.

▶ The variety of bites and stings that can occur and the signs and symptoms associated with reactions to bites and stings.

▶ The potential complications sustained by patients struck by lightning.

▶ The means to provide basic and specific medical support for environmental emergencies.

▶ Sick	▶ Not Yet Sick
• Observe patients closely for the development of shock. • Do not warm a frostbitten extremity if there is a possibility of refreezing or continued cold exposure. • Immediately begin cooling patients with heat exhaustion or heat stroke. • The best treatment for altitude-induced emergencies is descent to lower atmospheric levels.	• Ensure personal safety before entering the environment. • Protect patients from further exposure. • Ask the patient if they've ever had a reaction to bites or stings or been bitten or stung before.

Introduction

Environmental emergencies are medical conditions that are induced by the interactions of physical, chemical, and biologic factors with a susceptible individual. In a sense, all medical conditions that do not originate from within (such as genetic and degenerative diseases) are environmental diseases. This would, of course, include all trauma, infectious diseases, and toxic exposures. For the sake of this discussion, however, the focus will be on some of the principle types of environmental emergencies typically associated with outdoor surroundings, including heat-related illnesses, cold-related illnesses, bites and envenomations, dysbarism, illnesses of high altitude, and lightning injuries. DOT 5-10.1, 5-10.6

Human beings can survive only in a relatively narrow span of physical conditions. In some cases, an individual can adapt to adverse conditions; in other cases, supporting equipment can make an inhospitable environment tolerable. Homeostasis is a reasonably stable state of equilibrium in the environment. Attaining homeostasis within physiologic boundaries affords protection from environmental insults.

For the prehospital provider, environmental conditions may present unique challenges. Not only can environmental conditions create disease, but they can also affect triage, treatment, and transportation decisions and potentially can place rescuers at risk as well. DOT 5-10.7,5-10.12, 5-10.17 **Skill Sheet 12: Pulse Oximetry (and Step-by-Step 12) supports this chapter.**

Temperature-Related Illness

The number of annual heat-related deaths can vary greatly with the magnitude of heat stress. During "non-heat wave" years, there has been an average of 179 deaths in the United States from heat illness. However, this number has risen to over 800 during years of extreme heat.[1] Further, there are probably at least 10 times as many "heat-aggravated illnesses" (e.g., myocardial infarction and cerebrovascular accident). Although there are multiple risk factors for heat-related death, athletes and soldiers are at particular risk, given the degree of their exertion in hot environments (Box 38-1). In fact, heat-related deaths are the third leading cause of death among American athletes, following head and spinal cord injuries and cardiac arrest.[2] DOT 5-10.3

At the other end of the temperature spectrum, there are over 700 deaths from hypothermia in the United States annually. Approximately half of those occur in people over the age of 65.[3] There are multiple risk factors for cold-related illnesses (Box 38-2). The incidence of frostbite in the United States is unknown, partly because there is no standardized reporting system. A nationwide study of hospital admissions in Finland, however, estimates 2.5 cases of frostbite per 100,000 inhabitants.[4] The incidence of nonfreezing cold injuries is even harder to estimate.

Metabolism is an exothermic (heat generating) process. The basal metabolic rate of human beings

BOX 38-1 Risk Factors for Heat Illnesses

Ambient temperature greater than 95 degrees F

Relative humidity greater than 60%

Exertion

Dehydration

Extremes of age

Medical and physiologic conditions

Fever

Hyperthyroidism

Infections

Seizures

Drug or alcohol intoxication

Malnutrition

Obesity

Impaired sweating ability

Medications that inhibit sweating (including anticholinergics, antidepressants, antihistamines, antispasmodics, diuretics, lithium, MAO inhibitors, phenothiazines)

Heat stress prior to acclimatization (particularly within the first 10 to 20 days)

Heavy clothing DOT 5-10.4

BOX 38-2 Risk Factors for Cold Illnesses

Heat loss

Radiation from uncovered skin (inadequate clothing)

Conduction to cold objects (worse in immersion accidents)

Convection to a windy environment

Evaporation from the skin and lungs in a low humidity environment

Diminished heat production

Lack of exertion

Dehydration

Shock

Extremes of age

Medical and physiologic conditions

Hypothyroidism

Infections

Drug or alcohol intoxication

Malnutrition

Medications that interfere with central temperature control (benzodiazepines, barbiturates, opiates, phenothiazines) DOT 5-10.55

---

generates 50 to 60 kcal/hr/m^2 of body surface area (approximately 100 kcal/hr for a 70 kg person).[1] However, this can increase by as much as 20 times during strenuous exercise.[5]

Heat transfer can occur in a combination of four mechanisms: conduction, convection, radiation, and evaporation (Figure 38-1).

- **Conduction** refers to heat transfer from warmer to cooler objects by direct physical contact.

- **Convection** is the transfer of heat from a warm object into the surrounding atmosphere. The amount of heat dissipated by convection is directly proportional to the temperature gradient between the object and the environment. Therefore, heat loss through convection drops as air temperature approaches skin temperature. However, convective heat loss varies directly with wind velocity, meaning more heat will be lost with increased wind speeds.

- Heat transfer by electromagnetic waves is **radiation.** It is a major source of heat loss or gain.

- The **evaporation** of liquids is an endothermic (heat consuming) process. The evaporation of 1 mL of sweat will cool the body by 0.58 kcal.[5] Evaporation

of sweat from the skin is the dominant mode of cooling in hot conditions.

The physiology of heat regulation requires three components working together: thermosensors, the central integrative area in the CNS, and thermoregulatory effectors.

- **Thermosensors** are temperature-sensitive neurons located in the skin, spinal cord, limb muscles, and the anterior hypothalamus. There are approximately 10 times more "cold" thermosensors as "hot" thermosensors on certain parts of the skin.[6]

- The **central integrative area** in the CNS interprets input from the thermosensors and regulates the thermoregulatory effectors to maintain a set point temperature.

- The **thermoregulatory effectors** carry out heat loss or conservation primarily through skin blood flow (by vasoconstriction or vasodilation), sweating, and shivering.

If these adaptations cannot keep up with the environmental demands, temperature-related illnesses result. If, for example, volume depletion from increased

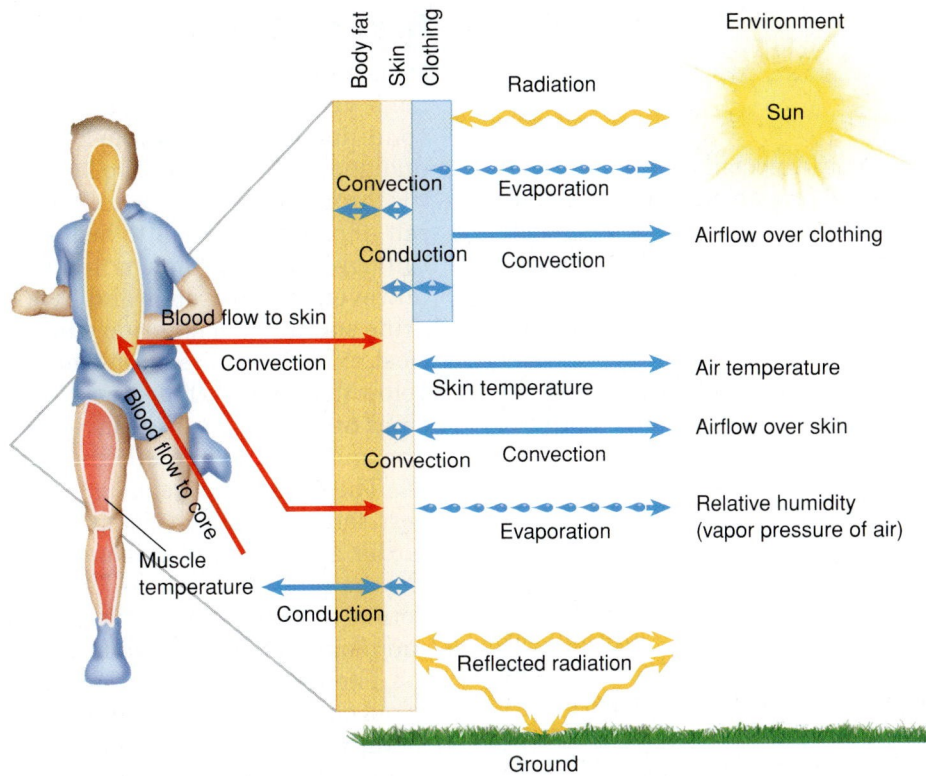

Figure 38-1 Heat transfer occurs four ways: conduction, convection, radiation, and evaporation.

sweating in a hot environment combines with inadequate fluid replacement, heat exhaustion (heat prostration) results. If the homeostatic thermoregulatory mechanisms fail, however, heatstroke may be the outcome with an extreme elevation of the core temperature. DOT 5-10.10

Minor heat illnesses include heat cramps, heat edema, heat syncope, and prickly heat. Continuing along a spectrum, the next more severe heat illness is heat exhaustion. Heatstroke is the most severe heat illness.

Cold illness can be a local injury, such as trench foot, chilblains, or frostbite. It can also be an illness affecting the entire body, causing hypothermia. Within the category of hypothermia, it is useful to talk about mild, moderate, severe, and profound hypothermia because the characteristics of the disease response change as the temperature lowers and the recommended treatment also varies. DOT 5-10.5-10.13,5-10.14, 5-10.15, 5-10.16

Heat-Related Illness

There are multiple steps in maintaining a constant core temperature in the setting of environmental heat stress. A failure in any one of these can cause heat illness.

The body has the ability to acclimatize to hot environments by decreasing heat production and increasing heat loss efficiency. This process takes from 10 to 60 days. During acclimatization, skeletal muscle mitochondria increase, as do glycogen stores, allowing less heat production for a given amount of work. Aldosterone secretion is enhanced, which helps conserve sodium by changing the composition of sweat and urine so that less salt is lost. Aldosterone also acts to increase extracellular volume. The volume of sweat that is produced is increased, and the temperature at which sweating starts is lowered.

Heat Cramps

Unacclimatized people who exert themselves in hot environments may produce large quantities of sweat in the body's attempt to accelerate heat dissipation through evaporation. If allowed adequate access, the individual takes in large quantities of water (hypotonic) to replace the volume loss (isotonic). The result is salt loss. Fatigued muscles seem to be particularly vulnerable to sodium fluxes, and the resulting brief, intermittent muscle cramping of the most-worked muscles is known as **heat cramps.** This syndrome can be largely prevented by assuring adequate salt intake as well as adequate water intake.

The treatment for heat cramps is refraining from exertion in the hot environment and sodium replacement, either orally or parenterally, in severe cases. Orally, salt-containing sport drinks or 56 to 112 mEq (one-quarter to one-half teaspoon of table salt per liter of water) is recommended. Isotonic normal saline

(0.9% NaCl) is the intravenous solution that should be used in severe cases.

Heat Edema

Unacclimatized individuals, especially the elderly, may develop foot and ankle edema in hot environments. Usually, the edema is minimal and resolves after acclimatization in a few days. The pathophysiology is likely related to peripheral vasodilation, capillary permeability, and the rise in aldosterone in response to heat stress.

The treatment of heat edema involves elevating the legs or wearing support hose. Diuretics have not been found to be effective and may place individuals at greater risk for more severe heat illnesses.

Heat Syncope

As a response to heat stress, peripheral vasodilatation can result in a drop in central venous pressure and cardiac filling. This can result in inadequate cardiac output to adequately perfuse the brain. With a lack of perfusion, loss of consciousness (syncope) is the result. Persons most at risk are the elderly, those who stand up abruptly (orthostatic), and those who are standing still for long periods of time (the soldier at attention). Often a prodrome of light-headedness, vision loss (scotomata or tunnel vision), nausea, vomiting, and diaphoresis precede the loss of consciousness.

The condition is usually self-limited in that the victim falls to the ground, and cerebral perfusion is reestablished in the recumbent position. Prevention is adequate hydration and avoiding a prolonged standing-still posture. Be aware that during the syncope, patients may sustain injuries in their fall to the ground.

Prickly Heat

Prickly heat is an acute inflammatory skin disorder that occurs in tropical environments. It is also known as miliaria rubra, lichen tropicus, or heat rash. It is manifested by intensely pruritic (itchy) vesicles (fluid filled bumps) on an erythematous (reddened) base, usually in clothed areas. The pathophysiology involves the obstruction of sweat gland pores and subsequent staphylococcal infection. It may progress to form a deeper sweat gland obstruction with the formation of keratin plugs and a deeper vesicle, the profunda vesicle. At this stage, it is not pruritic but can become a chronic dermatitis.

Prevention of prickly heat involves wearing light, loose fitting, clean clothing and avoiding talcum powder. The acute phase can be treated with topical antibacterials. The profunda stage requires oral antibiotics.

Heat Exhaustion

Heat exhaustion (heat prostration) is a result of intravascular volume depletion, brought on by heat stress. The condition can occur through water depletion in which oral intake is inadequate to keep up with losses, primarily through sweating. Another, less common cause is salt depletion. Similar to heat cramps, more salt is lost through sweating than is replaced. In this condition, however, hyponatremia and hypochloremia result. The urine sodium and chloride concentrations are also low. Heat exhaustion based on salt loss takes longer to develop than heat exhaustion based on water loss. Most cases of heat exhaustion have a mixture of water depletion and salt depletion (Figure 38-2).

The signs of heat exhaustion include malaise, weakness, fatigue, headache, nausea, vomiting, vertigo, tachycardia, and impaired judgment. Sweating continues and may be profuse. The core body temperature is usually normal or only mildly elevated (less than 40°C [104°F]), and major CNS dysfunction (seizures, coma) is absent.

The treatment of heat exhaustion includes rest in a cool environment. Volume replacement is the primary therapy. This can be done orally with salt-containing solutions in mild cases or may require parenteral treatment in more severe cases. Patients with severe volume and electrolyte disturbances should be admitted for cautious correction of their deficits. Admission is also advised for elderly patients and those with cardiovascular disease.

Heatstroke

At the most serious end of the heat illness spectrum is **heatstroke.** In this condition, the body's compensatory mechanisms for handling environmental heat stress

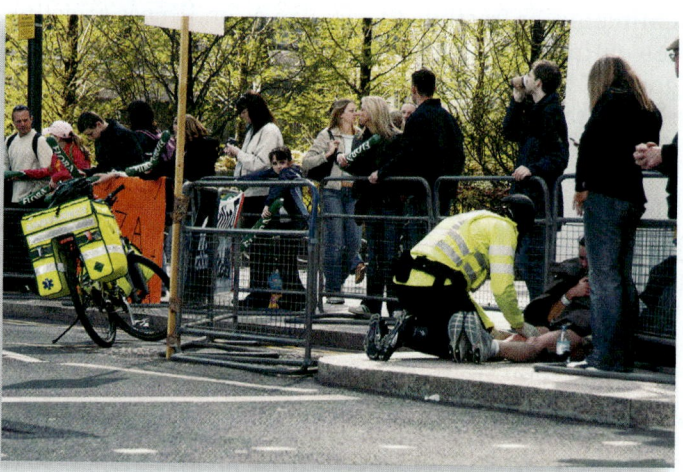

Figure 38-2 Marathon runners are prone to heat exhaustion.

fail. The result is a severely elevated core body temperature (greater than 40.5°C [104.9°F]) and multisystem dysfunction. Realize, however, that the maximal core temperature may have been attained prior to the medical assessment and may have fallen as much as 3.3°C prior to arrival at the hospital.[7] Neurologic dysfunction is a necessary feature of heatstroke, but other systems, such as cardiovascular, hepatic, and gastrointestinal, are affected.

Heatstroke is different from **hyperpyrexia** (fever). By definition, hyperpyrexia is a core temperature greater than 41°C. There are many potential reasons for hyperpyrexia, including fever as a response to infection. The mechanism of fever involves a resetting of the hypothalamic thermostat to a higher point. However, temperatures greater than 42°C (107.6°F) are most often noninfectious. Heatstroke is one such cause of severe hyperpyrexia. Other causes include head injury, drug ingestion, and malignant hyperthermia.

There may be prodromal symptoms as the victim passes from heat exhaustion to heatstroke. In most cases, however, the onset of heatstroke is sudden and marked by an alteration of consciousness. Although the cessation of sweating has been observed in heatstroke victims, it is a late and variable finding.[8,9,10]

Organ and tissue damage seems to be related more to the duration of the elevated temperature than the magnitude of the elevation. Other factors, such as age, prior health, and degree of exertion also play a role.

Two forms of heatstroke have been described: exertional and classical. In **exertional heatstroke,** the victims are usually young and healthy (i.e., athletes and military recruits) (Figure 38-3). In the **classical** form, the victims tend to be elderly, debilitated, or living in underventilated dwellings without air conditioning (Figure 38-4). They often suffer from chronic diseases or are taking medications that impair adaptation to heat stress. The different characteristics of exertional and classical heatstroke are listed in Table 38-1.

Heatstroke patients are critically ill, and regardless of the cause, the key to treatment is rapid cooling. This should be initiated in the prehospital setting by removing the patient from the hot environment, removing their clothing (radiation), and starting active cooling

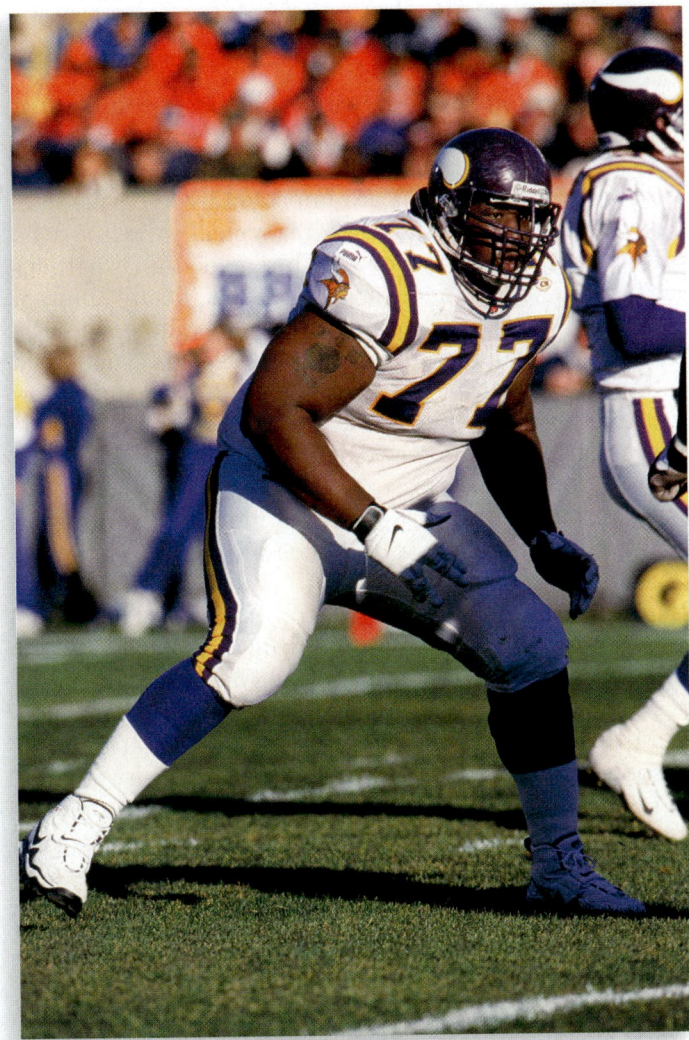

Figure 38-3   Korey Stringer, offensive tackle for the Minnesota Vikings, collapsed from heatstroke on August 2, 2001, after football practice in 90°F weather. His body temperature was recorded as 108°F; he lost consciousness and died early the next day.

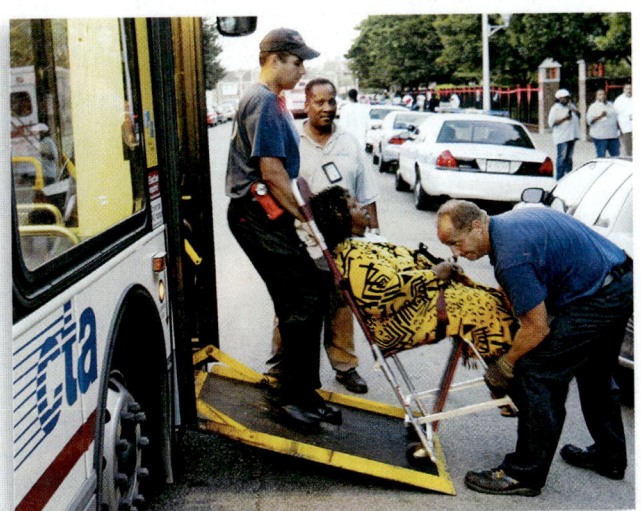

Figure 38-4   With a record high of 106°F, the 1995 Chicago heat wave was deadly. While no official death toll was published, statistics show that 739 more people than normal died during the peak week. Most of the deceased were elderly living in the heart of the city with no air conditioning.

TABLE 38-1 Usual Characteristics of Heatstroke

Exertional	Classical
Healthy	Predisposing factors or medications
Younger	Older
Exercise	Sedentary
Sporadic occurance	Heat wave occurrence
Diaphoresis usually present	Anhidrosis (lack of sweating)
Hypoglycemia	Normoglycemic
Disseminated intravascular coagulation	Mild coagulopathy
Rhabdomyolysis	Mild creatinine kinase elevation
Acute renal failure	Oliguria
Marked lactic acidosis	Mild acidosis
Hypocalcemia	Normocalcemic

Source: From Table 135-1 in B. Yarbrough, and S. Vicario, "Heat Illness," In *Rosen's Emergency Medicine: Concepts and Clinical Practice,* 5th ed., J. Marx, R. Hockberger, and R. Walls, eds. (St. Louis, MO: Mosby, 2002), p 2004.

by fanning (convection), wetting the skin by tepid water mist (evaporation), and applying ice packs, especially to the groin, axilla, and neck (conduction), if available (Figure 38-5). Ice water immersion is an extremely rapid cooling technique but has the practical limitation of limited immediate availability and concern for the ability to perform other resuscitative treatments in the prehospital setting. Generally, the most practical and efficient cooling method is evaporative cooling. If patients shiver in response to cooling, benzodiazepines or phenothiazines may be administered to minimize the shivering as shivering serves to increase heat production. This is not often seen because the hypothalamic set point is not altered; this is as opposed to patients with a fever, in which that thermostat set point is raised. Care should be taken to not

cause **overshoot hypothermia.** This is accomplished by stopping the active cooling measures when a patient's core temperature falls below 39°C.

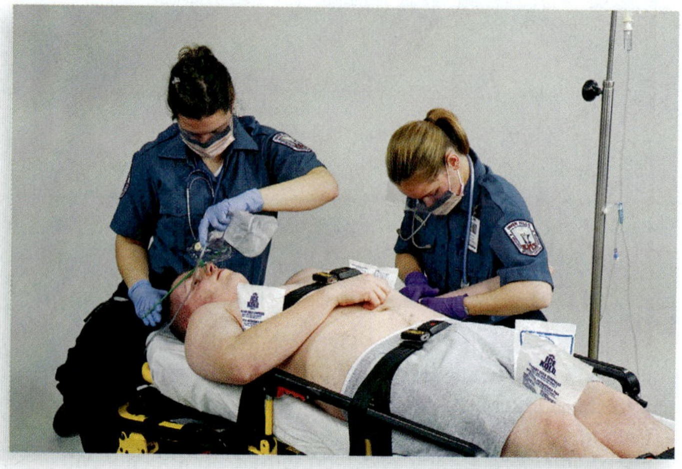

Many organ systems are impacted by hyperthermia. The most sensitive is the CNS. It is typically the first to be affected and the last to recover. The cerebellum is particularly vulnerable. The liver is also specifically injured. Similarly, the kidneys are at-risk for acute tubular necrosis and for myoglobinuric renal failure.[11] Death is usually due to multiple organ failure, including disseminated intravascular coagulation (DIC), acute renal failure, liver failure, and acute respiratory distress syndrome (ARDS).[12]

Aspiration, seizures, pulmonary edema, and hypoxia are common in heatstroke victims. Prompt airway management may be necessary. Hypotension is common and may be related to a combination of dehydration and peripheral vasodilatation. The blood pressure usually rises with cooling. Intravenous fluid therapy is often necessary, but the volume required for resuscitation is hard to ascertain without invasive monitoring. Overaggressive volume administration is associated with the development of pulmonary edema. It is best to begin with a bolus of 250 to 1000 mL of normal saline over the first hour of initial cooling and monitor the vital signs. Similarly, pressors can exacerbate the core temperature rise and should be reserved for cases in which either invasive monitoring has been established or the patient has been adequately cooled (core temperature between 37°C and 39°C) and their intravascular volume has been restored. Seizures prevent effective cooling and should be controlled promptly with benzodiazepines. Therapies that are not recommended include atropine, antipyretics, and alcohol baths. DOT 5-10.8, 5-10.9, 5-10.11, 5-10.18, 5-10.19, 5-10.20, 5-10.21, 5-10.22, 5-10.23, 5-10.24, 5-10.25, 5-10.26, 5-10.27, 5-10.28, 5-10.29, 5-10.30, 5-10.31, 5-10.32, 5-10.33

Figure 38-5 Rapid cooling is the key to treatment of heat stroke.

Cold-Related Illness

Cold illnesses can be local tissue injuries (frostbite, frostnip, chilblains, trench foot) or systemic alteration (hypothermia). Although both local and systemic injuries can occur simultaneously, the homeostatic response to cold is primarily designed to maintain the body's core temperature. This is accomplished through cellular metabolism, muscular activity and shivering, vasoconstriction, and shunting. Cellular metabolism in the heart and liver are responsible for the greatest amount of exogenous heat production.

Hypothermia

By definition, **hypothermia** occurs when the core temperature drops below 35°C. Hypothermia has been classified as **primary** (usually the result of an environmental exposure) or **secondary** (occurring in patients with a predisposing illness, frailty, or intoxication). Secondary hypothermia has also been called "urban" hypothermia because of its frequency in urban environments. It is more common at the extremes of age. Diseases associated with decreased heat production include hypopituitarism, hypoadrenalism, hypothyroidism and myxedema, severe malnutrition, and hypoglycemia. Increased heat loss can be seen in a variety of skin diseases, ethanol and drug intoxication, and Wernicke's encephalopathy (Box 38-3). Thermoregulation can become impaired with a number of diseases and conditions (Box 38-4).

Another way of classifying hypothermia is by severity: mild (core temperature 35° to 32.2°C), moderate (core temperature 32.2° to 28°C), and severe (core temperature less than 28°C). This method of organizing hypothermia makes the most sense because signs, symptoms, and treatment change with the severity of the condition (Table 38-2). In addition, some have sorted hypothermia by duration into acute (less than six hours in onset) and chronic (greater than six hours in onset).

Mild Hypothermia

As the core body temperature falls toward 35°C, thermosensors in the skin, spinal cord, and gastrointestinal tract become active and stimulate the hypothalamus. In response, the hypothalamus sends vasomotor and hormonal signals that increase heat production and heat retention. The effects are an increase in the endogenous metabolic rate, primarily in the heart and liver, cutaneous vasoconstriction (with shunting of blood toward the core), piloerection (which increases skin insulation), and shivering. Shivering can increase heat production two- to fivefold.[13] However, maximal heat production can only last for a few hours due to glycogen depletion and fatigue.[14]

Mild hypothermia has been described as the excitatory phase. At this point, the body's physiologic adaptations are maximally effective. The patient will have the perception of being cold. Pulse, blood pressure, and respiratory rate may be elevated. There may be some subtle mental status changes with lethargy, apathy, confusion, and slurred speech. Cold, dry air, in particular, can induce bronchospasm, bronchorrhea (secretions in the bronchi), and cough. The victim may experience a cold-induced diuresis, probably on the basis of central

---

BOX 38-3 Wernicke's Disease and Korsakoff's Psychosis

Wernicke's disease and Korsakoff's amnesic state are common neurologic disorders that have been recognized since the 1880s. **Wernicke's disease** (originally called polioencephalitis hemorrhagica superioris) is characterized by nystagmus (rapid side-to-side eye movements), abducens (the sixth cranial nerve is damaged and the eyes cross) and conjugate gaze palsies (conjugate means moving together), ataxia (halting movements) of gait, and mental confusion. These symptoms develop acutely or subacutely and may occur singly or, more often, in various combinations. Wernicke's disease is due specifically to a deficiency of the vitamin thiamine and is observed mainly, though not exclusively, in alcoholics.

Korsakoff's amnesic state (Korsakoff's psychosis) is a unique mental disorder in which retentive memory is impaired out of proportion to all other cognitive functions in an otherwise alert and responsive patient. This amnesic disorder, like Wernicke's disease, is most often associated with alcoholism and malnutrition, but it may be a symptom of various other diseases that have their basis in lesions of the brain. In the alcoholic, nutritionally deficient patient, Korsakoff's amnesia is usually associated with and follows the occurrence of Wernicke's disease. The term **Wernicke's disease** or **Wernicke's encephalopathy** should be applied to a symptom complex of ophthalmoparesis (the thousand mile stare), nystagmus, ataxia, and an acute apathetic-confusional state. If the patient also has a learning or memory deficit, the symptom complex is appropriately designated as the **Wernicke-Korsakoff's syndrome**.[1]

BOX 38-4 Factors Predisposing to Hypothermia

Decreased Heat Production

Endocrinologic Failure

Hypopituitarism

Hypoadrenalism

Hypothyroidism

Insufficient Fuel

Hypoglycemia

Malnutrition

Marasmus (chronic undernurishment)

Kwashiorkor (failure to thrive in infants
from malnurishment)

Extreme exertion

Neuromuscular Inefficiency

Age extremes

Impaired shivering

Inactivity

Lack of adaptation

Increased Heat Loss

Environmental

Immersion

Nonimmersion

Induced Vasodilatation

Pharmacologic

Toxicologic

Erythrodermas

Burns

Psoriasis (chronic patchy, red, scaly skin disease)

Ichthyosis (chronic scaly skin disease)

Exfoliative dermatitis (flakey, peeling skin disease)

Iatrogenic (medically caused)

Emergency deliveries

Cold infusions

Heat stroke treatment

Impaired Thermoregulation

Peripheral Failure

Neuropathies

Acute spinal cord transection

Diabetes

Central Failure or Neurologic

CNS trauma

Cerebrovascular accident

Toxicologic

Metabolic

Subarachnoid hemorrhage

Pharmacologic

Hypothalamic dysfunction

Parkinson's disease

Anorexia nervosa

Cerebellar lesion

Neoplasm (tumor)

Congenital intracranial anomalies

Multiple sclerosis

Miscellaneous Associated Clinical States

Recurrent hypothermia

Episodic hypothermia

Sepsis

Pancreatitis

Carcinomatosis (widespread metastatic cancer)

Cardiopulmonary disease
    Vascular insufficiency

Uremia

Paget's disease (excessive bone resorption with
abnormal healing)

Giant cell arteritis (inflammatory disease of arteries)

Sarcoidosis (nodule in the lungs, liver, skin, and
lymphnodes)

Shaken baby syndrome

Source: From Box 134-1 in D. Danzl, R. Pozos, et al., "Accidental Hypothermia," *Rosen's Emergency Medicine: Concepts and Clinical Practice,*
5th ed. eds. J. Marx, R. Hockberger, and R. Walls (St. Louis, MO: Mosby, 2002), p 1984.

hypervolemia caused by peripheral vasoconstriction.[13] Laboratory values may be normal or may show minor changes, such as a respiratory alkalosis and increased hematocrit.

The treatment of mild hypothermia relies on allowing the body's compensatory mechanisms to correct the problem. This means removing the victim from the cold environment, removing wet clothing, and administering passive external rewarming by providing warm clothing or blankets. Core body temperature should rise back to normal quickly. Active external rewarming techniques, such as heating lamps, heating blankets, hot water bottles, and forced air warming systems (such as the Bair Hugger system) can also be used.

TABLE 38-2   Differentiating the Degrees of Hypothermia Severity

HYPOTHERMIA	Mild	Moderate	Severe
Core temperature range	35° to 32.2°C (95–90°F)	32.2° to 28°C (90°F–82.4°F)	Less than 28°C (<82.4°F)
Signs and symptoms	Apathy, hyperreflexia, disorientation, tachycardia, hypertension, tachypnea, bronchorrhea, bronchospasm, shivering, vasoconstriction, diuresis, decreased GI motility	Hyporeflexia, paradoxical undressing, hypotension, bradycardia, atrial dysrhythmia, diminished gag reflex, decreased oxygen consumption, decreased shivering, muscle spasm, GI erosions, pancreatitis, hepatic necrosis	Coma, areflexia, ventricular dysrhythmias, asystole, pulmonary edema, apnea, muscle rigidity, compartment syndrome, decreased renal blood flow, oliguria
Test results	Respiratory alkalosis	Hypoxia, metabolic and respiratory acidosis, increased hematocrit, hyperamylasemia, leukopenia, thrombocytopenia, ECG changes (bradydysrhythmia, atrial fibrillation)	Hypoxia, severe metabolic and respiratory acidosis, increased hematocrit, hyperamylasemia, leukopenia, thrombocytopenia, ECG changes (ventricular dysrhythmias, asystole), coagulopathy, hyperglycemia (or hypoglycemia), severe hyperkalemia
Treatment	Passive external rewarming: clothing, blankets	Active external rewarming: heating lamps, heating blankets, hot water bottles, hot packs, warmed IV fluids, forced air warming systems	Active internal rewarming: warm humidified oxygen (42° to 46°C), peritoneal lavage, bladder lavage, pleural lavage, extracorporeal blood rewarming (cardiopulmonary bypass, arteriovenous rewarming, venovenous rewarming, or hemodialysis)

Moderate Hypothermia

As patients become more hypothermic, they enter the range of moderate hypothermia, or the slowing stage. At this point, compensatory mechanisms begin to fail. Mental status changes accelerate, with judgment and coordination being particularly affected. At this stage, many patients exhibit "paradoxical undressing behavior." This is thought to be a result of a misperception of being overly warm, possibly brought on by further shunting of blood towards the core.[15] The EEG becomes progressively more abnormal, and patients may become hyporeflexive.

Similarly, the pulse and respiratory rate may slow during moderate hypothermia, and the patient may develop atrial dysrhythmia. Atrial fibrillation with a slow ventricular response is the classic cardiac rhythm described at this degree of hypothermia. Other ECG findings include PR, QRS, and QTc prolongation, a decrease in the P wave amplitude, nonspecific ST and T wave changes, and J waves or Osborn waves. Osborn waves are a slow, positive deflection at the end of the QRS complex. These waves, although characteristic of hypothermia, are neither pathognomonic nor prognostic.

The moderately hypothermic patient's blood pressure may drop and, in fact, may be unobtainable in the limbs. Shivering typically stops at this stage and heralds a rapid decline in core temperature. If kept at this stage long enough, many of these patients develop gastric erosions, hepatic necrosis, and pancreatitis.

Inadequate oral intake and cold-induced diuresis can render hypothermic patients hypovolemic. This condition may be difficult to diagnose because of the challenges in obtaining peripheral vital sign readings. If intravenous fluids are given, they should be warmed (43°C) so as to not make the situation worse. Furthermore, lactated Ringer's solution should probably be avoided because the hypothermic liver may not be able to metabolize lactate.

Since the body's compensatory mechanisms in moderate hypothermia begin to fail, the treatment requires the addition of exogenous heat. Remove the victim from the cold environment, remove wet clothing, and administer passive external rewarming; in addition, active external rewarming techniques, such as heating lamps, heating blankets, hot water bottles, and forced air-warming systems (such as the Bair Hugger system), should be used. The most efficient means of rapid rewarming is with immersion in warm water. However, for technical practicality and safety reasons, this is not often feasible.

Severe Hypothermia

One of the greatest challenges in assessing severely hypothermic patients is that the clinical signs can mimic the appearance of death. Patients may become areflexic and unresponsive. Their pupils may be fixed and dilated; they may have no measurable vital signs; they may have a degree of muscle rigidity that suggests rigor mortis. Further, most standard thermometers do not measure temperatures this low; without a means of accurately measuring the core temperature with a low-reading rectal thermometer, this degree of hypothermia may be difficult to appreciate.

The electrocardiogram undergoes characteristic alterations with progressive hypothermia. Initially, there is prolongation of the intervals: PR first, then QRS and QTc. J waves, or Osborn waves, then develop and are most commonly seen in leads II and V_6. As hypothermia becomes more severe, the Osborn waves become more pronounced in leads V_1 to V_4. Although neither pathognomonic nor prognostic, Osborn waves suggest a core temperature less than 32.2°C.

Ventricular and atrial dysrhythmias occur in hypothermia due, in part, to slowing of conduction. This slowing can be so profound in severe hypothermia that the myocardial conduction time is greater than the absolute refractory period. The ventricular fibrillation threshold is lowered. At temperatures less than 25°C, patients may experience ventricular fibrillation or asystole, either spontaneously or with minimal stimulation (such as intubation, nasogastric tube placement, or even rough handling during transportation).

A phenomenon of the core temperature of severely hypothermic patients dropping in a seemingly paradoxical fashion during rewarming efforts has long been recognized. This "core temperature afterdrop" is generally seen in circumstances of large temperature gradients between the core and "supercooled" extremities. As the periphery is warmed and vasoconstriction is lessened, colder venous blood may return to the central circulation, further reducing the core temperature. This effect is more pronounced in dehydrated, hypovolemic patients and in patients receiving active external rewarming to the limbs (as might happen in an attempt to treat frostbite prior to temperature stabilization of the core).

The goals of prehospital care in hypothermia are to rescue, examine, insulate, and rapidly transport. Active external rewarming techniques may be difficult to effectively apply in the prehospital setting. With the exception of heated, humidified oxygen inhalation (which requires special equipment), the majority of active internal rewarming techniques are impractical and risky outside of a hospital. CPR should be provided to hypothermic patients in cardiac arrest. Defibrillation is usually unsuccessful until the core temperature is above 28°C. In general, most cardiac drugs should be avoided in severely hypothermic patients.[13] The reason for this is that most of these drugs will not be effective at cold temperatures. Then, once the patient has been rewarmed, they may all exert their effects at the same time. Atropine is not indicated for hypothermia-induced bradycardia. Vasoconstrictors may promote dysrhythmias, and vasodilators can worsen core temperature afterdrop. Digitalis and calcium channel blockers are not warranted for hypothermia-induced atrial fibrillation (upon rewarming, these rhythms usually revert to sinus). Lidocaine and propranolol are ineffective. Procainamide lowers the fibrillation threshold. Quinidine, however, may be an effective antidysrhythmic agent in hypothermia.

Because there have been survivors of accidental hypothermia with core temperatures as low as 13.7°C and severely hypothermic patients have the appearance of death, the adage, "no one is dead until they are warm and dead," is good advice. This simply means that resuscitation measures and active rewarming should continue until the patient's core temperature is greater than 32°C. Of course, there are exceptions: patients who have sustained obvious fatal injuries or those in which an unreasonable risk to the rescuers would be imposed by attempting resuscitation should be pronounced dead.[13]

DOT 5-10.34, 5-10.35, 5-10.36, 5-10.37, 5-10.38, 5-10.39, 5-10.40, 5-10.41

Local Cold Injury

Local cold injuries include both freezing (frostbite) and nonfreezing syndromes (trench foot, chilblains). These syndromes may occur in isolation or in the setting of hypothermia. There are several risk factors for developing local cold injury (Box 38-5).

Frostbite

Frostbite is a tissue injury that results from macrovascular, microvascular, and direct cellular disruption from freezing. As tissue cools, ice crystals form in the extracellular fluids. These crystals create mechanical disruption of cells as they expand. They cause intracellular dehydration and electrolyte shifts, leading to further cell harm.

Inadequate clothing

Malnutrition

Previous injuries or illnesses (especially previous frostbite injury)

Decreased perfusion

    Tobacco use

    Vascular disease

    Restrictive clothing

Vasodilation

    Alcohol use

    Medication use

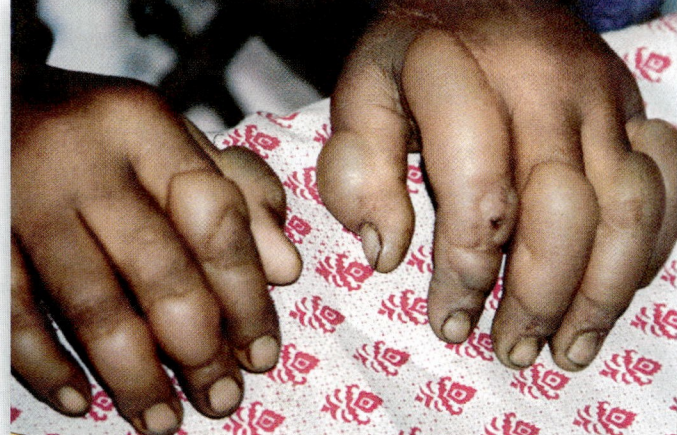

Figure 38-6   Superficial frostbite of the hands showing edema and fluid-filled blisters.

The endothelium of blood vessels, in particular, may become injured, leading to ischemia. In addition, vasospasm and the sludging of cold, viscous blood contributes to tissue hypoxia. After thawing, microemboli may further compound the extent of damage.

The extent of frostbite damage has been classified based on depth, from superficial to deep, in similar fashion to burn injury (Figure 38-6). The most superficial form has been called **frostnip.** After rewarming an area with frostnip, there is no discernible tissue loss. The next more serious degree is **superficial frostbite,** in which the dermis and portions of the subcutaneous tissues are damaged. Upon palpation, the skin may feel "doughy." In **deep frostbite,** subdermal and deep tissues are affected. The tissues feel hard and noncompressible. Differentiating superficial from deep frostbite may be the most straightforward after thawing (Table 38-3).

Chilblains (pernio) is a superficial injury that results from skin inflammation and tissue hypoxia from cold-induced vasoconstriction (Figure 38-7). The environmental conditions for pernio are dry, above-freezing temperatures, often with wind across exposed skin. Erythema, edema, and pruritus are common manifestations.

DOT 5-10.45, 5-10.46, 5-10.47, 5-10.48, 5-10.49, 5-10.50, 5-10.51

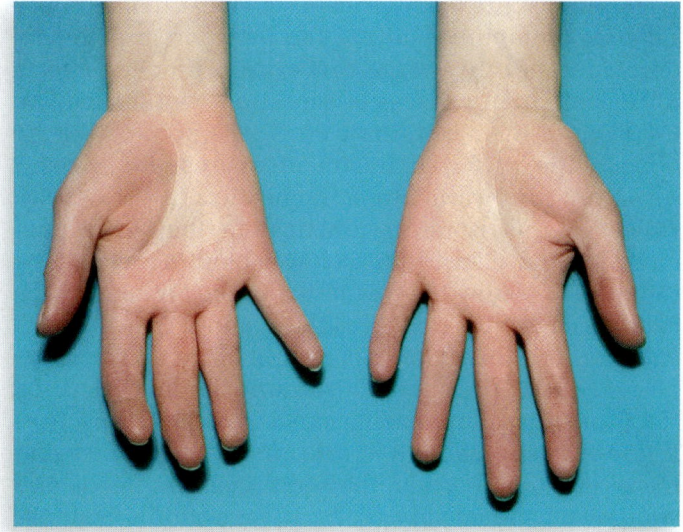

Figure 38-7   Chilblains.

Trench foot or **immersion foot** is a nonfreezing injury that results from prolonged contact with cold water (Figure 38-8). The soles of the feet become swollen, thickened, and fragmented. A noninfectious inflammatory response, vasospasm, intravascular thrombosis, and tissue necrosis can occur within 24 hours. Immersion foot is the most commonly encountered cold injury, particularly in homeless populations.

TABLE 38-3   **Differentiating Superficial from Deep Frostbite**

Superficial	Deep
Severe tingling, throbbing pain during rewarming	Cold, mottled, blue, or gray after rewarming
Edema accumulation within hours	Hard, black eschar within 9 to 15 days
Clear fluid-filled vesicles within 3 to 24 hours	Edema is slow to develop
Hard, black eschar within a week	Deep, blood-filled blisters form in one to three weeks

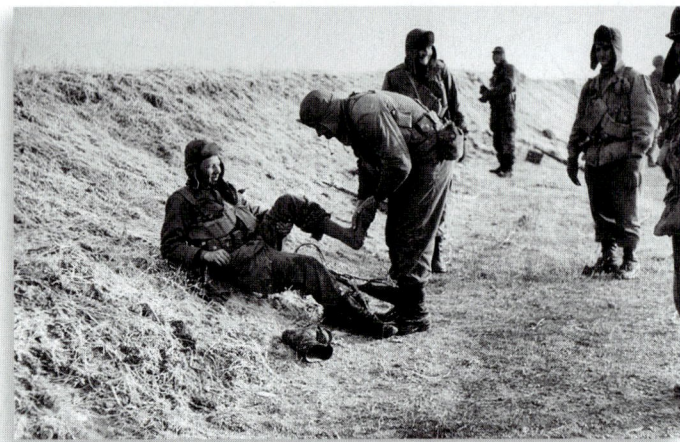

Figure 38-8 Trench foot was extremely common in soldiers unable to keep their feet dry and warm.

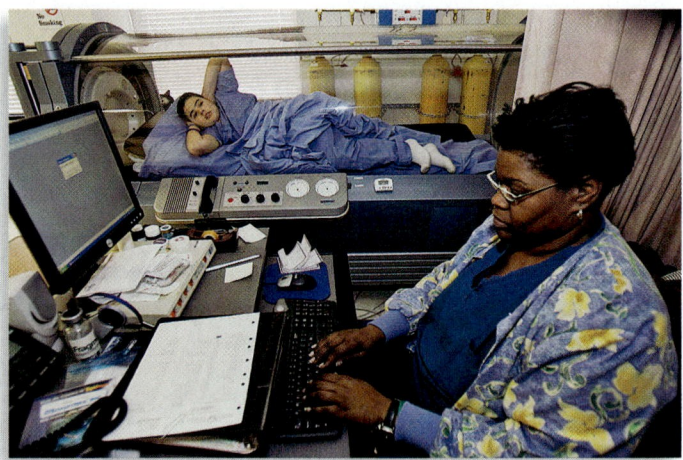

Figure 38-9 A hyperbaric oxygen therapy chamber.

Optimal prehospital care of local cold injury requires prompt recognition and transportation to a facility for rapid rewarming. Since one of the early effects of freezing injury is loss of sensation, victims may be unaware of their condition until it is pointed out by others. The preferred treatment of frostbite is rapid rewarming by warm water immersion (37° to 40°C). However, this is rarely practical in the prehospital environment. Constricting or wet clothing should be removed. Rubbing the frostbitten tissues is contraindicated because it is not efficacious, and it increases tissue loss. Frostbitten tissues should be kept away from heaters during transport. Rewarming should be delayed if a possibility of refreezing exists because the cycle of freeze-thaw-freeze-thaw creates more thrombosis and tissue necrosis. Further, thawed tissues are fragile and should be handled very gently. If, for example, a mountaineer with frostbitten feet must walk out to be rescued, it would be better to leave the feet untreated.

During rapid rewarming, pain is expected, may be severe, and may require parenteral analgesics. After thawing, the tissues are dressed and treated much as one would treat a burn. Adjunctive therapies including thrombolytic agents, low molecular weight dextran, anti-inflammatory drugs, alpha-blockers (phenoxybenzamine), calcium channel blockers, surgical sympathectomy, and hyperbaric oxygen therapy (HBO) have all been investigated in the hospital treatment of frostbite (Figure 38-9).

Dysbarism

Dysbarisms are conditions that result from exposure to increased ambient pressure secondary to volume-pressure changes within the air-filled cavities in the body and from increased dissolution of gasses, particularly nitrogen, in body tissues.

Amateur sport diving became feasible with the development of the _s_elf-_c_ontained _u_nderwater _b_reathing _a_pparatus (scuba) by Jacques-Yves Cousteau and Emile Gagnan in 1943.[16] Scuba requires a demand regulator and high-pressure air tanks that will allow the delivery of an air supply at an appropriate pressure for the depth of the diver.

It is estimated that there are currently up to 2.9 million active scuba divers in the United States. There are over 500,000 new diver certifications issued annually around the world. The risk of an accident during a dive is 1 in 250,000.[17] There are a number of conditions and behaviors that have been associated with an increased risk of developing dysbarism (Box 38-6).

BOX 38-6 Risk Factors for Dysbarism

Exceeding safe diving limits for depth or time

Not observing safe surface intervals between dives

Air travel after diving

Drug or alcohol intoxication

Dehydration

Difficulty with ear or sinus equilibration

Medical and physiologic conditions

    Ear or sinus infections or abnormalities

    Dental infections or new fillings

    Emphysema or asthma

    Coronary artery disease

    Patent foramen ovale

    Neurologic illnesses including seizures

Inexperience

Panic

Emergency ascent

Breath holding during ascent

Under standard conditions, the atmosphere exerts a pressure of 760 mmHg or 14.7 lb/in^2 (psi) at sea level. Another way of expressing this is one atmosphere (1 atm) of pressure. A diver's depth gauge reads pressure in addition to the pressure at sea level. Therefore, at sea level, a pressure gauge reads zero. The absolute pressure, or *atmospheres absolute,* is the total pressure on a diver, which is the addition of gauge pressure and atmospheric pressure.

The laws of physics determine the behavior of gasses and liquids under pressure and explain the pathophysiology of dysbarism (Box 38-7).

BOX 38-7 Laws of Physics Important for Dysbarism

Pascal's law: Pressure applied to any part of a liquid is transmitted equally throughout.

Boyle's law: At a constant temperature, the absolute pressure and the volume of gas are inversely proportional. As pressure increases, the gas volume is reduced; as the pressure is reduced, the gas volume increases.

Charles' law: At a constant pressure, the volume of a gas is directly proportional to the change in the absolute temperature.

Dalton's law: The total pressure exerted by a mixture of gasses is equal to the sum of the pressures (partial pressures) of each of the different gasses making up the mixture, with each gas acting as if it alone was present and occupied the total volume.

Henry's law: The amount of a gas that will dissolve in a liquid at a given temperature is directly proportional to the partial pressure of that gas.

The **general gas law** combines these concepts to predict the behavior of a gas when the factors change. The formula for expressing the general gas law is

$$P_1 \times V_1/T_1 = P_2 \times V_2/T_2$$

where

P_1 initial pressure (absolute)

V_1 initial volume

T_1 initial temperature (absolute)

P_2 final pressure (absolute)

V_2 final volume

T_2 final temperature (absolute)

BOX 38-8 Dysbaric Diseases

External, middle and inner ear barotrauma

Barosinusitis (sinus swelling and hemorrhage)

Facial barotrauma

Nitrogen narcosis

Oxygen toxicity

Decompression sickness

Pulmonary barotrauma

Arterial gas embolism

Pneumothorax

Pneumomediastinum

Subcutaneous emphysema

Alveolar hemorrhage

Alternobaric vertigo (vertigo due to unequal ear pressure)

Barodentalgia (pain due to air expansion under a dental filling)

Gastrointestinal barotrauma

Avascular osteonecrosis (blood vessel obstruction due to air emboli leading to bone death)

Pulmonary edema

Since there are a number of diseases associated with dysbarism (Box 38-8), it is extremely helpful in establishing a diagnosis to determine the timing of the initial presentation of a patient's symptoms. For example, onset of symptoms during descent is characteristic for ear barotrauma, facial barotrauma, and sinus barotrauma. Symptoms that begin at depth include nitrogen narcosis, hypothermia, oxygen toxicity, and contamination from the air supply. Symptoms occurring either during or after the ascent are features of alternobaric vertigo, arterial gas embolism, pneumothorax, pneumomediastinum, pulmonary hemorrhage, barodentalgia, GI barotrauma, and decompression illness (DCI).

One of the most helpful means for differentiating the dysbaric diseases in a particular diver is the focused dive history (Box 38-9).

Diseases of Descent

During descent, gas-filled structures are compressed by the increasing pressure of the surrounding water. By a depth of 33 feet in seawater, the pressure is twice what would be experienced on the surface. Therefore, without equilibration, gas-filled structures would have a

- When was the first onset of symptoms?
- What type of equipment was used, compressed air, mixed gas, enriched air, rebreather? What was the source of the gas?
- Did the dive approach or exceed decompression limits? Was a dive computer used?
- What were the number, depth, bottom time, total time, and surface intervals for all dives in the 72 hours preceding symptoms (the dive "profiles")?
- Were decompression stops used? Was in-water decompression attempted?
- What was the time delay from the last dive to air travel?
- Did the diver experience difficulty with ear or sinus equilibration? Did the pain occur on descent or ascent?
- Was the diver intoxicated? Dehydrated? Working strenuously?
- How long after the dive did symptoms present? Were they present at surfacing? Delayed? Progressive?
- Is a medical history of ear or sinus infections or abnormalities present? Emphysema or asthma? Coronary artery disease? Patent foramen ovale? Neurologic illness?

tendency to be "squeezed" into half their volume. **Middle ear barotrauma (MEBT),** also known as **barotitis** or **ear squeeze,** is the most common complaint of scuba divers. It is experienced by 30% of novice scuba divers and 10% of experienced divers.[18] There are several maneuvers that a diver can perform to force additional air through the eustachian tubes into the middle ear, maintaining an equal pressure across the tympanic membrane. However, if equilibration of middle ear pressure does not occur, the floppy medial third of the eustachian tube collapses shut, making any further attempts at equalization futile. Further pressure increases can cause the tympanic membrane to rupture. The pain may or may not resolve as the tympanic membrane ruptures. The ruptured tympanic membrane, however, exposes the middle ear to cold water, resulting in a caloric-induced nystagmus and vertigo.

External ear barotrauma (EEBT) is less common than MEBT. If air becomes trapped in the external ear canal because of obstruction from cerumen, stenosis, earplugs, or a tight-fitting wet suit hood, a relative negative pressure will develop in the external canal. Pain occurs as the tympanic membrane bulges outward.

Inner ear barotrauma (IEBT) is much less common than MEBT but has a greater associated morbidity. Initially, the mechanism is similar to MEBT in that a large negative pressure develops in the middle ear if the diver is unable to equalize pressure during descent. Sudden equilibration of pressure in the middle ear or a vigorous Valsalva maneuver may rupture the round window and may cause hemorrhage into the inner ear or tearing of the labyrinthine (Reissner's) membrane. The symptoms of IEBT include hearing loss, severe vertigo, nausea, tinnitus, and fullness in the affected ear. Signs include severe nystagmus, positional vertigo, ataxia, and vomiting.

The maxillary, frontal, and ethmoidal sinuses are all susceptible to the effects of increased pressure. Equilibration of pressure within the paranasal sinuses requires open nasal passages. Obstruction to this path can result in pain over the sinuses during descent or ascent. The pain of maxillary barosinusitis may be referred to the teeth. Epistaxis is a frequent finding.

Facial barotrauma results from compression of the air within a dive mask that is over the eyes and nose. If the pressure is not equalized by a forced exhalation through the nose, the pressure gradient can produce facial and conjunctival edema, diffuse petechial hemorrhages on the face, and subconjunctival hemorrhages of the sclera. Rarely, optic nerve damage can result from severe facial barotrauma.

These **squeeze syndromes** can be largely prevented by diving techniques. If they develop, the emergent treatment is primarily symptomatic. Symptoms of hearing loss, vertigo, tinnitus, or visual disturbances require evaluation in a hospital or clinic setting.

Diseases of Depth

Nitrogen narcosis, known as "rapture of the deep," results from the intoxicating effects of increased tissue nitrogen concentration at depth. As pressure on a diver increases, more nitrogen is forced into the tissues. Symptoms include euphoria, a false feeling of well-being, confusion, loss of judgment or skill, disorientation, inappropriate laughter, diminished motor control, and tingling and vague numbness of the lips, gums, and legs.[19] Although the effects of nitrogen narcosis resolve with ascent to shallower depths, the diver may drown because of poor judgment or seriously impaired motor skills in the face of a dive emergency. Because of the dangers of breathing nitrogen at increased partial pressures, the use of compressed air is not recommended for sport diving to depths greater than 120 feet.

At partial pressures exceeding 1.6 atmospheres absolute for extended periods of time, oxygen can be toxic to the CNS or lungs. Symptoms of CNS oxygen toxicity may be remembered by the following mnemonic: [19]

VENTIDC

V Visual symptoms (tunnel vision or blurred vision)

E Ear symptoms (tinnitus)

N Nausea or spasmodic vomiting

T Twitching and tingling symptoms (small facial muscles, lips, or muscles of the extremities)

I Irritability, confusion, agitation, and anxiety

D Dizziness, clumsiness, incoordination, and unusual fatigue

C Convulsions

Diseases of Ascent

One of the consequences of breathing compressed air under pressure is the formation of microbubbles of nitrogen gas in the venous system upon decompression.[20,21] This happens even if the diver does not exceed safe diving limits derived from tables or dive computers. Fortunately, in the vast majority of cases, these venous gas bubbles are asymptomatic and resolve spontaneously.

Decompression illness (DCI) results from the formation of small bubbles of nitrogen gas in the blood and tissues. These bubbles of nitrogen develop as the excess nitrogen forced into the tissues from increased pressure applied during descent now starts to come back out as the pressure on the diver decreases during ascent to the surface. Small, asymptomatic venous gas emboli are probably common in the ascending diver and are filtered by the lungs without apparent permanent damage.[22,23] The microbubbles can cause mechanical obstruction, ischemia, and tissue hypoxia as well as inflammation, platelet aggregation, and thrombosis. A patent foramen ovale (PFO) may be a risk factor for increased susceptibility to DCI because bubbles in the venous circulation may not be prevented from entering the arterial circulation by the vasculature of the lungs.

In order to reduce the risk of DCI, a diver should ascend in a slow, controlled manner, allowing the gradual release of nitrogen. Off-gassing continues after the diver has surfaced and may take up to 12 hours at the surface for nitrogen stores to return to normal sea level values. There are a series of dive tables (and submersible dive computers based on those tables) that estimate the amount of nitrogen that will accumulate in the body during a dive to a particular depth for a specific duration. These tables calculate a maximal dive time at a particular depth (called the no-decompression limit), which allows a return to the surface without sufficiently exceeding the solubility of nitrogen at sea level to produce a high risk of DCI. Repetitive dives within several hours result in accumulation of tissue nitrogen and shorter no-decompression limits. Sport divers are encouraged never to exceed the no-decompression limits on initial or repetitive dives. Because dive tables are based on several assumptions regarding nitrogen elimination, even strict adherence to these tables does not ensure that DCI will not occur. If the no-decompression limits are exceeded, underwater decompression stops are recommended.

The clinical manifestations of DCI have been divided into two categories, Type I and Type II. Type I DCI affects the musculoskeletal system, skin, and lymphatic vessels (so-called "pain only" DCI). Type II DCI involves any other organ system. Type I DCI is also called "the bends." It is manifested most commonly as pain near joints, especially the elbow and shoulder. Skin manifestations of DCI Type I may include pruritus, erythema, and marbling.

Type II DCI includes symptoms involving the CNS, the inner ear, and the lungs. The CNS is particularly susceptible to decompression illness because of its high lipid content. The spinal cord, especially the upper lumbar area, is more often involved than cerebral tissue. There may be limb weakness or paralysis, paresthesias, numbness, and low back and abdominal pain. Bladder symptoms, fecal incontinence, and priapism may occur. Mild to moderate headache, blurred vision, diplopia, dysarthria, unusual fatigue, inappropriate behavior, and a sense of detachment are characteristic of cerebral DCI. Loss of consciousness, however, is rare.

Inner ear DCI causes nausea, dizziness, vertigo, and nystagmus. It is commonly called **the staggers** due to the associated ataxia. Pulmonary DCI **(the chokes)** produces progressive dyspnea, cough, and chest pain. The progression of symptoms probably depends on the number and volume of bubbles in the pulmonary arterial circulation. The patient may have cyanosis and hypotension in association with increased central venous pressure and pulmonary arterial pressure, right-sided strain on electrocardiogram, and a decreased end-tidal CO_2 level. The condition may progress to respiratory arrest.

If air is trapped within the lungs during ascent, the pressure gradient can cause the lung volume to expand and can cause injury. This is often the case in a panicked diver who makes a rapid, uncontrolled ascent. **Pulmonary barotrauma** can result in five conditions: arterial gas embolism (AGE), pneumothorax, pneumomediastinum, subcutaneous emphysema, and alveolar hemorrhage.

The most severe form of pulmonary barotrauma is **arterial gas embolism (AGE).** AGE is the second leading cause of mortality of sport divers after drowning, accounting for approximately 30% of diving-related deaths.[24] With increasing pressure, air bubbles are forced across the alveolar-capillary membrane into the pulmonary venous circulation and then through the left atrium and ventricle and into the arterial circulation. AGE can also result from a right-to-left shunt of venous bubbles, such as in a diver with a PFO (patent foramen ovale in the heart).

Coronary and cerebral artery air emboli are associated with the most serious consequences. Cardiac ischemia, myocardial infarction, dysrhythmias, cardiac arrest, loss of consciousness, confusion, disorientation, headache, dizziness, convulsions, visual changes, or acute stroke may result. Pulmonary symptoms include dyspnea, pleuritic chest pain, and hemoptysis. Because alteration of consciousness is so common in AGE, a scuba diver who surfaces unconscious or who loses consciousness within 10 minutes of reaching the surface should be assumed to be suffering from AGE.

Damage to the lungs from pulmonary overpressure during ascent can cause **pneumothorax** or **pneumomediastinum.** A tension pneumothorax is a possible but rare complication. The symptoms and signs of a pulmonary barotrauma-related pneumothorax (chest pain, dyspnea, and tachypnea) are typical for a pneumothorax from any cause. The manifestations of pneumomediastinum may include fullness in the neck, palpable subcutaneous crepitance, and a change in voice quality or timbre. Pulmonary barotrauma can also cause alveolar hemorrhage. Hemoptysis occurs together with chest pain and dyspnea.

Management of Diving Injuries

The initial priorities of treating diving injuries are resuscitation and stabilization. Supplemental oxygen should

be administered to all patients, and airway control and cardiopulmonary resuscitation may be required for severe cases. Definitive therapy may require hyperbaric recompression in a hyperbaric chamber. Beyond the initial resuscitation measures, the most important decisions that a paramedic can make in managing a diving injury are determining which patients require recompression and how to arrange for the expeditious transport of the patient to an appropriate facility (Box 38-10).

The Divers Alert Network (DAN), located at Duke University in Durham, North Carolina, is a membership association that provides courses for both physicians and nonphysicians on the management of diving-related emergencies and collects and publishes data on diving accidents and fatalities. Clinicians can locate the nearest hyperbaric chamber by contacting the Divers Alert Network. DAN provides a 24-hour medical emergency hotline (919-684-8111).

Hyperbaric recompression is the only definitive treatment for DCI (Types I and II) and AGE. Field treatment should begin with the administration of 100% oxygen. This reduces the bubble size by increasing the differential pressure for nitrogen to diffuse out of the bubbles and speeds the "washout" of nitrogen from the tissues.[25] In-water recompression is extremely risky and should hardly ever be attempted.

Rapid transportation to a hyperbaric facility is important. Patients with AGE who are recompressed within five minutes of surfacing face a mortality rate

BOX 38-10   Diving Disorders that Do and Do Not Require Recompression Therapy

Diving Disorders that *Require* Recompression Therapy	Diving Disorders that *Do Not Require* Recompression Therapy
DCI Type I	MEBT (middle ear barotrauma)
DCI Type II	EEBT (external ear barotrauma)
AGE	IEBT (inner ear barotrauma)
Possibly contaminated air (carbon monoxide poisoning)	Barosinusitis
	Facial barotrauma
	Nitrogen narcosis
	Oxygen toxicity
	Pneumothorax
	Pneumomediastinum
	Subcutaneous emphysema
	Alveolar hemorrhage
	Alternobaric vertigo
	Barodentalgia
	Gastrointestinal barotrauma
	Avascular osteonecrosis

of 5%, with an extremely low risk of morbidity among the survivors. If recompression is delayed by five hours or more, the mortality rate climbs to 10%, with 50% of the survivors suffering morbidity.[26] Although spontaneous resolution of symptoms may occur in patients with AGE, all patients should be recompressed.

Monoplace hyperbaric chambers are compact, lightweight, and less expensive and may be more widely available than multiplace chambers. Unfortunately, because of their design, most cannot be pressurized beyond 3 atmosphere absolutes (ATA), nor can they deliver air-oxygen mixtures. The 3 ATA limit makes monoplace chambers unsuitable for certain recompression protocols. The small size of a monoplace chamber makes it a less optimal choice for the unstable patient who may need attendance within the chamber. The decision to bypass a monoplace chamber for a potentially more distant multiplace hyperbaric chamber must be weighed carefully. The DAN hotline may be helpful in locating the closest suitable chamber. DOT 5-10.70

Ground transport to a hyperbaric facility is preferred over air transportation, if at all practical, because air transport only serves to further decrease the external atmospheric pressure and potentially worsen the DCI. If air transportation must be used, it is important to maintain cabin (internal) pressure at less than 1,000 feet.

In addition to recompression therapy, several adjunctive treatments have been advocated in the treatment of DCI and AGE. Controlled hyperventilation may very transiently decrease intracranial pressure in patients with CNS symptoms but should not be maintained. Intravenous fluid administration to ensure a urine output of 1–2 mL/kg/hr may facilitate tissue perfusion. The treatment or prevention of hypothermia may also help perfusion and off-gassing.

There are no drugs that have been definitively proven to prevent or lessen the symptoms of DCI or AGE. Aspirin therapy (325–650 mg) is recommended by some due to the presumed contribution of platelet aggregation in DCI. Similarly, steroids (1,000 mg hydrocortisone, 125 mg methylprednisolone, or 6 mg dexamethasone) have been advocated in the adjunctive treatment of neurological DCI and AGE. Lidocaine has been speculated to be of use in the treatment of DCI, possibly because of reducing the cerebral metabolic rate, preserving cerebral blood flow, or reducing leukocyte adherence to damaged endothelium.

Cardiac dysrhythmias may be refractory to standard treatments until the diver is recompressed. Seizures may be managed with benzodiazepines; however, mannitol should be avoided. Spinal DCI patients with urinary retention should have a Foley catheter inserted. Of note, endotracheal tube and Foley catheter balloons should be inflated with water or saline (not air) before initiating recompression therapy. Transport of the patient with AGE in the supine position is recommended to maximize arterial-venous flow. The Trendelenburg position, once thought to reduce the degree of cerebral embolization, increases intracranial pressure and facilitates gas embolization to the coronary circulation.

A large number of diving injuries do not require recompression. The treatment of MEBT, EEBT, facial barotrauma, and barosinusitis is largely symptomatic. The treatment of IEBT, however, is controversial and may depend on the extent of damage sustained by the inner ear.

Nitrogen narcosis symptoms should resolve upon ascent. If neurologic symptoms persistent after surfacing, a search for other etiologies, such as DCS, cerebral AGE, contaminated air, and near-drowning, is indicated. DOT 5-10.56, 5-10.57, 5-10.58, 5-10.59

With the exception of AGE, none of the pulmonary barotrauma disorders (pneumothorax, pneumomediastinum, subcutaneous emphysema, and alveolar hemorrhage) require recompression therapy. Treatment with 100% oxygen may aid in the resolution of the disorders. Although tension pneumothorax is a rare condition, rescuers should be prepared to perform needle decompression in patients with loss of breath sounds, hypotension, increasing dyspnea, compromised ventilation, tachypnea, and tachycardia. Tracheal deviation and jugular venous distention are late and inconsistent signs of tension pneumothorax. If a patient with any size pneumothorax is to undergo recompression therapy for concomitant AGE or DCS, a chest tube is indicated prior to the recompression to prevent a tension pneumothorax from developing.

Treatment of pneumomediastinum consists of bed rest and 100% oxygen. Supportive therapy to correct hypoxia is indicated in the treatment of alveolar hemorrhage. DOT 5-10.52, 5-10.53, 5-10.54, 5-10.60, 5-10.62, 5-10.63, 5-10.64, 5-10.65, 5-10.66, 5-10.67, 5-10.68, 5-10.69, 5-10.71, 5-10.72, 5-10.73

Bites and Envenomation

Bites and stings can become medical issues by several means: trauma from the bite wound, toxic envenomation, allergic reactions, and infections. Bite wounds should receive meticulous wound care, including thorough irrigation and local exploration for foreign bodies (e.g., teeth) and damage to deep structures. For this reason, any bite that penetrates the dermis should be evaluated in a hospital or clinic setting. There are several species of biting animals that inject venom into the wounds that they create. For some of these toxins, specific antivenins are available; for others, supportive care is all that can be offered. There are also bites and stings in which the antigenicity of the venom may cause allergic reactions in a susceptible individual. Many bite wounds are also prone to infection. There are a number of risk factors for bites and envenomations (Box 38-11).

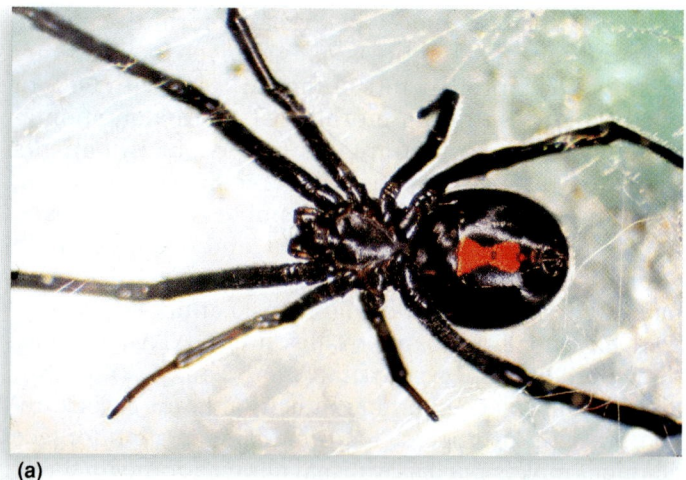

(a)

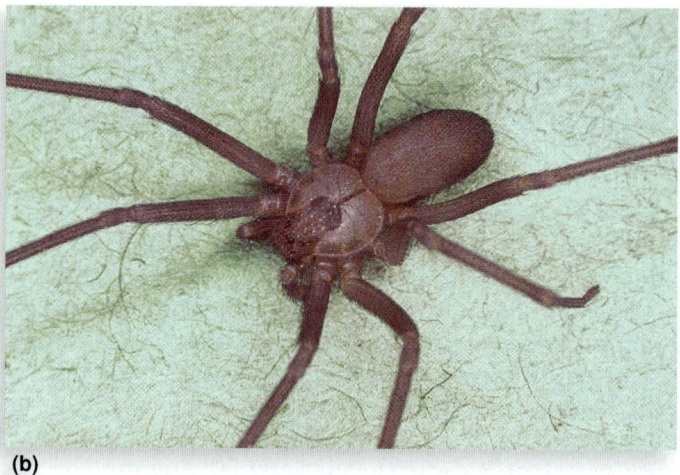

(b)

Figure 38-11 (a) Black widow spider. (b) Brown recluse spider.

By shear numbers of serious reactions and deaths, arthropods (including insects, scorpions, crustaceans and spiders) are the most dangerous group of animals.[27]

Insects

Hymenoptera (bees and wasps) account for the majority of serious reactions to insect stings (Figure 38-10). There are four types of reactions: toxic reactions, anaphylactic reactions, delayed reactions, and unusual reactions (Table 38-4).[28]

Prehospital providers should be prepared to treat the immediate anaphylactic reactions to hymenoptera venom.

CONNECTIONS See Chapter 32: Allergies and Anaphylaxis for additional information on managing patients with reactions to bites and stings.

In addition, removal of the bee stinger should be done as soon as possible because the venom sac may continue to pulse venom even after it has been detached from the bee. This is done by scraping the stinger out with a credit card rather than by pinching and plucking it with fingers or tweezers and risking the inadvertent injection of more venom.[28]

Spiders

All spiders possess venom. However, there are two spiders of particular clinical importance in the United States: Latrodectus (black widow) and Loxosceles (brown recluse or fiddleback) (Figure 38-11). The envenomation syndromes of these two spiders are quite distinct (see Table 38-5).

Mammals

Cat and dog bites make up the majority of nonhuman mammalian bites that receive emergency attention. These bites are capable of inflicting deep tissue injuries and introducing bacteria into the wound. Prehospital

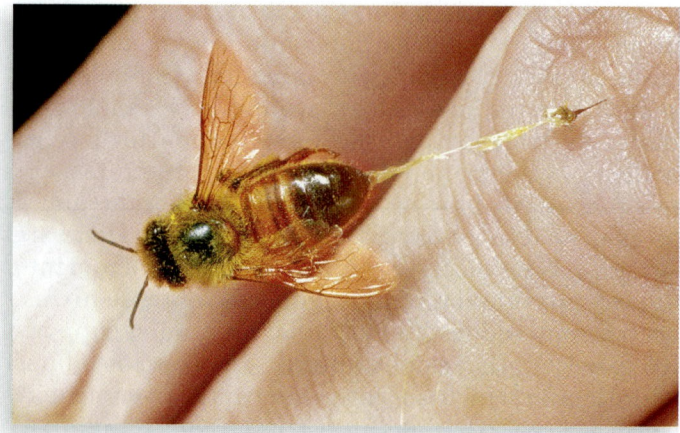

Figure 38-10 Bees (and wasps) account for the majority of reactions to insect stings. The stinger of bees is pulled from the insect, killing it, and the stinger often remains in the skin.

TABLE 38-4 **Reactions to Insect Stings**

	Toxic Reactions	Anaphlyactic Reactions	Delayed Reactions	Unusual Reactions
Description	Nonantigenic response to the venom	Most commonly seen in Vespidae stings (wasps, hornets, yellow jackets)	Serum sickness-like syndrome 10 to 14 days after the sting	Idiopathic reactions following envenomation
Presentation	Local irritation at the sting site, vomiting, diarrhea, light-headedness, syncope, headache, fever, drowsiness, involuntary muscle spasms, edema without urticaria, convulsions	Urticaria, angioedema, laryngeal edema, nasal congestion, gastrointestinal swelling, abdominal cramping, vomiting, flushing, headaches, hypotension, syncope, bronchospasm	Rash, joint inflammation, aseptic meningitis, fever, myalgias, adenopathy, vasculitis	Encephalitis, neuritis, vasculitis, and nephritis
Treatment	Supportive care, cool packs, analgesics	Intravenous fluids, epinephrine, antihistamines, corticosteroids, vasopressors, ventilatory support, inhaled beta agonists	Antihistamines and corticosteroids	Supportive care

CONNECTIONS: Chapter 32: Allergies and Anaphylaxis has more information on insect allergens (page 797).

TABLE 38-5 **Envenomations Syndromes for Black Widow and Brown Recluse Spiders**

	Latrodectus: Black Widow	Loxosceles: Brown Recluse
Markings on spider	Red hourglass shape on the ventral abdomen (♀)	Dark, violin-shaped spot anterodorsally
Presentation	Pain at the bite within one hour, target-shaped erythema, swelling, diaphoresis • Diffuse large muscle cramping, including the abdomen (which may mimic peritonitis) • Latrodectisima: characteristic facial muscle spasm, lacrimation, photophobia • Headache • Light-headedness • Nausea and vomiting Severe envenomations may result in dysphagia, hypertension, respiratory failure, shock, and coma	Typically, an initially mild bite characterized by erythema Bite becomes necrotic over two to four days Systemic reaction may occur in one to two days • Fever • Chills • Vomiting • Arthralgia • Myalgia • Hemolysis • Coagulopathy May result in renal failure and death
Treatment	• Wound care • Analgesics, benzodiazepines for spasm • Tetanus prophylaxis • Calcium gluconate (IV) provides only minimal (if any) relief and is no longer recommended • There is a horse-serum antivenin: administer a test dose and then, if no severe reactions, one to two vials over 30 minutes (somewhat controversial given the incidence of reactions to the horse serum)	• Wound care • Analgesics • Tetanus prophylaxis • Surgical debridement and possible grafting for lesions greater than 2 cm • Transfusion or dialysis, as necessary • Hyperbaric oxygen therapy, corticosteroids, and dapsone have been advocated by some, but there is no clear evidence of efficacy in humans • Currently, there is no commercially available antivenin

care includes hemorrhage control, irrigation, and splinting as necessary.

Human

In an urban practice, one of the most common bite wounds is that inflicted by another person. A particularly dangerous wound is the **fight bite** or **clinched fist injury (CFI)**. It occurs when the fist of one opponent strikes the teeth of a second opponent. This usually involves the knuckles of the dominant hand. The importance of this injury is that the laceration can involve the extensor tendon and its bursa, the superficial and deep fascia, and the joint capsule. These structures are contaminated with oral flora at the time of injury and are notorious for becoming infected. The most important issue related to these wounds involves recognition of the mechanism of injury and transport or referral to the ED for thorough exploration, irrigation, and antibiotic treatment.

Rabies

Rabies is a disease caused by an RNA rhabdovirus transmitted by inoculation with infected saliva. The virus primarily affects the central nervous system and is almost always fatal. In the United States, animal bites from skunks, raccoons, bats, foxes, and woodchucks should be considered highest risk. Treatment begins with a thorough cleansing of the wound. Postexposure prophylaxis in the hospital is a method of reducing the chances of contracting the disease by administering immunoglobulin and a vaccine (human rabies immunoglobulin and human diploid cell vaccine).

Marine Organisms

Jellyfish envenomate by injecting small harpoon-shaped spines (Figure 38-12). Physical or chemical stimulation may cause this discharge. Frequently, "undischarged"

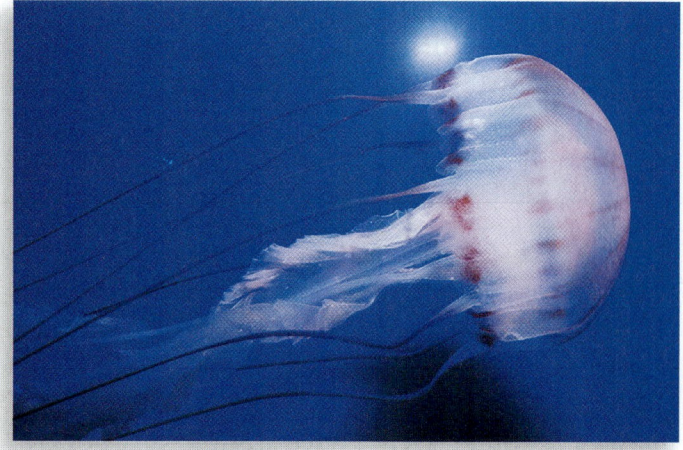

Figure 38-12   Jellyfish envenomate their victims with harpoon-shaped spines known as nematocysts.

nematocysts within the jellyfish tentacles remain in contact with the victim's skin. Acetic acid (vinegar) inhibits nematocyst discharge (it has no affect on those already discharged). If vinegar is not available, acidic drinks (soft drinks and fruit juices) may be tried. Although popular in folklore, urine has not been proven to inhibit nematocyst discharge and may actually stimulate nematocyst discharge.[28]

After acetic acid decontamination, immersion of the affected extremity in hot, but not scalding, water may be of some benefit. The nematocysts that remain in the skin can be removed by applying shaving cream, talc, baking soda, or flour and by shaving the area. Stings from sea anemones or fire coral may be treated in the same fashion. There is an Australian box jellyfish (*Chironex fleckeri*) antivenin available.

There are a large number of stinging fish. They all share a common characteristic of having heat-labile toxins in their venom. Embedded barbs and spines should be promptly removed. The venoms can be rendered nontoxic by placing the affected extremity of the victim (usually the foot) into hot water (less than or at 45°C) for 90 minutes.

There is a stonefish horse serum antivenom available. There are three places in the United States that stock it: Sea World San Diego, Sea World Ohio, and the Steinhardt Aquarium in San Francisco.

Snakes

In the United States, snakebites are uncommon and mortality is rare. In their 2003 report, the American Association of Poison Control Centers (AAPCC) documented 6,889 snakebites (venomous and nonvenomous), out of 94,247 bites and envenomations that they tracked. In 2003, there were two deaths attributed to snakebites in the United States (one from a rattlesnake, one from a poisonous exotic snake). Moderate or major sequelae were seen in 1,694 and 178 cases, respectively. The most common of these were from rattlesnakes (35%); the next most common were from copperheads (26.8%) (Figure 38-13).[27]

Even poisonous snakes do not always inject venom when they bite. In fact, as many as 20–25% of all bites from rattlesnakes in the United States do not result in envenomation ("dry bites").[28] Clinically, snakebites can be divided into four categories. The category of no envenomation consists of only fang marks. Minimal envenomation consists of fang marks and local swelling but no systemic symptoms. Moderate envenomation includes the above with the addition of nausea, vomiting, and mild changes in coagulation parameters. Severe envenomation includes all of the above with marked local swelling and signs of significant coagulopathy (e.g., subcutaneous ecchymosis or hematuria).[2]

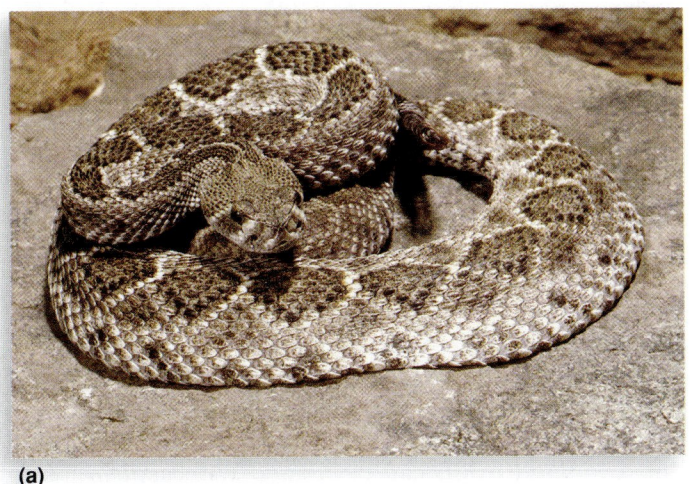

(a)

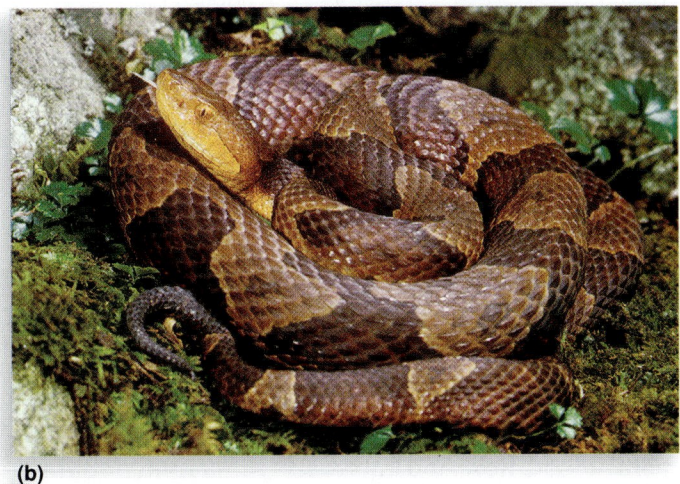

(b)

Figure 38-13 Poisonous pit vipers. (a) Rattlesnake. (b) Copperhead.

Quick observations helpful in determining whether rattlesnake envenomation has taken place include the presence of fang marks that ooze nonclotting blood with surrounding ecchymosis and severe burning pain. These signs, combined with microhematuria, are characteristic of severe envenomation and a poor prognosis.

There is an antivenin for rattlesnake bites, CroFab (Crotalidae Polyvalent Immune Fab by Altana, Inc). If it is to be used, it should be administered in a hospital setting. It is provided as a lyophilized powder and must be reconstituted (this takes 30 to 40 minutes).

Coral snakes, lacking fangs, envenomate by "chewing" the skin, so as many as 50% of their bites do not envenomate. In coral snake envenomation, there may be few signs at the bite site, and systemic signs may be delayed for as long as 12 hours. The earliest signs and symptoms to develop tend to be nausea, vomiting, headache, abdominal pain, diaphoresis, and pallor. Coagulopathy is not a feature of coral snake envenomation. Neostigmine (2.5 mg every 30 to 60 minutes) and equine antivenin (Wyeth Pharmaceuticals) are the treatments for coral snake envenomation.

There are several therapies for snakebite that are either harmful or are of dubious help. Incising the wound and attempting to extract the poison by oral suction (cut and suck), electric shock to denature the toxin proteins, carbolic acid, strychnine, enemas, urine, cauterization, prophylactic antibiotics, ice packs (cryotherapy), and arterial tourniquets are probably ineffective or harmful.[28] The use of constriction bands, splints, and venom removal with *The Extractor*™ (a mechanical suction device that produces about 1 atmosphere of negative pressure and may remove 30% of the injected venom if used within three minutes of the bite) are controversial, with proponents and opponents. The mainstay of treatment for snakebite envenomation in the prehospital setting is support and rapid transportation. DOT 5-8.58

High Altitude Illness

Altitude illnesses are due to exposure to a hypobaric hypoxic environment. Air contains about 21% oxygen (FiO_2 = 0.21). At sea level under standard conditions, the atmospheric pressure is 760 mmHg. Therefore, the contribution of oxygen to this pressure is 0.21 × 760 = 160 mmHg. This is called the partial pressure of oxygen. However, atmospheric pressure decreases as altitude increases. At approximately 5,800 meters (19,030 feet), the atmospheric pressure is half of the sea level value (380 mmHg) and so is the partial pressure of oxygen (80 mmHg). At the summit of Mt. Everest (8,850 meters; 29,035 feet), the partial pressure of oxygen is about 28% of the sea level value, or only 45 mmHg. The rule of thumb is that pressure drops about 1 inch of Hg (25.4 mmHg) for each 1,000 feet (304.8 meters) of elevation.

There are multiple respiratory, cardiovascular, and hematologic adjustments that the body makes over time in response to the lowered partial pressure of oxygen (PaO_2) at altitude. This process is known as acclimatization. Initially, there is an increase in minute ventilation (relative hyperventilation), lowering the partial pressure of carbon dioxide ($PaCO_2$) in arterial blood. As the $PaCO_2$ decreases, there is an increase in PaO_2. The increase in minute ventilation is induced by altitude (the hypoxic ventilatory response or HVR) and may be affected by several factors, including alcohol, sleep medications, caffeine, cocoa, prochlorperazine, and progesterone.[29]

Within two days of ascent, bicarbonate is excreted from the kidneys, compensating for the respiratory alkalosis brought on by the relative hyperventilation. As the pH drops back towards normal, the minute ventilation can continue to increase. This is maximal by six to eight days.

The relative hypoxia of increasing altitude causes an increase in heart rate, blood pressure, cardiac output, and venous tone. Pulmonary vascular resistance and pulmonary artery pressure increases. Cerebral blood flow increases, causing an increase in intracranial volume and possibly intracranial pressure.

Hypoxia also induces an increase in red blood cells and hemoglobin concentration. This effect begins as early as four days after ascent to altitude but takes up to two months to complete. In addition, there is an increase in 2,3-diphosphoglycerate (2,3-DPG), resulting in a right shift of the oxyhemoglobin dissociation curve. This promotes the release of oxygen from the blood to the tissues.

If acclimatization is inadequate for the hypoxic stress, physiologic factors such as pulmonary hypertension leading to pulmonary capillary leakage and pulmonary edema can result. Similarly, increased cerebral blood flow and increased intracranial volume, combined with an increased permeability of the blood brain barrier, can lead to cerebral edema. Clinically, this can be manifested as acute mountain sickness (AMS), high altitude pulmonary edema (HAPE), and high altitude cerebral edema (HACE).

AMS affects 18–42% of the 30 million annual visitors to the mountainous western states. However, only about 0.01% will develop high altitude pulmonary edema or high altitude cerebral edema.[30] Most victims of AMS experience only moderate incapacitation for one to three days before the resolution of their symptoms.[29] However, patients suffering from HACE who are in a coma face a mortality of over 60%.[31] Several factors have been identified as risks for altitude illness. (See Box 38-12 for risks of altitude illness.)

BOX 38-12   Risks for High Altitude Illness

Rapid ascent to altitude

Attaining altitudes in excess of 2,500 meters (8,200 feet)

Sleeping at high altitude

Previous episodes of altitude illness

Medical and physiologic conditions:

    Anemia

    Asthma or emphysema

    Coronary artery disease

    Sickle cell disease

    Smoking

    Exertion

    Drug or alcohol intoxication

    Dehydration

DOT 5-10.74, 5-10.75, 5-10.76, 5-10.77, 5-10.78, 5-10.82, 5-10.83, 5-10.84, 5-10.85, 5-10.86, 5-10.87, 6-4

Acute Mountain Sickness

Acute mountain sickness (AMS) is a syndrome of headache and at least one of the following: anorexia, nausea, fatigue, dizziness, or difficulty sleeping.

The symptoms usually develop within hours after arrival at high altitude (greater than 8,000 feet). Generally, symptoms are worst between 24 and 48 hours after ascent. Resolution usually happens by the third or fourth day at altitude; however, at higher altitudes, symptoms may persist for longer periods or even until descent.[32]

Mild cases of AMS do not require treatment beyond rest. Moderate AMS can be treated with aspirin, acetaminophen, or acetazolamide (a carbonic anhydrase inhibitor and centrally active respiratory stimulant that causes metabolic acidosis, thereby increasing ventilation and arterial oxygenation) and prochlorperazine (an antiemetic).[33] Some have advocated supplemental oxygen, 1 to 2 L/min, particularly for nighttime use. In severe cases, dexamethasone may help. Halting ascent or descending until symptoms resolve is recommended.

Preventing AMS is a matter of making a gradual ascent to allow time for acclimatization. A high carbohydrate diet and avoidance of alcohol or smoking may decrease the incidence, as well. Prophylactic acetazolamide or dexamethasone, begun prior to the ascent, has also been shown to be effective. Its use is indicated for rapid ascents and in patients with a history of recurrent AMS.[33] DOT 5-10.79

High Altitude Pulmonary Edema

High altitude pulmonary edema (HAPE) is a potentially life-threatening condition. It is rare below 8,000 feet. Most commonly, it occurs in individuals who have ascended above 14,500 feet. The onset of symptoms classically occurs during the second night at high altitude, but this can be variable.

The HAPE syndrome includes dyspnea at rest, cough, fatigue, headache, anorexia, cyanosis, rales, tachypnea, and tachycardia.[29]

The cough may become productive of clear, watery sputum or blood. Classically, the rales begin in the right middle lobe. Patients may be febrile, and the clinical picture may mimic pneumonia. Chest x-ray shows a noncardiogenic pulmonary edema.

The treatment of HAPE includes descent to lower altitudes, bed rest, and supplemental oxygen. Very mild cases of HAPE may recover with bed rest alone. However, these patients can deteriorate quickly, so they should be watched closely. Supplemental oxygen is indicated for moderate cases. These patients should also be monitored closely; any progression mandates descent to lower altitudes. Severe cases require descent; even descents of 1,500 to 3,000 feet have been associated with dramatic improvement. "Simulated descents" using supplemental oxygen and hyperbaric chambers have been used to treat AMS and HAPE. Portable, lightweight, manually pressurized, fabric hyperbaric chambers (the Gamow Bag) are capable of generating 103 mmHg (2 psi) above the ambient pressure. This increase in pressure is the equivalent of a descent of 4,000 to 5,000 feet at moderate altitudes (theoretically, use of such a chamber on the summit of Mt. Everest would simulate a descent of 9,000 feet).

A number of drugs have been put forth for the treatment of HAPE. Diuretics (furosemide, 80 mg twice daily) may help to diminish pulmonary blood volume. However, dehydration could occur. Similarly, morphine may lower pulmonary vascular resistance but could also decrease the ventilatory drive. Calcium channel blockers such as nifedipine (10 mg sublingually every four to six hours or 30 mg of a slow-release preparation once or twice daily), which is a pulmonary vasodilator, are effective in treating HAPE. Nifedipine, however, is not more effective than oxygen.

Prevention of HAPE involves gradual ascent to allow for acclimatization. At the first onset of symptoms of AMS the ascent should be stopped before HAPE develops. Patients with a history of HAPE may benefit from nifedipine and acetazolamide during their ascent. DOT 5-10.80

High Altitude Cerebral Edema

Most cases of **high altitude cerebral edema (HACE)** occur above 12,000 feet, but deaths have been reported as low as 8,200 feet.[34] It is usually associated with AMS or HAPE. The syndrome can take 12 hours to nine days to develop after the onset of AMS symptoms; most frequently, HACE occurs in one to three days.

The signs and symptoms of HACE include ataxia, severe headache, nausea and vomiting, altered mentation, seizures, and, finally, coma.

Early recognition of HACE is important because the mainstay of treatment is expeditious descent. High-flow oxygen should be administered if it is available. Steroids (8 mg dexamethasone) may help. Intubation and ventilatory support may be necessary. Loop diuretics (furosemide) and osmotic diuretics (mannitol) may decrease the intracranial pressure but risk causing or exacerbating hypovolemia. If immediate descent is impossible, hyperbaric therapy in a Gamow Bag may be lifesaving. DOT 5-10.81

Lightning and Electrical Injury

There are between 50 and 300 deaths in the United States from lightning strikes annually; four to five times that number suffer nonlethal injuries (Box 38-13).[35] How many of the 296,106,557 people living in the United States (U.S. Census Bureau estimate) were exposed to lightning conditions during that time? Nobody can know the answer to that question.

Lightning is a very high-voltage atmospheric electrical discharge. Technically, it is a unidirectional current impulse (not really direct current or alternating current). The amount of energy released is amazing: up to two billion volts and 300,000 peak amps. There is more electrical energy in a single lightning bolt than is produced by all of the electrical generators in the United States at that instant. However, since the duration of the strike is so short (0.1 to 1 millisecond), there is only enough total electrical energy to light a single light bulb for about a month, if it could be harnessed. This energy is dissipated as light, heat, sound, and radio waves.

Approximately two-thirds of the lightning flashes in the United States happen in the summer months (June, July, and August). Similarly, about two-thirds occur in the afternoon (from noon local time to 6 p.m. local time).[35]

For lightning to develop, there must be an area of charge separation. This typically begins with hailstones and raindrops settling at various rates within a convectively active cloud. Charged particles become stripped off, and the cloud becomes a dipole with a negatively charged base and a positively charged roof. A tripole phenomenon is also possible with a negatively charged base and roof and a positively charged center. In either case, the cloud becomes a large battery or capacitor. The charge separation (potential) can be as great as 7,500 volts per inch. The lightning strike begins with a "stepped leader," an ionized plasma channel that extends

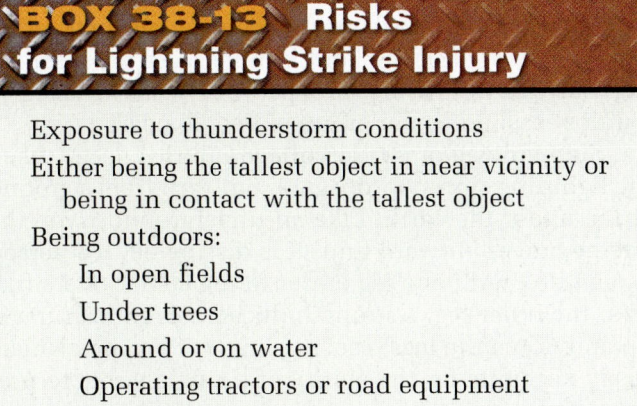

BOX 38-13 Risks for Lightning Strike Injury

Exposure to thunderstorm conditions

Either being the tallest object in near vicinity or being in contact with the tallest object

Being outdoors:

   In open fields

   Under trees

   Around or on water

   Operating tractors or road equipment

   On golf courses

downward in a series of zigzag, short, stepped branches. Simultaneously, there is a rising, positively charged "pilot stroke" coming up from the ground. The pilot stroke and the stepped leader meet at 50 to 100 meters above the ground, creating a connection that initiates the "return stroke." The return stroke is the high-voltage, high-current, high-velocity, rising discharge that we think of as the lightning bolt. Before the plasma channel dissipates, there is an average of four to five return strokes through it. The plasma channel is also extremely hot, up to 8,000° to 50,000°C (by comparison, the surface of the sun is about 6,000°C).[35]

Thunder is the noise that we associate with lightning. It is due to the sudden heating of the air, which creates a pressure rise of up to 10 atm. This causes an acoustic wave or thunder. It tends to have a lower pitch at greater distances and is rarely heard over 10 miles away.

There are several mechanisms for lightning strike injuries, including direct strike or contact, splash or side flash, step or stride voltage, blast trauma, secondary trauma, and fires.

Some **direct strike** victims experience a **flashover phenomenon** in which the current is conducted over the skin without deeper penetration. If this occurs, it lowers the mortality of a direct strike victim from 85% to 40%. However, the victim is standing in a very strong electromagnetic field. That field can cause apnea and asystole. Other evidence of the electromagnetic field includes the characteristic skin signs, described as ferning, arboration, fractals, or Lichtenberg's flowers. This arborescent superficial erythema is pathognomonic for lightning, but it is seen in only about 20% of confirmed lightning strike cases. The erythema is not a true burn and fades within hours. There may, however, also be partial thickness linear or punctate burns in moist skin areas, such as the axilla and groin. There may also be evidence of deeper burn penetration from surface objects (jewelry, belt buckles, and zippers) or around thin skin (eyes and ears). Clothing or nearby objects may ignite and cause secondary thermal burns.

Splash or **side flash injury** occurs when an object is struck (tree or building, for example), and the dissipating current, following the path of least resistance, "jumps" to a person or group of people nearby.

Step voltage or **stride voltage** injuries occur when the lightning current propagates outward from a ground strike under the earth. Like an underground river, the energy moves outward until it is dissipated. If a person is standing with one leg closer to the center of a strike than the other leg, a strong induced current can travel up and down the legs, causing injury. This mechanism likely accounts for the ability of a single strike to produce multiple victims.

Rescuers should keep in mind the violent nature of a lightning strike. Victims are at-risk for blast trauma, secondary trauma from falls (or objects falling on them), and burns from heated metal objects (zippers, jewelry, etc.) in contact with the skin and ignited materials close to the victim (clothing, trees, etc.) These forms of secondary trauma may be occult and difficult to diagnose initially.

Lightning is a rather inefficient killer with a mortality of 5–30%.[35,36,37] However, 70–75% of the survivors have some medical sequelae. Specific lightning complications can include injuries to the heart, lungs, central and peripheral nervous systems, ears, and eyes. Victims who receive a direct lightning strike experience a massive countershock; most are rendered asystolic and apneic. If they maintain their oxygenation, some will recover spontaneous circulation. If, however, they become hypoxic, they can deteriorate into ventricular fibrillation. Other cardiac findings can include nonspecific ST and T wave changes, ST elevation, and T wave inversions. Lightning survivors often experience a hyperadrenergic state manifested by tachycardia and hypertension. Rarely, myocardial infarction can be seen.

Lightning also affects the nervous system. Universally, direct strike victims are amnestic to the incident. Surviving victims may experience transient aphasia, vertigo, Horner's syndrome (loss of ocular sympathetic innervation secondary to a lesion within the sympathetic pathway), pupillary changes, EEG abnormalities, or extrapyramidal symptoms such as dystenic-like complaints. Further, they may have cerebral edema, seizures, ataxia, or coma. A variety of brain injuries, including intracranial hematomas, intraventricular hemorrhage, brain coagulation, skull fractures, and cerebral artery thrombosis, have been described.

An interesting finding is **keraunoparalysis** or **Charcot's paralysis.** This "lightning paraplegia" is characterized by the inability of the victim to move their extremities. It is accompanied by cool, pale skin and diminished peripheral pulses. The pathophysiology likely stems from severe vasoconstriction from the hyperadrenergic state and often resolves.

The blast trauma from the thunderclap can cause pulmonary injuries, including pulmonary contusions and hemorrhage, hemothorax, and pneumothorax. In addition, lightning victims are at-risk for prolonged respiratory depression and hypoxia.

Up to 50% of lightning victims experience tympanic membrane rupture from the thunderclap. Seven to twelve percent of victims have temporary hearing loss, and some have permanent hearing loss. Tinnitus is common but usually resolves over hours to days.

Electrical, thermal, or light energy from a lightning strike injures the eye in as many as 55% of victims. Twenty percent of victims will develop cataracts within three years. Others may experience ocular autonomic disturbances.

There are a number of psychiatric conditions associated with lightning strikes. These can include depression, psychosis, "storm apprehension," memory impairment, personality changes, and hysteria. These are usually transient, and children are more susceptible than adults. It is thought that many of these symptoms represent a direct injury to the limbic system rather than a posttraumatic stress disorder.

Essentially, only those who present in cardiac arrest are at-risk of dying, and bystander CPR doubles survivability from 24% survival without CPR to 50% survival with CPR. It is for this reason that lightning multiple casualty incidents (MCIs) are the exception to the usual triage rules. In the typical MCI, patients who are not moving and not breathing have low priority because they have little chance of survival, and they tend to shift resources away from salvageable victims. In contrast, lightning strike victims in cardiac arrest have a chance of recovery if treated early, and victims who have not arrested have little chance of dying. Therefore, the first triage priority in a lightning MCI goes to those who are not moving and not breathing. Some have called this the **Reverse Triage** principle.

Rescuers should not become victims. The belief that "lightning never strikes twice in the same place" is a myth. In fact, the conditions that made an initial lightning strike possible make subsequent strikes also possible. The Empire State Building in New York City, for example, is struck about 23 times a year; on one occasion, it was struck eight times in 24 minutes. Therefore, rescuers may be at-risk of injury or death by performing treatment on-scene under the same meteorological conditions. It may be prudent in some cases to quickly extricate victims to safer settings.

Submersion Incidents

Drowning is defined as death by suffocation after submersion. The term "near-drowning" is open to misinterpretation and is not preferred. The terminology recommended by the American Heart Association and the European Resuscitation Council is **submersion incident.** A person who suffers adverse affects from being submerged in water has experienced a submersion incident; this may or may not result in a fatal outcome. Submersion incidents can be classified based on the severity of cardiopulmonary findings (Box 38-14). The importance of this system lies with its correlation to mortality: near 0% for Grade 1 up to 93% for Grade 6.[38]

There were 3,447 unintentional drownings in the United States in 2002, not including drownings in boating-related incidents. In children 14 years of age and younger, nonfatal submersion incidents (near-drowning) are three times more common than fatal, although the true incidence may also be underreported.[39] Worldwide, there may be as many as 500,000 deaths from drowning annually.[40] However, this number is nearly impossible to ascertain accurately because of variable reporting.

Submersion incidents have a bimodal age distribution. There is one peak in children less than five years of age. Drowning is the second leading cause of injury-related death for children from one to fourteen years.[39] These incidents frequently happen in bathtubs and swimming pools. Small children (less than one year of age) most often drown in bathtubs, buckets, or toilets.[41] The second peak occurs in young adults of ages 15 to 25. The victims are more often male, accounting for 80% of the fatal drownings in the United States in 2002.[39] These incidents tend to occur in rivers and lakes and at

Nice to Know

Lightening Safety

You may reduce your risk of becoming a lightning strike casualty by doing the following:

1. Avoiding thunderstorms.
2. Avoiding being the tallest lightning "target" in the near vicinity.
3. Avoiding contact with "lightning rods," such as tall trees, fences, golf clubs.
4. Avoiding touching conductors, such as water pipes or electrical wires.
5. Seeking shelter indoors or in a car.
6. Placing your feet together and crouching down to reduce your stride potential.

BOX 38-14 Submersion Incident Classification

Grade 1: Normal examination with cough
Grade 2: Rales in some lung fields
Grade 3: Acute pulmonary edema
Grade 4: Pulmonary edema with arterial hypotension
Grade 5: Isolated respiratory arrest
Grade 6: Cardiopulmonary arrest

Source: A. B. Newman, "Submersion Incidents," In *Wilderness Medicine,* 4th ed., P. S. Auerback ed. (St. Louis, MO: Mosby, 2001), p 1341.

BOX 38-15   Risk Factors for Drowning

- **Male gender:** 80% of drownings in the United States are males.
- **Children:** second leading cause of injury-related death for children from one to 14 years.
- **Race:** the overall age-adjusted drowning rate for African Americans is 1.4 times higher than for whites; most likely, this is primarily due to socioeconomic factors.
- **Alcohol:** 25–50% of adolescent and adult deaths associated with water recreation also involve alcohol use.
- **Boating:** 70% of boating fatalities are caused by drowning.

Source: CDC, "Nonfatal and Fatal Drownings in Recreational Water Settings—United States, 2001–2002," Morbidity Mortality Weekly Report, 53(21)(June 4, 2004):447–452.

beaches.[42] Several risk factors for drowning can be identified (Box 38-15).

Obviously, human beings must breathe to survive. Through force of will, we can hold our breath for a period of time, which is quite variable among individuals and circumstances. Eventually, a "breakpoint" is reached at which a powerful involuntary drive forces inhalation.[43] If this gasp occurs underwater, the result is aspiration. Water enters the lungs and "washes out" surfactant, resulting in alveolar collapse, atelectasis, intrapulmonary shunting, ventilation-perfusion mismatch, pulmonary edema, hypoxia, and acute respiratory distress syndrome (ARDS).[42,44] Hypoxemia, in turn, produces effects in all of the tissues throughout the body.

Ten to twenty percent of drowning victims do not have evidence of a significant volume of aspirated water in their lungs at autopsy. These so-called **dry drownings** were once thought to be the result of severe laryngospasm that could lead to hypoxia and death without allowing water to enter the lungs. This notion has recently been questioned. It is more likely that dry drownings actually represent death by sudden cardiac standstill (as associated with patients with long QT syndrome or mutations in the KCNQ1 or KCNH2 genes).[45,46] The percentage of drowned victims with otherwise normal heart and lungs who do not have penetration of liquid into their airways is less than 2%.[45] Whether or not fluid is aspirated into the lungs would seem to be an important determinant of survival. However, it is nearly impossible in the prehospital environment to establish whether aspiration has taken place. Further, the success of the resuscitation is much more dependent on the rapid reversal of hypoxia rather than whether the drowning was "wet" or "dry."[38] Attempts to remove water from the pulmonary tree by means other than suctioning (such as the Heimlich maneuver) are not necessary, likely not effective, and not recommended.[47]

Most drowned victims aspirate less than 4 mL/kg.[48] However, aspiration of 1–3 mL/kg can lead to significant impairment of gas exchange in the lungs.[40] Aspiration of either freshwater or saltwater in these amounts produces similar effects on the lungs. In theory, aspiration of hypertonic fluids (saltwater) can lead to massive pulmonary edema and hypertonic serum; hypotonic fluids (freshwater) can lead to intravascular volume overload, dilution of serum electrolytes, and hemolysis. However, aspiration of more than 11 mL/kg is necessary before blood volume changes occur; aspiration of more than 22 mL/kg is necessary before electrolyte changes occur.[48,49,50] Therefore, the distinction between freshwater and saltwater drowning is not significant in the majority of cases. It is the amount of water aspirated, not the tonicity, that determines the effects on the lungs.

The signs and symptoms of submersion incidents can range from subtle to profound. The lungs are nearly always affected to some degree. However, other organ systems may also become involved (Table 38-6).

Immersion syndrome is sudden death upon submersion in very cold water (at least 5°C less than body temperature). The pathophysiology of this phenomenon is not well understood but is likely a result of vagal stimulation and subsequent cardiac arrest. It has been postulated that this is related to the **mammalian dive reflex.** This reflex is triggered by cold water stimulating receptors in the skin. Vasoconstriction then shunts blood away from the skin, mesentery, and extremities toward the brain and heart. Bradycardia results from vagal nerve stimulation in response to this increase in central blood volume. There is great individual variability in the strength of this reflex in human beings, and it is probably strongest in small children.

Immersion in cold water quickly induces hypothermia. Water has 25 times the ability to conduct heat as does air. Heat can be lost quickly through the skin. Further, swallowing or aspiration of cold water can also lead to very rapid core cooling. Significant cerebral cooling is likely in these patients, even before circulatory collapse.[51] This may have a protective effect through decreasing the oxygen demands of the brain. This phenomenon probably accounts for the rare cases of recovery in victims submerged under very cold water for 30 minutes or more. These patients are usually profoundly hypothermic and may appear to be dead.

It is generally considered prudent to continue resuscitation efforts until the victim has been warmed to at least a core temperature of 33° to 35°C.

TABLE 38-6   Common Symptoms and Signs of Submersion Incidents by Organ Systems

Organ System	Symptoms	Signs
Pulmonary	Coughing Choking Dyspnea	Apnea Hypoxia Cyanosis Tachypnea Rhonchi Rales Wheezing Pulmonary edema Aspiration pneumonia
Central nervous system	Lethargy Coma	Cytotoxic cerebral edema Increased ICP Decreased cerebral perfusion pressure
Renal	Nausea Vomiting	Acute renal failure*
Gastrointestinal	Palpitations Chest pain	Gastric distention Aspiration
Cardiac		Dysrhythmias Cardiac arrest Hypotension Cardiac ischemia Immersion syndrome
Hematologic		Acidosis (lactate) Coagulopathy DIC

*As a result from hypoxia, acidosis, or rhabdomyolysis.

The pathophysiology and treatment of hypothermia is discussed in the beginning of this chapter.

Postimmersion syndrome has been called "secondary drowning." It is the development of the acute respiratory distress syndrome hours or days after the initial resuscitation. It occurs in up to 5% of submersion patients.[52] The etiology is likely multifactorial and includes hypoxia, loss of surfactant, transalveolar fluid shifts, and aspiration of contaminants.

Prompt rescue breathing is the most important treatment for submersion victims. If it can be safely accomplished while the patient is being extricated from the water, it should be. Routine immobilization of the cervical spine is not necessary unless there is a history of diving, use of a water slide, signs of trauma, or signs of alcohol intoxication.[47] If any of those conditions are present, however, the patient should be suspected of having suffered occult trauma and should be treated accordingly. There is no need to clear the patient's airway of aspirated water. Due to buoyancy, in-water chest compressions are ineffective. However, they may be provided once the patient has been extricated, if necessary. Early intubation and the usual ACLS guidelines are recommended. The patient's wet clothing should be removed and the patient should be wrapped in blankets to prevent further hypothermia. All submersion victims, regardless of how minimal their resuscitation need, require monitoring and transportation to a medical facility.

Treatment in the emergency department is guided by the patient's signs and symptoms over the first six to eight hours. If a patient remains awake and alert, asymptomatic, and not hypoxic after that period of observation, the patient may be discharged. Supplemental oxygen, continuous positive airway pressure (CPAP), intubation, active or passive rewarming, CPR, cardiac resuscitation, or trauma resuscitation can be administered based on specific findings.

Several treatments for submersion victims have been studied, including, barbiturates, steroids, nitric oxide, therapeutic hypothermia, and vasopressin. To date, there is insufficient evidence to recommend any of them.[47] **E**xtra**c**orporeal **m**embrane **o**xygenation **(ECMO)** has been described in case reports in the treatment of young children with severe hypothermia after submersion. The early, quick actions of the prehospital providers to provide ventilation and treat hypothermia remain the most important therapies for submersion incident victims.

Summary

Environmental emergencies occur when changes in the environment or extreme environmental exposures challenge or overwhelm the body's ability to adapt or compensate for these exposures and the effects they bring about. Paramedics must understand normal body function and responses, how the body adapts and compensates, and the signs and symptoms of a body that is losing the battle to exposure. Simple measures to protect the patient and more complex and specific management options and the paramedic's familiarity with them will make a significant difference to these patients.

Notes

1. B. Yarbrough and S. Vicario, "Heat Illness," *Rosen's Emergency Medicine: Concepts and Clinical Practice,* 5th ed., J. Marx, R. Hockberger, and R. Walls, eds. (St. Louis, MO: Mosby, 2002), 1997.
2. J. Knochal, "Dog Days and Siriasis. How to Kill a Football Player," *Journal of the American Medical Association* 233(6)(1975): 513–515.
3. CDC "Hypothermia-Related Deaths—Vermont, October 1994–February 1996," *Morbidity and Mortality Weekly Report: Surveillance Summaries* 45(1996): 1093.
4. K. Juopperi, J. Hassi, et al., "Incidence of Frostbite and Ambient Temperature in Finland, 1986–1995. A National Study Based on Hospital Admissions," *International Journal of Circumpolar Health* 61(4)(2002): 352–362.
5. D. Robertshaw, "Factors in Heat Stroke," In *Heat Stroke and Temperature Regulation,* M. Khogali and J. Hales, eds. (New York, NY: Academic Press, 1983).
6. M. McKinley and V. D. O'Loughlin, *Human Anatomy* (New York, NY: McGraw-Hill, 2006), 569.
7. J. R. Sutton, "Heatstroke from Running," *Journal of the American Medical Association* 243(19)(1980): 1896.
8. M. G. Austin and J. W. Berry, "Observations on One Hundred Cases of Heatstroke," *Journal of the American Medical Association* 161(16)(1956): 1525–1529.
9. D. Richards et al., "Management of Heat Exhaustion in Sydney's the Sun City-to-Surf Run Runners," *The Medical Journal of Australia* 2(9)(1979): 457–461.
10. S. Shibolet et al., "Heatstroke: Its Clinical Picture and Mechanism in 36 Cases," *The Quarterly Journal of Medicine* 36(144)(1967): 525–548.
11. M. Weinmann, "Hot on the Inside," *Emergency Medical Services* 32(7)(2003): 34.
12. H. B. Simon, "Hyperthermia," *The New England Journal of Medicine* 329(7)(1993): 483–487.
13. D. Danzl, R. Pozos, and M. Hamlet, "Accidental Hypothermia," In *Rosen's Emergency Medicine: Concepts and Clinical Practice,* 5th ed., J. Marx, R. Hockberger, and R. Walls, eds. (St. Louis, MO: Mosby, 2002).
14. P. O. Granberg, "Human Physiology Under Cold Exposure," *Artic Medical Research* 50 (Suppl 6)(1991): 23–27.
15. B. Wedin, L. Vanggaard, et al., "Paradoxical Undressing' in Fatal Hypothermia," *Journal of Forensic Sciences* 24(3)(1979): 543–553.
16. A. Brylske, "A Brief History of Diving: Evolution of the Self-Contained Diver (Part 2)," *Dive Training* 4(1994): 20–26.
17. T. S. Neuman, A. A. Bove, R. D. O'Connor, and S. G. Kelsen, "Asthma and Diving," *Annals of Asthma* 73(1994): 344.
18. S. M. Green, S. G. Rothrock, et al., "Tympanometric Evaluation of Middle Ear Barotrauma During Recreational Scuba Diving," *International Journal of Sports Medicine* 14(7)(1993): 411–415.
19. *U.S. Navy Diving Manual, Revision* 4, Naval Sea Systems Command (United States Navy, 1999).
20. Z. Baj, R. Olszanski, et al., "The Effect of Air and Nitrox Divings on Platelet Activation Tested by Flow Cytometry," *Aviation, Space, and Environmental Medicine* 71(9)(2000): 925–928.
21. G. Masurel, "The Value of Ultrasonic Detection of Circulating Bubbles in Animal and Man—The Contribution to Physiopathogenesis of a Decompression Accident," *Schweizerische Zeitshrift fur Sportmedizin* 37(1)(1989): 41–44.
22. B. D. Butler and B. A. Hills, "The Lung as a Filter for Microbubbles," *Journal of Applied Physiology: Respiratory, Environmental, and Exercise Physiology* 47(3)(1979): 537–543.
23. T. J. R. Francis and D. F. Gorman, "The Pathogenesis of the Decompression Disorders," In *The Physiology and Medicine of Diving,* 4th ed. P. B. Bennett and D. H. Elliott eds. (Philadelphia, PA: WB Saunders, 1993).
24. R. H. Cales, N. Humphreys, et al., "Cardiac Arrest From Gas Embolism in Scuba Diving," *Annals of Emergency Medicine* 10(11)(1981): 589–592.
25. M. B. Strauss and R. C. Borer, Jr., "Diving Medicine: Contemporary Topics and Their Controversies," *The American Journal of Emergency Medicine* 19(3)(2001): 232–238.
26. A. J. Tomassoni, "Cardiac Problems Associated with Dysbarism," *Cardiology Clinics* 13(2)(1995): 266–271.
27. W. A. Watson, T. L. Litovitz, et al., "2003 Annual Report of the American Association of Poison Control Centers Toxic Exposure Surveillance System," *The American Journal of Emergency Medicine* 22(5)(2004): 335–404.
28. L. W. Shockley, "Bites and Stings," In *Emergency Medicine Secrets,* 3rd ed., V. J. Markovchick and P. T. Pons, eds. (Philadelphia, PA, St. Louis, MO: Hanley & Belfus, Mosby, 1993), 407–417.
29. P. Hackett and R. Roach, "High-Altitude Medicine," In *Wilderness Medicine,* P. S. Auerbach ed. (St. Louis, MO: Mosby, 2001), 2–43.
30. B. Honigman, M. K. Theis, J. Koziol-McLain, R. Roach, R. Yip, C. Houston, L. G. Moore, and P. Pearce, "Acute Mountain Sickness in a General Tourist Population at Moderate Altitudes," *Annals of Internal Medicine* 118(8)(April 15, 1993): 587–592.
31. C. Clarke "High Altitude Cerebral Edema," *International Journal of Sports Medicine* 9(2)(April 1988): 170–174.
32. I. Singh, P. K. Khanna, et al., "Acute Mountain Sickness," *The New England Journal of Medicine* 280(4)(1969): 175–184.
33. B. Honigman and M. Yaron, "High-Altitude Medicine," In *Rosen's Emergency Medicine: Concepts and Clinical Practice,* 5th ed., J. Marx, R. Hockberger, and R. Walls, ed. (St. Louis, MO: Mosby, 2002), pp. 2035–2050.

34. C. S. Houston and J. Dickinson, "Cerebral Form of High-Altitude Illness," *Lancet* 2(7938)(1975): 758–761.

35. M. A. Cooper, C. J. Andrews, R. L. Holle, and R. E. Lopez, "Lightning Injuries," In *Wilderness Medicine,* 4th ed., P. S. Auerbach, ed. (St. Louis, MO: Mosby, 2001), pp. 73–110.

36. M. A. Cooper, "Lightning Injuries: Prognostic Signs for Death," *Annals of Emergency Medicine* 9(1980): 134.

37. C. J. Andrews, M. Darveniza, and D. Mackerras, "Lightning Injury: A Review of Clinical Aspects, Pathophysiology and Treatment," *Advances in Trauma* 4(1989): 241.

38. A. B. Newman, "Submersion Incidents," In *Wilderness Medicine,* 4th ed., P. S. Auerbach, ed. (St. Louis, MO: Mosby, 2001).

39. "Nonfatal and Fatal Drownings in Recreational Water Settings—United States, 2001–2002," *Morbidity and Mortality Weekly Report: Surveillance Summaries* 53(21)(June 4, 2004): 447–452.

40. J. P. Orlowski and D. Szpilman, "Drowning. Rescue, Resuscitation, and Reanimation," *Pediatric Clinics of North America* 48(3)(June 2001): 627–646.

41. R. A. Brenner, A. C. Trumble, G. S. Smith, et al., "Where Children Drown, United States, 1995," *Pediatrics* 108(1) (July 2001): 85–89.

42. L. K. DeNicola, J. L. Falk, M. E. Swanson, et al., "Submersion Injuries in Children and Adults," *Critical Care Clinics* 13(3)(July 1997): 477–502.

43. M. J. Parkes, "Breath-Holding and Its Breakpoint," *Experimental Physiology* 91(1)(January 2006): 1–15.

44. J. J. Bierens, J. T. Knape, and H. P. Gelissen, "Drowning," *Current Opinion in Critical Care* 8(6)(December 2002): 578–586.

45. P. Lunetta, J. H. Modell, and A. Sajantila, "What Is the Incidence and Significance of 'Dry-Lungs' in Bodies Found in Water?" *The American Journal of Forensic Medicine and Pathology* 25(4)(December 2004): 291–301.

46. J. H. Modell, M. Bellefleur, and J. H. Davis, "Drowning Without Aspiration: Is This an Appropriate Diagnosis?" *Journal of Forensic Sciences* 44(6)(November 1999): 1119–1123.

47. "2005 American Heart Association Guidelines for Cardiopulmonary Resuscitation and Emergency Cardiovascular Care," 112 (24 Supplement) (December 13, 2005): IV–134.

48. J. H. Modell and J. H. Davis, "Electrolyte Changes in Human Drowning Victims," *Anesthesiology* 30(4)(April 1969): 414–420.

49. J. H. Modell and F. Moya, "Effects of Volume of Aspirated Fluid During Chlorinated Fresh Water Drowning," *Anesthesiology* 27(5)(September–October 1966): 662–672.

50. J. H. Modell, F. Moya, E. J. Newby, et al., "The Effects of Fluid Volume in Seawater Drowning," *Annals of Internal Medicine* 67(1)(July 1967): 68–80.

51. A. W. Conn and G. A. Barker, "Fresh Water Drowning and Near-Drowning—An Update," *Canadian Anaesthetists' Society Journal* 31(3 Pt 2)(May 1984): S38–44.

52. J. H. Pearn, "Secondary Drowning in Children," *British Medical Journal* 281(6248)(October 25, 1980): 1103–1105.

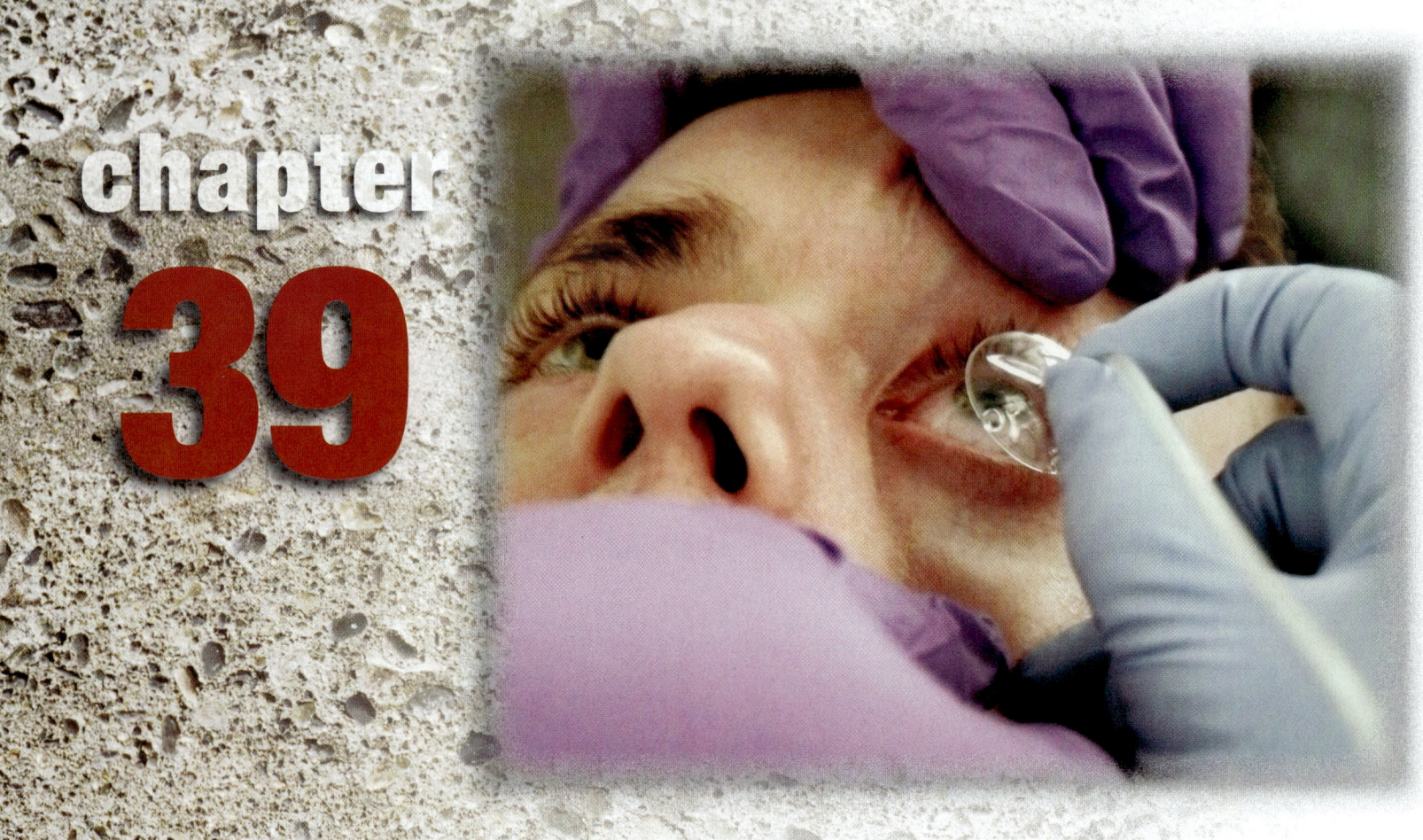

Eyes, Ears, Nose, and Throat

"See with your eyes, hear with your ears. Nothing is hidden."

—Tenkei

Need to Know

▶ Complaints about the throat, nose, eyes, and ears can range from mild and of little consequence to severe or life-threatening. Injury or illness to these structures can result in compromise to the airway and breathing.

▶ Loss of function in terms of speech ability, sight, or hearing can result in a lifetime of disability and may force a person out of their chosen career or seriously affect their interpersonal relationships.

▶ Long-term psychological impact is possible when an illness or injury results in permanent scarring or disfigurement.

▶ Sick	▶ Not Yet Sick
• Any airway compromise, whether actual or impending, requires prompt assessment, monitoring, and treatment.	• Ask the patient if any prior conditions involving the throat, nose, or eyes resulted in an emergent situation. Pay particular attention to any history of compromise of the airway or breathing.
	• Carefully screen the patient for any history of allergies, anaphylaxis, or hypersensitivity to allergens.

Introduction

The presenting signs or symptoms for throat, nose, eye, and ear complaints may be subtle and can belie serious illness or injury that threaten hearing, sight, speech, or even life. Whether injury or illness, vital senses that orient people to the environment and others they interact with, as well as the airway, can be affected by illness or an injury involving the eyes, ears, nose, and throat. Obtaining a careful history of the events precipitating the complaint and closely examining the head and neck for signs of significant pathology are essential. **Skill Sheet 56: Eye Drop Drug Administration and Skill Sheet 80: Eye Irrigation support this chapter.**

Primary Survey—Initial Assessment

The primary survey of patients with throat, nose, eye, and ear problems is directed at identifying any life-threatening injuries or illnesses that may require immediate intervention by the paramedic. Immediate problems that must be corrected involve the following:

■ Compromise to the airway and ventilation and traumatic injuries resulting in loss of blood or penetration of the head or neck. These situations include the following:

  • Patients complaining of difficulty speaking, inability to swallow, significant throat pain, or tightness demand immediate attention to airway patency.

  • Inflammation and swelling of the epiglottis can quickly lead to complete airway obstruction.

  • Foreign bodies can lodge in the throat, partially or fully occluding the airway.

  • Victims of inhalation burns may develop airway edema that is rapidly progressive.

  • Patients with exaggerated hypersensitivity (allergic) reactions and anaphylaxis are in danger of losing their airways from edema.

  • Patients with obvious nasal trauma have the potential for underlying serious intracranial, maxillofacial, or cervical spine injury.

  • Nosebleeds that cannot be controlled with compression of the nares.

■ Of secondary importance is loss of an organ or loss of function of the organ.

  • Significant eye injuries result from high-energy blunt trauma or penetration of the globe with sharp objects.

  • An ophthalmologic emergency that demands immediate intervention in the field is a chemical burn to the cornea.

  • Trauma to the external ear is common and can cause long-term cosmetic disfigurement.

  • Thermal injury to the ear often accompanies burns to the head and face and may be severe enough to cause necrosis and sloughing of the entire auricle.

  • Neck trauma may result in the inability to speak clearly and distinctly.

Throat Complaints

Any patient complaining of difficulty speaking, inability to swallow, throat pain, or tightness demands immediate attention to airway patency. Numerous processes can narrow or close the airway, including obstruction by a foreign body or swelling from allergic reactions, trauma, burns, or infection. The patient should be monitored constantly for signs of airway closure. Early intervention is essential to prevent death due to hypoxia or suffocation. DOT 2-1.1, 4-4.5

Clues to throat problems may be subtle, and a seemingly minor complaint can rapidly and unexpectedly deteriorate into an immediate life threat. If the patient is speaking in a normal voice, in full sentences, and with no sign of respiratory distress, the airway is patent for the moment. DOT 2-1.2

Applied Anatomy and Physiology of the Throat

The throat, or **oropharynx,** is the only anatomic conduit in which air drawn in through the nose or mouth can pass to the lower respiratory tract (Figure 39-1). Air must pass through the larynx to enter and exit the trachea. Intricately coordinated movement of small muscles and the **vocal cords** within the larynx generate phonation (speech) as air flows through the throat. DOT 2-1.3, 2-1.4, 4-5.25, 4-5.26, 4-5.27, 4-5.28

The throat is also the only anatomic route by which ingested food and liquid can pass from the mouth into the stomach. The muscular tongue is the most anterior

structure of the pharynx, and one of its main functions (in addition to aiding in speaking) is to direct the passage of liquid and chewed food to the back of the throat and into the esophagus. The esophagus is a collapsible muscular tube whose opening lies immediately behind the larynx. The superior opening of the larynx is protected by the epiglottis, a flap of soft tissue that folds over to seal the larynx during swallowing to prevent food and liquid from passing into the trachea. DOT 4-5.29, 4-5.30, 4-5.31, 4-5.32, 4-5.33, 4-5.34, 5-1.2

Pathophysiology of Throat Complaints

Any process that causes swelling within or around the throat can narrow the airway to the point of obstruction. Foreign body obstructions can quickly lead to death if not relieved. Blunt or penetrating trauma to the neck can cause bleeding and swelling of the soft tissues surrounding the throat, compressing the cavity and impeding airflow. Burns to the respiratory system can cause rapid life-threatening swelling. Allergic and certain drug reactions can cause a similar and very dangerous pattern of swelling.[1] A number of specific infections, including epiglottitis, laryngotracheitis (croup), and abscesses can lead to soft tissue swelling in or around the throat and can threaten the airway. DOT 2-1.23, 2-1.25

Primary Survey

The patient with significant or complete airway obstruction from any cause will have increasing hypoxia and may demonstrate panic and agitation before developing lethargy and coma. Rapid and labored respirations with obvious accessory muscle use may degenerate into complete apnea. The skin may appear cyanotic, but this is an ominous, late finding. The conscious patient with partial airway patency will speak in a muffled or distorted voice in one- or two-word, gasping sentences. As the obstruction worsens, speech may be altogether impossible. The patient will attempt to assume a position that maintains maximal airway patency, usually by sitting upright and forward with the neck slightly extended. This position is referred to as the **sniffing position** or **tripod position,** where the patient juts the jaw and lifts the chin slightly in an attempt to align the airway into a better position for breathing (Figure 39-2). DOT 2-1.24, 2-1.26, 2-1.27, 2-1.29

Less obvious signs may signify a partial narrowing of the airway with potential to progress to full obstruction. **Stridor** is a high-pitched whistling sound that results from air passing through an abnormally narrowed portion of the upper respiratory tract during inspiration. When severe, it is easily heard with each inspiration by the patient. Less pronounced stridor, however, may only be detectable through a stethoscope placed over the patient's anterior neck. Other important

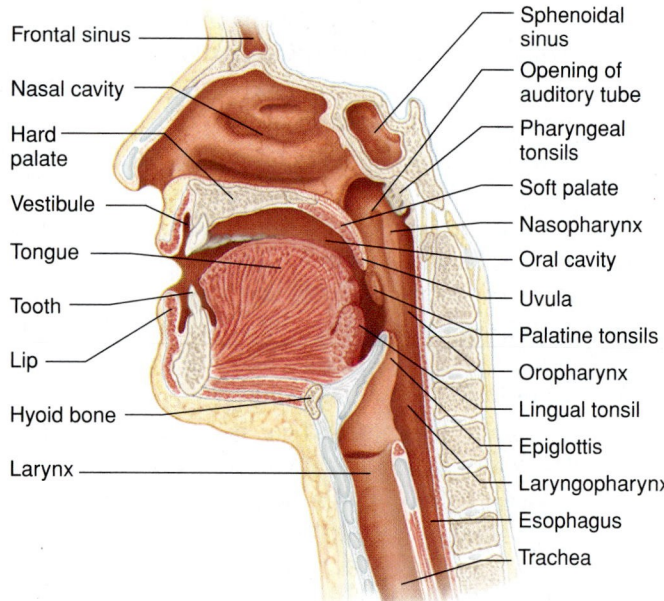

Frontal sinus
Nasal cavity
Hard palate
Vestibule
Tongue
Tooth
Lip
Hyoid bone
Larynx

Sphenoidal sinus
Opening of auditory tube
Pharyngeal tonsils
Soft palate
Nasopharynx
Oral cavity
Uvula
Palatine tonsils
Oropharynx
Lingual tonsil
Epiglottis
Laryngopharynx
Esophagus
Trachea

Figure 39-1   Anatomy of the throat.

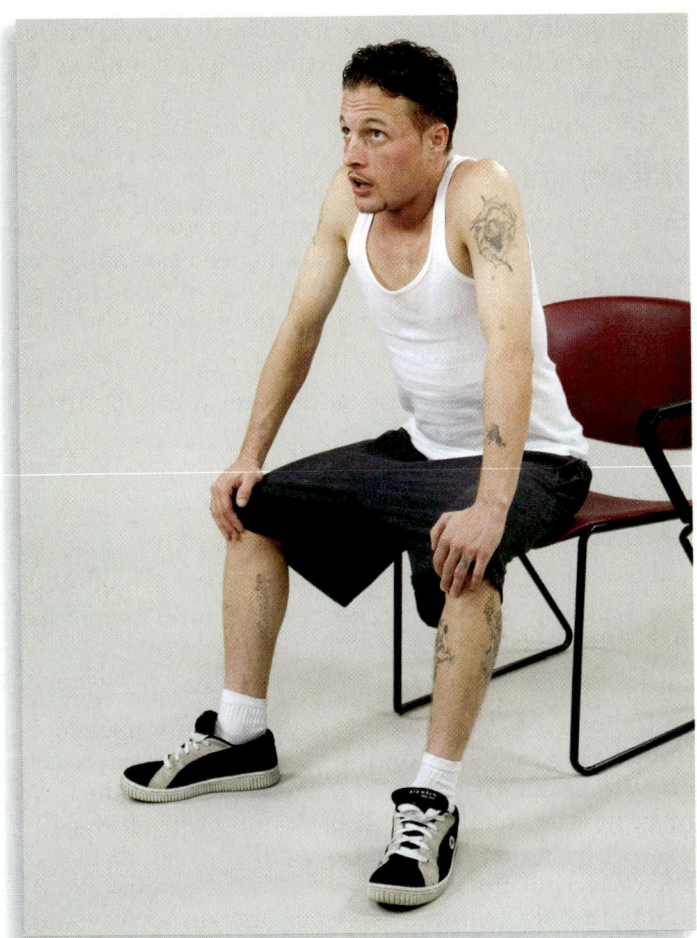
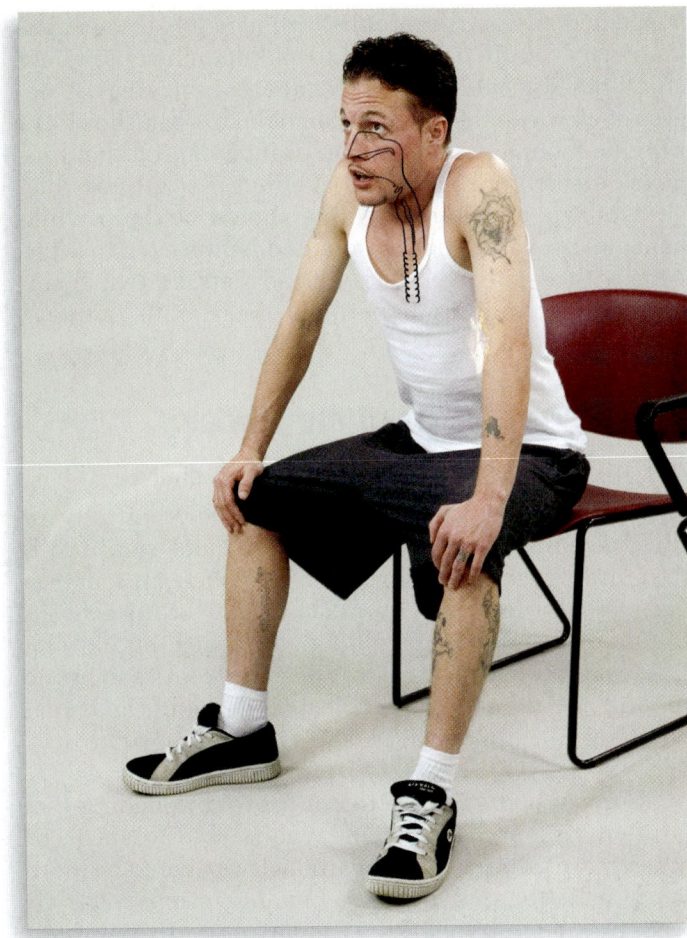

Figure 39-2   The tripod position. Note how the larynx and trachea align, allowing for better air flow.

clues to the threatened airway include changes in voice pitch or volume, drooling, or slight increases in the normal respiratory rate. DOT 2-1.55, 2-1.78, 3-2.8, 4-3.43

External signs and symptoms in the patient with throat pain or swelling may be few or may offer important clues to the nature of the underlying problem. If open wounds are present in the soft tissues of the neck, occlusive dressings should be applied immediately. Inhalation burns of the mouth, throat, and lower respiratory tract are often accompanied by obvious external findings of thermal injury. Facial burns, singed nasal hairs, or the coughing up of soot-laden sputum signify that damage to the tissues lining the upper airway has likely occurred and may progress to airway-threatening edema. In the setting of anaphylaxis, tongue and lip swelling is common, and the patient may also complain of hives or an urticarial rash.[1] DOT 4-3.17, 4-3.18, 4-3.32, 4-3.33

A patient with significant bacterial infection of the throat such as epiglottitis or parapharyngeal abscess will appear toxic with a high fever. Drooling is common because of the patient's inability to swallow secretions, and these individuals resist any effort or encouragement to lie supine because this often occludes the airway further. A patient with croup rarely appears toxic, but detectable stridor, increased work of breathing, and a barky cough should immediately alert the paramedic to the underlying disease process.[2,3]

Street Secrets

When a patient presents with obstructed respirations, you can determine the location of obstruction by whether the abnormal sounds are apparent on inspiration or expiration. If the patient has respiratory noises or wheezes on inspiration, the obstruction is in the upper airway. If the wheezes are expiratory, the problem is in the lower airway.

General Approach to Management of Throat Conditions

The approach to patients with throat pain or discomfort hinges on whether a threat to the airway is apparent or suspected. In the majority of cases, patients with suspected airway compromise who are breathing spontaneously should be allowed to maintain the position of comfort that enables them to maintain the greatest degree of airway patency. Supplemental oxygen should be provided, but any other action or intervention that provokes discomfort should be avoided if at all possible. Transport to a receiving facility should be rapid while constant preparation is maintained for the need to intervene with assisted ventilation or advanced airway management techniques if patients deteriorate. DOT 3-2.61, 4-3.46, 4-3.47

Specific Problems of the Throat
Foreign Body Obstruction

Foreign bodies can lodge in the throat, partially or fully occluding the airway. Toddlers and small children are particularly susceptible to such obstruction because of a tendency to place objects of all sorts in the mouth, a poorly developed gag reflex, and a relatively narrow upper airway. The elderly are also prone to food and other foreign objects lodging in the throat because of a diminished gag response. DOT 3-2.20, 3-2.22, 3-4.2, 4-3.44, 4-3.45

Foreign bodies in the throat provoke coughing that is often violent. The patient who is able to speak or muster a cough has at least partial airway patency. More ominous is the patient who is unable to move any air past the obstruction. Progression to frank cyanosis, coma, and full cardiopulmonary arrest may be rapid without prompt intervention.[2,4]

If a foreign body is suspected, allow the breathing and coughing patient to continue attempts to clear the airway, but be prepared to intervene quickly and decisively if fatigue or progression to complete obstruction precipitates complete respiratory failure. Clearing the airway of a foreign body is best accomplished with the foreign body airway obstruction (FBAO) maneuvers recommended by the American Heart Association.

Anaphylaxis

Signs of anaphylaxis include the following:

- Respiratory distress
- Laryngeal edema
- Intense bronchospasm
- Vascular collapse
- Shock
- Pruritis
- Urticaria
- Gastrointestinal manifestations, including nausea, vomiting, diarrhea, and cramps[5] DOT 5-5.1, 5-5.2

In the setting of an acute allergic reaction threatening the airway, the administration of epinephrine and diphenhydramine is indicated. Advanced airway management will be necessary if the patient continues to deteriorate.[4]

Trauma to the Throat

Injury to the throat may involve the upper airway, jaw, and neck. It is characterized by hoarseness, apnea or respiratory distress, stridor, or bubbling of blood during inspiration or expiration in open neck wounds or subcutaneous emphysema.

- Assume cervical spine compromise has occurred, and stabilize accordingly.
- Cover all open wounds on the skin of the neck with occlusive dressings.
- Dress all freely bleeding wounds.
- Use direct pressure to control external bleeding.
- Utilize suction as necessary to control secretions and blood.

The alert patient can often be given the suction device and allowed to self-suction any accumulating secretions or blood. Fracture of the mandible disrupts the structural integrity of the jaw and may permit the now unsupported tongue to fall back and obstruct the airway. Pulling the mandible forward is often all that is necessary to relieve the obstruction. Use airway adjuncts to help maintain an open, patent airway, and provide oxygen and ventilatory support, as needed. Airway management may require intubation or cricothyrotomy. If subcutaneous emphysema is present, assume a tracheobronchial or thoracic injury is also present.[6] DOT 4-6.3, 4-6.27

> **CONNECTIONS** Chapter 20: Head, Face, and Neck Trauma discusses head and neck trauma. Please refer to that chapter for additional information on managing throat injuries.

Respiratory Burns

Normally the oropharynx, nasopharynx, and upper airway regulate the temperature of inspired air and dissipate any excess heat, even in the presence of fire. However, dissipation of heat within the airway can result in significant thermal injury to the proximal portion of the tracheo-bronchial tree, causing life-threatening edema. Thermal injury manifests itself as edema, hemorrhage, and ulceration, and the swelling often progresses rapidly. True thermal damage to the lower airway is rare, unless exploding gasses or steam are inhaled directly. When present, these patients often die from untreatable asphyxia.[7] DOT 4-4.1, 4-4.2, 4-4.3, 4.4-4, 4.4-12, 4-4.13, 4-4.23–4-4.30, 4-4.57, 4-4.62, 4-4.67, 4-4.76, 4-4.79, 4-4.81

Patients with the greatest risk of airway obstruction within the first 24 hours following the injury are those injured in an explosion with burns to the face and upper thorax and also those unconscious in a fire in what is referred to as a **confined space situation.** These patients are at greatest risk of airway compromise within the first 24 hours following the injury.[7] Signs of respiratory burn include singed nasal nares, soot around the nares, carbonaceous sputum (sooty spit), hoarseness, stridor, and symptoms of respiratory distress.[6]

Patients suspected of respiratory burns should be intubated at the earliest sign of airway compromise, utilizing advanced airway techniques, including rapid sequence intubation, if necessary. Consider the need to use an ET tube smaller than expected (with standard measurement techniques) due to the swelling. A surgical airway such as cricothyrotomy may be required if intubation is not possible.[7] DOT 3-2.63, 3-4.1

CONNECTIONS See also Chapter 26: Burn Trauma for additional information.

Airway Compromise from Diseases

Epiglottitis. Epiglottitis is a bacterial infection of the epiglottis that is particularly hazardous because of that structure's strategic location at the opening of the larynx. Inflammation and swelling of the epiglottis can quickly lead to complete airway obstruction (Figure 39-3).

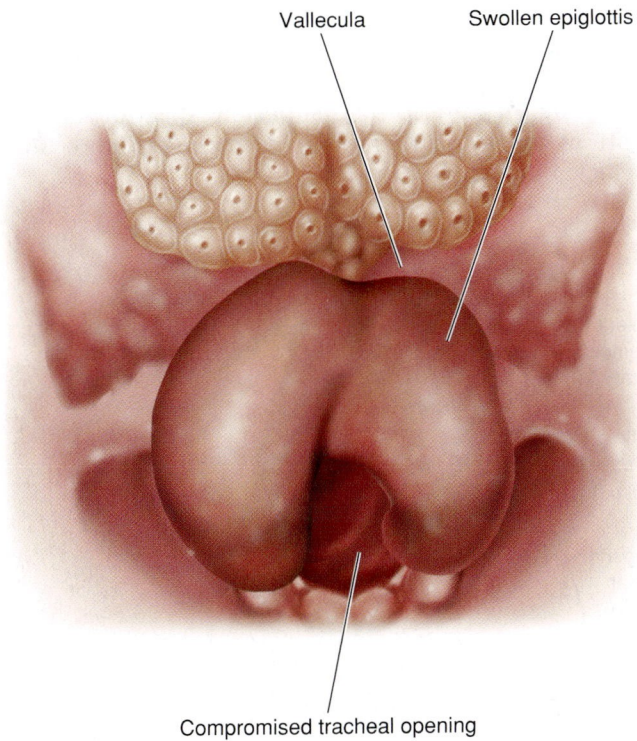

Vallecula   Swollen epiglottis

Compromised tracheal opening

Figure 39-3   View of epiglottitis. Note the small opening of the airway.

Moreover, the inflamed tissues of the epiglottis and the base of the throat are extremely sensitive to even the slightest irritation that can stimulate further swelling of the tissues within the larynx, closing the airway.[3]

Although epiglottitis can occur in any age group (including adults), at one time the median age was three years old. For years, the bacteria *Haemophilus influenzae* was the primary causative agent for epiglottitis. With the introduction and widespread use of immunization for *H. influenzae,* the groups most commonly affected now are older children and adults, and *H. influenzae* now accounts for less than 25% of all epiglottis infections. Currently gram positive organisms such as *Streptococcus pyogenes, Staphylococcus aureus,* and *Streptococcus pneumoniae* account for most cases of the disease found in immunized individuals.[8]

The signs of epiglottitis vary by the age of the patient. Adults and older children may have subtle signs and symptoms and may only complain of a sore throat. These patients may complain of severe tenderness upon manipulation of the hyoid bone which is located at the top of the larynx. As the infection and swelling progress, stridor may also be noted. These patients can often be handled as general "sick" patients unless airway compromise is present. Bag-mask ventilation can be performed, if necessary, but intubation or other aggressive therapy should be avoided unless the paramedic is proficient in handling difficult airways.[8] Swelling of the epiglottis distorts the visible anatomy and tissues during intubation thus making the procedure extremely difficult.

The classic signs of epiglottitis seen in younger patients are an abrupt onset of high fever, sore throat, stridor, and drooling. Cough is generally not a sign accompanying epiglottitis. If inflammation extends beyond the epiglottis, the voice pitch may be muffled or altered. Signs generally develop over several hours but may take one to two days to become severe. The child often appears very apprehensive and extremely sick. If able, the child will sit in the "sniffing" (tripod) position.[8]

When it occurs in children, epiglottitis can quickly lead to life-threatening complications due to edema and laryngospasm resulting in airway obstruction. Optimal management of pediatric patients with epiglottitis occurs in the operating room, not in the ambulance.[9] The child should be gently handled with the goal of maintaining the child in a calm state. For this reason, invasive procedures such as IV therapy and bag-mask ventilation should be withheld unless apnea occurs. Supplemental oxygen should be administered to all children with signs of respiratory distress.

CONNECTIONS See Chapter 43: Pediatric Patients for additional information on managing patients with epiglottitis.

Laryngotracheitis. Laryngotracheitis, or **croup,** is an infection of the tissues within and below the larynx. Nearly all cases of croup are caused by parainfluenza virus type I, II, and III, but it can also be caused by influenza A or B, respiratory syncytial virus (RSV), rhinoviruses, adenoviruses, and even the measles virus.

Croup is particularly common among children between the ages of three months and six years, with the peak incidence occurring between the ages of one and two years. Soft tissue swelling at and below the vocal cords accounts for the characteristic "seal-like" barky cough classically associated with croup. The cough generally lasts for three to four days and is worse in the late evening and at night and may even only occur at that time. If a fever is present, it is generally low-grade. Infants and small children are particularly vulnerable to airway narrowing from croup or other inflammatory processes due to the small airway size.

Although life-threatening complications with croup are rare, a child with signs and symptoms of croup should be handled gently. Humidified air is thought to soothe the throat but has not been shown to be effective in studies.[9] Keep the child with the parent to decrease agitation during transport for further evaluation. Blow-by oxygen can be administered if the child will tolerate it. Pulse oximetry should be monitored, but IV or IO rehydration is usually not required in the hospital setting, so it is reasonable to assume it is not required in the prehospital setting either.[9]

CONNECTIONS Chapter 43: Pediatric Patients contains additional information on croup.

Other Infections of the Throat. Infections in the tissues surrounding the oropharynx can lead to pus collecting to form an abscess in the parapharyngeal spaces. The signs and symptoms can be very similar to those of epiglottitis. The patient will complain of a sore throat, trouble swallowing, and fever. Difficulty handling secretions, resulting in drooling, may be noted. Unlike epiglottitis, there may be visible swelling of the neck or submandibular area. As the abscess expands, it can block the airway, leading to stridor and respiratory distress. Such abscesses are usually the result of the unchecked progression of severe dental and other oral infections.[2]

Most cases of abscess are treated in the hospital by needle or surgical aspiration or antibiotics. Prehospital treatment is aimed at transport for evaluation, and unless airway compromise is present, the transport is not emergent.[2,9]

Nose Complaints

Since the nasopharynx is a component of the airway, complaints of the nose are discussed next. The nose sticks out prominently from the head, rendering it particularly susceptible to trauma. The rich, vascular supply of the tissues lining its inner passages predisposes the nose to hemorrhage **(epistaxis)** that can occur spontaneously or from injury. Bleeding from the nasopharynx could compromise the airway, or if swallowed in quantity, can result in nausea and vomiting. DOT 4-4.5

Applied Anatomy and Physiology of the Nose

The nose serves to warm, humidify, and filter air drawn through its passages en route to the lower respiratory tract. Its structural integrity is maintained by cartilage and thin sheets of bone. Hair follicles and moist mucous membranes lining the internal surfaces of the nose trap particulate matter present in inspired air. The nasal septum divides the passages of the nose longitudinally, and each side of the nose contains convoluted channels for airflow formed by the nasal turbinates. Turbulent airflow through the turbinates slows air movement to allow time for warming by the highly vascular mucosa lining the nasal passages. Numerous arteries supply the nasal mucosa, the branches of many of which converge at a site along the anterior and superior aspect of the nasal septum known as **Kiesselbach's plexus** (Figure 39-4). DOT 4-5.20, 4-5.21, 4-5.22, 4-5.23, 4-5.24

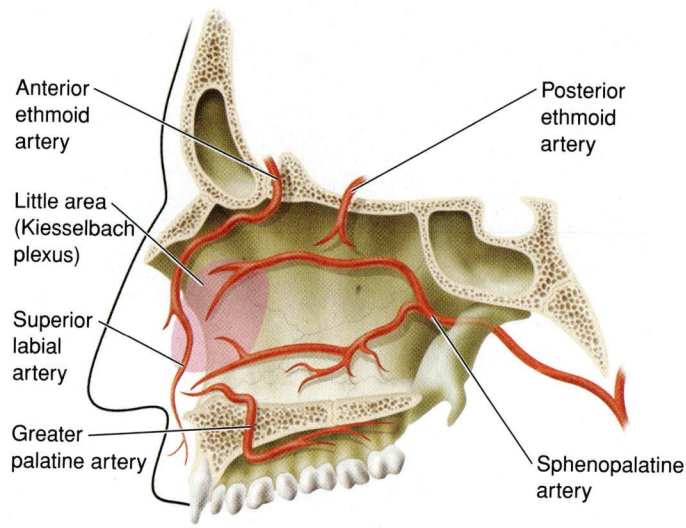

Anterior ethmoid artery

Posterior ethmoid artery

Little area (Kiesselbach plexus)

Superior labial artery

Greater palatine artery

Sphenopalatine artery

Figure 39-4 The arteries that supply the nasal mucosa.

Pathophysiology of Nose Complaints

Traumatic fracture of the nose is the most common of the head and neck fractures. It is often associated with septal fractures and epistaxis.[10,11,12] Although frequently the result of battery, a broken nose is most often not life-threatening. Significant functional impairment and physical disfigurement may result if a displaced fracture is not treated promptly.[11] The patient often presents with pain, periorbital ecchymosis (raccoon's eyes), displacement of the nose, and crepitus.

Edema following the injury is often extensive. The delicate bone structure fractures easily, and concomitant rupture of nasal blood vessels can cause bleeding that can range from trivial to profuse. Epistaxis can also occur spontaneously without precipitating trauma. A flow of copious clear fluid from the nose following head trauma may signify leakage of cerebrospinal fluid through a fracture at the base of the skull.

Young children commonly insert small foreign bodies into the nose, causing irritation, bleeding, and the potential for aspiration of the offending object into the lower respiratory tract. Nasal trauma in children is more often the result of accidental sports injury and play than from fights or battery. However, it is estimated that between 30% and 50% of all pediatric abuse victims present to the emergency department with maxillofacial injuries, including fractured nose.[11]

Primary Survey

Approach the patient with obvious nasal trauma with concern for the potential of underlying serious intracranial, maxillofacial, or cervical spine injury. Perform a thorough assessment to rule out concurrent injury to the eyes, teeth, and mouth.[11] Blood flowing from the anterior nose is obvious; however, inspect the posterior pharynx for evidence of bleeding as well. Ask all patients with epistaxis whether the event was spontaneous or precipitated by trauma, if any underlying medical condition exists that might predispose patients to bleeding, and whether they take anticoagulant or antiplatelet medicines. DOT 3-2.18

Management of Nose Complaints

Manage lacerations, contusions, or other superficial trauma to the nose with gentle pressure for bleeding control and standard wound care. Foreign bodies in the nose should be left in place and the patient transported to an appropriate receiving facility. Removal may require specialized equipment, and inappropriate attempts at extrication in the field may cause inadvertent aspiration of the object or additional soft tissue trauma.[13]

In 90% of the cases, bleeding from the nose originates from the rich vascular network of Kiesselbach's plexus.[12] Because of its relatively exposed position along the anterior wall of the septum, irritation caused by dry air, frequent nose blowing, or the insertion of a finger (also called "digital trauma") can spark hemorrhage. Nose bleeds originating in this area are classified as anterior and are usually readily controlled with digital pressure applied for ten minutes.[10] Although packing with nasal tampons or balloons is an effective hospital treatment, it has not been shown to be effective in the prehospital setting, so it is not recommended.

Bleeding can also emanate from the larger, more posterior arteries supplying the nasopharynx. Blood loss in such instances can be profuse and can flow down the posterior pharynx, threatening the airway and causing aspiration. Posterior epistaxis can occur without any inciting event, particularly among patients with bleeding disorders, poorly controlled hypertension, or those taking anticoagulant or antiplatelet medications such as coumadin and aspirin.[10,14] Successful management of posterior bleeding requires packing of both the anterior and posterior nasopharynx, which is not performed in the prehospital setting. Prompt transport of these patients is required.

Prehospital treatment of both anterior and posterior epistaxis entails sitting the patient upright (when possible) with the head tilted forward to prevent blood from coursing down the posterior pharynx.[10] Gentle pressure should be applied by pinching the proximal portions of the nostrils together while instructing the patient to breathe through the mouth (Figure 39-5). A number of commercial devices designed to clamp the nostrils closed are also widely available. Do not attempt to pack the nostrils in the field. Instead, reassure the patient, and

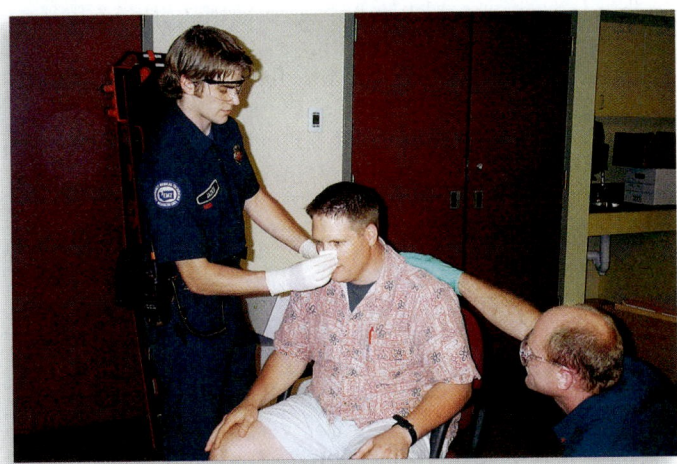

Figure 39-5 To treat a patient with epistaxis, sit the patient upright with the head tilted slightly forward, and gently pinch the nostrils together to apply external digital pressure.

ensure adequate breathing during transport. Although hemorrhagic shock is rare, monitor the patient closely and treat all signs of shock as appropriate.[14]

Eye Complaints

Acute injuries or afflictions that threaten the eye or compromise sight provoke extreme anxiety on the part of the patient. Proper field management of the patient with ocular complaints begins with an assessment and management of potential life-threatening conditions. Attention can then turn toward careful history taking and inspection of the eyes to determine the nature of the problem and whether or not a need for immediate intervention exists. In the vast majority of cases, the responsibility of the paramedic lies in the following:

1. Recognizing the signs or symptoms of a potential sight-threatening condition, and alerting hospital personnel of the need to mobilize specialized resources.

2. Taking careful steps to prevent further harm to the eye.

3. Providing comfort and support to the patient fearful of permanently losing vision. DOT 3-1.8, 4-4.5

Applied Anatomy and Physiology of the Eyes

The eye is a globe measuring approximately 3 centimeters in diameter (Figure 39-6). Each globe sits within a pyramid-shaped recess in the skull called the **orbit.** Thin bone forms the walls of each orbit. Within the orbit, numerous long, thin muscles are attached to the surface of the globe and are anchored to the orbital walls. These muscles rotate the globe, and it is the fine coordination of this movement within both orbits that allows for the complex act of visual tracking.

The **sclera** is a tough, fibrous coat that envelops most of the globe. It forms the "white" of the visible portion of the eye. The colored iris in the center of the anterior globe is protected by the **cornea,** a transparent sheet of tissue that is susceptible to scratches or the embedding of small foreign bodies. It is also quite sensitive—even the smallest corneal abrasion causes extreme pain, tearing, and sensitivity to light (photophobia) in the affected eye. The **conjunctiva** is a thin covering that extends from the inner aspects of the upper and lower eyelids and across the exposed portion of the sclera. It does not cover the cornea. Moistening of the conjunctiva with tears secreted by the **lacrimal glands** lubricates the surface of the eye and allows the eyelids to glide smoothly over the globe's surface.

Behind the cornea lies the **anterior chamber,** a space filled with circulating intraocular fluid called the **aqueous humor.** The posterior wall of the anterior chamber is formed by the **iris,** a colored ring of thin muscle. Contraction or relaxation of the musculature of the iris dilates or constricts the **pupil,** the central opening of the iris through which light enters the globe itself. The **lens** is situated immediately posterior to the pupil. Subtle changes in the shape of the lens focus entering light upon the **retina,** a thin sheet of richly vascularized and highly specialized nerve tissue that adheres to the posterior inner wall of the globe. The retina converts light images into neural transmissions interpreted as sight by the brain.

Pressure within the globe is maintained by a careful balance in the volume of aqueous humor circulating within the anterior chamber and the more gelatinous fluid known as **vitreous humor** that fills the eyeball itself. The integrity of the retina depends upon the maintenance of proper intraocular pressure (IOP) within a specific range. A sudden loss of IOP, such as might occur when the globe has been punctured or ruptured, can deform the globe and separate the retina from its attachment to the posterior wall of the globe, which may result in blindness. Conversely, sudden rises in IOP can disrupt the retina or, over time, compromise its blood flow, causing ischemic damage to this delicate nerve tissue.

Numerous conditions cause acute eye pain or compromise vision. Most important among these are chemical exposure, trauma, and certain medical conditions such as acute glaucoma or sudden compromise of the vascular supply to the eye.[15]

Primary Survey

Patients with problems affecting the eye usually complain of some combination of pain, visual change, eye redness and drainage, tearing, or photophobia. For the paramedic, the most important immediate task is to determine whether such symptoms stem from chemical damage, trauma, or a nontraumatic process affecting the eye. A focused history, if obtainable, followed by or in conjunction with a rapid but thorough inspection of the eyes will usually make that determination. DOT 3-2.13, 4-4.10, 4-4.11, 4-4.12, 4-4.13, 4-4.14

Proper inspection of the eyes requires a systematic approach and the use of an adequate light source such as a penlight. The eyelids, the orbits, and the tissue surrounding the eyes should be examined for bruises, lacerations, penetrating objects, redness, or swelling. The penlight should be used to examine the pupils for size, shape, symmetry, and reactivity to light. Inspect the conjunctivae and sclerae for any evidence of redness, pus, lacerations, or foreign bodies. Photophobia is

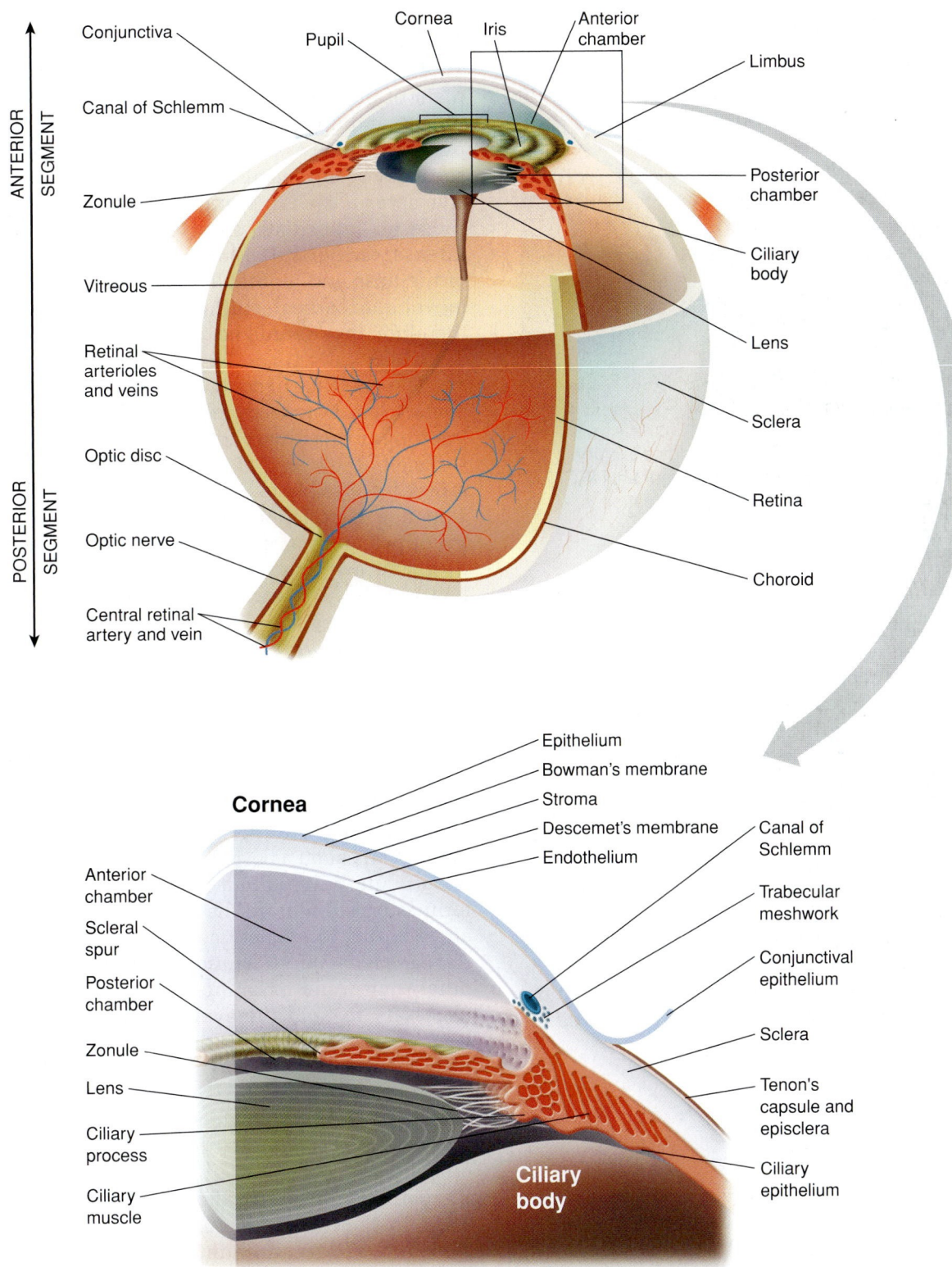

Figure 39-6 Anatomy of the eye.

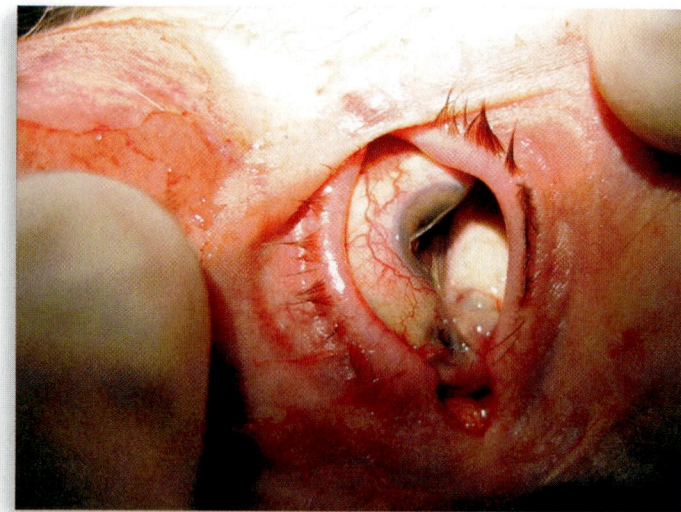

Figure 39-7   Eye injuries such as this open globe injury can be quite painful and can provoke significant anxiety. Providing topical anesthesia or anxiolytic medication is appropriate.

a common symptom of eye irritation, so be gentle when performing this assessment.

Assess eye movement by asking the patient to focus on your finger and follow it as you move the finger upward, downward, and from side to side. Some sense of the patient's visual acuity can be gained by covering one eye and testing the opposite eye by asking the patient to read print on a paper held approximately twelve inches in front of the face. This process is then reversed to test the contralateral (opposite) eye.

The pain and anxiety caused by a significant eye injury—and, of course, by the blindness resulting from subsequently bandaging both eyes—can cause significant patient agitation and movement. Emotional support and, if necessary, anxiolytic (anxiety relieving) medication are important elements of good patient care in this situation (Figure 39-7). DOT 4-3.50, 4-4.71, 4-4.72, 4-4.73

Specific Problems

Chemical Contamination

With the advent of more "do-it-yourself" projects at home, the incidence of chemical injuries to the eye is on the rise.[16] Chemical burns to the eye can erode the sclera and the cornea. Both acid and alkaline substances are caustic, and tissue damage begins immediately upon contact. Exposure to chemicals should be treated as a true ocular emergency.[17] Alkaline substances are generally more devastating to the eye.[18] Alkaline compounds penetrate the eye while acids burn the surface. Long-term blindness can result if both types of chemicals are not washed quickly and effectively from the surface of

the eye. DOT 4-4.31, 4-4.32, 4-4.33, 4-4.34, 4-4.35, 4-4.36, 4-4.37, 4-4.38, 4-4.58, 4-4.63, 4-4.68, 4-4.79, 4-4.82

Patients with caustic chemical exposure will complain of intense pain as well as blurred or diminished vision, photophobia, or a feeling that a foreign body is present. The eye will be red, and the surrounding tissues may be burned also. Riot control agents and defensive sprays, such as tear gas, mace, and pepper spray, cause an immediate onset of severe ocular burning, intense tearing, and irritation of the mucous membranes of the nose and mouth. These agents may denude (remove) the corneal epithelium and inflame the eye; therefore, they should be treated as chemical exposures as well.[19]

The presence of contact lenses should be noted. If a contact lens is present, it must be removed to prevent trapping any residual chemical between the lens and the surface of the eye. If attempted removal is too painful, it may be possible to float the lens from the eye during irrigation. If irrigation does not remove the lens, squeeze the opposite sides of the lens either with gloved fingertips or by exerting pressure and closing the upper and lower eyelids. This will bow the lens and break its seal from the cornea.

Treatment with copious irrigation should begin immediately. Lactated Ringer's solution is preferred for irrigation, but normal saline may be used also. Flow the fluid through standard IV tubing, and the use of a Morgan lens can be helpful (Figure 39-8). A minimum of 2 liters should be used to flush the chemical from the eye.[17] Ensure you protect your own eyes and skin from splash contact with the chemical by using proper BSI precautions such as eye or respiratory protection. This is particularly important if the chemical is in powder form as brushing it off the patient can place it into the air, resulting in inhalation. DOT 4-4.77

Never use any chemical substance or "antidote" other than water or saline to flush the eye. It is often necessary to hold the eyelids open during irrigation because of the natural inclination to close the eye in response to pain and irritation. A steady stream of irrigating fluid should be directed onto the medial surface of the exposed globe and allowed to run off the lateral aspect of the eye to avoid contaminating the opposite eye (Figure 39-9). If possible, turn the side of the patient's face with the eye to be irrigated downward to facilitate this run-off. Irrigation should be continuous for a minimum of 20 minutes, longer if the chemical is known to be alkaline. If both eyes have been exposed, alternate flushing between each of them frequently, and extend the overall time spent irrigating accordingly.[1]

In the hospital setting, testing of the pH of the eye will be used to determine if decontamination is complete. In the prehospital setting, this is not available, so irrigation should continue if the patient complains of additional

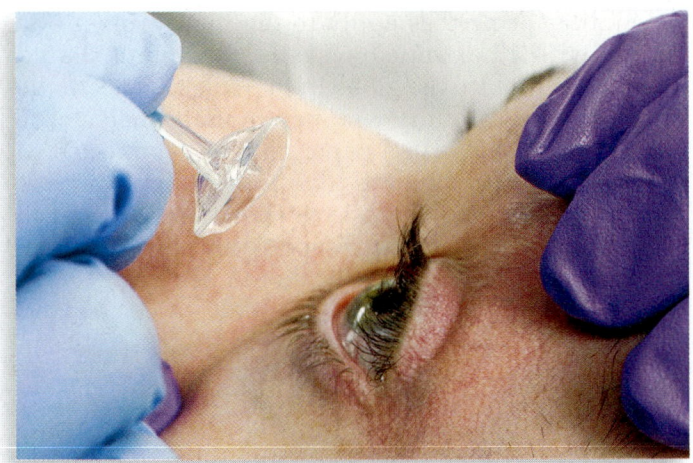

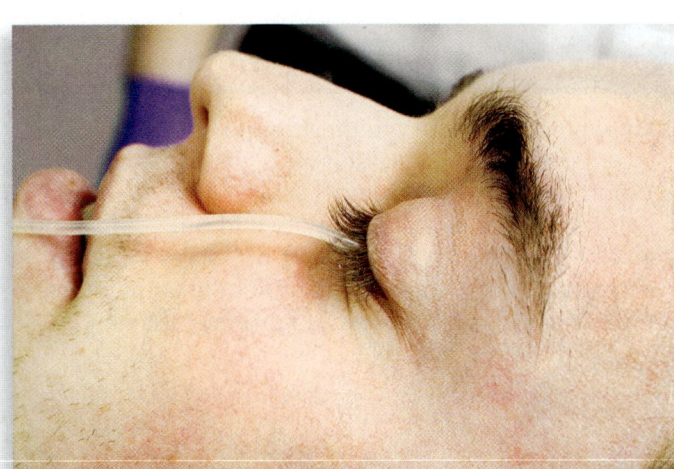

Figure 39-8   A Morgan lens and standard IV tubing for irrigation.

pain. The use of sedatives or analgesics may also be appropriate to help calm the patient or control pain.[10]

Trauma

Approximately 50,000 serious sight-threatening incidents occur every year in the United States. About one million Americans, comprised mostly of young men and children currently have visual loss from trauma, with 75% of those individuals blind in at least one eye.[16]

Eye trauma and severe pain can result from something as simple as a small foreign body on the surface of the cornea or conjunctiva. Dirt, sand, plant debris, or metal fragments frequently fall or are blown into the eye, causing irritation, tearing, and photophobia. Usually, tearing and blinking suffice to remove the foreign material, but particles may occasionally become embedded in the cornea. If a patient complains of something in

their eye and the history supports it, a foreign body is usually present on the cornea or under the upper lid.[15] Even if removed spontaneously, the foreign body may scratch the surface of the eye, causing pain and a persistent sense that the particle is still present.

More significant eye injuries result from high-energy blunt trauma or penetration of the globe with sharp objects. Blunt trauma can deform the globe, exerting pressure on the surrounding fragile orbital wall and often cause a fracture. Often, periorbital ecchymosis and edema are significant, and the eyes are swollen shut, making assessment difficult.[19] Do not force the eyes open to inspect them. DOT 4-3.15

If the musculature attached to the globe extrudes through the broken bone, motion of that eye may be compromised. When this occurs, the two eyes no longer move in tandem, causing the patient to complain of **diplopia,** or double vision (Figure 39-10). This type of fracture is called a "blowout" fracture. About one-third

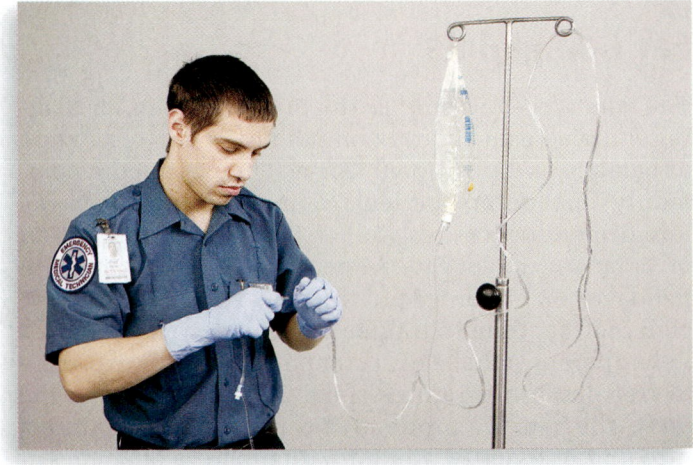

Figure 39-9   Irrigate for a minimum of 20 minutes.

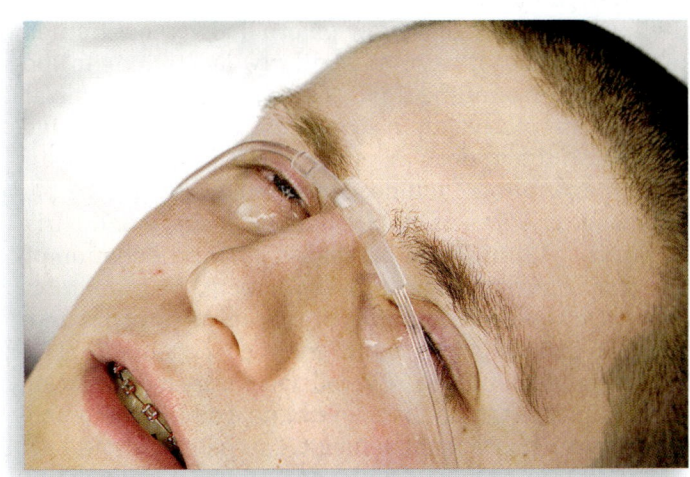

BOX 39-1 Hyphema

Hyphema is an injury to the anterior chamber of the eye that disrupts the vessels and results in bleeding. When the quantity is significant enough, the blood tends to form a layer, and gravity will cause it to pool and be visible as a blood level when the patient is sitting upright. Symptoms can include pain, photophobia, and blurred vision (Figure 39-10).

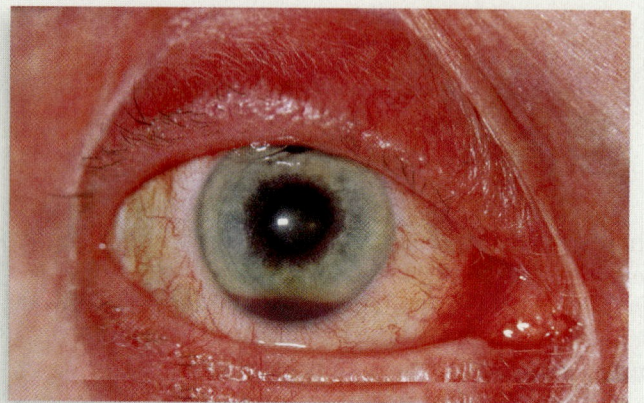

Figure 39-10 An hyphema. Note the pooled blood at the bottom of the iris.

of all blowout fractures are associated with other ocular trauma such as **hyphema** (Box 39-1), retinal tears, lens dislocations, and so on.[19] Higher energy transfer, as seen with major motor vehicle accidents, for example, may shatter the socket, avulse the eye, and, potentially, rupture the globe itself (see Figure 39-7, page 968).

Sharp objects may impale the globe, allowing vitreous humor to extravasate and deforming the eye to the extent that the integrity of the retina is compromised. Penetration of the globe may not be obvious, however. Penetration of the eyeball by small particles moving at high velocity may leave few external signs that trauma to the globe has occurred. Similarly, lacerations to the eyelids or surrounding soft tissue may appear superficial but in fact represent an injury of sufficient depth to have punctured the underlying eye. Subtle, indirect signs of globe penetration include decreased vision in the affected eye and loss of the normal round shape of the iris or pupil, resulting from decreased IOP and deflation of the globe.[20] When managing the patient, manipulation of the eye should be kept to a minimum as pressure may result in extrusion and loss of intraocular contents. The injured eye should be covered with a metal shield or paper cup and the opposite eye bandaged lightly to prevent consensual eye movement. The patient should be transported supine. The patient should be cautioned not to squeeze the eyes shut and to remain still.[15]

Similar principles apply to the management of a patient with an extruded eyeball. No attempt should be made to replace the globe in its socket. Instead, the eye should be carefully wrapped in moistened sterile gauze or covered with a paper cup and supported in its current position with the absolute minimal amount of pressure applied. Both eyes should be covered to prevent sympathetic eye movement. Transport to an appropriate receiving facility should be rapid.[21]

Nontrauma Causes of Eye Complaints

Nontraumatic causes of sudden eye pain or vision loss also prompt patients to seek emergent medical care. Acute glaucoma results from a rapid and abnormal increase in IOP due to a sudden imbalance between the production and drainage of aqueous humor in the anterior chamber. As IOP quickly increases, intense pain results. The eye appears red, and the affected pupil becomes nonreactive. The cornea may take on a cloudy appearance. Patients often complain of associated headache, nausea, and vomiting. If not corrected, the increased IOP compromises blood supply to the retina and damages its delicate nerve structures.[22] Glaucoma is the leading cause of blindness for Americans of African descent.[5]

Sudden loss of vision in one eye can result when the vascular supply to the nerves of the retina is acutely compromised. Most often, this is the result of a blood clot or a fragment of atherosclerotic plaque that has broken loose from the heart or a major artery to become lodged in the smaller vessels of the eye, impeding blood flow. This is usually a painless process, so patients will rarely complain of anything other than sudden blindness in the affected eye. It is important to remember that another cause of painless vision loss is a stroke that affects the visual center of the brain. All such patients must be transported expeditiously and closely monitored for other neurologic symptoms.[20]

Ear Complaints

The ears serve not only as the primary organ for hearing but also as a central component of the regulation of balance and positional sense. The paramedic commonly encounters patients complaining of hearing impairment or loss, as well as the sudden disruption of balance, or **vertigo.** Moreover, as protruding appendages on either side of the head, the ears are especially susceptible to trauma and the extreme changes in temperature that can accompany burns or exposure to freezing temperatures. Like all other parts of the body, the ears are prone to specific patterns of infection that frequently prompt patients to seek emergent medical care. DOT 4-4.5

Applied Anatomy and Physiology of the Ear

The **auricle**, also called the **pinna**, is the funnel-shaped external portion of the ear. A thin sheet of cartilage forms the distinctive shape of the auricle, and that cartilage is covered by tightly adherent and richly vascularized skin. The auricle channels sound waves from the surrounding environment into the **external auditory canal,** an s-shaped tube lined with a thin layer of skin. Cartilage forms the outer one-third of the external auditory canal before it tunnels into the bony structures of the skull for the remaining inner two-thirds of its length (Figure 39-11).

DOT 4-4.19, 4-5.15, 4-5.16, 4-5.17. 4-5.18

Sound passes through the external auditory canal to strike the **tympanic membrane** (TM), a drum-like fibrous membrane that forms the outer covering of the **middle ear.** The middle ear is an air-filled cavity within the petrous bone of the skull. That cavity is joined to the nasopharynx anteriorly by the **eustachian tube.** The **mastoid air cells** extend posteriorly from the middle ear into the base of the skull to form another cavity located just beneath the bony prominence behind each auricle. The middle ear contains the **auditory ossicles,** a trio of delicate bones (incus, stapes, and malleus) that conduct reverberating sound waves from the TM across the middle ear to stimulate specialized conducting nervous tissue in the **inner ear.**

The two major components of the inner ear are the **cochlea,** which contains auditory sensory receptors that convert conducted vibrations into neural impulses perceived and interpreted by the brain, and the **vestibular labyrinth.** The vestibular labyrinth consists of three semicircular canals oriented at right angles to one another and embedded in the bone at the base of the skull.

Shifting fluid within the semicircular canals that occurs with movement of the head sends neural signals to the brain that are coordinated with visual and other sensory input to maintain a proper sense of balance.

Pathophysiology of Ear Conditions

Trauma to the external ear is rarely life-threatening, but it can cause significant bleeding and long-term cosmetic harm.[23] Pressure waves generated by significant blunt trauma to the ear can traverse the external auditory canal to rupture the fragile TM and cause sudden hearing loss.[11] Blunt trauma is the most common cause of traumatic hearing loss. Motor vehicle crashes are the major cause of blunt head trauma and account for approximately 50% of all temporal bone injuries. Penetrating trauma is relatively rare, occurring in less than 10% of all cases.[11] Penetrating or blunt trauma that fractures the base of the skull can cause bleeding within the middle ear **(hemotympanum)** that, likewise, compromises hearing and may disrupt the normal sense of balance by damaging the vestibular labyrinth.

Thermal injury to the ear often accompanies burns to the head and face and may be severe enough to cause necrosis and sloughing of the entire auricle. Burns of the head and neck represent approximately 30% of all burns, and one study cited 42% of all patients with facial burns as also having burns to the ears.[23] The large surface area of the auricle is covered with thin skin and little subcutaneous tissue, which renders the external ear particularly susceptible to frostbite and freezing.[1]

Foreign bodies of all sorts can lodge in the external canal of the ear. Examples range from small pebbles or toy pieces self-inserted into the ear by toddlers and small children to insects that crawl into the canal of an unsuspecting adult. In the latter instance, movement by the insect within the ear and in close proximity to the TM is extremely disconcerting and uncomfortable for the patient. Supportive care and, if necessary, medication to control pain or anxiety is warranted.

Sudden hearing loss in the absence of trauma occurs as the result of infection, vascular and hematologic disease, drug toxicity, and autoimmune processes. Certain viral infections such as mumps may be associated with sudden hearing loss.[5] The delicate nature of the blood supply to the bone-encased inner ear can predispose patients to sudden deafness in the setting of certain leukemias, vascular malformations, and systemic inflammatory diseases. Drugs such as furosemide, aminoglycoside antibiotics, and antimalarial agents can damage the nerves of the inner ear in toxic doses, thus impairing normal hearing.[24,25]

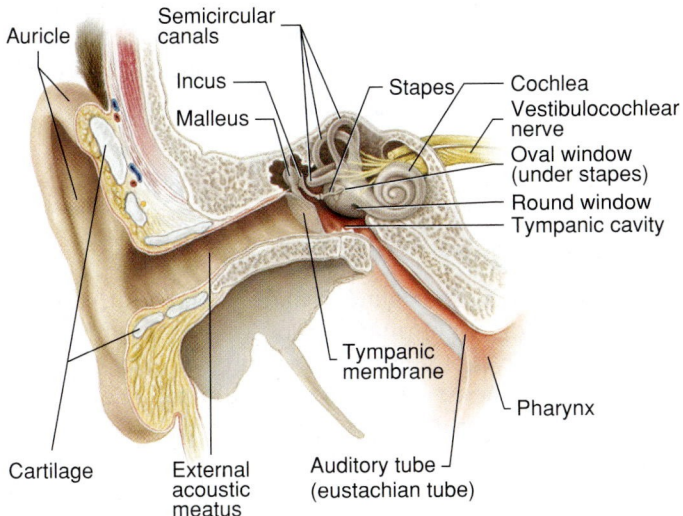

Figure 39-11   Anatomy of the ear.

Tinnitus is the abnormal perception of sound when no external stimulus is present. Patients will complain of a "buzzing" or "ringing" in one or both ears. Tinnitus is often caused by toxic blood levels of drugs such as aspirin, nonsteroidal antiinflammatory agents, and aminoglycoside antibiotics. Head trauma, neurologic diseases such as multiple sclerosis, and certain autoimmune conditions such as Ménière's disease can also cause patients to experience tinnitus.[26]

Vertigo, the abnormal perception by the individual that either they or the surrounding environment is in motion, can result from abnormalities of the inner ear or from disease processes of the brain, such as tumor or stroke. Inner ear problems that can cause vertigo include infections or injuries involving the vestibular labyrinth, toxicity from certain drugs, and Ménière's disease.[27,28]

Infection can invade any part of the ear. **Otitis externa** connotes infection of the auricle or the external auditory canal. This occurs most commonly when the integrity of the skin is compromised by minor scratches to the skin or when maceration and changes in its surface pH occur through frequent exposure to water, a condition known commonly as "swimmer's ear." Usually, the infection stems from bacteria already present on the skin invading the damaged tissue. One particularly virulent type of infection results when such invasion is by the bacteria *P. aeruginosa.* This malignant form of otitis externa tends to strike diabetics, the elderly, and others who suffer from some form of immunocompromise, and it may be life-threatening. **Otitis media** typically occurs when inflammation narrows the eustachian tube, trapping fluid and infectious organisms—typically viruses or bacteria—in the middle ear.[29]

Primary Survey

As with all patient encounters, the initial assessment of the patient with an ear complaint begins with a focused history while vigilance is maintained for other conditions that may threaten the airway, breathing, or circulation. Obvious trauma to the ear signals a potential for injury to the brain or cervical spine, and the patient must be quickly assessed for signs of trauma to other vital regions such as the neck and upper chest. When a non-traumatic etiology of the complaint is suspected, a rapid but thorough collection of information regarding the signs and symptoms experienced by the patient as well as any underlying medical conditions or medication use is essential. **DOT 3-2.16**

Assessment of the ear begins with inspection for bruising, lacerations, avulsions, burns, or other injury. While visualization of the entire external auditory canal requires the use of specialized equipment such as an otoscope, a penlight or other properly positioned light source can illuminate at least the outermost segment of the canal. Blood emanating from the canal may signify TM rupture and, potentially, an underlying fracture of the base of the skull. Copious clear fluid in the canal often represents leakage of cerebrospinal fluid through such a fracture as well. Bleeding from a basilar skull fracture may also fill the mastoid air cells, giving a bluish hue to the bony prominence behind the auricle **(Battle's sign).**[6]

When no trauma is present or suspected, inspect the auricle and the outermost aspects of the external auditory canal for signs of inflammation or infection. Redness, swelling, and tenderness may signify otitis externa. When the external auditory canal is involved, that inflammation and swelling may seal closed the outermost aspect of the canal. Any purulence or drainage should be noted as well.

Management of Ear Conditions

Traumatic ear injuries are managed in the same way as any soft tissue injury. Save any severed or avulsed portions of the auricle, and transport them with the patient in saline-soaked gauze.[30] When dressing an ear injury, placing a small amount of packing between the ear and the side of the head helps to support the auricle in its natural position. Bleeding or cerebrospinal fluid emanating from the external auditory canal should be absorbed with gauze placed at the opening of the external auditory canal, but the canal itself should never be packed. Similarly, never probe the canal or attempt to remove any foreign body as this may result in canal laceration.[11]

Prehospital management of most non-traumatic ear complaints centers on supportive care and expeditious transport to an appropriate receiving facility. Patients with significant ear infections may benefit from appropriate analgesic medications. Those with ongoing vertigo will often gain relief from antiemetic medication as well as treatment with a benzodiazepine such as diazepam.

Summary

Safe and effective management of the patient with throat, nose, eye, and ear complaints requires careful attention to presenting symptoms and thorough evaluation for the subtle signs of acute and serious pathology. Familiarity with the basic patterns of injury and illness involving these structures and competency in performing those interventions called for in the field may be lifesaving, or they may prevent permanent sensory impairment.

Notes

1. R. F. Edlich, T. L. Bailey, and T. J. Bill, "Thermal Burns," *Rosen's Emergency Medicine: Concepts and Clinical Practice,* 5th ed., J. A. Marx, ed. (St. Louis, MO: Mosby, 2002), pp. 801–812.

2. M. Manno, "Upper Airway Obstruction and Infection," *Rosen's Emergency Medicine: Concepts and Clinical Practice,* 5th ed., J. A. Marx, ed. (St. Louis, MO: Mosby, 2002), pp. 2245–2257.

3. M. F. Murphy and B. A. Kent, "Adult Epiglottitis," *The Clinical Practice of Emergency Medicine,* 3rd ed. (Philadelphia, PA: Lippincott, Williams, & Wilkins, 2001), pp. 90–93.

4. J. E. Clinton, "Nontraumatic Upper Airway Obstruction," *The Clinical Practice of Emergency Medicine,* 3rd ed. (Philadelphia, PA: Lippincott, Williams, & Wilkins, 2001), pp. 133–137.

5. D. L. Kasper, E. Braunwald, A. S. Fauci, S. L. Hauser, D. L. Longo, and J. L. Jameson, eds., *Harrison's Principles of Internal Medicine,* 16th ed. (New York, NY: McGraw-Hill, 2006).

6. C. K. Stone and R. L. Humphries, "Maxillofacial and Neck Trauma," *Current Emergency Diagnosis & Treatment,* McGraw-Hill's AccessMedicine (accessed October 5, 2006).

7. F. C. Brunicardi, D. K. Andersen, T. R. Billiar, D. L. Dunn, J. G. Hunter, J. B. Matthews, R. E. Pollock, and S. I. Schwartz, "Burns," *Schwartz's Principles of Surgery,* 8th ed., McGraw-Hill's AccessMedicine (accessed October 5, 2006).

8. J. E. Tintinalli, G. D. Kelen, J. S. Stapczynski, O. J. Ma, and D. M. Cline, "Upper Respiratory Emergencies," *Tintinalli's Emergency Medicine: A Comprehensive Study Guide,* 6th ed., McGraw-Hill's AccessMedicine (accessed October 12, 2006).

9. J. E. Tintinalli, G. D. Kelen, J. S. Stapczynski, O. J. Ma, and D. M. Cline, "Pediatric Airway Management," *Tintinalli's Emergency Medicine: A Comprehensive Study Guide,* 6th ed., McGraw-Hill's AccessMedicine (accessed November 15, 2006).

10. L. W. Way and G. M. Doherty, *Current Surgical Diagnosis and Treatment,* 11th ed. McGraw-Hill's AccessMedicine (accessed October 5, 2006).

11. A. K. Lalwani, *Current Diagnosis & Treatment in Otolaryngology—Head & Neck Surgery,* McGraw-Hill's AccessMedicine (accessed October 5, 2006).

12. J. E. Tintinalli, G. D. Kelen, J. S. Stapczynski, O. J. Ma, and D. M. Cline, "Nasal Emergencies and Sinusitis," *Tintinalli's Emergency Medicine: A Comprehensive Study Guide,* 6th ed., McGraw-Hill's AccessMedicine (accessed October 12, 2006).

13. J. E. Tintinalli, G. D. Kelen, J. S. Stapczynski, O. J. Ma, and D. M. Cline, *Tintinalli's Emergency Medicine: A Comprehensive Study Guide,* 6th ed., McGraw-Hill's AccessMedicine (accessed October 12, 2006).

14. T. C. Rothenhaus and I. D. Paul, "Nasal Hemorrhage," *The Clinical Practice of Emergency Medicine,* 3rd ed. (Philadelphia, PA: Lippincott, Williams, & Wilkins, 2001), pp. 107–110.

15. L. M. Tierney, Jr., S. J. McPhee, and M. A. Papadakis, eds., R. Gonzales, R. Zeiger, online eds., *Current Medical Diagnosis & Treatment* McGraw-Hill's AccessMedicine (accessed October 5, 2006).

16. P. Riordan-Eva and J. P. Whitcher, *Vaughan & Asbury's General Ophthalmology,* 16th ed., McGraw-Hill's AccessMedicine (accessed November 15, 2006).

17. K. J. Knoop, L. B. Stack, and A. B. Storrow, *Atlas of Emergency Medicine,* Chapter 4: Opthalmic Trauma, McGraw-Hill's AccessMedicine (accessed October 5, 2006).

18. J. E. Tintinalli, G. D. Kelen, J. S. Stapczynski, O. J. Ma, and D. M. Cline, "Caustics" *Tintinalli's Emergency Medicine: A Comprehensive Study Guide,* 6th ed., McGraw-Hill's AccessMedicine (accessed October 12, 2006).

19. J. E. Tintinalli, G. D. Kelen, J. S. Stapczynski, O. J. Ma, and D. M. Cline, "Ocular Emergencies," *Tintinalli's Emergency Medicine: A Comprehensive Study Guide,* 6th ed., McGraw-Hill's AccessMedicine (accessed October 12, 2006).

20. C. A. Marco, "Acute Visual Disturbances," *The Clinical Practice of Emergency Medicine,* 3rd ed. (Philadelphia, PA: Lippincott, Williams, & Wilkins, 2001), pp. 57–62.

21. B. E. Bledsoe and B. Ho, "Sight-Threatening Eye Injuries: Prehospital Management of Ophthalmological Emergencies," *Journal of Emergency Medical Services* 29(10)(October 2004): 94–106.

22. W. Bozeman, "Acute Angle-Closure Glaucoma," *The Clinical Practice of Emergency Medicine,* 3rd ed. (Philadelphia, PA: Lippincott, Williams, & Wilkins, 2001), pp. 62–70.

23. J. E. Tintinalli, G. D. Kelen, J. S. Stapczynski, O. J. Ma, and D. M. Cline, "Common Disorders of the External, Middle, and Inner Ear," *Tintinalli's Emergency Medicine: A Comprehensive Study Guide,* 6th ed., McGraw-Hill's AccessMedicine (accessed October 12, 2006).

24. J. Isaacs, "Acute Hearing Loss," *The Clinical Practice of Emergency Medicine,* 3rd ed. (Philadelphia, PA: Lippincott, Williams, & Wilkins, 2001), pp. 116–119.

25. R. M. Schears, "Acute Hearing Loss," *The Clinical Practice of Emergency Medicine,* 3rd ed. (Philadelphia, PA: Lippincott, Williams, & Wilkins, 2001), pp. 111–115.

26. R. W. Crummer et al., "Diagnostic Approach to Tinnitus," *American Family Physician* 69(2004): 120.

27. J. S. Olshaker, "Dizziness and Vertigo," *Rosen's Emergency Medicine: Concepts and Clinical Practice,* 5th ed. (St. Louis, MO: Mosby, 2002), pp. 123–130.

28. E. M. Raynor and R. D. Herr, "Vertigo and Labyrinthine Disorders," *The Clinical Practice of Emergency Medicine,* 3rd ed. (Philadelphia, PA: Lippincott, Williams, & Wilkins, 2001), pp. 120–126.

29. H. W. Severence, "Acute Otitis Externa," *The Clinical Practice of Emergency Medicine,* 3rd ed. (Philadelphia, PA: Lippincott, Williams, & Wilkins, 2001), pp. 129–132.

30. K. J. Knoop, L. B. Stack, and A. B. Storrow, *Atlas of Emergency Medicine,* Chapter 1: Head and Facial Trauma, McGraw-Hill's AccessMedicine (accessed October 5, 2006).

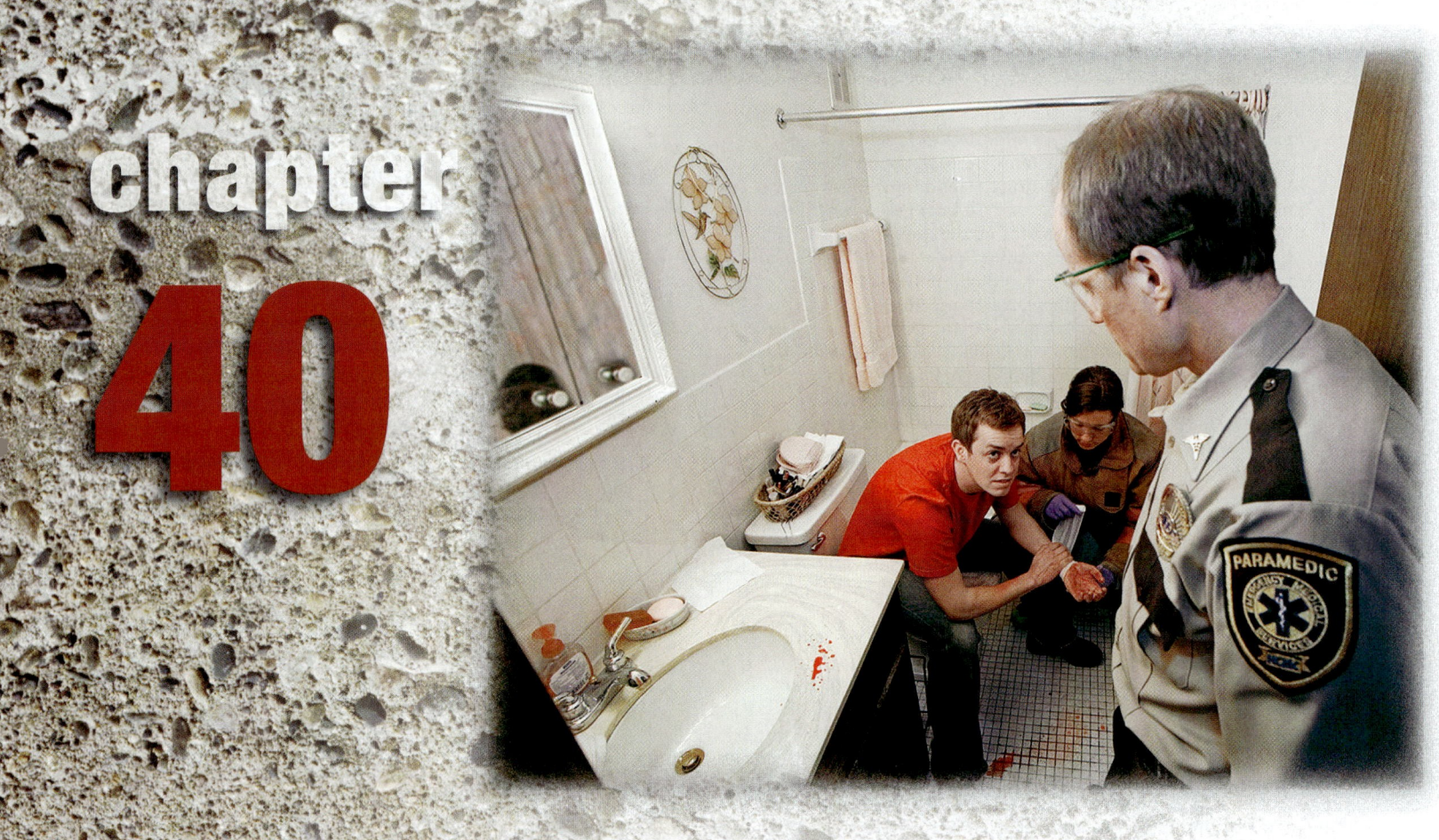

Behavioral and Psychiatric Disorders

"When written in Chinese, the word "crisis" is composed of two characters. One represents danger and the other represents opportunity."

—John F. Kennedy

Need to Know

▶ By definition, every 9-1-1 call can be considered a crisis of sorts. Crisis intervention skills can be used during every prehospital encounter.

▶ Altered behavior should be suspected from medical causes or external factors first and psychiatric (internal) causes last.

▶ EMS interventions, even for a very short duration, can be very therapeutic.

▶ Scene safety is critical; early identification of a patient's threat to themselves or others and effective de-escalation skills are essential.

▶ It is not necessary to accurately label or diagnose the exact nature of a psychiatric condition to provide good EMS care.

▶ EMS has a clear duty to intervene and attempt to prevent suicide.

▶ Mood disorders include depression and bipolar disorders; anxiety disorders include panic, phobic, obsessive-compulsive, and post-traumatic stress disorders; thought disorders include dementia, delirium, psychosis, and schizophrenia.

▶ Delirium is an abnormal mental state that impairs the patient's ability to think. This temporary condition usually presents suddenly and is reversible. Dementia is also a condition that impairs thinking, but it is a more permanent condition that involves a gradual decline in knowledge, memory, and ability to think.

▶ Schizophrenia is a progressive thought disorder marked by psychosis, hallucinations, delusions, and deteriorating thought and functioning. The median age of onset is mid-to-late 20s.

▶ A dystonic reaction is an involuntary contraction of muscles usually involving the face and neck. It appears similar to a seizure but is actually a reaction to some neuroleptic medications such as prochlorperazine (Compazine™), haloperidol (Haldol™), and droperidol (Inapsine™). Diphenhydramine (Benadryl™) will reverse a dystonic reaction.

▶ Sick	▶ Not Yet Sick
• Remain alert to the safety of EMS responders. Look for weapons or common objects that can hurt you. • Approach the patient calmly to de-escalate and to avoid a physical confrontation. • Observe the patient's movements, emotions, orientation, language, memory, and cognition. • Suspect a medical reason such as hypoglycemia, overdose, seizure, head injury, hypo- or hyperthermia, or hypo- or hypertension for the patient's symptoms.	• Is there specific intent to self-harm? Ask detailed questions about a plan. Is there a recent crisis? • Listen actively (summarize what you've heard, and identify emotions). Reflect the feeling back to the patient; if you are incorrect, let the patient correct you. • Be truthful with your patient, maintain good eye contact, and give your patient your full attention. • Focus on open-ended questions (questions that require more than a simple answer). • Define the problem, provide support, examine alternatives, make a plan, and get the patient's commitment.

Introduction

Eight of the 10 leading causes of disability are mental illnesses. In developed countries, the 10 leading causes for lost years of healthy life from ages 15 to 44 follow:

1. Major depressive disorder
2. Alcohol use
3. Road traffic accidents
4. Schizophrenia
5. Self-inflicted injuries
6. Bipolar disorder
7. Drug use
8. Obsessive compulsive disorders
9. Osteoarthritis
10. Violence[1]

Paramedics are often called to assess and care for people who are acting abnormally.[2] These common calls can be some of the most interesting, challenging, and dangerous encounters in EMS.[3] This chapter explores the paramedic's role in assessing and caring for patients with altered behavior and psychiatric emergencies. Major depression is the leading cause, followed by alcohol and drug use, schizophrenia, bipolar disorder, and obsessive compulsive disorders.[1] DOT 5-12.3, 5-12.4

In the prehospital setting, assessments need to be made in a limited amount of time, and patients may display very diverse behavior. It may be difficult to distinguish between the various forms of psychiatric illness, but it is often not necessary to pinpoint the exact condition. Behavioral emergencies should be approached in a systematic way, considering the most important and life-threatening conditions first. This chapter is presented in the same order that diagnostic concepts should be considered in the field.

Maintain a high level of awareness when approaching patients with behavioral emergencies. There are many reasons for altered behavior, and discovering the exact reason for the alteration can be challenging. Ironically, one of the most important lessons in this chapter is not about psychiatric (functional) causes of altered behavior. Your first and most important job is to consider medical (organic) causes of altered behavior.[4] Especially consider those that might be life-threatening.[5] Medical conditions such as low blood sugar (hypoglycemia), hypotension, alcohol intoxication, drug overdose, seizures, head injuries, and many others can present as altered behavior. These conditions can be lethal if they are not discovered in a timely manner. In some cases, a medical condition such as hypoglycemia can be easily discovered and quickly reversed in the field. Other times, differentiating between a medical and psychiatric cause can be more difficult.

Once a medical condition has been ruled out, assessment and care can focus on mental health issues. In many cases, identifying the underlying cause of the altered behavior may not be possible. Table 40-1

TABLE 40-1   Factors in Differentiating Organic and Functional Psychosis

"MADFOCS"	Medical or Reversible (Formerly Called Organic)	Psychiatric (Formerly Called Functional)
Memory deficits	Recent impairment	Remote impairment
Activity	Psychomotor retardation	Repetitive activity
	Tremor	Posturing
	Ataxia	Rocking
Distortions	Visual hallucinations	Auditory hallucinations
Feelings	Emotional lability	Flat affect
Orientation	Disoriented	Oriented
Cognition	Islands of lucidity	Continuous scattered thoughts
	Perceives occasionally	Unfiltered perceptions
	Attends occasionally	Unable to attend
	Focuses	
Some other findings	Age greater than 40	Age less than 40
	Sudden onset	Gradual onset
	Physical examination often abnormal	Physical examination normal
	Vital signs may be abnormal	Vital signs usually normal
	Social immodesty	Social modesty
	Aphasia	Intelligible speech
	Consciousness impaired	Awake and alert

Modified from D. S. Frame and E. E. Kercher, *Emergency Medicine Clinics of North America* 9(1991):123.
Source: J. A. Marx, *Rosen's Emergency Medicine: Concepts and Clinical Practice,* 5th ed., (St. Louis, MO: Mosby, 2002), p 1546.

discusses some causes of altered behavior using the following memory aid:

MADFOCS

M Memory deficits

A Activity

D Distortions

F Feelings

O Orientation

C Cognition

S Some other findings

There are three keys to good patient care for behaviorally altered patients:

1. *Be Safe!* Approach these situations with extreme caution and stay alert to potential threats throughout the encounter.

2. *Consider medical (reversible or external) problems first.* Rule out life-threatening and reversible causes before deciding that patients are suffering from a psychiatric disorder.

3. *Use standard crisis intervention techniques.* Pinpointing the exact mental illness is less important than therapeutically intervening using standard crisis intervention skills that are useful for all patient encounters. This includes the following:

   • Making sure that patients are not a danger to themselves or others.[5]

   • Using good communication skills.

   • De-escalating the situation.

   • Helping patients identify the most pressing issues, which can greatly affect patient outcome.[6]

   • Initiating therapeutic crisis intervention immediately.

What Is a True Behavioral Emergency?

Although some clinicians disagree over what constitutes normal versus abnormal behavior, it is clear that patients who are not acting within accepted societal norms or who present a threat to themselves or others must be carefully assessed. When altered behavior requires immediate attention to avert a serious outcome, it is considered an emergency.[7] Behavioral emergencies range in severity and include suicidal ideation, disruption in thought patterns such as schizophrenia, disruption in moods such as depression and mania, and addictive behaviors such as substance abuse. Less emergent mental health disorders include eating disorders such as bulimia, factitious disorders such as Munchausen syndrome, and anxiety disorders such as panic disorder, obsessive compulsive disorder, and post-traumatic stress. DOT 5-12.1, 5-12.2

This chapter explores crisis theory as a basis for understanding some of the psychosocial issues and intervention steps at the emergency scene. It also explores the important topics of suicide and mood and thought disorders.

Crisis Intervention in EMS

In general, people live in a state of balance. They go about their daily activities and routines, sometimes more effortlessly than at other times. As challenges appear, people use their coping skills to overcome them. Occasionally, people encounter an event that might be unfamiliar or more serious than anticipated. If normal coping strategies do not seem to work, this event can escalate and cause anxiety, fear, shock, and distress. Emotions can overpower an individual's sense of confidence and take away the ability to see options that might help resolve the problem. When this event overwhelms the ability to cope, it becomes a crisis. DOT 5-12.6

Most of the emergency requests for EMS involve some form of a crisis. In most cases, 9-1-1 has been called because someone perceives an urgent problem is beyond their ability to control or overcome. Sometimes this can be a simple emergency that might not seem serious to an EMS responder, such as a cut finger or persistent cough. Other times, the crisis is clear, poses an immediate threat to life, and requires rapid medical intervention. Someone in crisis is not necessarily mentally ill. They simply may have been presented with an unfortunate series of events that present both danger and opportunity for growth.

Crisis intervention is a short-term helping process that focuses on the immediate and temporary restoration of the patient's own balance (Box 40-1). The goal of crisis intervention is not psychotherapy, resolution of the crisis, or even identification of the underlying cause of the abnormal behavior. It is a brief intervention in which a crisis worker, such as a paramedic, can help the patient identify the elements of the crisis, provide support and empathy, and help the patient create a short-term plan to cope with the crisis. If the source of the crisis is rooted in a psychological (functional) cause, the paramedic can focus on referral and transport to an appropriate mental health or psychiatric emergency service center.[8,9]

Formal training in crisis intervention is available from various sources. The American Psychotherapy Association has a formal program involving three levels of certification.[10] Other programs are also available

BOX 40-1   Myths about People in Crisis

Myth: People in crisis cannot help themselves.

Fact: Most people have a desire to help themselves, and their capacity to grow from the crisis is usually enhanced with timely help from neighbors, family, friends, and trained crisis workers (Figure 40-1). Caregivers who try to "save" the patient and act as if the patient is not able to help themselves may be damaging a patient's prospects of resolving the crisis.

Myth: Only psychiatrists or highly trained therapists can effectively help people in crisis.

Fact: A great deal of crisis work has been done by lay volunteers, police officers, and other frontline workers, such as EMS personnel.

Myth: Crisis intervention is a mere bandage and is trivial in comparison to the real treatment carried out by professional psychotherapists.

Fact: Early intervention can promote more rapid improvement and decreased hospitalization. Techniques such as listening intently and giving feedback are used by therapists and crisis workers alike. Unlike psychotherapy, crisis intervention avoids probing into deep-seated psychological problems.

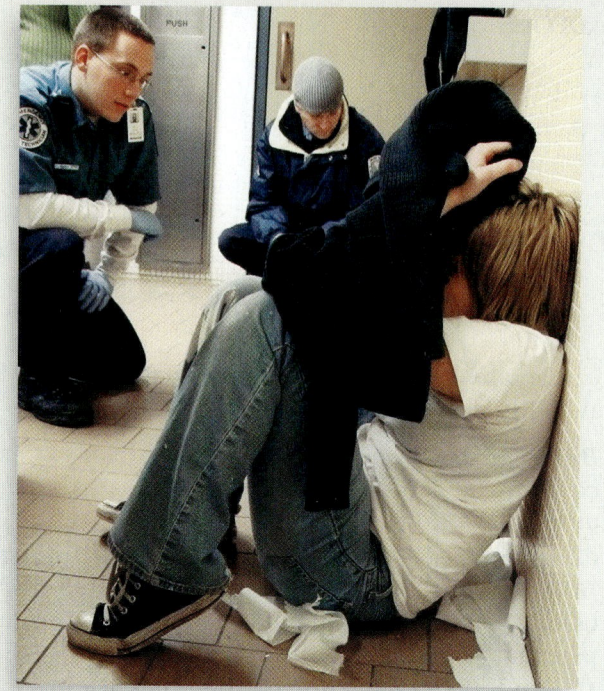

Figure 40-1   Patients in crisis may be embarrassed, frustrated, and afraid. Good communication skills and helping patients define their own problems are some of the keys to good patient care.

locally from crisis intervention centers and social service agencies.

Even without the presence of underlying mental health issues, the presence of a crisis that requires the patient or family members to call 9-1-1 is a stressful event.

Primary Survey

The initial approach to a behaviorally altered patient should focus on safety.[5] Maintain a high level of awareness for potential violence on every response you make. Before even making contact with the patient, look for factors that can predict potentially violent scenes, including police presence, past history of psychiatric disorders, possible presence of alcohol, drug use, or possible interpersonal violence.[11] As you approach the scene, try to have an unobstructed access and a way out (egress). If needed, as you enter, clear away objects that might block your path should you need to leave in a hurry. DOT 5-12.10, DOT 5-12.12, 5-12.14

CONNECTIONS   Scene safety is often thought of as a "safe" or "not safe" condition. In reality, scene safety can change in a matter of seconds and is more like a continuum. To read more about this, turn to Chapter 9: Safety and Scene Size-Up.

Street Secrets

Look for objects that could be used as a weapon against you. Simple objects such as pens, scissors, kitchen utensils, or hand tools can appear harmless but in the hands of an assailant may be deadly.[12]

Make sure that law enforcement officials are present to help secure the scene, and enough personnel are on hand to restrain a patient should the patient become violent.[2] If physical restraint is necessary, it should be performed as a last resort, and a minimum of five people should ideally be present (Figure 40-2).[2,7,13] Sometimes a show of force alone is enough to deter a confrontation.[18] In the field, each

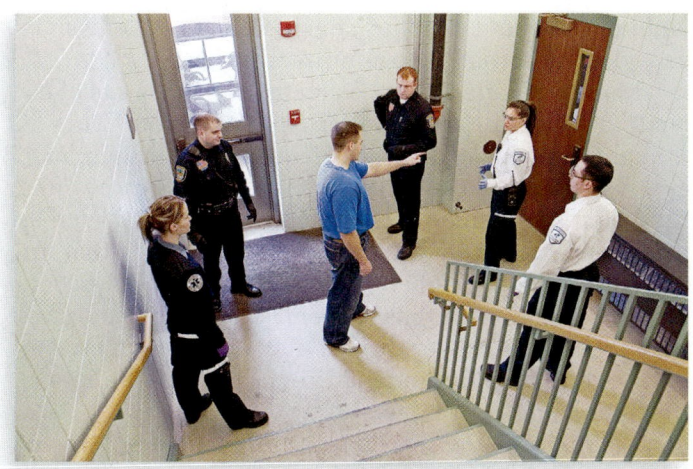

Figure 40-2   The paramedic taking the lead should communicate with the patient and attempt to de-escalate the situation before physical restraint is needed. Avoid becoming trapped in an enclosed space in close proximity to an angry patient. This situation is very dangerous, and your reaction time is very limited.

situation will present unique challenges and needs. Requesting additional assistance early is important.

Street Secrets

When a crowd of people is forming around your scene, your interview and care may become more difficult. Discretely enlist the help of other responders, such as law enforcement personnel, to dissipate the crowd. It is best to respectfully and professionally encourage on-lookers to leave.[7] DOT 5-12.11

Approach the patient in a nonthreatening manner, allowing as much personal space as possible (Figure 40-3). Take an open stance (palms facing out) with your hands out of your pockets, so the patient sees that you have nothing to hide. Stand sideways at a slight angle (bladed), so you are less imposing and a smaller target. Explain your intentions to help the patient calmly. Don't rush; allow time for the scene and the patient to cool down.[12,13,14]

The first step in crisis intervention is to define the problem. Is the patient a threat to themselves? To others? To you? Safety takes precedence over everything else. Take immediate steps to protect yourself or others if the situation is unsafe. Just as with any patient, assess the airway, the work of breathing, and perfusion first. Correct any problems in these areas quickly and before moving on to other secondary assessments.

Once safety is established, you must establish a positive rapport with the patient. Ask open-ended questions that allow the patient to explain the problem.

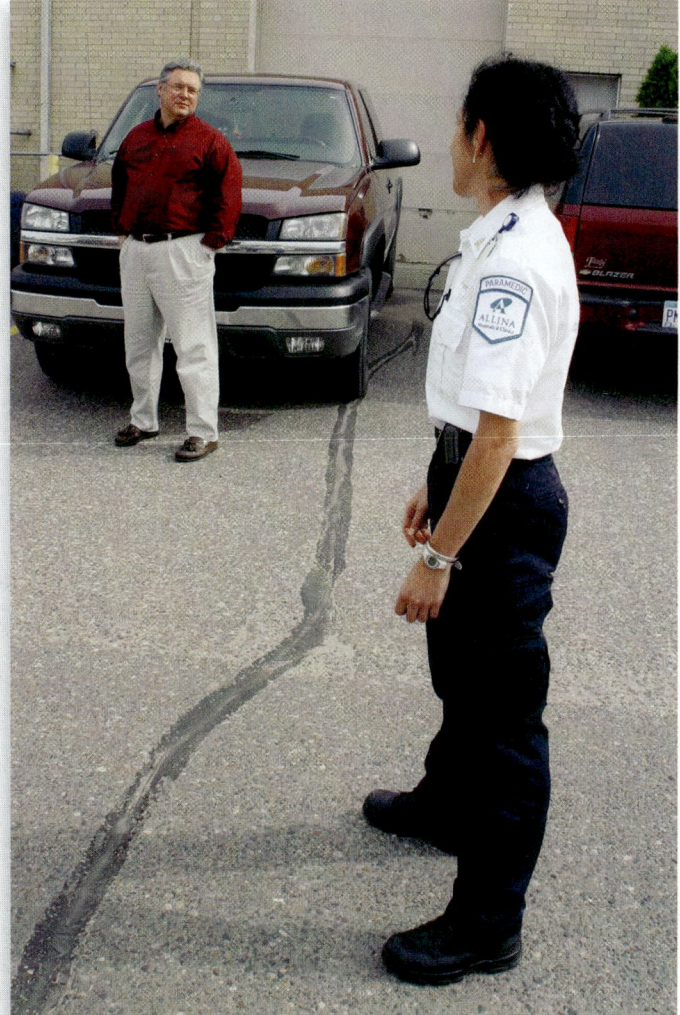

Figure 40-3   This paramedic has a bladed stance and is keeping her weight on the leg that is furthest from the patient. This allows her to turn and evade the patient should she need to make a quick escape. The patient has his hands in his pockets; this can be very dangerous. In this circumstance, ask the patient to please let you see his hands.

Remember to be friendly, listen actively, and be straightforward. During this first phase, it may be necessary to redirect the patient, so the focus stays on the important elements of the crisis. Medical (organic) causes of altered behavior should be considered until they can be definitively ruled out, usually in the hospital, after laboratory tests (see Table 40-1). A careful assessment of suicidal thoughts, suicide method, and the degree to which that method is lethal should be performed. DOT 5-12.8, 5-12.9

CONNECTIONS   Review Chapter 10: Therapeutic Communications and History Taking for more information on open-ended questions and establishing rapport.

While the patient is talking, observe the following:[5]
DOT 5-12.14

- **Movements.** Does the patient appear to make repetitive movements or not move at all?
- **Affect.** Does the patient express a high level of emotion or seem ambivalent (flat). Is the patient talking in a monotone voice or not interested in talking at all?
- **Orientation.** Is the patient awake, alert, and oriented to person, place, and time (AAOx3)? Does the patient understand the situation that is happening in the environment?
- **Language.** Is there slurred speech, or can the patient be understood readily? Is the pattern of speech logical, and does it make sense?
- **Memory.** Can the patient remember past history or their birth date (long-term memory)? Can the patient repeat three words immediately after you say them? Then five minutes later can the patient remember these same words (short-term memory)?
- **Cognition.** Is the patient making sense and able to organize thoughts?

All of these can be clues to help determine an accurate field impression.

Finally, before moving to a secondary assessment, make an initial determination of the overall acuity of the patient. Is the patient sick or not yet sick? Address primary survey problems immediately. Address airway, breathing, and circulation issues quickly. If the patient is aggressive or is creating a potentially unsafe environment, think of the patient as "sick" until you can determine a medical cause for the behavior or you can safely de-escalate or transport the patient.

Behavioral Emergencies

Suicide

Suicide is presented in this text before other emergencies because it is a common problem that can be present in any behavioral emergency and must be addressed as part of the primary survey of a behaviorally altered person. Suicide is one of the top 10 leading causes of death in the United States. It is a serious and common healthcare problem that not only involves the person attempting or completing the act but also the victim's surviving family and friends.[15] Although statistics are thought to be underreported, estimates are that 30,000 people will complete suicide each year and that attempts outnumber completions by a 40 to 1 ratio.[21] DOT 5-12.17

A common stimulus in suicidal patients is a desire to end extreme psychological and sometimes physical pain. The patient reaches a moment of generalized hopelessness and helplessness. Suicidal patients feel ambivalent about life and consider killing themselves as a viable alternative to continued suffering.[9,12,15]

Men, particularly Caucasian men over the age of 35, complete suicide more often than women. This is thought to be due to their use of more lethal means, such as guns and hanging. Women attempt suicide more often than men but commonly use less lethal means such as drug overdose or wrist slashing. Other groups that are at proportionately higher risk for suicide are adolescents ages 15 to 24, particularly teenage African American males, and adults over the age of 65. Native Americans have one to one and one-half times the suicide rate of the national U.S. average.[5,16]

There are many myths regarding suicide. Some of them are listed in Box 40-2. One common misconception is that a failed attempt at suicide is considered an attention-getting gesture.[9] It is important to remember that 90% of patients who complete suicide have previously attempted it.[15] In this context, every attempt should be assessed thoroughly and treated as seriously as possible. Paramedics, nurses, and physicians have been shown to have negative attitudes toward suicide attempters.[5,9] These attitudes have the potential to influence care and possibly encourage punitive practices.[5,9] These negative practices only reinforce the patient's own bad feelings and may cause more psychological harm.

Personal beliefs regarding suicide can vary, depending on religious, cultural, and moral beliefs. While it is

BOX 40-2 Suicide Myths

Myth: Talking about suicide with patients will put the idea into their head.

Fact: Most people who are depressed have thought about suicide. Patients may feel relief that you asked since suicide is considered a taboo subject, and talking about it will communicate that you are willing to listen to their true feelings.[16]

Myth: There is a link between suicides and winter holidays.

Fact: Research shows that suicide rates in the United States are lowest in winter and highest in the spring.[17]

Myth: Suicidal patients attempt to kill themselves when they are most depressed.

Fact: At the low point of depression, patients do not have the strength or will to kill themselves. Most attempts occur at a time of acute crisis when patients have more energy to harm themselves.[5]

TABLE 40-2 Suicide Lethality

Demographic or Social Profile	High Risk	Low Risk
Age	Older	Younger
Gender	Male	Female
Social history	Recent stress or instability: Divorce, death, isolation, criminal apprehension	Stable: Married, supportive family
Job status	Unemployed	Employed
Physical health	Acute or chronic illness	Good health
Mental health	Depression, schizophrenia, bipolar disorder, or panic disorder	Mild anxiety
Feelings	Hopeless	Hopeful
Suicidal ideation	Frequent, prolonged, specific, and realistic plan	Infrequent, low intensity, vague, or no plan
Suicide attempts	Repeated attempts, continuing wish to die	No prior attempts, wish to live
Other	Lack of concern	Good insight

Source: Adapted from J. Tintinalli, *Emergency Medicine, A Comprehensive Study Guide,* 6th ed. (New York, NY: McGraw-Hill, 2004), p 1815, Table 289-2.

important to be respectful of cultural beliefs, paramedics have a clear duty to intervene and attempt to prevent all suicides. Forty-nine states consider the act of suicide to be illegal, and most states consider EMS personnel to be mandated reporters of threats to self or others. At this time, only one state has sanctioned assisted suicide of terminally ill patients under very specific and controlled conditions. This was done by the state of Oregon in 1994.[4]

CONNECTIONS Provider attitudes about death, dying, and the paramedic's role in these cases can vary widely. Chapter 48: Patients from Diverse Cultures may be helpful in exploring issues related to death and dying.

Assessing Suicidal Risk

The treatment goal for suicidal patients is early identification of suicidal thoughts (ideation), potential risk (lethality) of a plan, and identification of anything they may have already done to try to hurt themselves. Risk factors include the patient's age, gender, ethnicity, health history, marital status, past attempts, and recent stressful events. (See Table 40-2: Suicide Lethality.) In general, the more specific and realistic the plan, the more lethal it is. Maintain a high index of suspicion. Even patients who may not appear initially to be depressed should be assessed for suicide risk. For example, you might be called to evaluate a laceration on the back of a hand because a patient put a fist through a window. The laceration is important to address, but investigating if the patient intentionally placed a hand through the window is also important. Be sure to ask specific questions regarding the method and plan for suicide. A vague statement like, "I wish I was dead" is considerably different from a statement such as, "I'm thinking of stepping in front of the 4 p.m. commuter train." DOT 5-12.16

Street Secrets

Specific = Lethal

Ask the patient to describe the suicide plan. The more specific and realistic it is and the more lethal the means, the higher the risk.

Patients who are experiencing a serious crisis have most likely considered suicide. Asking patients about this will not give them a new idea. It will likely be a relief to have the opportunity to talk about it. In cases where the risk and danger are obvious, it may be necessary to act rapidly and de-escalate the situation. It is always best if patients maintain some control over the choices they are making.[9,13] This empowers them and is part of the healing and treatment process.

Working in the Gray Zone

Whose Job Is It to Assess, Talk to, and Transport Suicidal People?

The practice of prehospital care varies greatly from one EMS system to another (Figure 40-4). Even within a single city or county, different fire, ambulance, and police departments or districts may have different policies about how to respond and transport patients who have altered behavior. Ideally, EMS and law enforcement agencies work together to ensure good patient care, but no formal research is available that might help guide best practices.

Some key issues to consider include: Law enforcement has the clear duty to ensure the safety of the patient, the public, and other responders, including your safety; EMS has a clear role in assessing the nature of a person's altered behavior. In many cases, it is probably best if a paramedic, rather than an EMT-basic, assesses the patient since an advanced level of assessment, knowledge, and judgment may be helpful in determining whether a medical reason may be the cause of the behavior.

You should prepare yourself to respond to all types of suicidal and behavioral emergencies. Just as you may call for police assistance if a scene becomes dangerous, the police are likely to call you for assistance in reasoning with a person who is imminently ready to complete the act of suicide. In June 1997, paramedic Peter Black received a special commendation for assisting the Minneapolis police in "talking a man down" from the wall of a freeway bridge. Paramedic Black is quoted as saying, "I relied on my training and making little deals with my patient until he walked off the bridge by his own power."

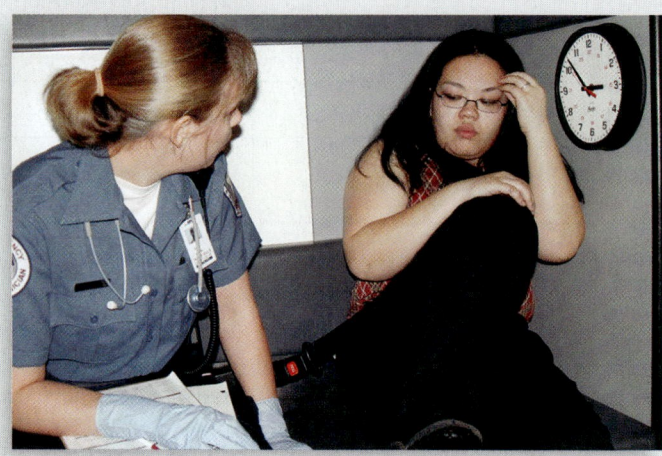

Figure 40-4   A patient who is paranoid or actively experiencing positive symptoms, such as hallucinations or delusions, may become afraid of you and react abruptly to routine questions. Any physical procedure or touch should be clearly explained and consented to before you attempt it. Maintain a high level of awareness for your safety.

Treating the Suicidal Patient

Once suicidal risk has been assessed, you can focus on keeping the patient safe and continuing to communicate with the patient therapeutically. Separate patients from the method they were intending to use to kill themselves. Enlist the assistance of law enforcement so that weapons, or potential (unconventional) weapons, are either confiscated or left at the scene. Often, active empathetic listening, paraphrasing, and reframing are enough to help a patient begin to manage their crisis (See Chapter 10: Therapeutic Communications and History Taking for additional tips).

CONNECTIONS For more information about the role of EMS and interfacing with other agencies review Chapter 52: Teamwork and Operational Interface.

While you will not be able to compromise on safety, giving patients some choices regarding their care will also help them feel as if they are regaining or maintaining control over their crisis.[9,18] Something as simple as, "Which shoes would you like to wear?" or "Which hospital would you like to be transported to?" can be helpful. It is helpful to make small contracts, especially for safety and cooperation.[5,9,19,20] These are small, short-term agreements that you can make with patients to enlist the patients' cooperation in their own care. An example of a contract would be for patients to promise that they will not attempt to flee or harm themselves while in your presence. Another mutually acceptable contract with patients might involve remaining cooperative en route to the hospital or agreeing to talk openly with caregivers in the emergency department.

Any patient who has suicidal thoughts (ideation) or who has just attempted suicide, no matter how minor the attempt, should be evaluated in the emergency department. If the patient is refusing and cannot be convinced to be transported voluntarily, you may need to enlist the assistance of other personnel that can issue a transportation or involuntary commitment order. In many states, a law enforcement official can assist you in lawfully transporting a suicidal person against the person's will. In some states, a mental health or emergency or transportation hold form is required. Mental health holds are valid for a brief period of time, usually less than 72 hours, and permit a patient to be held for transport to and evaluation at a medical facility. There are variations from state to state, but generally, police officers, physicians, psychologists, psychiatric nurses, and social workers are able to place a patient on a temporary or emergency hold until additional involuntary commitment orders are formalized. Extended commitment papers are a more formal process that require judicial court proceedings.[21] DOT 5-12.5, 5-12.13

Secondary Survey

Once the primary survey of a mental health emergency has been addressed, it is possible to perform a more focused assessment of the nature of the patient's altered behavior. DOT 5-12.7, DOT 5-12.18, 5-12.19, 5-12.20

The Diagnostic and Statistical Manual of Mental Disorders, fourth edition (text revision), commonly known as DSM-IV-TR is a concensus document from the American Psychiatric Association (APA). It contains a comprehensive list of every criteria and classification in the mental health field. The DSM-IV-TR has recently reclassified its categories into a multiaxial system. Each axis refers to a different domain of information as shown in Box 40-3. Familiarize yourself with the axes and terminology since you may be required to use it in the field during mental health emergencies.

The following are the most important causes of altered behavior with which a paramedic should be most familiar. With the exception of personality disorders at the conclusion of this section, all of these are axis I conditions.

Mood Disorders

Sadness and joy are part of everyday life, but these emotions can become debilitating and severely impair a person's ability to function. **Mood** or **affective disorders** are a grouping of illnesses that are characterized by a longer term sadness (unipolar) or a combination of sadness and mania (bipolar). Mood disorders can be caused by physiological factors, such as decreased metabolism from an abnormally functioning thyroid gland, or from a psychiatric origin. Regardless of the cause, these illnesses can be crippling and may even alter the way a person's brain manages it's neurochemical balance.

Depression

Depression is a progressive mood disorder that involves a persistent sadness, dysphoria, or loss of interest in usual activities.[5] Depression affects up to 10% of the U.S. population and causes an economic impact of billions of dollars annually.[22,23] Most people with depression do not seek treatment although the great majority can be helped.[15] There is a wide range of symptoms and severity of depression. Although there are times that depression can be transient and can be resolved by changing environment or utilizing a social support system, many times depression can become long-term. The mnemonic, "In SAD CAGES," is one way to remember the classic elements of depression.

In SAD CAGES

I   Interest (is lost)
S   Sleep (may be increased or decreased)
A   Appetite (usually decreased)
D   Depressed mood
C   Concentration (is decreased)
A   Activity (levels decline)
G   Guilt (increases)
E   Energy (is decreased)
S   Suicide (is considered or attempted)

A common misconception is to assume that people can simply "lift themselves" out of a depressive state. This may simply not be possible from a chemical standpoint. Prolonged stress, particularly when the origins appear hopeless, can lead to decreased levels of norepinephrine, dopamine, and serotonin in the brain. This leads to decreased levels of energy and interest and may be the reason why patients cannot improve their mood without using medications to alter their brain chemistry. This may also explain the success of selective serotonin reuptake inhibitor (SSRI) medications. These medications use the serotonergic neural pathways to boost levels of serotonin in the brain. This seems to enhance sleep-wake cycles and appetite and decrease aggressive behavior in animal research models.[4,23] Other medications, such as monoamine oxidase inhibitors and tricyclic antidepressants, work to block the reuptake of dopamine, norepinephrine, and serotonin in the presynaptic neurons of the brain.

BOX 40-3   The DSM-IV-TR

- **Axis I** refers to clinical mental health disorders.
- **Axis II** includes personality and development disorders.
- **Axis III** is general medical conditions.
- **Axis IV** is psychosocial and environmental factors.
- **Axis V** covers global and overall functioning.

Generally speaking, axis I and II conditions are the conditions that are most relevant to the paramedic. They include mood, thought, and anxiety disorders.

In addition to biochemical theories about depression, it is believed that cognition also plays a role. Depressed people feel guilty and helpless and blame themselves. This thinking has also been linked to learned behaviors and childhood development.[24]

Nice to Know

The theory of learned helplessness was developed in the 1960s when Martin Seligman subjected animals to electrical shocks if they attempted to leave their cages. Eventually, even when the cages were left open, the animals remained in the cage. Although some of the links between human and animal research have been questioned, current research confirms that depression causes a person to become hopeless and blame themselves for their problems. Even when options to help themselves are present, the depressed person may not see them or have the ability to take advantage of them.[24] This theory may also be applicable to survivors of domestic abuse.

CONNECTIONS To review domestic and other forms of abuse, visit Chapter 45: The Abused and Neglected.

Depression may also be caused by organic causes. Some examples of this include conditions such as hypothyroidism, drug side effects, or drug withdrawal. These patients experience a lower metabolic rate due to a medical condition. During the winter, it is possible that decreased daylight can cause seasonal affective disorder and depression.[25] Poor health and prolonged illness can also cause depression.

Bipolar Disorder

Bipolar disorder, formerly known as manic depression, is a condition characterized by extreme changes in mood, energy, thinking, and behavior.[4,26] Patients cycle through periods of very high energy (mania) and major lows (depression). Patients in a manic phase classically present with rapid, uninterrupted, and pressured speech as they describe racing thoughts and grandiose ideas. Patients may talk about "ending world hunger" or "making more money than all of Wall Street." Often, patients have unrealistic ideas about sweeping plans in work, wealth, or romance. Patients may perceive they have special abilities or that they are famous.[4,5] Mania that is untreated can be confused with and might even progress to a psychotic state.[15] Patients may become embarrassed, argumentative, or even hostile if their perceptions are proven wrong.[26]

Onset of bipolar disorder usually occurs around the age of 20 but is being diagnosed more and more in children. Depressive episodes are more common, and

patients often return to a fully functional baseline between episodes. As the patient ages, the time between episodes can tend to decrease. The more frequent the cycles from one extreme to the other, the poorer the prognosis for the patient.[26]

Long-term treatment of bipolar disorder includes pharmacological interventions. The most commonly prescribed mood-stabilizing agent is valproic acid (Depakote®), used 90% of the time, and, as a distant second, lithium (used 8% of the time).[6] These medications can sometimes take up to three weeks to be effective.

Street Secrets

Determine how long patients have been taking antidepressant medication and how compliant they have been. If they stopped, it is helpful to know when and why they stopped. It may take several days for the therapeutic level of the medication to wear off. Often, patients stop taking their medication because they don't think it is making a difference, when the medication has not yet reached therapeutic levels. Other patients may stop taking their medication because they start feeling better and believe they don't need it anymore.

Thought Disorders

Dementia and Delirium

Dementia is a condition in which there is a deficit of cognitive thought and reasoning. It involves disturbances in judgment, abstract thinking, personality, memory, and other higher brain (cortical) functions such as language. Dementia usually progresses slowly and is generally not life-threatening.[4] In the U.S., 20–40% of individuals over age 85 suffer from dementia.[27]

Delirium is also a disturbance in thought and reasoning but has a more rapid onset and is usually temporary. Approximately 15% of the U.S. population over the age of 65 has some form of cognitive failure.[28]

Street Secrets

Differentiating between dementia and delirium can be very difficult, even for experienced clinicians. One of the keys is to carefully evaluate the onset of symptoms. Patients with dementia are more likely to have suffered a gradual decrease of mental function over months or years.

Organic (medical or drug-induced) causes of altered mental status are important to suspect and rule out first (see Table 40-1).[6]

Psychosis

Psychosis is a state in which there is severe loss of contact with reality. Patients may have delusions, hallucinations, disorganized speech patterns, and bizarre or catatonic behaviors. Psychosis may be seen in manic or schizophrenic patients but can manifest itself in other conditions such as drug intoxication, drug withdrawal, and dementia.

Schizophrenia

Schizophrenia is a degenerative psychological disorder marked by a deterioration in thought and functioning. It is characterized by three types of symptoms:

1. *Thought disturbances:* problems forming logical thoughts and loss of contact with reality (psychosis).
2. *Positive symptoms:* bizarre behavior, false perceptions (hallucinations), and false beliefs (delusions).
3. *Negative symptoms:* restricted range of emotions (flattened affect) and social withdrawal.

Schizophrenia is poorly understood, and symptoms are highly variable from patient to patient. While patients tend to deteriorate gradually over time, many schizophrenic patients live healthy and productive lives, often with the assistance of antipsychotic medications. Approximately 1% of the worldwide population has this chronic illness, and it is 10 times more likely to occur in first-degree relatives of individuals with the disorder. Suicide is a major concern for patients diagnosed with schizophrenia.[29]

The onset of schizophrenia is also highly variable but typically occurs in adolescence or early adult life. The median age of onset for the first psychotic episode is early to mid-20s for men and late 20s for women.[26] Recently, it has been described as progressing along a continuum.[30] This continuum begins with depression or "negative" symptoms, continues into a bipolar phase, and ends in an "active" or psychotic phase.

Early in the disease process, patients may become withdrawn from social interactions and may neglect their personal appearance. Other negative symptoms include a diminished emotional response (blunted affect). Active symptoms typically appear later and include hallucinations, delusions, and grossly disorganized behavior. Patients can become withdrawn and rock or stare in a hypervigilant state. In some cases, patients may have a more sudden onset, traditionally described as a "psychotic break," marking the beginning of symptoms. The sudden appearance of voices that no one else can hear can be very frightening. Patients may be afraid to admit those symptoms out of fear that they are "going crazy" and fear of being involuntarily committed. Other schizophrenic patients may not seek care if they do not think they are acting abnormally.[4,5]

Subtypes of schizophrenia include the following:[26,29]

- *Paranoid:* grandiose delusions and hallucinations and feelings of persecution.

BOX 40-4 Typical Antipsychotic (Neuroleptic) Medications

Low Potency

Chlorpromazine (Thorazine)

Intermediate Potency

Loxapine (Loxitane)

Thioridazine (Mellaril)

Mesoridazine (Serentil)

Molindone (Moban)

Perphenazine (Trilafon)

High Potency

Fluphenazine (Prolixin)

Thiothixene (Navane)

Trifluoperazine (Stelazine)

Haloperidol (Haldol)

Source: Adapted from J. A. Marx, *Rosen's Emergency Medicine: Concepts and Clinical Practice,* 5th ed., (St. Louis, MO: Mosby, 2002), p. 1546.

- *Disorganized:* disorganized speech and behavior.
- *Catatonic:* physical symptoms of immobility or repetitive or excessive motor activity and bizarre postures.
- *Undifferentiated:* mixed symptoms.

Traditionally, schizophrenics are prescribed antipsychotic (neuroleptic) agents such as those listed in Box 40-4. During a psychotic exacerbation, it may be very difficult to tell schizophrenic patients from those who are bipolar in a manic phase.[30] Sometimes, patients' medications may be helpful in determining a past history of psychiatric problems. Patients may be taking a low or intermediate intensity antipsychotic medication such as chlorpromazine (Thorazine) or thioridazine (Mellaril).

Neuroleptic Medication Adverse Reactions

Dystonic Reactions

Neuroleptic agents alter levels of dopamine in the brain and have a high frequency of adverse effects. Watch for signs of a dystonic reaction: tongue protrusion and involuntary contraction of muscles in the face and neck (torticollis). These reactions can look like a focal motor seizure. The key is to elicit a good history.

Street Secrets

Reversing a dystonic reaction by giving diphenhydramine (Benadryl™) 25–50 mg IM or IV will usually improve dystonic symptoms and is the treatment of choice.

Neuroleptic medications can have other adverse and possibly more serious reactions. These are less common, but they can include orthostatic hypotension, tardive dyskinesia, and neuroleptic malignant syndrome (NMS). Orthostatic hypotension is defined as a drop in blood pressure of 20 mmHg or more on assuming an upright posture.[31] If symptomatic, treat it with oxygen, Trendelenburg's position, and IV fluids.[4]

High potency neuroleptic medications such as haloperidol (Haldol®), droperidol (Inapsine®), and thiothixene (Navane®) are recommended more for active psychosis and may be used for many psychiatric problems, not just schizophrenia.[4,5] When administering these

Working in the Gray Zone

Is droperidol a safe prehospital medication? For many years droperidol (Inapsine®) was successfully used in the prehospital setting for patients with acute agitation.[2] Droperidol, along with other drugs in its class (butyrophenones), causes a prolongation of the QT interval. In 2001, the Food and Drug Administration, in response to 100 adverse events following administration of droperidol, gave the drug a black box label.[32] The FDA label recommends a 12-lead ECG be performed prior to using droperidol, which may be hard, if not impossible, to accomplish on an agitated patient.[2] One subsequent prehospital study showed that using midazolam (Versed®) for out-of-hospital sedation increased the need for intubation and ICU admissions when compared to droperidol.[33] Droperidol also has antinausea properties and has been successfully used to decrease motion sickness in patients being transported in an ambulance.[34] Further research is needed to definitively address the use of droperidol in the prehospital setting.[35] Until that time, lorazepam (Ativan®), haloperidol (Haldol®), and possibly a combination of these drugs (consult your local protocols) can be used.[36]

CONNECTIONS To review prolonged QT syndrome, review Chapter 29: Cardiology, Section II.

medications in the prehospital setting, you should watch for adverse reactions, especially dystonic reactions such as those described previously.

Tardive Dyskinesia

Tardive dyskinesia usually appears after several years of neuroleptic medication treatment. It is characterized by involuntary movements, particularly of the face. Often a twisting and curling of the tongue will be noticed first. These movements are difficult to tell apart from an acute psychotic event. The definitive treatment is to reduce the dose or discontinue the neuroleptic medication that is causing it. If you cannot distinguish between a dystonic reaction and tardive dyskinesia, a trial dose of diphenhydramine (Benadryl®) 25–50 mg IM is an appropriate prehospital course of treatment.

Neuroleptic Malignant Syndrome

Neuroleptic malignant syndrome (NMS) is a potentially fatal side effect of neuroleptic medications. It usually occurs in the first few weeks of treatment. NMS is marked by hyperthermia, catatonic rigidity, altered mental status, renal failure, and seizures.[6]

Atypical Antipsychotic Medications

Today, you are more likely to encounter patients who are prescribed newer "atypical" antipsychotic agents such as risperidone (Risperdal®), olanzapine (Zyprexa®), clozapine (Clozaril®), and ziprasidone (Geodon®). These drugs work on both the negative (flat) symptoms and the positive (active) symptoms of schizophrenia. They act by blocking serotonin to a greater degree than they block dopamine. They have less extrapyramidal side effects such as muscle rigidity, tremors, or difficulty walking and moving. These drugs are also less lethal if a patient attempts to overdose using them. Atypical antipsychotic drugs take days to weeks to reach therapeutic levels and are not administered in the prehospital setting.

Note: You may also see these medications used in lower doses for children with attention deficit disorders, and they are used at subtherapeutic levels to help control behavior in children and adults with autism spectrum disorders.

Anxiety Disorders

Anxiety and Panic

Anxiety is an uneasy feeling that is commonly experienced when a person is fearful or anticipating harm, even if the fear appears irrational. It is more prevalent than any other mental health disorder.[4] Anxiety is commonly encountered in the emergency medical services setting and often accompanies medical and traumatic illness. In one emergency department study, as many as 42% of patients who were thought to have anxiety ended up being diagnosed with a problem that was medical in nature.[4] Anxiety is not a life-threatening condition itself, but you need to consider medical and environmental causes of anxiety that are possibly lethal and reversible.

The human body reacts to discomfort by engaging its fight or flight system, and the autonomic nervous system releases catecholamines to overcome the stressful challenge. Initially, anxiety can increase awareness and improve performance, but too much anxiety becomes overwhelming and dysfunctional.[37] In the prehospital setting, anxiety should be treated and minimized. Anxiety that is persistent and out of proportion to the presenting danger should be considered more pathological.

When anxiety becomes chronic and persistent for six months or greater, patients may be diagnosed with a generalized anxiety disorder.

A **panic attack** is a sudden onset of acute anxiety. There is acute apprehension, fear, and feelings of impending doom. Patients experiencing a panic attack will present with physical symptoms of palpitations, tachycardia, shortness of breath, diaphoresis, chest tightness, and other catecholamine-related symptoms. Most patients who have panic attacks will recover without treatment and do not go on to develop chronic panic disorder.[4,5] Patients who do develop a recurrent pattern of panic attacks over a period of six months may be diagnosed with panic disorder.[5] The patients worry constantly about when the next unexpected attack will come. When panic attacks become a more chronic problem, patients may be placed on antidepressant or benzodiazepine medications to reduce the anxiety.

Prehospital care for patients having anxiety or panic attacks centers around calming them and determining if there is a medical cause for the altered behavior. With limited time and complex scene dynamics, you may often not be able to conclusively determine whether the problem is medical or behavioral. These patients should be transported to an emergency department for further evaluation. Remember that hypoglycemia, hypoxia, and any cause of altered mental status may also present as anxiety. Administer oxygen, check blood glucose level, and perform a thorough exam to ensure you can discover any problems you will be able to address.

Obsessive Compulsive Disorder

Obsessive-compulsive disorder (OCD) is a condition in which intrusive ideas, strange images, or fears

bother the patient who cannot eliminate them. Patients may be aware that their worries have become excessive or unreasonable but cannot control them. Usual fears revolve around being the victim of violence, perverse sexual behavior, or germ contamination. The symptoms are relieved by rituals that attempt to compensate for the fears. Excessive washing, repetitive checking, or counting can occupy a great deal of time.[26]

Phobias

A **phobia** is a persistent and irrational fear due to an external factor. The affected person usually recognizes that the reaction is excessive and makes a conscious effort to avoid the cause of the fear. Common phobias revolve around specific fears such as heights, animals, storms, or small spaces. Agoraphobia is an irrational fear of open spaces or public places where it may be difficult to escape or to find help.[38]

Street Secrets

Do not confuse phobia with paranoia. These are different in that paranoia usually involves a delusion or hallucination. Paranoia is a general mistrust and feeling of persecution. Phobias are irrational fears about specific objects.

Posttraumatic Stress

Posttraumatic stress disorder (PTSD) is a disorder in which the memory of a previous overwhelming or traumatic event is repeatedly reexperienced. In between traumatic events, patients may experience periods of emotional numbness and emptiness. The memories are intrusive and cause intense fear, helplessness, and horror. Typically individuals who survive life-threatening events, assaults, fires, criminal violence, or national disasters are at most risk. A common behavior is to try to avoid any stimulus that triggers the intrusive memories. Since emergency workers are at-risk for developing this disorder, this topic is covered extensively in the chapter on the well-being of the paramedic (see Chapter 2: The Well-Being of the Paramedic).

It is important to note that, in the context of behavioral emergencies, PTSD is a diagnosis found in the DSM-IV-TR. It is not just a disorder that affects military veterans or EMS workers; the public is also vulnerable to its effects. Sleep disturbances, survivor guilt, night terrors, and substance abuse are common complications.[5,37]

Addictive Behavior

In the United States, an average of $240 to $500 billion dollars is spent each year for the pleasure of putting addictive substances into the body.[39] This includes the cost of alcohol, tobacco, and recreational drugs and the trickle-down effect on the criminal justice system and healthcare system. Legal and illegal drugs are big business. Alcohol alone is the third leading cause of preventable death in the United States, after smoking and obesity.[40] Excluding tobacco, 32 million people in the United States have some degree of serious dependency on drugs. About 1 in 13 people will have a drug abuse problem at some point in their lives, and 1 in 6 will have an alcohol dependency problem.[26] Studies performed in urban emergency departments indicate that up to 20% of patients may have problems with alcohol and that 40–50% of all highway deaths are alcohol related.[26,41]

Substance Abuse and Dependence

Substance abuse can best be defined as a chronic pattern of chemical use that leads to clinically significant impairment or distress. The DSM-IV-TR identifies four criteria for substance abuse. Over the course of a 12-month period, the person exhibits one or more of the following recurrent patterns:

1. Failure to fulfill major work, school, or home obligations.
2. Uses chemicals in situations that could be physically harmful such as driving or working machinery.
3. Repeated legal problems such as arrests for disorderly conduct related to substance use.
4. Continued use despite interpersonal problems with family, friends, and coworkers that are exacerbated by substance use.

People are thought to be dependent on chemicals when they become unable to stop using, have a repeated need to use a substance despite the negative consequences, need more of the chemical to achieve the same desired effect (tolerance), or have negative effects when use is discontinued (withdrawal). Substantial amounts of time and effort are placed on obtaining and using the substance, even though individuals may want to stop.

Treating Substance Abuse

Efforts to curb substance abuse date back to the Romans who tried to curb drinking by placing spiders in the bottom of wine cups.[42] Various models are used to treat addiction and dependence. They include behavioral, psychosocial, prescriptive, moral, and psychoanalytic.[24]

CONNECTIONS More information about the effects of substance use can be found in Chapter 35: Toxicology

The important concepts to remember about substance use in the context of a behavioral emergency include:

- The altered behavior could be caused by the substance intoxication or withdrawal.
- The substance in conjunction with an underlying mental health problem could be causing the altered behavior.

The direct effects of the substance abuse issue may be very reversible in the prehospital environment, such as a heroin overdose, but the underlying addiction or mental health problem needs to be addressed in the long term. When you are assessing patients with altered behavior, consider two possibilities:

- That drugs or alcohol are involved.
- That even if drugs or alcohol are involved, there could still be an accompanying behavioral problem.

It is dangerous to assume that the underlying behavior is related to the chemical intoxication or withdrawal alone. Examples of patients who were thought to be "just drunk" or under the influence but in fact had major medical problems are too common.[43,44,45] The best course of action is to assume that there may be both a medical or external cause and an internal or psychological cause of the behavior, and treat patients accordingly.

Psychosomatic versus Factitious Disorders

The DSM-IV-TR includes extensive definitions for a series of non-life-threatening disorders in which patients mistakenly believe they are having a medical problem and seek medical treatment for it but are later found to have no medical cause for their symptoms. These disorders can be separated into two main categories: somatoform (psychosomatic) and factitious. The main difference between psychosomatic and factitious disorders is whether the patients are consciously trying to deceive the caregiver.

In somatoform disorders, such as hypochondriasis and conversion disorder, patients consciously believe their physical symptoms are being caused by a medical problem. They seek the opinions of their healthcare practitioners and are convinced that they need medical help.

Patients with a factitious disorder are consciously and actively working to deceive their medical practitioners. In the more severe cases (Munchausen syndrome), patients may go to great extremes to seek hospitalization and painful medical procedures.[46] In Munchausen by proxy, patients fabricate symptoms in another person (such as a mother fabricating information about her child). Diagnosing a psychosomatic or factitious disorder in the field is generally not possible. These diagnoses are only made after every other possible option has been thoroughly investigated and ruled out. This is termed a diagnosis of exclusion. Focus on a thorough investigation of the patient's symptoms so that life-threatening conditions are not missed.

Street Secrets

It is better to treat for the worst and hope for the best. Assuming that the patient may be exaggerating or inventing symptoms can lead to disastrous consequences if you withhold care when someone, in fact, did need immediate intervention. The reverse case, where you assess, treat, and transport a patient who may not be ill or injured, is not nearly as dangerous. For example, checking someone's blood sugar has relatively low risk of complications when compared to missing a patient who is in insulin shock.[6]

Drug-Seeking Behavior

On occasion, a patient may present untruthful or exaggerated symptoms in an effort to trick medical professionals into giving mood-altering substances. Recent studies point to a serious lack of adequate analgesia in emergency rooms.[47] One part of this may be due to the exaggerated concern on the part of nurses, physicians, and paramedics over drug-seeking behavior. It is best, in this case, to err on the side of treating someone's pain and later find out that the patient may have been abusing the system than to withhold medication from someone who is in pain. A small amount of prehospital narcotics is not likely to cause, or to greatly worsen, a patient's addiction.

Personality Disorders

Personality disorders form a category of mental disorders characterized by long-lasting rigid patterns of thought and behavior. Over time, these inflexible and maladaptive patterns cause distress and impair social and occupational functioning.

The DSM-IV-TR lists ten personality disorders:

- **Cluster A:** Odd or eccentric disorders
  - Paranoid personality disorder
  - Schizoid personality disorder
  - Schizotypal personality disorder

- **Cluster B:** Dramatic, emotional, and erratic disorders
  - Antisocial personality disorder
  - Borderline personality disorder
  - Histrionic personality disorder
  - Narcissistic personality disorder
- **Cluster C:** Anxious or fearful disorders
  - Avoidant personality disorder
  - Dependent personality disorder
  - Obsessive-compulsive personality disorder (not the same as obsessive-compulsive disorder)

In-depth knowledge of personality disorders is not necessary for the paramedic, and definitions of each of these are beyond the scope of this text. You should, however, maintain an awareness of one personality disorder that presents special challenges in assessment and prehospital care.

Borderline Personality Disorder

Borderline personality disorder is a condition in which a person's mood, interpersonal relationships, self image, and identity are unstable. These patients may frantically try to avoid real or imagined abandonment and think in terms of extreme "black and white" relationships. Some patients have chronic feelings of emptiness marked with periods of intense irritability and anxiety. Recurrent suicidal behavior, suicidal threats, and self-mutilation are common (Figure 40-5).[48]

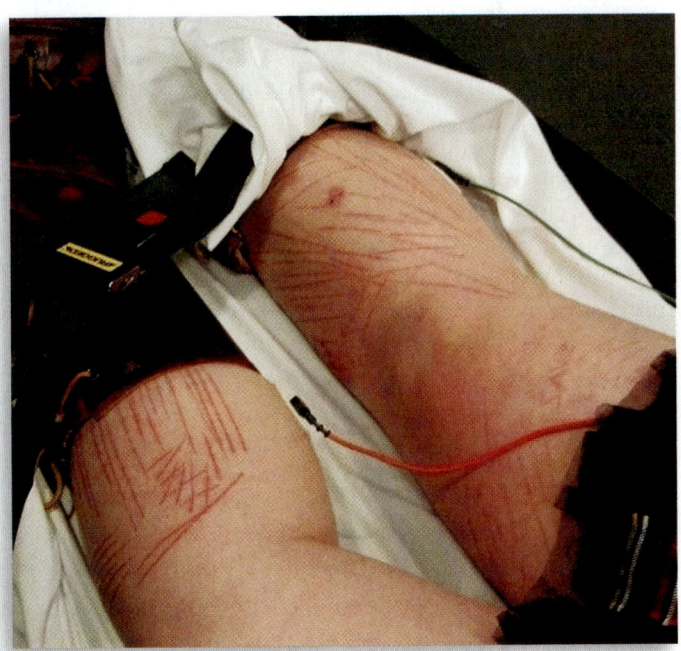

Figure 40-5   The teenage female cut herself repeatedly with a razor. Self-mutilation is highest among teenage females, patients diagnosed with borderline personality, and patients with dissociative disorder (multiple personality disorder). Over half of self-mutilators were sexually abused as children.[61]

Onset of this personality disorder occurs in early adulthood, and the majority of diagnosed cases appear to have been victims of childhood abuse. These patients may be challenging to manage at a prehospital scene. They may exhibit paranoid ideas, impulsive behavior, and angry outbursts of emotion. As their caregiver, it is important to stay objective, set appropriate limits on inappropriate behavioral outbursts, and expect extreme changes in the patients' moods.

Prehospital Care for Behavioral Emergencies

As discussed earlier in this chapter, your first priorities in a mental health emergency revolve around ensuring safety; ensuring an adequate airway, breathing, and circulation; ruling out reversible conditions; and using crisis intervention skills. You need to be constantly aware of your surroundings and potential risks. Carefully approach any scene where a patient is behaviorally altered. Creating a good rapport, building trust, and communicating effectively with the patient are essential in successfully managing behavioral emergencies[5,6]

DOT 5-12.15, DOT 5-12.21

A crisis is a dangerous time but one that may be a catalyst for health, self-evaluation, and linkage to the healthcare system and long-term care. Studies have shown that early identification and therapeutic intervention during a crisis can promote more rapid symptom control, reduce use of restraints, and shorten the length of stay for patients who are admitted. Poor management of the crisis patient can cause much harm.[9,20]

If the patient has physical symptoms, a focused assessment of the involved systems is important. Reversible causes of altered behavior, such as diabetic reactions, hypotension, substance abuse or withdrawal, hypoxia, or other medical causes, should be treated immediately. Any patient who is behaving inappropriately or was reported to have altered mental status prior to your arrival must be evaluated by a physician. Case reports are plentiful in which the patient died shortly after a paramedic decided that the patient was not having a medical problem and did not treat or transport the patient.[43–45,49–51] While keeping a high index of suspicion for reversible causes of altered behavior, use the following simple crisis intervention steps to assess and treat these patients:

1. *Define the problem.* Introduce yourself, build rapport, and actively listen to the patient. Ask open-ended questions, and help the patient identify the elements of their crisis. Paraphrasing these problems will help check back with the patient to ensure that you understand the true problem the patient is describing. Paraphrasing also lets the patient know you are listening and encourages the patient to divulge more personal information.

2. *Ensure patient safety.* Control the environment; if necessary, move to a safer location or reduce external stimuli (such as loud noise, televisions, or bystanders). Work with law enforcement to properly search and disarm the patient. Ensure proper separation from objects that can be used as nontraditional weapons, including your own scissors, pens, and multifunction tools clipped to your belt.

3. *Provide support.* Demonstrate empathy while not passing judgment. Provide for small comforts such as a tissue, towel, pillow, or seating. This can sometimes be enough to build a strong rapport and obtain the trust of your patient. Help the patient understand that they are not alone and that you can link them to caregivers who can help them create a long-term plan for mental health.

4. *Examine alternatives.* Give patients limited options that are realistic and therapeutic. Involving patients in decisions about their care will empower them to feel more in control of their own health. Identify and reinforce patients' strengths. Reframe or reorient the conversation so that key issues are summarized. In some cases, it may be necessary to distract patients momentarily to divert attention from an issue that seems overwhelming so that patients do not begin to escalate into more anxious behavior.

5. *Make a plan.* This is a mutually agreed upon plan that maps out a very short-term strategy to address the patient's concerns. The plan may be as simple as going in the ambulance and getting a ride to talk to a mental health practitioner at the emergency department. If the patient is not going to be transported by ambulance, talking to a supportive friend or getting the right phone numbers (and even appointments if possible) to a social service or mental health agency is very helpful.

6. *Obtain a commitment.* This last step may be small in the prehospital environment, but it is critical as it affirms the plan made in the previous step. It is a reaffirmation that the plan is mutually agreed upon and acceptable.[20]

There may be times when you will need to make a plan that is not mutually agreed upon, such as when you are forced to transport a patient who is suicidal, and the patient is refusing to go. It is important not to lie to the patient but rather to explain that even when transportation will be mandatory, the patient still has options (for example to cooperate and have a non-restrained ride to the hospital or to be forcibly restrained).

The Violent Patient

If patients show signs of threatening behavior or inability to control their language or patients are difficult to assess due to alcohol ingestion, you need to be hypervigilant about the potential for violence. Verbal de-escalation is essential. A show of force can sometimes deter violence before it begins. In this case, at least five people should be involved and should present a calm unified approach that is gradual and nonthreatening to patients. Law enforcement, fire department, and EMS staff may be able to deter a confrontation. DOT 5-12.23

If violence is imminent, then it may be necessary to anticipate the need to use physical or chemical restraint (Figure 40-6 and Figure 40-7). The steps to safe physical restraint are listed in Box 40-5. **Skill Sheet 65: Physical Restraints (and Step-by-Step 65) outlines a step-by-step procedure for patient restraint.**

Chemical Restraint

When confronted with an agitated or potentially harmful patient, interventions should begin with the least invasive possible.[2] The goal of chemical restraint is to use medication to mildly sedate the patient and control their agitation to achieve control of a violent and dangerous situation.[58] This endpoint is very important as over-sedation is dangerous and may increase the rate of

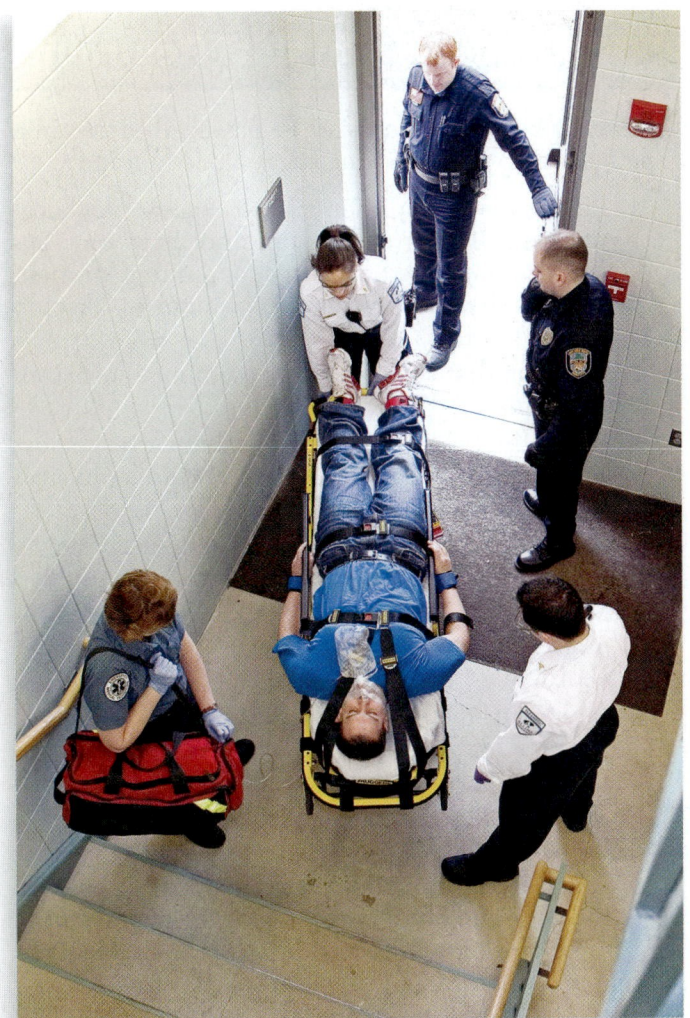

Figure 40-7   Illustration of a properly restrained patient. Law enforcement and EMS in this case have used seatbelts and soft Velcro® restraints to secure the patient to the stretcher. The oxygen mask helps ensure adequate oxygenation and decreases the risk of contamination if the patient spits.

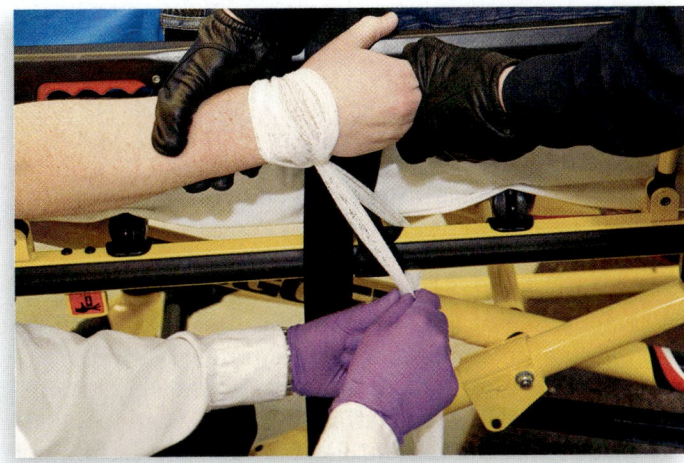

Figure 40-6   Familiarity with simple equipment that is readily available, such as Kling® or Kerlix® bandages, can become critical when emergency restraint is needed for the safety of the patient and the crew. Be sure you check distal circulation, motor function, and sensation after applying restraints.

hospitalization and length of stay. These are often associated with poor patient outcomes.[6] Paralytic agents are not appropriate unless indicated for an underlying medical or traumatic condition.[2]

Chemical restraint in the prehospital setting is usually accomplished with a benzodiazepine such as midazolam (Versed®) or lorazepam (Ativan®). In some systems, a butyrophenone such as haloperidol (Haldol®) is used alone or in combination with a benzodiazepine. Though chemically induced, some of the same principles as physical restraints apply in these cases as well. Documentation, continued monitoring, and humane care is just as important. Restraints of any kind should not be used to punish or teach the patient a lesson.

BOX 40-5   Physical Restraint — Clinical Pearls

When it becomes necessary to physically restrain a patient, keep the following suggestions in mind:

1. Before the case presents itself, know your local protocol. If your system does not have one, encourage your medical direction, administration, and quality improvement personnel to develop clear guidelines.[2]

2. Attempt first to de-escalate without the use of restraints.[12,13,14]

3. Enlist the help of law enforcement early; a show of force is sometimes enough to avoid a physical confrontation.[16,52]

4. Keep your cool; do not be affected by the patient's inappropriate language or behavior.

5. Make a plan, and act together as a team. A common phrase or code may be useful to initiate a coordinated physical approach.

6. Be sure to have enough people to safely overpower the patient; the safety of both the patient and providers is always the key priority.[5]

7. The stretcher should be placed in a lowered position as close to the patient as possible.

8. Grasp clothing and large joints, avoid pressure on the neck and chest, and do not restrict movement of the abdomen (excursion of the diaphragm) or impair breathing.

9. Use of soft restraints such as kerlix or leather is recommended.[2,53]

10. Seatbelts should be placed just above the patient's knees to prevent flexion and on the chest underneath the arms. Care should be taken not to tighten seatbelts so hard as to cause hyperextension of the patient's knees or breathing impairment.

11. Restraints on each limb should be placed one extremity at a time.[5]

12. The patient should be restrained face up (supine or semi-sitting);[54] never restrain a patient in the prone or face-down position.

13. Once applied, do not remove restraints until you have reached the hospital.

14. Continually reassess the patient's mental status, breathing, and circulation, including circulation, motor, and sensory functions of the hands and feet.[55]

15. Place the patient on 100% oxygen via mask; this helps shield rescuers from biting and spitting but more importantly improves oxygenation during a time of increase oxygen demand.

16. Check a blood glucose level, and administer dextrose if appropriate.

17. Detailed documentation is essential. Document assessment and reassessment findings before and after restraints. Be sure to include quotes from the patient and actions that made you believe there was danger to the patient or others on scene. Avoid using adjectives such as "combative" or "aggressive" as you may have to later explain their meaning in a legal proceeding.[56]

*Be sure to check your local protocols for approved methods of restraint in your EMS system.[57]

Summary

Psychiatric and behavioral emergencies should be considered medical problems first and treated with both caution for safety and compassionate care. Once scene safety, airway, breathing, and circulation have been addressed, formulating an accurate diagnosis in the field is not as important as ruling out reversible causes. Standard crisis intervention techniques can be used with any patient exhibiting altered behavior and can be very therapeutic. In a relatively short prehospital patient encounter, a paramedic can set in motion a healing process that may seriously improve a patient's outcome. Simple communication skills, definition of the problem, and working to empower the patient into regaining some control or perspective of their crisis are some of the keys to excellent care (Box 40-6).

Although it may sometimes appear as if patients in crisis will not benefit from the lifesaving services of a paramedic, remember that your observation of the patient's environment, your assessment skills, communication skills, and patient advocacy can make all the difference in a patient getting the right help. Any altered mental status patient should be evaluated by a physician.

Depriving a human being of the right to move is a serious matter and should not be taken lightly. Restraining a patient should only be done as a last resort. Be sure to practice this skill so that you can apply it safely and quickly in an emergency situation.

BOX 40-6 **Emergency Mental Health Services: A Future Role for Paramedics?**

Paramedics are uniquely suited to assess, triage, and care for behavioral emergencies.[9] The paramedic can perform both a medical and mental health assessment and can determine the best care for the patients. Some ambulance services have implemented mobile crisis teams staffed by paramedics. One such program exists in Santa Barbara, California, where selected American Medical Response (AMR) paramedics receive a specialized 45-hour mental health assessment training (MHAT) course.

The mobile crisis team responds to psychiatric emergencies in specially equipped Ford Explorers. They can be called to respond alone or in co-response with police, fire, or an ambulance. They assess, treat, and transport patients to appropriate mental health facilities thereby reducing the cost of care and transportation for these types of patients.[59]

Although no formal study of this EMS mobile crisis unit model is available today, similar approaches nationwide have been shown to decrease the severity of the crisis, reduce criminalization, and hospitalization. In Dekalb County, Georgia, a study showed less hospitalization rates and 23% cost decrease per case handled by the mobile crisis team. In the Dekalb model, police officers were specially trained and responded with a nurse between the hours of 3 p.m. to 10:30 p.m.[60] Patients seeking mental health services often use the 9-1-1 system and emergency department during evening hours when other psychiatric services are not available.[5]

Notes

1. C. J. Murray and A. D. Lopez, *The Global Burden of Disease* (Cambridge, MA: Harvard University Press, 1996), Table 5.4, p. 270.
2. D. F. Kupas and G. C. Wydro, "Patient Restraint in Emergency Medical Services Systems" (Position Paper, National Association of EMS Physicians, approved February 28, 2002), *Prehospital Emergency Care* (Philadelphia, PA: Hanley and Belfus, 2002), http://www.naemsp.org/Position%20Papers/restraint.pdf (accessed March 15, 2005).
3. J. T. Grange and S. W. Corbett, "Violence Against Emergency Medical Services Personnel," *Prehospital Emergency Care* 6(2002): 186–190.
4. J. A. Marx, ed. *Rosen's Emergency Medicine Concepts and Clinical Practice,* 5th ed. (St. Louis, MO: Elsevier Mosby, 2002), pp. 1543–1545.
5. J. Tintinalli, *Emergency Medicine, A Comprehensive Study Guide,* 6th ed. (New York, NY: McGraw-Hill, 2004), pp. 1807–1808.
6. M. H. Allen, G. W. Currier, D. H. Hughes, et al., "Treatment of Behavioral Emergencies: A Summary of the Expert Consensus," *Journal of Psychiatric Practice* 9.1 (2003): 16–38.
7. Z. Atakan and T. Davies, "ABC of Mental Health—Mental Health Emergencies," *British Medical Journal* 314, 6 (1997): 1740–1742.
8. D. C. Aguilera, *Crisis Intervention—Theory and Methodology,* 6th ed. (St. Louis, MO: CV Mosby 1990), pp. 21–25.
9. L. A. Hoff, *People in Crisis—Understanding and Helping,* 4th ed. (San Francisco, CA: Jossey-Bass, 1993).
10. "Emotional First Aid: American Psychotherapy Association," http://www.emotionalfirstaid.com/ (accessed March 16, 2005).
11. D. Houry, C. Parramore, et al., "Characteristics of Household Addresses That Repeatedly Contact 911 to Report Intimate Partner Violence," *Academic Emergency Medicine* 11.6 (2004): 662–667.
12. D. R. Krebs, K. C. Henry, and M.B. Gabriele, *When Violence Erupts, A Survival Guide for Emergency Responders* (St. Louis, MO: C. V. Mosby, 1990).
13. J. R. Petit, "Management of the Acutely Violent Patient," *Psychiatric Clinics of North America* 28(3)(September 2005): 701–711.
14. K. B. Dernocoeur, *Streetsense: Communication, Safety and Control* (Redmond, WA: Laing Communications Inc., 1996), pp. 67–69.
15. National Institute of Mental Health, "In Harm's Way: Suicide in America" (April 2004), http://www.nimh.nih.gov/publicat/harmaway.cfm (accessed March 16, 2005).
16. P. T. Pons and V. J. Markovchick, eds., *Prehospital Emergency Care Secrets: Questions You Will Be Asked—at the Scene, in the ED, on Oral Exams* (Philadelphia, PA: Hanley and Belfus, 1998), pp. 192–193.
17. Centers for Disease Control, National Center for Injury Prevention and Control (December 22, 2004), http://www.cdc.gov/ncipc/factsheets/suifacts.htm (accessed March 16, 2005).
18. B. Q. Hafen and K. J. Frandsen, *Psychological Emergencies and Crisis Intervention, A Comprehensive Guide for Emergency Personnel* (Englewood Cliffs, NJ: Prentice Hall, 1985), pp. 24–30.
19. R. Behrman, *Nelson Textbook of Pediatrics,* 17th ed. (Philadelphia, PA: Elsevier, 2004).
20. R. K. James and B. E. Gilliland, *Crisis Intervention Strategies,* 5th ed. (Belmont CA: Brooks/Cole, 2005), p. 21.
21. J. L. Jacobson and A. M. Jacobson, *Psychiatric Secrets,* 2nd ed. (Philadelphia, PA: Hanley and Belfus, 2001), pp. 479–480.
22. L. B. Andrew, "E-Medicine Emergency Medicine Textbook; Depression and Suicide" (June 2004), http://www.emedicine.com/emerg/topic129.htm (accessed March 16, 2005).
23. National Institute of Mental Health, "Depression" (September 2002), http://www.nimh.nih.gov/publicat/depression.cfm (accessed March 17, 2005).
24. K. Hahner, "Learned Helplessness: A Critique of the Research and Theory," Americans for Medical Advancement, http://www.curedisease.com/Perspectives/vol_1_1989/Learned%20 Helplessness.html (accessed April 5, 2005).
25. E. Weir, "Winter Needn't Be the SAD Season," *Canadian Medical Association Journal* 164(2)(January 23, 2001): 256.
26. R. Hillard and B. Zitek, *Emergency Psychiatry* (New York, NY: McGraw-Hill, 2004).

27. D. Venes and C. L. Thomas, *Taber's Cyclopedic Medical Dictionary,* 19th ed. (Philadelphia, PA: FA Davis Company, 2001).

28. M. H. Beers and R. Berkow, *The Merck Manual of Diagnosis and Therapy,* 17th ed., Section 14, Chapter 171, http://www.merck.com/mrkshared/mmanual/section14/chapter171/171a.jsp (accessed March 31, 2005).

29. M. H. Beers and R. Berkow, *The Merck Manual of Diagnosis and Therapy,* 17th ed., Section 15, Chapter 193, http://www.merck.com/mrkshared/mmanual/section15/chapter193/193b.jsp (accessed March 30, 2005).

30. C. M. Adler and S. M. Strakowski, "Boundaries of Schizophrenia," *Psychiatric Clinics of North America* 26.1 (March 2003).

31. M. H. Beers and R. Berkow, *The Merck Manual of Diagnosis and Therapy,* 17th ed., Section 16, Chapter 200, http://www.merck.com/mrkshared/mmanual/section16/chapter200/200a.jsp (accessed March 31, 2005).

32. "Droperidol Gets Second-Line, Narrowed Indication Due to Arrhythmia Risk," *The Pink Sheet* 63(2001):23.

33. M. Martel, J. Miner, R. Fringer, K. Sufka, et al., "Discontinuation of Droperidol for the Control of Acutely Agitated Out-of-Hospital Patients," *Prehospital Emergency Care* 9(1) (January–March 2005): 44–48.

34. L. Weichenthal and T. Soliz, "The Incidence and Treatment of Prehospital Motion Sickness," *Prehospital Emergency Care* 7(4) (2003): 474–476.

35. L. W. Kao, "Droperidol, QT Prolongation, and Sudden Death: What Is the Evidence?" *Annals of Emergency Medicine* 41(4)(April 2003): 546–558.

36. J. Alexander, "Rapid Tranquillisation of Violent or Agitated Patients in a Psychiatric Emergency Setting. Pragmatic Randomized Trial of Intramuscular Lorazepam v. Haloperidol Plus Promethazine," *British Journal of Psychiatry* 185(July 1, 2004): 63–69.

37. M. H. Beers and R. Berkow, *The Merck Manual of Diagnosis and Therapy,* 17th ed., Section 15, Chapter 187, http://www.merck.com/mrkshared/mmanual/section15/chapter187/187a.jsp (accessed April 10, 2005).

38. R. Albucher, "Phobic Disorders; Psychiatry Textbook" (March 13, 2005), http://www.emedicine.com/MED/topic1821.htm (accessed April 11, 2005).

39. H. E. Doweiko, *Concepts of Chemical Dependency,* 4th ed. (Pacific Grove, CA: Brooks/Cole, 1999), pp. 8–9.

40. W. Thompson, "Alcoholism," *E-medicine Psychiatry* (September 21, 2004), http://www.emedicine.com/med/topic98.htm (accessed April 11, 2005).

41. A. Cohagan, M. Plewa, and R. Worthington, "Alcohol and Substance Abuse Evaluation," *E-medicine Emergency Medicine—Psychosocial* (March 15, 2006), http://www.emedicine.com/emerg/topic20.htm (accessed April 11, 2005).

42. J. W. Smith, "Treatment of Alcoholism in Aversion Conditioning Hospitals." In *Encyclopedic Handbook of Alcoholism,* E. M. Pattison and E. Kaufman, eds. (New York, NY: Gardner Press 1982), pp. 874–884.

43. S. Silvestri, S. G. Rothrock, D. Kennedy, J. Ladde, M. Bryant, and J. Pagane, "Can Paramedics Accurately Identify Patients Who Do Not Require Emergency Department Care?" *Prehospital Emergency Care* 6(4)(October–December 2002):387–390.

44. "Assault Victim's Daughters Sue City; The Victim Died After Being Struck with a Bottle," *Providence Journal-Bulletin,* February 13, 1995.

45. R. Alford and J. Nirode, "Paramedics Refused to Carry Student; OSU Report," *The Columbus Dispatch,* June 4, 1998.

46. W. Ernoehazy and E. Frazer, "Munchausen Syndrome," *Emergency Medicine Textbook—Psychosocial* (December 7, 2004), http://www.emedicine.com/emerg/topic322.htm (accessed April 14, 2005).

47. T. Rupp, "Inadequate Analgesia in Emergency Medicine," *Annals of Emergency Medicine* 43(4)(April 1, 2004): 494–503.

48. American Psychiatric Association, *Diagnostic and Statistical Manual of Mental Disorders (DSM-IV-TR),* (Arlington, VA: American Pschiatric Publishing, 2000).

49. Shannon O'Boye, *Sun-Sentinel* (Fort Lauderdale, FL), "Grand Jury Says Simple Steps Could Have Saved Man Killed by Police Pepper Spray," March 4, 2004.

50. Shannon O'Boye, *Sun-Sentinel* (Fort Lauderdale, FL), "Paramedics to Be Fired for Inaction in Pepper-Spray Death," August 14, 2003.

51. S. Knight, L. M. Olson, L. J. Cook, N. C. Mann, H. M. Corneli, and J. M. Dean, "Against All Advice: An Analysis of Out-of-Hospital Refusals of Care," *Annals of Emergency Medicine* 42(5)(November 2003): 689–696.

52. G. W. Currier, "The Controversy Over 'Chemical Restraint' in Acute Care Psychiatry," *Journal of Psychiatric Practice* (Philadelphia, PA: Lippincott Williams & Wilkins, 2003), pp. 59–70.

53. N. G. Lee, *Legal Concepts and Issues in Emergency Care* (Philadelphia, PA: W. B. Saunders 2001), p. 123.

54. S. J. Stratton, C. Rogers, K. Brickett, and G. Gruzinski, "Factors Associated with Sudden Death of Individuals Requiring Restraint for Excited Delirium," The *American Journal of Emergency Medicine* 19(3)(May 1, 2001): 187–191.

55. T. Dick "Straight Shot, Use of Restraints Part 2," *JEMS: Journal of Emergency Medical Services* 28.1 (2003): 98–101.

56. D. Perry and T. Dick, "Count Your Fingers, More Stuff on Restraints," *JEMS: Journal of Emergency Medical Services* 28.5 (2003): 22–23.

57. W. A. Maggiore and R. B. Palmer, "Exercise Restraint," *JEMS: Journal of Emergency Medical Services* 27.3 (2002): 84–104.

58. M. H. Allen et al., "Use of Restraints and Pharmacotherapy in Academic Psychiatric Emergency Services," *General Hospital Psychiatry* 26.1 (2004): 42–49.

59. M. Nordberg, "Paramedics Provide Care to Mentally Ill," *Emergency Medical Services* 30.8 (2001): 25.

60. R. L. Scott, "Evaluation of a Mobile Crisis Program: Effectiveness, Efficiency, and Consumer Satisfaction," *Psychiatric Services,* 51.9 (2000): 1153–1156.

61. Health A to Z, "Self-Mutilation," http://www.healthatoz.com/healthatoz/Atoz/ency/self-mutilation.jsp (accessed October 5, 2006).

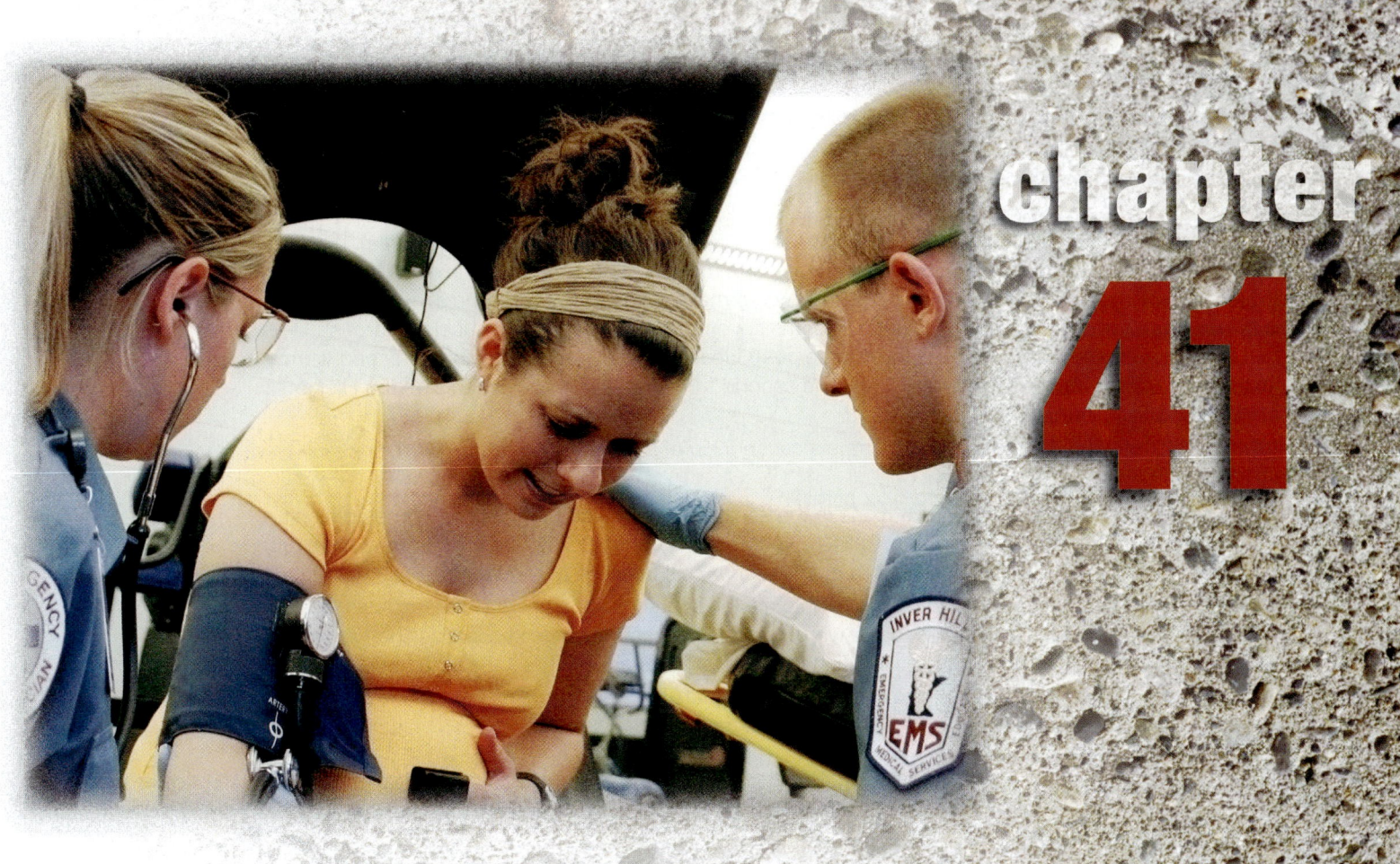

Obstetrics and Gynecology

*"**W**e have a secret in our culture, and it's not that birth is painful. It's that women are strong."*

—Laura Stavoe Harm

Need to Know

▶ Normal pregnancy is defined as lasting from the first day of the last normal menstrual period (LNMP) until the start of labor that brings forth the baby.

▶ Pregnancy that ends with labor anytime between 37 to 42 weeks is considered normal and called a term pregnancy.

▶ Pregnancy is divided into three trimesters: First trimester is weeks 1 to 12 (months one to three). A pregnancy test can show positive results within a week of a missed period. Second trimester is weeks 13 to 27 (months four to six). The uterus now has grown to make it palpable above the symphysis pubis (pubic bone). Third trimester is weeks 28 to 40 (months seven to nine). The uterus muscle enlarges 10 to 20 times its pre-pregnant size over the course of 40 weeks. Many women have experienced warm-up uterine contractions, some as early as during the second trimester; these are called Braxton Hicks contractions.

▶ Hemorrhage, ectopic pregnancy, and preeclampsia cause 59% of all maternal deaths in America.

▶ Stages of birth:

- First stage of labor: beginning of contractions in the early part of the first stage is sometimes difficult to distinguish from the uterine tightening, called Braxton Hicks contractions, the mother may have felt during her pregnancy. The first stage ends when the cervix has become fully dilated.

- Second stage is when the cervix is fully taken up into the lower uterine segment and is completely dilated, and the baby moves down into the birth canal with pushing. The second stage can last as short as one push or up to 2.5 hours, which is average in a first-time labor. This stage includes the birth of the baby.

- Third stage is timed from the birth of the baby to the complete delivery of the placenta, and this is the shortest stage of all, usually being completed within 30 minutes.

▶ Complications of birth include cord prolapse, breech presentation, compound presentation, multiple pregnancy, shoulder dystocia, bleeding, and embolism.

▶ Sick	▶ Not Yet Sick
• Look for hypertension (toxemia) or hypotension (bleeding). Provide fluids to support a BP of 90 systolic. • Heavy bleeding in the third trimester should be considered an emergency. • During childbirth, if the presenting part is anything other than the head, consider the birth to be complicated. In the case of a prolapsed cord and breech birth, you may need to insert a gloved hand into the mother's vaginal canal to help prevent birth, or form a "V" to help the baby breathe. • Monitor the patient's vital signs closely, especially blood pressure. Keep the pregnant patient on her left side. • Consider the mother's urge to push or feeling of a bowel movement as a sign of imminent birth. Check for crowning. Prepare for delivery.	• Births may rapidly change. Continuous monitoring of progress is necessary. • When was the patient's last menstrual period? Is there any chance the patient could be pregnant? You may need to be specific: Is the patient sexually active? What method of birth control is being used? • Is there vaginal discharge? If so, is it purulent? Is there blood present? Is there rectal discharge? • Investigate the location, severity, onset, and provocation of pain. Is it cramping pain? Is the pain constant? • Measure and record the duration, severity, and frequency of contractions. • Obtain gravity (number of previous pregnancies) and parity (number of live births). Were the births vaginal or cesarean? Were there other complications? Was there bleeding or hypertension?

Introduction

This chapter covers material in four categories: gynecological emergencies, pregnancy complications, out-of-hospital childbirth, and childbirth complications.

The assessment and care of women of childbearing age depends on your knowledge and understanding of the female reproductive system. It is essential that you gain a basic understanding of a woman's reproductive cycle

Working in the Gray Zone

It is important to note that in the prehospital environment it may be impossible to tell whether the patient is pregnant. Even patients who report that there is "absolutely no way I could be pregnant," have been caught by surprise when their method of birth control has failed. For this reason, you should suspect that a woman of childbearing years *is pregnant* until proven otherwise by a lab test or there is unquestionable evidence that she could not be pregnant (such as a complete lack of sexual contact or a hysterectomy). A woman may be very reluctant to report a sexual history, especially in the presence of family members or to a stranger. You should maintain a high index of suspicion since overlooking a pregnancy complication, such as an ectopic pregnancy (the egg is mistakenly implanted in the fallopian tube), can lead to a bad outcome for your patient.

and the physiology of pregnancy in order to properly care for these patients.

Instead of trying to memorize tables, charts, signs, and symptoms, you are encouraged to think of gynecological and obstetric problems in two main categories: the pregnant (or possibly pregnant) patient and the nonpregnant patient. This chapter is divided into these two

categories to help guide you in the practical application of your gynecological and obstetric knowledge.

It is also helpful to place your patient in a "reproductive timeline" or a continuum. This continuum begins with a nonpregnant patient having her normal menstrual period, continues into ovulation (ovary releases an egg), then, assuming the egg is not fertilized, the shedding of the lining of the uterus as the menstrual period begins again. Should the patient become pregnant, the fertilized egg will normally implant and grow in the uterus. The medical conditions and complaints your patient will have largely depend on the stage in the reproductive cycle or the stage of pregnancy the patient is in.

For example, a patient who is less than 14 days from her last menstrual period is more likely to have a gynecological problem (such as ovarian torsion) than a pregnancy-related problem.

Applied Anatomy and Physiology

The female reproductive organs become active at puberty when multiple physical and physiological changes happen in the body (Figures 41-1 and 41-2). Menarche, which is the term for the first menstrual cycle, on average, happens for girls between the ages of 12 and 13 years.[1] Menopause, the cessation of menses, happens between the ages of 45 and 52 years, on average. Women usually experience several months or years of perimenopausal signs before the last episode of bleeding.

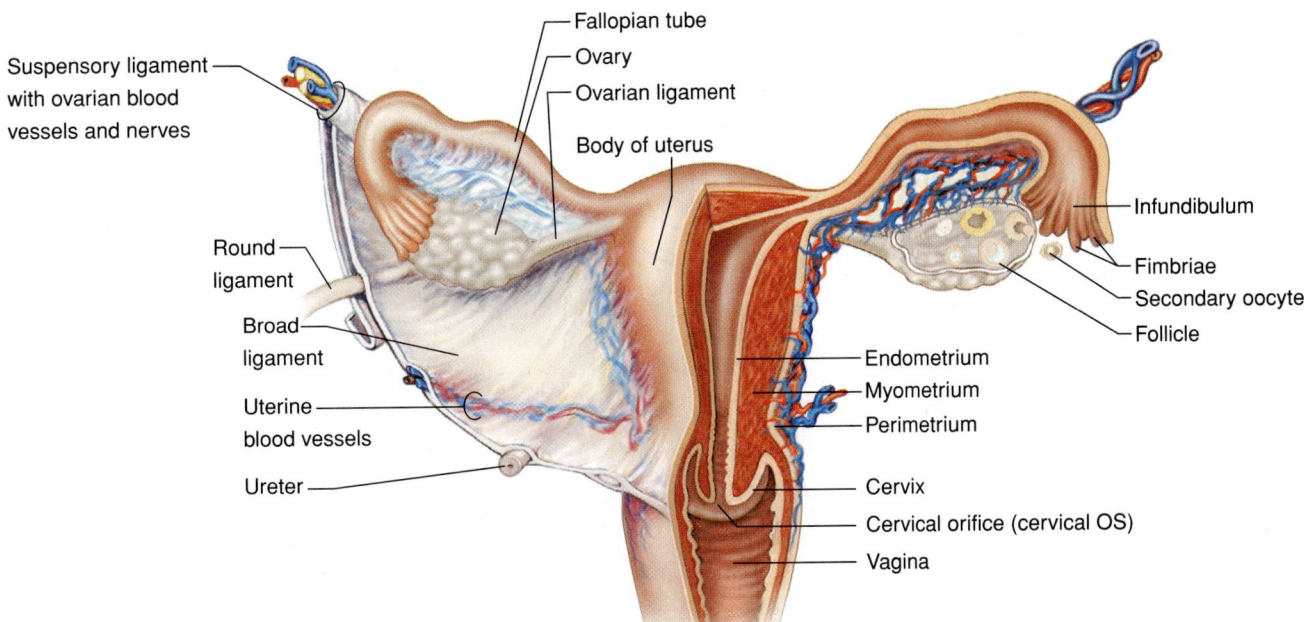

Figure 41-1 Anatomy of the female reproductive system.

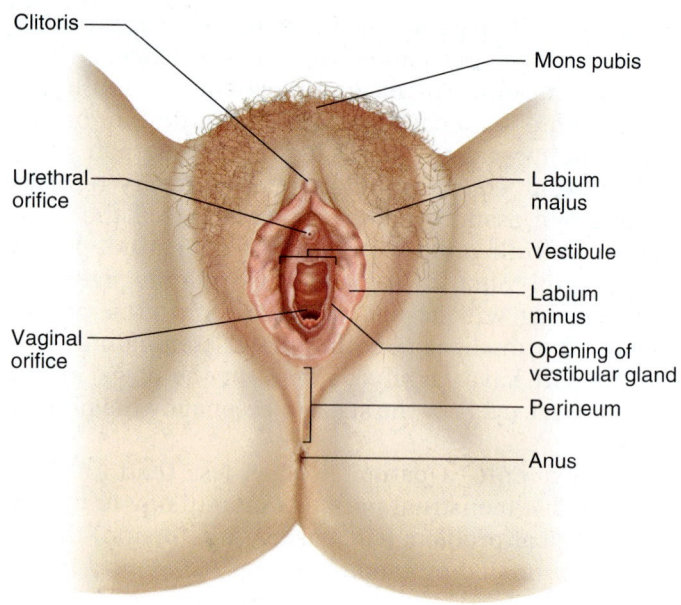

Figure 41-2   External genitalia of the female.

Menstrual cycles are usually 24 to 35 days in duration, with the average being 28 days (Figure 41-3 and 41-4).[1] The first day of bleeding is also known as the first day of the menstrual cycle. Flow varies in duration, with four days being average. The amount of blood lost is variable, with many women describing their "periods" as scant, light, medium, or heavy. Menstrual blood usually does not clot, and the total amount lost is 60–80 mL per cycle.[1] The menstrual bleeding indicates an unfertilized egg, and the blood indicates the uterine lining is being shed. Every month during a woman's reproductive years, the ovary prepares to release an egg, and a series of hormonal preparations are undertaken to increase the potential for successful pregnancy.[1] The pattern of hormone release affects the woman's entire body, and can impact her behavior, and her mood. The first part of the cycle, called the follicular phase, is when estrogen is released by the developing follicle (the ovum or egg). The follicular phase also prepares the woman for ovulation, receiving the sperm, and fertilization. Ovulation happens around the 14th

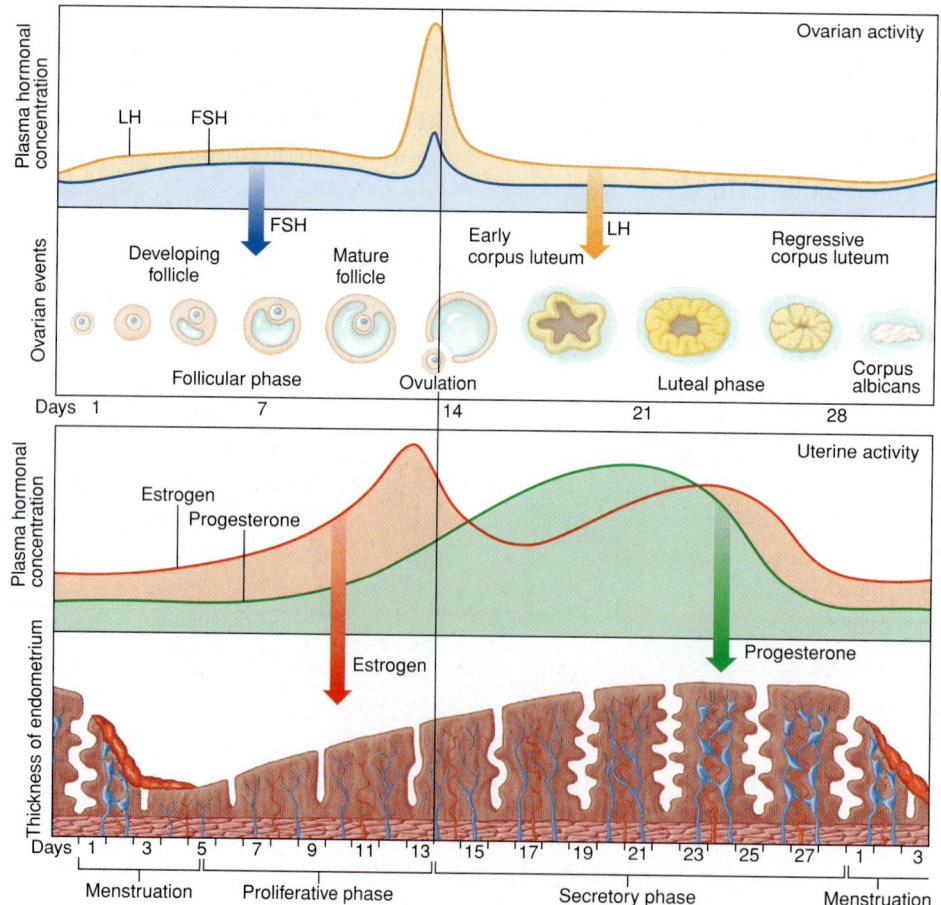

Figure 41-3   Menstrual cyle.

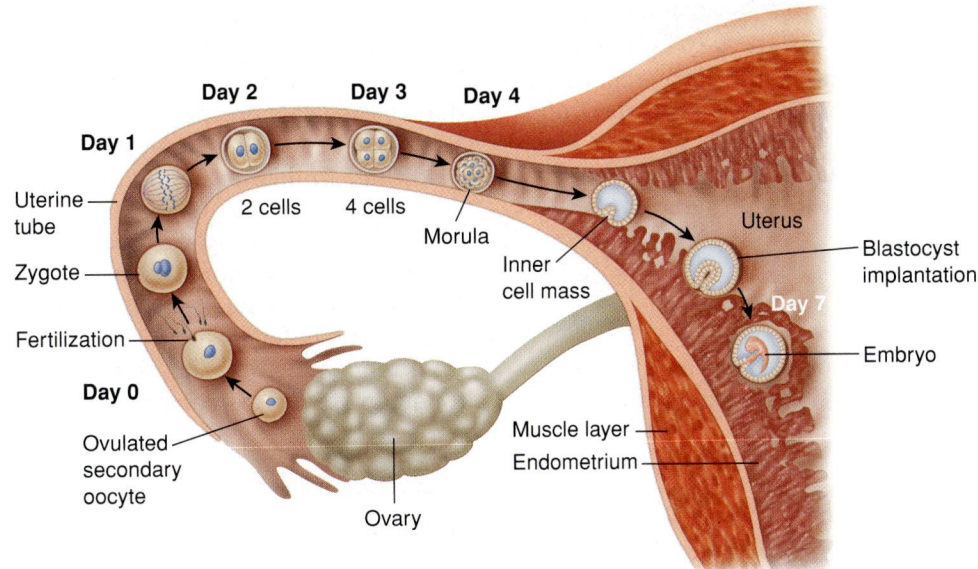

Figure 41-4 Pregnancy begins when an egg joins with a sperm cell. The fertilized egg passes from the fallopian tube into the uterus and implants in the wall of the uterus around day 7.

day after the first day of the menstrual period. Some women who are familiar with their cycles may notice an increase of clear, abundant mucus from the vagina at the time.

The second half of the cycle is called the luteal phase, which is progesterone-dominated and the time in which the body is preparing for pregnancy by promoting implantation and nurturing the conceptus after fertilization. If fertilization does not happen, the cycle ends in menstruation (in lay terminology, a woman's "period"), and the whole cycle begins again. DOT 5-13.2

Pathophysiology of Gynecological Disorders

Infectious Disorders

Infections of the female reproductive tract also include those found in the perineal and pubic regions, as well as internal organs and external genitalia. The most common infection is **candidiasis** or **"yeast."** However, this category of disease includes all nonsexually transmitted infections such as bacterial vaginosis and gardnerella and the sexually transmitted infections such as syphilis, gonorrhea, chlamydia, herpes, condyloma, human papilloma virus (HPV), molluscum contagiosum, and *Trichomonas vaginalis* (which can be nonsexually transmitted, too). The symptoms and treatment vary accordingly, and vaginal infections are the most common reason someone seeks out gynecological care. Common symptoms are pruritus (itching), pain, bleeding, vaginal discharge, and ulcerated lesions.[2]

CONNECTIONS Chapter 33: Infectious and Communicable Diseases covers these infections in more detail.

Pelvic inflammatory disease (PID) is a term used to describe a spectrum of infections in the female upper reproductive tract. It is estimated that 1.5 million cases occur in the United States each year.[3] As many as 25% of cases can result in long-term complications, including infertility, ectopic pregnancy, and chronic pain.[4] PID is caused by an infection that starts most often in the vagina but travels further up into the reproductive tract, involving the fallopian tubes, ovaries, and uterus. The main pathogens are usually *Neisseria gonorrhoeae* or chlamydia, both sexually transmitted and sometimes asymptomatic, which is why the infection goes untreated until it involves the reproductive organs and causes pain and fever. Not all causes of PID are from sexually transmitted infections.[2] Patients may report pelvic pain and discomfort, abdominal tenderness, and possibly signs and symptoms of fever. This disease is notorious for symptoms that can be confused with ectopic pregnancy, appendicitis, gastroenteritis, diverticulitis, and more.

CONNECTIONS To review these conditions, as well as assessment techniques for abdominal pain, see Chapter 34: Gastroenterology.

Specific risk factors for PID include late adolescence, multiple sex partners, frequent douching, recent IUD (intrauterine birth control device) insertion, prior history, and cigarette smoking.[4]

Purulent (foul smelling) vaginal fluid discharge and a history of painful intercourse should strengthen your suspicion of PID. This condition will typically also cause midline, diffuse, and cramping pain that is poorly localized (visceral pain similar to other conditions that stretch hollow organs).

Prehospital treatment is focused on assuring adequate hydration and pain relief, if protocols allow.

Ovarian Cyst

During the normal ovulation cycle, the follicle develops and releases an egg, and then is converted into a corpus luteum. If follicular development is stopped for some reason, the follicle or corpus luteum can become filled with fluid, and an ovarian cyst is formed.[5] If the cyst is formed early, within the first two weeks of the cycle (before ovulation), it is considered to be a follicular cyst (graafian cyst). If the cyst is formed later in the cycle, it is called a luteal cyst.

A ruptured cyst can lead to severe sharp pain and is localized to one side. Approximately 25% of menstruating women will experience this type of ruptured cyst. They are a relatively common finding, and most are benign.[6]

A ruptured ovarian cyst can become complicated by bleeding and may even become a life-threatening emergency.[7]

Increasing use of ultrasound has, not surprisingly, increased the discovery and diagnosis of asymptomatic cysts (adnexal masses).[6] Unilateral pelvic pain is the most common symptom of an enlarging cyst. Rupture may cause instant relief and usually produces no significant sequela.

Prehospital treatment includes careful assessment of vital signs and a high index of suspicion for hidden bleeding as well as the possibility of a missed ectopic pregnancy.

Ovarian Torsion

Cysts may also be complicated by torsion. **Torsion** of the adnexa (fallopian tube, ovary) is most often caused by rotation of the ovary due to cyst formation, resulting in 3% of emergency surgeries in women. About 20% of women diagnosed with torsion are also pregnant. Occasionally, only the fallopian tube is involved in the torsion. The progression of symptoms may be gradual over a number of hours to days. As the torsion twists the fallopian tube tighter, causing increased swelling,

eventually the blood supply is cut off, causing the patient to report a high degree of severe pain. Torsion occurs most often in women of childbearing years but does happen in postmenopausal women and children. Besides pain, patients may present with nausea and vomiting, unilateral abdominal tenderness or rigidity, diarrhea, constipation, dizziness and low-grade fever. A definitive diagnosis can be made with ultrasound imaging or exploratory surgery in the hospital. Women who are on medication to increase ovulation are at increased risk for torsion.[8]

Prehospital care involves monitoring the patient for signs of hidden bleeding as well as shock.

Uterine Conditions

Dysfunctional bleeding is irregular uterine bleeding that is different from the normal menstrual cycle. In this broad category, too little or infrequent menses is also considered "dysfunctional." **Menorrhagia** is a term used to describe a large amount, more than 80 mL, or prolonged, longer than 7 days, of menstrual bleeding. A woman saturating a menstrual pad in one hour or less can be suffering from menorrhagia. Although this guideline is very subjective, it may give you some idea of what to ask the patient. Clinically, lab work that detects anemia is used to diagnose true menorrhagia. The cause of dysfunctional bleeding includes clotting disorders, fibroids, cervical cancer, hormones, and thyroid conditions, among others.[9]

Uterine prolapse is one part of a multi-linked problem also known as pelvic organ relaxation. Uterine prolapse is when the cervix and neck of the uterus are seen in the vaginal canal or extending beyond the vaginal opening. Prolapse can be caused by overstretching or damage to the ligaments, muscles, and organs in the pelvis. Patients report some of the following symptoms: pelvic or vaginal pressure, heaviness in the lower abdomen, backache, and changes in urination or bowel habits. Less commonly, the prolapse happens abruptly after lifting heavy objects.[10] The diagnosis is confirmed by visualization of the uterus at or beyond the vaginal opening.

Conditions of the Vagina and Vulva

Bartholin's Abscess. The Bartholin's glands are really two ducts; their purpose is mucus secretion. These ducts are located at approximately four and eight o'clock on the labia majora; these glands can become obstructed and inflamed, which leads to cyst formation, usually unilateral. Most resolve on their own. On occasion, the cyst becomes infected, causing an abscess and resulting in swelling, extreme localized pain, localized erythema, and sometimes walking difficulties from the swelling and pain.[11]

Foreign Body. Any object that has been inserted into the vagina is considered a foreign body. Objects such as crayons or small toys are frequently found in children. In women, the most common foreign object is an unretrieved tampon. Scene removal of foreign objects is not recommended due to the increased risk of trauma and bleeding.

If a foreign body has been lodged for a longer period of time, a copious, foul-smelling vaginal discharge may be evident. Long-term consequences of untreated foreign body can cause permanent damage to vaginal and anal structures due to erosion of tissue.[11] As in all medical calls, courtesy and kindness to alleviate anxiety for the patient are essential.

Street Secrets

Foreign object placement may *not* have been consensual, and the perpetrator may have become worried enough to call for help. Do not make any assumptions, find a way to speak to the patient away from bystanders or family members to determine the circumstances of the foreign body placement, and ask her if she feels safe in her relationship. DOT 5-13.4, 5-13.5, 5-13.6

Primary Survey

The initial assessment of a female patient with abdominal pain, vaginal fluid, or bloody discharge should include a standard evaluation of the patient's airway and breathing. If these are compromised, the primary survey should be interrupted, and oxygenation and ventilation should be immediately treated, as noted in earlier chapters.

Evaluation of the circulatory status of your patient is essential and should be performed as part of the primary survey. Severe bleeding in the abdomen may not be immediately apparent or detectable and may be life-threatening. A weak and rapid pulse, along with other signs of shock, should alert you to the possibility of major blood loss.

If bleeding is severe or uncontrolled, you should consider the patient's condition to be sick and expedite transport. Treat blood loss according to standard protocols discussed in previous trauma, shock, and resuscitation chapters.

The evaluation of external bleeding in the vaginal area should be handled with as much privacy as possible, without compromising patient care. If vaginal bleeding is severe and there is trauma to the external genital area, direct pressure should be applied. If direct pressure does not control the bleeding and you suspect the bleeding is originating from an internal source, do not pack the vaginal area with gauze. Simply apply a trauma dressing to the external vaginal area, and focus on rapid transportation as well as fluid resuscitation for patients who are hemodynamically compromised (blood pressure below 90 mmHg).[4]

Table 41-1 summarizes causes of pelvic pain. **Skill Sheet 36: Abdominal Assessment includes assessment of the female patient with abdominal pain.**

Street Secrets

If the patient complains of a sudden onset of severe abdominal pain, you should suspect a life-threatening condition, such as organ rupture, and expedite transport. Though gradual onset of pain may also be life-threatening, acute obstruction, ischemia, and perforation of an organ are more commonly associated with a rapid onset of pain.[4]

The Pregnant Patient

Pregnancy

Normal pregnancy is defined as lasting from the first day of the last normal menstrual period (LNMP) until the start of labor that brings forth the baby. Pregnancy is also called the antepartal period or antepartum. Pregnancy normally lasts about 40 weeks or 280 days from the LNMP if a woman has an average 28-day menstrual cycle. Pregnancy duration is also approximately 38 weeks from known conception date. Pregnancy that ends with labor anytime between 37 and 42 weeks is considered normal and called a term pregnancy. While many women comment on how many months pregnant they are, it is more exact to date pregnancy by weeks. Pregnancy is divided into three trimesters.

First Trimester—Weeks 1 to 12 (Months One to Three)

During this time, the uterus grows and is contained inside the pelvic cavity. During this period of development, the fetus is most vulnerable to exposures to teratogens (a substance, medication, organism, or physical agent capable of causing abnormal fetal development).[12] The heart begins to beat at about six weeks after the LNMP but will not be detectable until about 10 to 12 weeks with an ultrasound device. Some 50–80% of women experience nausea and vomiting sometime after six weeks that usually lasts until about 13 weeks although it can continue throughout the pregnancy.[13]

Other normal signs of early pregnancy are cessation of menses (menstrual bleeding), breast tenderness, frequent urination, and fatigue.[14] The baby is active, moving around in its amniotic sac that is filled with fluid, but the mother will not be able to feel the movements

TABLE 41-1 Differentiation of Common or Potentially Catastrophic Causes of Pelvic Pain

	Pain history	Associated symptoms	Supporting history	Prevalence in ED	Physical examination	Useful tests	Atypical or additional aspects
Ovarian torsion	Acute onset of moderately severe lateral pain	Nausea and vomiting	History of ovarian mass	Uncommon	Adnexal tenderness, possible peritonitis, (+) cervical motion tenderness (CMT), adnexal mass	Ultrasound with Doppler flow studies, laparoscopy	Torsion can be intermittent
Appendicitis	Duration often less than 48 hours. Generalized followed by localized in RLQ	Low-grade fever, nausea, anorexia	Abdominal pain before vomiting, anorexia, migration of pain to RLQ	Common	RLQ tenderness with or without peritoneal signs	WBC often elevated, ultrasound or CT in equivocal cases	Early in course tenderness may be minimal or poorly localized
Ectopic pregnancy	Classically severe, sharp, lateral pelvic pain, but both severity location and quality often variable	Vaginal bleeding common	Missed period; history of previous ectopic, infertility, tubal ligation, or IUD use	Common	Very variable, classically lateral adnexal tenderness, (+) CMT, adnexal mass	Pelvic ultrasound, quantitative β-hCG, progesterone, laparoscopy	Cannot reliably exclude diagnosis based on history and physical; severe pain, hypotension, or peritonitis suggest rupture
PID/tubo-ovarian abscess (TOA)	Without TOA, pain usually bilateral. May present acutely within 48 hr or have more subacute presentation 1–2 wk of pain.	Fever, vaginal discharge	Vaginal discharge, prior history of PID, lack of nausea vomiting or anorexia	Common	Pus from cervical os, (+) CMT. If peritonitis present, usually bilateral adnexal mass with TOA	CBC, ESR, pelvic ultrasound, laparoscopy, cervical cultures, cervical smear looking for WBC	History and physical alone inaccurate, particularly in patients presenting subacutely
Ruptured corpus luteal cyst	Abrupt moderately severe lateral pain	Light-headedness if bleeding is severe; rectal pain from fluid in cul-de-sac		Uncommon	Hypotension and tachycardia if blood loss is significant, possible peritonitis	Pelvic ultrasound, CBC	Physical exam findings often do not correlate with volume of blood in pelvis at ultrasound

TABLE 41-1   *(continued)*

	Pain history	Associated symptoms	Supporting history	Prevalence in ED	Physical examination	Useful tests	Atypical or additional aspects
Nonruptured ovarian cyst or tumor	Lateral ache, gradual onset	Often minimal	Prior history similar pain	Common	Lateral pelvic tenderness, with or without a mass, (+) CMT	Pelvic ultrasound, CBC	
UTI	Pain with urination, usually not severe unless has flank pain from associated pyelonephritis	Urinary urgency and frequency; fever and vomiting if has associated pyelonephritis	Recent urologic procedure, prior history UTI	Common	Suprapubic tenderness, flank tenderness and fever with pyelonephritis	Urinalysis, urine culture	WBC can be present in urine with PID and appendicitis
Endometriosis	Unilateral or bilateral pelvic pain, often recurrent	Dysmenorrhea, dyspareunia	Prior history of same type of pain in association with the menstrual cycle	Common	Unilateral or bilateral adnexal tenderness, occasionally pelvic mass present, peritoneal findings uncommon	Pelvic ultrasound, laparoscopy	Symptoms can mimic other types of pelvic pathology, laparoscopy often needed for confirmation
Ureteral colic	Acute onset presents within hours, pain is lateral usually, moderate to severe, often radiates into the groin	Nausea and vomiting	Prior history of stones	Common	Patient often appears very uncomfortable, but PE can be otherwise unremarkable	Urinalysis hematuria present in about 90% of cases, abdominal CT	If stone is at junction of ureter and bladder, can have very localized tenderness that can mimic appendicitis or other acute pelvic pathology

CMT, Cervical motion tenderness; *RLQ,* right lower quadrant; *WBC,* white blood cell count; *CT,* computed tomography; *IUD,* intrauterine device; *β-hCG,* β-human chorionic gonadotropin; *TOA,* tubo-ovarian abscess; *PID,* pelvic inflammatory disease; *CBC,* complete blood count; *ESR,* erythrocyte sedimentation rate; *UTI,* Urinary tract infection.

until the second trimester. A pregnancy test can show positive results within a week of a missed period.[14] Ideally, in this first part of the pregnancy, a woman will seek prenatal care, which includes routine lab testing, determination of a due date, nutritional and lifestyle assessment, and evaluation of potential risk factors.[13]

Second Trimester—Weeks 13 to 27 (Months Four to Six)

Most women feel a renewed sense of energy at this point. Some of the minor discomforts of the first trimester have abated, and their pregnant abdomen is not so large as to interfere with activities. Prenatal care continues on a monthly basis, with some additional lab testing to rule out certain congenital anomalies (for example, trisomy 21 or spina bifida). The uterus now has grown to make it palpable above the symphysis pubis (pubic bone), and the woman starts to look pregnant. The uterus grows to the height of the mother's umbilicus by 20 weeks. From 20 to 36 weeks, the fundal height of the uterus corresponds with the weeks of gestation, plus or minus 2 cm.[13] When the woman is about 24 weeks pregnant, other people besides the mother can feel fetal movement through her abdomen, and by 26 weeks, the movement can be identifiable enough to guess if a movement was the head or a foot. Prenatal care is offered monthly for women at this point.

Third Trimester—Weeks 28 to 40 (Months Seven to Nine)

The uterus enlarges 10 to 20 times its prepregnant size over the course of 40 weeks, and by the start of the third trimester, the uterus reaches about halfway between the umbilicus and the xiphoid process. After 36 weeks' gestation, the uterus and abdomen fall slightly forward as the baby moves down into the pelvis, referred to as, "the baby has dropped." By the third trimester, some of the early pregnancy discomforts have returned such as frequent urination and fatigue. All babies born after 28 weeks' gestation have a good survival rate and, depending on their prematurity, may or may not need hospitalization.[15]

Women look for signs of impending labor, but its actual signal is still not completely understood. Losing the mucous plug, which is thickened cervical mucus in the cervical os, is a good sign that hormonal changes are happening. Many women have experienced warm-up uterine contractions, some as early as the second trimester; these are called **Braxton Hicks contractions.** It is common for women to have false labor pains, which are not "false," just not the kind of uterine activity that is going to bring forth the baby. Many healthy women who have enjoyed their pregnancies begin to feel a shift, and giving birth becomes preferred over continuing to be pregnant. For those getting regular prenatal care, they will be seen every other week starting at 28 weeks and then weekly from 36 weeks until birth.[13] At term, most women have a typical weight gain of 30 pounds, and the average baby will weigh between 7 and 8 pounds (Figure 41-5). DOT 5-14.1, 5-14.2

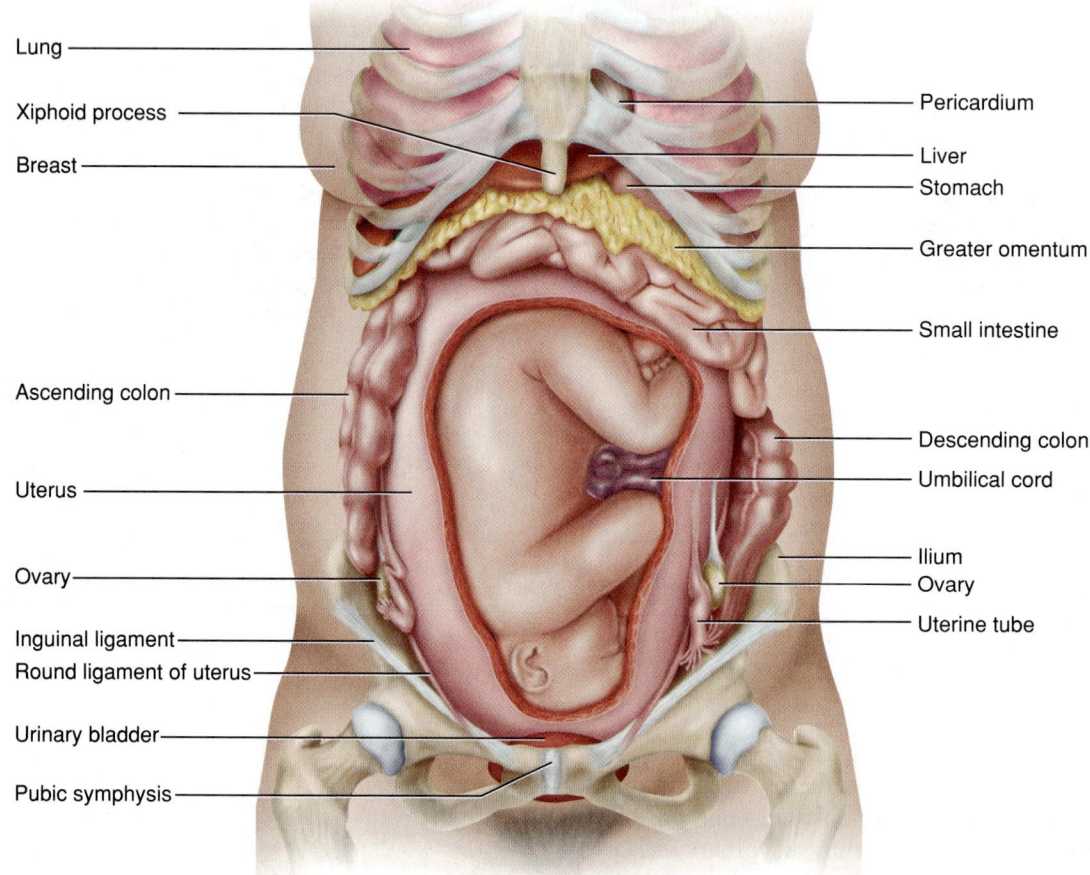

Figure 41-5   At term, the average fetus weighs 7 to 8 pounds, and the average woman has gained 30 pounds.

Complications of Pregnancy

In the U.S. the most frequent causes of pregnancy-related problems are spontaneous abortion, ectopic pregnancy, premature labor, hemorrhage, blood clots, high blood pressure or preeclampsia, infection, stroke, amniotic fluid embolism, diabetes, and heart disease.[16] Many problems are preventable, and others will have less harmful effects if preventative measures are taken.

Hemorrhage, ectopic pregnancy, and preeclampsia cause 59% of all maternal deaths in America.[17]

African American women die of pregnancy-related complications at a rate three times higher than their white counterparts (22 per 100,000 live births versus 7.5 per 100,000).[18] Pregnant Hispanic women and women of any race over 35 years of age double their risks of morbidity and mortality. Complications attributed to race are, in fact, related to psychosocial and economic issues including poverty, lack of insurance, poor nutrition, working or living in unsafe environments, and receiving medical services by staff that is insufficiently trained.[19] A woman in North America has a 1 in 3,700 chance of dying related to pregnancy and childbirth.[20]

Street Secrets

When assessing a patient who is pregnant, determining the age of the gestation (the duration of the pregnancy) may be very helpful in the creation of differential diagnoses. To help you more easily transfer the knowledge from this chapter into practical assessment and field application, the complications that follow are listed in the timeline (trimester) where they are most likely to occur.

First Trimester Bleeding and Abdominal Pain

Ectopic Pregnancy

The definition of the word *ectopic* is simply "away from normal position". An **ectopic pregnancy** simply means that a fertilized egg has implanted somewhere outside its normal position in the uterus. Ninety-eight percent of the incorrect implantations occur in the fallopian tube (Figure 41-6); however, implantation can happen on the ovary, cervix, and on abdominal organs.[13]

Implantations in locations other than the uterus rarely go to term and most often result in rupture of the structure unless diagnosed early enough. Ectopic pregnancy has a maternal death rate of about 10%.[21]

Repeated episodes of pelvic inflammatory disease (PID) as well as other illnesses and injuries that produce scarring in the fallopian tubes may cause blockage and prevent the fertilized egg from entering the uterus. If your patient has a history of PID, ovarian cysts, or previous ectopic pregnancies, their risk of an ectopic pregnancy rises significantly.[4,21]

Due to the catastrophic nature of, and possibly preventable death from, a ruptured ectopic pregnancy, any female patient of potentially childbearing age (ages nine to 60) complaining of abdominal pain should be presumed to have an ectopic pregnancy until proven otherwise.

Most often, patients will report vaginal spotting or bleeding sometimes thought to be just an unusual period.[13] Abdominal or pelvic pain can have a gradual onset, then rapidly escalate. Abdominal pain is reported in greater than 90% of ectopic pregnancies. A palpable mass is only identified in half of ectopic pregnancies.[21]

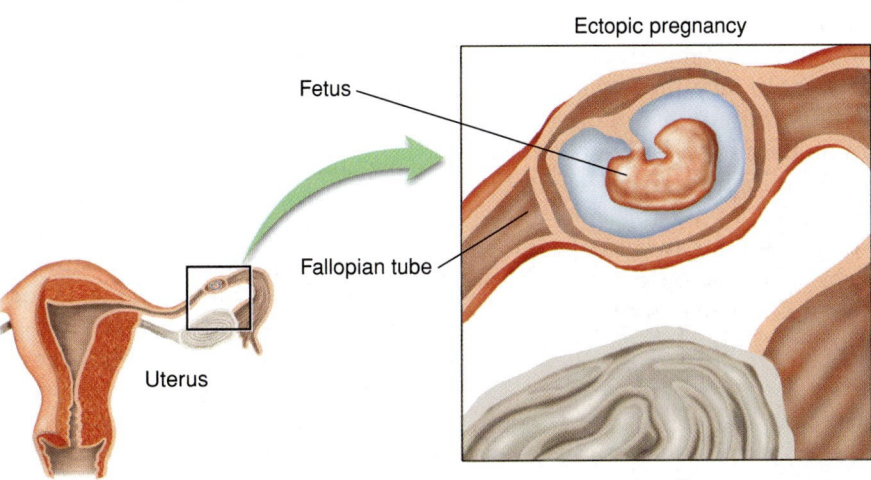

Figure 41-6 Ectopic pregnancy; the fertilized egg has implanted and is growing in the fallopian tube.

Ectopic pregnancy is usually diagnosed in the first trimester, often before six weeks gestation, as the fallopian tube cannot accommodate the growing conceptus.[13] One of the reasons ectopic pregnancies are so dangerous is that some women do not realize they are pregnant and may dismiss symptoms, such as abdominal pain, assuming these are due to menstrual cramps or even food poisoning.

Ideally, ectopic pregnancy is diagnosed before the growing conceptus causes tubal rupture and hypotension occurs.

Street Secrets

Some ectopic pregnancies may produce referred pain into the shoulder due to diaphragmatic irritation from blood that has spilled into the abdomen.[4]

Prehospital assessment and treatment for a suspected ectopic pregnancy are focused on early recognition and a high index of suspicion.

Determining the last normal menstrual period (LNMP) may help to narrow your list of differentials. If the patient believes she could possibly be pregnant, attempt to determine how many weeks.

A thorough medical history, especially if it includes risk factors such as pelvic inflammatory disease, previous ectopic pregnancy, ovarian cysts, endometriosis, or abortion, will help narrow the list of differentials, as well.

As was mentioned earlier, abdominal pain in a female of childbearing age should be considered to be a possible ectopic pregnancy. In similar fashion, unexplained hypotension and severe abdominal pain in a female of childbearing years should also be considered a ruptured ectopic pregnancy until proven otherwise in the emergency department. The onset of symptoms is often sudden and unexpected.

During the physical exam, gently palpate all four quadrants of the abdomen to determine tenderness or rigidity. Note the location and character. If the patient is bleeding, you should attempt to determine the quantity and duration. Although inaccurate, estimating blood loss from the number of menstrual pads that have been saturated may give the receiving caregivers a frame of reference.

Rapidly transport these patients to an appropriate facility. As with other shock states, fluid resuscitation with intravenous fluids should focus on maintaining a blood pressure of 90 mmHg systolic.

Abortion

Spontaneous abortion (SAB) is more commonly known as a **miscarriage.** One in four pregnancies ends in a miscarriage, defined as pregnancy loss occurring before 20 weeks gestation.[13] About 80% of miscarriages happen in the first trimester of pregnancy, at less than 12 weeks gestation.[13] The causes of miscarriage are multifactorial, but chromosomal abnormality is a likely explanation for a great percentage, especially those that terminate before eight weeks of completed pregnancy.[12] Patients will most often present with abdominal cramping, lower backache, and vaginal bleeding. Some women will report decreased symptoms of pregnancy. A patient may report the passage of clots, fetal or placental tissue, or other products of conception prior to notification of EMS. Whenever possible, save what has been passed, and transport such products with the mother to the hospital for evaluation as determination of whether the miscarriage is "complete" or that only parts of the developing fetus (called the conceptus) have passed will be helpful for an accurate assessment for the mother.

Not all bleeding results in the termination of a pregnancy. Some patients with bleeding during pregnancy are diagnosed with a "threatened abortion," meaning that they may lose the pregnancy, but have not yet. However, in many cases they are able to carry the pregnancy to term without further complications.

Therapeutic abortion (TAB) is defined as the deliberate termination of pregnancy before 24 weeks gestation.[22] Beyond 24 weeks, abortion is not legal in the United States unless it is to save the life of the mother. Maternal morbidity is lowest if the procedure is done before the mother is eight weeks gestation, and the leading cause of maternal death related to TAB is from general anesthesia.[6] Worldwide, illegal abortion is the fourth leading cause of maternal morbidity and mortality.[20] Legal abortion as performed in the U.S. is relatively safe and is accomplished using a variety of methods. The method selected is based on how far along the pregnancy has progressed.[20]

High-Risk Pregnancy

A pregnancy is considered "high-risk" when certain predisposing factors or complications have a likelihood to jeopardize the pregnancy. Certain lifestyle and environmental factors such as alcohol abuse, substance abuse, cigarette smoking, and exposure to toxic chemicals increase a woman's risk for complications in pregnancy and birth. Chronic illnesses such as diabetes, heart disease, cancer, or other medical history may require special monitoring. In addition to preexisting conditions, the mother may develop gestational diabetes, hypertension, or hypotension, which also categorizes the pregnancy as high-risk. Women who are older or pregnancies where the infant has been determined to have a congenital defect are also considered high-risk.[23]

Poor nutritional status and certain psychosocial factors are known to contribute to increased potential

OB/GYN Assessment Continuum
Consider OB/GYN problems in any female ages 9–60

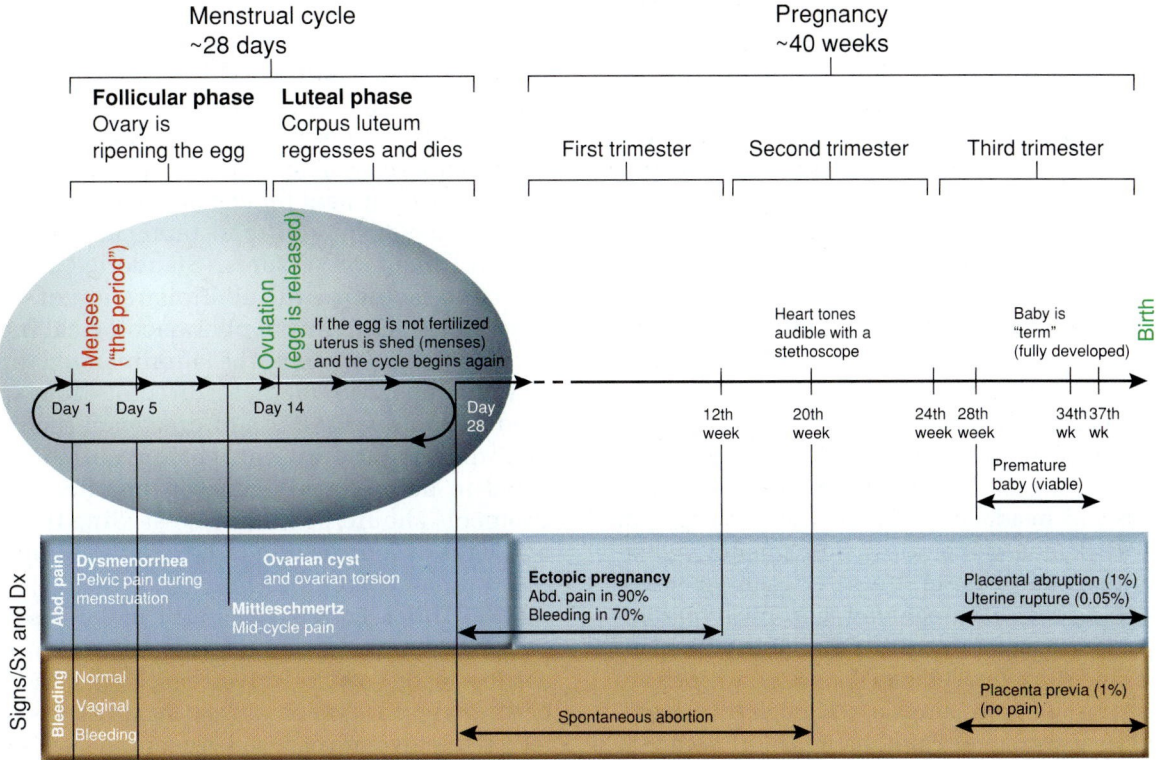

Figure 41-7   The OB/GYN assessment continuum.

Second Trimester

Pregnancy-Induced Hypertension (PIH), Preeclampsia, and Eclampsia

for problems. Risk assessment is an ongoing, dynamic process.[13] As a paramedic, you should be aware of the risk factors that make a pregnancy more dangerous than others. This is especially helpful if you are called to assess a patient who is in labor but may not have regularly visited her physician. If the patient's pregnancy is considered high-risk, referral and evaluation in a specialized hospital may be appropriate. You should consult your local protocols to discover what your medical director and local EMS system recommend.

Figure 41-7 is helpful in visualizing a timeline for the various stages of pregnancy and the possible complications that may occur.

High blood pressure is the most commonly identified risk factor during pregnancy and complicates 10% of all pregnancies or 13.2 million births a year; the association between hypertension and other pregnancy complications for mother and baby has been identified in several studies.[14]

Pregnancy-induced hypertension (PIH) is classically defined as blood pressure greater than 140/90 diagnosed on two or more occasions at least six hours apart. Some women enter pregnancy with a diagnosis of chronic hypertension while others develop the condition during pregnancy.

Street Secrets

Many healthy young women have normally low blood pressure such as 90/60. A second definition of pregnancy-induced hypertension (PIH), is more relative and is based on the patient's normal blood pressure. PIH in this case is determined after 20 weeks gestation and is defined as a systolic BP more than 30 mmHg over the woman's baseline and diastolic BP more than 15 mmHg over the base.[13]

If PIH is accompanied by edema or an increased excretion of proteins in the urine (proteinuria), it is defined as **preeclampsia** (also known as **toxemia**). The exact pathophysiology of PIH and preeclampsia remains unknown.[24] One theory is that dysfunction in the placenta causes a systemic spasm of the vascular system (vasospasm). This spasm, if severe, may lead to reduced blood flow to various organs and may result in damage to maternal organs. There is also a risk of thrombosis or embolism. The disorder affects all organs, including renal and liver functions, and causes protein excretion in the urine. Thrombocytopenia (abnormal decrease of platelets in blood) and ultimately neurological dysfunction may also occur.[13]

The term **eclampsia** is reserved for patients who have severe preeclampsia and are actively seizing or in a coma. The seizure activity is thought to be caused by hypertensive encephalopathy (swelling inside the brain due to high blood pressure).[24]

Preeclampsia is responsible for 15% of premature births, and 12.4% of infants born to mothers who have had preeclampsia will die within their first month of life.[25]

Preeclampsia is a disorder that only happens during pregnancy *and* postpartum. Elevated blood pressure, increase of swelling or a sudden weight gain, visual disturbances, and headaches may be the first signs or symptoms.[25] Risk factors include first pregnancy, maternal age less than 18 years and greater than 35 years, history of PIH in previous pregnancy, chronic hypertension or renal disease, multiple pregnancy, insulin-dependence, and diabetes. African American women are at an increased risk of preeclampsia.[25] Though preeclampsia can occur in any pregnant mother, it is more common in patients under the age of 20 years.[24]

PIH and preeclampsia are closely related, and medical diagnosis and management are essential to decrease the potential poor outcomes. Preeclampsia and eclampsia can cause placental abruption; hemorrhage; kidney, liver,

heart, brain, ocular, and lung damage and failure; stroke; blindness; paralysis; seizures; and death.[25]

Prehospital care for preeclampsia includes securing an IV line, monitoring the ECG, and administering oxygen. The patient should be transported in the left lateral position (Figure 41-8).[24]

If the pregnant patient is seizing, eclampsia should be considered as one of the primary differentials. Definitive treatment for eclampsia is the delivery of the fetus in the hospital. Prehospital care revolves around the treatment of seizures. Standard care for seizing patients, including the administration of diazepam or midazolam, is an initial pharmacological intervention. Since midazolam may be administered intramuscularly, some EMS medical directors may prefer this medication over the use of diazepam that requires an IV. Administration of magnesium sulfate is also indicated to help control some of the effects of toxemia. Protocols should be in place regarding the indications and dose of magnesium to be used. DOT 5-14.7

CONNECTIONS For a more in-depth review of seizures visit Chapter 30: Neurology. Also, you should be familiar with the antidote for any medication you are giving. In this case benzodiazepines—diazepam and midazolam—can be reversed with romazicon, and hypermagnesemia may be reversed with calcium gluconate; reviewing these and other medications is essential and should be done with a resource that is regularly updated. To review general pharmacology and the role of antidotes see Chapter 15: Pharmacology.

Third Trimester Bleeding and Pain

Abruptio Placenta

Abruptio placenta is more commonly called **placental abruption.** It happens when the placenta abnormally separates from the uterine wall before the birth of the baby. It can be partial or total. Placental abruption causes 30% of all reported antepartum bleeding.[10] Bleeding always occurs between the placenta and uterine wall with varying degrees of consequence to the mother and fetus. Fifty percent of abruptions happen after 30 weeks gestation, which is during the third trimester, and only 15% happen during actual labor and birth.[10]

The causes of abruption are not known; however, certain conditions and situations are highly suspect, and the most common link is maternal hypertension (defined as maternal blood pressure greater than 140/90).[26] Sometimes, abruption is diagnosed after the birth, when examination of the placenta reveals retroplacental clots on the maternal side of the placenta. This is another reason for bringing not only the mother and newborn to the hospital after an out-of-hospital delivery but also all other tissue such as the placenta that has passed. A large portion of the placenta separating from

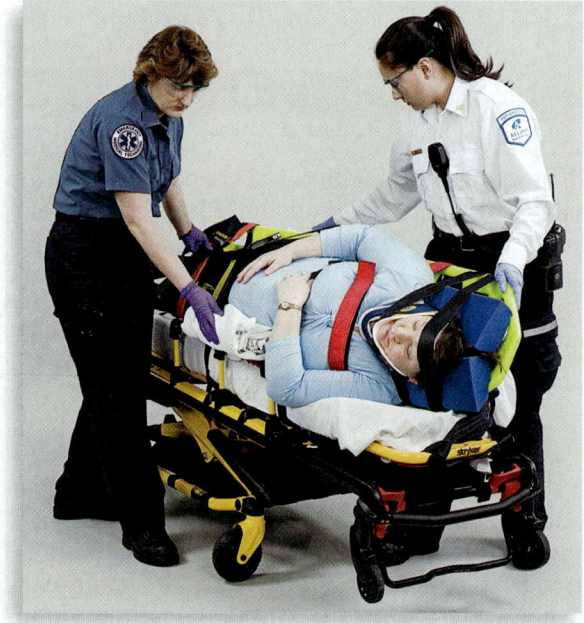

Figure 41-8 Pregnant women should be immobilized on a longboard tilted slightly to the left to relieve pressure on the inferior vena cava by the gravid uterus.

the uterine wall can cause premature birth, hypovolemic shock, disseminated intravascular coagulation disorder (DIC), and fetal compromise. Although you should be alert to hidden bleeding (20% of cases), 80% of abruptions will present with vaginal bleeding.[13] Maternal mortality varies from 0.5% to 5%, and fetal mortality occurs in about 35% of abruptions.[21]

> The combination of pregnancy beyond the first trimester, a firm uterus, and severe pain with or without apparent vaginal bleeding should make you think of placental abruption.

Other helpful assessment clues you will want to know follow:

- Has the mother been receiving routine prenatal care?
- Is there vaginal bleeding (present 80% of the time)?
- Abdominal tenderness or abdominal rigidity?
- Any substance use or abuse or any recent injury or trauma?
- Is the mother noticing uterine irritability (irregular uterine tightening)?

The mother may report that the baby was overly active and then became quiet prior to this episode.

Placental abruption is a life-threatening condition for both the mother and the baby. Your care should focus on rapid transportation. En route, establish IV therapy and guard against maternal hypotension.

Placenta Previa

Placenta previa occurs when the placenta implants over the cervical os (or internal opening of the cervix) connecting to the uterus. The condition accounts for 20% of bleeding episodes in the third trimester but usually resolves itself by the time of delivery.[27] Placenta previa at term is rare, occurring in 0.5% of pregnancies.[28] Placenta previa can be categorized into two different types: complete or partial (Figure 41-9). Complete placenta previa

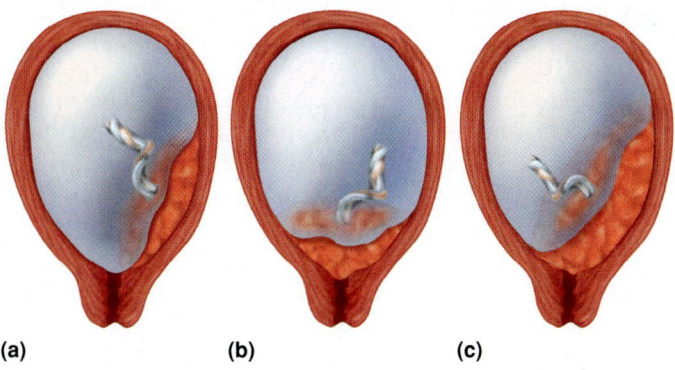

Figure 41-9 Placenta previa. (a) Low-lying previa. (b) Complete previa. (c) Marginal previa.

is the most life-threatening of the variations. In these cases, the placenta completely covers the cervical os. If the placenta is stretched (when there is cervical dilation such as will occur with labor) or the patient is examined by a healthcare practitioner who accidentally perforates the placenta, severe bleeding may occur. Patients with this condition require rapid surgical intervention.

Partial or marginal placenta previa occurs when only a portion of the placenta covers the cervical os or when the placenta just borders the os.

Shock and fetal death are due to the disruption of the oxygen supply to the baby via the placenta. Premature delivery accounts for 60% of fetal deaths. Early detection is the key to successfully managing this condition; in the hospital or clinic an ultrasound can accurately diagnose this condition about 95% of the time.[13]

Many undiagnosed previas are discovered when a woman seeks medical care for a bleeding episode, usually occurring during the second or third trimester. Bleeding associated with a placenta previa is usually bright red with *no pain*.

Street Secrets

To differentiate placenta previa from placental abruption, it is helpful keep in mind that *p*revia is usually *p*ainless, and *a*bruptio includes *a*cute pain 90% of the time.[13]

With complete placenta previa, cesarean birth is the only safe way to deliver the baby. With partial and marginal previas, vaginal deliveries may be allowed, depending on the circumstances associated with the labor and medical personnel on hand. Low-lying placenta, where the placenta has imbedded in the uterus near the cervix, is not to be confused with the variations of previa.

On occasion, placenta previa is complicated by not only location of implantation but also the depth of the implantation in the uterus. Placenta accreta, increta, and percreta are when the placental implantation has an abnormal invasion into the uterine wall. When one of these abnormal implantations has occurred, the placenta will not separate normally from the uterus. Two-thirds of women who have combined placenta previa and accreta end up with a hysterectomy as a last resort to deal with the ongoing hemorrhage that accompanies this condition.[28]

As a general rule, paramedics do not typically perform vaginal exams, which can be particularly dangerous in the case of placenta previa. A healthcare practitioner's digital exam can cause a catastrophic bleed.

It is important to determine the following:

- Whether the patient has previously had any spotting or bleeding in this current pregnancy.
- How far along the pregnancy is (measured in weeks and is usually second or third trimester or 24 to 40 weeks).
- Whether the patient has been seen for routine prenatal care.

Assess vitals. Assess vaginal bleeding, which is usually painless and bright red. No masses or tenderness will be palpated, but EMS providers will feel the abdomen to rule out other possible diagnoses. Start an IV, and transport to a medical facility.

Hyperemesis Gravidarum

Hyperemesis gravidarum is nausea and vomiting in pregnancy that lasts excessively long, sometimes throughout the entire pregnancy, or is severely pronounced and interferes with normal daily functioning.[14] The cause has not been determined, but continuation of elevated hormonal levels for pregnancy and psychological factors are implicated.[14] The effects can be profuse vomiting, poor or no appetite, and inability to keep food down so that nutritional intake suffers. The vomiting can cause dehydration and electrolyte imbalances with further chemical disturbances; this is considered a pathological situation for which medical treatment should be sought.[14]

Prehospital assessment of the patient's hydration and vital signs are helpful in guiding care. A dehydrated mother may have severe electrolyte imbalances that can put both her and the baby at risk. You should monitor the patient's ECG for irregularities due to conduction disturbances and dehydration. Establish an IV, and administer a fluid bolus if signs of dehydration or hypovolemia are present.

Normal Labor and Out-of-Hospital Birth

Although the thought of out-of-hospital (OOH) emergency childbirth may seem overwhelming and dangerous to a novice EMS provider, in fact, birthing complications are very rare. In much of the world, childbirth is accomplished without any medical provider present.[29] Normal labor and delivery is divided into three stages as outlined below and as illustrated by the birth shown in Figure 41-10.

First Stage of Labor

The early part of the **first stage of labor** is sometimes difficult to distinguish from the uterine tightening called Braxton Hicks contractions the mother may have felt during her pregnancy. Braxton Hicks contractions are a labor "practice," and help tone the muscles around the uterus for the day of delivery. Contractions associated with true labor may start slowly or may come on quickly. The difference between warm-up contractions and real labor is that, eventually, real labor contractions become increasingly more frequent and more intense and lead to delivery (Box 41-1).

The mother may notice that she has "lost her plug" or may see signs called "bloody show," both of which mean the mucous plug inside the cervix that protects the uterine contents has now come out, usually with pink or blood-tinged fluid or mucus. Likewise, the **amniotic sac** (commonly known as the **bag of waters**) may or may not break in the first stage of labor. A patient's water may break at any time, but it is more likely to happen during active labor, even more often with pushing during the second stage of labor. The first stage can take hours as the cervix needs to dilate in order for the baby to move from the uterus down into the birth canal.

Progress in labor is determined by paying attention to the mother's contraction pattern, breathing, and overall affect. There are many nonverbal cues as to birthing progress, and a wise paramedic can become very skillful at knowing where a woman is in the labor process. At this stage of labor, only healthcare practitioners trained in obstetrics should check the cervix for dilation. Cervical checks are uncomfortable for the woman, and the potential to introduce pathogens into the vagina increases with each exam.

During the first stage of labor, the mother's cervix progresses from 0 to 10 cm dilated. In addition, the first stage is usually divided further into two parts: **early labor,** approximately 0 to 4 cm cervical dilation, and **active labor,** which is 4 to 10 cm dilation.

When contractions are at least five minutes apart, lasting one minute, for one whole hour, you can assume that the mother has now started the active phase of labor and is probably between 4 and 5 cm dilated. This is normally when a patient should go to the hospital if the birth has been planned for the hospital.

BOX 41-1 Timing Contractions

How to time labor contraction: "How far apart" or frequency of contractions is measured by noting the time at the *beginning* of one contraction and then noting the time at the *beginning* of the next contraction; this will be stated in minutes. How long the contraction lasts is counted by observing the time at the start of a single contraction and the time when it ends. This time is usually counted in seconds, but when labor is intense and very active contractions lasting 90 to 120 seconds are common.

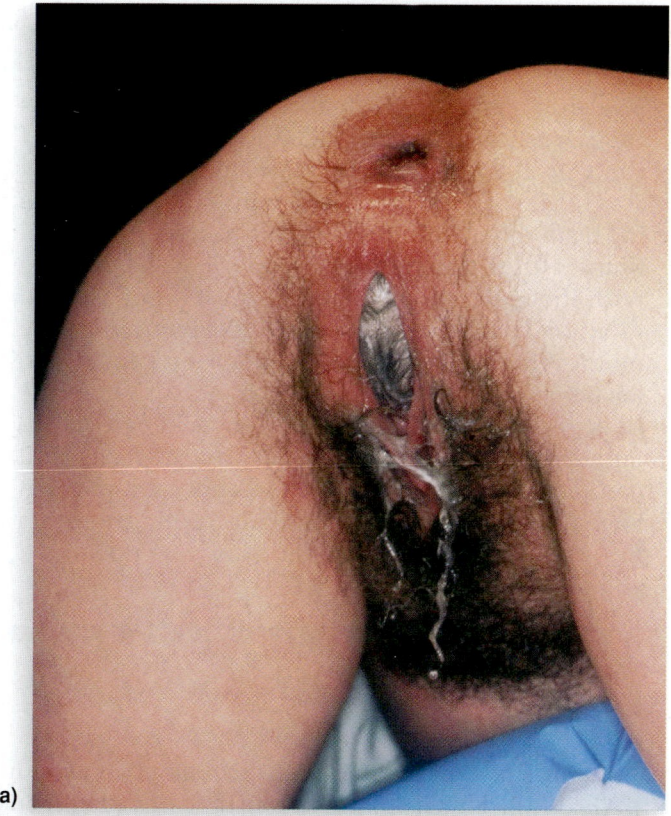

(a)

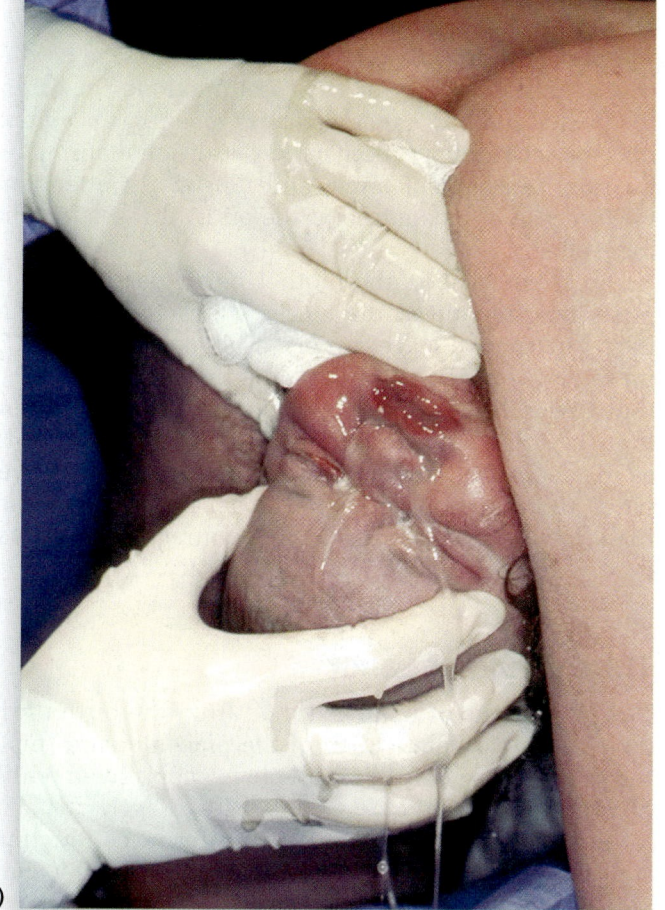

(b)

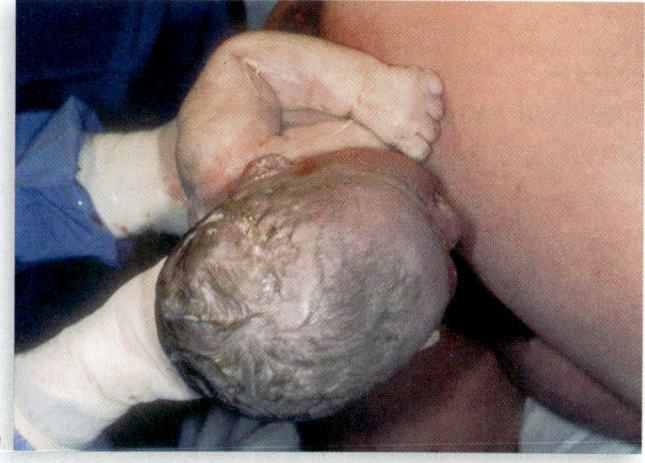

(c)

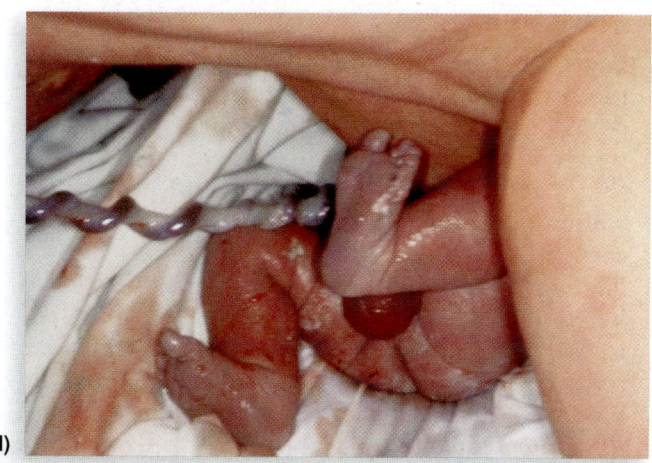

(d)

Figure 41-10   (a) "Crowning" of the fetus's head indicates that delivery is imminent (*Note:* mother is in a kneeling position). (b) Delivery of the head. (c) Delivery of the shoulders and chest. (d) Footling breach delivery.

By this point, the contraction pattern has a definite beginning, middle (peak of intensity), and end. As the active first stage progresses, the mother will need to focus on her contractions; she will talk less and may find her companions less amusing. As your patient works harder and harder with each contraction, she will get hot and may sweat. If you are working in a rural setting or transport is delayed, your patient should be reminded to continue emptying her bladder. As the mother approaches 8 cm dilation, she will be breathing more rapidly and may moan with her contractions. Contractions will last anywhere between 40 to 60 seconds in length. She may need to vomit, and the amount of discomfort will be peaking; this is called the **transition phase of labor,** going from 8 to 10 cm dilated. In a planned hospital birth, if the mom has missed other clues, it is time to get to the hospital.

Cervical Exam

While it is unlikely that you will be trained to perform a cervical check, knowing what this check entails and the results that may be reported to you by another healthcare provider will help you understand how far along your patient is in the birthing process. It is common for paramedics to transfer high-risk patients to a specialty center. An obstetrical nurse report should contain information about the cervical checks that have been performed so far.

Three things are checked in a cervical exam: effacement, station, and dilation. **Effacement** of the cervix is the thinning and stretching of the cervix. It is monitored by digital exam, and the number given is in percentage, with 100% being the thinnest the cervix can get. A long, thick, closed cervix is going to take longer to efface than one that has thinned out before labor has started.

A skilled birth attendant will also check the **station** of the baby to determine whether it has descended into the pelvis. Using the ischial spine as a landmark, the examiner scissors her fingers to feel where the head is in relationship to the spine. The ischial spines are considered 0 station. If the top of the baby's head is above the spine, it is noted in minus numbers; −2 means the baby is about 2 cm above the spine. When the top of the baby's head has moved past the spine, the station is then called "plus," with +3 being a particularly optimistic sign.

The **dilation of the cervix** means that the cervix changes from being closed to its widest, 10 cm; at that point, the woman is called "complete." Checking for dilation is done by using the two fingers of one hand in a scissor motion. The attendant determines how wide apart her fingers can reach from one side of the cervix to the other, with one finger roughly equivalent to 0.5–1.0 centimeter. Due to the wide variety of hands and finger sizes, this gauge is only a guide.

Transition is a time when many women express their frustration aloud and it is quite normal. "I can't do it," "Just get the baby out," and "I don't want to do this anymore," are familiar comments in the birth room. Your role is to listen, encourage, and remind the mother she is doing very well at coping with the hard work of labor. The last bit of cervical dilation is often the shortest, and reminding the mother that her baby will be here soon can help to keep her energy and spirits going in the right direction. As a paramedic, you may be faced with difficult decisions about when to stay on-scene and complete a birth and when to begin transporting. Each situation will be different. If the birth appears to be uncomplicated, it should not be considered an emergency.

vaginal orifice and the perineum is distended see Figure 41-10(a)). This is a sign that birth is imminent, and you should not attempt to transport the mother. It is best to set up for delivery in a place where the mother is comfortable or on your stretcher.

Some women may like the pushing stage as they can actually work with their contractions. In a non-medicated mother, a renewed burst of energy accompanies the second stage, triggered by additional hormones. Pushing is a primal force, and most birth attendants never cease to be amazed at the effort it takes to bring forth a baby.

In normal labor, the mother never has to actively push her baby out as the uterus is designed to do just that. The second stage can last as short as one push or up to an average of 2.5 hours in a first-time labor. Current research is supportive of *not* having women hold their breath and to forcefully, "PUSH, PUSH, PUSH" as it decreases oxygenation to the baby. However, when there is an urgent need to get the baby out fast, then the "cheerleader" style of encouragement to push hard with each contraction is necessary.

Second Stage of Labor

The **second stage of labor** is when the cervix is now completely dilated, and the baby moves down into the birth canal with pushing. Pushing eventually becomes involuntary, and nothing can or should stop the expulsive efforts. At this stage of labor, you will be able to see crowning (the fetal scalp is visible at the

Third Stage of Labor

The **third stage of labor** is timed from the birth of the baby to the complete birth of the placenta, and this is the shortest stage of all, usually being completed within 30 minutes. DOT 5-14.4

Immediately after the birth, the uterine contractions stop for a rest period. Try to cover the mother's vaginal

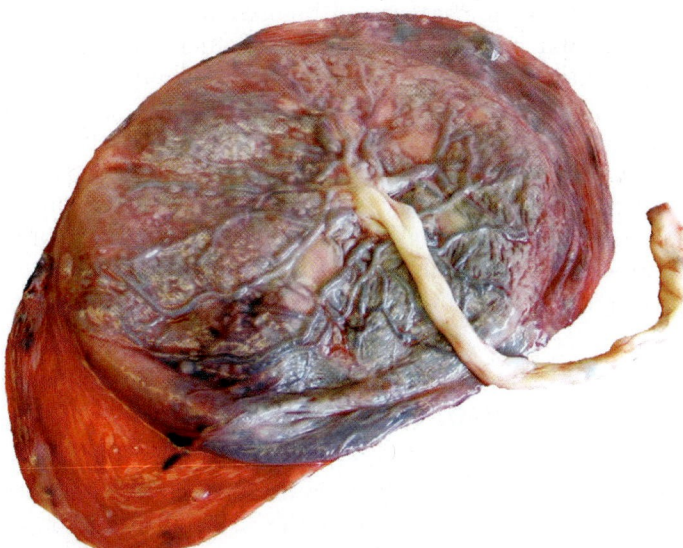

(a) Fetal side

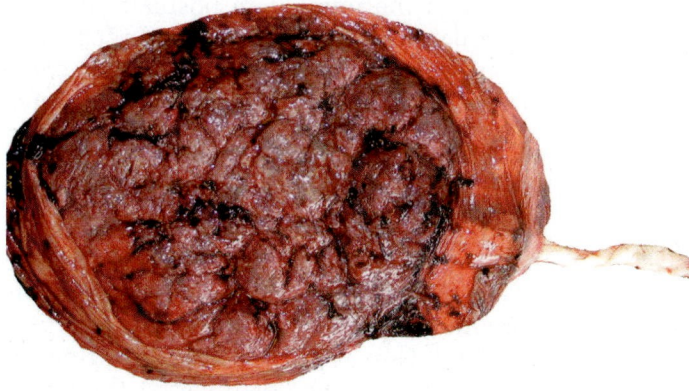

(b) Maternal (uterine) side

Figure 41-11 The fetal side (a) and maternal side (b) of the placenta.

area to give her privacy while waiting for the placenta. Monitor vaginal bleeding, and look for signs of placental separation. Contractions will resume, helping release the placenta from the uterine wall; these contractions are not as intense as labor pains. Figure 41-11 shows the maternal side and fetal side of the placenta.

Street Secrets

While some mothers worry that birthing the placenta is going to hurt, your reminder that the placenta is soft with no bones may put her at ease. Telling women that the placenta is like a big sponge coming down the birth canal to mop up after baby is descriptive and in actuality is exactly what the placenta is doing.

Assessment of the Pregnant Patient in Labor

After performing the primary survey and determining if there are any life-threatening concerns with airway, breathing, and circulation, you should turn your attention to a more focused assessment of labor. You will need to make a quick assessment of two key factors:

- First and most importantly, how far has labor progressed? Is birth imminent (contractions are strong, longer in duration, and regular, and you can see crowning), or will you have time to transport the patient to the hospital? Much of this depends on your service area, protocols, and even traffic and weather.

- Second, is the patient in a high-risk pregnancy category, and are there known problems that may complicate the birth? Risk factors such as the ones listed earlier in the chapter (hypertension, preeclampsia, premature labor, and abnormal bleeding) are predictors of possible complications with the baby. In this case, the patient and baby may be better off delivering in the ambulance, moving toward a hospital with a higher level of care and additional resources.

Box 41-2 presents an outline of the initial assessment of a patient in labor.

You will never be able to predict a normal birth with 100% certainty, and you should not delay transport if you think you can reach a hospital before the mother gives birth. However, rushing to the hospital with lights and siren for what appears to be an uncomplicated normal birth will expose the patients (mother and baby), your crew, and the public to unnecessary danger and risk.

Knowing that most births are normal should give you increased comfort that the primary focus will be to reassure the mother and those in attendance that this is what the female body has been designed to do.[29]

It will also be helpful to consider if this is a planned out-of-hospital birth and you were called because something has gone wrong or if circumstances have just caught the mother by surprise, and an out-of-hospital birth is unplanned.

Unplanned Out-of-Hospital Birth

In the best case scenario, an unplanned out-of-hospital (OOH) birth means that the labor is progressing so well that the mother has not had enough time to get to the hospital. This also means that there is a high probability that everything is going to proceed very well for both the mother and infant. You should continue to be alert for signals that the birth is not in the range of normal or that there might be a problem for the baby, but again,

BOX 41-2 Initial Birthing Assessment

1. Reason for the call?

2. Is the mother actively contracting? How far apart are her contractions? Can you observe a change in her breathing with a contraction? Is she able to talk during a contraction and through the entire contraction?

3. Are the contractions more than or about 5 minutes apart (regardless of how many seconds the contractions are lasting). If so, transport.

4. Are contractions less than five minutes apart? If she is a first-time mother (primipara), you should transport. She still has the second stage of labor (pushing), and that can take a couple of hours.

5. For any mother contracting less than or about 5 minutes apart, with the duration lasting 60 seconds or longer, transport, but be prepared for a birth.

6. Have there been previous pregnancies? For a mother with previous births (multipara) who is contracting less than 2 to 3 minutes apart with the duration 60 to 90 seconds, prepare for a birth.

7. Does the mother report strong pressure in her rectum or an urge to bear down? If yes, then prepare for the birth on-scene. DOT 5-14.8

in the normal case, this is one scenario where most often you will be able to look back and think that something really nice happened while working your shift.

Street Secrets

Be alert for possible deviations from normal. Is this a term pregnancy? Has the mother had routine prenatal care? Is the age of the mother greater than 15 years of age or less than 35 years of age? Is the mother healthy (no medical problems)? Is the baby healthy (no known defects or complications)? Is this a single pregnancy? If you can answer all of these questions with a "yes," the better the chances that an out-of-hospital birth will be uncomplicated.

When arriving on the scene, your most important contribution is to provide calm, confident care and *assist* the mother to birth her baby safely. Having only one paramedic give directions to the mother will be less confusing for her. Speak in a composed voice, and tell her you are here to help. You may find the mother in her

bathroom as the pressure of the baby moving down the birth canal mimics the feelings of an urge to have a bowel movement. If she is on the toilet, help her to get off immediately! You can expect to see stool as part of the birth process, but you cannot risk having the baby deliver in the toilet. In fact, the whole birth process involves a variety of bodily fluids and substances including amniotic fluid, mucus, blood, and possibly vomit, urine, and stool. You should expect this and take appropriate bodily fluid precautions.

Planned Out-of-Hospital Birth

If the OOH birth is intentional, then the paramedic needs to know if a skilled attendant is at the scene. The World Health Organization defines skilled attendant as "a health professional—such as midwife, doctor or nurse—who has been educated and trained in the skills needed to manage normal (uncomplicated) pregnancies, childbirth, and the immediate postnatal period, and in the identification, management, and referral of complications in women and newborns."[30] Most commonly in the United States, paramedics will encounter a midwife at a planned OOH birth. See Box 41-3 for further explanation on attendants and situations that may be found in planned OOH birth.

A skilled attendant will have experience and education in the area of maternity care. It is becoming more widespread for families to hire a doula to be with them for labor and birth. Doulas provide a supportive service for mothers. However, their role and training are not the same as midwives or doctors; therefore, they do not and should not provide clinical or diagnostic roles as part of their care for pregnant and laboring clients.

If you are called to a planned OOH birth that has not progressed or has become complicated, you should assess the patient just as you would normally, with a hightened index of suspicion for complications. The information you receive from the birthing attendant, no matter what their level of training or background, is critical to the smooth transfer and continued care of the patient. Sometimes the very idea that the mom is going to the hospital will be enough to encourage the progression of her labor with a baby arriving shortly after getting to the medical facility.

Childbirth is a uniquely special time for a family. Even while you prepare for transport and during transport, it is important to promote contact between mother and child. This bonding time is very important, and you can help as much as possible to create an environment that promotes healthy attachment for the mother and infant.[14] If both patients are stable, transport the infant on the mother's chest, dimming the lights and covering both patients. DOT 5-14.5, 11, 13, 14

BOX 41-3   Childbirth Choices and Birth Attendants

Certified Professional Midwife (CPM) is a knowledgeable, skilled, and professional independent midwifery practitioner who has met the standards for certification set by the North American Registry of Midwives (NARM), (Midwives Alliance of North America [MANA], 2005). Many states offer licensing (LM) or registration for midwives (RM) beyond the CPM credential.

Certified Nurse Midwife (CNM) are licensed healthcare practitioners educated in the two disciplines of nursing and midwifery. They provide primary healthcare to women of childbearing age including prenatal care, labor and delivery care, care after birth, gynecological exams, newborn care, assistance with family planning decisions, preconception care, menopausal management, and counseling in health maintenance and disease prevention (American College of Nurse Midwives [ACNM], 2003).

Lay Midwife "Traditional birth attendants (TBA) either trained or not, are excluded from the category of skilled health workers. Strictly the term TBA refers only to traditional, independent (of the health system), nonformally trained and community-based providers of care during pregnancy, childbirth, and the postnatal period" (WHO, 2004).

Naturopathic Doctor (ND) holds a doctorate in naturopathic medicine from an accredited naturopathic medical school. This degree confers the title of doctor and allows the holder of the degree to guarantee to the public that they possess the requisite didactic and clinical training to practice Naturopathic Medicine. (New York Association of Naturopathic Physicians [NYANP]).

Medical Doctor (MD) means a duly qualified doctor of medicine entitled under the laws of the province, state, or country where the services are rendered to practice medicine and surgery without restriction (PBC Health Benefits Society [PBCHBS], 1997–2003).

Doula is a Greek word meaning "woman's servant." In labor support terminology, a doula refers to a supportive companion (not a friend or loved one) professionally trained to provide labor support. She performs no clinical tasks (Doulas of North America, 1998). Doulas most often come to the laboring woman's home when she is in early labor and accompany her to the hospital, where they attend the birth with the mother in a continued supportive capacity.

Unassisted (UA) birth is where the mother or family plans to have an OOH birth without a skilled attendant. The mother is most often attended by her mate. Other planned UA births will have family members or friends on site.

Family-centered birth is an increasingly common choice for both hospital and OOH births. When children are present, if possible, EMS should provide some reassuring words to help all those at the scene better deal with the unexpected events.

Waterbirth EMS may be called to a planned OOH birth with a large water "birth tub" at the scene. Many families now are choosing water labor and waterbirth for OOH and in-hospital births.

Step-by-Step Instructions for a Normal Birth

Second Stage—Birth of the Baby

Also see Skill Sheet 41: Uncomplicated Birth.

1. *Establish body substance isolation (BSI)* practices. Wear a gown, gloves, glasses, and mask.

2. *Prepare a delivery area.* Find a comfortable and clean surface. Do not have the patient get into a recumbent position as it may be uncomfortable for her and the pregnant (gravid) uterus pressing down on her vena cava and could make her hypotensive and limit the oxygen available for the baby.[31] Semi-sitting or left side lying are most comfortable.

3. *Remove clothing.* If the patient's lower body is still clothed, remove her clothing from the waist down. Try to create as much privacy as the situation will allow.

4. *Open your OB Kit* Have your birth kit in nearby reach (Box 41-4).

5. *Place a fresh clean underpad* or sheet beneath her buttocks.

6. *Have a clean blanket* or other linens nearby, if possible, for warming the mother and drying the baby after the birth.

7. *During contractions,* encourage her to push only with the contractions.

8. *Give clear instructions.* Talk to her in a firm, kind voice, and remind her that her baby is almost here.

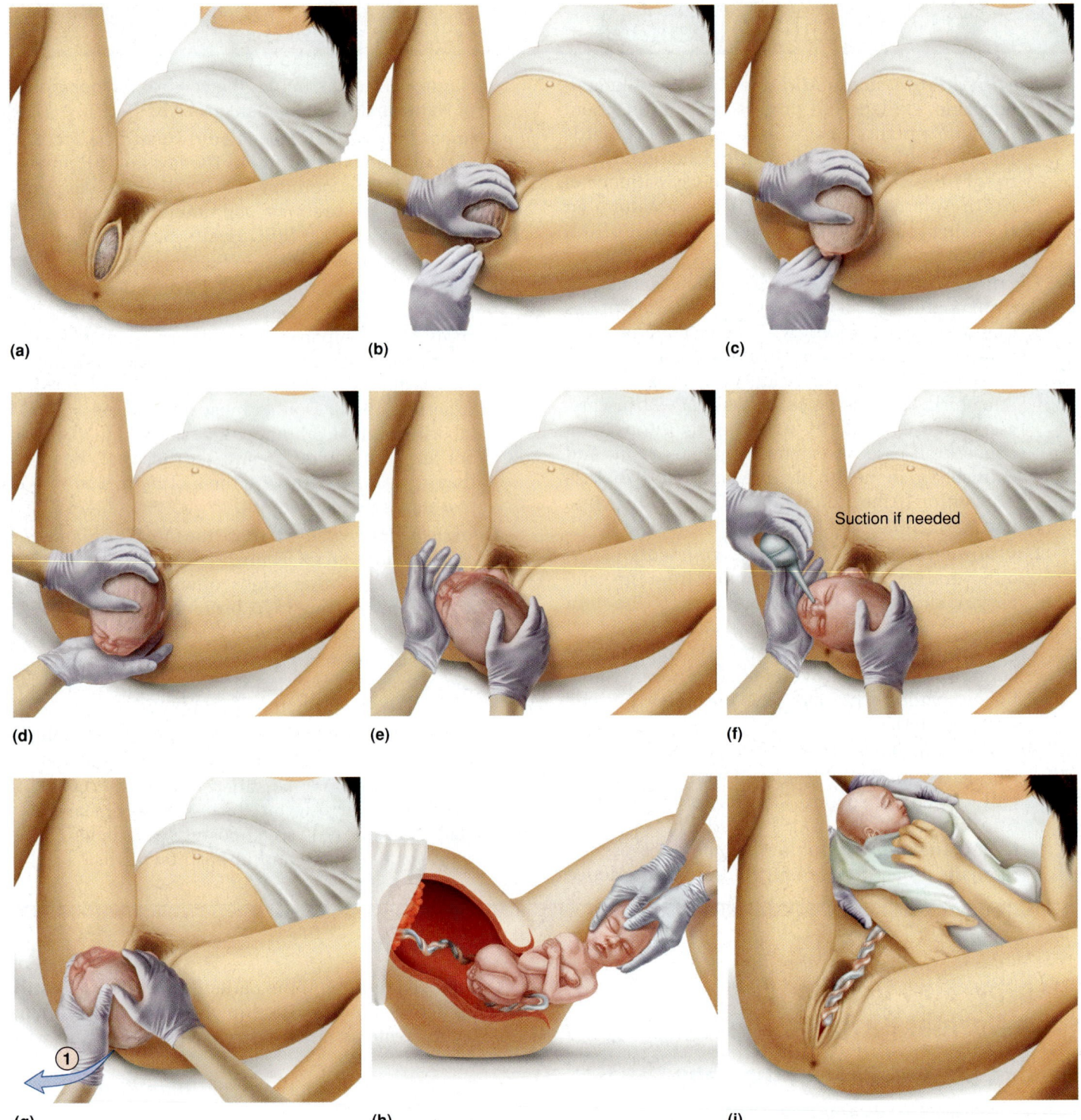

(a)

(b)

(c)

(d)

(e)

(f) Suction if needed

(g) ①

(h)

(i)

Figure 41-12 Birth sequence of the most common presentation—anterior—where the baby is born facing the mother's tailbone.

9. **Support the emerging head.** In between contractions, sometimes the emerging top of the baby's head slides back inside the vagina; this is normal (Figure 41-12(a)). This process is giving the mom's perineal tissue time to stretch, and it prevents tearing. With your top hand, support the emerging head, and with the other hand, support the tissue between her vagina and anus, which is called the perineum

BOX 41-4   A Basic Birth Kit

Sterile non-latex gloves

Sterile scalpel (for cutting the cord)

One OB disposable pad

Two packs of sterile pads

One bulb suction aspirator

One set of cord clamps (two clamps)

Three nonwoven towels (set up your instruments on these)

OB toilettes (for wiping off feces)

One plastic bag for the placenta (can use kidney basin or urine bedpan)

One plastic apron

Two twist-ties

Trash bag

APGAR score chart

One hat

One receiving blanket

Foil space blanket

If you can add to the kit, include more disposable underpads, sterile gloves, and another receiving blanket DOT 5-14.9

(Figure 41-12(b)). Once the top of the head appears and does not slide back inside, keep one hand on the perineum and the other hand gently supporting the head. This to keep you ready and to prevent the head (and slippery, wet infant) from barreling through on the next contraction. Some babies will attempt to burst forth and others will s-l-o-w-l-y emerge; both are normal variations.

10. *Deliver the head.* Usually with the next contraction, the head will be born. Most often, the head will be born with the face looking towards the mother's tailbone (Figure 41-12(c)). Posterior presentations, are also normal, just less common.

   a. Check for the umbilical cord around the neck while supporting the head with your nondominant hand; use your dominant hand's index finger and sweep most of the way around the baby's neck (Figure 41-12(d)). You are feeling for and looking to see if the umbilical cord is looped around the neck or shoulder; if you find one, it is called nuchal cord and, information of what to do is found in Nuchal Cord on page 1021. You are also looking and feeling for little fingers, a fist, elbow, or rarely a foot that might have come down with the head; this is called a compound presentation (see Breech Birth on page 1021).

   b. Next, the baby will turn its head and will look either right or left, at one of the mother's thighs (Figure 41-12(e)). Inside the mother, the shoulders are lining up, and the head is the outward movement of the internal process.

11. *Suction the nose and mouth.* Once the head has been born, suction the mouth and nose (Figure 41-12(f)). If a clean gauze pad or cloth is available, you can wipe off the baby's face of any mucus or blood.

   a. Traditionally, suctioning of the mouth and then the nostrils has been recommended with a bulb syringe. This common practice has not been assessed in any clinical trials, and its value is uncertain. If nasal and pharyngeal suctioning is used, care should be taken to minimize pharyngeal stimulation. Suction bulbs rather than catheters should be used because suction bulbs are less likely to induce cardiac dysrhythmias.[32]

12. *Remember,* this part of the birth can happen so quickly that the restitution and rotation may occur in one rapid movement. Be prepared because the baby can be completely born in one contraction. With the next contraction, while continuing to support the head with both hands, the paramedic gently moves the head down toward the mom's bottom (Figure 41-12(g)). Sometimes the maneuver has to be repeated a couple of times; gentle and firm touch with your hands is the expectation. Once a shoulder is released, remember the whole body can slip out quickly (Figure 41-12(h))!

13. *Keep* the neonate's head about the level of the vagina.

14. *When the baby is born* all the way, wrap the newborn in a sheet or blanket, and place the baby on the mother's belly (Figure 41-12(i)). (If the cord is too short, lay the baby across one of her thighs.)

15. *Note the birth time.*

16. *Assess the APGAR.* With your hand supporting the baby, until you are certain it is securely in the mother's care, and remembering baby is still connected via the umbilical cord, you or your partner will be doing the job of assessing the baby's one-minute and five-minute **APGAR score** (Box 41-5).

   a. If the baby is crying vigorously and is pink, your score is rather obvious, so you do not need to wait one whole minute to know that the baby's score is eight to ten.

BOX 41-5 APGAR Scoring

APGAR scoring is to be done at one minute and five minutes after birth. Assess the infant, and add the points from the column headings. Continue at five-minute intervals until the baby scores a seven or above. Review neonatal resuscitation steps.

APGAR	0 points	1 point	2 points
Appearance	Blue, pale	Body pink, extremities blue	Completely pink
Pulse	Absent	Less than 100	Greater than 100
Grimace or reflex	No response	Grimace	Cry
Activity and muscle tone	Limp	Some flexion of extremities	Active movement
Respiratory effort	Absent	Slow, irregular	Good, strong cry

17. ***Dry the baby.*** Simultaneously, you will be drying the baby off and replacing the wet linen with something dry.

18. ***Clamp and cut the cord*** at this time (Figure 41-13).
    a. Observe body substance isolation precautions.
    b. Equipment at hand includes one or two plastic cord clamps, one hemostat, and one blunt-tip scissors.

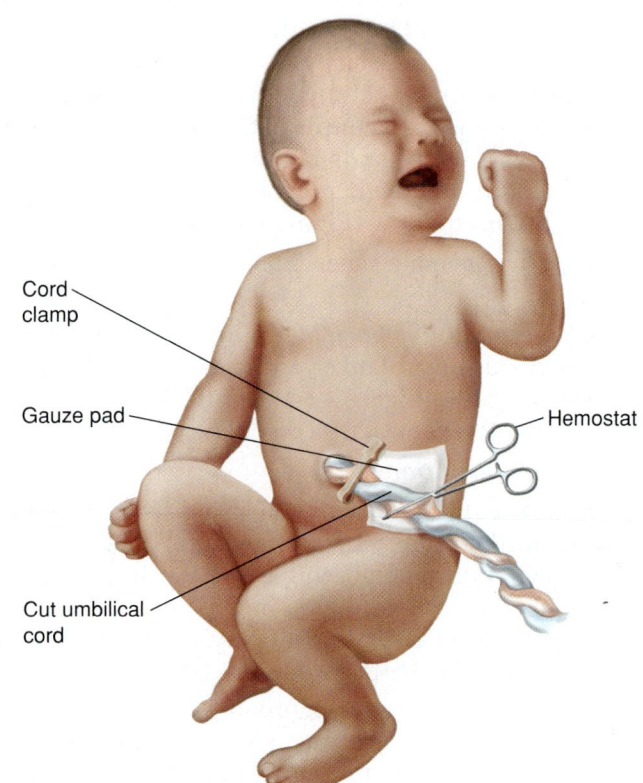

Cord clamp

Gauze pad

Hemostat

Cut umbilical cord

Figure 41-13 Cutting the cord.

c. Place first cord clamp about four inches away from where cord inserts into the abdomen of the baby.

d. Place hemostat or second cord clamp on the umbilical cord approximately one to two inches distal (further away from the baby) from the first cord clamp.

e. Place a sterile gauze under where you will cut as some blood will ooze out.

f. Place your fingers underneath the cord, holding the gauze in the smaller space between the two clamps. (In case you slip, you will cut your own fingers and not the baby!)

g. When you are certain that everything is positioned with your other hand, cut the umbilical cord.

h. Remember you have a living, wiggling baby to contend with. Sometimes it helps to have the mother or the second medic hold the baby's legs gently as they have the tendency to draw them to their belly, obscuring your sight.

i. Once the cord is cut, dab off any blood that may have landed on the baby with gauze.

j. Wrap the baby and mother together.

k. Transport the placenta to the hospital with mother and baby.

19. ***Keep the baby warm.***

20. ***Place the infant on the mother's chest.*** The mother is the best radiant heat source, so make sure to lift up the baby briefly and dry off the mother's abdomen, replacing the baby back on her; this is especially important if the initial placement of the infant has left the mom's abdomen wet with birth fluids. Both mom and baby should be skin-to-skin and wrapped in a blanket together. This is essential. If the mom is planning to breastfeed, remind

her that it is okay to do so now. Some experienced moms are going to offer the breast to their baby instinctively. Your reminder that it is a good time to nurse the baby serves multiple purposes:

a. Helps baby to settle and keep warm next to mother's skin.

b. Helps mother's uterus to contract and expel the placenta by releasing hormones.

c. Decreases postbirth bleeding.

Remember avoid cold stress and hypothermia in the baby!

21. *Assess vitals of the mother.*

22. *Monitor bleeding.* You will be paying attention to the blood loss that comes after giving birth. Put a clean underpad, linen, or newspaper beneath her so that it is easier to differentiate new (after baby) blood loss. Every birth is associated with some blood loss as the mother's blood volume has increased almost 40% during the pregnancy. An average amount lost is 250 ccs; there is usually more bleeding with or after the placenta than before.

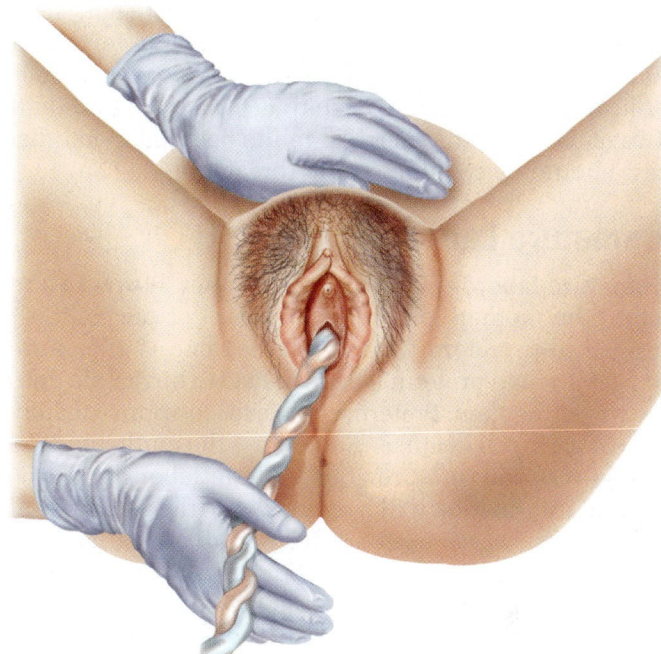

Figure 41-14   Guarding the abdomen while guiding the placenta out of the vagina.

Third Stage—Birth of the Placenta

1. Often, the paramedic will note that the placenta is ready because there will be a splash of new blood called the "separation gush."

2. Lengthening of the umbilical cord is another sign to watch for.

3. Alternatively, a mom might report that she is feeling "crampy;" if that happens, remind her that the placenta is ready to be born.

4. Helping mom sit up or give a little push may bring the placenta in further view at the vaginal opening.

5. With one hand supporting or guarding her lower abdomen and the other holding onto the cord, with the hemostat in your hand you can gently guide the placenta out (Figure 41-14).

6. You must *never* pull on the cord to get the placenta out.

7. You will see the placenta emerge and look either shiny or meaty (see Figure 41-11 on page 1013):

a. Shiny is the membranes or amniotic sac, the umbilical cord side.

b. The meaty side of the placenta is the maternal side.

8. Most often, the placenta comes out neatly with some blood and clots; place the placenta on an underpad or in a plastic bag.

9. You can now gently massage the mother's belly to make sure that her uterus contracts. It feels like you are squeezing a grapefruit for ripeness. The uterus should be firm and toward the middle of her abdomen; if it feels boggy or blood and clots are being passed out of

her vagina, continue to gently massage until the uterus becomes firm or until the bleeding stops.

10. Bring the placenta wrapped in an underpad or bag to the hospital with the mother; someone there will examine it for completeness.

11. Continue to monitor the mother's vital signs.

12. Continue to peek at the baby, making sure it has good color and is breathing.

13. Many mothers have uncontrollable shaking after the birth has been completed; this is normal.[14] DOT 5-14.16

Complications of Labor

For the small percentage of births where there is deviation from normal, your skills in identifying the problem and providing an appropriate response will allow the birth to be safe for both mother and child.

Fetal Distress

Fetal distress, which generally indicates that there is some problem affecting the fetus, is difficult to detect without advanced equipment. In the field, you may encounter a nurse, midwife, or physician who has already identified fetal distress at a planned OOH birth or clinic. Irregularities in the fetal heart rate pattern, tachycardia, bradycardia, deep variable decelerations, or late decelerations of the fetal heart rate, are all indicative of fetal distress. In many cases, treatment involves maintaining the mother's blood pressure, oxygenation and rapid transport to an appropriate hospital.[33] Other signs such as meconium (first tarry stool from baby) mixed in with the amniotic fluid seen at the time of delivery is indicative of fetal stress. The finding of meconium should always be reported on arrival to the hospital. Fetal distress should be considered life-threatening.

Premature Labor

Premature labor is labor that occurs after 20 weeks and before the mother completes 37 weeks of pregnancy.[14] Premature or preterm labor is not the same as premature birth. Although preterm labor can lead to birth, this does not always happen. Preterm birth leads to approximately 75% of perinatal deaths.[14] Sometimes the mother will be on bed rest due to a previous preterm labor diagnosis, and that information will be conveyed to the paramedics. Because the cervix does not have to dilate as far for a preterm baby to be born, the labor process usually happens faster than in a term pregnancy. There will also be a higher incidence of malpresentations and congenital problems for babies born preterm. Substance abuse, especially cocaine, is a known labor inducer.[14] Pregnancy violence or abuse can also bring on preterm labor.

Assessment of the preterm labor patient includes all of the same questions and exam as for the term labor patient.

Prehospital treatment for premature labor includes keeping the mother calm and avoiding any unnecessary jostling or moving. Administer oxygen and obtain IV access. In some systems, protocol includes the administration of tocolytics (medications that inhibit uterine contractions) such as terbutaline sulfate.

Premature Rupture of Membranes (PROM)

PROM is the spontaneous rupture of the amniotic sac when there are no signs of labor. In lay terms, the mom might report, "My water broke" or "my bag is leaking." Preterm premature rupture of membranes (PPROM) is when rupture of the amniotic sac occurs before 37 completed weeks of pregnancy. PROM or PPROM is not an emergency, but such cases should be transported for evaluation as the risk of infection involving the uterus and its contents is increased. At term, 69% percent of women will start spontaneous labor within 24 hours of rupture.[13]

Uterine Rupture

Uterine rupture is a very uncommon event, even with blunt trauma to the mother such as motor vehicle crash, and only occurs in 0.6% of all pregnancies.[34] Uterine rupture occurs when a scar from a previous uterine surgery, such as a cesarean section opens up and the contents of the uterus, amniotic sac and baby spill into the peritoneal space with extensive bleeding.

Uterine rupture is more likely to happen during labor, and induced or augmented labor increases the risk of rupture to 7.7 out of 1000.[13] Other causes for uterine rupture include prolonged, obstructed labor, uterine abnormalities, grand multiparity (more than five children), and invasive cervical or uterine manipulations.[35]

Death of the mother or baby can happen with uterine rupture due to severe bleeding in the mother and the disruption of oxygen supply to the baby.

You should suspect the possibility of uterine rupture in the patient who reports a sharp pain during a contraction and decreased fetal movement. Look for signs of hidden bleeding and shock related to the internal bleeding.[35]

Cord Prolapse

Cord prolapse occurs when the umbilical cord presents through the open cervix during labor but before the baby presents and is observed in the vagina or outside of the vagina (Figure 41-15). This complication is found in 3% of vertex births and 3.7% of breech births.[35,36] When the umbilical cord is not visible but is coming down the birth canal next to the baby, it is called an occult cord prolapse. The scenario of prolapse is often further complicated by a malpresenting baby. Associated complications are breech, prematurity, excessive amniotic fluid, and nonengagement of presenting part due to the size of the baby or congenital anomaly. Unsuspected cord prolapse becomes evident most often with the rupture of membranes, and in one study, 47% of cord prolapse happened within five minutes of rupture of the amniotic sac.[35] A cord prolapse is a serious complication, and an emergency cesarean birth is most often indicated to save the life of the infant. This is a life-threatening complication for the baby because as the baby moves down the birth canal, it compresses the prolapsed cord and prevents oxygen from being delivered. Perinatal

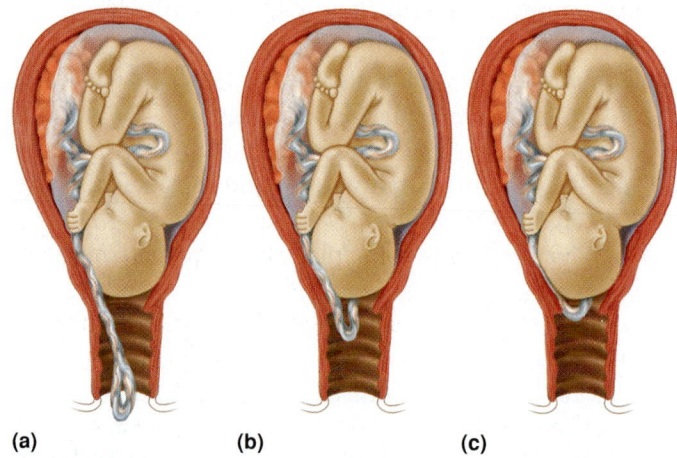

(a) (b) (c)

Figure 41-15 Prolapsed cord. (a) Cord visible outside the vagina. (b) Cord in the vagina. (c) Hidden prolapse.

mortality can be as high as 35%, depending on how long the compression goes on before the baby is delivered.[35]

Cord prolapse instructions for suspected or known cord prolapse follow:

1. Get the mother into knee-chest position; elevate her bottom as high as possible.

2. Insert a gloved hand into the vagina, and lift the presenting part off the cord. You must not take your hand out until you feel the baby being lifted out during the cesarean surgery. Under no circumstances should you give up this position. Do not compress the cord with your hand.

3. The mother should be given oxygen with nonrebreather mask at 10/lpm.[35] Transport emergently. Start an IV as soon as possible, but do not delay transport for this.

4. If equipment such as a Doppler is available, have someone monitor fetal heart tones as often as possible, right up to the surgical suite. Fetal heart tones in the 120 to 160 range is an excellent sign.

5. Do not allow mom to stand up or lay on her back.

6. Keep mom's bottom half covered with a sheet or blanket to keep her warm as involuntary shivering may occur.

Malpresentations

Breech Birth

A **breech presentation** occurs when the baby presents with their buttocks, foot, or knees first instead of the head. At term, breech births happen only 3–4% of the time.[37] Because 25% of babies are breech before 28 weeks, the biggest concern for breech birth is also prematurity.[38] All babies born preterm can sustain trauma based on their rapid descent through the birth canal; breech presentation exaggerates that potential. In about 6.3% of breech presentations, a congenital anomaly is the reason the baby does not present head first.[37] There are four classical categories of breech presentation (Figure 41-16):[37]

Complete breech

1. Baby sits cross-legged.

Incomplete breech

2. Extended or frank breech when the legs are bent at the hip and up to the face.

3. Footling when a foot or feet come first; this is not common.

4. Kneeling is much more rare, when the bent knees present first.

The good news about breech births is that they usually go very well, but when they do not, the results can

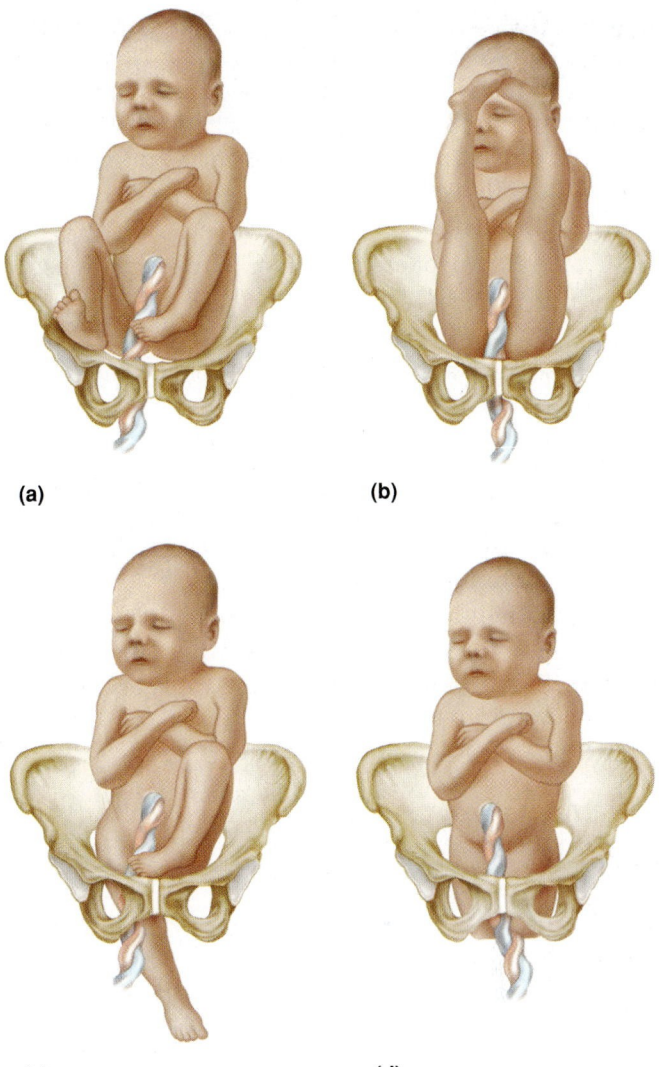

(a)   **(b)**

(c)   **(d)**

Figure 41-16 Breech presentations. (a) Complete. (b) Frank. (c) Footling. (d) Kneeling.

be catastrophic. Be suspicious of a breech presentation if you note fresh, thick, dark, tarry meconium stool from the vagina. Meconium passage may occur as the pressure of the vaginal walls squeezes the baby's rump and causes the bowels to release.[37] Box 41-6 describes the process of managing a breech birth.

Nuchal Cord

Nuchal cord occurs when the umbilical cord is wrapped around the infant's neck (Figure 41-17). It is not a true complication as cord around the neck happens in about 20% of *normal* births.[35] The problem with nuchal cord is that the cord may get too tight during the labor process and cause fetal distress. Sometimes the cord is so tight or short that it impedes the labor process, making labor longer but having a normal outcome. Most of the time, even when a loop of cord is seen wrapped tightly

BOX 41-6 Breech Birth Management

1. Shoulders, not the head, are normally the difficult part to deliver.
2. If delivering,
   a. Allow neonate to deliver to the umbilicus.
   b. With the legs clear, support the body in your palm.
   c. Extract approximately four- to six-inch loop of umbilical cord.
   d. Rotate the neonate for anterior-posterior shoulder positioning.
   e. Apply gentle traction until axilla is visible.
   f. Guide the neonate upward and deliver the posterior shoulder.
   g. Guide the neonate downward to deliver the anterior shoulder.
   h. Ease the head out; do not apply excessive manipulation.
3. If the head does not deliver,
   a. Form a "V" with fingers on the sides of neonate's nose to create airway.

BOX 41-7 Nuchal Cord Assessment and Instructions

1. Feel to see if there is enough slack in the cord to either pull it over the baby's head or permit delivery of the rest of the baby through the loop of cord.
2. If not,
   a. Immediately clamp the cord with two hemostats; be certain it is the umbilical cord.
   b. With round-tip or blunt scissors cut *between* the two hemostats.
   c. Unwind the cord before the body is born.

When a baby is born with the cord so tightly wrapped around the neck that you cannot fit a finger beneath the cord, you have to cut the umbilical cord.[35] Detailed instructions are given in a Box 41-7.

Intact Amniotic Sac

Occasionally, the fetus is born "in the caul," meaning the amniotic sac is intact after birth. Presentation will be a head being born that looks like it has been shrink-wrapped. The shiny amniotic sac may appear tightly adhered to the head or may contain visible amounts of amniotic fluid. It can look very much like a water balloon surrounding the head.[35] Delivery instructions are in Box 41-8.

Meconium

Meconium is the infant's first stool. Occasionally, an infant will pass its first stool while in utero. Meconium-stained amniotic fluids can be indicative of a compromised baby.[13] When a baby is born with meconium-stained

around the neck, if the attendant can slide a finger between the neck and the loop, it is considered loose enough. If some slack is available, you may be able to flip it over the baby's head or push the cord down the baby's shoulders while the head and body emerge.[35]

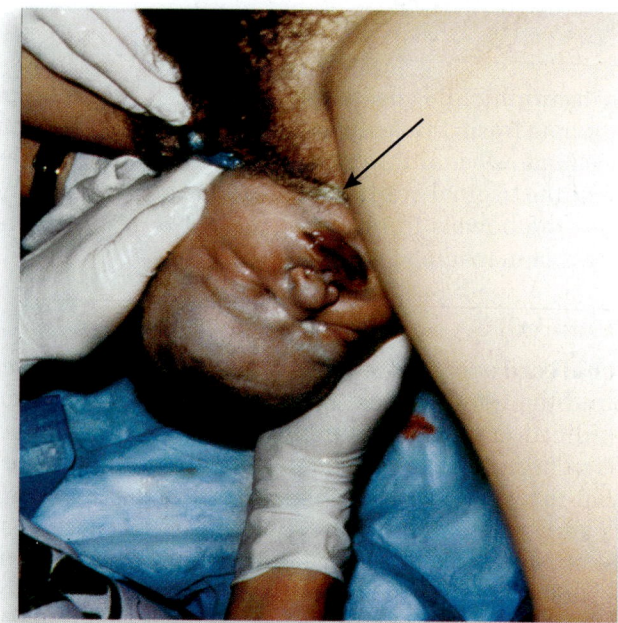

Figure 41-17 Nuchal cord (arrow).

BOX 41-8 Assessment and Instructions for Birth with an Intact Amniotic Sac

1. Identify the baby's face.
2. With your pinky finger, gently apply pressure into the baby's mouth.[35] That is usually enough to pop the bag.
3. Peel the sac back from the face.
4. If you missed it and the whole baby is born in the sac, follow the same procedures, and remove the infant from the sac.
5. At this point, wipe the face and dry the infant.

fluid, use the bulb syringe to suction the baby's mouth and nose after the head is born and before the body is born. Aspiration of meconium can lead to serious pulmonary complications for the newborn. Warn the mother beforehand, and tell her that you are going to ask her to pant and not push when the head is born because you need to suction the baby.

> The order for suctioning is mouth then nose; think of M before N in the alphabet to help you remember.

Squeeze the bulb, which deflates it, and insert the tip into the baby's mouth, being careful not to go too far back. Release the bulb slowly and that will suction up any secretions and meconium. Take the bulb out of the baby's mouth, squeeze the bulb onto the underpad, and note any meconium or mucus. If meconium is visible on the pad, deflate the bulb and insert into the baby's mouth again. Next, follow the same steps, one nostril and then the next. After the baby is born, you may choose to or need to suction the baby again. Be extra mindful when you listen to the baby's lungs postbirth to determine that they are clear. DOT 5-14.6, 10, 19, 20, 22

Multiple Pregnancy

A pregnancy of multiples can be previously diagnosed, or it can be a surprise finding at the time of birth. The challenging complication to a multiple pregnancy is the potential for the babies to arrive before 37 weeks gestation. In twin pregnancy, 40% have the additional consideration of one baby being breech.[37] Multiple pregnancy rates continue to increase due to infertility treatment options and, in these cases, are rarely surprise findings at the time of birth.[28] One complication associated with multiple pregnancy is placental abruption after the birth of the first baby, causing fetal distress or death for the second baby due to lack of oxygenation.[28]

If you are waiting for a placenta and the mom starts vigorously contracting and pushing or another amniotic sac breaks, think twin and not placenta. Undiagnosed twin is another reason not to aggressively manage placenta delivery. If it is determined or suspected that there is another baby, then the cord of the first baby must be clamped if it has not yet happened. If you are surprised by a twin birth, the best thing to do is to treat the situation as one baby and then one baby again. Remain calm and clearheaded. There is a greater likelihood for postpartum hemorrhage due to the increased placental diameters nourishing multiple babies, so be prepared.

Premature Birth and Babies

Premature babies are those born before 37 completed weeks of gestation. Premature babies are at-risk for many things, but respiratory distress syndrome (RDS) and asphyxia are notable complications.[14] RDS manifests itself as breathing difficulties such as nasal flaring, seesaw breathing with chest contractions, poor color, and rapid and irregular respiratory rate, all due to immature lungs.[28] Premature babies will be smaller, their head appears larger than their body, and they may have very little subcutaneous fat, which makes them vulnerable to cold stress and inability to maintain their body temperature. The skin of premature babies varies in its appearance, based on gestation, looking normal or red and thinner, with visible veins and fine downy hair; the skin is more fragile (Figure 41-18). DOT 5-14.23

"About 12 percent of babies in the United States are born preterm. Of those, the majority (84 percent) are born between 32 and 36 weeks of gestation. About 10 percent are born between 28 and 31 weeks of gestation, and about 6 percent are born at less than 28 weeks of gestation."[15] Identifiable risk factors for preterm birth are having a previous preterm birth, multiple pregnancy, being African American, and being less than 17 years of age or over age 35.[15] A long list of lifestyle and medical conditions can increase the chances for delivering preterm. Most preterm babies do very well, even though many end up having a stay in the Newborn Intensive Care Unit (NICU)."[39]

Postpartum Complications

Postpartum Hemorrhage

A hemorrhage after the birth of the fetus but before the delivery of the placenta is rare. After the placenta has been delivered, if the uterus does not contract, blood and clots

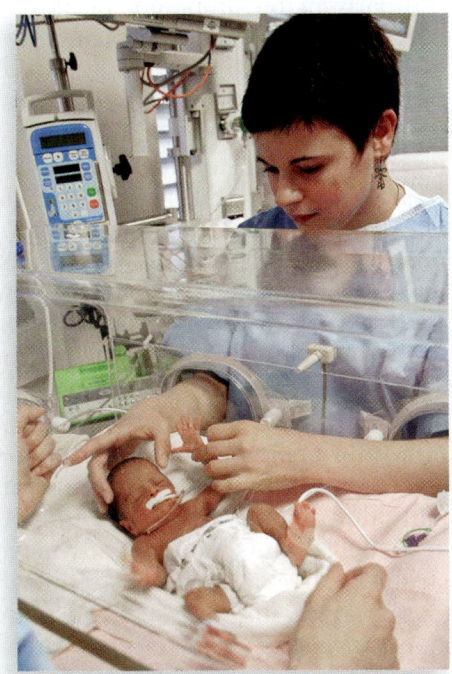

Figure 41-18 Premature infant being cared for in a neonatal intensive care unit (NICU).

may be observed coming from the vagina. The best thing to do is to massage the uterus externally until it becomes firm and feels like a large grapefruit in the abdomen. This procedure is called **fundal massage.** When performing fundal massage, be careful not to push too hard and cause the uterus to be pushed out of the vagina. Occasionally, after an overly long birth, and sometimes even after a rapid birth, the uterus forgets to stay firm and the attendant has to keep checking the uterus continually to keep it from getting "boggy." If the bleeding continues unabated, it may be due to lacerations of the perineum, vagina, or cervix, and compression techniques will not usually stop the bleeding.[35] Treatment will instead be focused on maintaining blood pressure and applying a pad dressing on the outside of the vagina.

All women continue to have some bleeding for up to six weeks postpartum; this is normal and is called lochia. At first the bleeding is heavier and red colored, as time passes it changes color and amount and may even begin to look creamy with mucus. Lochia is the evidence of the healing happening inside the uterus as it involutes to its pre-pregnant size. Most women have been advised to call their care-provider if they saturate a menstrual pad with blood in 30 minutes or less. However, if the bleeding continues the woman will be advised to call 9-1-1.

Delayed hemorrhage beyond the immediate postpartum period is defined as hemorrhage after the first 24-hours following delivery.[14] Causes of delayed hemorrhage can be retained uterine blood clots, placental fragments, hematoma, and infections. EMS may be called for excessive bleeding for days or even weeks postpartum. When EMS receives a call for excessive vaginal bleeding postpartum, be prepared for the signs and symptoms of shock and treat appropriately.

Embolism

An embolism is defined as the entry of foreign materials into the blood.[35] Pregnant and postpartum women are at-risk for **pulmonary embolism** due to the increased blood volume and hypercoagulability of normal pregnancy. Pulmonary embolism is more likely to happen to women who have a history of varicose veins or thrombophlebitis. Observe your patient for signs and symptoms of "air hunger," feelings of doom, rapid heart rate, and possible sharp chest pains.[14]

Amniotic fluid embolism (AFE), while extremely rare, is when amniotic fluid enters the maternal circulation, usually during labor or birth. The incidence is 1:8,000 to 1:30,000.[35] The woman's body may respond with catastrophic physical reactions similar to those seen in anaphylaxis and sepsis.[35] The patient may experience a devastating drop in blood pressure and decreased cardiac function, which leads to a maternal mortality rate of 60–80%.[35] Prehospital care is supportive with maintenance of oxygenation and blood pressure. DOT 5-14.21

Postpartum Infection

Puerperal infection is a bacterial infection that originates in the reproductive tract during labor or birth. Women who are at risk include those who had prolonged labor, prolonged rupture of membranes, hemorrhage with blood loss greater than 1000 mL, care that included breaks in aseptic technique, multiple vaginal exams, instrumental delivery (vacuum or forceps), or surgery.[14] Mothers will report flu-like symptoms, with fever, often abdominal or uterine pain and usually vaginal discharge with an obvious unpleasant smell. Puerperal infection is specifically defined as fever greater than 100.4°F and occurring after the first 24 hours postpartum up to ten days postbirth.[14]

Of the several infections that can manifest in postpartum, a common site is the internal layer of the uterus and is called **endometritis,** most often following a cesarean birth.[14] The infections can be found locally in any area of the mother's reproductive tract. Prehospital treatment is supportive with transport to the hospital for antibiotic therapy and usually inpatient hospitalization.

Summary

When caring for a pregnant, or possibly pregnant, patient, remain focused on providing a good assessment and recognizing potentially life-threatening conditions. Consider signs and symptoms of shock that may point toward bleeding, such as unexplained hypotension with accompanying abdominal pain. Toxemia should be considered in any pregnant patient with hypertension, headache, or blurred vision.

A good assessment should include a thorough history, including last normal menstrual period, past pregnancies and birth history, if applicable, and current prenatal care. The patient should be interviewed as privately as possible, away from other family or friends, so that truthful and confidential answers can be encouraged.

Consider any pregnant patient having contractions as being in labor until further evaluated by a specialized clinician. If contractions are strong and frequent and the patient has a strong urge to push, you should prepare for an imminent birth. Coach and reassure the patient through each stage of the birthing process.

Just as you would for any skill that is performed infrequently, it is important to review obstetric assessment and birthing skills on a periodic basis.

Although you may work your entire career without ever attending a prehospital birth, your role in a birth may be pivotal and very rewarding. Assuming there are no complications, childbirth is one of the few cases in emergency medical services where you are being called to assist in a normal and healthy part of new life. Your communications skills, your hands, and a warm blanket may be the only tools you really need to ensure a good outcome.

Notes

1. J. Coad, *Anatomy and Physiology for Midwives* (London: Mosby, 2001), p. 89.
2. I. K. Stone, "Sexually Transmitted Diseases," In *Obstetric and Gynecologic Emergencies,* G. I. Benrubi, ed. (Philadelphia, PA: J. B. Lippincott, 1994), pp. 211–232.
3. D. B. Rein, W. J. Kassler, K. L. Irwin, et al., "Direct Medical Cost of Pelvic Inflammatory Disease and Its Sequelae: Decreasing But Still Substantial," *The Obstetrician and Gynaecologist* 95(2000): 397.
4. J. Tintinalli et al., *Tintinalli's Emergency Medicine,* 6th ed., Chapter 109: Introduction (New York: McGraw-Hill, 2004), www.accessmedicine.com (accessed August 15, 2005).
5. A. Kazzi, "Ovarian Cysts," http://www.emedicine.com/emerg/topic352.htm (accessed February 6, 2006).
6. J. Ludmir and P. G. Stubblefield, "Surgical Procedures in Pregnancy," In *Obstetrics: Normal and Problem Pregnancies,* 4th ed., S. G. Gabbe, J. R. Niebyl, and J. L. Simpson, eds. (Philadelphia, PA: Churchill Livingstone, 2002). pp. 607–650.
7. D. McCormick, "His and Hers Abdominal Pain: Gender-Specific Factors," Emergency Medical Services; May 2005; Cygnus publishing. http://www.emsresponder.com/publication/article.jsp?pubId=1&id=1836 (accessed February 6, 2006).
8. C. J. Dunton, "Torsion of the Ovary," In *Obstetric and Gynecological Emergencies,* G. I. Benrubi, ed. (Philadelphia, PA: J. B. Lippincott Company, 1994), pp. 275–281.
9. S. J. Sondheimer, "Menorrhagia and Abnormal Vaginal Bleeding," In *Obstetric and Gynecological Emergencies,* G. I. Benrubi, ed., (Philadelphia, PA: J. P. Lippincott Company, 1994), pp. 251–262.
10. T. L. Callahan, A. B. Caughey, and L. J. Heffner, *Blueprints in Obstetrics and Gynecology* (Malden, MA: Blackwell Science, 1998).
11. B. J. Horowitz, "Vulvar and Vaginal Disease," In *Obstetric and Gynecological Emergencies,* G. I. Benrubi, ed. (Philadelphia, PA: J. B. Lippincott Company, 1994), pp. 233–249.
12. J. L. Simpson and J. R. Niebyl, "Occupational and Environmental Perspectives of Birth Defects," In *Obstetrics: Normal and Problem Pregnancies,* 4th ed., S. G. Gabbe, J. L. Simpson, and J. L. Niebyl, eds. (Philadelphia, PA: Churchill Livingstone, 2002).
13. L. V. Walsh, *Midwifery: Community Based Care During the Childbearing Years* (Philadelphia, PA: W. B. Saunders, 2001).
14. H. Varney, J. M. Kriebs, and C. L. Gegor, *Varney's Midwifery,* 4th ed. (Sudbury, MA: Jones and Bartlett Publishers, 2004).
15. March of Dimes Birth Defects Foundation, "Pre-term Birth" (2005), http://www.marchofdimes.com/prematurity/5196_5799.asp (accessed June 11, 2005).
16. Centers for Disease Control and Prevention, Division of Reproductive Health, "Safe Motherhood: Promoting Health for Women Before, During and After Pregnancy" (2004), http://www.amchp.org/aboutamchp/publications/maternaldeathandinjury.pdf (accessed May 5, 2005).
17. Gates Foundation, "Global Health: Reproductive, Child Health," http://www.gatesfoundation.org/GlobalHealth/ReproductiveChildHealth/Announcements/Announce-204.htm (accessed May 6, 2005).
18. U.S. Department of Health & Human Services, "Maternal Mortality Rate, by Race of Mother: 2000" (2003), http://www.mchb.hrsa.gov/chusa03/status.htm#maternal (accessed May 20, 2005).
19. M. Wagner (2003, May–June), "Real Revealing Risks: Obstetrical Interventions and Maternal Mortality-Pregnancy, Birth & Midwifery," *Mothering* (May–June, 2003), http://www.findarticles.com/p/articles/mi_m0838/is_2003_May_June/ai_102791856/pg_2 (accessed May 16, 2005).
20. Safe Motherhood, "Women's Risk of Dying From Pregnancy and Childbirth," http://www.safemotherhood.org/facts_and_figures/maternal_mortality.htm (accessed May 15, 2005).
21. J. L. Simpson, "Fetal Wastage," In *Obstetrics: Normal and Problem Pregnancies,* 4th ed., S. G. Gabbe, J. R. Niebyl, and J. L. Simpson, eds. (Philadelphia, PA: Churchill Livingstone, 2002), p. 743.
22. *Dorland's Illustrated Medical Dictionary,* http://www.mercksource.com/pp/us/cns/cns_hl_dorlands.jspzQzpgzEzzSzppdocszSzuszSzcommonzSzdorlandszSzdorlandzSzdmd_a_02zPzhtm#12101848 (accessed February 6, 2006).
23. The Thompson Corporation, "Definition High Risk Pregnancy" (1999), http://www.chclibrary.org/micromed/00051310.html (accessed June 8, 2005).
24. M. Brooks, "Pregnancy Preeclampsia," *Emergency Medicine,* http://www.emedicine.com/emerg/topic480.htm (accessed February 7, 2006).
25. Preeclampsia Organization, "What Is Preeclampsia?" (2000), http://www.preeclampsia.orgr/seattlemandate.pdf (accessed June 9, 2005).
26. B. M. Sibai, "Risk Factors for Preeclampsia, Abruptio Placentae, and Adverse Neonatal Outcomes Among Women with Chronic Hypertension," http://www.ncemch.org/alert091198.htm#4 (accessed June 10, 2005).
27. J. A. Marx, ed., *Rosen's Emergency Medicine Concepts and Clinical Practice,* 5th ed. (St. Louis, MO: Elsevier Mosby, 2002), pp. 2420–2422.
28. B. R. Sweet and D. Tiran, *Mayes' Midwifery: A Textbook for Midwives,* 12th ed. (London: Bailliere Tindall, 1999).
29. G. J. White, *Emergency Childbirth: A Manual* (Marble Hill, MO: NAPSAC Reproductions, 1994).
30. World Health Organization, "Definition of Skilled Attendant" (2004), http://www.who.int/reproductive-health/global_monitoring/skilled_attendant.htm (accessed June 10, 2005).
31. A. DeJonge, T. A. Teunissen, and A. L. Lago-Janssen, "Supine Position Compared to Other Positions During the Second Stage of Labor: A Meta-Analytic Review," *Journal of Psychosomatic Obstetrics and Gynaecology* 25 (2004): 35–45.
32. M. Enkin, M. J. Keirse, M. Renfrew, and J. Neilson, *A Guide to Effective Care in Pregnancy & Childbirth,* 2nd ed. (New York, NY: Oxford University Press, 1999).
33. J. T. Parer, *Handbook of Fetal Heart Rate Monitoring,* 2nd ed. (Philadelphia, PA: W. B. Saunders, 1997).
34. L. Doan-Wiggins, "Trauma in Pregnancy," In *Obstetrics and Gynecologic Emergencies,* G. I. Benrubi, ed. (Philadelphia, PA: J. P. Lippincott, 1994), p. 63.
35. A. Frye, *Holistic Midwifery: A Comprehensive Textbook for Midwives in Homebirth Practice. Volume II: Care of the Mother and Baby From Onset of Labor Through the First Hours After Birth* (Portland, OR: Labrys Press, 2004), p. 1136.
36. B. L. Morgan and M. G. Ross, "Umbilical Cord Complications" (May 14, 2003), http://www.emedicine.com/med/topic3276.htm (accessed May 25, 2005).
37. M. Banks, *Breech Birth: Woman Wise* (Hamilton, New Zealand: Birthspirit Books, 1998).
38. S. M. Lanni and J. W. Seeds, "Malpresentations," In *Obstetrics: Normal and Problem Pregnancies,* 4th ed., S. G. Gabbe, J. R. Niebyl, and J. L. Simpson, eds. (Philadelphia, PA: Churchill Livingstone, 2002), p. 482.
39. E. P. Tappero and M. E. Honeyfield, *Physical Assessment of the Newborn: A Comprehensive Approach to the Art of Physical Examination* (Pestaluma, CA: NICU INK, 1993).

part 5

Special Populations

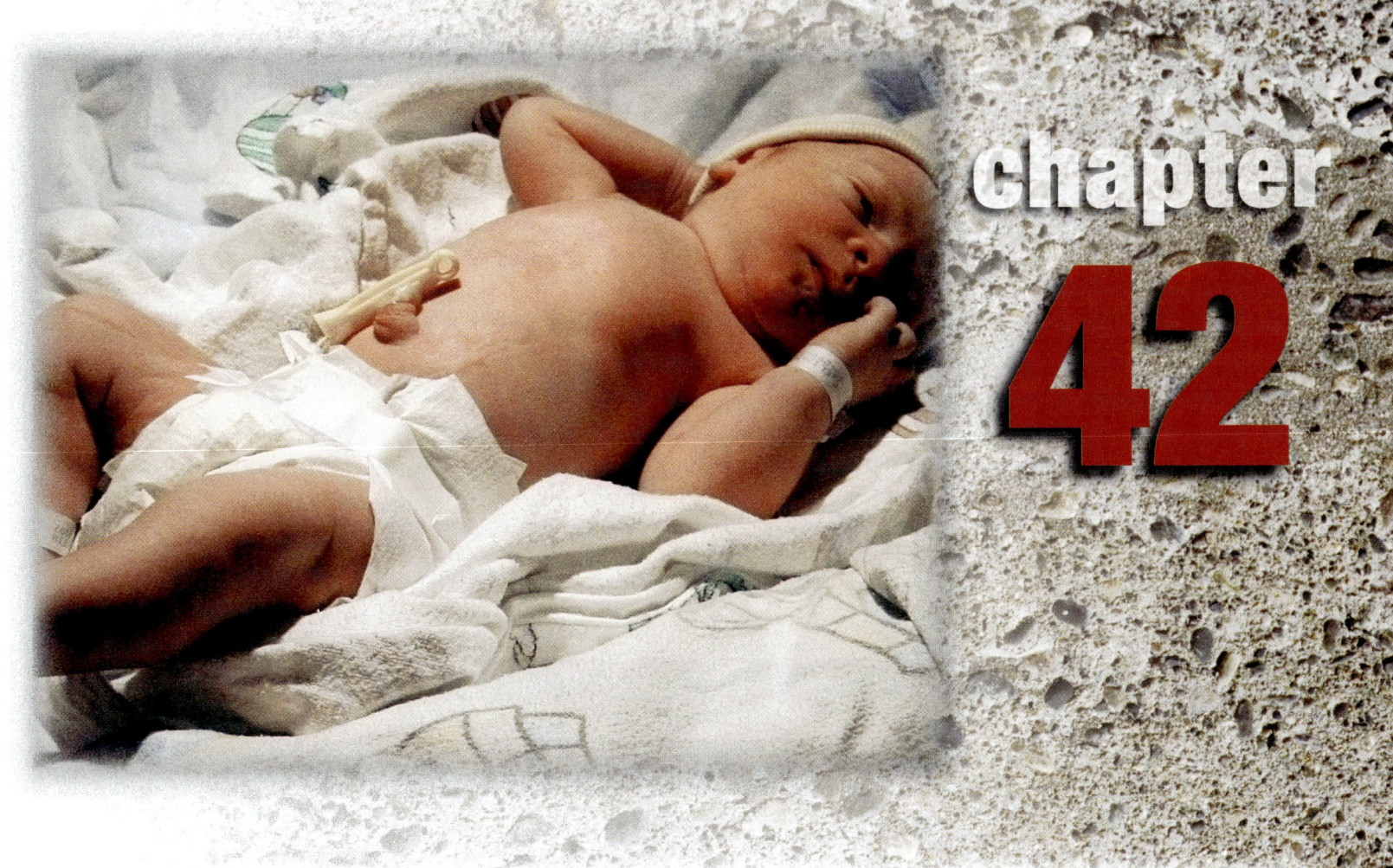

Neonatology

"*C*hildren are one-third of our population and all of our future."

—Select Panel for the Promotion of Child Health, 1981

Need to Know

▶ Neonatal resuscitation should follow a standardized approach that focuses on assessing the ABCs and providing standard treatments when abnormalities are detected.

▶ Most problems arising during childbirth have a respiratory cause, which is frequently corrected with blow-by oxygen administration or bag-mask ventilation.

▶ Only 1 of 10 out-of-hospital births requires resuscitation.
  • Of those, 1% (or 1 in 1000 total out-of-hospital births) has significant complications that require aggressive management.

▶ All treatments performed during neonatal resuscitation should be done for 30 to 60 seconds, and then the patient should be reassessed.

▶ The paramedic should move up or down within the neonatal resuscitation algorithm, one step at a time, depending upon how the infant is responding to treatments.

▶ Intubation should not be performed unless positive pressure ventilations (PPV) with a bag-mask unit have failed to increase the heart rate over 60, the infant persists with apnea despite PPV, or the infant is in cardiac arrest.

▶ Intubation for the purpose of meconium suction with a meconium aspirator and ET tube should be performed immediately after the child delivers if the meconium is thick. Intubation following the completion of meconium suctioning is not necessary in most cases.

▶ Sick

• Any neonate with a heart rate of 60–100 BPM needs PPV bag-mask ventilations. Reassess after every 30 seconds, and determine if this is still needed.

• Any neonate with a heart rate less than 60 needs PPV and, if they do not improve, PPV and CPR.

• Use of naloxone or other narcotic antagonists should not be first-line therapy; manage the patient with oxygen and ventilatory support first, and consider naloxone when respiratory depression persists after the heart rate is within the normal range of greater than 100 bpm.

• Secondary apnea requires PPV ventilatory support because the infant is too tired to overcome the problem on their own.

• Central cyanosis is always an abnormal finding. It should begin clearing up if the patient is responding well to oxygenation and ventilation.

▶ Not Yet Sick

• Determine if the baby is breathing and crying at least 30 to 60 times a minute; if not, intervention is required.

• Determine if the heart rate is at least 100 per minute; if not, intervention is required.

• Obtain an APGAR score at one and five minutes. Determine if the baby has good muscle tone.

• Infants with a RR of 30 to 60 are not sick; however, infants with rates in the low end of normal (30–40) with acrocyanosis (blue arms and legs) need blow-by oxygen and perhaps PPV.

• Infants with a heart rate greater than 100 are not sick.

• Infants with a heart rate between 60 and 100 are not sick if they are responding to oxygen and ventilatory support with an ever increasing heart rate and respiratory rate.

• Primary apnea can be treated with blow-by oxygen and should resolve after the infant has recovered from the stress of the birthing process. If unrecognized or left untreated, it can develop into secondary apnea.

• Infants with APGAR scores above seven are not sick.

• Acrocyanosis is normal when the infant continues to respond favorably to treatment.

• Ask about prenatal care, anticipated complications, and whether this is a single or multiple birth event.

• Ask if the baby was at or near term.

• If not witnessed, ask if the amniotic fluid was clear of thick meconium, thin meconium, or any signs of discoloration that might indicate infection.

Introduction

Precipitous deliveries are those that occur spontaneously or away from the setting for which they were intended, which is usually the hospital labor and delivery unit. It is estimated that less than 1% of deliveries in the United States happen outside an appropriate medical birthing facility.[1] This number includes planned home deliveries, a popular trend in America. Often, these planned deliveries are attended by midwives or other trained healthcare professionals instead of EMS providers. This makes the numbers of precipitous births attended to by paramedics even less prevalent than the 1% overall statistic.

Anxiety may be experienced by the prehospital provider during active labor and immediately following birth because of unfamiliarity with these situations and because of the acute awareness of serious complications that can occur with the newborn, especially if the child is premature. This chapter will focus on the basics of newborn management and resuscitation that every prehospital provider will need to know to be comfortable with deliveries. It will discuss how to manage the newly born infant during the transition to the hospital setting.

Neonatology Terminology

Newborn

A **newborn** is an infant who was just delivered from the mother's body. The photograph on the chapter opener shows a newborn just a few minutes old. The term "newborn" can be used as either a noun or an adjective; "Is this your newborn?" or "This infant is newborn." Either way, it is placing a time frame on the child as having just been born. It does not make a distinction as to the length of the gestational time frame. Gestation is the length of time the baby spends growing and developing inside the uterus. DOT 6-1.2

Fetus

Fetus is the term used to describe the infant while it is still living inside the uterus of the mother. The fetus (Figure 42-1) is totally dependent upon the maternal circulation for the delivery of oxygen and nutrients and the removal of all wastes. The fetus is connected to the mother through the placenta, which is attached to the inside of the uterus.

Full-Term Infants

The normal length of gestation during pregnancy is 40 weeks. Newborns at 40 weeks' gestation are described as **full term.** Often, the gestational time frame is estimated because it is not always possible to pinpoint the exact date that conception took place. Estimates of this date are made from information gathered from the mother, comparisons with the timing of her menstrual cycle, evaluation of the changes occurring to the mother, and the size (growth rate) of the uterus during the pregnancy.

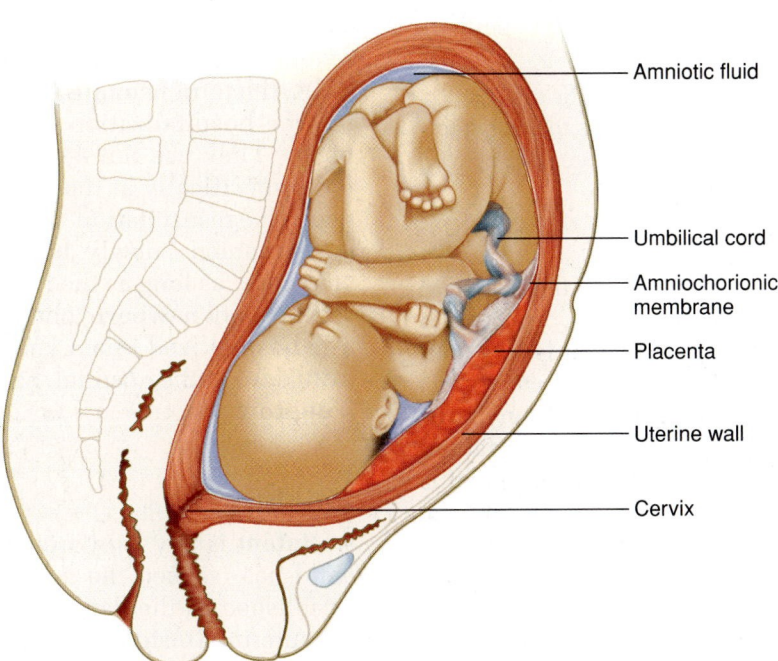

- Amniotic fluid
- Umbilical cord
- Amniochorionic membrane
- Placenta
- Uterine wall
- Cervix

Figure 42-1   The fetus is connected to the mother via the placenta. This full term fetus is in the vertex position and is ready for delivery.

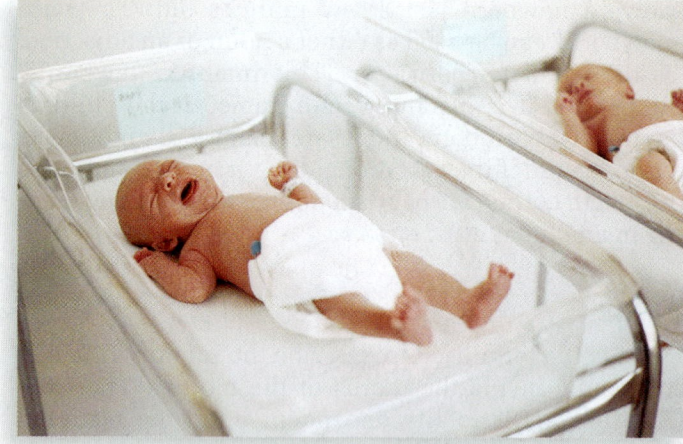

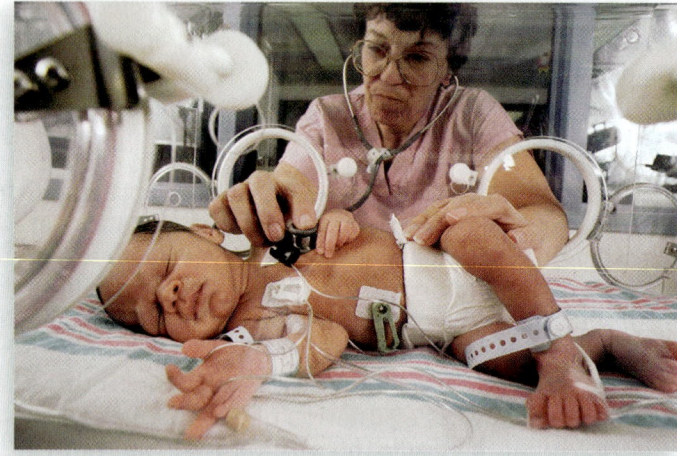

Figure 42-2 Premature infants are often smaller, less able to regulate body temperature, and their lungs are less developed than term infants.

CONNECTIONS Return to Chapter 41: Obstetrics and Gynecology. Figure 41-5 (on page 1004) shows the enlarged uterus and organ displacement of a full-term pregnancy.

Premature Newborns

Although terminology varies, according to the Neonatal Intensive Care Unit at the University of Chicago Comer Children's Hospital, a **premature newborn** is less than 37 weeks' gestational age while a "full-term newborn" is 37 weeks of gestation and above. Premature newborns with a body weight between 700 and 1,000 grams (about 1.5 to 2.2 pounds) survive, but the rate of survival in this group is approximately 80%.[2] Figure 42-2 shows the difference in size between a term newborn and a premature newborn. Premature infants have difficulty maintaining their body temperature, and hypothermia is likely, even when appropriate steps for normal-sized newborns are used. DOT 6-1.6, 6-1.51

Advances in science have increased the rate of survival for premature infants so that some children born

as young as 20 weeks of gestation (five months) have survived. These children have significant hospital stays of up to a year or longer and often have developmental disabilities or significant health problems. However, some of these premature children survive with surprisingly few long-term complications.[4]

Neonates, Newly Born Infants, and Newborns

The terms *neonate* and *newborn* traditionally implied that the child was less than one month old from the date of birth. Unfortunately, these terms have not always had a clear definition, which has lead to confusion. The American Heart Association 2005 Guidelines redefined these terms somewhat. According to the AHA, the term **neonate** is best used for any infant during the hospitalization phase immediately following birth.[3] They use the term **newly born** to identify infants specifically at the time of birth. In other words, once the resuscitation phase is complete, the previously named "newly born" infant is now called a "neonate" as long as the infant remains in the hospital setting and **newborn** once he or she is sent home. The hospitalized infant keeps the term neonate for up to 30 days in the hospital, but they could keep it longer, if appropriate. DOT 6-1.2, 6-1.3

Infants

An **infant** is any baby from the time of birth until the child has reached the first birthday. The birth date is established as the date the fetus transitioned from the intrauterine (inside the uterus) environment to the extrauterine (outside the uterus) environment, independent of whether or not the infant was at the 40-week mark of gestation. For infants that are significantly

Nice to Know

Unfortunately, there is no clear guidance on when the term newborn ceases to apply, but in many settings that ends at the 30-day mark. Although this sets some measurable points to use for terminology purposes, it is still not without potential confusion. Fortunately, the term "infant" is appropriate at all times during the first year of life.

premature (again, not easily defined or consistently applied), time may be marked by the date they were expected to reach their 40 week gestation point as well as the actual date they were born. This information is important to the hospital personnel treating the infant and perhaps to the parents, but is usually not of great importance in the prehospital setting.

Knowing an infant is premature may help the paramedic understand why the infant is very small or why the child has certain medical complaints such as respiratory problems or developmental issues, which are consistent with prematurity.

Overdue Infants

Some infants are born after their expected due dates. This could be from a simple miscalculation of the expected due date, it could have no known cause, or it could be due to a medical problem. Often late-term infants are larger than normal.

Street Secrets

If the infant is significantly over the due date, they may have severely irritated skin if the mother's immune system has begun to "attack" the infant as a foreign body.

The birth process may be complicated by the large size of the fetus. The birth of an overdue fetus may require forceful measures such as drug-induced labor or cesarean section. **Cesarean section** is surgical removal of the baby from the uterus. Neither cesarean section nor drug-induced labor should be performed outside the appropriate medical facility.

Prenatal Care

If a pregnant patient has received appropriate prenatal care, she may be aware of expected complications. It is also important to determine when she is due and whether or not multiple births are expected.

Street Secrets

It is helpful to know if she is a first-time mother or if she has delivered other children as the labor process often takes longer with the first pregnancy. All of this information can help guide you in the decision to attempt a field delivery versus performing a rapid transport.

CONNECTIONS Chapter 41: Obstetrics and Gynecology discusses child birth from the perspective of the mother in labor. It provides additional history questions and maternal assessment tips. It also discusses delivery and obstetrical complications such as placenta previa, uterine rupture, and other emergency situations and postdelivery care for the mother.

Epidemiology of Resuscitation

The most likely complication to arise during vaginal childbirth is related to breathing. Why this occurs will be discussed in greater detail along with information regarding how to treat this problem.

Approximately 10% of all newly born infants require some assistance in breathing, with a majority responding appropriately and faring very well with just a few minutes of respiratory or ventilatory assistance. However, 1% of the sub-group of 10% requires additional and extensive resuscitative efforts just to survive.[5] This means that nine out of 10 births are without complications while one of 10 will have some problems, and most of those problems are tied to the respiratory system. Of the one in 10 problem births, 1% of those require aggressive resuscitation measures. This means that one of every 100 problematic births needs significant resuscitation efforts. Aggressive measures include positive pressure ventilation with the bag-mask unit; performing tracheal suctioning; and initiating IV, IO, or umbilical lines for fluid or medication administration. Chest compressions and intubation may be required for a severely bradycardic heart rate or a cardiac arrest situation.
DOT 6-1.39

Nice to Know

Of all births, 10% have complications, and 1% of the 10% have significant complications. So for every 1,000 births, 100 will have a problem; 99 of the 100 will fair pretty well with respiratory support measures, and one of that 100 will require significant interventions just to survive.

TABLE 42-1 Antepartum and Intrapartum Factors

Antepartum Factors	Intrapartum Factors
Smoking	Abnormal fetal presentation (any non-vertex)
No prenatal care	Premature labor
Illicit drug use or medications	Precipitous labor (both out-of-hospital and rapid)
Mother's age (less than 16 or more than 35)	Prolonged rupture of membranes (over 18 hours)
Medical conditions	Prolonged labor (beyond 24 hours)
• Hypertension	Use of narcotics within the past four hours
• Diabetes	Meconium stained amniotic fluid
• Renal disease	Prolapsed cord
Multiple gestations	Abruptio placentae (placenta breaks off uterine wall)
Trauma	Placenta previa (placenta implanted in lower uterine segment)
• Maternal distress	
• Premature rupture of membranes	

Birth Weight Complications

As previously discussed, prematurity can cause problems. But it is not only the gestational age of the infant that determines complications; birth weight can cause complications as well. There is only a partial relationship between birth weight and the rates of complications.

About 80% of newborns weighing less than 1,500 grams (1.5 kg or 3.3 pounds) at the time of delivery require some sort of resuscitation.[1]

Many low birth weight babies simply need extra attention to preserve body heat and fare well with the application of oxygen. Some require more aggressive measures such as those outlined previously. DOT 6-1.30, 6-1.48, 6-1.49, 6-1.50, 6-1.51

Antepartum and Intrapartum Factors Causing Problems with Delivery

There are many factors, known as antepartum and intrapartum factors, that cause low birth weight or premature delivery before 37 weeks of gestation. **Antepartum factors** are variables that are present before labor begins. **Intrapartum factors** are defined as variables that occur during labor or the birthing process. Common variables are listed in Table 42-1. DOT 6-1.4, 6-1.5

Pathophysiology of Circulatory Changes during Birth

The newborn heart rate is known to be the most sensitive indicator in evaluating physiological distress.[6] Since the neonate has a fixed stroke volume, the cardiac output depends solely on the heart rate. Bradycardia is caused by hypoxia, and hypoxia is the result of poor respiratory circulation. DOT 6-1.44, 6-1.45

The most exceptional physiological change required of the newborn occurs during the transition from the intrauterine to the extrauterine environment. During this change, the cardiovascular and respiratory systems transition from the placenta-dependent fetal circulation to the autonomous first breath and self-support systems.

During fetal life, the lungs are essentially nonfunctional. Complete support comes from the mother via the placenta that is attached to the inner surface of the uterus (Figure 42-3). Typically, the newborn's metabolic system begins to change over from maternal support to self-support as the chest emerges from the vaginal canal. This squeezing phenomenon prepares the lungs for the first breath by pushing some of the amniotic fluid out of the nose and mouth. Air enters the upper airway to replace the lost fluid during the brisk recoil of the thorax as the chest emerges from the vagina. This is why it is important to try to clear the airway while the head is still protruding from the birthing canal before the shoulders and chest emerge.

If the amniotic fluid is stained with thick, chunky meconium, tracheal suction will need to be performed with a meconium aspirator. Meconium, which is fetal fecal matter (or stool), acts like tar and will plug the bronchi and coat the inner surface of the alveoli, causing their walls to stick together when they deflate. Managing

Nice to Know

The optimal position for the infant to be born in to allow for the immediate resumption of self-supported metabolic processes is the head first, face down position, which promotes drainage of secretions from the mouth and nose. This position is called the **vertex position.** (Refer back to Figure 42-1.)

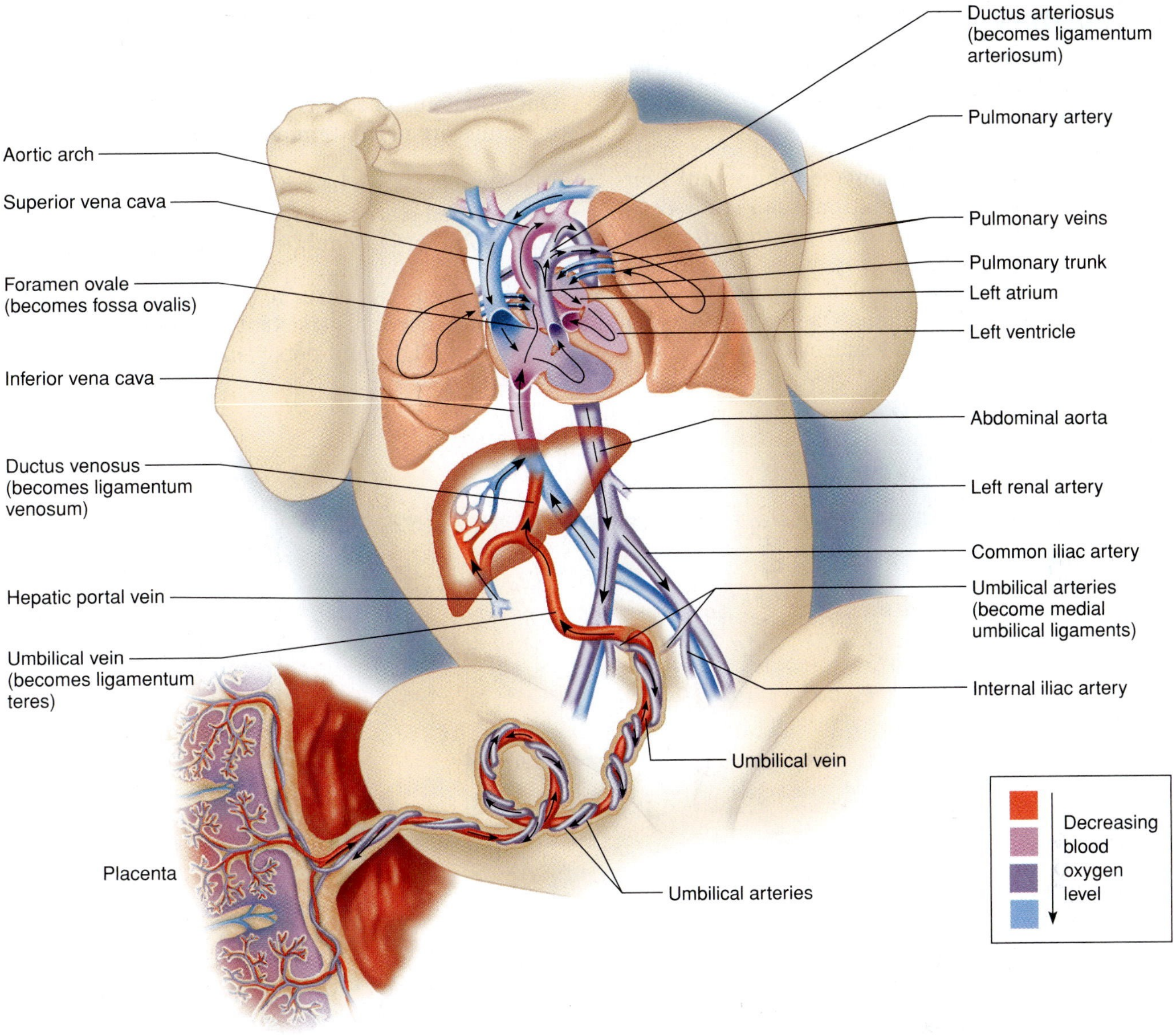
Ductus arteriosus
(becomes ligamentum
arteriosum)
Pulmonary artery
Aortic arch
Superior vena cava
Pulmonary veins
Pulmonary trunk
Foramen ovale
(becomes fossa ovalis)
Left atrium
Left ventricle
Inferior vena cava
Abdominal aorta
Ductus venosus
(becomes ligamentum
venosum)
Left renal artery
Common iliac artery
Hepatic portal vein
Umbilical arteries
(become medial
umbilical ligaments)
Umbilical vein
(becomes ligamentum
teres)
Internal iliac artery
Umbilical vein
Decreasing
blood
oxygen
level
Placenta
Umbilical arteries

Figure 42-3 Fetal circulation. The two umbilical arteries and one umbilical vein make up the umbilical cord. This cord links the placenta to the fetus. The umbilical cord attaches directly into the liver.

infants with meconium will be discussed in greater detail later in this chapter.

The First Breath

After the newborn is delivered, the first breath happens within seconds. Two factors initiate this response:

1. *Chemical factors,* which include low oxygen levels in the hemoglobin (hypoxemia), high levels of carbon dioxide, and a low (acidic) pH level. This combination stimulates the respiratory center in the medulla.
2. The *thermal factor* stimulates the respiratory center as the body responds to the air temperature. This happens when the fetus leaves the warm environment of the uterus and enters the cool environment of the delivery area.

With the first breath, oxygen-enriched air rapidly rushes into the alveoli, displacing the fluid and inflating the sacks. With every newborn breath, the oxygen concentration is increased in the blood, starting a chain of circulatory events. A chemical substance that is produced by the body, called surfactant, aids in the ease with which the alveoli reinflate after they empty. Surfactant production begins during the final weeks of gestation and is typically not present in infants born prior to the 37th week. These infants require ventilatory support to prevent permanent alveolar collapse, and their lungs are often described as "stiff" and noncompliant to ventilatory efforts. They must be handled carefully as too forceful a ventilation can result in barotrauma (pressure caused damage) while breaths that are not forceful enough will not allow for ventilation.

The Circulatory Transition to Self-Support

As the infant continues to breathe more and more air, pulmonary arterioles start to dilate, allowing more oxygen to enter the pulmonary bloodstream. This increased oxygen supply stimulates the closure of the fetal shunting system that connected the infant's circulation to the maternal circulation (see Figure 42-3). These shunts are the *foramen ovale, ductus arteriosus,* and *ductus venosus.* When they were functioning, these shunts allowed the blood to bypass the lungs and supply the rest of the fetus's body with oxygen from the placenta. Figure 42-4 schematically describes the fetal circulation. DOT 6-1.8

Problems Preventing the Transition to Fetal Circulation

Once the fetus becomes a newborn, normally functioning lungs are needed immediately.

The oxygen-enriched blood will start to close the shunts that were required for fetal circulation, forcing the blood into the pulmonary circulatory system.

Two problems can occur to prevent this smooth transition from occurring: persistent pulmonary hypertension-newborn (PPHN) and persistent fetal circulation (PFC). DOT 6-1.40

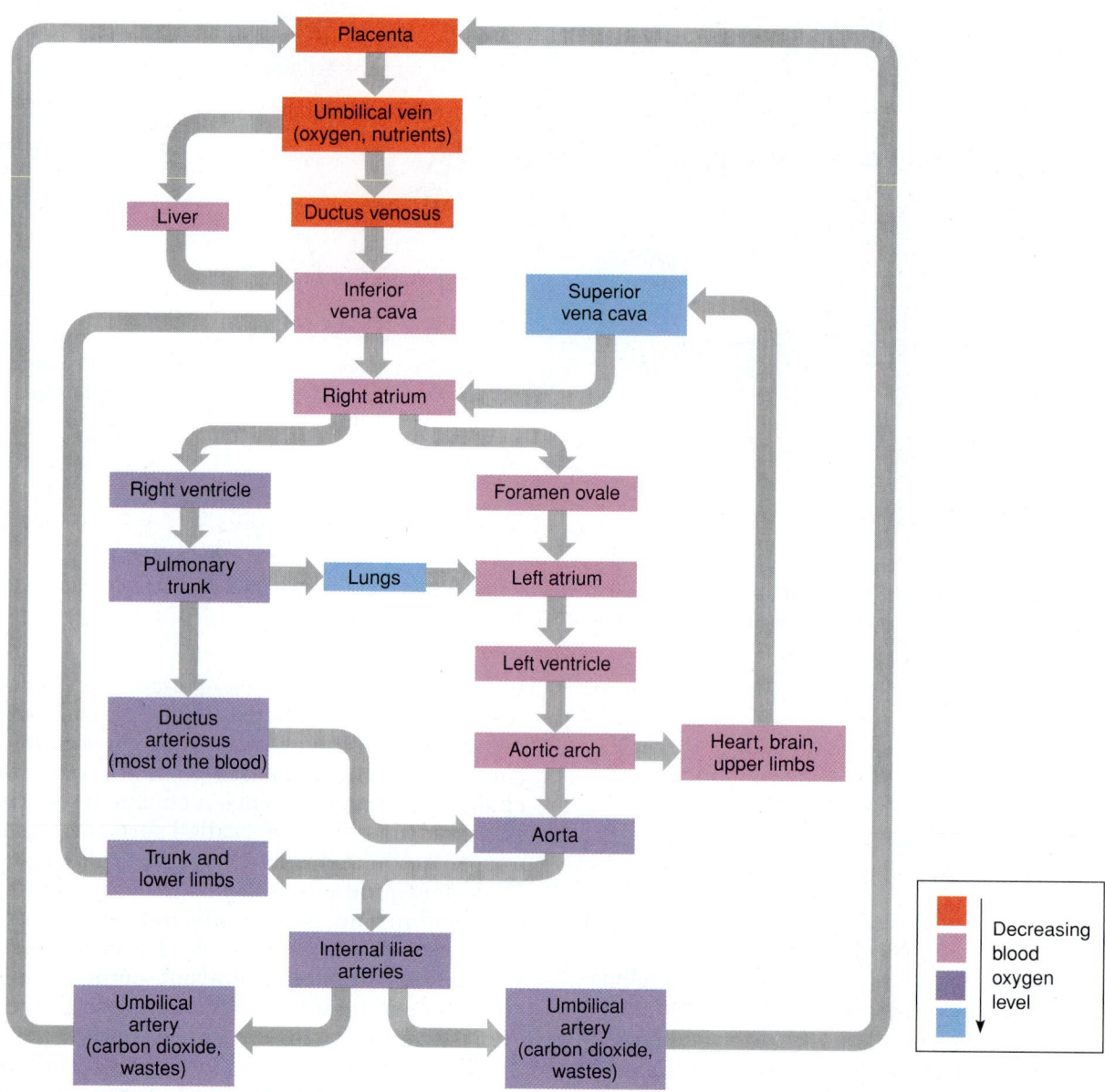

Figure 42-4   The general pattern of fetal circulation shown schematically.

Persistent Pulmonary Hypertension-Newborn

If the newborn has meconium-filled alveoli, normal expansion cannot take place. This causes an increased pressure within the chest that will keep blood from flowing to the lungs. Blood being shunted away from the lungs causes a hypoxemic (low blood oxygen level) state. This condition is known as **persistent pulmonary hypertension-newborn (PPHN)**. Infants in this state are not able to oxygenate their own blood, and if uncorrected, death will occur. Suctioning the trachea and bronchi can help correct this problem. DOT 6-1.13

Persistent Fetal Circulation

The infant may maintain a metabolic acidosis state if the infant is allowed to become hypothermic. The infant has little body fat, and the energy reserves deplete quickly. This leads to increased levels of acid accumulating in the blood. As the infant's glucose levels deplete, hypoglycemia develops. These reactions worsen the acidotic state, putting additional stress on the infant. DOT 6-1.13

A persistent acidotic state can retrigger the resumption of fetal circulation and cause a condition known as **persistent fetal circulation (PFC)**. This reopens the fetal shunts that were closing and decreases the flow of blood to the lungs. Eventually, the oxygen supply decreases, ending in a vicious, revolving cycle. If the blood flow through the placenta has ceased, the infant will no longer be getting any more oxygen from the mother.

Street Secrets

Not properly drying and rewarming the infant quickly results in the burning of brown fat to preserve body heat.

Preventing PPHN and PFC

The paramedic can help prevent both PPHN and PFC. If meconium-stained fluid is present, early tracheal suction should be performed. The infant should also be provided with a warm environment. The newborn should be kept dry and out of wet towels.

Primary and Secondary Apnea

The respiratory system is the first system to fail when the newborn is compromised. According to the American Academy of Pediatrics, "Respiration is the first vital sign to cease when a newborn is deprived of oxygen."[7] This is evident when explaining primary and secondary apnea.

Primary apnea is the newborn's futile attempt to compensate when fatigued (tired). Primary apnea will manifest as a period of rapid respirations followed by a period of apnea. This apnea is treated through stimulation activities such as tapping the feet, drying with warm towels, or gently rubbing the back. There will be no changes in heart rate or blood pressure during episodes of primary apnea. That is why it is important to watch the patient closely and not rely on monitors as the sole source for information. Untreated primary apnea episodes will continue until the newborn cannot compensate any longer. DOT 6-1.14, 6-1.40, 6-1.42

Primary apnea leads to secondary apnea. **Secondary apnea** occurs when the infant ceases to breath and there is a considerable drop in both heart rate and blood pressure (Figure 42-5). DOT 6-2.7

Simple stimulation will not correct secondary apnea episodes. The paramedic needs to assist ventilations. Fortunately, neonates respond well to this procedure. Use an appropriately sized bag-mask system that is connected to supplemental oxygen. Provide just enough positive pressure to visualize the rise of the chest.

Positive pressure ventilation (PPV) will increase the heart rate, blood pressure, and the oxygen saturation rate. Perform the bag-mask ventilations at a rate of one per second or one per 1.5 seconds (40 to 60 per minute) for one minute and reassess. Continue as needed until the infant responds with an appropriate rate of their own. Blow-by oxygen administration may be needed to replace PPV once the infant can sustain a respiratory rate of 30 to 60. DOT 6-1.52, 6-1.53, 6-1.54, 6-1.55

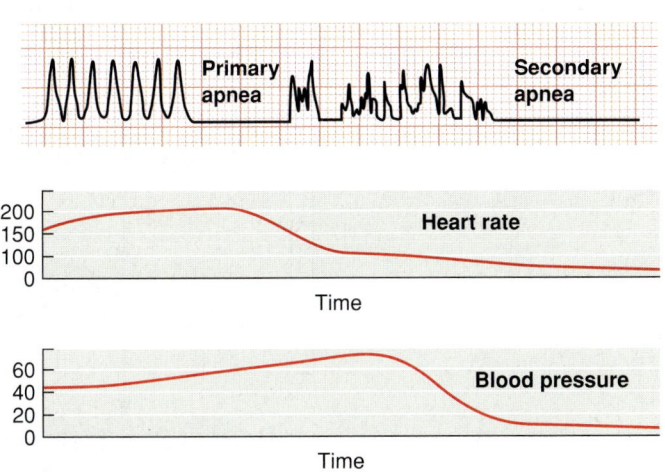

Figure 42-5   Fetal monitor tracing showing the effect of primary and secondary apnea on heart rates and blood pressure.

The AHA Initial Resuscitation Algorithm for Newborns

The previous portion of this chapter focused on neonatal resuscitation from the perspective of physiology by discussing what is occurring as the fetus transitions during the birthing process. Each part describes how a paramedic can respond to abnormal findings to try to improve the infant's vital signs. Thus far, this discussion has not provided a step-by-step process to work through in performing the neonatal resuscitation which we will now review.

The American Heart Association has an algorithm for the resuscitation of newborns that follows a logical progression based upon assessment findings, treatments, and reassessment (Figure 42-6).

As you progress through this algorithm, it is important to perform each intervention and treatment for approximately 30 seconds and then reassess the infant.

If the infant responds appropriately, there will be an improvement in skin color and an increase in respiratory rate and heart rate.

The optimal respiratory rate is 30 to 60, and the optimal heart rate is greater than 100.

Neonatal Flow Algorithm

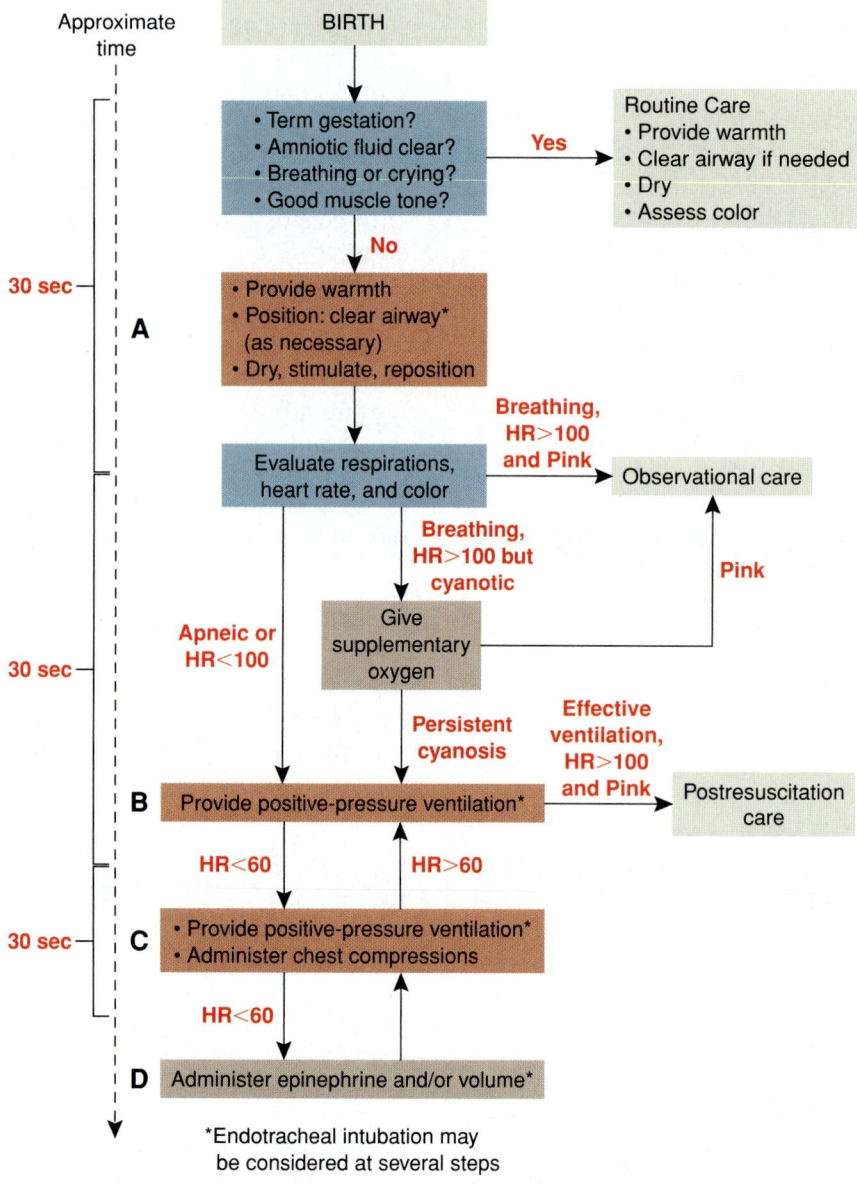

Figure 42-6 Neonatal resuscitation algorithm.

When the infant does not meet these target rates, interventions must be performed until these rates are met. DOT 6-1.10

Stimulate and Check for Responsiveness

As the infant's head emerges, suction the mouth (first) and nose (second) with the bulb syringe. This should occur prior to the shoulders and thorax emerging. If the infant has completely emerged, perform bulb suction only if spontaneous respirations have not yet started or the infant's breathing sounds "wet." The infant's head and neck should always be supported in a neutral alignment, and the infant should be handled gently. DOT 6-1.9

Stimulate the infant, and check for responsiveness (Figure 42-7). Rubbing the soles of their feet will result in movement of the legs and flaring of their toes and also stimulates the child to breathe and cry. Rubbing their back will cause the infant to slightly arch their back. They dislike the gentle rubbing along their spine, and it will trigger breathing and crying. It is never appropriate to dangle children upside down or slap their bottom.

The act of drying also stimulates the infant to cry and breathe. Be careful not to place too much pressure on the top of the head or to rub too vigorously. Discard the last wet towel, and wrap the infant in a clean, dry towel to conserve body heat. Cover the head as this area can be a significant source of heat loss and can lead to hypothermia. DOT 6-1.64

> If thick meconium is present, tracheal suctioning with a meconium aspirator is the first step in the resuscitation process. This will be discussed later in this chapter.

Street Secrets

It is unnecessary to immediately clamp or cut the umbilical cord once the infant is born. However, an uncut cord does restrict how much movement you have, so it should be cut as soon as practical, but it should not take priority over resuscitation efforts. Until the cord is cut, you should hold the infant higher than the cord. Clamp the cord at least 5 to 7 inches away from the infant's abdomen and then 3 inches beyond that point. The umbilical cord can be used to access the infant's circulation for up to seven days if the cord is not treated.

Skin Color Check

Normal newborns may be pink all over, or they may have a pink body and bluish colored extremities **(peripheral cyanosis).** Peripheral cyanosis, along with a pink core, is called **acrocyanosis.** This condition is considered a near-normal finding immediately following birth, and it indicates the infant has slow or sluggish circulation

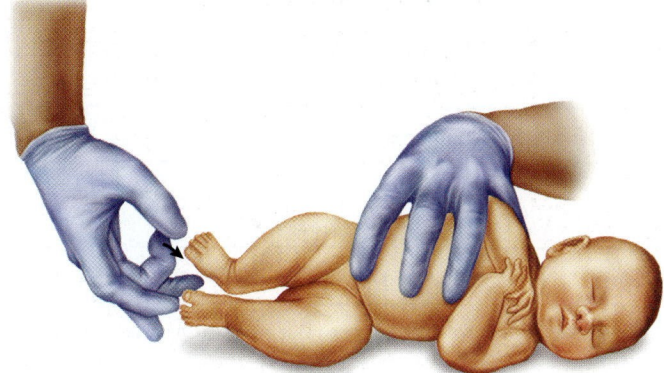

Figure 42-7   Stimulate the infant by flicking the soles of the feet or rubbing the back.

to the arms and legs. If it clears within a few hours, it is not considered a problem. To be considered an acceptable finding, the infant should still have a normal respiratory rate, grimace, activity level, and so on.

The combination of central and peripheral cyanosis is a problem. Central cyanosis accompanied by a bluish discoloration of oral mucous membranes and generalized body cyanosis is a critical finding and a late sign of infant respiratory distress syndrome or IRDS. It might be relieved when treated with supplemental oxygen via the blow-by method, but the newborn will tire quickly without any ventilatory support and will require positive pressure bag-mask ventilations. Central cyanosis can be seen 30 minutes to two hours after birth. The paramedic should keep this in mind if delivery happened prior to the prehospital team arrival.

Is Resuscitation Needed?

To determine if resuscitation is needed, ask yourself the following five questions:

1. Was the baby at or near term (37 to 40 weeks)?
2. Was the amniotic fluid clear of thick meconium, thin meconium, or any signs of discoloration that might indicate infection?
3. Is the baby crying and breathing at least 30 to 60 times a minute?
4. Is the heart rate at least 100 per minute?
5. Does the baby have good muscle tone?

If the answer to all of these questions is "yes," the infant will most likely not need any additional resuscitation efforts. As the infant begins to cry, you can position them high on the mother's abdomen with the head angled down towards the mother. This will help facilitate drainage. Continue to observe the skin color, breathing, and activity levels. An APGAR score can be obtained at one minute and five minutes after birth.

TABLE 42-4   The APGAR Assessment

	Appearance	Pulse	Grimace	Activity	Respiratory
0	blue, pale	absent	no response	limp	absent
1	pink body, peripheral cyanosis	below 100	grimace	some flexion	slow, irregular
2	pink body	above 100	cries vigorously	active flexion	crying lustily

Note: APGAR scores should be assessed at one and five minutes and as needed.

APGAR Scores

The **APGAR score** is a tool that quantifies the findings of the neonatal assessment, using easily understood criteria. APGAR evaluates the **a**ppearance (skin color), **p**ulse rate, **g**rimace (responses to stimuli), **a**ctivity level and muscle tone, and **r**espiratory efforts. Table 42-4 includes the criteria for the APGAR score. Current guidelines suggest obtaining APGAR scores at one and five minutes for all neonates. If the score is less than seven points on any single assessment, an updated score should be recorded every five minutes until twenty minutes have passed or a score greater than seven has been achieved. DOT 6-1.11, 6-1.12

Working in the Gray Zone

If a newborn requires resuscitative efforts, obtaining the APGAR score is not a priority. If desired, once the child is resuscitated successfully, the APGAR score can be reconstructed for documentation purposes.

Open the Airway

If the infant is not spontaneously crying and breathing, position the infant supine, and open the airway. Place a layer of padding under the shoulders and along the spine. This should position the child so that the head is neither hyperextended nor hyperflexed. Approximately one inch of padding is sufficient for a normal-sized newborn.

Clear the airway of any material that is present. Note if blood, mucus, or meconium is present. The act of clearing the airway will provide additional stimulation, which may trigger respirations.

Assess for Breathing

Assess the infant for respirations and crying. If a strong cry is present, further resuscitation efforts are not indicated. If the cry is weak or absent, perform a look, listen, and feel for 10 seconds to assess for spontaneous respirations (Figure 42-8). The respiratory rate should be between 30 and 60. If the rate is near 30, continue to closely monitor the infant and consider more aggressive treatment (like blow-by oxygen or bag-mask ventilations) if the respiratory rate does not begin to increase.

The respiratory pattern may be irregular during the first few hours after birth. Respirations are sufficient when central cyanosis is absent or it does not persist. If the infant is noted to occasionally gasp and normal breathing is not noted between the gasping efforts, additional resuscitation is required via blow-by and if no response, bag-mask ventilation. (This indicates primary apnea may be present.)

Check the Pulse

Feel for a pulse. Place a finger around the underside of the base of the umbilical cord where it attaches to the infant's abdomen. Once the umbilical cord is clamped, it will cease to be an appropriate location to determine the heart rate. It is best not to cut the umbilical cord until the heart rate is no longer felt in the cord.

Alternatives to the umbilical pulse are the apical and brachial sites. The apical pulse is assessed by

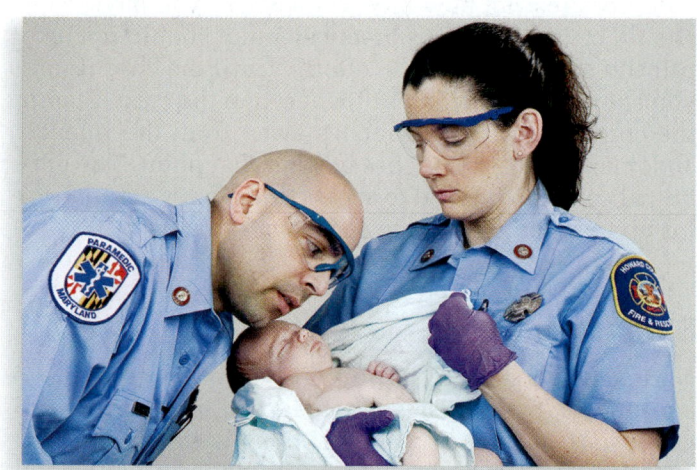

Figure 42-8   Perform the look-listen-feel for at least 10 seconds.

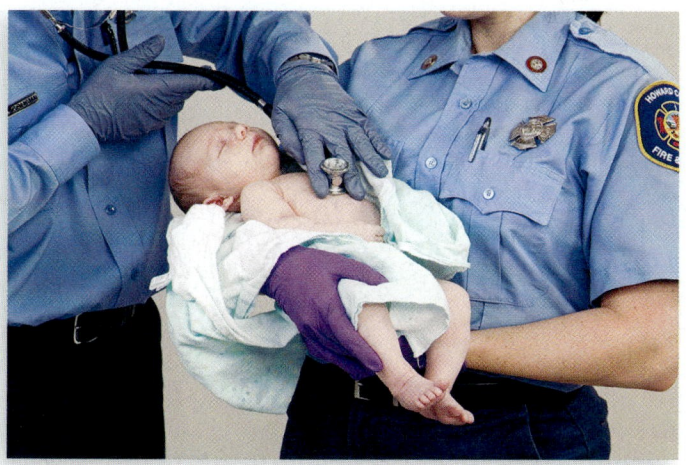

Figure 42-9 The apical pulse is measured by auscultating with a stethoscope directly over the heart.

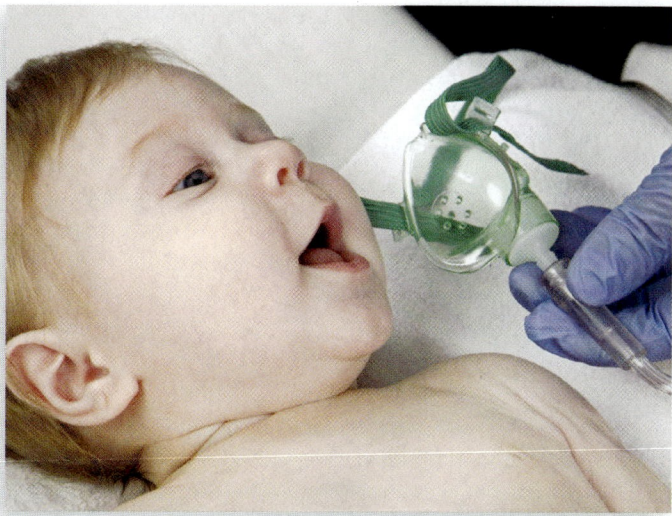

Figure 42-10 Do not chill the infant or flow the oxygen at too high of a liter flow rate as this may cause apnea.

placing the bell (the small piece) of the stethoscope directly over the heart and counting the beats (Figure 42-9). The apical pulse should only be used if the infant is pink or has other evidence of peripheral perfusion. The pulse can also be assessed by feeling for the brachial artery in the upper portion of the arm. Regardless of the location you palpate, the pulse should be greater than 100 beats per minute, or additional treatments are required.

If the infant is pink and has an adequate respiratory rate (30 to 60), and the heart rate is greater than 100 beats per minute, continue to observe the infant and care for the mother. No additional treatment is required for the infant as long as the respiratory and heart rates remain within normal ranges.

If the infant is breathing but the heart rate is between 60 and 100 and the skin color is abnormal, provide supplemental oxygen via the blow-by method. Blow-by oxygen administration is accomplished by holding an oxygen source next to the infant's face. Blow-by is low-flow oxygen, usually set at 0.5 lpm to 1 lpm. It is placed on the side of the newborn's face usually next to the cheek and is held between your index finger and thumb (Figure 42-10). Never put the oxygen directly on the face because this may make the child stop breathing. It needs to be on the side of the face or under the chin. Reassess after 30 seconds, and continue blow-by or provide positive pressure ventilations if the infant's condition is not improving. DOT 6-1.14, 6-1.24, 6-1.25, 6-1.46, 6-1.47

Provide Ventilations as Needed

If the infant is breathing but the heart rate is less than 60, quickly begin performing positive pressure ventilations. Reassess after 30 seconds, and depending upon the response, either provide blow-by oxygen (if the

response is positive), continue to perform bag-mask ventilations (if no change is observed), or add chest compressions (if the RR or HR is decreasing). DOT 6-1.26

If the infant is apneic (not breathing) and the heart rate is less than 60, provide bag-mask ventilations and chest compressions for 30 to 60 seconds and reassess.

Provide positive pressure ventilations with a bag-mask device. Place only enough air into the lungs to cause the chest to begin to rise. If the chest is not rising adequately, reposition the head, suction the airway (if needed), check the mask seal, and try again.

Lung compliance on a newborn requires only 15 to 20 cm H_2O. The lungs can easily be damaged if you are too excited or aggressive in supplying artificial respiration and the pressure valve (pop-off valve) is locked. Premature infants may only need 5–10 mL of air to support their lungs. Always count aloud when providing PPV to maintain a rate of 40 to 60 breaths per minute. DOT 6-1.14

Note that *initial* breaths may require a higher inflating pressure to overcome the resistance in small and fluid-filled airways. If the bag-mask device is equipped with a pop-off valve to regulate pressure, it may need to be disabled in order to allow for the additional pressures needed to ventilate the patient.

Assess the Response to Treatment

Reassess the infant after 30 to 60 seconds of bag-mask ventilations. If the heart rate and respiratory rate are improving, consider providing blow-by oxygen for an additional 30 to 60 seconds. Blow-by oxygen may be provided for the remainder of the transport, provided the infant remains pink and active, and is breathing well.

If the infant is not responding appropriately and the heart rate is less than 60, begin chest compressions

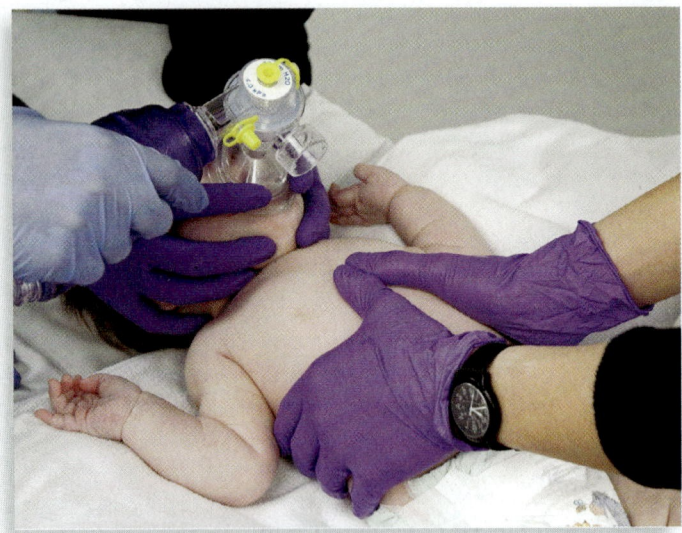

Figure 42-11   A commonly used technique for CPR during neonatal resuscitation is to place both thumbs on the chest and circle the hands around to the back.

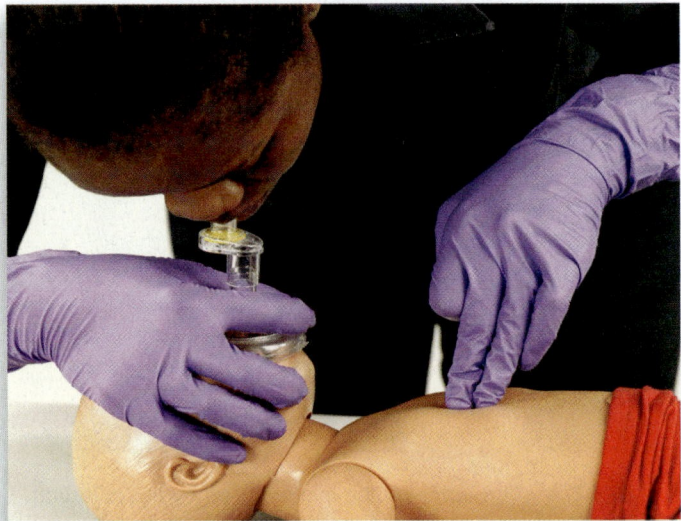

Figure 42-12   Two fingers can also be used to perform CPR.

at a rate of three compressions to one ventilation. Two techniques are recommended: two thumbs pressing the anterior chest with the fingers encircling the chest (Figure 42-11) or using two fingertips on the anterior chest (Figure 42-12). Both procedures should be performed on the lower third of the sternum. The two thumb technique has been shown to perhaps generate higher systolic and coronary perfusion pressures, so this technique is preferred. The anterior procedure may be preferred if access to the umbilical vein is needed. DOT 6-1.15, 6-1.16, 6-1.17

Compress the Chest

When the heart rate is less than 60 beats per minute and the infant is clearly not responding to bag-mask ventilations, begin chest compressions. If after 60 seconds the heart rate is 60 and rising, continue to provide bag-mask ventilations for another 30 to 60 seconds and reassess. Return to compressions any time the heart rate drops below 60. DOT 6-1.15

Chest compressions for the newborn are given in a ratio of 3:1, with three compressions followed by one ventilation. Try to give 120 total events of compressions plus ventilations per minute. Reassess the heart rate after every 30 to 60 seconds until the heart rate improves. As the infant improves, continue to perform PPV for another 30 to 60 seconds and reassess.

Properly utilizing the AHA neonatal algorithm requires that a reassessment occur after 30 to 60 seconds of intervention. When an infant begins to respond favorably, resuscitation efforts should not simply be stopped. For example, if the infant was apneic and the heart rate was 45, once the heart rate is 68, compressions will stop but PPV will not. As the infant continues to improve and

the HR approaches 100, PPV may stop but blow-by will not. DOT 6-1.29

> Move up and down within the algorithm one step at a time. Continue to reassess the child, and move forward or backward depending upon how the infant responds.

Additional Treatment for an Infant Not Responding to Interventions

If the infant is not responding to chest compressions and positive pressure ventilation, additional treatment is needed. Additional treatment includes drug or fluid administration and perhaps intubation. Drugs are rarely needed to resuscitate a newborn.[9] Epinephrine is the most common drug to use, but other drugs may be necessary, particularly if the infant is depressed because of the mother's use of sedatives or narcotics. Because narcotic antagonists like naloxone have not yet been shown to be effective in newborn resuscitation, caution should be used, and consultation should be obtained prior to their use. If fluid volume resuscitation is needed, give boluses at a volume of 10 mL/kg. This may be repeated one time. When using the umbilical vein or if the infant is premature, be careful not to give the fluid too fast. DOT 6-1.18

Umbilical Vein Cannulation

The umbilical vein is the largest hole in the umbilical stump of the three vessels that are there (Figure 42-13). The other two vessels are arteries. The vein is accessed with a 3.5 to 5 French umbilical catheter. This is a sterile technique and should only be attempted if properly trained. If the line is inserted too deeply it will enter into the liver, causing damage (Figure 42-14). When drugs are administered via the umbilical vein, the same dose and

Maternal blood
Umbilical arteries
Umbilical cord
Umbilical vein

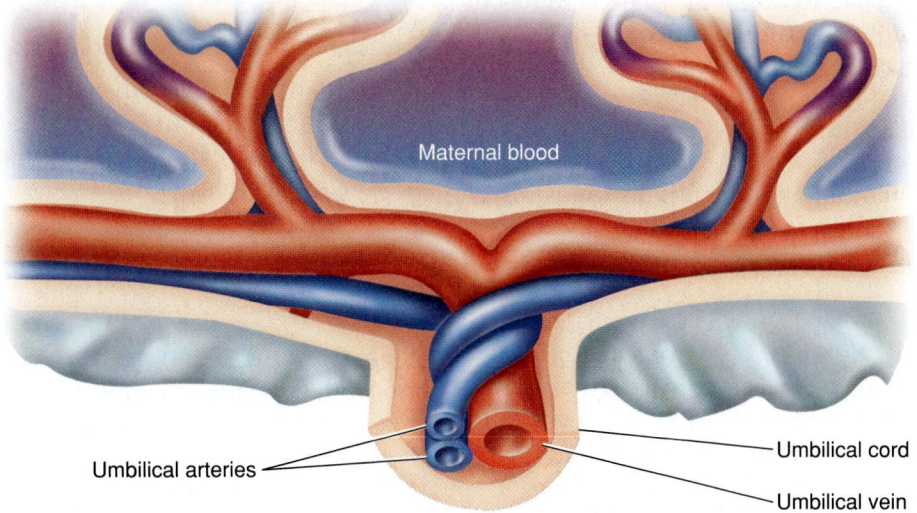

Figure 42-13 The umbilical cord has one vein and two arteries. The vein can be used to access fetal circulation.

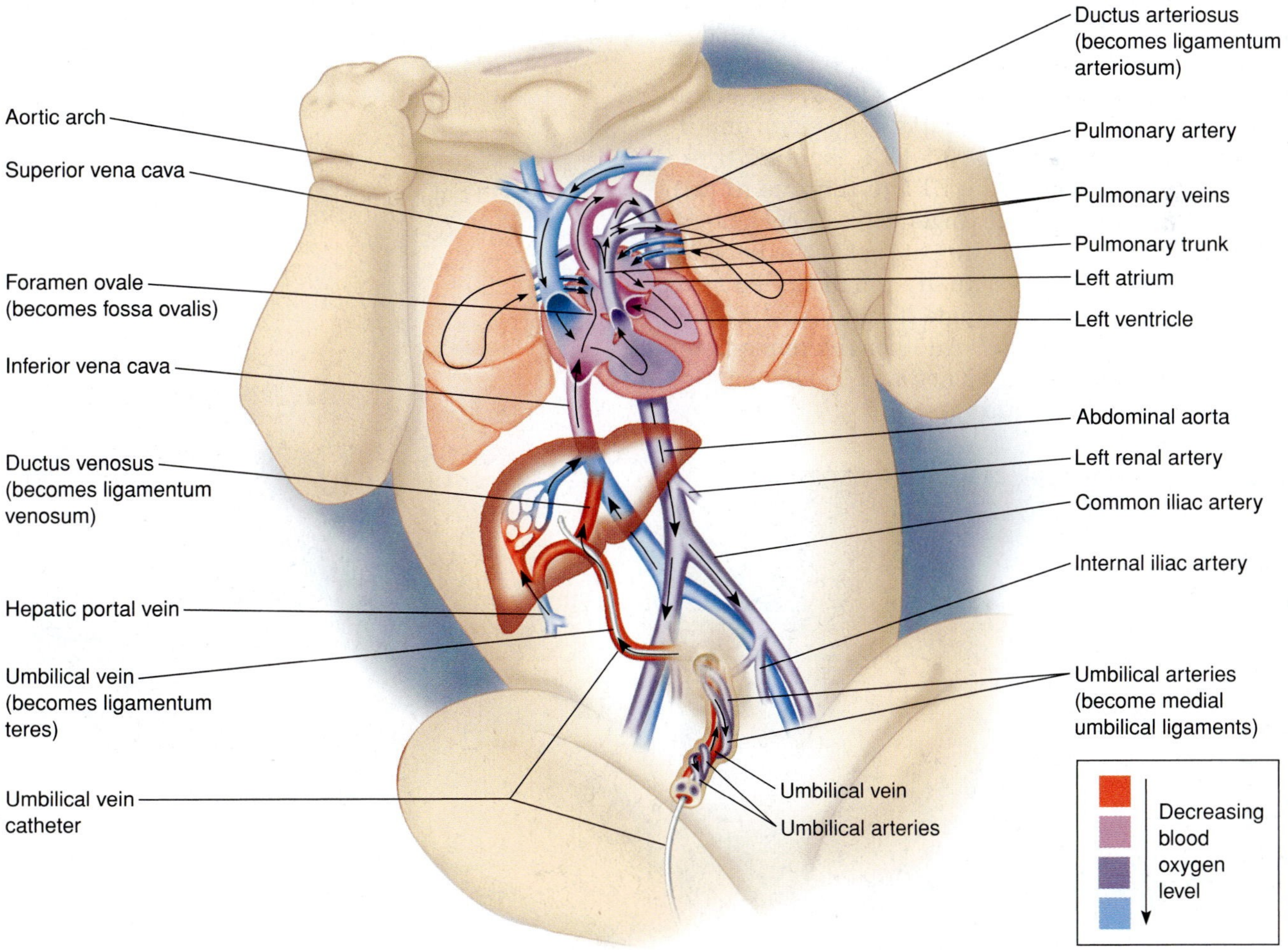

Aortic arch
Superior vena cava
Foramen ovale (becomes fossa ovalis)
Inferior vena cava
Ductus venosus (becomes ligamentum venosum)
Hepatic portal vein
Umbilical vein (becomes ligamentum teres)
Umbilical vein catheter
Ductus arteriosus (becomes ligamentum arteriosum)
Pulmonary artery
Pulmonary veins
Pulmonary trunk
Left atrium
Left ventricle
Abdominal aorta
Left renal artery
Common iliac artery
Internal iliac artery
Umbilical arteries (become medial umbilical ligaments)
Umbilical vein
Umbilical arteries
Decreasing blood oxygen level

Figure 42-14 Umbilical catheterization should only be performed by trained individuals. If the catheter is introduced too deep (as shown in this image), liver damage can occur.

flushing volume should be used as for the IV or IO routes. Care should be used not to instill the fluids too quickly. **See Skill Sheet 46: Umbilical Vein Cannulation.** DOT 6-1.22, 6-1.23

Endotracheal Intubation

Intubation should not be attempted until positive pressure ventilation has failed to result in any improvement in the respiratory rate or heart rate. DOT 6-1.18

CONNECTIONS   Recently, there has been a great deal of controversy surrounding the use of intubation in the prehospital setting, particularly in pediatric patients. Chapter 43: Pediatric Patients has a discussion on the issues surrounding pediatric intubation. DOT 6-1.21

To set up for intubation, make sure you have the appropriately sized equipment, and place a blanket roll under the shoulders and down the back taking care not to hyperextend the neck, which can impair visualization of the vocal cords. Straight laryngoscope blades are preferred and easier to use for pediatric patients.[10]

There are several tricks to determine the appropriate size of the endotracheal tube to use. A rule of thumb is to calculate the size based upon the gestational age. For example, if the child is 25 weeks, use a 2.5 ETT, if 28 weeks use a 3.0 (2.8 is not a size), and if the infant is 35 weeks use the 3.5 ETT. Another trick is to compare the bevel of the ETT to the size of the nare or fingernail on the little finger. If the bevel covers the nailbed or fits into (not snug or loose) the nare, it is the correct size. Do not actually touch the ETT to the child as this will contaminate it, but visualize the tube against these structures. Another reference is to consult prepared charts or devices such as the length-based measuring tape (Figure 42-15).

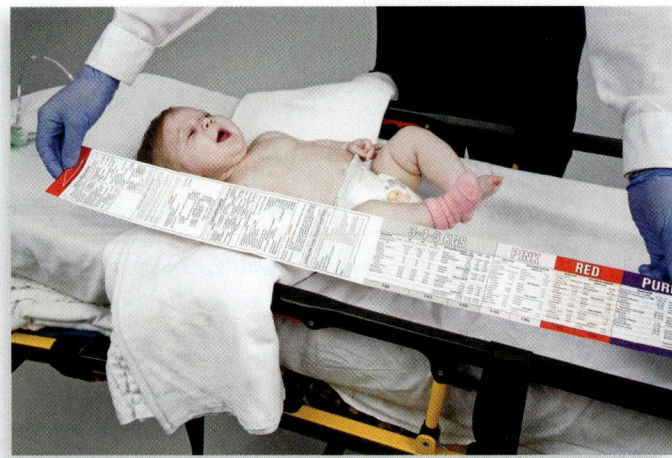

Figure 42-15   The Broselow® tape is a length-based measuring tape used to estimate infant body weight by measuring the infant's length.

Insert the ETT between the cords, visualize the chest rise and fall, and auscultate bilateral breath sounds (Figure 42-16). If the child has spontaneous respiration, it will be difficult to determine tube placement this way, so in conjunction with those methods, use a colorimetric CO_2 detector or an end-tidal CO_2 detector to verify tube placement (Figure 42-17). If a colorimetric device is used, make sure at least six ventilations are given before the colorimetric device is read. Secure the ETT using tape or other approved device. **See Skill Sheet 7 (and Step-by-Step 7): Endotrachael Intubation, Skill Sheet 9 (and Step-by-Step 9): Endotrachael Confirmation Techniques, and Skill Sheet 90: NREMT Pediatric Ventilatory Management.** DOT 6-1.19

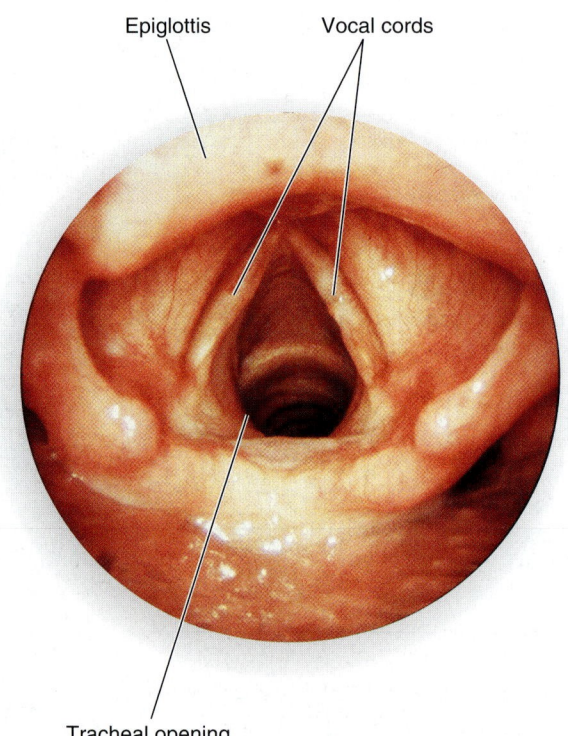

Epiglottis   Vocal cords

Tracheal opening

Figure 42-16   Laryngoscopic view of glottis, epiglottis, and trachael opening during endotracheal intubation of a single patient.

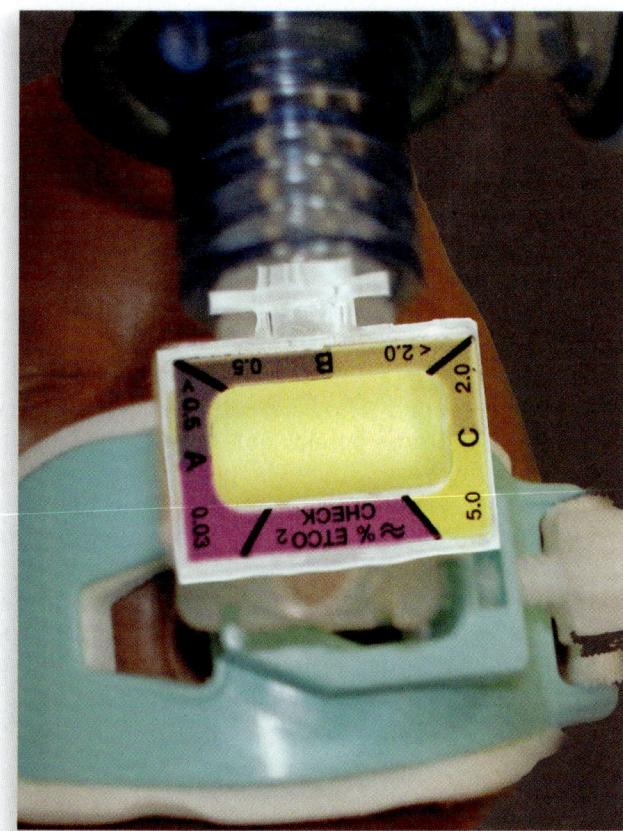

Figure 42-17 Pediatric colorimetric CO_2 detector.

Additional Challenges in Neonatal Resuscitation

Meconium Aspiration

Normally, amniotic fluid is clear and free of debris and particulate matter. Sometimes the mother's amniotic fluid sac has ruptured prior to your arrival, so ask the mother if her "water" was clear or if it was stained with any color (red, green etc.) and if it had any particles or matter in it. If the amniotic fluid is stained with black or green fluid, then it can be assumed the infant was under stress during labor. DOT 6-1.35, 6-1.36

Meconium is fecal matter released by the fetus while in the uterus. It is released when the infant is stressed before delivery. It occurs when the fetus is subjected to fetal asphyxia or other stressors that cause the anal sphincter to relax and pass stool. DOT 6-1.8

The problem with meconium is that it floats around inside the amniotic sac and enters the mouth and nose. If the meconium is thick and tar-like or if it contains chunks of any significant size, it will plug the bronchi if aspirated. Thin, watery meconium does not require aggressive suctioning. The infant will have respiratory compromise if thick meconium is not suctioned out with the meconium aspirator. This can cause foreign

body airway obstruction, PPHN, or aspiration pneumonia. **See Skill Sheet 22 (and Step-by-Step 22): Meconium Suctioning.** DOT 6-1.37

As discussed earlier in the chapter, the first breath occurs as the chest wall of the newborn passes through the vaginal opening, causing a change in pulmonary pressures. This high to low pressure change causes air to rush into the lungs, according to Boyle's law of pressure. Meconium that is thick is tenacious and obstructs the normal air flow and oxygen exchange. The infant's physiological response is to increase respiration, which causes more thoracic negative pressure, trying to get air to flow in. DOT 6-1.36

These infants will have tachypnea and will be severely hypoxic and neurologically depressed. When performing PPV on these infants, they will require high pressures to force air into their lungs. Barotrauma occurs which may result in pneumothoraces. DOT 6-1.37

Thick meconium should be immediately suctioned prior to performing any other resuscitation efforts. The mouth and nose should be suctioned extensively while the head is protruding from the vaginal opening and the chest is still inside the mother. DOT 6-1.38

Once the body is delivered, do not stimulate the child further until deep tracheal and hypopharyngeal suctioning is accomplished. Use a meconium aspirator attached to the endotracheal tube to perform suction. Suction on withdrawal of the ET tube for 10 to 15 seconds.

Working in the Gray Zone

Do not perform suction more than two or three times. Suctioning the first time will likely stimulate the infant into taking breaths unless the infant is extremely hypoxic and neurologically depressed. Care must be taken to balance the need to remove the meconium with the need to oxygenate the infant.

For the worst cases of meconium aspiration that survive the event, the infant is placed on ECMO in the neonatal intensive care unit (NICU). **ECMO** is a cardiopulmonary bypass machine as shown in Figure 42-18.

Narcotic-Addicted Infants

Narcotics have been used in a controlled manner in deliveries for many years, with very few consequences. This section will focus on a resuscitation situation when the mother is a habitual user. The two most common street narcotics used by mothers are heroin and methadone.[11] Both of these drugs have a low molecular weight and pass readily across the placental membrane into the fetus. Habitual use by the mother makes the fetus

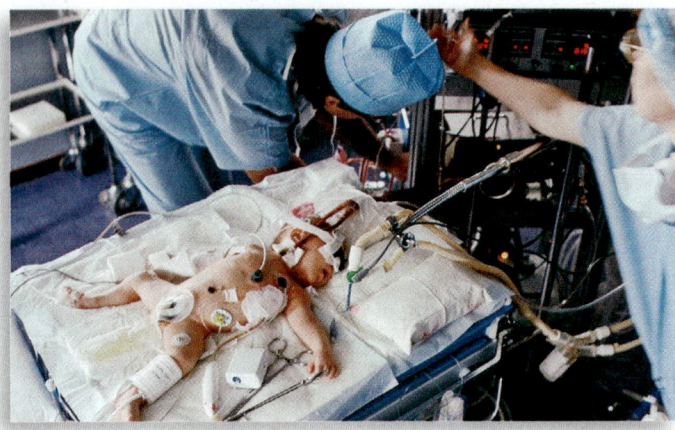

Figure 42-18 Patient on ECMO machine for meconium aspiration.

Working in the Gray Zone

A second rescuer can perform stimulation and can dry the infant while PPV is in progress. Expect the lungs to be stiff and noncompliant. Proceed through the neonatal algorithm, moving up or down based upon the heart rate, respiratory rate, and skin color. At a minimum, these infants should receive blow-by oxygen. They may not require intubation for the purpose of performing ventilations.

addicted as well. These infants are considered high-risk neonates. DOT 6-1.31

When delivery is imminent in the field setting, it is important to ask about prenatal care and social habits. At birth, the addicted infant might display respiratory depression along with a poor neurological response evidenced by weak, flaccid muscles.

Although naloxone is the treatment of choice for opiate overdose, it is not the first therapy to provide the narcotic-addicted newborn. It may be indicated if severe respiratory depression persists after PPV has restored a normal heart rate and normal color. The dose for naloxone is 0.1 mg/kg, and the route of administration is the same as in adults. DOT 6-1.32

Narcotic-addicted infants should be observed closely for the development of seizures if the mother has a prolonged history of narcotic use and naloxone is administered. The withdrawal signs are pronounced for 48 to 72 hours after administration and include the following:[8]

- Irritability
- Tachypnea greater than 60/min
- Tremors
- Excoriations (chafed or abraded skin) of knees and face
- Shrill crying
- Frequent sneezing
- Hypertonicity
- Vomiting
- Poor feeding
- Temperature instability
- Hyperactivity
- Diarrhea
- Little sleeping
- Convulsions
- Sweating

If the mother stopped using narcotics before delivery, withdrawal symptoms might not be seen for up to 10 days after delivery. Since the gastrointestinal system is involved, along with hyperthermia during withdrawal, any suspicion of dehydration needs to be evaluated further and treated by the paramedic with 10 mL/kg of crystalloid IV fluids. Dehydration quickly leads to hypovolemia in the neonate. They have good compensatory regulatory systems that may mask the severity of the problem until it is too late.

Hypovolemia

Shock in the neonate is caused by abnormal vasoregulation, not necessarily associated with hypovolemia, but when hypovolemia is suspected, dehydration is usually the leading culprit.[12] Hypovolemia is the leading cause of shock in the neonate, with dehydration being the leading cause of hypovolemia. Hypovolemia in the newborn and infant due to dehydration is discussed in Chapter 43: Pediatrics. This chapter focuses on newly born infants. The most likely cause of hypovolemia in these infants is from blood loss. An improperly clamped umbilical cord or cutting the cord before it has stopped pulsating could be the cause of the hypovolemia. DOT 6-1.72, 6-1.76

Signs of hypovolemia due to blood volume loss include pale color, cool skin, diminished peripheral pulses, delayed capillary refill time, lethargy, poor muscle tone, and later on, a lack of wet diapers. DOT 6-1.28

Hypovolemia is treated with isotonic fluid boluses of 10 mL/kg. After the bolus, reassess the infant and repeat, if necessary, a bolus of 5–10 mL/kg. Seek medical direction before infusing any more fluid into the newborn. The first bolus is given as fast as possible, depending upon the size of the catheter and the route of administration. If umbilical or peripheral access cannot be initiated, then an intraosseous (IO) site needs to be accessed.

Intraosseous Infusions

The IO procedure consists of inserting a rigid needle into the medullary cavity of a long bone. The proximal tibia is the most common place for neonatal IO insertion. When the IO is inserted, bone marrow may be aspirated (which looks like blood) or no blood may return. Marrow aspiration is not needed for confirmation of proper IO placement or for infusion of fluids. There has to be free-flowing IV fluid with no swelling in the extremity for the IO to be considered patent (Figure 42-19). **See Skill Sheet 45 (and Step-by-Step 45): Intraosseous Access and Drug Administration and Skill Sheet 91: NREMT Pediatric Intraosseous Infusion.**

Hypoglycemia

According to the *Journal of Endocrinology,* hypoglycemia is defined as a blood sugar reading less than 40 mg/dL in neonates. If the value is less than 45 mg/dL (2.5 mmoL/L), clinical interventions aimed at increasing the blood glucose concentration are indicated.[13] During the fetal stage of development, only 40–50% of maternal glucose passes through the placenta to the baby. The infant is unable to store much glycogen, and any reserve glucose is totally depleted within 12 hours of birth. Glucose is depleted even faster when the infant is stressed and is forced to try to warm themselves to try to prevent hypothermia. DOT 6-1.68

Illnesses and sepsis can also quickly deplete glucose from the newborn. Hypoglycemia conditions are also divided into other categories such as prematurity and small for gestational age (SGA). In these cases, the neonate has decreased glycogen storage abilities from the start. Other causes of hypoglycemia include being born to a diabetic mother. This is attributed to hyperinsulinism. DOT 6-1.69

The signs and symptoms of hypoglycemia are lethargy, irritability, apnea, tachypnea, cyanosis, hypothermia, seizures, and a high-pitched cry. The treatment of choice is an infusion of 10% dextrose at a dose of 2 to 4 mL/kg. Additionally, any cause of stress, such as hypothermia, should be treated or should be prevented from occurring. DOT 6-1.70, 6-1.71

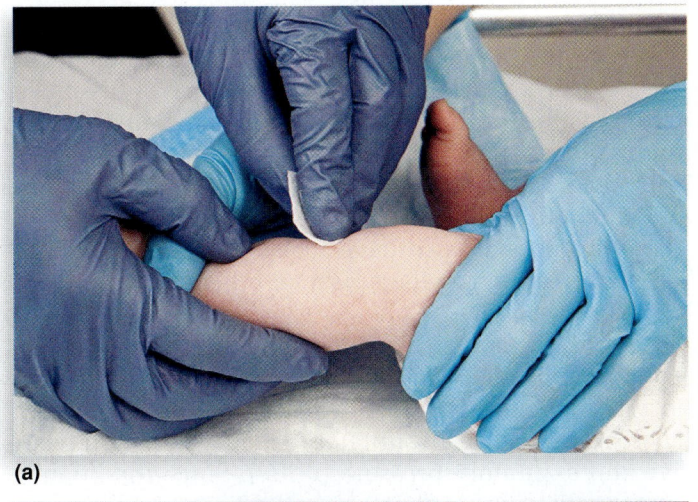
(a)

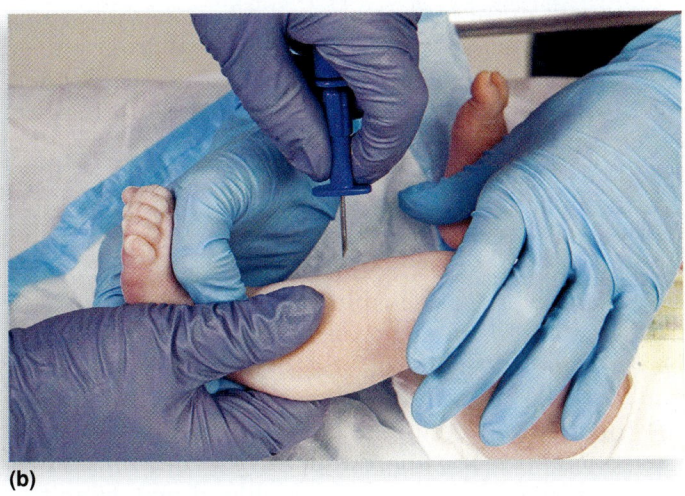
(b)

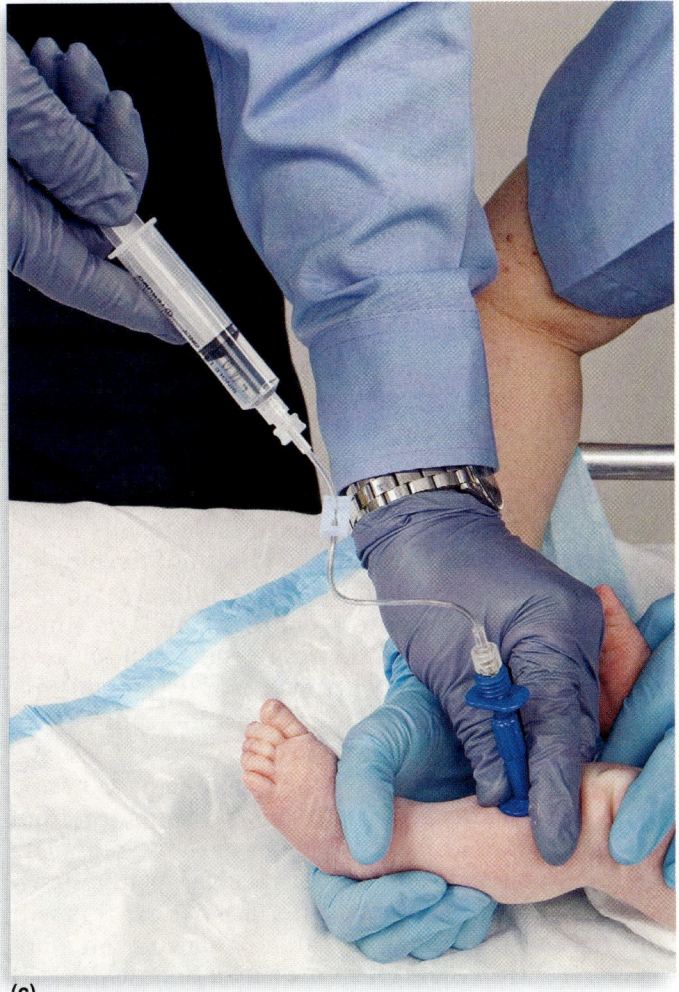
(c)

Figure 42-19   An IO offers venous access when IV and umbilical access is not possible.

Hyperthermia

The temperature of a newborn varies dramatically, and the environment can have a lot of impact upon their body temperature. Hyperthermia can pose a medical emergency in newborns. Temperature regulation of the newborn involves the measures taken at birth and in the first days of life to ensure that the newborn does not become either cold or overheated and maintains a normal body temperature of 36.5° to 37.5°C (97.7° to 99.5°F).

Hyperthermia, like hypothermia, is considered a medical emergency because the newborn cannot regulate temperature very well.[14] They do not perspire like adults. They release heat by increasing respirations and heart rate. Rates can rise as high as 70 breaths per minute and over 200 heart beats per minute. If this does not lower the temperature, then the child can have pyretic (fever-induced) seizures. DOT 6-1.61, 6-1.62, 6-1.63

Seizures occur during a fever as a last effort to lower the core temperature. When seizure activity is noted in the neonate, it is generally caused by underlying disease. The infant with hyperthermia should be suspected of being septic. Septicemia is a generalized bacterial infection in the blood stream. Meningitis, and other diseases, can cause septicemia.

Neonates are susceptible to disease because they have diminished nonspecific and specific immunity, especially if they are not being fed breast milk. Maternal breast milk supports IgA, IgM, and IgG antibodies, which help prevent infections.

Congenital Diaphragmatic Hernia

In the healthy newborn, the diaphragm separates the abdominal contents from the thoracic contents, allowing the lungs to inflate and deflate readily. The diaphragm sometimes does not develop while in utero, causing the intestines and stomach to enter the chest cavity and take up precious space. This results in the lung on the affected side of the chest not developing properly. The external chest wall will appear normal in shape and size, and the condition will go undetected until respiratory distress occurs. These newborns will have persistent pulmonary hypertension and will look cyanotic due to their poor pulmonary blood flow. DOT 6-1.43

The treatment for congenital diaphragmatic hernia is to intubate immediately.[5] This prevents air from entering the stomach and causing a greater tamponade effect. The neonate should not receive positive pressure bag-mask ventilation with a facemask as this will worsen the condition. PPV can also cause a pneumothorax. If this occurs, chest decompression will need to be performed. If the ambulance carries orogastric tubes, place one into the stomach via the mouth to help decompress the stomach. This infant should be transported rapidly for further evaluation and surgical correction of the problem. DOT 6-1.27

Transport of the Neonate

There are three types of patient transportation modalities for neonatal transport. The most common form of neonate transportation is via the standard ambulance. The next most common is helicopter and lastly the fixed wing aircraft. What mode of transportation is appropriate will depend upon the underlying condition, the urgency of the need to get the newborn to a tertiary care center, and the distance to that center. DOT 6-1.33

A newly born infant and mother from an uncomplicated delivery situation can be transported by any paramedic crew in a standard ambulance that contains standard supplies and equipment appropriate for a neonate. During a routine transport, it is important to keep the newborn warm (normothermic) and pink (with the application of oxygen, if needed), so the child does not become hypoglycemic during transport. DOT 6-1.34

If the birth was complicated or problems arise, more highly trained providers may be required to perform a secondary transport from the receiving facility to a tertiary care facility capable of managing the problems of the newborn. Specially equipped neonatal intensive care transport units may be found in some areas of the country. Transports in these vehicles are provided by critical care teams of experienced paramedics with additional continuing education beyond the entry level. These teams may also have registered nurses, neonatologists, respiratory therapists, or other specialty team members. DOT 6-1.34

Typically, a sick neonate requires transport in an **isolette** (a special size bed that is heated and has full access for monitoring and performing procedures). There must also be a ventilator to manage PIP and positive end expiratory pressure (PEEP). Since the infant's lungs work off of inspiratory and expiratory pressures and not volume, the ventilators must be appropriate for use on infants. There must be properly sized equipment for intubation, venous access, cardiac monitoring and other procedures. Depending upon the severity of the problems encountered in the mother and child, a separate ambulance crew may need to transport the mother while another crew attends to the neonate.

The ultimate destination for the sick newborn is important. Not every hospital is equipped to take care of neonates. Most newborns and their mothers can be transported to the closest facility that has labor and delivery services. However, in the event of a life-threatening situation, the receiving facility will coordinate the transportation of the newborn to a neonatal intensive care unit capable of managing the problem.

Summary

Resuscitation of the neonate can pose difficult challenges, particularly if the infant is premature or has a complication such as meconium aspiration, hypoglycemia, hypothermia, or a congenital diaphragmatic hernia. The AHA neonatal resuscitation guideline provides a standardized approach to resuscitation that moves through a basic assessment process and is followed by treatments and reassessments.

It is important to remember that a majority of the child birth situations are normal and without incident. When they are not, always make sure the airway is clear, especially if meconium is present, evaluate and support respirations if needed, and keep the child warm and dry. Hypothermia can cause hypoglycemia, bradycardia, and apnea.

Notes

1. S. C. Curtin, "Trends in the Attendant, Place and Timing of Births, and in Use of Obstetrics Interventions: United States, 1989–1997," *National Vital Status Report* 47(1999): 1–12.

2. J. F. Lucey, C. A. Rowan, P. Shiono, A. R. Wilkinson, S. Kilpatrick, N. R. Payne, J. D. Horbar, J. Carpenter, J. Rogowski, and R. F. Soll, "Fetal Infants: The Fate of 4172 Infants With Birth Weights of 401 to 500 Grams—The Vermont Oxford Network Experience (1996–2000)," *Pediatrics,* 113(2004):1559–1566.

3. American Heart Association, "2005 AHA Guidelines for CPR and ECC," *Circulation* (Suppl) 112(24) (December 13, 2005): IV-188.

4. J. E. Tintinalli, G. D. Kelen, J. S. Stapczynski, O. J. Ma, and D. M. Cline, *Tintinalli's Emergency Medicine: A Comprehensive Study Guide,* 6th ed., McGraw-Hill's AccessMedicine (accessed October 15, 2006).

5. American Academy of Pediatrics, *Textbook of Neonatal Resuscitation*, 4th ed. (Dallas, TX: American Heart Association, 2000).

6. M. A. Fletcher, *Physical Diagnosis in Neonatology* (Philadelphia, PA: Lippincot-Raven Publishers, 1997).

7. American Academy of Pediatrics, *Textbook of Neonatal Resuscitation,* 4th ed. (Dallas, TX: American Heart Association, 2000), Sections 1–7.

8. D. L. Wong and M. J. Hockenberry, *Nursing Care of Infants and Children,* 7th ed. (St. Louis, MO: Mosby, 1999).

9. J. M. Perlman and R. Risser, "Cardiopulmonary Resuscitation in the Delivery Room: Associated Clinical Events," *Archives of Pediatric Adolescent Medicine,* 13(1984):79–86.

10. American Heart Association, "Pediatric Advanced Life Support," *Circulation* 112 [Suppl I] (2005):IV-167–IV-187.

11. Robert W. Llewelyn, "Substance Abuse in Pregnancy: The Team Approach to Antenatal Care," *The Obstetrician and Gynecologist* 2(1) (2000):11–16.

12. I. Seri, "Circulatory Support of the Sick Newborn Infant." In *Seminars in Neonatology: Perinatal Cardiology,* M. I., Levene, N. Evans, N. Archer (eds.) (London: W.B. Saunders, 2001), pp. 85–95.

13. Marvin Cornblath, Jane M. Hawdon, Anthony F. Williams, Albert Aynsley-Green, Martin P. Ward-Platt, Robert Schwartz, and Satish C. Kalhan, "Controversies Regarding Definition of Neonatal Hypoglycemia: Suggested Operational Thresholds," *Pediatrics* 105(5)(2000):1141–1145.

14. World Health Organization, *Thermal Protection of the Newborn: A Practical Guide* (Geneva, Switzerland: WHO Press, 1997).

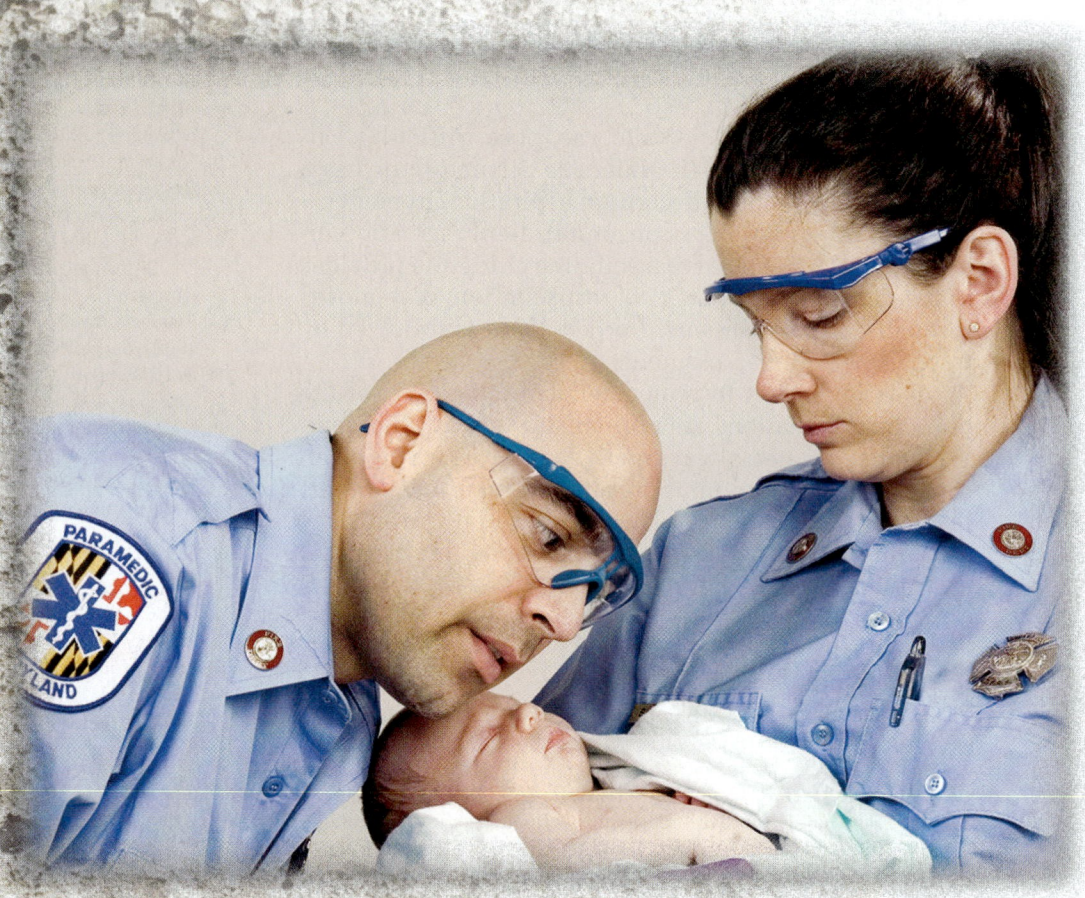

Pediatric Patients

"Children are NOT small adults."

—Anonymous

Need to Know

▶ Children have different developmental stages and physiologies and, therefore, different vital signs; different reactions to illness, injury, and pain; and different physiological responses.

▶ The importance of the role of the EMS professional in reducing morbidity and mortality rates in the pediatric population.

▶ The role of EMSC, its development, and its impact on reducing morbidity and mortality in the pediatric population since its inception.

▶ An understanding of injury prevention for children and the role of the EMS professional in promoting injury prevention.

▶ Sick	▶ Not Yet Sick
• Inactive, passive children should be considered ill or injured until it can be ruled out. • When the child's breathing catches your attention right away, it indicates respiratory distress. • Assess the skin; poor turgor or loose skin that "tents" when pinched indicates dehydration.	• Pay attention to how the child interacts with the environment and the people in it. • Pay attention to what irritates or pleases the child. • Take note of general appearance and hygiene of the child. • Be suspicious of signs of multiple injuries in varied stages of healing and histories that don't match the presentation. • Ask the family about when the child was last "well" and when they first noticed the child was not. • Ask the family about previous medical conditions and previous doctor or hospital visits. • Ask the family about siblings and any illness in the house. • Ask the family for history to describe injuries found during exam. • When interviewing children, ask simple questions calling for direct answers, not multiple choice questions. • Children that are still active, even if they are uncomfortable, are responding normally to exams. • Normally, breathing is unremarkable and effortless. • Pink, firm skin indicates adequate hydration. • Children that are not yet sick can transition very rapidly to being sick.

Introduction

Caring for a sick or injured child can be stressful and emotional for a variety of reasons. EMS providers may feel ill-prepared to manage a pediatric patient because of infrequent contact with children. The equipment, which is familiar in adult sizes, may be intimidating when scaled down to a pediatric size. The fragile appearance of a sick child or the small size of infants and young children may cause anxiety when the need for aggressive treatments such as IV therapy, needle decompression, or cardioversion arises.

Unfortunately, the best cure for this anxiety is experience in handling sick and injured children, and the "opportunity" infrequently occurs. Until you gain experience, the next best way to prepare is to learn as much as possible about children and their unique emergency healthcare needs. This chapter focuses on the assessment, care, treatment, and management of the sick or injured child in the prehospital setting.

What Is a Pediatric Patient?

An issue that continues to plague the medical community is the question, "What is a pediatric patient?" Is the definition of pediatrics based solely on chronological age? The U.S. Department of Health and Human Services (DHHS) defines "pediatric" as any person between the ages of zero and 21 years of age.[1]

The American Heart Association has used ages as low as eight years as the point between child and adult for the purpose of providing Basic Life Support by the lay (public) rescuer. However, the AHA guidelines for healthcare providers changed in 2005 to broaden the group of individuals called "children" to be from age one until the onset of puberty, which is between twelve and fourteen years of age.[2]

DOT 6-2.6

Should pediatric and adult distinctions be based on age, physical appearance, developmental stage, or some other criteria? Because final maturation of various organs and body systems, like brain development (which ends in the early to mid 20s) and sexual organ maturation and puberty (which occurs in the teens), occurs at different ages, what should be used to establish the transition points between childhood and adulthood? When does someone cease to be an infant and become a child or cease to be a child and become an adult? Many transition points are based on perceived or actual physiological differences that are detectable between the age groups. This accounts for some of the classification schemas currently in use.

Epidemiology of Pediatric Emergencies

Because it is difficult to pin down the age that is "pediatric," it is difficult to interpret statistics unless the age groups included within the statistics are provided. In 2003, there were 73 million children ages zero to 17 in the United States. They comprised 25% of the population. By 2020, children ages zero to 17 are projected to comprise 24% of the total population.[3]

An annual survey of parents is conducted by the Maternal Child Health Bureau in the United States.[4] In 2005, 8% of all children under the age of 18 were reported to have a chronic health problem that caused significant stress on their family unit. Fifteen percent were reported to have had at least one significant health problem in their childhood. When asked about dealing with specific chronic diseases, 16% of families with a child with asthma report their family was "affected a great deal" by their child's condition. Nearly 22% of all children did not receive routine preventative health visits, and up to 45% of all children had not had routine dental visits. In addition, 16% of children ages six to 11 were reported by their parents to be home alone for at least a few hours a week, and boys were more likely to be left alone than girls. All of these statistics point to some of the possible reasons ambulance transports may be required: the presence of chronic illness and families with limited resources to deal with the illness, lack of routine preventative measures, and children who are sometimes left unattended.

Pediatric patients (under age 18 years) account for approximately 5–10% of all EMS calls and 25–30% of all ED visits annually.[5] It is estimated that approximately six million children under the age of 18 are transported by ambulance each year in the United States. The most common age groups requiring ambulance transport are between the ages of zero to two years and greater than 10 years. Approximately 5–10% of all pediatric ambulance transports are for children deemed to be in serious or critical condition.[6]

Trauma remains the leading cause of death in children over the age of one year. DOT 6-2.35

Injuries associated with motor vehicle crashes account for the most traumatic deaths. Drowning, burns, and fire-related injuries account for a significant number of deaths as well, particularly in younger children.[7]

However, the frequency of the need for EMS services is nearly equally distributed between injury and illness.

Fewer children die from acute illnesses than injuries, but many more end up hospitalized from illness. The leading cause of illness-related EMS response is respiratory complaints and includes asthma, wheezing, and stridor. Seizures and altered mental status are also common medical reasons for EMS response.[7]

Although concern for cardiac arrest has been a major focus for many years, its occurrence in the pediatric population is uncommon. Unfortunately, survival from a cardiac arrest by a child is uncommon as well. Unlike adults where resuscitation has been shown to be beneficial if initiated within four to six minutes, cardiac arrest in children is most frequently a terminal event of a disease process or injury.[8] As a terminal event, it is likely the end product of a chronic problem instead of a sudden, and perhaps reversible, event such as the formation of a blood clot within a coronary artery.

In children, the most common reason they require aggressive resuscitation is respiratory compromise or arrest.[8] If treatment is initiated promptly, survival rates in the 60–70% range can be expected. If the prehospital care provided is not of the highest quality, the rest of the "continuum of care" that occurs in the hospital setting may not improve outcome. DOT 6-2.10, 6-2.11

CONNECTIONS Maintaining respiration and ventilation are critical for children at all ages. Chapter 42: Neonatology describes respiratory compromise as the most common reason a newly born infant requires resuscitation measures.[9]

Pediatric Care in Historical Perspective

In the past twenty years, several studies have been conducted to evaluate the effectiveness of pediatric care in the prehospital environment.[10–13] At least one of these studies showed that children cared for by EMS had a higher mortality rate than their adult counterparts.[1] One possible conclusion drawn from this was that prehospital pediatric emergency care was lacking throughout the United States. In the 20 years since these studies were conducted, things have improved. Recommendations from these studies have been implemented. Among the recommendations are the following:

- Prehospital providers must receive additional education and training related specifically to pediatric care.
- Prehospital providers need to be trained in and have access to pediatric-specific equipment.
- Prehospital providers must have protocols specific for pediatric patients.

Emergency Medical Services for Children (EMSC)

Legislation was passed in 1984 under Section 1910 of the Public Health Service Act, authorizing the development of the Emergency Medical Services for Children (EMSC) Program. Its purpose is to ensure that all ill and injured children and adolescents receive state-of-the-art emergency care, including primary prevention, prehospital care, acute care, and rehabilitation. The program is designed to reduce childhood death and disability from severe illness or injury. DOT 6-2.4

Emergency Medical Services for Children (EMSC) is a federally-funded, national program of the U.S. Department of Health and Human Services (DHHS), Health Resources and Services Administration (HRSA), and Maternal and Child Health Bureau (MCHB). It functions in collaboration with the U.S. Department of Transportation's (DOT) National Highway Traffic Safety Administration (NHTSA). Since 1984, the EMSC programs have made significant advancements in reducing pediatric morbidity and mortality rates.

In 1985, Congress appropriated $2 million dollars to the EMSC program to accomplish its mission. The first grants were given to four states (Alabama, California, New York, and Oregon), which saw the need to address the following:

- The lack of pediatric education for prehospital and emergency healthcare providers.
- The lack of knowledge or tools to properly assess critically ill and injured children.
- The lack of the establishment of data collection in order to identify major health problems specific to the pediatric population within the EMS system.
- The lack of strategies to address pediatric emergency care.

Over the next twenty years, all 50 states, the District of Columbia, and all five U.S. territories successfully implemented statewide EMSC programs. Since its inception and with the help of local, state, and national collaborations and partnerships, the program has allocated $138 million dollars to fund over 850 grant awards. DOT 6-2.5

Injury and Illness Prevention

Prevention—one of the first aspects of any healthcare system—is another of the many lessons learned from the EMSC program. The American College of Emergency Physicians (ACEP), the American Academy of Pediatrics (AAP), and the National Association of EMTs and others joined forces to initiate a wide variety of prevention programs.

Preventing illness and injury is far more effective in reducing death and disability in children than any treatment that can be offered. Illness prevention and public health activities are expanding roles within EMS, while injury prevention remains a mainstay of the EMS profession. DOT 6-2.36

Injury and illness prevention is critical. Each year more than 22 million children are injured, 20 million are treated in the emergency department, up to 6 million will be treated and transported by EMS, 780,000 will be hospitalized, and over 19,000 will die.[14]

The Centers for Disease Control and Prevention (CDC) cite the following leading causes of preventable injury that deserve attention: DOT 6-2.2, 6-2.3

- Child maltreatment
- Child passenger safety
- Fireworks-related injuries
- Playground injuries
- Poisonings
- Residential fire-related injuries
- Suicide
- Traumatic brain injury
- Water safety
- Young drivers
- Youth violence

Development of Infants and Children

Children, like adults, are individual and unique, and their rate of development is also unique. However, there are some fairly predictable trends. Therefore, "normal" values emerge for vital signs and developmental changes and milestones. Table 43-1 describes the various age and developmental stages of the pediatric patient, and Table 43-2 outlines normal weight ranges for children.

CONNECTIONS Be aware that not all children develop typically. Chapter 46: Patients with Special Challenges gives an overview of children with developmental disabilities such as Down's syndrome and autism.

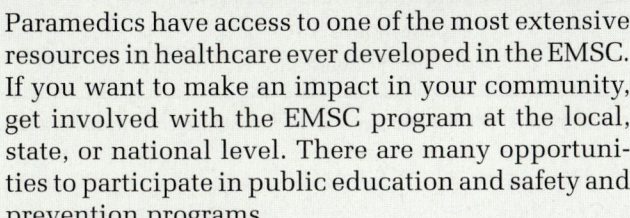

Nice to Know

Paramedics have access to one of the most extensive resources in healthcare ever developed in the EMSC. If you want to make an impact in your community, get involved with the EMSC program at the local, state, or national level. There are many opportunities to participate in public education and safety and prevention programs.

TABLE 43-1   **Developmental Aspects of Pediatric Patients** DOT 6-2.7, 6-2.9

Chronological Age	Characteristics	Interaction Pearls
Newborn (birth to one month)	Normally alert, looking around Focuses well on faces Keeps extremities flexed	Enjoys being held and kept warm Loud noises, bright lights should be avoided Pacifier or bottle may help comfort
Infant (one to 12 months)	Alert, looks around, attentive to activity around them Tracks paramedic with eyes Can straighten extremities, but may prefer flexed positioning Can rollover at three to six months Can sit up by self at six to eight months May be "clingy" to parents—separation anxiety May start walking	Wants to be held Typically wants parents close by or holding them Conduct toe-to-head assessment Use tools to distract—penlights, toys, stickers, etc.
Toddler (one to three years)	Normally alert and extremely active May be "clingy" to parents—separation anxiety Completely mobile by 18 months Inactivity may be critical sign or caused by fear of *you* May grab at penlight or push hand away	Engage in active assessment—game playing Make a game of assessment Use tools to distract—penlights, toys, stickers, etc. Conduct toe-to-head assessment Family-centered care during assessment may be helpful Respect modesty Keep child covered for warmth and modesty
Preschooler (three to six years)	Normally alert and interactive Inactivity may be critical sign or caused by fear of *you* Will usually cooperate once trust is established Can normally rationalize information and instructions Story telling is both a comforting tool and a method to explain what is not understood	Use simple language that is age appropriate Tell the child what will happen next *Tell the truth* Use tools to distract—story, penlights, toys, stickers, etc. Respect modesty Keep child covered for warmth and modesty
School-age child (six to 12 years)	Will usually cooperate once trust is established Often has fixation with death, even if this event is non-life-threatening Participation in assessment and treatments normally increase trust and allow a perception of control	Use simple language that is age appropriate Allow child to be actively involved in their care decisions Allow the child to participate in your assessment Keep child covered for warmth and modesty
Adolescent (12–18 years)	Has clear understanding of what they want to occur Must engage in the decision-making processes Must respect their views even if they are in opposition to your personal beliefs or concepts	Treat the child with respect Allow them to be actively involved in their assessment and treatment Explain what you are doing and why Respect modesty Keep child covered for warmth and modesty

Adapted from Paramedic TRIPP: Teaching Resource for Instructors in Prehospital Pediatrics (CD-ROM). (New York, NY: The Center for Pediatric Emergency Medicine, 2002).

TABLE 43-2   Normal Weight Ranges for Boys and Girls
Children's Weight by Age and Sex

Ages Two to 15 With a Valid Weight Measurement   *1998*

Weight (kg)	Age															Total
	2	3	4	5	6	7	8	9	10	11	12	13	14	15	
Boys															
Mean	14.0	16.4	18.5	20.5	22.9	25.9	29.0	31.6	36.5	40.5	44.6	51.7	56.5	62.2	32.7
5th percentile	11.2	13.7	14.9	17.0	17.7	19.7	22.4	23.9	27.7	28.6	32.6	35.4	42.9	46.3	14.1
10th percentile	11.8	14.2	15.5	17.6	18.9	20.5	23.3	25.0	28.8	31.6	33.6	37.5	45.2	47.2	15.8
15th percentile	12.4	14.6	16.2	18.0	19.9	21.2	23.7	25.7	29.9	33.1	34.9	40.4	46.6	49.1	17.3
Median	13.9	16.3	18.4	20.3	22.3	25.3	27.5	30.6	34.1	37.5	43.3	49.8	54.8	61.5	28.4
85th percentile	15.9	18.3	20.8	22.9	25.8	30.9	34.4	37.3	44.5	49.0	54.2	63.4	66.8	75.5	50.7
90th percentile	16.4	18.8	21.5	23.7	27.0	32.3	35.8	39.5	47.0	52.0	59.2	65.7	72.9	78.6	57.6
95th percentile	17.3	19.6	22.5	24.7	30.3	34.4	38.4	43.9	50.7	59.2	63.6	72.4	79.3	83.6	63.7
Girls															
Mean	14.0	15.9	18.6	20.3	22.7	26.0	28.9	33.7	36.5	43.6	48.5	53.4	56.2	60.0	33.8
5th percentile	11.6	13.2	15.1	16.0	17.0	19.8	20.8	24.0	26.6	29.3	34.3	38.3	42.2	44.5	14.0
10th percentile	12.0	13.6	15.6	16.9	18.0	20.8	22.4	25.3	27.9	31.2	36.3	41.2	44.6	45.8	15.5
15th percentile	12.4	13.9	16.0	17.4	19.3	21.6	24.0	26.1	28.9	32.2	37.6	43.3	45.5	47.3	16.9
Median	13.8	15.5	17.8	19.8	22.3	25.6	27.5	32.0	35.5	41.4	47.3	51.2	55.5	58.3	29.3
85th percentile	15.9	17.7	21.5	23.4	25.9	30.5	34.3	42.0	44.4	55.5	57.4	64.6	66.7	71.1	52.9
90th percentile	16.3	18.6	22.4	24.3	28.1	31.8	36.8	45.2	47.1	57.8	60.9	67.9	70.4	83.0	57.9
95th percentile	16.8	20.0	25.7	28.4	29.7	34.3	39.1	49.3	50.8	61.4	69.3	70.9	75.9	88.1	64.5

Source: http://www.dh.gov.uk/assetRoot/04/06/53/90/04065390.doc

Developmental Characteristics

During the first years of life, the pediatric patient will go through more physical, intellectual, emotional, and developmental hallmarks than during any other time in life. This first year of life brings forth physical growth that is unparalleled. Within these 12 months, the child will usually triple their birth weight, increase their height by approximately 12 inches, have teeth emerge in their mouth, and have a nervous system that has developed from reflex-based to consciously controlled. The subsequent stages are equally exciting from a developmental perspective. DOT 6-2.12

Children have a number of defensive mechanisms that are used during times of stress, fright, danger, illness, or injury. Table 43-3 provides some examples.

Newborns Ages Zero to One Month

Newborns (also called infants) are transitioning from total dependence to minor levels of self-sufficiency. Nutrition, warmth, oxygenation, waste removal, and movement, which were once effortless activities (in the uterus), must be learned and mastered by the organs and systems of their body. Suckling (feeding) is an example of one of the few instinctive skills innate to the newborn. If the newborn has a respiratory disorder, the body may have to choose between breathing and feeding as it may not be able to accomplish both at the same time. After a day or two of struggling, both processes may become compromised to the point that the child's overall health is at significant risk.

Newborns move their extremities in the first months of life, and this is their only mobility. Their relaxed position is flexed, and a **moro reflex** or **startle reflex** is a primitive reflex that occurs when newborns grasp anything placed into the palm of their hand (Figure 43-1). This reflex is often confused with deliberate movement. The other component of the moro reflex is having the appearance of being startled when the sense of falling is invoked or a loud, sudden noise is heard. For example, infants will appear to jump and may cry when a book is dropped onto a wooden table.

Newborns are alert and frequently look as if they are communicating with their eyes. They may look as if they are focused on objects, but their eyes will not track or follow when the object is moved away. Crying is an expression of hunger, fear, discomfort, or pain. Newborns begin to explore their environment by placing things

TABLE 43-3   **Defense Mechanisms of Children**

Mechanism	Definition	Example
Regression	Return to past behaviors or lack of progress on new ones	Child returns to pre-toilet-trained stages, i.e., is incontinent.
Repression	Blocking or forgetting uncomfortable behaviors	Child is unable to remember events that caused significant stress, pain, or abuse.
Rationalization	Converting unacceptable behaviors to acceptable	Child justifies or deflects actions such as biting another child because they took "my toy."
Fantasy	Creating a story or series of stories to buffer the impact of the objectionable behavior	The child creates a story to help buffer the impact of the event(s). Pretending they are a cartoon character or that one is with them is not uncommon.

in their mouths. Because they lack muscle tone and coordination, they may hit themselves in the head as they attempt to place objects into their mouths.

Infants (One to 12 Months)

At approximately two months, infants begin to focus on and follow moving objects. They also obviously smile in reaction to pleasure and react when the primary caregiver's (usually the mother) voice is heard. Months four through six bring increased motor activity and determined motion. The infant will reach for objects, roll over, respond to sounds and voices, sit up without assistance, and crawl.

By six months, mobility and independence are increasing along with the imitation of sounds and attempts at verbalization. "Mama" and "Dada" are common first words, as is the word "No." Separation anxiety becomes more common when strangers are present. These children will notice when strangers, including paramedics, are present and may react by crying and reaching for the

parent or other familiar individual. Crying remains a primary method of communication, usually indicating hunger, pain, fear, or needing a diaper change.

Older infants are beginning to build their basic "trust" senses. Normally, infants learn trust through the nurturing care provided by their parents or primary caregivers. Being loved, fed, clothed, warmed, cuddled, and comforted are all components of building a strong sense of trust. Depending upon where infants are in this development, they may allow you to handle them, or they may still protest (Figure 43-2).

Street Secrets

If you are loud or imposing, most likely the older infant will react with fear. Approach the child gently and cautiously. Use a "toe-to-head" approach. Start by evaluating the foot. You can assess alertness, temperature, capillary refill, and maybe even pulse from the foot. DOT 6-2.8

Toddler (One to Three Years)

From total dependence to the "terrible twos" on through the beginning of independence, the toddler years signify massive changes in both intellect and physical development. In the early years, the child is learning the art of walking and mobility, language and communication, and intellect and thinking. Regardless of the terrain, the toddler will work diligently to master flat surfaces, stairs, inclines and declines, and uneven surfaces. At this age, they are often referred to as being "in constant motion."

The two significant challenges presented with mobility that must be considered by the paramedic are the increased frequency of falls and the fact that restraining a child of this age will most likely result in a Houdini-like ability to squirm and escape from the best restraining techniques. Cuddling the child in a well-padded, warm, comfortable bundle may instill security and reduce or

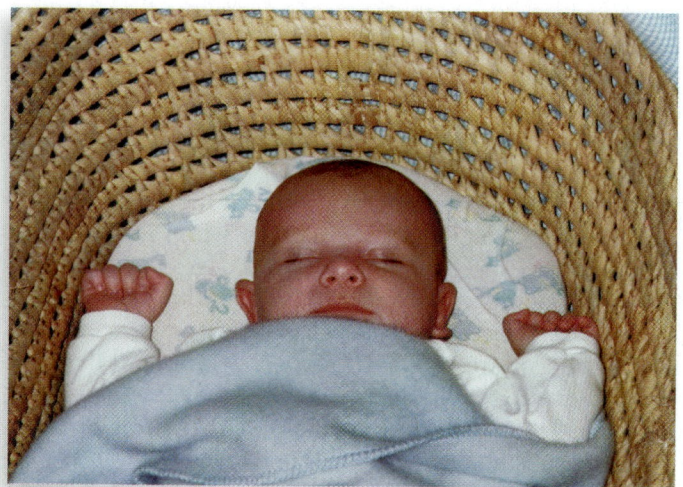

Figure 43-1   One-week-old infant asleep with arms flexed.

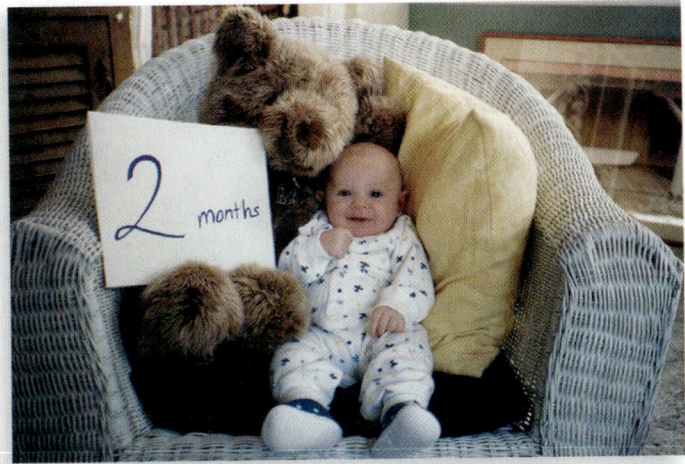

(a)

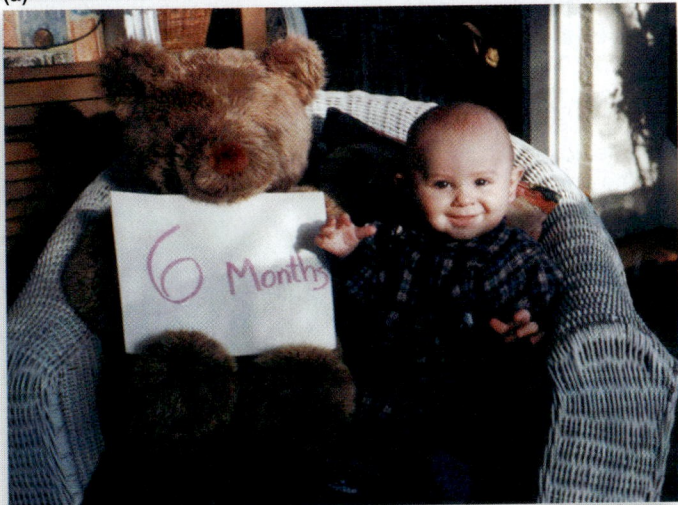

(b)

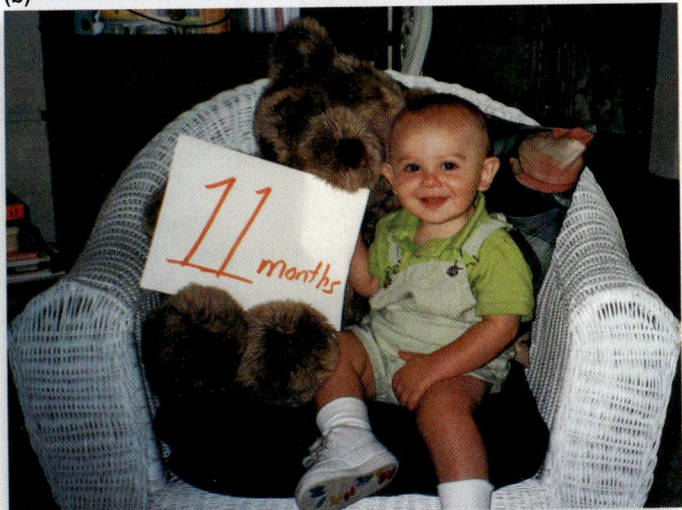

(c)

Figure 43-2   Infant at various stages of development. (a) At two months, he held his head up, but had to be propped up for the picture. He engaged with his parents during the picture-taking. (b) At six months, he could sit up with a little assistance and grabbed for the sign shortly after this picture was taken. (c) At 11 months, he was just about to start walking and talking. He had developed significant separation anxiety and reacted negatively to all strangers.

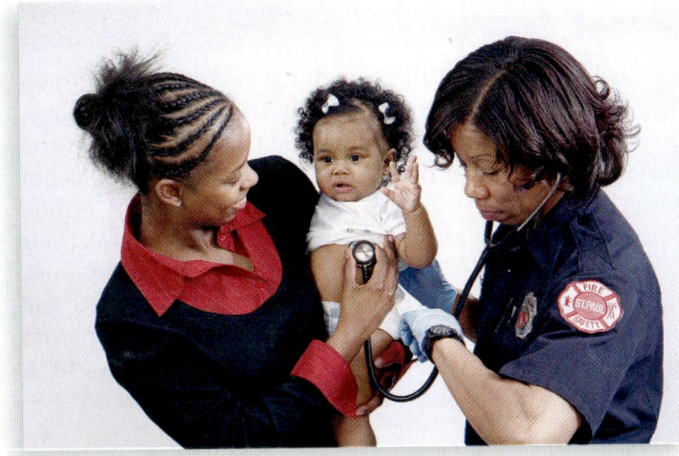

Figure 43-3   Assessing a toddler may be easier to perform if the parent is holding the child. Enlist the help of the parent to hold stethoscopes and place other diagnostic tools. Use simple words such as "stickers" for bandaids, ECG electrodes, or pulse oximeter probes.

eliminate the need for the child to move. If it is practical, a parent may be called upon the hold the child while you perform your assessment as well as some treatments such as blow-by oxygen administration (Figure 43-3).

Street Secrets

Although children this age are beginning to understand and reason, when they are stressed, they become overwhelmed as do adults. Pay close attention to what you are saying to them. Their imaginations do not understand when you "take" their blood pressure. They may ask you if you are going to "give it back" when you are done. Instead, tell them you are going to squeeze their arm or give it a tight hug. If you draw blood, they think they will lose it all and die. If the parents are calm and willing to assist, they can reassure the child that you are helping and not harming.

Since activity is the normal state for toddlers, anything less should cause concern. A child sitting calmly in the parent's lap may be a simple expression of fear, or it may be an indication that the child is in a more critical condition than thought. Observe the child closely for shock or respiratory distress.

Basic language skills are steadily increasing, as is their understanding of simple sentences and concepts. Reasoning abilities are being developed as language skills increase. Toddlers have active imaginations. Thinking capabilities, curiosity, independence, exploration, likes and dislikes, the ability to fear, and the ability to create stories about the known and the unknown are typical attributes in this age group.

Street Secrets

If possible, save painful procedures such as blood drawing or starting an IV until after the assessment is complete. Do not discuss painful procedures until right before you perform them. Never lie to the child that something is not going to hurt, but do not be dramatic about it either. Apologize to them for causing them pain. Do not ask their permission if "No!" is not an option. Do not prepare your equipment or supplies until just prior to performing the painful skill. Try to prepare the equipment away from their field of vision, so the child does not have to watch you as this will cause a lot of anxiety.

A child's ability to socialize also continues to increase. The paramedic's ability to gain the toddler's trust and involve them in appropriate care decisions may be successfully accomplished in a playful manner.

Preschooler (Three to Six Years)

Complete mobility, high activity levels, daily expressions of independence, conversational language skills, growing intellect, and peaked curiosity are a few of the attributes of the "preschool" aged child. Learning words, language, activities, colors, stories, socializing, independence, and motor skills are part of the daily routine for this child.

The cognitive capacity of preschoolers is concrete and literal, allowing them to think about words, symbols, and people. Their thought processes are still developing and may present challenges when assessing their medical needs. An example of this might be the child who crashed while learning to ride a bicycle. Injuries include a Colles' fracture of the right wrist, abrasions to the right forearm, and an abrasion hematoma on the right lateral chest with significant respiratory difficulty. You are focusing on the ABCs, specifically the chest injury and respiratory distress. As you assess the child, the chief complaint and attention is on the painful right wrist because it looks "funny." The association of pain with wrist injury overwhelms the child's reasoning ability about the magnitude of the chest injury. The child's complaint has a direct association with pain and appearance and does not match your concern that the chief complaint should be difficulty breathing (Figure 43-4).

Street Secrets

Because this age group has such an active imagination, their attention can be captured and diverted easily. If the child has an obvious injury that results in deformity, discoloration and bruising, or bleeding, cover it up as soon as you can. Although the pain will probably not go away, not seeing the injury can have a calming effect on the child.

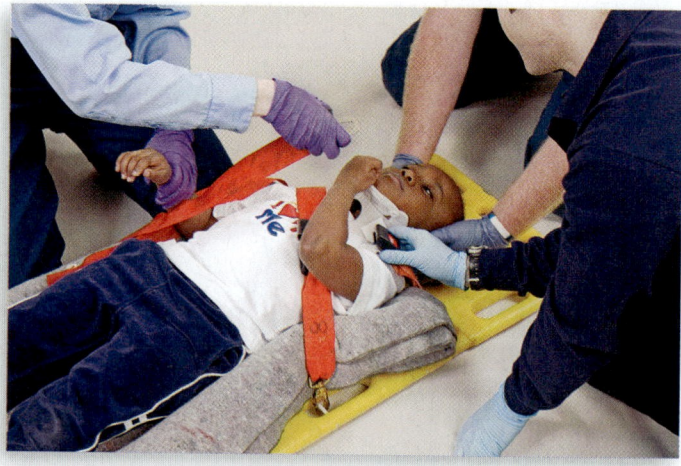

Figure 43-4   Explaining assessments and treatment in terms of games may help the preschooler feel less afraid and trust you. This child became cooperative after the paramedic explained that he would be safe and the game was a new kind of "elevator bed" the child could "surf" with. The paramedic also called the backboard straps "Seatbelts, just like the ones you wear when you are in your car."

Assessing the preschooler presents challenges because of their self-image and awareness. Their likes and dislikes are becoming more pronounced. The choice in clothing combinations, the clothing being worn, i.e., and modesty has become extremely important by age six. Having them take off a piece of clothing or cutting off a favorite pair of pants may invoke strong emotions and opposition.

Separation anxiety can make a trusting relationship with the child impossible. Some children need to be held by their parents; others might only need to have their parents hold their hands, touch their head, or be within visual contact. Using familiar items such as a blanket or favorite toy may provide some level of comfort.

Preschoolers have the ability to interact with others during play and while socializing. Preschoolers are becoming social creatures and practice their skills at every opportunity. They may initiate conversations, take control of the game, adapt the rules as they see fit, and desire to be the center of attention. Try to utilize play skills in an effort to reduce preschoolers' fears and increase their participation in the assessment and treatment process. Where possible, utilize the parent or caregiver during both the assessment and treatment phases of care.

Preschool-aged children are exploring and mastering complex mobility and coordination skills. The acts of running, skipping, riding a tricycle or bicycle, balancing on one foot, and throwing or catching a ball are all examples of complex activities that require higher neuromuscular system development. By age six, most children can ride a bike, play games that have rules or require coordinated bodily movements, dress a doll, and catch a ball. This age group can frequently make us think they are "small adults," yet they are still children.

School Aged Children (Six to 12 Years of Age)

The six-to 12-year-old age group continues to advance their understanding of the world and the concepts associated with it. Time association has advanced to understanding the past as well as the future. Discussions about what they did yesterday or when the pain started can occur. Conversations often become an engaged dialog with questions about every aspect of the assessment and treatment.

In the six-to eight-year group, death is a frequent fear or thought process. Regardless of the magnitude of the event, "Am I going to die?" or "Nobody will be my friend because I'm going to be ugly," are the type of statements frequently made. Because these children have a more advanced understanding of concepts and factual information, often their fears can be eliminated with simple, truthful responses.

Unfortunately school-age children seem to have an innate ability to sense fear, joy, anger, shame, truth, dishonestly, and emotional projections by others. This places the paramedic in a compromising situation if they attempt to be less than forthright with the child or their parents (Figure 43-5).

This age group continues to develop their ability to think and rationalize, which also brings forth the ability to make decisions. A common error in this and older age groups is the failure to talk directly with the child. Failure to communicate may result in a loss of trust and a conscious effort on their part not to respond, verbally or physically. Frequently, they are excellent historians and provide detailed information about their illness or injury, particularly a chronic one they have had for several years.

Modesty and self-image have become strong influences in their lives. Every effort must be taken to assure that medically appropriate assessments and treatments are conducted within the guidelines of respecting the child. If possible, a paramedic of the same sex should assess the child, particularly if clothing must be removed or the injury is in an intimate area of the body. If possible, have a parent or witness present during the examination.

Discussing what needs to be done, honoring their privacy and modesty, and engaging them in the health-care process are actions that will continue to build a trusting relationship. Treat the child with respect and professionalism.

Adolescents (12 to 21 Years of Age)

Adolescents (or teenagers) have developed to near-adult-like abilities to think, rationalize, and evaluate abstract thought processes and have mastered most of the neuro-muscular and coordination skills required for daily living. This group may appear adult in physical ways but still possesses thought patterns, emotions, and mannerisms of children. The single largest gap between this age group and adults is life experience. Hobbs described adolescence as the following:

> "Adolescent and teenage life is studded with milestones that are supposed to make us feel grown up, supposed to mark a transition from childhood into adulthood. Yet many of us reach our late 20s, 30s or even our 50s and 60s still feeling that we are children inside, with all the responsibilities and obligations that entails."[17]

From the quote, it is easy to see that the challenges of adolescence are similar to those of adulthood: confusion and emotional swings without predefined answers or solutions. To further complicate this stage of life, adolescence is considered by some to be cultural instead of biological and more specifically the "transition from childhood to adulthood."[16] Some believe that the proper term for the adolescent stage of life should be "young adult." Throughout the remainder of this chapter, we will refer to adolescents and teenagers as young adults, not because of one expert's opinion over another but because the respect projected can be extremely beneficial to all parties involved.

If culture is a determining factor of young adulthood, then depending on the environment in which children were raised, their understanding of right and wrong and moral and societal values will vary significantly. An example is the child raised in a nondisciplinarian household might have differing values than one raised in a strict disciplinarian household. The latter may speak to adults only by saying "Sir" or Ma'am"

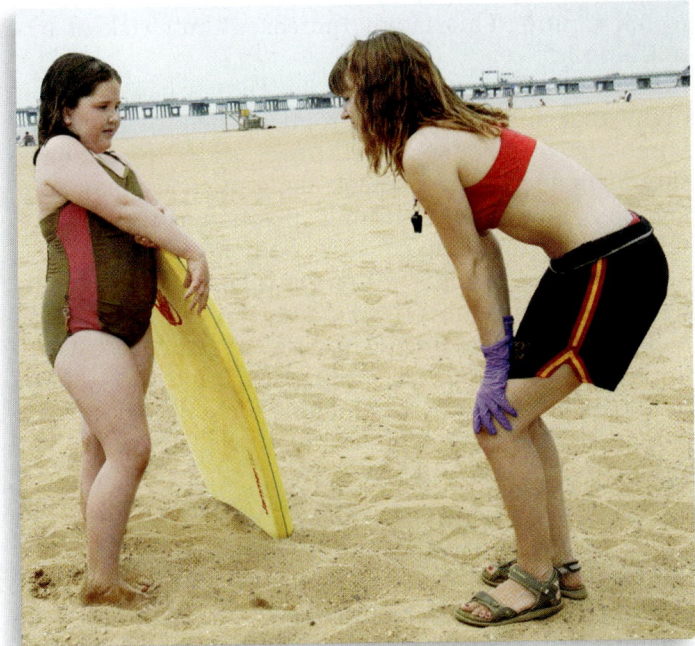

Figure 43-5 This lifeguard is listening attentively and allowing the patient to express her concerns prior to assessing her arm.

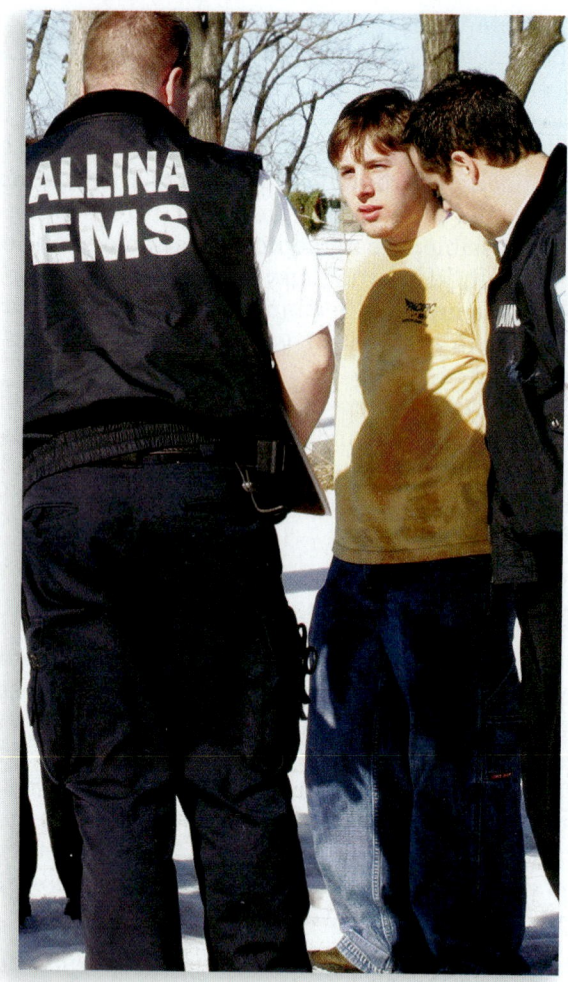

Figure 43-6 Teens appreciate being treated as adults. This teen was fearful and distrustful of the police but responded well to a friendly approach by the paramedic.

while the former may expect to call you by your first name regardless of your station or rank. Despite the variations, young adults should have firmly established determinations of right and wrong and good and bad. Young adults are often considered, "social animals," and often these social interactions have a greater influence on them than their families.

A significant skill set for the paramedic treating a young adult is to be able to discern between real and perceived issues. The fear of permanent disfigurement is frequently a topic of concern for the patient whether it is expressed or withheld. Young adults, regardless of gender, are significantly concerned about body image. This age group spends countless hours and millions of dollars on cultivation of their self-image.[14] Every child is concerned about his or her self-image.

The young adult has gained the ability to effectively communicate, has effectively mastered mobility, and has often increased their willingness to engage in risk-taking behaviors.

This age group is often sexually active, but they may be unwilling to disclose this information. You may not get a truthful response when asking a female patient if she is sexually active or pregnant, particularly if someone she knows is present at the time.

Your interaction with the young adult needs to be respectful and professional. Treat the person as you would want to be treated. Talk with them, listen to them, and allow them to be actively involved in their assessment and care. This will allow them to gain your trust as you gain theirs (Figure 43-6).

Anatomic and Physiologic Differences between Children and Infants

As children grow, their anatomy and physiology changes. In order to effectively care for this population, it is essential that the EMS professional have a solid understanding of these changes, when they occur during development, and how they impact care. Before you can understand the changes, you need to understand what represents *normal* anatomy and physiology. Both are described below and are summarized in Box 43-1. DOT 6-2.12

Head

The head-to-body ratio in pediatric patients is larger than in adults (Figure 43-7). This accounts for the high frequency of head trauma in falls, pedestrians hit by motor vehicles, and motor vehicle crashes. Pediatric patients also have an increased body surface area to mass ratio. This factor increases their risk of hypothermia.[15]

The occipital area is large, which may cause flexion of the neck and airway compromise when the patient is immobilized. Placing a small towel under the patient's shoulders and down the back along the body may help maintain a neutral or "sniffing" position as well as provide padding and help conserve body heat.

The bones of the skull of the infant have not completely fused together. Two large openings, called fontanelles, can be felt at the top of the head or on the back of the head (Figure 43-8). Depending on the age of the infant, the fontanelles are open. A bulging fontanelle is suggestive of increased intracranial pressure (ICP). A sunken fontanelle is a sign of dehydration.

Airway

Infants are obligate nose breathers. The oral cavity is smaller, with a larger tongue, and the larynx is higher and more anterior, which may make intubation more difficult. The epiglottis is larger and "floppier." The

BOX 43-1 Key Points of Pediatric Anatomy and Physiology

- Most true in infants, children's heads are proportionally larger than their body, making them at a higher risk for head injuries anytime they are victims of traumatic injury.
- The body surface area of the infant is large when compared to weight, making them susceptible to hypothermia.
- A complete set of brain cells are present at birth; myelinization and ongoing development occur throughout the first year of life.
- The anterior fontanelle and open sutures are palpable for up to 18 months.
- Children have higher metabolic rates, requiring greater caloric intake and greater oxygen requirements.
- The tongue is large relative to the size of the oral and nasal cavities and occupies most of the oropharynx.

- Until approximately age five, the short, narrow trachea increases their risk of airway obstruction.
- Until the approximate age of 12 years, a child's cardiac output is rate dependent. Stroke volume is relatively fixed.
- Blood volume is approximate 80 mL/kg.
- Tidal volume is 7 to 10 mL/kg.
- Until about the age of five years, children are diaphragmatic breathers. This places them at a greater risk for metabolic acidosis due to inefficient CO_2 exhalation, especially during events causing respiratory depression.
- Until approximately 10 years of age, children have a faster respiratory rate, lower lung volume, and smaller alveoli than adults.

airway is narrower in general. Implications for the EMS professional include the following:

- Keep the nares clear in newborns and infants less than six months of age.

- Narrower upper airways are more easily obstructed by flexion or hyperextension, foreign bodies, and swelling.
- Gentle suction with a bulb syringe can improve respirations significantly.

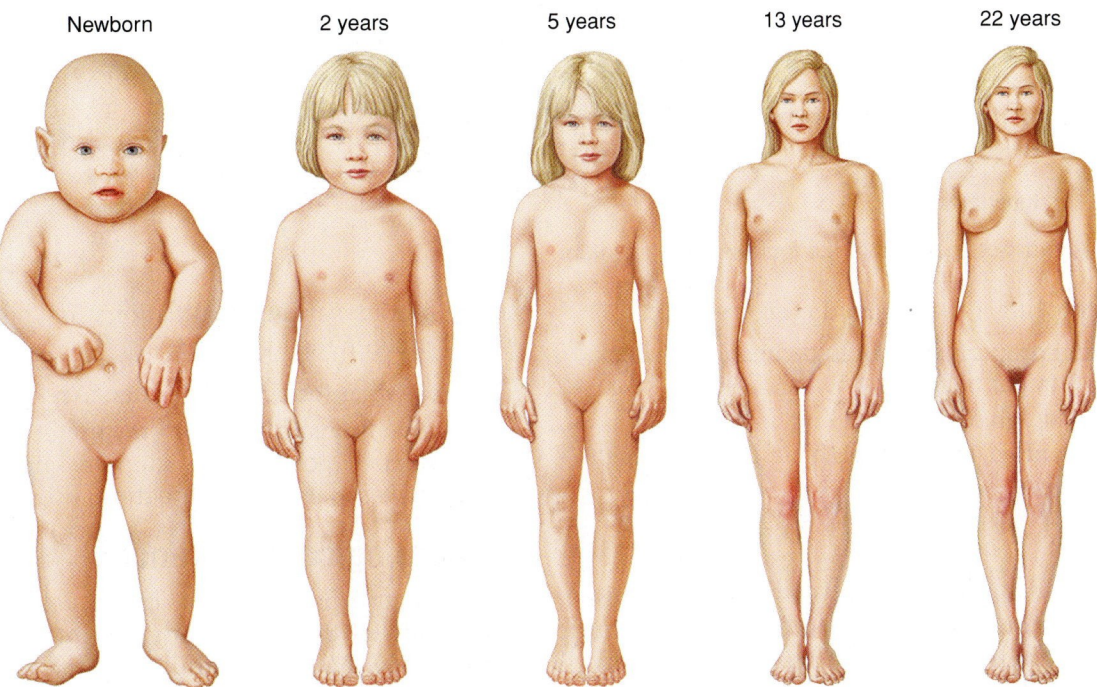

Newborn   2 years   5 years   13 years   22 years

FIGURE 43-7   Note the head-to-body ratio in children versus adults.

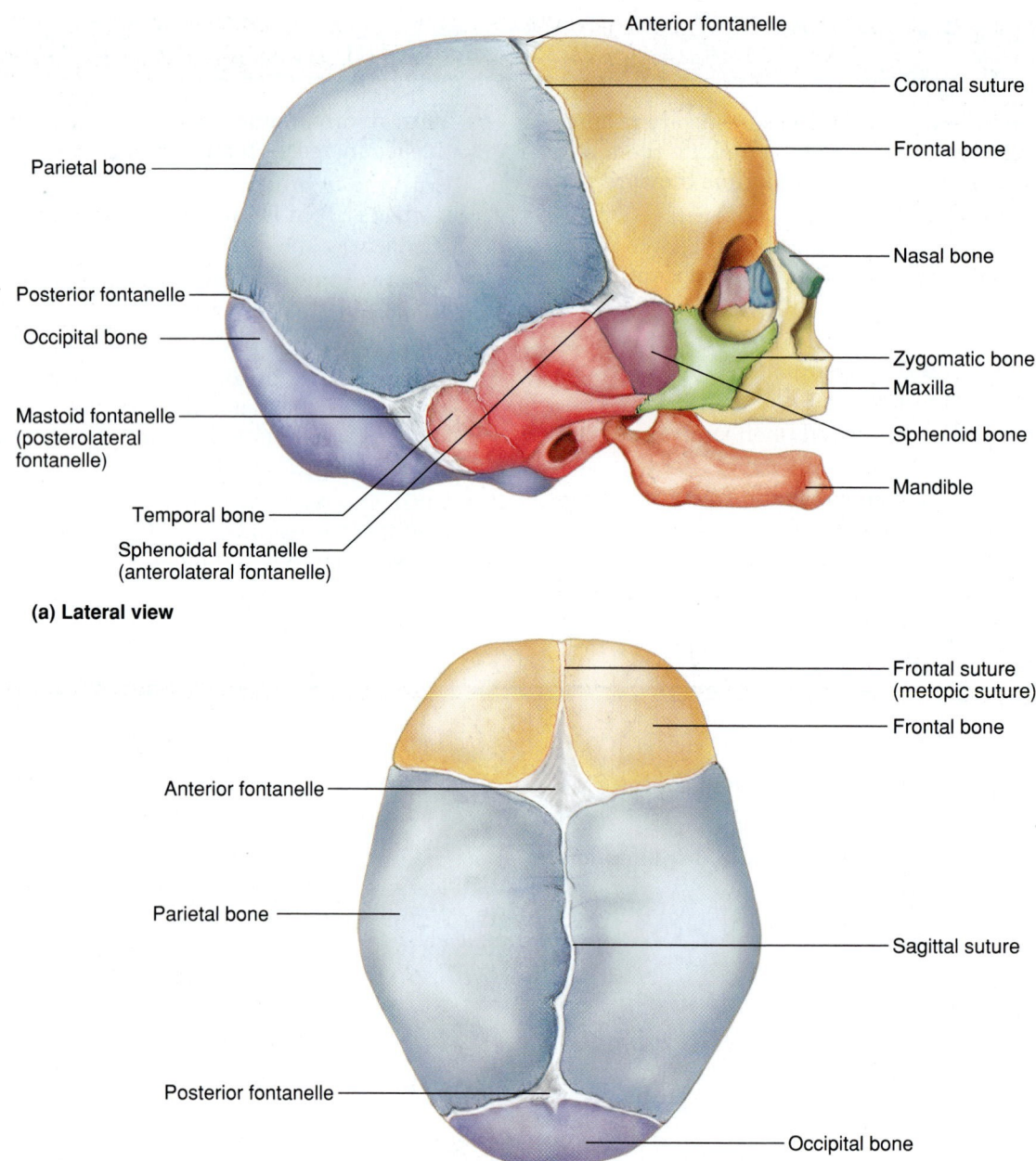

(a) Lateral view

(b) Superior view

Figure 43-8   Anatomical position of the fontanelles in an infant.

- When intubating, proceed gently (Figure 43-9).
  - Position properly; do not hyperextend the neck.
  - Use a straight blade.
  - Lift the epiglottis.
  - Use uncuffed tubes in patients less than eight years of age.

Respiratory

Pediatric patients' oxygen requirements are twice those of adults, and their oxygen reserves are smaller.[14,16] Due to these factors, these patients can rapidly become hypoxic. Children who develop hypoxia may compensate by becoming tachycardic then decompensate and become bradycardic. Implications for the EMS professional include the following:

- Close monitoring of the patient's respiratory status.
- Interventions to maintain respiratory sufficiency as indicated (positioning, supplemental oxygen, bag-mask ventilation, or intubation) (Figure 43-10).

Hematological Differences

The pediatric patient's total blood volume is approximately 8% of their total body weight compared to approximately 6% in the adult. The total blood volume, however, is less, resulting in greater consequences in children who experience blood loss. Blood loss is

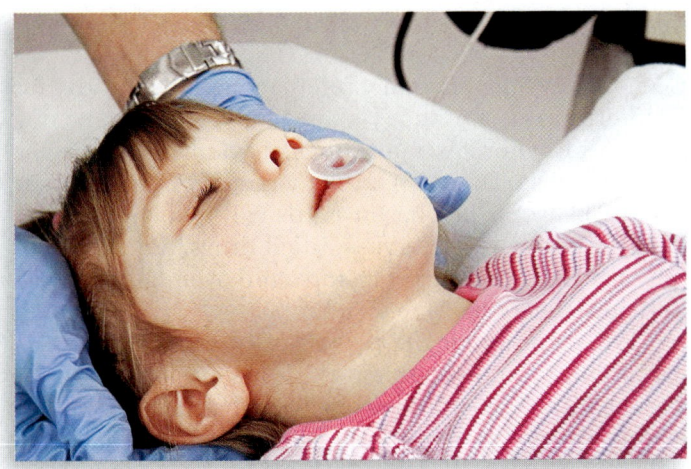

Figure 43-9 Select and carefully place an oral airway in an unconscious child. Proper positioning and simple airway adjuncts can ensure a patient's airway is cleared faster than any of the more advanced procedures, such as intubation.

initially compensated for by an increased heart rate.[16] Children can maintain their blood pressure longer than adults. Implications for the EMS professional include the following:

- If tachycardia is present, therapy must be initiated immediately and the patient monitored closely for signs of shock.
- Assess for other signs of shock (i.e., tissue perfusion), even in the presence of a normal blood pressure.
- If shock is suspected, early intervention is necessary in order to prevent progression to decompensated shock.

Cardiothoracic Differences

The pediatric patient's ribs are more pliable, resulting in fewer rib fractures. Conversely, because of their flexibility,

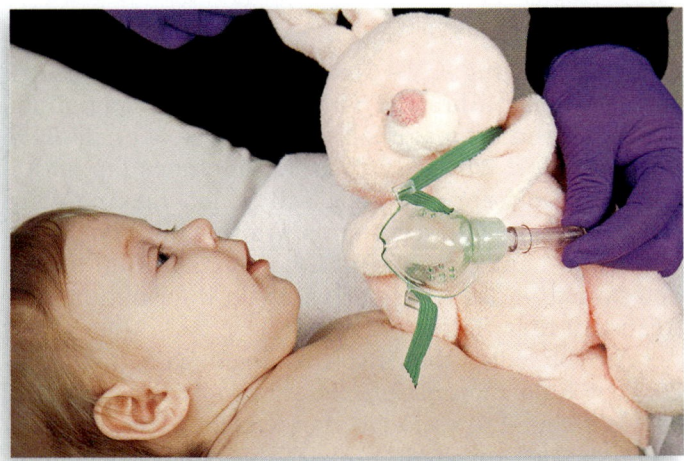

Figure 43-10 Sometimes using a familiar object, like a favorite stuffed animal, can distract the child. Placing oxygen on the object or having a parent hold it near the patient's face can be effective, too.

the ribs offer less protection to underlying organs. Muscles in the chest wall are not fully matured and fatigue easily. Lung tissue is more fragile. Implications for the EMS professional include the fact that significant internal injuries may have occurred in the absence of obvious external signs.

Abdomen

Abdominal muscles are not fully developed; thus, they offer less protection to the underlying organs. The diaphragm is positioned in a horizontal plane, causing the liver and spleen to be positioned anteriorly. The liver and spleen are large, and all of the organs are in closer proximity to each other (Figure 43-11). Implications for the EMS professional are that injuries to the liver and spleen are more common, as is the risk of multiple organ injury.[15]

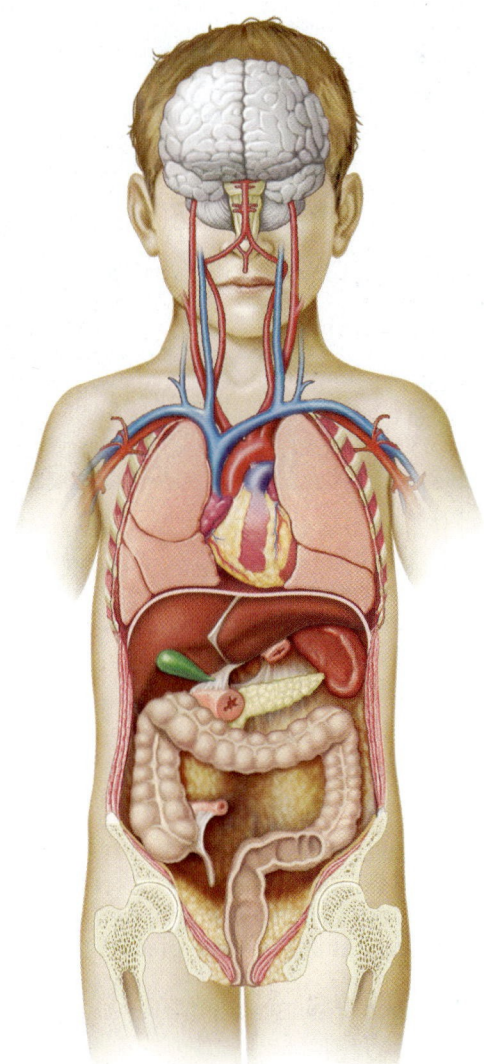

Figure 43-11 Because the diaphragm in a child is relatively flat, all of the abdominal organs are extremely close together. (The stomach has been removed to allow visualization of the pancreas and spleen.)

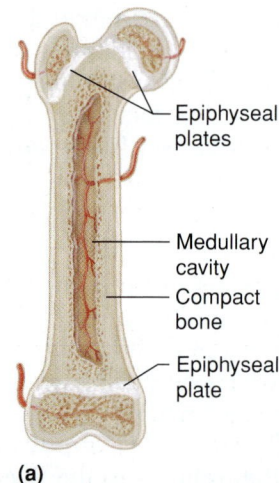

(a)

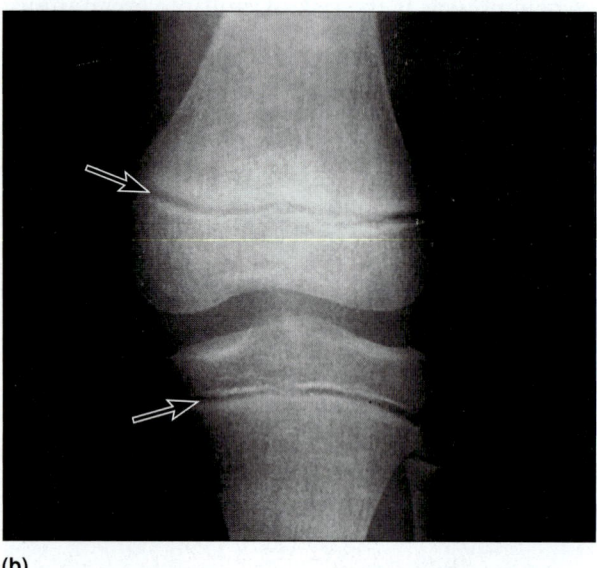

(b)

Figure 43-12 (a) Endochondral bone of a child. Note the epiphyseal growth plates. (b) Radiograph of child's bone showing growth (epiphyseal) plates (arrow).

Musculoskeletal Differences

Pediatric patients' bones are softer until young adulthood. If an injury occurs through a growth plate, growth may be disrupted. Implications for the EMS professional follow:

- Immobilize any injured extremity until a fracture can be ruled out.
- If intraosseous insertion is attempted, the epiphyseal (growth) plates should not be pierced (Figure 43-12).

CONNECTIONS Chapter 24: Skeletal Trauma discusses fractures in greater detail.

Nervous System

The nervous system is immature. The skull and spinal column afford less protection to the brain and spinal cord in pediatric patients than adults.

Assessment

Scene safety and personnel safety remain the priority for EMS. It is irrelevant that you are called to the home of a sick child; your safety and that of your partner comes before all else. Do not sacrifice yourself or change your normal behavior just because this call involves a child. Child abuse, domestic abuse, illicit drugs, and other potentially hazardous activity surround even the youngest patients. *Do not* become a victim.

When caring for the pediatric patient, you must be certain that your assessment skills are mastered. The assessment process provides you with the ability to understand problems as they present, detect problems that have not presented themselves in a conventional manner, discover problems that are responsible for comorbid complications, and discover the full gamut of medical issues that will need to be addressed. Without a proper and complete assessment, the ability to determine the correct treatment plan is nearly impossible.

In the pediatric population, the difference between medically stable (not sick) and critical (sick) is often only a few minutes of allowing the disease process or traumatic injury to progress. Small children have tremendous abilities to compensate, but when they decompensate, they decompensate and crash quickly. A poor assessment cannot be overcome by stellar technical skills. Being able to accurately read a 12-lead ECG is of no value if you failed to understand that the cardiac dysrhythmia was secondary to respiratory failure.

One of the best first steps in the assessment process is making an initial determination prior to touching the child, commonly called the "20 Foot Rule" or the initial impression:

20 Foot Rule: What does the child look like, act like, and sound like as you enter the room?

The 10-year-old boy who has audible wheezing at 20 feet is moving some amount of air but is working extremely hard to breathe, is burning excessive amounts of energy, and is most likely on the verge of crisis. The 3-year-old girl who is lying in her mother's lap, has a "glazed" look, appears pale, and is not tracking your presence is already in extremis. Waiting until you have laid your hands on the child to make your initial determinations is a loss of valuable information and treatment time (Figure 43-13).

As you enter the area and begin gathering your 20 Foot Rule information, be sure to utilize common courtesy and professional mannerisms to begin your initial assessment. First, properly introduce yourself to the child and the parents or caregivers. "Hello, we're paramedics. I'm Bob and this is my partner Isabel. And you are . . . ?" Out of respect, ask how they prefer to be addressed. Do not call patients, parents, or caregivers by

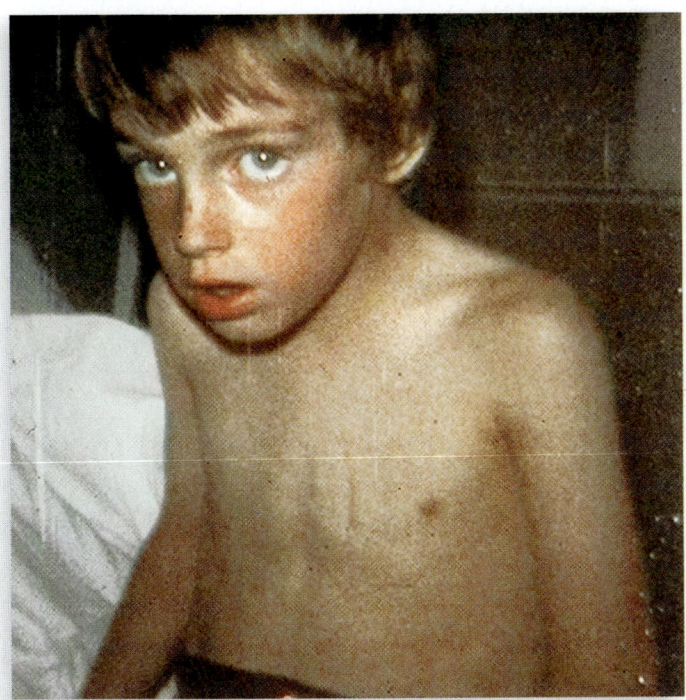

Figure 43-13   This child is clearly having difficulty breathing. As you look at him from across the room, look for signs of air hunger, intercostal and sternal retractions and his work of breathing.

cutesy titles you may use with friends and family. Names such as, "sweetie," "honey," or "buddy," are often taken as condescending and unprofessional. If the child or parent asks you to refer to them by a nickname, you may do so. Otherwise, professionalism must prevail.

Next, ask about the nature of the emergency and the patient or caregiver's impression of the problem. Many times, this seems like repeating an embarrassingly obvious statement, but the importance of hearing the patient's chief complaints will provide you with information that might otherwise be lost. "Ms. Lucero, what seems to be the problem with Kala today?" "Look at her! She can't breathe! And hasn't been able to since we came back from the ice cream store." Does the ice cream store add anything to your assessment? Maybe not, but if Kala has an allergy to nuts and ate a cross-contaminated ice cream cone, you may have the answer to the prime question, "What's killing her first?" During this time, you are conducting your initial assessment by evaluating Kala's ABCs, mental status, and appearance while simultaneously gathering additional historical information.

Using your assessment skills, thus far you have been able to assess the patients' airway, their breathing, circulation, mental status, and appearance twice, and you have also had two opportunities to begin formulating a treatment plan, once when you were 20 feet away and once while you were conducting your initial assessment. If you've discovered no issues that require immediate treatment, you can move on to the detailed assessment and focused history.

If you did find a life threat or have an impression that this child is medically unstable, focus your energies on eliminating the threat or at least reversing it.

Never, never convince yourself that further assessment or treatment is futile.

Trust yourself. Your first impression is most commonly correct, especially as you gain additional pediatric expertise. As you begin your initial assessment, you need to be assured that all life threats have been eliminated or reversed and that your treatment plan, including transport, is appropriate for this situation.

Primary Survey

The initial assessment for the pediatric patient is similar to that used for the adult patient with few differences. The objective is again assessment-based care: Discover, prioritize, treat, and reassess. One of the easiest methods to assure that you discover all that can be discovered is to think in terms of what is normal:

- What is this child's' normal physiology?
- What are this child's normal vital signs?
- What is this child's normal mentation?

If you have a clear understanding of "normal," the ability to discover abnormal is greatly increased (Table 43-4).

The American Academy of Pediatrics developed the Pediatric Assessment Triangle or PAT.[18] (Figure 43-14). The PAT is a simple equilateral triangle in which the peak is Appearance, the bottom right is Work of Breathing, and the bottom left is Circulation. This highly effective tool allows us to quickly determine if the child requires urgent intervention or not. The PAT helps us understand that the three sides of the triangle are equally important to the whole. If any of the three are compromised, the whole pediatric patient is compromised. Adults commonly have a single system complaint, and treatment is directed toward the system-specific issues. In children, they function as a whole unit. If one system begins to fail, the entire unit begins to fail. The child in respiratory distress will soon progress to respiratory failure, cardiac failure, and central neurogenic failure, and as time progresses, all other systems will fail. The PAT is a subtle way to remember what may need your full attention.

The initial assessment begins as you approach the patient by assessing the patient's mental status. The acronym AVPU (A = Awake; V = Verbal, responds to verbal stimuli; P = Painful, responds to painful stimuli; U = Unresponsive to all stimuli) provides a simple way to remember this complex tool. The Modified Glasgow Coma Scale is commonly assessed after the ABCs are addressed (Box 43-2).

TABLE 43-4   **Review of Normal Vital Signs for Pediatric Age Groups** DOT 6-2.13

		Pediatric Vital Signs			
AGE	**WEIGHT (Kg)**	**PULSE**	**RESP**	**SYST BP**	**DIAST BP**
Premature	1	145	< 40	42 +/− 10	21 +/− 8
Premature	1–2	135	—	50 +/− 10	28 +/− 8
Newborn	2–3	125	—	60 +/− 10	37 +/− 8
1 mo	4	120	24–35	80 +/− 16	46 +/− 16
6 mo	7	130	—	89 +/− 29	60 +/− 10
1 yr	10	120	20–30	96 +/− 30	66 +/− 25
2–3 yr	12–14	115	—	99 +/− 25	64 +/− 25
4–5 yr	16–18	100	—	99 +/− 20	65 +/− 20
6–9 yr	20–26	100	12–25	100 +/− 20	65 +/− 15
10–12 yr	32–42	75	—	112 +/− 20	68 +/− 15
Over 14 yr	> 50	70	12–18	120 +/− 20	75 +/− 15

Source: National Center for Emergency Medicine Infomatics at http://www.ncemi.org/cgincemi/edtable.pl?TheCommand=Load&NewFile=pediatric_vital_signs&BlankTop=1 (accessed October 12, 2006).

Airway and Breathing

Determine whether the airway is open and patent. If not, open it by repositioning the head (if no cervical spine trauma is present). The child's airway should be patent. If not, you must take appropriate steps to assure the patency. You need to assure that the child is ventilating adequately and is able to do so through continuous observations. Watch the respiratory processes including the rate of respirations, whether the chest is rising and falling (or abdomen in the younger child), the amount of chest rise and fall, the use of accessory muscles, the amount of accessory muscle

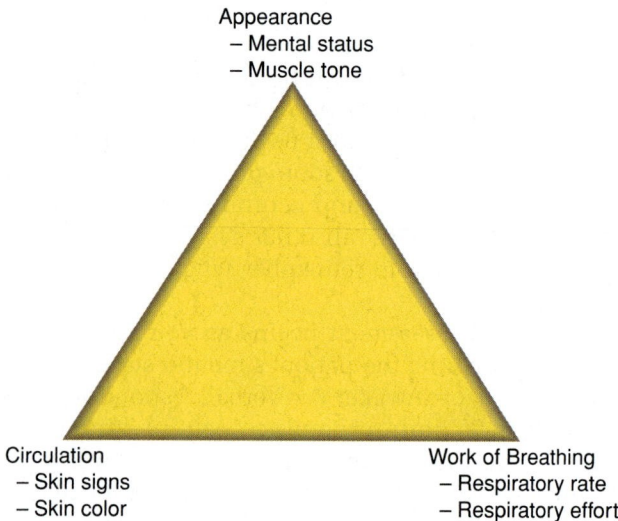

Appearance
– Mental status
– Muscle tone

Circulation
– Skin signs
– Skin color

Work of Breathing
– Respiratory rate
– Respiratory effort

Figure 43-14   Patient Assessment Triangle (PAT).

> **BOX 43-2   Modified Glasgow Scale**
>
> Any combined score of less than eight represents a significant risk of mortality.
>
> **Best eye response: (E)**
>
> 4. Eyes opening spontaneously
> 3. Eyes opening to speech
> 2. Eyes opening to pain
> 1. No eye opening
>
> **Best verbal response: (V)**
>
> 5. Infant coos or babbles (normal activity)
> 4. Infant is irritable and continually cries
> 3. Infant cries to pain
> 2. Infant moans to pain
> 1. No verbal response
>
> **Best motor responses: (M)**
>
> 6. Infant moves spontaneously or purposefully
> 5. Infant withdraws from touch
> 4. Infant withdraws from pain
> 3. Abnormal flexion to pain for an infant (decorticate response)
> 2. Extension to pain (decerebrate response)
> 1. No motor response

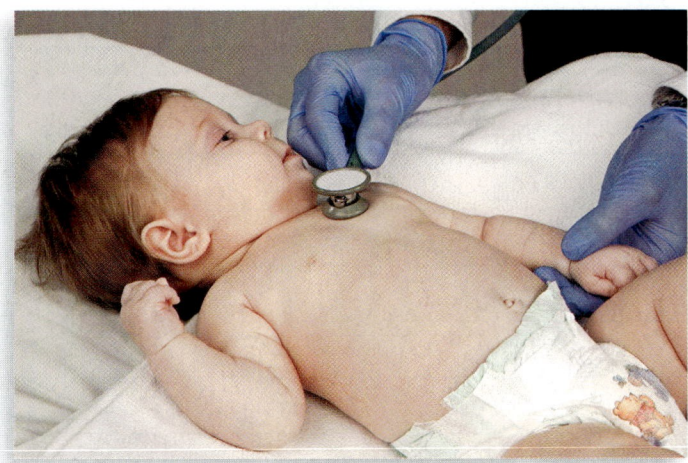

Figure 43-15 Careful assessment of lung sounds is essential. Note the towel under the child's shoulders to keep the baby's airway open.

use, nasal flaring, retractions, abnormal breath sounds (such as wheezing, stridor, grunting, snoring, gurgling), tripod positioning, head bobbing, and abnormal respiratory patterns (such as tachypnea, Cheyne-Stokes, Kussmaul's sign, or bradypnea) (Figure 43-15).

If a problem is discovered, corrective intervention is mandatory. If the child's respiratory status is compromised, immediate interventions are required. Your treatment plan should include supplemental oxygen, and any airway adjunct such as an oral airway, nasal airway, endotracheal intubation, and suctioning, as necessary.

Circulation

Assess for the adequacy of the child's circulation. Evaluate the child's skin condition, including color, temperature, and turgor. Determine the quality and quantity of the distal pulses. Finally assess the child's capillary refill time (Figure 43-16). All of these questions must be addressed quickly and accurately. Touching the child's skin will answer a number of these questions simultaneously. The skin condition combined with the appearance of the child will provide you with information that you will be validating as you complete your assessment. An example is the child who appears pale and lethargic at 20 feet, has an open airway with shallow respirations, and is warm to the touch. As a paramedic, you should already be thinking this child is sick.

Central and distal pulses should be checked simultaneously. In small, chubby children the carotid pulse may be difficult to find without obstructing the airway. Consider checking the femoral pulse. If either pulse site is diminished, poor circulatory status is obvious. The child is in a hypoperfusion state, and immediate treatment must ensue.

The PAT tells us that if the appearance is poor, the child should be considered critical until proven otherwise. What pulse rate would you expect to find? Pallor, lethargy, a decreased respiratory rate, and mental function compromise tell you the best case is the child will have an accelerated heart rate (compensating tachycardia), but equally likely is a slowed heart rate (decompensating bradycardia). The tachycardia is actually a better sign than the bradycardia, yet the bradycardia should be the expected rhythm. The entire treatment plan is being formulated for the more critical situation.

Airway, breathing, circulation, appearance, and mental status have now all been assessed. Any potential life threat should now be discovered and addressed. "What is killing the child first?" Table 43-5 list normal rates and ranges for pediatric patients.

The CUPS Assessment Scale developed by the Critical Illness and Trauma Foundation, Inc., is an assessment

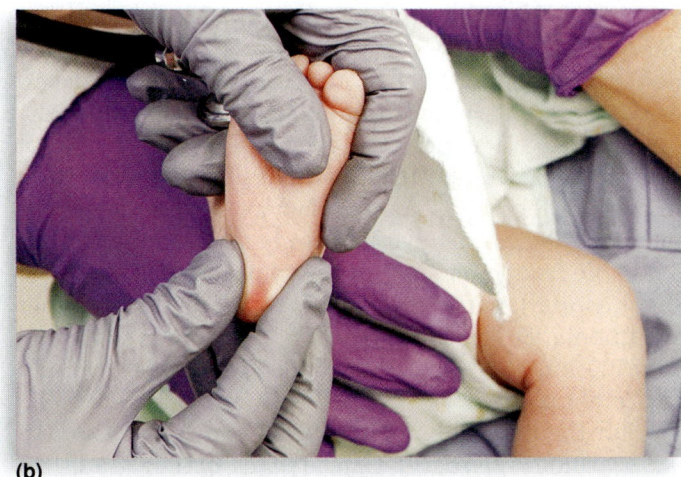

(a)   (b)

Figure 43-16 (a) Sometimes it is possible to palpate or auscultate (not shown) an apical pulse. Place two fingers slightly distal and lateral to the xiphoid area as shown. (b) Your lower limb assessment in a small child should include a good capillary blanch test. Firmly grasp the foot and press; then observe how quickly color returns to the area. Document the time duration on your care report form.

TABLE 43-5 Pediatric Vital Sign Normal Ranges DOT 6-2.13

Age Group	Respiratory Rate	Heart Rate	Low-Normal Systolic Blood Pressure	Weight in kilos	Weight in pounds
Newborn	30–60	100–160	> 60	2–3	4.5–7
Infant (one to 12 months)	20–30	100–160	> 60	4–10	9–22
Toddler (one to three years)	20–40	90–150	> 70	10–14	22–31
Preschooler (three to six years)	22–34	80–140	>75	14–18	31–40
School Age (six to 12 years)	18–30	70–120	> 80	20–42	41–92
Adolescent (13+ years)	12–20	60–100	> 90	> 50	> 110

Source: Modified from TRIPP Paramedic at www.cpem.org and http://emsresource.net/vitals.shtml (accessed October 12, 2006).

tool that can be used to assist in the determination of the criticality of the patient.[19]

CUPS determines rapidity of transport

C Critical
U Unstable
P Potentially unstable
S Stable

If you have performed your initial assessment and assessment-based care skills and nothing is a life threat, you can move on to the focused history.

Focused History

By the time you complete your paramedic training, you will be well briefed on the focused history. The differences in this process are specific for the age of the pediatric patient. It is of the utmost importance to understand that if the patient is unstable or critical, the opportunity to conduct a focused history may not present itself. On the other hand, if time allows, failure to acquire location sensitive or person sensitive information (information available only at the home or only available from a person not accompanying the child to the hospital) may result in inaccurate or improper treatments. The need to gather all of the child's relevant information is vital in order to develop an accurate treatment plan.

For the infant, the history must come from the parent or primary caregiver instead of the patient. Toddlers and preschoolers may be able to assist with certain aspects of the history, but frequently they cannot, especially if the situation is serious or critical. As children get older, their ability to assist with both the history and

treatment plan increases with age. By the time the older teens transition into adulthood, their ability to provide valued information is equal to that of most adults. From this chronological hallmark forth, the same principles apply for young adults and adults alike. The commonly used SAMPLE history mnemonic is as appropriate for children as it is for adults.

Detailed Physical Examination

As with the focused history, the detailed examination may never be performed if the child is unstable or critical. Instability requires that your full attention be focused on the lifesaving therapies that will make a difference. Do not be distracted by less important issues when a child needs your full and undivided expertise.

If the situation allows and you are to the point of performing the detailed physical examination, completeness is the benchmark. Again, the detailed physical examination is similar to that of the adult, yet there are specifics based on age for the pediatric patient.

In patients of all ages, the approaching paramedic increases the anxiety and fear already present at the emergency scene. The time-honored method to overcome these challenges in children is to conduct your assessment from the toes to the head. In addition, the toe-to-head method forces you to get down to the patient's eye level, which helps to reduce the child's anxiety. If a mother is holding a young child on her lap, you must kneel, putting you at or below the patient. If the patient is a young adult, you still have to kneel to start the assessment. Being at or below the patient's eye level is a key aspect to this method.

As you approach the patient, note any soft tissue abnormalities. Regardless of the area or region, soft

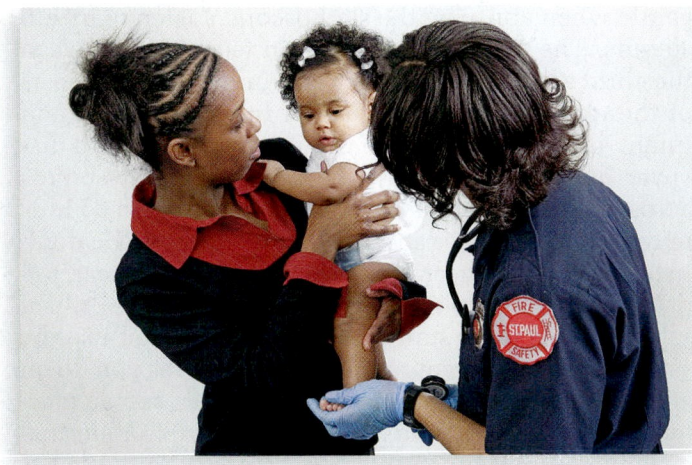

Figure 43-17   Gradually approach the child and begin by touching the feet or hands to develop trust and rapport.

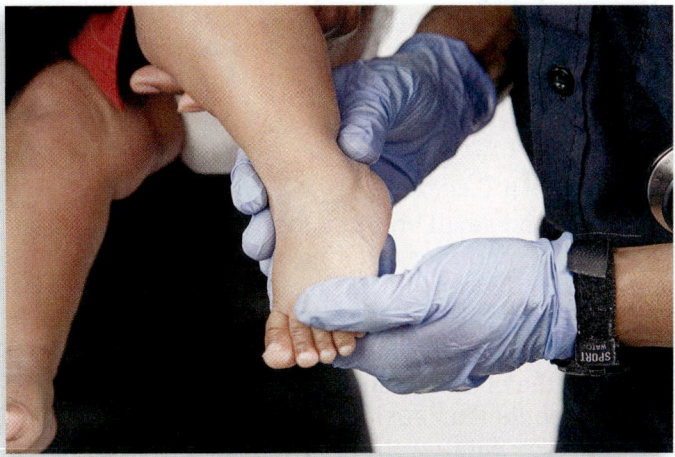

Figure 43-19   Assessment of a lower leg.

tissue injuries can be both informative and revealing. Understanding the mechanism that produced the injury and what additional injuries may have occurred is essential. If there is no concern for potential spine injury, assess the posterior aspects or the back of the patient. Examination of the back of the patient can frequently provide information that is otherwise lost.

The Feet

Starting your physical assessment from the toes allows for the trust relationship to begin in earnest (Figure 43-17). There is less anxiety generated from a stranger touching the toes or feet than there would be touching the "personal zone"—the nose down to the

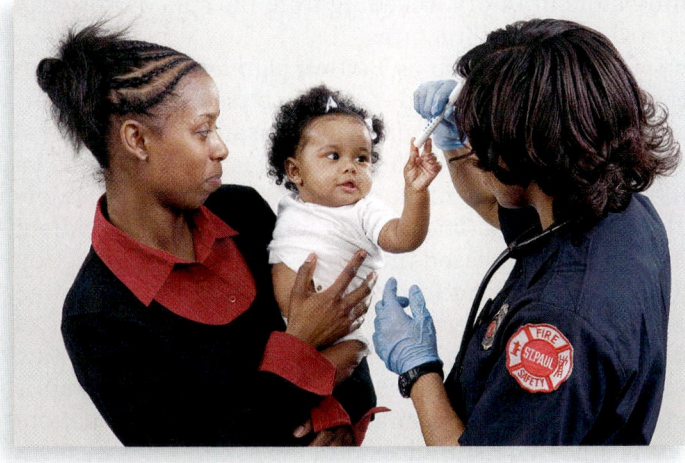

Figure 43-18   A playful child with good reaction time or one who is able to reach and touch your assessment tools is usually alert and has good neurological function.

symphysis pubis. While at the feet, the distal pulses can be assessed. If you have pulses at the dorsalis pedis or posterior tibialis, the child's circulatory status is within the "compatible with life" category. Bounding distal pulses indicate a higher cardiac output. Assessing the child's skin at the feet also provides a vast amount of information. Color, turgor, temperature, dryness, moisture, and warmth can be easily assessed and correlated to the quality of the sign at the body's core. While assessing the feet, you can watch the abdominal area to count respirations without causing a change in respiratory pattern or rate due to the patient's sense of someone staring at the chest. Audible breath sounds can also be listened to from this vantage point.

Finally, you are able to assess the patient's mental status simply by paying attention to the child's reaction to you as you proceed (Figure 43-18). If the child follows your movements, pulls away from you, or does not move as you touch the feet, the general mentation can be revealed. Finally, comparing the distal and central pulses can be completed prior to leaving the feet.

Lower Extremities and Pelvis

Next on the toe-to-head examination are the legs (Figure 43-19). Check for symmetry in circulation, motion, strength, and sensation. If the child has not sustained physical trauma to the pelvic region, evaluating the integrity of the pelvic ring is not necessary. If there has been trauma, a standard orthopedic examination should be conducted. Checking a femoral pulse may be appropriate at this juncture. Ask the child about any injury or illness to the organs in the pelvic girdle. Does the patient have any pain with palpation? Any problems with bowel or bladder function? Vaginal bleeding or discharge? Rectal bleeding? Bleeding at the urethral meatus? Is there any soft tissue injury(s) to the pelvic or genitalia region?

Abdomen

In infants and small children, observe the abdomen for signs of distention or swelling. Crying will sometimes cause the child to swallow considerable amounts of air. This problem may cause respiratory compromise due to the inflated stomach pressing up on the diaphragm and reducing the child's tidal volume. Before touching the patient's abdomen, look for any soft tissue injuries, and ask about any pain, swelling, or discomfort. This inquiry will allow you the opportunity to listen to the patient's concerns prior to inflicting any discomfort. The trust you have worked hard to build will be instantly destroyed if you touch the most painful area without the patient's understanding of why you would do so. In addition, stimulating a pain response prior to assessing the areas around the complaint will cause a conscious and unconscious muscular response that may mask the true magnitude of the problem.

Palpate the area of concern last, not first. When you do palpate, remember that every patient has four quadrants of the abdomen. A common error, especially in the obese child or young adult, is to palpate four locations above the beltline. When privacy permits, you must palpate the lower abdomen as well as the upper portion. Failure to palpate the lower abdomen is a life-threatening error waiting to happen, regardless of the patients' age. Observe and palpate the posterior abdomen (flanks) to be assured that the area is not forgotten once spinal immobilization or transport has begun.

Chest

Undress the child and visually inspect for signs of respiratory distress, such as retractions. As with the abdomen, look for any soft tissue abnormalities prior to palpation. Gentle palpation may reveal areas of tenderness, subcutaneous emphysema, or bony crepitus. Wheezing, rhonchi, rales, and stridor that are audible from a distance are of greater significance than similar lung noises that can only be heard with a stethoscope. A young child's ribs are soft and flexible and, therefore, less likely to break even when the blunt force trauma is significant enough to cause internal organ damage. If broken ribs are discovered in the younger child, the force involved is most likely extreme. Soft tissue and organ damage from this magnitude of trauma must be investigated with interventional treatments started. Listening to breath sounds is normally not considered palpation, but touching a tender area with the stethoscope may cause the child significant discomfort, so be

gentle when applying the stethoscope. Listen to breath sounds. The primary difference in technique between the child and the adult is to listen in the lateral aspects of the chest. Listen to the axilla in the newborn and infant, as this provides the greatest opportunity to discover an abnormality by hearing the breath sounds across the greatest distance. Diminished breath sounds may be as alarming as absent breath sounds. If you don't listen, you won't hear. If you listen and don't hear, the detailed assessment must cease, and immediate critical interventions must start instantly. Be sure you use the same technique on your pediatric patients as you do on adults, including listening to every patient so you master normal breath sounds and will recognize abnormal ones when present. Listen to heart tones in every patient you encounter. Again, the only way to understand abnormal is to master normal. DOT 6-2.14

Neck

The primary issues with the neck focus on the great vessels and trachea. Make sure that there are no soft tissue injuries or abnormalities that would interfere with respiration or circulation. In the absence of trauma, evaluate the neck for stiffness or rigidity. If the child is irritable, lethargic, appears sick, or presents with the nondescript "something is wrong," check for neck stiffness, fever, altered mental status, suprasternal retractions, and respiratory compromise. Infection or toxicity may be the cause.

Head

Look for soft tissue abnormalities. Any soft tissue injury or defect may be the initial indicator that a more ominous issue is present. Scalp injuries can bleed excessively and may be the origin for hypovolemic shock. Many of the common signs to look for, if present, are late indicators of injury. Bleeding from the ears or nose can be a sign of skull fractures.

Other signs such as Battle's sign and raccoon eyes typically take an extended time to be seen. If these signs are found, the patient may have sustained a fracture at the base of the skull. The fontanelles or "soft spots" of the newborn and infant are open until approximately 18 months of age. The anterior fontanelle is an excellent indicator of increased intracranial pressure or infection (bulging or elevated) or dehydration (sunken). Fontanelle status, temperature, and skin status are pieces of information that can quickly be gathered by evaluating the fontanelles (Figure 43-20). Evaluation of the pupils may require greater patience than in the adult patient but is otherwise similar.

Overall, the detailed physical examination is similar for pediatrics and adults. The specifics of age and development require adjustments. Reassessments should be

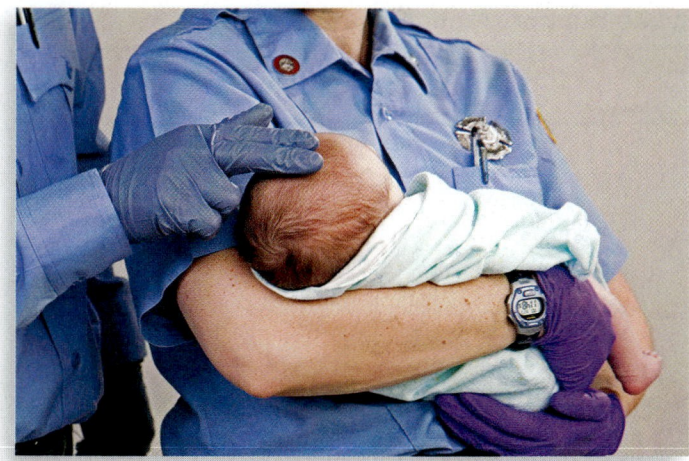

Figure 43-20 Gently touch the top of the baby's head to feel for either a depression (sunken) or a bulging fontanelle.

conducted on an ongoing basis. Some literature claims that reassessments should be conducted every 15 minutes for stable patients and every five minutes for unstable. These time factors are not based on any science and serve only as general guidelines. The condition of children will change drastically in an extremely short period of time. Waiting for a specific time interval to occur is a recipe for disaster. The reassessment process should be continuous and complete.

Reassess, treat, reassess, treat, reassess.

Procedures and Equipment

For many years, much of the equipment used in the prehospital setting for pediatric patients was actually designed for adults and merely made smaller. With the advent of EMSC and the numerous pediatric and emergency medical specialists who have dedicated themselves to increasing the quality of pediatric prehospital care, this is changing. Today, many of the devices and tools used are specifically designed to meet the anatomic and developmental requirements of the youngest patients. This section will describe a variety of equipment used during the care of children, how to properly size the equipment, and any special procedures unique to children. See Tables 43-6 and 43-7.

Airway Management

In general, the process of managing the airway of the newborn, infant, child, or young adult is similar to that of the adult. The major differences in airway management are in the size of the airway and adjunct equipment and in the variation of the procedures necessitated by the anatomical differences. Children with no oxygen

reserves are extremely sensitive to hypoxia and anoxia. Care must be taken to assure that oxygen is administered early in the course of prehospital care.

Supplemental Oxygen

In small children, use of the nasal cannula, simple mask, or the nonrebreather mask may prove to be a great struggle and, therefore, force the child to burn more oxygen than you are providing. This negative impact can change the child's condition from serious to critical or fatal. Utilizing blow-by techniques allows you to provide supplemental oxygen without increasing oxygen consumption. Use techniques such as holding the mask near the patient's face (pointing it toward the mouth and nose) or simply having the parent hold the oxygen tubing near the child's face. Some manufacturer's produce oxygen delivery devices that look like toys or may captivate the child's attention. When all else fails, simply placing the oxygen tubing close to the patient's face usually works well (Figure 43-21).

Airway Adjuncts

The primary airway adjuncts utilized in EMS include the following: DOT 6-2.15, 6-2.16, 6-2.17, 6-2.18

- **Suction devices.** Suction is the most forgotten of the critical procedures (Figure 43-22). Despite knowing that, every time airway management is needed, suctioning may be the difference between completing a procedure quickly and without complication and not being able to complete the procedure and having a patient, if the patient survives, with aspiration pneumonia. The use of hard tip versus soft tip catheters is situation specific. Determinations are similar to those in the adult patient.

- **Oral airways.** Oropharyngeal airways (OPA) come in a variety of sizes and can serve as a bite block for the child who begins to regain consciousness yet needs assistance maintaining their airway. Oral airways can be placed by using a tongue blade for a direct insertion approach, by starting at 90 degrees and rotating into proper position, or by starting at 180 degrees and rotating into proper position. Regardless of the technique used, be sure that the OPA does not push the posterior aspect of the tongue into the glottic opening.

- **Nasal airways.** Nasopharyngeal airways (NPA) are used in children when they are conscious and breathing but are unable to control their own airway. NPAs can be beneficial for the paramedic caring for a child who needs aggressive airway maintenance but needs to have both hands free for other procedures. The insertion technique is similar to that of the adult. Because the NPA can be irritating or painful, a water-soluble analgesic gel

TABLE 43-6 Pediatric Equipment and Supplies for Basic Life Support Ambulances

BLS Equipment & Supplies

ESSENTIAL

1. Oropharyneal airways (sizes 00–5)
   (a) infant
   (b) child
   (c) adult
2. Self-inflating resuscitation bag[*]
   (a) infant
   (b) child
   (c) adult
3. Masks for bag-mask device
   (a) neonatal (for delivery of premature infant)
   (b) infant
   (c) child
   (d) adult
4. Oxygen masks
   (a) infant
   (b) child
   (c) adult
5. Nonrebreathing masks
   (a) pediatric
   (b) adult
6. Stethoscope
7. Backboard
8. Cervical immobilization device (wedges, collars, etc., but not sandbags)
   (a) infant
   (b) child

   (c) adolescent
   (d) adult
9. Blood pressure cuffs
   (a) infant
   (b) child
   (c) adult
10. Portable suction unit with regulator
11. Suction catheters: rigid and 6F-14F flexible
12. Extremity splints: pediatric sizes
13. Bulb syringe
14. Obstetric pack (OB kit)
15. Thermal blanket[§]
16. Water-soluble lubricant

DESIRABLE

1. Infant car seat
2. Nasopharyngeal airways: sizes 18F–34F, or 4.5–8.5 mm[¶]
3. Glasgow Coma Scale reference
4. Pediatric trauma score reference
5. Small stuffed toy
6. Computer with CD-ROM capability (at base station)
7. EMSC CD-ROM training discs[**]

[*]A self-inflating resuscitation bag should be self-refilling, should have an oxygen reservoir and should not have a pop-off valve. A child bag has a reservoir of 450 mL; whereas, an adult bag has a reservoir of at least 1,000 mL.

[§]A thermal blanket may help minimize heat loss. Hypothermia will complicate many illnesses and injuries, particularly in infants and young children. The type of material used will depend on local preference, protocols, and procedures but may include Mylar, standard blankets, or aluminum foil for small infants.

[¶]A nasopharyngeal airway may be useful when the upper airway compromises respiration and an oral airway cannot be secured. Providers must be trained in its use and know the contraindications for insertion of this device.

[**]Contact: EMSC Clearinghouse, 2070 Chain Bridge Road, Suite 450, Vienna, VA 22182 (703-902-1203/1272), emsc@circsol.com or info@emscnrc.com; or visit the EMSC web site: http://www.ems-c.org.

Source: Seidel et al; "Committee on Ambulance Equipment and Supplies, National Emergency Medical Services for Children Resource Alliance," *Annals of Emergency Medicine* 28(6) (December 1996): 699–701.

should be used as both the lubricant and numbing agent. Extreme care must be taken to assure that the posterior tongue is lifted away from the back of the pharynx to ensure that it does not continue to partially obstruct the airway.

Endotracheal Intubation (ET)

Pediatric intubation is a procedure that has been the subject of a great deal of controversy over the past few years. The basis of the discussion is found in a large study conducted by Dr. Marianne Gausche from 1994 through 1997.[11] The study showed that the benefit of paramedic intubation of pediatric patients in the Los Angeles area was questionable and potentially detrimental. The study further found that the use of the bag-mask was at least as beneficial as endotracheal intubation and maybe of greater benefit. This study, the largest of its kind ever conducted, has limitations but does show that in the Los Angeles area, prehospital

TABLE 43-7   **Pediatric Equipment and Supplies for Advanced Life Support Ambulances**

ALS Equipment & Supplies

ESSENTIAL

1. Transport monitor
2. Defibrillator with adult and pediatric paddles[#]
3. Monitoring electrodes: pediatric sized and multifunction pads
4. Laryngoscope
   (a) straight blades 0–2
   (b) curved blades 2–4
5. Endotracheal tube stylets
   (a) pediatric
   (b) adult
6. Endotracheal tubes
   (a) uncuffed sizes 2.5–6.0
   (b) cuffed 6.0–8.0
7. Magill forceps
   (a) pediatric
   (b) adult

8. Nasogastric tubes: 8F–16F[**]
9. Nebulizer
10. IV catheters: 16 to 24 gauge
11. Intraosseous needles
12. Length/weight-based drug dose chart or tape (e.g., Broselow® Tape)
13. Needles 20 to 25 gauge and syringes 1 mL to 50 mL.
14. Resuscitation drugs and IV fluids that meet the local standards of practice

DESIRABLE

1. Blood glucose analysis system[††]
2. Disposable CO_2 detection device
3. Computer with CD ROM capability
4. EMSC CD-ROM Training set [++]

[#]A defibrillator should be able to deliver 5 to 360 joules. The addition of pediatric paddles may give the responding unit enhanced capabilities but is not essential for units that rarely use this equipment. The defibrillator may be equipped with only adult paddles/pads or pediatric paddles and adult paddles/pads. Units carrying only adult paddles/pads should insure that providers are trained in the proper use of adult paddles in infants and children. When the defibrillator cannot deliver a low dose of joules for infants, shock at the lowest possible energy level.

[**]Nasogastric tubes may be useful when the transport time is greater than 30 minutes in patients who have abdominal distention that may impede respiration.

[††]Many EMS systems estimate blood glucose in the field. The accuracy of any one blood glucose test is influenced by many factors such as the shelf life of the particular strip used, how the blood sample was obtained, and the education of the providers performing the skill. Quality improvement is an important component of any laboratory analysis and should be applied to this field procedure. Universal precautions must always be followed when blood is handled.

[++]Contact: EMSC Clearinghouse, 2070 Chain Bridge Road, Suite 450, Vienna, VA 22182 (703-902-1203/1272), emsc@circsol.com or info@emscnrc.com; or visit the EMSC web site: http://www.ems-c.org.

Source: Seidel et al., "Committee on Ambulance Equipment and Supplies, National Emergency Medical Services for Children Resource Alliance," *Annals of Emergency Medicine* 28(6) (December 1996): 699–701.

intubation of the pediatric patient may not be the "gold standard" of care. Dr. Gausche herself has been vocal in stating that EMS systems must evaluate their efficacy in pediatric intubation before changing protocols based solely on reading the study.[13,20]

The procedure of pediatric intubation is similar to that of the adult patient (Figure 43-23). Care must be taken to assure that, if intubation is going to be done, it is done effectively and efficiently. Remember that the child's anatomy varies by age. Consideration must be given to those differences (Box 43-3). A straight blade is recommended for children less than 2 years of age.[21] As soon as the ET is visually observed passing between the vocal cords, have your EMS partner or other qualified healthcare provider check breath sounds and gastric sounds for tube placement and apply an ETCO$_2$ detector for confirmation. DOT 6-2.19, 6-2.20

If the ET tube was not visualized passing between the vocal cords, the procedure should be considered a "blind intubation," and additional validation

measures must be taken. If the ET tube is visualized passing between the vocal cords, confirm breath sounds with bag-mask inhalations by listening over the epigastrum, left chest, and right chest. If the ET tube passed between the vocal cords, right mainstem bronchus placement is the most common location for an ET tube placed too deeply. Listening to the left chest allows the opportunity to hear breath sounds from a properly placed ET tube. Hearing no breath sounds in the left chest but having good chest rise on the right side, indicates the tube is advanced too far and in the right mainstem bronchus. While listening to breath sounds, the ET tube can be withdrawn slightly until breath sounds are heard in both lung fields. Be careful not to withdraw the ET tube out of the trachea.

End-tidal CO_2 detection is highly recommended to confirm proper tube placement.[22] The "gold standard" is electronic capnography. In the prehospital setting, use of the colorimetry device is the most common. Care

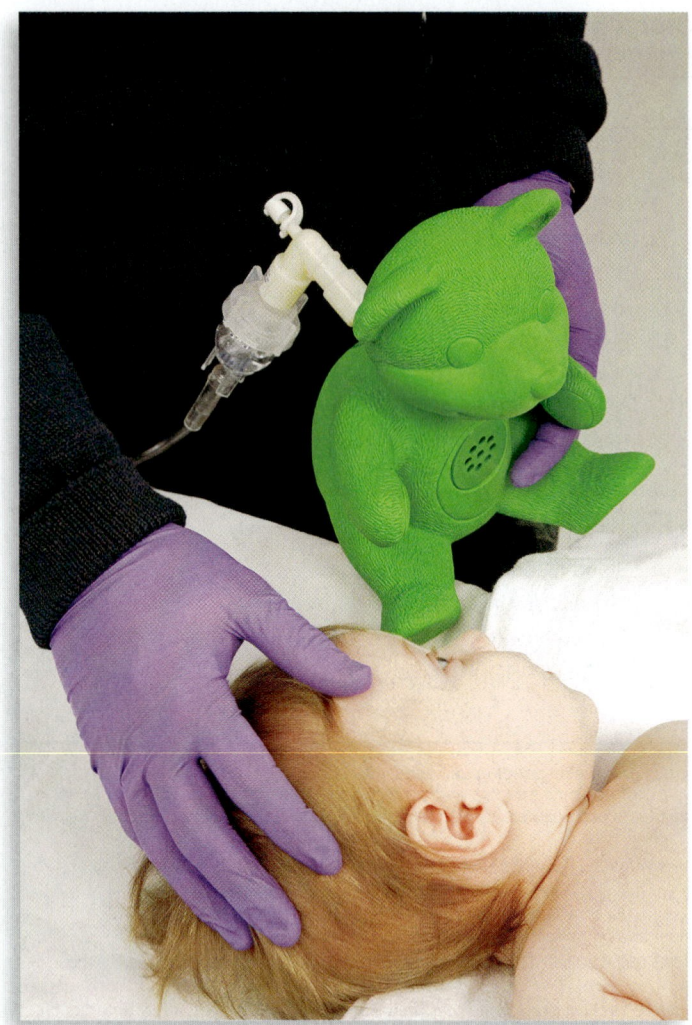

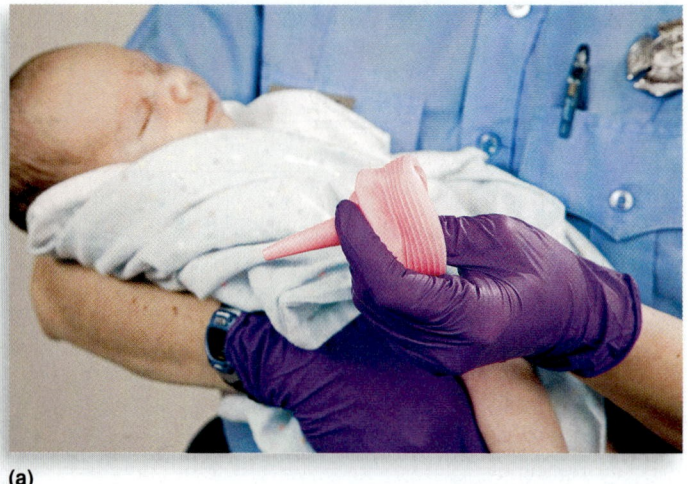

(a)

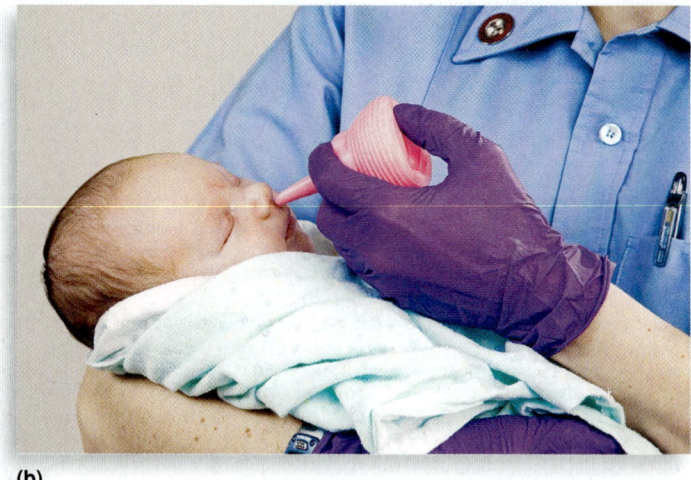

(b)

Figure 43-21 Some commercially available devices that look familiar to the child may assit treatment, such as this bear that is being used to administer a nebulizer treatment.

must be taken to use the pediatric-sized device in the small pediatric patient. The dead air space in the adult-sized devices may allow for false readings or facilitate retained CO_2 being delivered back into the child, resulting in a worsening hypercarbia or hypoxia. It is also worth noting that in cardiac arrest, the color change may suggest an improperly placed ET tube, not because the tube is placed in the esophagus, but because the CO_2/O_2 exchange in the lungs is minimal. In this type of situation, do not remove the ET tube solely on the colorimetry change or lack thereof.

The issue of how to best secure the ET tube is also one of debate. Several recent studies have shown the advantages of cervical collars for the nontraumatized intubated patient, along with the use of commercially available "tube ties or holders."[23] Regardless of whether the securing device is commercially developed or tape, the definitive answer is that the tube must be secured.

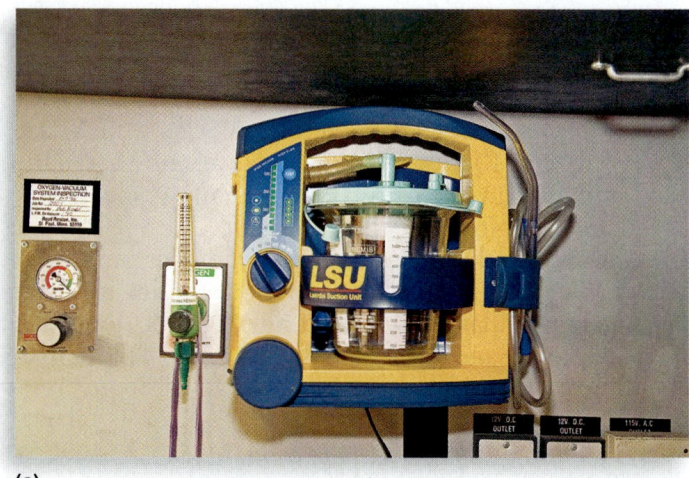

(c)

Figure 43-22 In smaller children, a bulb syringe may be useful in clearing small amounts of secretions. (a) Depress the bulb to expel the air. (b) Then insert the bulb in the nasopharynx or oropharynx and release your finger. (c) A suction unit with adjustable power should be available in the ambulance and be portable so that it can be brought to the patient's side.

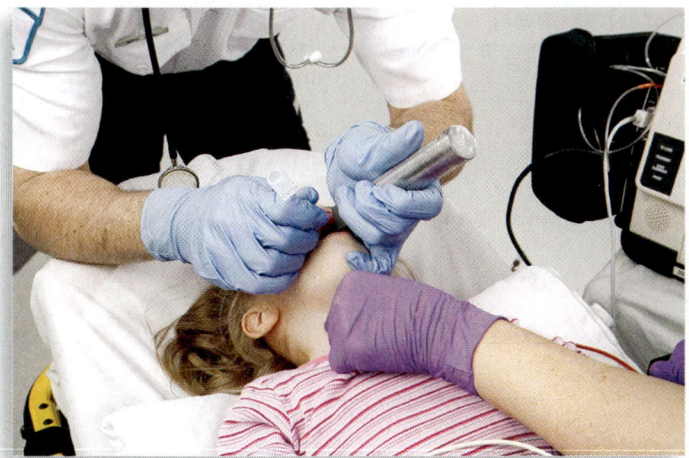

Figure 43-23   Use of a straight blade with a towel or blanket lifting the shoulders, as well as gentle cricoid pressure, will aid in visualizing pediatric cords and successful intubation.

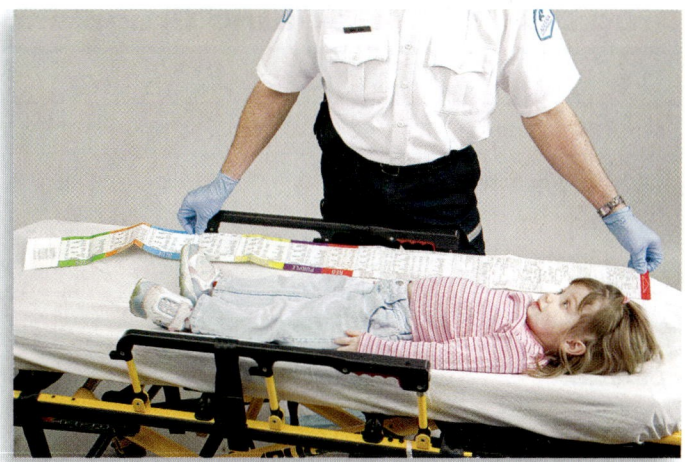

Figure 43-24   The Broselow® Tape can be useful for estimating weights, vital signs, and medication dosages in children.

Vascular Access

The use of intravenous (IV) therapy for the delivery of fluids and medications has become a mainstream skill for all ages of patients. Pediatric patients are often denied this potentially life-saving therapy simply because they are children. Basically, if the child needs an IV, start one. Do not let age distract from the treatment pathway.

IV access is generally achieved through venipuncture of the hand, radial, antecubital, medial cephalic, scalp, or the external jugular veins just as in the adult. (Note: Local protocols may dictate the inclusion or exclusion of specific sites.) The use of intraosseous (IO) access has become an accepted practice in many EMS systems. The primary difference between the pediatric and adult IV access is the size of the catheter used. DOT 6-2.31, 6-2.32, 6-2.33

Medications

The two most significant caveats relative to pediatric medication administration follow:

> Treat the cause first, *not* the symptoms.
> Length-based determinations of dosage are evidence-based; use the evidence.[25]

Pediatric patients are most often responsive to ventilation, oxygenation, and temperature regulation. Medications are utilized a small percentage of the time, especially when compared to the adult patient. That being said, when necessary, *do not* withhold medications from patients simply because they are children.

The primary medication given to children is oxygen. Oxygen, a medication with numerous indications, few contraindications, and fewer untoward side effects, is one of the most important therapeutic actions a paramedic can take while caring for the child in crisis. The second most common medication category administered to children is fluids, normal saline being the most frequently given. Drug Box 43-1 provides an overview of the principal medications and dosages used in the prehospital arena.[27]

Medication routes for the pediatric patient are similar to that of adults. They include inhalation (metered dose inhaler or nebulizer), intramuscular, intranasal, intraosseous, intravenous, oral, peripheral, rectal, subcutaneous, sublingual, and transmucosal. Depending on local protocols, utilization of each route will vary significantly.

BOX 43-3   Tube Size and Depth of Insertion by Age

Tube size approximation = diameter of the child's little finger

or

4 + (age in years / 4) = size in mm

Example for 6-year-old child:

4 + (6 / 4) = 5.5 mm

Depth of insertion = 3 × internal diameter of tube appropriate for age

Example for a 6-year-old child:

3 × 5.5 = 16.5 cm

Use a Broselow® Tape to determine which size equipment to use (Figure 43-24).[24,25,26]

Drug Box 43-1   Pediatric Drugs and Calculations   DOT 6-2.50

Drug	Dose	How Supplied	Remarks
Atropine sulfate	0.01–0.03 mg/kg IV	0.1 mg/mL	Maximum dose child: 1 mg
Benadryl (diphenhydramine HCl)	zero to one year: 1 mg/kg Max of 50 mg IM or IV	50 mg/mL	Over 1 minute, slow IV push or deep IM injection (contraindicated for asthmatics)
Calcium chloride	20 mg/kg/dose	100 mg/mL	Give slowly via IV
Dextrose			See Drug Box 43-2, page 1083
Dopamine	5–15 mcg/kg/min IV, alpha effects dominate at 10 mcg/kg/min	40 mg/mL	Dilute 200 mg in 250 mL D5W-800 mcg/mL *or* dilute 400 mg in 250 mL D5W-1600 mcg/mL
Epinephrine	1:10,000 0.01 mg/kg (0.1 mL/kg) IV		For bradycardia, cardiac arrest
Epinephrine	1:1,000 0.01 mg/kg (0.01 mL/kg) IM	1 mg/mL	For asthma
Furosemide (Lasix)	1 mg/kg IV	10 mg/mL	
Lidocaine	1 mg/kg IV	10 mg/mL (1%)	
Lidocaine drip	20–50 mcg/kg/min IV	10 mg/mL	Dilute 100 mg in 100 mL D5W
Narcan (Naloxone)	0.1 mg/kg IV, IM, nasal	0.4 mg in 1 mL ampule or 2 mg vials	Short half-life
Sodium bicarbonate	1–2 mEq/kg IV	1 mEq/mL	Should be diluted for newborns

General Principles of Patient Management

Respiratory System Issues

From birth until about 12 years of age the child's airway is constantly growing and changing. Because of this constant flux and physically smaller anatomy, children are persistently at risk for airway compromise or respiratory system complications. DOT 6-2.22, 6-2.23, 6-2.24, 6-2.53–6-2.5b

Apnea

The irregular, periodic breathing of the newborn must not be confused with apnea, and apnea *must not* be confused with irregular breathing patterns. **Apnea** is defined as, "transient cessation of respiration whether normal or abnormal."[28] The usual time factor included in the definition is that the episode lasts longer than 20 seconds. Apnea is one of the first signs of significant respiratory compromise. Apnea is commonly due to prematurity, toxicity, or ALTE (apparent life-threatening event).

Apparent Life-Threatening Event (ALTE)

An **apparent life-threatening event** is a period of apnea accompanied by other respiratory complications (such as choking or gagging), skin color change, or change of muscle tone. Some have referred to ALTE as "near miss SIDS," although an underlying organic origin is usually found. According to a recent study, up to 50% of the ALTEs can be attributed to digestive problems. Only 20% are correlated to respiratory problems, and a full 50% are idiopathic.[29] If you encounter a child with an ALTE type episode, supportive care and immediate transport are mandatory. DOT 6-2.34

Sudden Infant Death Syndrome

Sudden infant death syndrome or **SIDS** is the sudden, unexplained death of children under the age of one year. The incidence of SIDS is highest during the second through fourth months of life. The syndrome becomes uncommon after the sixth month of life, yet it may still occur. The presentations of SIDS are wide and varied. Prematurity, low birth weight, and exposure to passive smoke are a few of the potential risk factors. The treatment involves one of two pathways. First, if the parents have established the fact that their child has died and no further medical care is necessary, the parents become your patients, and care should be directed at providing them with needed emotional, mental, and spiritual support. If on the other hand, the parents are unaware or are not willing to accept that the child has died, a full resuscitation should be conducted. As a paramedic, you may fully understand the gravity of the situation, and your medical knowledge confirms that the outcome will remain the same; remember that the parents are now your patient. In the future, when the parents are working to heal from this terrible event, they will be able to look at themselves in the mirror and state, "Everything that could have been done, was." Neither this book nor any other can give you the exact best answer. Only you can do that when the situation occurs. Contact your local SIDS support group for the most up-to-date information on the syndrome.[30] DOT 6-2.43, 6-2.44, 6-2.77, 6-2.82, 6-2.83, 6-2.84, 6-2.85

Upper Airway Obstruction

Upper airway obstructions occur throughout the span of life, but are most common in the 14 years and younger age groups. The National Injury Prevention and Control Center provides us with the following facts:[31]

- In 2000, 160 children ages 14 years or younger died from an obstruction of the respiratory tract due to inhaled or ingested foreign bodies. Of these, 41% were caused by food items and 59% by nonfood objects.

- For every choking-related death, there are more than 100 visits to U.S. emergency departments. In 2001, an estimated 17,537 children 14 years or younger were treated in U.S. emergency departments for choking episodes.

  - Candy was associated with 19% of all choking-related ED visits by children ages 14 years or younger; 65% were related to hard candy; and 12.5% were related to other specified types of candy (chocolate candy, gummy bears, gum, etc.).

  - Coins were involved in 18% of all choking-related ED visits for children ages one to four years.

  - In 2001, 10.5% of children treated in the emergency department for choking episodes were admitted to the hospital or transferred to a facility with a higher level of care.

If the obstruction is above the trachea, the inspiration of air is affected. If the obstruction is below the trachea, generally the exhalation of air is affected. DOT 6-2.25

Foreign Body Obstruction (FB). Foreign body obstructions are most commonly caused by the aspiration of a foreign object into the child's airway. Despite being a possibility at any age, the more prevalent age range for this disorder is six months to four years. As a child develops and starts becoming mobile, there is a dramatic increase in oral exploration. For some infants, everything that touches their hands will be placed in their mouth. Presentation of an FB aspiration can vary from a sudden onset of coughing to complete airway obstruction.

It is also common that a child who aspirated a FB and had symptoms that prompted the parent to call 9-1-1, presents to the paramedic as a normal, healthy looking child. Either the FB was only partially obstructing the airway and became dislodged prior to EMS arrival, or the obstruction is still a threat but has changed the degree of obstruction enough for the child to be ventilating adequately. Unless the object was physically seen being dislodged, the child spit it out, or it was removed by the parent, the latter potential remains a high risk.

A coin is one of the easiest FBs to mentally visualize. A coin can rotate from a complete obstruction to a partial obstruction and back. Like a flutter valve, the FB itself can move and re-obstruct, or the subsequent edema around the FB can re-obstruct. Never take the chance that the patient has dislodged the object simply because the patient appears okay at your initial impression. A full respiratory evaluation must be completed, including breath sounds in both anterior and posterior lung fields and over the trachea. The absence of abnormal breath sounds does not confirm dislodgement.

Treatment for these patients is usually supportive and precautionary if the object has been removed prior to your arrival. Full assessment of the patient, their airway patency, breath sounds, and vital signs needs to occur. Supplemental oxygen, continuous vital sign monitoring, and transport for further evaluation may be required. If the patient remains obstructed, the degree of obstruction may be determined by the respiratory noises heard. Stridorous noises indicate a partial obstruction; whereas, silent or absent breath sounds and the inability to speak indicate a full obstruction. If the obstruction is present, standardized methods of intervention are immediately required such as abdominal thrust if the patient has lost consciousness or direct visualization and removal with a Magill forceps. If the Magill forceps are used, remember, if you cannot positively identify the object, *do not* blindly attempt to remove unknown objects as they may be a vital structure. In cases involving peanuts or other pieces of food (hot dogs, etc.) where the foreign object cannot be removed and the obstruction persists, consideration must be given to intubating and ventilating the child, even if doing so will push the object deeper into the lungs. Remember, having one mainstem bronchus obstructed is better than having the trachea obstructed. The American Heart Association recommendations for pediatric airway obstruction provide guidelines for managing these patients.[32]

Reactive Airway Disorders

Reactive Airway Disorders (RAD) occur when an irritant, bacteria, virus, or allergen invades the airway. RADs cause mucus production, inflammation, edema, and bronchospasm. They are typically self-limited and reversible and responsive to standard treatments.

Asthma. Asthma is a chronic reactive disorder that has plagued humans since ancient times. In modern times, this malady is responsible for a significant percentage of school absentees. With nearly 5 million children diagnosed with asthma, it remains one of the most common chronic conditions. Asthma is more prevalent in boys until they reach adolescence; then the occurrence is nearly equal between both genders. In the seven years between 1980 and 1987, the incident of asthma increased by 31%. The occurrence of a fatal asthma event is more common in adults than children, yet in 2002, 187 children lost their lives to this disease.[33]

This disease process produces three primary pathophysiological pulmonary changes. First, the bronchioles spasm and constrict in response to a "trigger" or stimulus. This causes a decrease in the diameter of the airways and an increase in airflow restriction. Second, mucus is secreted within the airway walls, in response to inflammation, which further restricts the airflow and begins to create obstructions or blockages at the alveolar level. The final change is a fluid shift within the cells of the airway wall, causing further restriction and increasing the potential of "air trapping."

Street Secrets

Persistent coughing is a sign of asthma.

Once alveoli or bronchioles become obstructed, the potential for collapse is significant. This collapse or atelectatic area continues to receive blood through the vascular system, but gasses are not exchanged. As a critical mass of alveoli are collapsed and the size of the atelectasis increases, so does the degree of hypoxemia. As unoxygenated blood continues to return to the heart and arterial system, the hemodynamic status of the child starts to deteriorate. It is easy to see why once this vicious cycle begins, aggressive therapy is required.

Treating the asthmatic patient may be as simple as providing a comfortable place to rest for a few minutes with humidified oxygen at 15 L/m via a nonrebreather mask or as complicated as a full resuscitation

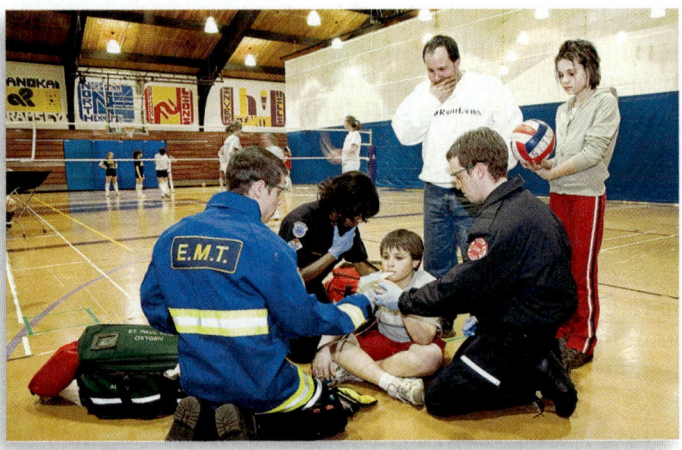

Figure 43-25 If the asthmatic patient is treated early, when the patient is still able to adequately breathe, nebulized albuterol may help avoid the need for more aggressive airway and ventilation procedures.

(Figure 43-25). The standards of ABCs, O_2, ECG, and vitals are necessary with every patient to assure that any hidden complications are discovered. If the basic treatments do not reverse the symptoms within one to two minutes, begin aerosolized beta$_2$ adrenergic agonist therapy immediately. The most common regiment is albuterol MDI. Provide one to two puffs several minutes apart, and be sure to use a spacer for increased delivery efficiency. If the symptoms are not resolved within a few minutes or the patient does not describe significant improvement, nebulized albuterol can be administered. The standard dosing follows:[34]

- Weight 10 kg or under the age of 12 months: 1.25 mg (0.25 mL) in 2 mL NS.
- Weight 10–35 kg or one year to 10 years: 2.5 mg (0.5 mL) in 2 mL NS.
- Weight greater than 35 kg or age over 10 years: 5.0 mg (1.0 mL) in 2 mL NS.

Subsequent doses may be given. Depending on your pediatric protocols, other medications may be given in conjunction with albuterol. These additional medications might include the following:

- Alupent (metaproterenol)
  - Six to 12 years: 0.1–0.2 mL diluted in 2.5 mL NS
  - 12 years or older: 0.2–0.3 mL diluted in 2.5 mL NS
- Atrovent (ipratropium)
  - Less than two years old: 250 mcg nebulized
  - Greater than two years old: 500 mcg nebulized
- Epinephrine (adrenalin)
  - 0.01 mg/kg [1:1000] SC or 0.1 mg/kg [1:10,000] IV push for critical cases (max dose: 0.3 mg)[27]

- Terbutaline
  - Greater than six years: 0.01 mg/kg SC or IV (max dose: 0.4 mg)
- Magnesium sulfate
  - 25–50 mg/kg IV over 10 to 20 minutes (2 gram maximum dose)[27]

CONNECTIONS Review Chapter 28: Pulmonary for more detailed information on asthma.

Bronchiolitis

Bronchiolitis is commonly confused with asthma. Inflammation of the bronchioles caused by **respiratory syncytial virus (RSV)** or other viruses can mimic asthma because of the wheezing it produces.[35] The primary differences are in the associated symptoms, dry cough, running nose, and fever, which are almost always present. Nasal flaring, tachycardia, tachypnea, inspiratory and well as expiratory wheezing, and rhonchi may also be present. Because the child may have been ill for several days, the potential for dehydration is real. A complete assessment of the respiratory system is essential to differentiate and properly treat bronchiolitis.

Depending on the severity of the disease and the general condition of the child, be prepared to provide simple supportive measures through advanced resuscitation. Humidified supplemental oxygen via a nonrebreather mask at 15 L/m may reduce the mild hypoxemia and decrease the respiratory distress. If signs and symptoms are more significant, nebulized albuterol may be required, as well as pulse oximetry and cardiac monitoring. If signs of dehydration are present, vascular access is recommended. Fluid boluses of 10–20 mL/kg should be given. If the child remains in shock, additional boluses may be required.

Croup (Laryngotracheitis)

Croup is a partial obstruction of the upper airway from the trachea to the bronchi caused by a viral infection, resulting in swelling of the upper respiratory tract. The most common cause is the parainfluenza virus, which accounts for 75% of cases of croup. The syndrome affects boys more than girls, and ages of risk are usually between three months and five years.[36] The primary signs of croup follow:

- **Stridor,** the high pitched musical noise created by the narrowed airway.
- The classic "seal bark" cough.
- Hoarseness.

The typical history is a child who has had "flu-like" symptoms, but seems okay at the end of the day. During the middle of the night, the entire household is abruptly awakened with the loud, barking cough. It is not uncommon for the events to replay themselves for one or more nights. If the parents take the child to the emergency department during the night, it is common for the child to be symptom free upon arrival. The "secret" treatment is cold air. The chilled air reduces the airway edema and decreases the symptoms. Because croup is normally a cooler weather syndrome, using cold air to your advantage is therapeutic and simple. The drawback is that the warm air of the ambulance may again worsen the condition. Croup is normally self-limited, and treatment will be supportive: humidified oxygen, pulse oximetry, and complete respiratory system assessment. If the croup syndrome has progressed to respiratory failure or respiratory arrest, immediate lifesaving measures must be taken.

Epiglottitis (Supraglottitis)

Epiglottitis is a disease syndrome that is a paradox within itself. The bad news is that the bacterium causing the disease has expanded its range of affliction from two to six years of age to all ages. Most often the *Haemophilus influenzae* type B (HIB) bacteria is responsible; however, streptococcus or staphylococcus can also be the culprit. The good news is that the HIB vaccine has dramatically reduced the number of cases. Immunization is making the difference.[37]

Epiglottitis is a serious disease that has the propensity to cause fatal airway obstruction (Figure 43-26). The signs and symptoms are the following:

- Rapid onset of distress.
- Drooling.

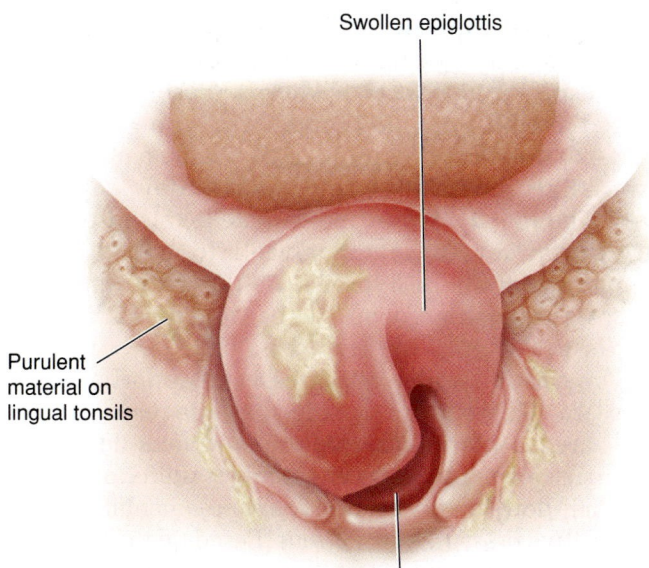

Swollen epiglottis

Purulent material on lingual tonsils

Compromised tracheal opening

Figure 43-26 Epiglottitis.

- Changes in the quality of the child's voice.
- Inability to speak.
- Moderate to extreme pain with swallowing.
- Frequently assumes the "tripod position."
- Inspiratory stridor.
- Deliberate mouth breathing.
- Fever—sudden onset high grade (102°F +).

Visual inspection of the oral cavity is strongly discouraged as doing so may trigger complete laryngospasm, and further swelling of the epiglottis, a fatal event if the patient cannot be ventilated or intubated.

The primary treatment concerns for the paramedic are to keep the patient in a comfortable, relaxed environment. Transporting the child to a definitive care facility is of critical importance yet should be performed without excitation. Smooth transport, no lights or siren, and no sudden starts or stops are highly recommended. Provide the patient with supplemental humidified oxygen via nonrebreather mask at 15 L/m. If the patient fights having the oxygen mask placed on them, provide it via blow-by. Keep the patient calm.

If the patient continues to deteriorate, the patient can usually be supported with bag-mask ventilation. Endotracheal intubation is typically extremely difficult to accomplish as the epiglottic swelling will distort the visible anatomy and intubation attempts may serve only to further increase the swelling.

Lower Airway Disorders

Neonatal respiratory distress syndrome, bronchopulmonary dysplasia, bronchitis, bronchiolitis, pneumonia, tuberculosis, and cystic fibrosis are examples of lower airway disorders. These disorders are the result of structural or functional problems in the lungs.[38] DOT 6-2.26

Neonatal respiratory distress syndrome (RDS) is often caused by hyaline membrane disease or meconium aspiration. These newborns present with decreased breath sounds, labored tachypnea rates of 70 to 120 breaths per minute, retractions, paradoxical respirations, grunting, cyanosis, and slow capillary refill. The inactivated or inadequate levels of pulmonary surfactant cause the alveoli to collapse and ultimately results in hypoxia. As the syndrome progresses, the alveoli die, only to become nonfunctional scar tissue.[39,40]

The treatment plan is aggressive; supportive therapies are focused on assuring that adequate oxygen levels are maintained during transport to a definitive pediatric care center. Treatment might include intubation; high-flow, high-concentration supplemental oxygen; and positive pressure ventilations. Based on the Gausche study, bag-mask ventilations with 100% oxygenation may be the most appropriate delivery method. You need to be comfortable with your newborn intubation

skills and protocols before encountering this type of critical condition.

Bronchitis and Bronchiolitis

Bronchitis and bronchiolitis are caused by inflammation of the bronchi or bronchioles. **Bronchitis** is normally a disease that is seen in combination with other respiratory illnesses such as croup. The symptoms include a coarse, hacking cough that worsens at night and may cause painful respirations or coughs simply due to the harshness of the coughing episodes. Bronchitis is typically self-limited, and treatment is supportive.

Bronchiolitis manifests itself similarly to other lower airway illnesses but may cause severe respiratory distress due to inflammation and obstruction of the affected structures. Primarily seen in infants and toddlers, bronchiolitis can become life-threatening if not treated aggressively.[41] Most commonly caused by the RSV, signs and symptoms initially include upper respiratory symptoms, cough, running nose or nasal congestion, and fever. After several days of symptoms, the illness progresses and begins to affect the lower airways as well. As the pulmonary system becomes more compromised, moderate to severe respiratory distress becomes apparent. Nasal flaring, deeper more frequent cough, refusal to eat, lethargy, and labored breathing are seen.

Treatment includes aggressive support of the airway and oxygenation. If the nasal cavity is clear, provide oxygen via nonrebreather mask at 15 L/m. Because the child may become agitated with the oxygen delivery system, utilizing blow-by techniques is acceptable. Transport to a definitive care facility is mandatory.

Pneumonia

An inflammation or infection of the lungs and alveolar spaces, this illness affects children of all ages. **Pneumonia** is caused by viral, bacterial, or mycoplasmal organisms. The signs and symptoms include cough, abnormal breath sounds, abnormal respiratory patterns, tachypnea, and elevated fever. Confirmation of the illness is done through radiographic studies, and prehospital treatment is focused on supportive measures to assure reduction or elimination of respiratory distress.[42]

Tuberculosis (TB)

Tuberculosis is an ancient disease caused by *Mycobacterium tuberculosis* and is spread through droplet transmission. Coughing and sneezing are the usual transmission vehicles. The rise in the number of cases seen in the U.S. has been dramatic since 1988.[43] Symptoms include a history of weight loss, fever, persistent cough, wheezing, and potentially decreased breath sounds. Treatment for TB is preventive and supportive. Preventing the patient from exposing the paramedic to the disease is pivotal. Simply putting a protective mask on the patient is a good first step. All EMS personnel must don appropriate personal protective equipment (PPE) and notify the receiving facility if any suspicion of TB exists. The supportive measures include oxygen administration for respiratory distress and hypoxia.

Cystic Fibrosis (CF)

Cystic fibrosis is an autosomal disorder of the exocrine glands, resulting in physiological changes in the respiratory, GI, integumentary, and muscoskeletal systems. This inherited disorder is found predominately in white children of both genders.[44] The primary clinical manifestation of CF is the thick, sticky production of mucus that obstructs the air passages in the lungs. Clubbed fingers and toes in the older child indicate the disease is progressing and chronic hypoxia has developed. Treatment by the paramedic is primarily supportive respiratory care. DOT 6-2.21

Hypoperfusion and Shock

Hypoperfusion or shock involves inadequate perfusion, inadequate oxygenation, inadequate waste removal, or any combination of the three. This highly complex pathophysiological process results in the body's inability to meet its metabolic demands, thereby ultimately facilitating cellular death. Hypoperfusion or shock is often thought of as the loss of bodily fluids, blood, or water, resulting in decreased blood pressure and increased heart rate.

Mechanisms of Hypoperfusion

Hypoperfusion has four primary mechanisms of origin: hypovolemic shock, distributive shock, cardiogenic shock, and obstructive shock.

Hypovolemic Shock. This occurs when the body's ability to distribute bodily fluids throughout the system is intact, yet there is a significant decrease in the amount of blood or fluids. This can be from events such as vomiting and dehydration or from acute events such as profuse bleeding. It can also be from metabolic disorders (metabolic shock), causing an increase in fluid requirements. A common cause of metabolic shock is osmotic diuresis secondary to hyperglycemia-induced dehydration. DOT 6-2.51, 6-2.58

Distributive Shock. Distributive shock is caused by an alteration in the relative size of the vascular system

relative to the amount of fluid. This can be caused by vasodilatation (an increase in the size of the vascular container) or by an increase in vascular permeability (leakage of vascular fluid into the extravascular space). Common forms of distributive shock are anaphylactic, septic, and neurogenic. Distributive shock in the pediatric patient presents similar to that seen in the adult.

Cardiogenic Shock. Cardiogenic shock is an inability of the heart to adequately pump blood. The primary difference between pediatric and adult cardiogenic shock is the etiology. In children, cardiogenic shock is most likely to occur secondary to hypoxia or acidosis rather than from an AMI as is adults.[45] Congenital anomalies are a likely cause, especially if there is a history of congenital complications or a relevant family history. Regardless of the child's age, never forget that if they appear to be having a "heart attack," an acute myocardial infarction is a strong possibility. If it looks like an AMI, it probably is. Children die of AMI as do adults.

Obstructive Shock. This is exactly what the name implies, an obstruction. Common causes of obstructive shock are pulmonary embolism, tension pneumothorax, and cardiac tamponade. Immediate transport for invasive therapy must be provided.

The Pediatric Response to Shock

The stages of shock begin with the compensatory phase, where the body attempts to maintain homeostasis through vasoconstriction and tachycardia. As the cause of the shock remains unabated, the child's compensatory mechanisms begin to fail. Signs and symptoms include anxiety, irritability, increases in both the heart and respiratory rates, a potential widening in the pulse pressure, peripheral shunting (strong central pulses and weakened or absent distal pulses), cooling of the extremities, and decreased urinary output.

As the child moves from failing compensation to decompensation, the signs and symptoms of distress become evident. Significant lethargy or coma, slowed heart and respiratory rates, dropping blood pressure, weak or absent central pulses, absence of urinary output, and mottled skin are common findings. Without the provision of respiratory and fluid resuscitation and transport to a definitive care facility, the child's expected survivability is greatly reduced.

The common causes of hypoperfusion are vomiting, diarrhea, blood loss, anaphylaxis, fluid shifts, organ failure, and infection—just as in the adult population. The primary difference is the prevalence and priority of each etiology.

What allows children to respond differently to shock? First, children have stronger, healthier cardiovascular systems that have a remarkable ability to respond to stress. In addition, their vascular systems have the profound ability to shunt circulation from the extremities to the central circulation. During times of extreme circumstance, both defense mechanisms engage in an attempt to ward off the detrimental effects of hypoperfusion. It is also important to understand that relative to adults, children have not had the opportunity to abuse their bodies with poor diet, lack of exercise, and "aging" as have their adult counterparts.

Second, since children have proportionally less blood volume, they typically present with signs and symptoms of shock at significantly lesser amounts of fluid loss.[45,46] Most adults will not show significant signs of shock (BP below 90 mmHg) until they have lost 25–40% of their fluid volume while children may become anxious or irritable and tachycardic with a volume loss as small as 5%.[46]

Third, the cardiac output capabilities of the child are dictated by their heart rate. Infants and young children do not have the ability to increase their contractility or stroke volume and, therefore, must rely solely on increasing their cardiac rate. A mild to moderate tachycardia is indicative of some form of hypoperfusion. It must be reiterated that once children begin to decompensate, their end-organ perfusion begins to drop dramatically and they "crash" quickly. DOT 6-2.59, 6-2.60

Management of the Hypoperfused Child

The primary therapeutic pathway for the hypoperfused child is to assure ventilation and oxygenation is adequate. Regardless of the respiratory rate, if the child is not adequately ventilating, decompensation will either occur or worsen. Go back to the "question" "What is going to kill the child first?" If the oxygenation and ventilation are adequate, then fluid status is the next point of concern. If shock is secondary to blood loss, bleeding control and intravenous or intraosseous therapy, and giving 20 mL/kg fluid boluses, become the next priorities. If the fluid loss is secondary to vomiting, diarrhea, or fluid shifts, intravenous therapy of 20 mL/kg fluid boluses must be initiated. If cardiac failure is present, consideration must be given to fluid resuscitation. A child will most commonly respond to fluid boluses. If the child is in crisis due to obstructive causes, such as tension pneumothorax or pericardial effusion, treatment of the mechanical threat must be addressed per local protocol. DOT 6-2.28

Altered Mental Status (AMS)

Altered mental status in the pediatric patient is sometimes difficult to determine. The two-year-old that has a ten-second attention span; the five-year-old who is fixated on a single topic; the 15-year-old who does not seem to recognize his parents, even when they are standing next to him all may be normal or may have a significant change in the level of consciousness. Altered mental status can be defined as a change in the normal level of consciousness and is usually evidence of a change in brain function. The challenge with children is that their level of consciousness and orientation varies with age, activity, and environment. Any time a child is suspected of having an altered mental status, the paramedic must determine if the airway is patent, if oxygenation is adequate, if ventilation is sufficient, and if perfusion is adequate. If any of the baseline parameters are changed, correction of the potential life threat is the top priority, and then a complete assessment to determine the origin of the alteration is required.

The neurological assessment for newborns or infants will focus on their response to discomfort or pain; observe for sadness, crying, laughing, smiling, or other physical activity. Assessing toddlers will include the physical appearance and behavior to answering simple questions. Some young children, especially those raised in a medically oriented home or those with chronic health disorders may be able to provide information well above their expected knowledge levels. Preschool and school-age children are typically able to discuss their illness or injury with a higher level of accuracy and completeness. Because infants and small children do not have large stores of glycogen, hypoglycemia must always be considered and the serum glucose checked. DOT 6-2.65, 6-2.66, 6-2.67, 6-2.68

The presentation of AMS in the young patient may well be chemically induced (illicit drugs, prescription medications, over-the-counter medications, alcohol, or other consciousness-altering substances), intentional, or unintentional. The U.S. Department of Health and Human Services, Substance Abuse and Mental Health Services Administration (SAMHSA) reports that 29% of young adults consume alcohol, 11.6% are currently using illicit drugs, with the 18- to 25-year-old group being the greatest offenders.[47] DOT 6-2.34

Street Secrets

If a child (particularly male) won't make eye contact with you, doesn't want to be touched, and is either talking nonstop or refuses to talk, he may have an autism spectrum disorder (ASD), not AMS. Ask the parents or caregivers if the child is exhibiting any neurological differences from their usual presentation. Review Box 46-5 (page 1143) in Chapter 46: Patients with Special Challenges for more information on children with ASDs.

The common causes of AMS may be remembered by using the following mnemonic.

AEIOU-TIPS

A Alcohol

E Epilepsy

I   Insulin - diabetes
O   Overdose
U   Unusual problems—metabolic
T   Trauma
I   Infection or Intracranial
P   Poisoning
S   Sepsis

Altered level of consciousness is a frequently seen medical condition in the pediatric population. It is important to determine if the alteration requires medical care or not. Behavioral causes may require mental health therapeutic pathways in addition to medical care.

Other Common Medical Complaints

For many years, the focus of prehospital pediatric care has been the resuscitation of the child in respiratory or cardiac arrest, yet the incidence of this type of call is relatively low. Even in extremely high-volume EMS systems, the opportunity to intubate, defibrillate, or administer resuscitation medications to children is uncommon.[11,12] Instead of focusing on the uncommon, it is important to ensure that the paramedic is prepared for the more common situations. This section will focus on the common medical complaints encountered in the prehospital setting.

Abdominal Pain

Abdominal pain in children may vary in its presentation simply because of the vast range of sensations it produces. "My tummy hurts" is also a frequent complaint that children provide and use as a response to myriad symptoms. As in the adult, signs and symptoms including onset, radiation, changes in mental status, abnormal vital signs, nausea and vomiting, feeding problems, changes in bowel habits, bloody vomit or stool, distension, and pain with palpation are all important considerations.

Infants.   Specific complications affecting infants include the following:

- **Colic.** A condition marked by recurrent episodes of prolonged crying and irritability in an otherwise healthy infant. Colic is of unknown cause and usually subsides after three to four months of age.
- **Hernia.** A protrusion of an abdominal organ through an opening in the abdominal wall. Femoral, inguinal, and umbilical hernias are common types in infants.
- **Intussusception.** The slipping of a length of intestine into an adjacent portion, usually producing obstruction on or blood in the stool.

Children.   Specific complications affecting children include the following:

- **Appendicitis.** An inflammation of the vermiform appendix.
- **Constipation.** The delayed or infrequent passage of dry, hardened feces.
- **Gastroenteritis.** An inflammation of the lining of the stomach or intestine presenting with vomiting and diarrhea.
- **Urinary tract infection.** An infection that can happen anywhere along the urinary tract—the kidneys, the ureters (the tubes that take urine from each kidney to the bladder), the bladder, or the urethra (the tube that empties urine from the bladder to the outside).

Young Adults.   Specific complications affecting young adults include the following:

- **Appendicitis.**
- **Constipation.**
- **Ectopic pregnancy.** A fertilized egg that has implanted outside the uterus. The egg implants in the fallopian tubes more than 95% of the time. This is why ectopic pregnancies are commonly called "tubal pregnancies." The egg can also implant in the ovary, abdomen, or the cervix, so you may see these referred to as cervical or abdominal pregnancies. Eggs that implant outside the uterus cannot survive and may rupture causing life threatening hemorrhage.[48]
- **Gastroenteritis.** Alcohol or chemical ingestion may be the cause in this age group.
- **Pelvic inflammatory disease (PID).** PID is a spectrum of infections of the female genital tract that includes endometritis, salpingitis, tuboovarian abscess, and peritonitis. PID affects over 1 million women per year and is responsible for nearly 250,000 hospitalizations. Ectopic pregnancy rates are 12–15% higher and chronic pelvic pain is 18% higher in women afflicted with PID. Although this malady can occur in any age women, young adults under the age of 25 years are at the greatest risk.[49]
- **Testicular torsion.** A urological emergency with life-changing implications if the correct diagnosis is delayed or missed. Occurring in approximately one in 4000 males in the 10 to 20 year age group, this emergency is the most common cause of testicular loss.[50] If proper diagnosis is made within six hours from onset, organ recovery is 80–100%. If the delay in diagnosis reaches the 12 hour mark, organ viability is nearly 0%. Testicular torsion is a malady seen in newborns as well.

Cardiac Abnormalities

As the fetus develops from the single-cell stage to the fully developed newborn, millions upon millions of cell divisions occur, each allowing for the slightest of errors. Normally, everything progresses without complications, but once in a while the process fails. While the incidence of anatomical abnormalities varies, EMS providers are frequently called when the anomaly first presents itself. This section will review several of the more common congenital heart defects you may encounter.[45,51] DOT 6-2.99

Aortic Valve Stenosis. Thickening or obstructing of the aortic valve. This malady occurs in approximately five in 10,000 persons, usually males, and may not present until later in life.

Atrial Septal Defect (ASD). A defect between the right and left atria, allowing oxygenated blood returning from the lungs to mix with the unoxygenated blood from the vena cava. ASD is present in four out of every 100,000 people. If there are no other defects, the child may be asymptomatic. Children with ASD are susceptible to infective endocarditis, atrial fibrillation, and heart failure. Symptoms include palpitations, shortness of breath, and difficulty breathing.

Patent Ductus Arteriosus. A congenital vascular remnant that connects the pulmonary artery and aortic arch, allowing oxygenated blood from the aortic arch to mix with unoxygenated blood from the right ventricle. There is a 10% prevalence of PDA in children with congenital heart disease.

Pulmonary Valve Stenosis. A defect causing a partial obstruction of the pulmonary valve, thereby restricting flow of blood to the lungs. There is a 10% prevalence of PVS in children with congenital heart disease. Symptoms include fatigue, shortness of breath, cyanosis, poor weight gain or failure to thrive, and chest pain.

Tetralogy of Fallot. A complex of abnormalities due to developmental failures of the ventricles. First described in 1888 by Fallot the defects include the following:

1. The walls of the pulmonary valve are thickened.
2. The right ventricular wall is hypertrophied.
3. The aorta is overriding the right ventricle.
4. There is a ventricular septal defect.

This congenital defect represents 10% of all congenital heart defects. Without definitive treatment, it is estimated that 25% of these patients will die in their first year of life, 40% by age four, 70% by age 10, and 95% by age 40. The relevant medical history will usually include cyanosis (especially with exertion, or when crying), difficulty breathing (worsening with exertion), a low birth weight, and small size for age.

Ventricular Septal Defect (VSD). A defect in the septal wall between the two ventricles. The size and location of the defect will dictate the significance of the clinical presentations. Approximately 1% of all newborns have VSD. In 80–90% of the cases, the defect is small and will repair itself as the infant grows.

Treatment for all of these congenital heart problems include aggressive primary support of the ABCs, venous access, full assessment and monitoring, and immediate transport to a definitive care facility.

Diabetes

Diabetes is one of the fastest growing medical conditions affecting school-age children in the United States. Approximately 13,000 children are diagnosed with Type I diabetes each year. The incidence is seven in 100,000 children under the age of four, 15 in 100,000 in the five-to-nine age group, and 22 per 100,000 in the 10- to 14-year-old group. Nearly 75% of all new cases of diabetes occur in pediatric patients under the age of 18 years. The two primary types of diabetes seen in the pediatric population are Type I and Type II.[52]

Type I diabetes is defined as the failure of the body to make adequate insulin. Type II is defined as the body's inability to adequately utilize insulin. Type I is often referred to as juvenile onset diabetes, whereas, Type II is commonly considered noninsulin-dependent diabetes. Although both types can affect people of any age, Type I occurs most frequently in children and adults less than 30 years of age. Type II is the most common form and can affect persons of any age, especially those who are obese. There is ongoing research into the effectiveness of Islets of Langerhans transplants, which is showing some promise for the future. Until then, children with Type I diabetes must take insulin injections, probably for the rest of their lives.

Type I diabetics are susceptible to further complications such as diabetic ketoacidosis (DKA) or diabetic coma. DKA occurs when the lack of insulin reaches a state when the body is forced into metabolizing fat. The by-products are organic acids (i.e., carboxylic, uric, and lactic) and ketones. The symptoms are typically acute and, frequently the child, young adult, or even the parent can identify a specific date when the child became ill. Early symptoms include increases in urination, thirst, and hunger; nausea; weakness; increased respirations; blurred vision; changes in mental status; and weight loss. As the illness progresses, the child may start showing signs of increasing severity dehydration; dry, warm to hot skin; flushed appearance; abdominal pain mimicking gastroenteritis; vomiting; more extensive changes in mental status and consciousness; obvious increases in respiratory status to the point of Kussmal respirations; tachycardia; and lethargy advancing to coma. The increasing levels of ketones and acids in the child's blood stream may cause an acetone or a sweet fruity or "Juicy Fruit™" gum smell on the patient's breath. Not everyone's olfactory senses are capable of making this distinction. Failing to smell acetone on a patient's breath does not rule out DKA.

The therapeutic pathway for the DKA child is support of primary ABCs; administration of high-flow, high-concentration oxygen with ventilation support, as necessary; documentation of the blood glucose levels through the use of a glucometer or collection of blood samples for future lab analysis; IV or IO access; infusion of 20 mL/kg NaCl or LR boluses until perfusion has stabilized (usually two to three boluses, depending on local protocol, is appropriate in the prehospital setting); full assessment and monitoring; and immediate transport.[53]

A diabetic may also present in insulin shock, which is a hypoglycemic state. Elevated levels of insulin or reduced levels of nutrients set the stage for a rapid onset of glucose insufficiency. This is a true life-threatening emergency. Signs and symptoms include diaphoresis, anxiety, tachycardia, weakness, confusion, altered mental status, seizure, or coma.

The therapeutic pathway includes aggressive intervention to assure the ABCs are adequately supported; administration of high-flow, high-concentration oxygen with ventilation support, as necessary; documentation of the blood glucose levels through the use of a glucometer or collection of blood samples for future lab analysis; IV or IO access; infusion of dextrose; full assessment and monitoring; and immediate transport as required by local protocol. The dose of dextrose is shown in Drug Box 43-2.[17,54]

In infants and children, the ability to differentiate between hyper- and hypoglycemia may be difficult. Keep in mind that, as a rule, hyperglycemia presents with warm, dry, flushed, skin with an extended onset of symptoms. Hypoglycemia normally presents with cool, clammy, diaphoretic skin and sudden onset. If for whatever reason, you are unable to differentiate between the two, immediate transport with attention focusing on the primary ABCs is appropriate.

Fever

Fever or pyrexia is one of the most common maladies seen in the pediatric population. An increase in body temperature is frequently a response to infection, a medication side effect or complication, an extended exposure to heat, or even stress. Fever may also be a response to healing processes, to teething in the infant, and as a protective mechanism against future allergies.[55] Fevers are divided into two major categories, low-grade, up to 102° F (38.8° C), or high-grade, greater than 102°F (38.8° C). If the increase in body temperature is caused by internal etiologies, the body normally restricts the thermoregulation system from going above 106°F (41.1° C). If the rise in body temperature is due to external variables, such as a child being left in a car on a warm day, the body has no natural protective mechanism beyond its response to heat exhaustion and heatstroke. If the rise in temperature is acute or rapid, the child may experience a febrile seizure.

Febrile seizures are a common reaction to a sudden or sharp rise in body temperature, and are most often seen in children less than six years of age. Signs and symptoms include a fever over 100° F (37.7°C), tonic-clonic seizure activity, and a short or absent postictal state. Most febrile seizures are considered simple seizures and require minimal support efforts. Occasionally, they can be more complex in origin and require aggressive, supportive care and transport. Complex febrile seizures present more like nonfebrile seizures with longer postical states and loss of bladder control, and they can occur more than once in a 24-hour period. In either case, supportive care and definitive evaluations must be done to assure that the cause is not more ominous.

The therapeutic pathway includes assuring the child is capable of maintaining the child's own airway or an adjunct used and that the child is ventilating adequately with supplemental oxygenation and consideration for passive cooling if the core temperature continues to be elevated. The use of anticonvulsants is withheld unless the seizure activity is prolonged,

Drug Box 43-2   Dextrose

Newborn: 5–10 mL/kg of $D_{10}W$ bolus (over five to 10 minutes) and flush access line
Infants: 0.5–1 G/kg of $D_{25}W$ bolus (over five to 10 minutes) and flush access line
Children: 0.5–1 G/kg of $D_{25}W$ bolus (over five to 10 minutes) and flush access line
Young Adults: 0.5–1 G/kg of $D_{50}W$ bolus and flush access line

the child has multiple seizures, or the child is in status epilepticus.

Hyperthermia and Hypothermia

Hyperthermia and hypothermia can be life-threatening situations typically brought on by environmental variables. Because children are more sensitive to and, therefore, more susceptible to heat- and cold-related injuries than adults, extreme caution must be exercised when responding to these emergencies.

CONNECTIONS Hyperthermia and hypothermia are discussed in detail in Chapter 38: Environmental Conditions.

Meningitis

Meningitis, inflammation of the meninges, is a medical emergency seen in children of all ages and is caused by bacterial, viral, and other organisms. The bacterial form of this disease can be life-threatening and is a major cause of death and disability in children worldwide; more than 1,000,000 cases and 200,000 deaths are estimated to occur each year. The prevalence of meningitis has forced many schools and universities to require HIB vaccination prior to admission.[56] The signs and symptoms in children vary by age. Infants may have elevated or bulging fontanelles and may be difficult to arouse, and they may feed poorly. During their awake periods, they may be irritable and nonconsolable. School-age children and young adults may have generalized body aches, an inability to find a comfortable resting position, and irritability.

Meningitis is spread through airborne droplets; therefore, personal self protection, mask, goggles, gloves, and gowns must also be of cardinal importance. The therapeutic pathway includes primary supportive care and continuous assessments to discover life-threatening complications before they become life-threatening.[57,58]

Osteogenesis Imperfecta

Osteogenesis imperfecta is a congenital birth defect, causing abnormally fragile bones. This autosomal dominant pattern has a 50% chance of being inherited. Signs and symptoms include a history of fractured bones at birth, ease of breaking bones, fractures from minor trauma, deafness, "blue" sclerae (instead of white), bowed legs, and pectus carinatum (unusual caving in of the sternal area).

Sepsis

Any infection that migrates to the bloodstream may be the origin of sepsis. Common causes in pediatric patients include infection of the urinary tract, soft tissue injuries, meningitis, pneumonia, and bacteremia. In severe cases, septic shock develops, requiring fluid support.

Syncope

A loss of consciousness resulting from insufficient blood flow to the brain is commonly referred to as syncope.[59] Normally lasting only a few seconds, the effects of this sudden drop in perfusion are accompanied by nausea, diaphoresis, pallor, generalized weakness, dizziness, and vision disturbances. Although paramedics are typically familiar with adult syncope, it is commonly confused with a seizure disorder in children. The origin of the complication may be founded in the cardiac, metabolic, orthostatic, respiratory, or nervous systems. As in adults, the cause of syncope needs to be determined in order to properly care for the child. Do not forget to provide primary supportive care, and be prepared to provide additional therapies if the cause is not readily corrected.

Sickle Cell Disorders

Sickle cell anemia is an inherited disorder in which the red blood cells become malformed. Instead of being uniformly rounded, they become sickle-shaped when the patient is hypoxic. The potential for vascular blockages and tissue damage increases as the cellular malformations increase. The therapeutic pathway includes aggressive management of the ABCs. IV infusion of fluids may be required to rehydrate the child or to maintain a medication route. Since fever is a common sign associated with sickle cell crisis, an antipyretic such as acetaminophen (Tylenol™) may be given. Transportation to a definitive care facility and frequent assessments are also required.

CONNECTIONS See Chapter 37: Hematology for more information on sickle cell disorder.

Chest Pain

Thoracic or chest pain is typically a confusing and confounding presentation in children. Chest pain in adult patients is quickly associated with cardiac problems, but a person of any age is susceptible, child or otherwise. The key to determining the cause and the implications is a good assessment. Be careful to allow children to explain their symptomology in their words. Do not give them multiple choice questions or leading questions that may alter their description of the problem. Remember that their sense of pain may escalate the drama to a sense of imminent doom and lead them simply to try to answer your questions as you want them answered. The single largest challenge in the pediatric patient is convincing yourself that if the history, assessment, and symptoms indicate cardiac origins, then the problem probably lies in the cardiac systems. The therapeutic pathway includes supportive care and preparation for invasive procedures if the situation dictates. IV access and oxygenation may facilitate a reduction in symptoms and physiological tissue damage. DOT 6-2.30

Trauma

Dr. Peter Rosen, considered by some as the "father of emergency medicine," often taught emergency care principles through "pearls." One of "Rosen's pearls" follows:

> "No one dies of an extremity injury before they die of a pelvic injury, no one dies of a pelvic injury before they die of an abdominal injury, and no one dies of an abdominal injury before they die of a chest injury."[60]

What Dr. Rosen engrained in his students was that injury (or illness) to the chest has the highest mortality rate. Focus on the critical issues, and keep your priorities straight. All the great vessels, the lungs, and the heart reside in the chest cavity, making it the most life-threatening area of the body when injured.

Motor vehicle crashes are one of the most common causes of injuries to the pediatric population.[61] The most significant difference between children and adults in trauma is the airway. Because of the proportionally larger head and tongue, anterior glottis, narrow cricoid ring, and prominant occipital skull, the potential for airway compromise is considerable. Younger children are more likely to sustain blunt force trauma; their older counterparts, young adults and adults, are more likely to receive penetrating injuries. Understanding mechanisms of injury and enhancing your evaluation of the emergency through a complete assessment allows you to understand the magnitude of the situation (Figure 43-27).

CONNECTIONS Review Chapter 18: Mechanism of Injury, especially the pediatric section, for additional information.

Internal organs can bleed excessively when damaged by blunt force trauma. In a child, the encapsulation of the organs frequently prevents blood loss or creates a tamponade, which reduces total blood loss. If the organ capsule tears or has been ruptured, the process of decompensation can occur rapidly.[62] The child's clinical presentation, including vital signs, may undergo subtle change during the compensating phase. Their ability to compensate despite ominous injury necessitates continuous reassessment and clinical monitoring. Failure to do so will result in unrecognized sudden, life-threatening changes, which will eventually become

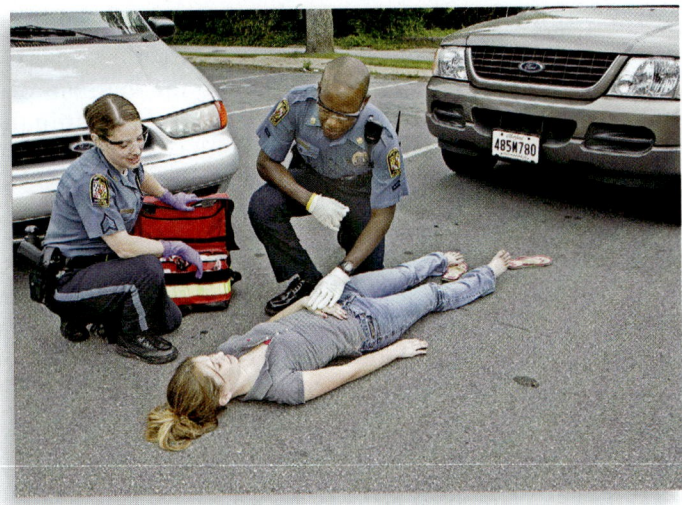

Figure 43-27   Trauma is the leading cause of injury and death in pediatric patients. Teens are more likely to receive penetrating injuries, whereas younger children are more likely to be injured in an MVC.

clinically obvious even to the untrained eye. Monitor and reassess the child constantly.

According to the Centers for Disease Control and Prevention, the leading causes of nonfatal injuries in the pediatric population are falls, being struck by or against another object (i.e., vehicles), overexertion, motor vehicle occupant, cuts or piercing, other assault, bite or sting, cycling injuries, unknown, and foreign bodies. The leading causes of fatal injury in the same age group are motor vehicle crash, homicide by firearm, suicide by firearm, drowning, poisoning, suicide suffocation, fire or burns, unintentional suffocation, homicide by cut or piercing, and homicide (unspecified).[61] As we can see, five of the nonfatal injuries are caused by blunt force trauma; only one in the fatal category is the result of blunt force trauma. DOT 6-2.69

Classic presentation of head injuries may be a fallacy in the child. Confusion, restlessness, lethargy, irritability, nausea, or vomiting may be the only indicator of brain trauma. Severe head trauma may cause a "talk and die" response. Typically the child is initially awake and alert and even has an acceptable assessment. Then, a sudden change in neurological status occurs, and the child may become restless or lethargic or may seize. This acute change is an indication that the injury is truly life-threatening, and aggressive supportive care must be provided. The presence or history of a seizure immediately after the traumatic event does not indicate an immediate life threat, but it provides indication and justification that the child must have a full assessment at a definitive care facility. DOT 6-2.70

Because children are generally "flexible," the potential for an actual spinal cord injury is less than that of their adult counterparts. Children represent only 5% of all spinal cord injuries.[63] Despite this, every precaution must be taken anytime the mechanism of injury or your assessment indicates potential spinal trauma.

CONNECTIONS Review Chapter 23: Spinal Trauma for more information.

Children of all ages can have the same life-threatening injuries to the chest as seen in adults. Because of a child's increased oxygen demand and lesser reserve capacities, hypoxia can occur quickly and without warning. The secondary effects of the trauma may also cause an increase in the work of breathing, which can intensify the respiratory distress syndromes.

Abdominal trauma has several unique characteristics in the pediatric population. It is more common for a child to have an abdominal injury secondary to or associated with skeletal and head injuries. Because the rib cage does not fully protect their liver and spleen, these organs are commonly injured. A groundbreaking study has shown that children with these otherwise life-threatening injuries to the solid organs of the abdomen often recover without surgical intervention.[62] Historically, child abuse has played a significant role in pediatric abdominal trauma. Proper assessment and history may indicate that the injury was not accidental. The paramedic must be keenly aware of the possibility for child abuse. DOT 6-2.71, 6-2.72

CONNECTIONS Review Chapter 22: Abdominal Trauma for additional information.

Appropriate equipment sizing and usage are necessary to properly care for children. For example, improperly sizing the cervical collar or assuming "one size fits all" may result in failure to stabilize a child's injured neck. This may also cause additional injury or complications such as external airway obstruction, respiratory compromise, partial great vessel obstruction, and unnecessary pain. The large occipital skull of infants and young children forces their necks to flex when placed supine on a hard surface (Figure 43-28). Placing a pad under the child's shoulder and down to their pelvis will lift their body up enough to maintain neutral alignment of the spine. Assurance that the spine is in a neutral position and the airway is unobstructed is of greater benefit to the long-term outcome of the child. Concerns about the padding allowing excessive movement of the vertebra have been shown to be unfounded. Although not designed to be utilized on pediatric patients, equipment such as the Kendrick extrication device (KED) and similar tools have also been shown to effectively immobilize children. DOT 6-2.37, 6-2.38

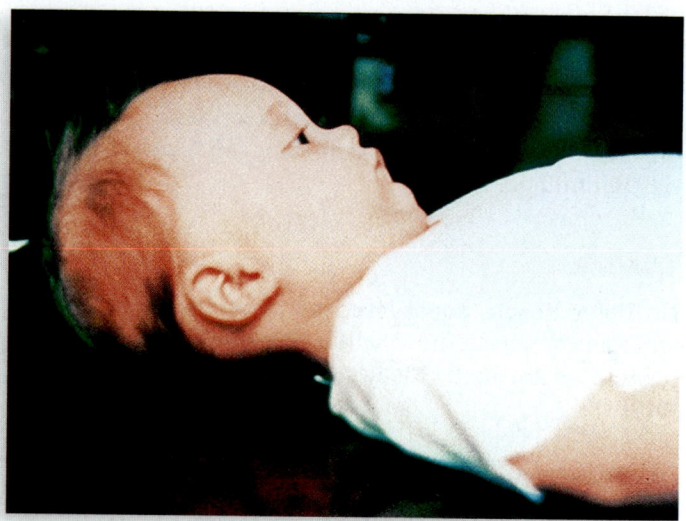

Figure 43-28   It is important to place an infant or toddler's head properly during airway management. EMSC Slide Set (CD-ROM), 1996. Courtesy of the Emergency Medical Services for Children Program, administered by the U.S. Department of Health and Human Services's Health Resources and Services Administration, Maternal and Child Health Bureau.

The care of burn injuries is extremely important because of the lifelong implications. In a child, the "rule of nines" remains the primary tool used to assess the extent of damage (Figure 43-29).[64] Unfortunately, the "rule of nines" has variations dependent upon the age of the child. The infant version places a value of 18% for the head and 13.5% for each leg. While most providers use these two tables, there are also tables for a child with a value of 12% for the head and 16.5% for each leg, and the adolescent version places a value

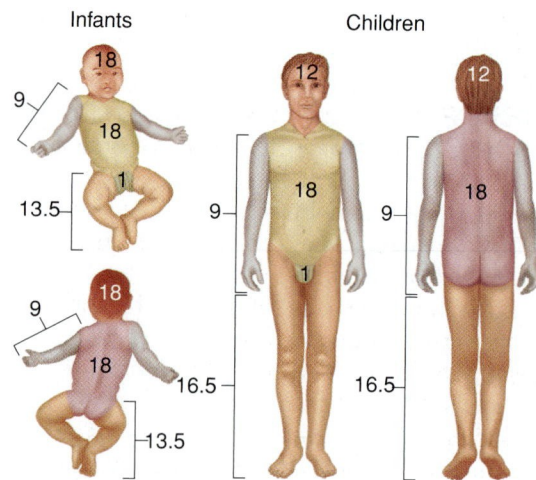

Figure 43-29   Rule of nines showing the difference in assigned percentages based upon age in the infant and child.

of 9% for the head and 18% for each leg. It can be difficult for providers to determine precisely which scale to use. One universally accepted estimate is to use the child's palmar surface (Rule of Palms) as an equivalent to 1% total surface area. Once an estimate of the total surface area burned is determined, a therapeutic pathway can be developed regarding the immediacy and method of transport to definitive burn care facility.

Therapeutic pathways include primary supportive care and aggressive assurances that the child's airway will remain open and patent. The appropriateness of prehospital pediatric intubation remains in question. The effectiveness of intubating the child in light of a respiratory burn injury is of great concern.[65] If intubation is not an option, remember that simple oxygenation or oxygenation via bag-mask may be more than adequate to maintain ventilations. Keep in mind, oxygen has some edema-reducing effect simply because of its cool, ambient temperature. IV or IO access may also be required to restore normal perfusion status and as a medication lifeline. If any signs or symptoms of shock are present, a 20 mL/kg fluid bolus should be administered. Subsequent boluses should be provided, dependent on local and burn unit protocols. DOT 6-2.39

CONNECTIONS Review Chapter 26: Burn Trauma page 533 for additional information on the pediatric version of the rule of nines.

A complete assessment and investigation for additional injuries or medical complications is mandatory. Inhalation or respiratory system involvement, fractures, and head trauma are common associated injuries seen in the injured child. Remember that the child may have sustained injuries other than just the dramatic burns.

Triage

The hysteria of a multiple or mass casualty event is magnified when the patient mix includes children. Unfortunately, unless the cause of the casualty event occurs strictly at an adult gathering, children will be typically involved. The Sacco Triage Methodology (STM) is an evidence based triage methodology recently developed. Dr. William Sacco and others developed STM in response to the need to maximize the number of expected survivors and to effectively utilize resources during mass casualty events.[66] The STM utilizes Respiratory Rate, Pulse Rate, and Best Motor Response (RPM) to determine the criticality of the patient at the time of the assessment. The RPM are assessed and each value is correlated to a coded value.

The respiratory rate (15 second count) and pulse rates (15 second count) are taken and the best motor response is determined (up to 10 seconds). The values of each are then converted to the coded values and added together to give the patient a point or Sacco score ranging from 0–12. Each Sacco score correlates to a specific level of criticality at the time the values were taken and also to the patient's expected survival to hospital discharge. Research (unpublished data) indicates that a simple adjustment based on age enables the Sacco Score to be a more accurate predictor of survival across the entire age range of victims. This allows the STM to be used as a stand alone, comprehensive triage method. Once patients are scored, they are grouped into score ranges at the scene, and they are dispatched from the scene in consideration of the timing and availability of transport and treatment resources. The priority assignment of patients is accomplished using optimal STM software or predetermined simulation-based triage rules.

In 1995, Dr. Lou Romig, a Board-certified pediatric emergency medicine physician, recognized that no published or commonly used triage protocol existed for children. Current protocols failed to address the unique anatomy and physiology of children as well as decision points for the many variations within this age group. Based on the START (Simple Triage and Rapid Transport) protocol, Dr. Romig devised "JumpStart." JumpStart is a pediatric-specific protocol that continues to evolve as evidence-based research becomes available. Dr. Romig implemented the protocol in a number of locations across America and in various foreign countries.[67]

CONNECTIONS For additional information on triage, see Chapter 50: Medical Incident Command.

Other scoring systems and triage tools have been developed and are used in various locations. Tools such as the Pediatric Trauma Score and Modified Glascow Coma Score are but two examples. One of the greatest challenges with these variations, regardless of how widespread their usage, is the ability to predict outcomes and survivability.

Children with Special Healthcare Needs (CSHCN)

The incidence of children surviving despite being afflicted with complex medical or traumatic maladies continues to grow. Research and healthcare advances have enabled children, who in years past would have otherwise died, to survive outside the hospital and integrate into their communities. Metropolitan, urban, suburban, and rural communities are now home to medically complex children: commonly referred to as children with **s**pecial **h**ealthcare **n**eeds (CSHCN).[68] CSHCN is defined as the following: DOT 6-2.45

- A child with a chronic illness.
- A child dependent upon technology or a technology **a**ssisted **c**hild (TAC). DOT 6-2.46
- A child with a congenital disability.
- A child with a developmental disability.[69]

The level of special needs can be as simple as the child with an inhaler or as complex as the child with all four disorders. It is becoming more common for the paramedic to walk into a home with intensive care-type equipment similar to or even more advanced than is found in their local hospitals. The parents of these technology assisted children are on duty continuously and have a vested interest in the care of their child. These parents or caregivers are actively involved in the concepts of "family-centered care," and it is to the paramedic's advantage to utilize this information resource before and during the provision of prehospital care.[70] Normal vital signs, communication abilities, and medical history will vary grossly with any child with special needs. Knowing what is normal for *this* child will allow you to understand what may have changed and what therapeutic pathways will need to be followed. DOT 6-2.78, 6-2.79, 6-2.80

The American Academy of Pediatrics (AAP) and the American College of Emergency Physicians (ACEP) joined forces to develop the Emergency Information Form (EIF) specifically to assist with the exchange of vital medical information anytime a CSHCN is contacted by healthcare professionals (Box 43-5). Although the EIF assists all levels of healthcare providers in their provision of care to these medically complex children, it is not a complete medical record. Additional history or specific changes since the last EIF update will need to be provided by the parents or primary caregiver. If local protocols and the situation allows, any member of the physician team can be contacted to enhance the therapeutic pathway. DOT 6-2.81

Street Secrets

If the medically complex child is going to be transported to a definitive care facility, it is valuable to take the patient's "go bag" with the patient. The "go bag" is similar to a baby's diaper bag in that it contains a supply of all the equipment that may be required while the child is away from the home, such as suction tubing and catheters, trach tubes, ostomy bags, nutrient solutions, airway devices including bag-mask, nasal cannulas, medications, monitoring devices, and additional batteries. If a specific piece of equipment is needed, the "go bag" probably contains it.

CSHCN are one of the most challenging circumstances a paramedic will ever encounter. The increasing survival rates of medically complex children provide unique challenges for the entire healthcare community. Complete assessments, including this child's "normals," pertinent chronic and acute history, and family-centered care facilitate quality patient care.

Summary

Children are a large part of society and a larger part of emotional foundation. Additional knowledge and skills are required to assure that this vulnerable group is properly cared for. Specific considerations must be given to anatomical, physiological, developmental, and emotional differences within the pediatric population and between pediatric and adult patients. As a paramedic, it is your responsibility to become a life-long learner of medicine, which includes pediatrics. Becoming an integrated member of the healthcare team will afford children their best opportunity to be cared for. Failure to do so may mean a lifetime of medical complications.

Notes

1. "The Do's and Don'ts of Transporting Children in an Ambulance," Washington, DC: U.S. Dept. of Health and Human Services, Maternal and Child Health Bureau, and the U.S. Department of Transportation, National Highway Traffic Safety Administration, December 1, 1999.
2. 2005 AHA Guidelines for Cardiopulmonary Resuscitation and Emergency Cardiovascular Care, Supplement to *Circulation* 112 (24) (December 13, 2005), IV-13.
3. http://www.childstats.gov/americaschildren/index.asp (accessed May 20, 2006).
4. U.S. Department of Health and Human Services, Health Resources and Services Administration, Maternal and Child Health Bureau. The National Survey of Children's Health. Rockville, Maryland: U.S. Department of Health and Human Services, 2005. The Health and Wellbeing of Children: A portrait of states and the nation 2005. www.mchb.hrsa.gov/thechildpdf/2child.pdf (accessed May 20, 2006).
5. R. A. Dieckman and R. W. Schafermeyer, "EMS for Children." In *Principles of EMS Systems,* W. R. Roush ed. (Dallas, TX: American College of Emergency Physicians, 1994).
6. "Overcrowding Crisis in Our Nation's Emergency Departments: Is Our Safety Net Unraveling?" *Pediatrics* 114(3)(September 2004): 878–888.
7. "Emergency Medical Services for Children," http://books.nap.edu/catalog/2137.html (accessed May 20, 2006).
8. Amelia G. Reis, Vinay Nadkarni, Maria Beatriz Perondi, Sandra Grisi, and Robert A. Berg, "A Prospective Investigation into the Epidemiology of In-Hospital Pediatric Cardiopulmonary Resuscitation Using the International Utstein Reporting Style." *Pediatrics* 109(2) (February 2002):200–209.
9. 2005 AHA Guidelines for Cardiopulmonary Resuscitation and Emergency Cardiovascular Care, Supplement to *Circulation* 112, (24) (December 13, 2005): IV-190.

BOX 43-5 Emergency Information Form

Emergency Information Form for Children With Special Needs

			Date form completed	Revised	Initials
American College of Emergency Physicians°	American Academy of Pediatrics		By Whom	Revised	Initials

Name: | **Birth date:** | **Nickname:**

Home Address: | **Home/Work Phone:**

Parent/Guardian: | **Emergency Contact Names & Relationship:**

Signature/Consent:*

Primary Language: | **Phone Number(s):**

Physicians:

Primary care physician: | **Emergency Phone:**
| **Fax:**

Current Specialty physician: | **Emergency Phone:**
Specialty: | **Fax:**

Current Specialty physician: | **Emergency Phone:**
Specialty: | **Fax:**

Anticipated Primary ED: | **Pharmacy:**

Anticipated Tertiary Care Center:

Diagnoses/Past Procedures/Physical Exam:

1.

Baseline physical findings:

2.

3.

Baseline vital signs:

4.

Synopsis:

Baseline neurological status:

*Consent for release of this form to health care providers

(continued)

BOX 43-5 *(continued)*

Diagnoses/Past Procedures/Physical Exam continued:

Medications:

1.

2.

3.

4.

5.

6.

Significant baseline ancillary findings (lab, x-ray, ECG):

Prostheses/Appliances/Advanced Technology Devices:

Management Data:

Allergies: Medications/Foods to be avoided   **and why:**

1.

2.

3.

Procedures to be avoided   **and why:**

1.

2.

3.

Immunizations (mm/yy)

Dates					Dates				
DPT					Hep B				
OPV					Varicella				
MMR					TB status				
HIB					Other				

Antibiotic prophylaxis: Indication: Medication and dose:

Common Presenting Problems/Findings With Specific Suggested Managements

Problem   **Suggested Diagnostic Studies**   **Treatment Considerations**

(continued)

BOX 43-5 *(continued)*

Comments on child, family, or other specific medical issues:

Physician/Provider Signature: Print Name:

© American College of Emergency Physicians and American Academy of Pediatrics. Permission to reprint granted with acknowledgement.

Source: http://www.aap.org/advocacy/eif.doc

10. K. D. Young, M. Gausche-Hill, C. D. McClung, and R. J. Lewis, "A Prospective, Population-based Study of the Epidemiology and Outcome of Out-of-Hospital Pediatric Cardiopulmonary Arrest. *Pediatrics* 114(1) (July, 2004):157–164.

11. M. Gausche and R. J. Lewis, "Out-of-Hospital Endotracheal Intubation of Children." *Journal of the American Medical Association* 283(21)(June 7, 2000): 2790–2792.

12. M. Guasche, R. J. Lewis, S. J. Stratton, et al., "Effect of Out-of-Hospital Pediatric Endotracheal Intubation on Survival and Neurological Outcome: A Controlled Clinical Trial." *Journal of the American Medical Association* 283(6) (February 9, 2000): 783–790. Erratum in *JAMA* 283(24) (June 28, 2000), p. 3204.

13. M. Gausche and J. S. Seidel, "Out-of-Hospital Care of Pediatric Patients." *Pediatric Clinics of North America* 46(6) (December, 1999):1305–1327.

14. Injury Prevention Fact Sheet, EMSC, www.ems-c.org/products/ (accessed October 12, 2006).

15. J. Ball and R. Bindler, *Pediatric Nursing—Caring for Children,* 2nd ed. (Norwalk, CT: Appleton and Lange, 1999).

16. "What Is Health? Defining Adolescence and Youth," www. distance.vic.edu.au/subschools/vcesubjectinfo/pdf (accessed May 20, 2006).

17. "Lecture," http://www.amritahobbs.com/presented March 16, 1999 (accessed February 18, 2007).

18. American Academy of Pediatrics, *Pediatric Education for Prehospital Professionals (PEPP),* 2nd ed. (Sudbury, MA: Jones and Bartlett, 2006).

19. N. S. Rahm, J. D. Hansen, and N. D. Sanddal, "Critical Trauma Care by the Basic EMT" (Bozeman, MT: Critical Illness and Trauma Foundation, Inc., 1997).

20. T. L. Sanddal, "Relative Stasis of Prehospital Provider Comfort Levels Concerning Pediatric Care [Abstract]" (Dallas, TX: 3rd ed., EMSC National Congress on Childhood Emergencies, 2002).

21. M. Rubin and N. Sadovnikoff, "Chapter 15: Pediatric Airway Management" in *Tintinalli's Emergency Medicine: A Comprehensive Study Guide,* 6th ed., McGraw-Hill's AccessMedicine (accessed February 10, 2007).

22. M. F. O' Connor and A. Ovassapiar, "Chapter 35: Airway Management." In *Principles of Critical Care,* 3rd ed., McGraw-Hill's AccessMedicine (accessed February 10, 2007).

23. M. J. Sagarin et. al., "National Emergency Airway Registry (NEAR) Investigators," *Pediatric Emergency Care* 18:417, 2002.

24. C. T. Neiman, C. F. Manacci, D. M. Super, C. Mancuso, and W. F. Fallon, Jr., "Use of the Broselow Tape May Result in the Underresuscitation of Children." *Academy of Emergency Medicine* (2006) 13(10): 1011–1019.

25. D. S. Lubitz, J. S. Seidel, L. Chameides, R. C. Luten, A. L. Zaritsky, and F. W. Campbell, "A Rapid Method for Estimating Weight and Resuscitation Drug Dosages from Length in the Pediatric Age Group." *Annals of Emergency Medicine* (1988), 17(6):576–581.

26. R. K. Cydulka, "Emergency Medicine: Use of the Broslow Tape May Result in the Underresuscitation of Children." Update to *Tintinalli's Emergency Medicine. A Comprehensive Study Guide,* 6th ed. (2004), McGraw-Hill's AccessMedicine (accessed February 10, 2007).

27. NAEMSP Model Pediatric Protocols, EMSC Partnership for Children, 2003, http://nedarc.med.utha.edu/nedarc/media/pdf/ModelPediatricProtocols.pdf (accessed October 12, 2006).

28. MedlinePlus Dictionary, http://www.nlm.nih.gov/medlineplus/mplusdictionary.html (accessed October 12, 2006).

29. K. L. Hall and B. Zalman, "Evaluation and Management of Apparent Life-Threatening Events in Children," *American Family Physician* (June 15, 2005), http://www.aafp.org/afp/20050615/2301.html (accessed October 12, 2006).

30. National Safekids Coalition, www.Safekids.com (accessed October 12, 2006).

31. Nation Center for Injury Prevention and Control Center, http://www.cdc.gov/ncipc/ (accessed October 12, 2006).

32. 2005 AHA Guidelines for Cardiopulmonary Resuscitation and Emergency Cardiovascular Care, Supplement to *Circulation* 112:24 (December 13, 2005).

33. Asthma Prevalence, Health Care Use and Mortality, 2002, http://www.cdc.gov/nchs/products/pubs/pubd/hestats/asthma/asthma.htm (accessed October 12, 2006).

34. Physicians Desk Reference (Boehringer Ingelheim Pharmaceuticals, Inc.).

35. T. J. Brousseau and N. Kissoon, "Chapter 117, Common Neonatal Problems." In *Tintinalli's Emergency Medicine: A Comprehensive Study Guide*, 6th ed., 2004. McGraw-Hill's AccessMedicine (accessed February 10, 2007).

36. Croup, http://www.healthopedia.com/croup/symptoms.html (accessed October 12, 2006).

37. R. K. Jackler and M. J. Kaplan, "Epiglottitis." In M. A. Papadikis and S. J. McPhee, eds., *2006 Current Consult: Medicine,* McGraw-Hill's AccessMedicine, Quick Access (accessed February 10, 2007).

38. H. Aly, "Respiratory Disorders in the Newborn: Identification and Diagnosis." *Pediatric Reviews* (2004) 25:201.

39. O. Flidel-Raman and E. S. Shinwell, "Respiratory Distress in the Term and Near-Term Infant." *NeoReviews* (2005) 6:e289.

40. M. G. Ross, "Meconium Aspiration Syndrome—More Than Intrapartum Meconium." *New England Journal of Medicine* (2005) 353:946.

41. M. Kou and T. Mayer, "Chapter 24: Pediatric Asthma and Bronchiolitis." In J. E. Tintinalli, G. D. Kelen, J. S. Stapczynski, O. J. Ma, and D. M. Cline, *Tintinalli's Emergency Medicine: A*

Comprehensive Study Guide, 6th ed., McGraw-Hill's AccessMedicine (accessed February 10, 2007).

42. K. Brown and W. Gilford, Jr., "Chapter 24: Pediatric Asthma and Bronchiolitis." In J. E. Tintinalli, G. D. Kelen, J. S. Stapczynski, O. J. Ma, and D. M. Cline, *Tintinalli's Emergency Medicine: A Comprehensive Study Guide*, 6th ed., McGraw-Hill's AccessMedicine (accessed February 10, 2007).

43. J. Stark, "Childhood Tuberculosis during the 1990s." *Pediatrics in Review* 1(3) (1992): 43–53.

44. Lung Transplantation in Cystic Fibrosis, http://www.fpnotebook.com/LUN120.htm (accessed October 12, 2006).

45. D. Markenson, *Pediatric Prehospital Care* (Upper Saddle River, NJ: Brady—Prentice Hall, 2002).

46. National Association of Emergency Medical Technicians, *Prehospital Trauma Life Support*, 5th ed. (St. Louis, MO: Elsevier Mosby, 2005).

47. Results from the 2002 National Survey on Drug Use and Health: National Findings, SAMHSA, http://www.oas.samhsa.gov/nhsda/2k2nsduh/Results/2k2Results.htm (accessed October 12, 2006).

48. Kids Health for Parents, Ectopic Pregnancy, http://kidshealth.org/parent/pregnancy_newborn/pregnancy/ectopic.html (accessed October 12, 2006).

49. eMedicine from WebMD, Pelvic Inflammatory Disease, http://www.emedicine.com/EMERG/topic410.htm (accessed October 12, 2006).

50. M. L. Stoller, C. J. Kane, and P. R. Carroll "Urology." In *Current Medical Diagnosis and Treatment 2007*. McGraw-Hill's AccessMedicine, (accessed February 10, 2007).

51. F. G. Cunningham, K. L. Leveno, S. L. Bloom. J. C. Hauth. L. C. Gilstrap III, and K. D. Wenstrom, "Chapter 13: Prenatal Diagnosis and Fetal Therapy." In *Williams Obstetrics*, 22nd ed., McGraw-Hill's AccessMedicine (accessed February 10, 2007).

52. R. S. Vasan, E. J. Benjamin, L. M. Sullivan, and R. B. D'Agostino. "Chapter 2: The Burden of Increasing Worldwide Cardiovascular Disease." In *Hurst's The Heart*. 11th ed., McGraw-Hill's AccessMedicine (accessed February 10, 2007).

53. American Diabetes Association, "Clinical Practice Recommendations," *Diabetes Care* (2002) 25 (Suppl 1): S1.

54. M. A. Papadakis and S. J. McPhee, eds., "Diabetic Ketoacidosis," *2007 Current Consult: Medicine*. McGraw-Hill's AccessMedicine (accessed February 10, 2007).

55. L. Williams, "News release, National Institute of Allergy and Infectious Diseases," *Journal of Allergy and Clinical Immunology* 113 (February 2004): 291–296.

56. O. O. Bilukha et al., Centers for Disease Control and Prevention (CDC). Prevention and Control of Meningococcal Disease. Recommendations of the Advisory Committee on Immunization Practices (ACIP). *Morbidity Mortality Weekly Report* (2005) 54(RR-7):1.

57. A. R. Tunkel et al., Treatment of Bacterial Meningitis. *Current Infectious Disease Reports*. (2002) 4:7.

58. Centers for Disease Control and Prevention, *Haemophilus influenzae* Type B Meningitis in Children, Eritrea, Durgadas G. Naik, and Melles Seyoum, www.cdc.gov/ncidod/eid/vol10no1/03-0132.htm (accessed March 10, 2007).

59. Merriam-Webster Online Dictionary, http://www2.merriam-webster.com (accessed October 12, 2006).

60. J. A. Marx, ed., *Rosen's Emergency Medicine Concepts and Clinical Practice*, 5th ed. (St. Louis, MO: Elsevier Mosby, 2002).

61. Centers for Disease Control and Prevention, 2002, http://www.cdc.gov/ncipc/wisqars (accessed October 12, 2006).

62. S. Stylianos, Outcomes from Pediatric Solid Organ Injury: Role of Standardized Care Guidelines. *Current Opinions in Pediatrics* 17(3) (June 2005):402–406.

63. "Pediatric Trauma," http://www.dscc.edu/crihfield/PediatricTrauma.htm

64. B. S. Atiyeh et al., "State of the Art in Burn Treatment." *World Journal of Surgery* (2005) 29:131.

65. American Burn Association, "Inhalation Injury: Diagnosis." *Journal of the American College of Surgeons* (2003) 196:307.

66. W. J. Sacco, M. Navin, K. E. Fiedler, R. K. Waddell, W. B. Long, and R. F. Buckman, Jr. "Precise Formulation and Evidence-Based Application of Resource-Constrained Triage," *Academic Emergency Medicine* 12 (2005): 759–770.

67. T. L. Sanddal, T. Loyacono, and N. D. Sanddal, "Effect of JumpSTART Training on Immediate and Short-Term Pediatric Performance." *Journal of Pediatric Emergency Care* (in press).

68. U.S. Department of Health and Human Services. *Healthy People 2010* (Conference Edition, in Two Volumes). Washington, DC: U.S. Department of Health and Human Services, January 2000.

69. The National Center of Medical Home Initiatives for Children with Special Needs, http://www.medicalhomeinfo.org/ (accessed October 12, 2006).

70. Family Centered Care Fact Sheet, EMSC, www.ems-c.org/products/ (accessed October 12, 2006).

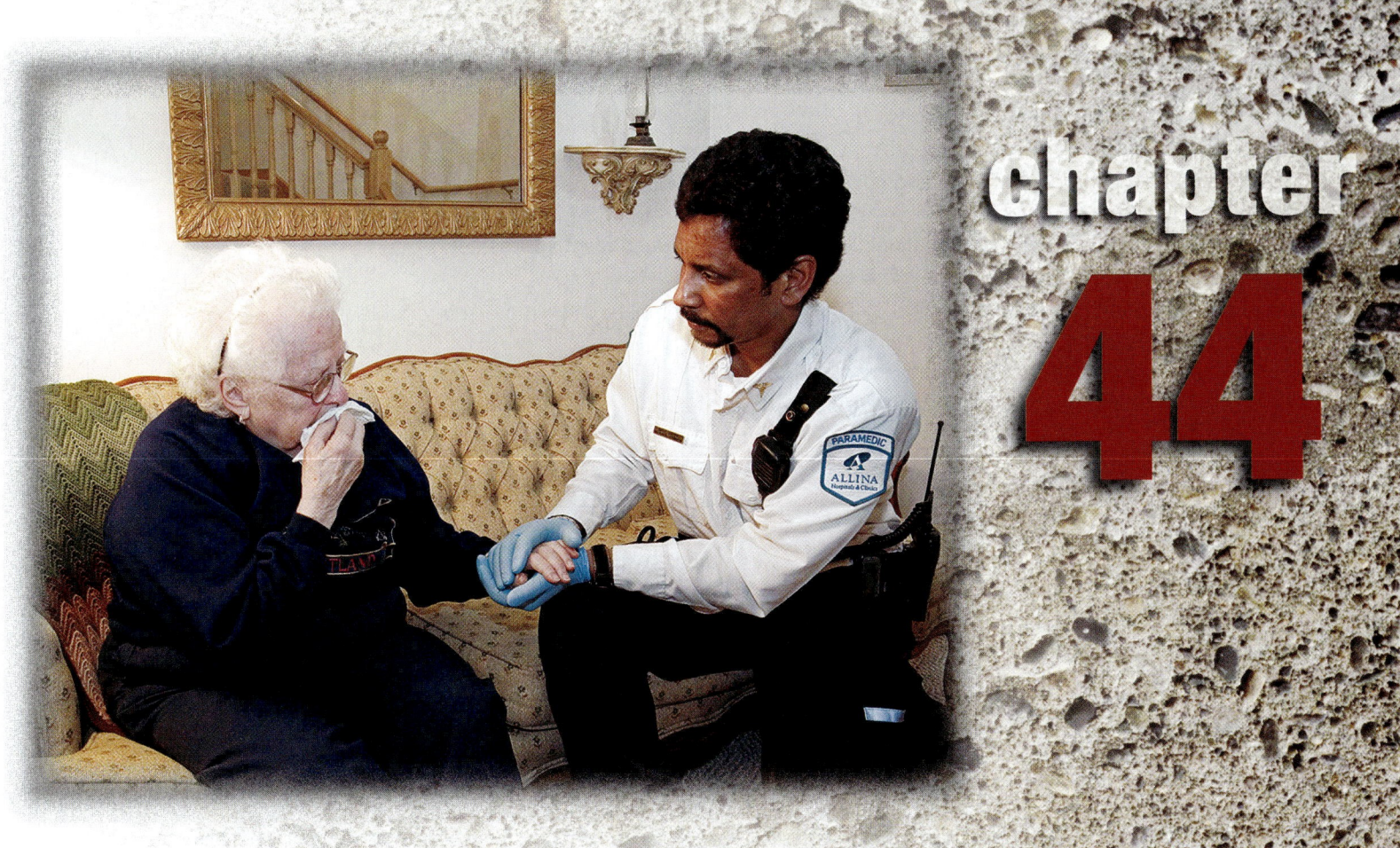

Geriatric Patients

"Youth, which is forgiven everything, forgives itself nothing: age, which forgives itself everything, is forgiven nothing."

—George Bernard Shaw

Need to Know

▶ The geriatric population is growing rapidly.

▶ The alterations in mobility geriatric patients may exhibit.

▶ The effects of aging on body systems and how that affects the way they describe or fail to describe their medical conditions.

▶ The types of medications that elderly patients may be on that affect patient assessment.

▶ The types of brain disorders that become more likely with age.

▶ How to approach confused and distrustful patients in a way that makes them more comfortable with your care.

▶ The types of fractures to which the elderly are prone.

▶ Methods of immobilizing elderly patients with deformed posture.

▶ Do	▶ Ask
• Treat elderly patients with respect.	• Ask elderly patients about their medications.
• Accommodate changes in your patient's mobility and positional discomfort.	• Ask your patients about their ability to move and painful positions.
• Look for medications or medication administration devices in the home.	• Ask your patients about their history, such as diabetes, cardiac disease, hypertension, pulmonary disease, and other problems.
• Be prepared for patients with deficits related to organic brain syndrome or Alzheimer's disease.	• Ask your patients simple questions relative to the present situation, and be considerate and helpful when patients exhibit frustration with their inability to remember or respond appropriately.
• Be cognizant of the patient's comfort and position, and immobilize the patient according to need and patient comfort.	• Ask the patients if it hurts when you move or reposition them.
• Be concerned about patients with dizziness, hypotension, shortness of breath, or signs of CHF. Geriatric patients present with classic AMI symptoms less than one-third of the time.	• Ask your patients if they have had similar episodes and if they have any other potential symptoms of AMI.

Introduction

Just as the pediatric population has unique characteristics, the older population has its unique characteristics. As people age, there are differences in the ability to respond to injury and illness. The normal aging process begins as the growth process ends. Beginning around age 30 years, the body's ability to respond to change demonstrates a very slow decrease from its optimal functioning that appears to be the result of gradual wear and tear.[1] The results of this process may be from changes in the mechanism of cell regulation, the impact of genetic and environmental factors, or degenerative processes. The cumulative effect impacts the life span, lifestyle, response to injury, and the development of disease in the older adult.

What Is Gerontology?

Gerontology is the scientific study of the process and problems of aging. Due to the growth in numbers of the older population, research, education, and clinical training programs in gerontology for all healthcare professionals have exploded.

In the U.S., population estimates for 2004 showed over 41 million people age 65 and older.[2] With the attention to healthy lifestyles, medications, and medical advances, the population over 75 years old is projected to be almost 25 million by 2025, with 6 million people older than 85 years of age. Life expectancy in the United States is 77.6 years, with women living until 80.5 and men until 75.4.[3] Within the geriatric age group, the oldest old, those over 85 years of age, are growing most dramatically. As this population grows, it will continue to account for an increasing number of emergency responses.

Since there are differences in patient presentation and therapeutic interventions, the need to identify proper care is shown by the increase in research focused on this age group and the development of continuing education courses tailored to the care of the geriatric population.

With this population increase, the need for Medicare, Social Security, and retirement benefits also grows.

The percent of state and national dollars dedicated to services for the elderly will need to increase. The problem will be a smaller population at work to support the needed tax base contributing to Medicare and Social Security. Local services such as county Office for Services for the Aging, day programs for adults with disabilities, hospice care programs, Meals on Wheels services for nutrition, and a variety of other programs become increasingly important. The elderly may continue to live independently at home, in retirement communities, assisted living facilities, or nursing homes, depending on their chronic and acute illnesses, disability, financial resources, and family support. Retirement may be forced on an individual by illness, injury, or mobility issues, or it may be a planned event. Others may desire or financially need to continue working (Figure 44-1).

Depending on societal and cultural beliefs, support for the elderly varies. For example, Denmark has health insurance for anyone who has lived in the country for seven years. Arrangements are made to allow the older adult to remain in the home setting with supportive services, including rehabilitation. The United States has a high number of uninsured people, leading to access to care issues. Without the resources for adequate housing, health care, or medications, the burden on the healthcare system increases dramatically.

Families in some cultures live together, combining the generations under one roof. Others provide care as long as possible and then need to place the ill adult in a nursing care facility. The current generation is often caught between raising children and caring for parents at the same time. DOT 6-3.1, 2, 3, 4, 5

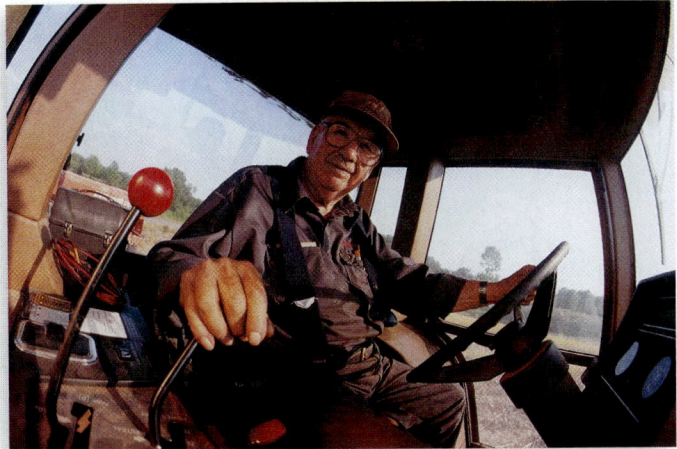

Figure 44-1 For some elderly people, retirement is not an option and they continue to work as long as they can.

Street Secrets

Do a little research to determine the demographics of your service area. Do you have a large elderly population? Can you get involved in local senior education to teach them about EMS and their own personal safety?

CONNECTIONS See Chapter 48: Patients from Diverse Cultures for more information on multigenerational families.

During the aging process, physiologic changes occur to everyone. This will occur at different rates, but it is occurring to everyone at some point after age 30. Disease may strike at any time, and the signs and symptoms may be different than in the younger adult. The older body's response to medications is different due to physiologic changes. Pain may not be felt, the body may not respond to infection with fever, and classic indicators may be absent. Multiple illnesses or conditions may exist simultaneously. These issues complicate the assessment, recognition, and the critical thinking process the paramedic uses in everyday practice.

Whether aging is a preprogrammed, cellular event or a genetic or environmental cumulative cause, there are common changes to expect. This happens on an individual basis as well as to each organ system that undergoes change on its own time schedule. Cardiac function decreases and the blood vessels become more rigid. The compensatory mechanisms necessary in shock are limited due to the cardiac changes and, often, medications taken on a daily basis. The ability to see, hear, taste, feel, and move decrease, leading to changes in mobility, nutrition, communication, and social interaction. Short-term memory is impaired. The loss of elasticity in the respiratory system and the decrease in the ability of the immune system to be protective invite infection and complications. Every system of the body has changes that lead to less than optimal functioning.

Outliving a spouse, friends, and family creates gaps in friendship, support, travel, and daily interaction with other human beings (Figure 44-2). Isolation leads to depression and often a decrease in nutrition, activity levels, and mental functioning. Social services may need to be contacted to provide evaluation and support for the elderly person. The cost of living, shelter, food, utilities, doctor or hospital bills, medications, and insurance, may exceed the resources saved for retirement. A choice may be made between heat and eating and taking an essential medication. Appropriate referrals to support services do make a difference in the lives of the older patient. Social and political changes will be required as the older segment of the population increases in numbers and requires additional programs and support.

Remember that aging and disease are not one and the same. The physiologic process of cell death and loss

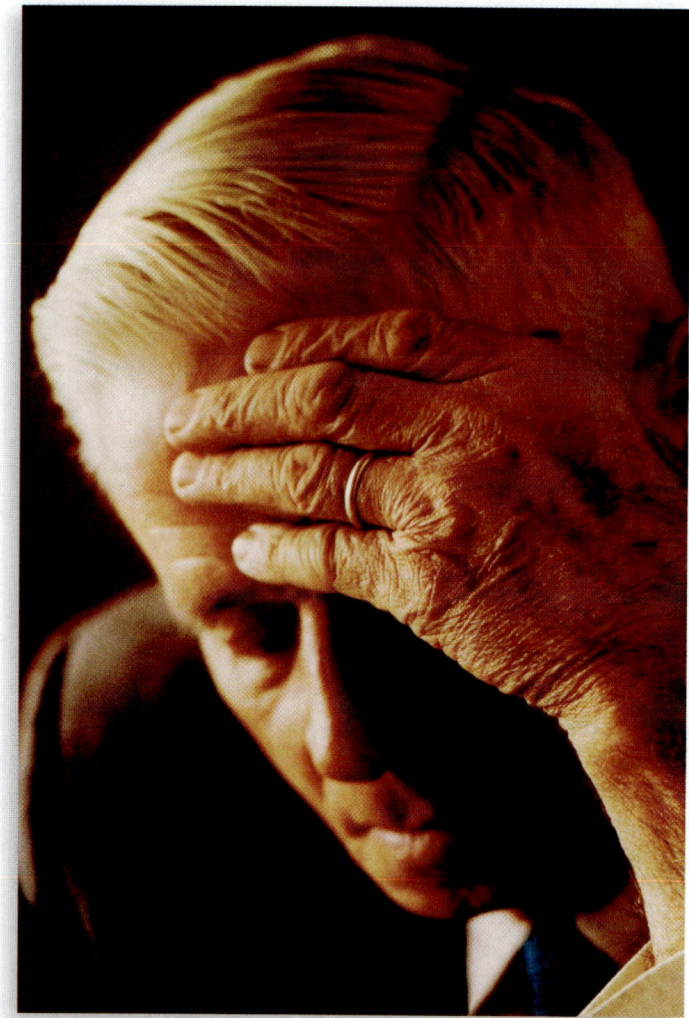

Figure 44-2 The death of a spouse can lead to isolation and depression.

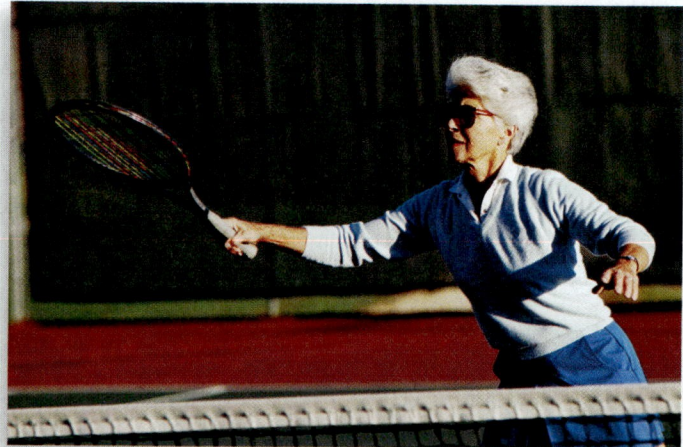

Figure 44-3 Exercise increases overall wellness in the elderly.

This impacts recovery time, and with prolonged loss of normal activities and contacts, the patient may become more isolated from family and friends.[1]

Health Promotion

The development of illness or injury may be influenced by promoting healthy practices that one can implement every day. Appropriate nutrition, including vitamin supplements, may require a referral to an agency for assistance such as Meals on Wheels, pastoral care, or other community resources. Encouraging participation in an exercise program including walking and strength training increases muscle strength, mental health, and overall wellness (Figure 44-3).[4] Injury prevention should be a part of each response to a home. Identify fall hazards; unhealthy situations; and lack of fire, smoke and carbon monoxide detectors, as well as heat and cooling devices. Be watchful for indications of elder abuse, and if found, report as required. After the emergency response is over, refer the patient to the appropriate support service.

Providing immunizations is a newer role for many EMS providers. Influenza and pneumococcal vaccines are important for this population, supported by the Healthy People 2010 goals for the over 65 population.[5]

of function occur on a very slow continuum. Illness may or may not occur. Unfortunately, there is a common misconception that all elders have illnesses and questionable mental function. The reality is that, in the absence of disease, the elderly are healthy and able to continue an active lifestyle with few changes or restrictions.

Challenges are presented with the geriatric patient when complaints are not clear and easily matched to a disease process. Patients may be unable to express more than that they do not feel right, they feel weak or dizzy, or they are not able to do their normal activities. Vague complaints may be the indicators of serious disease processes, such as myocardial infarction or sepsis, that do not have the classic signs and symptoms. Multiple disease conditions often exist concurrently, leading to a confusing picture at the time of an emergency. Diminished functional reserves complicate everyday life and contribute to the loss of compensatory mechanisms.

Nice to Know

Paramedics are exposed to geriatric patients that may need services not available from EMS. It is a good idea to be aware of senior services in your community in order to refer family and patients for assistance outside of your capabilities.

Anatomy and Physiology of the Elderly

Since the cumulative effect of cell and organ damage will progress at an individual rate, this discussion addresses general changes to each body system from the aging process. Understanding these changes will allow you to anticipate disease presentations that do not have the classic signs and symptoms as in the younger patient. In some cases, it is difficult to tell where physiologic change ends and pathology begins, so general trends in aging will be discussed. Pharmacologic interventions are sometimes different partially due to the changes in the clearing ability of the liver and kidneys. This requires an awareness of dosage changes and side effects of medications.

Respiratory System Differences

Over time, respiratory function decreases with an accompanying decrease in PO_2. With age, there is a loss of elastic recoil of the lungs, ossification of the ribs and joints, and a decrease in respiratory muscle strength. Stiffening of the chest wall results in a decrease in compliance and the reduction of respiratory capacity. This leads to a decrease in vital capacity although total lung capacity remains the same. (The residual volume increases.) This affects the reserve volume available during times of exertion and stress. The volume of air available for actual gas exchange is decreased. Decreases in the pulmonary capillary network and enlargement of the alveoli reduce the surface area available for gas exchange. These structural and mechanical changes impair gas exchange, resulting in a decrease in PO_2 while pH and PCO_2 remain fairly constant. For example, the PO_2 of an adult at sea level breathing room air is approximately 90 mmHg. At age 70, the PO_2 would be approximately 79 mmHg; at age 80, it would be 76 mmHg.[1]

The normal triggers to increase or decrease respiratory effort are also affected by age. There is less sensitivity to hypercapnia and hypoxia, leading to less effective compensation.

The ability of the respiratory system to compensate for increased body need and workload is decreased. During exertion, this limits the compensatory mechanisms that are available. The more active the individual, the more reserve capacity is developed and available. Beginning exercise at any point in time will strengthen respiratory muscles and increase endurance.

The protective ability of the lungs to prevent and fight infection is decreased by the loss of muscle strength in the cough and gag reflexes. The loss of cilia lining the respiratory tract decreases the amount of particles trapped and removed before they can cause harm. There is an impaired response to foreign antigens with the loss of lymphoid tissue, resulting in a less effective immune response.[1]

Prior respiratory conditions may reoccur. Infection is a danger. Influenza and pneumonia are serious diseases in this age group. Long-time smokers and those who worked in conditions of high toxic exposures will have more drastic respiratory system changes and a greater potential for respiratory infections and complications.

Cardiovascular System Differences

Cardiovascular disease is the most prevalent disease process seen in the older population.[2] The net effect of microvascular changes in the elasticity of vessels, patency of the lumen, and muscle strength is to decrease the resilience and ability of the heart, arteries, and veins to compensate during times of stress. Although there is tremendous variation in the development and manifestation of the physiologic changes, some patterns emerge. The heart enlarges or hypertrophies over time. This results from the loss of muscle cells and the harder workload of pumping against arteries that have stiffened. This stiffening may be due to the loss of elastin and collagen, leading to an increase in systolic blood pressure.

The ability of the baroreceptors that allow the body to compensate or adjust to changes in position from lying or sitting to standing appears to decrease with age.[1] This decrease leads to a slowing in the ability to signal an increase or decrease of heart rate to maintain blood pressure. With the slowed response, sudden position changes can result in dizziness or a fall.

Atherosclerosis, which begins early in life, is the quiet, progressive disabler and killer. This process of inflammation, atheroma, and plaque development can affect every vessel. It may show as peripheral vascular disease, coronary artery disease, angina, stroke, or myocardial infarction. It has an impact on every organ.

The heart at rest is able to function with only a slight impact from aging. The impact of the aging process truly shows when the body is under conditions of exertion. Whether it is exercise, stress, or the increased demand from illness or injury, the body is not able to draw on a reserve to compensate. This may lead to prolonged illness or recovery. Cardiac output decreases with a decrease in heart rate.[1] The loss of electrical conduction cells may lead to dysrhythmias, which also contribute to a decrease in cardiac output.

Gastrointestinal System Changes

The condition of the teeth and the ability to taste and smell have an influence on the desire to eat. Tooth decay and tooth loss impacts the chewing of food, which affects the ability to swallow and begin digestion. With aging, there is a decrease in saliva, which is also needed to begin digestion.[1] Motility in the GI tract begins to slow with age, often leading to slower gastric emptying and constipation. Gastric and digestive secretions, necessary for the breakdown of food as it moves in the gut, are reduced. This affects the absorption of nutrients, leading to deficits of important substances. The protective layer of mucus, which lines the surface of the GI tract to protect it from stomach acid, decreases. Even with less acid being produced, without this protective lining, ulcer disease can occur.

The liver plays a role in metabolism, synthesis of nutrients, and protection through its ability to remove foreign substances and bacteria. It also has a major role in detoxifying drugs. With aging, blood flow to the liver is decreased, and each function is less effective.[1]

Renal System Changes

With aging, there is a loss of the functional units of the kidney, the nephron. This leads to a decrease of 45–55 % in total body water over the aging process.[1] As the number of cells decrease, the body is less able to concentrate urine. The ability to compensate and regulate situations of over- or underhydration is affected, leading to overhydration or dehydration. Medication use can also affect the ability to maintain the correct electrolyte and fluid balance. Some medications affect sodium and water balance. Both aging and medications can affect the renal hormonal regulatory system. This involves vitamin D, necessary for calcium and phosphate; erythropoietin, the stimulant for the production of red blood cells especially when hypoxia has occurred; and atrial natriuretic peptide, a trigger to adjust salt and water amounts when the right atrial blood pressure is elevated. With the decrease in effectiveness, the body is less able to tolerate the impact of disease processes. There is decrease in the absorption of glucose as well.

Another important aspect of the renal system is its role in acid/base balance. As the third line of defense to pH changes, this process becomes less effective, prolonging the body's adjustment to minute changes.

Drug filtration and clearance slows, which can lead to the accumulation of a drug in the bloodstream. Without the ability to excrete a drug from the body, toxic amounts can accumulate. The knowledge of side effects from toxicity is necessary and should be considered during patient evaluation. By-products of metabolism fall into this arena as well. With the limited clearing ability, nitrogen waste products such as urea, ammonia, and creatinine will build up in the system.

Urinary incontinence, prostate enlargement leading to urinary frequency, and difficulty urinating, become increasingly prevalent concerns. The lifestyle changes that manifest this disruption to normal activities include the inability to sleep through the night, the fear of not getting to the bathroom in time, and the frequent number of trips to the bathroom that interfere with normal work and recreation patterns. DOT 6-3.10

Neurological System Changes

As the ability to remember, recall, and react all change, it is evident that there are decreases in the level of neurologic functioning of the older person. Short-term memory decreases, searching for the correct word increases, and slowed reflexes make it harder to do the activities of daily living. Brain weight and size decrease, myelin is lost, and the number of synapses decreases.

Some functional changes become obvious with age. Hearing diminishes, especially since high frequencies are lost, making it difficult to understand words and communicate. This may result from a disease process (Ménière's, diabetes, neoplasm), exposure to loud noises, the toxicity of certain medications, or it may be hereditary. The eye undergoes changes in the cornea, lens, and muscles needed for accurate vision. Glaucoma, cataracts, and visual acuity changes may occur. Near vision is impacted by the loss of the ability to accommodate or change the thickness of the lens, resulting in extending the arm to be able to read a paper. The amount of light needed to safely navigate and to retain mobility is increased. Colors become less vivid with the aging of the lens and its discoloration process makes it more yellow.

The ability to taste and smell has a direct correlation to appetite and adequate nutrition. When the flavor of food is decreased, enjoyment of eating also decreases. Eating is often thought of as a social event. The cumulative effect of the loss of flavor, difficulty chewing, fear of incontinence, and visual changes may result in the loss of enjoyment, isolation, and inadequate nutrition.

The ability to know what position the body is in and to maintain balance is essential in mobility and preventing falls. Due to aging or illness, there is a loss of tactile sensation and proprioception—the ability to know the position of the body. Neuropathies, inner ear disturbances, trauma, infection, and the degenerative process lead to inner ear dysfunction such as a loss of balance, gait changes, and vertigo. DOT 6-3.8, 9

Temperature regulation is the ongoing balance of metabolic, vascular, hormonal, nervous system, and muscular activities mediated by the hypothalamus. The mechanisms to respond to temperature extremes—heat and cold—are less efficient with age. A slower metabolic rate, decreased shivering, decreased vasoconstriction, thinning of the dermis, and less sensitive touch and nerve endings decrease the ability to maintain the body temperature within normal range. The elderly's inability to respond to hyperthermia or hypothermia conditions results in morbidity and mortality that could be prevented through adequate clothing, shelter, heating, and cooling.

Economic constraints may limit access to sufficient resources.

The body normally has a protective ability to generate a fever under conditions of infection. This beneficial mechanism deters bacterial and viral growth and replication, stimulates the immune response, and increases phagocytosis. With aging, these abilities are decreased or lost, often resulting in no fever response under times of severe infection. Without this protective action, morbidity and mortality increase.

Sleep patterns may be disrupted and become fragmented due to underlying medical problems or medications. Sleep disorders, depression, obesity, chronic pain, urinary frequency, and daytime napping can interrupt and change sleep patterns. The resulting fatigue can lead to daytime sleepiness and motor vehicle crashes and can complicate underlying medical conditions.

Musculoskeletal Changes

Many people assume a more sedentary lifestyle as they age, reducing muscle tone. The consequence to this action is less endurance and decreased metabolic rate. Bone density decreases with microscopic changes to the bone structure itself, often seen in loss of height and increased risk for fractures. Osteoporosis screenings and interventions attempt to prevent the fractures that occur, often from minor injuries or falls.

Street Secrets

Changes to the skeletal system include kyphosis, a curvature of the spine that causes the patient to appear hunched or stooped forward. When immobilizing geriatric patients to long boards, you will need to liberally pad the patient to accommodate curvatures in the spine.

Immune and Inflammatory Changes

Recent research identified the role of inflammation and immune response leading to vascular changes linked to increased risk of cardiovascular disease. Interleukin–6, C reactive protein, adipokins, and leptin are related to chronic inflammation and changes in the endothelial lining and cardiovascular disease, obesity, and insulin resistance. As the evidence base develops, interventions on weight, nutrition, and vitamin supplementation will be decided. It is known that many elderly do not receive adequate nutrition, and vitamin supplementation enhances the nutritional status as well as boosts the immune system.[4,5]

Since the skin and mucous membranes are the first line of defense against infection, it is apparent that the physiologic aging changes have a profound impact. The increasing thinness and permeability of the skin and the decrease in blood flow, secretory glands, and ability of the mucosal linings to protect cause the body to lose this protective ability. There is a decrease in lymphoid tissue in the mucosal linings, so identification and phagocytosis of foreign substances is much less efficient.

Summary of Changes in the Elderly

There are a variety of age-related physiologic changes that have significant consequences in geriatric patients, from changes in the endocrine system that increase glucose levels in response to illness to decreased cough reflexes that create micro aspirations and increase the potential for respiratory disease. Understanding these changes can increase the paramedic's index of suspicion when assessing geriatric patients.

DOT 6-3.11

Assessment of the Geriatric Patient

Building upon the information presented in earlier chapters about assessment of all patients, this section will address differences in assessment techniques and history taking for the elderly. When paramedics respond to calls at patients' homes, they are in a unique position to ascertain patients' living situations and needs and to communicate identified needs to the healthcare team. Observing and reporting living conditions, support systems, medications, fall hazards, and pertinent conditions provides the route for intervention, if needed (Figure 44-4).

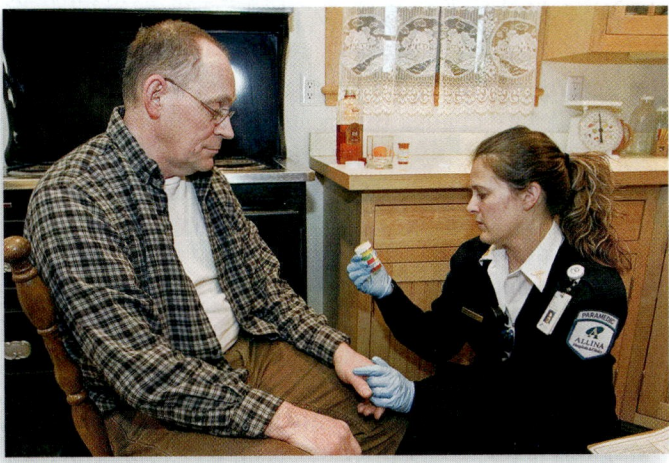

Figure 44-4 Carefully observe your patient's living conditions and report your findings to the hospital staff if the patient is transported.

Common Traits in the Geriatric Population

- The older adult will often not report symptoms to their healthcare provider for several reasons. There is the assumption that certain body changes will occur with aging and that these symptoms are not important and are "to be expected." Consequently, they do not receive evaluation and intervention even though there are many treatable conditions.

- Concurrent illnesses are often present. A chronic condition exists, and the acute presentation is difficult to differentiate from the presentation and complications of the underlying conditions. Multiple conditions can be occurring in the person, creating a complex picture.

- The adage that the symptoms can be understood by a single unifying diagnosis often does not apply.[7] The picture in the elderly is more complex. Often the presenting symptom is unrelated to the acute disease process but occurs in the organ system most prone to illness. The weakest systems are often the brain, lower urinary tract, cardiac, or musculoskeletal system. Associated presenting symptoms may be confusion, depression, urinary incontinence, falls, or syncope as the first signs that an acute illness is occurring—no matter what the cause of the disease process.

- Due to symptoms occurring simultaneously or the limited compensatory reserves, what would be a minor or moderate disease process in the young or middle-age person becomes a major event. DOT 6-3.13, 14

Assessment Pitfalls

- There is an erroneous theory that an elderly person is often a hypochondriac. On the contrary, the elderly person is more likely not to report symptoms than to complain. Many elderly have the false impression that changes in the ability to function occur naturally with aging and there is nothing to do for them. Any change that results in a loss of function is serious and must be evaluated.

- Classic symptoms are often not the presentation found in the aging. Vague feelings of not feeling well or weakness may often be the only presentation. Remember, the chief complaints often are not from the system causing the problem.[10]

- Do not attribute a new presentation to the chronic condition and overlook the acute problem. Do not be misled or underestimate the severity of disease. Investigate the sudden onset of new problems.

- Avoid disrespect, even though not intentional, by using familiar names when addressing the patient or not asking questions to the person directly.

- Do not have a lack of patience; allow time for the person to understand and answer your questions. Cognitive processing may take longer to understand information and formulate the answer.

Obtaining a History

As you begin to gather a history, identify obstacles in communication and remedy, if possible. If the patient uses a hearing aid and it is available, make sure it is in and turned on; find eyeglasses, if possible. Remember that background noises can be very distracting if there is hearing loss. When at all possible, decrease the noise level at the scene. Position yourself so the person can see your face clearly and make eye contact. Ensure adequate light. This makes it easier for those with hearing and visual deficits to focus on your questions (Figure 44-5).

Allow time for the person to answer the question. Gain cooperation, as undoubtedly you will be assessing as you ask questions. Make sure the person understands what you are going to do before you touch them. Obtaining necessary information regarding age, present and past medical history, and medication information is essential. The presence of advance directives is common, and if available, this document should accompany the person to the hospital. Advanced directives need to be communicated to medical command but they do not mean that interventions are not provided.

CONNECTIONS See Chapters 3: Professional Ethics and 4: Legal Issues for more information on advanced directives.

As you receive answers to questions, you will be formulating an opinion on the patient's mental state.

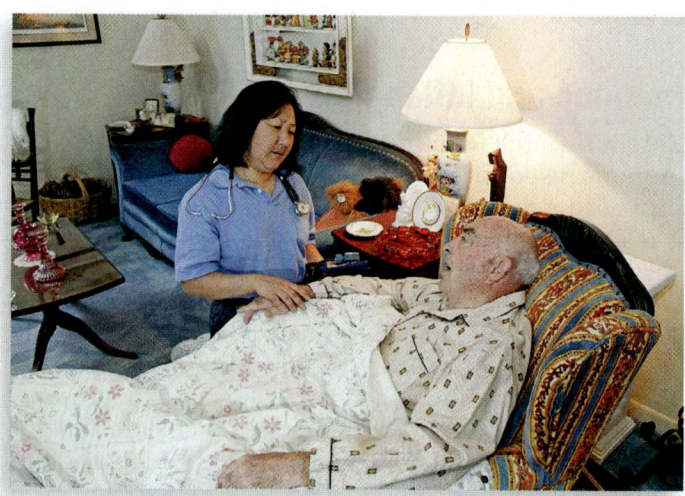

Figure 44-5 Make sure your patient can see and hear you well.

Approach the patient anticipating that they are intact neurologically since the majority of elderly do not have dementia. Listen closely for signs of confusion that may be from an underlying disease process or medication use. Depression is common, especially in the elderly facing hospitalization. Pay attention to appearance and hygiene. If there has been a change in these, it may be a clue to the severity of symptoms or depression.

It is a realistic fear that going to the hospital may result in not being able to return home. Additional care and assistance for activities of daily living may be required, making it impossible to return to the previous housing situation. Remember that the elderly may function every day on the edge of their physiologic ability, and illness may result in significant decompensation. DOT 6-3.12

Physical Examination

As you ensure the airway is patent, breathing is adequate, and circulation is intact, consider the physiologic differences previously discussed. Be careful not to hyperextend the head since occlusion of the airway can occur secondary to stiffening of the trachea, decreased gag reflex, or other central nervous system diseases. Observe posture; if kyphosis is present, there is an ongoing, existing reduction in ventilation, as well as more difficulty positioning the person in a comfortable position (Figure 44-6).

Anticipate decompensation even with vague symptoms. Obtain serial vital signs and watch for trends. Evaluate pulse pressure and mean arterial pressure. Obtaining vital signs in two positions (tilt test) may be helpful. Do not assume "normal" vital signs are stable. Evaluate medication use and the patient's usual range for vital signs, then relate those to the current vital signs. An example is use of a beta-blocker that decreases the pulse rate even under conditions of duress. Assessing hypothermia, which is common in this population, requires a thermometer capable of low readings. Respiratory rates over 25 breaths per minute have been found to be a reliable indicator of lower respiratory tract infections.[6]

Evaluating mental status is essential. Clues to the severity of a change may be found in the evaluation of confusion or any sudden changes in mental status. These may be the indicators of a disease process occurring since many of the traditional signs and symptoms will not be seen.

The head-to-toe survey is performed, as always, with attention to the total picture. Be careful not to be misled by vague symptoms. Subdural hematoma may occur without trauma secondary to cerebral atrophy, fragility of vessels, and coagulopathies. The chest wall is more fragile, leading to an increase in hidden injuries. Crackles heard in the lungs are abnormal at any age. Occasional premature atrial or ventricular contractions may be common without symptoms or progression to a problem. S_3 heart sounds are indicative of congestive heart failure. Changes may be subtle; have a high index of suspicion.

Medication Issues and Toxicology

The use of medications increases with age (Figure 44-7). It is estimated that older persons have four prescribed drugs and three over-the-counter medications that they take every day.[3,6,7] When eliciting a history, it is important to find out if they actually take their prescribed medications, and if so if they take them as ordered. Are there other supplements taken on a daily basis? Are there over-the-counter medications routinely used?

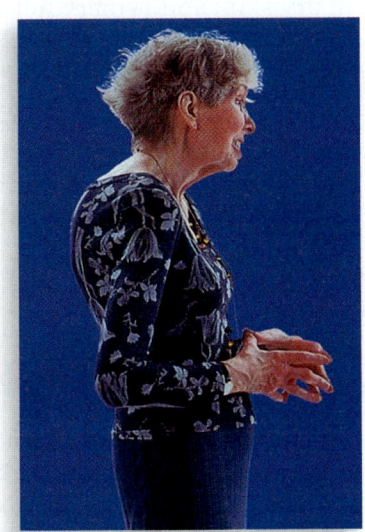

Figure 44-6   Kyphosis compromises ventilation and spinal immobilization.

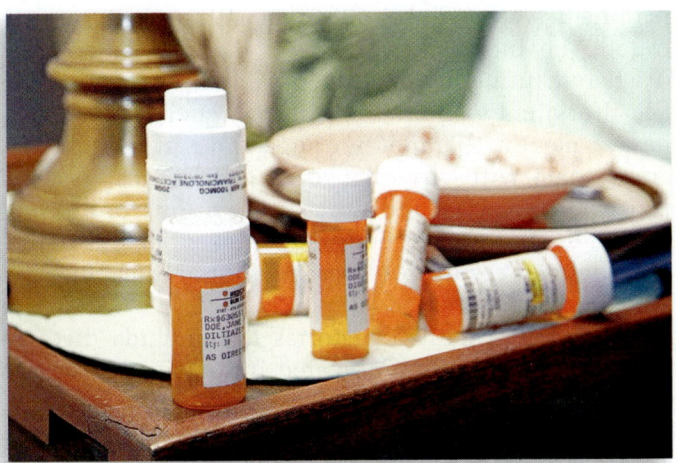

Figure 44-7   The average elderly person takes four prescribed and three over-the-counter (OTC) medications every day.

Medication regimes can be very complex, leading to difficulty understanding, remembering, and complying with the instructions. Starting or stopping a medication can affect the other medication levels. Based on principles of distribution, absorption, metabolism, and excretion, one medication can directly impact the level of another medication.

Look at the prescribing physician's name on the pill bottle. Is it the same prescriber on each? Are there multiple physicians ordering medications? Are they filled at different pharmacies? As it is common to have a specialist caring for a particular problem and many elderly have multiple problems, it is easy to understand how many different physicians can prescribe medications. This fragmentation becomes detrimental if there is no one evaluating the total picture for drug compatibilities and interactions. Many pharmacists will do this routinely, but this safeguard only works if all medications are obtained from one pharmacy.

This point is important as the effects of many drugs on the elderly population are not known. Research studies are usually conducted on patients younger than 65 years and, consequently, do not provide definitive information for the geriatric age group. Based on the limited research that has been done, the common practice is to begin a medication at the lowest dose possible and evaluate for effectiveness and side effects.[8]

It is known that adverse reactions to drugs occur more often in the elderly than in the younger patient. This may be a result of physiologic changes, disease to drug interactions, or drug to drug interactions. The likelihood of an adverse reaction is five times more likely to occur if the patient is on five or more medications.[7] Drug clearance is often reduced due to the decrease in renal plasma flow, glomerular filtration rate, and reduced hepatic clearance. Distribution of a medication is changed with the decrease in total body water, leading to water-soluble drugs becoming more concentrated; the increase in body fat leads to fat-soluble drugs remaining in the body longer with a longer half-life. Certain types of medications, such as digoxin, have a narrow therapeutic range and can quickly become toxic with any change in compliance, disease processes, lifestyle, additional medications, or discontinuation of a medication. Accidental exposures in the elderly often result from dosage errors rather than intentional exposures.

Be wary of patient histories that include digoxin since it is frequently implicated in toxicity. Anorexia, confusion, depression, and dysrhythmias can result from digoxin use. Administration of diphenhydramine, diazepam, sedatives, benzodiazepines, and barbiturates can also result in confusion.

Over-the-counter drugs for insomnia and nonsteroidal antiinflammatory drugs can interfere with control of high blood pressure and cause renal dysfunction and gastrointestinal bleeding. Gingko biloba may interfere with anticoagulants.

Many drugs have a paradoxical effect or produce complications such as the following:

- CNS depressants can result in agitation, delirium, or confusion.
- Lidocaine, an antidysrhythmic, can cause blurred vision, hypotension, ventricular tachydysrhythmias, CNS depression, and seizures. The dose in elderly patients should be reduced, especially in patients with hepatic and renal disease.
- Beta-blockers, used in hypertension, angina pectoris, and cardiac dysrhythmias, can result in a change in level of consciousness, AV blocks, hypoglycemia, seizures, hypotension, and tachycardia. Since the use of these drugs limits the body's ability to respond to shock by increasing the heart rate, when additional cardiac output is needed in times of exercise, hypovolemia, and stress, it cannot respond. Changing positions from lying or sitting to standing can result in postural hypotension.
- Calcium channel blockers can result in changes in level of consciousness, AV block, organ ischemia, hyperglycemia, and hypotension.
- ACE Inhibitors can cause an increased risk for angioedema, hyperkalemia, renal insufficiency, and hypotension.
- Antihypertensive and diuretic drugs can cause volume depletion, leading to postural hypotension, circulatory collapse, and potassium loss.
- Antipsychotics can have two different presentations of adverse effects. Some antipsychotic drugs cause a change in level of consciousness, miosis, and extrapyramidal reactions (dystonia, inability to sit still, parkinsonism). Others can cause physiologic stimulation, dry skin, and urinary retention.
- Antidepressants can result in a change in level of consciousness, drowsiness, and postural hypotension.
- Narcotic analgesics can cause sedation, mood changes, orthostatic hypotension, and respiratory depression. These effects result from the inability of the liver or kidney to process the drug as well as the changes in total water to body fat composition.

DOT 6-3.15, 16, 17, 18, 19

Street Secrets

Patient medications are not always kept where you would expect. Besides the medicine cabinet, check kitchen cabinets and refrigerators, and look for shoe boxes or other types of boxes on bedroom dressers and end tables. Be sure to bring all medications you find to the hospital.

Performing a Systems Review in the Elderly

Geriatric presentations reflect the combined physiologic changes of aging and chronic condition symptomatology complicated by the acute condition. It is often difficult to sort out this complex picture. Building on the pathophysiology and interventions presented in earlier chapters, this section will highlight specific presentations that commonly occur in the elderly population. Refer to the basics of these disease processes that have been presented in earlier chapters. This section will highlight specific differences in the geriatric population for your consideration.

Pulmonary Presentations

Normal lung aging is a benign process and has little impact on exercise tolerance in the elderly up to age 85. The factors that promote illness include environmental stressors such as smoking, concurrent illness, childhood infection, and lack of exercise. Elderly women are showing an increase in lung cancer and COPD.[6] In this population, respiratory problems often have an atypical presentation. Due to the blunting of certain responses such as fever, cough, and central nervous system responsiveness, the patient may present with confusion as the predominant sign.

Pneumonia

Pneumonia is the sixth leading cause of death, with the elderly accounting for the highest morbidity and mortality.[12,13] The typical signs and symptoms of fever, cough (productive in bacterial pneumonia), pleuritic chest pain, chills, and malaise occur in the younger person. The elderly may present after a fall or with confusion as the initial presentation, making diagnosis more complex (Figure 44-8).[10] Tachypnea, tachycardia, dullness to percussion, egophony, and crackles are often found on assessment. The fever response may be absent. The elderly with underlying medical conditions such as COPD, dementia, stroke, Parkinson's, heart failure, cancer, or diabetes are at greater risk. Those hospitalized or in long-term care facilities have a higher risk of developing pneumonia. Pneumonia is the most common reason to transfer a geriatric patient from the nursing home to the hospital.

Many different organisms cause pneumonia, with different types being found in the community versus those found in hospitalized or nursing home patients. Vaccines, both influenza and pneumococcal, are preventive measures against some of these organisms.

The extent of illness seen in pneumonia leads to an ineffectual cough, a decrease in vital capacity, and an increase in ventilation/perfusion mismatch. Consequences of pneumonia include hypoxia, hemodynamic

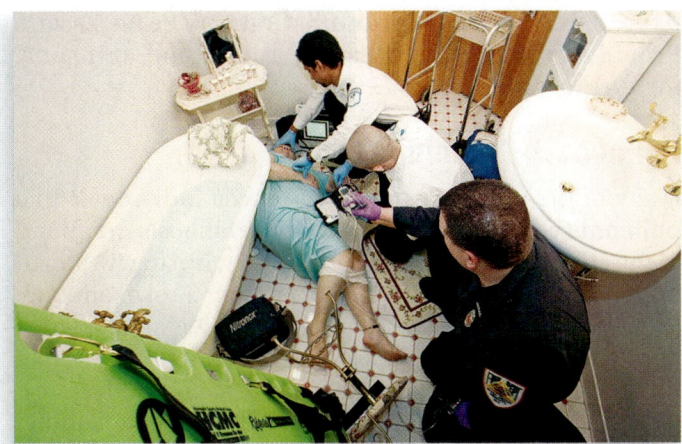

Figure 44-8 Pay attention to the circumstances of a fall to help determine the cause.

instability, and respiratory failure. Prevention by receiving the pneumococcal vaccine is essential.[6,8,9] Recovery from pneumonia, even for a healthy person, can be a very long process.

Airway management, cardiac monitoring, and IV fluid administration with possible use of bronchodilators are indicated based upon assessment and protocols. Administer IV fluid to assist in maintaining an adequate blood pressure. Once physician evaluation, chest x-ray, and sputum and blood cultures are obtained at the hospital, antibiotics are initiated. Good handwashing and attention to preventing the spread of infection are important for the prehospital provider.

Chronic Obstructive Pulmonary Disease (COPD)

Chronic obstructive pulmonary disease (chronic airflow obstruction), is the fourth leading cause of death in the United States, with cigarette smoking being a major risk factor.[3,10,11] Chronic bronchitis and emphysema increase after age 60 and are found equally in men and women. Long-term home oxygen has been useful in extending the quality and length of life. Daily medications such as bronchodilators, anticholineric agents, and beta agonists are commonly used. Of concern is the 40% of elderly who do not use metered dose medications correctly. Due to arthritis, coordination problems, or cerebral vascular disease, the actual delivered dose of medication may be less than optimal.[8] Provide education and coaching on the proper administration techniques at every opportunity.

Acute episodes often follow an infection or are the result of an exacerbation. Increased dyspnea and wheezing, tachypnea, tachycardia, and often a productive cough are seen. Hypoxemia and acidosis occur, often in association with decreased level of consciousness. Intervention includes airway support and correction of hypoxia. Provide supplemental oxygen. BiPAP, CPAP, or intubation may be necessary. Provide bronchodilator medications and transport for further intervention.

Pulmonary Embolus (PE)

Many of the conditions that predispose individuals to a **pulmonary embolus** or **deep vein thrombosis** are found in the elderly population. Major surgery, hip fracture, cancer, heart failure, myocardial infarction, stroke, and any cause of immobility are examples. Known as the "great masquerader," the diagnosis of PE is difficult. Older patients may complain of vague chest discomfort, dyspnea, tachypnea, and tachycardia. Pleuritic chest pain and hemoptysis may indicate a small embolus; dyspnea, syncope, hypotension, or cyanosis indicate a massive PE.

Since the signs and symptoms are similar to so many other disease processes, interventions are based on airway, breathing, and circulatory support. The earlier the diagnosis is made, the better the outcome. In-hospital care includes the possibility of thrombolytics, use of anticoagulants, and treatment of right heart failure. DOT 6-3.20, 21, 22, 23, 24, 25

Cardiovascular Presentations

Age-related changes reduce the cardiovascular reserve. Combined with other organ system changes, comorbid conditions, and multiple medications, there is an increased risk of complications.[7] Cardiovascular disease often presents with nonclassical symptoms in the older person and is the major cause of death and disability in the over 65 age group.

Myocardial Infarction (MI)

The classic symptom of chest pain from MI occurs less frequently in the elderly, being reported by less than one-third of patients over 85 years old.[6] The initial presentation may include dyspnea, exacerbation of heart failure, syncope, nausea and vomiting, confusion, or stroke. Symptoms are more likely to occur at rest or during sleep. Although unrecognized MI is more likely to occur in women, delay in diagnosis may exclude both men and women from the potential benefit of angioplasty or thrombolytic therapy. In addition to the normal risk factors you have learned, assess for concurrent medical or surgical problems that are associated with hypovolemia, blood loss, infection, or hypotension since these may be precipitating factors. Many elderly patients will present with non-Q wave infarctions. Due to preexisting bundle branch block, prior MI, left ventricular hypertrophy, or medication effects to name a few, the ST elevation and reciprocal T wave inversion patterns may not be present.[5]

With the atypical presentation and nondiagnostic ECG pattern, delayed or missed diagnosis can prevent optimal care. The possibility of MI should be high on the list of potential causes, and interventions should follow the priorities of airway, breathing, and circulation, with attention to careful monitoring and treatment for any dysrhythmias that develop. Transport for evaluation. DOT 6-3.26, 28

Heart Failure

Heart failure results from the inability of the left ventricle to fill or eject blood adequately. This is primarily a condition of the elderly. With the dramatic increase in the age group over 65 years, this condition will continue to be the most common cause of hospitalization in the Medicare age population.[12]

Early diagnosis is sometimes extremely difficult. It is not uncommon to have symptoms such as easy fatiguability, cough, dyspnea, and ankle swelling attributed to the normal process of aging. Failure to recognize these symptoms result in delayed evaluation and intervention. Coronary heart disease, hypertension, valvular disease, and dilated cardiomyopathy are the most common causes. Precipitating causes include conditions that lead to high output states such as thyrotoxicosis, anemia, or pregnancy.

Signs and symptoms include dyspnea and fatigue that can limit activity and cause exercise intolerance. Fluid retention leads to pulmonary congestion and peripheral edema. Insomnia, orthopnea, confusion, lethargy, anorexia, ascites, or nocturia may be noted. Patients with a history of heart failure often record daily weights to assist in evaluating fluid retention.

Treatment is aimed at identifying the underlying cause and precipitating causes in order to improve cardiac output. Immediate measures include airway, breathing, and circulation attention with pharmacologic support, as required. Depending on the level of distress, aggressive ventilatory support may be needed. Medications such as furosemide, nitroglycerin, morphine, ACE inhibitors, and antidysrhythmics may be necessary.

Dysrhythmias

The aging process leads to degeneration of the sinoatrial node, with approximately 10% of the pacemaker cells remaining at age 75.[7] Combined with atrial and ventricular myocardial changes, the results are increased ectopy and dysrhythmias. Bradydysrhythmias, such as sinus bradycardia, sinus pauses, and sinus arrest, and tachydysrhythmias, such as atrial fibrillation, atrial flutter, and atrial tachycardia, can occur. Sick sinus syndrome may present as either extreme or combined as a tachy-brady syndrome. Fifty percent of the pacemakers implanted in patients are required for sinus node disorders. Hypertension, hypothyroidism, hypothermia, and severe hypoxia are associated with SA node dysfunctions.

Dysrhythmias can occur without any symptoms, or they may be accompanied by palpitations, lightheadedness, or syncope. When syncope is from a cardiovascular cause, one year mortality rates have been found to be significant (24%).[6] Evaluate for concurrent injury from falls due to possible syncope. It is common to find PVCs and PACs in the elderly population. Atrial fibrillation is common and is a significant risk factor for stroke. Treatment follows the process identified in the cardiac chapter, with attention to assessment and perfusion of the brain. Pharmacologic dosages need to be tailored to decrease the likelihood of adverse reactions.

CONNECTIONS Treatment algorithms for Cardiac dysrhythmias are found in Chapter 29, Section II: Cardiovascular Diseases. DOT 6-3.27

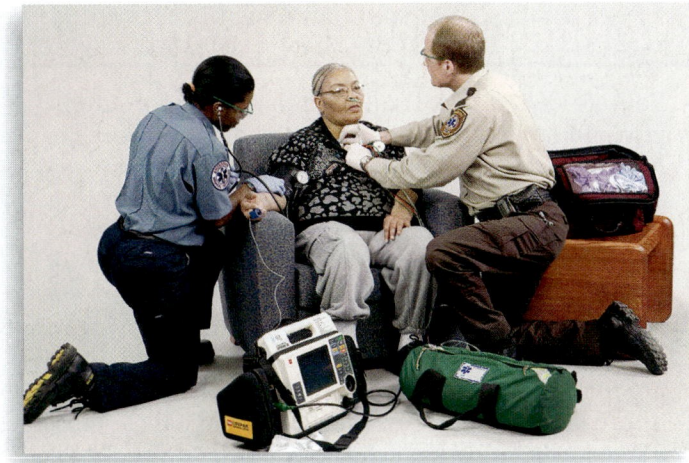

Figure 44-9 Hypertension is a major risk factor for cardiovascular and cerebrovascular disease.

Aortic Aneurysms

Aneurysm, a pathologic dilation or outpouching of the aorta, is commonly associated with atherosclerosis. Thoracic aneurysms in the ascending aorta and descending thoracic area, occur less frequently than do abdominal aneurysms. Symptoms of expanding lesions include chest pain, dyspnea, cough, dysphagia, heart failure, and venous congestion of the head, neck, and upper extremities.

Abdominal aneurysms occur more frequently in males and are found in 1–2% of men over age 50.[8] The majority of aneurysms related to atherosclerosis are located below the origin of the renal arteries. Often found on routine examinations, the aneurysm is measured and watched until it begins to expand. Expansion causes symptoms such as pain in the lower back, chest, or scrotum. A pulsatile mass may be felt in the abdomen. Any symptoms require immediate evaluation and surgical intervention. Rupture can occur with or without preceding symptoms and is a true emergency. Surgical intervention and graft placement for expanding, unruptured lesions results in mortality of 1–2%. If rupture has occurred, mortality is greater than 50%.[8] Prehospital intervention is grounded in the principles previously covered, airway, breathing, and circulatory support, based upon the patient presentation. Gentle but immediate transport is necessary to a facility capable of immediate operative intervention.

Hypertension

In the population 60 years and older, over 50% of noninstitutionalized people have hypertension (Figure 44-9). Hypertension, as discussed previously, is a major risk factor for cardiovascular and cerebrovascular disease. Obesity, lack of exercise, salt intake, and smoking combine to increase the risk of developing hypertension. New guidelines from the National Heart,

Lung, and Blood committee find that the risk of dying from ischemic heart disease increases progressively and linearly when blood pressure exceeds 115/75 mmHg.[13] Normal BP is now classified as under 120/80 mmHg, prehypertensive between 120/80 and 139/89, stage I hypertension between 140/90 and 159/99, and stage II above 160/100.

Aggressive treatment is called for in the prehypertensive category and higher. Initial lifestyle changes such as weight loss, reduced sodium intake, regular aerobic exercise, reduced alcohol intake, and careful monitoring need to be implemented. Since aging results in stiffness and damage to the arteries, these prevention measures are essential. It was found that having a normal blood pressure at age 50 still resulted in a 80–90% risk of having hypertension by age 80.[13] Lifestyle modifications are supplemented with medication administration such as thiazide-type diuretics and other antihypertensive therapy to gain control and reduce the blood pressure to less than 140/90. With diseases such as diabetes or renal disease, the desired blood pressure is less than 130/80.

Diabetes, renal disease, stroke, blindness, and aneurysms are examples of the multiple diseases that have increased complications from hypertension. The impact of this one disease affects every organ system.

Intervention includes treating the presenting symptoms such as headache, stroke, or epistaxis. Many vague symptoms occur and are often not attributed to hypertension. Nausea, vomiting, dysrhythmias, dizziness, and palpitations have many causes. Many people with hypertension have no symptoms. Of concern is the hypertensive patient who has had significant volume loss but on assessment has a blood pressure in the normal range. This patient is actually in shock based on the dramatic decrease from his normal hypertensive state. Airway, breathing, and circulatory support are essential. If your system permits antihypertensive medication

Working in the Gray Zone

You are called to a local church to care for an 86-year-old female who "passed out" during a service. As you enter the church with your partner, you see a group of people fanning the elderly woman in a chair near the rear of the church. Your initial impression is a syncopal episode, probably brought on by the press of people in the crowded church and the heat of the day. Her dizziness persists, however, even after you get her onto your stretcher and move her to the air-conditioned ambulance. She seems to improve a bit with the oxygen but seems a little short of breath and clearly does not feel well. Once placed on the monitor, you see that she has elevations in her ST segments.

The point to be reinforced here is the one made earlier in the text that less than one-third of patients over the age of 85 have classic AMI symptoms. It is important to have a high index of suspicion with a geriatric patient who has changes in LOC, shortness of breath, hypotension, or any other sign of decreased cardiac output.

initiation, titration infusion devices should be used to control the rate of delivery. Hypotension is not a desired effect!

CONNECTIONS Chapter 5: Clinical Decision Making contains discussion of situations when it may be difficult to determine if a patient is actually sick because they present with vital signs that are typically considered "normal" for patients of that age group. If you are still having problems understanding this concept please review Chapter 5 again.

Neurological Presentations

Major neurological disorders have been discussed previously in Chapter 30: This section will highlight conditions predominantly found in the elderly population.

Cerebrovascular Accident

Stroke is the leading cause of disability in the United States and the third leading cause of death. Of the 4 million people disabled by stroke, 70% are vocationally impaired.[6] With the incidence of stroke increasing with age, the best strategy remains prevention. Stroke screenings, including control of atrial fibrillation and evaluation of carotid stenosis, modification of hypertension and hyperlipidemia, anticoagulation, and stop smoking programs, all contribute to a decreased risk of stroke.

With the window of treatment time very narrow, it is essential that rapid recognition of a stroke and transport to a stroke center occur immediately. Evaluation and treatment at a specialized stroke center has been shown to reduce death or disability.[6]

Delirium

Cognitive impairment can result from delirium, dementia, or depression. Changes in level of attention and cognitive functioning are found in delirium. It is an acute presentation often seen in hospitalized patients or as the presenting symptom of a underlying medical disease. Sudden occurrence of inattention, disorganized speech, or altered level of consciousness is the leading presentation of an acute illness in at least 30% of older people.[6] Predisposing factors include dementia, severe illness, visual impairment, metabolic disorders, and dehydration. Any underlying medical condition can be a contributing factor to the development of delirium. The use of medications, especially multiple medications such as sedatives, hypnotics, narcotics, H_2 blockers, and drugs with an anticholinergic effect contribute to its development.

Delirium may be the presenting symptom in acute myocardial infarction, congestive heart failure, respiratory failure, and infection. Careful evaluation for signs of these conditions is required since chest pain and dyspnea may be absent. Unrecognized infections such as pneumonia, urinary tract sepsis, abdominal abscess, or septic arthritis may be the precipitating cause.

Delirium is a serious problem with increased morbidity, mortality, complications from the underlying conditions, and poor long-term prognosis. Although the pathophysiology is not clear in this disorder, it appears to be the end result of multiple insults to cerebral oxidative metabolism.[6] Considered a transient problem, it may last 30 or more days and have a prolonged recovery period before returning to the previous level of function.

Key signs and symptoms revolve around inattention, disorganized thinking, and an altered level of consciousness. These symptoms have the onset of hours to days and usually fluctuate over a 24-hour period, often with times of being coherent and oriented. There is a range of presentations from hyperactive, hyperalert states to hypoactive, hypoalert states. The elderly often present with the hypoactive, hypoalert, lethargic form that frequently is confused with dementia and not recognized.[7]

Inattention is the inability to focus, maintain, and shift attention. The inability to follow a normal conversation, becoming easily distracted, or needing repetition to understand directions to perform a task is common. Disorganized thinking results in rambling, incoherent, or inappropriate speech. Altered level of consciousness may vary from hyperacute and vigilant to hypoactive and lethargic. Agitation, hallucinations, paranoid delusions, emotional fluctuations, and sleep disturbances can occur.

Prehospital interventions include the following:

- Assess and manage the airway and breathing, especially if there is a decreased level of consciousness. Support ventilations to decrease hypoxia.
- Assess circulation and initiate IV fluid, as needed, to counter dehydration.
- Reduce anxiety and agitation by maintaining a calm presence. Decrease the number of people interacting with the person. Encourage a supportive family member to accompany or meet the person at the hospital.
- Maintain patient and personal safety, if severely agitated behavior exists and is a safety hazard to the person or staff, restrain the patient as needed following protocol. Assure a patent airway and adequate breathing throughout the restraint period.
- Sedate if directed or by protocol only if absolutely necessary. Remember, the patient's confusion will become worse.
- Altered level of consciousness requires exclusion of other causes. Assess for hypoglycemia and narcotic use; follow protocols for treatment.
- Continue to perform a complete assessment. Prescription and over-the-counter medications should accompany the patient to the hospital. Perform ongoing neurologic assessments and monitor vital signs en route to physician evaluation.

Dementia

Cognitive function deficits form a continuum from the normal processes of aging to the disease state of dementia in varying degrees. Mild cognitive impairment is demonstrated by memory problems and difficulty remembering where something is located but not to the extent of functional loss. For example, the patients may forget where they left the car keys, but they are still able to drive the car. There appears to be a link to the development of Alzheimer's disease over time. **Dementia** is a severe form of cognitive impairment, resulting in a progressive impairment spanning memory deficits and the inability to carry out motor functions, aphasia, inability to identify objects, and compromised higher level thought processes. These deficits lead to loss of daily functional ability. Since this is a gradual process, the decline may not be noticeable until strange behavior or safety issues arise. If the person lives at home, safety needs to be evaluated. Has the stove been left on? Does the person wander or get lost? Does the person forget where the car is parked? When family notices the extent of disability,

it is often not until functional and social skills have been lost or severely compromised. There is a direct benefit to intervention before the disease progresses to this stage. Late diagnosis results in further incapacitation, more burden on the family, and higher healthcare costs. Twenty-five percent to 40% of elders over age 85 living in the community have dementia, with 60–70% due to Alzheimer's disease.[14]

Alzheimer's disease is the most common form of dementia. Characterized by the loss of memory and inability to learn, this slow, progressive disease robs an individual of the ability to reason, make judgments, communicate, or carry out activities of normal day-to-day living (ADLs). Personality changes are common, including suspicion, hallucinations, agitation, and paranoia. As the disease progresses, help is needed with basic ADL functions such as eating, dressing, and personal hygiene, with constant supervision for safety. There is neural degeneration that, when seen on autopsy, confirms the diagnosis of Alzheimer's. The cause of this progressive loss of nerve cells in the brain and atrophy has not been identified. Research continues to explore risk factors. Increasing age and family history have the highest link to occurrence. Strategies to control high blood pressure, weight and cholesterol levels, and exercise and activities to promote mental alertness may reduce the risk of developing Alzheimer's disease. Research is ongoing into possible causes such as beta-amyloid proteins, reduction of acetylcholine, genetic disorders, and environmental influences.[14]

Symptoms begin with memory loss and progress to disorientation in time, to place, and lastly to person. The individual often does not realize these deficits are occurring, indicating the loss of the cognitive functions required to process information and reasoning ability. Language difficulties begin, subtle at first, progressing to total inability to talk. Visuospatial tasks are increasingly difficult, resulting in getting lost and wandering. Independent living becomes unsafe, and the move to a safe living environment with Alzheimer's resources is necessary. Progressive behavioral patterns are common, including apathy, irritability, or depression. In the moderate and advanced stage of disease, agitation and psychotic symptoms such as hallucinations, delusions, and paranoia are common. Verbally abusive and violent behaviors may be experienced. Interventions involve caregiver education and support, pharmacological support often with cholinesterase inhibitors to slow the progression of the disease, and medications to manage symptom presentations such as antipsychotics and antidepressants. In moderate and advanced stages, inpatient facilities may be required. Progressive loss of awareness and isolation occurs. Total care is required. Death is from the progressive loss of ability to eat and swallow or from aspiration or infection.

Emergency interventions follow the general guidelines as in dementia. Supportive care with attention to patient and rescuer safety is needed.

Parkinson's Disease

Parkinson's disease is a common brain disorder in which nerve cells are impaired or die, rendering the patient unable to produce dopamine, an essential chemical messenger that transmits signals through the brain structures. The signals promote coordinated movement, so interference with these signals allows unregulated action such as tremors at rest. Symptoms are evident with the death of 70% of the dopaminergic neurons.

This is a common disease in the age group above 60, where one in 100 people have Parkinson's disease. The age group younger than 40 accounts for 5–10% of patients with this disease. Reviewing the identified causes show a genetic cause for some, environmental toxicity for some, and infection for some, but current theories suggest a combination of genetic and environmental factors. No one factor has consistently demonstrated a link.

Symptoms are tremors, often beginning in one limb, slowness of movement, stiffness or rigidity, and difficulty maintaining one's balance. Progressive involvement includes loss of facial expression, slowing of speech, stooped posture, and balance instability, leading to maximum loss and bed or wheelchair dependence. Interventions reflect the standard treatment protocols, including anticipation of respiratory difficulty due to the effect of postural changes and frequency of respiratory infection. Dysphagia is common; be mindful of choking and aspiration. Postural hypotension results from autonomic dysfunction. With postural instability, fall prevention is important.

Endocrine Presentations

The physiologic changes of aging combined with the insult of obesity, alcohol use, diet, environmental factors, and often a genetic factor can result in deficiency or excess of various hormones.

Diabetes Mellitus

With beta cell function declining with age compounded by obesity, changing levels of activity, and loss of muscle mass, **diabetes** is found in 20% of the over 65 population. Of concern is the fact that half of this number are undiagnosed.[6] Another 20–25% have carbohydrate disorders that fall into the impaired glucose tolerance category.

An increasing number of people over age 65 with diabetes will have hypertension. Deaths from diabetic ketoacidosis increase after age 75. Hyperosmolar nonketotic coma is predominantly found in the elderly, resulting from diuresis due to hyperglycemia, leading to dehydration. Legal blindness is found in a significant portion of those with diabetes. The incidence of stroke is twice as common in those with diabetes. The rate of infection for diabetics is greatly increased. Renal failure, retinopathies, and neuropathies are common. This combination of associated problems and diabetes has been shown to reduce lifespan by three to five years, depending on the age when diagnosed with diabetes and how long diabetes has been present.[6]

The elderly have risk factors that may complicate the course of diabetes. Living alone, obesity leading to not being able to take care of their feet, vision changes that make identification of medication or drawing up a dose of insulin difficult, concurrent infection, and underlying diseases all increase the risk of complications. Anticipate multiple healthcare issues needing intervention.

Assessment and intervention revolve around life threats and multisystem problems. Maintain airway, breathing, and circulatory support. Assess for ketones. Blood glucose levels determine the need for IV dextrose.

Thyroid Disease

Aging leads to atrophy and fibrosis of the thyroid gland, resulting in disorders of hypo- and hyperthyroid states. **Hypothyroidism** is common, with more presentations in the subclinical range. The symptoms found in the younger person, such as fatigue, weight gain, and cold intolerance, are often thought to be part of the normal aging process. Onset is over months or years, with the elderly often presenting with only fatigue or weakness, cold intolerance or weight gain, or there may be no symptoms. Presenting signs may include hypertension, bradycardia, or tachydysrhythmias. Depression, dementia, poor memory, constipation, and facial edema may be found. Because of the frequency of this disease in the elderly, hypothyroidism should be suspected in every patient contact.

Hyperthyroidism is less common, again with many cases being in the subclinical range. Atrial fibrillation, osteoporosis, loss of muscle, weight loss, poor appetite, confusion, and congestive heart failure may be the presenting signs. Any patient on thyroid hormone replacement therapy for an underactive thyroid should be evaluated for hyperthyoidism. This may result from the aging effect on the ability to metabolize the hormone, leading to accumulation of toxic levels.

Intervention is focused on treatment of specific presentations such as angina, dysrhythmias, heart failure, infection, or hypoglycemia and supportive care. Physician evaluation after stabilization of the presenting symptoms includes treatment options such as hormone replacement medication, radioactive iodine therapy, thyroid gland ablation, or infrequently, surgery.

CONNECTIONS Endocrine disorders are discussed in detail in Chapter 31: Endocrine, Electrolytes, and Acid/Base.

Gastrointestinal Presentations

There is an increase in certain abdominal disorders found in the elderly. Gastric ulcers increase with age. The results of atherosclerotic vascular disease contribute to ischemic bowel disease. Gastrointestinal bleeding is more common as are certain malignancies such as colon cancer. Reflux esophagitis and difficulty swallowing are common. Even swallowing pills, especially if lying in bed, can present a problem.

Common complaints include constipation and incontinence. There is 40% more constipation reported in the elderly than in middle age. Incontinence of urine or feces can occur although incontinence is not a normal consequence of aging. When these conditions occur, evaluation and intervention are needed for symptomatic relief as well as diagnosis of cause. Possible causes include infection, tumor, enlargement of the prostate, diabetes, and other neurologic diseases.

Gastrointestinal Hemorrhage

The most common causes of hemorrhage are peptic ulcer disease, gastritis, esophagitis, and diverticulitis. Peptic ulcer disease results from nonsteroidal anti-inflammatory drug (NSAID) use and *Helicobacter pylori*. *H. pylori* is found in increasing numbers; over 50% of adults over age 60 carry this organism. The use of NSAIDs contributes to the decreased health of the gastric mucosa. With concurrent health problems, the elderly are frequent users of NSAIDs for pain relief. Complications range from severe hemorrhage to perforation or obstruction of the stomach or bowel. The sensation of abdominal pain may not occur in up to 50% of the elderly.[5]

Signs and symptoms include **hematemesis** (vomiting bright red blood), coffee ground emesis, or **melena** (black stools). With significant blood loss, syncope, confusion, or shock may present. Orthostatic vital signs may provide a clue to hypovolemia, with the pulse being more sensitive than blood pressure changes.[5] Assessment will include determining medication use such as NSAIDs, aspirin, or anticoagulants.

Interventions are based upon patient presentation and degree of acuity. Life threats need rapid airway, breathing, and circulatory support with transport to the hospital.

Bowel Obstruction

Causes for bowel obstruction range from a hernia with trapping of the intestine through the abdominal muscle or inguinal ring, tumor growth blocking the lumen, torsion, and adhesions from previous surgeries, to paralytic ileus from peritonitis, pneumonia, or ischemic bowel disease. Symptoms begin with colicky pains that intensify with peristalsis, followed by pain free intervals. There may be associated sweating, nausea, and hypotension. The pain may change in character; strangulation leads to constant severe pain as ischemic bowel begins to die. Depending on the location of the obstruction, vomiting and distention occur. In small bowel obstruction, vomiting of either clear gastric juice or bile-stained fluid with mild abdominal distention is seen. Large bowel obstruction has greater distention with less vomiting, but the emesis contains fecal material. If the obstruction is partial, diarrhea or constipation may occur. If complete constipation develops, the patient is unable to pass any feces or gas.

Intervention involves assessing for dehydration, electrolyte imbalances, metabolic alkalosis or acidosis, infection, hypovolemia, and shock. Treatment is based upon maintaining the airway, breathing, and circulatory status. In-hospital interventions include a nasogastric tube, volume replacement, and surgery, if required.

Musculoskeletal Presentations

With the decrease in muscle mass and changes in bone density, it is easy to understand why almost everyone will develop symptoms of musculoskeletal disease. Osteoarthritis, osteoporosis, and resulting fractures are projected to increase in the coming years.[6,7] The effect of chronic pain can result in loss of normal activities and sleep and can lead to depression and isolation. Reducing the loss of mobility through fall prevention is important. While you are in a home, assess for fall hazards and medication interactions and effects that lead to sub-optimal functioning.

Osteoporosis

Low bone mass and density, combined with microarchitectual deterioration, result in the increase of bone fragility and the occurrence of fractures. There are typically no signs or symptoms until a fracture occurs, often in the vertebrae, hip, wrist, proximal humerus, pelvis, or femoral area. Occurring more frequently in women with accelerated bone loss during the postmenopausal period, an estimated one out of two women will have a fracture due to **osteoporosis**.[6] Men reportedly have a 25% likelihood of having a fracture due to osteoporosis, and this number is increasing.

Symptoms of vertebral fractures can range from back pain, postural changes such as kyphosis, and loss of height to no symptoms at all. Hip fractures, especially at age 75 or older, result in significant mortality. Returning to previous levels of functioning is often impossible.

The best intervention is prevention. Dietary supplements of calcium and vitamin D, pharmacologic agents to decrease bone resorption, and possibly hormone replacement therapy are prescribed. Fall prevention is essential. Prevention of postural hypotension through control of coexisting diseases reduces the likelihood of dizziness and syncope leading to fracture. Encourage exercise, especially weight-bearing activities. Prehospital intervention focuses on treatment of the presenting problem such as hip fracture and stabilization with transport. Of concern is the elderly person living alone who falls and cannot reach the phone to call for help. Pain and dehydration may precipitate multisystem involvement, requiring complex medical care. Kyphosis will complicate spinal immobilization, requiring additional attention to immobilization of the cervical spine and appropriate padding.

Osteoarthritis

The cumulative effect of wear and tear of the cartilage leads to erosion of the articular surfaces, resulting in painful joint motion. This process develops over the years, resulting in almost everyone by age 70 having at least one painful, stiff joint. With progressive disease, the affected joint may become increasingly stiff and deformed, resulting in loss of function. Normal day-to-day activities become difficult. Interventions include acetaminophen, nonsteroidal antiinflammatory agents, weight loss to reduce the burden on a joint, and low-impact exercise. Surgical options include arthroscopy to remove cartilage, joint fusion, and total joint replacement procedures.

Integumentary Presentations

As the skin becomes thinner, loses part of its immune response ability, and has a reduced blood supply, infection becomes more prevalent. Venous stasis ulcers (as in the diabetic patient), pressure sores or decubiti, skin cancers, and infections occur. Immobility, poor nutrition, long-term steroid use, sun exposure, and infection increase the likelihood of skin disorders. Trauma to the skin is more likely with the loss of elasticity and thinness. The loss of thermal regulation increases the risk of hypothermia or hyperthermia. Care must be taken in simple procedures such as moving the patient from bed to stretcher, dressing a wound, and any action that results in pulling of the skin and causing friction or shearing.

Pressure Ulcers

Pressure or **ischemic ulcers** develop in areas with a lack of blood flow usually due to pressure preventing adequate circulation. These are often over bony prominences such

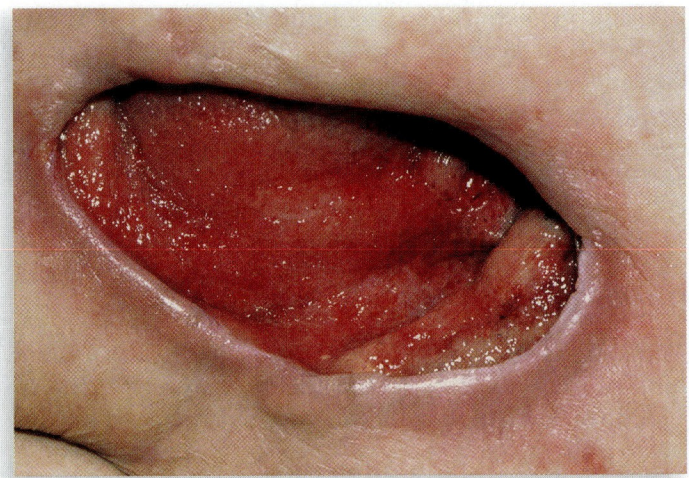

Figure 44-10   The damage of pressure ulcers begins at the epidermal layer, followed by dermal damage, and then damage of the subcutaneous tissues.

as the sacrum, heels, or greater trochanter (Figure 44-10). Risk factors for development of ulcers are the elderly in hospitals or nursing homes, immobilization, incontinence, or neurologic diseases such as spinal cord trauma, stroke, or dementia. The term decubitis ulcer refers to pressure ulcers that develop during periods of long-term bedrest.

Chronic venous insufficiency, especially with injury, will begin the inflammatory process and will lead to an ulcer. Beginning as a reddened area, if blood flow is not reestablished, progressive tissue breakdown happens. Epidermal damage followed by dermal damage will continue and involve the subcutaneous and deeper tissues without adequate intervention. Pressure ulcers, venous stasis ulcers, and diabetic ulcers have different etiology but can result in cellulitis, osteomyelitis, or gangrene. Interventions include relieving the pressure at the site, dressing the wound, and preventing or treating infection. Surgical options are more effective in the younger patient than the elderly patient.[6]

Environmental Presentations

Temperature regulation is compromised in the elderly. With slowed blood circulation, skin changes, and functional deficit in thermal regulatory mechanisms, the elderly have lost many of the protective responses that enable the body to adjust body temperature.

Hypothermia

The elderly have less ability for thermal perception, and they have underlying disease processes that may lead to immobility and difficulty regulating heat generation or conservation. These deficits include the inability to shiver, reduced body fat, and inability to increase heart rate. The number of elderly becoming hypothermic increases with psychiatric illness, dementia, underlying medical conditions, and socioeconomic factors. Conditions that increase the risk of hypothermia include hypothyroidism, hypoglycemia, stroke, Parkinson's disease, malnutrition, sepsis, shock, immobility, and medications such as alcohol, barbiturates, and phenothiazines.[10] Although outdoor exposure is a common cause in the younger population, it is less likely in the elderly unless there is significant alcohol use or conditions that lead to wandering. Socioeconomic factors include the cost of heating on a limited, fixed budget, living alone, lack of support network, and lack of adequate nutrition.

Presenting signs and symptoms include apathy, impaired judgment, ataxia, slurred speech, hallucinations, and progressive change in mental status. Severe hypothermia may present with coma or cardiac arrest. Interventions follow the guidelines in the environmental emergencies chapter with supportive measures until rewarming and evaluation occur at the hospital.

Hyperthermia

Although this condition occurs less often than hypothermia, it will occur in weather conditions such as a heat wave that lasts several days or more. With the loss of ability to regulate heat through sweating and loss of heat perception, the patient becomes hyperthermic. Medical conditions such as Parkinson's disease, stroke, or head injury increase the risk of hyperthermia. Medications such as anticholinergics, diuretics, monoamine oxidase inhibitors, tricyclic antidepressants, and amphetamines all contribute to hypothermia.

Presenting signs and symptoms span the categories of heat cramps, heat exhaustion, and heatstroke. Interventions have been previously discussed. Of note, hyperthermia does not respond to antipyretics.[8]

The category of malignant hyperthermia occurs because of a genetic defect that, combined with certain anesthetics (e.g., halothane) or succinylcholine, creates an elevated temperature, rhabdomyolysis, muscle rigidity, acidosis, and cardiovascular instability. This presentation is often fatal.

Behavioral Presentations

Depression

Once considered common in the older population, major depressive disorder has been found to be less likely with aging than in the younger population.[6] Those reporting depressive symptoms, however, account for 10–15% of the aging population. There is the theory that the present group of those over 65 are different from previous and future generations. Speculation is that this group has lived through hard times during the Depression and World War II. The quality of life since

that time is greatly improved. Adapting to change may be easier for them. Future generations that have had a higher standard of living and less chaos while young may find more difficulty adapting to old age and may have higher rates of depression.[6] The rates of depression increase for the elderly who are hospitalized or living in nursing homes.

Preexisting diseases such as Parkinson's, Alzheimer's, stroke, AMI, metabolic disorders, cancer, and multiple chronic diseases can contribute to depression. Medication use is associated with depression. Examples include antianxiety medications, antihypertensives, chemotherapy drugs, and others that have a central nervous system effect. Multiple causes including genetic, biological, and psychosocial factors and physical illness, especially those that lead to brain atrophy, disability, or chronic pain, have been linked to the development of depression.

To review, the signs and symptoms of depression include the following:

- Weight loss
- Insomnia
- Loss of interest
- Inability to concentrate
- Fatigue
- Irritability
- Hopelessness
- Feeling worthless
- Thoughts of suicide
- Isolation

Often overlooked and not diagnosed, your assessment may be complicated by these symptoms.

Interventions to identify depression and to obtain medical evaluation are essential. Medication use or abuse and attempts or thoughts of suicide are necessary to assess. A thoughtful, caring approach may allow the patient to voice fears or concerns. Assess carefully for concurrent underlying medical conditions. As always, relay information about living conditions to the emergency department staff to facilitate appropriate social service interventions. DOT 6-3.6

Suicide

The rate of suicide increases with age, the over 65 years old group has the highest age-specific rate of suicide. In the over 65 years old group, older men are more likely than women to commit suicide, many using a firearm. Risk factors include being male, increasing age, marital status (divorced, separated, or single), alcohol or substance abuse, severe stress, physical illness, and previous suicide attempts. If depression exists with other mental illness, the risk increases even more. It has been found that many elderly patients have seen their primary physician in the weeks before the suicide attempt and that this may be the first diagnosed episode of depression.[15]

Careful assessment includes asking directly about thoughts of hurting or killing themselves, and if so, do they have a plan to do so. Determine if there are weapons in the home or if drugs have been stockpiled to use. Safety for all must be considered, and law enforcement assistance may be required at the scene. Patients expressing a plan to commit suicide must be evaluated by the emergency department and psychiatric crisis workers for determination of appropriate intervention.

> The cardinal rule is to stay with the patient at all times; do not allow the opportunity for a suicide plan to be carried out.

Substance Abuse Presentations

The negative consequences of alcohol and substance abuse span the gamut from medical problems, family relationships, legal consequences, and economic loss to social and psychological issues. It is estimated that 17% of older adults report alcohol or substance abuse or misuse.[10] Alcoholism is the third most common psychiatric disorder in the older population.[7] Many cases of alcoholism are not diagnosed, even in hospitalized patients. Research is needed to study the rates of illicit drug use in the elderly. Little data is available, but it is thought that the amount of use is low.

Alcohol use presents added concern due to the change in pharmacokinetics with aging. There is a decrease in the volume of distribution of water-soluble substances, especially with the decrease in total body water and change in body fat. This leads to higher blood alcohol levels with less intake. Alcoholism results in changes to multiple systems. Central nervous system impact, unsteady gait, risk of falls, emotional fluctuations, and memory loss are compounded by the physiological changes of aging. Nutritional deficiencies occur with chronic alcohol use. Wernicke-Korsakoff syndrome should be suspected in anyone with alcoholism. Anemia may occur from insufficient folic acid. Overall nutritional status is often compromised.

The combination of alcohol, illicit drugs, prescription drugs, and over-the-counter drugs is dangerous. Of major concern is the interaction between these substances. Approximately one-half of the 100 most commonly prescribed drugs have adverse reactions when combined with alcohol.[10] Some medications report increased effects, such as antianxiety drugs, sedatives, antidepressants, and antipsychotic medications. Alcohol interferes with diabetic medications. The effect of anticoagulants and seizure drugs changes. Antibiotics taken at the same time demonstrate side effects. Acetaminophen and alcohol lead to a negative interaction.

Awareness of the multiple causes of dementia, confusion, emotional changes, osteoporosis, hip fractures, and occult head injury allow the paramedic to explore drug and alcohol use. Direct questioning is flawed; most people underreport use. Assess the home for clues as you care for the patient. If the patient is a smoker, ask about alcohol use; there is a high correlation between these two. Interventions follow the previously discussed patterns for life threats and supportive care.

Presentations Involving the Special Senses

The loss of the senses leads to major changes in lifestyle. If vision or hearing is impaired, the pleasure of social interaction, independence, ability to communicate, and happiness are affected. Safety issues result: vision impairment leads to difficulty with accurate medication administration, and hearing loss increases the risk of not hearing smoke detectors or an oncoming vehicle when crossing a street.

Vision Presentations

From age 40 on, there are progressive changes in the ability of the eye to accommodate and adjust to the dark, and there is a decrease in visual acuity, color vision, and the ability to recover from glare. Common conditions found are macular degeneration, cataracts, diabetic retinopathy, and glaucoma. **Cataracts** are found in 45% of the population over age 52.[6] Risk factors for the lens becoming opaque include exposure to sunlight, smoking, high cholesterol and triglycerides, diabetes, and eye injury. Cataract surgery is a common procedure performed in the outpatient setting.

Glaucoma presents with increased intraocular pressure, optic disk changes, and visual field loss. The increased pressure leads to damage to the optic nerve. Without early intervention, the vision loss is permanent. Depending on the type of glaucoma, there may or may not be pain, halos noted around lights, blurred vision, and redness of the eye. Diagnosis of glaucoma through periodic screenings prior to reaching the point of symptoms may preserve sight. Treatment is through medication and topical agents. Laser surgery may be a possibility in certain cases.

One in three people over age 75 have **macular degeneration,** leading to blurred vision and loss of central vision. Peripheral vision may be retained, allowing for careful ambulation. Retinopathy is a common cause of vision loss in diabetics due to the small vessel disease and occlusion. Achieving maximum blood glucose control on a long-term basis helps to improve vision outcomes in the diabetic. The ability to see an insulin syringe and measure the correct dosage is an obstacle to consistent treatment and control.

Hearing Presentation

Hearing loss presents in 33% of the over 65 years old population. Often, this loss involves high frequencies and then the speech frequencies, resulting in impairment to hearing speech. This leads to social and emotional isolation. In addition to aging, viruses, tumors, and certain medications may result in hearing loss. Hearing aids, cochlear implants, and assistive listening devices may improve communication. Be sensitive to communication issues and use appropriate volume, pitch, and clarity. DOT 6-3.9

Trauma Considerations

Trauma to the elderly accounts for about 12% of all trauma events, affecting males and females equally.[9] Although the incidence is less than in other age groups, the elderly are more likely to have severe consequences from trauma than other age groups. This results in the highest population-based mortality rates of any age group, making trauma the seventh leading cause of death in the elderly. An important point to remember is that the physiologic reserve of the elderly is compromised from the aging process and concurrent diseases. With less ability to compensate, the elderly function on the edge in normal circumstances. Traumatic injury pushes them over the edge, prolonging recovery and leading to increased morbidity and mortality.

Mechanisms of Injury and Pathophysiologic Changes

The mechanism of injury is similar to other age groups with differing patterns of injury. Falls, motor vehicle crashes, and burns are the most common causes of injury (Figure 44-11). Other causes of trauma include acts of violence such as robbery, assault, abuse, and suicide.

Falls account for the most common cause of injury, with many elderly experiencing repeated falls. The elderly often fall on a level surface, with a resulting isolated extremity fracture. Falls are more common due to the age-related changes in balance, stability, muscular strength, coordination, and postural hypotension. Diminished vision contributes to fall hazards. Underlying medical conditions can predispose the person to falls. Syncope has many causes, including dysrhythmias, hypoglycemia, hypoxia, postural hypotension, and volume depletion. Substance use and abuse, as well as prescription medications, contribute to gait problems.

Motor vehicle crashes (MVC) and pedestrian injuries account for the second leading cause of trauma. Crash injuries result in more fatalities in the elderly than in any other age group. Slower reaction times, visual and hearing deficits, memory, and judgment impairment

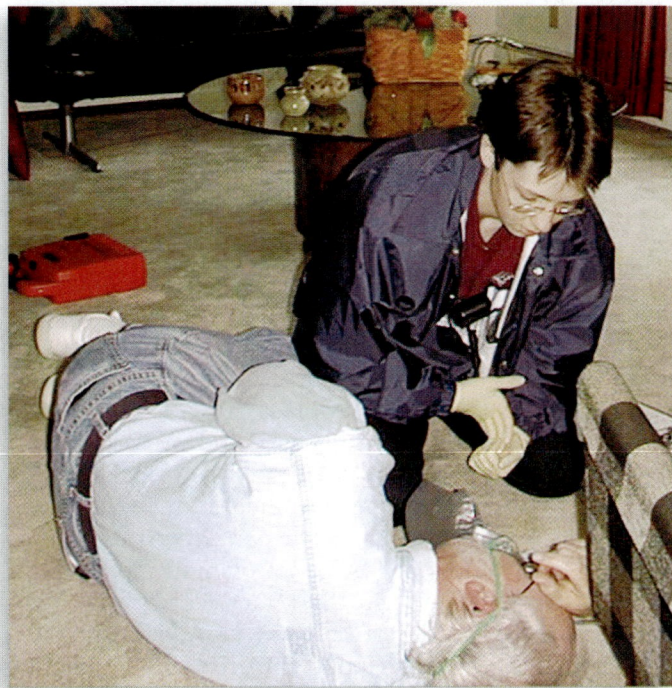

Figure 44-11 Falls are one of the more common mechanisms of injury in the elderly.

contribute to the rate of crashes. Twenty-two percent of pedestrian-automobile fatalities occur in the elderly. The slower pace of walking, vision and hearing deficits, judgment impairment, and kyphosis limitations to posture contribute to the incidence.

Burns in the elderly account for 20% of burn unit admissions. Most injuries occur at home from smoking and associated flame injury, cooking, or hot water scalds. There is a definite correlation between age and mortality—the older the patient, the greater risk of death.[9] Physiologic changes underlie the increasingly dismal outcome from these injuries. Events considered minor often result in significant injury due to the loss of muscle, decreased bone density, decrease in pain sensation, and loss of physiologic reserve.

CONNECTIONS See Box 26-1 (page 529) in Chapter 26: Burn Trauma for a discussion of the Baux score, which provides an estimate of burn injury mortality based on age and criticality of the burn. Remember: the rate of mortality rises with each successive year of age.

History and Assessment Challenges

The history is not just a list of problems to be recorded. It is increasingly important in the elderly to search for a medical cause for the traumatic event and vice versa. Due to the complexity of presentation, never consider the elderly person as having an isolated injury until that is proven to be true. The goal of assessment is twofold:

- To discover or exclude injury or a medical cause for the symptoms.
- To identify the degree of clinical compromise that is masked by the physiologic changes associated with aging.

After obtaining the patient history and assessing vital signs, it is important to review the geriatric basics. Multiple medications are more common than not, so what class of drugs are being taken, and why is the patient taking that drug? Almost 70% of the elderly have hypertension. Evaluate the blood pressure; findings in the normal range may not be normal for that patient! We know cardiac output is reduced and the normal tachycardic response to pain, hypovolemia or anxiety, may be lost or blunted. Common medications such as beta-blockers can mask tachycardia. With aging and the shrinkage of brain tissue, loss of muscle strength, and weakened bone integrity, the protective resources that worked to prevent or compensate for many injuries during the younger years are lost or may be blunted by medication use.

Trauma protocols exist to ensure that patients are appropriately triaged and transported to trauma centers for optimal care. These protocols have the component of age as a factor in the scoring and decision-making process. It is important to anticipate the extent of physiologic reserve lost and to realize that the cumulative effect of seemingly minor injuries can be deadly to the elderly person. The change from stable to unstable and critical can occur very quickly, without the vital signs changes one would expect.

Head Injury

Evaluating mental status becomes more challenging with the subtle changes in thought process, memory, coexisting diseases, and medications. It is important not to attribute deficits in mental status to dementia or underlying disease without further confirming information. Due to brain atrophy, there is an increase in subdural hematomas. The amount of time it takes before becoming symptomatic from an intracranial hemorrhage can increase due to the added space within the skull, masking the accumulation of blood. It has been found that 35–50% of patients with a subdural hematoma have no documented history of trauma. Alcohol use, dementia, and conditions that impair memory account for most of these situations. A fall may have occurred but is not remembered. Carefully assess and document any loss of consciousness.

Cervical Spine Injuries

Cervical spine injuries are more common in the elderly than the younger population. Loss of bone density and

osteoarthritis can predispose the person to spinal injuries. Based on mechanism of injury or the presence of neck pain, careful immobilization without hyperextension of the neck is necessary. Occlusion of the airway secondary to stiffening of the trachea and CNS diseases that affect the tongue, swallowing, or gag reflex demand added attention to cervical spine immobilization principles. Kyphosis requires adaptation of basic principles to maintain normal alignment.

Another hyperextension injury that can occur is central cord syndrome. As discussed earlier, suspect this when the arms show greater weakness and sensory loss than the legs.

Chest Injuries

The chest wall is more fragile, leading to increased likelihood of rib fractures and damage to the underlying organs. With the baseline PO_2 level being decreased with aging and the loss of physiologic reserves, any insult to the respiratory system will increase hypoxia and respiratory distress. Associated injuries such as pulmonary or cardiac contusion, pneumothorax, hemo-pneumothorax, and flail chest can quickly lead to decompensation and respiratory complications. Hypoxia and infection require aggressive interventions to prevent further multisystem organ involvement.

The myocardium is less able to respond to hypoxia and acidosis. Dysrhythmias increase in frequency and cardiac output decreases. Silent myocardial infarction may occur. Evaluate any elderly patient who presents with confusion for MI. Traumatic aortic aneurysm may result due to trauma but may be difficult to recognize due to chronic pain and beta-blocker use.

Abdominal Injuries

Abdominal assessment is one of the more unreliable parts of the examination in the geriatric patient. Thirty-five percent of trauma patients have abdomen injuries but many have a normal examination.[9] There are limited signs of peritoneal irritation found. Suspect abdominal injury whenever you find pelvic or lower rib area injuries.

Musculoskeletal Injuries

Mortality from pelvic fractures reaches 90% for those with open fractures and 50% for those with closed fractures. Severe blood loss can result from pelvic fractures as well as femur fractures. Blood loss, immobility, loss of physiologic reserve, and complications such as infection or sepsis, adult respiratory distress syndrome, clotting disorders, and renal failure demonstrate the multiple organ system failure syndrome process.

Commonly occurring fractures include the hip, femur, tibia, humerus, and radius. Osteoporosis contributes to the occurrence of fractures. Fall prevention is an important role for all healthcare providers. The loss of independence, complications, and need for supportive services dramatically increase when falls occur. Remember that pain perception is decreased. During examination, pain may not be elicited, leading to the mistaken assumption of the bony structure being intact. Attention to body positioning, neurovascular findings, and mechanism of injury are important.

Trauma Interventions

Rapid assessment of life threats is done for every patient. Geriatric trauma differences include particular attention to airway positioning (watch for dentures), adequacy of breathing, and circulation. Hypoxia and hypovolemia are not tolerated for very long by the older person. Even brief episodes lead to ischemia of vital organs. Vital signs can be misleading. Suspect shock with "normal" vital signs. Fluid resuscitation is best provided by the principle of bolus fluid administration using 250–500 mL. Reevaluate blood pressure and lung sounds; bolus again and reevaluate. Fluid overloading is to be prevented while maintaining adequate volume. Attention to temperature is necessary. Prevent hypothermia by covering the patient whenever possible and administering warm fluids. Ideally, rapid transport would allow the patient to be in a trauma center quickly where red blood cell transfusion can begin. Limiting crystalloid infusion and switching to blood products will enhance oxygen delivery and minimize ischemia.

Positioning requires added padding and postural support (Figure 44-12). Kyphosis and posture changes create gaps that need to be padded to enable secure stabilization and safe transport. Since most trauma patients are stabilized on a long spinal board, consideration for those patients with COPD and respiratory difficulty needs to be addressed. Due to spinal injury concerns, sitting up is not an option. It is possible, depending on the blood pressure, to elevate the head of the long board to ease respiratory effort.

Prevention is the key to avoiding these injuries. Monitoring and education about daily medications and their effects, setting the hot water heater temperature at 120° to 130°F, fixing fall and tripping hazards, and installing smoke and carbon monoxide detectors are all steps of prevention. When prevention fails, a high index of suspicion, combined with good assessment and management, can reduce the likelihood of long-term disability, complications, and death. The goal is to return the elder trauma patient to the preexisting level of functioning.

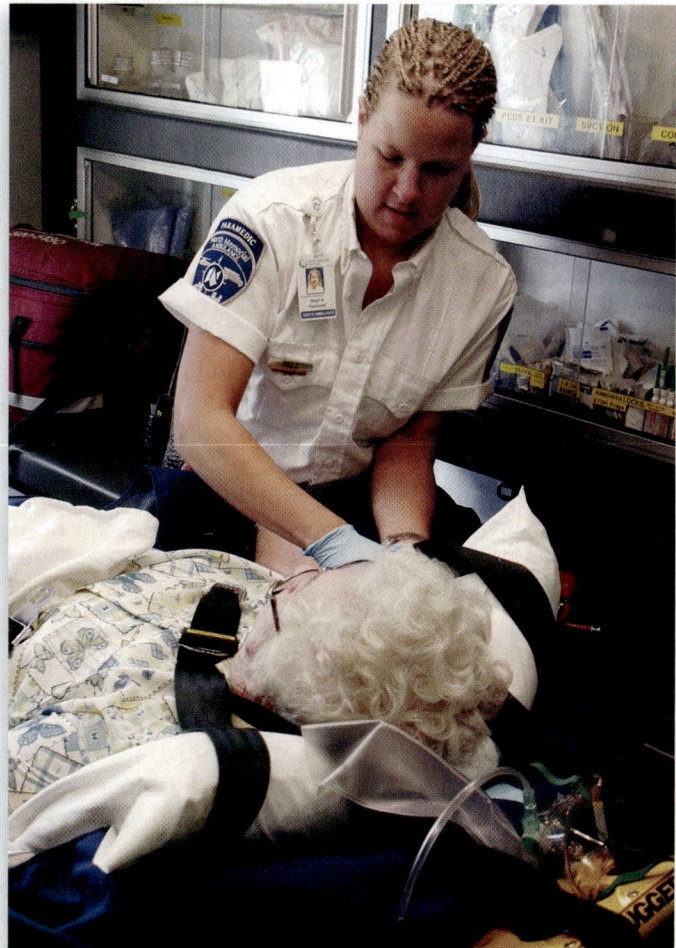

Figure 44-12 Use extra padding for postural support, and keep your elderly patient warm by covering with blankets to prevent hypothermia.

Elder Abuse and Neglect

With the increase in the number of older people, the incidence of elder abuse and neglect rises. As in other forms of abuse, this is often hidden from view and is underreported. Many barriers to disclosure exist, including fear of retribution, social isolation, and shame. Whether the adult is in a home situation or nursing home, each has the same risk factors for mistreatment. Cognitive impairment, inability to defend oneself, and reliance on others for adequate food and shelter put the elder at risk.

CONNECTIONS Chapter 45: The Abused and Neglected offers additional information on this topic.

Passive and active neglect are types of abuse that can occur. In active neglect, the caregiver intentionally fails to meet the physical, social, or emotional needs of the elder person. In passive neglect, the caregiver unintentionally neglects the person, often due to being overloaded or stressed or having lack of knowledge. Physical abuse is intentional. Injuries can range from improper restraint, slapping, or beating to unexplained injuries. Financial abuse occurs with expenditures in excess of the needs to care for the person. Theft of money from bank accounts, forcing someone to sign legal documents to change wills or power of attorney, and theft of personal belongings all occur. Psychological abuse can range from insults to verbal threats. Sexual abuse occurs when sexual acts are committed without the elder's consent. Neglect is the more common form of mistreatment, accounting for 70% of all cases.[7]

During evaluation the elder may present with physical signs of injury such as scratches, bruises, fractures, pressure ulcers, burns, or restraint marks. Behavioral signs may include fear of strangers, agitation, passive behaviors, hypervigilance, or confusion. Genital trauma, venereal diseases, and infection may be indicators of sexual trauma. Malnutrition, dehydration, and poor hygiene are also indicators of neglect. Self neglect is another category, often reflecting the inability to care for oneself in independent living situations.

Assessment of the home environment, evaluation of the interaction with the caregiver, and careful physical examination are essential. Document all findings. Report findings to the receiving personnel at the hospital, and follow through with reporting to adult protective services as required by your state. Law enforcement needs to be involved if there is immediate danger to the person. Interventions will be based upon the assessment findings, addressing life threats, and supportive care.

Summary

In the age group 65 years and older, there is tremendous variation in the physiological effects of aging. Different organ systems age at different times. The physiologic ability to compensate in disease states has very narrow limits and is exceeded quickly. The impact of multiple deficits leads to a complex picture of multisystem involvement. Hypoxia and ischemia are not tolerated in the elderly. Consequences of illness or injury more frequently lead to prolonged hospitalization and recovery, disability, or death. The goals of care need to be focused on prevention, immediate aggressive treatment, and at the end of life, compassionate care. With many productive years of life remaining at age 65, the older years need to be approached with knowledge. Prevention is an essential role. When prevention fails and illness or injury occurs, intervention tailored to the physiologic changes and needs is required. Expert assessment and anticipation of ongoing physiologic changes is the key to adequate treatment. **DOT 6-3.7**

Notes

1. S. E. Huether and K. L. McCance, *Understanding Pathophysiology*, 3rd ed. (St. Louis, MO: Mosby, 2004).

2. U.S. Census Bureau, Population Estimates, http://www.census.gov/popest/states/asrh/tables/SC-EST2004-01res.pdf (accessed August 13, 2005).

3. National Center for Health Statistics, Life Expectancy Hits Record High, http://www.cdc.gov/nchs/pressroom/05facts/lifeexpectancy.htm (accessed September 14, 2005).

4. N. Jitramone, "Evidence-Based Protocol. Exercise Promotion: Walking in Elders," *AHRQ, National Guideline Clearinghouse* (2001), http://www.guideline.gov (accessed August 13, 2005).

5. U.S. Department of Health and Human Services, *Healthy People 2010 Understanding and Improving Health*, 2nd ed. (Washington, DC: U.S. Government Printing Office, 2000).

6. C. K. Cassel, R. M. Leipzig, H. J. Cohen, E. B. Larson, and D. E. Meier, *Geriatric Medicine: An Evidence Based Approach*, 4th ed. (New York, NY: Springer, 2003).

7. C. S. Landefeld, R. M. Palmer, M. G. Johnson, C. B. Johnston, and W. L. Lyons, *Current Geriatric Diagnosis and Treatment* (New York, NY: McGraw-Hill, 2004).

8. D. L. Kasper, E. Braunwald, A. S. Fauci, S. L. Hauser, D. L. Longo, and J. L. Jameson, eds., *Harrison's Principles of Internal Medicine*, 16th ed. (New York, NY: McGraw-Hill, 2006).

9. J. E. Tintinalli, G. D. Kelen, J. S. Stapczynski, O. J. Ma, and D. M. Cline, *Tintinalli's Emergency Medicine: A Comprehensive Study Guide*, 6th ed., McGraw-Hill's AccessMedicine (accessed October 13, 2006).

10. Substance Abuse & Mental Health Services Administration, http://www.samhsa.gov/aging/age_05.aspx (accessed September 14, 2005).

11. Health and Age, Alcoholism, http://www.healthandage.com/html/well_connected/pdf/doc56.pdf (accessed October 13, 2006).

12. S. A. Hunt, W. T. Abraham, M. H. Chin, A. M. Feldman, G. S. Francis, T. G. Ganiats, M. Jessup, M. A. Konstam, D. M. Mancini, K. Michl, J. A. Oates, P. S. Rahko, M. A. Silver, L. W. Stevenson, and C. W. Yancy, "ACC/AHA 2005 Guideline Update for the Diagnosis and Management of Chronic Heart Failure in the Adult: Summary Article: A Report of the American College of Cardiology/American Heart Association Task Force on Practice Guidelines (Writing Committee to Update the 2001 Guidelines for the Evaluation and Management of Heart Failure)," *Circulation* (2005): 112, 1825–1852.

13. A. V. Chobanian, G. L. Bakris, H. R. Black, et al., "National Heart, Lung, and Blood Institute Joint National Committee on Prevention, Detection, Evaluation, and Treatment of High Blood Pressure. National Heart, Lung and Blood Institute; National High Blood Pressure Education Program Coordinating Committee. Seventh Report of the Joint National Committee on Prevention, Detection, Evaluation, and Treatment of High Blood Pressure," *Hypertension* 42 (2003): 1206-1252.

14. Alzheimer's Association, Fact Sheet: Experimental Alzheimer Drugs Targeting Beta-amyloid and the "Amyloid Hypothesis," http://www.alz.org/Resources/Factsheets/FSBetaAmyloid.pdf (accessed October 13, 2006).

15. National Center for Injury Prevention and Control, Suicide: Fact Sheet, http://www.cdc.gov/ncipc/factsheets/suifacts.htm (accessed September 9, 2005).

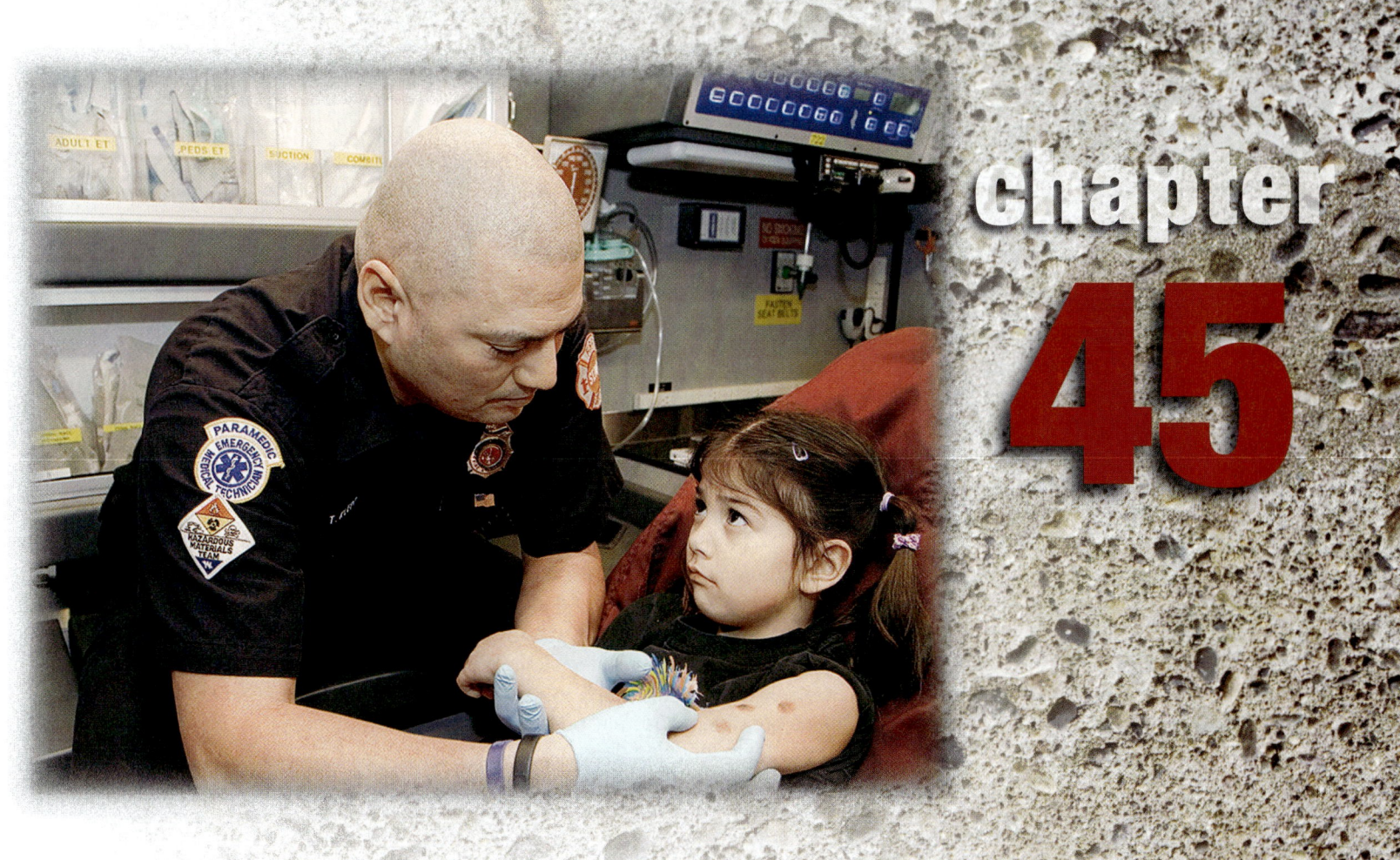

The Abused and Neglected

*"**T**hose who aspire to greatness must immerse themselves in the agonies of their times."*

—Oliver Wendell Holmes

Need to Know

▶ The most consistent finding of abuse is a history that does not match the clinical examination.

▶ When you suspect potential child, domestic, or elder abuse, communicate your concerns and findings to the hospital personnel. Your assessment of the home situation and family dynamics may be invaluable in recognizing abuse.

▶ Carefully document all findings—statements from patients themselves, injuries noted on exam, environmental findings, the current living situation, as well as your concerns.

▶ Child abuse and neglect is defined as any recent act or failure to act on the part of a parent or caretaker, which results in death, serious physical or emotional harm, sexual abuse, or exploitation, or an act or failure to act, which presents an imminent risk of serious harm.

▶ Shaken baby syndrome is a severe form of child abuse that frequently results in death or serious, permanent, neurological disability. The sickest infants most commonly present with seizures or respiratory distress from intracranial bleeding.

▶ Neglect is the most common form of elder maltreatment; it is defined as the refusal or failure to fulfill any part of a person's obligations or duties to an elderly person.

▶ Domestic abuse cases are common in EMS. They are very dangerous scenes. Safety is of utmost concern for you and the patient. Never promise the victim a guarantee of safety. Frequently, assailants will be released from police custody within hours and the victim may be in a very dangerous situation.

▶ While the definition of sexual assault varies from state to state, it generally refers to any genital, anal, oral, or manual penetration of the victim's body by way of force and without the victim's consent.

▶ While attending to the patient's physical and emotional needs, take steps to preserve any evidence from the crime scene. Disturb the crime scene as little as possible, especially prior to the arrival of law enforcement. Do not allow the patient to drink, brush teeth, shower, defecate, or urinate.

▶ Do	▶ Ask
• Treat ABCs and assess for medical and traumatic injuries as well as emotional needs.	• Where is the assailant? What types of weapons or assault methods were used?
• Look for unusual injuries that do not match the mechanism.	• Ask yourself, "Does the story match the injury?"
• Look for signs of malnutrition, dehydration, or burns in a shape or pattern.	• Has anyone hurt you?
• Try to preserve evidence (place clothes in paper bag, do not cut through bullet or other holes).	• Has anyone touched you without your consent?
• Look for soft tissue injuries at various stages of healing.	• Have you gone without food or medicines?
• Be respectful of a victim's personal space, and ask permission to touch the victim even for routine procedures such as vital signs.	• Limit your history-taking to questions that allow you to provide emergency medical care; the patient will be asked the specifics of the assault many times at the hospital and by law enforcement.
• Look for environmental signs that may indicate abuse, including lack of food in the home, unsanitary living conditions, prescription medications that have gone unfilled, and hazards to younger or older patients.	
• Be sure to tell the victim, "This is not your fault, no one has the right to do this to you."	
• Documentation of the assault should be factual, direct, and nonjudgmental.	

Introduction

Interpersonal violence, abuse, and neglect may be regarded as the epidemic of the 21st century. Violence against family members has been an aspect of Western society for generations and the problem is not decreasing. Prehospital providers will deal with victims of interpersonal violence on a regular basis, including victims of child abuse, partner abuse, elder abuse, and sexual assault. This chapter will define types of interpersonal violence and abuse, list characteristics of abusers and victims, discuss the assessment and documentation of abused patients, and address legal aspects of the care of an abused patient. **Skill Sheet 33 (and Step-by-Step 33): Secondary Survey, Skill Sheet 63: Verbal Communication, and Skill Sheet 64: Documentation support this chapter.**

Scene Safety and Personal Safety

As discussed in other chapters, scene safety and personal safety are paramount in any call related to intentional injuries or violence. If it is known from dispatch information that the scene is one of domestic violence, law enforcement personnel should be summoned, and the EMS crew should not enter the scene until it has been secured. If intimate partner violence is discovered once on scene, maintain caution when dealing with any potential assailant. Domestic violence (DV) abusers can be violent, erratic, and aggressive and may demonstrate an "If I can't have her, no one can" attitude concerning their victims. These scenes have historically been extremely dangerous to police and EMS responders.

Child Abuse and Neglect

As an EMS provider, you are in a unique position to recognize child abuse and neglect. You have the opportunity and responsibility to prevent children from sustaining further harm. Abused and neglected children rarely receive routine medical care; thus, episodic care in emergency settings may be their only contact with the medical community. Prehospital providers are one of the few healthcare professionals who enter the environment where abuse and victimization occurs. The home environment may reveal a family in desperate need of intervention and support services. DOT 6-2.73

What Is Child Abuse and Neglect?

Each state is responsible for defining child maltreatment and neglect although federal legislation does set minimum standards. The majority of states recognize four major types of maltreatment:

1. Neglect
2. Physical abuse
3. Emotional abuse
4. Sexual abuse

Child abuse and neglect, at a minimum, can be defined as any recent act or failure to act on the part of a parent or caretaker, which results in death, serious physical or emotional harm, sexual abuse, or exploitation, or an act or failure to act which presents an imminent risk of serious harm (Figure 45-1).[1] DOT 6-2.41, 6-2.42

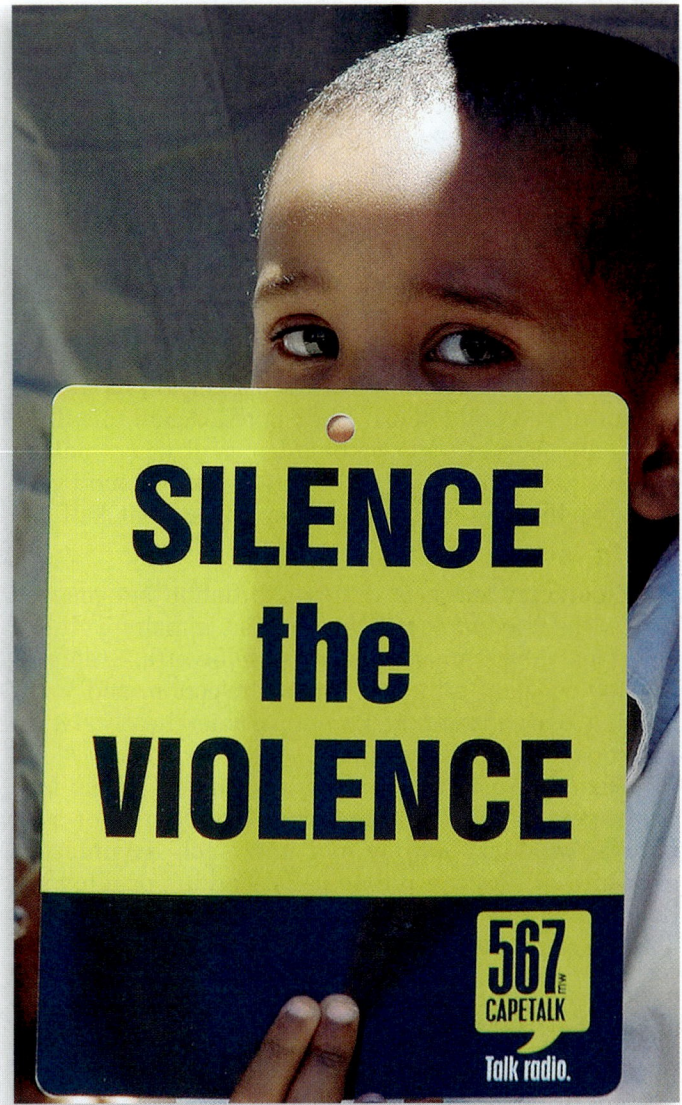

Figure 45-1 Educating the public about abuse is an important step toward prevention and recognition of the problem as well as healing the abuse victims.

Neglect is defined as failure to provide for a child's basic needs. Examples of neglect may include the following:

- Physical neglect (failure to provide food or shelter or lack of appropriate supervision).
- Emotional neglect (inattention to a child's emotional needs or failure to provide basic emotional support)
- Medical neglect (failure to provide medical or mental health treatment)
- Educational neglect (failure to educate the child or attend to special education needs)

Physical abuse is physical injury of a child at the hands of their caregiver. Injury can range from minor bruises to fractures and can be the result of punching, beating, kicking, shaking, throwing, choking, hitting, or burning. Any such injury is considered abuse in most states, regardless of whether the intent was to harm the child.

Street Secrets

Some cultures practice rituals and customs for treating sickness that are not in keeping with Western medicine practices. Some treatments leave behind discolorations on the skin. Coining and cupping are two such practices. Each results from the rubbing of skin or placement of devices that draw blood to the surface of the skin. Neither results in permanent damage to the patient and should not be considered child abuse when noted. Again this illustrates the need to remain nonjudgmental when making observations and treating patients in the field. Report your objective findings to the emergency department staff.

Emotional abuse is difficult to define but may be viewed as a *pattern* of behavior that impairs a child's emotional development or sense of self-worth. Examples include constant criticism, threats, rejection, and withholding love and support. Emotional abuse nearly always accompanies other forms of abuse.

Sexual abuse includes *physical acts* such as fondling, genital or oral stimulation, intercourse, or sodomy as well as *nonphysical acts* such as indecent exposure or obscene phone calls. Forcing or allowing children to engage in prostitution or pornography is defined as **sexual exploitation.** DOT 6-4.2, 4.5

Child Abuse Statistics

In 2003, nearly 3 million referrals concerning the welfare of 5.5 million children were made to local child protection agencies for investigation of abuse or neglect. Reports from medical personnel accounted for 8% of reports. Two-thirds of reported cases were investigated, and over 900,000 cases of abuse or neglect were substantiated. It is important to note that unsubstantiated cases are not to be considered "false reports"; further information in the future may allow for identification of an abused child. Neglect accounts for 60% of child abuse cases; 20% of cases involved physical abuse, and 10% of cases involved sexual abuse. Young children (under age three) are the most likely to be abused. The rate of abuse is also higher in children of Pacific Islander, American Indian, Alaska Native, and African American descent.[2]

The National Child Abuse and Neglect Data System (NCANDS) reported approximately 1,400 child fatalities in 2002 as a result of abuse or neglect. However, most authorities believe that child abuse fatalities are seriously underreported due to varying definitions of "child homicide" or "child abuse." Additionally, deaths attributed to accidents or to sudden infant death syndrome may actually be the result of abuse or neglect. Recent reports indicate that 50–60% of child maltreatment-related deaths are not recorded as such on death certificates. Fatalities due to abuse and neglect are most frequent among young children; children under the age of one account for 40% of fatalities, and children under the age of four account for 75% of all child abuse-related fatalities. Infant boys have the highest rate of fatalities, nearly 18 deaths per 100,000 infants. Repeated physical abuse (battering) or a single incident (such as drowning, suffocating, or shaking) may result in a child's death. In addition, a caregiver's failure to act may result in fatal neglect; the neglect may be chronic (extended malnourishment) (Figure 45-2) or acute (an infant drowning in a tub due to lack of supervision).[3] DOT 6-2.73, 6-4.1

Risk Factors for Child Abuse

The multifactorial theory of child abuse proposes that three things are necessary for the development of an abuse episode: the right parent, the right child, and the right day.[4]

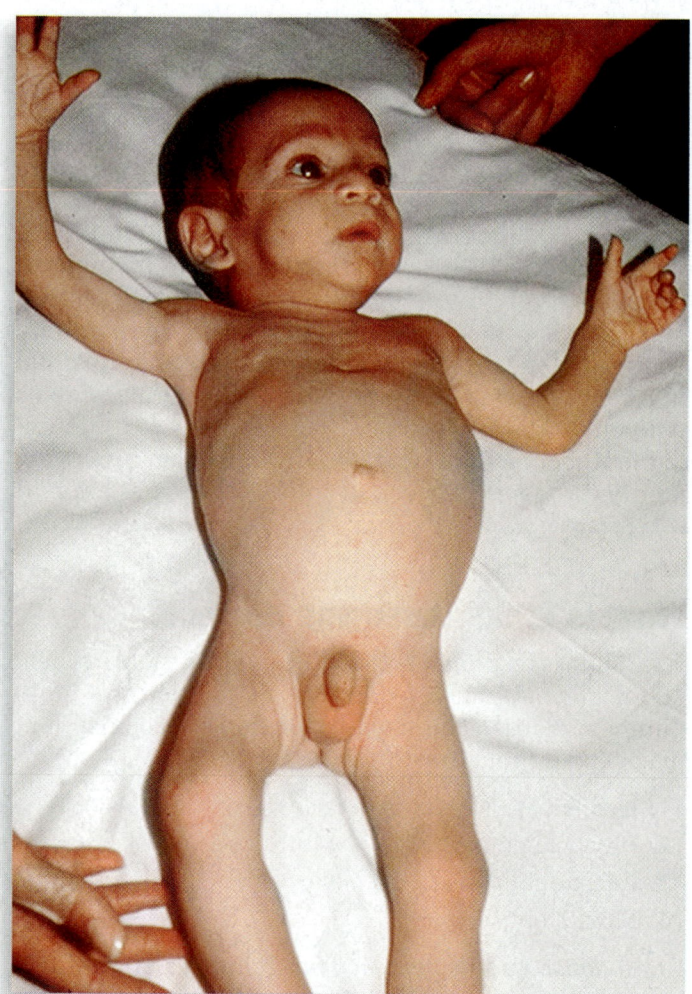

Figure 45-2 Physical neglect is the failure to provide appropriate food, shelter, and supervision. Note the lack of fat on the arms, legs, chest and face of this malnourished child.

Eighty percent of child abuse victims are abused by their parents.[5] ("Parents" includes birth parents, adoptive parents, and stepparents.) Certain characteristics in a parent or caregiver increase the risk of abuse occurring. Drugs or alcohol in the home greatly increase the risk for abuse; over half of all child abuse cases involve substance or alcohol abuse by the perpetrators. Abusers often have rigid, unrealistic expectations of their children and have limited knowledge of normal childhood development and capabilities. They are unable to cope with children who do not meet their expectations, regardless of the child's developmental stage. For example, the normal difficulty a three-year-old may have in toilet training is viewed by parents as willful disobedience and may be punished harshly. The parents often were abused or neglected themselves as children and have no successful parental role models.[6] While it is important to remember that child maltreatment occurs in all socioeconomic levels, the disadvantaged are at greater risk due to increased stress, life crisis, and limited resources.[7] DOT 6-2.74

Certain characteristics may place a child at increased risk for abuse. Children with developmental delays, cognitive delays, or special needs are at high risk. These children can be very frustrating to interact with on a day-to-day basis. Caregivers without adequate support services or adequate coping skills may respond to these demands with abusive or neglectful behaviors. Children with young, single, nonbiological parents may also be at increased risk.[6] DOT 6-2.75

Episodes of abuse may be triggered by a situation that overloads the caregiver's coping mechanisms. As mentioned above, drugs and alcohol compound the risk of loss of control in the caregiver. Domestic violence in the home clearly increases a child's risk of abuse or neglect. The presence of significant stressors such as homelessness; joblessness; isolated families; multiple, unintended pregnancies; and young families may also precipitate a crisis and lead to abuse. DOT 6-2.76, 6-4.9

Recognizing Child Maltreatment

Clues in the Caregiver or Parent's Behavior

Child abusers are often described as emotionally immature, self-centered, with low self-esteem, and are frequently critical of the child. They may demonstrate little insight into how a child may feel and seem unconcerned about the child's injury or treatment. Occasionally, abusers will blame the child for the injury and may show little guilt or remorse when their child is injured.

Clues in the Child's Behavior

Familiarity with normal child development and age-appropriate behavior is essential when evaluating any child, and it is critical to the recognition of child abuse or neglect.

Child abuse or neglect should be considered when a child exhibits any of the following behaviors:

- Excessively passive behavior, especially if the child is under the age of six
- Excessively aggressive behavior, especially in children over the age of six
- Children who cry hopelessly during treatment or children who cry very little, even with painful procedures
- Children who do not mind if their parents or caregivers leave the room
- Children who do not look to the parents or caregivers for reassurance
- Children who are wary of physical contact
- Children who appear extremely apprehensive
- Children who are constantly on the alert for danger

Clues in the Home Environment

You will often be the only medical provider to observe the home environment and to observe the child in their own home environment. Look for signs of a recent fight or signs of drugs and alcohol. Try to determine if the environment is safe for children. Does there appear to be adequate shelter, food, and basic necessities of living? Is there evidence of infestations or rodents? Is adequate supervision evident? Are the interactions between the child and the family reassuring? Be sure to communicate your impressions regarding the safety and appropriateness of the child's home environment to hospital staff. DOT 6-4.9, 4.13

Street Secrets

As you gain experience in the field, you will enter many homes with different degrees of cleanliness and living conditions. You may have senior partners who are accustomed (or you may become accustomed yourself) to seeing home environments that are not ideal for children. While you should remain respectful of those who are financially disadvantaged or simply have different styles of living, it is important to keep a high index of suspicion for abuse. You may be the only person who can, by simply reporting your observation, help a child who is in a dangerous situation.

Secondary Survey

Injuries during childhood are very common and are usually unintentional. Identifying abuse and neglect can be difficult at times, but maintaining a high degree of suspicion for the presence of abuse can prevent a child from suffering further harm or even death. A careful history should be taken from the parent as well as from the child (if the child is able to give a history).

The most consistent finding of abuse is a history that does not match the clinical examination.

Histories that should be concerning include the following:

- A history that does not match exam findings
- Details of the history that change over time
- A significant delay between the time of injury and when the parent seeks medical care for the child.
- Injuries that are blamed on a younger sibling or younger playmate
- A minor trauma mechanism as an explanation for a significant injury
- Injuries where the parent simply cannot provide an explanation as to how the trauma occurred
- A child is developmentally incapable of the specified mechanism (e.g., a nine-month-old who fell off a tricycle; a four-week-old who rolled off the bed)

Strong indicators of physical abuse on examination include the following:

- A physical exam that is not consistent with the history given
- Bruises in unusual locations (inside of arms, inside of thighs, outside of mouth)
- Bruises in a nonambulatory infant ("you have to cruise to bruise")
- Bruises with a characteristic pattern (belt mark, hand mark, loop mark)
- Cluster of bruises or bruises of varying age
- Burns in a "stocking-glove" pattern (Figure 45-3)
- Burns of the perineum
- Burns that are small and round suggesting a cigarette as the cause
- Femur fracture in a nonambulatory child
- Significant injury ascribed to minor trauma (Of note, the literature suggests that children who fall from a bed or sofa never sustain a serious injury beyond a simple fracture or bruising; a fall of greater than 4 feet is required to result in a significant closed head injury.[8])

Shaken Baby Syndrome (Acceleration/Deceleration Injury)

Shaken baby syndrome is a severe form of child abuse that frequently results in death or serious, permanent, neurological disability. The infant most commonly

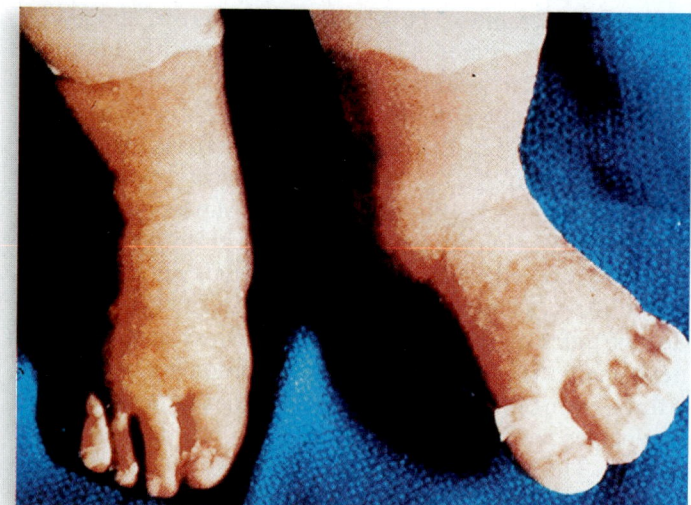

Figure 45-3 "Stocking-glove" pattern burns caused by dipping the child into scalding water.

presents with seizures, coma, or respiratory distress from intracranial bleeding. Initially, a history of shaking may not be provided by the parent or caregiver. The typical scenario is an infant with inconsolable crying who is then repeatedly and violently shaken. Fractures of the ribs or lower extremities can be seen when infants are squeezed tightly about the thorax or shaken back and forth while being held by the legs.[9]

Field Evaluation and Treatment

In order to increase the recognition of child abuse victims, consider the possibility of abuse in each and every child you are called to evaluate. Distinguishing between an intentional injury and an authentic accident can be challenging. The most important clues are obtained by observing the child and the child's relationship with the parent or caregiver and in matching the history of the event to the injury. Consider whether the history is consistent with the injuries you are seeing. Maintain a high index of suspicion; you may be able to prevent further injury to an infant or child.

The field evaluation and treatment of an abused child obviously depends on the presenting complaint. Manage physical injuries and medical complaints according to standard practice for those problems. Frequent reassurance of the child and attention to any emotional needs are important. Maintain a neutral, professional, calm attitude to any caregivers who may be present; your responsibility is not to assign blame for the abuse. Be sure to communicate your observations and findings to the appropriate authorities, even in uncertain and unclear cases. Sometimes a "gut feeling" that something is not right can be a very important clue.

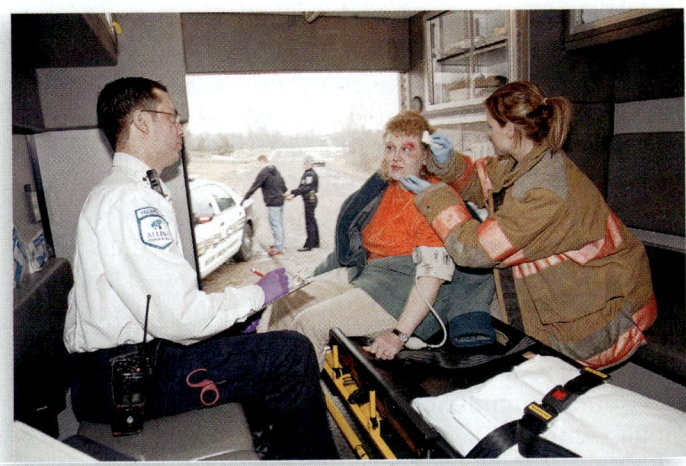

Figure 45-4   Approximately one-quarter of all women will experience domestic abuse during their lifetimes.

Domestic Violence

The term **domestic violence (DV)** most commonly refers to violence and abuse between intimate partners (Figure 45-4). However, domestic violence in a broad sense may refer to intimate partner violence, spousal abuse, elder abuse, and child abuse. For the purposes of this chapter, DV refers to violence between intimate partners, usually male to female, but it can also involve female to male, male to male, and female to female. The more specific term **intimate partner violence (IPV)** will also be used.

What Is Domestic Violence?

The Family Violence Prevention Fund defines IPV as "a pattern of assaultive and coercive behaviors, including physical, sexual, and psychological attacks, as well as economic coercion, that adults or adolescents use against their intimate partners."[10] IPV includes physical acts, such as battering and sexual assault, and nonphysical acts such as verbal abuse, emotional abuse, economic abuse, isolation from friends and family, threats to harm children and property, and prevention of access to healthcare or prenatal care. Most battered women state that the nonphysical abuse is more humiliating and distressing to them than the physical injuries.[11] DOT 6-4.2, 4.3

The medical effects of IPV are far-reaching and include soft tissue injuries, fractures, miscarriages, infertility, sexually transmitted diseases, unwanted pregnancies, poor prenatal care, concussions, neurological deficits, poorly managed chronic illnesses, alcoholism, drug abuse, mental illness, and homelessness.[12,13,14]

Intimate Partner Violence Statistics

Approximately 1.3 million women are victims of IPV each year; on average, a victim suffers 3.4 separate assaults per year.[14] CDC studies indicate that approximately 25% of all women will experience some form of IPV during their lifetime.[6,15] Thirty percent of Americans state that they know a woman who has been physically abused by her husband or boyfriend in the past year.[15] Abuse rates in emergency department populations tend to be higher, with more than 50% of women reporting a history of partner abuse.[16] Approximately 10% of women who present to an emergency department for treatment on any given day are there due to abusive situations.[17] Many battered women first access medical care via the 9-1-1 system. One-half of all homeless women and children are homeless due to domestic violence. The healthcare-related costs of rape, physical assaults, and homicide by intimate partners exceed five billion dollars each year.[15]

Intimate partner violence is primarily a crime against women. Women account for 85% of victims of IPV while men account for approximately 15% of victims.[18] Males report domestic assault at a very low rate, possibly due to humiliation, guilt, or fear of their assailant. While men are more likely than women to be the victim of a violent crime overall (usually from a stranger assailant), women are five to eight times more likely to be abused by an intimate partner. Women are seven to 14 times more likely than men to report suffering severe physical assaults from an intimate partner and are more likely to be killed by an intimate partner.[19] In 2000, over 30% of murdered women were killed by an intimate partner; intimate partner homicide accounts for less than 4% of the murders of men.[18]

Research reveals racial and ethnic differences in IPV rates. American Indian and Alaska Native women are most likely to report physical assaults and sexual assaults while Asian and Pacific Islander women are least likely to report physical and sexual victimization. Hispanic women are also less likely to report rape victimization than non-Hispanic women. In addition, DV may be underreported in same sex relationships. However, it is unclear if the differences in prevalence rates are due to differences in actual violence experienced or differences in victim willingness to disclose physical and sexual assaults.[19] DOT 6-4.1

Cycle of Violence

Some experts believe that domestic violence follows a cycle of three phases (Figure 45-5).

- Phase 1 is a "tension-building phase." Arguing and an increase in verbal or minor physical abuse occurs during this phase, along with a breakdown of communication. Often, the victim will feel the need to keep things calm.
- Phase 2, the "crisis phase," involves the actual battering episode.
- Phase 3 is often described as the "honeymoon phase," where denial and then apologies occur.

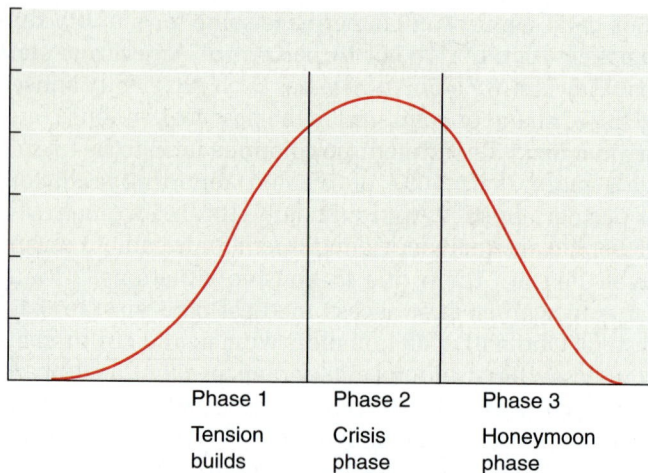

Phase 1 | Phase 2 | Phase 3
Tension builds | Crisis phase | Honeymoon phase

Figure 45-5 The three-phase cycle of domestic violence.

The assailant may deny that the abuse took place or downplay the seriousness of the event, and may blame drugs or alcohol as the reason for the assault. The abuser may then become contrite, apologetic, and state that it will never happen again.

Typically, the cycle repeats itself over and over, increasing in frequency and severity if no intervention occurs. Intervention during phase 2 or 3 has the best chance for a positive outcome.[13]

Street Secrets

As a paramedic, you will often arrive just after violence has occurred. In this transition between violence and honeymoon, the victim may feel a sense of relief that the violence is over. The victim may also feel renewed hope and love, as well as a conflicting sense of fear should the abuser perceive the victim as a threat. The victim may act aggressively toward authority figures, including EMS. This can be frustrating for you as you are only trying to help and the victim appears to reject your help. It is very important that you stay in a therapeutic role and repeat key messages that should be helpful to the victim. Statements such as, "No one has the right to hurt you," and "This is not okay," even if they appear to be rejected at the moment, may later be remembered and may help the victim seek intervention.

Characteristics of Persons in an Abusive Relationship

Women who experienced childhood physical abuse are at-risk of being involved in an abusive relationship during adulthood.[20] Similarly, neglected children are at increased risk of becoming violent as adults. Certain personality traits may be seen in either the abuser or the victim; these include low self-esteem, intense need for love or affection, uncontrolled temper, jealousy, insecurity, and an unrealistic expectation of a relationship. Persons with disabilities are at increased risk of abuse as are the elderly. Other populations at-risk for abuse include pregnant women, individuals who abuse drugs or alcohol, and individuals whose partners abuse drugs or alcohol.[14,20] The most significant risk factor for becoming a victim or abuser is witnessing or experiencing violence as a child; the cycle of intergenerational violence continues.

Domestic violence occurs in all racial, ethnic, religious, and socioeconomic populations. Households with financial stress, job insecurity, or legal difficulties are at increased risk of abuse. The presence of a firearm in a household with a history of intimate partner violence significantly increases the risk of a homicide occurring.[21] DOT 6-4.7, 4.11

Recognizing Intimate Partner Violence
Barriers to Disclosure

Victims of intimate partner violence may be difficult to recognize. Many legitimate barriers exist to prevent open dialogue concerning the violence. Victims are frequently fearful of potential retaliation from their abuser if the violence is disclosed. Victims may feel humiliated or shameful that abuse is occurring, or may feel the need to protect their partner. Although sometimes difficult for caregivers to understand, the feelings of love are still present and strong, even if the relationship is unhealthy. Belief that EMS and law enforcement will not understand and cannot help may also prevent open disclosure.[22]

Street Secrets

Sometimes disclosure may not be needed for you to link the victim with helpful resources. One approach may be simply to apologize if you are misperceiving the situation since you may see so much violence and to suggest that help is available from a specific location, crisis phone number, or individual. A victim may be in the habit of having to memorize conversations because the abuser requires them to report, verbatim, what has been said to others. If you simply say a phone number, a name, or a location where help is available, that may be enough for the victim to remember. Another more risky approach that some ambulance services have attempted is to carry business cards. To protect the patient, the cards should only have a phone number or information that the abuser may not immediately identify as a threat should the card fall into the wrong hands.

Barriers to Inquiry

Healthcare providers also have difficulty inquiring about potential intimate partner violence. They may have preconceived notions that abuse cannot occur in this patient, that whatever occurred is a "private matter," or that the patient provoked the abuse by the actions. Other barriers to inquiry include the belief that the victims could simply leave if they wanted to, that the violence should be disclosed without questioning, or that it is the job of others to identify intimate partner violence. Other practical and structural barriers to recognition of DV include the lack of privacy to conduct an interview, the presence of the perpetrator at the scene, or the need for a translator who may be a friend or relative of the victim or abuser.[22]

Concerning Presentations

Despite these barriers, the paramedic should maintain a high level of suspicion and should try to directly inquire about abuse whenever possible. Concerning clues in the patient's history include a conflicting account of what occurred, a history that is not consistent with the physical examination, or a significant delay in seeking medical attention for a serious injury. The partner's behavior may also be a red flag. Abusers may seem overly concerned for the victim and may hover, refusing to leave the patient's side and answering all questions for the patient. Alternatively, the companion may be hostile to you or to the patient, refusing to assist EMS or refusing to permit evaluation or transport. There may be evidence of a recent fight or of drug and alcohol abuse.[11]

Street Secrets

The presence of alcohol intoxication can seriously impair your ability to evaluate and care for a domestic violence victim. You should keep in mind that no one deserves to be abused, even if they have made bad choices in partners or use mood-altering substances. If you can separate the victim from the abuser and find a safe place for them until they can become sober, this may be enough to break the cycle of DV and get them to seek additional help.

Presenting complaints obviously include injuries. Be wary of injuries sustained during pregnancy and of genital injuries. Multiple injuries in various stages of healing and "accidental" injuries in unusual locations (inner aspect of thighs for example) are also of concern. A significant percentage of women in abusive situations experience strangulation and choking at the hands of their abusers. If the injury does not match the history given, further inquiry is warranted. Victims of domestic violence can also present with non-traumatic complaints.

Depression, alcohol use, and drug abuse, as well as suicide attempts often have their roots in a history of intimate partner violence. Abusers may prevent their partners from seeking care for chronic medical conditions or for prenatal care; therefore, maintain a high level of suspicion when caring for women who have had no prenatal care or who present frequently with complications due to noncompliance with medical therapies.[22]

The Patient Interview

Sample questions when interviewing abused patients might include the following:

- What happened? Were you hit, kicked, or punched by someone?
- Has any household member physically hurt you?
- You seem frightened. Has anyone hurt you?
- We often see people with injuries such as yours that have been caused by someone else. Is this happening to you?
- Many patients tell me they have been hurt by someone close to them. Is this what happened to you?
- Are you afraid of anyone in your household?
- Do you feel safe at home?

Maintain a nonjudgmental attitude, and avoid comments such as "What did you do to make him so mad or upset?" or "Why didn't you leave?" It is important to maintain a supportive attitude and not to minimize the situation.[22]

Street Secrets

In some cases, you may be called repeatedly to the same home for continued abuse. In these cases, you may find it difficult to understand why the victim does not accept your help or leave. It is especially important that you set aside your own feelings and that your interview, demeanor, and intervention stay focused on positive and therapeutic actions. You never know when your words will finally be heard and the victim will accept help.

Safety Planning

Not uncommonly, victims may decide to decline treatment and transport or to stay with the abuser. As an adult, it is important to respect the victim's final decision; only she can assess the risks of leaving her abuser at the current time. The most dangerous time for a victim of intimate partner violence is the time frame after she has left the relationship. No police system or social service system can fully guarantee her safety. Many EMS systems provide victims information on safety planning, community resources, and shelter or hotline numbers for patients who elect not to be transported. This information should be relayed to the patient in private; any written information should be on a small, easily concealed card.[13] DOT 6-4.14

Legal Considerations

While mandated reporting laws vary from state to state, most states require that physical assault be reported to the police. Regardless of the relationship between assailant and victim, it is a crime to assault another individual. In uncertain or highly suspicious cases, be sure to communicate your concerns to hospital personnel. Domestic violence assaults may be categorized as a misdemeanor or a felony, depending on state law, severity of injuries, and devices used in the assault. Frequently, assailants will be released from police custody within hours on their own recognizance. If early release from custody is likely, the victim may be in a very dangerous situation. Violence often escalates, following police or medical interventions. Encourage your patient to take personal safety precautions, especially if the patient is not transported to the hospital.

Working in the Gray Zone

Your EMS documentation may play a key role in the legal system. Whether your patient later seeks a restraining order or the abuser is on trial, your written words will be carefully inspected and interpreted. You may even be summoned to court to elaborate or substantiate your words. Be sure you are as complete, detailed, and factual as possible, and do not assign blame or report any personal opinions. Even if you think you know what happened, you may only have been given partial information. Documentation of a victim's refusal of patient care and transportation can be particularly problematic. The mere fact that the patient did not go to the hospital may be used in court to show that she was not really injured. Again, reporting as factually as possible is essential. If alcohol is involved, you should be very specific about the patient's level of orientation as this may be a key factor in determining if she is capable of making decisions on her own. While being respectful of the patient's right to refuse and the importance of a victim to have control over her decisions, every effort should be made to transport the patient. This may help link the victim with additional help and provide some time and space for a safety plan to be made.

Elder Abuse

Elder abuse affects hundreds of thousands of elderly persons each year in the United States. The true incidence and prevalence of elder abuse is difficult to quantify due to significant underreporting, varying definitions, and the lack of a national tracking system. The best available data suggest between 1 and 2 million Americans ages 65 and older have been injured, exploited, or otherwise mistreated by someone on whom they depend for care and protection. The frequency of elder abuse ranges from 2–10%; it is estimated that only one in 14 incidents of elder abuse is reported. Financial exploitation is similarly underdetected; experts state that only one in 25 cases of financial abuse victims is identified.[23]

What Is Elder Abuse?

The National Center on Elder Abuse defines several different types of **elder abuse** (Figure 45-6):

- Physical abuse
- Sexual abuse
- Emotional abuse
- Financial exploitation
- Neglect
- Abandonment
- Self-neglect[24]

Neglect is the most common form of elder maltreatment; it is defined as the refusal or failure to fulfill any part of a person's obligations or duties to an elderly person. Typically, neglect means failure to provide necessities such as food, water, clothing, shelter, personal

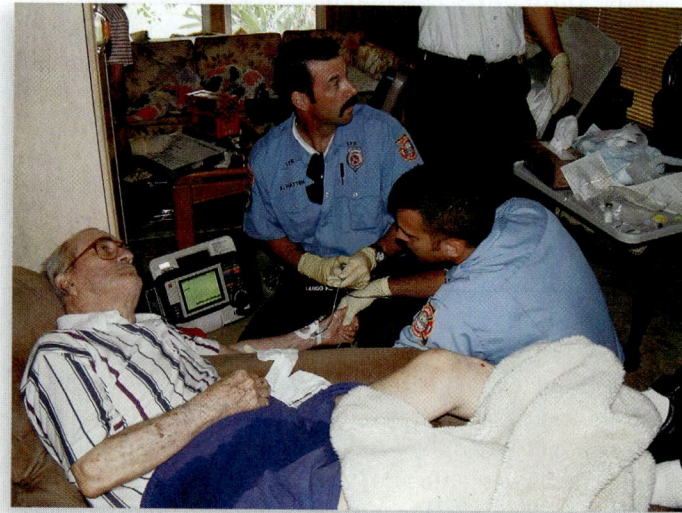

Figure 45-6 Besides physical abuse, the elderly may fall victim to sexual or emotional abuse as well as neglect or abandonment.

hygiene, medicine, or comfort. Signs and symptoms include dehydration, malnutrition, untreated bed sores, poor personal hygiene, unattended health problems, unsanitary and unclean living conditions, or hazardous or unsafe living conditions.

Physical abuse is the use of physical force, resulting in bodily injury, physical pain, or impairment. Examples include slapping, shoving, shaking, pinching, burning, force-feeding, or unreasonable physical or chemical constraint. Signs and symptoms of physical abuse may include signs of an assault (bruises, welts, fractures, lacerations, sprains, etc.), broken eyeglasses, signs of being subjected to physical punishment, signs of being restrained, and laboratory findings of medication overdose or underuse of medication.

Sexual abuse is nonconsensual sexual contact with an elderly person. Physical exam may reveal bruises around breasts or in the genital area, unexplained vaginal or anal bleeding, or torn, stained, or bloody underclothing.

Emotional abuse is the infliction of anguish, pain, or distress through verbal or nonverbal acts. It often involves verbal assaults, insults, intimidation, humiliation, harassment, or threats to institutionalize an elder. Treating an elder like an infant, isolating the elderly person, or giving an older person the "silent treatment" are other examples of emotional abuse.

Financial and material exploitation is defined as illegally or improperly using an elder's funds, property, or assets. Examples include theft of social security checks, embezzlement, or the use of threats to enforce signing or changing legal documents.

Abandonment is desertion of an elderly person by an individual who has physical custody of the elder or who has assumed responsibility for providing care to the elder. Elders may be deserted at a hospital, nursing facility, clinic, shopping mall, grocery store, or other public location.

Self-neglect is a concept unique to elder abuse; it describes behaviors of competent elderly persons that threaten their health or safety. It may be difficult to distinguish between elders who are choosing inappropriate behaviors and elders whose health has deteriorated so much that they are no longer able to manage on their own. Examples include dehydration, malnutrition, untreated or improperly attended medical conditions, poor personal hygiene, and unsafe living conditions. In either case, further investigation and intervention are warranted. DOT 6-4.2, 6-4.4

Elder Abuse Statistics

Approximately two-thirds of elder abuse victims are female; the average age is 78 years. More than two-thirds of the perpetrators are family members; adult children are the most frequent abusers of the elderly

(approximately 38%). Other family members and spouses account for about 25% of perpetrators. The overwhelming majority of victims live with their abusers. There is an equal distribution between male and female perpetrators of elder abuse.[25] Elders at risk for abuse include elders with multiple medical problems or cognitive impairment or dementia, socially isolated individuals, and elders who are financially dependent on their caregivers. Elderly persons who live with a nonvoluntary caregiver or a caregiver who has a mental illness or substance abuse problem are at high risk for abuse.[26] DOT 6-4.1, 4.12

Several theories exist regarding the etiology of elder abuse. Until recently, the most common theory was that frail, dependent, cognitively impaired elders would be abused by their stressed caregiver. However, recent literature has not supported this conclusion. Increasing impairment of an elderly person does not directly correlate with the risk for abuse. The social learning theory proposes that children who grew up in violent and abusive households will be abusive to their own children as well as their elders. Other experts believe that a pathological characteristic of the abuser leads to the abuse.[27] Research does indicate that a significant number of abusers suffer from substance abuse, mental illness, depression, or cognitive impairment or are financially dependent on the elder they are abusing.[26] DOT 6-4.8

Institutional Abuse

Elderly individuals may also be abused in nursing homes and other healthcare facilities by paid staff and caregivers, professionals, and other residents. Physical abuse, sexual abuse, neglect, and financial and emotional abuse can all occur in an institutional setting. Risk factors for institutional abuse include poor working conditions; inadequate training, experience, and supervision of staff; poorly paid staff; and high patient-to-staff ratios. Maintain a high level of suspicion when you evaluate elders in a nursing home setting who have unexplained physical injuries, dehydration, malnutrition, or poor personal hygiene or who appear to live in unsanitary and unclean conditions.

Recognizing Elder Abuse

As with the other forms of interpersonal violence, recognition depends on maintaining a high level of suspicion. Be cautious and thoughtful when evaluating elders with any traumatic injuries.

Concerning Histories

Is the exam consistent with the history given? Was this a witnessed "accidental fall," or was it only reported as such? Was there a significant or unexplained delay in seeking care? Are the interactions between the patient and the caregiver reassuring, or does the elder seem frightened of the caregiver? Is the elder referred to as accident prone? If mentally competent, is the patient allowed to explain the situation to you and to answer questions unsupervised? Are there signs of drug or alcohol abuse in the caregiver? Does the environment seem adequately clean, safe, and appropriate for the elder's level of function? Is an impaired or frail elder presenting for care alone?[26]

Physical Exam Indicators

Physical exam indicators of elder abuse include multiple injuries in various stages of healing, inconsistent injuries, unusual patterns of injury, restraint marks, gag marks, evidence of sexual abuse, and unexplained injuries. Signs of neglect include dehydration and malnutrition; signs that the patient has been laying in urine and stool; inappropriate clothing for the weather; soiled, torn, stained, or bloody clothing; recurrent calls for untreated medical conditions; and unkempt, dirty, unshaven elders.[26]

Assessment and Management

Treat any injuries or medical complaints as needed based on your usual trauma or medical protocols. Elderly patients who are competent and who retain decision-making capacity should be allowed to accept or refuse interventions (Figure 45-7). The patient's autonomy should be respected and supported when appropriate.

Elderly patients are four times more likely to present to the emergency department via ambulance than

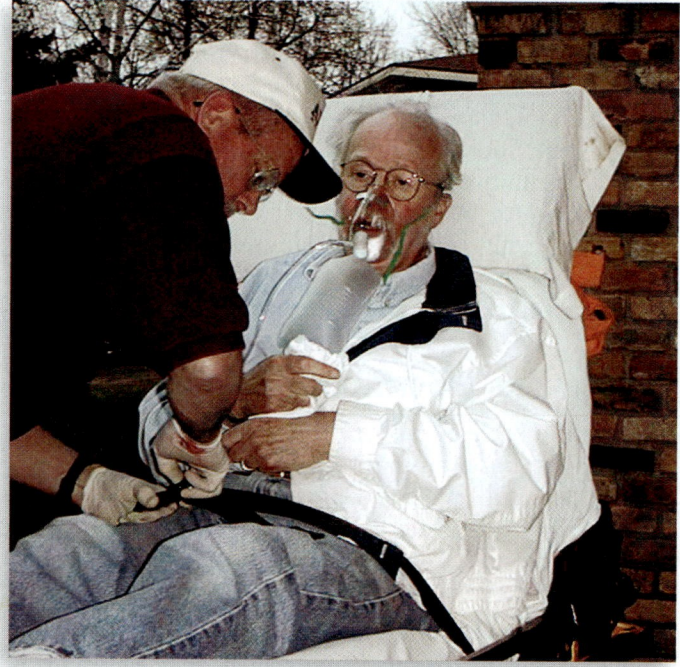

Figure 45-7 Competent elderly patients should be allowed to accept or refuse interventions.

Working in the Gray Zone

Competent adults of any age have the right to refuse medical care. As long as the patient is alert and oriented, understands the consequences of their decision, and is still refusing care, the patient's right to refuse should be respected. In patients older than age 64 years, recent studies point to negative outcomes within 72 hours of these patients having been seen by an EMT or paramedic.[28,29,30] One of these recent studies showed that older patients refused care not only because they did not want it, but because a significant number were worried about the cost of care (40%), and of more concern, because the paramedics implied that the patient did not need care (20%).[30] In this same study, 50% of the elderly patients interviewed said they would have changed their minds if they had spoken to a physician. Paramedics are significantly influential in the patient's decision to be transported.[31] As a paramedic, you are in a position of authority and respect, and patients will listen closely to your advice. If you are not able to convince a patient to go to the hospital with you, try placing the patient on the telephone with a base station medical control physician. This may help convince the patient.

nonelderly patients. When you suspect potential elder abuse, communicate your concerns and findings to the hospital personnel. Your assessment of the home situation and family dynamics may be invaluable in recognizing elder abuse. Without appropriate input regarding an elder's home situation, patients may be discharged to an unsafe and dangerous environment. DOT 6-4.14

Legal Considerations and Documentation

Most states require that intentional injuries (assault) be reported to the police. All 50 states have elder abuse statutes, and in most states, reporting of suspected abuse is mandatory. Suspected abuse or neglect should be referred to Adult Protective Services. Carefully document all findings: statements from the patient themselves, injuries noted on exam, environmental findings, the current living situation, as well as your concerns. DOT 6-4.15, 4.17

Sexual Assault

What Is Sexual Assault?

While the definition of **sexual assault** varies from state to state, it generally refers to any genital, anal, oral, or manual penetration of the victim's body by way of force and without the victim's consent. Individuals who have an impaired mental function due to alcohol, drugs, sleep, or unconsciousness are unable to give consent. The more traditional term **rape** is defined as forced vaginal, anal, or oral intercourse; force includes both psychological coercion and physical force. This definition includes attempted rapes, male and female victims, and heterosexual and homosexual rape. DOT 6-4.2, 4.6

Sexual Assault Statistics

Every two and one-half minutes, somewhere in America, someone is sexually assaulted.[32] Over recent years, an average of 223,280 victims of rape, attempted rape or sexual assault were reported to law enforcement.[33] However, research indicates that only 40% of sexual assaults are reported to law enforcement.[34] Approximately 18% of women have experienced a completed or attempted rape at some point in their lives, and 3% of American men report a completed or attempted rape during their lifetimes. Of women who report being raped, 54% were under the age of 18 when they were victimized. Rape in America has been termed a "tragedy of youth." Women who are sexually assaulted as children and adolescents are at greater risk of being sexually assaulted as an adult. While most victims of sexual assault are women, men can be assaulted by other men, and occasionally, women perpetrate sexual assaults against other women or men. The vast majority of sexual assaults (80%) are perpetrated by someone whom the victim knows.[35] DOT 6-4.1

Vulnerability Factors

While anyone may suffer sexual violence, certain factors increase the likelihood that an individual will suffer harm. Poverty makes the daily lives of women and children more dangerous (e.g., walking alone at night, less parental supervision) and may increase their risk for sexual assault. In addition, the economic status of poor women forces them into certain high-risk occupations, including prostitution. As mentioned above, young women are at higher risk of being raped compared to older women. Recreational drug use also increases the likelihood of rape. American Indian and Alaskan Natives report rape significantly more often than African American or Caucasian women.[35]

Characteristics and Consequences of Sexual Assault

Rape is a crime of violence and control, not a crime of passion. Thirty-two percent of women over 18 who are sexually assaulted report being injured in the assault, and 36% seek some type of medical treatment. General body trauma occurs more frequently than genital trauma. Injuries may include abrasions and bruises on the arms, head, and neck; signs of restraint (such as rope burns or mouth injuries); broken teeth; fractured nose or jaw from being punched or slapped; and muscle soreness or stiffness from restraint in positions allowing sexual penetration.[36] Between 4% and 30% of rape victims contract sexually transmitted diseases, including HIV, and it is estimated that over 32,000 pregnancies result each year from sexual assault. Victims of sexual assault exhibit a wide variety of psychological responses, including agitation, distress, hysteria, crying, calmness, and overly controlled responses.[35]

Assessment and Management

Not uncommonly, sexual assault results in traumatic injuries. The patient's medical needs should be attended to first and foremost. After managing any traumatic complaints, the paramedic should provide emotional support. A nonjudgmental, supportive attitude is essential; tact, kindness, and a compassionate manner will help ease the victim's distress. Move the patient to a private area before obtaining a history or performing a physical exam, and provide a blanket or sheet to cover the victim, if needed. A paramedic of the same sex as the victim should attend to the patient, if possible.

History

Limit your history-taking to questions that allow you to provide emergency medical care; the patient will be asked the specifics of the assault many times at the hospital and by law enforcement. Ascertain the following:

- What type of sexual assault occurred? (Vaginal, anal, or oral? Digital penetration? Foreign body?)
- Was there any type of physical assault?
- Was the victim punched, kicked, strangled, or forcibly held down?
- Was a weapon used?

Working in the Gray Zone

It has been said of sexual assault that it is the only crime in which the victim is expected to fight back before the victim is truly considered to be a victim. This expectation is unrealistic, unacceptable, and should not be considered when caring for a victim of sexual assault.

- Was there any loss of consciousness?
- What physical symptoms is the victim experiencing now? (Abdominal pain, pelvic pain, vaginal bleeding, etc.)
- General past medical history, especially if the patient is pregnant.

Physical Exam

Your physical examination should be aimed at identifying any physical trauma, outside the pelvic region, which may require attention. Facial fractures; fractures of the arms, wrist, and hands; chest trauma; abdominal trauma; and human bites are not uncommon. In general, examination of the genitalia and perineum is not necessary in the field unless the patient complains of severe pain or significant bleeding.

Evidence

While attending to the patient's physical and emotional needs, take steps to preserve any evidence from the crime scene. Disturb the crime scene as little as possible, especially prior to the arrival of law enforcement. Do not allow the patient to drink, brush the teeth, shower, defecate, or urinate. The victim should not change clothes, and clothing should be handled as little as possible. If evidence needs to be transported to the hospital (i.e., the victim's original clothing, condoms, tampons, towels, etc.), paper bags, not plastic bags, should be used.

CONNECTIONS For more information about how to handle crime scenes and potential evidence, review Chapter 52: Teamwork and Operational Interface.

Regardless of the patient's decision to file a police report or to pursue charges, and regardless of law enforcement's decision to request a forensic examination, hospital or clinic personnel should evaluate all sexual assault patients. Specially trained sexual assault nurse examiners may be used in certain areas of the country. All victims should be examined and treated for any traumatic injuries. It is important to transport these patients so that they may be treated prophylactically for sexually transmitted diseases and for pregnancy, if needed. DOT 6-4.14

Legal Considerations

While statutes vary from state to state, sexual assault is a crime, and law enforcement should be notified whenever you care for a victim of sexual assault. Local and state laws also vary with respect to the confidentiality of minors who have been assaulted; some areas allow minors to seek care and be treated for a sexual assault without obtaining parental consent.

In all situations, remember that sexual assault and rape are legal terms. The medical community should not try to decide if the victim is telling the truth or if the rape really happened. Patients presenting with a history of sexual assault should receive professional, competent, nonjudgmental care without personnel beliefs influencing the paramedic's actions. DOT 6-4.15

Documentation

Documentation of the assault should be factual, direct, and nonjudgmental. Lengthy comments concerning the patient's demeanor (hysterical, crying, overly calm) or detailed discussion of the sequence of events are not necessary. Discrepancies between the various medical and law enforcement records may unfairly jeopardize a victim's case in court. Utilize a straightforward description of the presenting complaint ("patient states she was vaginally and orally assaulted by two men") along with appropriate physical examination findings. Avoid the term "alleged sexual assault," which carries a negative connotation; "sexual assault by history" is preferred. DOT 6-4.17

CONNECTIONS Review Chapter 17: Documentation and Communication for more information on writing appropriate reports.

Giving care to patients who have been assaulted or abused can be stressful. You may be witness to some of the most aggressive, offensive, and abusive human behaviors in our culture. You may also find it difficult to care for someone who is injured or vulnerable but may be rejecting your help. Additionally, you may find yourself feeling upset and powerless to change or prevent this kind of violence. It is important to recognize that these feelings are normal reactions to stressful events. Some EMS providers may appear to be calloused or hardened as they try to shield their emotions from repeated exposure to such cases. Taking good care of yourself at these times is essential to staying healthy.

Summary

Abuse and neglect occur in every potential patient population and in every socioeconomic group. The paramedic should be vigilant for signs of abuse and neglect and be compassionate and professional when caring for victims. It is of equal importance that the paramedic's documentation is complete and consistant and that proper reporting is done in accordance with the law and the best interest of the patient.

Notes

1. National Clearinghouse on Child Abuse and Neglect, "What Is Child Abuse and Neglect?" (Washington, DC: 2004), http://nccanch.acf.hhs.gov/pubs/factsheets/whatiscan.cfm (accessed August 5, 2005).

2. National Clearinghouse on Child Abuse and Neglect, "Child Maltreatment 2003: Summary of Key Findings" (Washington, DC: 2005). http://nccanch.acf.hhs.gov/pubs/factsheets/canstats.cfm (accessed August 5, 2005).

3. National Clearinghouse on Child Abuse and Neglect, "Child Abuse and Neglect Fatalities: Statistics and Interventions" (Washington, DC: 2004). http://nccanch.acf.hhs.gov/pubs/factsheets/fatality.cfm (accessed August 5, 2005).

4. C. H. Kempe and R. E. Helfer, *Helping the Battered Child and his Family* (Philadelphia, PA: JB Lippincott, 1971).

5. U.S. Department of Health and Human Services, Administration on Children, Youth and Families, "Child Maltreatment 2003," (Washington, DC: US Government Printing Office, 2005), http://www.acf.hhs.gov/programs/cb/publications/cmreports.htm (accessed August 5, 2005).

6. National Center for Injury Prevention and Control, Center for Disease Control, "Child Maltreatment: Fact Sheet" (Atlanta, GA), http://www.cdc.gov/ncipc/factsheets/cmfacts.htm (accessed August 5, 2005).

7. J. A. Marx, ed., "Child Abuse," *Rosen's Emergency Medicine Concepts and Clinical Practice,* 5th ed. (St. Louis, MO: Elsevier Mosby, 2002).

8. D. L. Chadwick, S. Chin, C. Salerno, et al., "Deaths From Falls in Children: How Far is Fatal?" *The Journal of Trauma* (31) (October 1991): 1353–1355.

9. J. M. Whitworth, "Child Abuse." In *The Clinical Practice of Emergency Medicine,* 2nd ed. A. L. Harwood-Nuss, ed. (Philadelphia, PA: Lippincott-Raven, 1996).

10. A. L. Ganley, "Understanding Domestic Violence," In *Improving the Health Care Response to Domestic Violence: A Resource Manual for Health Care Providers,* 2nd ed., D. Lee, N. A. Durborown, and P. R. Salber, ed., The Family Violence Prevention Fund (1998). www.endabuse.org. (accessed October 18, 2006).

11. P. Salber and E. Taliaferro, "The Physicians Guide to Domestic Violence" (Volcano, CA: Volcano Press, 1995), http://www.volcanopress.com/bookprofile.cgi?stockno=P2900&cat=DV&backmsg (accessed October 18, 2006).

12. J. Abbott, "Injuries and Illnesses of Domestic Violence," *Annals of Emergency Medicine,* 29 (6) (June 1997): 781–785.

13. L. B. Burnett, "Domestic Violence," In eMedicine, S. A. Conrad, F. Talavera, R. C. Harwood, et al., eds., www.emedicine.com/emerg/topic153.htm (accessed August 1, 2005).

14. National Center for Injury Prevention and Control, "Intimate Partner Violence: Fact Sheet," www.cdc.gov/ncipc/factsheets/ipvfacts.htm (accessed August 1, 2005).

15. Family Violence Prevention Fund, "The Facts on Domestic Violence," http://endabuse.org/resources/facts/DomesticViolence.pdf (accessed August 1, 2005).

16. J. Abbott, R. Johnson, J. Koziol-McLain, et al., "Domestic Violence Against Women. Incidence and Prevalence in an Emergency Department Population," *Journal of the American Medical Association* 273 (22) (June 14, 1995): 1793–1797.

17. K. M. Feldhaus, J. Koziol-McLain, H. L. Amsbury, et al., "Accuracy of Three Brief Screening Questions for Detecting Partner Violence in the Emergency Department," *Journal of the American Medical Association* 277 (17) (May 7, 1997): 1357–1361.

18. Bureau of Justice Statistics Crime Data Brief, "Intimate Partner Violence, 1993–2001" (February 2003), www.ojp.usdoj.gov/bjs/pub/pdf/ipv01.pdf (accessed October 18, 2006).

19. P. Tjaden and N. Thoennes, "Prevalence, Incidence, and Consequences of Violence Against Women: Findings from the National Violence Against Women Survey," *National Institute of Justice and Centers for Disease Control* (November 1998), http://ncjrs.org/pdffiles/172837.pdf (accessed October 18, 2006).

20. National Institutes of Justice Research in Brief, "Violence Against Women: Identifying Risk Factors" (November 2004), http://www.ncjrs.org/pdffiles1/nij/197019.pdf (accessed October 18, 2006).

21. A. L. Kellermann, F. P. Rivara, N. B. Rushforth, et al., "Gun Ownership as a Risk Factor for Homicide in the Home," *The New England Journal of Medicine* 329 (15) (October 7, 1993): 1084–1091.

22. P. R. Salber and E. Taliaferro, "Domestic Violence." In *Emergency Medicine: Concepts and Clinical Practice*, 4th ed., Rosen and Barkin, eds. (St. Louis, MO: Mosby 1998), pp. 2908–2921.

23. National Center on Elder Abuse Fact Sheet, "Elder Abuse Prevalence and Incidence," http://www.elderabusecenter.org/pdf/publication/FinalStatistics050331.pdf (accessed August 2, 2005).

24. National Center on Elder Abuse: The Basics, "Major Types of Elder Abuse," http://www.elderabusecenter.org/default.cfm?p=basics.cfm (accessed August 2, 2005).

25. National Center on Elder Abuse, "National Elder Abuse Incidence Study: Final Report," Washington, DC: United States Department of Health and Human Services, Administration on Aging, 1998, http://www.aoa.gov/eldfam/Elder_Rights/Elder_Abuse/ABuseReport_Full.pdf (accessed October 18, 2006).

26. D. Anglin and H. R. Hutson, "Elder Abuse and Neglect." In *Rosen's Emergency Medicine: Concepts and Clinical Practice*, 5th ed., Marx, ed. (St. Louis, MO: Mosby 2002), pp. 875–882.

27. National Center on Elder Abuse Commissioned Review of Research, "Domestic Abuse in Later Life: Causation Theories," http://www.elderabusecenter.org/pdf/research/risks.pdf (accessed August 2, 2005).

28. S. Moss, T. Chan, J. Buchanan and J. Dunford, "Outcome Study of Prehospital Patients Signed Out Against Medical Advice by Field Paramedics," *Annals of Emergency Medicine* 31(2) (February 1998).

29. S. Knight et al., "Against All Advice: An Analysis of Out-of-Hospital Refusals of Care," *Annals of Emergency Medicine* 42(5) (November 2003).

30. Gary M. Vilke et al., "Follow-Up of Elderly Patients Who Refuse Transport After Accessing 9-1-1," *Prehospital Emergency Care* 6(4) (October/December 2002).

31. L. Bultman, J. Ho, and D. Page, "Undesignated Patients: Where Do They Go and Why?" Presented at the National Association of EMS Physician meeting Naples, Florida, January, 2005; *Prehospital Emergency Care* (January/February 2005).

32. RAINN Statistics, "Rape, Abuse, and Incest National Network (RAINN), Calculations Based on U.S. Department of Justice National Crime Victimization Survey 2003," http://www.rainn.org/90seconds.html (accessed October 18, 2006).

33. Bureau of Justice Statistics, U.S. Department of Justice, "National Crime Victimization Survey 2003" (Washington, DC), http://www.ojp.usdoj.gov/bjs/pub/pdf/cv03.pdf (accessed August 2, 2005).

34. Rape Abuse Incest National Network, "The Facts About Rape" (Washington, D.C.), http://www.rainn.org/statistics.html (accessed August 3, 2005).

35. National Center for Injury Prevention and Control, Centers for Disease Control, "Sexual Violence: Fact Sheet," http://www.cdc.gov/ncipc/factsheets/svfacts.htm (accessed August 4, 2005).

36. N. Riggs, D. Houry, G. Long, et al., "Analysis of 1.076 Cases of Sexual Assault," *Annals of Emergency Medicine* 35(4) (April 2000): 358–362.

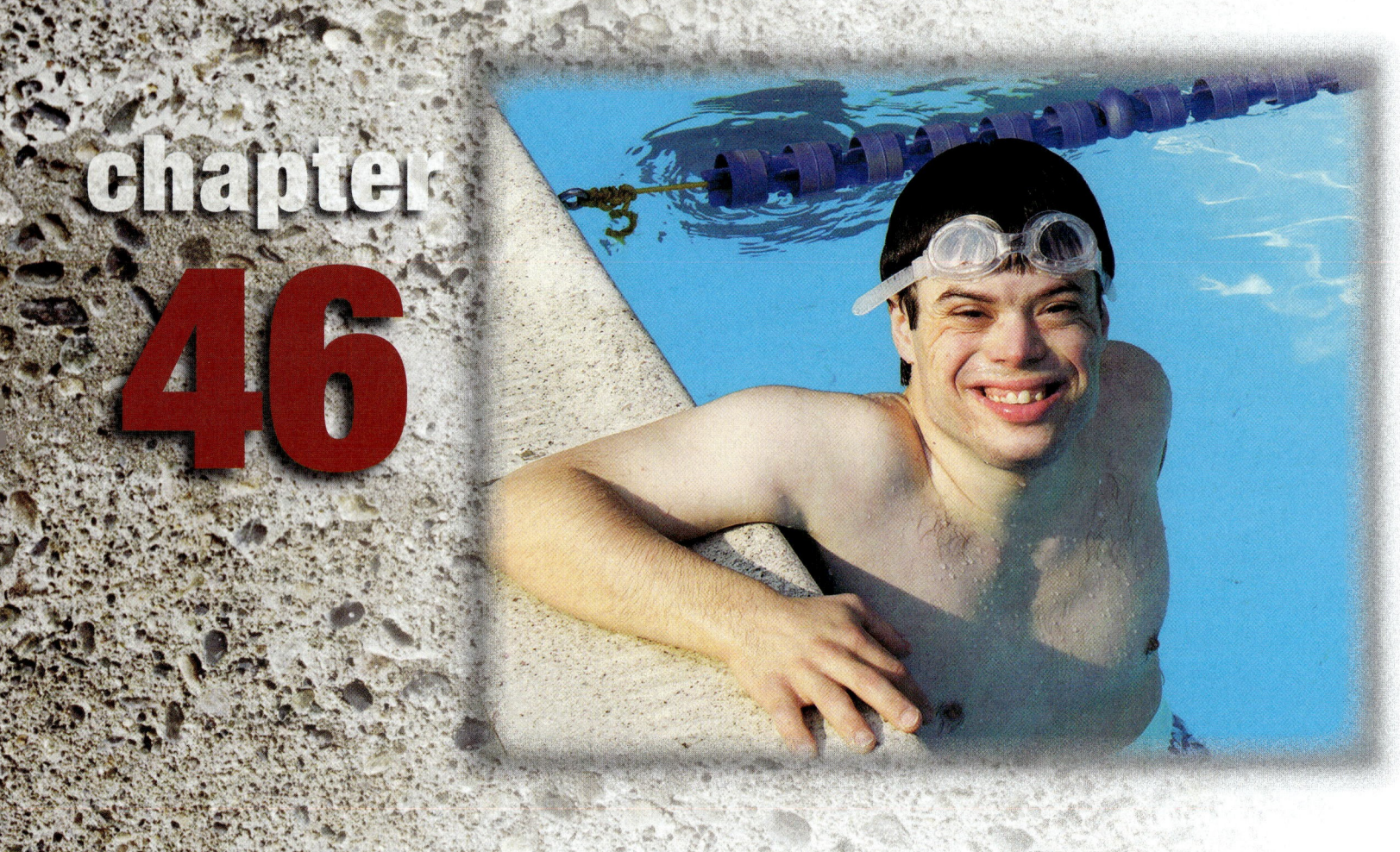

chapter
46

Patients with Special Challenges

"When we lose the right to be different, we lose the right to be free."

—Charles Evan Hughes

Need to Know

▶ The variety of special needs that patients may present with.

▶ The skills for communicating with patients having communication disabilities.

▶ The options concerning bariatric patients.

▶ How to safely care for patients with varying degrees of paralysis.

▶ How to safely and humanely work with patients suffering emotional and behavioral difficulties.

▶ How to care for patients with pathologic and psychiatric disorders.

▶ How to care for patients suffering from chronic diseases with potentially progressive disabilities such as neuromuscular disease, cystic fibrosis, and patients with chronic pain.

▶ How to compassionately care for patients suffering from cancer.

▶ How to care for patients with crippling birth defects.

▶ How to care for and protect patients with autoimmune disorders and depressed immune systems.

▶ Do	▶ Ask
• Familiarize yourself with facilities that care for special needs patients.	• Ask patients about their special needs and how they can help you care for them best.
• Identify special needs patients in your service area.	• Ask family members about the history of your patient and how they can help you care for the patient.
• Learn about special needs patients with whom you may need to change your typical response to medical situations and injuries.	• Ask special needs patients if they understand you and what you are doing. If not, you'll need another method of communication.
• Ensure that scenes are safe when dealing with emotional or behavioral emergencies.	• Ask for help when the size and weight of the patient exceeds your immediate ability to handle them safely.
• Treat bariatric patients with respect while taking special care to do so safely.	• Ask family members to be involved, when possible, showing them compassion and understanding as well.
• Show compassion for patients with a chronic debilitating disease or injury.	• Ask patients and family about their practices in caring for and protecting the patient.
• Become familiar with autoimmune disorders and immunosupressed patients in order to protect them while in your care.	• Ask patients and family what positions are most comfortable and what positions are uncomfortable or dangerous due to their condition.
• Give care and comfort to patients with physical impairments, paying special attention to comfort.	

Introduction

Paramedics are often called upon to care for a patient who presents special challenges. These challenges may be the reason that EMS was summoned, or they may be totally unrelated and just a normal part of the patient's life. A patient may have a physical challenge such as difficulty hearing or seeing, have a mental or emotional challenge, have a preexisting illness or disease, or have some other challenge that the patient must deal with on a daily basis.

Physical Challenges

Hearing Impairments

Hearing loss is the inability to recognize a range of sounds normally heard by someone without the deficiency. Hearing certain frequencies may be more difficult, or there may be equal loss at all frequencies. This deficiency can range anywhere from mild impairment to complete loss of hearing. The extent of the patient's impairment directly relates to the difficulty in the patient's ability to communicate.

The inability to hear is called **deafness.** A person may be partially or completely deaf and may be deaf in one ear or in both. The condition may be present at birth due to a congenital anomaly or injury during the birthing process, or it may occur later in life as a result of illness, injury, disease, or the aging process.

Over 25 million Americans have some degree of hearing loss, and as the population continues to age, this number will continue to rise.[1] Hearing loss can occur suddenly or gradually. See Skill Sheet 63: Verbal Communications.

Types of Hearing Loss

There are two main types of deafness: conductive hearing loss and sensorineural hearing loss.

Conductive Hearing Loss. Conductive hearing loss results from damage to the middle or outer ear. This type of hearing loss is often mechanical in nature and can sometimes be corrected by medicine or surgery. The cause may be as simple as a buildup of earwax or other matter, causing blockage in the ear canal, or it may be caused by injury to the middle or outer ear.

The most common cause of conductive hearing loss in children is otitis media, an infection in the middle ear. Ear infections are relatively common in children, usually caused by an upper respiratory infection that spread to the middle ear via the eustachian tube. A build-up of fluid in the middle ear impedes transmission of sound, causing hearing loss. Otitis media is usually treated with antibiotics. Surgery is sometimes performed for persistent infections and is highly successful.

Otosclerosis is the most common cause of conductive hearing loss in adults. The loss is caused by fixation of the stapes, the third bone in the middle ear. This fixation prevents the transmission of sounds, resulting in hearing loss. It is thought to be an inherited condition, affecting approximately 10% of the population, and only 10% of those with otosclerosis suffer from hearing loss.[1] Surgical removal of the stapes (stapedectomy) is very effective in treating otosclerosis.

Sensorineural Hearing Loss. Sensorineural hearing loss is usually the result of damage to the cochlea or auditory nerve, causing inability of nerve impulses to reach the auditory center in the brain, or it may be due to brain damage itself. The loss may be described as mild, moderate, severe, or profound and is measured in decibels. This type of hearing loss is often permanent.

There are numerous causes of sensorineural hearing loss (Box 46-1). It may be a congenital anomaly (present at birth) or an inherited condition. Some infants and children may be at-risk for sensorineural deafness, including preterm infants, neonates with severe respiratory problems, infants treated with ototoxic drugs such as furosemide or gentamycin, and those exposed to certain diseases, such as cytomegalovirus or rubella, in utero early in the pregnancy.

Hearing loss in adults results from a wide variety of causes, including infection, injury to the inner ear, or certain diseases. High doses of ototoxic drugs in adults can also result in sensorineural hearing loss. For example, aspirin toxicity often presents with **tinnitus,** or "ringing in the ears." Hearing impairment may also be caused by a tumor in the brain or middle ear. Acoustic neuroma is a benign tumor, causing hearing loss from pressure on the auditory nerve. Early detection and removal of the tumor may prevent future hearing loss.

Other causes of sensorineural hearing loss include injury to the brain or to the ear itself and chronic expo-

---

BOX 46-1   Causes of Hearing Impairment

Conductive Deafness (Curable)

- Infection
- Injury
- Impacted earwax, water, or other irritant

Sensorineural Deafness (Many Incurable)

- Congenital
- Birth injury
- Disease
- Medication-induced
- Viral infection
- Tumor
- Prolonged exposure to loud noise
- Aging

---

sure to loud noises such as heavy machinery, jack hammers, lawn mowers, and chain saws, as well as explosives and gunfire. Listening to loud music for prolonged periods of time can also lead to an impairment.

Presbycusis, or age-related hearing loss, is a progressive loss of the ability to hear high frequencies as people get older. The disorder occurs in about 25% of people aged 65 to 75 and in 70% to 80% of those over the age of 75.[2]

Nice to Know

Environmental-Induced Hearing Loss

How loud is too loud? Sounds above 90 decibels may cause such intense vibration that the inner ear is damaged, especially if the sound is prolonged. A decibel (dB) is a measurement of the loudness of a sound or strength of its vibration.

- 90 dB is about the loudness of a large truck about 5 yards away. Motorcycles, snowmobiles, and similar engines range around 85 to 90 dB.
- 100 dB is reached by some rock concerts.
- 120 dB is a jackhammer from 3 feet away.
- 130 dB is a jet engine from 100 feet away.

As a general rule of thumb, if you need to shout to be heard, the sound is loud enough that it can result in hearing loss.

Recognizing Hearing Impairment

It is essential to recognize hearing impairment early in an assessment and to make accommodations to ensure accurate assessment and treatment of the patient. The most obvious sign of hearing impairment is the use of a hearing aid or the use of sign language (Figure 46-1).

A patient with hearing impairment may exhibit behaviors that can be mistaken for head injury, such as the following:

- Speaking with poor diction
- Repeatedly asking questions
- Responding inappropriately to questions or commands
- Misunderstanding questions or responses to questions

Patients with hearing impairment may also exhibit an inability to respond to verbal communication in the absence of direct eye contact. If the patient is looking directly at the paramedic's lips while listening, it is important not to block the patient's view.

Accommodating Patients with Hearing Impairment

Accommodating patients with a hearing impairment may be as simple as finding their hearing aid or other listening devices. Family members may be helpful in identifying that a patient uses a hearing aid as well as locating it. If no family members are around, ask patients if they wear a hearing aid and where it might be, and then attempt to find it. Pen and paper may be a useful tool in communicating with the patient. Write directions, draw simple illustrations, and let the patient do the same.

When communicating with patients with hearing impairment, identify yourself and make sure patients know you are speaking to them. Get patients' attention by tapping them on the shoulder or moving directly in front of them so they can read your lips. Speak using a

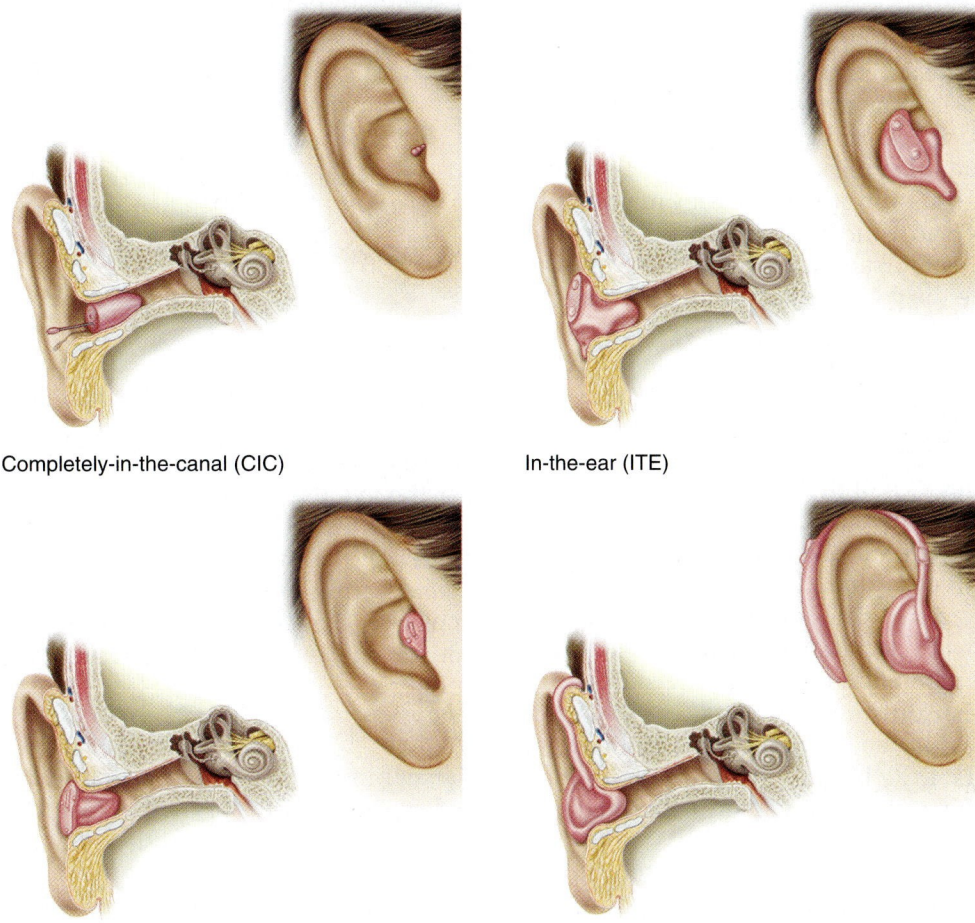

Completely-in-the-canal (CIC)

In-the-ear (ITE)

In-the-canal (ITC)

Behind-the-ear (BTE)

Figure 46-1 Various types of hearing aids.

normal voice. Although you may need to speak loudly into a patient's ear, do not shout. Since 80% of hearing loss is related to the loss of high-pitched sounds, use low-pitched sounds directly into a patient's ear canal. Eliminate any background sounds that may interfere with communication such as a television or radio.

Street Secrets

When using an interpreter, make sure you maintain eye contact with the patient instead of speaking to the translator.

If the patient uses sign language and there is no family member present to assist with interpretation, use some other means of communication, such as pen and pencil, until an interpreter can be found. Notify the receiving hospital as soon as possible so that they can have an interpreter present to assist in communicating with the patient. DOT 6-5.1, 6-5.2

Street Secrets

A patient with hearing loss or deafness may be mistaken as someone with a head injury or a patient who is mentally challenged. It is your responsibility to determine the patient's working level of communication and act accordingly. Patients may need an interpreter, writing board, or keyboard (possibly a TTY), or they may simply need to be able to read your lips or have a hearing aid in place. If a hearing aid cannot be located, try placing your stethoscope in the patient's ears and speak into the diaphragm.

Visual Impairments

Proper vision requires all of the structures of the eye to work perfectly to adapt to light and dark, perceive color, and accurately evaluate an object's location in space. The eyes are sensitive to differences in contrast and can provide detailed vision, which is measured as visual acuity, with "normal" visual acuity reported as 20/20. Legal blindness is defined as uncorrected visual acuity of 20/200. This means that a person with 20/200 vision can see at 20 feet what the "normal" eye would see at 200 feet. Although legally blind, some individuals may still be able to use vision to do certain things. Others have no vision at all.

It is estimated that 10 million people in the United States are blind or visually impaired.[3] Visual impairments result from numerous causes, including injury, disease, congenital anomalies, infection, and degeneration of the eyeball, optic nerve, or nerve pathways (Box 46-2).

BOX 46-2 Causes of Visual Impairment

Injury to Eye, Optic Nerve, or Brain
- Blunt trauma
- Penetrating trauma
- Burns (chemical or thermal)

Disease
- Diabetic retinopathy
- Glaucoma (increased intraocular pressure on the optic nerve)
- Stroke

Degeneration (Commonly Caused by the Aging Process)
- Lens
- Retina
- Optic nerve
- Nerve pathways

Congenital Disorders
- Cerebral palsy
- Premature birth

Infection
- Cytomegalovirus (CMV), causing inflammation of the retina (often seen in patients with AIDS)

Injury

Injury to the eye can result in permanent loss of vision. Injury could include a penetrating injury to the orbit, muscles, and tissues surrounding the orbit, optic nerves, or the eye itself, all of which can result in varying degrees of visual impairment. Chemical or thermal burns to the eyes can also cause loss of vision, which may be temporary or permanent. Corneal abrasion from a foreign object or a chemical burn associated with deployment of an airbag can result in temporary loss of vision.

Disease

Visual impairment can be caused by a disease process of the eye itself, or as the result of another disease process such as diabetes that affects the eye.

Glaucoma. Glaucoma is a group of eye diseases that causes gradual visual impairment. Vision loss is caused by damage to the optic nerve. Once thought to be caused primarily by high intraocular pressure (IOP), which damages the optic nerve, persons with "normal" IOP can also experience vision impairment from glaucoma.

There are two main types of glaucoma: open angle glaucoma and angle closure glaucoma. Open angle glaucoma is the most common form, affecting about 3 million persons in the U.S. It is caused by prolonged elevation of IOP of the inner eye due to clogging of the eye's drainage canals. There are often no warning signs and no symptoms of open angle glaucoma, with the exception of gradual loss of vision. It usually responds well to medication if diagnosed and treated early.

Angle closure glaucoma, also known as acute glaucoma or narrow angle glaucoma, is much less common. It differs from open angle glaucoma in that the eye pressure usually increases rapidly, causing the drainage canals to get blocked, similar to a clogged sink drain. With angle closure glaucoma, the space between the iris and cornea is not as wide open as it should be. The outer edge of the iris bunches up over the drainage canals when the pupil enlarges too much or too quickly. This can happen when entering a dark room. Symptoms of angle closure glaucoma include headaches, eye pain, nausea, rainbows around lights at night, and very blurred vision. Treatment of angle closure glaucoma usually involves medication and sometimes surgery to remove a small portion of the outer edge of the iris to unblock the drainage canals.

Glaucoma can occur as the result of an eye injury, inflammation, tumor, or in advanced cases of cataract or diabetes. It can also be caused by certain drugs such as steroids. This form of glaucoma may be mild or severe. The type of treatment depends on whether it is open angle or angle closure glaucoma.[4]

Cataracts.   A cataract is a film that clouds the lens of the eye, causing impaired or blurred vision. The lens is responsible for focusing light and producing sharp images. It is contained in a sealed capsule, and when old cells die, they become trapped in the capsule. Over time, the dead cells accumulate to form a cloudy film, resulting in blurred vision. For many, cataracts are a normal part of the aging process. In fact, cataracts are the leading cause of visual impairment in persons over the age of 55. Cataracts can also be caused by injury to the eye, medications, and certain diseases.[5]

For the person with cataracts, everything looks cloudy (Figure 46-2). Treatment is usually surgery to remove the clouded lens.

Diabetic Retinopathy.   Diabetic retinopathy is a complication of diabetes resulting from damage to the tiny blood vessels inside the retina. The retina is the light-sensitive tissue at the back of the eye that is necessary for good vision. At first, there may be no noticeable change in vision. Over time, however, the retinopathy can get worse, resulting in visual impairments. Most

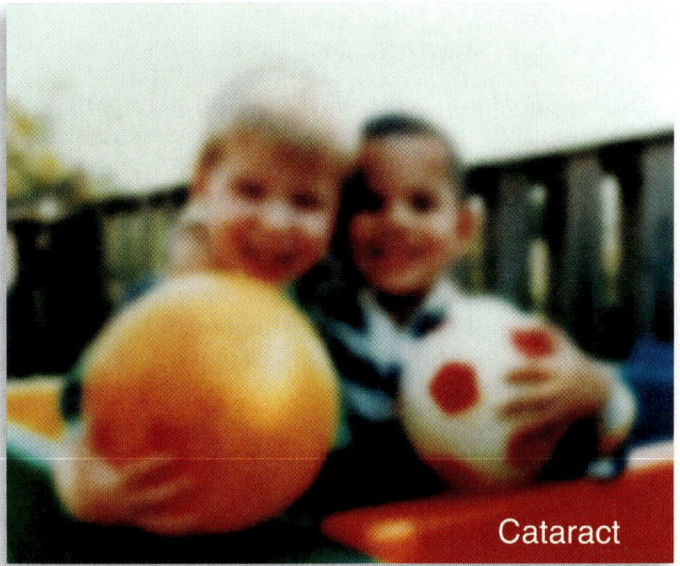

Figure 46-2   This is what a person with cataracts might see.

patients develop diabetic changes in the retina after approximately 20 years of the disease. Diabetic retinopathy usually affects both eyes.

According to the American Diabetes Association, diabetes is the leading cause of new cases of blindness among adults 20 to 74 years old, with diabetic retinopathy causing 12,000 to 24,000 new cases of blindness each year.[6]

Retinal Detachment.   Retinal detachment occurs when the retina inside the eye detaches from the outer scleral layer. The typical characteristics are sudden onset of what the patient describes as "a curtain falling down over the vision," sudden onset blurriness, "floaters" across the field of vision, spots, and flashing lights when eyes are closed. Rapid assessment and laser repair can save the sight but timing is critical. Immediate transport while calming the patient is all that is required. The patient will likely be scared and anxious, particularly if vision is lost or disrupted. Maintain constant contact and touch to reassure the patient.

Recognition of Patients with Visual Impairments

Recognizing that a patient may suffer from a visual impairment may be difficult unless the patient is completely blind. Many patients with visual impairments live active, independent lives. Even patients who are blind can live independently with the use of tools such as a walking stick or service dog. When assessing a patient, it is important to determine if the visual impairment is a permanent disability or a new symptom of illness or injury.

Accommodating Patients with Visual Impairments

As you approach a patient with a visual impairment, make certain to identify yourself so the patient knows you are there. Take extra measures to describe everything that you are doing as you do it. If the patient has special devices to assist with sight (glasses, a magnifying glass, a walking cane, etc.), retrieve the items for the patient. If the patient is ambulatory, guide the patient by leading them rather than by pushing or pulling. Allow the patient to hold onto your arm, rather than you holding onto the patient's arm.

If the patient has a service dog, *do not* pet or disturb the dog without the patient's permission. Based on local protocols, transport the dog to the hospital with the patient. DOT 6-5.4, 6-5.5, 6-5.6

Working in the Gray Zone

Consider a patient who has multiple sensory impairments, unable to hear, unable to see, and is a passenger in a vehicle that has flipped over on its roof. Recognizing this patient's impairments as soon as possible is important, but your response is equally important. Contact is imperative. Picture yourself in this situation. Everything is out of position. You can't hear or see. You are in pain, and you know something horrible has happened. Contact would be important, letting the victim know that someone knows about the bad situation and is working to help. Just holding a hand could make the difference.

Speech Impairments

Speech impairments include disorders of language, articulation, voice production, and fluency (Box 46-3). The type of impairment is often related to the area of the brain affected as identified in Figure 46-3.

Communication disorders, also known as **aphasia,** result from damage to the language centers of the brain. They usually occur as a result of brain injury, tumor, or a CVA. Aphasia involves the loss of communication skills previously learned and commonly occurs following strokes or in people with brain tumors or degenerative diseases that affect the language areas of the brain. This term does not apply to children who have never developed communication skills. In some cases of aphasia, the problem eventually resolves itself, but in others, the condition is permanent.

Dysarthria or articulation disorders are caused by the inability of an individual to produce sounds. Speech

BOX 46-3 \ Causes of Speech Impairment

Language Disorders
- Stroke
- Head injury
- Brain tumor
- Delayed development
- Pervasive development disorder
- Hearing loss
- Lack of stimulation
- Emotional disturbance

Articulation Disorders
- Damage to nerve pathways
- Delayed development

Voice Production Disorders
- Disorder affecting vocal cords
- Hormonal or psychiatric disturbance
- Severe hearing loss

Fluency Disorders
- Etiology is not fully understood

can be slurred, indistinct, slow, or nasal. Dysarthria usually results from damage to the nerve pathways from the brain to the muscles of the larynx, mouth, or lips. It may be caused by brain injury or by certain diseases including multiple sclerosis and Parkinson's disease. In children, it may result from hearing problems. Degenerative neurological disorders affecting the cerebellum or brainstem can also cause dysarthria, as can stroke and any facial weakness, such as Bell's palsy or tongue weakness. It may also be caused by excess medications such as narcotics, phenytoin, or carbamazepine or by alcohol intoxication.

Voice production disorders are characterized by hoarseness, harshness, inappropriate pitch, and abnormal nasal resonance. DOT 6-5.30, 6-5.31, 6-5.32e

Recognition of Patients with Speech Impairments

Language Disorders (Aphasia). Patients may demonstrate aphasia by slowness to understand speech and difficulties with vocabulary and sentence structure. Aphasia can affect children and adults, resulting in difficulties in an individual's ability to speak or comprehend words (written or spoken).

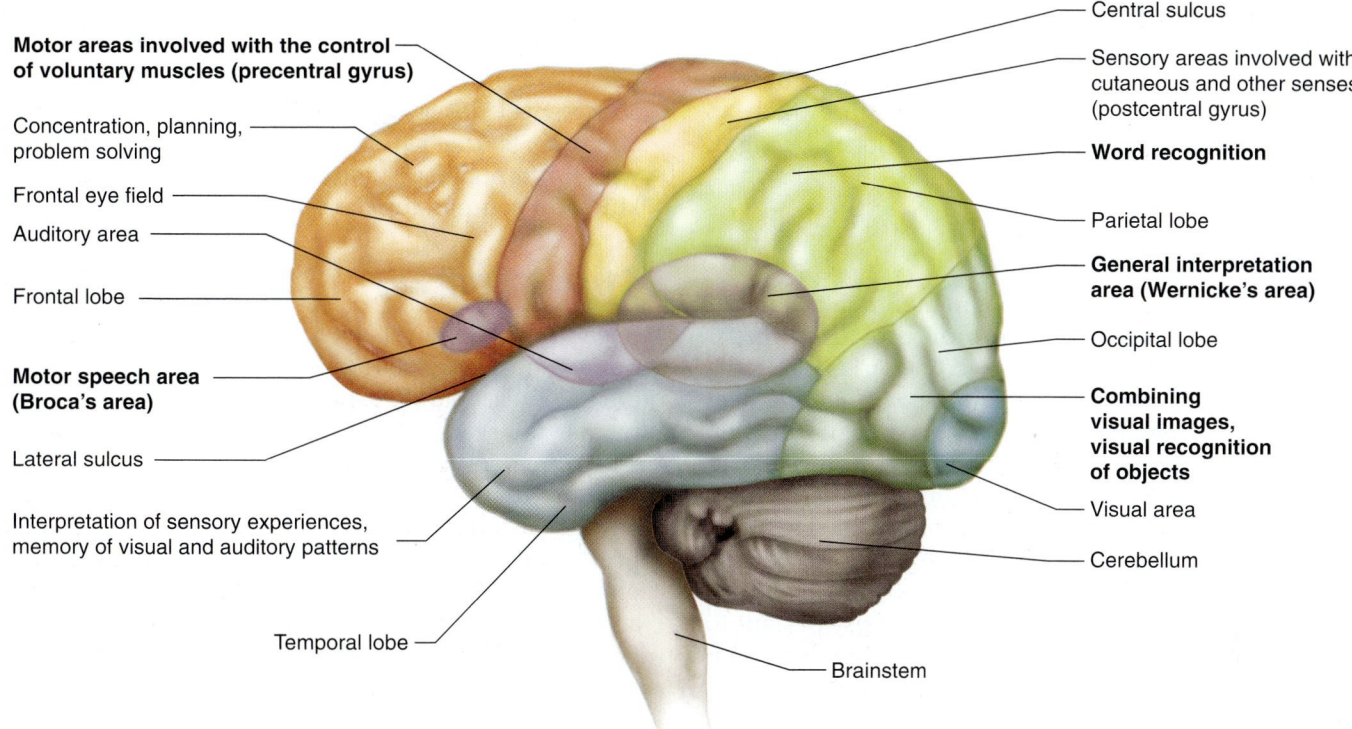

Figure 46-3 Anatomy of the brain.

Articulation Disorders (Dysarthria). Patients with dysarthria often exhibit speech that is slurred, indistinct, slow, or nasal. It is generally apparent in daily conversation where there is difficulty expressing certain sounds or words.

Voice Production Disorders. A patient with a voice production disorder may complain of hoarseness as a result of speaking. In addition, their speech tends to be harsh, with an inappropriate pitch or abnormal nasal resonance.

Fluency Disorders. The primary identifying factor of a fluency disorder is stuttering.

Accommodating Patients with Speech Impairments

Patients with speech impairments are often frustrated by their difficulties in communicating easily. Patience is essential when dealing with this type of patient. Allow the patient time to respond to questions and provide aids, such as pen and paper to write out responses to questions, whenever possible. DOT 6-5.7, 6-5.8, 6-5.9

Obesity

More than half of the people in the U.S are overweight. Being obese, however, is different from simply being overweight. An adult female is considered obese when her weight is 25% more than the maximum desirable weight for her height. A male is considered obese when his weight is more than 20% over the maximum. Anyone more than 100 pounds overweight is considered morbidly obese.

Alarmingly, the rates of obesity are climbing, and even more concerning is the fact that the number of children and adolescents who are obese has doubled in the last 20 years.[7]

There are various reasons for obesity, including the following:

- Consumption of more food than the body can use
- Excess alcohol intake
- Sedentary lifestyle
- Low basal metabolic rate
- Genetic predisposition

The most common reason for obesity is eating too much of the wrong foods and not getting enough exercise. The body cannot store protein or carbohydrates, so any excess protein or carbohydrate intake is converted to fat for storage. One pound of excess weight represents approximately 3,500 excess calories.

In addition to decreased mobility and chronic hypoxemia due to inadequate ventilation, obesity increases a person's risk of illness, including diabetes, hypertension, depression, osteoarthritis, coronary artery disease, stroke, high cholesterol, and kidney and gallbladder disorders and may increase a person's risk for some types of cancer.

Genetic factors also contribute to obesity. In fact, children of obese parents are 10 times more likely to be obese than children with parents of normal weight. DOT 6-5.30, 6-5.31, 6-5.32b

Accommodating Obese Patients

The main responsibility of the paramedic in caring for an obese patient is to provide professional and thorough emergency care. Regardless of the cause of the condition, it is essential to obtain a complete medical history, which may be extensive since obesity is often associated with other chronic medical conditions.

When assessing the patient, determine if symptoms are new or part of a chronic condition. This may be difficult at times, however, since an obese patient often blames aches, pains, and difficulties on the excess weight. Just moving can cause an obese patient to become short of breath. Difficulty breathing, however, may also be caused by any number of serious medical conditions. As such, it is essential to adequately assess each symptom to identify and treat any life threats. Determine if any preexisting symptoms have been more severe than usual, and if so, for how long.

Flexibility in assessment, performing vital signs, and actually transporting an obese patient is key. When performing a physical assessment, use appropriately sized diagnostic devices such as an extra large blood pressure cuff. It may be necessary to place ECG electrodes on the patient's arms and thighs rather than on the chest if excessive adipose tissue presents a problem. If the patient is so obese that he or she cannot lean forward to listen to lung sounds posteriorly, listen anteriorly.

Determine what medications the patient is taking. An obese patient may be taking a large number of medications due to the number of associated complications. Also, determine if the patient has recently tried any fad diets or taken dietary supplements.

Transporting an obese patient may be particularly problematic. Most stretchers are not designed to accommodate an obese patient. Make certain to request enough manpower to lift the patient. *Do not* risk personal injury. Inform the emergency department of the need for additional resources as well. Make sure that both side rails on the stretcher are up and locked and that the patient is strapped to the stretcher before moving. Otherwise, the patient's weight may shift during transport, causing the stretcher to topple. If there is a possibility of cardiac arrest, place a backboard on the stretcher first.

Consider keeping the stretcher in a low position while moving an obese patient. If that is not possible, ensure additional EMS providers are placed around the stretcher to serve as "spotters" while the stretcher is moved.

At all times, it is essential to maintain professionalism when caring for an obese patient. Put aside any personal feelings, and treat the patient with the dignity and respect deserved. Finally, try not to draw undue attention to the patient. Obesity is a sensitive issue, which often causes embarrassment to the patient. Be kind and compassionate. DOT 6-5.10, 6-5.11

Street Secrets

Recently, there have been a number of people who have undergone gastric bypass surgery and related procedures. These patients have limited intake of food at regular intervals during the day, usually no more than 4 ounces at a time. After surgery, the stomach can hold no more than 1 cup of food. These patients usually do not eat and drink at the same time, but rather wait approximately 30 minutes after eating to drink, and then only take small sips. They also take supplements and are limited in the types of medications they may ingest. For example, they are not permitted to take aspirin or ibuprofen, but rather only acetaminophen for pain.

Paralysis

You may respond to a call for assistance and find the patient is unable to move some or all of their extremities as a result of a previous traumatic event or medical condition. In this situation, the paramedic must assess and treat the patient's chief complaint while making accommodations for the fact that the patient is paralyzed.

Paralysis is the complete loss of muscle function, which can affect a small area (localized) or be widespread (generalized). Paralysis is a major medical event that can result in severe depression. Paralysis can be temporary or permanent, one-sided (unilateral) or two-sided (bilateral), and can affect the lower extremities (paraplegic) or upper and lower extremities (quadriplegic). Paralysis can also be an indication of an acute life-threatening problem such as Guillain-Barré syndrome.

Paralysis generally takes two forms, paraplegia and quadriplegia. A **paraplegic** patient is paralyzed from the waist down as a result of injury to the spinal cord below the seventh cervical vertebrae. **Quadriplegia** is paralysis of both arms and legs as well as the trunk and is caused by injury to the cervical spinal cord. Injury to the spinal cord at or above the level of C4 vertebrae will also result in paralysis of the muscles needed for respiration, thereby requiring artificial ventilation via a ventilator for the patient to remain alive.

In the case of stroke, paralysis may be more localized such as paralysis of some facial muscles, causing facial drooping or hemiplegia, where there is paralysis on only one side of the body.

BOX 46-4 Causes of Paralysis

- Cerebrovascular accident (stroke)
- Bell's palsy
- Spinal cord injury
- Poliomyelitis (polio)
- Amyotrophic lateral sclerosis (ALS)
- Botulism
- Paralytic shellfish poisoning
- Guillain-Barré syndrome

In the U.S., the majority of paralysis results from stroke (cerebrovascular accident, CVA) or from trauma, such as a fracture of the spine in the back or neck. Paralysis is usually irreversible. Other causes of paralysis include infectious diseases, genetic diseases, autoimmune diseases, and toxic conditions (Box 46-4).

If cranial nerves are damaged, the patient may have difficulty with chewing and swallowing. Prolonged immobility can cause serious complications, including skin sores, infections, and muscle atrophy. The use of splints may help prevent muscle contractions.

Patients who are paralyzed are very susceptible to secondary infections, especially UTIs, which are often accompanied by fever and associated with in-dwelling foley catheters. Even quadriplegics can sense the onset of an infection. If the patient tells you he feels like he has a UTI, he most likely does.

Street Secrets

Always maintain the Foley catheter collection bag below the level of the bladder. This prevents backflow of urine, which leads to infection.

Accommodating the Paralyzed Patient

If the patient is on a home ventilator, it is essential to maintain a patent airway and assist with ventilations during care and transport. The patient's ventilator may be transportable, or the ambulance may have one on board. If taking the patient's ventilator, ask a family member how it works or ask them to accompany the patient in the ambulance. Always have a bag-mask and oxygen equipment readily available in case the ventilator fails. Notify the hospital of the need for ventilatory assistance upon your arrival. If the patient has a tracheostomy, keep suction equipment readily available since obstruction from mucus is fairly common. These pa-

tients are often extremely anxious, so spend extra time reassuring the patient prior to changing any of the patient's life support system.

If the patient's injury was recent, he may have an external spine immobilizer (commonly called a "halo" because of a metal ring that encircles the patient's head) in place. If so, it is important to stabilize the device prior to transport. The patient and family are most likely well versed in dealing with the immobilizer. If you are unsure of how to move the patient, call the patient's physician.

The patient may also have a **colostomy** or **ileostomy** if the patient does not have normal bowel or bladder function. Take extra supplies with you in the ambulance in case you need to change the ostomy bag. Take care when moving the patient.

Patients who have lived with paralysis for some time have a good handle on their illness and treatment, as well as the best way to move themselves with assistance. The patient may have a trapeze over the bed to help with movement. For transfer from a bed to a stretcher, a transfer board is often used, as well as a drawsheet. Ensure that there is adequate assistance for transfer of the patient, and transport any ambulatory assistance devices with the patient (wheelchair, cane, walker, etc). DOT 6-5.12, 6-5.13

Once the patient is transferred to the ambulance cot, insure there are no wrinkles present in the sheet or blankets under the patient as these can cause pressure sores. If the transport is long, make sure the patient is repositioned to allow circulation to continue in dependent places on the body. Inspect the heels and calves as well as the buttocks and shoulders for pressure sores.

Street Secrets

A paralyzed person sometimes suffers from sudden leg spasms in one or both legs. This can be relieved by placing gentle, firm, direct, downward pressure on the patient's kneecaps, by holding the legs still on the bed, or by applying downward pressure along the side pieces of a wheelchair.

Mental and Emotional Challenges

Mental illness includes any form of psychiatric disorder including anxiety, depression, paranoia, schizophrenia, phobias, bulimia, anorexia, obsessive-compulsive disorder, and a large list of other disorders. EMS may be summoned because of the patient's mental illness or because of a different chief complaint. It is important to recognize that patients with mental impairments may be taking a large number of medications and may have other physical problems as well. It is important to recognize that a disorder such as anorexia or bulimia can cause serious complications including dehydration and electrolyte imbalance, resulting in possible cardiac problems.

Patients with emotional or mental impairments may be incapable of caring for themselves. They may appear unclean or malnourished. They may be depressed or even suicidal. Attempt to determine if they have taken their prescribed medications on a regular basis, or whether they have been drinking alcohol, which often intensifies the effects of medications.

Etiologies of Mental Illness

Mental illness is generally divided into two groups: psychoses and neuroses. Psychosis is caused by a complex, biochemical disease of the brain and is characterized by thought disorders. This type of disorder generally includes schizophrenia, bipolar disorder (formerly called manic-depressive disorder), and organic brain disorder. Many patients with psychosis do not know they are ill.

Neuroses, on the other hand, are diseases related to personality. Patients with neuroses generally remain "in touch" with reality and are aware of their disorders. Major neurotic disorders include obsessive-compulsive disorder (OCD), phobias, and depression.

CONNECTIONS Specific mental and emotional disorders are covered in detail in Chapter 40: Behavioral and Psychiatric Disorders.

Accommodating Patients with Mental Illness

Personal safety and the safety of the crew are the top priorities in any emergency situation. When caring for a patient with mental illness, it is important to always be prepared for any potentially violent behavior and to take steps to ensure your safety. Never allow the patient to stand between you and the door. Evaluate the patient's behavior. If there is any evidence of violent behavior, leave the scene immediately and summon police assistance. It is not abandonment to leave a potentially hazardous environment to summon additional help. Go to the ambulance, move a safe distance from the scene, and summon assistance.

Assess the patient as much as possible. Identify medications the patient may be taking. A patient with mental illness may take numerous medications. Patients who have been on medication for prolonged periods of time may have lists already prepared for you. If not, just take all the prescription bottles with you to the hospital. Determine the last dose(s) the patient has taken and, if appropriate, why the patient is taking the medication.

If a patient is considered a threat to self or others, it is possible to "involuntarily commit" the patient. This requires use of the "mental health hold" process. While EMS personnel are often called to assist with taking a mentally ill patient to the hospital, ultimate responsibility usually rests with law enforcement. If you do not feel safe transporting the patient, refuse to do so or insist the police officer accompany you and the patient in the back of the ambulance. Patients in police custody handcuffs or plastic ties should be accompanied by law enforcement in the back of the ambulance whenever possible. DOT 6-5.14, 6-5.15, 6-5.16, 6-5.17, 6-5.24, 6-5.25, 6-5.26, 6-5.27, 6-5.28, 6-5.29

Street Secrets

Treat a patient with mental illness as you would any patient. Patients with mental illness also experience myocardial infarctions, hypoglycemic episodes, dislocated shoulders, and other illnesses and injuries.

Developmental Disabilities

A developmental disability involves impaired or insufficient development of the brain, resulting in the inability of an individual to learn and function at a usual rate. There are various causes for developmental disabilities, including genetic problems such as Down syndrome or the result of brain injury due to trauma or hypoxia. Brain injury can occur before, during, or after birth.

Many patients with developmental disabilities function in normal day-to-day activities in school and society in general. They might live with their families, in residential facilities, or in group homes, depending on the severity of their disabilities. DOT 6-5.18, 6-5.19

Autism Spectrum Disorders

Pervasive development disorders (PDDs) are neurobiological disorders that are present from birth. PDD comprises five disorders: autism, Asperger's syndrome, PDD-Not Otherwise Specified (PDD-NOS), Rett's disorder, and childhood disintegrative disorder. The last two are quite rare. The PDDs are often called **autism spectrum disorders (ASD)**. They affect the brain's normal development of social, communication, and sensory skills.

The exact number of people with ASDs is not known. However, it is estimated that as many as one in every 150 children are affected by the disorder, and boys are three to four times more likely to be affected than girls.[8] This makes ASDs more common than childhood cancer, Down syndrome, muscular dystrophy, or cerebral palsy.[9] Symptoms of these disorders appear in the first three years of life although they are sometimes diagnosed much later.

Common presenting features of ASDs vary from mild to severe and include impaired social interactions, impaired verbal and nonverbal communication, and restricted and repetitive patterns of behavior (Box 46-5). Most children and adults with ASDs look "normal."

BOX 46-5   Characteristics of Autistic Spectrum Disorders

Communication

- Is unable to start or sustain a social conversation
- Exhibits slow or nonexistent language development (autism)
- Talks nonstop about a favorite topic (Asperger's syndrome)
- Uses **echolalia** (repetitive words or memorized passages, like commercials)
- Does not refer to self correctly (for example, says "You want water" when the child means "I want water")
- Communicates with gestures instead of words

Social Interaction

- Appears withdrawn
- Prefers to spend time alone rather than with others
- May not respond to eye contact or smiles
- May avoid eye contact (eye contact is described as "painful" by some with ASDs)
- Shows a lack of empathy
- Does not make friends

Response to Sensory Information

- Has heightened sensitivity to sight, hearing, touch, smell, or taste
- Exhibits a heightened *or* diminished response to pain

- May withdraw from physical contact because it is overstimulating or overwhelming
- Does not startle at loud noises *or* may find normal noises painful and hold hands over ears
- Rubs surfaces, mouths or licks objects

Play

- Shows little pretend or imaginative play
- Does not imitate the actions of others
- Prefers solitary or ritualistic play

Behaviors

- Has a short attention span
- Uses repetitive body movements
- Shows a strong need for sameness and does not handle change well
- "Acts up" with intense tantrums
- Has very narrow interests
- Demonstrates perseveration (gets stuck on a single topic or task)
- Shows aggression to others or self
- Is overactive or very passive
- Lacks fear of risky situations

Those on the mild end of the spectrum often appear as only eccentric or quirky. People with **Asperger's syndrome** have at least average intelligence and have no delay in language acquisition. Those with **autism** have delayed language skills (although most are verbal), and most (70%) also have mental retardation. Very few people have the most severe form of autism. Those who do tend to be nonverbal or have very limited language, and the paramedic would need to rely on the autistic patient's caregiver to help with communication.[10]

These conditions appear to be linked to abnormal biology and chemistry in the brain; however, the exact cause of ASDs is unknown. Genetics is thought to play a role in their development, and the effects of the environment on development of ASDs are being studied.[10]

Recognizing a Patient with ASD

Symptoms of ASDs often present by the time a child is 18 months of age and generally involve difficulties in verbal and nonverbal communication, social interactions, and pretend play.

Patients with an ASD may perform repeated body movements, show unusual attachments to objects, or have unusual distress when dealing with change. They may exhibit unusual or extreme sensitivities in sight, hearing, touch, smell, or taste. For example, a child with autism might refuse to wear "itchy" clothes or a shirt with a string hanging from it and may become unduly distressed if forced. Some combination of the factors outlined in Box 46-5 will be present in varying degrees.[11]

Accommodating a Patient with Autism

Caring for a sick or injured child with an ASD can be difficult. While autistic children are alike in many ways, they also differ in many ways. Therefore, each situation could be different, depending on the child. The parent or caregiver of the child is the best source of information for the paramedic because they know their child the best. As such, one of the first things a paramedic should do is to ask the parent if they can offer any help in calming the child. This is true regardless of the age of the child (Box 46-6).

BOX 46-6   A Boy with Asperger's Syndrome

Will is 6 years old and has Asperger's syndrome. He is first and foremost a bright, happy boy. He has just finished kindergarten in a mainstream classroom. He has friends, he loves to ride his scooter and play soccer, and he swims like a fish.

He is different from his typical peers in that he can be quite rigid; he likes things done the same way every time—drive the same route, line up the toys in the same order, and so on. Social interaction with children did not come naturally to him; he had to be taught how to play with others. He can get overwhelmed by groups—even at his own birthday parties—but has learned to take a break in his room when he starts feeling stressed. He has good eye contact with people he knows, but he has to be reminded to make eye contact when he meets someone new.

Will has a lot of special interests, and they bring him great joy. His particular favorites are clocks, trains, and the solar system. He will talk nonstop about his favorite subjects, and he has to be reminded to let other people have a turn to talk.

He would be frightened of being cared for by a paramedic. He overreacts to pain, so being in pain from an injury or illness would be especially hard for him. He has extremely sensitive hearing, so the ambulance sirens would be excruciating to him. But if his mother or father were present, his beloved blanket was brought along, and he was allowed to tell the paramedic all the planets in order, he would cooperate.

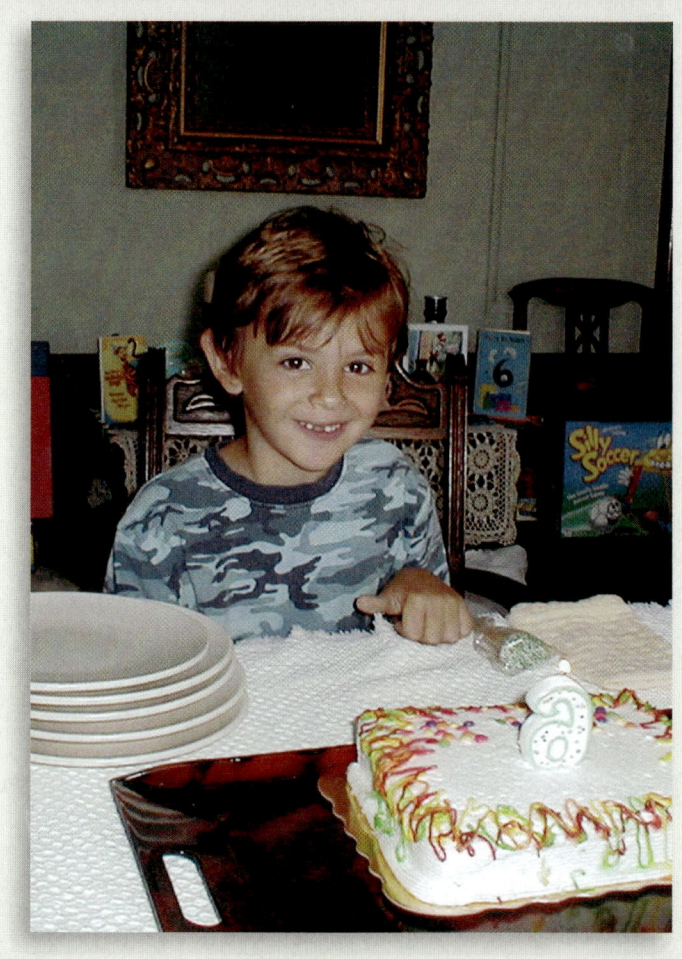

In general, autistic children are fearful of strangers and of change, and many dislike being touched (because they are hypersensitive), so an encounter with a paramedic can be extremely difficult for them. Whenever possible, gain their trust: Explain what you are doing and why you are doing it. Ask them how they prefer to be handled. Many children with ASD have a favorite object (blanket, toy, etc.) or subject they like to discuss. Allow them to keep their object or discuss their special interest; it is soothing to them. Use restraint as a last resort. If a child is hypersensitive, restraint is painful and frightening.

Street Secrets

If an IV is absolutely necessary in the prehospital environment, have the mother hold the child on her lap while wrapping her legs around the child's legs and holding one arm. Have another person hold the arm being used for the IV. The paramedic can then attempt IV insertion.

If emergency care is necessary and restraint of the child is not possible, consider contacting medical command for authorization to administer a sedative such as midazolam per local protocols.

Most adults with ASDs have learned coping skills as they have matured, and therefore aren't particularly difficult to work with although you may have to be extra patient and accommodate their special needs or interests.

A paramedic's first responsibility is personal safety and then safety of the crew. If you do not feel safe while caring for a patient with autism, leave the scene and summon assistance.

For additional information on autism spectrum disorders, visit the Autism Society of America (www. autism-society.org), Online Asperger Syndrome Information and Support (www.udel.edu/bkirby/asperger/), and Dennis Debbaudt's website, (www.autismriskman agement.com/index.htm), which includes video clips for training police officers on interactions with people with ASDs.

Down Syndrome

Down syndrome, also known as **trisomy 21,** is a chromosome abnormality due to an extra copy of the 21st chromosome. This syndrome usually, although not always, results in mental retardation. It is the most common single cause of human birth defects with an occurrence in one out of every 660 births, and an increased incidence in babies born to women over the age of 40.

Individuals with Down syndrome have a widely recognized characteristic appearance (see chapter opening photo (page 1132) and Box 46-7). The head may be

---

BOX 46-8 Physical Characteristics of a Patient with Down Syndrome

- Eyes that slope up at outer corners
- Folds of skin on either side of the nose, covering the inner corners of the eye
- Small face and features
- Large and protruding tongue
- Flattening on back of the head
- Short and broad hands

---

smaller than normal (microcephaly) and abnormally shaped. Prominent facial features include upward slanting eyes. Retardation of normal growth and development is typical, and most affected children never reach average adult height. While some individuals may be severely mentally retarded, many are only mildly impaired. The IQ of these patients varies from 30 to 80. An average IQ of 80 to 120 is considered "normal." See Box 46-8 for additional physical characteristics of a patient with Down syndrome.

Individuals with Down syndrome often have other medical conditions as well, including congenital heart defects (25% of the cases); gastrointestinal abnormalities, including obstruction of the esophagus, duodenum, and GI tract; and a higher incidence of acute lymphocytic leukemia (ALL). (See Box 46-9 for additional complications associated with Down syndrome.)

BOX 46-7 A Young Man with Down Syndrome

Jason is 25 years old and has Down syndrome. Jason graduated from high school at age 21 and now works full time at a hotel in the housekeeping department. He is an excellent and reliable worker. Jason lives at home with his mother, has a girlfriend (who also has Down syndrome), and enjoys an active social life with friends, extended family, and his younger siblings.

Jason is a sports fanatic, both as a participant with Special Olympics, and as a fan of the Baltimore Orioles and Baltimore Ravens. He reads the sports section of the newspaper daily to keep up with his favorite teams.

Jason has some of the typical health problems associated with Down syndrome but overall is a happy, healthy, productive young man.

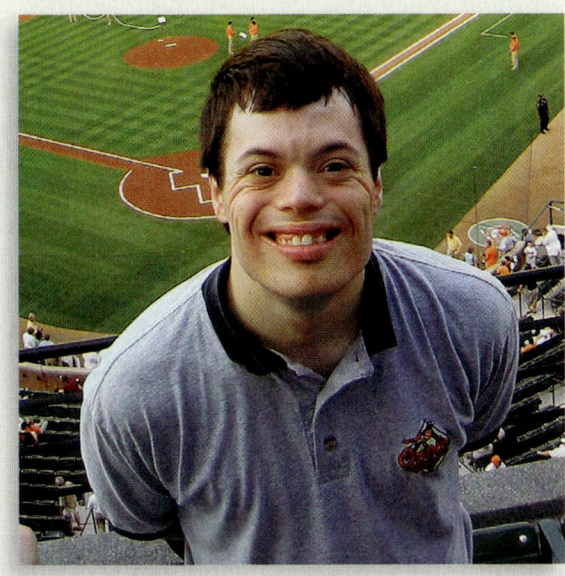

BOX 46-9 Complications Associated with Down Syndrome

- Hearing loss
- Problems with vision
- Cardiac abnormalities
- Increased incidence of acute leukemia
- Frequent ear infections
- Increased susceptibility to infections
- GI disorders (imperforate anus, esophageal atresia, duodenal atresia)
- Blocked airway during sleep
- Dementia in older patients
- Compression injury of the spinal cord

Street Secrets

Because of anatomical differences in individuals with Down syndrome, managing the airway may be difficult. Remember that the tongue may take up a greater amount of space in the oropharynx than in patients without Down Syndrome.

The normal life span of an individual with Down syndrome is usually shortened due to the associated complications. Since the mental retardation varies from person to person, some adults with Down syndrome are able to live independent and productive lives.

For additional information on Down syndrome, visit the website of the National Down Syndrome Congress (http://www.ndsccenter.org).

Accommodating a Patient with a Developmental Disability

Depending on the severity of the disability, much of the information regarding a patient's history and symptoms may need to come from someone other than the patient. This may be a family member or someone else who cares for the patient. It is important to take the time to establish rapport with the patient prior to touching. Take extra care, and remember that although the patient may be "slow" to learn, he or she often understands what you are doing and saying. Treat all patients with the dignity, privacy, and respect that they deserve.

Ask family members for assistance when necessary. They know the patient best and know how to communicate and understand the patient. If the patient seems slow to understand you during attempts to communicate, keep directions and questions as simple as possible. When transporting a patient with a developmental disability, it may be necessary for the primary caregiver to accompany the patient to the hospital. The patient will most likely be anxious, confused, and scared, and having a familiar face may be helpful. DOT 6-5.20, 6-5.21, 6-5.22, 6-5.23

Pathological Challenges

Arthritis

Arthritis is inflammation of a joint, characterized by pain, stiffness, swelling, and redness. It is a chronic condition that affects people of all ages, including children. It affects 70 million Americans or in every people.

There are more than 100 different types of arthritis, and the cause of most is unknown. The most common types of arthritis include the following:

- Osteoarthritis (most common)
- Rheumatoid arthritis
- Juvenile rheumatoid arthritis
- Lupus
- Gout
- Polymyalgia rheumatica

For additional information on specific types of arthritis, visit The Arthritis Foundation's website (http://www.arthritis.org).

The severity of arthritis can range from mild discomfort to debilitating pain, making it difficult to perform the normal activities of daily living such as climbing stairs, opening a jar, or bending over to pick up something. For some, the simple task of walking is difficult for a patient with severe arthritis.

Recognizing a Patient with Arthritis

Specific symptoms of arthritis depend on the type but generally include the following:

- Pain (constant or occasional), which can be local or systemic in nature.
- Stiffness in joints.
- Occasional swelling or redness of the skin (may be warm to touch).
- Decreased range of motion (more pronounced in the morning or after periods of inactivity).
- Fatigue, poor appetite, or fever may be present with some types of arthritis.

Medications used to help alleviate some of the symptoms of most types of arthritis include aspirin, nonsteroidal antiinflammatory drugs (NSAIDS), and corticosteroids. Various pain medications are also used to treat the pain associated with different forms of arthritis.

EMS may be called to care for conditions caused by side effects of the medications regularly taken by patients with arthritis. For example, aspirin can cause stomach pain, heartburn, nausea and vomiting, and GI bleeding. NSAIDS can cause problems with the stomach, including vomiting, ulcers, and gastric discomfort. Corticosteroids can cause hyperglycemia, bloody emesis, and decreased immunity.

Accommodating a Patient with Arthritis

Because of the joint pain and swelling, decreased range of motion is normal and may limit a complete physical examination and make moving or immobilizing the patient more difficult. Specific points to consider when caring for a patient with arthritis include the following:

- Allow the patient to move at his own pace, whenever possible.
- Be sensitive to the patient's pain and discomfort.
- Make the patient as comfortable as possible. Allow the patient to find a position of comfort.
- Use pillows to elevate affected extremities.
- Limit touching the patient. Assessment may be difficult since many areas of the body are in constant pain. However, the patient knows his or her own body and will know if something is different. Ask the patient to identify any new pain, and perform a focused assessment in that area.
- Make modifications to patient care in order to accommodate the mobility of the patient. Make equipment fit the patient's needs and not vice versa. Pad all voids. DOT 6-5.30, 6-5.31, 6-5.32a

Cancer

Cancer is the second leading cause of death in the United States. Over one million people are diagnosed with cancer each year. Approximately one of every two men and one of every three woman in the U.S. will develop cancer during their lifetimes. Although anyone can get cancer at any age, approximately 77% of all cancers are diagnosed in people age 55 or older. Today, millions of people are living with cancer or have had cancer in the past.[12]

Cancer develops when cells in the body grow out of control. Normal cells grow, divide, and die. Cancer cells grow and divide and then grow and divide into new abnormal cells, which invade into and outlive the normal cells. The process continues until the abnormal cells replace normal cells.

Cancer cells develop because of damage to DNA. This usually occurs through heredity or exposure to something in the environment such as smoking or radiation.

Cancer usually forms tumors but can be a systemic problem such as leukemia, which affects the blood and blood-forming organs. Cancer cells often travel to other parts of the body, where they begin to grow and multiply and ultimately replace normal tissue. This process is called **metastasis.** The more cancer cells metastasize, the more difficult it is to "cure."

There are numerous types of cancer, but they all originate due to the abnormal growth of cells. Specific types of cancer are named for the place of their origin. Different types of cancer behave very differently. They grow at different rates, spread to different areas, and respond differently to various types of treatment. Prognosis for patients with cancer is directly related to the type of cancer they have.

There have been thousands of books, articles, and papers written about cancer. It is impossible for this chapter to cover everything the paramedic could learn on the subject. The focus here is to identify key points the paramedic should focus on when dealing with a patient who has been diagnosed with cancer. For more information on a specific type of cancer, visit The American Cancer Society's website (http://www.cancer.org).

Recognizing a Patient with Cancer

Signs and symptoms of cancer generally depend on the size and location of the cancer and how much it affects the surrounding organs and structures. If a cancer has metastasized to other organs, symptoms may be widespread (Box 46-10).

As a cancer grows, it begins to push on nearby organs, blood vessels, and nerves. This pressure creates some of the signs and symptoms associated with cancer. If the cancer is in a critical area, such as certain parts of the brain, even the smallest tumor can produce early symptoms. However, these symptoms often mimic other diseases (such as Alzheimer's disease) and may be misdiagnosed.

Some forms of cancer occur in places where symptoms may not be evident until the cancer has grown quite large. For example, cancer of the pancreas usually does not result in a tumor large enough to be felt on physical examination. As such, pancreatic cancer may not produce symptoms until it is large enough to obstruct nearby bile ducts or to cause pain. Unfortunately, by the time a pancreatic cancer causes these signs or symptoms, it has usually reached an advanced stage where a "cure" is unlikely.

A cancer may also cause generalized symptoms such as fever, fatigue, or weight loss. This may be caused by cancer cells releasing substances that change the body's metabolism, or the cancer may cause the immune system to react in ways that produce such symptoms.

Sometimes, cancer cells release substances into the bloodstream that cause symptoms not generally thought to result from cancers. For example, some cancers of the pancreas can release substances that cause blood clots to develop in veins of the legs. Some lung cancers produce hormone-like substances that affect blood calcium levels, affecting nerves and muscles and causing weakness and dizziness.

Cancer treatment depends on the specific type of cancer present but may include any or all of the following:

- Surgery to remove the tumor
- Chemotherapy to kill cancer cells in and around the tumor
- Radiation to kill cancer cells in a specific area

While it may be difficult for the paramedic to identify a patient with cancer, signs of cancer treatment

BOX 46-10   Signs and Symptoms of Cancer

General Signs and Symptoms

- **Unexplained (unintentional) weight loss:** Loss of greater than 10 pounds may be the first sign of cancer, particularly cancers of the pancreas, stomach, esophagus, or lung.
- **Fever:** Fever is very common with cancer, more often in advanced disease, but may also be an early sign of cancer, such as with Hodgkin's disease.
- **Fatigue:** Fatigue may be a significant symptom as the cancer progresses but may occur early, if the cancer is causing a chronic loss of blood, as in some colon or stomach cancers.
- **Pain:** Pain may be an early sign with some cancers, such as bone cancers or testicular cancer. Most often, however, pain is a symptom of advanced disease.
- **Skin changes:** In addition to cancers of the skin, some cancers can produce visible skin signs such as darkening (hyperpigmentation), yellowing (jaundice), reddening (erythema), itching, or excessive hair growth.

Specific Signs and Symptoms

- **Change in bowel habits or bladder function:** Chronic constipation, diarrhea, or a change in the size of the stool may indicate colon cancer. Pain with urination, blood in the urine, or a change in bladder function (such as more frequent or less frequent urination) could be related to bladder or prostate cancer.
- **Sores that do not heal:** Skin cancers may bleed and resemble sores that do not heal. A persistent sore in the mouth could be an oral cancer and should be dealt with promptly, especially in patients who smoke, chew tobacco, or frequently drink alcohol.

Sores on the penis or vagina may either be signs of infection or an early cancer.

- **Unusual bleeding or discharge:** Unusual bleeding can occur in early or advanced cancer. Blood in the sputum (phlegm) may be a sign of lung cancer. Blood in the stool could be a sign of colon or rectal cancer. Cancer of the cervix or the endometrium (lining of the uterus) can cause vaginal bleeding. Blood in the urine is a sign of possible bladder or kidney cancer. A bloody discharge from the nipple may be a sign of breast cancer.
- **Thickening or lump in breast or other parts of the body:** Many cancers can be felt through the skin, particularly in the breast, testicle, lymph nodes (glands), and the soft tissues of the body. A lump or thickening may be an early or late sign of cancer.
- **Indigestion or difficulty swallowing:** While they commonly have other causes, these symptoms may indicate cancer of the esophagus, stomach, or pharynx (throat). In esophageal cancer, by the time one experiences difficulty swallowing, the cancer would need to obstruct the esophagus by one-half (5 mm).
- **Recent change in a wart or mole:** Any change in color or shape, loss of definite borders, or an increase in size should be reported to your doctor without delay. The skin lesion may be a melanoma, which if diagnosed early, can be treated successfully.
- **Nagging cough or hoarseness:** A cough that does not go away may be a sign of lung cancer. Hoarseness can be a sign of cancer of the larynx (voice box) or thyroid.

---

are usually easily spotted. These may include the following:

- **Alopecia** (hair loss) resulting from chemotherapy
- Weight loss associated with loss of appetite and vomiting due to chemotherapy
- Ink marking on the skin indicating positioning sites for radiation therapy
- Physical markings from surgery to remove tumors (e.g., removal of a breast or insertion of a drainage tube for a tumor in the jejunum)

Street Secrets

Patients with cancer may have pathological fractures. The cancer process can result in a loss of calcium from the bones which can make them brittle and prone to fracture with little stress. Move cancer patients carefully and gently. Weight bearing may not be possible as cancer advances so assist the patients in ambulating if they tell you they want to walk to the ambulance cot.

Accommodating a Patient with Cancer

Management of patients with cancer can present challenges for the paramedic. Patients who undergo chemotherapy become neutropenic (deficient in neutrophils), which places patients at extreme risk for developing infections. Many patients die not from the cancer itself, but from a secondary infection such as pneumonia, which the body cannot fight in its weakened state.

When caring for a patient with cancer, it is essential to reduce any exposure to infection. Always assume that a cancer patient is neutropenic. Due to the body's inability to fight bacteria and other infectious organisms, a neutropenic patient can go into septic shock within hours of developing an infection. Always put a mask on the patient and on yourself to reduce exposure to infectious agents. In addition, wear gloves when touching the patient, and take extra precautions when prepping the skin prior to inserting an IV and when administering IV fluids. Ensure sterile techniques are used at all times.

Another challenge presented by patients with cancer is that their veins may have become scarred as a result of frequent IVs, blood tests, and caustic chemotherapy. In addition, weight loss and dehydration can make IV access very difficult. Some patients will present with an implanted vascular access device (VAD), which involves a catheter implanted into a larger vein in the chest, neck, or arm. The port is used for chemotherapy treatment, IV therapy, and sometimes for infusion of nutrients (total parenteral nutrition or TPN). These ports should not be used by the paramedic unless local protocols allow and the paramedic has received special training in the use of such devices.

Cancer patients are often in a great deal of pain and sometimes take extremely high doses of pain medication. The patient may not be coherent, in which case the paramedic must rely on family members for information regarding history of illness. Since the pain medication may mask certain symptoms, it may be difficult to obtain an accurate assessment.

Street Secrets

Be careful when administering naloxone to patients on long-term opiates for pain control. Naloxone will restore breathing but it could also precipitate a seizure in these patients. Also be careful if the patient is wearing a fentanyl patch. Fentanyl is a potent opiate. Several small children have died after ingesting used fentanyl patches or playing "patient" and placing them on their skin. If a fentanyl patch is removed it should be placed into the sharps container to prevent accidental exposure to the medication.

When caring for a patient who receives chemotherapy in the home, take extra precautions to avoid any direct contact with the drug or even indirect contact from urine, blood, vomit, or sputum. These drugs can be hazardous to healthcare workers as follows:

- They can cause abnormal changes in DNA **(mutagenic).**
- They may alter development of a fetus or embryo, leading to birth defects **(teratogenic).**
- They may cause another type of cancer **(carcinogenic).**
- Some may cause localized skin irritation or damage.

When self-administering chemotherapy at home, the patient should be using separate plastic containers to dispose of sharp items, syringes, IV tubing, and medication bags. Gowns and gloves should also be disposed of in special bags.

Above all, when caring for a patient suffering from cancer, show compassion and empathy. Recognize that the patient is in pain and is most likely extremely scared of what tomorrow will bring. Include them in their prehospital care as much as possible, for they have lost much control over their lives as a result of the cancer and the ensuing treatment. DOT 6-5.30, 6-5.31, 6-5.32b

Street Secrets

Some patients with breast cancer have had lymph nodes in their armpits removed. The arm that had the lymph nodes removed may have significant swelling due to lymph accumulation. Do not attempt to obtain a blood pressure in a swollen arm in which the tissue was removed.

Cerebral Palsy

Cerebral palsy is a blanket term used to describe a group of chronic conditions affecting body movements and muscle coordination caused by damage to the cerebrum either in utero or as a result of trauma during the birthing process.

Cerebral refers to the brain and *palsy* to a disorder of movement or posture. People with cerebral palsy are not able to use some of their muscles in a normal way due to injury to the brain. Children with cerebral palsy may not be able to walk, talk, eat, or play in the same ways as most other children (Figure 46-4).

The United Cerebral Palsy Association estimates that more than 500,000 Americans have cerebral palsy. Approximately two to three in every 1,000 children over the age of three have cerebral palsy. Despite advances in the prevention and treatment of certain causes of cerebral palsy, the number of persons it affects has remained essentially unchanged or has risen slightly over the past 30 years. This is due in part to more premature and frail infants surviving as a result of improved intensive care.[13]

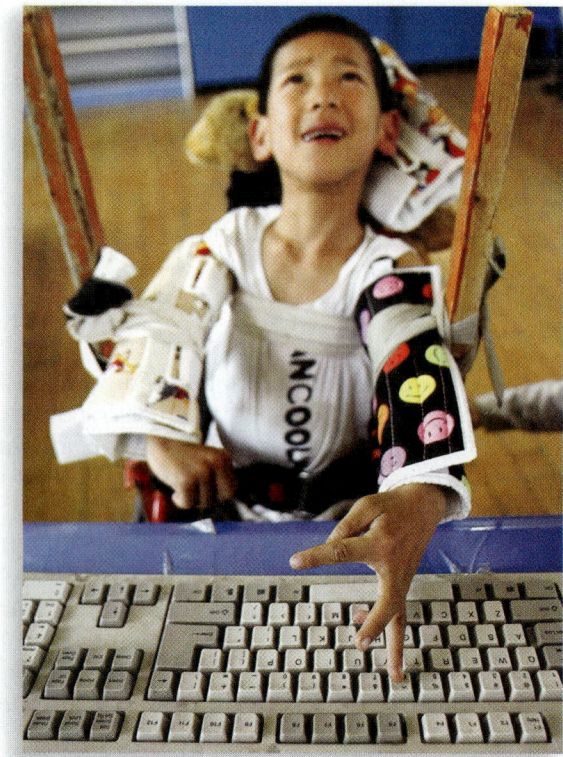

Figure 46-4 A child with cerebral palsy.

Cerebral palsy is neither progressive nor communicable. The condition is not "curable," although education, therapy, and applied technology can help persons with cerebral palsy lead productive lives. Many children with cerebral palsy have other problems that require treatment, including mental retardation, learning disabilities, seizures, and vision, hearing, and speech problems.

Cerebral palsy is classified into four broad categories based on the type of movement disturbance: DOT 6-5.30, 6-5.31, 6-5.32c

- **Spastic Paralysis** affects 70–80% of patients and is a condition where the muscles are stiffly and permanently contracted. Spasticity refers to the inability of a muscle to relax and is identified by the limbs involved (hemiplegia, diplegia, or quadriplegia). Hemiplegia is cerebral palsy that involves one arm and one leg on the same side of the body; whereas, diplegia involves both legs. When the knees are turned inward, it causes a characteristic "scissor gait." Quadriplegia refers to a pattern involving all four extremities as well as trunk and neck muscles.

- **Athetoid** affects about 10–20% of patients and is characterized by uncontrolled, slow, writhing movements of the hands, feet, arms, or legs and, in some cases, the muscles of the face and tongue, causing grimacing or drooling.

- **Ataxic** affects 5–10% of patients and presents as difficulty with balance and depth perception. Affected persons often have poor coordination, walk unsteadily with a wide-based gait, and experience difficulty when attempting quick or precise movements, such as writing or buttoning a shirt.

- **Mixed Forms** are combinations of two or more forms of cerebral palsy. The most common mixed form includes spasticity and athetoid movements, but other combinations are also possible.

In about 70% of cases, cerebral palsy results from events occurring before birth that disrupt normal development of the brain. Contrary to popular belief, according to a 2003 report by the American College of Obstetricians and Gynecologists (ACOG) and the American Academy of Pediatrics (AAP), lack of oxygen reaching the fetus during labor and delivery contributes to only a small minority of cases of cerebral palsy. A small number of babies also develop brain injuries in the first months or years of life that result in cerebral palsy.

In many cases, the cause of cerebral palsy in a child is not known.[14] Some of the known causes of cerebral palsy, however, include the following:

- **Infections during pregnancy.** These include rubella, cytomegalovirus and toxoplasmosis, and maternal infections involving the placental membranes and urinary tract infections.

- **Insufficient oxygen reaching the fetus.**

- **Prematurity.** Premature babies who weigh less than 3.3 pounds are up to 30 times more likely to develop cerebral palsy than full-term babies.

- **Asphyxia during labor and delivery.** It is estimated that fewer than 10% of the type of brain injuries that can result in cerebral palsy are caused by asphyxia.

- **Blood Diseases.** Rh incompatibility between the blood of the mother and her fetus can cause severe jaundice and brain damage, resulting in cerebral palsy.

- **Severe jaundice.**

- **Other birth defects.**

- **Acquired cerebral palsy.** About 10% of children with cerebral palsy acquire it after birth due to brain injuries that occur during the first two years of life, most commonly meningitis or head injury.

Recognizing a Patient with Cerebral Palsy

Cerebral palsy is characterized by an inability to fully control motor function, particularly muscle control and coordination. Depending on which areas of the brain have been damaged and the severity of the damage, one or more of the following may occur:

- Muscle tightness or spasm
- Difficulty with fine motor tasks, such as writing or cutting with scissors
- Difficulty maintaining balance and walking
- Involuntary movements, such as uncontrollable writhing motion of the hands or drooling
- Abnormal sensation and perception
- Impairment of sight, hearing, or speech

The symptoms differ from one person to the next and may even change over time in the individual. Some people with cerebral palsy are also affected by other medical disorders, including seizures or mental impairment. Contrary to common belief, however, cerebral palsy does not always cause impairment of intelligence. Some degree of mental retardation does occur in approximately 75% of people with cerebral palsy; however, many people with athetoid and diplegic cerebral palsy are highly intelligent.

Accommodating a Patient with Cerebral Palsy

When caring for a patient with cerebral palsy, keep in mind that many of these patients rely heavily on special devices to help them with mobility. When dealing with a severe handicap, ask family members the best way to move the patient. If the patient is immobile, additional resources may be necessary to facilitate transport.

When assessing the patient, do not assume mental retardation. As already stated, some individuals with cerebral palsy are highly intelligent. Ask questions as if this were any other patient. If a patient does have difficulty communicating, ask a caregiver to assist with the assessment process.

When transporting patients with cerebral palsy, make accommodations, as necessary, to prevent further injury. If contractures are present, do not force the extremities to move. Rather, pad any voids with pillows and blankets. In addition, have suction readily available, as increased oral secretions may require suctioning.

Cystic Fibrosis (Mucoviscidosis)

Cystic fibrosis (CF) is a genetic disease that most commonly affects breathing and digestion. CF affects approximately 30,000 children and adults in the United States. It occurs in approximately one of every 3,500 live births, with about 1,000 new cases being diagnosed each year. More than 80% of patients are diagnosed by the age of three; however, nearly 10% of newly diagnosed cases are age 18 or older.

Advances in medical treatment continue to improve the outlook for affected children and adults. However, there is no cure. Most affected individuals survive to about age 30 though some die in childhood and others live to age 40 or beyond.

CF is an inherited disease caused by an abnormal protein that does not allow the normal passage of chloride (which, along with sodium, makes up salt) into and out of certain cells, including those that line the lungs and pancreas. As a result, these cells produce thick, sticky mucus and other secretions that can do the following:

- Obstruct air passages in the lungs and lead to life-threatening lung infections.
- Obstruct the pancreas, preventing digestive enzymes from reaching the intestines to help break

down and absorb food. These individuals have big appetites but gain weight slowly.
- Block the bile duct in the liver, eventually causing permanent liver damage in approximately 6% of people with CF.

More than 10 million Americans are unknowing, symptomless carriers of the defective CF gene. An individual must inherit two defective CF genes, one from each parent, to have CF. Each time two carriers conceive, there is a 25% chance that their child will have CF, a 50% chance that the child will be a carrier of the CF gene, and a 25% chance that the child will be a noncarrier.

Some children with CF are well enough to attend school, participate in some exercise and recreational activities (though stamina is generally reduced), and go on to college and rewarding careers. Others, however, are too ill to attend school regularly.

The treatment of CF depends upon the stage of the disease and the organs involved. Clearing mucus from the lungs is an important part of the daily CF treatment regimen. Chest physical therapy is a form of airway clearance done by vigorous clapping on the back and chest to dislodge the thick mucus from the lungs. Other types of treatments include antibiotics to treat persistent lung infections and pancreatic enzyme supplements to help with the absorption of food in the digestive tract.

According to the CF Foundation's National Patient Registry, the median age of survival for a person with CF is in the mid-30s. As more advances have been made in the treatment of CF, the number of adults with CF has steadily grown. Today, nearly 40% of the CF population is age 18 and older. Adults, however, may experience additional health challenges including CF-related diabetes and osteoporosis. CF can also cause reproductive problems. In fact, more than 95% of men with CF are sterile; however, with new technologies, some are becoming fathers. Although many women with CF are able to conceive, limited lung function and other health factors may make it difficult to carry a child to term.[15]

DOT 6-5.30, 6-5.31, 6-5.32d

Recognizing a Patient with Cystic Fibrosis

Although symptoms vary from person to person, due in part, to the more than 1,000 mutations of the CF gene, generally people with CF have a variety of symptoms including the following:

- Very salty-tasting skin
- Persistent coughing, at times with phlegm
- Wheezing or shortness of breath
- Repeated lung infections
- An excessive appetite but poor weight gain
- Greasy, bulky stools

Accommodating a Patient with Cystic Fibrosis

Individuals with cystic fibrosis have been chronically ill their entire lives and may resist prehosptial care. As such, treatment can be difficult for both the patients and the caregivers.

Because of the high probability of respiratory distress in patients with CF, when caring for the patients it is necessary to provide oxygen therapy, including administering oxygen by whatever means the patients will tolerate, and suctioning to clear thick secretions in the airway.

Make certain to document any medications the patients are currently taking. Patients with CF often take antibiotics, inhalers, or mucomyst to thin secretions.

For additional information on Cystic Fibrosis, go to the Cystic Fibrosis Foundation's website (http://www.cff.org).

Multiple Sclerosis

Multiple sclerosis (MS) is a progressive disease of the CNS whereby scattered patches of myelin in the brain and spinal cord are destroyed as a result of repeated inflammation of the myelin sheath. Myelin is the tissue that covers and protects nerve fibers. When this occurs, nerve impulses to the affected area are blocked. Thus, a person with MS experiences varying degrees of neurological impairment, depending on the location and extent of the scarring.

The exact cause of multiple sclerosis is unknown; however, it is considered to be an autoimmune disorder. Onset usually occurs between the ages of 20 and 40. Although there is no known cure for MS, individuals with MS often live productive lives for 50 years after initial onset of symptoms.

At present, there are 350,000 to 500,000 people in the United States who have been diagnosed with multiple sclerosis. MS is more common in women and appears more frequently in whites than in Hispanics or African Americans. Ninety percent of MS patients diagnosed are between the ages of 16 and 60, but MS can make its first appearance in early childhood or after age 60.[16]

Management of MS has changed dramatically. More than two-thirds of those with MS are still walking 20 years after developing the disease. Forty percent of persons diagnosed with MS experience little or no disruptions of normal activities, and 75% never need a wheelchair. With appropriate management, including medical, rehabilitative, and psychological approaches, much can be done for the patient with MS.

Recognizing Patients with Multiple Sclerosis

The onset of multiple sclerosis is slow, with minor numbness or tingling in the affected area or a slight change in muscle strength. Signs and symptoms of MS may be persistent or may cease from time to time. Because the signs and symptoms that define the clinical picture of MS are the result of nerve lesions causing disturbances in electrical conduction in one or more areas of the central nervous system, the nature of the symptoms that occur is determined by the location of the lesion.

If the brain is affected, the patient may exhibit the following:

- Fatigue
- Vertigo
- Muscle weakness
- Slurred speech
- Ataxia
- Blurred or double vision
- Numbness, weakness, or pain in the face

If the spinal cord is affected, the patient may exhibit the following:

- Tingling, numbness, or the feeling of constriction in any part of the body
- Extremities that feel heavy and become weak
- Spasticity

The initial signs of MS are usually temporary; however, they become progressively more frequent and long lasting. Eventually, the symptoms become more permanent, leading ultimately to extreme weakness of the extremities or complete paralysis.

Accommodating a Patient with Multiple Sclerosis

It is important to recognize the characteristic presentations of multiple sclerosis. Since MS is a progressive disease, patients may eventually become bedridden and exhibit the following complications:

- Painful muscle spasms
- Urinary tract infections
- Respiratory infections
- Constipation
- Skin ulcerations
- Mood swings from euphoria to depression

When preparing to transport a patient with MS, ensure adequate assistance to move the patient to the stretcher. Do not expect the patient to walk to the stretcher. Ensure the patient is transported in the most comfortable position possible. Whenever possible, bring any supportive aids, such as a cane or walker, to the hospital.

In addition to comfort and supportive care, it is important to treat the patient for any signs or symptoms that are present. A patient with MS may have respiratory infections that require oxygen therapy and perhaps additional intervention. DOT 6-5.30, 6-5.31, 6-5.32e

Muscular Dystrophy

The muscular dystrophies (MD) are a group of genetic diseases characterized by slow but progressive weakness and degeneration of the skeletal muscles that control movement. There are nine forms of muscular dystrophy, some noticeable at birth (congenital muscular dystrophy) and others in adolescence (Becker MD). The three most common types of MD are Duchenne, fascioscapulohumeral, and myotonic. These three types differ in terms of pattern of inheritance, age of onset, rate of progression, and distribution of weakness.

Duchenne MD

- Primarily affects males.
- Results from mutations in the gene that regulates dystrophin, a protein involved in maintaining the integrity of muscle fiber.
- Onset appears between three and five years of age and progresses rapidly.
- Leads to progressive muscle weakness in the legs and pelvis.
- Generally causes paralysis by the age of 12.
- Ultimately affects the respiratory muscles and heart.
- By the age of 20 usually requires the use of a respirator to breathe.
- Death occurs at an early age.

Fascioscapulohumeral MD

- Causes progressive weakness in facial muscles and certain muscles in the arms and legs.
- Onset appears in adolescence.
- Progresses slowly.
- Can vary in symptoms from mild to disabling.

Myotonic MD

- Varies in the age of onset.
- Is characterized by the following:
  - Myotonia (prolonged muscle spasm) in the fingers and facial muscles.
  - A floppy-footed, high-stepping gait.
  - Cataracts.
  - Cardiac abnormalities.
  - Endocrine disturbances.
- Individuals have long faces and drooping eyelids
- Men have frontal baldness.

There is no specific treatment for any of the forms of MD, but ongoing therapies may include the following:

- Respiratory therapy.
- Physical therapy to prevent painful muscle contractures.
- Use of orthopedic appliances for support.
- Corrective orthopedic surgery to improve the quality of life in some cases.
- Use of a pacemaker to manage certain cardiac abnormalities.
- Use of medications to slow the rate of muscle deterioration.

The prognosis for patients with MD varies according to the type and progression of the disorder. Some cases may be mild and progress very slowly over a normal lifespan while other cases may have more marked progression of muscle weakness, functional disability, and loss of the ability to walk. In Duchenne MD, death usually occurs in the early 20s.

Accommodating Patients with Muscular Dystrophy

Because muscular dystrophy is a genetic disorder, a complete family history may prove useful. During assessment, it is important to identify the specific muscles that have been affected by the disease and plan care accordingly. Do not expect these patients to walk to a stretcher or even assist with movement. Ensure adequate assistance, and request additional help, if necessary. In later stages of the disease, respiratory support, such as oxygen and even intubation, may be necessary. DOT 6-5.30, 6-5.31, 6-5.32f

Poliomyelitis

Poliomyelitis (polio) is a highly contagious, viral disease that can involve the nervous system and cause paralysis. It once affected mostly infants and children; however, although it is no longer a common disease, it occurs more often in people over 15 years old. It is more common in the summer and fall. Adults and young girls are more likely to be infected, but infection in young boys is more likely to result in paralysis.

Polio occurs worldwide. However, because of the widespread use of polio vaccination, the disease is very rare in developed countries. In fact, other than cases involving the vaccination itself, there have been no cases of polio reported in the United States since 1979. However, there are individuals with polio in the U.S. who contracted the disease prior to development of the polio vaccine in the 1950s. In developing countries, where vaccination use is not as common, the disease is still prevalent.

The poliovirus is usually contracted from an infected person through direct person-to-person contact, by contact with infected secretions from the nose or mouth, or by contact with infected feces. The virus enters through the mouth and nose, multiplies in the throat and intestinal tract, and is then absorbed and spread through the blood and lymph system.[17] As long as the virus is contained, it usually results in only mild illness. In more serious cases, however, it attacks the CNS and alters nerve cells, which can result in paralysis or even death.

The majority of individuals infected with the poliovirus have few or no symptoms. Others have short-term, "flu-like" symptoms including headache, fatigue, fever, muscle ache, and stiff neck and back. If the nervous system becomes infected, however, permanent paralysis can occur, usually of the legs. Paralysis of the respiratory muscles is also possible, necessitating artificial ventilation.

Recognition of Patients with Poliomyelitis

There are three basic patterns of polio infection: subclinical infections, nonparalytic, and paralytic. Approximately 95% of these are subclinical infections, many of which go unnoticed.

Subclinical infection

- No symptoms, or symptoms lasting 72 hours or less
- Slight fever
- Headache
- General discomfort or uneasiness (malaise)
- Sore throat
- Red throat
- Vomiting

Nonparalytic poliomyelitis

- Symptoms last one to two weeks
- Moderate fever
- Headache
- Vomiting
- Diarrhea
- Excessive tiredness, fatigue
- Irritability
- Pain or stiffness of the back, arms, legs, abdomen
- Muscle tenderness and spasm in any area of the body
- Neck pain and stiffness
- Pain in the front part of neck
- Back pain or backache
- Leg pain (calf muscles)
- Skin rash or lesion with pain
- Muscle stiffness

Paralytic poliomyelitis

- Fever, occurring five to seven days before other symptoms
- Headache
- Stiff neck and back
- Muscle weakness, asymmetrical (only on one side or worse on one side)
  - Rapid onset
  - Progresses to paralysis
  - Location depends on where the spinal cord is affected

- Abnormal sensations of an area
- Sensitivity to touch, mild touch may be painful
- Difficulty beginning to urinate
- Constipation
- Bloated feeling of abdomen
- Swallowing difficulty
- Muscle pain
- Muscle spasms, particularly in the calf, neck, or back
- Drooling
- Breathing difficulty
- Irritability or poor temper control
- Positive Babinski's reflex

Accommodating a Patient with Poliomyelitis

EMS may be summoned for a variety of reasons. These may or may not be related to poliomyelitis itself. Box 46-11 lists many of the complications that can be associated with polio.

Lifesaving measures, particularly assistance with breathing, may be necessary in severe cases. If the patient is on a ventilator in the home, transport cannot occur without manually or mechanically providing artificial ventilations during transport. Narcotics are not usually given to patients with polio because of an increased risk in breathing difficulty. If it is necessary to

---

BOX 46-11 Complications of Poliomyelitis

EMS could be summoned for one of the many complications of polio, including the following:

- Spread of infection to other nonimmunized persons
- Permanent muscle paralysis, disability, deformity
- Pulmonary edema
- Shock
- Complications of immobility and respiratory involvement
- Aspiration pneumonia
- High blood pressure
- Urinary tract infections
- Kidney stones
- Paralytic ileus (loss of intestinal functioning)
- Myocarditis
- Cor pulmonale (right heart failure due to increased pulmonary pressure)

administer narcotics in the field, take care to monitor the patient's breathing.

A tracheostomy may also be necessary in certain cases of respiratory paralysis. Cases of lower extremity paralysis may require catheterization.

The application of moist heat (heat packs, warm towels, etc.) may reduce muscle pain and spasm.

Activity is limited only by the extent of discomfort and muscle weakness. Do not expect the patient to ambulate to the stretcher. Obtain additional help, as needed. Take any assistive devices (cane, crutches, brace, etc.) with the patient to the hospital.

The outcome varies with the form and the site affected. If the spinal cord and brain are not affected, which is the case over 90% of the time, complete recovery is likely.

Brain or spinal cord involvement is a medical emergency that may result in paralysis or death (usually from respiratory difficulties with lesions occurring high in the spinal column). DOT 6-5.30, 6-5.31, 6-5.32h

Previous Head Injury

A patient who has sustained a previous head injury, resulting in traumatic injury to the brain, may present with various cognitive, physical, and psychological challenges. There may be difficulties in balance and coordination, fine motor skills, or ambulatory skills as well as in communication skills, including language, memory, perception, and the processing of information, depending on the area of the brain that was injured.

Head injuries may result in irreversible brain damage, often due to bleeding inside the brain or by damage directly to the brain itself. These injuries can also result in the following:

- Changes in personality, emotions, or mental abilities
- Memory loss
- Speech and language problems
- Loss of sensation, hearing, vision, taste, or smell
- Seizures
- Paralysis
- Coma
- Angry outbursts or irrational thought processes

Depending on the extent of the injury and the area of the brain injured, assessment and patient care may be difficult. Some patients may require restraint. Follow local protocols. Involve family members whenever possible as they know how to handle the patient best. Ask family members if certain behaviors or symptoms are new or worse than usual.

When caring for these patients, remain calm and professional at all times. Extra time on the scene may be necessary to adequately assess and care for a patient with the special challenges associated with head injuries. DOT 6-5.30, 6-5.31, 6-5.32j

Spina Bifida

Spina bifida (SB) is a neural tube defect (a disorder involving incomplete development of the brain, spinal cord, or their protective coverings). It is caused by the failure of the fetus's spine to close properly during the first month of pregnancy.

Infants born with SB sometimes have open lesions on their spines where significant congenital abnormalities of the nerves and spinal cord have occurred. Although the spinal opening can be surgically repaired shortly after birth, the nerve damage is permanent, resulting in varying degrees of paralysis of the lower limbs. Even when there is no visible lesion present, there may be improperly formed or missing vertebrae and accompanying nerve damage. In addition to physical and mobility difficulties, some individuals have some form of learning disability.

The four types of spina bifida in order of decreasing severity follow:

- *Myelomeningocele.* The spinal cord and its protective covering (the meninges) protrude from an opening in the spine (Figure 46-5).
- *Meningocele.* The spinal cord develops normally, but the meninges protrude from a spinal opening.
- *Closed neural tube defects.* The spinal cord is marked by a malformation of fat, bone, or membranes.
- *Occulta.* One or more vertebrae are malformed and covered by a layer of skin.

The cause of spina bifida is unknown; however, genetic, nutritional, and environmental factors may play a role. Since nerve tissue cannot be repaired or replaced, there is no cure for the disorder. Treatment may include surgery, medication, and physiotherapy.

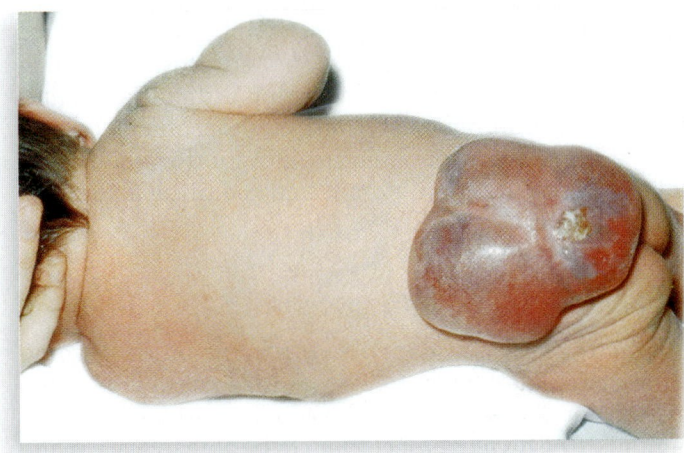

Figure 46-5 An infant with myelomeningocele.

Many individuals with SB will need assistive devices such as braces, crutches, or wheelchairs. Ongoing therapy, medical care, or surgical treatments may be necessary to prevent and manage complications throughout the individual's life. Surgery to close the newborn's spinal opening is usually performed within 24 hours after birth to minimize the risk of infection and to preserve existing function in the spinal cord.

The prognosis for individuals with SB depends on the number and severity of abnormalities. Prognosis is poorest for those with complete paralysis, hydrocephalus, and other congenital defects. With proper care, however, most children with spina bifida can walk, usually with assistive devices, and live well into adulthood.[18]

Recognition of Patients with Spinal Bifida

Depending on the type of spina bifida, symptoms can vary from person to person and range from minor physical problems to severe physical and mental disabilities. Individuals with occulta often have no outward signs of the disorder. Closed neural tube defects are often recognized early in life due to an abnormal clump of hair or a small dimple or birthmark on the skin at the site of the spinal malformation.

Meningocele and myelomeningocele generally involve a fluid-filled sac that is visible on the back and protrudes from the spinal cord. In meningocele, the sac may be covered by a thin layer of skin; whereas, in most cases of myelomeningocele, there is no layer of skin covering the sac, and a section of spinal cord tissue usually is exposed. The patient may have paralysis of both lower extremities and bowel and bladder dysfunction.

Most people with spina bifida are of normal intelligence although children with both myelomeningocele and hydrocephalus may have learning disabilities.

One complication associated with spina bifida is Chiari II malformation, commonly seen in children with myelomeningocele, in which the rear portion of the brain protrudes downward into the spinal canal or neck area, leading to compression of the spinal cord. Chiari II malformation can cause a variety of symptoms, most concerning of which are feeding, swallowing (which can lead to choking), and breathing difficulties. Chiari II malformation may also cause hydrocephalus (excessive accumulation of cerebrospinal fluid in the brain), putting pressure on the brain and requiring a shunt to help drain excess fluid.

Accommodating Patients with Spina Bifida

As many as 75% of patients with spina bifida develop allergies to latex. Therefore, assume a latex allergy when caring for these patients. Although most patients are ambulatory, do not expect them to be able to walk to the ambulance. Ensure adequate resources, as needed, and transport any assistive devices (braces, crutches, walker, etc.) with the patient to the hospital. DOT 6-5.30, 6-5.31, 6-5.32i

For additional information on spina bifida and other neurological disorders, look at the National Institute of Neurological Disorders and Stroke's website (http://www.ninds.nih.gov/disorders/spina_bifida/detail_spina_bifida.htm).

Myasthenia Gravis

Myasthenia gravis is an autoimmune disease in which the immune system attacks the body's own tissues. The disease is characterized by chronic weakness of voluntary muscles and progressive fatigue. It most commonly affects muscles of the eyes, face, throat, and extremities.

The cause of myasthenia gravis is unknown although it is suspected that viruses or bacteria may trigger the autoimmune response. The thymus gland may also play a role in development of the disease. There also appears to be a genetic predisposition to the disease. The condition results from a problem with neurotransmitters that block nerve signals from reaching muscles.

Myasthenia gravis can appear at any age but is more common in women younger than 40 and in men older than 60. It is one and one-half times more common in women than in men and usually reaches maximum severity within one to three years of onset. Estimates of the number of people with this disorder vary because it can be difficult to diagnose, but it likely affects between two and three people per every 10,000 in the United States.[19] With proper treatment, people with the disease can remain physically active. Progression to the point of needing a wheelchair is rare.

Weakness associated with myasthenia gravis may vary over time and during the course of a day. Individuals are usually stronger in the morning, with weakness increasing after prolonged use of affected muscles. In addition, symptoms may worsen with stress, systemic illness, fever, surgery, menses, pregnancy, thyroid dysfunction, and use of certain drugs.[20]

Recognition of Patients with Myasthenia Gravis

Patients with myasthenia gravis generally present with the following symptoms:

- Partial paralysis of eye movements, causing drooping eyelids, double vision
- Difficulty speaking
- Weakness and fatigue in the neck and jaws, causing problems in chewing, swallowing, and holding up the neck
- Difficulty in moving the extremities
- Weakness of respiratory muscles

Accommodating Patients with Myasthenia Gravis

Patients with myasthenia gravis present in various ways. Accommodation varies based on the specific presentation. Evaluate for airway patency, respiratory rate and effort, the presence of any cough or increased oral secretions, cardiac status, skin color and temperature, speech effort and quality, and mental status.

If respiratory problems are present, take measures to ensure airway patency. In severe cases, a patient may experience paralysis of respiratory muscles, leading to respiratory arrest. Administer oxygen, intubate, and assist with respirations, as necessary. If the patient is unable to swallow effectively, use suction, as needed, and elevate the head and shoulders. If foreign body obstruction is suspected, perform appropriate maneuvers to relieve the obstruction.

Street Secrets

If the patient with myasthenia gravis requires aggressive airway control, choose to sedate the patient if needed but avoid the use of paralytics.

Use caution when assessing a patient with myasthenia gravis. Avoid lengthy questioning as it can lead to undue fatigue. Since symptoms may worsen with emotional upset, take steps to reassure the patient and eliminate stress as much as possible. Maintain a calm and peaceful atmosphere. Use caution when administering narcotics to patients with myasthenia gravis as their use may worsen symptoms and further compromise breathing. Finally, do not expect the patient to walk to a stretcher. Ensure adequate help is present to transport the patient. DOT 6-5.30, 6-5.31, 6-5.32g

Terminally Ill Patients

Terminally ill patients are those in an advanced stage of disease where the prognosis is grim or there is no known cure. Caring for terminally ill patients can be extremely emotional. Many terminally ill patients make the decision to die at home, but then when something happens, the patient or family member calls 9-1-1.

In general, a person who is on hospice care has made a conscious decision to die at home or in a hospice facility. As such, they generally will not call for emergency care. In fact, if they do go to the hospital for emergency care, they are taken off hospice. You may, however, encounter a situation where the patient is prepared to die, but a loved one is not prepared to deal with the death. This creates an emotional and legal challenge.

If the patient has an advance directive or Do Not Resuscitate (DNR) order, honor the directive in the event the patient goes into cardiac or respiratory arrest while in your care. Keep in mind, however, that patients do have the right to change their mind. If the patient wishes to have care withheld, however, and the spouse or other family member wants emergency care provided, you must respect the wishes of the patient.

CONNECTIONS Review Chapter 3: Professional Ethics and Chapter 4: Legal Issues to learn more about advanced directives.

Caring for terminally ill patients is a very emotional time that requires a great deal of empathy and compassion for both the patients and their loved ones. If emotions run too high at the scene, it is the paramedic's responsibility to take control of the situation and calm all individuals involved. Above all else, provide the emotional support necessary as everyone is going through a very difficult time. If possible, offer to phone a family member, clergy, or a good friend to be with a loved one.

The paramedic should obtain a complete medical history and identify any changes in the patient's condition, specifically, the reason EMS was summoned. Determine if the patient has an advance directive or DNR order. Obtain documentation of any such orders. If you have any questions about an advance directive or DNR order, discuss such with medical direction.

Care of the terminally ill patient is often one of providing supportive measures. Pain assessment and management is an important aspect of care. Sometimes the amount of pain medication patients are on is so extreme that they are no longer mentally competent. Obtain a complete history of the patient's pain medication and look for the presence of any transdermal drug patches or other pain-relief devices the patient may be wearing. After assessing the patient's vital signs, LOC, and history, medical direction may order the administration of analgesics or sedatives such as morphine or midazolam to ensure the patient's comfort. DOT 6-5.37

Patients with Communicable Diseases

Infectious diseases can pose a significant health risk to EMS providers. As such, it is essential to take appropriate precautions to ensure personal protection on every emergency call. BSI precautions are based on the disease, mode of transmission, and risk. For example, if blood may splatter, the paramedic should wear a gown and goggles. At a minimum, gloves should be worn during *every* patient encounter.

Withhold any prejudices you may have as you are a professional. With certain infectious diseases, patients may be emotional and sometimes embarrassed. This is especially true for patients with AIDS. Recognize that the patient is a person who should be treated with respect and dignity. Maintain a professional behavior while ensuring personal protection. DOT 6-5.38, 39, 40

CONNECTIONS Specific communicable diseases, including etiologies and treatment, are covered in Chapter 33: Infectious and Communicable Diseases.

Patients with Financial Challenges

During your EMS career, you will most likely encounter a diverse group of patients. Some may be extremely affluent, others of middle class, some poor, and others homeless. The key to caring for all of these patients is to treat them in the same professional manner.

It is estimated that one-third of the population in the U.S. live in poverty and have no health insurance. Some of these individuals are homeless. In general, the homeless have numerous health problems, including chronic illness, frostbite, leg ulcers, respiratory infections, substance abuse, and psychiatric illness. They often have poor personal hygiene and poor nutrition. They are at a greater risk for trauma and are often at greater risk of HIV, TB, and other communicable diseases. Regardless, these individuals deserve to be treated with respect and dignity.

A patient's ability to pay for services should play absolutely *no* role in emergency care. EMTALA requires that hospitals and clinics provide evaluation and life-saving care to patients who do not have insurance or financial means. Patients who are financially challenged are often apprehensive about seeking medical care. Try to calm the patient's fears by discussing the situation and providing any information possible. Federal law mandates that medical screening be provided regardless of a person's ability to pay for services. Research your area to identify local hospital policies regarding care provided to patients with little means.

Summary

Paramedics will encounter many different types of patients who present special challenges. Whether there is a communication barrier due to a visual, hearing, or speech impairment; a challenge with movement, such as with paralysis, arthritis, muscular dystrophy, multiple sclerosis, or other physical diseases; a mental challenge, such as with persons with mental illness, emotional problems, Down syndrome, or autism; or a host of other issues that a patient deals with on a daily basis, for the paramedic, the goal is always the same. Take whatever steps are necessary to accommodate the situation; think

outside of the box, and identify the best way to assess and care for the patient, and above all else, treat the patient with the respect and dignity he or she deserves.

Notes

1. V. M. Bloedel Hearing Research Center, "Hearing Loss," http://depts.washington.edu/hearing/Hearing%20Loss.html (accessed June 12, 2005).
2. Medline Plus, "Age Related Hearing Loss," http://www.nlm.nih.gov/medlineplus/ency/article/001045.htm (accessed July 14, 2005).
3. American Foundation for the Blind, "Statistics and Sources for Professionals," http://www.afb.org/section.asp?Documentid=1367 (accessed June 12, 2005).
4. Glaucoma Research Foundation, "What Is Glaucoma?" http://www.glaucoma.org/learn/ (accessed June 12, 2005).
5. St. Luke's Eye, "Cataracts," http://www.stlukeseye.com/Conditions/Cataracts.asp (accessed July 15, 2005).
6. American Diabetes Association, "National Diabetes Fact Sheet," http://www.diabetes.org/diabetes-statistics/national-diabetes-fact-sheet.jsp (accessed June 12, 2005).
7. Medline Plus, "Obesity," http://www.nlm.nih.gov/medlineplus/ency/article/003101.htm (accessed June 12, 2005).
8. Centers for Disease Control, "How Common Are Autism Spectrum Disorders (ASD)?" www.cdc.gov (accessed October 18, 2006).
9. Patricia Romanowski Bashe and Barbara L. Kirby, *OASIS Guide to Asperger Syndrome*, 2nd ed. (New York, NY: Crown Publishers, 2005).
10. Autism Society of America, www.autism-society.org (accessed October 18, 2006).
11. Medline Plus, "Autism," http://www.nlm.nih.gov/medlineplus/ency/article/001526.htm (accessed July 15, 2005).
12. American Cancer Society, "What Is Cancer?" http://www.cancer.rg/docroot/CRI/content/CRI_2_4_1x_What_Is_Cancer.asp?sitearea (accessed July 15, 2005).
13. National Institute of Neurological Disorders and Stroke, "Cerebral Palsy: Hope Through Research," http://www.ninds.nih.gov/disorders/cerebral_palsy/detail_cerebral_palsy.htm#12053104 (accessed July 15, 2005).
14. March of Dimes, "Cerebral Palsy," http://www.marchofdimes.com/pnhec/4439_1208.asp (accessed July 15, 2005).
15. Cystic Fibrosis Foundation, "About Cystic Fibrosis," http://www.cff.org/about_cf/what_is_cf/ (accessed July 15, 2005).
16. Multiple Sclerosis Foundation, "MS Info: FAQs," http://www.msfacts.org/info/info_faq.html (accessed July 15, 2005).
17. Medline Plus, "Poliomyelitis," http://www.nlm.nih.gov/medlineplus/ency/article/001402.htm (accessed July 15, 2005).
18. National Institute of Neurological Disorders and Stroke, "Spina Bifida," http://www.ninds.nih.gov/disorders/spina_bifida/detail_spina_bifida.htm (accessed July 15, 2005).
19. Mayo Clinic Medical Services, "Myasthenia Gravis," http://www.mayoclinic.com/invoke.cfm?id=DS00375 (accessed July 15, 2005).
20. Myasthenia Gravis Foundation of America, Inc., "Emergency Management of Myasthenia Gravis," http://www.myasthenia.org/information/emergency.pdf (accessed July 15, 2005).

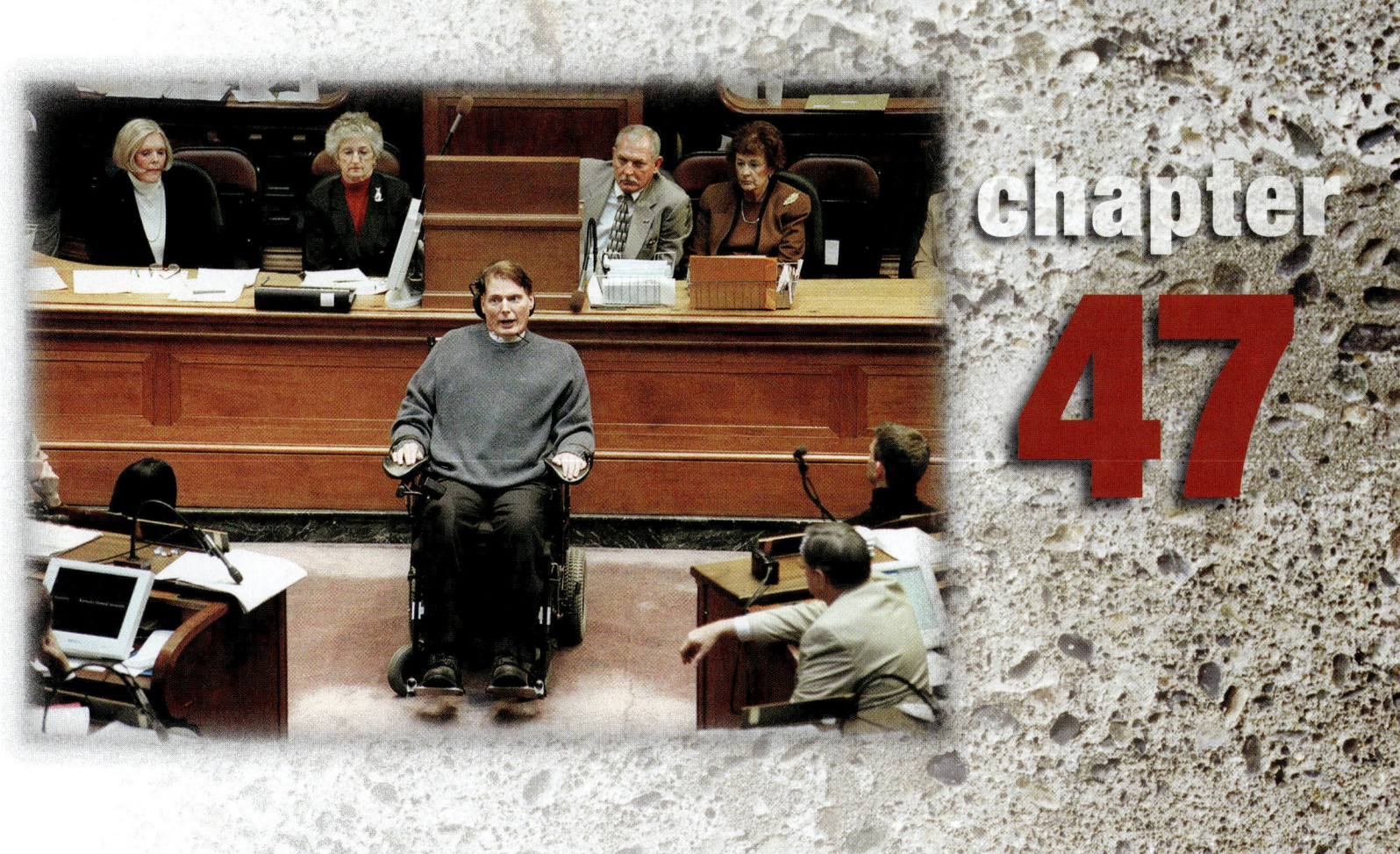

Patients with Chronic Illnesses

"*Your body is not who you are. The mind and spirit transcend the body. I think a hero is an ordinary individual who finds the strength to persevere and endure in spite of overwhelming obstacles.*"

—Christopher Reeve, referring to the number of disabled patients he met when he was first injured.

Need to Know

▶ That patients are being discharged with continuing medical needs, dependent on technology and technicians to keep them as healthy and comfortable as possible.

▶ EMS system policy regarding accessing ports or using devices that are in place on patients.

▶ The typical complications in a variety of home health and hospice situations.

▶ That patients have rights and that they may choose no care or limits to the care provided.

▶ The psychosocial needs of patients being cared for at home.

▶ Do	▶ Ask
• Familiarize yourself with system protocols regarding home healthcare patients.	• What is your system's policy toward home health and hospice patients?
• Become familiar with home care and hospice patients in your community.	• Ask home care technicians about the patient's history, treatments provided, and devices in place.
• Determine what, if any, dialysis centers may be in your community, and review possible complications patients using these centers might develop.	• Discuss with dialysis patients when their last treatment was and what their typical treatment schedule is.
• Be familiar with skin care problems typical of ostomy patients.	• Question ostomy patients about recent drainage history.

Introduction

A paramedics is one of the few medical professionals who makes house calls. However, there is another field of medicine that has well-established roots in the home. This field is home healthcare, a profession that treats patients at home for medical problems that were once only treated in the hospital setting. Home healthcare, along with the technical devices seen in the home healthcare environment, is a flourishing industry. Home healthcare has been around for many years, but due to a number of factors such as the increasing cost of hospitalization and the advances in automation of medical equipment, there has been a dramatic expansion in this field of patient care (Box 47-1).

Patients who once had lengthy hospital stays are now being discharged earlier to their homes to recuperate, undergo infusion therapies, or continue treatments for their medical conditions. As a result of the increasing acuity of patient conditions seen in the home healthcare setting, the paramedic will encounter a number of medical devices used to treat these conditions. Whether troubleshooting problems with these devices or maintaining the use of these devices during the evaluation, care, and transport of these patients, the paramedic of the present and the future must have a basic understanding of these devices to ensure optimal patient care. DOT 6-6.39

This chapter will discuss the expansion of the home healthcare industry, the advantages and disadvantages of home care, as well as the different types of healthcare providers caring for these patients. We will review frequently encountered devices found in the out-of-hospital environment and how to use and troubleshoot them. Different types of home care, including palliative care, hospice care, and comfort care, will be discussed. Finally, because there cannot be a field of medicine without legal, ethical, and moral concerns, we will cover some of the medical, legal, and emotional aspects of home care and hospice care. **The following Skill Sheets support this chapter: Skill Sheet 1: Airway Positioning and Maneuvers (and Step-by-Step 1), Skill Sheet 6: Foreign Body Airway Obstruction Removal—Advanced Techniques (and Step-by-Step 6), Skill Sheet 8: ALS Airway Adjuncts, Skill Sheet 10: End Tidal Capnography, Skill Sheet 11: Endotracheal Suctioning (and Step-by-Step 11), Skill Sheet 12: Pulse Oximetry (and Step-by-Step 12), Skill Sheet 23: Suctioning of Stoma (and Step-by-Step 23), Skill Sheet 24: Evacuation of Gastric Contents (and Step-by-Step 24), Skill Sheet 43: Intravenous Access Using Saline Lock (and Step-by-Step 43), Skill Sheet 47: Central Line Access for Fluids and Drug Administration, Skill Sheet 60: Putting On and Removing Gloves, and Skill Sheet 61: Handwashing (and Step-by-Step 61).**

History of Home Healthcare

Home healthcare began in the United States in the late 1700s in Boston. The original home healthcare workers were provided by the church to care for the poor in their homes when they became ill.[1] It was not until 1877 in New York City that licensed nurses played a role in the home healthcare setting.[2] During the 1900s, a steady expansion was seen in the role of licensed nurses in the home healthcare setting. However, during the 1980s the home healthcare industry experienced remarkable

BOX 47-1   Christopher Reeve

Christopher Reeve may have acted the part of Superman in his days as a film star, but he became a true hero after a tragic equestrian accident left him paralyzed in 1995. Reeve was thrown from his horse, landing on his head. Though his helmet protected his brain, he fractured his first and second cervical vertebra and was instantly paralyzed and apneic. Paramedics on the scene ventilated him and rapidly transported him to a Level I Trauma Center.

Reeve, like many other disabled and ventilator-dependent patients, required skilled care in order to stay alive. A mechanical ventilator supported his breathing. Like many patients who are paralyzed, Reeve eventually developed a pressure wound that became infected. The infection in this wound became systemic, causing septic shock.

Reeve was a strong supporter of EMS and safety. He died October 10, 2004, one month before he was scheduled to address the Virginia state EMS conference as the keynote speaker. His speech was written in honor of the EMS personnel who he credited for saving his life.

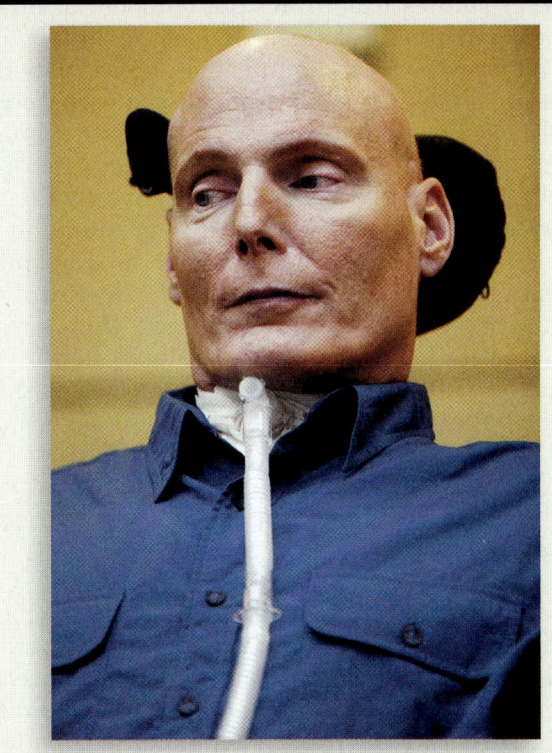

growth when the federal government changed legislation to control cost inflation in healthcare, and hospitals were no longer able to charge in a manner that assured them payment for services rendered.

Under the new system, hospitals would be paid a set amount for specific medical conditions based on **diagnosis-related groups (DRG).** This value, established by the government, specified a range of treatments and dictated the number of hospital days permitted for established conditions. If their costs exceeded the Prospective Payment System (PPS) DRG amount, the hospital would end up writing off those costs.[3] As a result of these new regulations, patients were discharged from hospitals "sicker and quicker." For example, patients admitted to the hospital with a diagnosis of acute myocardial infarction spent an average of 11.7 days in the hospital between 1986 and 1988 compared to an average of 5.9 days between 1997 and 1999.[4] These factors were instrumental in the rapid expansion of the home healthcare industry.[5] In 1997, while Medicare reimbursements were cut under the enacted Balanced Budget Act, home healthcare continued to grow due to its popularity and cost effectiveness.[6]

Home Healthcare Today

With the changes in hospital billing practices and, in turn, the dramatic decrease in the length of hospital admissions comes a dilemma for the patient, the family, and the interdisciplinary team charged with caring for the patient: Where is the patient going to be cared for when discharged from the hospital? The answer is specific to each patient and is based on multiple factors pertaining to each individual. These factors include the nature of the patient's hospitalization and the acuity of the patient at the time of discharge; the patient's financial status, including insurance and monetary capabilities; the options for care that are available in the area in which the patient lives; the patient's desire for care; the amount of care that is needed (can the patient's needs be met in several hours by a home care aide on a daily basis, does the patient require 24-hour nursing care, or is there some middle ground that fits the patient's needs the best?); and the informal support network for the patient once they are discharged.

Patients in need of more assistance than can be provided by their immediate support network, consisting typically of family or friends, are usually discharged to a **skilled nursing facility (SNF)** or to the home setting where they are given the services and equipment needed to provide for their needs. As previously mentioned, the factors that determine the type of care required by each individual are unique to the individual; however, recent research suggests that certain medical conditions may respond better to the treatment rendered in particular types of discharge settings as opposed to others.

Several studies examining the outcome of home healthcare patients discharged from the hospital with a respiratory diagnosis found that these patients appeared to benefit greatly from this type of post-hospital care. For example, Stewart and Vandenbroek and their colleagues discovered that "High risk patients with a discharge diagnosis of congestive heart failure were shown to have a significant reduction in unplanned readmission to the hospital, total hospital stay, hospital based costs, and mortality when enrolled in a home-based intervention program."[7] Similar results can be found regarding home healthcare interventions for patients with conditions such as chronic atrial fibrillation. "The benefits of home-based intervention (for patients with chronic atrial fibrillation) was associated with a trend towards prolonged event-free survival and fewer fatal events (than patients who received the usual post-discharge care)."[8]

A number of researchers support the use of home healthcare for patients who have suffered a cerebro-vascular accident (CVA); however, others suggest that placement into the hospital or an SNF for acute rehabilitation of a stroke patient may be more beneficial. Ozdemir, Birtane and others state: "Intense inpatient (either hospital or SNF) rehabilitation for stroke survivors provided significantly more favorable functional and cognitive outcomes with relatively low complications than did nonintense rehabilitation efforts in the home setting."[9] This is not to say that all CVA patients should receive their rehabilitation in a SNF or that all patients discharged from the hospital should receive their care at home. The point is that there are multiple options available to patients once they are discharged from the hospital. The issue of importance to paramedics is that they understand and are able to care for the conditions that these patients have and the medical devices used to care for these patients. DOT 6-6.26

The Complexities of Home Healthcare

The complex needs of the new generation of home care patients introduces the challenge of caring for them without the luxuries found in the hospital. This task is accomplished by advances in training and patient care, as well by advances in medical equipment designed to care for patients in the out-of-hospital setting. Many devices used in the hospital for treating critically ill patients have been adapted for use in the home. Mechanical ventilators and infusion pumps are just two examples of these devices.

Patients with serious, long-term physical conditions such as severe strokes, or amyotrophic lateral sclerosis (ALS) (Lou Gehrig's disease) who need

prolonged ventilatory assistance were at one time without options as to where they received their care. The availability of ventilators designed for use in the out-of-hospital setting, along with highly trained home healthcare professionals, affords the ventilator-dependant patient a variety of options concerning the location of their ongoing care.

Similarly, patients requiring chemotherapy, parenteral nutrition, or IV antibiotics are being treated in the out-of-hospital setting with a variety of different vascular access devices. A discussion of the use and trouble-shooting of a variety of medical devices that are being used in the out-of-hospital setting will be presented later in this chapter. DOT 6-6.1, 6-6.2, 6-6.23, 6-6.34, 6-6.38

Types of Home Healthcare

Just as some hospitals specialize in one area of medicine (e.g., trauma), some home healthcare agencies and extended care facilities cater to specific patient populations (e.g., patients who have dementia). On the other hand, just as some hospitals provide care to patients with varying medical conditions, so do various out-of-hospital care providers. In fact, many of the services available in the hospital setting are now offered to patients at home or in an extended care facility. For example, some home healthcare and extended care facilities offer services by physicians, nurse practitioners, pharmacists, registered nurses, licensed vocational nurses, certified nursing assistants, home health aides, social workers, physical and occupational therapists, respiratory therapists, speech language pathologists, medical equipment and supply dealers, and volunteers, to name a few.[10]

Home extended care facilities are very similar to the hospital when it comes to their reasons for existence. All of these medical care providers have several goals in common, but the primary objective that tops the list of importance and extends to all types of healthcare is providing the best quality medical care possible.

When discussing the objectives of the home care professional versus the caregiver who works in an extended care setting, many similarities and one major difference are discovered. The workers in the home healthcare environment are not only faced with the challenge of the treatment or maintenance of the patient's medical condition, but they are also faced with the task of supporting the patient's family, maintaining the home, and maintaining the patient's independence by preventing the patient from being admitted to an extended care facility.

Early hospital discharge of patients with high acuity medical conditions increases the possibility that the patients' conditions may deteriorate once they return home. Even the best efforts of a highly skilled healthcare provider cannot prevent some patients from taking an unfortunate turn for the worse and requiring emergent care. It is at this juncture that the worlds of the home healthcare providers and the emergency medical service (EMS) workers meet.

The Objective of Home Healthcare

The objective of the healthcare provider that works in the acute care setting (typically the emergency department or the in-patient hospital setting) is not different from the out-of-hospital healthcare setting (home care or SNF) or the EMS prehospital setting. The objective in all of these settings is the treatment of the patient's medical condition and improving or maintaining the patient's overall health.

The EMS field has many similarities to the acute care setting, especially the emergency department (ED). Just as the name implies, the ED deals with life-threatening and emergent conditions. The difference between ED and EMS professionals relates to level of training, scope of practice, and site of practice. In fact, the two fields are so similar that EMS workers (paramedics and emergency medical technicians) frequently work in EDs. Healthcare workers in the acute care (in-hospital) setting differ from the ED or EMS worker because they are charged with the task of taking these acutely ill patients once they have made their way from the EMS worker's environment, through the ED, and into the next stage of care. In this area, the healthcare provider works in conjunction with a physician and other healthcare specialists to continue the stabilization and treatment of patients until such time as they can be discharged home or to an out-of-hospital healthcare setting. DOT 6-6.35

Home Healthcare Professionals

Because there are a number of different healthcare professionals that the paramedic will encounter in the out-of-hospital setting, the roles of some of the most frequently encountered individuals as well as the level of training that they must have to function in their capacity are discussed next.

The following are general examples of training standards and roles and responsibilities for the different healthcare workers found in the out-of-hospital setting, and they may differ from state to state. For training standards and scope of practice specific to your state, contact the certifying or licensing organization in your area. Some of the workers in the home care or extended care setting (personal care aides, attendants, homemakers, and companions, or sitters) do not provide direct patient care. These workers provide support to people in need through assistance with house chores, childcare, and cooking. For the most part, these workers are not licensed or regulated. DOT 6-6.27, 6-6.32

Home Health Aides (HHA)

The **home health aid (HHA)** assists healthcare professionals such as nurses with the care of patients in the home care setting. HHAs do house chores, take care of children, and provide assistance to patients who could not otherwise live at home without their assistance.

The following are a few of the duties that an HHA may perform: assisting the patient with bathing, toileting, dressing, basic bandage changes, cooking, laundry, and emotional support, and assistance in maintaining independence.

The requirements to become an HHA are completion of a 120-hour home health aide certification course. The course teaches basic nutrition; meal planning and preparation; home cleaning tasks; and techniques for bathing, turning, and transferring a patient. The training covers emotional problems caused by illness, the aging process, and the behavior of the elderly. The training can be taken at a community college or vocational school and does not require completion of high school as a prerequisite.[11]

Certified Nursing Assistant (CNA)

Certified nursing assistants (CNA), also known as nursing aides, assist other healthcare professionals (especially nurses, physical therapists, and occupational therapists). Their duties include taking vital signs and assisting the patient with their **activities of daily living (ADL),** which include bathing, toileting, dressing, feeding, and assisting with house chores. CNAs observe the overall status of the patient and report any changes to the healthcare professionals that they are working with.[12] CNA training consists of approximately 200 hours of theory and clinical instruction, including personal skills, communication skills, rehabilitation skills, patient rights, prevention and management, body management, medical and surgical asepsis, patient care procedures, vital signs, nutrition, emergency procedures, long-term care, observation and charting, death and dying, elder abuse, dementia, and cultural awareness.

Licensed Vocational Nurse (LVN) and Licensed Practical Nurse (LPN)

An **LVN** is an entry-level nurse who provides basic nursing care under the direction of a physician or a registered nurse. **LPNs** provide patient care to the sick and the injured as well as the physically and mentally disabled. Some of their responsibilities include obtaining vital signs, administering injections, administering certain medications, applying and changing dressings, and assisting patients with their ADLs. The training for the LVN and LPN consists of approximately 1,530 hours that include around 576 hours of theory (54 of which are dedicated to pharmacology) and about 954 hours of clinical experience. The course usually takes 12 to 18 months. A high school diploma or equivalent is a prerequisite for entry into an LPN program.[13]

Registered Nurse (RN)

An **RN** is a healthcare professional who provides direct patient care under the direction of a physician, works in conjunction with other healthcare professionals (such as physical and occupational therapists), and directs the care provided by HHAs, CNAs, LVNs and LPNs, Some of the responsibilities of the RN include assessing patients, administering medications, performing dressing changes, administering injections, monitoring patient condition and advising the physician of any pertinent changes, documentation of care provided, and changes in patient condition.

A registered nurse must complete a state-approved nursing program. Typical options for becoming an RN include attending a community college and obtaining a two-year (associate's) degree or attending a four-year college and obtaining a bachelor's degree in nursing. Upon completion of the requisite training, the individual must take and pass a state licensure examination. In addition to the process discussed, the nurse must (in many states) get fingerprinted and undergo a criminal background check at the state or federal level.

Hospice Worker

Another healthcare professional that can be found in the out-of-hospital environment is the hospice worker. The professionals that make up hospice are a diverse and well-respected group of individuals. Their responsibilities range from providing medical care and pain relief to helping the patient and their family prepare for what

is to come. The members of the hospice team include physicians, nurses, social workers, religious or spiritual personnel, pharmacists, medical equipment and supply providers, volunteers, and many more. The objectives of the hospice worker focus on providing comfort to patients at the end of their lives, assisting patients and their family in getting all of their affairs in order, and maintaining the functioning of the household.[14] Further discussion of hospice care will take place later in this chapter.

With exposure to the serious acuity of patients that the paramedic will encounter in the out-of-hospital setting comes an understanding of the possibilities of all that can go wrong with these patients. A baseline comprehension of the conditions that these patients may have and, equally important, a knowledge of the medical devices that will be used to treat these patients, is critical in the age of early hospital discharge and expanding out-of-hospital care. DOT 6-6.3, 6-6.4, 6-6.5, 6-6.6, 6-6.7

Medical Devices Seen in the Out-of-Hospital Setting

Before discussing some of the medical equipment that the paramedic will encounter in the out-of-hospital setting, some of the basic concepts of dealing with these devices will be discussed.

First and foremost, if it is not broken, do not fix it. If it is broken and you do not know how to fix it or you are not permitted to use or troubleshoot such a device in the scope of practice of your state or region, leave it alone. Changing settings in general is always risky.

If possible, turn it off or otherwise discontinue its use. If you do not know how to turn it off, ask the person in charge of the patient's care. If they do not know how to fix it or discontinue its use, contact medical control, the manufacturer of the equipment (if their contact information is available) or the company that sold or rented the equipment to the patient.

Ultimately, if you are not specifically trained on how to repair a piece of medical equipment, do not try to fix it.

Your attempts to fix such equipment could have a negative effect on the patient, and if that is the case, the detrimental effects on the patient may be serious, if not fatal.

When you are faced with a malfunctioning piece of equipment, do not overthink the situation. Keep it simple and return to the basics. Assess and manage the

Nice to Know

Background and criminal checks are occurring for all levels of health care workers and may even be required prior to your admission to a clinical site as a paramedic student.

ABCs. No matter what is broken or how serious the situation, the bottom line is, first do no harm.

The content of this section is designed to give paramedics a basic understanding of some of the devices that they may encounter in the out-of-hospital setting. It is not a substitute for the in-depth training that should take place if your provider agency utilizes some or all of these devices. The fact that you have gained a basic knowledge of these devices does not change your scope of practice. If you are not approved to utilize these devices or if you are unable to obtain information on what to do in the event that you encounter any of these devices (in the policies and protocols that govern your EMS system), contact medical control for guidance. DOT 6-6.13

Airway Management and Oxygen Delivery Devices

Many home care patients are on some form of oxygen. The types of oxygen delivery systems seen in the home care setting are similar to those seen in the hospital and in the EMS field. The major difference between these settings is not necessarily the device that delivers the oxygen to the patient but the source of the oxygen. Where hospitals have oxygen plumbed into the walls and utilize portable oxygen tanks with regulators, oxygen for use in the home care setting typically comes in three forms (Figure 47-1):

1. Liquid oxygen
2. Oxygen concentrators
3. Compressed oxygen stored in tanks

The need for acute interventions in the home care setting surrounding oxygen use does not typically involve sources of oxygen or delivery systems; it involves patients who have acute presentations of respiratory distress, exacerbations of existing respiratory conditions, or any other conditions in which the patients are not receiving or distributing oxygen in a manner that will ultimately support life. This is not to say that you will never be called to assist a patient who has run out of oxygen or has a malfunctioning oxygen concentrator, but these situations are not in the scope of this discussion.

Ventilators

What Is a Mechanical Ventilator?

Mechanical ventilators are machines that allow for a specific concentration of oxygen to be warmed, humidified, and delivered in a specific volume to patients who are not able to breathe on their own or have an impaired ability to breathe in a manner that will sustain them (Figure 47-2).

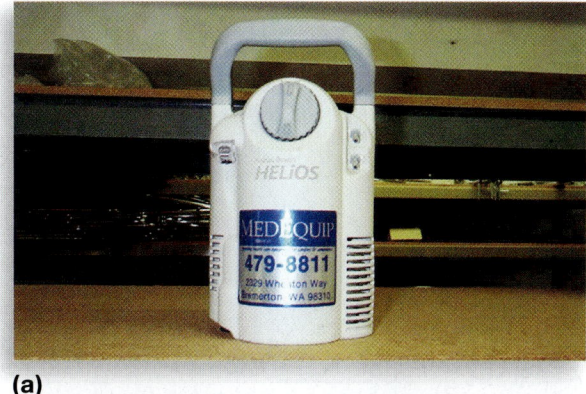

(a)

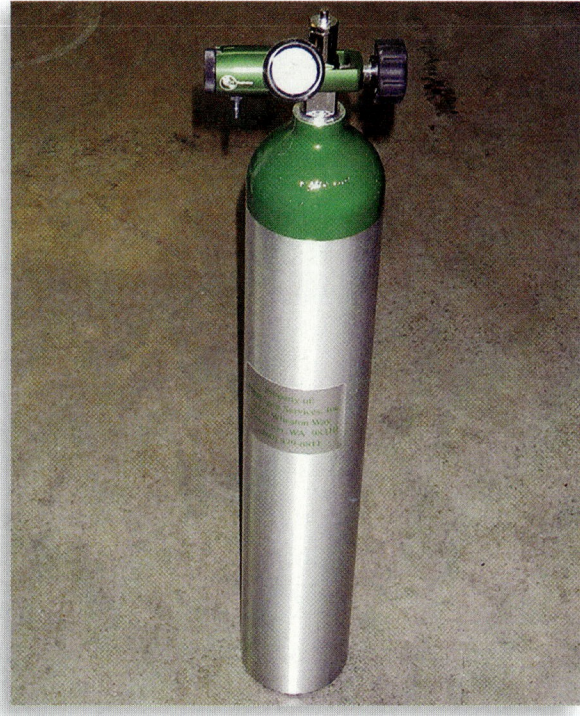

(b)

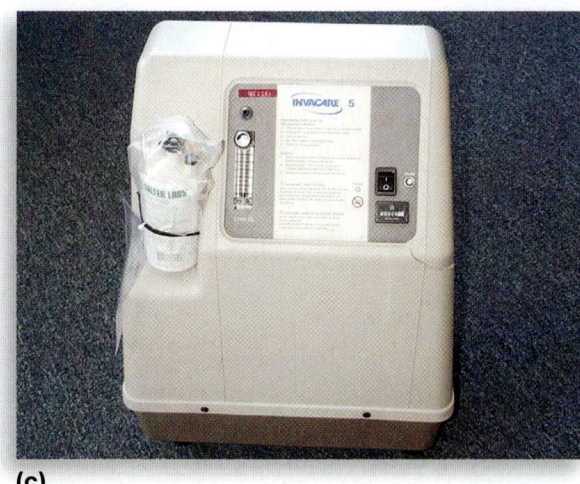

(c)

Figure 47-1   Oxygen for home care use. (a) Liquid oxygen machine. (b) Compressed oxygen stored in tank. (c) Oxygen concentrator.

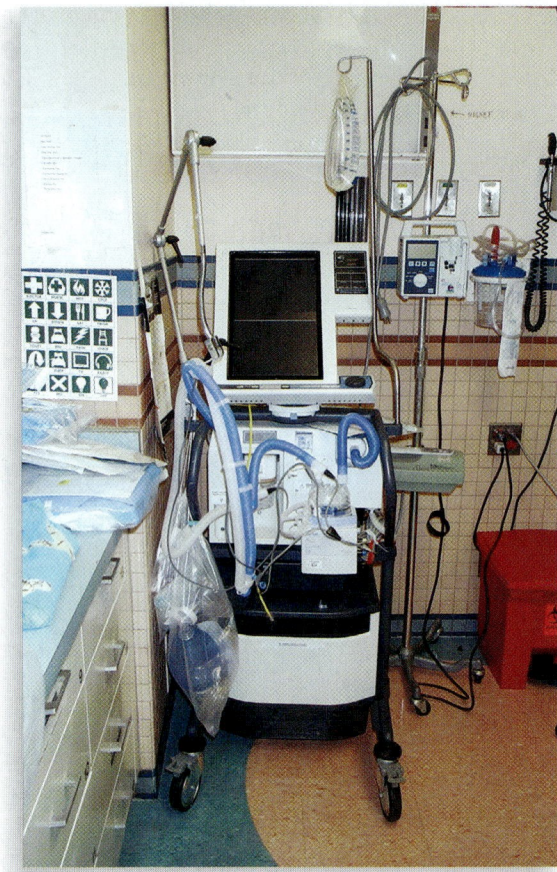

Figure 47-2 A mechanical ventilator.

TABLE 47-1 Frequently Used Mechanical Ventilation Abbreviations and Terms

Abbreviation	Term
A/C	Assist/control
CMV	Controlled mandatory ventilation or conventional mechanical ventilation
CPAP	Continuous positive airway pressure
SIMV	Synchronized intermittent mandatory ventilation
FiO$_2$	Fractionalized inspired oxygen concentration or functional concentration of inspired oxygen
I:E	Inspiratory to expiratory ratio
PEEP	Positive end expiratory pressure
PIP	Peak inspiratory pressure
V$_T$	Tidal volume

Ventilators can be reduced to a number of components: "A source of oxygen and air, warming and humidification system, valves controlling and monitoring gas flow, a user interface, a breathing circuit of plastic tubing and mechanisms for patient monitoring with alarm systems."[15] Table 47-1 lists frequently used ventilator terms and abbreviations.

When it comes to ventilators, remember the previously mentioned advice to keep it simple. If you are not familiar with ventilators, a call to treat a patient on a ventilator can be intimidating. In this situation there are several things to keep in mind:

1. When there is a malfunction with a ventilator, there is usually an alarm that sounds to let you know that there is something wrong. In most modern ventilators, the alarm will direct you to the source of the ventilator malfunction.

2. If the patient is in a home care or extended care facility, there is usually a caregiver that can help troubleshoot and, in many instances, correct the problem. (knowing the capabilities of the healthcare professionals that you are working with and being open to making the care of the patient a collaborative effort will likely provide the patient with the best care possible.)

3. If the problem cannot be resolved despite your best efforts and the best efforts of the healthcare worker(s) in charge of caring for the patient, the best course of action is once again to return to the basics. Turn off the ventilator or disconnect the patient from the ventilator, assess the patient's ABCs, and provide ventilatory assistance to the patient with a bag-mask device (in fact, if the troubleshooting of the problem is not accomplished almost immediately, disconnect the patient from the ventilator, assess the ABCs, and provide ventilatory assistance while further troubleshooting takes place). Do not overthink the situation. Keep it simple and use the bag-mask device if the ventilator is malfunctioning. Further discussion of troubleshooting of a malfunctioning ventilator will be discussed later in this chapter. DOT 6-6.16, 6-6.31

Patients Who Require a Ventilator

Most patients who require mechanical ventilation for acute medical conditions will be cared for in the hospital. In the hospital, when patients have been intubated and placed on a ventilator for an acute condition or an exacerbation of a chronic condition and their situation doesn't improve, patients may receive another type of advanced airway adjunct to allow for long-term ventilatory assistance. The airway of choice for prolonged airway management during ventilatory assistance is the tracheostomy tube.[16] The patient that has a tracheostomy tube and requires mechanical ventilation is the most likely case that the paramedic will encounter in the out-of-hospital setting. Examples of patients that may require the insertion of a tracheostomy tube and prolonged mechanical ventilation are patients with cerebrovascular accidents affecting the brainstem and the respiratory regulating portion of the brain, patients with traumatic brain injury, patients with a spinal injury to the cervical region that has caused a loss of diaphragmatic function, and patients with medical conditions such as amyotrophic lateral sclerosis (ALS) (Lou Gehrig's disease). Tracheostomy tubes are discussed in detail in the next section.

What You Need to Know about Mechanical Ventilators

The focus of this section is the delivery of care to patients who are experiencing trouble with their mechanical ventilators in the out-of-hospital setting. The depth of the information regarding ventilators will be specific to basic ventilator modes, alarms, and basic troubleshooting in the event of a ventilator alarm and possible ventilator malfunction.

A patient receiving mechanical ventilation in the out-of-hospital setting should have preestablished ventilator settings that have been tested and are appropriate for use on that individual patient. There are several different ventilator *modes* that may be chosen when the patient is initially placed on a ventilator. The modes are typically chosen based on the presentation of the patient and their underlying medical condition. Table 47-2 discusses the basic ventilator modes and examples of the type of patient that would be expected to use each of the modes.[16]

In addition to the selection of the mode of ventilation, there are several *parameters* that need to be selected for each individual patient. Table 47-3 outlines the basic ventilator parameters.[17]

Patients are placed on a ventilator in a manner that will assure that their respiratory and physiologic needs are being met. The mode of ventilation and the parameters used on each patient are assessed following their implementation to assure that they are appropriate for that patient. There are several means of assessing the

TABLE 47-2   Basic Ventilator Modes

Ventilator Modes*	Used for
CMV (Controlled mandatory ventilation)	The mode that is used when the patient is not breathing. The ventilator does all of the work of breathing for the patient.
CPAP (Continuous positive airway pressure)	The ventilator applies pressure during the entire respiratory cycle. This mode is used for patients who are breathing on their own but would benefit from positive pressure to expand atelectasic lungs, to ease the work of breathing, or as a weaning mode.
A/C (Assist/control)	Often used as the initial mode of ventilation in patients who are breathing but are tired from the work of breathing. It can also be used if the patient cannot initiate their own respiration. The ventilator can sense the patient's attempt to breathe as a negative pressure and will trigger the ventilator to deliver a prescribed volume of air. The patient can breathe at a rate faster than the set rate of the ventilator, and the machine will assure that the prescribed volume is delivered with each ventilation.
SIMV (Simultaneous intermittent mandatory ventilation)	Combines spontaneous breathing with A/C mode. The ventilator will function at a set SIMV rate, and if the patient breathes faster than the set rate, there will be no assistance from the ventilator. The mandatory ventilations that take place at the set rate will be volume assisted ventilations triggered by the patient's inspiratory effort. If the patient does not take a breath within a reasonable time frame, the ventilator will initiate a breath on its own. This is a useful mode for patients who have a normal respiratory drive but weak or fatigued respiratory muscles; to prevent atrophy of the respiratory muscles caused by prolonged ventilator use; and to assist in weaning a patient from the ventilator.
PEEP (Positive end expiratory pressure)	PEEP is the maintenance of pressure in the lungs at the end of the inspiratory cycle by preventing lung emptying. PEEP is indicated for any respiratory condition that is accompanied by alveolar collapse.

*(The manner in which the ventilator and the patient interact is based primarily on the respiratory effort and the underlying condition of the patient.)
Source: Adapted from R.L. Boggs, "Airway Management," *AACN Procedural Manual for Critical Care,* 3rd ed. (Philadelphia, PA: W. B. Saunders, 1993).

TABLE 47-3   **Basic Ventilator Parameters**

Sensitivity	• Specifies the effort required to trigger a breath when the ventilator is in the A/C, CPAP, or SIMV mode.
FiO$_2$	• Concentration of oxygen delivered with each ventilation • Initially set between 80–100% and decreased in increments of 10% until it is less than or equal to 50% based on pulse oximetry (an FiO$_2$ greater or equal to 50% is considered toxic if applied for an extended time).
V$_T$	• The amount of air inspired and expired with each breath • Normal spontaneous tidal volume 5–6 mL/kg ideal body weight* • Ventilator tidal volume should be approximately 6–8 mL/kg ideal body weight or approximately 10mL/kg actual body weight
Ventilatory rate	• The number of breaths delivered each minute • Usually between eight and 12 per minute (consider minute ventilation [Ve])
I:E ratio	• The amount of time spent in the inspiratory cycle compared with exhalation • The normal I:E ratio is 1:2, but patients with a prolonged expiratory phase (e.g., asthmatics) may need an I:E ratio of 1:3 or 1:4

*Ideal body weight is calculated as follows:
Men: 106 lb + 6 × (height in inches − 60)
Women: 105 lb + 5 × (height in inches − 60)

Source: Adapted from C. Spritzer, "Unraveling the Mysteries of a Mechanical Ventilator: A Helpful Step-by-Step Guide," *Journal of Emergency Nursing* 29 (2003): 29–36.

benefits of the chosen ventilator settings. The combination of multiple assessment tools, the constant reassessment of the ventilator settings, and the patient's physiologic status lead to the ventilator settings used by each individual patient in the home setting.

No matter where you find your patient requiring mechanical ventilation, there should be a readily accessible document that lists the patient's prescribed ventilator settings. This is nice to have, but keep in mind that the settings listed on this document are always subject to change. Remember that changes in patient status due to a number of factors may necessitate the alteration of the settings of the ventilator, and these changes are beyond the scope of this chapter. The steps that need to be taken in the event that there are changes in the patient's physiologic status, and in turn, changes in the patient's ventilatory needs, will be discussed in the following section.

Responding to Ventilator Alarms in the Out-of-Hospital Setting

In reality, most of the situations that involve ventilator alarms in the out-of-hospital setting will be assessed and easily corrected by the healthcare professionals who care for the patient on a regular basis. It is gradual or abrupt changes in the patient's condition that result in the need for involvement of EMS workers in the care of the ventilator patient. It does not matter why paramedics are called to assist the patient requiring mechanical ventilation;

it is important that they have a basic understanding of what to do in the event that a ventilator alarm sounds.

The paramedic's approach to ventilator alarms is quite simple. The overall concern of the paramedic is not the alarm, but the patient.

Treat the patient, not the alarm.

The advice to keep it simple has never been as valuable as when you are faced with a ventilator that is alarming.

This is what you need to do:

1. Remain calm.
2. Assess the patient for any signs of obvious changes in respiratory status (in other words, assess the patient's ABCs).
3. If there is any question concerning the patency of the patient's airway or their oxygenation status, disconnect the patient from the ventilator and assure that the airway is patent, and if it is, provide high concentrations of oxygen via a bag-mask device until the problem with the ventilator can be addressed.
4. If the problem cannot be addressed, if there is not a back-up ventilator, or if the reason for the ventilator alarm was a deterioration in the patient's respiratory or physiologic status, continue your interventions and transport the patient to an appropriate hospital.

Table 47-4 discusses some of the ventilator alarm situations that may be encountered by paramedics in the out-of-hospital setting.[18]

TABLE 47-4   Common Ventilator Alarm Situations and What to do

Alarm	Troubleshooting Actions	Corrective Action
Low pressure	1. Check to make sure that the patient is connected to the ventilator. 2. Check for leaks in or disconnection of the ventilator tubing. 3. Check for leaks in the airway or the airway balloon.	1. Be prepared to ventilate the patient with a bag-mask device and O_2. 2. Replace any leaking equipment and reconnect any disconnected tubing. 3. Be prepared to replace the airway if defective.
High pressure	1. Check for secretions or obstructions in the airway. 2. Check placement of the airway and displacement of the airway balloon. 3. Check for kinks in the ventilator tubing. 4. Check for water in the tubing. 5. Assess the patient who is coughing. 6. Assess the patient for anxiety level.	1. Be prepared to suction the airway or relieve an obstruction. 2. Be prepared to ventilate the patient with a bag-mask device and O_2. 3. Be prepared to remove the existing airway and replace it with another airway. 4. Remove any kinks, and if necessary, replace kinked ventilator tubing. 5. Remove the patient from ventilator and drain H_2O from the tubing. 6. If the patient is coughing, suction the patient, and if coughing persists, consult medical direction. 7. If the patient becomes anxious, assess the patient for signs of hypoxia, or need for suctioning and incorporate calming measures; if anxiety persists contact medical direction for sedative medication order.
Apnea	1. Determine if the patient is breathing. 2. Check for leaks. 3. Check sensitivity setting to assure that the ventilator is able to detect the patient's respiratory effort. 4. Check the apnea alarm time interval.	1. Treat the patient. 2. Be prepared to ventilate the patient with a bag-mask device and O_2. 3. Replace any leaking equipment. 4. Work with the caregiver on the scene and the physician to set the appropriate parameters.
Power input	1. Check the power source. 2. Check the ventilator fuse or circuit breaker supplying the room. 3. Try pressing the reset button.	1. Be prepared to ventilate the patient with a bag-mask device and O_2. 2. Try another power outlet. 3. Replace the fuse or reset circuit breaker (make sure circuit is not overloaded with electric devices).
Inoperative ventilator	1. Assure inoperative ventilator alarm.	1. Be prepared to ventilate the patient with a bag-mask device and O_2. 2. Turn the ventilator off and on again.
Low tidal volume	1. Check to make sure that the patient is connected to the ventilator. 2. Check for leaks in, or disconnection of the ventilator tubing. 3. Check for leaks in the airway or the airway balloon.	1. Be prepared to ventilate the patient with a bag-mask device and O_2. 2. Replace any leaking equipment, and reconnect any disconnected tubing. 3. Be prepared to replace the airway if defective.
Low F_IO_2	1. Check the oxygen (air) source for proper functioning or supply.	1. Be prepared to supply O_2 or to ventilate the patient with a bag-mask device and O_2.

Source: Adapted from J. N. Cairo and S. Pilbeam, *Respiratory Care Equipment,* 7th ed. (St. Louis, MO: Mosby, 2004), p 378.

When an airway device that is being used for ventilating a patient becomes obstructed or, for whatever reason, is no longer effectively protecting the patient's airway, suctioning of the airway by normal means should be attempted. If suctioning does not adequately clear the patient's airway, then the airway adjunct may need to be removed, usually after discussion with medical control. If you are faced with an issue surrounding ventilator settings or advanced airway issues, contact medical direction for consultation.

DOT 6-6.17, 6-6.18

Street Secrets

When confronted by equipment you are unfamiliar with, go with what you know. Use your own equipment rather than something you are not comfortable with.

Tracheostomy Tubes

A **tracheostomy** is a surgical opening in the neck that extends into the trachea (Figure 47-3). The tracheostomy is frequently seen in conjunction with a **tracheostomy tube,** a curved tube that is inserted into the surgical incision, also called a **stoma,** and comes in varied angles and multiple sizes.[19] Because tracheostomy tubes are the preferred airway for use in patients that require prolonged mechanical ventilation, it is important that the paramedic has a basic understanding of the tracheostomy tube and problems that are frequently associated with them.

A basic understanding of the physiologic changes that occur as a result of tracheostomy tube insertion are helpful to understand when caring for problems associated with tracheostomy tubes. The major changes in physiology resulting from tracheostomy tube insertion are as follows:

1. Several functions specific to the upper and lower airways (warming, humidifying, and filtering of the air that is breathed) are altered or bypassed, which leads to a decreased ability of these check and balance systems to prevent infections. Because the upper airway is bypassed, the air that the tracheostomy patient breathes is colder, dryer, and lacking the filtration of larger particles typically provided by the upper airway. A combination of these factors leads to considerably thicker secretions in the lower airway and an increased chance of developing respiratory infections and pneumonia. [20]

2. The fact that tracheostomy patients suffer from a decreased ability of the cilia that line the lower airway to clear particulate matter is a contributing factor to increased infection rates.[20]

3. The materials that tracheostomy tubes are made of (plastic and metal) are viewed by the body as foreign substances. The body's response to this foreign substance is increased mucus production. This is another reason for increased infection rates, as well as atelectasis formation among tracheostomy patients.[21]

4. Because the tracheostomy patient is not able to generate enough pressure to initiate a strong cough, another means of airway clearance is hampered, and the chances of developing respiratory infections increase.

5. As a result of the insertion of the tracheostomy tube, the motor and sensory functions that coordinate the ability to swallow are affected, and the chance for aspiration increases.[21]

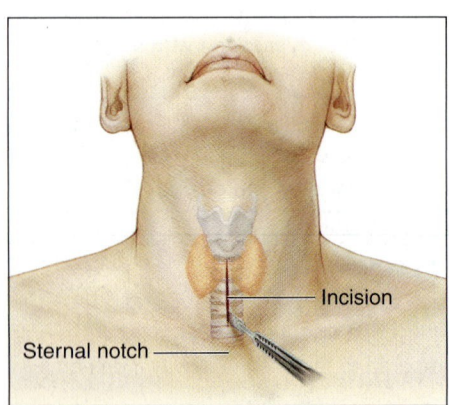

① Incision is made superior to sternal notch. Thyroid isthmus may have to be cut as well.

Incision
Sternal notch

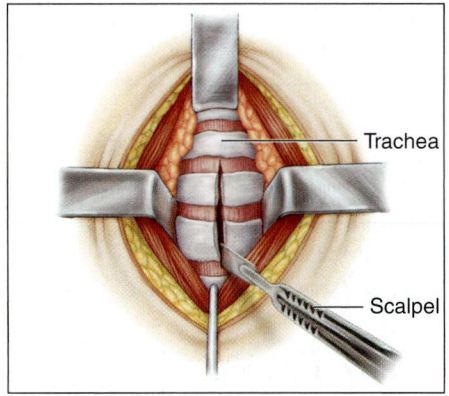

② Retractors separate the tissue, and an incision is made through the third and fourth tracheal rings.

Trachea
Scalpel

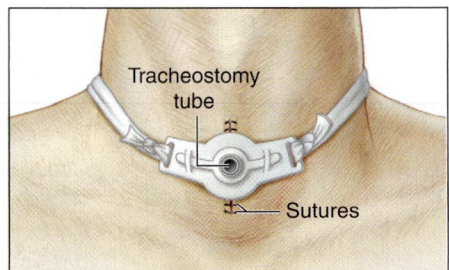

③ A tracheostomy tube is inserted, and the remaining incision is sutured closed.

Tracheostomy tube
Sutures

Figure 47-3 Tracheostomy procedure.

Tracheostomy Tubes

There are several types of tracheostomy tubes available for use on a variety of different patients (Figure 47-4 and Table 47-5). They can be made of plastic or metal. They come in a variety of sizes similar to endotracheal tubes. The average male size is 8 mm, and the average female size is 6 mm. The optimum size tracheostomy tube is one that has a small external diameter that will not cause tracheal stenosis and the largest possible internal diameter to decrease airway resistance.

The focus of this section is the acute care of the tracheostomy patient. The treatment for tracheostomy emergencies is the same, whether or not the patient is ventilator dependent.

Tracheostomy Mucous Plug

Because of some of the physiologic changes that take place when a tracheostomy tube is inserted into a patient, there is an increase in the production of mucus in the airway. Because the filtering, warming, and humidifying functions of the upper airway are bypassed and the patient has a decreased ability to cough and clear these secretions, the tracheostomy patient is not only at increased risk for developing respiratory infections, but also at-risk for developing mucous plugs.

If excess mucus is produced and not cleared from the patient's airway (through ciliary action, coughing, or by suctioning of the secretions), the passage of non-humidified air into and out of the tracheostomy with normal inspiration and exhalation will eventually lead to accumulation of dried thick mucus (otherwise known as a mucous plug). Patients dependent on a mechanical ventilator are fortunate that most ventilators have components that provide humidification, filtration, and warming of the air that is delivered through the tracheostomy. But, even with frequent suctioning and the benefits of advanced ventilator functions, the tracheostomy patient remains highly susceptible to mucous plug formation.

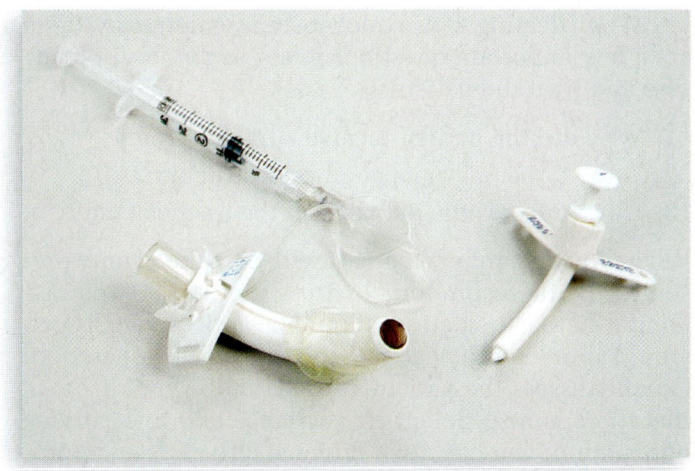

Figure 47-4 Tracheostomy tubes.

TABLE 47-5 Tracheostomy Tubes

Type	Use
Cuffed	• Must be used on a patient that requires mechanical ventilation. • When inflated, isolates the airway. • When used on spontaneously breathing patients, it may remain deflated except when the patient is being fed.
Uncuffed	• Typically used in patients who have permanent tracheostomies or patients who are being weaned.
Single cannula	• Available, but not frequently used.
Double cannula	• Inner cannula is used for easy removal and cleaning, which helps maintain a patent airway. • Outer cannula is the portion that contains the cuff in cuffed tubes and the portion that comes in contact with the trachea.

Fenestrated	• A tube that has holes in it to allow air to pass into the upper airway.
	 • Used on spontaneously breathing patients who have a patent or partially patent upper airway.
	 • Comes with two inner cannulas:
	   • A fenestrated cannula that allows air to pass through the tube and the holes in the tube.
	   • A nonfenestrated tube that allows for suctioning without inadvertent passage through fenestrations and subsequent tissue damage.

Non-fenestrated	• Used on patients requiring mechanical ventilation or patients who lack patency of their upper airway.

Source: Adapted from L. Tamburi, "Care of the Patient with Tracheostomy," *Orthopaedic Nursing* 19(2) (2000): 49–57.

When dealing with a tracheostomy emergency, there are a few important questions to ask as you begin to assess and treat the patient:

1. Why did the patient receive a tracheostomy?
2. Is the upper airway patent or obstructed?
3. How long has the patient had the tracheostomy?[22]

When you encounter a patient with a tracheostomy presenting with respiratory distress, anxiety, or altered mental status, the patient should be approached as you would approach any patient with the same presentation. Quickly assess the patient's ABCs, and if you discover that there is insufficient air exchange or a total airway obstruction, you have two options. If there is an appropriately sized sterile suction catheter readily available, you may quickly attempt to insert the catheter into the tracheostomy tube and suction the airway. If suction equipment is available and the catheter meets resistance when it is inserted into the tracheostomy tube, the inner cannula of the tracheostomy tube should be removed. If there is no suction equipment readily available, immediately remove the inner cannula of the tracheostomy tube. This by itself will frequently resolve the problem because it is typically the inner cannula that becomes obstructed with a mucous plug. Upon removal of the inner cannula, reassess the ABCs to see if the issue has been resolved. If the patient continues to present with the same signs and symptoms, continue your attempts to relieve the obstruction.

CONNECTIONS An in-depth discussion on sterile suctioning technique and tracheal suctioning is located in Chapter 12: Airway Management, Ventilation, and Oxygenation.

If the patient has a patent upper airway and the emergency was not abated with the removal of the inner cannula (if the tracheostomy tube is cuffed), deflate the cuff and again reassess the patient's airway. If deflation of the cuff permits the passage of air through the upper airway, then the outer cannula is the problem. Attempt to pass a sterile suction catheter through the lumen of the outer cannula, and if you continue to meet resistance in the tracheostomy tube, then the outer cannula is obstructed. While you are working with the home health-care professional on correcting the issue with the outer cannula, place the patient on high-flow oxygen by non-rebreather mask. Because the outer cannula is likely obstructed, it needs to be removed and possibly replaced.[23] The standard of care for patients with a tracheostomy is that two emergency backup tracheostomy tube sets are kept readily available. One set should be the same size as the tracheostomy tube that is being replaced, and one set should be the next smaller size.[23] To remove the outer cannula of the tracheostomy tube, make sure that the balloon is completely deflated,

quickly remove or cut the tracheal tie, and with suction standing by, gently remove the tracheostomy tube.

If the tracheostomy is new, the stoma has a greater chance of closing up when the outer cannula is removed, and if the tracheostomy is old, the stoma opening may become smaller over time, and the same size tracheostomy tube may not be able to be reinserted. If this situation should arise, use the next size smaller tracheostomy tube, and if one is not available or you are unable to insert the smaller tracheostomy tube, then an endotracheal tube that is one-half size smaller than the tracheostomy tube that was initially removed may be inserted in the stoma to a depth approximately the same as the tracheostomy tube that was removed.

The procedure for insertion of a tracheostomy tube is similar to the placement of an endotracheal tube in that they both have similar components, and they are both inserted with the aide of a device that is temporarily inserted into the lumen of the tube. The tracheostomy has a device that aids in its insertion in similar fashion to a stylette used to insert an endotracheal tube orally. The device used to assist in the insertion of a tracheostomy tube is called an **obturator,** and like the stylette used in endotracheal intubation, the obturator needs to be removed as soon as the tracheostomy tube is inserted in order for air to effectively pass through the lumen.

Once the tracheostomy tube has been replaced, the cuff needs to be inflated and correct placement confirmed. Appropriate physiologic response to the correction of the airway emergency should result in improved oxygen saturations, and appropriate carbon dioxide levels should follow. Because it is always a good idea to transport a patient to the emergency department following an airway emergency, proper tracheostomy placement can be confirmed by x-ray once the patient arrives at the hospital.

Decannulation or Displacement of a Tracheostomy Tube

Another acute intervention in the home care setting that may be encountered on a patient with a tracheostomy tube is the assessment and treatment of the displaced or decannulated tracheostomy tube.

Although this is a relatively rare situation, when it does occur, it can be fatal if not quickly and appropriately corrected (see discussion in Working in the Gray Zone on page 1173). The following are several of the factors that can lead to tracheostomy tube displacement or decannulation:

- Forceful coughing (especially against an obstructed tracheostomy tube)
- Obese patients with thick necks are more prone to tracheostomy tube displacement

Working in the Gray Zone

If your local or state EMS regulatory agency has policies and protocols governing the actions that a paramedic is permitted to take in the event of tracheostomy emergencies, follow these guidelines. If you have a situation that falls outside of the guidelines established by the EMS governing body, contact medical control for consultation and direction. If you are unable to contact medical direction, use your best judgment and follow national standards for advanced airway management. Above all, do what is best for the patient while staying within the paramedic scope of practice.

- Loose or absent tracheal ties
- Placement of the stoma low in the trachea
- Ventilator tubing pulling on the tracheal tube
- Excessive, quick, or forceful patient movements
- Ventilation of a patient with noncompliant lungs using a bag-mask device or a mechanical ventilator [24]
- Patient self-extubation secondary to hypoxia, anxiety, or tube obstruction

Because the dislodged tracheostomy is a true medical emergency, the response to this situation must be rapid, well orchestrated, and deliberate. In the event that you are faced with this situation, several things need to be done simultaneously. As with any other airway emergency, the ABCs need to be rapidly assessed, and the three previously mentioned questions (for patients with tracheostomy emergencies) need to be answered:

1. Why did the patient receive a tracheostomy?
2. Is the upper airway patent or obstructed?
3. How long has the patient had the tracheostomy?

If the tracheostomy is new, it has a greater chance of closing up if the tracheostomy tube is removed (tracheostomy stomas are particularly susceptible to closure within the first 72 hours), and if it is older, the stoma opening may have become smaller and, as before, the same size tube may not fit in the stoma.[22]

Remember that if the patient has a complete obstruction of the upper airway (no air exchange is possible through the mouth or nose), the gravity of the situation is tremendous, and the immediate reestablishment of a patent airway is critical. If the patient has a patent upper airway, supplemental oxygen may be delivered by non-rebreather mask, or by bag-mask (placing an occlusive dressing over the tracheal stoma), depending on the patient's level of respiratory distress and the patient's ability to breathe without assistance.[24]

If the stoma is open in the patient who has decannulated their tracheostomy tube and there is no passage of air through the upper airway, you may optimize the position of the airway for immediate ventilation and subsequent reinsertion of a tracheostomy tube by placing a pillow or towel roll under the patient's shoulders to extend the neck and place the patient in a "sniffing position." Use caution not to hyperextend the neck. At this point, if the patient is in need of ventilatory assistance, you can use a pediatric or a neonatal mask attached to a bag-mask device to ventilate the stoma while you prepare to reinsert a new tracheostomy tube. If the tube has a cuff, make sure that you test the cuff prior to insertion, and make sure that the cuff is completely deflated before you reinsert it into the tracheal stoma (Figure 47-5).

After you have tested the cuff on the tube and the patient is well oxygenated, remove the inner cannula from the tracheostomy tube and insert the obturator into the lumen of the outer cannula with a sterile gloved hand. With your dominant hand, place your thumb over the proximal end of the obturator and your pointer and middle fingers under the swivel neck plate (the hub) of the tracheostomy tube, and reinsert the tube into the tracheal stoma, following the path of the tube that was removed. The reinsertion should occur without any resistance. If there is resistance or if the stomal opening is too small for the same size tube, perform the same procedure using the next smaller size tracheostomy tube. Once the tube is in place and the hub is laying against the surface of the neck, remove the obturator and insert the inner cannula. Inflate the cuff of the tracheostomy tube, and confirm appropriate tube placement. Secure the tracheostomy tube with new tracheal ties. The patient can be transported to the closest, appropriate receiving hospital for further evaluation and confirmation of proper tube placement by x-ray.

If there is no new tracheostomy tube to replace the decannulated one, you may use an endotracheal tube (ETT) of like size until the patient is transported to the hospital or a new tracheostomy tube can be obtained. The ETT should be inserted approximately the same distance as the tracheostomy tube, and confirmation of tube placement should be similar to confirmation of an orally placed ETT. Once confirmation of proper placement is determined, secure the tube with tape and provide appropriate oxygenation and ventilatory support.[22]

Bleeding from a Tracheostomy Tube

Patients with tracheostomy tubes may call for medical assistance as a result of bleeding from a tracheostomy tube. In most cases, this bleeding results from irritation and erosion of tissue from the tracheostomy tube. However, the internal end of the tracheostomy tube often is

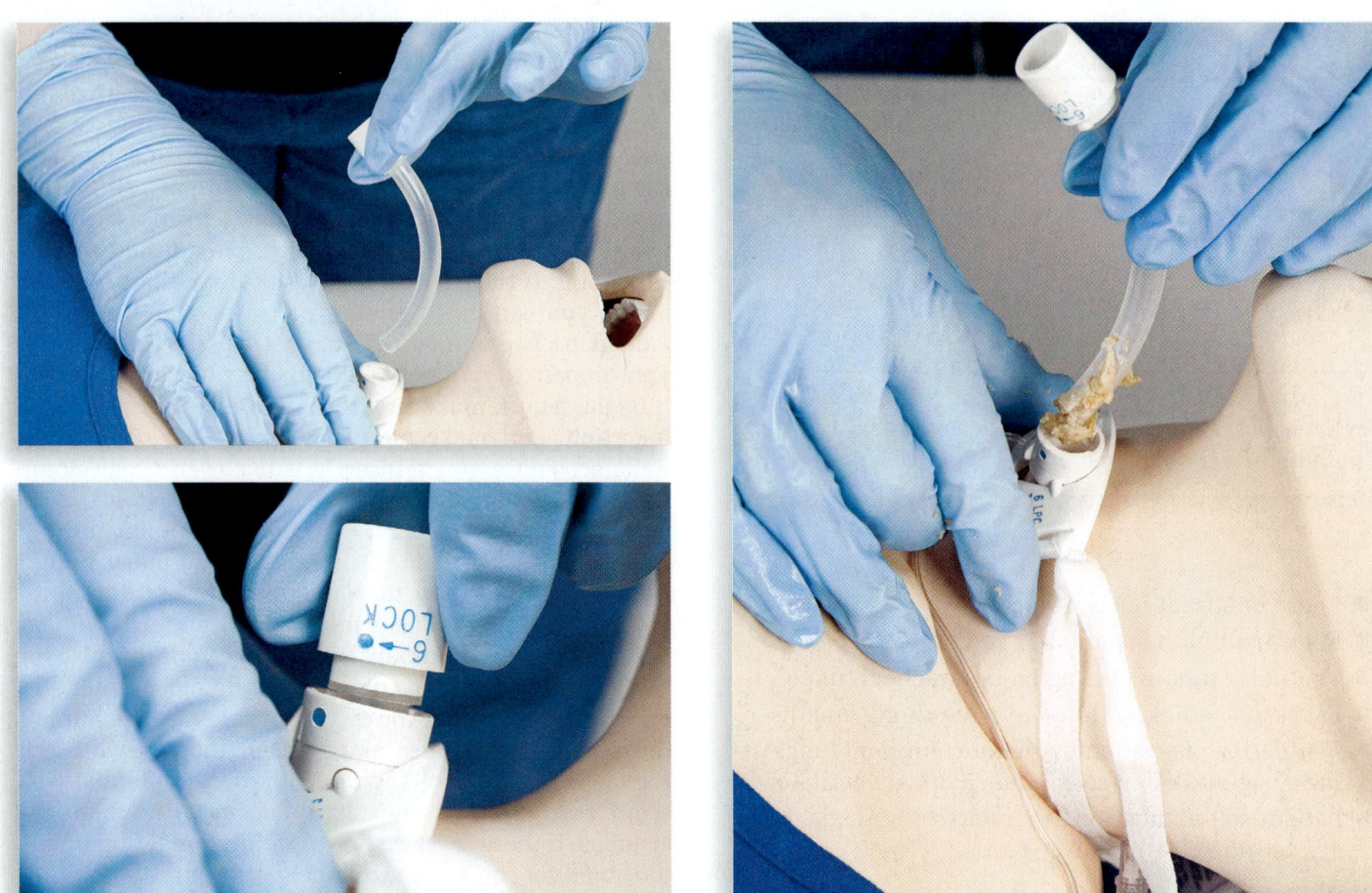

(a)   **(b)**

Figure 47-5   (a) Inner cannula of a tracheostomy tube. (b) A plugged inner cannula of a tracheostomy tube.

located adjacent to one of the major arteries coming off of the aorta and, over time, may gradually erode into the vessel. Patients often present with what appears to be a minor hemorrhage initially only to sustain a major, life-threatening bleed hours or days later. All patients who present with complaints of bleeding from a tracheostomy tube should be transported to the hospital for evaluation.

Gastrointestinal and Genitourinary Devices

Nasogastric (NG) Tubes

Nasogastric (NG) tubes can be used for several reasons in the home care setting. The most likely reason is to aid in the delivery of medication and formula to patients that are unable to receive their medication or nutrition by mouth. NG tube use is usually performed on a short-term basis due to the irritation that it can cause if left in place for extended periods of time.

Paramedics are rarely called to assist in resolving issues with NG tubes unless it comes to dealing with a patient on continuous NG formula feedings who has aspirated formula. In this case, you will be called upon to perform advanced life support techniques to secure the patient's airway and transport the patient to the hospital.

The first task the paramedic must perform when caring for a patient who has aspirated formula from a continuous tube feeding is to turn off the feeding pump. Locate and turn off the power to the pump or unplug the pump. If this does not turn the pump off, then remove the tubing from the pump and close the roller clamp.

The second task is to disconnect the NG tube from the feeding pump and clamp off or plug the proximal end of the NG tube. Due to the fact that the NG tube can easily be displaced, it is important to confirm the location of the distal end of the tube. Determining the location of the distal end of the NG tube could become problematic if the wrong method of confirmation is chosen. For example, the use of a 60-mL syringe to instill air into the tube may lead to further complications. If the distal end of the tube is located in the lungs, or even if it is located in the stomach, adding volume in the form of air can force more formula into the lungs.

In the event that the patient is in need of advanced airway management, the best course of action is to visually confirm NG tube placement while intubating the patient. If you see that the NG tube is in the trachea, it will have to be removed. It is prudent to first aspirate the contents of the NG tube with a 60-mL syringe, no matter where the distal end is located. If the NG tube is in the trachea or the lungs, aspiration will help clear some of the formula and, hopefully, will help with improving gas exchange in the lungs. If the NG tube is in the stomach, aspirating will decrease the volume of formula in the stomach and will help prevent further aspiration of stomach contents.[19]

Percutaneous Endoscopic Gastrostomy (PEG) and Gastrostomy (G) Tubes

Percutaneous endoscopic gastrostomy tubes (PEG tubes) and **gastrostomy tubes (G tubes)** are surgically inserted tubes that extend from the surface of the abdomen into the stomach and are used for long-term nutritional support in individuals who are not able to obtain their nutrition by mouth. There are very few acute interventions that a paramedic would perform on home care patients specifically related to their G tube. The most likely acute intervention related to a patient with a G tube would be a scenario similar to the continuously formula fed NG tube patient and the possibility of aspirating formula. The standard practice related to the care of a patient who receives continuous formula feedings from a feeding tube is as follows:

1. The patient needs to be placed in a semi-Fowler's position with the head of the bed elevated at least 30 degrees.
2. The stomach contents need to be aspirated prior to initiating the feeding.
3. If there is an excess of approximately 150 mL of stomach contents aspirated, then it should be returned to the stomach and given time to be absorbed.
4. If the residual is less than 150 mL, then the formula feedings may be implemented at a rate prescribed by the patient's physician.
5. During formula feedings, whether bolus or continuous, the residual volume needs to be reassessed on a regular basis, and if it is in excess of the prescribed residual volumes, then the feeding should be stopped.

If a patient with a PEG tube presents with signs and symptoms of aspiration while they are being given a formula feeding, the treatment of the patient is very similar to that of the NG tube patient on a continuous formula feeding:

1. First, stop the feeding.
2. Assess the patient's airway, and prepare to provide needed airway and ventilatory support, including suctioning and endotracheal intubation.
3. Manual aspiration of the stomach contents and positioning of the patient in a sitting position (if condition permits) is beneficial and should be attempted.
4. The need to confirm placement of the G tube in this situation is not critical because there is no chance that the tube has been inadvertently placed in the trachea.

Other complications that involve gastrostomy tubes and may require acute intervention by the paramedic involve the care, or lack thereof, of the insertion site or the displacement of the gastrostomy tube. Improper care of the surgical site may lead to complications such as ulcerations or infections. Site infections may become systemic infections that may lead to septic shock. Infections are not uncommon, but if proper care of the site is practiced and early identification of signs and symptoms related to infection are noted, then the patient can be treated without the threat of life-threatening infection. Patients with dislodgement of a gastrostomy tube should receive supportive care and transport to a hospital where they can be treated by a physician. In some cases, reinsertion of a gastrostomy tube can be performed by a paramedic, but due to the possibility of complications, it is preferable that the patient be assessed and treated by a physician.

Foley Catheters

The most likely reason for urinary catheterization in the home care setting is urinary retention. In women, urinary retention is most frequently associated with a failure of the bladder to contract (detrusor failure), and in men, it is most frequently associated with an enlarged prostate gland. Some other reasons for urinary retention include urethral strictures, calculi, tumors, medications, strokes, spinal cord injuries, and neuropathies caused by diabetes. One might think that urinary retention is not a serious problem, but if it goes untreated, it can lead to UTIs, stone formation, and potentially long-term structural damage to the bladder, ureters, or kidneys. The patient who is experiencing urinary retention may complain of an overwhelming need to urinate, restlessness, sweating, anxiety, bladder pain, and a feeling of bladder fullness.[19]

Insertion of Foley Catheters

The insertion of a urinary catheter is a procedure that exposes the patient to some risk. Possible complications associated with this procedure include infection (there is a high risk of urinary tract infection [UTI] in patients who receive urinary catheters); tissue trauma (can be caused by oversized catheters, friction caused by movement of the catheter, force applied when inserting the catheter, and accidental removal of the catheter while the balloon is inflated), which can lead to hematuria; and allergic reactions (on a local or systemic basis) in patients that have an allergy to latex.[25]

To prevent the potential for long-term damage and to provide comfort for the patient, the paramedic that is trained in the procedure should insert a urinary catheter in the patient either under standing orders or following the consultation of medical direction. Remember that the procedure for urinary catheter insertion is a sterile one. Failure to perform the procedure in a sterile manner may lead to UTIs and possibly urosepsis. If Foley catheter insertion is not an approved procedure, the patient should be transported to the hospital. DOT 6-6.28, 6-6.29

CONNECTIONS For a description of urinary catheterization, see Chapter 36: Urology.

Colostomies, Ileostomies, and Urostomies

Colostomies, ileostomies, and **urostomies** are designed to collect waste products from the body when the regular collection or excretion organs (the colon, the ileum, and the urinary bladder or urethra, respectively) are malfunctioning. The surgical opening, or **ostomy,** that is created between the surface of the body and the colon, ileum, or urinary bladder is an avenue by which fecal or urinary waste is emptied, typically into a collection pouch, and then discarded on a regular basis (Figure 47-6).

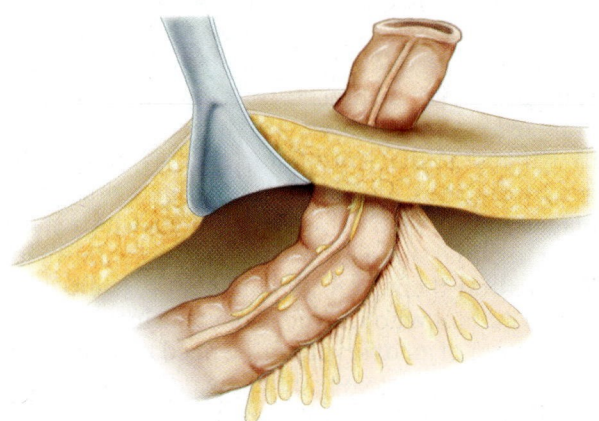

Figure 47-6 Surgical procedure for creating a colostomy.

Most of the complications seen in colostomy patients are seen in the relatively early postoperative period and include the following:

1. Suture line leakage with local or generalized peritonitis
2. Hemorrhage
3. Stomal necrosis
4. Retraction
5. Prolapse
6. Stenosis

Complications for the ileostomy patient are also relatively rare and are most frequently seen in the early postoperative period. The most frequent complications seen in the ileostomy patient include the following:

1. Intestinal obstruction (caused by obstruction of the lumen, food, adhesions, or stomal edema)
2. Hemorrhage
3. Hypoxia
4. Fluid and electrolyte imbalance[25] DOT 6-6.30

There are several types of urinary diversion procedures **(urostomies).** The common thread among these procedures is the creation of an ostomy on the surface of the abdomen that diverts urine from the urethra and sometimes the urinary bladder. Frequent complications following urinary diversion surgery include the following:

1. Hematuria
2. Stenosis of the stoma
3. Infection
4. Electrolyte imbalances
5. Difficult catheterization
6. Occlusion of urinary drainage device[25]

There is little that the paramedic can do for the patient with complications associated with ostomies other than to provide supportive care (oxygen, IV access, assistance with pain management), treat for shock should hemorrhage become uncontrolled or infection become systemic, and transport to a hospital for definitive care. DOT 6-6.33

Preexisting Vascular Access Devices

Patients who have renal failure or renal insufficiency are frequently treated with one of two forms of dialysis (hemodialysis or peritoneal dialysis).

Hemodialysis

Hemodialysis is a medical procedure that removes blood from a surgically constructed blood vessel, cleans the blood (removes metabolic wastes and excess water through a process of filtration, diffusion, osmosis, and pressure gradients) with an artificial kidney (the dialysis machine), and returns it to the patient through another peripheral vein or the same surgically created blood vessel. Anticoagulant therapy usually accompanies dialysis to prevent the coagulation of the blood as it passes from the patient, through the machine, and back to the patient.[26]

CONNECTIONS See Chapter 31: Endocrine, Electrolytes, and Acid/Base for a review of dialysis.

As previously mentioned, a surgically created blood vessel comes in two forms:

1. *Arterio-venous (A-V) fistulas* are created by anastomosing (surgically connecting) a peripheral artery with a peripheral vein and creating a pseudoaneurysm at which point vascular access for outflow can be created (inflow is typically accomplished by accessing a peripheral vein distal to the fistula).

2. *Arterio-venous (A-V) grafts* are the most frequently used dialysis access device. The A-V graft is created by inserting a Gortex™ tube into the chosen limb and anastomosing a vein and an artery to the ends of the tube. Blood flows through the tube and allows for access of both an outflow and an inflow needle.[27]

Patients in the home care setting who have renal failure and undergo hemodialysis are not usually in need of acute intervention by paramedics because they have an A-V fistula or an A-V graft. The only times that the A-V fistula or A-V graft may need intervention by a paramedic are when there is uncontrolled bleeding from the access site or the device becomes obstructed.

In the event that the patient has a bleeding disorder or the patient's anticoagulants are overused, then the possibility of hemorrhage from the access site is likely. If this situation should occur, use dressings and apply only enough pressure to control the bleeding without occluding the device (bleeding from an A-V fistula or an A-V graft should be treated similar to an arterial bleed).[26] Depending on the patient's hemodynamic status and the amount of blood that has been lost, IV access and fluid replacement may be necessary (remember that fluid replacement in the dialysis patient should take place in small increments with frequent reassessment of hemodynamic status and respiratory status).

An IV should be established in a peripheral vein, preferably in an extremity other than the one in which the dialysis access device is located. In the event of obstruction or occlusion of the dialysis access device, transport the patient to the hospital for the appropriate physician intervention. In a life-threatening emergency, the dialysis access site may be used for venous access if this procedure is approved by your local EMS agency, and if you have been trained in it. If in doubt, contact medical direction for advice.

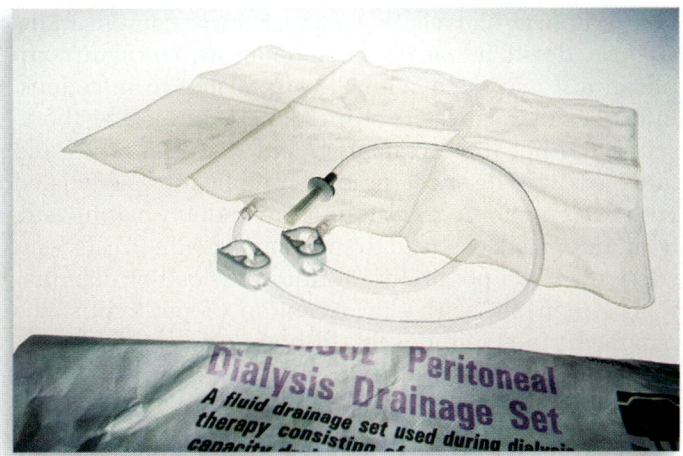

Figure 47-7 Peritoneal dialysis drainage set.

The true life-threatening emergencies that the dialysis patient will experience are not typically related to the patient's access device (A-V fistula or A-V graft) but rather conditions such as an excess or deficit of fluid and electrolytes. These emergencies are exacerbated by comorbid conditions frequently seen in dialysis patients, such as a history of myocardial infarction (MI) or congestive heart failure (CHF). The combination of these factors along with the primary causes of renal failure (hypertension [HTN], diabetes, etc.) can result in a patient with life-threatening systemic problems.

Peritoneal Dialysis

Peritoneal dialysis is a form of dialysis that allows patients to receive their treatment in the home setting (Figure 47-7). It involves the introduction of a sterile dialysis solution into the abdominal cavity through an implanted catheter. This form of dialysis uses the semipermeable peritoneal membrane and the vasculature that covers and transports blood to the abdominal organs to perform dialysis on a regularly prescribed schedule. This form of dialysis is accomplished through osmosis, diffusion, and active transport. Patients who are candidates for this type of dialysis are listed in Table 47-6.

TABLE 47-6   Indications for Peritoneal Dialysis

- Renal insufficiency or failure
- Hemodynamic instability
- Poor vascular access
- Patients with severe cardiac disease
- Volume overload
- Electrolyte imbalances
- Clotting disorders
- Contraindications to hemodialysis

Source: Adapted from L. A. Thelan, L. D. Urden, et al., *Critical Care Nursing—Diagnosis and Management*, 3rd ed. (St. Louis, MO: Mosby, 1998), pp 900–901.

Peritoneal dialysis (PD) has far fewer complications associated with it than does hemodialysis. The main complications associated with PD are related to infections. Infections of the exit site or the catheter tunnels by themselves are not life-threatening, and they can be treated fairly easily. The most serious complication associated with PD is peritonitis. Peritonitis is extremely painful and, if left untreated, can lead to sepsis and death. PD also carries with it the possibility of fluid overload or dehydration. All in all, with the exception of peritonitis, the paramedic interventions for the home care patient receiving PD are minimal and supportive in nature.[27]

Central Venous Access Devices

Central venous access devices come in many different forms. The choices regarding central venous access devices for patients in the home care setting have increased with the acuity of patients being cared for in this setting. The central venous access devices that have been used in the hospital for years (Broviac®, Groshong®, and Hickman®) are now being used in the home healthcare setting, but the device that has become the leader in home care central vascular access is the **peripherally inserted central catheter (PICC)** (Figure 47-8). Another new catheter to the home care setting is the midline catheter, which has proven to be a cost effective option for home healthcare patients. **DOT 6-6.41**

Both PICC lines and midline catheters look very similar from the outside and are both inserted in the antecubital (AC) area, but their similarities end there. PICC lines are inserted under fluoroscopy, are threaded through veins in the AC area (the cephalic, the basilic, or the median cubital vein), and end up with the distal tip positioned in the same place that most other central venous catheters terminate, in the superior vena cava. The midline catheter, on the other hand, is not a central line. It is a peripheral line that has a 3- to 8-inch long catheter. As previously stated, it is inserted in the AC area and terminates at or below the area of the axillary line (placement above the level of the axillary line is associated with a higher risk of thrombosis). Advantages of the midline catheter include lower risk of phlebitis and infection as compared to a standard peripheral catheter, and the midline catheter can remain in place for up to six weeks; whereas, the standard peripheral IV catheter should be in place no longer than six days.[28] Table 47-7 discusses the differences between peripheral venous access and central venous access.

When dealing with patients in the home care setting, it is important to be aware of the possible complications associated with central venous access devices. Table 47-8 describes some of the most common complications seen with central lines and the actions that should be taken when they occur.[29] Do not attempt to manipulate any of these devices unless you are approved to do so

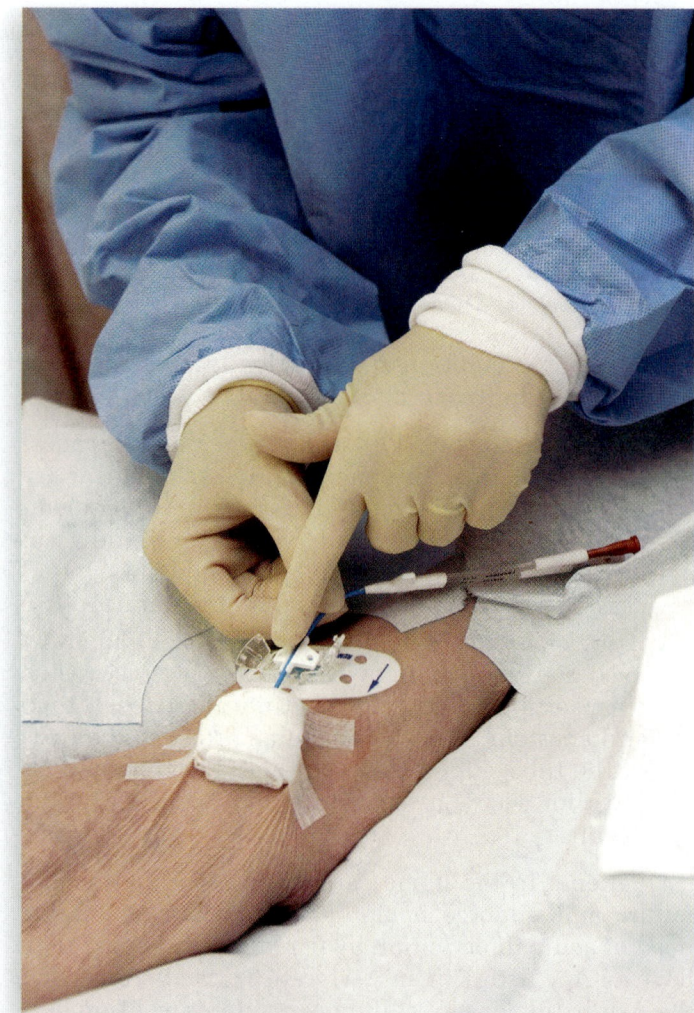

Figure 47-8   Peripherally inserted central catheter.

within your paramedic scope of practice, you have been trained in their use, or you have been instructed to do so by medical direction. Discovering and treating problems associated with central vascular access devices is not an easy task in many situations. If you are not sure how to treat the patient who is experiencing problems with a central venous access device, consult the patient's regular caregiver (if possible) and medical direction for assistance.

It is far more likely that you will be called to the home care setting for the condition for which the patient received the central venous access device in the first place rather than issues with the device itself. If this is the situation, you will likely need to rely on your ALS paramedic assessment and treatment skills to care for the patient.

In an emergent situation, you may need to utilize the patient's central venous access device to deliver IV fluids and medication to treat the patient's condition. Accessing a central venous access device is not a difficult procedure but one that the paramedic needs to be

TABLE 47-7   Central Versus Peripheral Venous Access

	Central Venous Access	Peripheral Venous Access
Duration of catheter placement	Months to years	• Less than six days with standard catheter • Two to six weeks with a midline catheter

Infusion properties	• Continuous vesicant chemotherapy
	• Parenteral nutrition formulas with:
	  • Greater than 10% dextrose
	  • Greater than 5% protein
	  • Solutions or medications with pH less than 5 or greater than 9
	  • Solutions or medications with osmolarity greater than 500 mOsm
	• Vein irritating solution administration (e.g., potassium)
	• Antimicrobial medications (e.g., vancomycin)
		• Most medications that fall outside of the restrictions of the previous column

Bleeding disorders	PICC lines should be avoided in patients with low platelet counts.	Use with caution in patients with bleeding disorders.
Cost	Cost effective for patients in need of long-term central venous access.	The midline catheter is the most cost effective vascular access device for patients who need IV access for the administration of nonvein-irritating medications for a two to three week period.
Blood sampling	Commonly used	Not recommended
Immunosuppressed patients	Infections can occur with any type of catheter insertion. Adhering to infection control guidelines, site assessment, and site care, extreme care and sterile technique when performing dressing changes, flushing of the vascular access device, administrating solutions or medications, and changing injection cap will provide for the greatest chance of preventing infections. PICC lines and midline catheters are associated with relatively low infection rates.	

Source: Adapted from L. A. Gorski and L. M. Czaplewski, "Peripherally Inserted Central Catheters and Midline Catheters for the Homecare Nurse," *Home Healthcare Nurse* 22(11) (2004): pp 760–764.

trained in and approved to perform by the state and local EMS governing entities. DOT 6-6.25

Because there are so many varieties of central venous access devices, it is beneficial to understand similarities and differences between the different device:

1. Hickman and Broviac® catheters are tunneled under the skin before accessing the venous system. These devices incorporate a Dacron® cuff in the portion of the catheter that is tunneled through the skin. This serves to create another barrier to prevent infection and permit the ingrowth of tissue around the cuff to help stabilize the catheter. PICC lines use sutures to affix the catheter in place. Central venous access devices come with one, two, or three access ports (the more ports, the greater incidence of infection).[30]

2. Some central venous access devices have external access ports (Hickman and Broviac® catheters, PICC lines) while others have ports that are surgically implanted under the skin (medi-ports, port-a-caths, etc.) and require special needles (Huber needles) to access them. The implanted central venous access devices are used primarily for medication administration. Attempts to access these devices with anything other than a Huber needle will destroy the device.

3. Although all central venous access devices need to be flushed on a regular basis, the decision regarding whether to use saline or heparin to maintain patency and prevent thrombus formation is up to the manufacturer and each healthcare provider agency. Heparin is recommended for use in central vascular access devices (VAD) in a concentration that prevents thrombus formation but does not interfere with systemic clotting factors. A common dose of heparin used to maintain the patency of central VADs is 2–3 mL of 10 or 100u/mL per day. Some

TABLE 47-8 Central Venous Catheter Complications and Treatments

Complication	Patient Presentation	Treatments
Phlebitis	• Erythema at site • Pain • Streak formation • Palpable venous cord • Purulent discharge	• Transport patient for evaluation at the hospital.
Catheter occlusion	• Unable to aspirate blood • Resistance to flushing • Sluggish infusion • Unable to flush or infuse	• Transport patient for evaluation at the hospital for treatment with thrombolytic drug, if thrombosis is suspected, or radiographic studies of catheter placement.
Catheter-related thrombosis	• Swelling in the arm, shoulder, or neck on the placement side of the catheter • Increased arm circumference • Pain—chest, jaw, earache	• Transport patient for evaluation at the hospital.

Infection	• Catheter-related sepsis
	  • Fever, weakness, chills, malaise
	• Local
	  • Erythema, tenderness, induration, purulent discharge at site
		• Transport patient for evaluation at the hospital.
		• If patient presents with systemic infection and signs or symptoms of shock, establish another IV and use that access site for treatment.
		• *Do not* use the infected access device unless it is the only possible access and you have been approved by medical direction to do so.

Catheter migration	• Change in length of catheter extruding from exit site
	• Change in ability to aspirate blood
	• Subjective complaints
	  • Palpitations or chest pain
	• External migration
	  • Increased risk of catheter-related thrombosis; increased risk of chemical-related phlebitis
	• Internal migration
	  • Hypotension, increased central venous pressure, tachycardia, loss of consciousness secondary to movement of catheter into the right atrium, ventricle, or the pulmonary artery
		• Treat patient per local protocols.
		• Never attempt reinsertion in the field.
		• Contact medical direction for consultation.
		• Transport patient for evaluation at the hospital.
		• Cover the catheter with a sterile occlusive dressing and transport.

Catheter fracture or embolism	• Crack or hole noted in catheter • Leaking	• Discontinue the infusion of medications or fluid of any kind. • Clamp off catheter between the damaged area and the skin if possible. • Transport patient for evaluation at the hospital.
Air embolism	• Chest pain • Shortness of breath • Shoulder or low back pain • Cyanosis • Hypotension • Tachycardia • Altered level of consciousness	• Place patient in a left lateral position with head lower than the heart; stop entry of air, fluid, etc; support ABCs; establish other IV access; rapidly transport patient to the hospital. • Place patient on 100% oxygen.

Source: Adapted from M. Marks, "The Management of the Difficult Peripherally Inserted Central Venous Catheter Line Removal," *Journal of Intravenous Nursing* 18(5) (1995): 246–249.

manufacturers of central VADs state that the use of saline to maintain the patency of the device is sufficient.[28] A question that your local agency will need to answer, if you are permitted to access central VADs in the EMS setting, is whether you need to aspirate the contents of the line or flush the line with saline (to assure patency) prior to utilization.

No matter what type of central VAD you encounter, make sure that you are approved to use it and that you are trained in its use prior to attempting to troubleshoot problems with it or before you attempt to access it for your own use. DOT 6-6.19, 6-6.20, 6-6.21

Patient-Controlled Analgesia (PCA) Pumps

Another device seen in the home healthcare setting that the paramedic should be aware of is the **patient-controlled analgesia (PCA) pump** (Figure 47-9). PCA pumps are designed to allow patients to deliver their own IV pain medication, according to their perceived level of discomfort, with the touch of a button.

The PCA pump has a locked medication chamber and control panel that can only be accessed and programmed by a healthcare professional. The reason for these security measures is to assure that patients do not accidentally overmedicate themselves. Because the medications most frequently used in a PCA are opioids, an accidental overdose could have life-threatening repercussions.

In fact, according to a report from the Center for the Advancement of Patient Safety of the U.S. Pharmacopia (USP), "Patient-controlled analgesia (PCA) pumps, while proven effective in pain management, continue to be a factor in harmful medication errors." From September 1998 through August 2003, 5,377 errors were reported to the USP's medication error database with 7.9% of them classified as having caused harm (in general, the percentage of medical error that causes harm is approximately 2%). Of these errors, 38.9% were related to improper dosage administration, 18.4% were related to the administration of an unauthorized medication, and 17.6% were errors of omission.[31]

PCA pumps have a lockout interval that prevents the patient from activating the PCA for a set time once the patient has activated the pump. This is another safety mechanism that prevents accidental overdose. The PCA pump can be programmed to deliver a set dosage in a certain time period so that the patient can activate the pump as much as they want until they have reached the prescribed dosage, and then the pump will prevent the patient from administering another dose of the medication until the prescribed time has lapsed.

There are many different possibilities for use of a PCA pump, and all of them are designed to reduce the likelihood of an accidental overdose. Furthermore, there

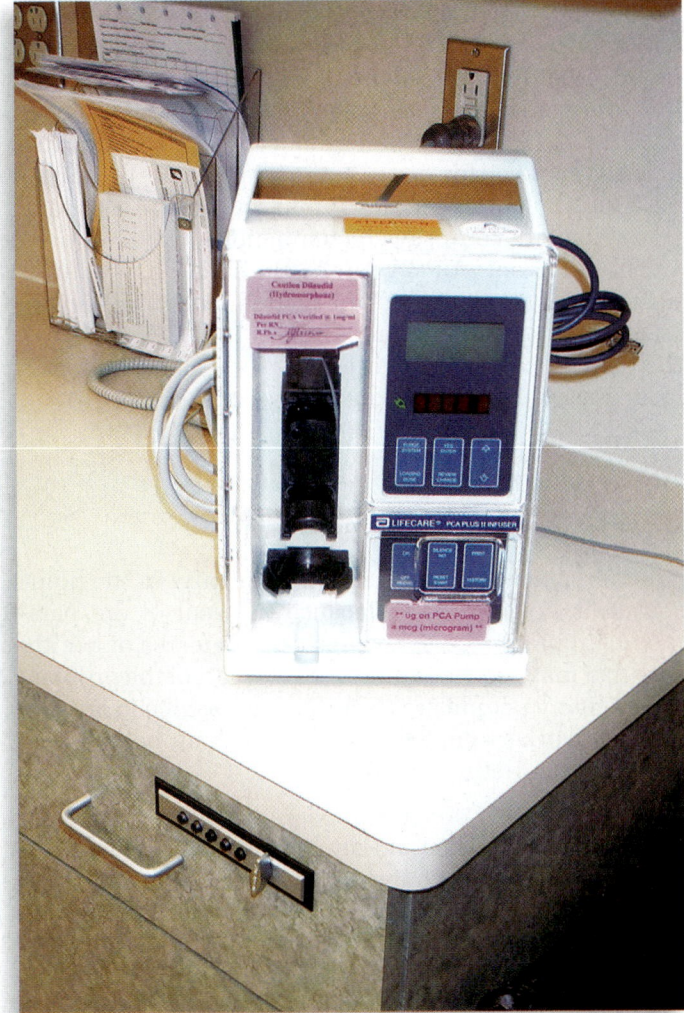

Figure 47-9 PCA pump.

are modes of operation for a PCA pump to deliver a baseline amount of medication to patients so that they do not underdose themselves and experience unnecessary pain.[19] Keep in mind that the PCA pump is designed for use by patients and not family or medical personnel who think that patients look like they are in pain. The only time that someone other than patients should activate a dose of medication is when patients request that you administer a dose and they are unable to deliver the dose themselves.

The critical interventions that the paramedic may experience in the out-of-hospital setting in relation to the PCA pump are typically related to overdose and pump malfunction. In the event of an overdose, turn off the pump, clamp the IV tubing, or disconnect the PCA IV tubing from the main IV tubing. Because most of the medications administered through a PCA are opioids, and morphine is the most common analgesic administered through a PCA, assess and treat your patient based on your protocols for opioid overdose.[19]

Assure that the patient is adequately oxygenated and ventilated, and be aware that rapid reversal of an opioid overdose in a patient who has been receiving long-term opioid analgesia may lead to symptoms of withdrawal and could precipitate a seizure. Contacting medical control for consultation, or slowly titrating a narcotic antagonist medication to reverse the signs and symptoms of overdose is recommended.

In the event of PCA pump malfunction or failure, turn off the pump, contact the manufacturer or the medical supply company that supplied the PCA, and treat the patient for pain or symptoms of overdose (per your local protocols), as previously described. DOT 6-6.8, 6-6.24

Hospice Care, Palliative Care, and Comfort Care in the Home

Another area of healthcare seen frequently in the home setting is hospice care. Because the goal of the paramedic is curative care, hospice care is an area of healthcare that may seem counterintuitive. Part of the problem is that many people are unsure what hospice is or what hospice workers do (Table 47-9). The National Hospice Organization defines **hospice** as

> A coordinated program providing palliative care to terminally ill patients and supportive services to patients, their families, and significant others 24 hours a day, seven days a week. Comprehensive case managed services based on physical, social, spiritual, and emotional needs are provided during the last stages of illness, during the dying process, and during bereavement by a

medically directed interdisciplinary team consisting of patients and their families, healthcare professionals, and volunteers. Professional management and continuity of care is maintained across multiple settings including homes, hospitals, long-term care and residential settings.[32]

Palliative care, also called **comfort care** (the major component of hospice care), is defined by the World Health Organization as

> The active total care of patients whose disease is not responsive to curative treatment. Control of pain, of other symptoms, and of psychological, social, and spiritual problems is paramount. The goal of palliative care is achievement of the best quality of life for patients and their families. Many aspects of palliative care are also applicable earlier in the course of the illness, in conjunction with anticancer treatment. Palliative care affirms life and regards dying as a normal process, neither hastens nor postpones death, provides relief from pain and other distressing symptoms, integrates the psychological and spiritual aspects of care, offers a support system to help patients live as actively as possible until death, and offers a support system to help the family cope during the patient's illness and in their own bereavement.[33]

Based on the premise of hospice care and palliative care, there is little that a paramedic can do to care for the hospice patient other than provide supportive care such as pain management. One of the most likely scenarios a paramedic will encounter when called on to care for a hospice patient is when there is a failure in

TABLE 47-9 Differences between Curative Care and Palliative Care

	Curative	Palliative
Goal	Cure	Symptom control
Approach to care	Analytical and rationalistic	Subjective
Basis of care	Based on diagnosis	Based on symptoms
Process of providing care	Scientific and biomedical	Humanistic and interpersonal
Focus of care	Aimed at disease process	Aimed at comfort
Approach to patients	Views patients as parts	Views patients as a whole
Treatment	Based on "hard" science	Based on "soft" social sciences
Patient care	Impersonal care	Individualized care
Healthcare team	Hierarchical	Interdisciplinary
View of death	Seen as failure	Accepted as normal

Source: Adapted from K. K. Kuebler, et al., *End of Life Care—Clinical Practice Guidelines* (Philadelphia, PA: W. B. Saunders, 2002), p 28.

communication or there is a change of heart by the patient or a family member when the end of the patient's life is near. When faced with a situation where a hospice patient, or an immediate family member of a hospice patient, has a change of mind about the decision to decline lifesaving measures at the end of life, the paramedic may be faced with a medical-legal/moral-ethical dilemma.

There is more than one way to manage this type of situation, and no single method is better than another.[34] If the EMS system has been activated, you will have to respond and deal with this situation to the best of your abilities. If you have any doubt about what you should do in this situation, do the following:

- Always err on the side of doing what is best for the patient.
- Maintain the practices of your state, the local EMS agency, and your employer.
- Begin performing basic life support.
- Contact medical control for consultation as quickly as possible.

CONNECTIONS For more discussion on the legal and ethical issues, review Chapter 3: Professional Ethics and Chapter 4: Legal Issues.

Most hospice organizations are very good at making sure that all of the appropriate medical-legal paperwork has been taken care of and is readily available when the patient dies. They also prepare the patient and their family for, and support them through, the end of life process. DOT 6-6.10

Summary

The landscape of the out-of-hospital setting has changed considerably over time and will undoubtedly continue to change. Whether in the home care setting, the skilled nursing facility setting, or any other out-of-hospital setting, the knowledge that the paramedic must possess in order to adequately assess and treat these high acuity patients and the medical devices used in their care has expanded on a gradual basis and will likely continue to do so. DOT 6-6.11, 6-6.36, 6-6.37

Notes

1. K. Buhler-Wilkerson, "Left Carrying the Bag: Experiments in Visiting Nursing," *Nursing Research* 36(1) (1986): 42.
2. M. Mundinger, *Home Care Controversy: Too Little, Too Late, Too Costly* (Rockville, MD: Aspen Systems, 1983).
3. M. Rappaport, *Remodeling Home Care, Making the Transition from Fee-For-Service to Managed Care* (New York, NY: Garland Publishing, 2000), p. 17.
4. F. Spencer, D. Lessard, et al., "Declining Length of Hospital Stay for Acute Myocardial Infarction and Post-Discharge

Outcomes," *Archives of Internal Medicine* 164(7) (2004): 733–740.
5. R. Rice, "Historical Perspectives and Philosophy of Care." In *Home Care Nursing Practice: Concepts and Application,* 3rd ed. (St. Louis, MO: Mosby, 2001), p. 31.
6. D. Nugent, "Providing Solutions for the Growing Trend Toward Home Healthcare," *Health Management Technology* 9 (1999): 28.
7. S. Stewart, A. J. Vandenbroek, et al., "Prolonged Beneficial Effects of a Home-Based Intervention on Unplanned Readmissions and Mortality Among Patients with Congestive Heart Failure," *Archives of Internal Medicine* 159(3) (1999): 257–261.
8. S. Inglis, S. McLennan, et al., "A New Solution for an Old Problem? Effects of a Nurse Led, Multidisciplinary, Home-Based Intervention on Readmission and Mortality in Patients with Chronic Atrial Fibrillation," *Journal of Cardiovascular Nursing* 19(2) (2004): 118–827.
9. F. Ozdemir, M. Birtane, et al., "Comparing Stroke Rehabilitation Outcomes Between Acute Inpatient and Non-Intense Home Settings," *Archives of Physical Medicine and Rehabilitation* 82(10) (2001): 1375–1379.
10. National Association for Home Care, "How to Choose a Home Care Provider" (1996), http://www.nahc.org/Consumer/wphc.html (accessed April 22, 2005).
11. California Employment Development Department, Labor Market Information Division, Information Services Group, "Home Health Aide Certification" (2005), http://www.labormarketinfo.edd.ca.gov/cgi/databrowsing/occExplorerQSDetails.asp?searchCriteria=Clerk&careerID=&menuChoice=occExplorer&geogArea=0601000000&soccode=311011&search=Explore+Occupation (accessed April 1, 2005).
12. Associated Affiliations American Nursing Assistants Association, "Certified Nursing Assistant Responsibilities" (2005), http:/www.Healthprofessions.com (accessed April 1, 2005).
13. California Board of Vocational Nursing and Psychiatric Technicians (BVNPT), "Licensed Vocational/Practical Nurse Fact Sheet" (2005), http://www.bvnpt.ca.gov (accessed April 1, 2005).
14. S. Connor, *Hospice: Practice, Pitfalls, and Promise* (Washington, DC: Taylor & Francis, 1998), pp. 7–8.
15. I. Greenwald and S. P. Rosonoke, "Mechanical Ventilation-Understanding Respiratory Physiology and the Basics of Ventilator Management" (December 2003), http://www.jems.com (accessed April 1, 2005).
16. R. L. Boggs, "Airway Management," *AACN Procedural Manual for Critical Care,* 3rd ed. (Philadelphia, PA: W. B. Saunders, 1993), pp. 1–65.
17. C. Spritzer, "Unraveling the Mysteries of a Mechanical Ventilator: A Helpful Step-by-Step Guide," *Journal of Emergency Nursing* 29 (2003): 29–36.
18. J. M. Cairo and S. Pilbeam, *Respiratory Care Equipment,* 7th ed. (St. Louis, MO: Mosby, 2004), p. 378.
19. P. Evans-Smith, *Taylor's Clinical Nursing Skills—A Nursing Process Approach* (Philadelphia, PA: Lippincot, Williams & Wilkins, 2005), p. 544.
20. K. L. McCance and S. E. Huether, *Pathophysiology: The Biologic Basis for Disease in Adults and Children,* 3rd ed. (St. Louis, MO: Mosby, 1998).
21. L. Tamburi, "Care of the Patient with a Tracheostomy," *Orthopaedic Nursing* 19(2) (2000): 49–57.
22. S. J. Seay, S. L. Gay, et al., "Tracheostomy Emergencies-Correcting Accidental Decannulations or Displaced Tracheostomy Tube," *American Journal of Nursing* 102(3) (2002): 59.

23. S. Sell and F. J. Tasota, "Action STAT—Tracheostomy Mucus Plug," *Nursing* 34(10) (2004): 88.

24. B. Eisenhauer, "Action STAT-Dislodged Tracheostomy Tube," *Nursing* 26(6) (1996): 25.

25. J. M. Black, J. Hawks, et al., *Medical-Surgical Nursing: Clinical Management for Positive Outcomes,* 6th ed. (Philadelphia, PA: W. B. Saunders, 2001).

26. I. M. Martinson, A. G. Widmer, et al., *Home Health Care Nursing,* 2nd ed. (Philadelphia, PA: W. B. Saunders, 2002).

27. L. A. Thelan, L. D. Urden, et al., *Critical Care Nursing— Diagnosis and Management,* 3rd ed. (St. Louis, MO: Mosby, 1998).

28. L. A, Gorski and L. M. Czaplewski, "Peripherally Inserted Central Catheters and Midline Catheters for the Homecare Nurse," *Home Healthcare Nurse* 22(11) (2004): 758–759.

29. M. Marks, "The Management of the Difficult Peripherally Inserted Central Venous Catheter Line Removal," *Journal of Intravenous Nursing* 18(5) (1995): 246–249.

30. J. Gabriel, "PICC Securement: Minimizing Possible Complications," *Nursing Standard* 15(43) (2001): 42.

31. D. Sofer, "PCA Pumps: An Illusion of Safety?" *American Journal of Nursing* 105(2) (2005): 22.

32. *National Hospice Organization: Standards of a Hospice Program of Care* (Arlington, VA: National Hospice Organization, 1993).

33. World Health Organization, *Cancer Pain Relief and Palliative Care* (Technical Report Series 804) (Geneva, World Health Organization, 1990).

34. K. K. Kuebler et al., *End of Life Care—Clinical Practice Guidelines* (Philadelphia, PA: W. B. Saunders, 2002), p. 28.

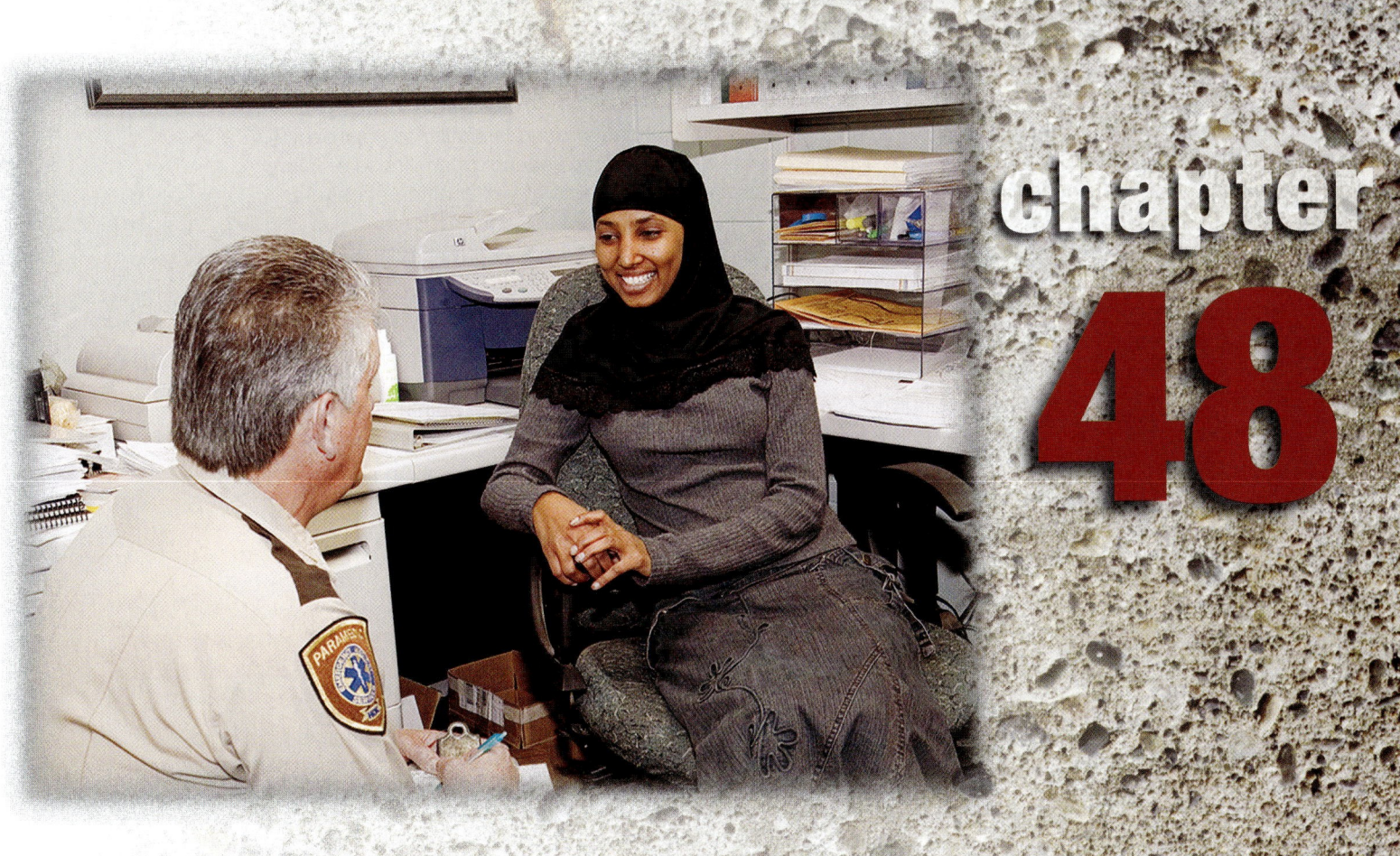

Patients from Diverse Cultures

"**M**y message is the practice of compassion, love and kindness. Compassion can be put into practice if one recognizes the fact that every human being is a member of humanity and the human family regardless of differences in religion, culture, color and creed. Deep down there is no difference."

—The Dalai Lama

Need to Know

▶ Culture impacts every patient interaction.[1] When a patient's cultural background is similar to your own, you will obviously feel more comfortable dealing with the mental and emotional aspects of an illness or injury.[1,2] However, as a frontline medical practitioner, you must often manage patients of vastly different cultures and upbringing.

▶ Every culture perceives disease and death differently.[2,3] Recognizing and addressing these differences requires you to adapt your treatment plan accordingly.[1]

▶ Although you must continue to treat every patient with appropriate medical interventions, your approach must also include a respectful awareness of how a patient's presentation, your treatments, and the outcome will be perceived by the patient as well as the patient's family and community.[1,2,4]

▶ Patient presentation changes across cultures.[2] Some cultures consider the display of pain a sign of weakness while other cultures encourage the expression of pain.[5]

▶ Cultural responses to the medical needs of women vary considerably.[2] Cultural boundaries in some communities may prevent women from seeking medical attention or being attended to by men.[2]

▶ Many cultures continue to rely on traditional medicine, ritual, and prayer as primary means to prevent disease and manage ill health.[2]

▶ Do	▶ Ask
• Recognize differences in culture, and adapt your approach to the patient and family appropriately. • Use translation help whenever a communication barrier exists. • Research the cultures and populations in the service area where you respond. • Seek out other emergency responders with different cultural backgrounds from your own, and learn from each other.	• Ask questions and explain your treatments with your patient's cultural background and biases in mind.

Introduction

Differences in people, their beliefs, behaviors, and social structures are present in every community in the world.[2] These differences will also be present in nearly every call to which you respond as a paramedic (Table 48-1). In many ways, issues of culture and cultural difference are more pronounced in the prehospital setting than in other healthcare settings. Unlike a physician or nurse who can often take time to prepare before walking into a patient exam room, paramedics respond to cases at a moment's notice with no warning about the patient's social group or language. You will also encounter patients in *their* own environments instead of having them come to an office or hospital.[4] Physically, the patient may be only blocks from your station, but they may

TABLE 48-1 Changing Demographics in the United States

Racial groups (in millions)	1990	2000	2010	2020	2030	2050
Total population	249	275	298	323	347	394
Hispanics	9.0	11.4	13.8	16.3	18.9	24.5
Non-Hispanic blacks	11.8	12.2	12.6	12.9	13.1	13.6
American Indians and Alaskan Natives	0.7	0.7	0.8	0.8	0.8	0.9
Asians and Pacific Islanders	2.8	3.9	4.8	5.7	6.6	8.2
Non-Hispanic whites	75.7	71.8	68.0	64.3	60.5	52.8

Source: U.S. Census Bureau, 1999.

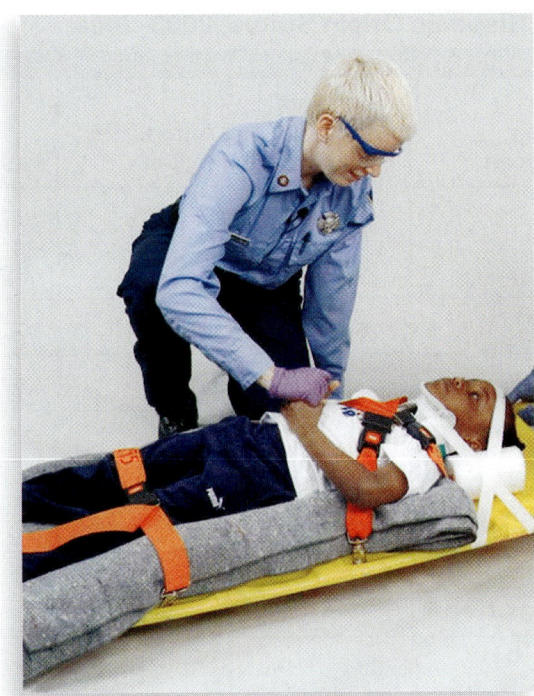

Figure 48-1   The response to illness or injury will depend on the cultural background of the patient. Knowledge and understanding of the patient's responses will facilitate the paramedic's ability to manage these cases.

be a million miles from your own cultural background (Figure 48-1). DOT 6-5.35

Patients who walk into a hospital or clinic have made a decision about the kind of healthcare they are seeking. In the prehospital environment, your patient will likely have had little to say about the request for 9-1-1 help and may not know what you do.[4,6] Your patient may not even want your assistance. One of the great challenges and privileges of working as a paramedic is that you will serve anyone who requests assistance, including patients from all cultural backgrounds living in diverse neighborhoods, and enter their homes in order to render urgently needed aid, treatment, and transport.[4]

If you are respectful of the beliefs and values of your patients and perform your job professionally in their time of crisis, your actions will speak volumes about both your capabilities as a paramedic as well as the entire medical and public health system you represent.[2]

Cultural Bias

As a medical professional, your attitudes toward illness and death may be quite different from some of the attitudes of the patients, families, and communities with which you will interact.[2] Your personal beliefs and values are based on your own cultural background as well as the experiences that have shaped your views over time. Together these form your own "cultural bias," which you use in social situations and when making judgments.[7] Your

approach to patients from other cultural backgrounds, however, will require both sensitivity of and a respect for beliefs, values, and experiences that may be significantly different from your own.[2]

In the minds of your patients and their families, you are not just a "healer" or medical professional.[8] Your uniform represents authority and is often viewed in similar fashion to those of other government representatives (such as law enforcement officers). Paramedics are often extensions of the local government and medical establishment, so your behavior represents more than just your own opinions.[8] You are showing the public what it can expect from mainstream ideas of medicine and healthcare. This makes you a role model in addition to a caregiver.

Evidence continues to grow demonstrating inequality among the degrees of healthcare sought by and made available to various population groups.[2,9] In some cases, cultural biases may shun the use of modern healthcare or favor "traditional" alternatives such as acupuncture, herbal remedies, or even prayer-based or spiritual healing.[5] In most cases, these lines of inequality reflect responses to both socioeconomic status and culture.[1,7] Many low-income and minority populations are simply unable to afford or fail to recognize the need for preventive healthcare altogether (Table 48-2).[10] The problem may be partially related to the fact that minorities are largely underrepresented in many key healthcare professions.[2,9]

According to the Sullivan Commission on Diversity in the Healthcare Workforce, this lack of cultural diversity in the medical workforce translates directly into cultural indifference, unequal treatment, communication barriers, and an overall lack of access to healthcare.[10] Unfortunately, for many minority groups this translates to worse health outcomes (Figure 48-2).[1,7] The National Center for Cultural Competence states that African Americans are 1.7 times more likely to have diabetes than whites. Latino/Hispanic Americans are 2.0 times more likely, and both Alaskan Natives and Native Americans are 2.8 times more likely to have diabetes than whites. Similar trends exist in cardiovascular diseases, respiratory diseases, cancers, and infant mortality (Figure 48-3).

Working in the Gray Zone

Many believe the best solution to managing cultural diversity in the field is to continue to encourage diversity in the EMS workforce. As EMS becomes more culturally diverse, the ability to understand and respond to different cultures and belief systems will improve. Others argue that, since many cultures do not value western medicine, both EMS and other medical professions will continue to fail miserably at diversifying. Still others feel that every medical professional must be trained to handle diversity appropriately. What do you think?

TABLE 48-2   **Key Indicators of Child Well-Being by Race and Hispanic Origin Status, 2003–2004**

Indicators	Total		White, Non-Hispanic	African American	Asian and Pacific Islander	American Indian	Latino
% low-birthweight babies	2003	7.9	7	13.4	7.8	7.4	6.7
Infant mortality rate	2003	6.9	5.7	14	3.8	7.8	5.8
Child death rate	2003	21	19	29	16	30	20
Teen death rate	2003	66	63	80	38	97	67
Teen birth rate	2003	42	27	64	17	53	82
% teens who are high school dropouts*	2004	8	6	8	3	13	15
% teens not attending school and not working*	2004	9	7	12	5	17	14
% children living in families where no parent has full-time/year round employment*	2004	33	27	50	32	51	39
% children in poverty*	2004	18	11	36	14	31	29
% children in single-parent families*	2004	31	23	64	15	47	35

*For this measure, the data for whites, African Americans, Asians, and American Indians are for persons who selected only one race. Data for African Americans, Asians, and American Indians Include those who are Hispanic/Latino.

Diversifying the healthcare workforce will take time.[2,9] Until that happens, both the federal government and advocacy groups are actively working to improve the quality and availability of healthcare for all cultural and socioeconomic populations.[10] At the same time, medical practitioners at all levels are learning to understand and respectfully interact with patients of various cultures.[10] Paramedics are no exception.[1,7] The National Association of EMS Educators recommends cultural awareness and diversity training for EMS providers.[1,7] Remember, in the eyes of most first responders as well as the public, a paramedic is the highest medical authority outside of a hospital. When dealing with cultural issues, patients will no doubt hold today's paramedic to the same standards as emergency department physicians.[1,7]

What Is Culture?

The Merriam-Webster dictionary defines culture as "the customary beliefs, social forms, and material traits of a racial, religious, or social group."[5] A culture does not necessarily imply a different country, skin tone, or foreign language. A variety of cultures and subcultures exist in both urban environments as well as small rural towns. A gang, a church group, or a particular corporate office and its employees are examples of subcultures with strong influences on beliefs, behaviors, and traditions.[5] Cultures will vary a great deal. They may be defined by ethnicity, national origin, spoken language, race, religion, age, sexual orientation, physical challenges, or any combination of these or other unique characteristics.[1,7] In addition, some people are strongly influenced by more than one culture. For example, a deaf Muslim may identify with and reflect the values and behaviors of both deaf culture and the Muslim community.

When attempting to define a culture, it is entirely too easy to use stereotypes kept alive by the media and long-standing social prejudices. A **stereotype** is an incomplete or oversimplified attempt to draw conclusions about groups of people with a particular defining characteristic.[5] Stereotypes are invalid because they fail to take into account variability within any given culture. For example, different young people of African or Asian descent may have quite different belief systems and social traits based on where they were raised, their parents' cultural ties and language preferences, the influences of peer groups, economic status, and so on.

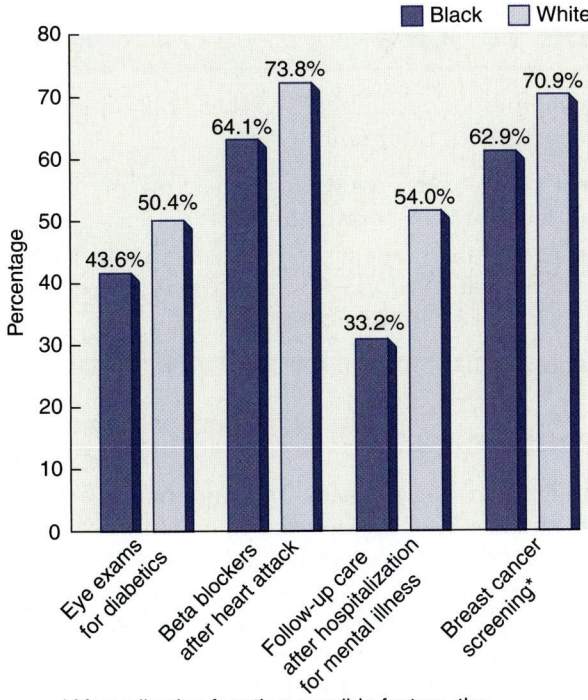

*After adjusting for other possible factors, the disparity was not statistically significant.

Figure 48-2 A study by the American Medical Association concluded that for 305,574 patients covered by one Medicare-managed health plan, blacks received poorer quality care than whites.[11]

As a paramedic, one of your responsibilities is to become familiar with the various cultures you will encounter while at the same time avoiding stereotypes. A much better alternative to ethnic or racial stereotypes is to learn the core values and beliefs of a culture.[1,7] By learning the basic differences between your cultural framework and another, you will create an understanding for yourself, and you can grow as you encounter the spectrum of variation within a cultural group. To the street-savvy paramedic, this base knowledge about a culture will be more useful than any stereotype ever could be.[1,7] DOT 6-5.34

Communicating with Diverse Populations

According to the U.S. Census Bureau's 2004 report, 12% of the American population is foreign born, and 18.7% of the population speaks a language other than English.[5] Of those who speak a language other than English, nearly half (45%) have at least some difficulty communicating in English (Table 48-3).[5] Obviously, at some point in your career as a paramedic, you will face a situation where you urgently need to communicate with and understand a non-English-speaking patient or family member. Knowing the languages that you are likely to encounter, identifying available resources, and planning ahead will allow you to continue to give the best possible patient care despite the language barrier.[2,9]

By far, the best and most rewarding approach is to learn another language.[5] For the most common languages, there are many self-directed audio and instructor-taught courses from which to choose, some with an emphasis on medical communication. Community colleges frequently offer beginner-level language classes, and some offer healthcare-specific courses such as "medical Spanish."

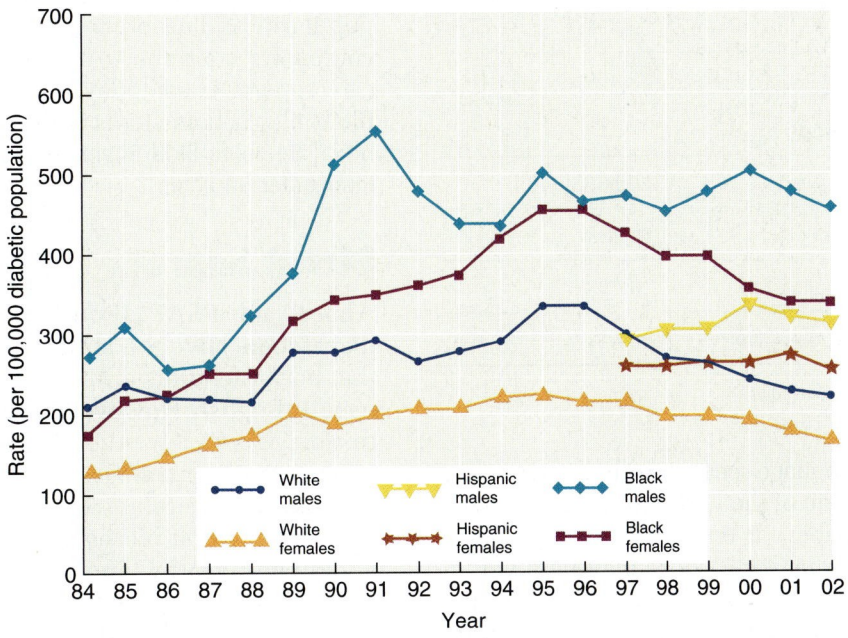

Figure 48-3 Incidence of end-stage renal disease in patients with diabetes, broken out by race, ethnicity, and sex in the United States from 1984 to 2001. Note that black men have the highest incidence and white women have the lowest.

TABLE 48-3   Selected Social Characteristics of U.S. Population

Selected Social Characteristics	2004 Percent Distribution
Place of Birth	
Total population	285,691,581
Native	88%
Foreign born	12%
Year of U.S. Entry	
Population born outside the U.S.	37,825,141
Native	9.4%
Foreign Born	34,279,756
Entered U.S. 2000 or later	18.3%
Entered U.S. before 2000	81.7%
World Region of Birth of Foreign Born	
Foreign-born population excluding population born "At sea"	34,279,584
Europe	14.3%
Asia	27%
Africa	3.3%
Oceania	0.6%
Latin America	52.4%
Northern America	2.4%
Language Spoken at Home	
Population 5 years and over	265,683,349
English only	81.3%
Language other than English	18.7%
Speak English less than "very well"	8.4%

Source: U.S. Census Bureau, Census 2004.

If learning a new language seems too challenging, you may want to consider one of many different pocket-sized translation books available for emergency response personnel. These instant translation books may help you to communicate with non-English speakers. Remember, any effort you make to improve communication across a language barrier will show both your patients and their families your commitment to the best possible patient care.[2,9]

Nice to Know

Most emergency medical services offer educational incentives for their employees.

- Do you know what languages you are likely to encounter in your community?
- Are there language courses available in your area that could improve your ability to communicate with your patients?

Street Secrets

Although learning to speak *and* understand a new language such as Spanish in order to communicate during a medical crisis may seem like a sizeable task, learning to speak a few basic phrases in a language can be extremely useful. For example, learning to ask the patient if they have pain requires only a yes or no response or gesture from the patient. Similarly, learning to ask a patient to point to the pain requires no language comprehension at all to understand the answer.

In addition, many dispatch centers have the ability to patch in a "language line" with a translator who can help with communication between you and the patient or family member. This service is available for more than 150 different languages.[5] Finally, many police departments and first response agencies are beginning to use handheld language computers that can translate between English and various languages while on-scene.[5] As the popularity and usability of these devices improve, and as computers continue to replace the paper-based patient care reports used today, these translation devices will likely also become tools in the paramedic's language toolbox.[3] **See also Skill Sheet 62: Communication Challenges—Interpreter Services.**

Street Secrets

Almost all PSAP (Public Safety Answering Point) dispatchers have the ability to patch in a language line that performs translation from one language to another, usually English. However, depending upon the language, this may take a few minutes for the dispatcher to set up. Often a family member nearby may be able to translate for you. Always remember to take into account the age, sex, and cultural biases of the translator as well as the patient and nearby family.

The ability to communicate with foreign-language patients will often rely on more than just being able to translate words to and from English.[5] In many situations, you are likely to find at least one person who speaks English, however poorly, and who can function as a translator.[5] Obviously, there are advantages to using on-scene resources to help with communication, including speed and availability. In this case, there is no need to set up a language line or pass a phone, radio, or computer between you and the person with whom you are trying to communicate. However, there are drawbacks to this approach as well.[2] Based on the translator's bias or beliefs and the relationship to the patient or family, the translator may not translate every communication with its original form or meaning intact.[2,9] There may also be privacy or confidentiality issues to consider as well as limits to what this person is capable of translating.[2,9]

When you are trying to communicate across a language barrier, consider the cultural values system of the person with whom you are communicating. Many Asian cultures, for example, believe it to be impolite to answer in the negative.[5] In these cultures, even a misunderstood or confusing communication may result in a "yes" gesture or verbal response. Answers that should clearly be "no" will instead be given as "maybe" or "perhaps." Nonverbal communication skills will also be a factor. For example, many northern European and Asian cultures and most Americans consider staring impolite; whereas, *not* making continuous direct eye contact with a Southern European or an Arab male may be perceived as disrespectful.[2,3,9] In addition, families in some cultures may designate and rely on a spokesperson based on gender or generational role.[5] Ignoring this family spokesperson may insult the entire family.[5]

Always consider the cultural implications of your communication, both in the questions you need to ask and the statements you make.[2,9] The various cultures you encounter as a paramedic will approach issues of gender, privacy, and sexuality very differently.[10] At any given scene, will you complete your patient assessment with family nearby or in the privacy of your ambulance?[2] Will you rely on a family member or friend to translate, or will you use other resources at your disposal? When will it be more appropriate to have your male or female partner ask the questions instead?[2] Your decisions in these situations will depend a great deal upon your sensitivity to these and other cultural issues.[2,9] DOT 6-5.35

Illness and Pain across Cultures

Culture groups also vary in their responses to illness and injury.[2,9] While some may favor stoicism and avoid showing or acknowledging pain altogether, others consider an overt display of pain appropriate before seeking help or medical attention. For example, Latino/Hispanic, Jewish, and Iranian cultures seem to encourage expressions of pain; whereas, many Asian

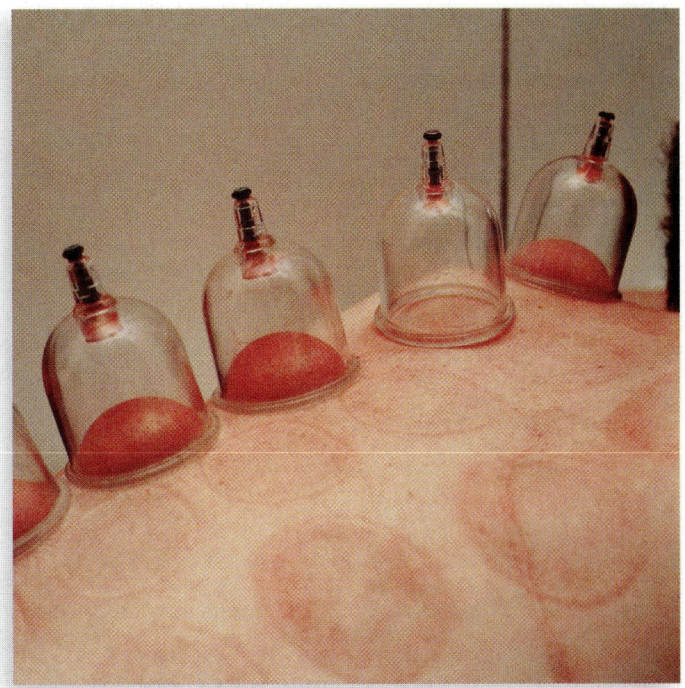

Figure 48-4   The practice of cupping leaves circular bruises on the affected area.

and Germanic cultures consider showing pain a weakness of character.[2,5,12]

Cultural rituals and traditions also play an important role in how patients think about, grade, and express pain. For example, many Native American cultures rely on some kind of physically demanding rite of passage in order to mark the transition from a boy to a man and harden away fearful reactions to pain or death.[5] Some African cultures continue to perform ritualistic clitoral circumcision on countless women each day with the belief that, despite the debilitating and painful consequences of this procedure, women with unaltered genitalia will become too promiscuous.[5,13] When Hmong children are ill, home remedies may include dietary changes; herbal medicines; ceremonies; wearing religious symbols to prevent soul loss; "cupping," which applies suction to the affected area of skin (Figure 48-4); and "coining," where warm oils or gels are applied to the skin and vigorously rubbed, both of which frequently bruise children's skin (Figure 48-5). Awareness of these and other cultural traditions and their consequences factor into your understanding of how an individual of that culture may tolerate or relate to injury and pain.[5]

Management of a patient's pain is an important aspect of being a paramedic, but appropriate management requires accurate assessment. Because cultural variations make a subjective assessment of pain more challenging, a paramedic should always gauge each patient's response to pain individually.[5] Although cultural views of illness and injury may partly obscure a patient's level of pain,

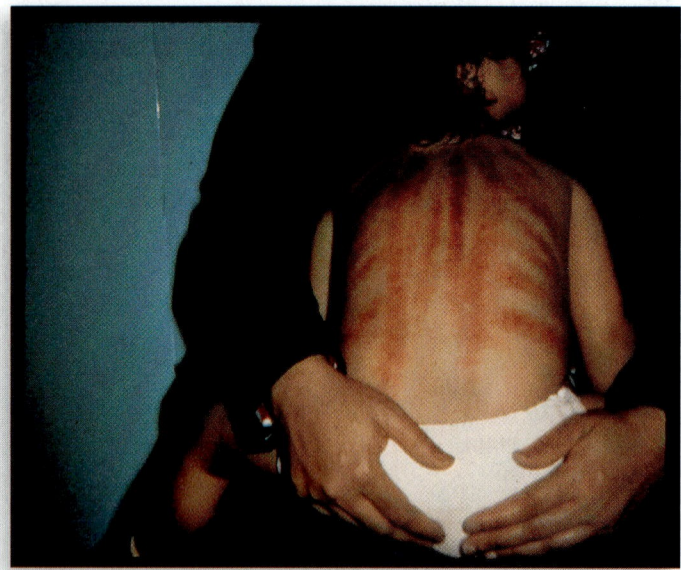

Figure 48-5 The practice of coining leaves striated bruising.

observing a patient during an obviously painful procedure (such as an IV start) may help to identify that particular patient's pain threshold and pain response. This will help you treat your patient's pain appropriately and with confidence.[2,9]

Healthcare in Other Cultures

Traditional healing methods, healing rituals, and herbal remedies continue to play an important role in many cultures throughout the world (Box 48-1).[5,10] According to the World Health Organization, in many African countries over half of all children with a high malaria-induced fever are treated at home with simple herbal remedies.[5] Likewise, the Chinese continue to rely heavily on traditional herbal preparations for up to half of all their medicinal needs.[5] In fact, artemisinin, perhaps the most effective antimalarial drug ever developed, comes from a medicinal herb used in China for over 2000 years to treat fevers.[5] While many herbal remedies have consistently been shown to help when used appropriately, other healing traditions can seem questionable at best. For example, some African tribal communities still believe ritualistic teeth pulling to be therapeutic for a number of childhood illnesses, including diarrhea.[5]

BOX 48-1 Traditional Medicines and Therapies

- **Acupuncture** attempts to manipulate specific energy channels in the body in order to elicit the desired response. Acupuncture, extremely popular in Asian cultures, is perhaps one of the most well-studied practices of traditional medicine.[5]

- **Chiropractic** treatments focus on joint manipulation in order to treat a variety of problems. Its popularity has waxed and waned over the years due to conflicting scientific data on the efficacy of chiropractic procedures.[5]

- **Herbalism** is the study and use of plant-based and mineral-based remedies. In fact, herbal remedies helped give rise to the modern pharmaceutical industry (one-quarter of all modern medicines are made from plants first used traditionally). Herbalists argue, however, that the isolated and manufactured clone of the functional part of a plant is missing essential components of the original plant.[5]

- **Holistic therapies** are those that focus on the mind-body connection and recognize that disease is an imbalance that includes both psycho-emotional and physiological components. Modern healthcare as a whole is now moving toward a more holistic direction, accepting that the treatment course of any patient can and should address the mental and emotional aspects of healing as well.[5]

- **Homeopathy** is the study and use of substances designed to elicit and amplify the symptoms produced by the body's own immune response in order to help the body fight disease. Homeopathic practitioners believe that the body's response to an invader or disease is the same response needed to cure it.[5]

- **Osteopathy** emphasizes the body's innate ability to heal itself, and osteopaths focus their efforts accordingly. Although Doctors of Osteopathy are fully licensed physicians who can prescribe medication and perform surgery, the fundamental philosophy of osteopathy is that the body contains its own best medicine.[5]

- **Shamanism** relies on the innate ability of a shaman (medicine man) to transcend the visible world and manipulate invisible lines of force in order to diagnose disease and induce healing. Many people from India rely on shamanic practices to maintain good health and cure illness.[1,7]

- **Therapeutic Massage** is the practice of using "healing touch" to manipulate muscle and body parts to facilitate healing and relieve stress. This is also a rapidly growing area of interest in modern healthcare, and many hospitals are now utilizing therapeutic massage to accelerate the healing process.[5]

Street Secrets

Many practitioners of western medicine are including nontraditional and eastern medical practices out of respect for the patients they are treating.

As a paramedic, you should understand that in certain cultures, disease is not an immediate reason for seeking medical attention or pharmaceutical interventions.[5] For many people, the traditional medicinal techniques used for many generations are both familiar and effective for most of their healthcare needs.[5] Today, even mainstream American families are beginning to experiment with and use traditional alternatives to modern medicine.[5]

Some cultures acknowledge a need for modern medicine and oppose only specific interventions. For example, both Jehovah's Witnesses and the Hmong associate special meaning with blood. Some Jehovah's Witnesses may not agree to receive a blood transfusion but usually have little problem with blood being drawn for testing.[5] In contrast, the Hmong generally believe that the body contains a finite amount of spirit and vitality represented by circulating blood, and they may hesitate at having their blood drawn for fear of losing or wasting this precious life energy.[5] Still other cultures and religions prefer faith and prayer to any medical intervention. For example, Christian Scientists believe that both the universe and the human being are perfectly designed and capable of limitless self-healing. A Christian Scientist believes they can correct whatever imbalance is preventing good health with prayer and mindfulness.[5]

Working in the Gray Zone

Christian Scientists and Jehovah's Witnesses argue that their reason for denying certain forms of medical care is a natural extension of their devout religious beliefs. More than once, this has resulted in the death of an individual whom modern medicine would have considered a "likely save." Doctors, with the support of the legal system, have often placed children in protective custody in order to treat life-threatening conditions despite the obvious violation of their parents' religious beliefs.

Because the appeal of traditional medicine affects nearly every culture you will encounter, there is a strong possibility that traditional medicine of some kind has been tried and has failed when you arrive at the scene of a life-threatening illness or injury.[3] You should, therefore, gather a history that specifically asks about any traditional therapies used on or by your patient, including any herbal remedies or other interventions tried to that point.[1,7] As you become familiar with the various cultures that you serve, you will also become more familiar with traditional therapies that they prefer for specific illnesses and injuries.

Remember to consider, in the case of immigrant populations, how far removed your patients are from their culture of origin. For example, when treating a young teenager in a multigenerational immigrant family, you can expect that the teen will probably be much more mainstream than will the eldest grandparent. The tendency of young people to lose touch with their culture is a source of continuous strain on these families and their expectations.[5] When treating a patient in a multigenerational environment, you should expect your patient and each generation of family onlookers to hold different beliefs and viewpoints.

Death and Dying

The "appropriate response" to death will vary a great deal from one culture to the next (Figure 48-6).[5] When you are required to give the notification of death, you can expect, for example, that a Somali family's response will not be the same as that of a Native American family.[1,7] Every culture has different beliefs about death.[3] This is especially true when a culture defines itself, at least in part, by common religious beliefs (Box 48-2).[5]

Most cultures have traditional views on the appropriate handling and aftercare of a lifeless body, but the specific rituals and customs vary from culture to culture.[5] In addition, the responses of those witnessing the passing of a loved one will be at least partly influenced by what is considered culturally appropriate at that time.[5] A paramedic should expect and allow for different reactions when a patient dies.[5] Becoming

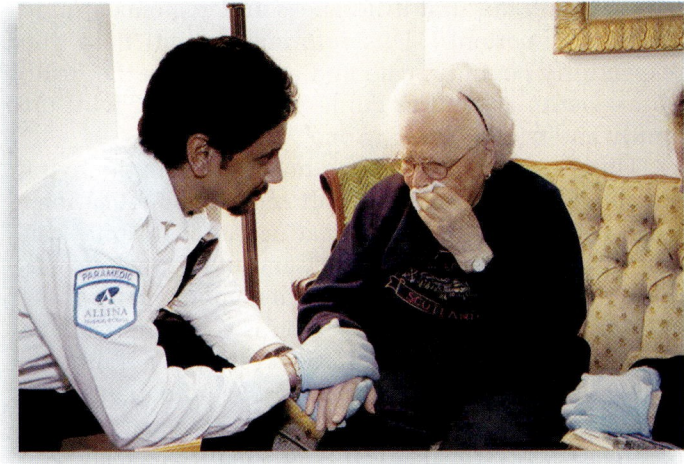

Figure 48-6 The response to death and dying will vary depending on the cultural background of the patient. Knowledge and understanding of these responses will help the paramedic deal with the patient's family and loved ones.

BOX 48-2 Various Cultural Responses to Illness and Death

- *Asian* culture views illness as involving the whole family. Decisions about treatment and patient handling go through the extended family. Many Asians prefer that caregivers avoid communicating news of a serious illness or disease directly to the patient for fear that this news itself will further burden the patient's health. This is especially true of the elderly, whom Asian communities hold in the highest regard. In death and dying, both the patient's wishes and the impact to the family are equally considered.[2,9]

- *European* cultures vary considerably. However, with the exception of Eastern European countries, most seem to generally mirror the range of contemporary western views on illness and death.[5] Unlike western views around patient autonomy, however, Eastern European cultures (as well as Russian culture) are frequently accustomed to accepting illness or injury at face value and relinquishing patient care decisions to whatever medical authority is in charge. These cultures view this as "unburdening" both the patient and family from having to make caregiving decisions.[5]

- *Hispanic/Latino* cultures consider patient care decisions and outcomes as they impact not only the patient but the entire family, and the family usually has considerable say in all patient care decisions.[11] However, Mexican Americans, for example, typically respect the caregiver-patient relationship and expect caregivers to interact directly with the patient first and the family second.[2,9] Rooted in the annual celebration known as the Day of the Dead, the Mexican culture maintains a very comfortable relationship with death and dying, viewing illness and death as natural and inevitable processes.[3,5]

- *Middle Eastern* views of illness and dying vary depending upon the faith. In illness, the Jewish culture tends to demonstrate overt displays of symptoms; whereas, the Muslim culture encourages denial and stoicism, especially in public or with strangers.[5] In dealing with death and dying, both faiths believe in and respect the autonomy of the patient and their wishes.[2,9] Both Jewish and Muslim faiths have very specific requirements when dealing with the body of a recently deceased loved one.[2,9]

- *Native American* cultures consider the spoken word to be very powerful and may refuse to acknowledge a negative diagnosis out of a concern that the spoken words will help manifest a negative outcome. In addition, Native American cultures place a high value on positive thinking and expect that all patient caregivers will use positive thinking while treating them and expect fundamentally positive outcomes from all treatments performed. Death is viewed as an inevitable reality not to be feared but also never to be openly discussed or planned for until after it has occurred.[5]

familiar with cultural differences and customs around death is important.[5] This information will help you respectfully communicate and acknowledge the death of the victim as well as guide you in dealing with the family and friends looking on.[5]

Until recently, training on how to inform the living about a death has not been part of medical education.[5] However, success rates for treating out-of-hospital cardiac arrests are still quite poor, and unfortunately, cardiovascular disease rates are higher among many of the culturally diverse population groups you will treat.[14] In addition, there are some situations, such as a traumatic arrest, where you may decide never to start patient care.[5] Although local protocols vary, it is generally the paramedic's responsibility to notify family present at an emergency scene that resuscitation efforts are not being effective and that you will be discontinuing efforts, as well as informing them of the death itself once you have stopped (Box 48-3). This is especially true when the resuscitation attempt is in progress and efforts are about to be stopped. The 2005 American Heart Association guidelines for resuscitation recommend that paramedics give family members the option to remain with their loved ones during emergency care.[15] Other groups, including the Emergency Nursing Association, also recommend this approach.[2,9] Studies suggest that family members, especially parents of young children, want to be present during both emergency procedures and resuscitation.[2,9,16,17]

Summary

Cultural diversity is a factor in every patient encounter. Because many of your patients' cultural beliefs, values, and customs may be significantly different from your own, you should try to learn as much as you can about the culture of the population groups you will serve. Only then can you expect to interact with and treat patients of different cultures effectively.

BOX 48-3   Step-by-Step Guide to Death Notification

1. ***Identify family members*** or other survivors who are present at the scene and must be notified of the death.[5] This may sound simple, but 9-1-1 calls attract many concerned neighbors, friends, and bystanders. It is critical to identify, gather, and attempt to provide some privacy for the family or people closest to the patient. In general, blood relatives and immediate family members are the most important people to gather and isolate. In some cases a family friend, clergy, alternative healer, or fiancée might be the appropriate person with whom to interact.

2. ***Assess any issues or cultural beliefs*** that might help predict the grief reaction or guide the way you should interact with the family. Issues such as a prolonged illness, terminal disease, old age, or cultural acceptance of death might make the event less traumatic for survivors. Generally speaking, the more unexpected, sudden, and violent the death, especially in a younger person, the more acute the grief reaction is likely to be.

3. ***Attempt to provide an area of privacy*** where the family can be away from the deceased. Have everyone sit down, including yourself. Sitting will set a tone of de-escalation and lessen the likelihood that family members might hurt themselves if they suddenly lose their balance or faint upon hearing the bad news.

4. ***Prepare the survivors*** for the notification. The family may view your resuscitation attempts as "lifesaving." The implication is that there is still "life" to "save." It is important to realize that the patient who is getting CPR is pulseless and apneic, in other words, clinically dead. If possible, the EMS team should inform the family of the progress of the resuscitation during the event. Simple words such as, "Your wife's heart has stopped and she is not breathing," can set the stage so that the family views the resuscitation as an attempt to revive, restart the heart, or bring their loved one back to life. This may help communicate how serious the condition is and lessen the chance that a failed resuscitation attempt will be seen as a negligent error on the part of the caregivers. Giving periodic updates will allow the family to mentally prepare for a negative outcome should the patient not be revived.

5. ***Keep it simple.*** Introduce yourself; be empathetic, caring, and direct. Use plain language and simple terms to explain your care and the patient's response. Say that the patient, using the patient's name, "has died." Then wait in silence for at least 30 to 60 seconds. Although this may seem abrupt the first time you do it, euphemisms and medical terms can be very confusing. Do not say the patient has "passed away," "is in a better place," or "is deceased." These terms may be misunderstood by a family member and only serve to make further interactions more difficult.

Notes

1. J. South-Paul, S. Matheny, and E. Lewis, *Current Diagnosis & Treatment in Family Medicine,* Chapter 54: Cultural Competence (New York, NY: McGraw-Hill, 2004).

2. G. Galanti, *Caring for Patients from Different Cultures,* 3rd ed. (Philadelphia, PA: University of Pennsylvania Press, 2004).

3. H. Perkins and J. Cortez, "Cross-Cultural Similarities and Differences in Attitudes About Advanced Care Planning," *Journal of General Internal Medicine* 17(2002): 48.

4. National Association of EMS Educators, *2002 National Guidelines for Educating EMS Instructors,* Module 21, http://www.nhtsa.dot. gov/people/injury/ems/Instructor/instructor_ems/2002_national_ guidelines.htm (accessed February 8, 2006).

5. L. Gerace and S. Salimbene, "Cultural Competency for Today's Nurse 3: Cultural Factor in Pain Management," http://www. nursingspectrum.com (accessed February 8, 2006).

6. "Paramedic Job Profile," http://www.jobprofiles.org/ (accessed February 8, 2006).

7. Cultural Bias, http://en.wikipedia.org/wiki/Cultural_bias (accessed February 9, 2006).

8. S. Stewart, *Customer Satisfaction in the Metropolitan Ambulance Service* (Australia: Victoria Graduate School of Business, 2001).

9. M. Fleming and K. Towey, *Delivering Culturally Effective Health Care to Adolescents* (Washington, DC: Maternal and Child Health Bureau, U.S. Department of Health and Human Services, 2001).

10. J. A. Marx, *Rosen's Emergency Medicine: Concepts and Clinical Practice,* 5th ed. (St. Louis, MO: Mosby, 2002).

11. E. C. Schneider, A. M. Zaslavsky, and A. M. Epstein, "Racial Disparities in the Quality of Care for Enrollees in Medicare Managed Care," *Journal of the American Medical Association* 287 (2002): 1288–1294.

12. V. Diaz, "Cultural Factors in Preventive Care: Latinos," *Primary Care* 29(3) (2002): 503–517.

13. L. Wallis, "When Rites Are Wrong," *Nursing Standard* 20(4) (2005): 24–26.

14. D. Perina, "EMS and Cardiac Arrest," http://www.emedicine. com/emerg/topic710.htm (accessed February 8, 2006).

15. American Heart Association in Collaboration with the International Liaison Committee on Resuscitation, "Guidelines 2000 for Cardiopulmonary Resuscitation and Emergency Cardiovascular Care," *Circulation* 102 (Suppl) (2000): I-1–I-374.

16. H. Bauchner, C. Waring, and R. Vinci, "Parental Presence During Procedures in an Emergency Room: Results from 50 Observations," *Pediatrics* 87(4) (April 1991): 544–548.

17. A. Sacchetti, R. Lichenstein, C. A. Carraccio, et al., "Family Member Presence During Pediatric Emergency Department Procedures," *Pediatric Emergency Care* 16 (2000): 85–87.

part 6

Operations

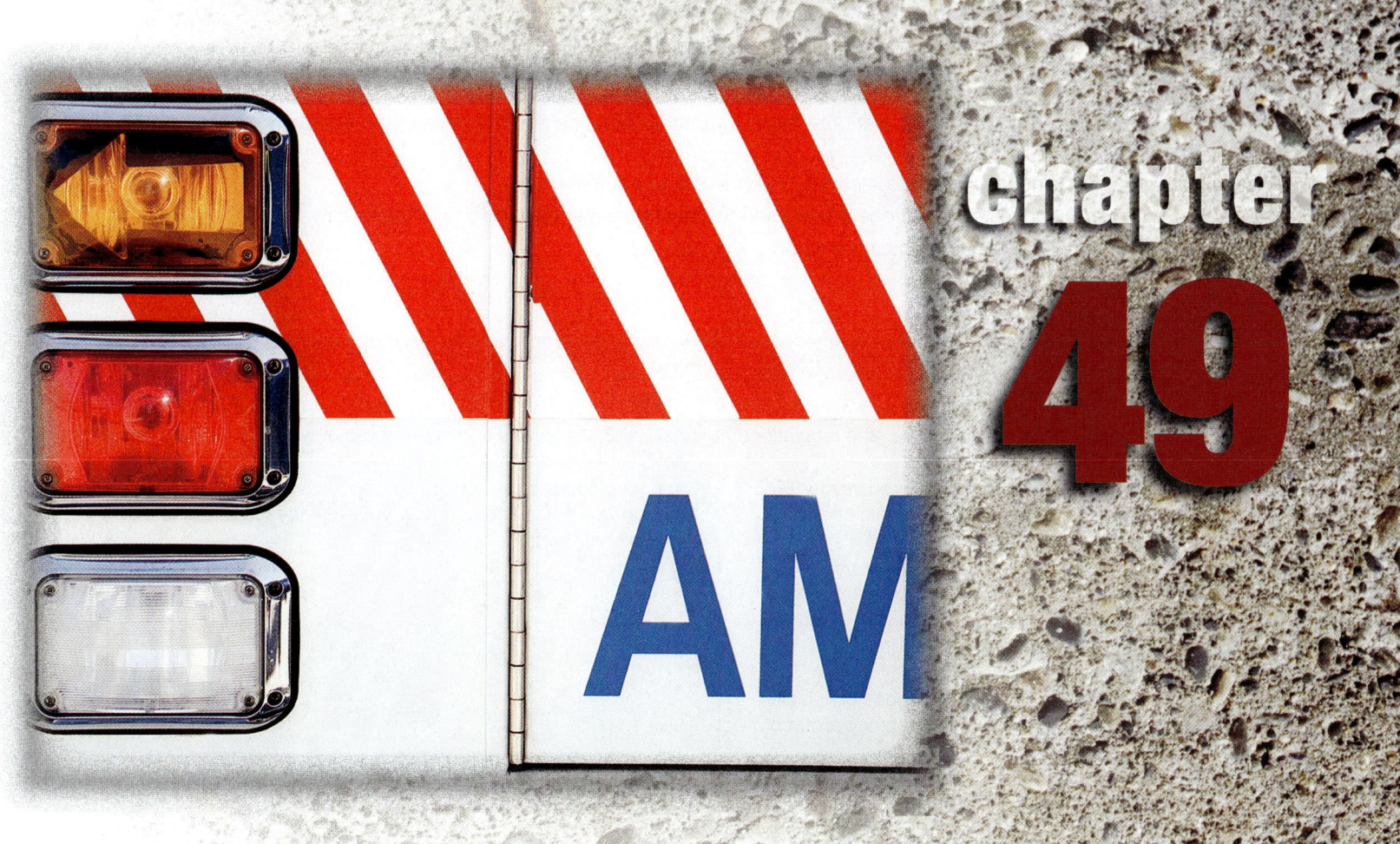

Ambulance Operations

"When written in Chinese, the word crisis is composed of two characters. One represents danger, and the other represents opportunity."

—John F. Kennedy

Need to Know

▶ The national, state, and local standards that determine paramedic practice and the design and equipping of ambulances.

▶ The importance of documenting daily inspections of vehicles and equipment.

▶ The various ways ambulances are positioned to provide the best possible response to a community.

▶ The limitations and benefits of aeromedical transport.

▶ Do	▶ Ask
• Review national, state, and local laws, rules, and regulations that describe and define your practice. • Become familiar with the documentation used in your EMS system that confirms inspections of EMS vehicles and equipment. • Become familiar with your agency's response to the demands of your service area (i.e., fixed positions, system status management, etc.). • Understand your EMS system's policies regarding aeromedical transport. • Perform daily and other scheduled inspections of vehicles and equipment according to system and agency protocol.	• Ask your instructors and supervisors at work about the rules and regulations that govern your agency's operation. • Ask your supervisors about how requests for ambulance response are handled and how your agency responds to multiple requests.

Introduction

Ambulance operations encompass all of the regulations and practices applicable to running a professional and accountable EMS agency. Professionally competent EMS requires commitment from every EMS agency and each of its providers and other employees. As a paramedic, you will be making a commitment to understanding the rules and regulations of your practice, ensuring that your vehicles and equipment are where they are supposed to be and in working order and that you are personally prepared to do your job. As you go about your job with attention to detail, you will serve as a role model for anyone who has the opportunity to work with you. DOT 8-1.7, 8-1.8

Local and State Ambulance Standards

There are a variety of standards and recommendations regarding ambulance specifications and the equipment carried. Local and state EMS authorities may have different specifications regarding ambulance standards. Many authorities have adopted the federal KKK-A-1822 specifications and the American College of Emergency Physicians/American College of Surgeons (ACEP/ACS) equipment recommendations, making additions or deletions where they felt necessary and incorporating them into their rules and regulations.[1,2]

National ambulance standards build upon three ambulance vehicle platforms, Type I, II, or III (Figure 49-1).

■ Type I ambulances are truck chassis with modular or box patient compartments (Figure 49-1(a))
■ Type II is the standard van-type ambulance (Figure 49-1(b))
■ Type III ambulances are van chassis with modular or box-type patient compartments (Figure 49-1(c))

The ACEP/ACS recommendations for equipment, however, are not binding on local and state governments. While the ACEP guidelines provide a framework for selection of necessary supplies and equipment, local and state authorities that oversee EMS can choose to adopt their own specifications, researching and writing specifications for vehicles and minimum levels of equipment and supplies.

To further complicate matters, EMS providers and local governments that contract for service may decide on their own to adopt differing specifications for vehicles, equipment, and supplies that are written into policy, procedure, and contract details. While they can decide to adopt a higher standard, they cannot adopt anything lower than the minimum specification designated by the regulatory authority. DOT 8-1.1

Regardless of where the regulations originated, it is important to know what your agency requirements are for equipping and stocking your vehicle.

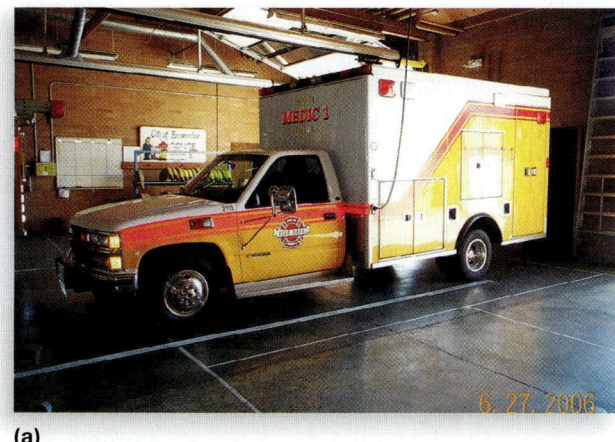

(a)

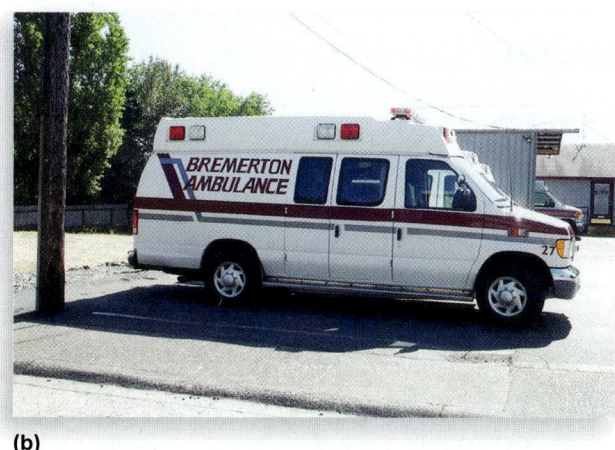

(b)

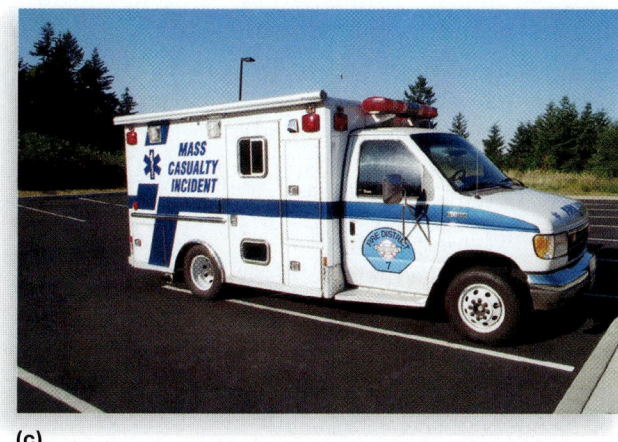

(c)

Figure 49-1 Ambulances. (a) Type I. (b) Type II. (c) Type III.

Phases of EMS Response

There are nine distinct phases of an EMS response:

1. Preparation
2. Dispatch
3. En route
4. Arrival on scene
5. Transfer of patient to the ambulance
6. Transport
7. Arrival at receiving facility
8. Return to station
9. Postrun

Preparation

Checking the ambulance at the beginning of the shift is a required ritual for EMS teams across the country. At the beginning of your shift, you should perform a complete check of your vehicle and equipment. Being prepared is the key to success for an EMS provider, and it is one of the most important tasks to undertake.

Equipment Check

Having a properly equipped vehicle means that you are ready to respond to any emergency. The last thing you would want to do is get into the driver's seat, respond to a call, and then find out in front of the patient and their family or friends that you do not have the proper equipment or that the equipment you have is not in working order.

Check-sheets listing the required equipment and supplies along with a par-level are the norm. Par-levels tell the EMS team how much of a particular item they should have in their vehicle or contained in a bag or box that they will bring to the patient's bedside. DOT 8-2.2

Par-levels generally indicate the minimum levels of supplies, but for larger pieces of equipment where space is at a premium or for supplies that are infrequently used and apt to expire, they may also be stated as the maximum number of a particular item. Every item needs to be checked for completeness and working order.

The following items, while not a complete list, are representative of the detail required to check and ensure operability. For the complete list of materials, see the ACEP/ACS document *Equipment for Ambulances.*

- *Oxygenation and airway equipment.* Advanced airway equipment poses some unique stocking issues. You need to have additional batteries for laryngoscope handles if handles and blades are not disposable. You should also have adequate numbers of the correct size replacement bulbs. Colorimetric CO_2 detectors, used to confirm endotracheal tube placement, whether they are stand-alone or incorporated into a bag-mask, are only good for four hours after they are removed from their packages. Unless you are going to use a colorimetric device immediately, do not open it. Quantitative CO_2 detectors require the appropriate adapters to be placed for either sidestream or in-line samples.

  Portable oxygen units and on-board oxygen systems need to be checked: Are they full? Do their regulators work? Can you adjust the liter flow without difficulty? It is crucially important to keep the regulators and the oxygen cylinder heads free of dirt, dust, and oil. Pressurized gases release a certain amount of heat and may ignite a dirty cylinder head or regulator causing serious injury.[3] Oxygen delivery devices must include infant, child, and adult Venturi masks, nonrebreather oxygen masks, simple masks, and nasal cannulas. You will also require bag-masks in various sizes, including adult, pediatric, and infant. You will also need the appropriate oxygen reservoirs, supply tubings, and masks. Any equipment that is reusable will have to be appropriately cleaned after an emergency response. Airways should be stocked in various sizes for oral, nasopharyngeal, and laryngeal airways. An adequate quantity of each ALS airway device (endotrachael tubes, laryngeal mask airways, and blind airway insertion devices) must also be assured. Portable and on-board suction units will have to be checked and should generally operate to a vacuum of 300 mmHg when the tubing is clamped between your fingers.

Various rigid and soft suction catheters, as well as disposable suction containers, need to be stocked. Again, if you are not using disposable containers, how will your aspirate containers be cleaned and ready for the next assignment, and who will clean them? See Box 49-1 for a more complete list of recommended airway and ventilation equipment.

- **Bleeding control.** Bandages, dressings, saline, and sterile water for irrigation have expiration dates. Are they satisfactory, or are they due to expire? If the package is damaged, you need to replace the item.
- **Vascular access and medications.** Are your medications stored in a temperature-controlled area? Extreme temperatures can cause some medications to become ineffective. Medications, IV fluids, advanced airway adjuncts, IV catheters, and tubing need to be checked for expiration dates and to ensure the packaging is intact. In addition, IV fluids and medications need to be examined for discoloration of the fluids and particulate matter floating in the vials or bags. See Box 49-2 for a more complete list of recommended vascular access equipment.

CONNECTIONS For a more complete list of recommended medications to carry in your Drug Box see Chapter 15: Pharmacology.

- **Cardiac monitor/defibrillator/pacer.** For battery-powered items, such as your cardiac monitor, you need to turn the device on to see if it will generate

BOX 49-1 Recommended Airway and Ventilation Equipment

1. Laryngoscope handle in adult and pediatric sizes with extra batteries and bulbs
2. Laryngoscope blades in sizes 0, 1, and 2, straight and sizes 3 and 4, straight and curved
3. Endotracheal tubes in sizes 2.5–6.0 mm uncuffed and 6.5–8.0 mm cuffed (two each); other sizes optional
4. Meconium aspirator
5. 10-mL non-Luerlock syringes
6. Stylettes for endotracheal tubes in adult and pediatric sizes
7. Magill forceps in adult and pediatric sizes
8. Lubricating jelly (water soluble)
9. Nasogastric tubes in pediatric sizes 5F and 8F and Salem sump sizes 14F, 16F, and 18F
10. 50 or 60 mL tapered tip syringes for NG tubes
11. End-tidal CO_2 detectors
    - Colorimetric or quantitative

BOX 49-2 Recommended Vascular Access Equipment

1. Intravenous administration equipment (fluid must be in bags not bottles)
2. Crystalloid solutions, Ringer's lactate or normal saline solution (four 1,000-mL bags), and 5% dextrose in water (optional)
3. Antiseptic solution (alcohol wipes and povidone-iodine wipes preferred)
4. IV pole or roof hook
5. Intravenous catheters 14G–24G, 1 inch long
6. Intraosseous needles
7. Tourniquet and rubber bands
8. Syringes of various sizes, including tuberculin
9. Needles in sizes 19G–25G
10. Intravenous administration sets (microdrip and macrodrip), Burretrol, and in-line blood pump (as differentiated from intravenous tubing with an in-line blood filter)
11. Intravenous arm boards in adult and pediatric sizes
12. Rigid sharps disposal container

Source: ACEP/ACS "Equipment for Ambulances (June 2000)" www.acep.org.

BOX 49-3 Recommended Cardiac Equipment

1. Portable, battery-operated monitor and defibrillator
   - With print capability or recorder, defibrillator pads, quick-look paddles or multifunction patches, ECG leads, adult and pediatric chest attachment electrodes, adult and pediatric paddles, with capability to provide electrical discharge below 25 watt-seconds.
2. Transcutaneous cardiac pacemaker
   - Either stand-alone unit or integrated into monitor or defibrillator

BOX 49-4 Recommended Infection Control Equipment*

1. Eye protection (full glasses or goggles, face shield)
2. Masks
3. Nonsterile gloves
4. Jumpsuits or gowns
5. Shoe covers
6. Disinfectant hand wash and commercial antimicrobial towelette, spray, or liquid
7. Disinfectant solution for cleaning equipment
8. Standard sharps containers
9. Disposable trash bags (identifiable color such as red)
10. N-95 HEPA mask

*Latex-free equipment should be available.

a tracing. Charge the defibrillator to be sure it will charge to the highest energy level. Check the battery indicators to show that you have sufficient power to care for a patient and be sure you have an adequate number of spare charged batteries. Look at your on-board charger to assure that it is working. Examine the patient cables for fraying. Do you have adequate numbers of electrodes and gel for defibrillation? Ensure that you have the proper cables and supplies for pacing and hands-free defibrillation. See Box 49-3 for recommended cardiac equipment. DOT 3-5.30

Street Secrets

Never discharge a defibrillator into the air to check it. Use the appropriate tester to ensure that it is working properly.

- **Personal protective equipment (PPE).** You also want to make sure that your personal protective equipment is easily accessible and adequately stocked. Carry gloves, masks, face, and eye protection on your person. Additional materials must be readily at hand in the cab and the patient compartment as well as in the trauma and medical bags. See Box 49-4 for recommended infection control equipment.
- **Miscellaneous.** Other items that need to be examined include spinal immobilization devices, extrication equipment, and additional PPE. Check turnout gear, chemical protective suits, escape hoods, self-contained breathing apparatus and powered air purifying respirators (PAPRs). Note that these may be stored in an outside compartment because of lack of

space. If you are responding to a chemical spill, while dispatch may tell you the correct route to approach the scene safely, you should stop and get your gear out ahead of time. During the Tokyo subway sarin attack, emergency responders were overwhelmed by people who were contaminated and left the scene, only to stop emergency responders several city blocks away from the subway station.

Supply, equipment, and vehicle checkout lists are quite extensive. If your unit and equipment are well maintained and kept stocked, this is not as daunting a task as it appears.

In addition to checking your equipment list, you should also receive a report from the off-going crew as to any deficiencies in the vehicle, its equipment, and the supplies. Did they leave any equipment at the hospital? Are there any devices that are damaged and need to be replaced? Even though the off-going crew provides a vehicle status report, you will still need to do a complete vehicle check. However, their report will allow you to concentrate on missing critical supplies, so in the event that you are dispatched on an emergency prior to completing your checkout, you will at least have enough equipment and supplies to complete several emergency assignments before having to go back to headquarters. You should also perform the narcotic count in front of the off-going team. Any discrepancies in the count will need to be rectified before they go off duty.

While this list is by no means complete, it is meant to give you an idea of what needs to be checked and determined to be in good working order prior to leaving the station.

Street Secrets

When you report to work and are assigned your vehicle, it is your ambulance. As a professional paramedic you are accountable for your own performance and the vehicle and equipment you bring to the scene. Do not rely on the competency of the crew prior to you. Ensure that the vehicle and the equipment on board are prepared to help you give your best effort for your patient.

Ambulance Inspection

You check the equipment and supplies for the patient; you inspect the ambulance for yourself and your partner. An unchecked vehicle may cause more problems than it can solve. The vehicle check includes the following:

- All vehicle fluids (oil, transmission, brake, radiator, windshield washer) need to be checked and filled if needed. Most EMS operations have fluid for use by the staff for the vehicles.
- Parking brakes should be checked on an incline, with the vehicle placed in neutral. If they hold the vehicle, they are fine; if they do not, they must be fixed.
- All glass (mirrors, windshields and windows) should be clean, inside and out.
- All lights—headlights, parking lights, hazards, and emergency lights—need to be tested to ensure that they are working properly, including high beams on the headlights, spot lights, grill lights, intersection lights, side warning lights, and any rotating lights. Some of these lights use bulbs that are easy to change; other lights, such as strobe lights, may require service by a mechanic.
- Tire pressure and tread depth need to be assessed. If you operate in a part of the country where snow is common, will you need chains and do you have them?

Dispatch

Emergency medical dispatch (EMD) has come into its own over the course of the past 25 years.[4] Prior to the birth of EMD, dispatchers for EMS were assigned based on a variety of different local factors. Sometimes a dispatcher might have been an EMT or paramedic who wanted a break from being in the field or someone who was on light duty because of an injury. Sometimes it was anyone who answered the job announcement.

Since then, the EMD has become a valuable member of the EMS team. Through pre-arrival instructions and telephone interrogation, they provide first aid to the patient by instructing the caller on appropriate steps to take and how to assess for any potential hazards, update dispatched units with additional information, and request additional resources or assistance when needed.

There are different programs for training and certifying EMDs, but most programs consist of 40 hours of training in the basics of emergency services telecommunication and interrogation. In addition, EMDs will receive another 40 hours of instruction relevant to telephone triage and pre-arrival instructions. This will usually be in addition to any other training that is required by their jurisdiction.

The EMD is unique. While physicians and paramedics are trained to evaluate patients using all of their senses, the EMD is at a disadvantage. They cannot use their sense of sight, smell, and touch, but instead they use their hearing and interrogation to gather the information required to dispatch the appropriate units and provide the appropriate pre-arrival instructions. The most important information the EMD can ascertain includes the following: DOT 3-5.1

- The location of the incident
- Name of the caller and a call-back number
- The location of the patient(s) (what floor the patient is on)
- Age, sex, and chief complaint of the patient
- Hazards in the roadway or at the scene

All of this occurs in the first 30 seconds to one minute of a 9-1-1 phone call. In some cases, if the local community is equipped with an enhanced 9-1-1 system, some of the information, such as the call-back number as well as the address associated with that call-back number, will be automatically displayed on the dispatcher's computer terminal (Box 49-5).

The EMD then needs to prioritize the assignment of EMS units, based on the information that they have determined from further interrogation of the caller. Then, the EMD communicates this information in a concise, efficient manner to the EMS unit that will respond. The job of the EMD is not over at this point. Depending on the chief complaint, the EMD now will give pre-arrival instructions. What the EMD is actually doing is turning the caller into a first-responder.

The EMD's job is crucial. Without pre-arrival instructions, it could mean the difference between a patient who has a chance at survival and one who will not survive at all, regardless of scene and transport times. DOT 3-5.28

BOX 49-5   Public Safety Answering Point and Public Safety Dispatch Point

The public safety answering point (PSAP) is where the initial call for 9-1-1 is answered. The call taker frequently performs the initial interrogation to determine the person's location and problem. They may then forward the call to a public safety dispatch point (PSDP) for further interrogation and dispatch of appropriate resources.

Sometimes the PSAP is a particular public safety agency. In New York City, the PSAP is the City of New York Police Department. They will determine the initial location of the emergency and the chief complaint of the person who is calling. If they require police assistance, they will keep the caller on the line and ascertain additional information. If the call requires the assistance of fire or EMS, the PSAP operator will instruct the caller to stay on the line and transfer the caller to the PSDP for fire or EMS. They will remain on the line until they ascertain that the PSDP operator has the caller.

Not all locations use the police department. Summit, New Jersey, about 20 miles east of New York City, uses the Summit Fire Department as their PSAP.[5] St. Charles, Missouri, uses their Division of Emergency Management.[6] In San Francisco, California, an Emergency Communications Department handles all the work of the PSAP and functions as the PSDP for police, fire, and EMS.[7]

The PSDP is where additional interrogation occurs and, in the case of EMS, where the caller will receive prearrival instructions from the EMD.

Deployment

Ambulances, like EMS systems, are stationed using a variety of different methods. Essentially, there are two types of ambulance deployments: static and dynamic. DOT 8-1.3

Static.   In a statically deployed system, ambulances are based at fixed locations such as hospitals, fire stations, or other types of quarters. They are then dispatched to assignments closest to them. Ambulances may be moved around in a system like this, but generally, when the unit is done with its call, it goes back to its station. Where the ambulances are stationed never changes, so the drawback to this system is that some units are busier than others.

Dynamic.   Dynamic deployment is used in a variety of ways.

- In the private sector, some systems use **system status management (SSM)**. In SSM, historical data drives unit deployment. Data over the prior 20 weeks is analyzed, and ambulances are deployed based on the anticipated need. The ambulances are staffed for shifts and deployed based on this historical analysis. They may be dynamically deployed to other areas based on increases in demand or because of analysis of patterns of request for service. Many systems use SSM successfully. When a system is new to SSM, it usually requires fine-tuning as they work out the bugs and decide on the best numbers for staffing and deployment.

- Another method for determining where to station ambulances uses a *demand profile* of the EMS system. A demand profile is a breakdown of the number of requests for EMS, by day of the week, hour of the day, and priority. This gives an EMS manager an idea of how many ambulances will be needed at different times of the day to manage workload. Then, using computer programming, it can be determined where to station those ambulances so as to ensure rapid emergency response.

- Other systems use a **global positioning system (GPS)** and **automatic vehicle locators (AVL)** instead of or to supplement their SSM. GPS uses satellites to give an exact position of a GPS unit within about 100 feet anywhere on earth. It finds its position based on information from three satellites continuously orbiting the earth, which then triangulates the unit's location. GPS hardware works with AVL software to show the EMD the location of all of the ambulances on a map. The AVL software will work with dispatch software to send the closest available EMS unit to the next emergency assignment.

Communication

Emergency medical services, like many other areas of medicine, rely on communication and, specifically, telecommunication. Equipment such as the radio and telephone is essential. Communication between the caller and the PSAP (Public Safety Answering Point), the PSAP/PSDP (Public Safety Dispatch Point) and the ambulance, the ambulance and another ambulance, the ambulance and the base station, the ambulance and the hospital, or a handheld radio and the dispatch center are just some examples of essential telecommunication.

Interagency communication is also important, not only for mass-casualty incidents, but also for everyday radio communications where police, fire, and EMS may all be responding to the same incident. In those instances, you want to make sure that if you are going to transmit on another agency's frequency, you abide by that agency's policy and radio procedure.

There are many types of communication systems. Some EMS systems employ a single system, but frequently a combination of communication systems is used.

If using a common frequency, refrain from using numeric codes unless you share the same codes with the other agency. If you do not share the same numeric codes, stick to common radio procedure words, and use plain language to describe anything else. In fact, the National Incident Management System strongly encourages the use of plain language instead of radio codes to avoid any confusion or miscommunication.

CONNECTIONS For more complete information about the National Incident Management System, look at Chapter 50: Medical Incident Command.

Radio Equipment. There are essentially three types of two-way radio equipment (Figure 49-2).

- **Base station.** Generally in a fixed location, some base stations are small enough to fit on a desktop, or some are so large that they require banks of consoles to contain them. They have larger antennas and more power than portable or mobile radios. This enables them to transmit over greater distances.

- **Mobile.** Mobile radios are radios mounted in a vehicle. They have more power and a larger antenna than a portable radio.

- **Portable.** Portable radios are lightweight, handheld communication devices. What you gain from a lighter weight, smaller device, you sacrifice in range and power. Portable radios have shorter transmission ranges than mobiles and base stations because they have less power and shorter antennas.

All radios have a push-to-talk (PTT) button on the microphone. It is necessary to press in the PTT button when you want to transmit a message and remember to release the button when you are through.

Street Secrets

As long as the button is depressed, it will transmit *everything* that is within your earshot. *Do not forget to release the button.* Failure to release the button may tie up radio transmissions for other EMS units in the field and may transmit information that you do not want transmitted. DOT 3-5.29

Communication Systems. Some examples of different types of communication systems include the following:

- **Simplex.** A simplex system is a single channel, one-way communication mechanism. This system utilizes one frequency to both transmit and receive radio traffic. A simplex radio system allows only one person to speak at a time. In this type of communication, it is

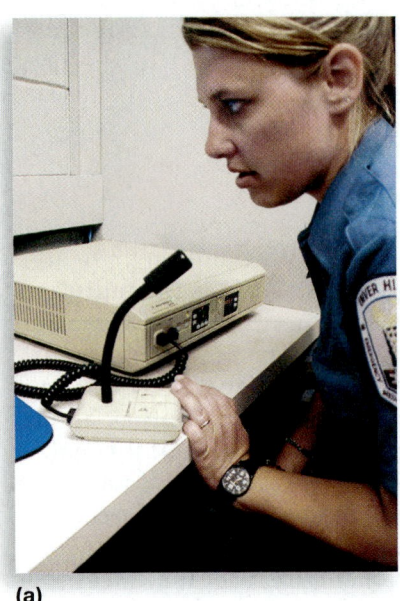

(a)

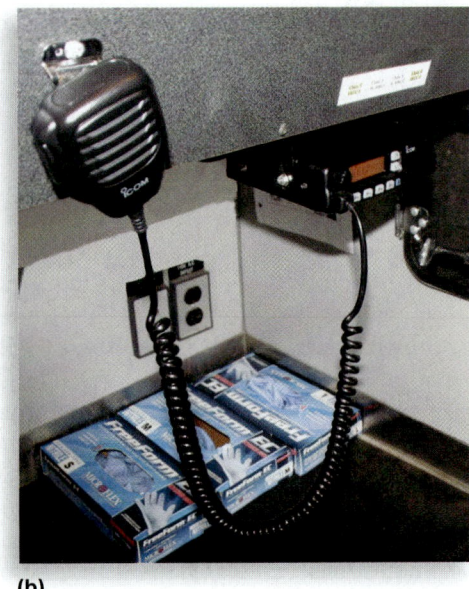

(b)

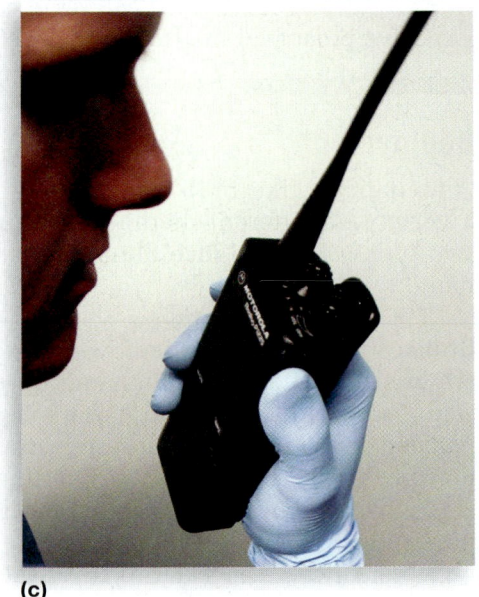

(c)

Figure 49-2 Two-way radio equipment. (a) Base station. (b) Mobile. (c) Portable.

necessary to end your transmission or statement with a common radio procedure word such as "over" to indicate to the other user that you have finished speaking. For example, EMS unit College 102 wants to contact its base station for some information:

"Base Station from College 102, OVER"

"College 102, this is Base Station OVER"

"Base Station from College 102, is Route 80 open to traffic? OVER"

"College 102 from Base Station, NEGATIVE, Route 80 is still closed to traffic, OVER"

"Base Station from College 102, ROGER, College 102 OUT"

In the previous transmission, placing "Base Station" first in the transmission alerts the radio operator that someone is attempting to contact them. The radio procedure word "OVER" lets the operator who is receiving the message know that College 102 has completed transmitting. "ROGER" is another procedure word that means affirmative and "OUT" means that College 102 is done transmitting.

- **Duplex.** A duplex system like a telephone allows simultaneous radio transmission between two people. Instead of making you wait for a break in the conversation, a duplex radio system lets you just interrupt the person making the transmission. This type of transmission requires two frequencies, one to receive and one to transmit.

- **Multiplex.** A multiplex system allows simultaneous transmission of multiple, different radio transmissions over one radio frequency. Think of the FM radio in your car. The right channel is actually on one frequency, and the left channel is on another. These two channels are then combined and transmitted to you in your car. You don't have to tune into separate frequencies to get the right and left channels; you just set your radio to one frequency, and the right and left channel are separated in your car radio and play over your stereo. Data terminals allow the entry of text messages or queries of databases. Using a multiplex radio system, simultaneous transmission of voice and data can occur at one time.

- **Trunked.** Larger organizations, which may have many users at one time, frequently use trunked radios. Trunked radios use a computer to switch users from one frequency to another automatically. Since there is a limited number of frequencies, trunks allow for more efficient use of the radio. The switching of frequencies is automatic and transparent to the individual radio operators. Trunked radio systems utilize one or more "control" channels. The control channel instructs each radio in the system which frequency to switch to in order to remain on the selected channel.

- **Digital.** Digital communications may be accomplished over radios, phone lines, and the internet. Digital communications take voice, data, and biomedical telemetry and convert them into binary code. They are then broken down into smaller packets for transmission. Digital communications can then be transmitted at very fast rates over radio frequencies as individual packets. Data and voice transmission packets can be mixed together and then reassembled on the receiving end, resulting in clear decipherable communication. By its nature, digital communications are encrypted, so eavesdropping by people outside your organization is impossible.

- **Cellular telephones.** The cell phone is considered an essential part of the communication system for many different types of agencies. Cellular phone technology works on a system of geographically separated zones called cells. Each cell site has its own "base station" that both receives and transmits radio signals. When a call is placed from a cell phone, a signal is sent from the cell phone antenna to the closest, available cell base station antenna. The base station responds to the cellular phone signal by assigning the phone an available radio frequency (RF) channel. When the RF channel is assigned, radio signals are simultaneously received and transmitted, allowing voice signals to be carried between the cell phone and the base. The base station then transfers the call to a switching center, where the call can be transferred to a local telephone carrier or another cell phone. There are limitations to cell phones. In urban areas, there are usually more cell sites. When you have more cell sites, you have better coverage and better cell phone service. Where there are fewer cell phone sites, such as in suburban and rural areas, coverage can get spotty and may not be as reliable. Since the mid-1990s all cellular service providers have gone to digital networks, so most cell phone coverage is secure. The only exception is that if you are using an older analog cell phone, it may be possible for people to electronically eavesdrop on your conversation.

Street Secrets

During disasters, people will frequently tie up cell sites with calls to family, friends, and 9-1-1. Since cell phones are so numerous, this creates competition for available cell sites between the general population and emergency services workers, making communication over these devices difficult at best. Public safety agencies, including EMS, can apply to the FCC to obtain priority access to cell sites in the event of an emergency.

- *Fax machines.* Fax machines are used extensively in emergency service communications centers and hospitals. Many of the newer, portable 12-lead ECG machines have built-in fax machines that allow for ECGs to be sent over cellular or standard phone lines to hospital emergency departments. Stand-alone fax machines are not common in ambulances.
- *Computers.* From the dispatch center, to data logs, to patient care, the computer has revolutionized EMS. Computers allow the EMD to collect information and track dispatch times. They can also send text messages to units in the field. Computers are also used to document patient information and look up medications and other information in databases. DOT 3-5.3

Federal Communications Commission

The Federal Communications Commission (FCC) is an independent United States government agency charged with oversight of interstate and international communications by radio, television, wire, satellite, and cable. The FCC has jurisdiction over the 50 states, the District of Columbia, and all U.S. possessions. They assign radio frequencies for use by emergency service organizations, as well as designate the rules and regulations for speaking on the radio.

Street Secrets

One FCC regulation makes it a crime to knowingly transmit a false radio report. Another regulation states that you may not use foul or inappropriate language on the radio.

Another responsibility of the FCC is to deal with issues arising from interference when one radio frequency or station interferes with the transmissions of another. This has come into the forefront with cellular phones and 900 mHz public safety radio frequencies. The FCC is attempting to work with both groups to ensure public safety while maintaining the needs of private industry.

The FCC also works with other federal departments and organizations such as the Commerce Department, Association of Public-Safety Communications Officials International (APCOI), National Association of State 9-1-1 Administrators, National Emergency Numbers Association, and the National Academy of Emergency Dispatchers, to ensure that issues relevant to public safety are addressed.

One issue arises when the FCC releases new radio frequencies. The release of new frequencies causes competition between private industry and the public sector. The FCC ensures that an adequate number of frequencies are reserved for public safety communication. DOT 3-5.25

En Route

In the early times of EMS, the driver of the ambulance usually was the person who had the most experience, and driving an emergency vehicle was not taken lightly. Later, after the initiation of emergency care training programs, the most experienced person was typically found in the back of the ambulance caring for the patient. Now we place equal emphasis on caring for the patient as well as operating the ambulance.

In many EMS organizations, local jurisdictions require completion of an emergency vehicle operators course (EVOC) prior to employment. Other organizations provide driver training during the training or orientation phase of employment.

Always review state and local laws, regulations, or ordinances in the area where you will be working, including, but not limited to the following:

- Vehicle parking or standing
- Procedures at red lights, stop signs, and intersections
- Regulations regarding speed limits
- Direction of flow or specified turns
- Emergency or disaster routes
- Use of audible warning devices
- Use of visual warning devices
- School buses

Some locales will give carte blanche to the operation of an emergency vehicle, and others will treat emergency vehicles just like any other vehicle under the law.

There are some things to keep in mind before getting behind the wheel. First, never drive an emergency vehicle or provide emergency care if you are taking medications that will slow your reaction time. These include prescription narcotics, cold remedies, and tranquilizers. If there is a concern about a medication, ask your medical director, pharmacist, or personal physician. Never get behind the wheel or provide patient care if you have consumed alcohol.

Emotions play a key role in operating an emergency vehicle. If you are upset, just got into an argument, or have just received bad news, for example, refrain from driving.

Emotions run high during an emergency response, and people will state that they or their partners become "different people" behind the wheel while on an emergency response. If this is true for you, then you should not be the individual driving.

CONNECTIONS Chapter 9: Safety Scene Size-Up provides additional statistics on ambulance crashes.

Basic Principles of EMS Vehicle Operations

EMS vehicles are usually much larger and heavier than your own private vehicle. They take a longer distance to stop after they get up to speed, and they are more prone to skidding during turns. Even among the various types of ambulances, there are differences (see Figure 49-1 on page 1199). Type II or high-top van ambulances have a higher center of gravity and are more prone to swaying and tipping. Type I and III ambulances, while having a lower center of gravity, are much heavier than Type II and require increased braking distances.

Become familiar with the different characteristics of the vehicles in your service before going on an emergency response. This should be part of your initial training and orientation.

Anyone operating an EMS vehicle is subject to the law of due regard. Regardless of the emergency nature of the medical crisis, the driver must perform driving tasks safely and with consideration (due regard) for the people both in the emergency vehicle and in surrounding traffic. Driving blindly through intersections, lights flashing and sirens wailing, failing to yield the right of way, speeding, and following too closely are all examples of failure to follow the law of due regard. The operator of an emergency vehicle is not exempt from traffic laws and may be criminally or civilly liable if death, injury, or property damage result from a crash.

Know the appropriateness of using lights and sirens. Never self-dispatch or self-upgrade your response to an emergency assignment. If you are closer to an assignment than the ambulance assigned, advise the communications center, and have them assign the call to you. Remember, the communications center will know who is responding to the location and can alert you to the response of other emergency units. An ambulance response with lights and siren is like a loaded gun. It should never be taken lightly.

If, after you arrive on the scene, you feel that the patient needs an upgraded or downgraded transport to the hospital, it is within your responsibility to make that decision. If you transport someone with a minor complaint with lights and siren and then are involved in an accident, the law will not look favorably on you.

Every time you activate the lights and siren, the reaction of the general driving public is unpredictable. In America, the law requires drivers to pull to the right and stop. Some drivers will stop regardless of where they are in traffic, some drivers will pull over to the left, and others will try to race ahead of the emergency vehicle. Some do as the law requires and will pull over to the side of the road and stop.

A crash may occur at any time; that is why it is critically important for the operator of the emergency vehicle to drive defensively. Emergency vehicle crashes cause loss of life and health, destruction of expensive equipment, and erosion of the public's trust in EMS providers' mission to "do no harm."[8] If a pedestrian is hit and killed by an EMS unit responding to a call that is minor in nature, the repercussions are widespread. When an EMS unit uses emergency mode to transport a patient from the scene to the hospital for a minor emergency, and there is a collision, public confidence is eroded.

Street Secrets

The EMD will prioritize the emergency assignment based on the information collected. This reduces the number of times ambulances are dispatched with lights and siren, and creates a safer environment for all.

Emergency vehicles are bigger and heavier than your standard car or sport utility vehicle (SUV). With this in mind, remember it takes longer to bring them to a complete stop. You will have to apply your brakes earlier to stop sooner.

While negotiating curves and turns, you will have to slow down going into those turns. Centrifugal force makes heavier objects track to the outside edge of a curve, making emergency vehicles prone to skidding. Avoid braking when going into a turn. Brake prior to heading into the turn and ease off the gas while making a turn.

Controlled braking can only occur on a straightaway or while traveling in a straight line. The same is true for acceleration. Accelerating or braking while making a turn or a curve may result in a loss of control and a collision.

Intersections pose another hazard for emergency response. Motorists arriving at an intersection as the light changes may not stop. Multiple emergency vehicles may be following each other closely and the waiting motorist, not expecting more than one emergency vehicle, might proceed after the first one goes by. A driver of a vehicle in the right lane whose vision is obstructed by vehicles in the left lane may not see the oncoming emergency vehicle. All of these are prescriptions for disaster.

As you approach intersections, if you have your partner in the front seat, use your partner as a spotter. Two pairs of eyes visually clearing the intersection, the driver checking the left and the partner checking the right, and attempting to make eye contact with drivers in the other vehicles, will help reduce intersection collisions.

Maintain a safe following distance, whether you are following another emergency vehicle or not. Never tailgate in an effort to pull someone over. With the advent of new and improved soundproofing in

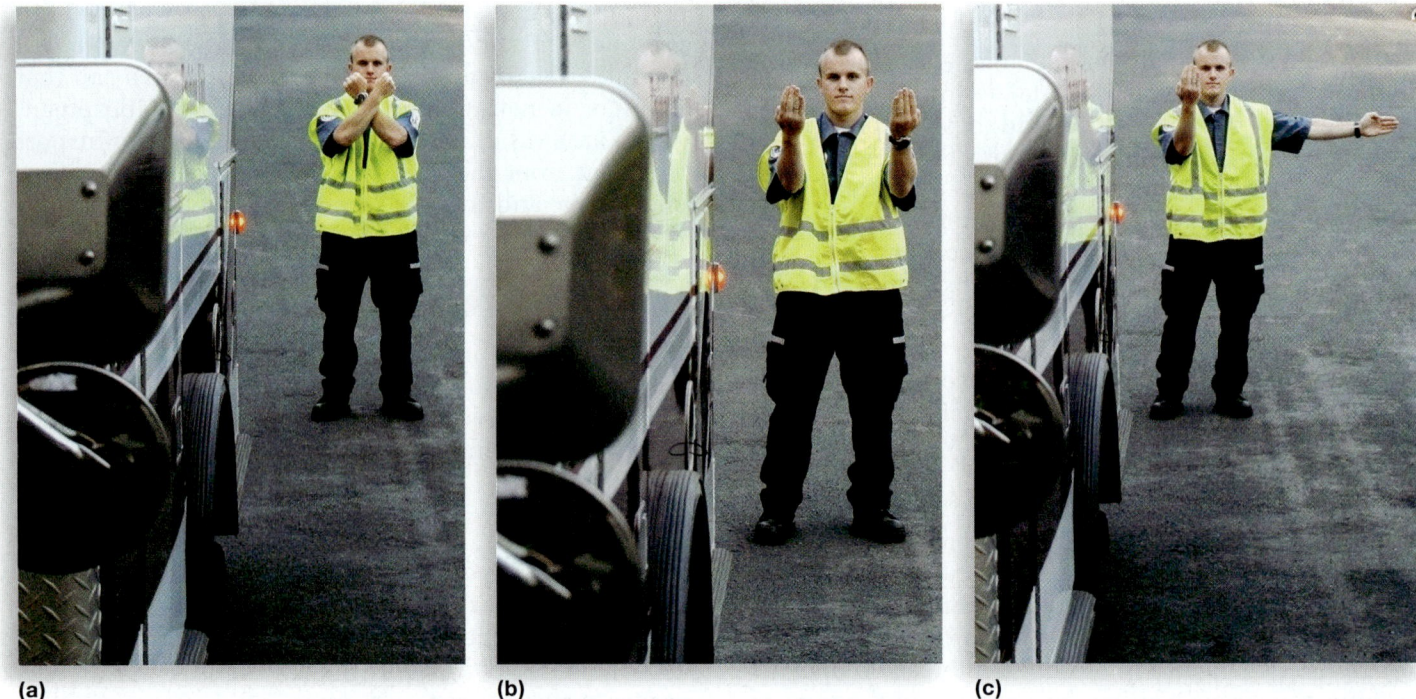

(a)   (b)   (c)

Figure 49-3   Spotter should stand 8–10 feet behind the ambulance. (a) Stop. (b) Move straight back. (c) Move toward the left.

today's automobiles, combined with the latest in digital audio equipment, it is quite easy to sneak up on and scare a driver into an erratic reaction that could prove fatal.

Any time you need to back up your vehicle, it is good to use a spotter. Generally, the spotter should stand 8 to 10 feet behind the vehicle on the driver's side, visible in the driver's side mirror, and watch for any hazards. The spotter should use hand signals to tell you to turn, stop, and back up (Figure 49-3).

If you have a patient on board, you are arriving at a hospital, and you cannot have a spotter exit the vehicle to back you up, have someone look out the back window or door. There will be hazards that you cannot see that a spotter will note looking out from a rear window or door.

Always select the appropriate route, the one that will bring you to the patient's side safely and quickly. Keep this in mind when transporting the patient to the hospital as well.

Other Issues

Prior to arrival on-scene, discuss with your partner what equipment each of you will get. This will minimize the chance that you will forget something. Discuss who will contact, question, and examine the patient, who will talk with family, bystanders, and other public safety responses, and who will maintain vigilance for scene safety issues. One of the most disconcerting things for patients is to have two people attempting to question them at the same time. You may need to change roles once on-scene; some patients may relate better to your partner, and vice versa. Being flexible is important.

CONNECTIONS   Chapter 9: Safety and Scene Size-Up describes contact and cover when interacting on a scene.

Have whoever is not driving monitor the radio for updates. The patient location may have changed from the time of initial dispatch, there may be hazards in the roadway, or the approach to the scene could be difficult. DOT 3-5.1

Arrival On-Scene

Notify dispatch when you arrive at the scene. If you are directed somewhere other than where you were initially dispatched, update the communications center as soon as possible and be specific. If the situation deteriorates and you need help with the patient or your life is in danger, the dispatcher will send help to your last reported location. DOT 8-1.6

As you are pulling up, determine if the scene is safe. If you were dispatched to a man with shortness of breath and there is a man standing out front with a handgun and another man lying in a pool of blood, unless the armed person is the police, the scene is not safe.

If you are dispatched to a motor vehicle crash where there is a cloud of purple-colored smoke leaking from a van involved in the collision, and people are lying on the ground not moving, the scene isn't safe.

Do you see a downed power line? Any other hazard present on the scene that may pose grievous harm to you, your partner, any other emergency responders, the public, and the patient must be noted and appropriate precautions must be taken.

For safety at the scene of suspected hazardous materials, park uphill and upwind from leaking hazards and at least 100 feet from wreckage.

Once you arrive on-scene, set the parking brake. Avoid parking in a location that will hamper your exit from the scene or impede the arrival of other emergency units. Shut off headlights unless there is a need to illuminate the scene. Leave the appropriate visual warning devices on unless you are at a scene that the police need to keep low-key. Park the vehicle in such a manner that you may exit without being in jeopardy from other traffic.

CONNECTIONS Review Chapter 9: Safety and Scene Size-Up for more information on safe parking.

Additional traffic safety devices may need to be placed out on the roadway to provide safety once on-scene. Avoid using road flares when there are flammable substances on the road; instead, use reflective triangles or other nonflammable warning devices.

If you are responding to a motor vehicle crash, park either well before or beyond the wreckage.

Never leave a running emergency vehicle unattended. They have been stolen, even from in front of a patient's address. Even at the emergency department, ambulances have been stolen. If your vehicle has an antitheft device that allows you to keep the vehicle running but prevents someone from driving away with the vehicle, use it. Otherwise shut down your vehicle or, if you cannot turn it off, leave someone in attendance (police, fire, EMS, or other public employee).

Update dispatch as soon as possible as to the number of patients, whether you will require additional resources, or other hazards that you have encountered.

When you arrive on-scene, always exit the vehicle with a patient carrying device and patient care equipment. For some patients, the minute you take to go back to the vehicle for something may be the last minute that they have. If you need additional equipment, or perhaps the situation dictates the use of a different carrying device, it is acceptable to go back and get the requisite carrying device or patient care equipment. The appropriate carrying devices can be anticipated based on the initial dispatch information.

Street Secrets

It is paramount to your credibility that when you exit the vehicle, you exit ready to go to work. Nothing says this better than walking up to the patient or the scene with all of your gear in hand.

Carrying Devices

Carrying devices should be selected and initially brought to the patient depending on the situation: DOT 8-1.9

- ***Reeves stretcher.*** Use this for an unconscious, unresponsive patient; an overdose; a stroke; bed-bound elderly patients; patients with a decreased level of consciousness such as those suffering from diabetes, seizure disorders, choking, unknown, respiratory or cardiac arrest, shooting, stabbing, and *trauma not involving the head, neck, or spine.*

- ***Stair chair.*** Use for stable patients with chest pain, respiratory distress, medical emergencies, or anaphylaxis, as well as wheelchair-bound patients (Figure 49-4).

- ***Long backboard.*** Use for a trauma patient who has sustained a fall; was struck by a motor vehicle; or who is suffering from an assault to the head,

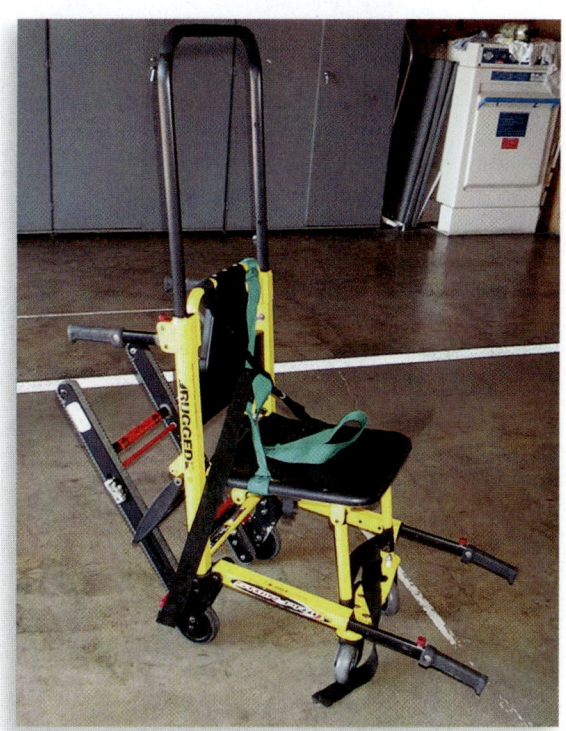

Figure 49-4 Stair chair.

neck, or spine by either blunt force trauma or penetrating trauma from a knife, gun, or any other object or any injury to the head, neck, or spine. The long backboard should also be used anytime you need to move a patient in a basket stretcher, using ropes to raise or lower a patient, or if necessary to "stand the patient up" while moving through narrow areas that would otherwise make it impossible to lay the patient flat while being carried. Any patient with a traction splint device must be transported or moved on a long backboard (Figure 49-5).

■ ***Orthopedic stretcher (Robinson stretcher).*** The orthopedic stretcher is an excellent carrying device and can be used as a backup to the Reeves stretcher if there are multiple patients who need to be carried lying flat. *It must never be used* for patients with head, neck, or spine injuries or injuries of the arms and legs that require a splint because the orthopedic stretcher does not protect or support the spinal column.

Again, if the device brought to the patient's bedside is not appropriate, you can always return it to the ambulance and retrieve the correct device.

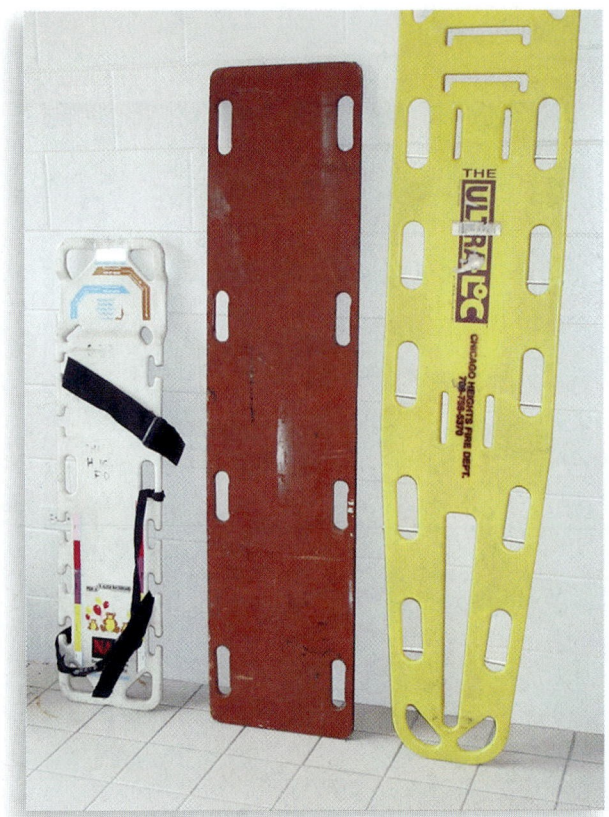

Figure 49-5 Examples of long backboards.

Patient Care Equipment

The following pieces of patient care equipment should be brought to the patient's side when exiting the ambulance:

■ ***Oxygen/medical/trauma bag.*** The oxygen/medical/trauma bag containing the necessary patient care equipment will always be removed from the ambulance when exiting to provide patient care. The oxygen/airway unit always leaves the ambulance with the team. Either the trauma or medical bag is selected based on the initial dispatch complaint.

Never leave the vehicle without patient care equipment.

■ ***Cardiac monitor/defibrillator/pacer.*** Delay in application and use of the monitor/defibrillator/pacer dramatically affects patient outcome. To increase the likelihood of successful defibrillation, based on the initial dispatch information, the monitor/defibrillator/pacer must be brought to the bedside of all patients, including, but not limited to the following:
  • Unconscious patients
  • Patients in cardiac arrest
  • Patients in respiratory arrest
  • Patient complaining of chest pain
  • Patient complaining of shortness of breath
  • Overdose patients
  • Seizure patients
  • Patients in anaphylactic shock
  • Drowning patients
  • Patient with AMS (altered mental status)
  • Diabetic patients
  • Chronic renal failure patients

- *Splints.*   Initially, splints should be removed from the ambulance in a variety of sizes to accommodate the patient's injuries. The exception to this rule would be if you were treating and assessing the patient in close proximity to the ambulance.
- *Suction.*   Protection of the airway is of key importance. Suction must be brought in the following situations:
  - Unconscious patients
  - Patients in cardiac arrest
  - Patients in respiratory arrest
  - Overdose patients
  - Seizure patients
  - Patients in anaphylactic shock
  - Drowning patients
  - Patients with altered mental status

Transfer of Patient to the Ambulance

Prior to lifting and moving the patient, make sure that the path to the ambulance is clear of obstacles. Has the cot been pulled out of the ambulance and is it waiting for you at the bottom of the stairs?

When you exited the ambulance with your carrying device, did you bring a sheet or blanket? You need something to cover the patient, regardless of temperature. A light sheet is acceptable in summer; use a sheet and a blanket in winter. You need to concern yourself with maintaining patient modesty as well as keeping the patient warm.

Lifting Patients into Ambulances

Safely lifting patients into ambulances requires an understanding of the cot or stretcher you are using and good body mechanics. Older style stretchers require medics to lift the stretcher from each side and pass the stretcher into the ambulance. Proper positioning is important so that there is no twisting of your back as the stretcher is slid into the ambulance. Newer varieties of so-called "one man" stretchers can be pushed into the ambulance with the stretcher and floor of the ambulance carrying the load. Still others have motors and hydraulics that assist in carrying the weight. Whatever stretcher you use, it is important to use it as it is intended to ensure the safety of the patient and the rescuers. Specific techniques are covered in the workbook that accompanies this text.

Take one last look around. Ensure that all the equipment brought into the scene is retrieved and accounted for. Check to see if there is anything else you need to get prior to leaving, such as prescriptions, medications, clothes, assistive devices such as eyeglasses, house keys for the patient, or any other important papers. Remove all of your used biohazard materials and sharps and dispose of them properly.

Once the patient is in the ambulance, are there any critical interventions that require completion, such as chest decompression, needle cricothyrotomy, or some other procedure? Are your IVs still in place? If the patient is intubated, check tube placement as moving and lifting patients is a high-risk time when potentially life-saving, endotracheal tubes often become dislodged. Remember to document this on your run sheet.

Transport

After getting the patient secured in the vehicle and checking that all devices are secure, prepare to notify the hospital. The driver of the vehicle needs to drive the shortest, most direct route to the hospital. Notify dispatch of the destination hospital, the number of patients you are transporting, and the priority (whether you require lights and siren). Regulate the temperature in the back of the ambulance to ensure the comfort of the patient.

Reevaluate your patient and obtain an updated set of vital signs. Determine if you need to provide additional treatment. Medical patients may receive the bulk of their care on-scene while trauma patients will receive minimal care on-scene and essentially all advanced life support measures in the back of the ambulance en route to the hospital. Determine the following:

- Does the patient have an increase or decrease in pain?
- Are symptoms relieved or are they getting worse?
- How does the patient look? Is the skin still pale or has the color improved? Does the patient look anxious or comfortable?

If you are transporting the patient to the hospital using lights and siren, tell the patient this so that it will not be a surprise and increase the patient's anxiety. Also, let the patient know that you will be calling the hospital to let them know that you are coming and that you will tell the hospital what the patient complained of, what you found, what treatment you provided, and how the patient responded. You do not want to surprise the patient, and the information you provide the hospital should not be the first time the patient hears it.

Street Secrets

Remember to talk to the patient during the ride to the hospital. It is acceptable to write your report while you are en route to the hospital; just don't forget about the person sitting or lying less than 2 feet away from you. The patient will probably be worried, and may have concerns or questions that you can address while you are going to the hospital.

CONNECTIONS More information about communicating with the patient can be found in Chapter 10: Therapeutic Communications and History Taking.

Aeromedical Transport

There are several advantages to air medical evacuation, the first of which is speed. When time is something the patient has very little of and the patient's condition is critical, the speed of the helicopter cannot be underestimated. There are disadvantages, however. It takes time for the helicopter to respond to your location and to perform the patient hand-off. If you can transport the patient to a hospital before the helicopter can arrive, there is no reason to wait on-scene just to use the helicopter. In many cases, weather will affect the ability of the helicopter to respond as well.

In some areas of the United States, air medical transport is the only way a patient will get to the hospital. In the majority of the United States, though, air medical transport is reserved for the critical medical and trauma patient, the inter-facility transfer of patients who require specialized care, and when time and the patient condition are paramount.

For trauma patients, use this rule of thumb:

If transport time by ground to the trauma center is less than 20 minutes, transport the patient via ambulance.

Setting up a landing zone and dispatching the helicopter take time to accomplish. If the patient is loaded in the ambulance and you are ready, drive to the trauma center.

DOT 8-1.4, 8-1.5

If the transport time is 20 to 30 minutes by ground, consider using air medical transport, especially if there are factors that will affect efficient transport. These factors include weather, road conditions, traffic, and on-scene time (prolonged extrication or other issues delaying access to the patient). If the transport time will exceed 30 minutes, helicopter transport will often be much faster.

Other issues to consider when requesting air medical transport include the following:[9]

- Try to use a predesignated landing zone (LZ). Predesignated landing zones will be well known to the pilot and have been picked because they are generally free of most obstacles that would be dangerous. They will also be easy to find as most flight programs will have the predesignated LZ programmed into flight computers with the appropriate GPS settings.
- If a predesignated LZ cannot be used and it is imperative that an LZ be picked close to or at the scene, keep these key facts in mind (Figure 49-6).
  - The LZ should be a minimum of 100 feet by 100 feet. Some air medical programs use smaller

helicopters and, therefore, may be able to use a smaller LZ. Find out what they require, but as a general rule 100 feet by 100 feet is adequate for most helicopters.
  - A thorough check of the area is required. Walk the landing zone and look for holes, remove all garbage and debris, and look for any overhead hazards (wires, trees, etc.) and anything that can be a danger to the helicopter. Overhead hazards are particularly dangerous, as what is readily seen from the ground is typically invisible from the sky, especially at night.
  - Mark the landing zone with flares, cyalume light sticks, or vehicle headlights at the corners of the landing zone.
  - Secure flares or cyalume light sticks as they will easily blow away with the force of the rotors.
  - Have the fire department (FD) on-scene with a charged line during landing and takeoff. The FD can depart after the helicopter is no longer visible or audible.
  - Have the police department provide perimeter control. Curiosity seekers and small children will flock toward a helicopter.

Street Secrets

Remember the tail rotor is going in excess of 1600 rpm. It is nearly invisible and always fatal if someone walks into it.

- Do not approach the LZ while the helicopter is landing and departing.
- Do not approach the helicopter on your own. Make visual contact with the pilot first and use hand signals to indicate that you want to approach the ship.
- Approach the helicopter from the front or side. If the helicopter must land on a slope, always approach from the down-slope side. Never approach from the uphill side.
- When approaching the helicopter, walk in a crouched position. The blades of the helicopter are extremely flexible and on some models will dip down to about 4 feet as the helicopter turbines slow down.
- Always take sheets off the stretcher before approaching the aircraft. Helicopters can generate hurricane force winds.
- Never leave a stretcher unattended near the landing zone.
- Do not wear hats around a running aircraft. If wearing a rescue helmet, make sure your chinstrap is buckled.

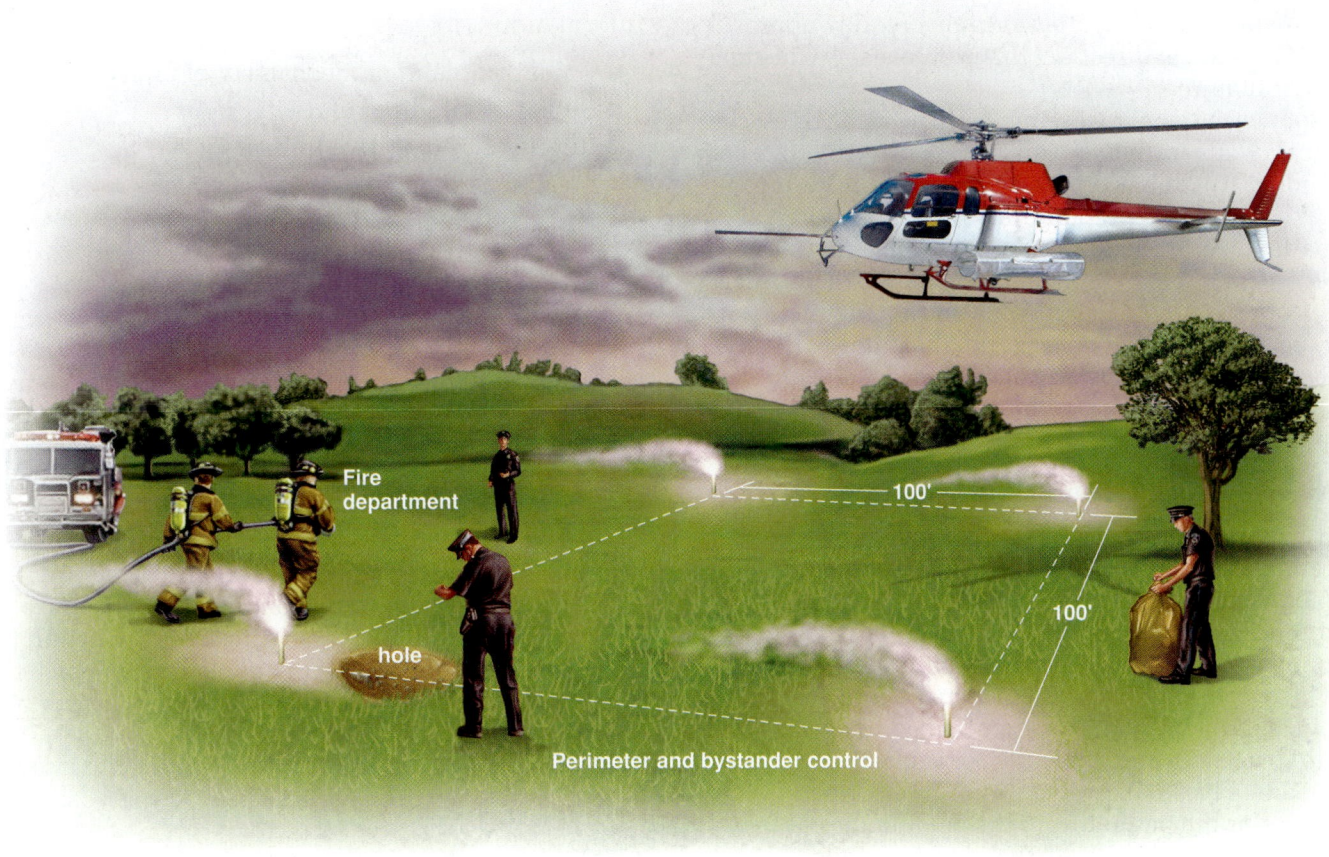

Figure 49-6 A helicopter landing zone requires at least 100 × 100 feet.

- Never walk under the tail of the helicopter.
- Never walk behind the helicopter.
- No smoking within 100 feet of the aircraft.
- Never shine bright lights or headlights at the aircraft during landing or liftoff.
- Do not carry IVs above your head or use an IV pole.
- No ambulances or other vehicles are permitted within 50 feet of the aircraft.
- Keep bystanders back an additional hundred feet from the landing zone. In case of an undesirable event on the field, objects can be hurled from the site and cause serious injury or death.

Whenever possible, helicopters land and takeoff facing into the wind. Some flight programs may ask you to mark the wind direction. Be familiar with the flight programs in your area and what they require.

Hospital Notification

The hospital will need to prepare a room to receive your critical patient. Advise the emergency department of the number of patients that you have and the cause of injury or chief complaint.

Remember that there are other EMS units in the system and they may also be transporting emergency patients to the same hospital, as well as anyone who walks up to the emergency department requesting care. All of these things may play a role in the availability of space at the receiving hospital.

In the case of trauma, the hospital will also need to assemble the trauma team. The sooner you can notify them, the better. Tell the receiving hospital the mechanism of injury, current vital signs, the injuries you have found, and what you have done to treat the patient.

If there are procedures that you perform that require approval of on-line medical direction, this would also be the time to ask or inquire.

For medical notifications, chief complaint or onset, current vital signs, *relevant* past medical history, and treatment should be communicated. It would include any existing medical conditions and medications that the patient is currently taking to treat them for diseases related to the patient's chief complaint.

Advise on-line medical command what treatments you initiated according to your standing order protocol and how the patient responded. Be prepared to begin additional treatment en route to the hospital. Again, if there are procedures you perform that require approval of on-line medical direction, this would also be the time to ask or inquire.

Contacting the receiving facility also gives the medical command physician the opportunity to order additional treatment or ask additional questions and to make additional preparations prior to the arrival of the patient. As an example, some hospitals have established stroke and heart attack centers. In many institutions, after a certain time in the evening, staff may be on call. Contacting the hospital will give them adequate time to call back the needed resources. DOT 3-5.24, 3-5.26

Arrival at Receiving Facility

Notify the communications center that you have arrived. Prepare the patient for leaving the vehicle. This may include moving the patient from on-board oxygen to a portable oxygen unit, moving IVs and cardiac monitoring equipment onto the cot, and checking stretcher belts.

Once you have moved the patient into the emergency department, you may be directed to a triage station to speak with the triage nurse or you may be directed to a bed in a particular room.

Transfer the patient from the ambulance cot to the hospital gurney. Check all IV lines and endotracheal tubes. Assist with placing the patient on cardiac monitors, noninvasive blood pressure monitors, pulse oximetry, and capnography, if time and local protocols permit (Figure 49-7). Provide a complete verbal report to the staff member (MD, nurse, physician's assistant [PA], or nurse practitioner [NP]) who will

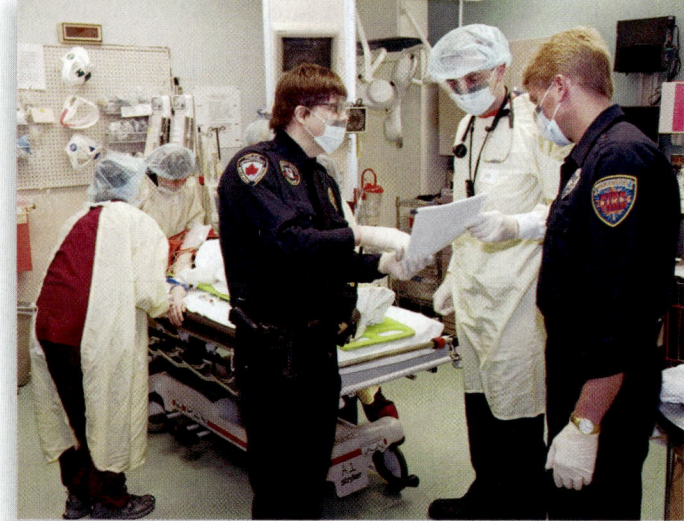

Figure 49-7 Your job is not finished until you have assisted the hospital personnel with transferring your patient and given a complete verbal report.

receive the patient from you, including the following information: DOT 3.5-1

- Chief complaint or mechanism of injury
- Subjective findings and vital signs
- Injuries and objective findings
- Treatment and response to treatment
- Past medical history
- Allergies
- Medications
- Last meal

Prior to leaving the hospital, complete your written patient care report. When you are done, make sure that you provide a copy of your written report to the emergency department staff. This becomes part of the patient's medical record, and is important to the care of the patient. It is important to understand that this report is a legal document, the terminology used should be appropriate, and the content should be complete to reflect the patient's experience under your care. Data collection that is used to determine the future of paramedic practice is also pulled from these reports. DOT 3-5.10, 3-5.11, 3-5.12, 3-5.27

CONNECTIONS Written and verbal reports are discussed in detail in Chapter 17: Documentation and Communication.

If it is permissible, restock your vehicle at the hospital. Also, clean and disinfect any surfaces that require attention. You should have disinfectant and cleaning supplies on your vehicle. You may be dispatched on another assignment, so the inside of your vehicle has to be ready to go.

Return to Station

Contact the communications center, and advise them that you are available to return to service, or that you are not available and need to return to headquarters to get more supplies and replace equipment.

You should have a list of materials that you need to restock the ambulance (if you could not accomplish this at the hospital). You should also replace any equipment that may have been damaged or destroyed on the last assignment.

This is also a good time to talk with your partner about the past assignment, discussing what procedures went well and what could have gone better.

Post-Run

Notify dispatch as soon as you are in your response area or your headquarters. You will want to refuel the ambulance and file any reports. Complete the restocking of your vehicle and finish cleaning and disinfection procedures that you were not able to accomplish at the hospital.

Summary

This chapter has described how EMS is built upon national standards and is further regulated at state and local levels. The phases of an ambulance response, from making sure the individual and the equipment are prepared to respond, to returning to service for the next request, have been described.

While this chapter has described typical ambulance operations, much of what you will learn about ambulance operations is specific to your individual service and the governmental agencies responsible for regulating EMS in your local setting. This chapter has laid a foundation on which the paramedic must build to learn how EMS functions where they are employed.

Notes

1. General Services Administration, "Federal Specification for the Star-of-Life Ambulance: KKK-A-1822E" (June 1, 2002), http://www.gsa.gov/gsa/cm_attachments/GSA_BASIC/ambulanc_R2E-r-eW_0Z5RDZ-i34K-pR.pdf (accessed October 24, 2006).

2. "Equipment for Ambulances: Joint Statement by the American College of Surgeons and the American College of Emergency Physicians" (June 2000), http://www.acep.org/NR/rdonlyres/AE62E47D-4700-4AD8-8A7B-3D168BDFFF29/0/ambulance_equip.pdf (accessed October 24, 2006).

3. FDA And NIOSH, "Public Health Advisory: Explosions and Fires in Aluminum Oxygen Regulators" (February, 1999), http://www.fda.gov/cdrh/oxyreg.html (accessed October 24, 2006).

4. J. J. Clawson and K. Boyd Dernocoeur, *Principles of Emergency Medical Dispatch,* 3rd ed. (Salt Lake City, UT: National Academies of Emergency Dispatch, 2000).

5. J. Houck (Battalion Chief, Summit Fire Department), July 2000.

6. S. Makky (ENP, St. Charles County, Missouri, Division of Emergency Management, Bureau of 911), November 2001.

7. L. M. Gerard (Public Safety Communications Dispatcher, City and County of San Francisco), February, 2005.

8. C. B. Custalow and C. S. Gravitz, "Emergency Medical Vehicle Collisions and Potential for Preventative Intervention," *Prehospital Emergency Care* 8(2) (April/June 2004).

9. "Federal Aviation Administration Advisory Circular 135-14A," http://www.airweb.faa.gov/Regulatory_and_Guidance_Library/rgAdvisoryCircular.nsf/0/152cbeb414a7ae42862569eb006cf424/$FILE/ac135-14a.pdf (accessed October 24, 2006).

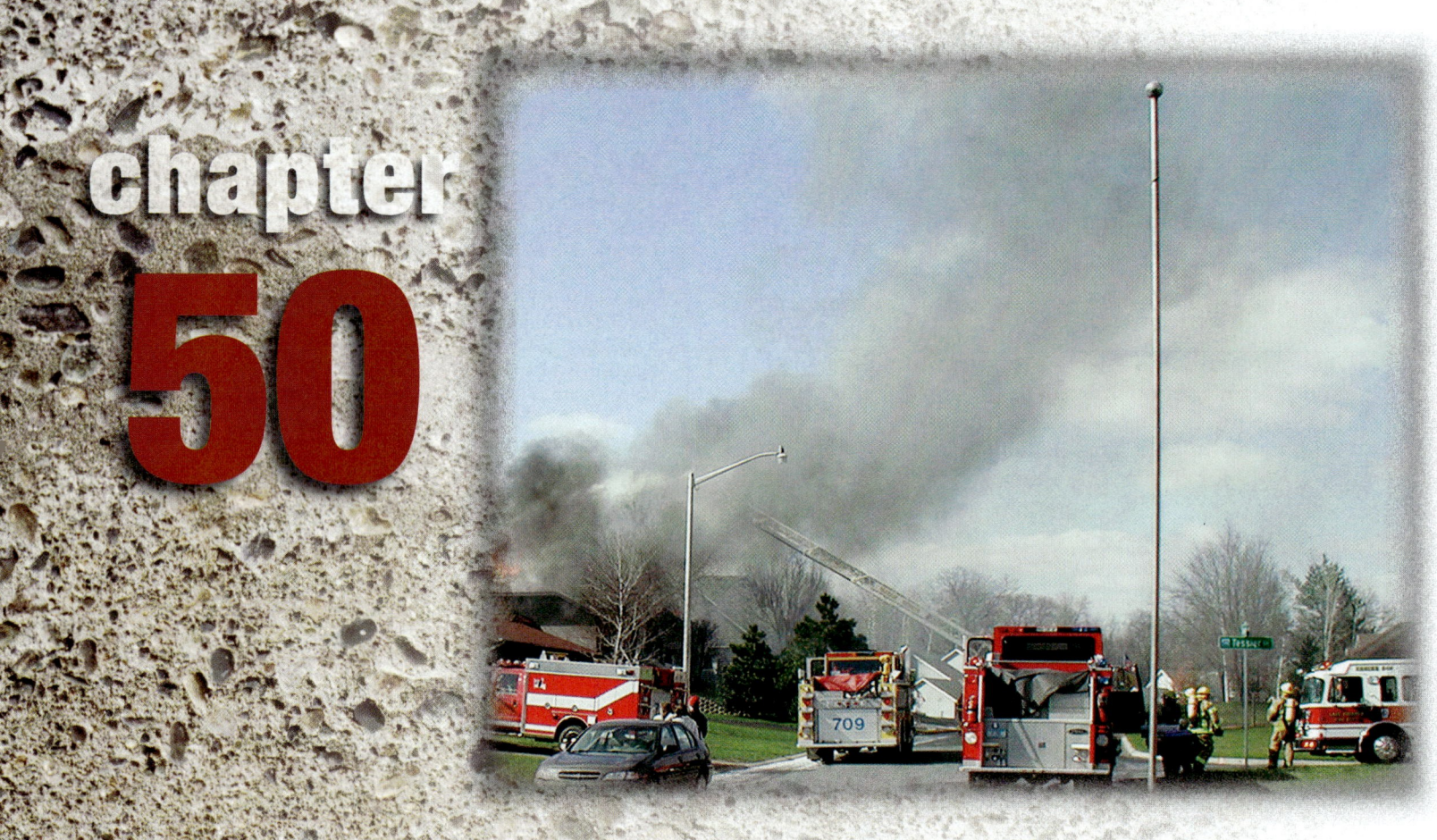

Medical Incident Command

*"**G**ood order is the foundation of all things."*

—Edmund Burke, British statesman, 1729–1797

Need to Know

▶ The National Incident Management System and the Incident Command System and be able to adapt your particular role and expertise to the appropriate organizational element.

▶ The functional components of an incident command system.

▶ The difference between singular and unified incident command.

▶ Unity of command.

▶ Your local Emergency Response Plan and your agency's role when participating.

▶ How to establish initial incident command when first on the scene of an event, and the importance of performing a scene size-up.

▶ The procedure to transfer command.

▶ How to adapt an incident management system to small or large events.

▶ Do	▶ Ask
• Become familiar with local, regional, and agency-specific emergency plans. • Be able to identify your role in the incident command structure. • Participate in disaster, multiple casualty incident, and mass casualty incident planning and drills in order to enhance your ability to respond when called upon. • Practice applying incident command principles to small and large scenarios. • Go to online federal resources from the NIMS and ICS and take the free online courses that are offered there.	• Learn about the EMS system emergency response plan. • Ask your supervisor about your agency's emergency response plan and your operational role.

Introduction

Emergency service providers respond to a wide variety of incidents. Citizen requests for help can vary from a simple investigation by a single unit to an incident that requires the involvement of multiple private and local, state, and federal organizations. Every incident—no matter how large or small—must be managed by implementing an incident command system. The 2005 and 2006 disasters on the Gulf Coast of the United States have underscored the importance and complexity of emergency planning and incident command. EMS systems need to be prepared when usual resources are overwhelmed, used up, or unavailable, and must be able to adapt to a variety of situations (Figure 50-1).

For the last few decades, disaster researchers have echoed the views of on-scene providers that a unified approach to incident management is a critical administrative component that has been lacking. The need for a universally accepted incident management system has been further accentuated by the increasing threat of potential large-scale incidents that could have a devastating and broad impact on the health and safety of the public. Additionally, the ability to coordinate

prevention activities for these incidents requires a degree of interagency cooperation that has not previously been attained.

The History of Incident Management Systems

The development of incident management systems largely began in the early 1970s, emerging from a need for a new approach to the problem of rapidly moving wildfires.[1] Throughout the years, several systems have been developed and implemented. Two widely accepted systems came out of those early efforts:

1. The National Interagency Incident Command System (NIICS), developed by a multiagency taskforce that included the California and U.S. Forest Service and the FIRESCOPE Task Force.

2. The Fire Ground Command (FGC) system developed by the Phoenix, Arizona, Fire Department.

In 1991, the National Fire Service Incident Management System Consortium Model Procedures Committee (NFSIMSCMPC) was formed, and soon after these two systems merged into a set of model procedures for both

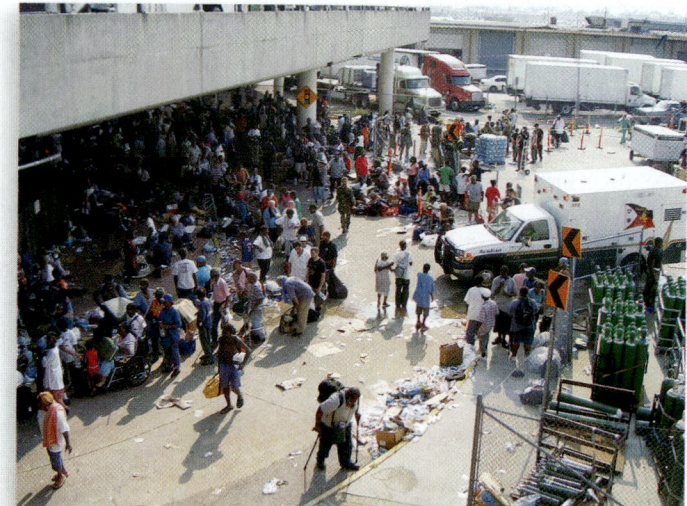

Figure 50-1   By August 30, 2005, it is estimated that over 10,000 refugees from Hurricane Katrina were living in the Superdome in New Orleans.

structural firefighting and EMS.² This system was widely used by fire, EMS, and hazardous materials agencies.

The National Incident Management System

On February 28, 2004, a Presidential Directive to the Department of Homeland Security created the **National Incident Management System, or NIMS.**³ This system is responsible for developing a process that creates a clear chain of command and a consistent approach for federal, state, local, and tribal governments to work together. It provides an orderly and systematic planning process with a common flexible management structure. It also establishes a consistent incident management system called the Incident Command System or ICS that uses common and consistent terminology. Emergency operations centers' (EOCs) structures and functions are outlined within the NIMS as well.

The government mandated that all federal departments adopt the NIMS system and made adoption of the NIMS system by state, local, and tribal agencies a condition for receiving federal preparedness assistance grants and resources.⁴ This meant that incident command systems were now essential for all domestic emergency response agencies. DOT 8-2.1

Overview of Incident Command Systems

An **incident command system (ICS)** starts when the first arriving unit communicates a scene size-up and then establishes command. The **incident commander**

(IC) establishes the ICS structure that best fits the needs of the incident. The IC has overall responsibility for managing an incident. According to the NIMS structure, the incident commander is the only position that is always staffed in every incident. Other positions are implemented as the need arises. In addition to directing operations on a scene, the incident commander is also responsible for planning, including preparing the incident action plan (IAP), logistics, and finance. ICS uses a management-by-objectives approach that has distinct steps that will be discussed later in this chapter. DOT 8-2.12

ICS is designed for use in all types of incidents, including the following:

- Structural fires and wildfires
- Natural disasters
- Human and animal disease outbreaks
- Search and rescue
- Hazardous materials incidents
- Criminal acts and crime scene investigation
- Terrorist incidents, including weapons of mass destruction (WMD)

ICS Key Concepts and Principles

The incident command system relies on several principles to provide structure. The concept of chain of command is in place to provide an orderly line of authority. Although the ICS establishes a single IC for each incident, the IC is allowed to delegate duties and responsibilities as the situation requires. The unity of command principle states that each individual worker on a scene is accountable to only one supervisor. Unity of command is different from unified command. Unified command allows for the sharing of the incident command function by two or more agencies or jurisdictions. DOT 8-2.8

As already mentioned, the ICS uses common terminology in organizational function, resource descriptions, incident facility types, and position titles. ICS is also designed to meet the needs of any size incident. The flexible structure allows the command structure to expand and contract as needed. It allows personnel to communicate and interact. It allows the appropriate stakeholders to interact in the decision-making process. ICS provides logistical and administrative support to operational staff who are performing the on-scene operations. It is also designed to be cost-effective by eliminating redundancy that occurs when multiple agencies work independently. DOT 8-2.9

Street Secrets

For more information and online training, visit the FEMA Web site (http://www.training.fema.gov).

Incident Command Facilities

Every incident will have an **incident command post** (ICP). This is where the IC oversees all incident operations. Only one ICP is allowed per incident. The ICP should be positioned outside the incident location. The ICP should be identified by the name of the incident, for example, Columbia Wildfire ICP or Chicago Heights Flood ICP. DOT 8-2.14

Staging areas are temporary locations, where personnel and equipment are kept until they are needed on the scene. The status of all personnel, equipment, and supplies in the staging area is "available." It is acceptable to have more than one staging area on an incident. DOT 8-2.15

Bases are the locations where primary logistical and administrative functions are coordinated and administered. The base may be co-located with the ICP. There should only be one base per incident. Resources located at the base are always designated as "out of service."

Camps are locations where resources are kept to support the incident operations. They may be needed to replace a base on an incident because of location, terrain, or accessibility. Camps are temporary. They are used to provide food, shelter, water, sleeping areas, and sanitation to the workers on the incident. Multiple camps are acceptable. Camps are designated by geographical location, for example, South Ridge Camp or Green Street Camp, or they can have a numerical designation. Not all incidents need camps.

Helibases are locations for helicopter operations. They function like the camps described above. These are required in many long-term events. **Helispots** are temporary locations and function as landing zones (Figure 50-2). There can be more than one helispot at an incident.

Emergency operations centers, or EOCs, are not actually a component of the NIMS, but because there are many EOCs operating across the country, the operation of the EOC during an incident was merged into the NIMS ICS structure. The EOC is required to use ICS management principles and terminology. An EOC is typically not located at an incident scene as many EOCs are already established at fixed locations around the country. The EOC is a multiagency coordination body that provides support to the on-scene responders. Many EOCs already have mutual aid agreements worked out that can be helpful to the ICP and IC. DOT 8-2.15

The Incident Action Plan

Every incident requires an **incident action plan (IAP)**. The IAP is an oral or written plan that contains the general objectives and reflects the overall strategy of managing the incident. The only type of incident that must have a written IAP is a hazmat incident. All other types of incidents may operate with either an oral or written plan.

The IAP describes the goals and objectives for the time frame it covers, which is called an operational period. The IAP typically spans a time frame of 12 hours, but it could cover more or less time. The IAP should be reviewed and updated at the conclusion of each segment of the operational period.

The IAP should outline the following:

- What needs to be done
- Who is responsible for doing it
- How communications are accomplished
- The procedure if someone is injured

The Incident Commander

In the NIMS structure, every incident must have an incident commander (Figure 50-3). In addition to overall management of the incident, the IC has three key

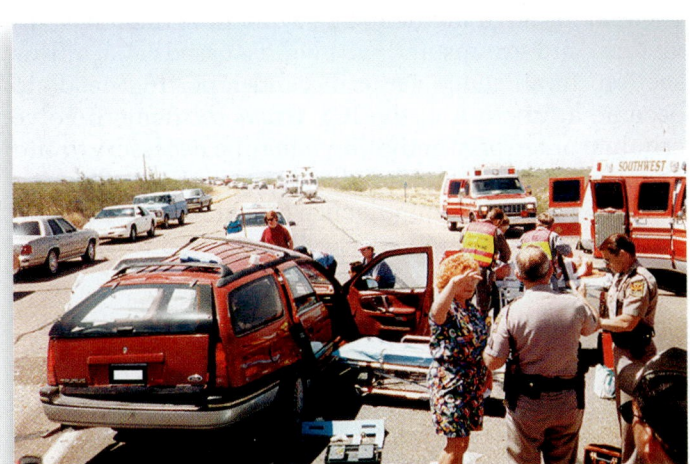

Figure 50-2 At a multiple casualty incident, such as the motor vehicle accident shown here, multiple helicopters may be required to transport patients and would land at a designated helispot.

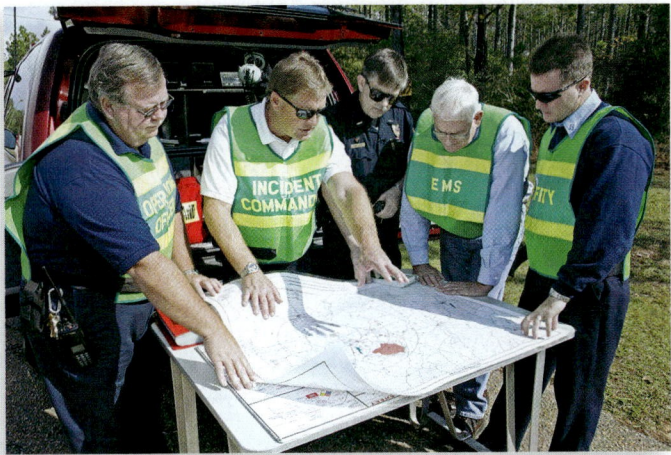

Figure 50-3 The IC ensures scene safety, provides information services to internal and external stakeholders, and establishes and maintains liaison with other agencies participating in the incident.

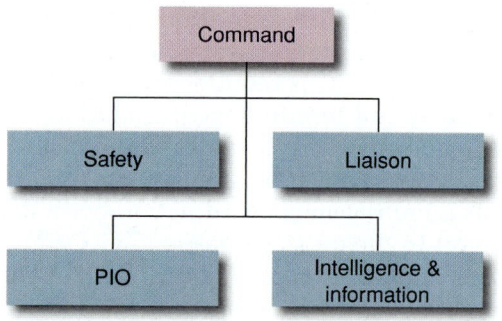

Figure 50-4 The command staff includes the safety officer (SO), public information officer (PIO), liason officer (LNO), and, in this example, an intelligence officer.

responsibilities: ensuring scene safety, providing information services to internal and external stakeholders, and establishing and maintaining communication with other agencies participating in the incident.

For most routine incidents, a single incident commander is sufficient. Depending on the size and magnitude of an incident, command can be shared by more than one commander. When command is shared by two or more agencies or jurisdictions, each jurisdiction is allowed a single representative, and this individual is also designated as incident commander. In this situation, the term that applies to this shared command structure is called *unified command*. Unified command allows each agency to retain its autonomy and also allows the agencies to work together to solve problems. Each IC in a unified command structure is required to work with the others in a single incident command post.

Command Staff

One of the key concepts in the incident command process is that a person has a manageable number of people directly under them. This **span of control** has established through research and practical experience, that the number of people one supervisor can effectively manage is between three and seven. The recommended ratio of supervisors to reporting elements is one supervisor to five reporting elements. Expansion and consolidation will allow these numbers to remain fairly constant. DOT 8-2.11

An incident commander can designate individuals to function as **command staff.** These people provide

information, safety, and communication services, and they report directly to the IC. The three common individuals are the **public information officer (PIO), safety officer (SO),** and **liaison officer** (Figure 50-4). The PIO serves as a conduit for information to internal and external stakeholders, including the media. The SO monitors the safety conditions and develops measures to ensure the safety of the workers on the scene. The SO also has emergency authority to stop or prevent unsafe acts during incident operations. The liaison officer serves as the primary contact for supporting agencies assisting in the incident. DOT 8.2-13

General Staff

As the operational objectives of an incident grow, there may be a need for other functions to be put in place. Large-scale incidents will often require four functions to be established:

1. Operations
2. Planning
3. Logistics
4. Finance and administration DOT 8-2.7

The term **general staff** refers to the individuals in charge of each section (Figure 50-5). The person in charge of each section is called a *chief*. The responsibilities of these section chiefs are described below. Remember, the ICS terminology is different from the daily operations of an agency or jurisdiction. The person who holds the title of chief in that setting may not have the same title during an incident. Also, people who have never had a title in their regular job may have the temporary title of chief during an incident if they are assigned to a general staff position.

Several types of modular, organizational elements can be established throughout the ICS structure, as needed, for large incidents. They include branches, divisions, and groups and will be discussed later in this section. Intelligence gathering and reporting needs to become a function of the ICS when incidents involve criminal or terrorist activities. It may be necessary to add an intelligence group to the operations or planning section or to add an intelligence officer to the command staff, similar to a safety officer (Figure 50-6).

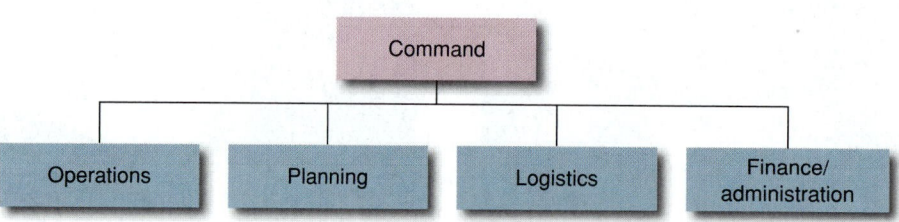

Figure 50-5 The incident commander (IC) and the section chiefs (the general staff) of the four main functions of ICS.

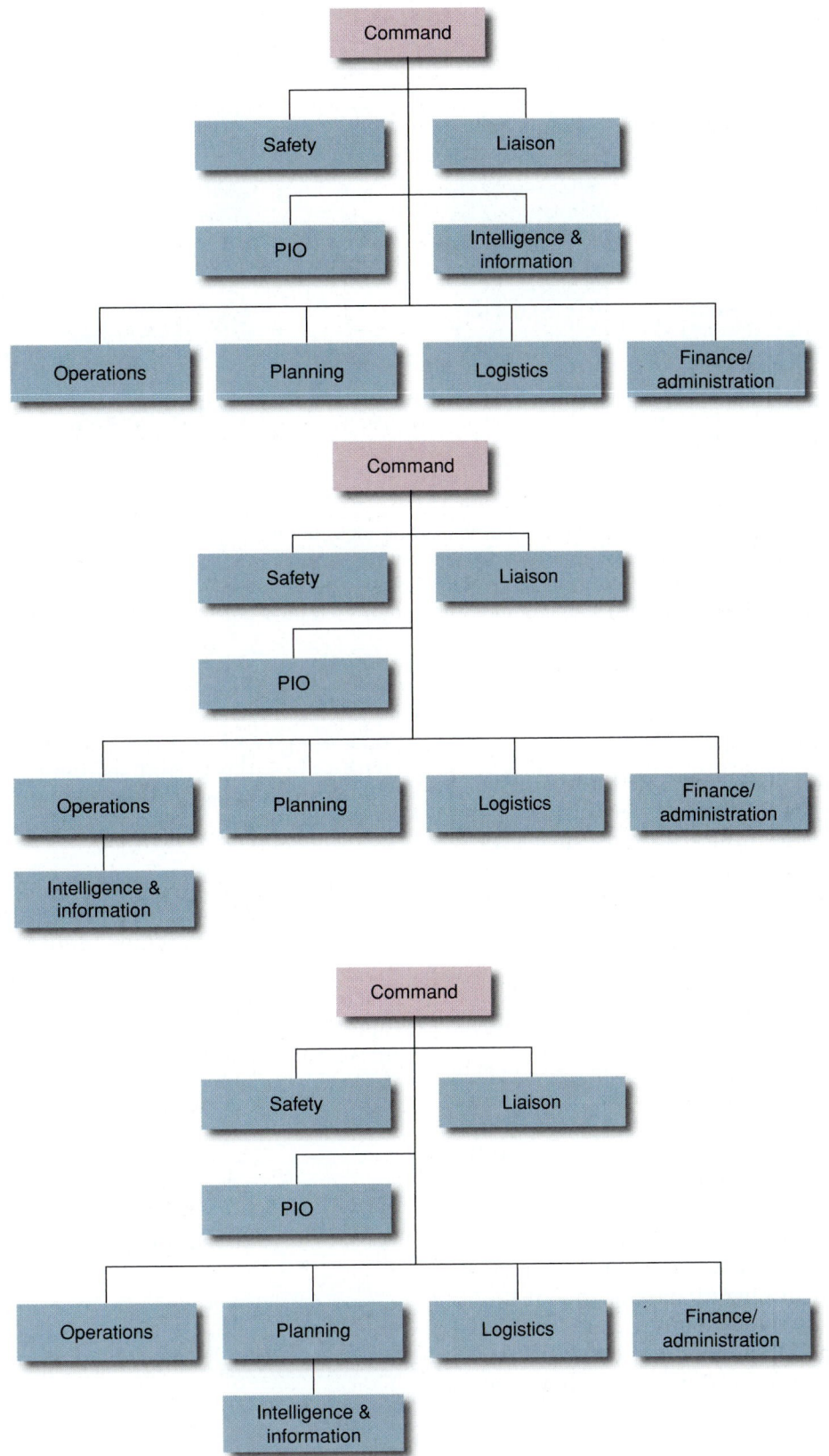

Figure 50-6 An Intelligence resource can be added as an advisor in the command staff or a branch or group within the operations or planning section.

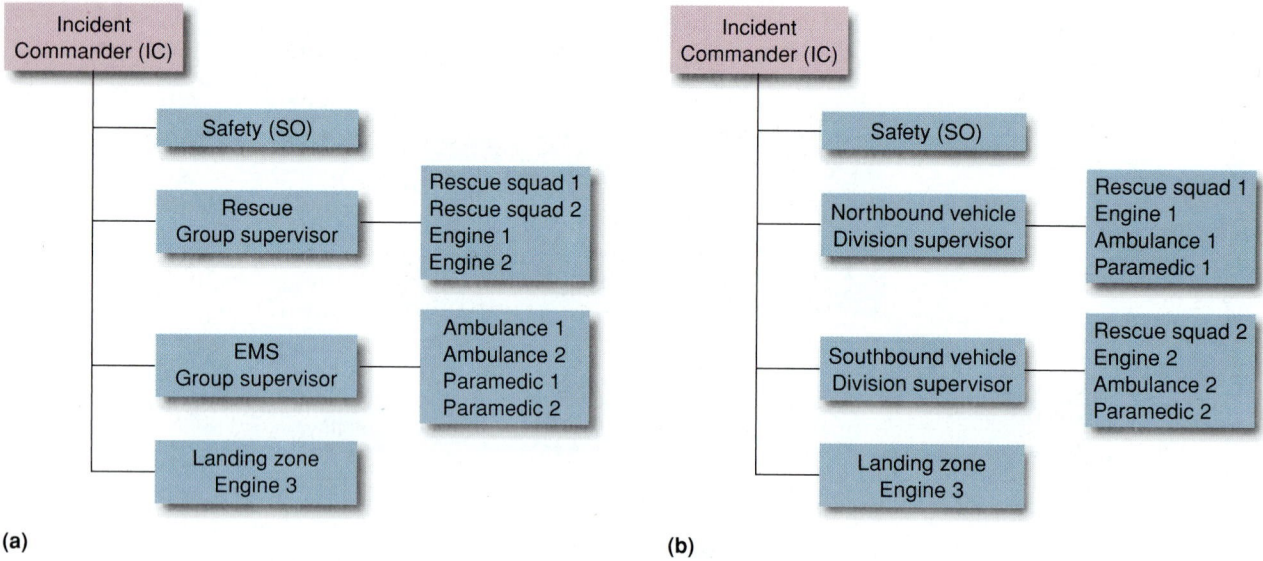

(a)   (b)

Figure 50-7   (a) An ICS structure with groups established based on their functions. This is a typical ICS structure for a fairly common emergency incident such as a motor vehicle crash with two patients entrapped. Notice that each supervisor is assigned a number of subordinates within his or her effective span of control. Also note that only functions that require multiple resource units are made into groups. (b) An alternative ICS structure with established divisions based on 'geographic' considerations.

Operations Section

The operations section is responsible for the management of tactical operations. These operations are intended to save lives and property and to successfully mitigate the emergency incident while maintaining safety and control of emergency service providers. In smaller incidents, the IC typically commands the three to seven groups performing operational objectives. **One of the operational areas will be EMS. An EMS specialist will direct the EMS portion of operations** (Figure 50-7).

For larger incidents, the operations section is established and commanded by an operations section chief. If the operational requirements of the incident call for the involvement of several different agencies, the operations section chief can establish one or more deputy section chiefs. These deputies are usually senior officials for their agencies (Figure 50-8).

Once there is an established operations section and chief to oversee tactical operations, the role of the IC changes. It becomes a more strategic role, providing direction to the general staff for the other main ICS functions (if established), overseeing the allocation of incident resources, and reviewing and evaluating the incident action plan.

The operations section can be organized in many ways. The attributes of the specific incident will dictate the most appropriate ICS structure. Factors that will affect this include the incident type, specific strategies for intervention, number and type of involved agencies,

incident geography, and jurisdictional boundaries. The NIMS gives the IC and section chiefs the flexibility to determine the most appropriate ICS structure for any given incident.

Staging. Typically, unless a staging area is established by the IC or operations section chief, incoming units will stage in an uncommitted position until they receive an assignment. Once a staging area is established, staging becomes a functional unit under the operations section, and all incoming units must check in with the staging supervisor. Units are then called up from the staging area, as needed, for the incident. The staging supervisor should assure that equipment can

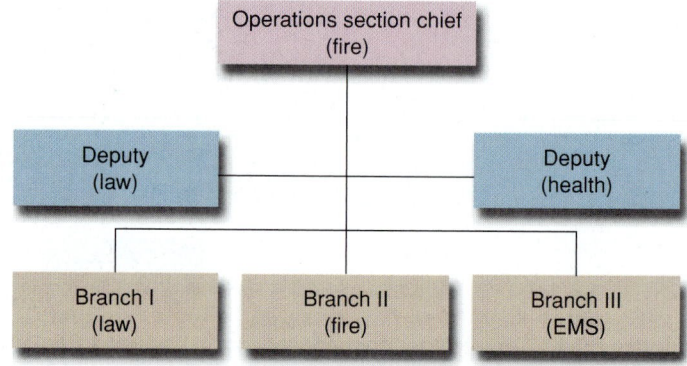

Figure 50-8   An example of an operations section structure for an incident requiring the involvement of several different agencies utilizing deputy section chiefs.

be efficiently deployed from the staging area and confer with the IC as to what resources are needed at the incident scene and what resources remain in the staging area. DOT 8.2-13

A Sample Sequence of Progression for the Structure of a Typical ICS.   Refer to Figure 50-7(b) for a graphic of the progression for the structure of a typical ICS.

■ Units are dispatched for a high-speed motor vehicle crash involving two vehicles on Interstate 13.

■ Ambulance 1 is the first to arrive at the scene, and the company officer of the ambulance gives this radio message: "Ambulance 1 is on location with a two-car, head-on crash with significant damage to both vehicles. It appears we have two critical patients entrapped in separate vehicles. Ambulance 1 will have initial 'Interstate 13' command. Ambulance 1 will be the command post. Command is requesting an additional rescue squad, engine, and paramedic unit."

■ The crew from Ambulance 1 begins patient triage while the company officer, who is now the IC, begins to gather information required to develop an incident action plan. Considerations might include an evaluation of scene safety concerns, the need for additional resources, anticipated apparatus positioning and assignments, the condition of the two patients, the proximity to a trauma center, the weather conditions, and where to locate a helicopter landing zone for medical evacuation.

■ Engine 1 then arrives on location. The company officer from Engine 1 confers with the initial IC face-to-face, and a **transfer of command** takes place. The CO from Engine 1 gives a radio message like this: "Captain from Engine 1 is assuming 'Interstate 13' command. Have all units come straight in to the scene. Rescue Squad 1 will have the northbound facing vehicle and Rescue Squad 2 and Engine 2 will have the southbound facing vehicle." The initial IC returns to the assignment as the company officer of Ambulance 1 and begins providing patient care with the crew. DOT 8-2.10

■ As other units arrive on the scene, the new IC gives them assignments. Because there are two active working rescues, the IC designates the captain from Engine 2 as the safety officer. The IC also designates the officer from each rescue squad as a division supervisor for the assigned vehicles. This is done by a radio message: "Command to Rescue Squad 1. You are now Northbound Division supervisor. You have Rescue Squad 1, Engine 1, Ambulance 1, and Paramedic 1 assigned to you." The company officer on Rescue Squad 1 acknowledges this assignment.

■ When the battalion chief arrives, the IC confers face-to-face and transfers command. This transfer of command is then announced over the radio. The Engine 1 captain returns to operate with the crew.

■ As the incident is resolved, the IC places units in service. When the incident is complete, the IC terminates "Interstate 13" command.

Planning Section

When implemented, the planning section consists of four units and a number of technical specialists. It is this section's responsibility to develop and document the IAP, which should include the operational objectives and strategies established by the IC or UC (unified command). The IAP should also address tactical and support requirements and is typically broken down into operational periods of 12 hours each. Documentation of incident activities and planning for demobilization are also responsibilities of this unit (Figure 50-9).

Technical specialists can be assigned as required for a specific incident. These are individuals who are specially certified in their fields or professions and are only activated when needed. They can be assigned anywhere in the organization, including the command staff. Their role is based on what is most appropriate for a given incident. For instance, the role of a cost analysis technical specialist may initially be part of the planning section but can be expanded to an entire finance and administration section if management of the incident makes it necessary.

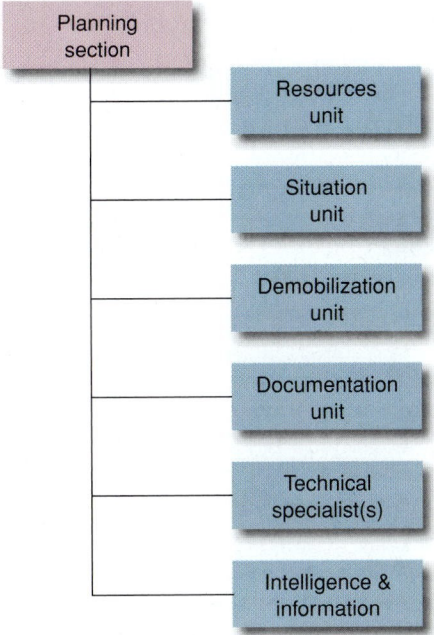

Figure 50-9   The planning section with intelligence group established.

Logistics Section

The logistics section is responsible for acquiring and coordinating required support resources. This could include obtaining and providing supplies, facilities, equipment maintenance and fuel, communications and information, technology support, food and water, and medical care to emergency service providers (Figure 50-10). **EMS personnel may be involved in this section to ensure the EMS response is adequate in human and physical assets.**

Logistics Section Medical Unit

The medical unit of the logistics section is responsible for developing an incident medical plan for incident personnel. This plan may need to provide rehabilitation, inoculations, vector control, crisis intervention, and medical care and transport and may even assist in coordinating personal affairs. All activities must be well documented and conducted with a focus on confidentiality and privacy. EMS providers may be specifically assigned to the medical unit.

Personnel assigned to rehabilitation should make efforts to secure a location that offers shelter and facilities. In extreme heat or cold, this function can be resource intensive, making early planning vital. DOT 8.2-13

Mental Health and Stress Monitoring

Personnel assigned to the health unit should actively monitor incident personnel for signs of stress. Signs of stress include emotional outbursts, inability to focus, and inability to function as directed. Workers can exhibit these from fatigue as well, so it is critical for workers to cycle in and out of work zones and take appropriate breaks. Many of the fundamental services provided by the logistics section (food, water, and shelter) will help to meet the basic needs of the providers. However, emergency response providers should be monitored for their own emotional responses to the incident, including confusion, disorganization, apprehension, frustration, irritability, apathy, and loss of objectivity.[5] Emergency service providers should have access to mental health professionals during and after major incidents. DOT 8.2-27, 8.2-28

Finance and Administration Section

An incident that requires extensive management resources, including finance and administrative support, may require a finance and administration section. This could occur if management of the incident spans several days. This section is responsible for cost analysis, compensation, procurement, and tracking personnel and hours of work. DOT 8-2.7

Modular Resource Components

Several types of modular organizational elements can be established throughout the ICS structure, as needed, for large incidents. They include the following:

- Branches
- Divisions or groups
- Units
- Strike teams or task forces

There can be up to five branches established in each section. Each branch can have up to five divisions or groups. Each division or group can have up to five resource units. A resource unit usually refers to a company or crew of an ambulance, fire engine, or rescue squad. In larger or specialized incidents, a resource unit could consist of uniquely qualified personnel or specialized equipment (Figure 50-11). DOT 8.2-30

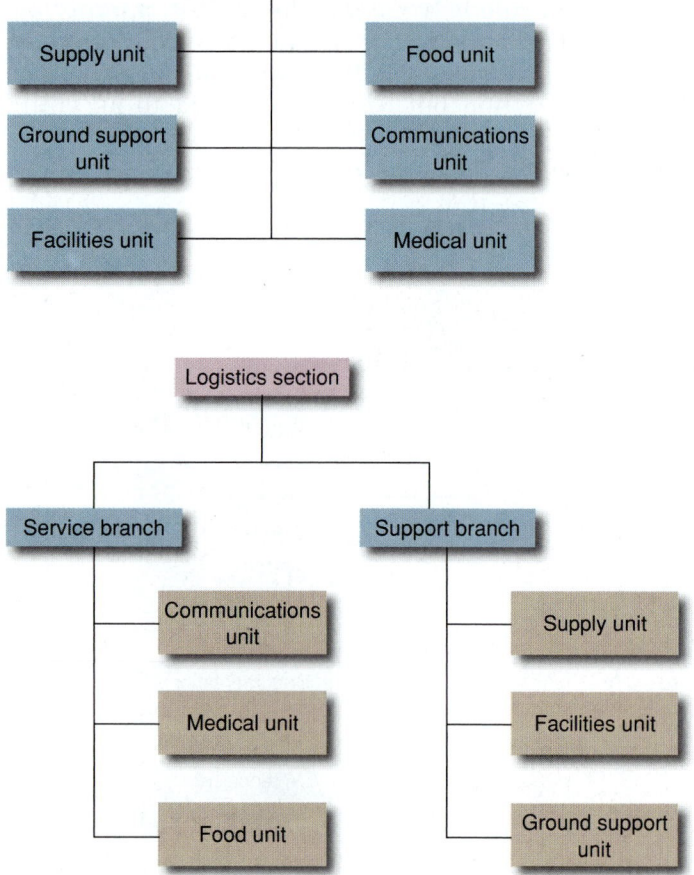

Figure 50-10 Two possible ICS structures for the Logistics section. If the number of resources within the section becomes extensive, two branches can be established in order to lessen the span of control of the logistics section chief.

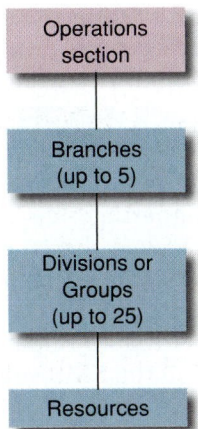

Figure 50-11 The modular resource components of the NIMS ICS. Branches, groups, divisions, or resource units (ambulances, fire engines, rescue squads, etc.) can be established within each main section.

Branches

Branches are typically established when the number of groups or divisions exceeds the recommended 1:5 span of control ratio for the IC or section chief. The single biggest reason to establish branches during an incident is because the span of control is exceeding recommended ratios. For this reason, branches often develop after divisions and groups.

The IC can establish up to five branches in each section as the number of required resources for incident mitigation grows. Branches are commanded by branch directors. Directors may have deputy directors to serve them directly. Branch directors can command up to five divisions or groups. An example of an incident that might require branches is one where there are multiple agencies involved, and each agency has different tasks to accomplish (Figure 50-12).

Divisions

An IC or section chief can establish a division in order to control assignments within a designated geographic area. In the case of the operations section chief, this could be one floor of a multistory building fire or one side of a train derailment or river, or it could be one of several parking lots where affected patients are exiting a complex (Figure 50-13). Divisions are used to divide an incident across geographical boundaries.

Groups

An IC or section chief establishes a group in order to control assignments that are related to a specific function. In operations, the function could be broad, such as a "medical group," which might comprise units with personnel performing triage, treatment, and transport. For larger incidents, when the number of resource units exceeds the span of control for one supervisor, the groups could be more specialized, such as "triage group," "treatment group," and transport group." This would typically be the case during a medium-sized multiple casualty incident (Figure 50-14).

Strike Teams and Task Forces

Like branches, groups, and divisions, strike teams and task forces can also be added to the ICS structure. Strike teams consist of a set number of the same type of resource. Task forces are any combination of resources put together to accomplish a specific mission. Both groups operate under a designated leader and have common communications between them. They are useful as they can be quickly deployed and do not require other changes to the ICS structure.

Guiding Concepts of NIMS

Agencies, jurisdictions, regions, and states should participate in the development of disaster plans. Every member of the EMS team has a role to play. Often, the actual patient care provider has insight into problems and solutions that may not be apparent to the administrators operating at the "30 thousand foot level." Every planning process should involve a review and comment phase before the plan is finalized. If the street-level EMS provider has not had an opportunity to provide

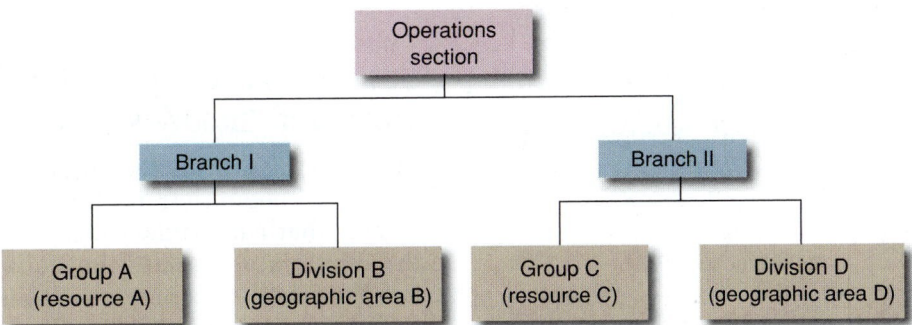

Figure 50-12 Branches, groups, and divisions can be established within each main section, in this case the operations section. Each supervisor can manage up to five branches, groups, divisions, or resource units.

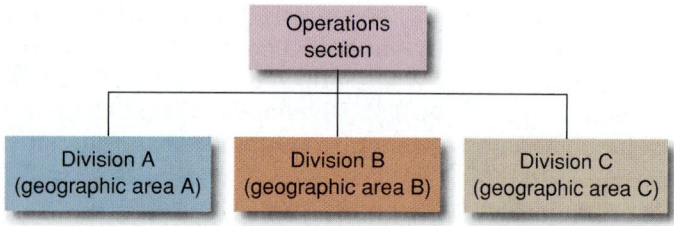

Figure 50-13 An operations section structure with the use of divisions to control geographically separate areas of an incident.

input prior to this phase, this is the optimal time to do so. DOT 8-2.5

It is also important for EMS providers and public safety workers at all levels to participate in disaster drills and tabletop exercises. These exercises allow exploration of the plan and provide an opportunity to test various components. This is a critical activity to help ensure that the plan will work in an actual disaster. Drills should be both small- and large-scale. Agencies should familiarize themselves with their own plans and then work with adjacent agencies to drill and practice. This allows the workers to integrate and learn each others' roles and tasks. Without drills and tabletop exercises, the people expected to utilize the disaster

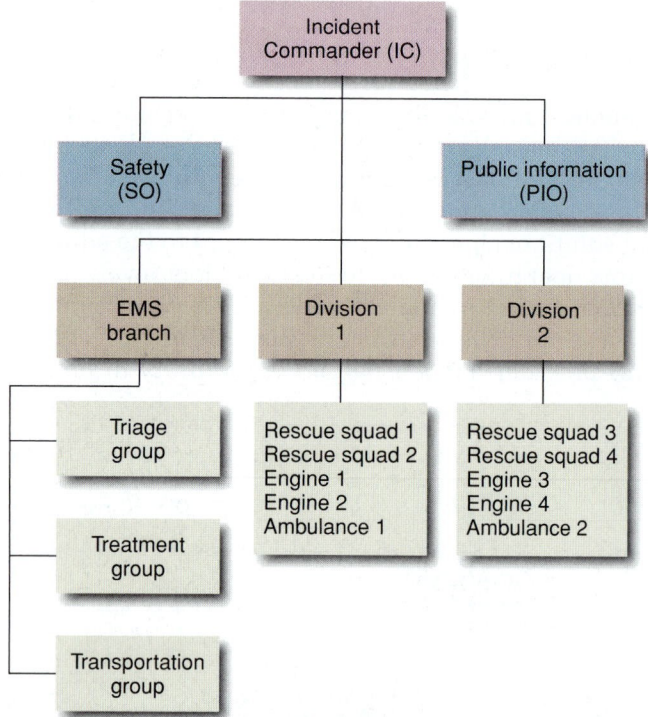

Figure 50-14 One possible ICS structure for a vehicle crash, for instance a bus crash, that produces multiple extrications and a multiple casualty incident with 25 to 35 patients.

plan will not be familiar with the components or their roles in the plan. DOT 8-2.29

Street Secrets

Encourage your administrators to practice the triage component by designating one day a month on a rotating shift basis to use the triage system. On this day, all patients are triaged using the procedures and equipment that would be used during a disaster. This allows the providers to remain familiar with the tools, their location on the EMS vehicle, and their use, and it helps them stay sharp in performing this task. DOT 8-2.34

The NIMS requires that field command and management functions be performed in accordance with a standard set of ICS organizations, doctrine, and procedures.[6] This commonality regarding the management of incidents is the strength of NIMS. It allows diverse organizations to come together and effectively manage an emergency incident.

The NIMS system has a flexible and scalable, modular, organizational structure that is designed to enable effective and efficient incident management. It can be expanded from the top down by adding functional modules, as required, to manage an incident. It begins with the establishment of an incident commander.

The system is designed so that it can be utilized for every incident regardless of size. At its smallest it may be one individual performing an investigation. Even in this circumstance certain fundamental procedures should be followed. The system is designed to facilitate a rapid expansion of objectives should it become necessary.

At its largest it serves as a set of common command and management procedures among any conceivable number of agencies and organizations that might participate in the mitigation of a complex incident.

A breakdown of any of the fundamental guiding concepts will erode the effectiveness of incident management.

Concept #1: Command Is Established Early and Includes an Incident Size-Up

"The command function must be clearly established from the beginning of incident operations."[6] The agency that has primary jurisdictional authority over the incident designates the individual who is authorized to establish command. This individual is responsible for the initial command functions, which include an incident size-up and official establishment of the ICS. DOT 8-2.3

The first unit on the scene should establish command. This may require the incident commander to handle multiple tasks:

- Ensure safety of personnel
- Utilize resources efficiently

The IC is responsible for developing and implementing an incident action plan (see Concept #3 below) and ensuring that these paramount objectives are being achieved. An early decision must be made as to whether additional resources will be required to mitigate the incident. If the incident is unstable and could become more extensive or generate more patients, the probability of needing additional resources is high. If the incident is stable, additional resources may or may not be necessary, depending on the size of the dispatched response. DOT 8-2.11

If quick action can make a difference to the outcome of the incident, ICS allows for the incident command to be flexible. The IC can elect to "pass command" to the second arriving unit if immediate action is necessary to positively affect the outcome of the incident.[2] An example of this situation would be the need to make a rapid rescue of a victim who is in immediate danger. The IC must weigh the benefit of immediate action against the cost of not being able to begin establishing incident management objectives. Adequate crew accountability is particularly at risk in this situation. Generally, passing command is not recommended.[2] If the IC still elects to pass command following incident size-up, incoming units should be clearly advised. DOT 8.2-10

The scene size-up is a brief report that summarizes the observations of the first arriving unit. It usually includes the designation of the company arriving on the scene, a brief description of the incident situation, any obvious conditions or safety concerns, a declaration of the strategy to be used, the assumption of command, and the designated location of the command post.[2]

The IC should give periodic updates of the status of the incident. Any change in the status of the event and any response to the efforts of the responders should be included in the reports. There are reports that go up and down the chain of command, and while the content may be similar, the focus may be different depending on the perspective or needs of the recipient.

Concept #2: There Is a Clear Chain of Command and Unity of Command

A chain of command is an orderly line of authority. Paramount to this concept is "unity of command," which means that throughout the management structure, every individual has just one supervisor at any given time. At the top of the line of authority is the

incident commander. At the fundamental level, the company officer is responsible for the resource unit and crew, whether it is an ambulance, fire engine, rescue squad, or some other special resource. (Refer to Figure 50-14.) DOT 8-2.8, 8-2.9

Street Secrets

It is important to work within your piece of the structure. The system counts on everyone reporting to the appropriate authority. The system breaks down when people freelance or work on their own plan.

When there are multiple agencies involved in incident management, there are a few options that can be implemented to increase management efficiency. The IC can place ranking officials from other agencies within the command staff so that they can be involved in incident management. Alternatively, the IC may elect to establish a unified command (UC). In this case, there is not one incident commander but rather an incident management team made up of agency officials who use a collaborative approach to formulating an incident action plan and evaluating incident management objectives. By using this method of command, the flow of information between agencies is optimized, and no single agency's legal authority is likely to be compromised.

Unified command is usually conducted with all participating individuals at the same location. There are complex procedures for effective use of a unified command that serve to ensure that the guiding principles of ICS, including "unity of command," are preserved. DOT 8-2.8

If several ICS structures exist within close proximity to each other, as might occur if there were several complex incidents at various locations around a city, **area command** is another type of command that can be established. Area command provides oversight to management of the various incidents, providing a kind of "umbrella command." It is particularly applicable when the management of multiple incidents will be competing for the same type of resources. Each incident IC would then be in close communication with an area commander in order to coordinate resources on a wider scale. This does not interfere with the "unity of command" principle. This sort of expansion of the ICS structure from the bottom up is only implemented when necessary. This could become necessary following a widespread terrorism event or hazardous materials release.

Area command can be physically established at a jurisdictional EOC as there are usually ideal facilities and coordination resources cached at those facilities. While it provides ideal physical facilities for an area command post, the usual purpose of an EOC differs.

Upon activation, an EOC coordinates support functions and provides resources and support for larger or long-duration incidents. EOC activation is particularly appropriate for management of a disaster, as the added problems of broken and overwhelmed infrastructure make mobilizing resources more difficult than usual. In addition to the continuing management of emergency incidents, disaster management also involves mobilizing resources to provide basic essential services, distributing relief supplies, and gathering information for disaster welfare systems. DOT 8-2.12, 8.2-15

Concept #3: There Is an Incident Action Plan Emphasizing a Management-by-Objective Approach

It is the responsibility of the IC to develop an IAP. This process includes gathering and analyzing information, establishing incident objectives and strategies to accomplish them, determining resource requirements for the plan, evaluating progress, and revising the plan if necessary. In the case of larger incidents, this process can be delegated to a group in the planning section. This group must have a clear line of communication with the IC.

Concept #4: Transfer of Command

Typically, the initial IC will not remain the IC for the entire incident. As the incident dictates, or when there is an expanding ICS, the initial IC may transfer command to a later arriving individual. The arrival of a higher-ranking officer does not imply an automatic transfer of command.[2] The transfer of command is a process that must include a briefing that incorporates all essential information for continuing safe and effective operations. It is best done face-to-face but can sometimes be accomplished over the radio, if necessary. Command should not be passed to a responder who is not on the scene unless absolutely necessary to facilitate addressing a critical task. When command is correctly transferred, all personnel on the scene should be advised that a command transfer has taken place. If an incident management worksheet has been initiated, which is recommended, that should also be passed to the new IC. Once the transfer of command has taken place, the initial IC could become a section chief or group supervisor or return to the company again as a company officer. DOT 8-2.10

It is recommended that a tactical worksheet of some sort be used to document and assist the IC and other supervisors in organizing the resources of the incident. Because the ICS is modular in design, supervisors can start with the same blank worksheet since they are each tracking only the three to seven resources that are assigned specifically to them. Tactical worksheets help supervisors visualize the scene, provide cues for critical

functions, document incident progress, and facilitate the transfer of command (Figure 50-15).

Concept #5: Each Supervisor Has a Manageable Span of Control

By expanding the ICS in functional modules, it ensures that no single supervisor is given more subordinates than they can effectively and safely control. This number is usually between three and seven, depending on the level of supervision required, the presence of hazards, other safety concerns, distances between personnel and resources, and whether or not a preexisting working relationship was in place prior to the incident. Once the number of resource units or tasks that any one supervisor has to manage exceeds the effective span of control, the IC can establish additional functional units (branches, groups, or divisions), each with its own supervisor. For example, for an incident such as a motor vehicle crash with two patients entrapped in separate vehicles, the IC may wish to divide supervision by function, establishing a rescue group and an EMS group (Figure 50-7(a)). Alternatively, the IC could divide supervision by geography, establishing a "vehicle one" division and a "vehicle two" division (Figure 50-7(b)).

Street Secrets

The key here is that the size of the command structure should be appropriate to the event. It is a mistake to have a command structure that uses up too much personnel, making it unsafe or impractical to execute the plan and rescue efforts. On the other hand, in larger events with multiple hazards, it is important that each functional group has a focus.

Concept #6: All Agencies Use Common Terminology

It is important that all personnel involved in an incident understand and use common terminology in their communications with each other and other agencies, both person-to-person and over the radio system. The use of codes violates this principle as all agencies may not use the same code meanings. It is for this reason that a "clear text" approach is needed for effective ICS. It is helpful to make radio communications two-way, where the receiving parties repeat information in order to confirm accuracy.

The NIMS defines common terminology for ICS organizational functions, resource descriptions, and incident facilities. It supplies extensive guidelines for the categorization of area resources for possible use in

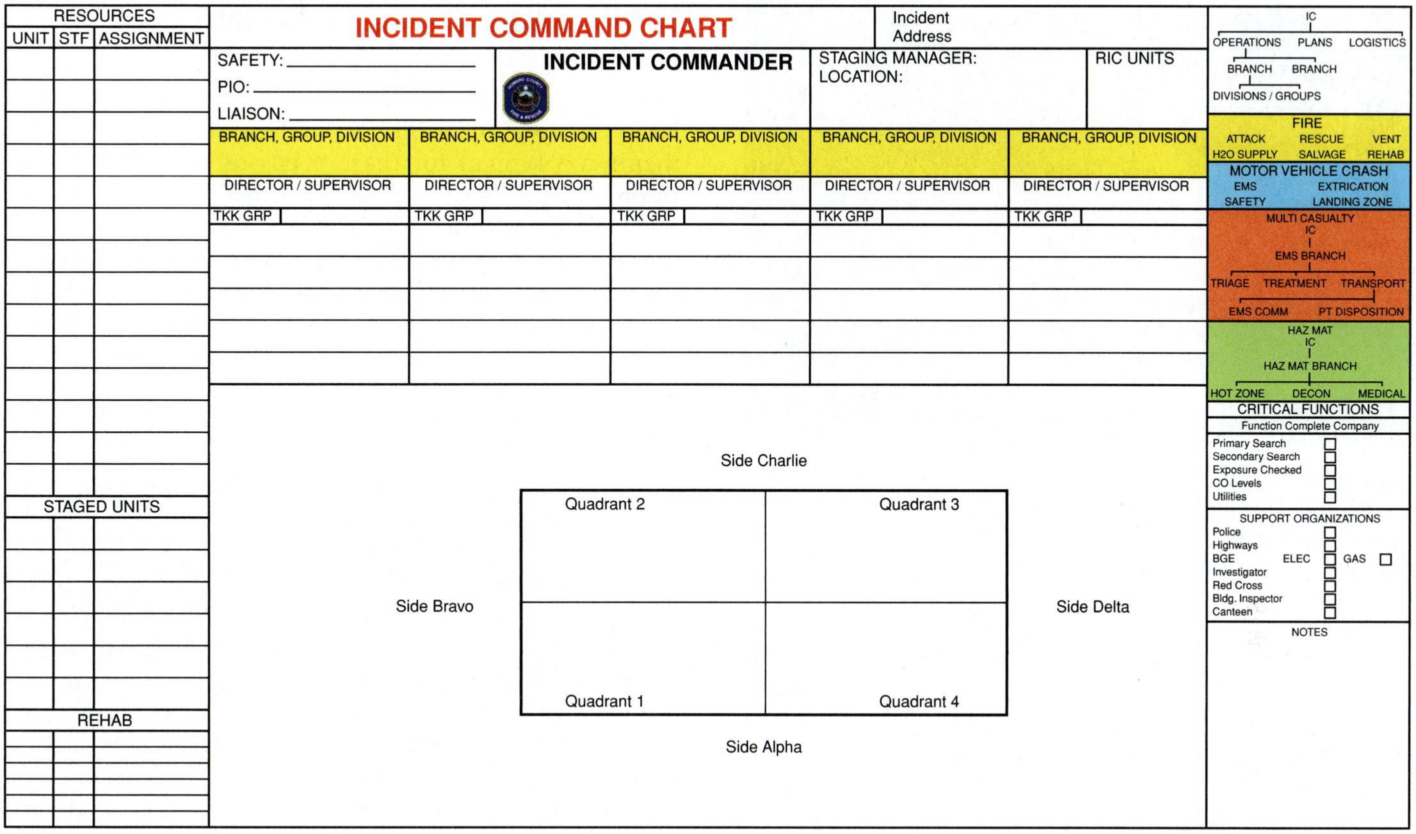

Figure 50-15 An example of an incident command tactical worksheet. This chart allows the IC, section chief, or group supervisor to sketch the incident; provides cues for critical functions; and provides suggested ICS structures for certain types of incidents. It is intended to be printed to an 8.5 by 17-inch size. *Source:* Developed by Deputy Chief Richard Freas, Howard County Department of Fire and Rescue Services.

an emergency. Though not outlined specifically by NIMS, the efficiency and safety of operations can be enhanced when agencies collaborate and implement standardized elements of ICS that have been for the most part universally accepted as the best practice. For instance, it is generally accepted that the areas of a structure be defined by designating the front of the structure as "side alpha," and going clockwise around the structure, the sides are designated as "bravo," "charlie," and "delta"[2] (see Figure 50-15). DOT 8.2-33

Concept #7: All Emergency Service Agencies Will Use the NIMS-Designated Position Titles

Position titles for the various ICS functions and resources are designated by NIMS. All agencies should be familiar with the NIMS position titles and should utilize them for all incidents when they are established. Individual titles within an agency do not carry forward to the NIMS structure, so a deputy chief on an incident may have a different rank than they usually carry on the job. The use of vests, hats, or other means of identification can be very helpful in identifying the

IC, command staff, general staff, and officers of the general staff.

Concept #8: Communications between Participating Agencies Are Integrated

Incident communications must be technically possible between agencies that are involved in incident mitigation. This implies that all communications follow a common communications plan that has been adopted by all involved agencies. This implies, at a minimum, that all resources and units operating on the scene have the technical capacity for radio communications with their ICS supervisor (Figure 50-16). DOT 8.2-31

Multiple Casualty Incidents (MCI)

A **multiple casualty incident (MCI)** is defined as an emergency incident that produces more patients than a jurisdiction is *routinely* capable of handling.[2] However, during a multiple casualty incident, the number of patients and the severity of their injuries do not exceed the capacity of area medical systems, hospitals, and facilities to render care. As a result, while it may require an uncommon mobilization of resources, patients with multiple system trauma or life-threatening illness are still treated first.[7] DOT 8-2.2

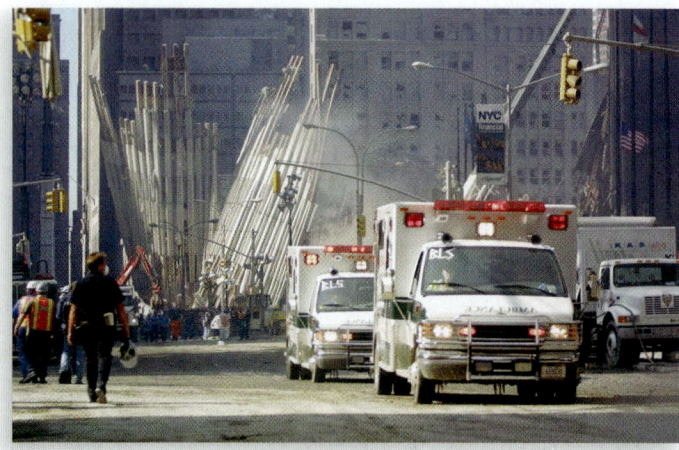

Figure 50-16 In critiques of the response to the World Trade Center incident on September 11, the inability of a variety of agencies to communicate with one another hampered efforts and may have contributed to casualties.

By contrast, a **mass casualty incident** is different. In a mass casualty incident, the number of patients and the severity of their injuries exceed the capacity of area medical systems and facilities. This situation forces an allocation of resources that allows the patients with the best chance of survival who require the least expenditure of time, equipment, supplies, and personnel to be managed first.[7] DOT 8-2.2

A mass casualty incident with overwhelmed resources both on-scene and at the receiving facilities is the typical definition of a **disaster.** Disaster management can be accomplished by utilizing the NIMS ICS structure. DOT 8-2.3

Management of multiple casualty incidents and mass casualty incidents should be planned well in advance. Emergency agencies should work to establish solid management plans for specific target hazards and potential situations that could occur within their jurisdictions. Coordination with surrounding jurisdictions and emergency management agencies is imperative. Administrative preparation should include the development of policies, procedures, standards of performance, and administrative conventions. Practical preparation should include provider training, using practice with tabletop and partial to full-scale MCI exercises, equipment acquisition, preincident surveys, and resource deployment. Planning activities should be accomplished well in advance of any potential incident. DOT 8-2.5, 8.2-29

Street Secrets

When an agency frequently uses the ICS on small incidents, they are used to it and they are better equipped to implement it easily during a large incident. DOT 8-2.30

Establishing an ICS for an MCI

It is extremely important to establish an ICS early in both mass and multiple casualty incidents as they require large numbers of resources. Certain ICS structural elements are typical for these types of incidents. Functional groups within the operations section that will need to be established include triage, treatment, and transport. Other needed groups, divisions, or branches could include disposition, morgue, medical supply, decontamination, search, rescue, and fire suppression (Figure 50-17). DOT 8-2.30

Multiple Casualty Incident Scene Size-Up

The initial IC should always communicate a scene size-up on arrival. In the case of a multiple casualty incident, the size-up should include all of the normal elements of a scene size-up and should also include a declaration that the incident is a multiple casualty incident. The report should include the results of a hazard assessment as well as a description of the incident and estimated number of patients. Local or regional policies may provide specific guidance for providers to follow regarding the classification of multiple casualty incidents. A physical location for a command post should be designated immediately, and the request for additional resources should be initiated. DOT 8-2.4

The speed and accuracy with which the scene size-up is performed will set the tone early for smoother operations. If the ICS is implemented immediately on arrival of the first units on scene, resources can be mobilized sooner, and the scene can be set up to best manage the patients. DOT-2.32

Triage

Triage is the prioritization of patient care based on the severity of illness, prognosis, and availability of resources.[8] It is implemented when the resource needs for patient care overwhelm the routine capabilities of the prehospital emergency medical system. The purpose is to accomplish the most good for the most number of patients. During the triage phase, resuscitation and definitive care are not appropriate. Patient care is limited to quick interventions that can save lives, such as manually opening an airway or controlling severe external hemorrhage.

There are many different methods that can be employed in triaging patients. Triage efficiency and consistency can be improved by training providers to use a uniform triage system. There are several systems in existence. Each is based on the rapid evaluation of a patient using criteria that are quickly and easily assessed and implies a certain severity of injury and prognosis for survival.

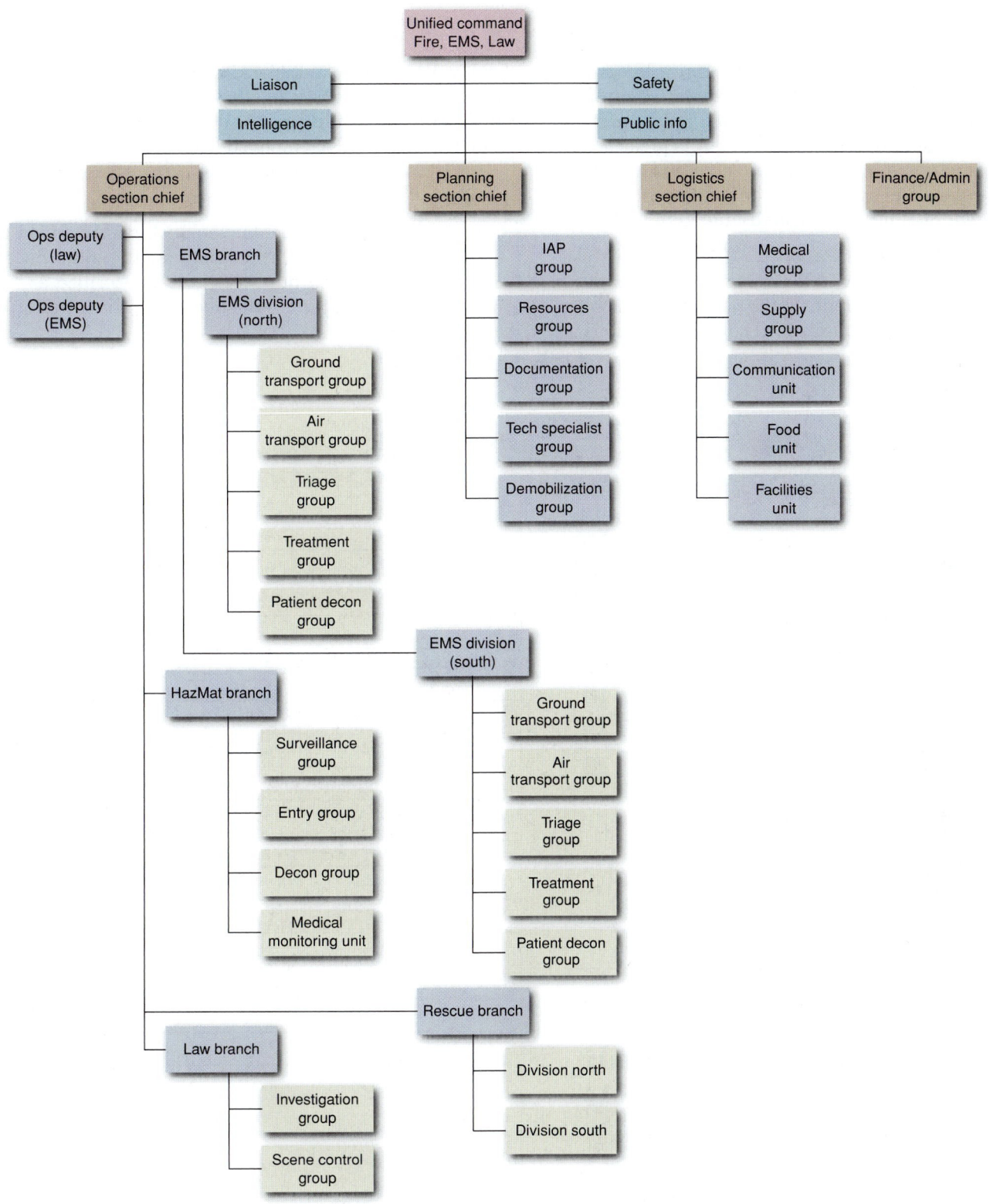

Figure 50-17 The ICS structure for a complex incident involving a large number of casualties at two different locations from a hazardous materials release. This example assumes participation from three agency types: fire, EMS, and law enforcement. Both unified command and operations section deputies have been established as a result. Also note the establishment of two EMS *branches,* in order to accommodate multiple *groups* operating at geographically separate locations. Two rescue *divisions* each oversee multiple *units* at two geographically separate locations. Despite the complex incident, the assigned number of subordinates is within each supervisor's effective span of control.

Just as is the case with ICS, the multiple casualty and triage methods and procedures for a jurisdiction are usually dictated by agency policies and procedures and a local or regional disaster plan. There is great benefit in having regional plans, given the increased likelihood that more than one agency will be participating in the management of a multiple casualty incident.

Triage Classification of Patients.   Triage systems classify patients into categories for treatment. Many systems use a color code to differentiate the patient treatment categories. The most commonly used color designations are red, yellow, green, and black. Colored tags or ribbons are attached to the patient, and these can be seen at a distance of several yards, allowing the stretcher bearers to quickly identify who is to be removed from the scene first.

Virtually all triage systems categorize patients as follows:

- *First priority*—patients who will likely survive but have immediate life threats; usually coded by the color red. This group can also be described as "immediate" in regard to the need for transportation off of the scene.

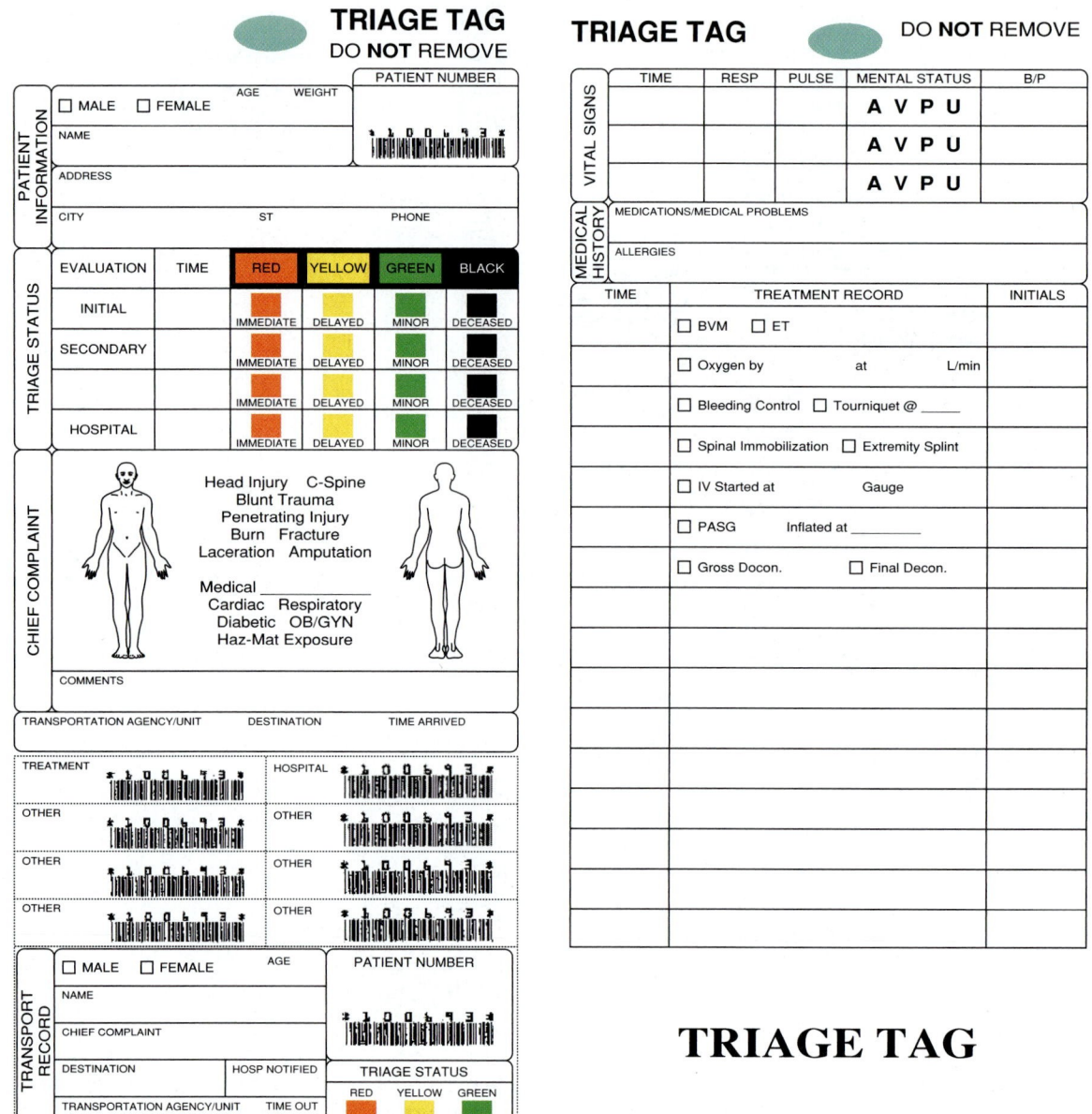

Figure 50-18   An example of a triage tag. This tag has tear-off stickers for patient numbers and for transport records, which facilitate patient tracking and documentation.

- *Second priority*—patients who have existing injuries that could become life-threatening but can tolerate a short delay in receiving care; usually coded by the color yellow. This group can also be described as "delayed," which means they should follow the immediate group off of the scene.

- *Third priority*—patients who have nonurgent and localized injuries without systemic implications; usually coded by the color green. The group is often referred to as the walking wounded, and they frequently self-extricate from the scene. The people in this group can be called upon to monitor patients and aid in treatment in some cases. This group is also described as the "hold" group, which means that transport off of the scene is not an urgent matter, unless the scene is unsafe.

- The last category is for patients who are dead or catastrophically injured and extremely unlikely to survive. This category is usually represented by the color black. This category is sometimes referred to as the "expectant" category. This group will typically be the last group removed from the scene and it is often labeled the "deceased" group. DOT 8-2.20

Triage Tags.   Many triage systems employ "triage tags" as a means to visually designate patient priority and to serve as ongoing documentation of patient assessment and care. Triage tags allow the assignment of a patient tracking number and facilitate the many transfers of care that occur between providers throughout the multiple casualty incident. They are designed to allow rapid documentation of injuries and treatments (Figure 50-18).

Many systems also utilize a length of colored plastic tape in place of triage tags during the initial triage phase. EMS providers simply tie an 18- to 24-inch length of red, yellow, green, or black plastic tape around the extremity of a triaged patient. This serves as a quick way to visually designate a patient priority. Patients will then receive a triage tag during a secondary triage phase or when they reach the treatment area (Figure 50-19). DOT 8.2-17, 8.2-20, 8.2-21

START Triage.   One widely used triage method is the simple triage and rapid treatment, or START system (Figure 50-20). START was developed in California in the early 1980s by Hoag Memorial Presbyterian Hospital and the Newport Beach Fire Department.[9] This easy-to-use system is effective as a primary triage method, where quick assessment of patients is important. The method begins by having all patients capable of walking proceed to a designated minor (green) treatment area. The remaining patients are then evaluated using the mnemonic "RPM." With the RPM system, the R stands for respiration, P stands for pulse, and M stands for mental status. Using the system's given parameters, any

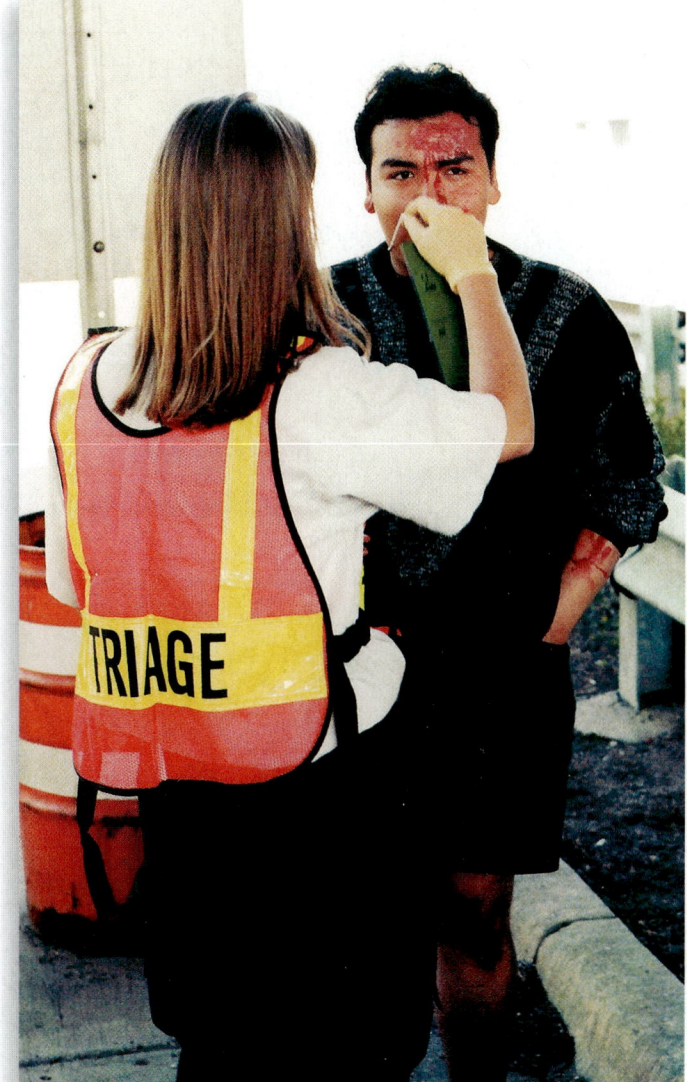

Figure 50-19   Patient receiving a green triage tag during the initial triage phase.

victim whose Respiration is absent or above 30, Perfusion is compromised (absent radial pulses or capillary refill time over two seconds), or Mental status is unconscious or unable to follow commands gets categorized to the immediate (red) treatment section. The remaining patients are usually categorized as delayed (yellow) or nonurgent (black). DOT 8-2.18

The order in which patients are removed from the scene by the stretcher bearers should reflect their color status, with red coming out first, followed by yellow, and then black. Of course, the green-tagged individuals self-extricate. Sometimes patients will be removed when their location is an impediment to rescue operations. For example, if two patients with a yellow-colored tag are blocking access to a red-colored tag, the yellow-tagged patients may be removed first.

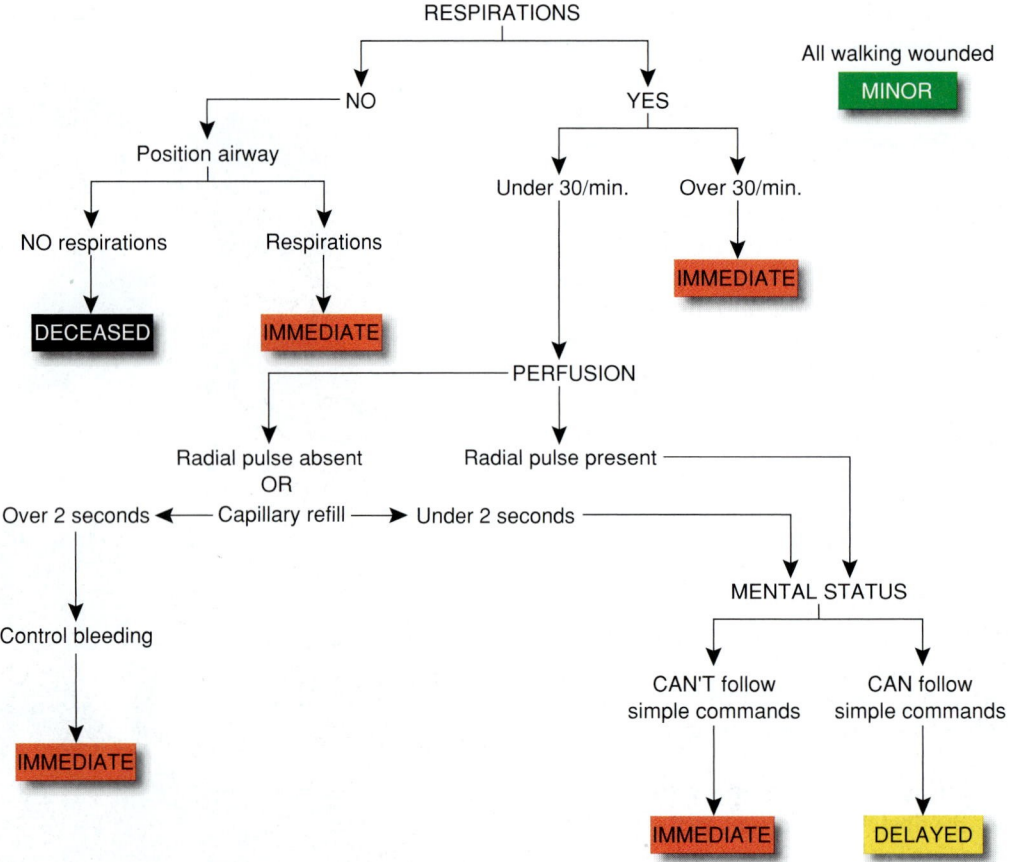

Figure 50-20   The START triage algorithm.
Source: G. Super, S. Groth, and R. Hook, et al., *Start: Simple Triage and Rapid Treatment Plan.* (Newport Beach, CA: Hoag Memorial Presbyterian Hospital, 1994). Graphic from http://www.citmt.org/start/images/flowchart2.jpg.

JumpSTART Triage. JumpSTART triage is a pediatric adaptation of the START method (Figure 50-21). Designed for triage of pediatric patients, it calls for giving five rescue breaths if a pediatric patient has a pulse but is not spontaneously breathing. It also modifies the parameters for the RPM assessment to accommodate pediatric differences. Using the system's given parameters, any pediatric victim whose respiration is below 15 or above 45, perfusion is compromised (using just absent radial pulses), or mental status is unconscious or demonstrates an abnormal response to pain is categorized to the immediate (red) treatment section. Remaining patients are categorized as delayed (yellow). The JumpSTART triage method was developed in 1995 by Dr. Lou Romig from Miami Children's Hospital in Miami, Florida.[10] DOT 8.2-18

Victim Decontamination

In some cases, there may be a need for decontamination of patients. In this scenario, triage crews might also be in protective clothing and require decontamination. Prior to patients entering a treatment area, they should be decontaminated. Gross decontamination with copious amounts of water may need to be initiated immediately.

CONNECTIONS See Chapters 33: Infectious and Communicable Diseases, 53: Hazardous Materials Incidents, and 55: Responding to Weapons of Mass Destruction for more information of decontamination of both patients and crew.

Typical ICS Groups for Multiple and Mass Casualty Incidents

Triage Group

The function of the triage group is to locate and quickly assess all patients of the incident. When determining the appropriate number of personnel to assign to triage, consider that it takes about 60 seconds for a responder to triage each victim to determine their primary triage designation. Transporting nonambulatory patients to the treatment area is labor-intensive and will usually require at least twice as many personnel as the number performing triage. For most mass and multiple casualty situations, the task of triage will likely need to be made a functional group and be given a supervisor. DOT 8-2.17

Once all patients are triaged, the personnel assigned to the triage group usually begin to transport patients to

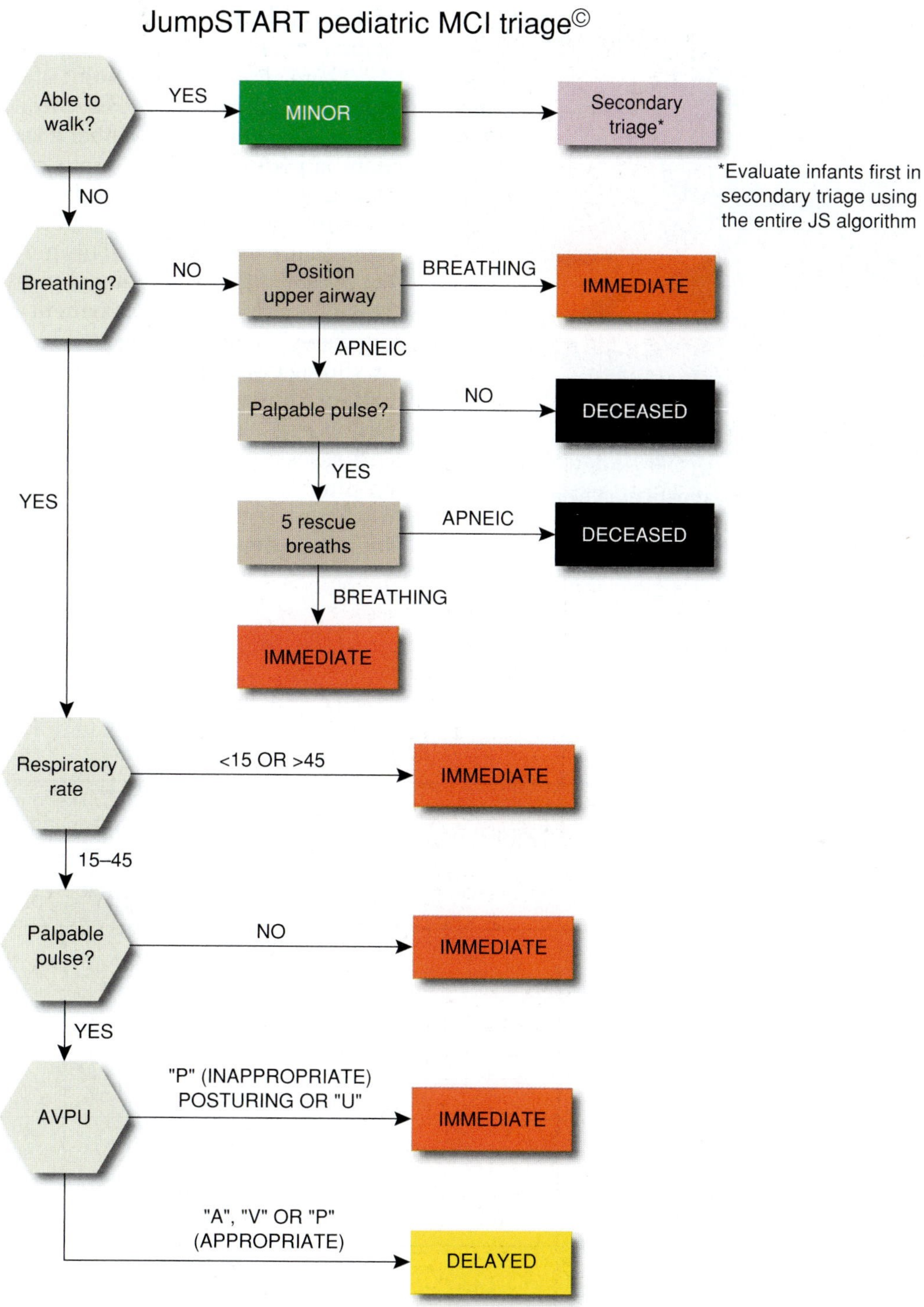

JumpSTART pediatric MCI triage©

Figure 50-21   The JumpSTART triage algorithm for pediatric patients.
Source: JumpStart developed by Dr. Lou Romig, MD, FAAP, FACEP, Miami Children's Hospital, Miami, FL. Graphic from http://www.jumpstarttriage.com/TheJumpSTARTAlgorithm.html.

the designated treatment area (Figure 50-22). If the situation allows, it is common to employ many long spine boards, cervical collars, and straps during this activity as this equipment is best applied to patients before they are moved to the treatment area. It helps stabilize them during the lifting and moving action that often occurs over uneven terrain.

Treatment Group

Designating areas for treatment should be established early in the incident. If possible, it is good practice to designate treatment areas visually, either with a colored tarp, a flag, or by priority number. Assigning a patient tracking number and logging each patient's entry and

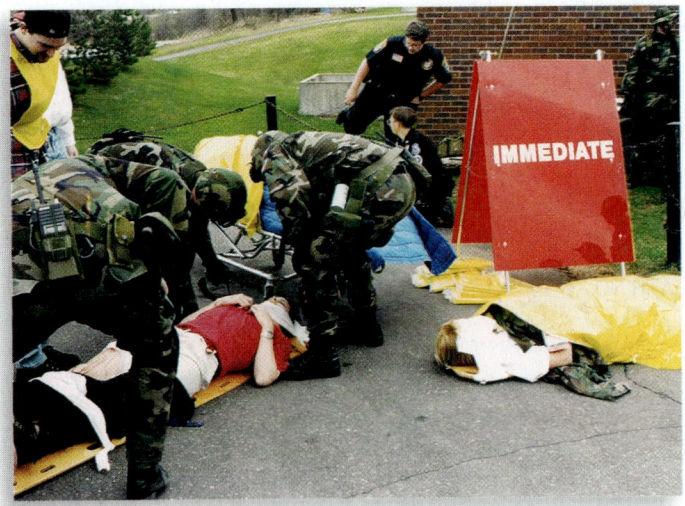

Figure 50-22 A well organized treatment area clearly designates where each group of patients belongs.

exit should also be accomplished. This is best done using a tracking form (Figure 50-23). DOT 8.2-13

There should be one point of entry and one point of exit from each treatment area. On entry, the treatment area supervisor should ensure that a secondary triage assessment is performed. This one is more thorough than the primary triage assessment and may include taking a blood pressure, pulse, and respiratory rate, and performing a rapid trauma assessment. This may result in recategorizing of the patient and removal to another treatment area. This is not uncommon as patient status is dynamic and can easily change as time goes by during an incident.

Supervisor duties, in addition to logging each patient's entry and exit, include assigning crews to care for patients, monitoring patient and provider safety, and assessing the need for additional resources. It is helpful to organize and cache medical supplies for the treatment sections in advance. Items should include such supplies as a multiple outlet oxygen supply,

Howard County DFRS

Treatment/Transportation Area Tracking Form

Date: _____ / _____ / _____   Incident: _____   Page _____ of _____

| TREATMENT AREA LOG | | | | | | | TRANSPORTATION AREA LOG | | |
| TREATMENT SUPERVISOR | | | | INTAKE COORDINATOR | | | TRANSPORT SUPERVISOR | COMMUNICATIONS | |
TIME IN	PT NAME	AGE	RACE	SEX	PT NUMBER (STICKER or "INITIALS + #")	TREATMENT AREA (CIRCLE)	TRANSPORTED BY UNIT	TRANSPORTED TO	TRANS TIME
	1					■ ■ ■ ■ 1 2 3 4			
	2					■ ■ ■ ■ 1 2 3 4			
	3					■ ■ ■ ■ 1 2 3 4			
	4					■ ■ ■ ■ 1 2 3 4			
	5					■ ■ ■ ■ 1 2 3 4			
	6					■ ■ ■ ■ 1 2 3 4			
	7					■ ■ ■ ■ 1 2 3 4			
	8					■ ■ ■ ■ 1 2 3 4			
	9					■ ■ ■ ■ 1 2 3 4			
	10					■ ■ ■ ■ 1 2 3 4			

Figure 50-23 An example of a patient flow worksheet form that could be used in the treatment area or the transportation area to track patient identification and flow.

oxygen masks, basic and advanced airway adjuncts, IV supplies and fluids, bandages, burn sheets, and spinal immobilization equipment.

Patients who have not yet been assigned a triage tag should be assigned one on entry into the treatment section. Any assessments and interventions that occur from this point forward should be documented on the triage tag. DOT 8.2-22, 8.2-26

The red, immediate, or "first priority" treatment area is the area where the most critically injured patients will be treated. It is also the first area that begins to receive nonambulatory patients from the triage crews who directed them to that location. Patients can benefit from the increased experience and expertise of physicians, and if the physicians are part of the jurisdictional EMS system, they can serve as on-site medical direction for EMS providers. DOT 8.2.16

The yellow, delayed, or "second priority" treatment area should be located in proximity to the red treatment area in order to facilitate sharing of equipment and resources. It will also usually require the assignment of ALS providers and equipment.

As time permits, the ambulatory patients should receive screening. Many of these patients have not been tagged with either tape or a triage tag because they walked out of the scene. An initial assignment by ALS providers should be performed on all these patients. The green, minor, or "third priority" treatment area will generally require only basic life support providers and supplies. The early designation of a treatment area for ambulatory patients, usually the nonurgent (green) area, is important. If this is not done quickly, the ambulatory patients will scatter and become difficult to locate. Some may even get into vehicles and drive away. While it may not sound like such a bad idea for nonurgent patients to get away from a multiple casualty scene, it becomes problematic when there has been a toxic exposure or poisoning (including food poisoning). They could be in need of decontamination, or as they develop symptoms, they could become sick while driving and create numerous emergency calls on area roads and highways. They could also spread the contaminating agent to others. DOT 8-2.23

In the case of hazardous materials exposure, gross decontamination of ambulatory patients with copious amounts of water can usually begin quickly. However, it may be necessary to designate an area for grossly decontaminated ambulatory patients to wait while further decontamination resources are set up. Choose an area that is somewhat sheltered, if possible. This area is best located immediately in front of the treatment areas, so patients can be moved quickly from one area to the other. Care must be taken to prevent cross contamination. Providers should not move between the established zones during the incident unless directed to do so.

CONNECTIONS   Chapter 53: Hazardous Materials Incidents discusses common duties and responsibilities of medical personnel present on hazmat scenes.

The black, expectant, or "fourth priority" treatment area sometimes also functions as a morgue. However, if the triage plan in effect classifies catastrophically wounded patients to this area, ALS resources with the ability to administer analgesics should be assigned. The manager of this area may need to work closely with the jurisdictional medical examiner, coroner, and law enforcement. Screening should be set up to allow patients as much privacy as possible. A separate area may also be set up near this area to allow family members to have private time with loved ones. Law enforcement should be present, particularly if the incident will be investigated for criminal activity. DOT 8.2-13

Working in the Gray Zone

Working with expectant patients can be very difficult emotionally for EMS providers who are used to providing maximum resuscitative efforts in managing patients. The National Disaster Management System, or NDMS, is another federal program that will work closely within the NIMS ICS structure during a national disaster. The NDMS provides for the mobilization of special teams called Disaster Mortuary Operational Response Teams, or DMORTs. The members of these DMORTs are typically better equipped emotionally to work with the dead patients, but they may also not be well equipped to work with dying patients. Make sure mental health professionals are available for any rescuer exhibiting stress from working in the disaster zone.

Transportation Group

One goal in the management of any multiple casualty incident is to get patients to definitive care as quickly as possible. Determining how and to which medical facility patients will be transported is accomplished within the transportation area. Communication with area medical facilities is established, and a determination is made as to their capacity for receiving patients. It is also important to determine which type of patient can be transported to the facility. For example, a hospital may not be able to handle a large number of contaminated patients.

Air and land resources must also be coordinated. A staging area for patient transportation resources may need to be established (Figure 50-24). Helispots may be required. Finally, patients must be physically moved to a transport unit. DOT 8.2-13

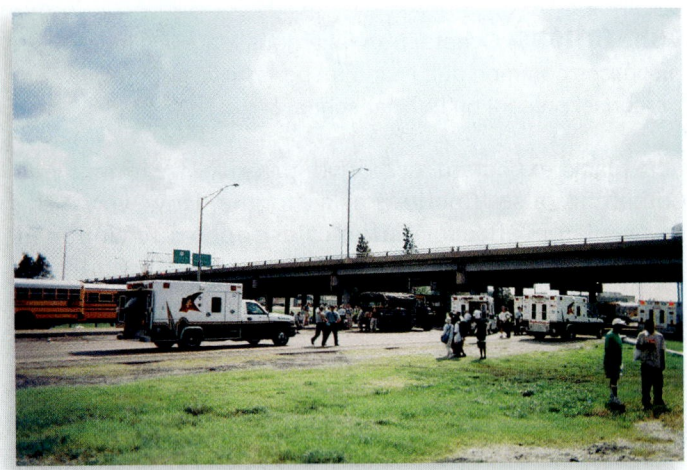

Figure 50-24   One of the transportation areas for victims of Hurricane Katrina. © Acadian Ambulance Serria/Dr. Chuck Burnell, photographer.

Transportation resources may consist of agency ambulances, mutual aid ambulances, private ambulances, medical and nonmedical helicopters, airplanes, and even passenger vehicles or buses for certain ambulatory patients. If possible, the transportation area should be close to the treatment areas. Additional needs include easy access, both into and out of this area, for transportation vehicles, and a means to communicate with area medical facilities.

The transportation area supervisor must assign workers under their command to supervise communications and patient disposition (in other words, to track their destination). For most incidents, patients can be moved directly from the treatment areas into transport units. However, if the incident size dictates a separate transportation area, there should be a single point of entry, and each patient entry should be logged. Additional duties of the transportation area supervisor include advising the treatment areas when transportation is available and for what type of patient, requesting transport units from the staging area, coordinating patient loading, and ensuring the ongoing medical monitoring of patients who are staged within the area.

The worker designated to coordinate transportation communications should quickly establish communication with area medical facilities. Area facilities should be advised of the incident and number of patients and their general mechanisms of injury. They should be updated as the incident progresses and informed when it is over. The communications coordinator should generate a written log, indicating the number and type of patients that each medical facility is capable of receiving and then immediately communicate this to an individual coordinating patient disposition. DOT 8.2-13, 8-2.24, 8.2-25

The individual coordinating patient disposition ultimately determines to what destination a patient will be transported. Once the patient is loaded, the transport unit should communicate with the disposition coordinator, so the patient number, name, and receiving facility can be logged.

It is beneficial if a one-way flow of vehicle traffic can be established up to and away from the transport site. The transportation group supervisor should be kept in the loop of communications between the workers supervising transportation and disposition, and should be updated frequently on the activities by these two workers. DOT 8.2-23, 8.2-24

Extrication or Rescue Group

For incidents where there are difficult extrication or rescue operations, a separate division, group, or even a branch may be established by the IC or operations section chief. The director or supervisor of a branch, division, or group should ensure the safety of personnel and work closely with the patient care teams in the planning and implementation of any extrication or rescue. Unique or specialized rescues could require the use of specially trained personnel and could require special vehicles and equipment. Units, strike teams, or task forces may be called in to perform heavy lifting operations, to provide structural integrity during the operation, or to perform other duties as assigned. DOT 8.2-13, 8.2-14

Summary

The national incident management system and incident command system are designed to establish order, maintain worker safety, and ensure that resources are allocated properly. In order for these systems to work, all of the participants need to understand the structure and function of the systems. It is important to understand the basic NIMS and ICS principles as well as the terminology used for the various sections within the ICS structure. Paramedics should participate in planning and exercises that will ensure familiarity with ICS principles. Once an incident occurs, the ICS structure needs to be implemented early. It is important for paramedics to understand that if they arrive first on the scene, their actions can help to assure the success of the operation.

Notes

1. National Wildfire Coordinating Group, "Incident Command System National Training," *Curriculum* (1994), http://www.NIMSonline.com/ics_training_docs/ICS_history.pdf (accessed June 6, 2005).

2. National Fire Service Incident Management System Consortium Model Procedures Committee, *Model Procedures Guide for Structural Firefighting*, 2nd ed. (Stillwater, OK: Fire Protection Publications, Oklahoma State University, 2000).

3. The White House of the United States of America, "Homeland Security Presidential Directive HSPD-5: Management of Domestic Incidents" (February 28, 2003), http://www.NIMSonline.com/docs/hspd-5.pdf (accessed June 30, 2005).

4. The White House of the United States of America, "Homeland Security Presidential Directive HSPD-8: National Preparedness" (December 17, 2003), http://www.NIMSonline.com/docs/hspd-8.pdf (accessed June 30, 2005).

5. J. T. Mitchell and H. L. P. Resnik, *Emergency Response to Crisis* (Upper Saddle River, NJ: Prentice-Hall, 1986).

6. U.S. Department of Homeland Security, "National Incident Management System" (2004), http://www.dhs.gov/interweb/assetlibrary/NIMS-90-web.pdf (accessed April 28, 2005).

7. American College of Surgeons, *Advanced Trauma Life Support Instructor Manual*, 6th ed. (Chicago, IL: American College of Surgeons, 1977).

8. E. K. Noji and G. D. Kelen, "Disaster Medical Services." In *Emergency Medicine: A Comprehensive Study Guide,* J. E. Tintinalli, G. D. Kelen, and J. S. Stapczynski, eds. (New York, NY: McGraw-Hill, 2004).

9. G. Super, S. Groth, R. Hook, et al., *START: Simple Triage and Rapid Treatment Plan* (Newport Beach, CA: Hoag Memorial Presbyterian Hospital, 1994).

10. L. E. Romig, "JumpSTART Pediatric Triage Tool" (2001), http://www.jumpstarttriage.com/TheJumpSTARTAlgorithm.html (accessed June 30, 2005).

chapter
51

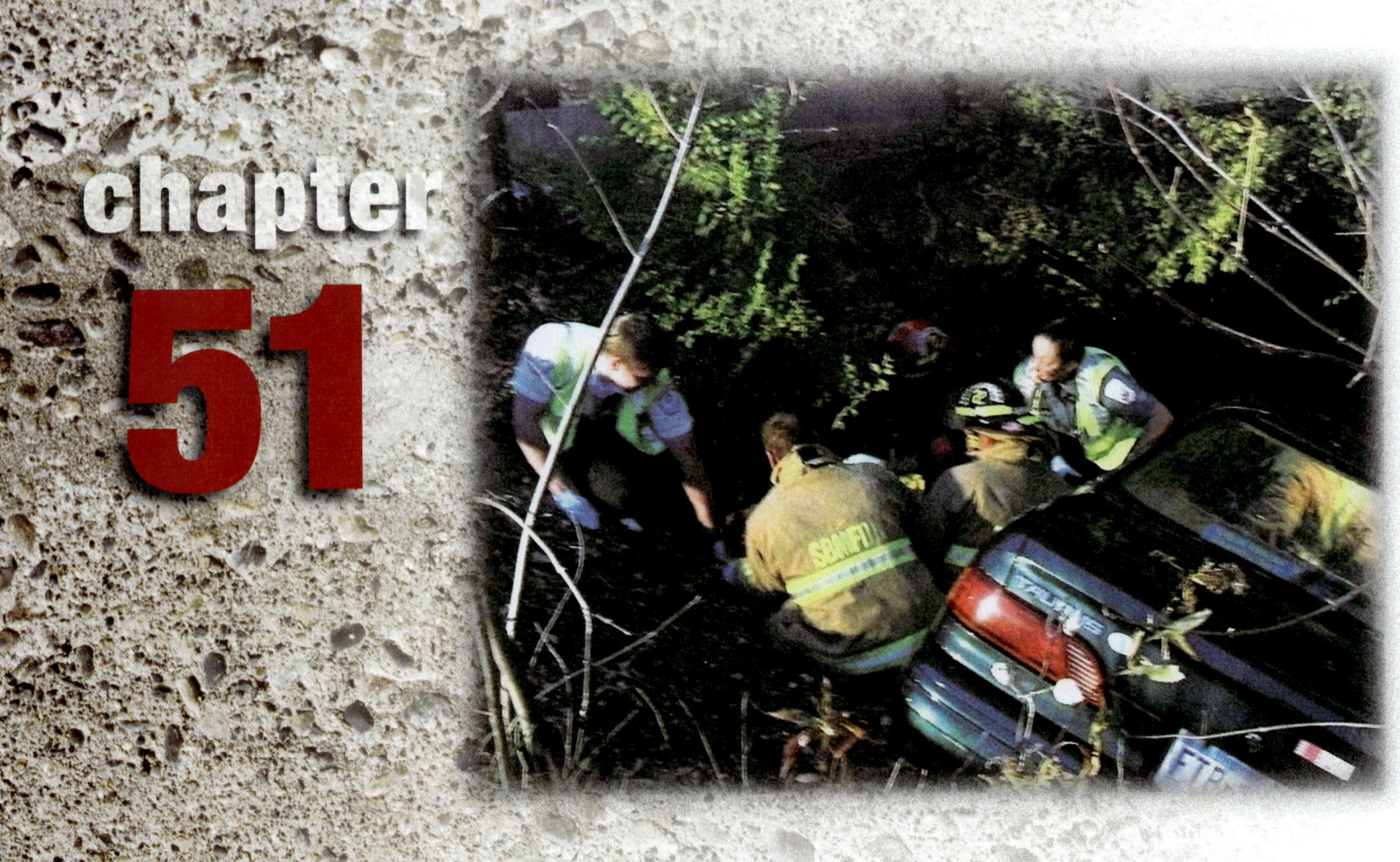

Rescue Awareness

"**C**ourage is not the absence of fear, but rather the judgment that something else is more important than fear."

—Ambrose Redmoon

Need To Know

▶ Safety is the first concern at rescue operations; this includes scene safety as well as crew safety, bystander safety, and patient safety.

▶ In most cases, specially trained technicians will perform the rescue while granting access to paramedics to provide care, or they will deliver the patient to the paramedic as soon as the patient is extricated from the hazard.

▶ Protective clothing appropriate to the rescue situation should be worn.

▶ Water rescue presents specific hazards including dangers beneath the surface of flat water and moving water.

▶ Water rescue requires specialized training and even with that training, actually going into the water is the last resort.

▶ A variety of hazards, including fire, chemical, and environmental, call for special technicians to secure the environment before patient contact can be made.

▶ Typical vehicle construction and methods for removing patients from crashed vehicles.

▶ The special hazards presented by hybrid vehicles.

▶ The challenges of high- and low-angle rescue.

▶ The extreme dangers present in trench rescue operations.

▶ The variety of specialty rescue stretchers and winching systems available for rescue operations.

▶ Do	▶ Ask
• Wear protective clothing appropriate to the operation. • Become familiar with operations employed by rescue teams you will be working with. • Evaluate all scenes for possible hazards. • Call for help (additional resources) if you are the first on the scene of a rescue situation. • Enter scenes only after specialists have instructed you that it is safe to enter. • Practice securing patients for movement over uneven terrain.	• Ask fire and rescue personnel if the scene has been made safe. • Ask dispatch for any information they may have about the scene while en route. • Question your supervisors and administrators about the rescue resources available to you. • Learn about equipment that might be available on other vehicles. • Request guidance and assistance when moving patients in difficult situations.

Introduction

The Webster's Dictionary's definition of rescue is "to free from confinement, danger, or evil." The two key words are confinement and danger. Most calls for EMS providers involve being able to immediately access and treat the patient in a fairly controlled environment. However, in a rescue situation this is usually not the case. In the rescue scenario, there will be medical procedures and mechanical extrication techniques being performed, often simultaneously. Paramedics, along with the other responders responsible for rescue efforts, must be able to deal effectively with the varied situations that can occur. For medical providers in the prehospital setting, an understanding of rescue is a must if they are to operate safely while involved in the rescue scenario. DOT 8-3.1, 8-3.2

Working in the Gray Zone

Rescue technician training is beyond the scope of the entry level training program for most paramedics. This chapter provides an overview, or awareness, of the concepts of rescue only. It **does not** enable you to perform rescue operations. Paramedics should not attempt rescue operations until they have taken additional specialty training as directed by their jurisdiction or agency. Paramedics who have not received specialty training may be able to work in a safe zone, receive patients directly from rescuers, or assess rescuers who are entering and exiting the work zone for fitness to perform rescue operations.

General Considerations

Incident Command System

Most, if not all, rescue calls involve complicated and dangerous situations, potentially requiring specialized equipment and personnel resources. As with anything the paramedic encounters, provider and patient safety is paramount. Thus, a formal incident management system like the incident command system (ICS) as specified by the National Incident Management System (NIMS) should be used on every rescue call. All responders to a rescue call should be familiar with the components and terminology of the ICS. The use of the ICS accomplishes three basic things: command, control, and coordination. Today, a standardized ICS system is required by the National Incident Management System. Moreover, the use of an ICS system in rescue helps to accomplish the cornerstone of any rescue call: safety.[1,2]

CONNECTIONS Refer to Chapter 50: Medical Incident Command for more information on NIMS and the ICS.

The Role of the Paramedic as a Medical Provider

The paramedic is a very important member of the team in the rescue setting. You will be directly responsible for the assessment and care of the patient during this process. You may also be tasked with assessing the vital signs and general fitness for duty of the team members working with the patient. To work effectively in these stressful environments, you need to be in good physical condition. You should determine ahead of time if you are able and willing to perform in these conditions. If you feel you cannot adequately care for a patient in these circumstances, you should alert your team members so that someone else can provide care to the patient. DOT 8-3.3

Assessment and Treatment Modifications to Fit the Environment

Entrapped Patients

The assessment and care of patients in the rescue environment will sometimes have to be modified to fit the circumstance (Figure 51-1). For instance, you may not be able to access all parts of an entrapped patient. This will limit your ability to assess and care for all life-threatening injuries that may be present. It may be difficult to control bleeding. The condition of the patient may dictate, to a certain extent, how the extrication process is approached. For example, it may be necessary to rapidly remove a patient from an unstable environment without ensuring that spinal precautions are established. DOT 8-3.35

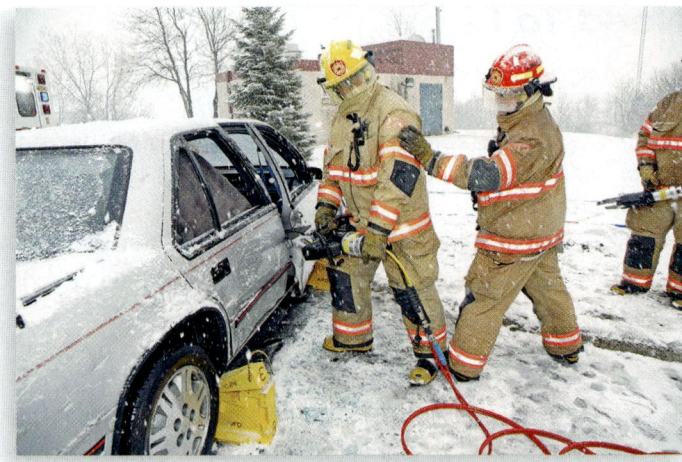

Figure 51-1 EMS crew extracting an entrapped victim from a crashed car. Note that the car has been stabilized.

Weather

Often you will have to operate in extreme weather situations. You will have to balance the need to protect the patient from the elements with the need to provide adequate assessment and treatment (Figure 51-2). DOT 8-3.39

Remote Locations

In remote locations, your regular equipment may not be sufficient to meet the patient's needs. You should carefully consider the equipment that you might require and whether it can be carried with some ease. It is a good idea to keep an "off-road" or wilderness pack of basic equipment for remote locations (see Box 51-1).

During the removal of a patient from a remote location, perform periodic reassessments to assure there

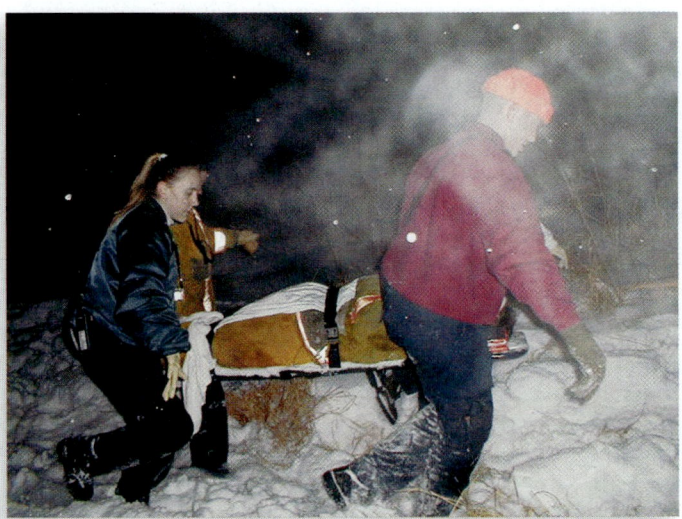

Figure 51-2 Balancing the need for treatment versus protecting a patient from the elements can be difficult.

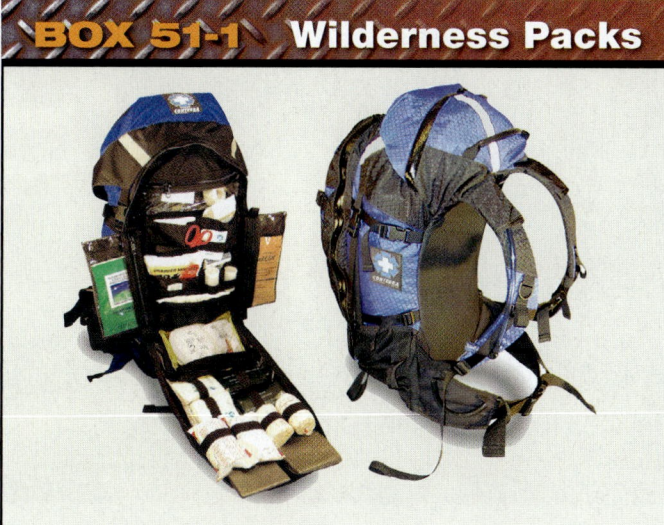

BOX 51-1   Wilderness Packs

- Triangular bandages
- 2-inch adhesive tape
- Band-Aids
- Oral airways
- Assorted sterile compresses
- Pocket knife
- Paramedic shears
- Rubber gloves
- Pocket mask
- Instant glucose
- SAM™ splint
- Blood glucose test strips DOT 8-3.36
- Epi-Pen™ and diphenhydramine

have not been any changes. The emphasis should be on BLS skills and maintaining the patient's ABCs. Remember, you may be with the patient for hours or even days in a remote location, and you have to plan accordingly. Carrying food and shelter may be as important in these circumstances as carrying medical supplies.

Improvised Patient Care

You may have to improvise and alter the treatment of your patient to fit an extended care scenario. For example, you may have to splint a patient's injured leg by tying it to the uninjured leg.

Street Secrets

Remember, newspapers and magazines can be used for splints, and coats on wooden sticks or tree branches can make a stretcher. Improvising in these situations calls for making the best use of what is available to you.

Patients who are entrapped for long periods of time may need on-scene pain management. Specialty teams may be required to perform surgical amputations in order to free an entrapped patient. Other long-term care requiring improvisation might include the following:[3] DOT 8-3.37, 8-3.38, 8-3.41

- Repositioning or reducing dislocations
- Cleansing and care of wounds, including suturing
- Removing impaled objects
- Rewarming the patient
- Treating crush injuries
- Terminating resuscitative efforts

CONNECTIONS Pain management is discussed in detail in Chapter 15: Pharmacology and Chapter 24: Skeletal Trauma.

Protective Equipment

Head Protection

Your choice of a protective helmet should be suited to your task. In general, the interior of all helmets should have a four-point harness system. This system is designed to withstand a greater force of impact and will provide greater protection than construction-type helmets. DOT 8-3.5

Most fire helmets that comply with National Fire Protection Association (NFPA) standards serve well in vehicle rescue situations. However, these can be cumbersome and are not recommended for use in other specialized environments such as rope work, confined space work, or swift water rescue. There are helmets that are lighter and smaller in size and are specifically designed for such applications. No matter which helmet you choose, it has to meet all applicable regulations and standards of the Occupational Safety and Health Administration (OSHA), American National Standards Institute (ANSI), or the NFPA (Figure 51-3).

Face Protection

Proper face protection usually includes some form of goggles or a helmet face shield. Goggles should be ANSI approved and should provide both front and side protection from flying objects. Remember, because they are designed with open sides, face shields on most helmets will not provide complete protection for the rescuer in the event of flying glass or other objects. Goggles should always be worn in addition to the face shield when there is the potential for flying debris.

Hearing Protection

Hearing protection comes in the form of either ear plugs or earmuffs. The primary factor in selecting this protection is practicality related to the application and

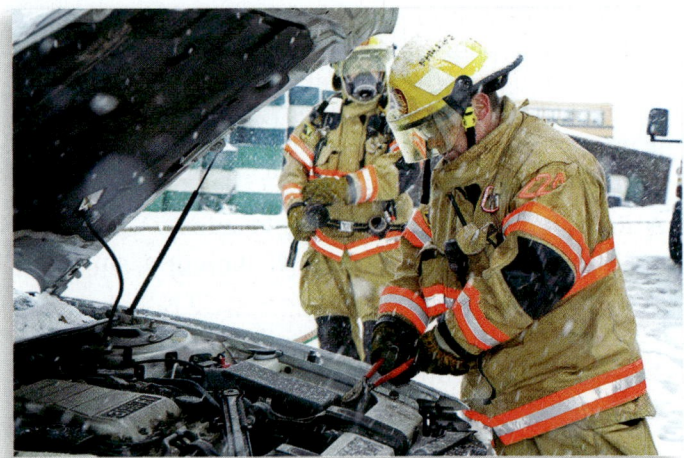

Figure 51-3 Full protective gear should be worn during any extrication activity. Note that the firefighter in the background has a charged line and is standing by in case any extrication activity ignites a fire.

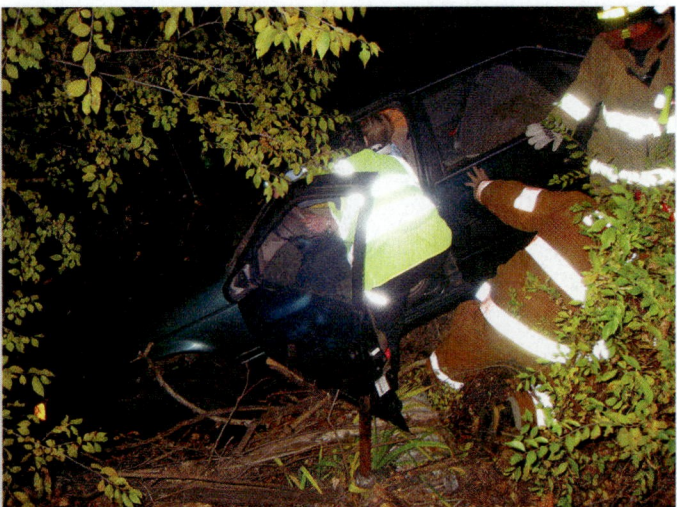

Figure 51-4 Wearing high visibility protective clothing is SOP for most departments.

convenience for the rescuer. For instance, earplugs with an attached band can easily be hung around the neck when not needed.

Respiratory Protection

The N-95 masks used for normal respiratory protection or commercial-grade dust masks will provide sufficient protection in most situations. However, it is imperative to remember that these masks will not provide protection in toxic or oxygen-deficient environments such as those found during confined space rescue.

It is also important to read the accompanying literature for the mask to determine the amount of time the mask will provide protection. Many masks cease to function after approximately 30 minutes of continuous use. As moisture collects from exhaled air, the filters become saturated with water and the masks lose effectiveness.

Body Protection

Body protection comes in the form of suitable clothing to protect the torso and extremities from sharp edges, flames, or flashes of heated air or liquid. Structural firefighting gear (or turnouts) has traditionally filled this role but is cumbersome and can be exhausting for responders to wear in hot weather. Today, lightweight jumpsuits of special material can serve in place of turnout gear in some circumstances. All protective gear should be made of a flame-retardant material such as Nomex™ or PBI® if there is a risk of fire or explosions.

The protective clothing should be highly visible for nighttime operations (Figure 51-4). Departments should have standing operating procedures (SOPs) in place that mandate the use of acceptable reflective materials that ensure optimal visibility of personnel in dark

conditions. Calls involving motor vehicle accidents where responders will interact with hazards such as those found on streets and highways call for high-visibility protective clothing.

Leather and porous materials such as cotton cannot be decontaminated, but they may be able to be cleansed of certain materials like dirt and soot. It is important to clean contaminated protective clothing as recomended by the manufacturer. Clothing that is heavily soiled or contaminated with certain substances such as hazardous materials must be properly disposed of and replaced.

Hand Protection

Wear gloves to protect your hands. This sounds simple enough, but the responder must remember that there are gloves made for specific purposes. Heavy insulated gloves, such as firefighting gloves, are suitable for vehicle extrication because they provide protection from punctures and cuts by sharp objects. During rope operations, a leather glove that is softer, lighter, and protects the hands from chafing by the rope while still allowing the rescuer to feel the rope is suitable. It is important to choose gloves appropriate for the task.

Foot Protection

For situations where there are sharp edges or where falling objects could be encountered, a boot that is steel-toed and steel-shanked (for ankle and arch support) will provide ample protection from cuts and punctures. Additionally, boots should have a sturdy sole that provides good traction. If the rescue is in a remote area that will involve varied terrain, a boot that is lighter and provides better support for the ankle is preferable.

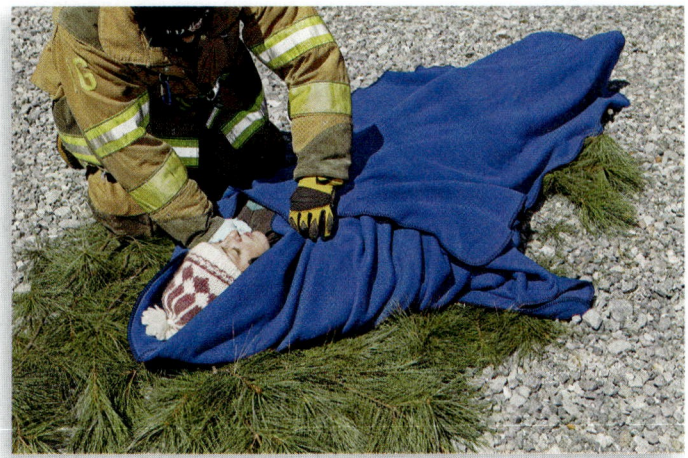

Figure 51-5 Patients should be covered to protect them from the elements. If feasible, place a barrier (such as these pine boughs) between the patient and the ground to provide comfort and warmth.

Patient Protection

It is important to remember that if the rescuer needs protection, the patient often will need some of the same protective equipment, such as helmets, eye protection, hearing protection, shielding, and thermal protection in cold environments (Figure 51-5). Observation shows that rescuers are very good at remembering their own safety but often are less attentive to the patient for whom they are caring.[4] Remember the objective of any rescue call is to do no further harm to either the rescuers or the patient being rescued. DOT 8-3.5

Phases of Rescue Operations

Rescue operations typically have five phases:

- Assessing the scene (or the scene size-up), which includes hazard identification and abatement
- Gaining access to the patient to begin assessment and treatment
- Disentangling the patient from the environment
- Removing the patient from the environment
- Providing emergency care and transport of the patient to a facility capable of providing definitive care DOT 8-3.4

Assessment of the Scene Via the Scene Size-Up

The first phase of any potential rescue call begins when the call comes into dispatch, not when the responders arrive on the scene. Although not always successful in obtaining information, the dispatch center will attempt to determine the nature of the incident, the potential number of patients involved, and any associated hazards.

The first crew to arrive should establish the incident command system (ICS) and begin initial triage if there are no hazards that would prevent this. Additionally, the initial incident commander (IC) should begin to assess the need for additional resources and notify the dispatch center of the initial findings. The initial report should include a basic summary of the incident and the environment, the number and position of patients, hazards found, and the need for any additional specialized resources.

Proper identification of the type of rescue needed and the timely request for appropriate resources are critical to a positive outcome for the patient. Now is not the time for jurisdictional squabbles concerning who is in charge or who should perform what aspect of the rescue. Assignment of resources should be based on technical expertise and specialty, not specific agency association. It is important to know the types of resources available in your response area. Also, it is important to understand the amount of time that it will take to get each resource to the incident. Remember that it is always better to request more resources than you anticipate needing. Any personnel or equipment not needed for your incident can be canceled. DOT 8-3.4

Hazard Identification and Abatement

Prior to any attempt to access and treat the patient, all known and potential hazards must be identified and controlled. It is important to remember that you may not be able to control all of the hazards present. For instance, if you encounter fumes indicating a hazardous materials incident, it would be prudent to back away, begin to isolate the incident site, and call for a hazardous materials team. Additional hazards such as gas leaks, explosive devices, downed electrical lines, and radioactive materials will require specialized resources beyond your capabilities.

When hazards are identified that are beyond your ability to handle, the most important thing to do is to ensure the safety of the arriving responders and bystanders in the area. This is accomplished by establishing a safe zone or perimeter that is outside of the hazard zone. If there are bystanders or individuals on the scene who are not following your instructions, make sure law enforcement is on the way to help control the scene. Emotions can run high during this time, and it may take law enforcement presence to ensure people respect the boundaries that have been established.

CONNECTIONS Chapter 53: Hazardous Materials Incidents has additional information on operating within a hazardous materials scene.

The environment in which you are working must be evaluated for hazards. Low light conditions and night-time darkness offer hazards as do low visibility conditions such as fog. Weather is always a factor in outdoor and even some indoor EMS responses. Be aware of any adverse conditions in the area in which you are operating such as lightning, hail, rain, snow, and ice. Often weather conditions will greatly impact the ability of the rescue personnel to operate safely and effectively. Other hazards include incidents that occur on highways and the traffic that may be present during rescue operations. Finally, if you are operating in remote locations, always be aware of the possibility of a vertical slope, rock slides, mud slides in rainy weather, cave-ins around trenches, and avalanches if there is snow present in mountainous areas.

Gaining Access to the Patient

Once all noted hazards are satisfactorily controlled, you can begin to formulate a plan to access the patient. Your ICS should already be in place by this point, and all the on-scene responders should be briefed as to everyone's specific responsibility. The briefing should be formal and should include all key personnel involved in the rescue operation.

This now begins the technical phase of your rescue operations. The personnel involved should be trained in rescue procedures and should be adept at the technical rescue skills being employed. All safety equipment should be in place, and all safety procedures should be followed. A scene safety officer should be designated, and this individual along with the rescue crew, should perform a quick inspection to ensure that the operation can still proceed. During the process of gaining access to your patient you should always be aware of any changes in the conditions around you and the patient. Should any safety concerns arise, it is always best to stop operations and address these immediately. The safety officer may also call a halt to the operation, even in the middle of performing a step, if a safety hazard is identified. This individual has absolute authority to stop a task in progress, so all crew members should be alert to the safety officer's commands.

Once the patient is accessed, the rescue team will determine if it is safe for an EMS provider to enter the scene. If it is and the EMS provider is wearing the appropriate protective clothing, the EMS provider will be given access to the patient. If it is not safe to enter, or the scene is unstable or dangerous, the initial assessment will likely be performed by the rescue crew, and a report of patient status will be relayed to the paramedic. The EMS crew will then be directed to wait in a designated area to receive the patient once the disentanglement phase is finished and the patient is removed from the environment.

Disentanglement of the Patient

This phase of rescue involves releasing the patient from the mechanism of entrapment, such as a wrecked vehicle, a collapsed structure, a trench, or a confined space. It can also involve removal of the patient from a dangerous height, side of a cliff or structure, or other position from which the patient cannot be easily removed.

The first phase of disentanglement is referred to as gaining access. The idea is for the rescue specialists to gain access to the patient for the paramedics. Paramedics may actually be able to get into the space to care for the patient while the vehicle is removed from around them. At the very least, access for some patient care should be provided as soon as possible, particularly in extended extrication situations.

Patient access and care will often take place simultaneously with the disentanglement process (Figure 51-6). For example, you might be assigned to assess and care for a patient during vehicle extrication. You cannot enter the scene unless you are wearing the appropriate safety clothing. You must be prepared to operate in the confined and noisy work environment. You may be covered up with a blanket or other protective covering and may stay with the patient during the rescue procedure. You will need to remain calm and reassure the patient throughout the process. Explaining to the patient what is occurring as the operation proceeds can provide reassurance and help keep the patient calm.

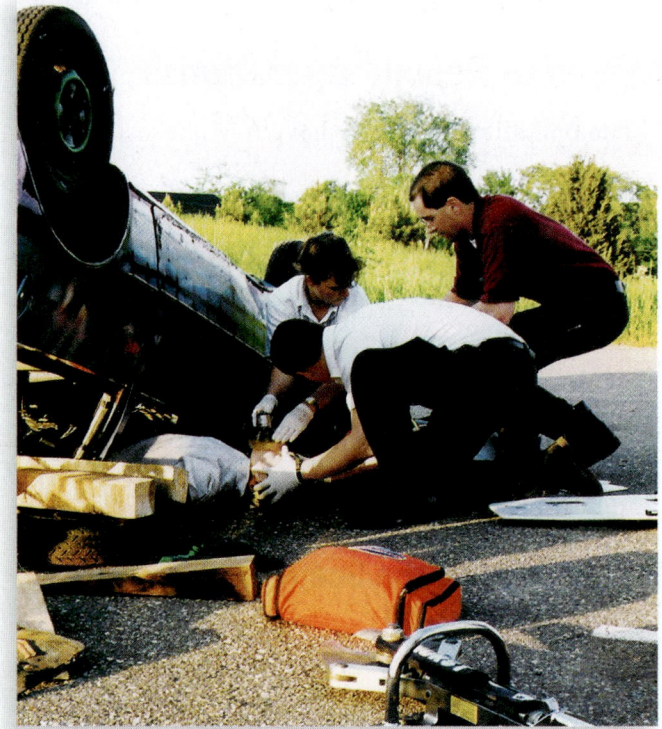

Figure 51-6 Paramedics treating a patient who is entangled in his vehicle.

Working in the Gray Zone

Paramedics providing emergency care have an obligation to wear the appropriate safety clothing and use the correct safety gear and equipment when they are in the rescue environment. If the rescue crew or fire department is wearing helmets, turnouts, ear protection, and gloves, the EMS crew should be dressed in a similar manner. Protect the patient as much as possible during the rescue and disentanglement process. Remain by the patient's side and provide comfort and reassurance as long as your presence does not interfere with the rescue operation. Tell the patient what is happening, and provide reassurance that the patient will be out of the environment as soon as possible.

During the process of disentanglement, you must constantly assess the safety situation for yourself and for the responders and patient. There must be a balance between patient care and the mechanical operations taking place to free the patient. Sometimes rescue operations will have to be stopped in order for you to properly care for the patient. An example would be if you need to perform suction to keep the airway clear. Effective and coordinated communications among all personnel involved in this process is essential.

Patient Packaging and Removal

This phase of the rescue can often be one of the most time-consuming tasks to accomplish. If you are operating in a remote environment or on a vertical slope, you must be prepared to care for the patient for an extended period of time. It is important to have a coordinated effort from all responders to design a plan for removing the patient to a transport unit. Decisions will have to be made regarding ground transportation, air transportation, or carryout by the rescue team members. Factors such as availability of insertion sites for helicopter rescue teams, distance to available transportation, and the condition of the patient should all be considered. Remember the goal is to present the patient to a definitive care facility safely in as short a time as possible.

Vehicle Rescue

Paramedics respond to vehicle crashes far more frequently than any other type of rescue situation, and vehicle rescue can be one of the most hazardous kinds of rescue. Highway operations must be approached in a systematic manner, just as any other rescue scenario would. Considerations specific to operating around moving traffic must be accounted for. It is important for paramedics to understand scene hazards, vehicle anatomy, basic initial stabilization techniques, and basic entry techniques for gaining access to patients.

Scene Hazards

There are many hazards associated with a response to a traffic accident. You must be able to recognize these issues and understand the methods used to reduce the danger. Below is a list of the basic hazards involved in motor vehicle crashes:

- *Traffic.* This is an inherent danger when working at a motor vehicle crash scene. You will often find yourself working on busy streets or interstate highways. There are several things that you can do to reduce this hazard:
  - *Vehicle placement.* You should place traffic cones in a manner that will divert traffic away from the area in which the rescue crews are working. This includes removing traffic from the area where ambulances are being loaded with patients (Figure 51-7).
  - *Scene lighting.* Too many emergency lights on a scene are just as bad as no lights. It is recommended that all vehicle headlights be turned off. At night, if you have access to high wattage light towers, take advantage of them. Extra lighting can also be obtained by strategic parking of the ambulance and using the scene lights on the side of the vehicle.
  - *Reflective clothing.* During both daytime and nighttime operations, you should wear a reflective vest or other uniform apparel with reflective tape sewn on the garment.
  - *Cones and flares.* These can be used to direct traffic away from your working area. Use caution with flares; they can ignite gasoline vapors. DOT 8-3.20, 8-3.21

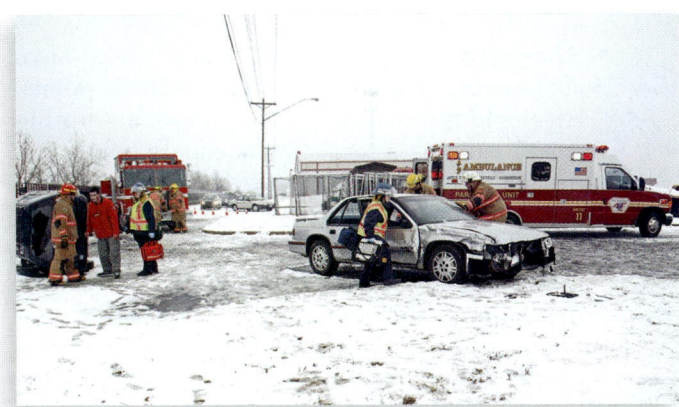

Figure 51-7 Place the ambulance and other rescue vehicles so that traffic is diverted from the scene.

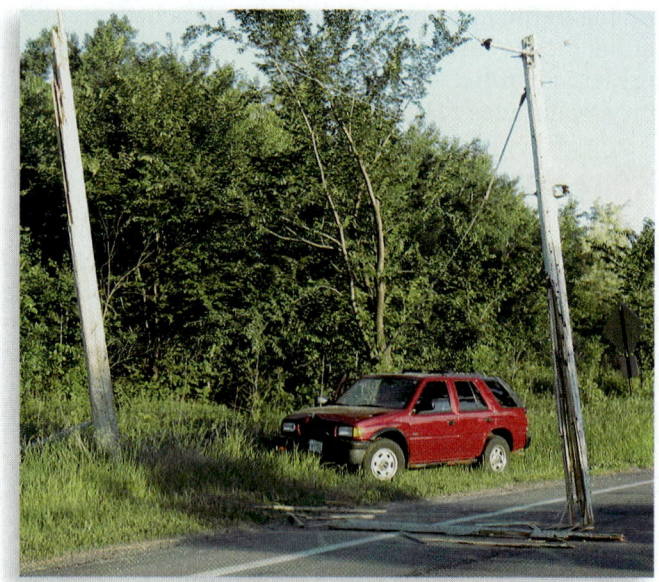

Figure 51-8 Never approach a vehicle in contact with power lines.

■ *Other hazards.*   Other common hazards related to vehicle crash scenes include the following:

• *Electrical hazards.* These can come in the form of downed electrical lines, broken utility poles, or ground-mounted electrical boxes (Figure 51-8). You should never attempt to approach a vehicle when there are downed lines of any sort. Always assume that they are live until the power company arrives and assesses the situation. This is true even if the downed lines are motionless as they can still be energized. The other not-so-obvious hazard is the ground-mounted electrical box. You will find some locations where these boxes are low enough for a vehicle to come to rest on top of one. Always be aware of this possibility when approaching an accident scene. If you suspect that the vehicle is in contact with a ground-mounted electrical box, do not approach it. Request the power company to assist you. DOT 8-3.25

• *Aboveground gas mains.* Many areas have aboveground natural gas mains or transfer points. A vehicle can override one of these, disrupting it and causing a leak. If this occurs, never approach the gas main directly; stage your vehicle a safe distance away in case of fire or explosion. It is easy to miss a gas line if the crashed vehicle is resting directly on top of it.

• *Bystanders.* Bystanders may not seem like much of a risk, but should a crowd form in the area of an accident, they can become a hindrance to safety and effective operations (Figure 51-9). Well-intentioned bystanders can get in the way or become injured by wandering into traffic.

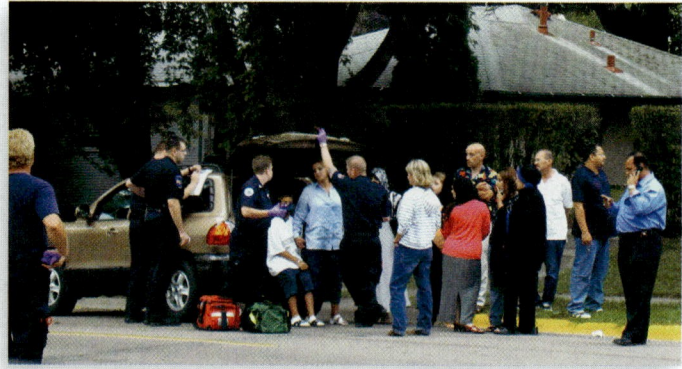

Figure 51-9 Bystanders can be a hindrance.

Crowds have also been known to turn hostile toward responders. This can happen if the incident occurs close to a family member's home and the family comes to the scene. While these issues do not usually come to the forefront, it is always prudent to be aware that this could become a concern at any rescue scene.

Vehicle Hazards

There are many vehicle hazards, and paramedics must have at least an awareness of them when responding to accident scenes: DOT 8-3.22

■ *Fuel leaks.* Be very careful when operating around a vehicle when a fuel leak is suspected. Notify fire officials immediately so that fire suppression measures can be taken in the event of a fire. Never park your vehicle in the area of a fuel leak or downhill from crashed vehicles. Finally, ensure that no bystanders are smoking in the area.

■ *Catalytic converters.* Any vehicle produced since 1970 will have this piece of equipment on it. These operate at very high temperatures and can be very hazardous to responders should there be a fuel leak. Do not drive your ambulance over or through a puddle of spilled fuel as this can ignite a fire. They can also cause severe burns should you come into contact with one on an overturned vehicle.

■ *Stored energy.* Energy is stored when a motor vehicle crash occurs and metal and other components on a vehicle are altered. Stress is put on metal as it is bent out of shape and then held in place by other bent pieces of the vehicle. The release of this stored energy occurs during the extrication process when components of the vehicle, such as a door, are opened or removed. When the tension is released from a door it can cause a sudden movement. As the crumpled metal springs back toward its original shape, it quickly releases the stored energy. This explosion of energy can injure anyone who happens to be in the way. Always be aware of your surroundings when working in the action area during an extrication process.

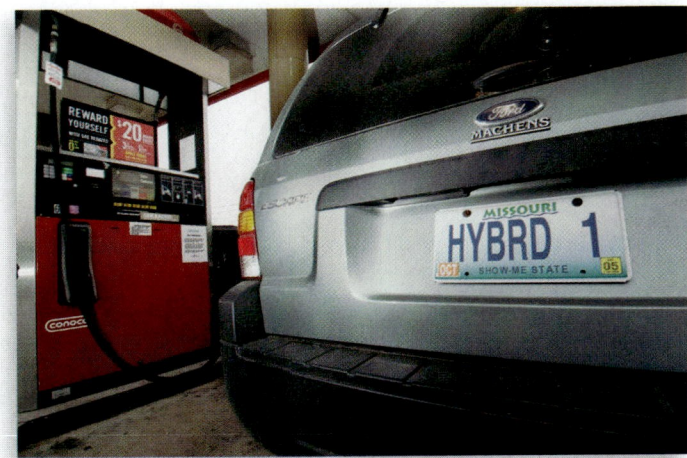

Figure 51-10 Hybrid gas/electric vehicles pose specific threats. Many more vehicles today are being manufactured using high voltage electrical systems along with conventional fuels or alternative fuels such as natural gas or hydrogen. These gasses are stored in high pressure cylinders and can pose a significant threat to responders if they are involved in a fire.

- *Alternative fuel systems.* Many more vehicles today are being manufactured using high-voltage electrical systems along with conventional fuels or alternative fuels such as natural gas or hydrogen. These gasses are stored in high-pressure cylinders and can pose a significant threat to responders if a fire occurs (Figure 51-10). Hybrid gas or electric vehicles also pose specific threats. Batteries, which are frequently located under the back seats, and high-voltage cables running along the outer edges of the floorboards can cause significant discharge of electricity if breeched (Figure 51-11). Cables can run inside the car frame along the door posts

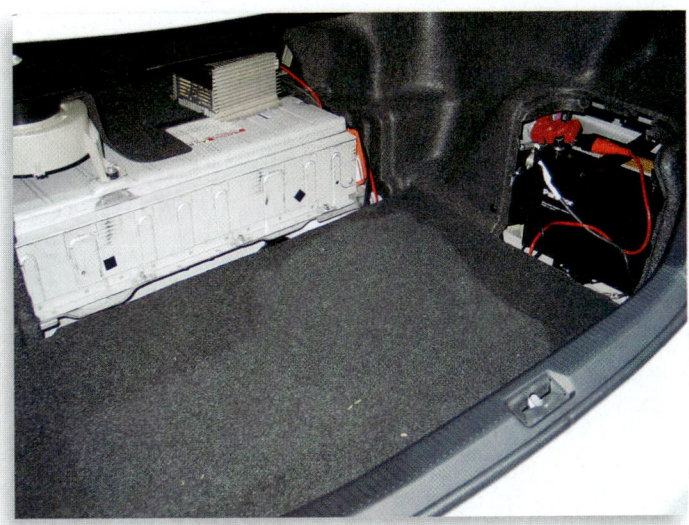

Figure 51-11 The battery compartment is in the trunk of this hybrid car.

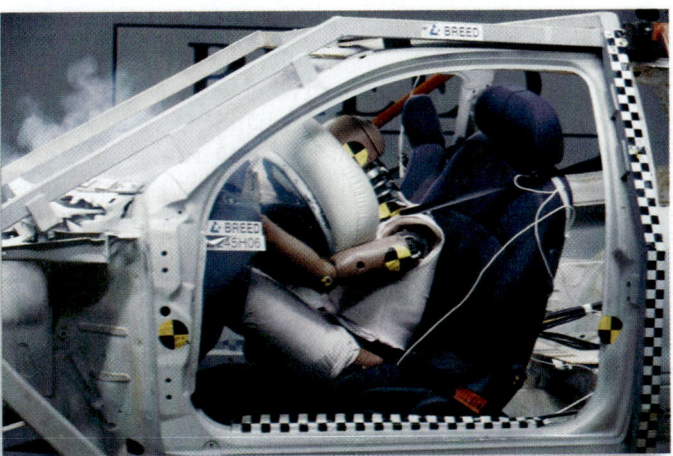

Figure 51-12 Undeployed airbags pose a significant threat.

as well, so care must be taken when cutting apart the car.

- *Airbag systems.* When this type of restraint system first arrived in vehicles, it came in the form of a single bag stored in the steering wheel column. Today, airbag restraint systems are becoming more and more complicated. Currently, there are vehicles with as many as 13 separate airbags located in the dashboard, door frames, and even the roof of the car (Figure 51-12). If the airbags are still undeployed, they can cause severe injury or even death to a rescuer who is directly in the path of one that unexpectedly deploys. Airbag systems must be deactivated prior to the disentanglement phase of the extrication process. This is usually accomplished by disconnecting the battery. **DOT 8-3.28**

- *Energy-absorbing bumpers.* These bumpers are designed to withstand a slow speed impact by utilizing a piston-like mechanism to absorb the impact and return the bumper to its original position. Sometimes these bumpers become loaded (they move in towards the vehicle) but do not return to their original position. Studies have shown that the risk of a sudden release is small; however, it is always wise to recognize the problem and avoid the area of the bumper if at all possible.[5]

Street Secrets

Paramedics don't usually have reason to approach a vehicle from the front or rear because they are often focused on the patient inside the vehicle. If it becomes necessary to approach from the front or rear, caution should be exercised around the bumpers.

- *Hazardous cargos.* If you arrive on any scene involving a commercial vehicle, particularly a transport vehicle such as Global Express, FedEx, or UPS, always suspect the possibility of a hazardous materials issue, even if the vehicle is not placarded (see Chapter 53 for additional information). All chemicals require some level of identification when they reach a specific weight or volume, but most chemicals can be legally transported without placards or warnings if they are under the specified weight. There are also few regulations governing which chemicals can or cannot be transported together. In the normal course of business, many different chemicals can be transported inside nonplacarded vehicles, so always use caution when you see any sort of cargo in a vehicle crash.

Anatomy of Vehicles

There are many components of a vehicle with which paramedics need to be familiar when participating in highway rescue operations. DOT 8-3.23

Basic Design

All vehicles come in either unibody or frame design. Most vehicles produced today are the unibody design type. The exception is light trucks, which still use frame designs. Unibody vehicles must have all working components intact in order to maintain their integrity. This includes the roof, floor pan, firewall, windshield, and roof supports. If these areas are severely damaged, the overall integrity of the vehicle will be compromised. If you should have to cut any part of a vehicle with a unibody construction, you can potentially reduce its integrity.

Firewall

The firewall in a vehicle separates the vehicle's engine compartment from the passenger compartment. Often, this is a source of entrapment in the vehicle when the patient's feet become entangled between the wall and the pedals.

Glass

All vehicles have two types of glass in them. The front windshield is made of a three-layer system of glass, called plastic laminate, and it is designed not to shatter in the event of a crash (Figure 51-13). This glass has to be cut out using commercial "glass master" tools or reciprocating saws. Be sure to cover your patient with a blanket or protective covering prior to cutting the glass because it can produce dust and small shards of glass during the removal process.

Tempered glass is designed to shatter into many small beads of glass (Figure 51-14). This flying glass is frequently a source of injury to both the patient and the rescuers if it is not removed prior to the disentanglement process. While specialized cutting tools are used for safety glass, a simple center punch or tapping the glass with a hammer or axe in a corner will shatter tempered glass into tiny pieces. Patients must also be protected from this glass type. DOT 8-3.26

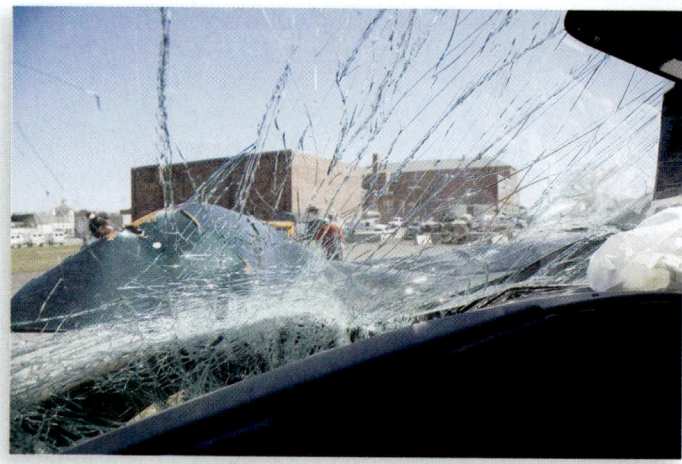

Figure 51-13   Plastic laminate windshields do not typically come apart when they break.

Doors

Doors generally have some common, basic components. At the front of the door, toward the front of the vehicle, are the hinges. At the rear of the door, on the opposite end of the hinge side, is a safety latch called the Nader pin. The Nader pin is a solid steel pin that latches the door to the door frame in order to keep the door closed in a crash. This pin is made of hardened steel and is not easily cut or manipulated. If the door hardware is mangled and the frame is bent too much, it may prevent the door from opening. You may be able to pry it open with a pry bar, but often a hydraulic spreader will be required because of the strength of the Nader pin.

Street Secrets

Do not forget to check all the doors to see if access can be gained or another door can be used to extricate the patient.

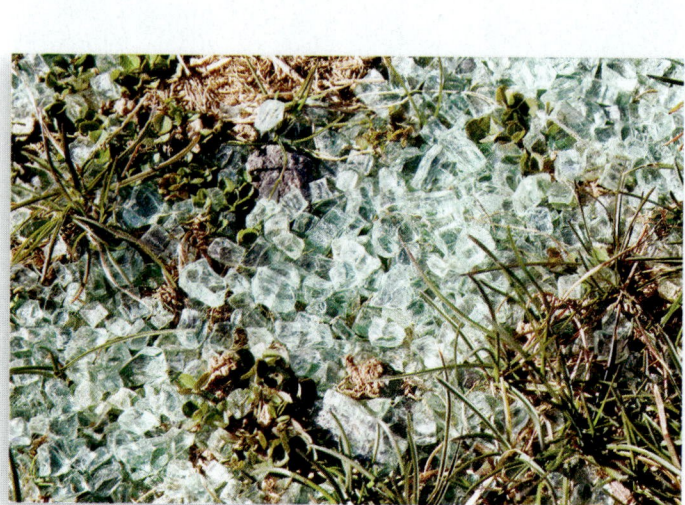

Figure 51-14   Tempered glass shatters into small, sharp edged beads and cubes.

In newer vehicles, there are often reinforcing bars placed in the door. These bars add structural strength, which lessens the likelihood that the door will be bent into the passenger compartment. Prior to this reinforcement, doors were basically two sheets of steel with a hollow core. They would buckle upon direct impact bending into, or intruding into the patient compartment. These bars, which help the doors absorb more energy, allow for less deformity of their shape. It does, however, make it difficult to remove the door and gain access to the patient. DOT 8-3.23, 8-3.27, 8-3.34

Rescue Strategies

The strategy for performing vehicle rescue follows the same, basic, step-by-step process that was outlined earlier for other rescues:

- *Scene size-up.* You will need to determine the nature of the incident, make an initial count of patients, and call for needed resources. Cut-resistant protective clothing should be worn along with leather or heavy duty work gloves and proper footwear. Helmets and eye protection are also required. It should be considered for the patient as well as the EMS crew.

- *Stabilization.* Before paramedics can safely access patients in a vehicle, the stability of the vehicle needs to be determined. The goal of stabilizing an unstable vehicle is to maximize vehicle contact with the ground. Generally, trained road rescue technicians will stabilize the vehicle and provide access to patients. This is accomplished through the use of cribbing, spare tires, or other car parts. Other examples of stabilization follow: DOT 8-3.24

  - *Vehicle on its side.* Cribbing is a useful tool. Cribbing is nothing more than hardwood lumber of various widths cut into various lengths that is used to stabilize a vehicle and keep it from rolling over or moving around (Figure 51-15). Sometimes cribbing is lashed together into various shapes, particularly wedge shapes. Other useful tools include cables, come-alongs, or winches. Come-alongs are winch systems that provide leverage through a handle that is pulled once the system of cables and riggings is put into place. They serve as a fulcrum to pull heavy weight or to pull and bend metal.

  - *Vehicle on its wheels.* Besides using cribbing, the air can be let out of the tires to bring more of the vehicle into contact with the ground and to prevent the vehicle from rolling (Figure 51-16). Do not simply cut the valve stems of the tires, however, as the tires can be reinflated once the rescue is complete so the vehicle can be more easily removed from the scene.

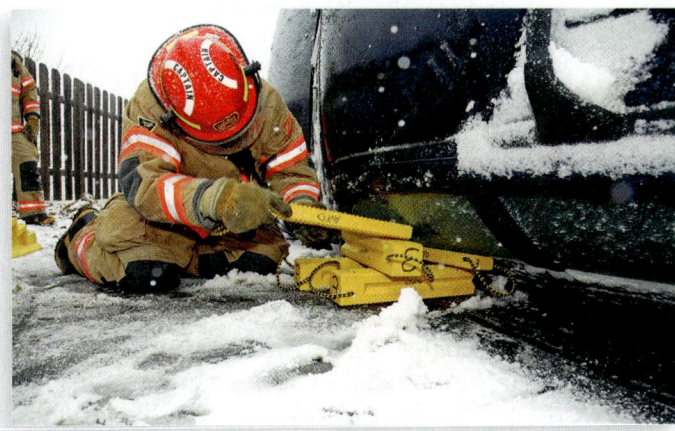

Figure 51-15   Stabilizing a vehicle on its side.

- *Vehicle on an incline.* It must be stabilized in a manner that ensures it will not move down the slope. Using emergency brakes, ensuring that automatic transmissions are in park, tying the vehicle to the ambulance bumper or trailer hook, and cribbing the wheels are useful techniques.

- *Vehicle on its roof.* Cables, cribbing, lengths of lumber, spare tires, other car parts, winches, or come-alongs can be used (see Figure 51-6). A vehicle on its roof is very unstable, and damage to the vehicle may bring about further collapse of the roof, intruding into more of the passenger compartment. Do not break out windows as these can actually be helping to support the frame, and breaking them can weaken the roof structure even more. It is important for trained road rescue personnel to ensure that the vehicle is stable prior to patient access. Trained technicians may employ hydraulic rams and other devices to support weakened structures.

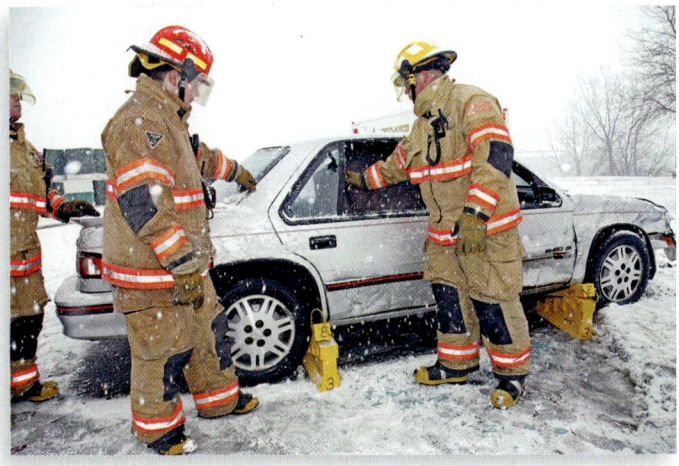

Figure 51-16   This vehicle has been adequately stabilized.

Special Access

While patients are usually removed through opened doors, some situations will require special access and removal options.

- Access through the floor is complex and requires technical training. Specialists are trained to recognize what parts of the vehicle are safe to cut away and which tools can be used to gain access through the vehicle's floor.

- Access through the trunk is difficult due to the small space, but some vehicles have fold-down access from the trunk into the passenger area. In vehicles with no built-in access, trained technicians may be able to cut into the passenger compartment; however, this is not the best approach, and it should be used only when there is no other option.

- Access through the roof can be accomplished by cutting the A and B posts that attach the roof to the body, removing or cutting the top portion of the windshield away from the roof, and rolling the roof back toward the rear of the vehicle. If all the posts are cut, the roof can be lifted off the vehicle. Cutting tools that are used include reciprocating saws (Sawzalls™), air-powered cutting tools, and more sophisticated extricating tools. The posts on all vehicles are consistently labeled, starting from the front of the vehicle. The A post is the post that attaches the windshield to the car. The B post is the next post behind the A post, and so on, down the length of the vehicle. DOT 8-3.23

- If the patient is trapped under the dashboard, the dash can be rolled up and out of the way by using hydraulic rams to push it up and forward off of the patient. Come-alongs, winches, and cables can also be used to pull the dash up and forward. Specialized extrication spreading tools may also be used.

- Steering wheels can be removed or pulled up and forward off of the patient using cables, come-alongs, or winches. Specialized extrication tools such as spreaders may also be used. Check the steering wheel to see if it is designed to move. You may be able to move it several inches so you can extricate the patient by relocating the steering wheel instead of having to cut it. DOT 8-3.45

- ***Determine if your patient is entrapped.*** Time is of the essence when you are caring for a critically injured patient. You must quickly determine if you will be able to free the patient yourself. It is always a good idea to try opening the doors on the vehicle first as you may find that the door is simply locked. Check the doors all the way around the vehicle as sometimes one is unlocked while the rest are locked. This is especially true for older model cars without power locks. If you cannot open the

---

Working in the Gray Zone

Move patients to the ambulance as quickly as possible to protect them from the weather, environment, and prying eyes of the media or bystanders. Also, moving patients into the ambulance places them close to your equipment and supplies. Many EMS providers think of their ambulance as their "office" and then attempt to get patients into their office as soon as possible so they can get more work done.

---

door to access the patient, call for the appropriate rescue resources.

- ***Assist in the treatment and removal process.*** The patient may require stabilization and immobilization. It is also important to ensure that a thorough assessment has been performed, and repeat the ABC assessment before moving on to any other patient care activities.

Water Rescue

Water rescues occur in many locations, including places that normally do not have water such as streets or culverts during flooding conditions. You will more than likely be involved in some sort of water rescue event during your career. It is important to have a basic understanding of the types of water you will encounter, the risks associated with these bodies of water, and how to approach a rescue in this environment.

Types of Water

There are two basic types of water: surface water and swift water. Each has its own unique characteristics with which you should be familiar.

Surface Water (Flat Water)

Surface water comes in the form of pools, ponds, lakes, quarry pits, or any other form of water that is not rapidly moving. The danger here is that because the water is calm, it does not appear to be a threat. It is well documented, however, that most drownings take place in surface water. These drownings are often associated with injury or some other complication.[6]

CONNECTIONS Chapter 38: Environmental Conditions has more information on the various types of drowning and management strategies for handling drowned patients.

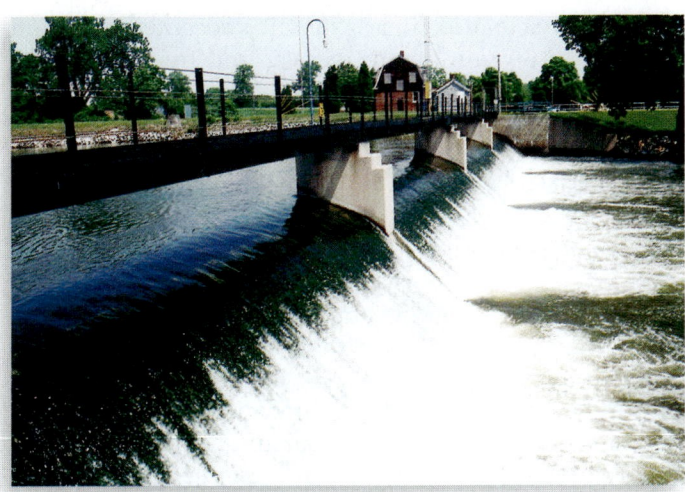

Figure 51-17 The swift water above and below a low-head dam is extremely hazardous.

Swift Water (Moving Water)

Swift water comes in the form of rivers, streams, flood control systems, low-head dams, and even flooded streets (Figure 51-17). Swift water is more hazardous than flat water. The force of moving water can easily deceive a rescuer, and you can be swept into the current and not be able to recover your balance or footing.

You should have training in swift-water rescue prior to any participation in an actual rescue. This training will provide you with an in-depth knowledge of the hazards, entry techniques, self-rescue techniques, rescue techniques, and rope techniques needed to work safely in moving water. DOT 8-3.6, 8-3.10

The following is an overview of the various types of swift-water situations. This is meant to provide a basic overview and awareness of moving water hazards.

- **Strainers.** This occurs when water moves through an obstruction such as downed trees, grates, or any other obstruction found either above or below the surface of the water. The force of the current will push you into the obstruction and make it nearly impossible for you to free yourself if you become trapped. These can be especially dangerous if water is flowing through an underwater object such as a drain. You can be trapped under water and will not be able to free yourself if the current is strong enough.
- **Hydraulics.** This occurs when water is flowing over an object such as a large boulder or a low-head dam. As the water tumbles over the object, it will create a circulating effect behind the object and will trap any object caught in its current, including rescuers. The water will circulate in a rolling motion, pulling you from the surface down in a loop and up again. Drowned victims sometimes cannot even be recovered from hydraulic boils because of the force of the

movement of the water. This type of scenario is especially dangerous when making rescue attempts because the rescuers can become trapped as well.

- **Dams and hydroelectric sites.** These can create many of the same problems as mentioned above both as strainer and as recirculating currents.
- **Low-head dams.** There is no safe approach to low-head dams without specialized training and equipment. Swift-water rescue teams use boats, ropes, and secure methods to ensure the safety of rescuers. DOT 8-3.9

Rescue Considerations

The first consideration for a water rescuer is personal safety. Being able to swim and being trained and able to swim while rescuing someone are two entirely different skills. No one should ever enter the water to perform a rescue unless trained as a rescue swimmer. The sequence to follow when performing a water rescue can be remembered by the following mnemonic:

Reach-Throw-Row-Go

- **Reach.** Use a pole or other object to reach out to the victim. Make sure you retain your balance, and do not allow yourself to fall in. Consider having another rescuer secure you by holding onto your belt or tying something around your waist.
- **Throw.** Throw a rope, some type of floating object, or both out to the victim. Be careful you do not strike the victim with the object.
- **Row.** Use a boat to row out to the victim. Make sure the boat is wide enough that it will not tip over as the victim attempts to climb in. Canoes and kayaks are usually not appropriate. It may only be possible to allow the victim to hold onto the boat and paddle them towards additional rescuers who can assist in lifting them from the water or into a shallow area where the victim can stand up and walk out.
- **Go.** Only trained rescue swimmers should ever attempt to swim out to the victim.

Before attempting a rescue, the rescuer must don a personal flotation device (PFD). PFDs should be worn by anyone working close to the water. Additionally, even if you do not have specific water rescue training, you should be familiar with rope throw bags and you should practice using them. These can be invaluable in keeping you or anyone else from having to enter the water. If you should have to enter the water, you will be subject to the same factors that the patient has been exposed to and will, therefore, be at greater risk of injury or death than you would have been by performing shore-based rescue efforts. DOT 8-3.11, 8-3.12

Self-Rescue

Every precaution should be taken to assure rescuer safety including the use of PFDs and shore rescue techniques. However, should you find yourself in swift water, there are techniques you can use for self-rescue:

- Protect your head and face as you enter the water.
- Do not attempt to stand up. This can cause a foot entrapment.
- Roll onto your back and hold your feet up out of the water. Angle yourself so you float toward the nearest shore if you come to calmer water.
- Look for calm places in the water where you might be able to reach the shore.
- Always be alert for any objects, such as the strainers discussed previously, that could cause you to become entrapped. DOT 8-3.14

Patient Factors in Water Rescue

Survivability Profile

Many factors can affect the ability of a person to survive a water incident: age, physical condition, amount of time submerged, water temperature, the presence of flotation devices, and more. Using these and any other factors present will assist you in determining whether you need to focus on the response as a rescue effort or as a body recovery. Remember also that any person recovered should not be declared dead until the person has been rewarmed if the submersion occurred in cold water. DOT 8-3.13

Cold Water

As mentioned in Chapter 38: Environmental Conditions, a person who is submerged in cold water has a greater chance of survival due to an effect known as the mammalian diving reflex. This occurs when a person is submerged in water colder than 70°F. Water temperature, particularly in very large bodies of water such as lakes, rivers, and the ocean, is vastly different than the water temperature that is encountered in pools and water parks. It is likely that even in the middle of summer, the water temperature in a natural body of water (and also man-made lakes) is 20° to 30°F colder than the air temperature, particularly in the northern part of the United States.

When the mammalian diving reflex is triggered, the parasympathetic nervous system is stimulated, causing the heart rate to slow rapidly and the blood pressure to drop. Shunting occurs, diverting more blood to the heart and the brain. It is also possible that laryngospasm occurred, closing the vocal cords and preventing water from actually entering the lungs. Patients in these situations quickly lose consciousness and are unable to effect self-rescue.

In this scenario, it is generally accepted that you have up to 60 minutes to recover and treat most submerged victims.[7] It is important to make attempts to establish a submersion time. If in doubt, remain in rescue mode, and make every attempt to find and treat the patient. DOT 8-3.7, 8-3.8

Hazardous Terrain

Outdoor activities are becoming increasingly popular, including sports such as hiking, mountain biking, and rock climbing. Paramedics will often be among the first responders on the scene should an accident happen. Paramedics must have a proper understanding of the types of terrain encountered and knowledge of how to approach a rescue in these situations. Medical responders will be interacting with specialized rescue teams in these instances and sometimes will be performing patient care during phases of the rescue.

Street Secrets

Some of these "outdoor" activities are taking place in urban settings as well as rural ones. Some adventurers play golf in and around construction sites, jump off of high buildings (called "base jumping"), and "rock" climb up the outside of buildings.

Types of Terrain

There are three types of terrain that can be encountered, and you should be able to differentiate between them. This is important because the type of terrain encountered will dictate the type of response needed and the procedures followed to safely access, treat, and remove your patient.

Flat Terrain

This is terrain that can be traversed without the aid of external rope systems. Angles range from completely flat (or level ground) to mild inclines of up to 15 degrees. Rescuers carrying a Stokes basket* or other patient carrying or moving device will be able to walk upright while looking out for obstacles or other trip hazards. Additionally, the litter bearers will not need to be tied to the Stokes basket in order to maintain their balance. Finally, no technical gear or other expertise is required to remove a patient from flat terrain. Some carrying devices can have a single wheel or set of wheels attached to the bottom of the device, which can make moving the patient much easier. Any level of EMS provider should be able to traverse this type of terrain. DOT 8-3.30

---

* The Stokes basket is the most widely used litter for rescue. They will be discussed in more detail later in this chapter.

Low-Angle

Low-angle terrain is often encountered in off-road scenarios. Angles encountered in this instance are up to 40 degrees from horizontal. An example would be an off-road embankment that is steep enough that rescuers must use a rope system in order to assist them in supporting the load of the Stokes basket as they remove the patient. The responders would be able to carefully walk down to access a patient, but they should be attached to a rope system to protect them from falling. While the rescue crew would not be directly hanging onto and totally dependent on the haul system, this scenario would still require a special rigging system and some problem-solving skills. It should not be attempted by untrained rescuers.

High-Angle

High-angle or vertical rope rescue involves working on slopes that approach 90 degrees, both natural and manufactured (Figure 51-18). In these situations, there will be only one to two responders interacting with the patient, while many others will be supporting them and monitoring their rigging and rope systems. The rescuers are totally dependent on the rope system to descend to the patient and to remove themselves and the patient from the slope. The responders will not bear the weight of the Stokes basket and will focus completely on patient care during removal.

In this scenario as well as in the low-angle scenario, the rescuers directly involved in the removal of the patient must have specialized training as outlined in NFPA 1983 and 1670.[8,9] This includes complete knowledge of knots, hauling systems, belay systems, and patient packaging techniques. Only specialized technical rescue teams should attempt high-angle rescues.

When working in a rescue environment such as this, medical personnel may hear terms with which they are unfamiliar. Box 51-2 lists some of these terms.

Patient Packaging

Proper patient packaging in the rescue environment is very important and should be done correctly and completely. There are several factors that should be considered when preparing a patient for removal:

- **The medical condition of the patient.** It is important that no further harm comes to the patient during the removal process. Note whether you might need

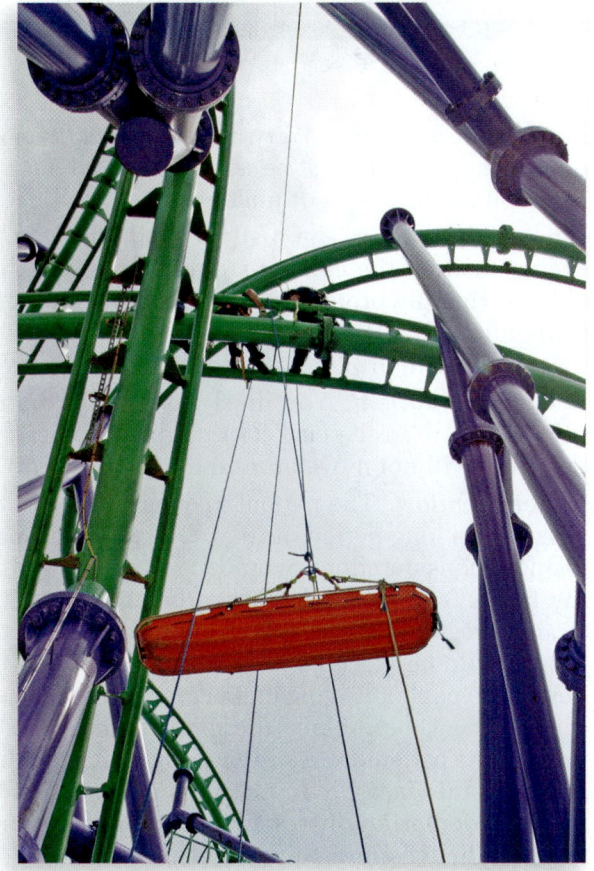

(a)   (b)

Figure 51-18   (a) and (b) High-angle rescue from a rollercoaster.

BOX 51-2 Terminology Used in High-Angle Rescues

- **Anchor.** A secure point of attachment for the rope system during a high-angle rescue.
- **Belay.** The belay line is the safety backup for the system. It protects against the fall of a rescuer and the patient by managing an unloaded rope in the event of a main line failure.
- **Loaded and unloaded rope.** When a rope or rescue line is slack and is not holding any weight it is called "unloaded." By contrast, a "loaded" rope has weight on it, and it is pulled tight.
- **Rappel.** This is a controlled descent on a rope. It is accomplished by using a friction device that controls the rate of decent.
- **Haul Team.** These people raise the load via a haul system.
- **System.** This is the combination of components used during a high-angle rescue to construct a functioning unit that is capable of supporting the patient, patient carrying device, and rescuers. DOT 8-3.29

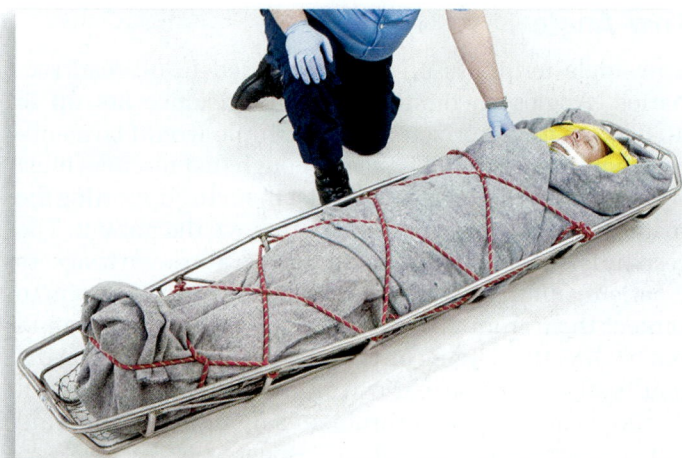

Figure 51-19. Patient properly stabilized in a Stokes basket.

to access and secure the airway or whether there are other injuries that must be accommodated such as unstable fracture sites or uncontrolled bleeding.

- ■ **The environment.** The patient will need to be protected from the elements and from any falling objects. Hearing protection and eye protection may be required. Blankets may be needed to prevent heat loss and also to provide padding or protection.

- ■ **Secure the patient.** You must ensure that the patient is secure in the basket or carrying device and that they will not move around during transport.

- ■ **Patient comfort.** The patient may have to be in the basket for a long period of time. One of the primary comfort considerations would be padding behind the knees to keep the legs from being locked in a straight position. If possible, an entire layer of padding should be placed between the patient and the device the patient is lying in. Make sure that the padding does not compromise the ability of the device to prevent the patient from slipping out. Using padding and any other measure to make the patient comfortable, particularly if it restricts further movement, may also help control pain to some degree.

Consider the types of equipment available for packaging the patient for a safe evacuation. The Stokes basket is

the most widely utilized litter for this type of rescue (Figure 51-19). The first Stokes baskets were made of wire mesh over a tubular frame that did not accommodate a long spine board. Today's Stokes baskets are made with a heavy-duty plastic bottom and steel frame. These devices have been enlarged and will accept many rigid-backboards. They are versatile devices and can be used to immobilize and transport a patient safely in any type of terrain.

The primary concern in using these baskets is the patient restraint system. Most Stokes baskets come with straps with a buckle that is inadequate for safe handling in low-angle and high-angle environments. The straps stretch a little under excessive strain, and the buckle can fail if too much stress is put on it. Additional steps must be taken to ensure that your patient is properly secured in these situations. DOT 8-3.30

Patient Evacuation

Rough or Flat Terrain

If you are working in flat or rough terrain, the stretcher can be carried by a team of no less than four rescuers. As the terrain roughens or becomes steeper or if the patient is large, additional rescuers are needed. It is important to remember that this will be a very strenuous activity even in the best of circumstances. Use team members who are in good physical condition, and have additional personnel available to rotate carry-out teams. In addition to the team, it is best to have someone act as a safety officer and look out for any trip-and-fall hazards or other unusual terrain features. It may be appropriate to have members of the team scout out the best route while other members of the team access and stabilize the patient.

There are a variety of devices available to assist the carry-out teams. For example, you can use webbing laced through the top rail of the stretcher and around the shoulders of the rescuer to assist in weight distribution. It is important to remember to match carry-out teams for height; this will keep any one person from bearing more weight than the other members of the team. DOT 8-3.32

Low-Angle Terrain

As previously mentioned, this type of rescue requires specialized training and should not be attempted by untrained rescuers. Information is included here for informational purposes only.

Low-angle terrain usually will require that the Stokes basket and the rescuers be tied into a fall arrest or haul system. This can be accomplished by using a two-rope system, where one rope is the main, weight-bearing line and the other is a belay (or safety line) used in the event of a main line failure.

All commands used in the raising and lowering of the system should be clear, consistent and understood by all involved in the operation. It is a good idea to practice these commands ahead of time. Do not use new commands or train personnel on the scene in these rescue techniques. DOT 8-3.31

High-Angle Evacuation

The basic system setup in the high-angle environment is similar to low-angle terrain. However, there is greater risk involved in high-angle rescue because the rescuers are totally dependent on the fall arrest and hauling systems. Additionally, the rescuer will not be directly attached to the litter. Instead, a point of attachment directly to the hauling system just above the Stokes basket is chosen in order to tend the stretcher and the patient during the haul (pulling up) or lowering of the basket.

As an alternative to traditional rope systems, many fire departments have access to aerial units. These are special pieces of fire apparatus that can telescope up from the ground at various angles and heights. These are usually employed in urban settings where tall buildings are involved. When using this method, the patient should still be secured in the Stokes basket, and a belay should be used when placing the patient on the bucket (the upper portion of the unit the rescuer is standing in) of the aerial unit. The Stokes basket should always be securely attached to the bucket. It is not appropriate to simply hold the basket in place during the lowering procedure. Box 51-3 gives tips for low-angle and high-angle rescues. DOT 8-3.33, 8-3.43

Confined Spaces

Confined spaces might be a trench, a silo, an underground tunnel, a vehicle tanker, or a manhole (Figure 51-20). Many of these will appear harmless to the untrained responder but can be immediately life-threatening should

---

BOX 51-3 Tips for Low-Angle and High-Angle Rescues

- **Protecting your patient**
  1. Line the inside of the litter with material, such as blankets, to secure the patient and provide additional padding.
  2. Provide protection from cold weather by wrapping a blanket around the patient, including the spine board, if it is to be used. Pile additional blankets on top of the patient.
  3. Protect the patient's eyes, face, and head by using either goggles or a commercial-grade face shield if your Stokes basket is equipped with one.

- **Securing your patient**
  1. Patients must be secured lengthwise so that they cannot slip out of the end of the stretcher. This is accomplished by applying clove hitches to the patient's feet as part of the webbing system used for security.
  2. If there are lower extremity fractures, then step 1 will not be feasible. A simple seat harness will be acceptable in these situations.
  3. Webbing should be used to secure the patient from the feet to the chest in conjunction with step 1 above. It is important to remember not to lace the webbing up to the upper chest or neck in case the patient does slide down. This could cause the patient to be strangled on the upper portion of the webbing.
  4. Your patient generally should have at least two points of attachment to the stretcher or haul system as an added safety measure. DOT 8-3.42

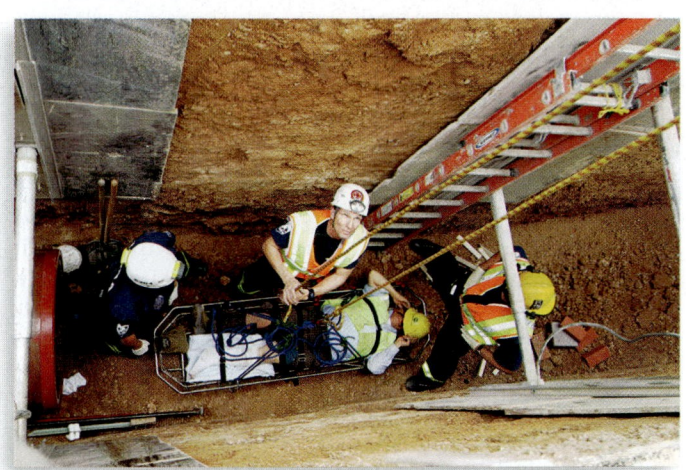

Figure 51-20 Trench rescues require proper training and equipment.

entry be made without proper preparation and protective equipment.

No matter the specific type of space, all confined spaces share certain characteristics as outlined in OSHA 1910.146. A confined space must meet the following criteria:[10,11]

- It must be large enough so that entry can be made and work performed.
- It must have limited access and egress.
- It must not be designed for continuous occupancy. DOT 8-3.15

Types of Hazards in Confined Spaces DOT 8-3.16

Oxygen Deficiency

Oxygen deficiency is one of the most common hazards associated with confined space rescue. Responders who are not trained in confined space rescue may not readily think of a lack of oxygen as a concern when approaching this type of rescue situation and may be unaware as oxygen deficiency develops. This deficiency is an invisible threat and should always be checked for prior to entry into any confined space, even if the victim is visible within the space. This monitoring should be done by personnel specifically trained in the use of air monitors. A normal range of oxygen concentration for safe operation within a confined space is 19.5–23.5%. Anything below this range is considered to be an oxygen-deficient environment and SCBA or other air- or oxygen-supplying devices are required for the rescuers. DOT 8-3.17

Chemicals: Toxics and Explosives

As oxygen is depleted from an environment, carbon dioxide is building up. Remember that carbon dioxide can reach toxic levels and represents a toxic hazard just as any other chemical. Other chemicals can be present in confined spaces and will present the rescuers with a toxic or explosive environment. A toxic atmosphere is one in which there are gasses, vapors, or fumes that have the potential to be harmful to the patient and rescuers. It is important to remember that the involved chemicals will often reach a toxic level before reaching an explosive level. Thus, as part of atmospheric monitoring, the rescue personnel on the scene must monitor for any potential toxic chemicals in addition to explosive potentials and oxygen irregularities.

Chemicals also carry a significant explosive risk if they are present in a high enough quantity relative to the confined space. A confined space will have flammable or explosive potential if the vapors present exceed 10% of their lower explosive limit (LEL). An oxygen-enriched environment (above 23.5%) will also increase the potential flammability of any chemicals present. There are several chemicals that are common to confined spaces:

- Hydrogen sulfide (H_2S)
- Carbon dioxide (CO_2)
- Carbon monoxide (CO)
- Methane (CH_4)
- Ammonia (NH_3)
- Nitrogen dioxide (NO_2) DOT 8-3.18

Engulfment Hazards

Should the rescue occur in areas such as farm silos or other storage facilities, there is a potential for materials to be present that can bury rescuers. Such materials include grains, dirt, sand, corn, and others. Grains that are stored for long periods of time compact and settle into a fairly solid mass. Mice and other grain-eating animals will enter the silo and eat some of the grain. Also, some of the grain will deteriorate as it ages. The compacted grain forms a crust on the top that appears to be solid, but underneath in the mass of the grain are pockets of air where the grain has been eaten or deteriorated. If enough weight is added to the crust, it can collapse inward, dragging whatever was on top into the mass. This can cause suffocation. Along with the risk of being buried, dust and debris in the air from the grain shifting around can ignite and explode.

Electrical Hazards

In many confined spaces, either an electrical supply can harm a rescuer or the electrical source supplies a mechanical hazard as described below. This hazard must be mitigated prior to entry. This can be accomplished by shutting off the power supply to the entire facility, but more often, this can be accomplished by shutting off power to the immediate area or machinery where the rescue is taking place. This power switch should have a visual warning attached to it in addition to the mechanical device that restricts power restoration. Many facilities have procedures in place specific to the types of equipment present, and the personnel who work in these areas should be utilized to assure that no further complications arise from the improper shutdown of machinery.

Mechanical Hazards

These might be blades, shredders, gears, augers, or conveyer belts within the space where the rescuers are working. These hazards must be locked off from their power supplies prior to entry into the space, and some sort of identification should be used to clearly indicate that the power is supposed to remain off. This lockout or tag out method will prevent the machinery from accidentally being restarted. The FEMA website, (http://www.fema.gov) has more details on lockout and tag out procedures.

Site Safety Procedures for Confined Space Entry

Federal and state regulatory oversight for industries that must operate in confined spaces is very stringent. Regulations require that educational programs be in place for these employees and that employers ensure that their trained employees are available to supplement your rescue team in the event of an emergency. This can be a very valuable resource for EMS responders.

Operating within a confined space requires a special permit. Regulations require that businesses and industries demonstrate that safety precautions and certain components are in place prior to being issued any permits that allow confined space operations to take place. Precautions include atmospheric monitoring, proper rescuer PPE, supplied air systems, and personnel retrieval systems. Backup teams are required as support for the initial rescuers.

It is important to remember that dealing with a confined space is a very dangerous operation. The rescue operation will be a very methodical and often lengthy process that is best left to properly trained personnel. DOT 8-3.17

Trench Operations and Cave-Ins

Construction site trenches are often the site of a rescue after a collapse has occurred. Collapses can occur even when OSHA-mandated stabilizing devices and appropriate safety measures are taken, but most collapses occur when procedures are not followed correctly. Working in and around a trench is not an easy task, and the risk of a secondary collapse is of primary concern to rescuers. Therefore, if you arrive on the scene first, your primary concern is to isolate the area, get any would-be rescuers out of the trench if they are attempting to rescue a victim, and await the proper specialized rescue services. Never attempt to approach and enter a trench unless it has been properly shored and you have had the appropriate operational and technical training.[10] DOT 8-3.19

Summary

All rescue operations should be performed in a methodical way by rescuers specially trained to understand the hazards specific to each type of incident. The rescuers must have an understanding of proper personal protective equipment and hazards associated with the different situations, and they must use alternative approaches to assessment and treatment in each situation.

The primary concern during rescue calls is the safety of the responders. As a member of the rescue team, you need to be aware of the situation that you and your fellow responders are in. This is true whether you are participating in the rescue operation or standing by to receive a patient once they are disentangled. You should be able to communicate effectively and quickly should you become aware of a safety concern.

Even if you are not participating in the rescue operation, in some situations you may be directed into the scene to perform patient care. You should be mentally and physically prepared to participate. In these circumstances, you will be responsible for establishing and maintaining care during all phases of the rescue, and you will accompany the patient from the scene to definitive care. During this process you will have to work closely with other members of the rescue team to assure the best possible outcome for your patient.

Skill Sheets that support this chapter include: Skill Sheet 31: Trauma Scoring, Skill Sheet 63: Verbal Communications, Skill Sheet 66: Bleeding Control and Shock (and Step-by-Step 66), Skill Sheet 68: Seated Spinal Immobilization (and Step-by-Step 68), Skill Sheet 70: Supine Spinal Immobilization (and Step-by-Step 70), Skill Sheet 72: Rapid Extrication, Skill Sheet 79: Crush Injury Management, Skill Sheet 83: NREMT Patient Assessment Skill Trauma, Skill Sheet 92: NREMT Spinal Immobilization (Seated Patient), Skill Sheet 93: NREMT Spinal Immobilization (Supine Patient), and Skill Sheet 94: NREMT Bleeding Control/Shock Management.

Notes

1. C. Merrick, ed., *Rescue Technician: Operational Readiness for Rescue Providers* (St. Louis, MO: Mosby, 1998).
2. FEMA Independent Study Program: IS-100 Introduction to Incident Command System, http://www.training.fema.gov/EMIWeb/IS/is100.asp (accessed April 10, 2006).
3. R. Worsing, ed., *Basic Rescue and Emergency Care* (Park Ridge, IL: American Academy of Orthopaedic Surgeons, 1990).
4. AAOS and the National Ski Patrol, *Outdoor Emergency Care* (Sudbury, MA: Jones and Bartlett, 2003).
5. J. Gargan and H. Grant, *Vehicle Rescue* (Upper Saddle River, NJ: Prentice Hall, 1997).
6. Ellis and Associates, *Aquatic Rescue Professional* (Sudbury, MA: Jones and Bartlett, 2000).
7. D. Smith and S. Smith, *Water Rescue: Basic Skills for Emergency Responders* (St. Louis, MO: Mosby, 1994).
8. S. Hudson and T. Vines, *High Angle Rescue Techniques* (St. Louis, MO: Mosby, 1999).
9. National Fire Protection Association, "1670 Standard on Operations and Training for Technical Rescue Incident," "1983 Standard on Fire Department Life Safety Rope and System Components," "1582 Standard on Medical Requirements for Firefighters," (Quincy, MA: NFPA).
10. M. Roop, T. Vines, and R. Wright, *Confined Space and Structural Rope Rescue* (St. Louis, MO: Mosby, 1998).
11. OSHA, "29—Labor, Code of Federal Regulations—Permit Required Confined Spaces, Excavation Requirements 1926.650, Respiratory Protection 1910.134, Personal Protective Equipment 1910.132," http://www.osha.gov/comp_links.html (accessed February 18, 2007).

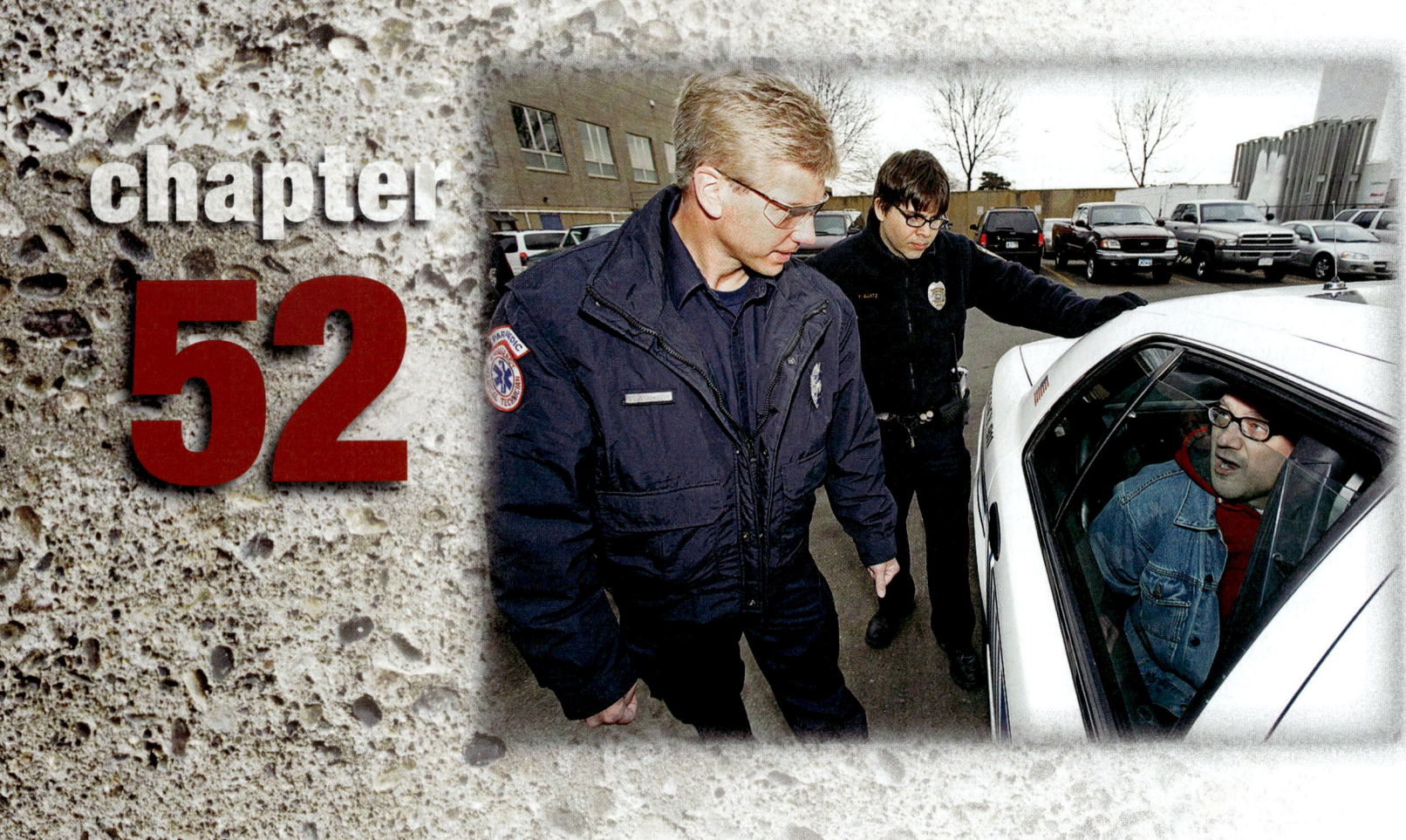

Teamwork and Operational Interface

*"**T**here is nothing more terrifying than ignorance in action."*

—J. Von Goethe

Need To Know

▶ A working knowledge of all of the governmental, public health, and legal entities with which you will work.

▶ The role of the paramedic in interfacing with these agencies regarding management of scenes, handover of patients, continuous quality improvement, and planning.

▶ The role of these agencies in emergency operational plans.

▶ A working knowledge of tactical operations and how patient care in tactical situations is affected.

▶ A minimum awareness level training in the National Incident Management System provided through the Department of Homeland Security.

▶ An awareness of crime scene issues and that a patient's needs remain a priority.

▶ The dangers inherent in criminal activity involving violent individuals or the response to locations such as methamphetamine labs.

▶ Do	▶ Ask
• Identify the various emergency response organizations with which you will be working. • Participate in education and hands-on training involving local and regional emergency operational plans. • Work with local police agencies to review practices at crime scenes. • Consider the risks inherent in scenes where any criminal activity has occurred. • Review and practice techniques for dealing with violent patients. • Consider the role of EMS in public health surveillance, and report trends concerning patient complaints to administrators, medical directors, and public health agencies.	• Other agencies involved with an incident for their assessments. This information will determine the safety and security of the scene and help with history and MOI in patient assessment. • Your supervisors about your agency's disaster plan and how it fits into the area's unified command plan. • Police at crime scenes about critical aspects of the scene that should not be disturbed, and protect the scene as much as possible without limiting patient care. • Police officers to assist with uncooperative or violent patients. • Police to identify hazards at scenes of criminal activity.

Introduction

Throughout your career as a paramedic, you will have the opportunity to interact with many other areas of public, legal, and governmental service. Your knowledge, understanding, and prior preparation for this interaction will leave a strong impression of you and your agency in the eyes of others. Although many of the points in this chapter may seem like common sense, it is always interesting to critique a multiagency incident afterwards to see how many of these points are misunderstood, miscommunicated, or simply forgotten.

Interfacing with Emergency Response Organizations

Most EMS personnel will respond at some time in their careers to natural disasters, such as tornadoes, hurricanes, floods, and earthquakes, or even terrorist incidents, such as bombings, fires, or other forms of attack that can result in varying numbers of casualties. Additionally, many civil disturbances and simple 9-1-1 calls for medical assistance require the interaction of more than one profession or agency. Most such incidents are managed by jurisdictions at the local level, and EMS agencies usually have the primary responsibility for patient care and transport. Depending on the size and scope of an incident, other emergency response and management organizations may also be involved, and paramedics frequently will work in coordination with these agencies.

Federal Emergency Management Agency (FEMA)

FEMA is the lead federal agency responsible for emergency management activities after natural and terrorist disasters. FEMA assists state and local organizations to prepare for, respond to, mitigate, and recover from emergencies. The agency also provides funding for many disaster responses.[1] FEMA assistance includes equipping local and state emergency preparedness agencies, coordinating the federal response to a disaster, training emergency managers, supporting the nation's fire service, and administering the national flood and crime insurance programs.[2]

National Response Plan

The Department of Homeland Security has created the **National Response Plan (NRP),** which establishes a comprehensive, all-hazards approach to enhance the ability of the United States to manage domestic incidents. The plan incorporates best practices and procedures from incident management disciplines such as homeland security, emergency management, law enforcement, firefighting, public health, emergency medical services, and others and integrates them into a unified structure.[3] The NRP supersedes all previous national response plans in the United States. All federal departments and agencies will use the NRP in their response to natural disasters or terrorist attacks. FEMA's Emergency Management Institute offers an online course designed to introduce the National Response Plan to responders.[4,5]

State and Local Emergency Management Agencies

Most states have emergency management offices, which exist to provide their citizens with advanced public safety information and assistance as well as to support the response activities of involved public safety agencies. In the event of an incident, whether man-made or natural, it is important for EMS personnel to be familiar with individual emergency and disaster plans in their state as they vary greatly depending on state resources and funding. Likewise, many county, parish, and city jurisdictions develop, operate, and maintain departments of emergency management to respond to incidents at the local level. Paramedics should seek and receive training in the incident command structure and standard operating procedures of the agencies in the area where they work.

CONNECTIONS For more complete information on the organization and structure of the National Incident Management System and Incident Command Structure, go to Chapter 50: Medical Incident Command.

Fire Agencies, Operating on the Fire Ground

Fire and EMS Interactions

There are numerous models of EMS delivery in the United States. These include but are not limited to

private sector, police, fire, public utility, and military.[6] Perhaps the two models that are most prevalent are the *Third-Service EMS Model* and the *Fire-Based EMS Model.* The term *Third Service* represents an EMS service that is separate from either police or fire (considered the first two public services) and may be operated by a private or public entity. Fire-based models are exactly that: paramedic services operating within the organizational structure of the local fire department. This model usually uses cross-trained firefighters as paramedic providers.

Fire and EMS Structure

Depending on the service model, your interaction with a fire agency may be limited or continual. A fire-based EMS model will, by definition, immerse the EMS provider in the culture of the fire service. Generally, the fire service tends to be a paramilitary style organization, with a rank structure and chain of command. Additionally, the fire service is the birthplace of the incident command system, a scalable management system that can be used on emergency incidents of any magnitude; thus, the fire service tends to follow this style of management at most incidents, including EMS calls.[7] This system allows for a single incident commander (IC) with personnel or other managers reporting to the IC for orders.

CONNECTIONS Chapter 50: Medical Incident Command provides a detailed discussion of ICS.

Multiple Agency Responses

If you work in a third-service EMS model system, you may or may not have frequent interaction with the fire service depending on the response structure in place in your EMS system. For instance, if your community uses the fire service as EMS first responders, you will likely interact with them on almost every call. Local protocols will dictate your interactions with the fire service in this situation. Generally, on a medical incident, the highest medical authority (likely EMS) will usually take over leadership of the situation.

There are a multitude of incident management systems; they range from a single page to hundreds of pages. Figure 52-1 shows a simple, tri-fold card devised by Minneapolis-St. Paul paramedics that outlines the EMS response to a multi-casualty incident.

Police and Tactical EMS, Operating in a Tactical Environment

You will likely have many interactions with law enforcement agencies during your career. Paramedics and police are often simultaneously dispatched to

ADDITIONAL ACTIONS / CONSIDERATIONS FOR EMS BRANCH DIRECTOR

Consult with Supervisor/Manager for the following:

• Need to operate entirely under Written Medical Protocols?
• Consider need for all non-event crews to transport to nearest emergency receiving hospitals (advise MRCC and On-Call M.D.)

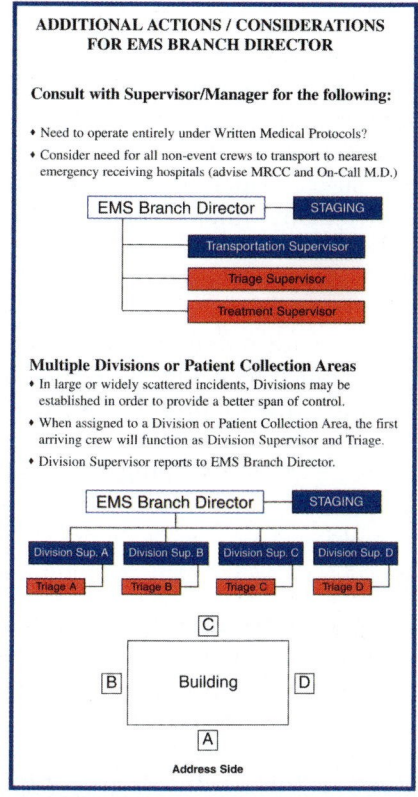

Multiple Divisions or Patient Collection Areas

• In large or widely scattered incidents, Divisions may be established in order to provide a better span of control.
• When assigned to a Division or Patient Collection Area, the first arriving crew will function as Division Supervisor and Triage.
• Division Supervisor reports to EMS Branch Director.

ON DUTY SUPERVISOR / MANAGER
(White Vest-Reports to Incident Command)

Responsible for all EMS Command and Control Activities, and for continued operation of the Department until delegated.

EN ROUTE

• Ensure sufficient response based on initial reports.
• Consider need to hold off going crews and staff.
• Confirm activation of emergency notification plans.
• Contact MRCC/Medical Control to place hospitals on MCI alert status.

ON ARRIVAL

• Scene safety size-up (HAZMAT, secondary hazards).
• Ensure safety of initial crew deployment.
• Report to EMS Branch Director and discuss assignments and event needs.

WHEN ASSUMING EMS BRANCH DIRECTOR

• Broadcast change in EMS Director.
• Reestablish contact with Incident Command.
• Initiate Special Response Guidelines, as needed.
• Do hazard assessment with Incident Command.
• Ensure crews are wearing proper protective equipment.
• Update Communication Center frequently.
• Reassess resource needs.
• Consider the need for multiple Divisions. (Multiple sites/patient collection areas).
• If the Command Post is distant from the incident site, consider establishing an Operations Section.
• Consider off-site **Staging** and **Staging Supervisor**.
• Consider MCI Trailer/additional supplies.
• Consider additional management staff (outside agency support).

Coordinate with Incident Command for the following:

• Buses for transport or shelter.
• Red Cross, Salvation Army, and other volunteer agencies.
• Long Term Operations such as Relief / Rehab.

EMERGENCY MEDICAL SERVICES INCIDENT RESPONSE PLAN

EVENT GUIDELINES:

• Most incidents can be handled by the first responding crew, supervisor, and system resources.
• Incidents with large numbers of patients (typically >30) may need additional command positions, multiple sectors, patient collection sites, and/or exceed readily available system resources.
• **If potential exists for patients to self transport, immediately contact the Communication Center to alert MRCC/Medical Control who will contact the appropriate hospitals.**
• **FIRST ARRIVING CREW:** (Refer to Panels A & B) Establish EMS Branch Director/Expedite Patient Transport.
• **2nd IN or LATE ARRIVING AMBULANCES:** (Refer to Panel C) Report to Staging.

EVENT COMMUNICATIONS:

• Crews will initially contact the Communication Center of the agency controlling the event.
• Use plain English instead of 10-codes, e.g. "agency name" to Communication Center "agency name".
• Once on scene the crew announces their arrival and establishes contact with EMS Branch Director.

Refer to agency specific guidelines for special incidents: HazMat, Police Tactical Operation, Fire Standby, Water Rescue, etc.

HAZMAT RESPONSE

• Identify safe access routes and staging areas.
• Ensure proper use of protective equipment.
• Consult with Incident Command to establish cold zones and decontamination process.
• Collection of patients in Cold Zone is preferred.
• Decontaminate patients prior to triage and transport.
• Check Temp., Humidity, Wind speed & direction.

Revised: April - 05   Release Date: June-04

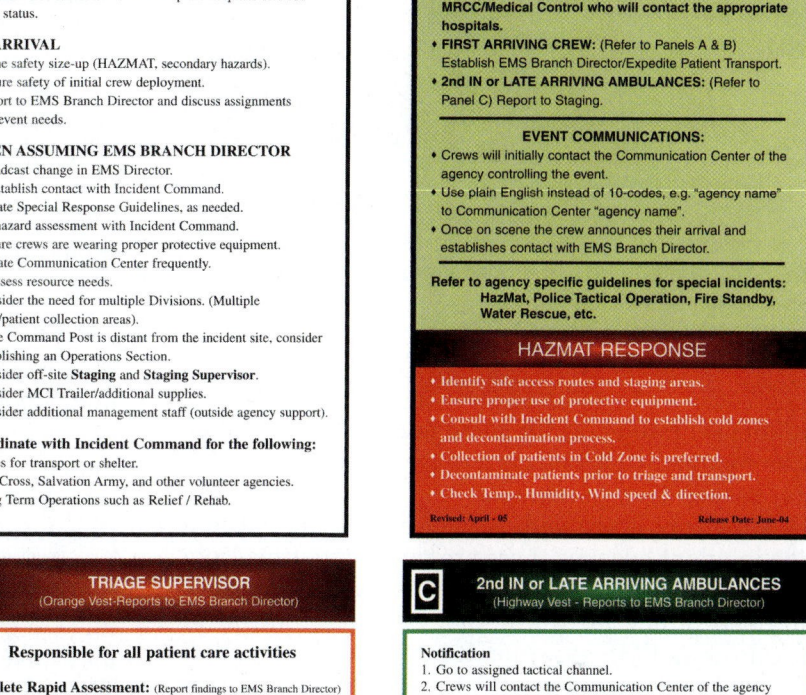

A EMS BRANCH DIRECTOR/TRANSPORTATION
(Blue Vest - Report to Incident Command when appropriate)

SCENE SIZE-UP

• Number of patients: _____
• Types of injuries: _____
• Severity of injuries: _____
• Best route in: _____
• Best route out: _____
• Staging location (if needed): _____
• Advise if there are multiple patient collection sites.
• Coordinate with Triage Supervisor.
• EXPEDITE TRANSPORT

Obtain triaged patient information from Triage Supervisor

G_____ Y_____ R_____ B_____

Is Operations Supervisor assuming EMS Branch Director?

Yes— Assume role of Transportation Supervisor or other duties as assigned.

No— Remain EMS Branch Director and maintain responsibility of the Transportation Supervisor.

TRANSPORTATION SUPERVISOR
(Blue Vest - Reports to EMS Branch Director)

• Coordinate ambulance movement and loading.
• Keep In/Out Routes open.
• Keys remain in ignition.
• Expedite Transport of Patients.

If large incident with delay in moving patients (>30 patients), consider need for Staging and Treatment Supervisors. Establish Patient Collection Area.

B TRIAGE SUPERVISOR
(Orange Vest-Reports to EMS Branch Director)

Responsible for all patient care activities

Complete Rapid Assessment: (Report findings to EMS Branch Director)
• At small incident, primary role is to identify critical patients.
• Identify and corral "walking wounded."
• Prepare patients for rapid transport.

Organize Patient Care Activities
• TRIAGE patients, consider triage tags for >10 patients.
• Perform life-saving treatments only.
• Early transport of critical patients.
• Direct First Responders caring for multiple patients.
Coordinate with Transportation Supervisor and transport crews to expedite patient transport.

TRIAGE

GREEN
• "Walking Wounded" or injuries treated by first-aid alone.

YELLOW
• Follows simple commands.
• Minor injuries but unable to ambulate.

RED
• Unable to follow simple commands.
• Respiratory Distress.
• Signs of Shock.

TREATMENT SUPERVISOR
(Orange Vest - Reports to EMS Branch Director)

• Triage Supervisor assumes role of Treatment Supervisor unless it is assigned to someone else.
• Organize medical care in treatment area.
• Determine need for supplies and staff in treatment area.
• Provide for medical need of all "walking wounded."

C 2nd IN or LATE ARRIVING AMBULANCES
(Highway Vest - Reports to EMS Branch Director)

Notification
1. Go to assigned tactical channel.
2. Crews will contact the Communication Center of the agency controlling the event.
3. Once on scene the crew announces their arrival and establishes contact with EMS Branch Director.
4. Mutual Aid crews use "Dept Name & Crew #" to identify themselves.
5. Approach scene using designated route to avoid hazards.

Arrival at the Scene
1. Leave keys in ignition.
2. Stay inside ambulance at Staging Area until assigned.
3. Remember other vehicles, do not block entry/exit routes.
4. Quickly load patients and provide treatment en route!

Leaving the Scene
1. Notify EMS Branch Director of the number of patients you have when leaving the scene.
2. Contact MRCC/Medical Control for destination hospital. Give name, age, gender, triage category, and chief complaint. Be brief!
3. Contact your Communication Center and advise them of your status. Do NOT use the tactical channel for this.
4. Before clearing hospital, crews must contact MRCC/Medical Control and give patient names and/or identification if not previously given en route.
5. When clearing hospital, contact your Communication Center for assignment.

STAGING SUPERVISOR
(Blue Vest - Reports to EMS Branch Director)

• Respond to requests for ambulances from EMS Branch Director.
• Direct movement of ambulances from staging area to Patient Collection site(s).
• Keep EMS Branch Director updated on resources in staging.
• In large incident, no difference between ALS and BLS.

Figure 52-1 Emergency Medical Services Incident Response Plan from Minneapolis-St. Paul.

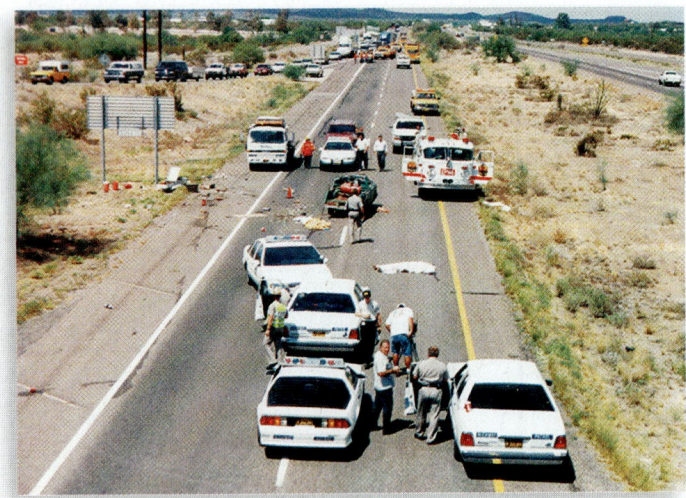

Figure 52-2 Paramedics and police must work cooperatively during large incidents.

incidents (Figure 52-2). In some communities, police are the medical first responders and may even be the initial responding paramedic for the community. In other situations, paramedics may be dispatched to a police incident because there are injured victims from a violent situation. In vehicle collisions, paramedics often need police for traffic or bystander control. In your role as an EMS provider, it is important to understand the line between medical care and law enforcement. Unless you are functioning in your community in a dual role as a sworn police officer and an EMS professional, you should not attempt to function as both.

On certain calls, it is necessary to have law enforcement personnel present. The literature documents that EMS personnel are at substantial risk for encountering violence directed at them while on duty.[8,9] It is never a good idea to be first on the scene of an assault, only to find yourself confronting the assailant still on the premises. Your agency should have a policy in place to dictate your actions on such calls. Most agencies have a policy in which EMS units stage a safe distance from the scene until police personnel have secured the scene. Generally, when there is known or suspected violence associated with your medical call, law enforcement should be allowed to arrive first and make the scene safe for you to enter. Keep in mind that most EMS providers wear uniforms and duty belts and arrive in marked emergency vehicles as do law enforcement officers. Many laypeople cannot tell them apart, especially in a stressful situation. To avoid being mistaken for a law enforcement officer with all of the accompanying potential violence that it can bring, it is best to be absolutely certain that the scene is safe before entering. DOT 8-5.1

Tactical Forces

Another area of EMS interaction with law enforcement is in the tactical arena. Law enforcement tactical operations occur during higher risk situations such as hostage rescue, sniper situations, high-risk search warrants, and active shooter scenarios. Depending on your community, these teams have many different names such as Special Weapons and Tactics (SWAT), Special Operations, and Emergency Response. These teams are found in many municipal and regional law enforcement agencies and are also found within federal enforcement agencies as well. Some tactical teams include specially trained medical personnel. If responding in a back-up role to tactical operations, paramedics should stage at a safe distance and await patients being brought to them for treatment.

Tactical Operations

To understand this operational interface, you must understand the basics of a tactical operation. In any tactical situation, a perimeter is established by law enforcement. Inside this perimeter is the area of interest, which also corresponds to the area of highest risk. Depending on the situation, this perimeter may be quite small (e.g., a search warrant for a home may have a perimeter that is only as large as the home), or it may be huge (e.g., pursuing an active shooter in a wooded area may have a perimeter that is several miles in diameter). The rationale of the perimeter is to contain the situation within it and also to have a built-in buffer of safety so that anyone outside the perimeter does not get hurt. For example, in a sniper situation, the sniper would be in the center of the perimeter, and since a sniper with a rifle can shoot people at a great distance, the perimeter would be large enough to ensure that people outside the perimeter could not be shot. Nonessential persons within the perimeter theoretically would be evacuated from the area for the duration of the incident. At the edge of the perimeter, law enforcement will typically set up a command post in a safe area where the IC can be found. Most law enforcement agencies use the incident command system or a similar variant, so having some familiarity with this system will be helpful during this type of situation. DOT 8-5.5

Tactical EMS Response

Typically during tactical operations, an EMS unit will be asked to "stand by" in case there are injuries. The expected response would be for the EMS unit to proceed to a safe staging area to await further orders from the incident commander (IC). This staging area is usually at or near the command post. Once there, you should check in with the IC and be ready to receive further direction as well as patients. If this is a large-scale incident, this is an appropriate time to take stock of your available resources and request additional help, if needed. It is also a wise time to advise the local receiving hospital or trauma center of the operation so that they can be ready. It is imperative to understand that in this situation only specially trained personnel should be operating within the perimeter. This includes EMS. Therefore, if there are patients to care for, they will either need to be brought to you, or you will need to wait to go to them until after the situation has been made safe.

Tactical Paramedics

During a tactical event, if there are injured people requiring medical attention, EMS must rely on law enforcement to evacuate the patients to the safe staging area for treatment (Figure 52-3). However, it is often difficult for law enforcement to disengage from what they are doing to form an evacuation or transportation team, especially if the perimeter is quite large or if there is an active, hostile situation unfolding (e.g., pursuing a shooting gunman through a populated high school). In response to this need for closer EMS involvement, the specialty of Tactical EMS has developed and is a growing area of interest within the EMS and law enforcement communities.[10]

Tactical EMS involves providing medical support within the perimeter of high-risk law enforcement operations. Having this capability available obviates the need for resource-draining evacuations to EMS personnel waiting outside the perimeter. Many law enforcement agencies are meeting the need for specialized medical care at these potentially dangerous situations in novel ways, including training local EMS personnel in law enforcement operations and techniques, or by

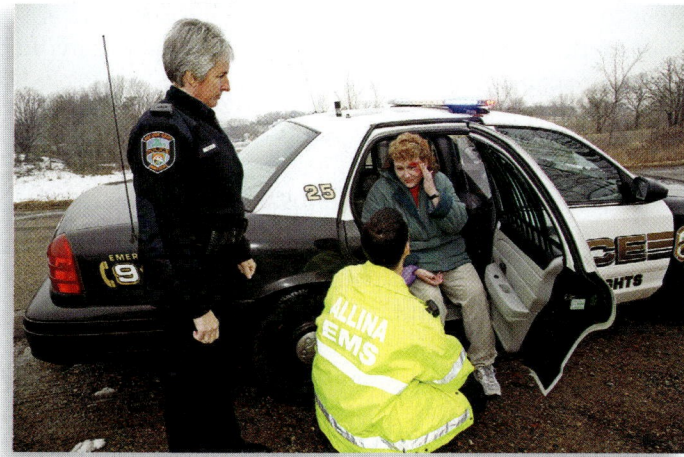

Figure 52-3 Paramedics must be able to assess and prioritize the needs of law enforcement duties with the best interest for medical care. The patient may also have different ideas about needs and refuse EMS assistance due to complicated legal and personal fears.

training police officers in EMS. Additionally, the tactical EMS provider may take on other healthcare roles within the team such as advising the IC on issues such as proper nutrition and hydration during an extended operation, tracking and providing for personnel rotations to avoid weather-related casualties, advising of the nearest trauma center and fastest evacuation method (air, ground, etc.), and maintaining team health records and fitness.

Tactical paramedics train with their respective teams on a regular basis, not only providing treatment of injuries incurred during training but also instructing law enforcement personnel in basic first aid, self-care of injuries or other illnesses, and extrication techniques for removing injured people safely while under fire or in danger. Often, the EMS member of the tactical team will provide care more frequently to officers during training than during actual missions since training exercises can last many hours or days while missions may be completed in only minutes. Tactical paramedics may also provide advice to canine handlers or actually help care for the dogs, keeping them well hydrated and treating or preventing injuries to their feet from trauma or extremes of temperature.

Crime Scene Awareness and Preserving Evidence

As an emergency responder, you will likely encounter crime scenes on a regular basis. You will need to take appropriate measures to protect and preserve investigative evidence. This is an important step in maintaining the integrity of the investigative process within the legal system. Failure to do so can result in misleading and even incorrect investigative conclusions. DOT 8-5.7

Locard's Principle

The most important concept for preserving evidence is named for Dr. Edmond Locard, a historical authority of investigative science. This principle is the foundation for all of forensics. It is obvious yet easily forgotten by EMS personnel.

Locard's Principle

Every contact leaves a trace, and there is something left to be found.[11]

Locard's Principle in the EMS realm means that, for every scene entered and for every patient cared for, paramedics will leave their mark. Although it is important to attempt to preserve evidence for the purposes of criminal investigation, your first and foremost responsibility is to ensure adequate and safe patient care (Figure 52-4). However, with a little forethought and planning, both goals can often be accommodated.

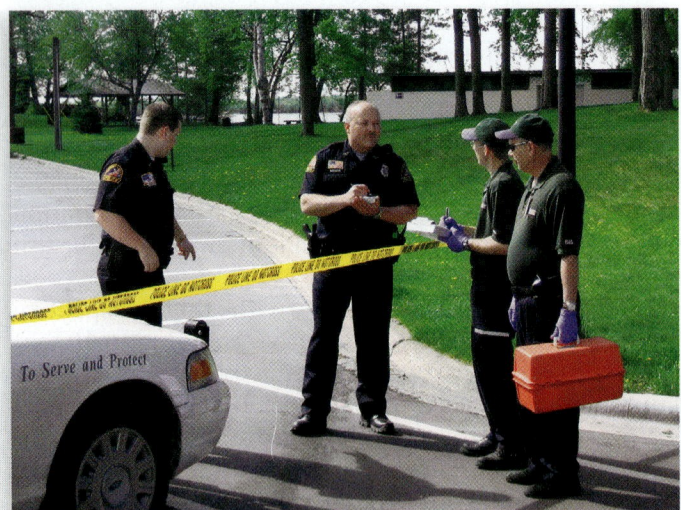

Figure 52-4 Remember Locard's Principle whenever approaching a crime scene.

Street Secrets

If your patient has been the victim of a stabbing or gunshot wound and clothing removal is required for exposure, you should avoid cutting through the knife hole or bullet hole in the clothing. The goals of exposure and evidence preservation are thus met.

Paramedics and the Crime Scene

The question of how to handle evidence with which the paramedic comes in contact needs to be addressed. If something comes into your possession that you believe represents evidence of a crime (such as drugs or a weapon), you should document the circumstances of how, when, and why it came to be in your possession. Attention to detail in this documentation will be important in helping investigators to recreate the custodial chain that this evidence followed. You should also protect the evidence from damage or additional handling, and you should alert law enforcement to its presence so that they can take it into their custody. However, as always, patient care is the first priority of EMS personnel (Box 52-1). DOT 8-5.7

Recognizing and Preserving Evidence

Paramedics may be requested by law enforcement personnel to secure paper bags over the hands of suspects or victims of suspected gunshot or explosive injuries in order to minimize the contamination or loss of trace evidence of gunpowder or powder burns. You may comply with this request unless exposing the hands or wrists is necessary for the treatment of the patient. In the case of an extremely unstable patient, it may not be appropriate to delay treatment or transport while you bag and tape the hands, but do take care to avoid unnecessarily contaminating or removing trace evidence.

Crime Scene Risks

Paramedics should be extremely careful to touch objects in the crime scene as little as possible. Not only does this prevent unnecessary contamination or alteration of the scene, but it also may prevent injury to the paramedic. Buildings or locations used for drug production or sales may be booby-trapped by their occupants to prevent rivals from intruding or to injure those who do. Pressure switches rigged to bombs or alarms may be placed under rugs or mats and are triggered when stepped on. Sawed-off shotguns are sometimes rigged in drawers to fire when the drawer is opened. Mercury switches may detonate explosives placed in the bodies of flashlights, insulated drink containers, or toys. Even light bulbs may be drilled and filled with explosive or flammable substances detonated by turning on the power. Paramedics should avoid unnecessary walking about, moving items at the scene, and even touching the surroundings. Constant scene awareness on the part of the paramedic is necessary to avoid injury or scene contamination.

BOX 52-1   Caring for Patients at a Crime Scene

There are a few standard procedures that you should carry out when caring for patients at a possible crime scene:

- Bring only absolutely necessary equipment into the crime scene.

- Always wear gloves, not only for self-protection against infectious hazards, but also to eliminate the possibility of leaving fingerprints at a scene.

- Report and document any pertinent or unusual observations made during the time at a crime scene.

- Document in quotes any declarations or pertinent comments made by patients, and note the time and location as well.

- Appropriate officials should be notified of dying declarations, admissions, or information leading to the discovery of possible other victims, in accordance with privacy regulations.

Blast Scenes

If called to the scene of a possible suicide bombing or terrorist attack, do not approach the suspect or the suspect's body or body parts until given clearance by law enforcement. There may be undetonated or partially detonated explosives or secondary devices present on or near the body. Wait until given clearance by law enforcement officials on the scene before approaching, touching, or moving the suspected bomber, whether they are alive or dead. Additionally, leave emergency vehicles that may have been driven into the inner perimeter of the blast scene in place until the bomb squad or other law enforcement officials can determine not only if they are safe to move but also if moving them will destroy key evidence.[12] Inform law enforcement officials of any suspicious packages or items you may find at the scene so they can be inspected.

Even if there has already been an explosion of a device, the placement of secondary devices designed to injure or kill first responders is a favorite technique of terrorist bombers and must be considered before entering a scene.

Methamphetamine Labs

Special attention should be paid to the dangers involved in working around methamphetamine labs (Figure 52-5). In a study of injuries related to methamphetamine labs from 1996 to 1999 in the *Morbidity and Mortality Weekly Reports,* 51% of reported injuries were suffered by first responders, law enforcement officers, or EMTs and paramedics.[13] There has been exponential growth in the numbers of methamphetamine labs since 1999, especially in rural America, and paramedics must be vigilant to avoid injury to themselves or others. Common chemicals found at methamphetamine labs include acetone, sodium hydroxide, hydrochloric acid, and anhydrous ammonia. All of these are toxic. If faced with a collection of burners, glassware,

chemicals, or suspicious containers, paramedics should immediately remove themselves and any patients from the area without touching anything. Not only does this reduce the risk of contaminating evidence, but it may also reduce injury or death due to burns, chemical exposure, respiratory problems, or explosions. DOT 8-5.5c

As a general rule, it is appropriate to avoid touching anything not related to the patient, patient care, or extrication. It is not always possible to know immediately which items at a scene are important as evidence, nor is it always evident which items may be dangerous. For these reasons, it is best to act quickly but with great caution when at the scene of a possible crime, moving or touching surrounding objects as little as possible. If in doubt, ask law enforcement personnel on the scene for advice. Paramedics should always place necessary, emergent patient care first but should also keep in mind Locard's Principle and ensure that they always operate to minimize contamination of a crime scene and the evidence that it contains.

Treating Prisoners

Basic Principles

There are many occasions when paramedics evaluate, treat, and transport prisoners of law enforcement agencies (Figure 52-6). The prisoner may be a newly captured

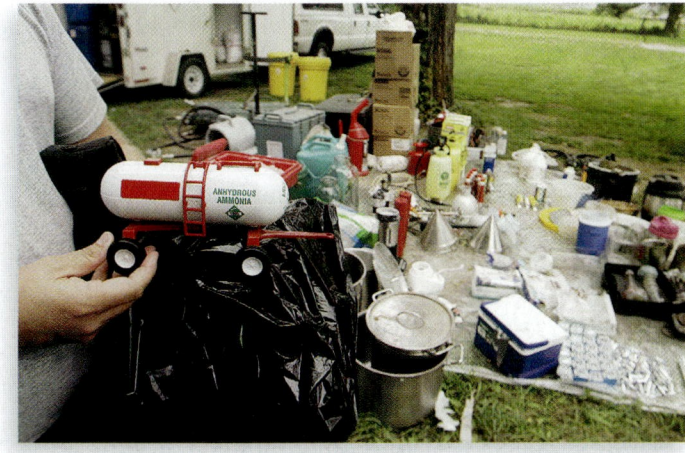

Figure 52-5   Meth labs are dangerous places. Immediately remove yourself and your patient without touching anything.

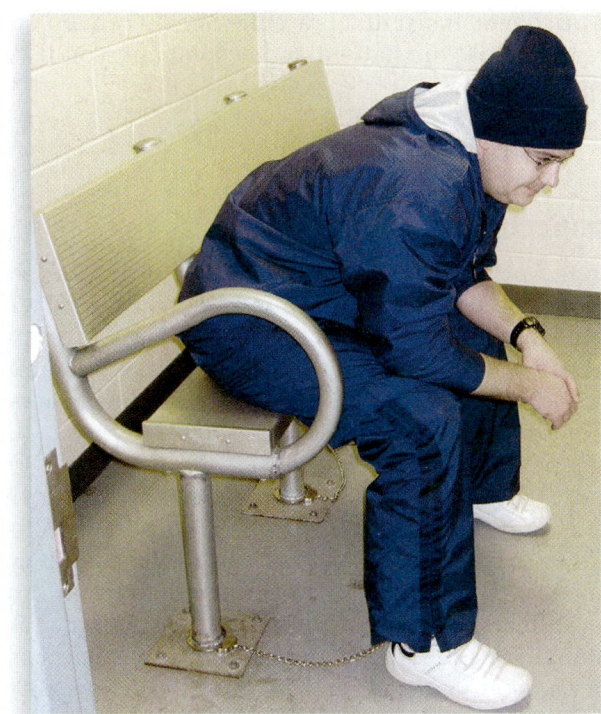

Figure 52-6   As a paramedic, you will be called to evaluate prisoners in a jail cell. This presents unique challenges in assessment and interface with law enforcement officials.

suspect who has sustained injuries in a motor vehicle collision or during a chase. They may have been injured in an altercation or may have symptoms of medical illness at the time of capture. Paramedics are also frequently called to jails, prisons, or detention centers to attend to prisoners with injuries and medical problems, such as chest pain, diabetic emergencies, suicide attempts, and assaults. While the medical evaluation and treatment of these problems are the same whether the patient is a civilian or a prisoner, there are special considerations to keep in mind when responding to a request for service for prisoners.

When called by law enforcement to evaluate a prisoner, the EMS crew must respond as they would for any other patient. If the call is to a crime scene, the paramedic must first determine that the scene is safe to enter. Scene safety is the responsibility of law enforcement officers as is the appropriate disarming, securing, and restraining of the patient. However, the paramedic should also conduct a brief search of the patient's clothing and body for weapons or other objects that could be used as a weapon. If called to a jail or prison, the EMS crew will likely be escorted by the jailer to the location of the prisoner. In both cases, police should continually remain with the paramedics while the patient is evaluated and treatment is initiated.

Street Secrets

Paramedics should never allow themselves to be alone with prisoners. Insist that law enforcement remain with you as you treat the patient and accompany you if you transport.

Transporting Prisoners

Once the prisoner has been evaluated and stabilized, the paramedic must determine, in consultation with law enforcement officers at the scene, the appropriate method of transport to the hospital, assuming transport is necessary. There are occasions when it is preferable that the prisoner be transported to the emergency department in the back of a police car. Obviously, the prisoner must be in stable condition with little or no chance of a change in condition before deciding to transport in the back of a squad car. If ambulance transport is needed, one or more law enforcement officers should accompany the prisoner and paramedic in the back of the ambulance. Some jurisdictions, such as the U.S. Marshals Service, also require another officer to follow the ambulance in a squad car and be available for moving the prisoner from the ambulance to the emergency department.[14]

Restraints and Security

Depending on the type of prisoner, the escape risk, and the law enforcement department's policies, patients being transported in an ambulance may require restraint with handcuffs, leg irons, or waist chains. The decision to restrain or not rests with officers of the jurisdiction in consultation with the lead paramedic. Prisoners should never be handcuffed, restrained, or chained to the ambulance cot unless a key to unlock the handcuffs is immediately available. If the prisoner's medical condition necessitates immediate removal of the restraints, the accompanying officer should have keys available to open every restraint device on the patient. If for any reason an officer does not accompany the paramedic in the patient compartment of the ambulance, the paramedic should be given the keys.

CONNECTIONS See Chapter 40: Behavioral and Psychiatric Disorders for additional information on properly restraining patients.

Transport Precautions

The safety of the paramedic and accompanying officer (if present) in the patient compartment of the ambulance deserves special discussion. While it may be tempting to lock the doors of the compartment to prevent the escape of the prisoner, locking the doors could result in the paramedic being unable to successfully flee should the prisoner become violent. On the other hand, if the doors remain unlocked, the prisoner being transported could potentially jump out of the ambulance, resulting in escape or possibly injury or death if the vehicle is moving or is in heavy traffic. The prisoner could also throw the paramedic out of the ambulance, with similar disastrous consequences. In general, the doors of the ambulance patient compartment should remain unlocked, and the prisoner should be adequately restrained and guarded by law enforcement officers if thought to be an elopement risk.

Military Assistance

On rare occasions, paramedics and EMS agencies may be dispatched to assist units of the U.S. military. Likewise, there may be occasions when local units of the military are called out to assist EMS agencies in response to disasters, such as floods, tornadoes, hurricanes, large-scale fires, riots, or terrorist attacks. These units may be active duty, National Guard, or reserve units, and they may function to evacuate victims of disaster by ground or air, conduct search and rescue operations, or provide security or protection in the aftermath of an incident (Figure 52-7). Often, the interactions between EMS providers and units of the United States military are

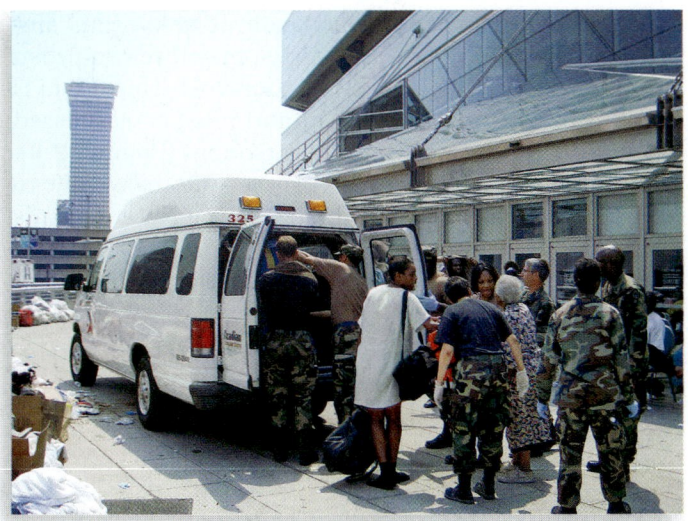

Figure 52-7 The National Guard was called to the Superdome in New Orleans during Hurricane Katrina.

governed by and described in the local, regional, or federal emergency management plans. Paramedics should be familiar with the military units in their area, as well as the recent history of interactions with these units during incidents and disasters.

Responding to Military Operations. When a civilian EMS unit is called upon to assist the United States military, most likely it will be in response to the previously mentioned natural disasters or terrorist incidents as opposed to an offensive military operation. While the military units will function under their own long-established and practiced incident command system, local EMS units called in to assist or accompany military units may need to be familiar with the particular IC system under which they are functioning. Military commanders may provide some direction regarding possible hazards that are likely to be encountered, give directives regarding scene safety, or give specific information about the injuries or illnesses the paramedic may encounter. The paramedic, meanwhile, should continue to provide appropriate medical care according to the previously established guidelines and protocols of the EMS agency's medical director.

Operating within Unified Command Situations

Unified Command

Most calls for emergency medical service involve a single ill or injured person. Frequently, additional first responders are dispatched to assist paramedics in caring for the patient. Law enforcement officers with oxygen and automatic external defibrillators may respond. Occasionally, several persons may be injured in a motor vehicle crash or other type of emergency. In many jurisdictions, law enforcement agencies, rescue squads, hazmat teams, or fire departments may also be dispatched to these incidents to provide assistance with patient care, traffic control, hazardous material containment, or fire suppression or prevention. Each agency carries out its task and duties in coordination and cooperation with the others, communicating as needed to ensure the quick and efficient extrication, evaluation, and transport of patients from the scene while minimizing or neutralizing other scene hazards, clearing debris, and routing traffic or onlookers away from the area. Whether it is formal or not, in most cases an incident command system is instituted and utilized to coordinate and direct the responders and resources in the most efficient manner to manage the situation.

In cases of mass-casualty incidents, large or dangerous hazardous material spills, or complicated incidents involving multiple risks, such as floods, fires, or tornadoes, a formal command system is necessary to coordinate large numbers of personnel from multiple agencies. In these instances, the incident command system may be expanded to a **unified command system** (UCS), which allows all agencies with geographical or functional responsibilities to determine objectives and strategies for managing the incident. Unified command also provides a forum for these agencies to make and relate consensus decisions.

CONNECTIONS Refer to Chapter 50: Medical Incident Command for a more complete discussion on the unified command system.

The Paramedic and the UCS

Frequently, the first paramedic on the scene assumes the role of lead EMS officer at the command post. A supervisor or other designated paramedic may be assigned to relieve the first arriving paramedic at the command post, depending on the type of situation or the duration of the incident. Rotation of paramedics may be necessary, depending on the duration of the incident. Patient care is delivered according to the protocols and standing orders of the EMS agency unless deviations are called for by the situation. Whether working as the EMS commander or as a responding paramedic you must have prior knowledge of incident command and unified command systems for an operation to proceed smoothly.

EMS and Public Health Agencies

Public Health Emergencies

Emergency Medical Services are very often among the first agencies to respond to incidents that ultimately prove to broadly threaten the public health. Frequently, the exact nature of the threat is not immediately apparent, resulting in exposure of paramedics to health risks and dangers that may only become evident over time. Public health emergencies can involve mass casualties from explosions, fires, earthquakes, tornadoes, or hurricanes. Though rarely encountered, accidental radiation leaks, nuclear blasts, or terrorist dirty bombs may occur. Chemical emergencies, such as anhydrous ammonia releases or nerve gas attacks, may threaten urban and rural populations alike. The threat of bioterrorism is a fact of life in the 21st century and must be addressed in planning and training EMS personnel (Figure 52-8). Most commonly, infectious disease outbreaks due to common agents such as influenza or more rare agents

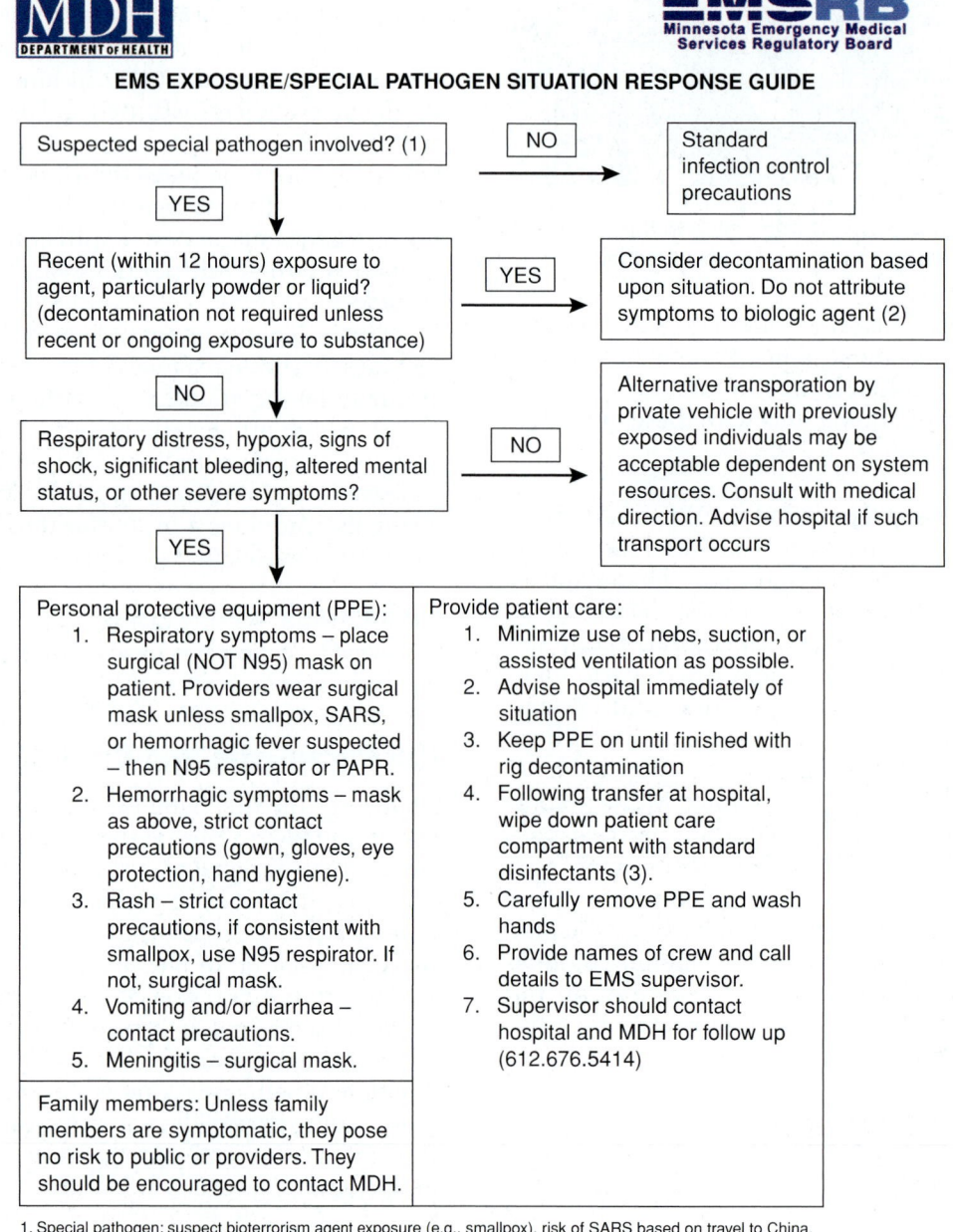

Figure 52-8 This situation response guide was prepared by the Minnesota Department of Health and the Minnesota Emergency Medical Services Regulatory Board.

such as severe acute respiratory syndrome (SARS) or the bird flu virus occur.

The EMS Response

An adequate response to a public health emergency must be planned, practiced, and constantly refined in order to be effective when an actual incident occurs. Mutual aid agreements with surrounding EMS jurisdictions should be in place, and staff should be familiar with the means to mobilize these additional agencies if they are needed. Paramedics should be familiar with the incident command system (ICS) used in the case of a multiagency, multijurisdictional incident. It may be necessary to call the National Guard for assistance, and though an individual paramedic will likely not be responsible for making the call or the decision, the procedure for doing so should be familiar. Standard triage and transport protocols as outlined in local or regional disaster plans should be followed.

Facility Capacities

Because large numbers of patients may require transport to hospitals, EMS agencies must know which facilities can and will accept patients or persons requiring quarantine, and there must be a mechanism for communicating this information to paramedics in the field. During an influenza outbreak in Los Angeles in 1997, investigators found that diversions of ambulances away from hospital emergency departments unable to accept any more patients rose dramatically. Over a three-month period during the peak of the outbreak, diversion hours rose from 15,844 to 25,584.[15] Ever decreasing hospital bed capacities and emergency department overcrowding in America contribute to the increase in diversions in both day-to-day operations and surges caused by large-scale public health emergencies.

Summary

There are numerous other agencies and teams with whom the paramedic will interact over the course of a career. Whatever the nature of the incident or the makeup of the responding agencies, cooperation between paramedics responsible for administering care and transport to ill or injured persons and other emergency response agencies is crucial. With the increasing likelihood of terrorist attacks, mass casualty incidents, or natural disasters, now more than ever before, paramedics must be aware of these other agencies, their responsibilities, and their capabilities. Almost certainly, new response agencies will be formed in coming years.

It is the responsibility of paramedics not only to know how to evaluate and treat victims of these incidents but also to know how to interact with law enforcement, fire, military, and other disaster response teams. Without cooperation, coordination, and communication, the complex response interactions necessary to manage these events will not be successful.

Notes

1. C. H. Schultz, "Disaster Response Organizations," *Rosen's Emergency Medicine: Concepts and Clinical Practice* (St. Louis, MO: Mosby, 2002), p. 2638.
2. United States Federal Emergency Management Agency, "About FEMA: What We Do" (October 22, 2004), http://www.fema.gov/about/what.shtm (accessed March 5, 2005).
3. Department of Homeland Security, "Homeland Security," February 18, 2005, http://www.dhs.gov/dhspublic/interapp/editorial/editorial_0566.xml (accessed February 18, 2005).
4. Emergency Management Institute, "National Response Plan (NRP) An Introduction," http://www.training.fema.gov/emiweb/IS/is800.asp (accessed February 18, 2005).
5. *National Response Plan Brochure* (Washington, DC: Department of Homeland Security, 2004).
6. A. E. Kuehl, ed., *Prehospital Systems and Medical Oversight* (Dubuque, IA: Kendall/Hunt Company, 2002), pp. 33–81.
7. National Interagency Fire Center, "Incident Command System," http://www.nifc.gov/fireinfo/ics_disc.html (accessed March 18, 2005).
8. E. F. Mock et al., "Prospective Field Study of Violence in Emergency Medical Services Calls," *Annals of Emergency Medicine* 32.1 (1998): 33–36.
9. J. T. Grange and S. W. Corbett, "Violence Against Emergency Medical Services Personnel," *Prehospital Emergency Care* 6.2 (2002): 186–190.
10. K. J. Rinnert and W. L. Hall, "Tactical Emergency Medical Support," *Emergency Medicine Clinics of North America* 20.4 (2002): 929–952.
11. N. C. Chamelin, C. R. Swanson, and L. Territo, "The Evolution of Criminal Investigation and Criminalistics." In *Criminal Investigation,* 8th ed. (New York, NY: McGraw-Hill, 2003), pp. 19–20.
12. Rescue Training and Resource Guide, "Emergency Response to Suicide Bombers" (January 20, 2005), http://www.techrescue.org/modules.php?name=News&file=article&sid=393 (accessed March 28, 2005).
13. "Public Health Consequences Among First Responders to Emergency Events Associated With Illicit Methamphetamine Laboratories—Selected States, 1996–1999," *Morbidity and Mortality Weekly Reports* 49(45): 1021–1024 (November 17, 2000), http://www.cdc.gov/mmwr/preview/mmwrhtml/mm4945a1.htm (accessed March 28, 2005).
14. U.S. Department of Justice/Office of the Inspector General, "United States Marshals Service's Prisoner Medical Care" (February 2004), http://www.usdoj.gov/oig/audit/USMS/0414/app5.htm (accessed April 1, 2005).
15. C. A. Glaser et al., Center for Disease Control, "Medical Care Capacity for Influenza Outbreaks, Los Angeles." *Emerging Infectious Diseases* 8 (6) (Atlanta, GA: United States Government Printing Office, 2002).

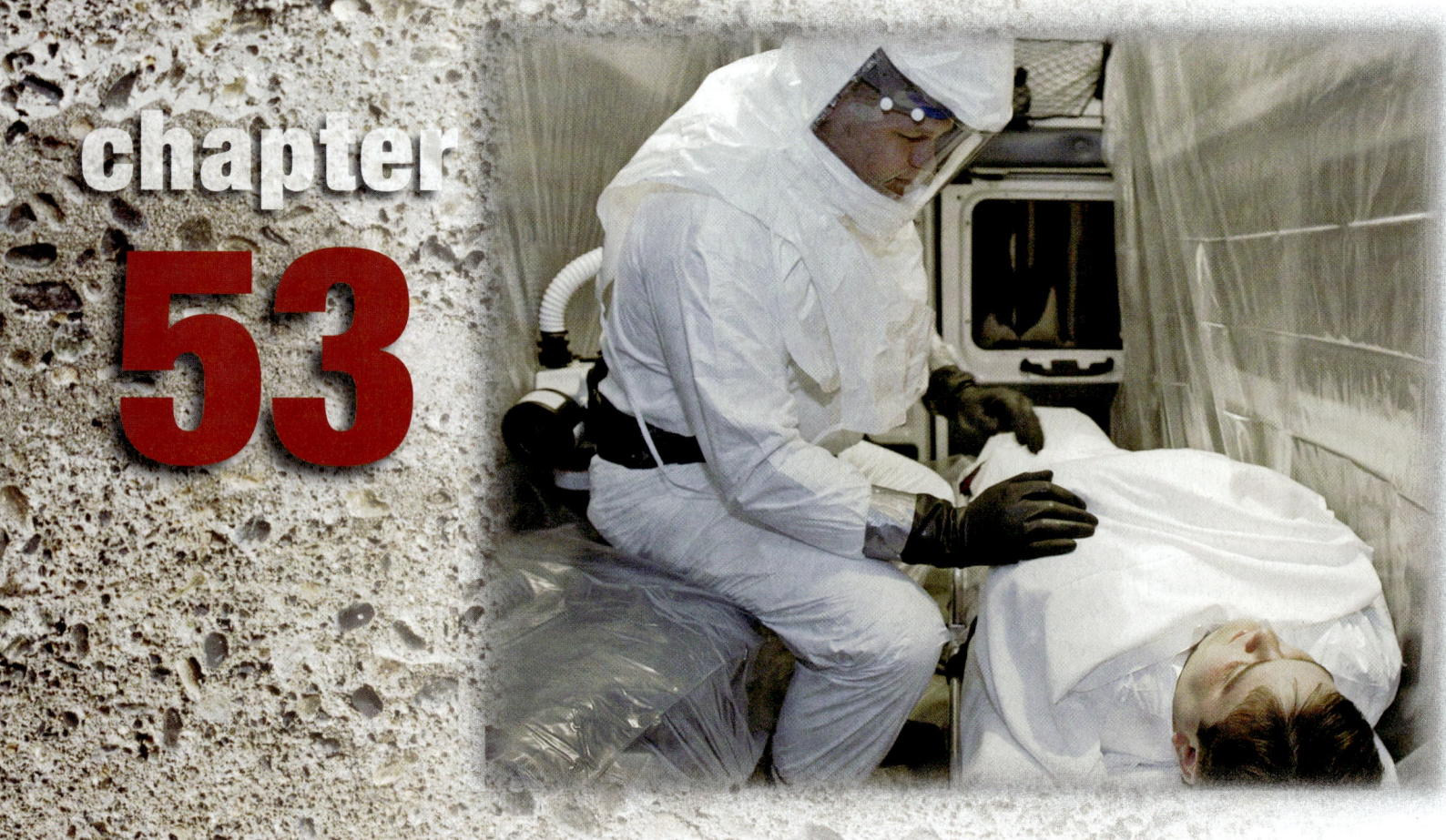

Hazardous Materials Incidents

*"**N**othing in life is to be feared, it is only to be understood. Now is the time to understand more, so that we may fear less."*

—Marie Curie

Need To Know

▶ Working around hazardous materials (hazmat) is all about safety.

▶ Recognize potential hazardous materials incidents and prevent self-exposure.

▶ Dealing with hazardous materials requires special training. Hazardous material responders are trained to four levels: awareness, operations, technician, and specialist.

▶ EMS providers are typically trained to the awareness level with emphasis on the medical implications for hazardous material response.

▶ Treating patients exposed to hazardous materials must first involve decontamination.

▶ Most hazardous materials only require treatment of symptoms.

▶ In some cases, antidotes are available, and paramedics should be familiar with the medications they carry that can be used in these exposures (e.g., organophosphates and cyanide).

▶ Do	▶ Ask
• Stay far enough away (upwind) from any scene that poses a danger to you. • Attempt to identify all of the materials that may be involved in the incident. • Determine whether specialized response such as the hazmat team is needed. • Do not enter the scene until hazardous materials incident command has cleared your entry. • Treat patients *after* they are decontaminated. • Communicate with the receiving hospital to ensure they are prepared with appropriate levels of personal protective equipment (PPE).	• Get as much information as possible from dispatch about the nature of the scene. • Request additional resources and specialized responders as required.

Introduction

Hazardous materials incidents can occur at anytime and anywhere in the world. It is only a matter of time before you respond to your first hazardous materials incident. The proliferation of increasingly diverse and numerous hazardous materials increases the chances and risk that you will be involved. The potential for exposure to a hazardous material exists on every scene to which you respond. You should be prepared to recognize a hazmat situation and take appropriate actions to protect yourself and the community.

Hazardous materials may be released prior to your arrival, on your approach, or as you are assessing patients. EMS personnel are tasked with multiple challenges at a hazardous materials event: ensuring the health, safety, triage, and medical care of both the community and the responding personnel. This is made more difficult by the many variables and complexities of hazardous materials threats, evolving strategies and operational techniques for managing these events, teams with varying levels of training, and available resources. The nature of the hazard will dictate the needed protective equipment, operational approaches, skills, and attitude. An orderly scene assessment is imperative. Both federal and state laws regarding the handling and disposal of dangerous materials will also need to be followed.[1] **The following Skill Sheets support this chapter: Skill Sheet 32: Primary Survey (and Step-by-Step 32), Skill Sheet 59: Autoinjector Drug Administration Device, Skill Sheet 60: Putting On and Removing Gloves, Skill Sheet 61: Handwashing (and Step-by-Step 61), Skill Sheet 63: Verbal Communications, and Skill Sheet 80: Eye Irrigation.**

Hazardous Materials Zones

Hazardous materials incidents have three specific areas referred to as the hot zone, warm zone, and cold zone. This information will be covered in greater detail later, but a brief description is provided here to help clarify the descriptions of the various awareness, operations, and technician levels of hazardous materials providers.

The hot zone is defined as the area of contamination. It is also called the exclusion zone. No one is allowed into the hot zone unless they have proper training and appropriate protective equipment and unless they are accompanied by a partner (called a buddy) with similar equipment and training. EMS involvement in this zone is uncommon except for hazardous materials technicians who also happen to be cross trained as EMS providers.

The warm zone is also called the contamination reduction zone. This is the area surrounding the hot zone that serves as a safety buffer area between the public and the hazardous material. It typically serves as the decontamination area and has an access and egress point established for the hot zone. Entrance into this zone requires proper training, proper personal protective equipment, and the use of the buddy system. Awareness level providers should not work in this zone.

The cold zone is also called the support zone. This area is safe and isolated from contamination. The command post, staging area, and treatment areas are located in the cold zone. This zone should be upwind, uphill, and upstream from the hot zone whenever possible in case the hazardous material spreads. This is the zone where EMS providers are most likely to be found unless they have training beyond the basic awareness level.

What Are Hazardous Materials?

There are many agencies involved in the regulation of hazardous materials. Each has jurisdiction over a chemical at various stages of manufacture, storage, transportation, or use.

- The Environmental Protection Agency states that a hazardous material is a chemical or agent that is potentially harmful to the public health or welfare when discharged into the environment.
- The Department of Transportation defines a hazardous material as any substance or material regardless of state or quantity that poses a risk to safety, health, and property while in transport.
- The American Conference of Governmental Industrial Hygienists does not define hazardous materials. However, they have identified levels of exposure that do not cause permanent injury. These values guide industry in setting limits on exposure.
- OSHA and the National Institute for Occupational Safety and Health (NIOSH) identify situations or conditions in the working environment that may cause injury or death.[2]

The most useful definition is probably the simple definition:

A hazardous material is any solid, liquid, or gas that, when released, is capable of harming people, the environment, or property.

Victim count can range from zero to entire communities, with scene times extending from minutes to months.[3]

Incidence

Hazmat incidents may occur anywhere hazardous materials are manufactured, processed, used, transported, or stored.

- ***Fixed facilities and storage.*** Seventy-five percent of all hazmat incidents (excluding fuel spills) occur in fixed facilities where the material is made, used, or stored. These incidents result in injury or death almost 1.5 times more frequently than transportation incidents.[4]
- ***Transportation.*** Government and hazardous materials industry officials estimate that there are more than 800,000 hazardous materials shipments daily in the U.S. This translates into the transport of more than 3.1 billion tons of hazardous materials annually.[5] Hazardous materials are transported by air, water, road, rail, and pipeline. Most hazardous materials transportation accidents involve flammable or combustible liquids such as gasoline and fuel oil. The second most frequent type of incident involves corrosive materials (Figure 53-1).
- ***Waste sites.*** Hazardous materials waste sites may take the form of abandoned dumps, municipal landfills, industrial ponds, storage piles, and military bases. The most common contamination at these sites is toxic **leachate.** As rainwater percolates through a landfill, leachate carries soluble toxic and hazardous materials through the soil and potentially into public water sources.

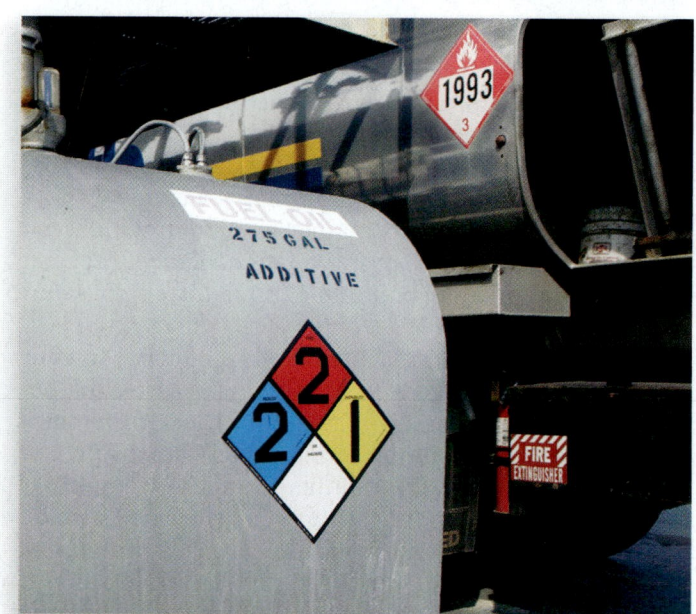

Figure 53-1   A placard is a diamond-shaped sign that is displayed on trucks, railroad cars, and large containers carrying hazardous materials.

- *Medical facilities and hospitals.* Radiation exposure occurs in diagnostic x-rays and radiopharmaceuticals. Prescription, over-the-counter, and herbal medications have toxic effects if inappropriately used. Medical gasses and flammable liquids are also present in healthcare facilities.

- *Households.* Most victims of chemical emergencies are injured at home. Such injuries often result from ignorance or carelessness in using flammable or combustible materials. In an average city of 100,000 residents, 23.5 tons of toilet bowl cleaner, 13.5 tons of liquid household cleaners, and 3.5 tons of motor oil are discharged into city drains each month, making even household sewage dangerous with various levels of toxins of unknown concentration.[6]

- *Naturally occurring toxic substances.* Radiation occurs naturally from cosmic radiation, the earth, and building materials. Radon is a colorless, odorless gas that comes from the decay of uranium found in nearly all soil. Trace amounts of radon can be found in human tissues.

- *Organic fuel combustion.* Engines emit nitrous oxides (one source of "acid rain"), carbon monoxide, and particulates.

- *Soil.* Soil may be contaminated by dumping and spills with potential contamination of groundwater. Contaminants in topsoil may be ingested after entering the food chain or absorbed through the skin during work or play.

- *Air.* Room or environmental air may be contaminated from exhaust (from burning or combustion) or the off-gassing of toxic chemicals following an initial liquid exposure. Off-gassing occurs when the material evaporates from a liquid state to a gas.

- *Water.* Wells, open water, and pools may be contaminated from spills or leaching.[7]

Regulations and Standards

Each employer must develop a safety and health program and provide for emergency response. While training and certification requirements vary from city to city and department to department, there are several health, safety, and performance standards that regulate minimum standards for EMS. In addition to medical training, emergency medical technicians and paramedics who, in the course of their regular duties may be required to respond to hazmat incidents, should have training that meets or exceeds these standards.[8]

OSHA 29 CFR 1910.120: Hazardous Waste Operations and Emergency Response (HAZWOPER) regulates EMS response by requiring that training be appropriate to the duties and functions performed by each responder of an emergency response organization.

BOX 53-1 NFPA Recommendations

- NFPA 472: Identifies the levels of competence required of all responders to hazardous materials incidents.
- NFPA 473: Identifies the levels of competence required of EMS personnel who respond to hazardous materials incidents, with specific requirements for reducing accidents, exposure, and injuries.
- NFPA 1561: Provides the template for organizing responders and reducing fatalities and injuries by using the ICS for all emergency incidents.

HAZWOPER also requires use of the National Incident Management System (NIMS), a written response plan that includes personnel roles, chain of command and communication, a safety officer, emergency alert procedures, and appropriate protective equipment. Safe response requires that individuals be trained and mentally prepared.[9]

CONNECTIONS See Chapter 50: Medical Incident Command for a detailed description of the NIMS.

OSHA regulations are law while standards such as NFPA 472, 473, and 1561 are recommendations, which may or may not be adopted by a jurisdiction. Box 53-1 describes the NFPA recommendations.

Certification Levels

There are many levels of training for hazardous materials responders regulated by OSHA (29 CFR 1910.120q):

DOT 8-4.1

- *First responder awareness level.* First responders at the awareness level have an increased chance of witnessing or discovering a hazmat release and are trained to initiate an emergency response by notifying the proper authorities. They should take no additional action. Awareness-level providers are not trained to enter the warm or hot zones. Awareness-level responders should be able to do the following:
  - Understand what hazardous materials are and the associated risks
  - Understand the potential outcomes of hazmat emergencies
  - Recognize and identify hazardous materials

- Understand their role in an emergency, which is mostly to support operations taking place in the cold zone (outside of the exposure range of the hazardous material)
- Realize the need for additional resources and notify the appropriate people
- Understand and use the North American Emergency Response Guidebook (ERG)

■ *First responder operations level.* Those at this level respond to releases or potential releases of hazardous materials as part of the initial response, with the goal of protecting persons, property, or the environment from the effects of the release. Training is limited to taking a defensive position without attempting to stop the release. The goal is to contain the release from a safe distance, keep it from spreading, and prevent further exposure. Operational level responders should be able to do the following:

- Know basic hazard and risk assessment techniques
- Select and use proper personal protective equipment (PPE)
- Understand basic hazmat terminology
- Perform basic control, containment, and confinement operations
- Implement basic decontamination procedures
- Understand relevant standard operating procedures (SOPs) and termination actions

■ *Hazardous materials technicians.* These technicians respond to releases or potential releases with the goal of stopping the release. They assume an aggressive role and approach the point of release in order to plug, patch, or stop the release of a hazmat. Hazardous materials technicians should be able to do the following:

- Perform at the *first responder operations level*
- Implement the company or agency emergency response plan
- Classify, identify, and verify known and unknown materials using instrumentation
- Select and use proper, advanced PPE
- Understand hazard and risk assessment techniques
- Perform advanced control, containment, and confinement operations
- Understand termination procedures
- Implement decontamination procedures
- Understand basic chemical and toxicological terminology and behavior

■ *Hazardous materials specialists.* Specialists provide support to hazardous materials technicians. Duties require specific knowledge of various materials. The hazardous materials specialist acts as the site liaison with federal, state, local and other government authorities. Hazardous materials specialists should be able to do the following:

- Perform at the *hazardous materials technician level*
- Know details of the state emergency response plan
- Understand detailed hazard and risk assessment techniques
- Perform specialized control, containment, and confinement operations
- Determine and implement decontamination procedures
- Develop a site safety and control plan
- Understand chemical, toxicological, and radiological terminology and behavior
- Act as liaison between various teams and responders

■ *Incident commanders.* ICs assume control of the incident scene and should be able to do the following:

- Perform at the *first responder operations level*
- Implement the NIMS Incident Command System
- Oversee the development of the written incident action plan (IAP) as required by the NIMS standards
- Implement the company emergency response plan
- Understand the hazards and risks associated with working in chemical PPE
- Implement the local emergency response plan
- Understand the state and federal emergency response capabilities
- Understand the importance of decontamination procedures[10]

There are three levels of hazardous materials training specific to EMS.

■ *Awareness and recognition.* Responders who, in the course of their normal duties, may be first on the scene of an emergency involving hazardous materials should have this training. EMS responders at the awareness level work only in the cold zone. Any responder who might be first on the scene is required to have a minimum of awareness level training. Awareness level providers should be able to do the following: DOT 8-4.1

- Recognize the presence of a hazardous material
- Know how to protect their own safety
- Call for technical support
- Secure the area

■ *EMS Level I responders.* Level I responders work only in the cold zone. They are healthcare professionals who are expected to provide care for patients who are no longer at significant risk for secondary contamination. EMS Level I providers should do the following: DOT 8-4.1

- Have EMT-B training or higher,
- Have hazmat awareness level training
- Know specialized topics such as hazardous materials toxicology[11]

■ *EMS Level II responders.* Level II responders are expected to perform decontamination in the warm zone and provide care for victims who still pose a significant risk of secondary contamination. EMS Level II providers should do the following:

- Perform at the *EMS/HAZMAT Level I*
- Analyze and determine the magnitude of problem areas at any scene involving hazardous materials incidents including criminal and terrorist incidents and weapons of mass destruction
- Plan an EMS response, and provide the appropriate level of emergency medical care and decontamination to victims
- Provide medical support to hazardous materials response personnel[11]

Initial Response

Planning

For many years, fire services have been using plans to identify locations that are a potential safety or security risk. Areas typically at risk include laboratories, factories, farm and paint supply outlets, and construction sites. Typically, planning includes identifying entrances (also called access points) and exits (also called egress points), specific hazardous materials kept at the site and their locations in the building, structural information that will help predict collapse, ventilation options, electrical panels, gas lines, sprinklers, and occupancy and hours of operation. Planning is the first step toward both prevention and recognition of a hazmat incident.

Responsibility for planning does not belong only to the fire department. All responders should be aware of the potential safety risks in their communities and consider those risks while en route to every call. Awareness of factors such as time of day, route, vehicle position, wind speed, topography, scene lighting, and other hazards will assist in everything from keeping a patient blanketed on a windy day and loading the stretcher with ease, to determining whether you should evacuate or defend in place in the event that the scene becomes unsafe as a result of assault by chemicals or violence.

On approach to every scene, look around, listen carefully, and approach slowly with caution. Dead animals or fish, fire, and irritation to the skin or eyes suggest the presence of hazardous materials. Many hazardous materials have a noticeable odor, even at nontoxic levels, or have visible smoke, liquid, vapors, or gas. Smell, however, is not a reliable indicator of toxicity, but it can alert you to the possible presence of toxins. Some chemicals impair the sense of smell (e.g., hydrogen sulfide) while others have no smell (e.g., carbon monoxide). If an odor is detectable, you may be too close, and you should evacuate immediately. Listen for high-pitched noises (a leak under pressure) and other sounds that may indicate an ongoing spill. Maintaining a watchful, vigilant attitude is critical and should continue until the incident is over.[12] DOT 8-4.2a

Recognition

Early recognition and accurate identification of hazardous materials is the first and most important thing that you can do to ensure safety while minimizing patient injury. If you do not recognize the presence of a hazard, you cannot take appropriate action, nor can you solve the problem. If you are not aware of the problem, it is likely that you will become part of the problem rather than part of the solution.[13]

Traditionally, EMS providers are trained to administer immediate care and rapid transport. Hazmat incidents are different. Rescue of injured patients should be attempted only after the risk for exposure and injury to responders is reduced or eliminated. Request additional support, as needed. (See Figure 53-2 for a sample decision tree for chemical incidents.)

Standard operating procedures (SOPs) need to be developed and implemented to safely and efficiently direct patient care and scene management. Only through education and training will responders recognize a dangerous scene and apply SOPs. DOT 8-3.1, 8-4.14, 8-4.18

Senses: Sights, Sounds, Smells

The caller or dispatcher may not always know the whole story before your arrival or before action is required. However, clues may help you to identify a hazardous materials incident based on information from the dispatcher, knowledge of the response area, and visual, auditory, or olfactory clues. Watch for smoke, vapor clouds, fire, and the sound of explosions and high pressure leaks. Look for discoloration of grass or trees and dead birds and other animals. Check flags, smokestacks, or vapor clouds for wind direction.

Many hazardous materials have odors or produce vapor clouds. While some materials have an odor at very low and even nontoxic levels, this is not a reliable indicator of potential toxicity. Many toxic, hazardous materials produce no detectable odor, and may lead to **olfactory fatigue** when your senses become accustomed to the smell and no longer perceive its presence. Olfactory fatigue instills a false security. Most importantly, if an odor is detectable, you may be too close, and you should retreat.

How many victims are there? Demographics of the incident may have implications for potential scope and severity of injuries. A release of a hazmat at a nursing home may have different implications than it would at an

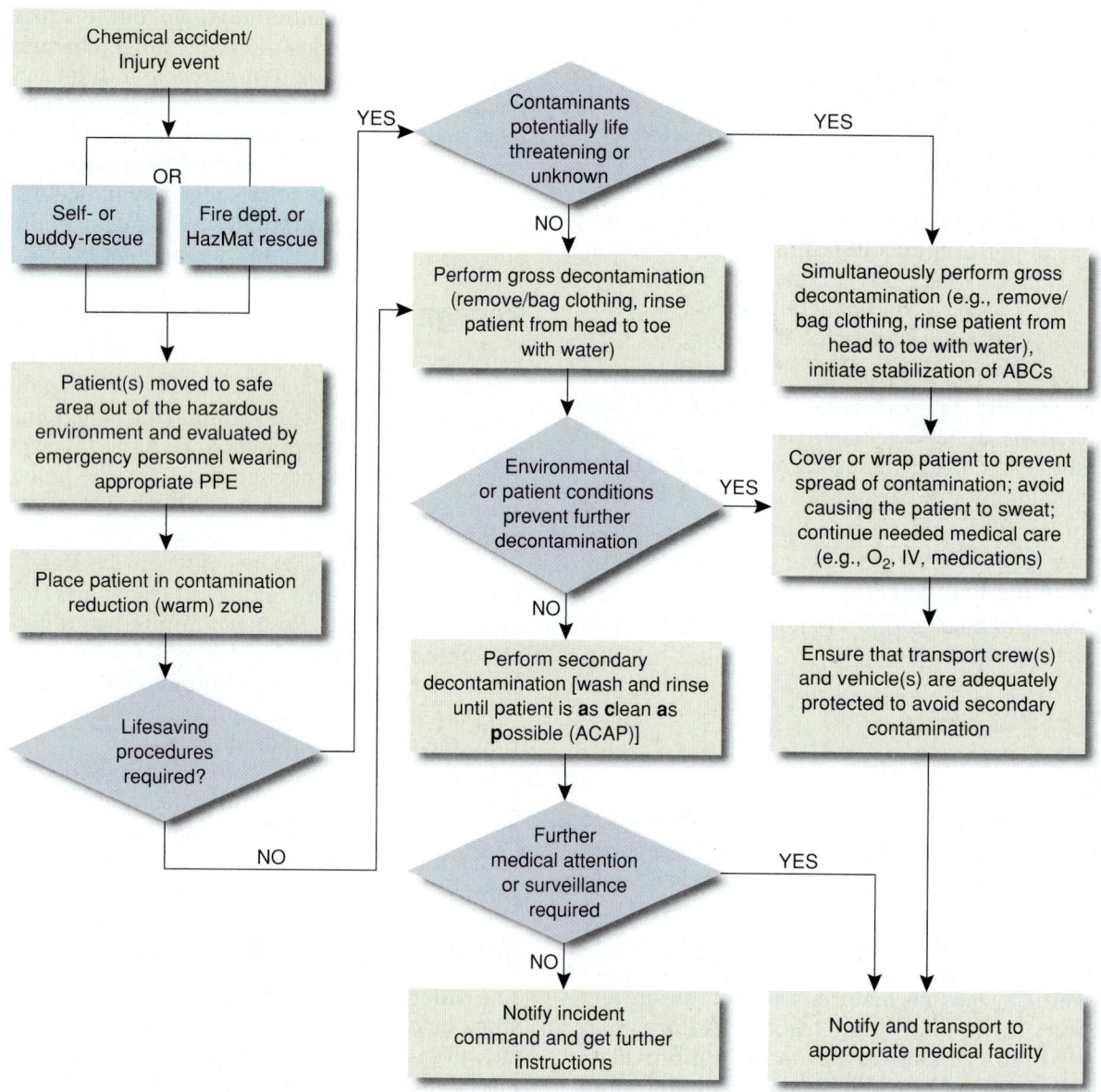

Figure 53-2 Sample EMS decision tree for chemical incidents.

elementary school or shopping mall.[14] Alert the occupants in the area. The concentrations of dense gasses or vapors are not diluted as they disperse or spread. High concentrations may persist. While evacuation is necessary for some materials and incidents, other scenes require occupants to shelter in place (go inside and close doors, windows, and air intakes into air distribution systems until the hazard has dispersed or been removed). Do not enter the contaminated area. Do not attempt to rescue contaminated victims. Many chemicals require specialized personal protective equipment and training.[15]

Incident Organization

Paramedics should be trained and prepared to care for patients in diverse situations. Hazmat incidents may not result in any injuries or may cause mass casualties. Even

a small spill can quickly overwhelm a small fire department or ambulance service, both of which may have little hazmat training and experience. The dynamic nature of the scene will impact the response and command structure.[16] Large incidents attract the media and many other people, including responders and equipment. These factors complicate the efforts to minimize contamination, injuries, death, and property and environmental damage. The incident commander (IC) is responsible for controlling the scene, defining control zones, establishing the level of protection, and decontamination. DOT 8-4.28

The National Incident Management System (NIMS) recommends using unified command if there is more than one agency responding or when incidents cross jurisdictional boundaries. Unified command recommends that designated officers of each agency work together to analyze intelligence information and establish common objectives and strategies to form one incident action plan (IAP).[16] NIMS guidelines always require a written IAP for hazardous materials incidents.

As the first responder on the scene, you may be expected to temporarily establish incident command (IC). Once the command structure is established and victims have been extricated, decontaminated, and moved to a central collection point (large incidents may have many collection points), you can then focus on the following:

1. Triage, treatment, and transport of patients
2. Medical surveillance of responders, including pre- and postentry examinations, with attention to physiological and mental stressors **DOT 8-4.1**

Hazardous Materials Work Zones

Establishing a safe perimeter is a priority. The **initial isolation distance** is the distance to which all occupants should be evacuated in all directions from the site of the spill or leak.[17] It may not be obvious what to secure, especially if the hazmat or size of the release is unknown. It is usually best to overestimate because it is much easier to make the perimeter smaller than larger. When setting up a perimeter and determining evacuation sectors, do not expose yourself by entering areas downwind or below grade. Remember, winds may shift. Changing wind direction warrants reassessing risk and the potential adjustment of the perimeter. Park vehicles pointed away from the scene to allow for a rapid departure. Stage vehicles and personnel a safe distance from the release area since vehicles can be an ignition source.

Many organizations (NIOSH, OSHA, U.S. Coast Guard, and the EPA) recommend dividing the scene into zones, establishing access and egress control points, and designating a contamination reduction corridor (Figure 53-3). Access to zones should be tightly controlled and limited to as few locations as possible. Wind direction, wind speed, and terrain topography (grade) are important considerations when establishing zones. Due to these variables, the zone is seldom round in shape but is more commonly elliptical.[15]

- ***The Hot Zone.*** The hot or exclusion zone surrounds the site of the hazardous materials release and should encompass all known or suspected hazards. Only trained and protected responders should be allowed access into this area.

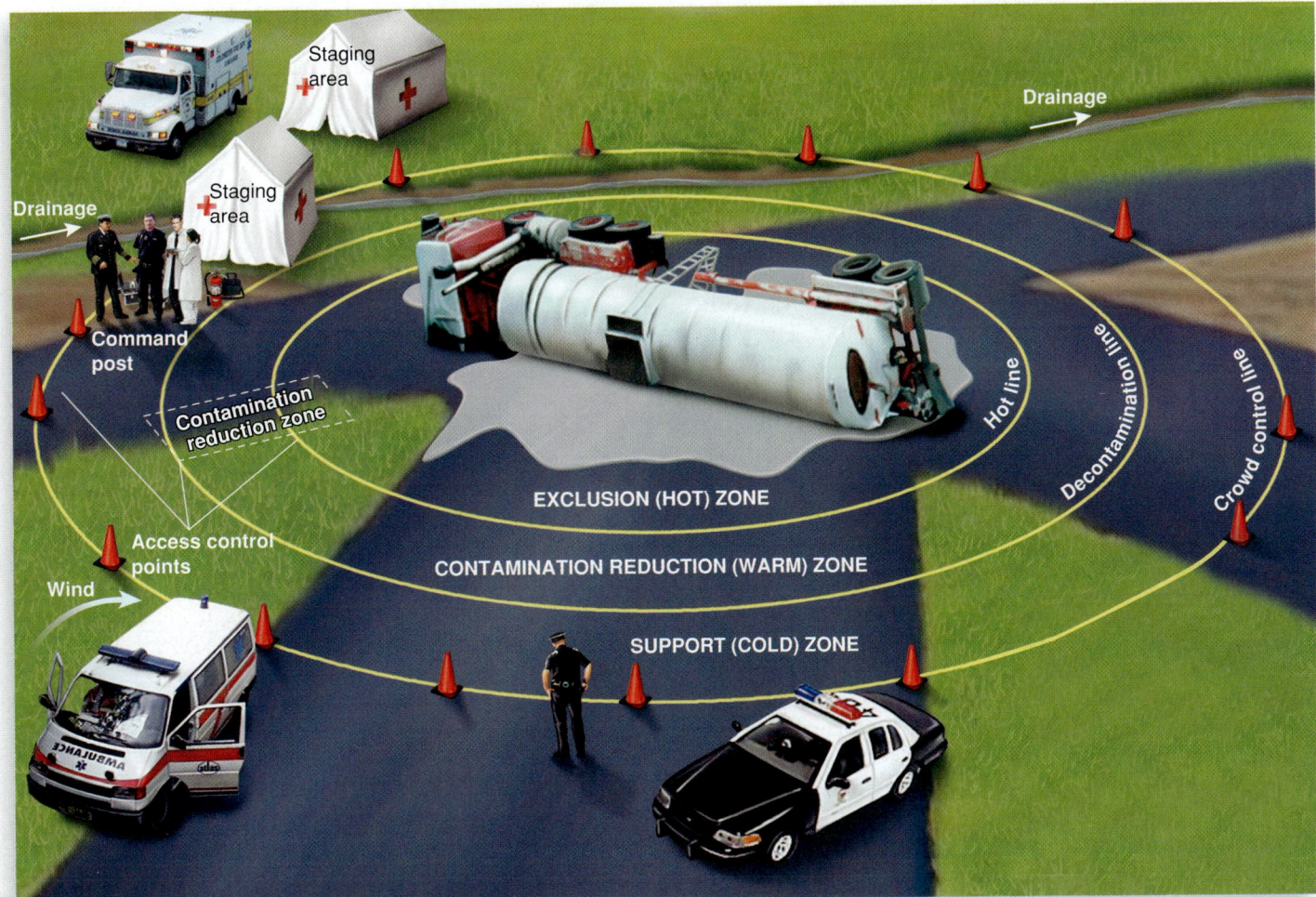

Figure 53-3   Illustration of work zones.

- ***The Warm Zone.*** The perimeter of the contamination reduction (or warm) zone is determined by the length of the decontamination corridor. It contains the "decon" stations and functions as a safety buffer between the hot zone and the cold zone.
- ***The Cold Zone.*** The support (or cold) zone should be "clean" and free of hazmat contamination, including discarded protective clothing and respiratory equipment. The incident command post and staging areas for support equipment that may eventually be needed should be kept in staging areas beyond the crowd control line.[14]

Identification of Hazards

Placards, container labels, shipping documents, Rail Car and Road Trailer Identification Charts, and hazardous materials experts are valuable information sources for identification of a hazmat. Additional information from the shipper or obtained from material safety data sheets (MSDS), the Department of Transportation (DOT) Emergency Response Guidebook (ERG), and <u>chem</u>ical <u>tr</u>ansportation <u>e</u>mergency <u>c</u>enter (CHEMTREC) can help identify health hazards, anticipated injuries, routes of exposure, level of PPE required, the size of the evacuation zone, and other dangers such as explosion or fire.[19]

Material Safety Data Sheets and Shipping Papers

Documents can help you identify and make the right decision about patient care and potential hazards. Health and safety decisions should be based on examining at least three resources. Material safety data sheets (MSDS) should be available at fixed facilities (Figure 53-4). While in transit, shipping papers should be available. These are usually located in the cabs of trucks, the first engine of freight trains, the bridge of ships, and in marked tubes on the decks of barges. Unfortunately, incidents that occur during transport often render shipping papers inaccessible. Identification of materials can become extremely difficult, especially when a variety of chemicals are in the same vehicle. This situation is referred to as a "mixed load." Until all materials are identified, a scene should be treated as if uncontrolled and hazardous.[14]

Colors and Placards

Markings on containers, buildings, or facilities may also provide material identification information. All markings should be observed from a distance. Using binoculars will help keep you safe and facilitate identification and scene size-up.

The National Fire Protection Association fire diamond (NFPA 704) placard system is used to immediately and easily identify hazardous risks. The placard uses a diamond shape divided into four areas (Figure 53-5). Each area represents a specific hazard:

1. MATERIAL SAFETY DATA SHEET	
PRODUCT NAME:	CAS #
CHEMICAL NATURE:	
% ACTIVITY:	

2. PHYSICAL DATA			
BOILING POINT, 760 MM HG		FREEZE POINT	
SPECIFIC GRAVITY		VAPOR PRESSURE AT 20 C	
VAPOR DENSITY		SOLUBILITY IN H_2O	
PER CENT VOLATILES BY WEIGHT		IONIC NATURE	
APPEARANCE AND ODOR			

3. CHEMICAL INGREDIENTS		
MATERIAL	%	TLV (Units)

4. FIRE AND EXPLOSION HAZARD DATA					
FLASH POINT (test methods)		AUTOIGNITION TEMPERATURE			
FLAMMABLE LIMITS IN AIR, % by volume		Lower		Upper	
EXTINGUISHINNG MEDIA					
SPECIAL FIRE FIGHTING PROCEDURES					
UNUSUAL FIRE AND EXPLOSION HAZARDS					

5. HEALTH HAZARD DATA	
THRESHOLD LIMIT VALUE	
EFFECTS OF EXPOSURE	
EMERGENCY AND FIRST AID PROCEDURES	

6. REACTIVE DATA			
STABILITY		CONDITIONS TO AVOID	
UNSTABLE	STABLE		
COMPATIBILITY			
HAZARDOUS RECOMPOSITION PRODUCTS			
HAZARDOUS POLYMERIZATION		CONDITIONS TO AVOID	

7. SPILL OR LEAK PROCEDURES	
STEPS TO BE TAKEN OR MATERIAL IS RELEASED OR SPILLED	
WASTE DISPOSAL METHOD	

8. SPECIAL PROTECTION INFORMATION				
RESPIRATORY PROTECTION				
VENTILATION	LOCAL EXHAUST		SPECIAL	
	MECHANICAL		OTHER	
PROTECTIVE GLOVES			EYE PROTECTION	
OTHER PROTECTIVE EQUIPMENT				

9. SPECIAL PRECAUTIONS	
PRECAUTIONARY LABELING	
OTHER HANDLING AND STORAGE CONDITIONS	

Figure 53-4 Material safety data sheet (MSDS).

1. Blue indicates health hazard
2. Red indicates flammability
3. Yellow indicates reactivity
4. White advises special information

NATIONAL FIRE PROTECTION ASSOCIATION (NFPA) Fire Diamonds					
Degrees of Health Hazards Color Code: BLUE		Degrees of Flammability Hazards Color Code: RED		Degrees of Instability Hazards Color Code: YELLOW	
Degree of Hazard		Degree of Hazard		Degree of Hazard	
Signal		Signal		Signal	
4	Materials that, under emergency conditions, can be lethal	4	Materials that will rapidly or completely vaporize at atmospheric pressure and normal ambient temperature, or that are readily dispersed in air and burn readily	4	Materials that in themselves are readily capable of detonation or explosive decomposition or explosive reaction at normal temperatures and pressures
3	Materials that, under emergency conditions, can cause serious or permanent injury	3	Liquids and solids that can be ignited under almost all ambient temperature conditions. Materials in this degree produce hazardous atmospheres with air under almost all ambient temperatures or, though unaffected by ambient temperatures, are readily ignited under almost all conditions	3	Materials that in themselves are readily capable of detonation or explosive decomposition or explosive reaction but that require a strong initiating source or must be heated under confinement before initiation
2	Materials that, under emergency conditions, can cause temporary incapacitation or residual injury	2	Materials that must be moderately heated or exposed to relatively high ambient temperatures before ignition can occur. Materials in this degree would not under normal conditions form hazardous atmospheres with air, but under high ambient temperatures or under moderate heating could release vapor in sufficient quantities to produce hazardous atmospheres with air	2	Materials that readily undergo violent chemical change at elevated temperatures and pressures
1	Materials that, under emergency conditions, can cause significant irritation	1	Material that must be preheated before ignition can occur. Materials in this degree require considerable preheating under all ambient temperature conditions before ignition and combustion can occur.	1	Materials that in themselves are normally stable but that can become unstable at elevated temperatures and pressures
0	Materials that, under emergency conditions, would offer no hazard beyond that of ordinary combustible materials	0	Materials that will not burn under typical fire conditions, including intrinsically noncombustible materials such as concrete, stone and sand	0	Materials that in themselves are normally stable, even under fire conditions

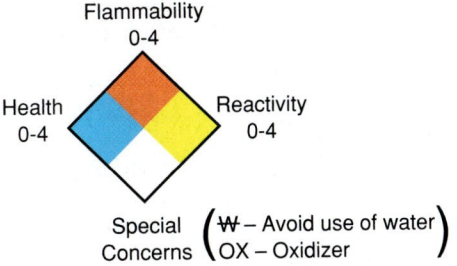

Figure 53-5   NFPA 704 Fire Diamonds.

A number ranging from zero through four indicates the severity of the hazard. Zero is low-risk and four is high-risk. This placard system only describes the risks associated with the chemical. It does not give specific information about the actual chemical.[18]

Street Secrets

You should maintain a high index of suspicion and caution with any vehicle or device that appears to carry a hazardous substance. If you do not see a placard, there may still be hazardous substances present. Placards are not always found where they should be. If the vehicle rolled over, placards may have broken off or been damaged. Also, the amount of hazardous material may be too small to meet the minimum DOT requirements for placarding. Another problem may occur if two or more hazardous substances are mixed together. The placard may not reflect this "mixed load" or any added dangers due to the substances interacting. Remember also that this placard system only works when the transporter of the hazardous material is complying with the law. Always expect the unexpected, and keep looking until you are satisfied that you see the whole picture.

Department of Transportation (DOT) Hazardous Materials Classifications

Once you have located a placard, the DOT Emergency Response Guide (ERG) helps you quickly identify specific or generic hazards of the material (Figure 53-6). The ERG suggests appropriate protection for responders and the general public while waiting for experts to arrive. It describes recommended isolation zones and also provides duplicate information in several formats; alphabetical, by numerical designation, and by degree of danger of the substance. The guide contains contact information for CHEMTREC in numerous locations throughout the book.

The ERG provides worst-case scenario information for the initial response (first 30 minutes of the incident). It does not provide specific information about the physical or chemical properties of dangerous goods. As hazard-specific information becomes available, the response should be tailored to the situation. The Department of Transportation (DOT) mandates use of DOT markings and identification numbers for all transportation vehicles. Delivery trucks and vans that regularly carry hazardous materials are required by law to be marked as well.

DOT placards provide information using colors, symbols, and either hazard class wording or a four-digit identification number. The placard is found above an identification number. The number is the United Nations (UN) number for the material contained in the vehicle and can be used to identify the material or class of material. Hazardous materials are grouped based on the chemical and physical properties of the product (hazard class). Each class has a symbol that suggests the primary type of hazard it poses. There are nine DOT hazard classes:

- Class 1—explosives
- Class 2—gasses
- Class 3—flammable liquids (and combustible liquids [U.S.])
- Class 4—flammable solids; spontaneously combustible materials; and dangerous when wet materials
- Class 5—oxidizers and organic peroxides
- Class 6—toxic materials and infectious substances
- Class 7—radioactive materials
- Class 8—corrosive materials
- Class 9—miscellaneous dangerous goods

Each of these classes is then divided into subsets.[19] Box 53-2 describes how the ERG is organized and used.

Location

The type of building, its location in the community, and the place within the building where a hazardous material is located provide clues to determining what type of hazards are present. A home, cooperative, manufacturing facility, or oil refinery may contain different hazards or multiple hazards.

Container Shape and Construction

If you can see the shape or silhouette of an individual container, you may have a clue to the chemicals with which you may be dealing. While the shape will not provide a specific chemical name, it will help to identify the general type of material. Container construction is also an important factor. A container made of polyethylene is more likely to contain a corrosive material while an open-ended drum is more likely to contain a solid than a liquid. Rounded ends on a truck suggest the material inside is under pressure. While boxes usually have powders, stainless steel containers usually contain either foods or corrosives. Glass holds corrosive liquids.

Chemistry Overview and Toxicology

Toxicology is the study of the nature, effects, and detection of poisons in living organisms. Every chemical has unique physical and toxicological properties with different onset, duration, and severity, depending on the toxicity of the chemical, route and duration of exposure, and health of the victim. In order to anticipate and treat signs and symptoms, we must understand basic principles and terminology of toxicology.

HAZARD CLASSIFICATION SYSTEM

The hazard class of dangerous goods is indicated either by its class (or division) number or name. For a placard corresponding to the primary hazard class of a material, the hazard class or division number must be displayed in the lower corner of the placard. However, no hazard class or division number may be displayed on a placard representing the subsidiary hazard of a material. For other than Class 7 or the OXYGEN placard, text indicating a hazard (for example, "CORROSIVE") is not required. Text is shown only in the U.S. The hazard class or division number must appear on the shipping document after each shipping name.

Class 1 - Explosives

Division 1.1	Explosives with a mass explosion hazard
Division 1.2	Explosives with a projection hazard
Division 1.3	Explosives with predominantly a fire hazard
Division 1.4	Explosives with no significant blast hazard
Division 1.5	Very insensitive explosives with a mass explosion hazard
Division 1.6	Extremely insensitive articles

Class 2 - Gases

Division 2.1	Flammable gases
Division 2.2	Non-flammable, non-toxic* gases
Division 2.3	Toxic* gases

Class 3 - Flammable liquids (and Combustible liquids [U.S.])

Class 4 - Flammable solids; Spontaneously combustible materials; and Dangerous when wet materials/Water-reactive substances

Division 4.1	Flammable solids
Division 4.2	Spontaneously combustible materials
Division 4.3	Water-reactive substances/Dangerous when wet materials

Class 5 - Oxidizing substances and Organic peroxides

Division 5.1	Oxidizing substances
Division 5.2	Organic peroxides

Class 6 - Toxic* substances and Infectious substances

Division 6.1	Toxic* substances
Division 6.2	Infectious substances

Class 7 - Radioactive materials

Class 8 - Corrosive substances

Class 9 - Miscellaneous hazardous materials/Products, Substances or Organisms

* The words "poison" or "poisonous" are synonymous with the word "toxic".

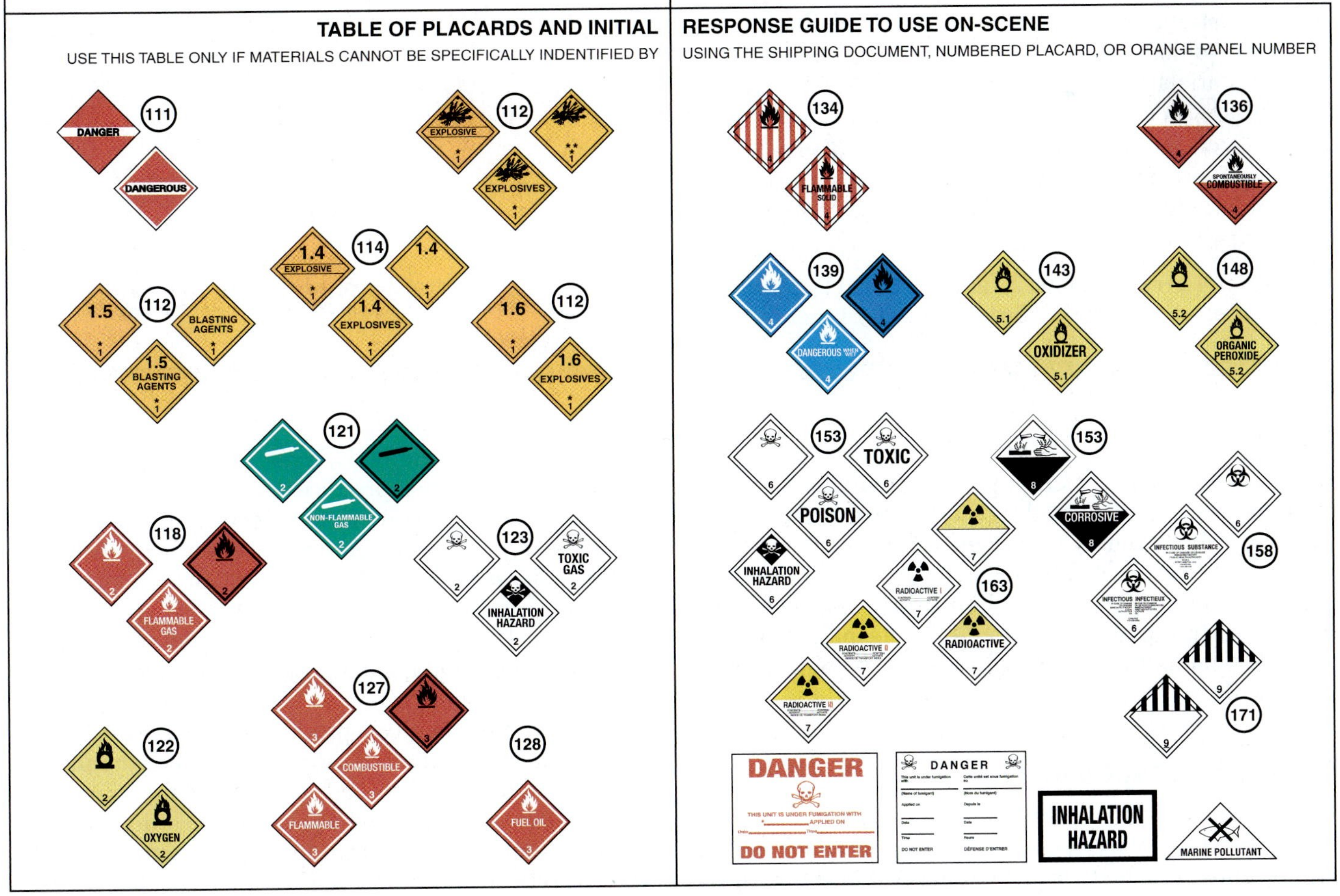

TABLE OF PLACARDS AND INITIAL

USE THIS TABLE ONLY IF MATERIALS CANNOT BE INDENTIFIED BY

RESPONSE GUIDE TO USE ON-SCENE

USING THE SHIPPING DOCUMENT, NUMBERED PLACARD, OR ORANGE PANEL NUMBER

Figure 53-6 The DOT ERG is the recommended source of information for identifying hazardous materials.

BOX 53-2 / Emergency Response Guidebook Contents

Chapter 1/yellow border: The four-digit ID number is listed in numerical order, followed by the emergency response guide assignment and material name.

Chapter 2/blue border: Materials are listed alphabetically, followed by the emergency response guide assignment and four-digit ID number.

Chapter 3/orange border: Provides safety recommendations and emergency response information (fire situations, spill or leak incidents, and first aid). Each guide is designed to cover a group of materials that possess similar chemical and toxicological characteristics. Each guide is divided into three main sections:

1. This section describes hazards in order of potential. It provides vital information to facilitate decisions regarding the protection of the responders and occupants.

2. This section provides general information about initial isolation of the incident site, recommends the type of protective clothing and respiratory protection, and suggests evacuation distances for small and large spills and fire or explosive situations. It also prompts the consultation of the tables listing toxic inhalation hazard (TIH) materials and water-reactive materials (green chapter), as needed (yellow and blue chapters).

3. This section lists emergency response actions and general first aid, with special precautions for incidents involving fire, spills, or chemical exposure.

Chapter 4/green border: A table displays ID number; TIH, including certain chemical warfare agents; and water-reactive substances. The table provides two different safe distances: initial isolation distances and protective action distances. Distances for both small and large spills are listed with day and night differentials (atmospheric conditions affect the potential size of the incident). Day and night affects the safe distances due to different mixing and dispersion conditions in the atmosphere. At night, the air is generally calmer, causing gasses and vapors to disperse less, thus increasing concentrations above the levels that would occur during the day. DOT 8-4.10, 8-4.17, 8-4.27

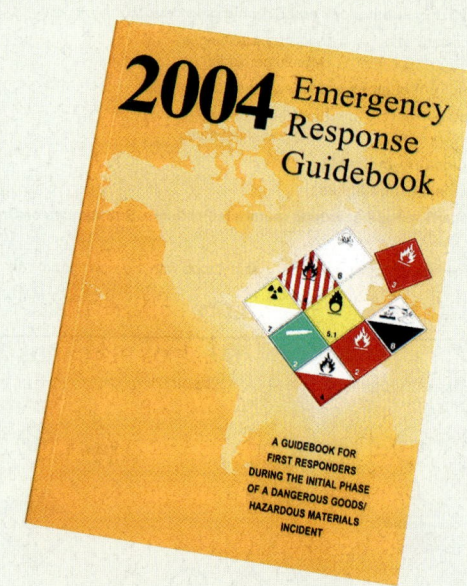

Source: U.S. Department of Transportation, *Emergency Response Guidebook*, 2004 ed., (Washington, DC: Government Printing Office, 2004).

Identifying hazmat incidents does not require extensive knowledge of chemistry or toxicology; however, a basic understanding can assist prehospital medical professionals in recognizing hazards associated with chemical family characteristics and provide safe treatment of patients while protecting responders.[20] It is important for paramedics to maintain and increase competence through aggressive continuing education.

Dose and Response

Toxic chemicals often produce effects or injuries where they contact the body. A chemical injury localized to the site of contact is called a local toxic effect. A chemical may also be absorbed into the bloodstream and distributed throughout the entire body, most often to target organs. This distribution then produces systemic effects.

Route of exposure is an important factor when considering the amount of the chemical absorbed. **Dose response** is a critical concept in toxicology. As the dose increases, the severity of the toxic response increases. Dose response values are often found on material safety data sheets (MSDS) and other sources of health information.

Hazardous chemicals produce a wide range of symptoms. A complex relationship exists between the amount of the compound absorbed (dose) and the concentration in the environment. The dose is seldom known. Factors such as concentration of the chemical, route, and duration of exposure all contribute to the dose received and will assist in estimating the response.

Routes of Entry

Personal protective equipment is designed to provide emergency medical personnel with protection from hazardous materials that can enter the body by inhalation, ingestion, direct contact absorption, and injection. DOT 8-4.5, 8-4.6

- Inhalation allows toxic compounds to enter the respiratory system. Water-soluble gasses are easily absorbed through mucous membranes. Non-water-soluble substances may be deposited in the lungs, causing local toxicity. Respiratory protection should be appropriate for the hazard and should be properly sized. For example, a typical N-95 mask is not a replacement for a self-contained breathing apparatus (SCBA). The mask should also be well-maintained. Respiratory protection may include dust masks, N-95 masks, purified air-powered respirators (PAPR), or bottled air (e.g., SCBA). The appropriate mask should be worn for each situation and should only be worn for the recommended amount of time. For example, the N-95 mask will not protect a person from the corrosive effects of a cloud of gas, but an encapsulated suit may.
- Ingestion is a less common route of exposure for responders. Chemicals may splash or spray on the mouth or nose. Improper decontamination followed by hand-to-mouth contact, eating, drinking, or swallowing saliva and mucus containing trapped airborne contaminants can cause exposure.
- Direct contact exposures occur when a chemical contact touches the skin or eye. Some chemicals are readily absorbed through the skin. The rate of absorption is increased when the skin, the body's protective layer, is opened by cuts or abrasions. Skin may be shielded by protective clothing, and full face respirators protect against direct contact and splashing or droplets.
- Hazardous materials may enter the body by accidental injection or wounds. Exposures from injection enter the blood almost immediately.[21]

CONNECTIONS Chapter 35: Toxicology has additional information on poisonings and how chemicals interact with bodily tissues.

Exposure Limits

Exposure limits are based on time-weighted average limits, ceiling values, or ceiling concentration limits to which a worker can be exposed without adverse effects.

- **Immediately dangerous to life and health (IDLH):** concentration of toxin that causes immediate threat to life.

- The effects may be immediate or delayed and often are irreversible.
- May interfere with person's ability to self-rescue.
- Lethal concentration or **lethal dose (LD):** concentration or dose of toxin that results in death of a defined percentage of test subjects.
  - LCt50 = concentration in air that kills 50% of test subjects.
  - LD50 = ingested, injected, or absorbed dose that kills 50% of test subjects.
- **Permissible exposure limit (PEL):** the maximum amount or concentration of a chemical that a worker may be exposed to under OSHA regulations.
- **Recommended exposure limit (REL):** the highest allowable airborne concentration that is not expected to injure a worker; expressed as a ceiling limit or time-weighted average for an eight- or 10-hour work day.
- Threshold limit value/**time-weighted average (TWA):** maximum concentration of toxin a person can be exposed to eight hours a day, 40 hours per week without suffering adverse effects.
  - **Threshold limit value/short-term exposure limit (TLV/STEL):** maximum concentration of toxin a person can be exposed to for 15 minutes without suffering adverse effects. (Not to be exceeded or repeated more than four times daily, with 60 minute rests between each exposure).
  - **Threshold limit value/ceiling level (TLV/CL):** maximum concentration of a toxin that should *never* be exceeded, even for a moment. DOT 8-4.16, 8-4.6

The above values are used as benchmarks for determining relative toxicity, and should be used to help select appropriate levels of PPE. Limit values are only useful if monitoring equipment is available to measure the concentration of the hazard. EMS personnel should have a working understanding of exposure limits because they will be referenced on documents that will suggest PPE, decontamination, and patient treatment based on the concentration.[4] Box 53-3 lists some additional hazmat terminology.

Responding to an Incident

Notification and Communication

Early and effective communication is essential to controlling an incident. Early communications with other agencies should indicate that the incident management system—incident command system (ICS) has been established and should advise the safest route of approach, known hazards, and the estimated number of

BOX 53-3   Hazmat Terminology

Other terms you may encounter that will increase your understanding and performance include the following:

- **Alpha particle**—A positively charged particle emitted by radioactive atoms. Alpha particles travel less than one inch in the air and are stopped by a thin sheet of paper. Ingestion is the primary route of exposure.
- **Beta particle**—Very high-energy particle that can penetrate a few centimeters of tissue.
- **Boiling liquid expanding vapor explosion (BLEVE)**—A container failure with a violent release of energy, followed by ignition.
- **Boiling point**—Temperature at which a liquid becomes a gas (temperature at which a substance's vapor pressure equals atmospheric pressure).
- **Catalyst**—A substance that accelerates chemical change yet is not permanently affected by the reaction.
- **Degradation**—A chemical action involving the molecular breakdown of protective clothing material due to contact with a chemical or molecular breakdown of the spilled or released material to render it less hazardous.
- **Emulsifiers**—Substances that help in mixing liquids that don't normally mix (e.g., soap acts on oil and water).
- **Flash point**—The lowest temperature at which a liquid generates enough vapor to ignite in air.
- **Flammable or explosive limits**
  - Lower explosive limit—Lowest concentration of chemical that burns in air.
  - Upper explosive limit—Highest concentration of chemical that burns in air.
- **Gamma radiation**—A high-energy photon (ray) emitted from the nucleus of certain radioactive

atoms, best stopped by dense materials such as lead.

- **Heavy metals**—A group of elements (such as chromium, lead, copper, and zinc) that can be toxic at relatively low concentrations and tend to accumulate in the food chain.
- **Ionizing radiation**—The release of energized particles that can produce charged particles (ions) in any material it strikes, causing damage to molecules, cells, or tissues.
- **Ignition temperature**—Lowest temperature at which a liquid will give off enough vapors to support ongoing combustion. Slightly higher than flash point.
- **Persistence**—The ability of a chemical to remain in the environment for longer than 24 hours. Liquids and solids are more likely to be persistent.
- **Reactive**—A class of compounds that are normally unstable and readily undergo chemical change, may react violently with water, can produce toxic gasses with water, or possess other similar properties.
- **Specific gravity**—Density of a liquid compared to water (water = 1).
  - Specific gravity greater than 1—Liquid sinks in water.
  - Specific gravity less than 1—Liquid floats on water.
- **Vapor density**—Measures the weight of a vapor or gas compared to air (air = 1).
  - Vapor density greater than 1—Gas sinks.
  - Vapor density less than 1—Gas rises.
- **Vapor pressure**—Measures the rate at which a liquid evaporates or changes into a vapor or gas. (Higher vapor pressures = Rapid evaporation).

DOT 8-4.15

---

injuries. A dedicated radio frequency may facilitate distribution of critical information.

Communication between EMS and medical control and receiving facilities should be established early, with updates as needed to reflect changes in patient numbers and severity. Early notification will facilitate hospital preparedness. Important information includes the following:

- Your identification
- Actual or estimated number of victims
- Number of victims in each triage category
- Decontamination status of victims

- Identity of contaminant
- Estimated time of arrival at the receiving facility[19]

Personal Protection Equipment

Some paramedics may never train with or use personal protective equipment (PPE) other than PPE that is used for infection control. However, all emergency responders should have an understanding of the different types of PPE available and when it is appropriate to wear them. This understanding will help the paramedic understand why various levels of PPE are used on a scene, as well as the stressors and limitations that responders will be subjected to.

Training is essential before any individual attempts to use PPE.

CONNECTIONS Chapter 9: Safety and Scene Size-Up discusses general PPE that is required for use on routine EMS calls.

There are several routes of exposure in which a hazardous agent may cause you significant distress, injury, and death. The respiratory system is by far the most vulnerable body system and is one of the fastest routes of exposure for most agents. By inhaling certain agents, you are more likely to become sick much faster than by other routes such as ingestion or absorption. Thousands of emergency personnel become injured as a result of respiratory injuries or exposures. Many of the exposures are the result of improper use, or lack of use, of SCBA during fire ground operations. DOT 8-4.7

Respiratory Protection

In addition to surgical masks, N-95 masks are used to filter certain larger particles and for infectious disease control.

There are two basic types of respirators: atmosphere-supplying and air-purifying. Atmosphere-supplying respirators include the self-contained breathing apparatus (SCBA) and supplied-air respirators (SAR). OSHA 29 CFR 1910.134 specifies mandatory legal minimum respiratory protection standards. NIOSH certifies specific respiratory protection equipment.

Personnel using respiratory protection must be fit-tested. The same style or design of a mask comes in a variety of sizes and shapes. EMS providers will try on a variety of sizes and will be evaluated for proper fit. This generally involves donning the mask and placing a hood over the head. A strong, odor-producing, nontoxic chemical such as peppermint oil is placed into the environment, and the provider is asked to breathe deeply and report if they smell the chemical. Proper fit is achieved when the odor is not detected. Providers must be trained and drilled in how to properly put on and securely tighten the mask. Stored equipment must be routinely inspected to ensure that it is still packaged correctly and is undamaged. DOT 8-4.9

Atmosphere-Supplying Respirators. Atmosphere-supplying respirators consist of the self-contained breathing apparatus (SCBA), which contains its own air supply, and the supplied-air respirator (SAR), which depends on an air supply provided through a line linked to a distant, ambient air source.

Positive Pressure Self-Contained Breathing Apparatus (SCBA). Also known as an airpack within the fire service, the SCBA supplies air to a facemask from a tank. Most SCBA systems fit the wearer with a full-face piece and a nose cup that helps improve visibility and reduce fogging. The SCBA provides the highest level of respiratory protection; if a leak develops, contaminants are forced out by the pressure in the supplied air. The SCBA is equipped with multiple fail-safe systems that ensure ample exit time from a hazardous situation. Use time is limited by the amount of air in the tank.

Supplied-Air Respirator (SAR). With an SAR, air is supplied to a facemask through a hose line connected to a source at a remote location. The large remote air source allows the wearer to work for a longer period of time without bottle changes, reduces bulk and weight, and increases agility. However, the hose line limits distance and restricts mobility around obstacles.

Air-Purifying Respirator (APR). Also called cartridge respirators or powered air-purifying respirators (PAPR), the APR does not provide a presupplied source of air. Instead, ambient air is filtered through hazard specific cartridges or canisters before inhalation. APRs increase mobility by reducing weight and eliminating a hose line. However, they require an atmosphere of at least 19.5% oxygen and the absence of hazards that cannot be filtered out by the mask. The APR is not as safe as the SCBA. Its use is reserved until after proper air monitoring has been accomplished and levels within the work zone are designated safe for APR use. The powered air purifying respirator (PAPR) is a motorized system that filters ambient air through hazard-specific cartridges or canisters before inhalation under positive pressure.[20]

Skin Protection

Second only to respiratory protection, protecting your skin from dangerous agents is best accomplished with the protective clothing available to emergency responders. Hazardous materials protective clothing comes in a variety of shapes, styles, and sizes. Chemical protective clothing is broken down into levels by the degree of protection that each offers. The levels range from A to D, with Level A affording the wearer the most protection and Level D the least protection (see Table 53-1 and Figure 53-7).

- **Level A** protection is the highest level of respiratory, skin, eye, and mucous membrane protection. It consists of a fully encapsulating, chemical-resistant suit and self-contained breathing apparatus (SCBA).

TABLE 53-1 Personal Protection Equipment

Level of Protection	Features	Indications	Advantages	Limitations
Level A	• Highest level of skin and respiratory protection • Chemical, vapor, and gas protective suit that is fully encapsulating • Self-contained breathing apparatus	• Anytime there is an unknown chemical or substance • Highest level of respiratory protection needed (based on chemical and physical properties of material) • Highest level of skin protection required • Highest level of eye protection required • Constant high concentration exposure • Skin absorbable chemicals • Suspected or confirmed carcinogens • Entrance into confined space of unknowns	• Virtually eliminates possibility of any contact with environmental hazards; it is its own environment • Best known protection • Provides limited thermal protection	• Bulky • Physically stressful; does not allow cooling • Psychologically stressful • Reduced mobility and dexterity; increases time to perform jobs • Makes communication difficult • Expensive
Level B	• Chemical resistant clothing • Self-contained breathing apparatus	• Incident when the highest level of respiratory protection is necessary but a lesser degree of skin protection needed • Chemical or agent is mainly a respiratory hazard	• High level of respiratory protection • Increased mobility and dexterity compared to Level A • Somewhat cooler • Compliant garments may have good penetration characteristics • Less expensive than Level A suits	• Not designed to protect from vapor or gas • Noncompliant suits may leak in liquids • Noncompliant suits provide no thermal protection
Level C (NFPA guidelines)	• NFPA 1993 garments made for support zone activities such as decontamination and remedial site mitigation • Air-purifying respirator	• Reduced level of respiratory protection needed • Well characterized and measured agents • Splashes or incidental contact with agent will not cause harm to skin or be absorbed	• Tested against penetration and liquid integrity • Lightweight and less physical stress • More comfortable • Designed to be disposable	• Can only be used in controlled situations • Greatly reduced flammability rating—no flash protection • Reduced strength from the typical Level B suit
Level D	• Eye protection • Coveralls • Boots or shoes that are chemically resistant and steel toed and shanked • Hard hat • Gloves	• Atmosphere contains no known hazard • Work activities preclude splashes, immersion, or the potential for unexpected inhalation or contact with hazardous materials	• Allows more efficient work activities in nonemergency situations	• No respiratory protection • Minimal skin protection

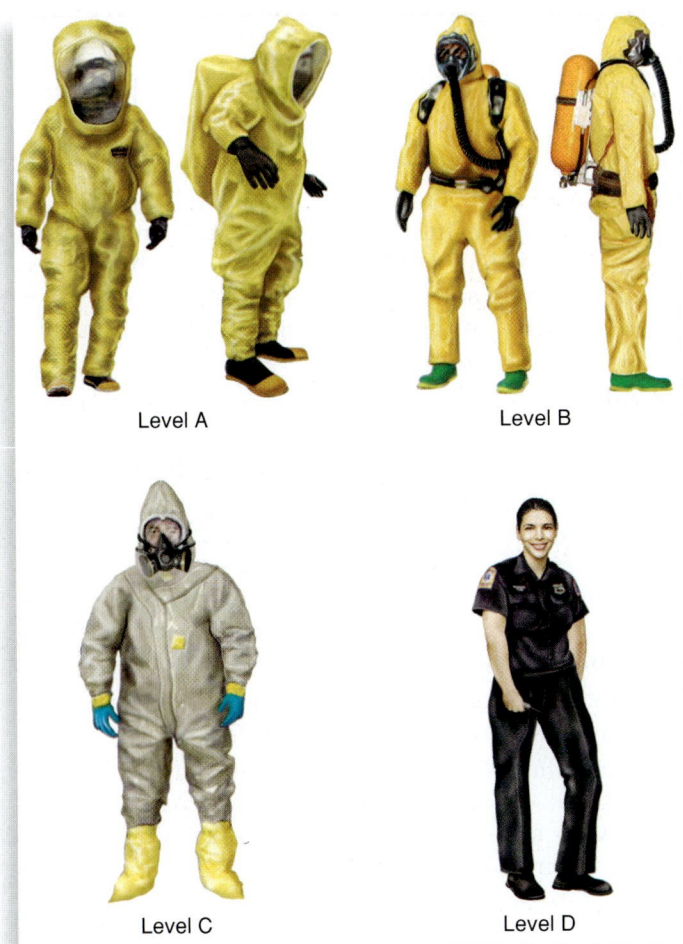

Figure 53-7   PPE examples.

PPE minimizes heat stress, physical and psychological stress, impaired vision, impaired mobility, and impaired communication ability. Users should be working close to a partner via the buddy system and should be monitored by a safety officer. An agreed-upon distress signal should be used if an emergency develops.[4] DOT 8-4.9

Protective clothing is impermeable to moisture, thus limiting the transfer of heat from the body through natural evaporation. This is a particularly important factor in hot environments or for strenuous tasks since such garments increase the likelihood of heat-related injuries. Proper boot and glove selection is also important. Choose outer boots and gloves that will resist the hazards that will be encountered. Inner boots should be chemical-resistant with a steel toe and shank. Multiple layers of gloves, while necessary, will impair obtaining vital signs, assessing patients, and performing simple skills.

The effectiveness of protective clothing is reduced by the following:

■ **Degradation.** Degradation occurs when the protective qualities of the material are altered through contact with chemical substances. Structural changes in the clothing (cracking and brittleness) increase permeability to chemical hazards.

■ **Permeability.** Permeability is the ease with which a chemical can pass through the barrier. It is affected by the specific properties and concentrations of the chemical, the type of protective barrier selected, and its integrity.

■ **Penetration.** Penetration occurs when the barrier is punctured or breached or when seams or openings allow the hazard to enter the suit.[4] DOT 8-4.9

Decontamination

Decontamination is the process of removing or reducing hazards that have accumulated on people or equipment to eliminate or reduce the toxic effect.

Street Secrets

Paramedics should adhere to both their level of training and their assigned role in the command structure. Paramedics should not engage in decontamination procedures unless their certification is hazmat EMS Level II and they have the PPE necessary to do so safely. An awareness-level provider is not equipped to perform decontamination at a hazardous materials incident.

Early decontamination can prevent secondary contamination and may make the difference between a minor injury and death. The most important and most effective

---

■ **Level B** protection uses the highest level of respiratory protection but offers less skin and eye protection. In conjunction with SCBA, it provides splash protection by use of chemical-resistant clothing.

■ **Level C** protection is for known airborne substances, with continuously monitored concentrations. Criteria for air-purifying respirators (APR) must be met, and skin and eye exposures must be unlikely. It provides the same level of skin protection as Level B but a lower level of respiratory protection.

■ **Level D** is a work uniform. It provides no respiratory protection and minimal skin protection. This is the appropriate level for awareness-trained individuals.

There is no universally appropriate equipment that provides adequate protection from all hazards. PPE should protect you from anticipated hazards while minimizing injury from incorrect use or malfunction. Inadequate training or improper use of equipment increases the risk of exposure and injury. Selecting appropriate

decontamination is done immediately after exposure. This is personal decontamination, and it can be performed by the victim. It occurs as the victim strips off contaminated clothing and places it inside a large trash bag. Ambulatory victims should be told to leave the hot zone and further decontaminate themselves by showering under the direction of the decontamination team. This will allow responders to concentrate on those unable to evacuate and decontaminate themselves. DOT 8-4.4

Formal decontamination is an enormous task. The process requires large numbers of responders, time, and resources.[21] Some incidents may require multiple stages of contamination reduction. Gross decontamination removes or chemically alters the majority of the hazard, but some residual contamination may remain. Secondary decontamination further reduces, or alters, contamination. DOT 8-4.8

Complete decontamination is an unrealistic expectation for a decontamination corridor with large numbers of casualties. Effective decontamination means making the patient as clean as possible. It is important to remember that even if a substance has been removed from skin tissue, some chemicals may be found in bodily fluids and exhaled air.[14] Therefore, remove what you can, and contain what you cannot. Some chemicals, such as strong alkalis, require copious amounts of flushing with an appropriate solution (usually water will suffice), reducing the concentration and therefore the hazard. Other chemicals, such as carbon monoxide, are off-gassed with no risk of secondary contamination. Two methods can be used to determine if contamination reduction is effective:

- Qualitative methods require a subjective decision about whether all harmful contaminants have been removed from responders, victims, and clothing. This usually involves a visual inspection.
- Quantitative methods use meters with objective environmental sampling techniques that can detect liquid and gases in small, quantifiable amounts to determine reduction effectiveness. Technology enables detection and measures contamination levels and then prompts the user to make a decision regarding a course of action, increasing responder and patient safety.[22]

At a minimum, gross decontamination should occur on-scene regardless of weather or temperature. However, the aggressiveness of contamination reduction should be based on the nature of the contaminant, the form of the contaminant, the patient's condition, environmental conditions, and available resources. Liquids and solids are the only materials that can be effectively removed from the skin. It is generally not possible or necessary to decontaminate skin after a vapor only exposure. Extricating a victim from a vapor atmosphere is the only decontamination usually needed.[21]

Decontamination should generally follow these steps:

- If clothing has been contaminated, remove all contaminated patient clothing and jewelry and double-bag all items using clear plastic bags. Label bags that contain patient clothing and jewelry. These items must remain at the decontamination site. They may be returned to the patient later if they can be successfully decontaminated.
- Advice should also be sought on how to preserve evidence for law enforcement.
- Clothing contaminated with dust should be removed dry, with care taken to minimize any dust becoming airborne. If circumstances, time, and practice allow, a dust mask or respirator should be place over the victim's nose or mouth prior to removing the clothing. Dust should be brushed off the face prior to fitting the mask or respirator.
- Contamination reduction should begin at a victim's head and move toward the feet.
- A contaminated, isolated extremity can be cleaned without decontaminating the entire patient. However, be aware of where fluids are draining to avoid secondary contamination.
- Then flush the entire body with plain water for two to five minutes.
- Use warm, never hot, water. Hot water increases tissue absorption of chemicals.
- Wash contaminated areas gently, using a soft sponge and mild soap, if appropriate.
- Be careful not to contaminate open wounds, mucous membranes, eyes, and body orifices. Flush exposed eyes and other body surfaces with copious plain water for two to five minutes. Eye irrigation should continue for at least 10 to 15 minutes. Normal saline solution is the preferred solution for flushing the eyes.
- If the contaminant is sticky, oily, or greasy, soap and shampoo may be used, followed by additional water flushing.
- Particular attention must be given to difficult-to-clean areas such as the scalp and hair, ears and nostrils, axillae, any folds of skin, under the fingernails, the navel, groin, buttocks, breasts, genitalia, behind the knees, between the toes, and under the toenails. DOT 8-4.23
- Clean under the fingernails and toenails with a scrub brush or plastic nail cleaner.
- If possible, contain runoff water for proper disposal; if not possible, runoff should be diluted with additional water.

Nice to Know

Remember, leather and other porous materials cannot be decontaminated. Consider removing your belt and work boots (replace them with rubber boots) before entering a cold zone.

Successful decontamination reduces the chances of secondary contamination to the community, responders, ambulances, equipment, hospitals, and the environment. Avoiding direct contact with contaminated victims eliminates risk and the need for decontamination. If contamination is unavoidable, then proper decontamination or disposal of the worker's outer gear is recommended. Sometimes it is necessary to dispose of equipment as well if complete decontamination cannot

be accomplished.[20] Box 53-4 lists some common terms used in decontamination.

Street Secrets

Awareness-level EMS providers will typically be staged within the cold zone and will receive decontaminated patients from the hazmat team. It is important to ask the team if they felt the decontamination efforts were successful. You should ask what the patient was contaminated with and what you might expect to find if the chemical continues to harm them. You should also ask what risk the chemical poses to you. For example, if the patient complains of renewed burning on their skin, you may need to pull the ambulance over and flush them again, provide analgesics or other medications to counteract the chemical, or alert the receiving facility and expedite the transport. You may also need to ventilate the patient compartment or wear protective equipment.

BOX 53-4 Common Terms Used in Decontamination

- **Dry decontamination**—Is contaminant-specific; uses hydrocarbon and halogenated hydrocarbon compounds, and is therefore used only for equipment.
- **Wet decontamination**—Uses copious flushing in emulsification and dilution operations. Water and water and soap solutions work by physical removal or dilution of agents. However, some hazards require a specific solvent in order to be rendered safe.
- **Emulsification**—Suspends immiscible (i.e., gasoline or toluene) and insoluble solids (i.e., iodine crystals) using an emulsifying agent such as a surfactant, soap, or detergent.
- **Neutralizers**—Negate the destructive forces of either an acid or a base (caustic or alkaline). Heat may be generated with risk for burns.
- **Chemical reaction or degradation**—Chemically alters the contaminant. Not recommended for use on living tissue.
- **Disinfection**—Removes the biological hazards by destroying microorganisms and their toxins. Bleach and hydrogen peroxide are commonly used. Removal may occur through either a wet or dry method.
- **Dilution**—Uses copious amounts of solution to reduce the concentration of contaminants. Most often used for those substances that are miscible

or soluble. If possible, identify the hazard before dilution to avoid activating solutes.
- **Absorption**—Moves a liquid or gas into another substance such as a sponge. Often used for decontamination of the scene.
- **Adsorption**—Refers to the formation and maintenance of a condensed layer of a substance, such as a chemical agent, on the surface of a decontaminant. In emergency situations, dry powders such as soap or detergents, earth, and flour may be useful.
- **Removal**—Removes hazard mechanically by pressure or vacuum, water, brushes and wipes, and air. Scraping with a wooden stick removes hazards and usually works well regardless of chemical structure. Knowledge of the specific contaminating agent or agents is not required.
- **Heat and radiation**—Uses heat and autoclaving on nonliving items. Solar, ultraviolet radiation is effective but difficult and not practical. DOT 8-4.12, 8-4.21, 8-4.22

Sources: US Fire Administration, Emergency Management Institute, "An Orientation to Hazardous Materials for Medical Personnel" http://training.fema.gov/EMIWeb/downloads/is346.pdf (accessed June 12, 2005).

C. G. Hurst, "Textbook of Military Medicine," *Decontamination,* http://www.nbc-med.org/SiteContent/HomePage/WhatsNew/MedAspects/Ch-15electrv699.pdf (accessed June 12, 2005).

Radiation Decontamination

Decontamination of victims exposed to radiation depends on the type of radiation and the route of contamination.

- External irradiation occurs when the victim is exposed to penetrating radiation from an external source. There is a difference between exposure and contamination. A person who has been exposed but has not been contaminated is *not* radioactive, presents no danger to responders, and does not need decontamination.
- External contamination occurs when radioactive gasses, liquids, or solids contaminate skin and clothing. PPE and decontamination are needed. External contamination is the easiest to remove.
- Internal contamination occurs when radioactive materials move through a "portal of entry" (e.g., mouth, nose, eyes, wounds, or other skin breaks). Intact skin forms a good barrier to most forms of radioactive materials.
- Incorporation occurs when radioactive materials are taken into cells, tissues, and target organs such as bone, liver, thyroid, or kidney. This is the most difficult type of contamination to remove.[21]

CONNECTIONS For more specific information on radiological and nuclear incidents, look in Chapter 26: Burn Trauma and Chapter 55: Responding to WMD Events.

Mass Casualty Decontamination

How to maintain control of a large, anxious crowd requiring decontamination before corridors are established is a daunting thought. Immediate decontamination is essential to diffuse panic, reduce secondary contamination, and facilitate treatment. Some fire departments may use water from hose lines, decon trailers, or aerial ladder trucks and nozzles to provide gross and secondary decontamination for a large group. After decon has been performed, towels, blankets, or paper jump suits will help protect modesty and provide some protection against the weather en route to shelter and the treatment sector.[4]

Decontamination of Prehospital Personnel

EMS personnel will not normally need decontamination. On rare occasions, EMS workers who inadvertently enter the hot zone or care for a victim who was not properly decontaminated should consider themselves contaminated. If in doubt, immediately report this to your supervisor and prepare to be sent to the decontamination station. Box 53-5 lists additional resources for hazard identification, decontamination, and treatment.

BOX 53-5   Resources for Hazard Identification Decontamination, and Treatment

- Always consult your *standard orders or protocols* and consult with *medical control.*
- *Emergency response guidebook (ERG)* is used by responders who arrive at a scene of a transportation incident to facilitate quick identification of the hazard and provide information about initial actions that protect initial responders and the public (http://hazmat.dot.gov/pubs/erg/gydebook.htm).
- *Poison control centers* offer specially trained nurses, pharmacists, and physicians who provide 24-hour information regarding poisoning (National phone 1-800-222-1222) (http://www.1-800-222-1212.info/poisonHelp.asp).
- *Material safety data sheets (MSDS)* are provided by manufacturers and blenders of chemicals with information about chemical composition, physical and chemical properties, health and safety hazards, emergency response, and waste disposal of the material as required by OSHA 29 CFR 1910.120.

- *Computer-aided management emergency operations (CAMEO)* is a tool to assist chemical emergency responders by integrating a chemical database, air dispersion models, and mapping. (www.epa.gov/ceppo/).
- *Chemical transportation emergency center (CHEMTREC)* Twenty-four-hour telephone hotline for chemical and emergency information that connects manufacturers and shippers. It provides advice on handling, PPE, and decontamination requirements (1-800-424-9300).
- *Agency for toxic substances and disease registry (ATSDR)* Twenty-four-hour emergency number for health-related support in hazardous materials emergencies, including on-site assistance (1-404-639-6360).
- *Toxicology data network (TOXNET)* is an online database of toxicology and hazardous chemicals compiled by the National Library of Medicine (http://toxnet.nlm.nih.gov/). DOT 8-4.3

Patient Triage

Upon receipt of the decontaminated patient, immediately assess the victim's airway, breathing, and circulation and perform appropriate BLS interventions while maintaining immobilization of the cervical spine if trauma is suspected. This function can be performed by responders working in the warm zone as they prepare victims for decontamination. Hazardous materials technicians who are not EMS providers may need some coaching on this process. Viable victims with significant illness or injury require rapid decontamination and transport. However, it is imperative that initial stabilization and at least gross decontamination be done prior to transport. The receiving facility should always be alerted that they are receiving a patient from a hazmat incident as they may reroute the ambulance to their own decontamination site prior to allowing the patient entrance into the hospital.

Victims with apparently minor symptoms may not be safe from injury. Triage may be complicated by delayed onset of signs and symptoms. Many toxic substances have delayed onset, and effects may be noted well after a victim has refused care and transport. Always consult with a physician or poison control to determine if delayed signs and symptoms of exposure are likely and for guidance on triage of asymptomatic or mildly symptomatic exposure victims. Anyone suspected of being exposed should be evaluated by emergency department staff.

Mass Casualty Triage

Triage is an organized system used to sort patients when the number of injured victims exceeds available resources. Large incidents may produce large numbers of patients with real or perceived exposures. Strictly following triage protocols will help identify priority patients and identify a need for more decontamination corridors due to a high volume of critical patients. A second triage done after decontamination helps track changes in patient presentation and validate the accuracy of the initial triage.

CONNECTIONS To learn more about triage, turn to Chapter 50: Medical Incident Command.

Patient Assessment and Treatment

PPE must be used by all responders until decontamination status is known and hazards are not a threat. Unfortunately, the use of PPE makes the performance of medical interventions much more difficult and time-consuming. Cervical spine stabilization and ABC assessment and treatment should occur simultaneously with decontamination. After the ABCs are assessed and treated, secondary patient assessment can begin.

Secondary surveys and continuous monitoring should be performed as conditions allow, with particular attention paid to any chemical-specific information available from the hazardous materials resources. Treatment of signs and symptoms should consider both preexisting conditions of the patient as well as the physiological response to the exposure.

Oxygen should be administered using a nonrebreather mask or bag-mask with a bag reservoir instead of corrugated plastic tubing reservoir. These devices will minimize mixing contaminated air with inhaled air. Invasive procedures (e.g., IVs, injections, or intubation) should only occur in the cold zone after decontamination as invasive procedures may act as a direct route for introduction of the hazmat into the patient. While some cases may require treatment with antidotes, most cases will be handled by treating any symptoms as they arise. Incidents involving agents with delayed onset require frequent reassessment of the patient. DOT 8-4.11

Antidotes

There is no antidote for most chemical exposures. Treatment will primarily be supportive after removal from any ongoing exposure. If an antidote is available and within your scope of practice, administration requires that providers are familiar with the antidote and its indications, contraindications, dose, route, side effects, and mechanism of action. Table 53-2 lists some hazardous chemicals that have specific antidotes.

TABLE 53-2 Hazardous Chemicals and Antidotes

Chemical	Antidote
Organophosphate pesticides	Atropine and pralidoxime chloride (2-PAM chloride)
Carbamate pesticides	Atropine
Cyanide	Cyanide antidote kit
Hydrogen sulfide	Amyl nitrite
Methemoglobinemia	Methylene blue 1%
Certain ingested substances	Activated charcoal
Hydrofluoric acid and hydrogen fluoride gas	Calcium gluconate (gel and IV)
Carbon monoxide	Oxygen, hyperbaric chamber

CONNECTIONS Specific treatment for these and other exposures can be found in Chapter 35: Toxicology.

Pediatric Population

Children needing decontamination and treatment complicate an incident for many reasons. Responders in PPE and the high level of energy surrounding a hazmat incident may be frightening for pediatric patients. Keeping parents and children together will reduce anxiety and make decontamination and assessment easier for both patients. If separation is necessary, reassurance and compassion will be required. Reuniting the parent and child should be done as soon as it is safe to do so. Family members should be transported together whenever possible.

Children are generally more susceptible to toxic exposure and are more likely to receive a higher dose relative to body weight than an adult patient. Causes for this follow:

- Pediatric patients are shorter, and heavier air toxins are concentrated close to the ground. Younger children can be crawling on contaminated ground or putting things into their mouth, which increases the likelihood of a higher dose exposure.
- The immature central nervous, liver, and renal systems increase susceptibility to injury with increased clearance times. This means it takes longer for their body to detoxify the chemicals.
- Their pulmonary system has a greater total surface area and tidal volume relative to their size when compared to an adult. This means they will have more exposure to the chemical than an adult, even if they are both in the environment for the same amount of time. The pediatric alveoli, which are healthier and often less burdened by disease, usually absorb better than those of an adult.
- Children have a larger skin surface for their body size compared to adults. They also have more effective dermal absorption than adults.[4]

Patient Transport

As in any incident, documentation is important. Before leaving the scene, document all available and pertinent information, including hazards, known toxicology, degree of patient exposure, decontamination, and treatments as well as specific patient information (i.e., name, date of birth, vital signs, SAMPLE history information, etc.). DOT 8-4.26

Decontaminate the victim at the scene prior to transport. If decontamination is inadequate but immediate transport is required, attempt to limit the spread of contamination. The vehicle and equipment must be

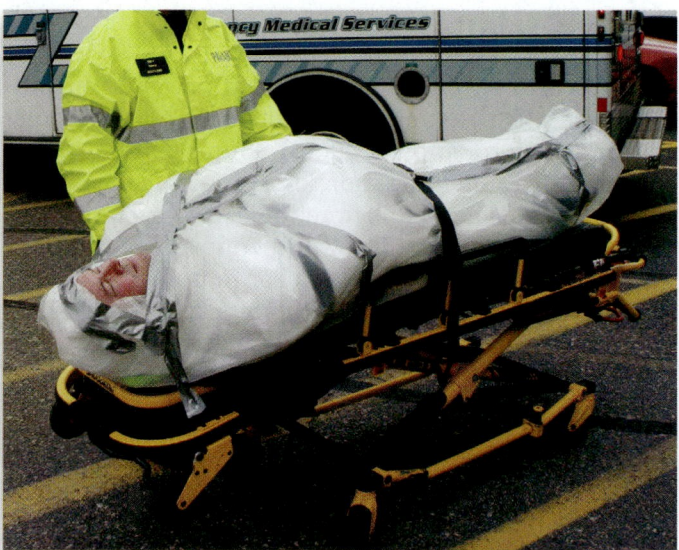

Figure 53-8 Cocooning the patient helps decrease the exposure of equipment and other responders to a contaminated patient.

protected, and personnel must be properly fitted and trained with appropriate PPE. When transporting a contaminated patient by ambulance, special care should be used to prevent secondary contamination. Either the patient should be cocooned (totally wrapped up), or the patient compartment should be enveloped. An enveloped patient compartment provides a barrier between the patient and the equipment cabinets. This protects the contents from secondary contamination. DOT 8-4.20

Cocooning allows airway maintenance but may inhibit detailed patient assessment and treatment. Cocooning a patient is not a difficult procedure; it entails wrapping a patient in heavy plastic after gross decontamination has been performed (Figure 53-8).

- Ensure gross decontamination by removing patient clothing.
- Place the patient on a backboard to facilitate lifting and moving the patient.
- Wrap the patient in blankets to facilitate absorption of any fluids, especially under the backboard where fluids may drain.
- Wrap the patient in plastic sheeting or place the patient in a body bag leaving the face exposed.

Cocooning a patient may exacerbate chemical absorption by the body due to increased body temperature. In this case avoid cocooning. Cocooning will also trap secretions and bodily fluids, which may risk recontamination of the patient.

Enveloping the patient compartment promotes detailed patient care but suggests the need for an increased level of PPE for the ambulance personnel. If the patient requires further decontamination avoid aggressive invasive patient management in the prehospital setting, if possible.

Treatment en route will depend on the contamination reduction performed, equipment, and protocols. Provide other patient care according to patient condition and local protocol.

- Provide fresh air ventilation by opening vents or windows.
- Prepare to contain secretions that may contain chemicals that pose a threat of secondary exposure.
- Monitor the airway and watch for respiratory distress; administer oxygen as needed.
- Irrigate eyes as needed.

Contact the receiving hospital as soon as possible or according to protocol to allow them to prepare to receive the patient. Ambulance parking should be in an area away from the emergency room or preferably in a parking area that will further limit exposure to hospital facilities and the community. In order to protect staff and other patients, the patient should not be brought into the emergency department or hospital decontamination area before receiving permission from hospital staff. DOT 8-4.13

Personnel, the ambulance, and equipment must be clean or made clean prior to returning to service. Equipment that came into contact with the patient should be segregated for disposal or decontamination. Contaminated equipment should be double bagged. The ambulance should not go back into service unless the vehicle is clean.

> If the patient is clean, then the vehicle will not become contaminated; therefore, the ideal situation is to fully decontaminate the patient prior to transport.[4]

Air Transportation

Transportation of contaminated patients by air is dangerous and not recommended due to the difficulty of confirming complete decontamination. The risk of the flight crew experiencing breathing or sight impairment leading to a flight accident is too large. Furthermore, the approach and landing of the crew (or media) can endanger the scene by flying through airborne gasses or vapors or can create air currents, which change the distribution of the hazard.[12]

Medical Surveillance and Rehabilitation

Historically, rehabilitation, or rehab, is associated with fire scenes because of the physical nature of firefighting. Rehab should be used for any incident where the

environmental dangers of heat, cold, humidity, physical exertion, psychological stress, impaired vision, limited mobility, and communication difficulties put the health and safety of responders at risk. Responders who are not allowed adequate rest, rehydration, and nutrition are at increased risk for illness or injury and become a threat to the safety of others. Their reaction time is impaired, and their ability to make critical decisions diminishes. Rehab is designed to ensure the physical and mental health of responders. This is particularly important for rescuers who are working in hazmat PPE Levels A, B, or C. These suits do not permit the usual cooling measures of sweating and evaporation. Thus, it is extremely common for rescuers in PPE to develop heat-related illness.

CONNECTIONS Chapter 2: The Well-Being of the Paramedic discusses wellness and provides tips and advice on how to develop a healthy lifestyle. EMS providers who work with hazardous materials need a high level of wellness in order to manage the stress that this type of work places upon the body.

In addition, rehabilitation is important to prehospital care providers who are subject to extreme circumstances or extended duration. It is easy to become engaged in the activities of a busy scene and disregard your own personal safety. This safety includes proper use of PPE, hydration, nutrition, and rest.

The incident commander should declare that a rehab sector be established when rest and rehab are needed. The rehab officer will usually report to the logistics section.

Location

Ideally, the rehab sector should be located in the cold zone away from the incident or environmental hazards. An ideal location might be a shady and cool area or a warm and dry place depending upon the season. A location away from the sights and sounds of ongoing operations promotes genuine rest while the workers can be monitored. The area should be accessible to EMS rescue personnel, equipment, supplies, transportation, SCBA refilling, and food and water. The location should also allow prompt reentry into the emergency operation upon complete recuperation.

Rehab Entrance and Exit Evaluation

Responders should be encouraged to report to the rehab sector if they are experiencing weakness, dizziness, chest pain, muscle cramps, nausea, altered mental status, or difficulty breathing. Even if symptom-free, responders should report to the rehab sector after extremely

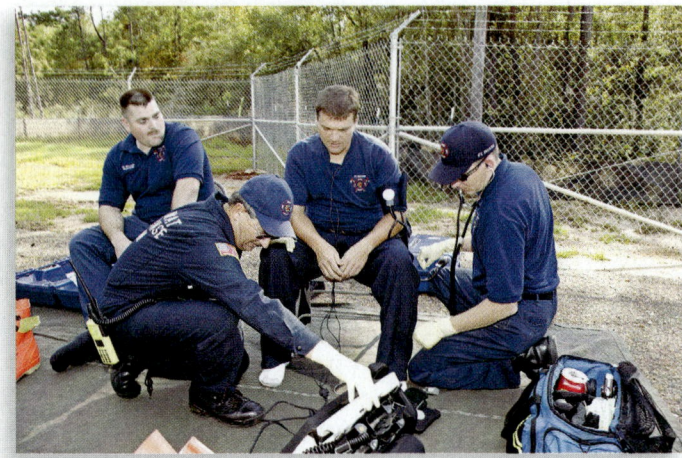

Figure 53-9 Paramedics working in a rehab area and evaluating a hazmat specialist during an incident.

strenuous activity, using two SCBA bottles, 30 minutes in a hazardous environment, or failure of their PPE. When evaluating responders, it is important to remember that a responder may have a preexisting health condition that may not interfere with their normal duties but may be exacerbated under stressful conditions or extended work duration. Some prescription or OTC medications may alter the body's response to prolonged, stressful events as well.[23] DOT 8-4.24

- **Heart rate and body temperature.** Check the heart rate and temperature as soon as the responder enters rehab. Elevated heart rate and temperature are indications of stress. If the heart rate is 110 beats per minute or higher or if the oral temperature exceeds 100.6°F, detain the responder until the vital signs stabilize. Always consider transport for assessment by a doctor. Body temperature should be lowered slowly using misting systems or fans. Air conditioning is only acceptable after a cooling period at ambient temperatures with sufficient air movement. Aggressive cooling is dangerous and may cause the patient to begin shivering, which could result in an increased body temperature (Figure 53-9).[23] DOT 8-4.25

- **Respiratory rate and quality.** Check during each assessment. Responders with a respiratory rate greater than 24 breaths per minute should be detained until the rate returns to normal. Comparing the entry and exit assessments of lung sounds and pulse oximetry may be valuable in helping you to determine their fitness to return to duty.[14]

- **Blood pressure and capillary refilling time.** These are linked to heart rate and are indicative of heart and vascular health. They are also warning signs of excessive stress, fluid imbalance, and temperature extremes. Both systolic and diastolic pressures should be obtained and compared to the responder's normal values.

- **12-lead ECG.** A 12-lead ECG tracing should be obtained if the patient reports chest pain or has an irregular heart rate. Any ongoing chest pain, dysrhythmias, or ST changes should exclude the responder from duty. Dysrhythmias should be treated according to protocol and assessed by a physician.[14]

- **Body weight.** Weigh rescuers in their full PPE before they enter the work zone and upon exit. Significant changes in weight are indicated by a loss of greater than 5% of their starting weight. This indicates significant dehydration has occurred, and appropriate rehydration measures should be started immediately.[24] Oral fluids may need IV supplementation if the workers have altered mental status or other signs of significant heat stress or electrolyte imbalance. Oral fluids should not be used if a significant altered mental status exists.

Hydration and Nourishment

Fluids and food should be available at all scenes with extended duration. Emergency personnel should be encouraged to drink fluids even if they deny being thirsty. Maintenance of water and electrolyte levels is critical to maintain homeostasis. As water is depleted, it must be replaced. During strenuous activities, at least one quart of water per hour should be consumed. This should occur regardless of absence or presence of thirst or ambient temperature reading.

While plain water is good, there is risk for developing hyponatremia if only plain water is consumed. Consider rehydrating with a 50/50 mixture of water and commercially prepared activity or sports drinks. It should be served at a temperature of no more than about 40°F. Ice cold is contraindicated. Hydration should occur regardless of ambient temperature. Heat stress can happen during any strenuous and stressful activity when PPE is used. Alcohol and caffeinated beverages cause diuresis and altered mental status and should be avoided. Nutritious food will replenish vitamins, minerals, and energy used. Avoid fatty or salty foods. DOT 8-4.25

Rest Cycles

Rest periods should last 10 to 20 minutes at a minimum. Vital signs should return to near normal or preincident levels before the rescuer is allowed to return to activity. However, the nature of the incident and available manpower may dictate shorter or longer rest periods. Medical evaluations should be documented, including name, complaints, vital signs, and time. After being cleared by rehab, responders should report to staging for their next assignment.

Critical Incident Stress

Incidents with large numbers of injured and dead patients and dangerous scenes may result in critical incident stress. Reducing the impact of these scenes requires immediate defusing and debriefing soon after the incident.[4]

Summary

Hazardous materials incidents present profound challenges to any emergency responder. It is not the intent of this chapter to provide all the information an EMS provider needs to work in hazardous materials incidents. It is instead meant to provide an overview of some of the concepts of working in hazardous materials incidents and to provide necessary information that protects paramedics and their patients.

Paramedics must first ensure that they do not put themselves, their partners, or bystanders at-risk by entering a hazardous environment. Firefighters and specially trained technicians will identify and secure hazardous materials scenes. They will then deliver decontaminated patients to the paramedic for treatment and transport. Paramedics must be prepared to treat these decontaminated patients according to the symptoms brought on by the exposure. Paramedics should avail themselves of training that will raise their awareness level in dealing with the potential for hazardous materials.

Notes

1. Federal Emergency Management Agency (FEMA), *Guidelines for Haz Mat/WMD Response, Planning and Prevention Training*, April 2003 ed. (Emmitsburg, MD: FEMA, 2003), p. 4.
2. Federal Emergency Management Agency, *Hazardous Materials Response Technology Assessment*, February 2000 ed. (Emmitsburg, MD: FEMA, 2000), p. 5.
3. P. Currance and A. C. Bronstein, *Hazardous Materials for EMS: Practices and Procedures* (St. Louis, MO: Mosby, 1999), p. 3.
4. Agency for Toxic Substances and Disease Registry, "Managing Hazardous Material Incidents, Volume II, Section 1" (2001), http://www.atsdr.cdc.gov/mhmi.html (accessed June 12, 2005).
5. Office of Hazardous Materials Safety, "Hazardous Materials Shipments," http://hazmat.dot.gov/pubs/hms/hmship.htm (accessed June 12, 2005).
6. Federal Emergency Management Agency, "Hazardous Materials Accidents," http://www.tallytown.com/redcross/library/FS-HazardousMaterialsAccidents.pdf (accessed June 12, 2005).
7. Emergency Management Institute, "FEMA IS Course Material Download: IS-5 An Introduction to Hazardous Materials," http://training.fema.gov/EMIWeb/IS/is 51st.asp (accessed June 12, 2005).
8. U.S. Environmental Protection Agency, "SARA Overview, Superfund, US EPA," http://www.epa.gov/superfund/action/law/sara.htm (accessed June 12, 2005).
9. Occupational Safety and Health Administration, "Safety and Health Topics: Emergency Preparedness and Response," http://www.osha.gov/SLTC/emergencypreparedness/responder.html (accessed June 12, 2005).
10. Occupational Safety and Health Administration, "Hazardous Waste Operations and Emergency Response," http://www.osha.gov/pls/oshaweb/owadisp.show_document?p_table=STANDARDS&p_id=9765&p_text_version=FALSE (accessed June 12, 2005).
11. South Dakota Office of Emergency Management, "Guidelines for Haz Mat/WMD Response, Planning and Prevention Training" (April 2003), http://oem.sd.gov/forms/curriculum_guide.pdf (accessed June 12, 2005).
12. Federal Emergency Management Agency, United States Fire Administration, "General Approach to a Hazmat Incident." In *Hazardous Materials Guide for First Responders*, http://www.imputsolutions.com (accessed October 31, 2006).
13. F. L. Fire, *The Common Sense Approach to Hazardous Materials*, 2nd ed. (Saddle Brook, NJ: Fire Engineering Books and Video, 1996), p. 2.
14. R. Stilp and A. Bevelacqua, *Emergency Medical Response to Hazardous Materials Incidents* (Albany, NY: Delmar Publishers, 1997), p. 39.
15. Agency for Toxic Substances and Disease Registry, "Managing Hazardous Material Incidents, Volume I, Section 3" (2001), http://www.atsdr.cdc.gov/mhmi.html (accessed June 12, 2005).
16. National Incident Management System (NIMS), "An Introduction IS-700 Self-Study Guide," *FEMA* (August 2004), http://www.training.fema.gov/emiweb/downloads/NIMS-Self-Study%20Guide.pdf (accessed October 31, 2006).
17. U.S. Department of Transportation, *Emergency Response Guidebook*, 2000 ed. (Washington, DC: Government Printing Office, 2000), p. 4.
18. Department of Health and Human Services Agency for Toxic Substances and Disease Registry, *Managing Hazardous Materials Incidents* (Atlanta, GA: Public Health Service, 2001).
19. U.S. Fire Administration, Emergency Management Institute, "An Orientation to Hazardous Materials for Medical Personnel," http://training.fema.gov/EMIWeb/downloads/is346.pdf (accessed June 12, 2005).
20. R. Burke, *Hazardous Materials Chemistry for Emergency Responders*, 2nd ed. (Boca Raton, FL: Lewis Publishers, 2003), p. 15.
21. C. G. Hurst, "Textbook of Military Medicine," *Decontamination*, http://www.nbc-med.org/SiteContent/HomePage/WhatsNew/MedAspects/Ch-15electrv699.pdf (accessed June 12, 2005).
22. D. F. Peterson, "How Clean Is Clean? Assuring Decontamination Efforts Are Adequate," http://cms.firehouse.com/content/article/printer.jsp?id=36029 (accessed June 12, 2005).
23. Federal Emergency Management Agency, United States Fire Administration FA-114, "Emergency Incident Rehabilitation" (July 1992), http://www.usfa.fema.gov/downloads/pdf/publications/FA-114.pdf (accessed October 31, 2006).
24. NFPA 473, *Standards for Compentencies for EMS Personnel Responding to Hazardous Materials/Weapons of Mass Destruction Incidents*, 2008 ed., Standard 5.5.3.

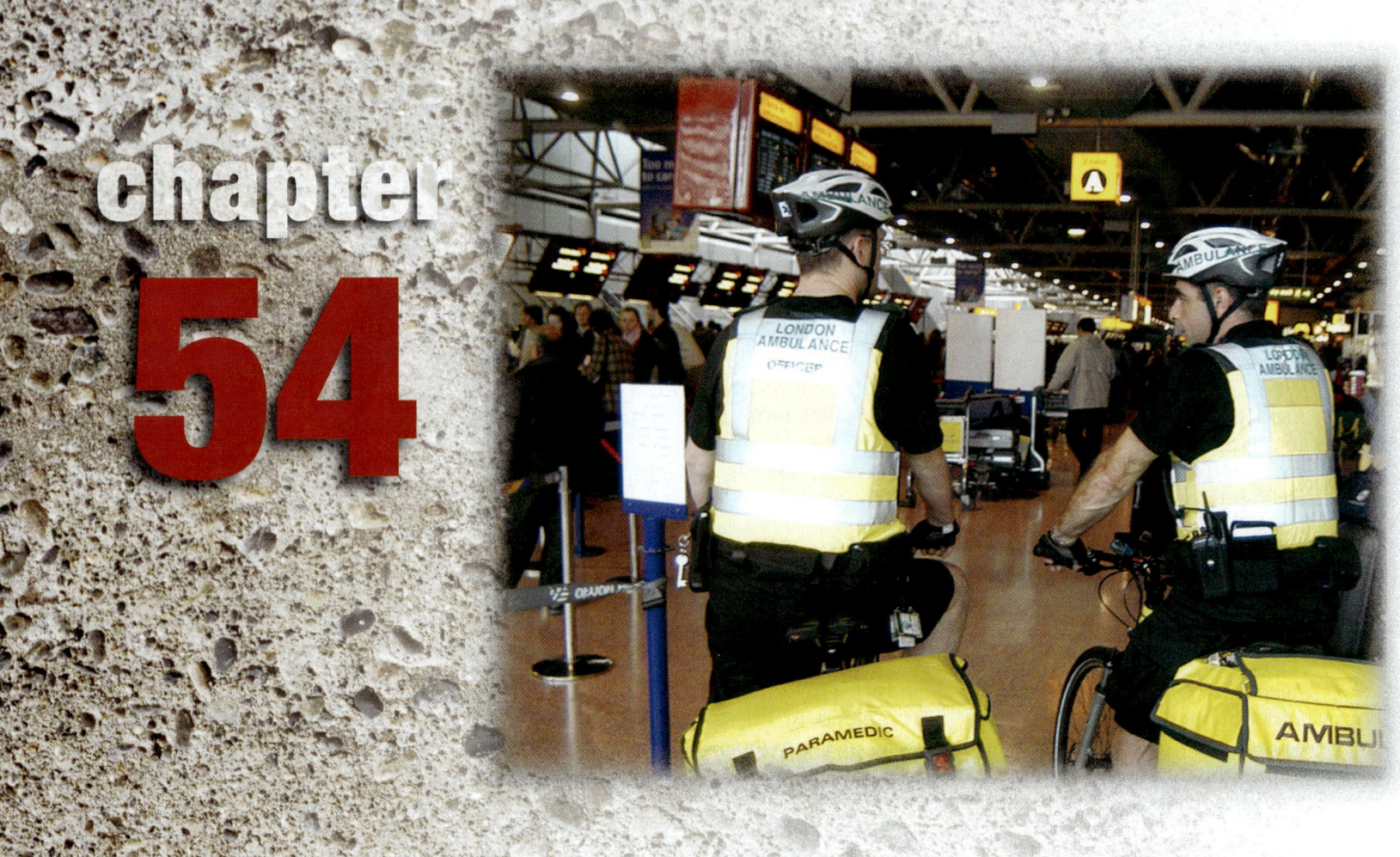

Special Events and Mass Gatherings

"One of the chief objects of medicine is to save us from the natural consequences of our vices and follies."

—H. L. Mencken

Need to Know

▶ EMS operations at mass gatherings involve the basic actions of disaster management planning, which include the following four phases: planning, response, mitigation, and recovery. This model provides a good framework for planning and executing large-scale events.

▶ The *planning* phase involves a complete assessment of the geography and occupancy, the number of expected people and their activity during the event. Protocol review will also be important as new protocols may need to be developed to care for people at the scene prior to release from the field or transport to other medical facilities.

▶ The *response* phase includes the deployment of equipment and personnel before the event begins as well as additional resources brought in to assist.

▶ The *mitigation* phase occurs during the event. It includes establishing the incident command post and the operational duties of the personnel and resources during the event.

▶ The *recovery* phase includes a return of the site to its pre-event condition and release of EMS personnel and equipment back to service with their regular jobs.

▶ The National Incident Management System provides the framework for establishing an incident command system for the event.

▶ An event-specific medical operations plan should be developed that can be used to guide the incident commander and medical response personnel during the mass gathering event.

▶ Do	▶ Ask
• Determine the existence of, or establish command at, a mass gathering using the framework provided by the NIMS ICS. In the event problems develop during the event, the framework for ICS will already be established. • Determine changes in traffic patterns relative to the event. • Participate in planning mass events to ensure EMS services are included, and know about these events ahead of time. • Make sure the mass gathering event will not deplete the normal EMS operating resources. If it will, use mutual aid agreements to obtain additional support for the infrastructure within your service area during the mass event.	• When responding to a mass gathering, determine whether your response is emergency or nonemergency, and respond accordingly. • Ask who the incident commander is, ensure you follow appropriate chain of command, report your arrival on-scene, and obtain your duty assignment.

Introduction

Humanity's desire to socialize leads to many types of gatherings, from small family occasions to colossal crowds of hundreds of thousands. Mass gatherings, generally defined in the medical literature as any event with more than one thousand persons, are common occurrences that present uncommon challenges to emergency medical services systems.[1,2]

Specific areas of concern for mass gatherings include the type and location of the venue, the composition of participants and attendees, the appropriate composition of the healthcare staff, access and transportation within and from the venue, and protocols for treatment and transportation. Some venues and types of gatherings can present additional challenges, ranging from difficulties of topography to coordination with multiple governmental agencies to developing systems to protect the health and safety of political dignitaries.

It is a challenge to create one guideline that can address all issues of any specific mass gathering. However, application of certain principles can increase preparedness. Disaster management principles comprise four phases for preparing for disasters: planning, responding, mitigating the event, and recovering from the event. This chapter will focus on these key topics. They will help the paramedic better understand and prepare for the delivery of EMS at mass gatherings.

Members of the event planning team should include a medical director in addition to police, fire, and other public safety representatives. Resources for guidance for the overall planning of mass gatherings include publications by the National Association of Emergency

Medical Services Physicians in 2000 and the American College of Emergency Physicians in 1996.[1,3]

Planning for Mass Gatherings

Venue Reconnaissance

Mass gatherings occur in a wide variety of venues. The overall medical operations plan for each event will take into account factors such as environment (whether indoor or outdoor), location, accessibility, and existing aid and emergency facilities (Figure 54-1).

Environmental emergencies are an important subset of the problems that mass gathering participants tend to report.[4–9] Venues are varied, and events take place in any season. Emergencies range from heat exhaustion and heatstroke to hypothermia and frostbite, as well as envenomations by snakes, arthropods, and marine life. Paramedics preparing for mass gatherings, particularly those in outdoor or remotely located areas, need to be familiar with the types of emergencies that may be caused by the environment and specific location.

Whether the event is held in a stadium with multiple levels, grandstands, and accessways or an outdoor area dotted with rivers, bridges, and hills, each venue has unique access and egress difficulties. These routes require preevent planning to ensure paramedics will be able to rapidly locate a patient and determine the best route for evacuation, if needed.

Many events occur in fixed locations with an infrastructure already in place to manage human needs such as food, water, shelter, and waste management. Stadiums, concert halls, and convention centers are examples of facilities specifically designed to host mass gatherings. Many have permanent locations for first aid centers, emergency response vehicles, and on-site medical staffing. These locations often have plans in place that include interfacing with local emergency services. These plans may identify key personnel to contact in the event of an emergency, or they may indicate the optimal access and egress routes. Contractual arrangements may be in place with off-duty local EMS personnel to provide on-site, stand-by assistance. Preexisting mutual aid and special response agreements (such as hazmat and tactical responses) may also be in place. Familiarity with preexisting plans will be helpful in the event an outside EMS response is required.

Legal and Political Reconnaissance

Although much of the legal and political work surrounding mass gatherings will not directly involve the paramedic (unless serving on a steering committee or directing the preparation for an event), a brief discussion of these concerns may help facilitate a better understanding of certain protocols and perceived barriers to response and patient care.

It is important to be aware of the multitude of agencies that may have a role in medical planning for a particular event. In addition to EMS, fire, and police agencies with which the paramedic is already familiar, planning for larger events may involve input from emergency managers, public health personnel, and government agencies at local, state, and federal levels. In particular, political events or events with high-profile participants may have separate response plans to ensure the safety of the attendees.

Event Timing

An event's timing also has an effect on the medical response. This is true both for time-of-year effects because of weather and time-of-day effects because of traffic patterns and hospital utilization.[5,10] These effects are likely to be included in the event medical operations plan. Paramedics should be prepared for on-site emergencies related to weather, as well as delays and access difficulties induced by poor weather or traffic. Additionally, alternative methods of access necessitated by adverse conditions will be discussed later in this chapter.

Street Secrets

As you plan to support a mass gathering event, explore alternative transportation routes to help prepare for unexpected emergencies. Also, make sure you take along extra water, snacks, foul weather clothing, and even a change of clothing to use while you are standing by at the event. If the event is occurring over a long period of time, there could be drastic changes in the temperature and you should be prepared. A spare roll of toilet paper should be kept with your supplies as well.

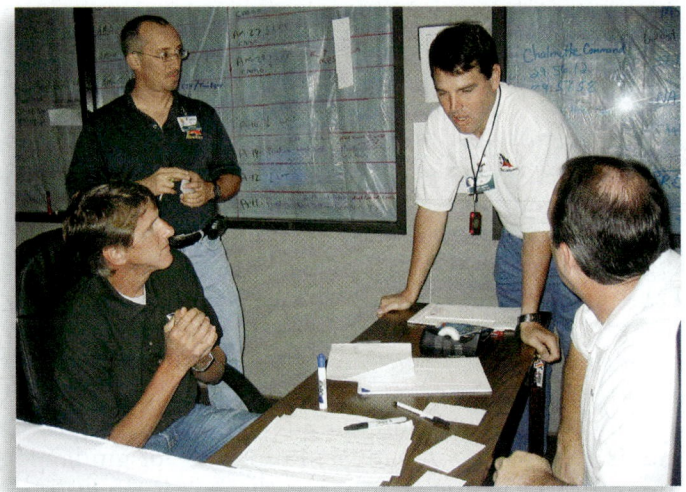

Figure 54-1 Planning for mass gatherings is essential.

Event Security and Safety Concerns

In recent years, the threat of terrorism and deployment of weapons of mass destruction have become very real concerns. Large-venue or heavily attended mass gatherings are targets for those who wish to impact the most people with the least amount of effort. All members of the medical response team have a duty to be aware of threats relevant to the mass gathering. Preparedness is improved through participation in disaster drills and other mass casualty and all-hazards training provided by local agencies.

Security and safety concerns may be more evident at some events than others. For example, events such as the Olympics, presidential inaugurations, and political conventions are classified as National Special Security Events (NSSE) in the National Incident Management System. NSSEs fall under the jurisdiction of the United States Secret Service. Local paramedics may be asked to provide support at these events. All participants providing support will be subject to background, credential, and identification checks prior to and during such an event. Appreciating and being prepared for this will save misunderstanding and the loss of critical time during an emergency response.

Using Existing Laws, Regulations, and Rules in the Planning Process

The medical operations plan for a mass gathering must be consistent with state laws specific to mass gatherings and with general laws regarding the provision of medical care. Few states currently have specific laws regarding mass gathering medical requirements; however, this is beginning to change.[11] Federal law does not provide specific guidance for mass gatherings although new post-9/11 requirements, such as use of the National Incident Management System (NIMS), will strongly influence the development of future operations plans.

CONNECTIONS See Chapter 50: Medical Incident Command for a review of NIMS.

Paramedic-related legal issues that should be planned for include liability coverage, jurisdictional authority, and billing and reimbursement procedures. These issues should be handled prior to the occurrence of any event. It may involve input from the medical director, state EMS lead agency, lawyers, union representative, and others. While an in-depth discussion of these issues is beyond the scope of this chapter, it is important for paramedics participating in a mass event to make inquiries and understand the measures in place to deal with these issues. Paramedics should understand that these complex issues may impact their work from time to time, most often through additional documentation requirements.

Event Participant Diversity

Events that draw large numbers of people vary in many ways besides the location of the venue. Different events tend to draw different crowds. It would be difficult to imagine the audiences at a trade convention, a political debate, and a rock concert being very similar. However, this can be misleading. Spectators at any given event tend to be a microcosm of the community at large. The participants are drawn from a wide range of people, who can have a variety of preexisting diseases, illnesses, and special medical needs (Figure 54-2).

Thus, although it is thought that different events have one particular sort of spectator, this is an overgeneralization that fails to recognize the variety of individuals within a group. Moreover predictions about the demographics of attendance may be wrong. For example, rock concerts do not draw only young, presumably healthy people. Certain musicians or bands may draw an older crowd with an increased prevalence of underlying diseases such as cardiac disease, diabetes, or hypertension.

Certainly, it is wise to prepare for the expected demographic of an event. For example, you should be familiar with event protocols for treatment and possible observation or transport of patients under the influence of intoxicating substances if a young, rowdy crowd is expected. Further, if spectators are expected to present under the influence of alcohol, narcotics, or amphetamines, the medical operations plan may need to include extra supplies of antidotes such as naloxone, IV fluids, or benzodiazepines for seizure control. Paramedics are cautioned to be ready for the full range of ages and medical pathology at any mass gathering, regardless of other circumstances.

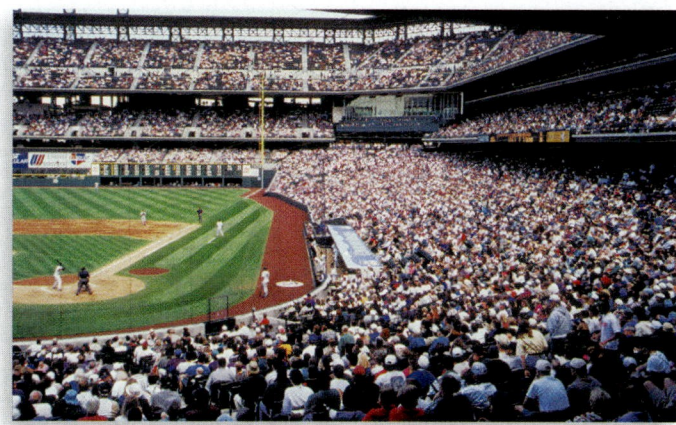

Figure 54-2 Events such as baseball games, other sporting events, and concerts result in the gathering of large numbers of participants of varying ages and medical conditions.

Street Secrets

Certain events may also be more likely to attract people with linguistic and physical barriers. For example, festivals celebrating holidays from other parts of the world or cultural music festivals may attract large groups of people for whom English is not the primary language or not understood at all. Special Olympics events or those that target certain diseases may have a large group of individuals attending that require intensive medical assistance if they have a medical emergency.

Featured guests at mass gatherings such as high-profile sports figures, politicians, and dignitaries, for example, may be "off-limits" to the paramedic. These individuals may have their own medical response teams accompanying them who will attend specifically to their needs. Alternatively, the paramedic may find that a celebrity is being treated by a dedicated physician and requires transportation under that physician's continued supervision. As previously discussed, paramedics must coordinate their efforts with other agencies, including law enforcement.

Anticipated Types of Emergencies

The medical operations plan must take into account the most likely conditions that will be encountered. This generally includes headache, gastrointestinal upset, mild dehydration, and minor trauma. The plan should also consider the management of life-threatening conditions. Even though situations such as cardiac arrest, anaphylaxis, and major trauma have a low expectation of occurrence, they require an immediate response and should be planned for. Equipment, supplies, and the skills required for rapid intervention and evacuation in critical situations must be immediately available.

Medical Personnel and Response Team Configuration

The medical response team for a specific event may include personnel with basic first aid training, EMTs, paramedics, nurses, nurse practitioners, physician assistants, physicians, and other allied health professionals. Although current research provides a range of opinions on ideal staffing ratios, the medical response plan for a particular event will consider the information discussed earlier in this chapter in determining the appropriate team composition for the event. Historical information from similar events may also be helpful in planning for the amount and types of emergencies encountered.[12–17]

Appropriate composition of the team depends on several factors. One of these is the positioning of response teams within the actual venue.[18] Many venues have fixed facilities for providing aid. These facilities can often serve as a "station" from which to respond and in which to provide aid. If a physician is part of the response team, this is often a logical place to base the physician. Paramedics often staff these locations, sometimes working under off-line treatment protocols.[6,15] However, although it is tempting to rely solely on these preexisting locations, it is important to consider the specifics of the event to determine if these facilities are sufficient and appropriate for the expected needs.

Event Resources and Equipment

Make sure to explore the impact to your infrastructure during the planning process for the event. Depending on the size and duration of the event, it may be appropriate to use existing mutual aid agreements to backfill stations within your response area if a significant number of resources will be devoted to supporting the event.

The paramedic's expertise in field operations will be of use to the planning team when choosing equipment for a particular venue and event. At a minimum, it would be wise to refer to the local agency requirements for response vehicles. Although exceptions may exist for vehicles that are not technically ambulances, patient safety will be enhanced and potential liability minimized by adhering to the recommended supplies as closely as possible. Special attention should be paid to supplies for common and critical conditions, as previously discussed. Additionally, if room is available, mitigation supplies discussed earlier such as water and blankets may be appropriate on response vehicles, particularly if those vehicles are based away from the main aid station.

Medical Equipment and Supplies for the Event

Whatever the plan for response and transportation, it is evident that the paramedic must be familiar with the vehicles and equipment to be used. For example, it would be less than ideal to station personnel who are unable to ski on a mountain slope in winter or to place personnel unfamiliar with ATVs on those vehicles. Further, the paramedic must remember that appropriate role modeling for the public, as well as personal safety, demands the use of appropriate safety equipment on all types of vehicles, whether this includes seat belts, life vests, or helmets.

Depending on the scope of the event and budgetary concerns, not all supplies are likely to be available to all vehicles and facilities at all times. Accordingly, it is probable that the paramedic will need to be familiar with the location within the venue of rarer pieces of equipment. Part of the medical operations plan must address the positioning of equipment within the venue. Specific items to address include placement of automated external defibrillators, including whether to make them accessible to the public and on which vehicles to place them, as well as the placement of surgical equipment for larger events with on-site physicians who may be providing surgical airways, central venous access, and other emergent procedures.[18–21]

Additional Resources Available during the Event

Community resources may be available to assist with equipment deployment, particularly with regard to nonperishable items such as gauze, bandaging and dressing material, splints, and backboards. If the response plan includes on-site participation by local ambulances, many items will become available because they are routinely stocked on the units.

Event Communication Equipment

A vital piece of equipment with which the paramedic must become familiar prior to the event is the venue communications gear. Many venues are equipped to participate in local 800 MHz trunking systems. If so, the paramedic will need to determine appropriate dispatch and tactical workgroups and frequencies. Other venues may rely on walkie-talkies, cellular phones, landlines, or pagers for communication. It is critical that the paramedic be able to easily use the available equipment to avoid delays in dispatch and treatment (Figure 54-3).

Protocols

Dispatch, treatment, and medical control policies and protocols for a particular event are often the same as, or heavily borrowed from, those of the local EMS agency. However, the nature of mass gatherings often causes important deviations from everyday policies and protocols with which the paramedic must become familiar. Typical examples of variations from protocol are treat-and-release protocols and transport deviations.

Treat-and-release protocols will allow the paramedic to provide specific types of care, such as dextrose for diabetic patients, and then will allow the paramedic to release the patient without transporting them to the hospital. These protocols will provide the critical decision points when a release is authorized and when it is not advisable. For example, if the patient has low blood sugar but has not been diagnosed as a diabetic, the treat-and-release approach would not be appropriate.

Treatment protocols for mass gatherings are highly dependent on the level of medical control, the composition of the response team, and the capability of available aid stations and transportation resources. Many events have benefited from off-line protocols for common conditions that would normally require transportation, such as heat exhaustion, headache, and minor trauma (Figure 54-4).[6,15]

Unusual protocols such as treat-and-release or field triage to atypical destinations such as clinics or rehydration units require careful education prior to the event, preferably with concurrent oversight, as well as post-event quality improvement evaluations. Additionally, an on-site physician or physician extender may be present to handle minor conditions such as laceration repair or minor foreign body removal. These individuals may greatly reduce the need for off-site transportation.[12,14,16]

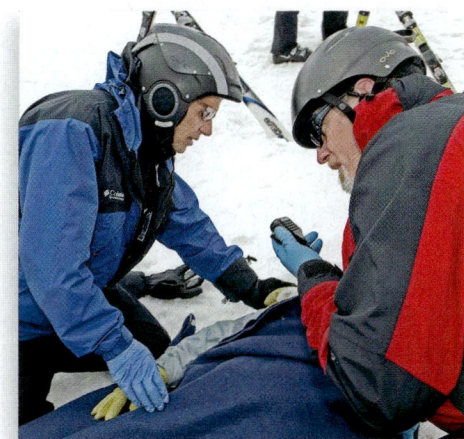

Figure 54-3 Practice with your communication equipment so that you can use it easily when needed.

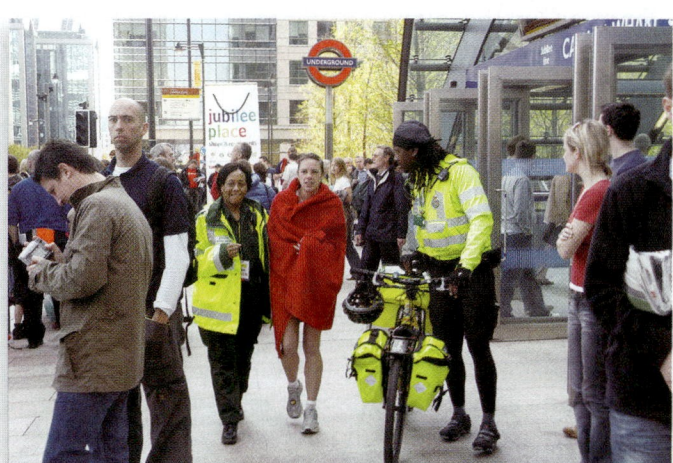

Figure 54-4 Treat-and-release protocols are necessary for mass events such as marathons.

The specifics of any treatment protocols beyond or different from local EMS procedure are a key issue for the mass gathering paramedic to know and understand. Local and state laws may place limitations on the extent to which a paramedic's scope of practice may be expanded, such as requirements for on-line medical control, physician presence and availability, transportation requirements, and exclusions of paramedic-only care for certain conditions.

As with the community at large, the attendees at mass gatherings may be appropriate candidates for treat-and-release protocols or may wish to refuse care. Both of these contingencies should be addressed in the comprehensive medical operations plan developed for that event.

Medical Control during the Event

Medical control should be available during the event to help determine the appropriate disposition for any individual patient. Although medical control may be provided off-line in the form of advanced treatment protocols and standing orders, large events are often better served by the continual availability of on-line medical control. For particularly large gatherings or those that attract a large proportion of persons with underlying disease processes, an on-site physician should be available for secondary assessment and additional treatment. The plan should also include information on diversion of patients to alternate receiving facilities (e.g., clinics) or using alternative transportation methods if they are permitted.[12,14,16]

The Responding Phase: Immediately Prior to the Event

Immediately before the event is held, the resources identified in the planning phase are assembled and brought to the venue. The final version of the medical response plan should be distributed, and all parties involved should read the document carefully and understand their roles and responsibilities as outlined in the plan.

The incident command system should be started and the incident command post established. The communications system should be checked, and agencies or personnel placed in the standby mode should be alerted that the event is ready to commence. Any personnel on the scene should be assembled and briefed. This is the final opportunity for questions to be asked and answered prior to the kick-off of the actual event. Responders should be staged, and all of their equipment and supplies should receive a final inventory before the event begins. DOT 8-2.30

The Mitigation Phase: Responding during the Event

Many of the health concerns discussed earlier in this chapter may afflict event participants. Examples include dehydration in actively exercising participants or thirsty spectators (especially those who may be consuming large quantities of alcohol or caffeinated beverages), environmental emergencies in outdoor settings (including insect bites and stings), drug and alcohol intoxication, and the potential for multiple patients with traumatic injuries (Figure 54-5).

As part of the medical response plan, paramedics may be called upon to assist with mitigation of known health hazards in an attempt to lessen their impact on the mass gathering. Although this public health aspect of emergency medical services is fairly unusual in the traditional setting, in the mass gathering situation paramedics performing these duties can have a significantly positive effect on the continued health of not just their patients but also the community at large. Possibilities for hazard mitigation include staffing rehydration units, providing information on safe rides and designated driver programs, and distributing blankets during outdoor winter events.[8] Many of these roles may be filled by community volunteers or the local Red Cross; however, paramedics may be needed to provide support, depending on the scope of the event.

The Public Safety Answering Point

The public safety answering point (PSAP) for the venue must work with medical control and be familiar with the capabilities of the response team. As many spectators may access 9-1-1 via wireless communications, ideally

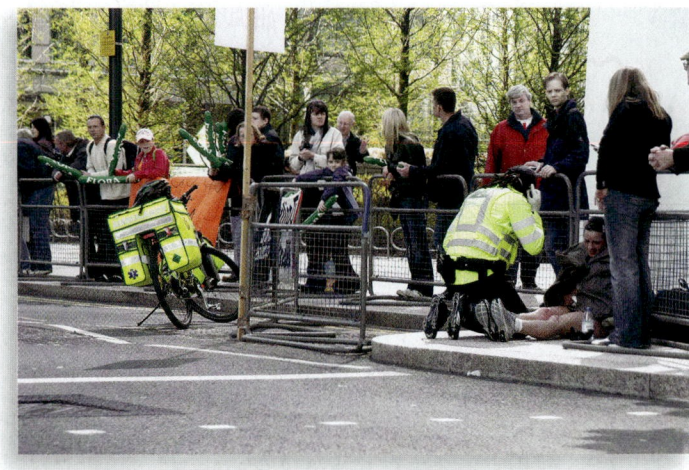

Figure 54-5 Dehydration of participants in sporting events is common.

the PSAP should be able to handle wireless 9-1-1 communications and to locate mobile phone users rapidly. If a tiered response is possible and permitted, the PSAP should be capable of employing a dispatch protocol to determine the best level of response. Research is lacking with regard to specific prearrival instructions in the setting of mass gatherings; however, paramedics should make themselves familiar with any dispatcher-directed care that may have been rendered prior to their arrival. Additionally, the protocol must include capacity for priority communications to request additional resources. Most calls, however, are unlikely to require an emergent response with maximal resources.

Maintaining a Safe Environment

Paramedics attending mass gatherings should be on high alert and scan the crowd constantly for evidence of danger or foul play. Additionally, careful observation on the part of paramedics may provide the necessary clues to uncover more subtle forms of attack (most notably bioweapons), presenting as clusters of patients with similar complaints. In some settings, public health authorities may call upon paramedics to assist in gathering biosurveillance data.

CONNECTIONS See Chapter 55: Responding to WMD Events for more on this topic.

Transportation of Patients during Events

Transportation deviations will allow for alternative locations to take patients. For example, a special treatment area may be established during an event to prevent overwhelming the local resource infrastructure. Another example is when patients are allowed to select their destination instead of using the local resources. Any special protocol or deviations will be outlined and approved in advance of the event.

Response to calls for aid is a frequent area of deviation from local protocol. Although small venues may receive a typical EMS response for every emergency call, most venues are expected to handle the majority of responses using preestablished, intravenue resources. Regardless of the specifics of the response, it is vital that the response contingencies be integrated into the overall plan for care. Some response deviation examples include sending a nurse to the aid station where a patient is waiting, dispatching a paramedic on a bicycle to an unconscious spectator, or deploying a physician or paramedic team on a boat to rendezvous with a rescue craft at the scene of a racing boat collision.

Documentation of Care during Mass Gatherings

Inherent in medical work is the need for documentation. Paramedics should be aware that responses within a venue, particularly for minor complaints that do not require transportation, still need a minimum level of documentation. Depending on how the plan is structured, a full patient care report may not be specifically required by the medical response plan. Documentation and patient care report types should be discussed prior to the event. All laws, rules, and regulations regarding the privacy of patient records still apply in mass gatherings. DOT 3-5.8 **See also Skill Sheet 64: Documentation.**

Unforeseen Situations Arising during an Event

Despite the best efforts at planning, unforeseen situations can arise during an event. For example, the venue itself may create artificial barriers to access. It may not be possible to cross a racetrack during a race to get to the aid station. In this case, it would be important to position response teams on both sides of the barrier. Also, tiered levels of care may be appropriate for venues with larger audiences or areas. These may range from having scattered first aid stations with one central secondary care area (perhaps staffed by a physician) to a network of secondary care areas that have the capability to stabilize seriously ill patients and transfer them to a tertiary-level field hospital (which may in turn transport some cases off-site).

The barriers to access and idiosyncrasies unique to the venue often lead to unusual methods of response and transportation. These range from foot patrols, motorized vehicles such as the Segway™, golf carts, and bicycle patrols to boats and all-terrain vehicles (Figure 54-6). Clearly, a vehicle designed for rapid access through difficult terrain or narrow, crowded passageways may not be ideal for transporting patients. Paramedics are an ideal resource for discussing these contingencies prior to the event with the medical response planning team, given their experience with the realities of patient treatment and transport in field conditions.

Street Secrets

The quickest way to access some patients during mass gatherings is by having bystanders bring the patient out of the crowd to the rescuers. If the crowd is under control and willing to assist, you can direct them as to what needs to be done to bring the patient to you.

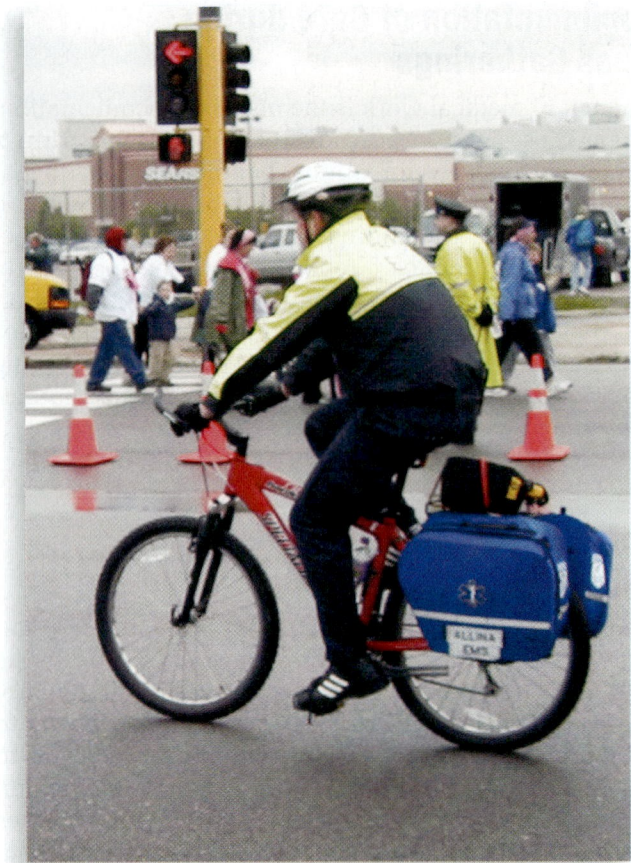

Figure 54-6 Bicycles are fast and nimble and allow the paramedic to carry necessary equipment.

After the Event: The Recovery Phase

After the mass gathering is concluded, the paramedic's experiences with preparation, mitigation, and response can provide valuable lessons for future events. In addition to standard postshift activities such as equipment cleaning and storage, restocking, and documentation, the paramedic may be asked to participate in debriefing and afteraction report meetings. Such activities help in planning for future events.

Postevent evaluations are an opportunity to provide quality assurance. Although ongoing events may have continual quality improvement schemes integrated into the medical operations plan, single-day or short-term events may focus on discussion of particular items of concern. The paramedic should be encouraged to participate in a dialogue on items for improvements in response, treatment, and patient safety.

Summary

EMS at mass gatherings can be a well-organized, planned event or an unanticipated response nightmare that cripples the existing jurisdiction's infrastructure. In the case of a planned event, all of the public safety agencies should be involved in planning for the event.

The four phases of disaster management—planning, response, mitigation, and recovery—provide a framework for approaching mass gathering management. The NIMS incident command structure provides additional information.

Well-planned events include medical direction and medical response teams. Responders on these teams should be briefed on their roles and responsibilities and should understand how their normal operating procedures, including protocols, are altered during this special detail. Paramedics who understand the plan and know their role in it will have the best experience at mass gatherings, and their patients will benefit.

Notes

1. D. Jaslow, A. Yancy, and A. Milsten, "Mass Gathering Medical Care; National Association of EMS Physicians Standards and Clinical Practice Committee," *Prehospital Emergency Care* 4(4) (2000): 359–360.
2. R. A. De Lorenzo, "Mass Gathering Medicine: A Review," *Prehospital Disaster Medicine* 12(1) (1997): 68–72.
3. American College of Emergency Physicians Emergency Medical Services Committee, "Provision of Emergency Medical Care for Crowds" (1995–1996), http://www.acep.org (accessed August 13, 2005).
4. P. Arbon, "The Development of Conceptual Models for Mass-Gathering Health," *Prehospital Disaster Medicine* 19(3) (2004): 208–212.
5. P. Arbon, F. H. Bridgewater, and C. Smith, "Mass Gathering Medicine: A Predictive Model for Patient Presentation and Transport Rates," *Prehospital Disaster Medicine* 16(3) (2001): 150–158.
6. M. J. Feldman, J. L. Lukins, et al., "Half-a-Million Strong: The Emergency Medical Services Response to a Single-Day, Mass-Gathering Event," *Prehospital Disaster Medicine* 19(4) (2004): 287–296.
7. R. B. Leonard, "Medical Support for Mass Gatherings," *Emergency Medical Clinics of North America* 14(2) (1996): 383–397.
8. J. L. Lukins, M. J. Feldman, et al., "A Paramedic-Staffed Medical Rehydration Unit at a Mass Gathering," *Prehospital Emergency Care* 8(4) (2004): 411–416.
9. S. D. Salhanick, W. Sheahan, and J. J. Bazarian, "Use and Analysis of Field Triage Criteria for Mass Gatherings," *Prehospital Disaster Medicine* 18(4) (2003): 347–352.
10. A. D. Perron, W. J. Brady, et al., "Association of Heat Index and Patient Volume at a Mass Gathering Event," *Prehospital Emergency Care* 9(1) (2005): 49–52.
11. D. Jaslow, M. Drake, J. Lewis, "Characteristics of State Legislation Governing Medical Care at Mass Gatherings," *Prehospital Emergency Care* 3(4) (1999): 316–320.
12. M. F. Boyle, R. A. De Lorenzo, and R. Garrison, "Physician Integration into Mass Gathering Medical Care; The United States Air Show," *Prehospital Disaster Medicine* 8(2) (1993): 165–168.
13. A. Flabouris and F. Bridgewater, "An Analysis of Demand for First-Aid Care at a Major Public Event," *Prehospital Disaster Medicine* 11(1) (1996): 48–54.
14. J. T. Grange, G. W. Baumann, and R. Vaezazizi, "On-Site Physicians Reduce Ambulance Transports at Mass Gatherings," *Prehospital Emergency Care* 7(3) (2003): 322–326.

15. C. C. McDonald, M. D. Koenigsberg, and S. Ward, "Medical Control of Mass Gatherings: Can Paramedics Perform Without Physicians On-Site?" *Prehospital Disaster Medicine* 8(4) (1993): 327–331.

16. S. J. Parrillo, "Medical Care at Mass Gatherings: Considerations for Physician Involvement," *Prehospital Disaster Medicine* 10(4) (1995): 273–275.

17. A. B. Sanders, E. Criss, et al., "An Analysis of Medical Care at Mass Gatherings," *Annals of Emergency Medicine* 15(5) (1986): 515–519.

18. L. S. Binder, P. J. Willoughby, and L. Matkaitis, "Development of a Unique Decentralized Rapid-Response Capability and Contingency Mass-Casualty Field Hospital for the 1996 Democratic National Convention," *Prehospital Emergency Care* 1(4) (1997): 238–245.

19. A. Kuehl, ed., *Prehospital Systems and Medical Oversight*, 3rd ed. (Dubuque, IA: Kendall Hunt, 2002).

20. T. J. Crocco, M. R. Sayre, et al., "Mathematical Determination of External Defibrillators Needed at Mass Gatherings," *Prehospital Emergency Care* 8(3) (2004): 292–297.

21. P. Trites and D. Stephenson, "Preparing a Field Hospital for a Mass Gathering," *Canadian Nursing* 80(11) (1984): 48–50.

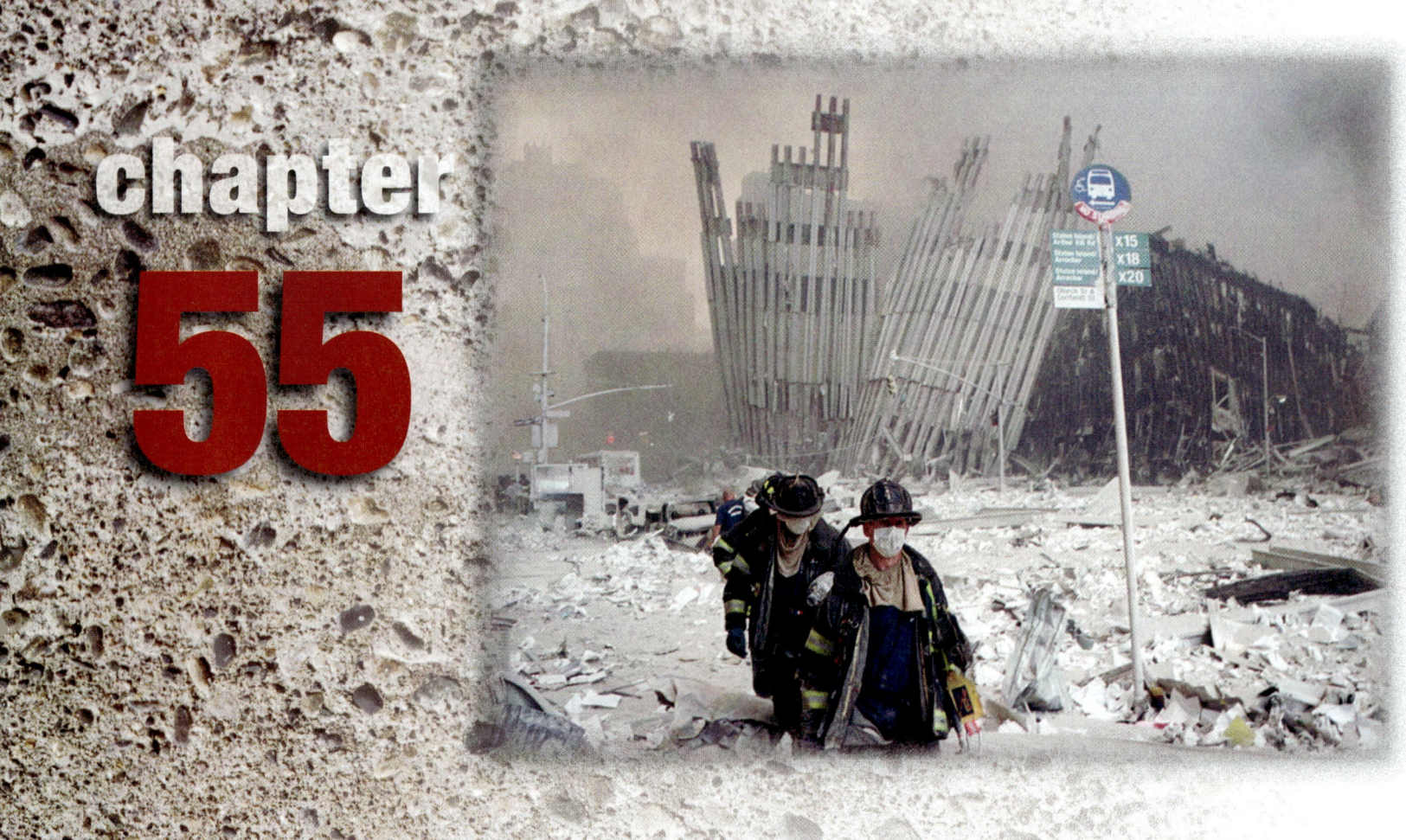

Responding to WMD Events

"Two conditions render difficult this historic situation of mankind: It is full of tremendously deadly armament, and it has not progressed morally as much as it has scientifically and technically."

—Pope John Paul II

Need to Know

▶ The history and future potential for WMD events.

▶ The different nature of chemical warfare agents, including nerve agents, vesicants, pulmonary agents, and riot control agents.

▶ Biological agents including bacteria, viruses, and toxins.

▶ Radiologic and nuclear devices and incendiaries and explosives.

▶ How WMD events are a variation of response planning for natural disaster emergency management and planning.

▶ Do	▶ Ask
• Review your agency's disaster planning with special attention to incidents involving WMD. • When called to an event, safety is the first concern. • Work within the level of your training and your immediate assignment. • Participate in postevent debriefings or critiques. • Attend training and courses on WMD and disaster management.	• Get as much information as possible while en route as to the size and nature of the event and the particular staging area. • Get as much information as possible from rescuers as patients are received in order to determine MOI and possible exposure.

Introduction

While historically weapons of mass destruction (WMD) have been used in nation-versus-nation warfare, recent history has seen WMD capability used by terrorists against civilian populations. Our awareness of WMD has to take into consideration the manufacture, transport, and deployment of these implements of destruction in places we may not have considered in the past. The elements that can be used as WMD are referred to as chemical, biological, radiological, nuclear, and explosive (CBRNE). While specialists will be called upon to respond to suspected or deployed CBRNE or WMD, every paramedic must have an understanding of the types of mass destruction devices that might be used by anyone with the objective of causing harm.

History and Current Threats of WMD

Weapons of mass destruction are designed to kill large numbers of people, induce fear, create havoc, and overwhelm response systems. Types of weapons in this class include biological, nuclear (including radiological weapons), chemical, and explosive weapons. Some types of WMDs are considered to have more of a psychological impact rather than a strict military usefulness. The use of weapons of mass destruction is not entirely new. Germany used mustard gas, phosgene, and chlorine during World War I; however, historical accounts of WMD go back much further. The first known use of biological warfare was in 1346 at Kaffa (now Fedossia, Ukraine), where the bodies of Tartar soldiers who had succumbed to plague were catapulted over the walls of the besieged city.[1] Smallpox, historically one of humankind's most devastating diseases, was used as a weapon several times during the 15th and 18th centuries. In the 15th century, Pizarro presented indigenous peoples of South America with smallpox-contaminated clothing. During the French and Indian War in the late 1750s, Sir Jeffrey Amherst ordered the provision of smallpox-laden blankets to indigenous Indians loyal to the French.[2] During World War II, the infamous Japanese Unit 731 conducted extensive biological warfare testing on human subjects. The unit was responsible for the only confirmed air attack using biological weapons when it dispersed plague-contaminated rice and fleas over Chinese cities.

To combat the proliferation and use of WMDs, specifically biological weaponry, the international community drafted the Convention on the Prohibition of the Development, Production, and Stockpiling of Bacteriological and Toxin Weapons and their Destruction, otherwise known as the 1972 Biological Weapons Convention. The agreement prohibited nations from conducting research on or producing biological agents for offensive or hostile purposes. Although 140 nations signed and ratified the 1972 Biological Weapons Convention, problems related to verification and interpretation of "defensive" research has limited its effectiveness. The Center for Nonproliferation Studies at the Monterey Institute of International Studies has identified 31 nation states that have or had chemical or biological weapons programs and have catalogued at least 46 instances of their use.[1]

Recent terrorist events have put the world on notice that WMD attacks can occur with massive and dire consequences. Over the past two decades, acts of terrorism have included the dissemination of aerosolized anthrax spores, intentional food product contamination, release of chemical weapons in major metropolitan subway systems, and suicide attacks using explosive devices. Unfortunately, predicting the exact time and location of such events is impossible. Since the bombing attacks at the World Trade Center in New York in 1993, the Federal Building in Oklahoma City in 1995, U.S. embassies in Kenya and Tanzania in 1998, and recently in Saudi Arabia and Morocco and the release of weaponized anthrax spores using the U.S. Postal System during the autumn of 2001, large-scale terrorist attacks on civilian populations using WMD no longer seem in the realm of the fantastic.[3] Preparing the health and medical systems in the U.S. may seem like a difficult undertaking; however, neglecting to prepare for such a challenge could prove devastating. EMS providers must be prepared to treat illness and injuries associated with a WMD event and understand the severe consequences such an attack could have on the nation's health and medical infrastructure.

Dissemination Methods of WMD Weapons

The number and type of dissemination methods for WMD agents is limited only by a terrorist's imagination. Most dissemination devices are classified in three categories: spraying devices, breaking devices, and bursting or exploding devices.

Spraying Devices

Spraying devices come in two forms: line source and point source. Examples of potential line source-generating devices might include an aircraft designed for crop dusting or the exhaust system of an automobile. Any line source spraying device poses a significant downwind hazard. Point source devices may include items such as aerosol cans and garden sprayers. Their reach is smaller and more focused, but they still pose a moderate downwind hazard.

Breaking Devices

Breaking devices enclose an agent and release it when the device is broken. Commonly found items such as vacuum bottles, balloons, and light bulbs could be used by inserting the agent and sealing the device. Chemical agents would be most effective to use with breaking devices because of the potential for evaporation. Breaking

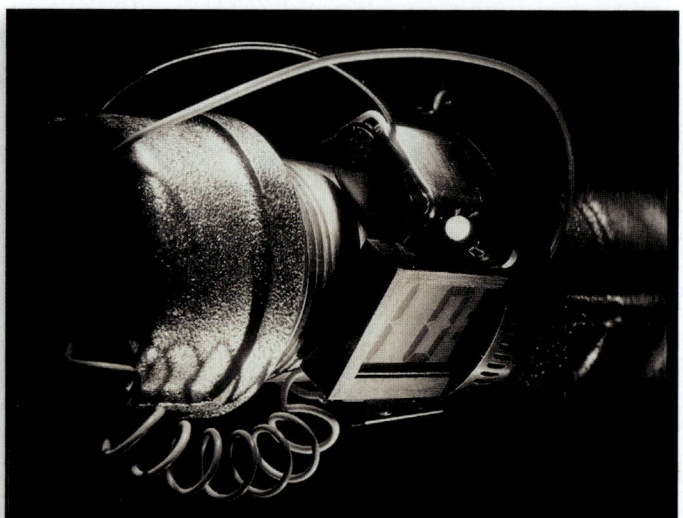

Figure 55-1   This pipe bomb is an example of a bursting or exploding device. These types of devices may be discovered by bystanders and rescuers because they are generally placed and left at the target.

devices provide point source dissemination of an agent and may create a downwind hazard to those individuals who are nearby.

Bursting or Exploding Devices

Bursting or exploding mechanical devices employ an explosive to break the agent container and disperse the agent (Table 55-1). These devices pose both an explosion risk and a downwind exposure threat to patients. Bursting or exploding devices may be more easily detected by bystanders and rescuers because they are generally placed and left at the target (Figure 55-1). Bystanders witnessing the use of a bursting or exploding device may be able to provide critical information to dispatch prior to the arrival of EMS.

TABLE 55-1   Impact of Dissemination Devices

Device	Downwind Hazard	Type of Agent
Spray	Moderate (point source) Significant (line source)	Biological or chemical
Breaking	Minimal/moderate	Chemical
Bursting	Moderate	All
Explosive	Moderate	Radiological (chemical/ biological possible)

Chemical Warfare Agents

Chemical agents may exist as solids, liquids, or gasses, depending on temperature and pressure. Chemical agents can be disseminated in aerosol form, defined as a collection of very small, solid particles or liquid droplets suspended in a gas. Chemical agents that are liquids are, to a certain extent, volatile; that is, they evaporate just as water or gasoline do and form an invisible vapor. A vapor is the gaseous form of a substance at a temperature lower than the boiling point of that substance at a given pressure. Volatility is thus inversely related to persistence because the more volatile a substance is, the more quickly it evaporates and the less it tends to stay or persist as a liquid and contaminate materials to which it is exposed. The accepted division between a persistent and nonpersistent chemical agent is 24 hours, meaning that a persistent agent will, by definition, constitute a liquid hazard and contaminate surfaces for 24 hours or longer.

Some chemical agents are said to have characteristic odors; however, such findings are not adequate warning properties to protect EMS workers. By the time a paramedic detects a chemical agent odor, a dangerous exposure would have already occurred. Upon arrival at a potential WMD scene, conscious patients may be able to provide information relevant to an agent odor that might aid EMS in identification.

Nerve Agents

Commonly used **nerve agents** include tabun (GA), sarin (GB), soman (GD), and VX. Nerve agents are the most toxic of all the man-made chemical agents and yet exist in commonly used forms such as organophosphates and other domestic insecticides. Nerve agents, like other organophosphate substances, block the action of acetylcholinesterase, an enzyme present in tissues and blood. As a result of the inhibition of acetylcholinesterase, the neurotransmitter acetylcholine accumulates to overstimulate the organs it normally activates in the nervous system. This causes hyperactivity in these organs, including tearing, salivation, urination, secretions in the respiratory and gastrointestinal tracts, diarrhea, vomiting, muscle twitching, and seizures.

Nerve agents are easily absorbed through the skin, eyes, or lungs and can cause a sudden loss of consciousness, seizures, apnea, and death. The paramedic's suspicion of nerve agent exposure will be derived from observation of patient symptoms. Patients may show signs of limited exposure, usually involving only one organ system, such as miosis, or more systemic exposure, involving multiple organ systems, such as vomiting and seizures. The combination of pinpoint pupils

and muscle fasciculation is the most reliable sign of nerve agent poisoning.

Volatile nerve agents, such as sarin, are nonpersistent chemicals that pose primarily an inhalation hazard because they convert to a gas relatively quickly (Figure 55-2). Symptoms of exposure are primarily dependent on the duration of exposure. Those patients that self-evacuate or are moved from the scene expeditiously will experience limited exposure and symptoms; however, those that inhale a larger dose or have prolonged exposure will have the highest mortality rates. Since chemical agents such as sarin are highly volatile, first responders and medical personnel are at risk of becoming secondarily contaminated from agent off-gassing. **Off-gassing** can occur when the chemical agent is trapped in a patient's clothes and it converts to a gas. It poses a serious inhalation hazard when EMS providers are not wearing appropriate

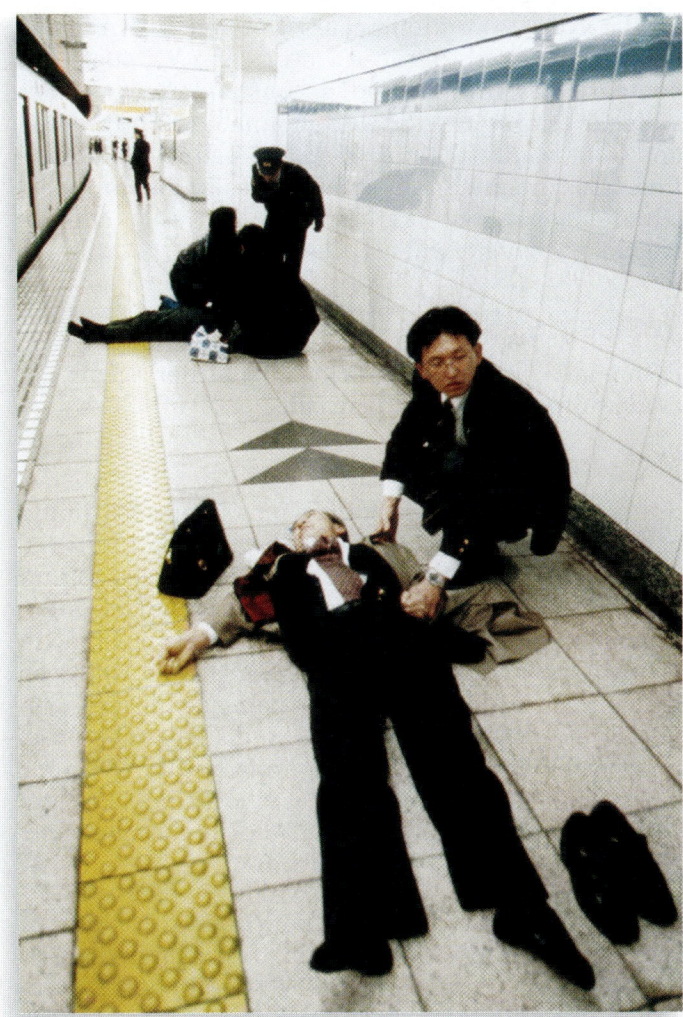

Figure 55-2 Sarin is a nonpersistent chemical nerve agent that poses an inhalation hazard as it converts to a gas relatively quickly, as in the Tokyo subway exposure.

respiratory protection and are caring for the contaminated patient. Symptomatic individuals require immediate treatment, including airway management and antidote therapy with atropine and pralidoxime (2-PAM), as well as decontamination.

Street Secrets

The doses of atropine that organophosphate-exposed patients may need exceeds normally lethal doses. Consequently, they will need more atropine than the typical paramedic drug box contains. Hazmat medical response kits are designed to have drugs in the quantities these patients will need.

Nerve agents such as VX are very persistent oily agents, do not readily vaporize, and pose primarily a liquid threat. The symptoms from such contamination may be delayed for minutes to hours, depending on the concentration, dose, and location of the contaminant on the skin (absorption occurs more readily on moist areas of the skin). Because victims of a VX attack are contaminated with a liquid, decontamination becomes a higher priority to limit the amount of agent absorbed and to minimize the risk of spreading the contamination. Decontamination should ideally be provided simultaneously with antidote administration and airway management, when necessary.

Vesicants (Blister Agents)

Commonly recognized **vesicants**, or **blister agents**, include **sulfur mustard** and **lewisite**.

Mustard

Sulfur mustard can pose both an inhalation and a liquid contact hazard, causing injury to the eyes, skin, airways, and some internal organs. The damaging effects of sulfur mustard exposure may not be evident for hours. Unfortunately, exposure to sulfur mustard causes no immediate pain, skin discoloration, or eye irritation. However, the exposed patient will later experience blisters, temporary blindness, and respiratory distress. The onset time for clinical effects ranges from two to 48 hours, most commonly between four and eight hours. Organ systems directly affected by mustard are the eyes, skin, respiratory tract, and bone marrow.

Eyes. Damage to the eyes from mustard exposure ranges from mild conjunctivitis to corneal ulceration or perforation, depending on the severity of the exposure. Even with the potential for serious eye damage, the documentation for World War I mustard victims indicates that over 95% of those sustaining eye injuries from the agent developed only mild to moderate

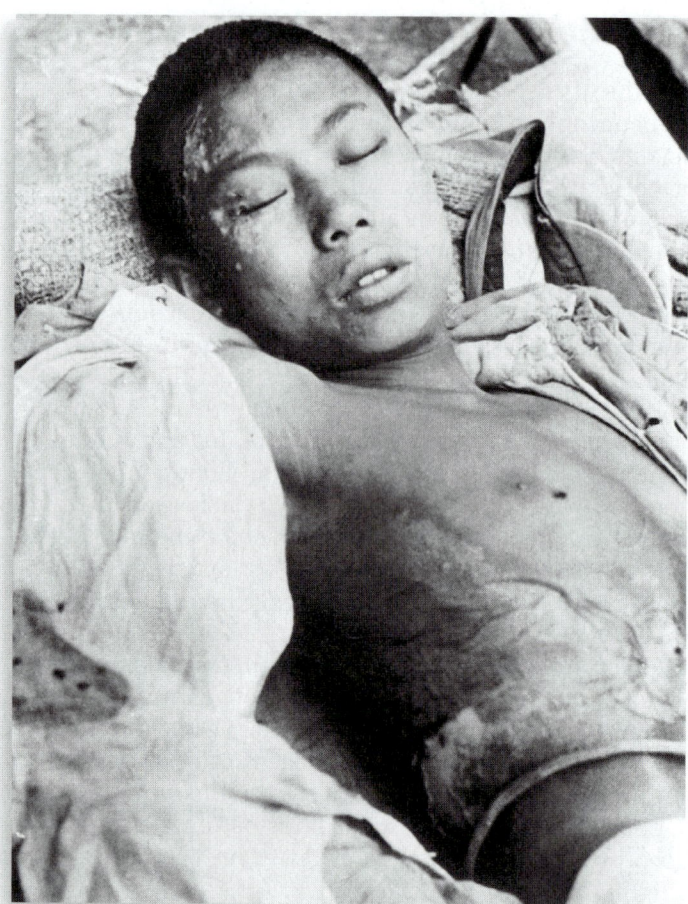

Figure 55-3 Damage to the skin from a mustard gas exposure ranges from mild erythema to blister formation to full thickness damage, depending on the severity of the exposure.

conjunctivitis and that less than 1 percent experienced permanent corneal injury. Prehospital treatment of mustard exposure to the eyes consists primarily of irrigation with saline or water.

Skin. Mustard effects related to skin exposure begin hours after exposure with erythema, followed later by the development of blisters (Figure 55-3). The size and depth of the lesion depends on the amount of exposure and whether exposure was by vapor or liquid. Treatment is largely supportive since there is no antidote for the effects of sulfur mustard. Decontamination consists of physical removal of any residual agent, beginning with removal of all clothing, rings, and jewelry, followed by decontamination using copious amounts of water to flush contaminated skin. Decontamination must be done as quickly as possible since cellular damage occurs in less than one minute. Decontamination of the patient 5 to 10 minutes or more after contact with mustard will not change the clinical course of the patient's illness but is effective in preventing cross contamination of providers.

Airway.   Mustard damages the mucosa or lining of the airways. This damage begins in the upper airways and descends down the air passages in a dose-dependent manner to the smallest bronchioles. Upper airway symptoms may include mild to moderate pharyngitis with an accompanying cough or voice loss. Severe mustard exposure may involve lower airways, causing dyspnea and a productive cough. Prehospital treatment of mustard exposure of the airway includes supplemental oxygen administration and positive pressure ventilation. Early endotracheal intubation may be indicated before laryngeal spasm or edema makes it difficult. The administration of bronchodilators may be helpful in treating bronchospasm.

Bone Marrow.   Sulfur mustard also has serious systemic toxicity. The most serious is damage to the bone marrow, which results in the inability to manufacture white blood cells leading to susceptibility to infection.

Lewisite Effects

Lewisite is a vesicant that is rapidly absorbed by the eyes, skin, and lungs. The chemical agent produces blisters similar to sulfur mustard; however, lewisite is highly irritating on initial exposure, causing pain and producing visible lesions more quickly. In addition, lewisite causes greater skin damage than sulfur mustard, presenting initially as an area of gray skin and quickly progressing to blisters and severe tissue necrosis. Patients exposed to lewisite experience immediate irritation to the nose and sinuses. Patients who immediately evacuate the area of contamination may prevent more severe lung damage. Lewisite causes increased capillary permeability, leading to volume depletion and hepatic and renal injury. Lewisite exposure will necessitate skin decontamination at the earliest possible opportunity to minimize the potential injury. Under emergency circumstances, dilute bleach, soap and water, or copious water are all acceptable decontaminants. The most important factor for lewisite treatment initially is decontaminating patients as soon as possible with whatever decontamination solution is available.

Pulmonary Agents

The pulmonary agents include phosgene, chlorine, and ammonia. Pulmonary intoxicants cause severe, life-threatening lung injury after inhalation. These effects are generally delayed for several hours after exposure.

Phosgene

Phosgene is a colorless gas that has a characteristic odor of freshly mown hay; it is four times heavier than air. It is a gas above 47° F and is principally a hazard by inhalation. The Bhopal, India, disaster of 1984 at the Union

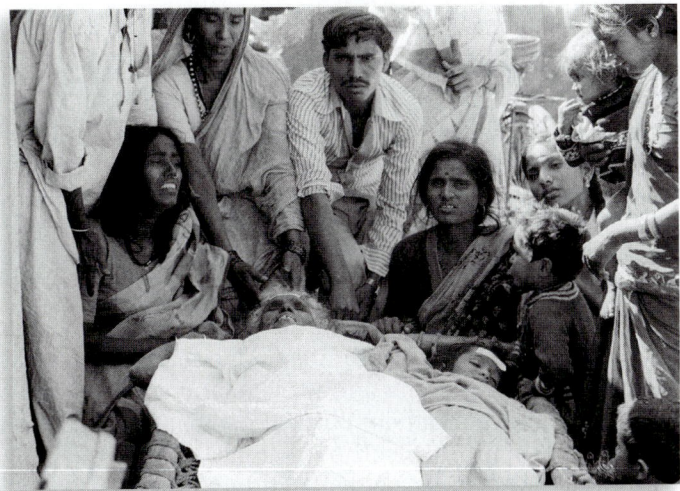

Figure 55-4   The Bhopal, India, disaster of 1984 at the Union Carbide plant involved the release of 50,000 pounds of methylisocyanate—a chemical composed of phosgene and methylamine.

Carbide plant involved the release of 50,000 pounds of methylisocyanate, a chemical composed of phosgene and methylamine. There were 150,000 people affected, 10,000 severely injured, and 3,300 killed. The effects of the release were due to a combination of isocyanate and phosgene (Figure 55-4).

Phosgene dissolves slowly in water to form carbon dioxide and hydrochloric acid (HCl). In contact with the conjunctiva and upper airways, HCl causes irritation of the eyes, nose, sinuses, and throat. It can also irritate the upper airway and bronchi, causing a dry cough. Because the upper respiratory tract is little affected, warning signs of exposure are slight, and symptoms may not appear for two to 24 hours after exposure. However, hydrochloric acid in the lungs causes pulmonary edema; in severe cases, death may result within 36 hours. The leakage of fluid in the lungs may be massive and cause severe volume depletion. After immediately removing patients from the source of exposure, victims must be kept quiet and not be allowed to ambulate. All patients with suspected phosgene exposure should be transported by stretcher. Decontaminate by removing clothing prior to transport. Although the patient clinically looks like traditional heart failure, do not use diuretics. These patients are volume depleted, and hypotension should be treated with fluid resuscitation. Some patients may require intubation and positive pressure ventilation.

Street Secrets

Phosgene and cyanide are two of the elements from which smoke inhalation victims may suffer when removed from fire ground situations.

Anhydrous Ammonia

Anhydrous ammonia is not a military chemical agent but is included because it can be used by a terrorist as a weapon. It is very damaging to human tissue and is widely available. Anhydrous ammonia is not to be confused with the household cleaning chemical ammonia. Anhydrous ammonia is much more toxic and has a pungent odor.

Ammonia is corrosive to the skin, causing pain, erythema, blisters, and tissue necrosis. If ingested, it severely damages the gastrointestinal tract. Exposure to the eyes causes burning and tearing, and a large exposure can cause permanent corneal damage. Airway exposure will manifest itself by dyspnea, coughing, and irritation. Severe exposures may induce chemical pneumonia with hemorrhage. After removing the patient from the area of exposure, clothing should be removed and decontamination initiated with large amounts of water for approximately 15 to 20 minutes. Burns can be treated with sterile dressings, and eye injuries can be treated with irrigation using water. The victims quickly develop shortness of breath and laryngeal swelling, so early intubation should be considered to protect the airway.

Chlorine

Chlorine is a greenish-yellow gas that has a characteristic pungent odor that is irritating to the nasal mucosa. It is commonly used in manufacturing chemicals, plastics, and paper, in addition to its use in swimming pools. Normally, chlorine is transported as a liquid and, when released, converts to a gas that has the potential of producing large numbers of casualties. It is toxic to any body surface it contacts, including the eyes, skin, respiratory tracts, and GI tract.

Chlorine injures cells by reacting with water, producing hydrochloric acid (irritating) and free oxygen radicals. This combination is 30 times more irritating to the respiratory mucosa than hydrochloric acid alone. After an exposure, patients may experience noncardiogenic pulmonary edema. Supplemental oxygen administration is recommended, and endotracheal intubation with assisted ventilation may be required. Toxicity to the eyes and skin should be treated with copious flushing with water.

Street Secrets

When evaluating patients for exposure to water-reactive chemicals, look for burns in moist areas of the body. Certainly look around the face, but look also under the arms, in the groin, and in any area where the patient may have had sweat with which the chemical could react.

Nice to Know

Bitter almond is the taste sensation associated with cyanide ingestion.

Cyanide

Several **cyanide** compounds could serve as WMD agents, most notably hydrogen cyanide and cyanogen chloride. Both of these compounds exist as a gas, with hydrogen cyanide smelling of bitter almonds to the 50% of the population that can detect it. Both of these compounds are very toxic, causing rapid onset of symptoms following any significant exposure. Low concentrations may produce symptoms of headache, weakness, dizziness, and ataxia. Higher concentrations may cause seizures, loss of respiration, and cardiac arrest. Treatment involves safe removal of the patient from the area of exposure, clothing removal, and decontamination using copious amounts of water. Supplemental oxygen administration and immediate transport to a receiving facility that is prepared to administer antidote therapy is required. The antidote for cyanide poisoning involves the administration of amyl nitrite, sodium nitrite, and sodium thiosulfate, but these must be administered in a hospital in a very timely manner to be effective. Recently, hydroxocobalamin was approved to treat cyanide poisoning and may become available as a prehospital treatment.

Riot Control Agents

Riot control agents such as mace and pepper spray are carried by most law enforcement agencies in this country. Such agents produce eye, nose, mouth, skin, and respiratory tract irritation (Figure 55-5). The effects of riot control agents are usually limited to 30 minutes after initial exposure. Medical treatment for those

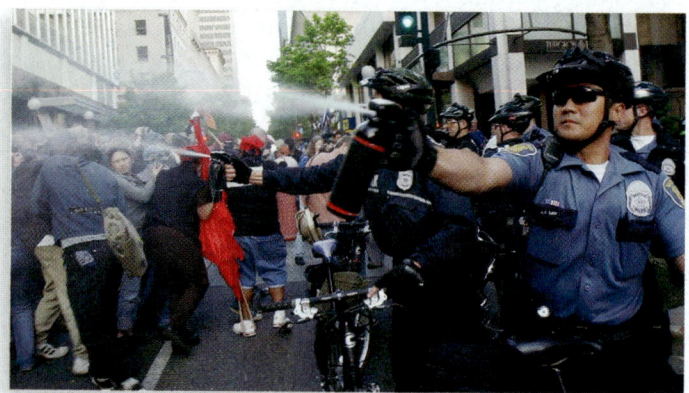

Figure 55-5 Mace and pepper spray produce eye, nose, mouth, skin, and respiratory tract irritation.

exposed to riot control agents involves the effects on the eyes, respiratory tract, and skin.

Eyes should be irrigated copiously with water or saline. Remove contact lenses. Treat bronchospasm with bronchodilators, and provide oxygen therapy, as needed. Most symptoms should improve within one to two hours. Most skin exposures require little more than reassurance; however, with prolonged pain, decontamination with soap and water may be helpful.

Biological Agents

The most effective biological weapon is delivered via aerosol and contains particles that are in the 1–5 micron size range. Particles of this size behave similarly to a gas and can travel to the end bronchioles and alveoli during respiration, where they can be deposited in order to produce the desired pathological effects. Larger particles either quickly fall out of the biological aerosol or become trapped in the upper airway. Smaller particles are breathed into the lungs but expired again without being retained. The identification of this ideal size range was a major advance in the development of biological weapons. After the discovery of the particle size/infectivity relationship, the next significant advance in biological warfare was the development of biological agent in freeze-dried powder formulations. Although the manufacturing of these weapons was both technically difficult and dangerous, their low refrigeration requirement, ease of dissemination, and high concentration made such weapons attractive.

The EMS provider will probably not immediately know that a biological attack has occurred as the presentation of symptoms indicating exposure is both delayed and nonspecific.

Nice to Know

Prehospital providers should increase their index of suspicion that a biological attack has occurred when any of the following are present:

- An abnormally high number of patients complaining of respiratory symptoms that are associated with an unprecedented mortality rate.
- EMS agencies within geographical proximity are also experiencing similar increases in patient volume and respiratory complaints.
- Sick or dead animals of multiple types are encountered.
- Prior intelligence reports or claims by attackers of a biological weapons attack.

Recognizing clues or patterns of illness will alert EMS personnel to question patients and their families to obtain useful epidemiological information. If a paramedic suspects the use of biological weapons, the provider should attempt to obtain the patient's infectious contacts, employment, recent history of travel, and activities over the preceding days or even weeks prior to the development of symptoms. Some biological agents such as smallpox have a prolonged incubation period of more than two weeks. EMS is a critical piece of effective disease surveillance and should report suspicions of unusual illness or infection to the receiving hospital. Three types of biological agents are normally recognized: bacteria, viruses, and toxins.

Bacteria as Biological Agents

Bacteria are single-celled microorganisms that vary in size and shape. Cocci are spherical-shaped cells that are approximately 0.5–1 micron in size, while bacilli are rod-shaped and vary between 1 and 5 microns. Bacteria are self-sustaining organisms that do not require a host to survive. These organisms contain DNA, cytoplasm, and a cell membrane that functions to keep the bacteria alive. Certain bacteria also have the ability to transform themselves into spores, which enables them to withstand cold, heat, and chemical exposure. Most spores are dormant but can easily germinate under the right conditions. Bacterial biological agents include anthrax, plague, tularemia, Q fever, and brucella.

Anthrax

Bacillus anthracis is a spore-forming, rod-shaped organism. Once **anthrax** is inhaled, it is ingested by macrophages, which are then transported to lymph nodes where toxins are produced, causing edema and tissue necrosis. Once anthrax enters the regional lymphatic system, the exposure can lead to toxemia and death. Anthrax is a naturally occurring bacterium that infects animals such as sheep, cattle, and horses. Humans may be "naturally" exposed to anthrax when handling contaminated animal fluids or hides, and consequently, this exposure has been historically referred to as woolsorter's disease. Cases of anthrax exposure are relatively rare in most industrialized countries because of the availability of vaccines for both animals and humans. There are three primary routes of exposure to anthrax. Anthrax can gain entry by contact with open and minor wounds. An anthrax skin infection has a 20% mortality rate if left untreated (1% if treated) (Figure 55-6). Anthrax can also be ingested or inhaled. The inhalation route remains the most probable to be used in a bioterrorism attack as a spraying device could easily disseminate anthrax. Inhalation anthrax historically carries a mortality rate approaching 90%.

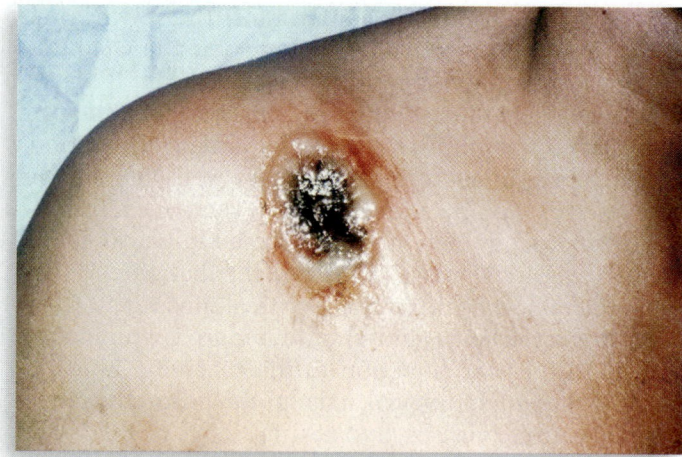

Figure 55-6 An anthrax skin infection has a 20% mortality rate if left untreated (1% if treated).

Street Secrets

The potential for exposure to these types of agents is another reason for paramedics to ensure that sores, cuts, or any breaks in the skin are covered to limit their potential for exposure to anything with which patients may be contaminated.

Inhalational Anthrax

Symptoms of inhalational anthrax develop within two to six days of exposure and include fever, generalized muscle aches, cough, and fatigue. The patient's condition appears to improve during the next few days, when abruptly respiratory distress, shock, and death within 24 to 36 hours are experienced. Physical findings of inhalational anthrax are usually nonspecific.

Gastrointestinal Anthrax

Although gastrointestinal anthrax has a mortality rate approaching 80–90%, large amounts of anthrax spores must be ingested to cause the disease. Initial symptoms of gastrointestinal anthrax exposure include fever, nausea, vomiting, abdominal pain, bloody diarrhea, and occasionally ascites. The disease presents in a similar fashion to an acute abdomen.

Anthrax Treatment

Cutaneous transmissions of anthrax have occurred; however, no documented cases exist of person-to-person transmission of inhalational anthrax. Universal precautions must be maintained for patients with both cutaneous and inhalational anthrax. Prehospital treatment is primarily supportive, with the administration of antibiotics in the hospital as the definitive treatment.

Plague

Yersinia pestis is a gram-negative, rod-shaped organism that is nonmotile and does not sporulate. The organism is killed when exposed to sunlight and temperatures above 72°C for 15 minutes but is resistant to near freezing temperatures and can remain viable in dry sputum, flea feces, and buried bodies. Fleas living on infected rodents such as rats, mice, and squirrels can pass the disease to humans in the naturally occurring form of the disease. All human populations are susceptible to the plague, and recovery from the disease may be followed by temporary immunity. *Yersinia pestis* is the most invasive bacterium known to medical science and is spread to humans from either the bite of an infected flea or by inhaling the organism.

The **plague** has been the cause of a number of devastating epidemics, including the "Black Death" during the 14th century in Europe, which caused the death of over 25 million people (Figure 55-7). In 1900, an epidemic of plague originating in China and carried aboard steamships to San Francisco caused disease transmission into the surrounding rodent population.

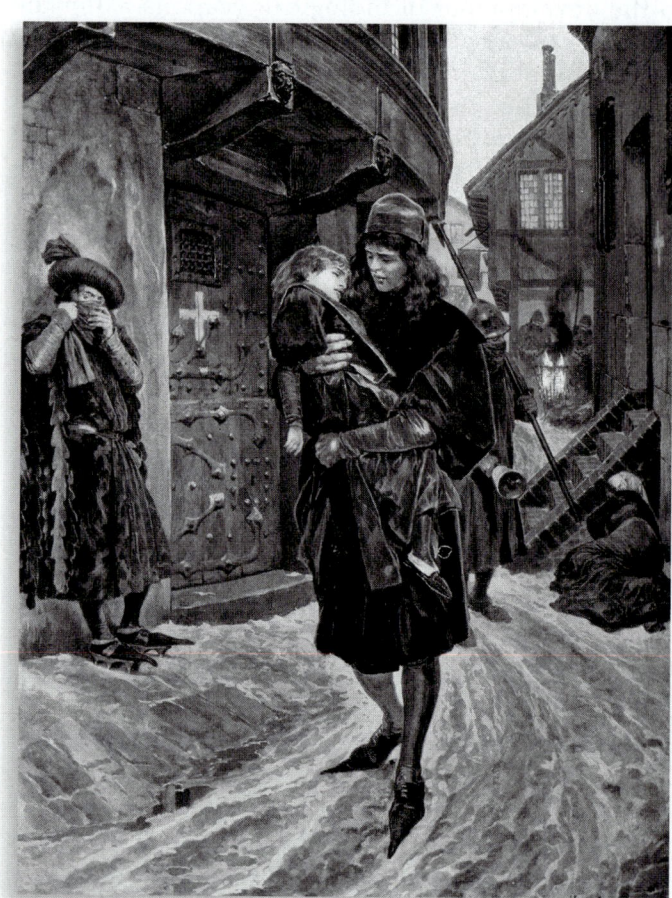

Figure 55-7 Plague, which killed millions of people in Europe in the 14th century, remains endemic in many areas of the world, including the southwestern United States where an average of 10 cases per year are reported.

Since this epidemic on the west coast, plague has spread as far east as Texas. Plague remains endemic in many areas of the world, including the southwestern United States, where an average of 10 cases per year are reported. Plague is primarily a disease of rodents but can be transmitted to humans through the bite of infected fleas (the most common route), through direct contact with infected animals, or via inhalation of respiratory droplets from an infected person with pneumonic plague. Experiments with primates have confirmed that an infectious aerosol of *Yersinia pestis* can be created. Inhalation of the agent would probably be the most likely form if used as a biological weapon.

Infection results in three types of disease: bubonic, which involves lymph nodes closest to the bite site from infected fleas; pneumonic, which is an infection of the lungs; and septicemic, which is a generalized infection in the blood from the bacteria escaping through the lymph nodes or lungs. Following inhalation, bacterial multiplication begins, causing infection in the lymph nodes followed by systemic infection. After skin inoculation, the bacteria are consumed by dermal macrophages that transport the organism to regional lymph nodes and then into the blood to infect organs such as the lungs, spleen, liver, and brain.

Bubonic Plague

Bubonic plague normally occurs from the bite of an infected flea. Initial symptoms develop acutely after an incubation period of two to three days and include erythema, fever, and swollen lymph nodes commonly referred to as buboes.

Bubonic plague may progress spontaneously to the septicemic form with organisms spreading to the central nervous system (CNS), lungs, and beyond. Bubonic plague is not usually transmitted directly from person to person unless there is contact with pus draining from buboes. EMS personnel should practice universal precautions when treating patients with suspected bubonic plague.

Pneumonic Plague Signs and Symptoms

Two or three days after inhaling the plague organism, the patient will develop high fever, myalgias, chills, headache, cough with bloody sputum, and signs of pneumonia. Pneumonia progresses rapidly, causing dyspnea, and cyanosis. Eventual respiratory failure and circulatory collapse develop. Pneumonic plague is highly communicable. For patients with suspected or confirmed pneumonic plague, respiratory droplet isolation with precautions against airborne spread is required. Vaccine is ineffective against aerosol exposures to plague.

Plague Treatment

Respiratory isolation and secretion precautions are mandatory for the first 48 hours of treatment of bubonic or pneumonic plague. Treatment must be started within 24 hours of the onset of symptoms to impact patient survival in the pneumonic form of the disease. Prehospital treatment for suspected plague is primarily supportive, with the administration of antibiotics as the definitive treatment. After antibiotic treatment is started, the swollen tissue typically resolves on its own. A vaccine is available, which is effective in preventing bubonic plague but not the pneumonic form.

Viruses as Biological Agents

Certain viruses have characteristics that make them particularly well suited for use as biological agents. Of the potential viral agents, we will be focusing on smallpox and the viral hemorrhagic fevers (VHF).

Viruses are the simplest type of microorganism and are composed of only genetic material (RNA or DNA) surrounded by a protein coat. Viruses are much smaller than bacteria and lack a system for their own metabolism, needing a host cell to survive and reproduce. This host can be plant, animal, bacteria, or human. Many viruses attack a specific type of cell, causing disease. Few antiviral medications are available; vaccination is the most effective means of preventing infection.

Smallpox

Smallpox is caused by the variola virus, an orthopox virus, which produces both a major and minor form of the disease. The smallpox virus only causes overt clinical disease in humans, and no animal reservoirs of the virus exist in nature. This was the major reason why the disease was selected for global eradication. Smallpox was declared eradicated in 1980 and is the only disease to date that has earned this distinction. The U.S. stopped its civilian vaccination program in 1981. Despite eradication of the clinical disease, concerns over remaining stockpiles of smallpox virus persist. The issue of destruction of U.S. laboratory stocks of the virus is under review. The smallpox virus has an extremely low, natural biological decay rate and a high secondary infection rate. It can easily be manufactured in large quantities. These factors make smallpox an ideal biological warfare agent when used against a nonimmune human population.

Smallpox would most likely be deployed as an aerosol during a biological attack. Then the disease would spread via person-to-person transmission. Smallpox is highly infectious; less than 10 virions are sufficient to cause infection, and exposure for less than 15 minutes is sufficient.

The secondary attack rate, person-to-person transmission, has been estimated to be between 25% and 40% in unvaccinated contacts. Higher rates of transmission are found during cool, dry conditions. Historically, three to four contacts were infected for every one carrier although it may be as high as 10 to 20 in unvaccinated populations. In determining infectiousness, the smallpox rash is the marker. Infectiousness begins approximately one day before the rash and peaks during the first week of rash. However, it is possible to be a smallpox carrier without a rash. Some data show the virus is detectable in saliva of contacts who never become infected. It is unclear if they can transmit the infection, but it is theoretically possible. Infectious materials include saliva, vesicular fluid, scabs, urine, conjunctival fluid, and possibly blood.

As mentioned earlier, there are several forms of clinical smallpox. Thus far, we have only discussed the variola major form. There is a "rule of threes" that is conventionally taught when referring to smallpox. Approximately one-third of the patients exposed to smallpox will acquire the illness, and approximately one-third of those who acquired the illness will die. Bear in mind that nearly all of our experience with smallpox is via the natural route of infection, which is by aerosolized oropharyngeal secretions from an infected individual, and does not take into account the possible weaponization and mass aerosolization of smallpox. The rule of threes has been traditionally taught, but some believe that the fatality rate may indeed be higher and will certainly vary with the underlying health and age of the patient. Unfortunately, patients who have been vaccinated do not enjoy 100% protection. Even though the one-third fatality rate drops to approximately 3% in patients who have been vaccinated against smallpox, they still have a risk of death. The other forms of smallpox include variola minor, which has a similar rash although much less severe. The variola minor smallpox is considered to be a milder strain of smallpox. This underscores the importance of the strain of the biological agent used. Consistent with this milder strain is a relatively low mortality in the 1% range.

There are three stages of the smallpox disease. The first, incubation, normally lasts between seven and 17 days, during which the patient is asymptomatic. The second, prodromal, normally lasts between two to four days, where the patient experiences a nonspecific, febrile illness and flu-like symptoms. Lastly, the eruptive stage, normally lasts between 10 to 14 days. This is when the patient has the characteristic smallpox rash (Figure 55-8). Scabs then separate between 14 to 28 days later. The smallpox rash follows predictable stages of development. All lesions in one region are at the same stage. Deep, tense vesicles develop by day two of the rash, turning into round, tense, deep pustules. Pustules dry to scabs by day nine; scabs then separate between 14 to 28 days later. Scab separation marks the end of the period of infectiousness.

Smallpox Treatment.   Treatment is supportive. Before smallpox was eradicated, the protocol for postexposure

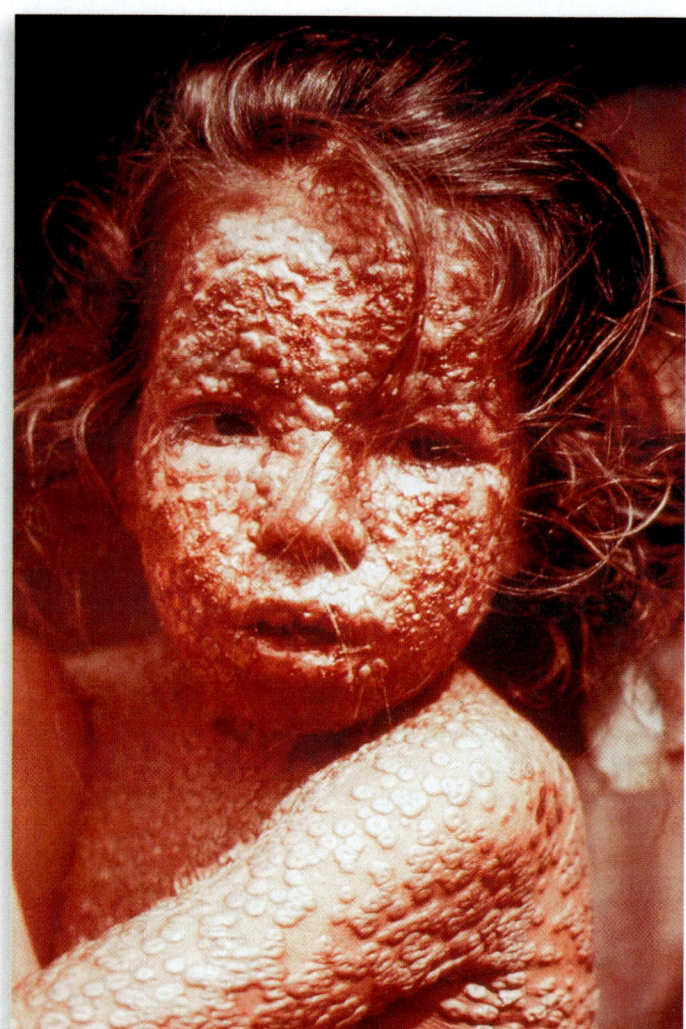

Figure 55-8   Smallpox presents with deep, tense vesicles that develop by the second day of the rash, turning into round, tense, deep pustules.

prophylaxis was to give the live vaccine to healthy patients up to one week postexposure, and to give the vaccine and vaccinia immune globulin (VIG) postexposure to those at risk of vaccinia complications, such as patients who were pregnant; had a history of eczema, psoriasis, unhealed burns, or other exfoliative skin disorders; or were immunocompromised. If the disease were to reappear, there is no consensus on post-exposure prophylaxis to severely immunocompromised patients, such as HIV-infected patients or organ transplant patients, but VIG alone would be a reasonable approach. The World Health Organization (WHO) warehouses approximately 20 million doses of the vaccine.

Prevention of Secondary Infection.   Smallpox historically has a secondary infection rate of 30%, which makes it less communicable than measles or influenza. However, the seriousness of the disease in unvaccinated individuals makes it mandatory that all close contacts be quarantined for at least 17 days, vaccinated, or treated with VIG, and the index case must be kept in isolation until all scabs have healed over. Scab material is infectious and should be handled as a biohazard. Infected patients have live virus in the lungs and are infectious before skin lesions appear. Appropriate respiratory, droplet precautions must be used when caring for these patients. Field care consists of supportive treatment.

Viral Hemorrhagic Fevers

The **viral hemorrhagic fevers** are a diverse group of illnesses caused by a variety of RNA viruses with a wide range of morbidity and mortality. Each of these viruses has a unique history of transmission and clinical presentation. The clinical syndrome these viruses cause in humans is called VHF.

Patients with VHF present initially with fever, myalgias, and prostration. Clinical evaluation may reveal conjunctival injection, petecchial hemorrhages, and hypotension. Full-blown cases will evolve into shock and generalized mucous membrane hemorrhage, with involvement of the respiratory, hematopoietic, and central nervous systems. There are differences between the numerous VHF strains; what is consistent among each of these viruses is that the target organ is the vascular bed, which causes widespread microvascular damage and changes in vascular permeability.

Ebola and Marburg can be transmitted by bodily fluids, and aerosol transmission has been documented in animal models. The highest risk for secondary transmission is in the later stages of the disease when viral titers in the body are high and patients may exhibit vomiting, bloody diarrhea, shock, and hemorrhage. Transferring patients may increase the potential for secondary transmission. Ebola and Marburg viruses are inactivated with routine disinfectant solutions. In previous outbreaks, simple barrier protection was sufficient to reduce the healthcare provider infection rate to zero. Accidental exposures are a serious consideration with Ebola and Marburg. Again, no recognized vaccine or antiviral treatment is available, and it has been calculated that a single viral particle may be enough to initiate an infection in humans.

The Marburg VHF has a seven- to 10-day incubation period, after which victims will experience the sudden onset of back and generalized muscle pain, headache, sore throat, and nausea. A papular or macupapular skin rash will subsequently develop, followed by jaundice and the bleeding abnormalities characteristic of VHF (Figure 55-9). Pulmonary and gastrointestinal hemorrhage will progress to fatal severity, with encephalitis and fulminant hepatitis also likely.

VHF Treatment. Treatment is largely supportive and typically requires intensive care monitoring to avoid

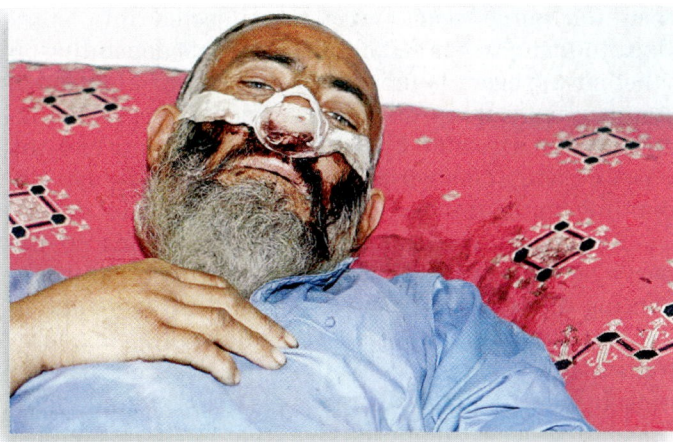

Figure 55-9   Marburg VHF causes papular or macupapular skin rash followed by jaundice and the bleeding abnormalities characteristic of VHF, such as this patient with epistaxis.

fluid overload while maintaining hemodynamic stability and providing appropriate comfort measures (sedation and pain medication). The acquired coagulopathy is typically difficult to counter. At this time, there is no approved antiviral medication for Marburg or Ebola virus infections and an effective vaccine awaits development.

Toxins as Biological Agents

A large variety of lethal biological toxins exist. The agents that will be discussed in this section are those that were found to have the necessary manufactured stability and effectiveness to effect a large area attack and cause mass casualties. These toxins include botulinum toxin and ricin. These two toxins produce disease effects by different mechanisms. Botulinum toxin acts to block nerve conduction while ricin is a potent cytotoxin, which inhibits normal protein synthesis in human cells.

Biological toxins are nonliving, poisonous, chemical compounds that are produced by living organisms (animals, plants, and microorganisms). These agents are hundreds to thousands of times more lethal than standard chemical agents but, unlike chemicals, are not typically volatile or able to cause illness through skin absorption. As a result, toxins are not prone to person-to-person transmission and are not very persistent when released. The toxicity of these agents varies by the route of entry (inhalation versus ingestion versus injection).

Botulinum Toxin

Botulinum toxin is a neurotoxin produced by the bacteria, *C. botulinum,* which causes the disease **botulism.** This toxin is the most lethal known compound per weight and is approximately 15,000 times more toxic than the nerve agent VX when injected into mice. Botulinum toxin has different dose effects depending on whether the agent is inhaled or ingested or inoculated. Aerosol exposure is much less effective at causing fatalities than exposure by the other routes. However, the onset of symptoms varies between hours and days, depending on the route of exposure and the initial dose.

Botulinum works by irreversibly binding to the nerve endings at the neuromuscular junction and preventing the release of acetylcholine (Ach) there and at cholinergic autonomic sites. This interruption of neurotransmission causes both bulbar palsies and skeletal muscle weakness. A bulbar palsy is a loss of function in the cranial nerves that originate from the brain stem.

Botulism Signs and Symptoms. After exposure to the toxin, a descending paralysis (head-to-toe) and bulbar palsies become the characteristic symptoms. Initial symptoms include blurred vision, mydriasis, diplopia, ptosis, photophobia, dysphagia, and dysphonia. The symptoms then progress to involve the skeletal muscles, including the muscles of respiration, which can lead to respiratory failure or arrest.

The limited differential diagnosis for botulism includes myasthenia gravis, which would have a sustained response to anticholinesterases; Guillain-Barré syndrome, which would involve an ascending paralysis with paresthesias; stroke, which would likely be asymmetric and have associated abnormalities on brain imaging; tick paralysis, which would develop ascending paralysis and paresthesias with the presence of a tick; and poliomyelitis, which would be asymmetric and follow a preceding viral illness. In addition to the neurologic syndrome, there are often other features present, depending on the route of intoxication.

Botulism Diagnosis and Treatment. Diagnosis is made from the unique clinical presentation of bulbar palsies and descending paralysis. Food-borne outbreaks are rare, and these occur in small clusters. An epidemic should therefore arouse suspicion of an intentional release.

Treatment is supportive and may require intubation and prolonged mechanical ventilation. An antitoxin is available from the CDC and should be administered as early as possible. The antitoxin is a horse serum product and, consequently, may be associated with serum sickness or anaphylaxis. A vaccine is currently being investigated for protection against Botulinum toxins.

Ricin

Ricin is a lethal cytotoxin that is derived from castor beans and is a byproduct of castor oil production. Over a million tons of castor beans are processed yearly into castor oil, and the Ricin by-product is 200 times more toxic by weight than VX nerve agent. Ricin is an extremely stable compound and is toxic by multiple routes of exposure. It can be dispersed as an aerosol and is effective orally or by injection. Direct exposure on the skin is ineffective.

Ricin Signs and Symptoms. After inhalation, victims begin to experience fever, chest tightness, cough, shortness of breath, nausea, and joint pain within four to eight hours of exposure. Ricin causes necrosis of the lower airway epithelium and severe pulmonary edema following inhalation. Death may occur in 36 to 72 hours. If Ricin is ingested, victims often develop rapid onset of nausea, vomiting, severe diarrhea, and gastrointestinal hemorrhage with necrosis of the liver, spleen, and kidneys. Shock typically ensues, with death occurring within three days. By injection, Ricin causes necrosis of muscles and lymph nodes near the site of injection along with multiple organ failure, leading to death within several days.

Ricin Treatment. Treatment is primarily supportive with supplemental oxygenation and hydration, if indicated. Gastric lavage and activated charcoal are probably indicated following accidental ingestion. No antitoxin or vaccine is currently available. If death has not occurred within three to five days, the patient usually recovers. **DOT 5-11.12**

Radiological and Nuclear Devices

Terrorist use of radioactive materials or a nuclear device constitutes a plausible threat. The medical consequences will depend on the type of device used in a terrorist event.

Basics of Radiation

Ionizing radiation can occur naturally, can be machine-generated (i.e., x-rays), or can come from radioactive atoms. The basic building block of all matter is the atom. The atom consists of a central nucleus with shells of electrons orbiting around this nucleus. The nucleus is made up of neutrons and protons. Each element has a defined number of protons. These protons, which are positively charged, have the tendency to repel each other. There is an average ratio of protons to neutrons for stability of an element. When an element is radioactive, usually there is an imbalance of this ratio of protons to neutrons; often the imbalance is due to an excess of neutrons.

In such a case, an unstable nucleus can become stable by changing a neutron into a proton with the ejection of a negative bit of matter (a beta particle or electron); conversely, a proton can change into a neutron with the ejection of a positively charged bit of matter (a positron or positively charged electron). The nucleus of large, unstable atoms can reach stability by ejecting larger particles that consist of two protons and two neutrons (an alpha particle). The nucleus of an unstable atom usually has an excess of energy. This excess is given off as electromagnetic energy of very short wavelength. It is called gamma radiation. When all the excess energy and mass is given off, the resultant element finally becomes stable.

The most common types of ionizing radiation are alpha particles, beta particles, gamma rays, x-rays, and neutrons. X-rays, like gamma rays, are electromagnetic energy of short wavelength. X-rays and gamma rays are sometimes referred to as photons.

Effects of Ionizing Radiation on Humans

The basic building block of any tissue is the cell, and damage to components of the cell may change its chemistry or DNA. The chemical damage from radiation is instantaneous, but the clinical manifestation of this damage can take hours to years to be evident. High doses of radiation delivered over a short period of time can result in clinical effects within hours (acute radiation syndrome or ARS). However, at lower doses, even with doses too low to cause acute effects, there is the probability, although low, of developing a radiation-induced cancer 20 to 30 years later. Other problems that may be observed weeks or months after an acute exposure include infertility, thyroid dysfunction (hypothyroidism), and cataracts. Cataract formation requires a prompt dose of about 200 rem to the lens of the eye. It has been shown that neutrons are more effective in producing this type of injury. Japanese children who, as a result of radiation from the atomic bomb explosions, received greater than 50 rads while in utero had congenital defects including low birth weight, small head size, and mental retardation.

Alpha Radiation

Alpha particles are composed of two neutrons and two protons. Alpha particles do not penetrate the skin and can be shielded by a thin layer of paper or clothing. Because the outer layer of skin is dead and several microns thick, the alpha particle is unable to penetrate through the dead layers of skin to reach the lower layers of living cells and generally will not cause any skin damage. If, however, an alpha emitter gets inside the body through inhalation, ingestion, or a wound, the alpha emissions are near live tissue, and localized damage could occur. Alpha radiation is therefore an internal hazard only.

Beta Radiation

Beta radiation may travel meters in air and is moderately penetrating. Beta radiation can penetrate human skin to the germinal layer, where new skin cells are produced.

If beta-emitting contaminants are allowed to remain on the skin for a prolonged period of time, they may cause skin injury. Contaminants emitting beta particles may be harmful if deposited internally. Beta radiation is both an external (primarily to the skin and lens of the eye) and internal hazard.

Gamma Rays (Photons)

Gamma radiation is able to travel many meters in air and many centimeters in human tissue. It readily penetrates most materials and is sometimes called penetrating radiation. X-rays are similar to gamma rays. They, too, are penetrating radiation. Radioactive materials that emit gamma radiation constitute both an external and an internal hazard to humans; x-rays are primarily external hazards since they are usually machine-produced. Dense materials such as lead are needed for shielding from gamma radiation and will prevent contamination of the skin by these materials. Gamma radiation frequently accompanies the emission of alpha and beta radiation.

Neutrons

Neutrons are neutral particles emitted from the nucleus of an unstable atom. Neutrons lose most of their energy through collisions with other atomic nuclei. An analogy that could be used is the billiard ball effect (i.e., when one billiard ball strikes another, energy is transferred from one ball to the other). Under certain circumstances, neutrons can be captured by a stable nucleus, making the nucleus radioactive. The process is called activation. An example of this is Na-23 being changed (transmutated) into Na-24. Neutron radiation is an external hazard.

Radiation Units

The basic unit for measuring radiation is the rad (**r**adiation **a**bsorbed **d**ose). The rad is defined as the deposition of 0.01 joule of energy per kilogram (kg) of tissue. To quantify the amount of damage that is suspected from a radiation exposure, rads are converted into rems (which at one time stood for **r**oentgen **e**quivalent **m**an). The rem is adjusted to reflect the type of radiation absorbed and the likelihood of damage. In most cases, the rad and rem will be equivalent (1 rem = 1 rad; 1,000 millirem = 1,000 millirad). Newer nomenclature has renamed the rad as the gray and the rem as the sievert.

For example, a standard x-ray machine was used to deliver 100 rads of radiation and to compare the biological endpoint with other types of radiation. It was found that 100 rads of gamma and beta radiation produced the same effect as 100 rads of x-rays. However, it was found that only 20 rads of neutrons and five rads of alpha radiation were needed to produce the same effect as 100 rads of x-ray. Therefore, neutron and alpha radiations were more potent and required fewer rads to produce the same effect.

Radiation Doses in Perspective

Radioactivity has existed for millions of years in the crust of the earth, in building materials, in the food we eat, in the air we breathe, and in virtually everything that surrounds us. Radiation from these materials, as well as cosmic radiation from the sun and universe, makes up the natural background radiation to which we are constantly exposed.

Most individuals are exposed to about 360 millirems per year from natural and man-made sources. Smoking 1.5 packs of cigarettes a day for one year produces a cumulative radiation dose of 16 rem to the bifurcation of the bronchus. If an individual is exposed to more than 100 rads at one time, predictable signs and symptoms will develop within a few hours, days, or weeks, depending on the dose. Fifty percent of individuals exposed to a single dose of 450 rads of penetrating radiation will die without medical intervention within 60 days. This is known as the LD 50/60, meaning the lethal dose of radiation in 50% of the people exposed within 60 days. EMS personnel must familiarize themselves with the radiation guidelines of time, distance, and shielding.

- **Time.** The shorter the time in a radiation field, the less the radiation exposure. WMD personnel must work quickly and efficiently. A rotating team approach can be used to keep individual radiation exposures to a minimum.
- **Distance.** The farther a person is from a source of radiation, the lower the radiation dose. Do not touch radioactive materials. Use shovels, brooms, and the like to move materials to avoid physical contact.
- **Shielding.** Although not always practical in emergency situations, shielding offered by barriers can reduce radiation exposure.

Types of Radiation Exposure

Regardless of where or how an exposure to radiation happens, three types of radiation-induced injury can occur: external irradiation, contamination with radioactive materials, and incorporation of radioactive material into body cells, tissues, or organs.

- **External irradiation.** External irradiation occurs when all or part of the body is exposed to penetrating radiation from an external source. During exposure, this radiation can be absorbed by the body, or it can pass completely through as it does during an ordinary chest x-ray. Following external exposure, an individual is not radioactive and can be treated like any other patient.

- **Contamination.** Contamination means that radioactive materials in the form of gasses, liquids, or solids are released into the environment. People who have radioactive materials on or in their bodies are said to be contaminated, and if radioactive materials get inside the body through the lungs, gastrointestinal tract, or wounds, the contaminant can become deposited internally.
- **Incorporation.** Incorporation refers to the uptake of radioactive materials by body cells, tissues, and target organs such as bone, liver, thyroid, or kidney. In general, radioactive materials are distributed throughout the body based upon their chemical properties. Incorporation cannot occur unless internal contamination has occurred.

These three types of events (i.e., external irradiation, contamination, and incorporation) can happen in isolation or in combination and can also be complicated by physical injury or illness. Irradiation of the whole body or some specific body part in most cases does not constitute a medical emergency, even if the amount of radiation received is high. The effects of irradiation usually are not evident for days to weeks and while medical treatment is needed, it is not needed on an emergency basis. On the other hand, contamination accidents must be considered medical emergencies since they might lead to internal contamination and subsequent incorporation. Incorporation can result in adverse health effects several years later if the amount of incorporated radioactive material is high.

Dispersion of Radiation

Radiation can be dispersed two ways.

Simple Radiological Device

This is the deliberate act of spreading radiation without the use of an explosive device. An example would be the placement of a high-activity radioactive isotope in a public place, exposing passing individuals to various levels of radiation. An example of this occurred in Brazil in 1987, when a hospital radiotherapy source was stolen by two scrap dealers. The source, Cesium-137, was broken up and dispersed. The incident was not detected for 15 days. It resulted in 249 people being contaminated, four deaths, and 112,800 people requiring monitoring. The medical response and clean-up phases took several months to complete. In this case, there was both an exposure and a contamination problem.

Explosive Device

In the western world, the probability of terrorism involving a nuclear reactor is low. This is due to the high security surrounding a reactor together with the safety systems incorporated into the reactor. There is extensive shielding around a reactor; therefore, a significant amount of explosives would be required to breach this containment. This is a low probability event. It is thought that the major effect of a nuclear reactor explosion would be psychological.

A radiologic dispersal device is, however, considered to be a very plausible scenario. Such a device involves taking radioactive material and using an attached explosive to disperse the radiologic source over a large area such as many city blocks. While the radiation exposure risk would likely be relatively small, the psychological impact would be large. In addition, there would be extensive economic and environmental clean-up costs.

Finally, terrorist use of an actual or improvised (home-made) nuclear weapon is thought to be unlikely, although certainly not impossible. Such a device would result in large numbers of casualties and have a massive impact on society.

In the event of a radiologic incident, the responding paramedic should assume all property and personnel to be contaminated. Ambulances should be positioned 150 feet upwind (2,000 feet or more in a nuclear explosion). A radiological survey should be performed to assess for the degree of contamination. All responding personnel should have dosimeters and should don appropriate PPE before rescue.

Scene Assessment

A scene evaluation (hazard analysis) should be performed immediately by the first responding personnel, using the information provided by bystanders and dispatch. Identify all hazards, including fire, explosion, toxic fumes, electrical, structural collapse, or their potential. Use radiation survey instruments, if available.

Establish a Hot Line and Decontamination Area

If the identity of the radioactive source is unknown, the limits of the contamination must be found using survey meters, so a hot line can be established. The hot line will separate the clean and contaminated sides of the release area for all responding personnel. A decontamination area should also be set up, preferably upwind and upgrade (uphill) from the release area and near the treatment station. While the hot line is being established, begin attending to accident victims.

Acute Radiation Syndrome

Acute radiation syndrome (ARS) is an acute illness that follows a roughly predictable course over a period of time, ranging from a few hours to several weeks after exposure to ionizing radiation. The acute radiation

syndrome is produced if enough radiation reaches enough sensitive tissue in a short enough period of time. Important factors are high dose, high dose rate, whole body exposure, and penetrating irradiation. In addition, other factors need to be taken into consideration, such as age, sex, genetics, and preexisting medical conditions. The source of radiation (i.e., reactor, nuclear weapon, industrial source, or medical therapy source) does not matter if the dose is high enough; it will produce the same effect. The signs and symptoms that develop in the ARS occur in four distinct phases:

- **Prodromal phase.** Depending on the total amount of radiation absorbed, patients may experience a variety of symptoms, including loss of appetite, nausea, vomiting, fatigue, and diarrhea. After high radiation doses, additional symptoms such as prostration, fever, respiratory difficulties, and increased excitability may develop. This is the stage at which most victims seek medical care.

- **Latent phase.** This is a transitional period in which many of the initial symptoms resolve. This period may last for up to three weeks, depending on the original radiation dose. This time interval decreases as the initial dose increases.

- **Illness phase.** This is the period of time when overt illness develops, often characterized by infection, bleeding, electrolyte imbalance, diarrhea, changes in mental status, and shock.

- **Recovery or death phase.** This follows the period of overt illness, which may take weeks or months to resolve.

Severity of Radiation Injury

In general, the higher the dose, the more severe the early effects will be and the greater the possibility of delayed effects. It is important at this stage to briefly discuss the effect of radiation on the cell. Obviously, one can increase the dose until the cell is killed outright. However, it is found that a much lower dose can stop cell division (sterilization). For example, if we consider the hematopoietic system, an individual hematopoietic stem cell has the capability of producing millions of mature cells. The death or sterilization of division means the loss of these cells. The importance of this is that a sublethal dose produces these effects. Two important organ systems that have rapidly dividing cell lines are the hematopoietic and gastrointestinal systems (small intestine).

Radiation Casualty Classification, Treatment, and Disposition

EMS personnel should be prepared for a radiologic incident. It will present many unique challenges to EMS personnel. A radiation-contaminated patient should be handled in the same manner as any hazardous materials accident victim. In some respects, these victims have an advantage over other hazardous materials-contaminated patients because they can be surveyed with instruments to determine if they are truly contaminated or not. In any case, there is minimal risk to responding and treating personnel if the victims are properly handled.

Once the radiological survey and decontamination procedure is complete, patients may be classified into one of three categories:

- Those receiving less than 100 rads can be classified as survival probable.
- Those receiving between 200–800 rads are listed as survival possible.
- Those receiving greater than 800 rads are listed as survival improbable.

Carefully evaluating the initial presenting signs and symptoms (such as nausea, vomiting, diarrhea, changes in mental status, shock, and lymphocyte count over the first 48 hours) becomes the most reliable indicator of the radiation dose and the patient's ultimate prognosis. Since no antidote exists for radiation exposure, treatment, after surface decontamination if necessary, is primarily supportive, with more specialized care directed towards patients with high-dose irradiation and those with internal contamination.

Incendiary and Explosives

Mechanical Explosion

Mechanical explosion is the result of increased pressure inside a container that exceeds the pressure limits of the container. Examples include the failure of a steam boiler or pressure cooker.

Chemical Explosion

Chemical explosion is characterized by the rapid conversion of a solid or liquid explosive compound into a hot, gaseous compound, having a much greater volume than the substances from which it was generated. Examples include gunpowder, dynamite, and plastic explosives.

Nuclear Explosions

Nuclear explosions may be generated by fission or by fusion. In a fission reaction, a heavy atom (such as uranium) is split into two or more smaller atoms. In contrast, a fusion reaction involves the joining of two smaller atoms to make a heavier one with the release of energy.

Bomb Blasts

Bombs are composed of a variety of explosive materials. When bombs are detonated, the reaction produces an instantaneous chain of events in which the explosive material is rapidly converted into a gas under extremely high pressure and temperature. This sudden conversion to expanding gas is transmitted to the surrounding medium as a blast wave (or shock wave) that travels outward from the explosion (Figure 55-10). After the explosion occurs, a mass of air (blast wind) is displaced by the explosive products traveling at speeds that can exceed hurricane proportions. This blast wind may be as damaging as the original explosion.

High-energy explosives (such as plastic explosives, TNT, diesel fuel, and fertilizer) detonate faster than the speed of sound. Low-energy explosives (i.e., gunpowder and dynamite) react slower than the speed of sound. It must be remembered that even a low-energy explosive can release devastating energy.

If a solid structure such as a wall or building is present in the path of the explosion, the blast wave will rebound off this structure and generate a reflective force that is magnified up to nine times its original strength. As a result, victims caught between the blast and a building may suffer injuries two or three times greater than expected for the amount of explosive detonated and the distance from the explosion.

Dynamite

Dynamite is the explosive most widely used for blasting operations throughout the world. In the past, dynamite has been relatively easy to obtain by theft or through legal purchase and has consequently been one of the explosives most frequently used by criminal bombers.

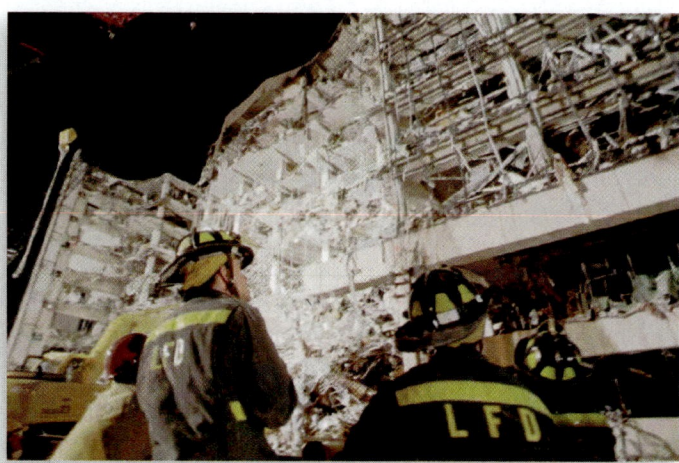

Figure 55-10 High-energy explosives (such as plastic explosives, TNT, diesel fuel, and fertilizer) detonate faster than the speed of sound as in the explosion at the Murrah Federal building.

Most commercial dynamites are made of liquid nitro-glycerin, oxidizers, and a binder material.

Ammonium Nitrate/Fuel Oil (ANFO)

Ammonium nitrate is the least sensitive and most readily available secondary high explosive. It is usually found in the form of small, compressed pellets or pills and is used in the manufacturing of certain dynamites. ANFO is produced by combining ammonium nitrate with fuel oil, most commonly diesel fuel. ANFO was the explosive used in the Oklahoma City bombing.

Blast Pressure

When a bomb detonates, several waves of pressure are produced that affect those exposed to the blast. With the initial and sudden conversion of the solid explosive material into an expanding gas, there is a large and rapid increase in pressure (blast overpressure). This sudden increase in pressure compresses hollow objects in its path. If one of those objects is a person, hollow organs, such as the eardrums, lungs and bowel, are compressed and potentially injured. In addition, the sudden pressure wave will displace anything in its path, throwing objects about. As the energy from the explosion is expended, all of the air that was displaced comes rushing back as there is now an area of relatively low pressure created in the void from which all this air was moved.

Blast Wave

There are several blast wave properties that relate to injury. First, the injury will depend on the size of the blast overpressure. Second, the duration of the positive pressure phase, including the relationship of the blast to reflecting surfaces and whether the blast occurred in closed or open space, will determine the severity of the injuries. Last, the distance from the explosion will determine the number and severity of injuries. Primary blast injury involves the direct effect of the blast wave on tissue and organs, primarily the hollow organs mentioned previously. Secondary blast injury involves objects striking the victim and often results in penetrating trauma (Figure 55-11). Tertiary blast injury involves victims striking a stationary object and often causes blunt trauma.

Bomb Blast Special Considerations

In a terrorist bombing, the potential for secondary contamination with WMD agents should always be considered. If contaminants are found or suspected, victims should be decontaminated with soap and water. At a minimum, their clothing should be removed, double-bagged (paper bags for explosives, paper bags into plastic bags for chemicals and explosives) and their wounds irrigated with sterile water (if available) and covered

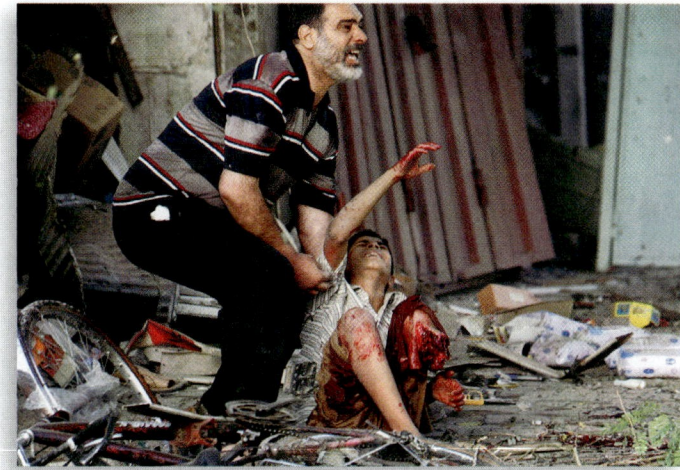

Figure 55-11   The secondary blast injury involves objects striking the victim and often involves penetrating trauma.

with a sterile dressing prior to hospital transport. This is especially true in unstable, multiple trauma victims who are potentially contaminated with WMD agents. Contaminated foreign bodies that remain in the wound require emergency surgical intervention and removal.

A bombing site should be secured and declared free of any additional explosive, chemical, or radioactive materials before unprotected emergency responders are allowed to enter the scene. A secondary explosive has been frequently used by terrorists in Ireland and Israel and, most recently, in the U.S. (Atlanta, Georgia and New York, New York). The presence of radiological materials (alpha, beta, and gamma) can be quickly determined by using survey meters such as an alpha meter or a Geiger counter. This should be considered a routine practice at any bombing site. The responding hazardous materials response team (HMRT) should also undertake a routine survey for chemical contamination. If biological weapons are suspected, routine protective gear worn by first responders (fire, EMS, law enforcement) will be adequate if it includes gloves and respiratory protection such as high-efficiency particulate arrestor (HEPA) filter-style mask or an air-purifying or atmosphere-supplied respirator.

Fragmentation

Fragmentation can be the most destructive characteristic of a bomb. The blast itself can create craters and blow down walls and buildings, but the concentrated power of a fragment can force penetration deeply into a target, tearing and shredding as it goes. Fragment velocities may range from 500 to 1500 meters per second.

Incendiary or Thermal (Heat)

In general, a low-energy explosive will produce a longer incendiary thermal effect than will a high-energy explosive. If a high-energy explosive is placed on a section of earth covered by dry grass and detonated, only a vacant patch of scorched earth will remain. However, if a low-energy explosive charge is placed on the same type of earth and detonated, more than likely a grass fire will result.

WMD Scene Assessment

Throughout your career as a paramedic, you will likely hear the words "personal safety" about as many times as you will hear the words "intubation" or "defibrillation." In fact, this should be the basis for every call to which you respond from now until the time you retire. Personal safety involves a multitude of factors and actions that, as a prehospital provider, you will most likely learn and perform through personal experience. It is what will allow you to respond to the next call for service and is what will allow you to go home at the end of each and every shift.

When responding to a weapons of mass destruction event, the paramedic will face even greater challenges to their personal safety. The persons responsible for a WMD attack have several objectives that they try to accomplish. The primary objective with the release or detonation of a WMD agent is to produce large numbers of casualties. With large numbers of casualties obviously comes a large response from police, fire, and EMS. The second objective that terrorists are known for trying to accomplish involves the strategic planting of secondary explosive devices in places where public safety personnel are likely to initially respond. It is imperative that public safety responders be diligent in looking for these devices during their response.

Once police, fire, and EMS have arrived on-scene, they immediately begin assessing the scene and considering the additional resources that they will need. This is obviously a very important component of scene management. However, it is also important that responders consider the type of personal protective equipment that they will need to use in order to remain safe on the scene, so they can continue to render aid throughout the duration of the incident. This section will focus on the types of PPE available to emergency responders and the issues surrounding contamination that can cause disastrous effects for these personnel.

Contamination

Public safety personnel face many challenges on any scene, as mentioned previously. Of the challenges faced, none is more important than prevention of secondary contamination. Secondary contamination occurs when a clean object or person comes into contact with a contaminated object or person. This is usually the result of well-meaning responders rushing into a scene, using poor scene management, inadequate pro-

cedures, or procedures that were not followed at all. DOT 8-4.1,2

Decontamination

To avoid secondary contamination, it is imperative that all prehospital providers understand and be proficient at performing decontamination. Decontamination is the process of removing contaminants from objects or persons who have or may have come into contact with a hazardous agent. The function of decontamination on any scene is important to ensure responder safety as well as the welfare of the clinical staff that awaits your arrival at emergency rooms. Consider the delay in patient care that will be unavoidable since the patient will now have to be decontaminated at the arriving facility. In addition, your crew, equipment, and vehicle will have to remain out of service until they can be thoroughly decontaminated.

EMS workers can observe several safety principles that will ultimately reduce their need for self-decontamination and save valuable time and energy that are often lost on hazardous materials and WMD incidents. These principles include the following:

- Practice avoidance. Staying clean is ultimately the best type of decontamination. Depending upon your role in the incident, you may or may not have direct contact with the hazardous materials.
- Remain aware of the location of the hazardous materials, and limit your exposure.
- Use disposable over-garments (gloves, boots, aprons, etc.). This can reduce the overall problem by simply removing contaminated articles.
- Only enter zones where you and your equipment are properly protected.

There are two distinct types of decontamination and multiple procedures that are used to perform each. The two types of decontamination are emergency decontamination and technical decontamination.

Emergency Decontamination

Emergency decontamination procedures are designed to decontaminate an injured person or crewmember as quickly as possible to enable medical staff to perform lifesaving interventions. Individuals who qualify to receive emergency decontamination are those who cannot wait for technical decontamination to take place. This concept of emergency decontamination is based on speed, not neatness. This process usually involves the use of hose lines from fire apparatus and water alone. However, a responder may use whatever steps or agents are necessary in order to ensure that the person being decontaminated is clean enough to safely begin treatment.

Technical Decontamination

Technical decontamination is the planned and systematic removal of contaminants from equipment, personnel, and anything else that has come into contact with the hazardous agent. Most agencies employ a formalized set of approved policies and procedures that are designed to progressively clean individuals and equipment. Technical decontamination also takes into consideration protecting those individuals who are performing decontamination in the warm zone of incidents.

Technical decontamination is time-consuming and the equipment used typically takes time to ready for use. Many agencies have invested in manufactured equipment whose sole purpose is technical decontamination. These products are expensive, and their functionality and efficiency has yet to be determined. The important aspect to remember is that technical decontamination is a necessity any time responders and patients have the potential to be contaminated or exposed to a product or agent with known life hazards.

As a paramedic, it is imperative that you ensure that your patient has been decontaminated before entering your ambulance. This will reduce secondary contamination and drastically reduce the amount of time that your unit will be out of service for decontamination.

Personal Protective Equipment

Some of you will work for paramedic services whose only personal protective equipment are gloves and safety glasses. These two pieces of protective equipment are important and will most likely suffice for the majority of your career. The rest of you may currently be, or at some point in time may become, employed by the fire service. Regardless, all emergency responders should have an understanding of the types of personal protective equipment available to them. This section will cover the types of personal protective equipment with which you, as emergency responders, may come into contact and could eventually have to use yourself on a given scene.

There are several routes of exposure by which a WMD agent may cause you significant distress or death. The respiratory system is by far the most vulnerable body system and is one of the fastest routes of exposure for most agents. By inhaling certain agents, you are more likely to become sick much faster than by other routes (i.e., absorption, ingestion, etc.). Thousands of emergency personnel become injured on-duty due to respiratory injuries or exposures. DOT 8-4.7,8

Self-Contained Breathing Apparatus

The positive pressure self-contained breathing apparatus (SCBA) is also known as an "airpack" within the fire service. This tool has become a mainstay for emergency

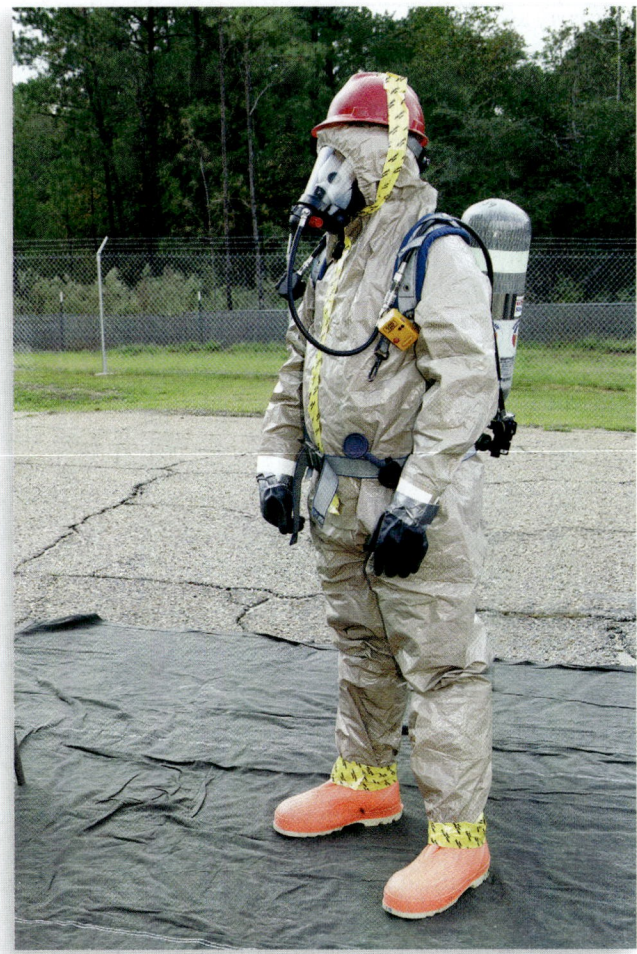

Figure 55-12 The SCBA provides personnel with the absolute highest level of respiratory protection available.

responders across the nation.[4] Most SCBA systems fit the wearer with a full-face piece and nose cup that helps to improve visibility and reduce fogging (Figure 55-12). The SCBA provides personnel with the absolute highest level of respiratory protection available. The SCBA is equipped with multiple fail-safe systems that ensure that if a problem occurs with the unit, the wearer will have ample time to exit the hazardous condition.

Advantages to positive pressure SCBA include the following:

- Most fire service responders are proficient in its use.
- It is readily available.
- It provides the highest level of respiratory protection against airborne contaminants and oxygen deficiency.

Limitations to positive pressure SCBA include the following:

- It is bulky and heavy.
- The limited air supply restricts work duration, although this may actually be an advantage.

- It may impair movement in confined spaces.
- Its resistance to chemicals is unknown.

Air-Purifying Respirators

Otherwise known as "cartridge respirators," the air-purifying respirators (APRs) do not provide a presupplied source of air like the SCBA. Instead, the outside air is filtered when the wearer inhales through their face piece. These protective tools are certainly not as safe as SCBAs and are typically recommended for use only after proper air monitoring has been accomplished and levels within the work zone are deemed safe for APR use.

Advantages of the APR include the following:

- Enhanced mobility (no weight or air lines) of the user.
- Lighter weight than the SCBA.
- Increased work duration.
- Less physical stress on the user.

Limitations of the APR include the following:

- Cannot be used in IDLH or oxygen deficient (less than 19.5%) atmospheres.
- Protects only against specific chemicals up to specific concentrations (proper cartridge must be selected).
- Limited duration of protection; it may be hard to gauge safe operating time in field conditions.
- Its use requires constant monitoring of contaminants and oxygen levels.
- Can be used only for gas and vapor contaminants with adequate warning properties or for specific gasses or vapors provided that the service life is known and a safety factor is applied or if the unit has an **e**nd of **s**ervice **l**ife **i**ndicator (ESLI).
- Face pieces must be fitted to each individual user to ensure proper seal (no positive pressure).

As you can see, the APR contains more limitations than the SCBA and is considerably less safe to wear in certain conditions.

Protective Clothing

Second only to respiratory protection, protecting your skin from dangerous agents is best accomplished with the protective clothing available to emergency responders. WMD and hazardous materials protective clothing comes in various shapes, styles, and sizes. One distinct difference is how this protective clothing is classified. Chemical protective clothing is broken down into levels by the degree of protection that each offers. The levels go from A to D, with Level A affording the wearer the most protection and Level D the least protection. One thing that should be noted is that anytime a wearer, commander, or safety officer is unsure of the level of protection needed for responders, the level affording the wearer with the most protection should be worn.

To simplify the process, we will begin with the suit that provides the least protection and work our way into suits that offer increased protection.

Level D Protection

Usually recognized as regular clothing, Level D protection should be the most readily identifiable form of protection available to you as a responder. In other words, the responder's uniform is considered to be Level D protection, with safety glasses and a hard hat or helmet. The Level D suit (or uniform) affords the user virtually no respiratory protection and minimal skin protection.

Features of Level D Protection

- Eye protection
- Coveralls
- Boots or shoes that are chemically resistant and have steel toes and shanks
- Hard hat
- Gloves (when appropriate)

Indications for use of Level D Protection

- Atmosphere contains no known hazard
- Work activities preclude splashes, immersion, or the potential for unexpected inhalation or contact with hazardous materials
- *There is no emergency!*

Level C Protection

The Level C protective specifications vary depending upon the organization that publishes the guidelines. This chapter will reference NFPA (National Fire Protection Association) guidelines to distinguish between Level C and Level B protection.

According to the NFPA, Level C protection affords the user the required amount of protection dependent upon the "known" chemical. This level of protection is worn when the agent is known to the responders and the agent that the suit is being exposed to will not penetrate through the material. This form of protection also affords the wearer an increased level of respiratory protection by providing the responder with an APR (Table 55-2).

Indications for use of Level C Protection

- Reduced level of respiratory protection needed
- Well characterized and measured products

TABLE 55-2 Level C Protection

Advantages	Limitations
Tested against penetration and liquid integrity	Can only be used in very controlled situations
Lightweight and less physical stress	Greatly reduced flammability rating; no flash protection
More comfortable	Reduced strength from the typical Level B suit
Basically designed to be disposable (no reuse)	

- Splashes or incidental contact with product will not cause harm to skin or be absorbed
- NFPA 1993 garments made for support zone activities, such as decontamination, and remedial site mitigation

Level B Protection

This level of protection gives the user the highest level of respiratory protection available (SCBA) and protection against accidental exposure to spills and splashes of a chemical. Most organizations whose employees have the potential for exposure to hazardous material spills provide Level B protection to employees.

This form of protection will suffice for most incidents. The only instances where Level B protection is not advised are when the wearer is working with an "unknown chemical" or when the product the wearer is being protected from is a gas or vapor (Table 55-3).

Indications for use of Level B Protection

- When the highest level of respiratory protection is necessary, but a lesser degree of skin protection is needed.
- Probable exposure to low concentrations—incidental splash
- Chemical or agent is mainly a respiratory hazard

Level A Protection

Level A protections affords responders with the highest level of both skin and respiratory protection. In order for a responder to be considered protected with Level A protection, the suit they wear must be fully encapsulating. This means that the responder has a chemical, vapor, and gas protective suit that covers the person and provides for their respiratory protection (most often an SCBA, see Figure 55-12).

This level of protection should be used any time responders are working with unknown chemicals or substances. Once the type of chemical is identified, the wearer should downgrade to the appropriate level of protection (Table 55-4).

Indications for use of Level A Protection

- Highest level of respiratory protection needed (based on chemical and physical properties of material)
- Highest level of skin protection is required
- Highest level of eye protection is required
- Constant high-concentration exposure
- Skin absorbable chemicals present
- Suspected or confirmed carcinogens present
- EPA recommends Level A protection for entrance in confined space of unknown content.

TABLE 55-3 Level B Protection

Advantages	Limitations
High level of respiratory protection	Noncompliant Level B suits may leak in liquids
Increased mobility and dexterity (compared to Level A)	Noncompliant Level B suits provide no thermal protection
May be cooler (compared to level A)	
Compliant garments have good penetration characteristics	
Cost—ranges from $45 to $1,500	

TABLE 55-4   Level A Protection

Advantages	Limitations
Can virtually eliminate contact with environmental hazards (it is basically its own environment)	Bulky
Best protection known at this time	Physically stressful; does not allow for cooling
Limited thermal protection	Psychologically stressful ("body bag with windows")
	Reduced mobility and dexterity; increases time needed to perform job
	More difficult to put on and take off
	Communication may be difficult
	Expensive — $1,000 to $4,000

As a paramedic, you will hopefully not encounter too many instances where protective suits are required. However, you have a responsibility to your coworker(s), family, and patients to recognize when a higher degree of protection may be required. It is important for you to know the differences between the levels of protection and what the different types of suits look like. DOT 5-11.13, 8-4.9

This chapter is supported by the following Skill Sheets: Skill Sheet 59: Autoinjector Drug Administration Device, Skill Sheet 60: Putting On and Removing Gloves, Skill Sheet 61: Handwashing (and Step-by-Step 61), Skill Sheet 63: Verbal Communications, and Skill Sheet 80: Eye Irrigation.

Summary

This chapter provides an overview of the various WMD, the damage they can cause, how rescuers might approach these events, and how paramedics can expect to respond. It becomes clear that training in hazardous materials and disaster planning dovetails with management of WMD events. Paramedics must be aware of the potential for these events, be familiar with their role in local and regional disaster planning and response, and continue to educate themselves about the devices and substances to which responders may be exposed.

Notes

1. R. Howard and R. Sawyer, *Terrorism and Counterterrorism: Understanding the New Security Environment* (New York, NY: McGraw-Hill, 2003).
2. D. Noah et al., "The History and Threat of Biological Warfare and Terrorism," *Emergency Medical Clinics of North America* 20 (2002): 255–271.
3. E. Noji, "Introduction: Consequences of Terrorism," *Prehospital Disaster Medicine* (July–September 2004): 163–164.
4. International Association of Fire Fighters, *Training for Hazardous Materials Response: Technician* (Washington, DC: IAFF, 2005).

Glossary

A

abandonment initiating patient care and then leaving the patient (or leaving the patient with a lesser-trained individual)

ABC the basic mnemonic of patient care: airway, breathing, circulation

ABCDE mnemonic to describe an expanded primary survey: airway, breathing, circulation, disability, expose and re-cover; also used as a mnemonic for strategy for handling shock: airway, breathing, circulation, oxygen delivery, achieving end points

abdominal aortic aneurysm (AAA) dilation of the abdominal aorta with resulting weakness of the aortic wall that can lead to leakage or frank rupture with massive intraabdominal hemorrhage; occurs in 2–13% of men and 6% of women over age 65

abduction a movement away from the body center or midline

aberrant ventricular conduction the abnormal conduction of a cardiac impulse through the ventricular conduction system resulting in a widened QRS complex, usually associated with a premature supraventricular beat, usually temporary, may be confused with ventricular dysrhythmias

abruptio placentae (placental abruption) occurs when the placenta separates prematurely from the uterine wall before the birth of the baby; it can be partial or total; can cause premature birth, hypovolemic shock, disseminated intravascular coagulation disorder (DIC), and fetal or maternal compromise or death

absence seizure seizure characterized by a loss of interaction, staring off into space, and returning to normal with no memory of the event, repetitive behaviors like lip smacking or continuous eye blinking may be noted

absolute refractory period part of the cardiac cycle; once the cell is in the depolarized state, the electrical gradient is such that no matter how strong an impulse is, the cell is not capable of responding to it; it is noted as occurring from the beginning of the QRS wave to the middle of the T wave

absorption the process by which chemicals can enter the body through the skin or mucous membrane; the movement of a medication through the skin or mucous membrane into the body cells, tissues, organs, and structures underneath

accelerated idioventricular rhythm (AIVR) abnormal heart rhythm that occurs when a ventricular pacemaker experiences increased automaticity (>50 and <100), commonly seen in reperfusion dysrhythmias and inferior or anterior infarctions

accelerated junctional rhythm resembles the junctional escape rhythm, but rhythm fires at a rate of greater than 60 but still less than 100

access entrance point into an area, a component of scene safety that asks the EMS provider to consider the safest entry point

accessory pathway (AP) additional pathway into the ventricles from the atria other than the normal electrical circuit

acetabulum the portion of the pelvic bone that articulates with the femoral head to form the hip joint

acid-base balance the control of the acid-base concentration in the blood and body fluids that allows cells to function normally within a narrow range of pH in the body

acidemia a drop in blood pH and a condition in which plasma pH or cellular pH falls below 7.35

acidosis a drop in blood pH and a condition in which plasma pH or cellular pH falls below 7.35

acoustic neuroma a benign tumor of the auditory nerve causing hearing loss from pressure on the auditory nerve

acquired immune deficiency syndrome (AIDS) a viral disease that results in low CD4 white blood cell count and the presence of opportunistic infections signifying the defect in cell-mediated immunity

acquired phimosis condition that occurs when the foreskin tightens, preventing it from being drawn back over the glans penis

acrocyanosis peripheral cyanosis

actin protein found in muscle fibers

action potential electrochemical signals that cause the cells to change their resting membrane potential

activated charcoal (AC) a pharmaceutical that adsorbs ingested poisons, most commonly used method of gastric decontamination

active labor the second part of the first stage of labor when the cervix dilates from 4–10 cm; when contractions are at least 5 min apart, lasting for 1 min, for 1 whole hour, the mother has now started the "active" phase of labor and is probably 4–5 cm dilated

active listening interactive listening that requires the listener to pay attention to both the content and the emotions the speaker is expressing

active transport (facilitated diffusion) diffusion of a substance such as glucose through a cell membrane that requires the assistance of a "helper," or carrier protein

activities of daily living (ADL) include bathing, toileting, dressing, feeding, house chores, etc.

acupuncture traditional healing therapy of Eastern medicine that attempts to manipulate specific energy channels in the body in order to illicit the desired response

acute adrenal crisis a life-threatening condition caused by insufficient levels of cortisol, a hormone that is produced in the adrenal gland

acute appendicitis condition caused by an inflammation of the appendix

acute bacterial prostatitis infection of the prostate characterized by chills, fever, pain in the lower back, perineum, base of the penis or genital area, urinary frequency or urgency, dysuria, and white blood cells and bacteria in the urine

acute coronary syndromes (ACS) a spectrum of disease caused by inadequate blood flow in the coronary arteries, includes acute myocardial infarction (AMI) and unstable angina (UA); most common cause of sudden cardiac death

acute mountain sickness (AMS) syndrome of headache and at least one of the following: anorexia, nausea, fatigue, dizziness, or difficulty sleeping that usually develops within hours after arrival at high altitude (greater than 8000 feet); treated with descent from the altitude and support of any symptoms that arise

acute myocardial infarction death of heart muscle from a coronary artery blockage manifested by chest pain unrelieved by rest, oxygen or nitroglycerin and lasting longer than a few minutes

acute pulmonary edema (flash pulmonary edema) rapid fluid increase within the pulmonary interstitium and alveoli, resulting in rapid onset of shortness of breath, hypoxia, pulmonary rales, a "frothy" cough, and usually tachycardia with hypertension

acute radiation syndrome (ARS) an acute illness that follows a roughly predictable course over a period of time ranging from a few hours to several weeks after exposure to ionizing radiation

acute renal failure (ARF) deterioration of renal function over a period of hours or days that results in the accumulation of metabolic waste products, primarily nitrogenous compounds, in the blood

acute respiratory distress syndrome (ARDS) noncardiogenic pulmonary edema; condition that may occur when alveoli become damaged by inflammatory cells in the body, resulting in alveolar wall swelling and leaking, with fluid collecting within the alveoli

Adam's apple (thyroid cartilage) a component of the trachea that is visible as a protruding structure on the front of a patient's neck

adaptive immunity in response to an antigen entering the body, the immune system attempts to recognize the antigen from its list of known "hostiles" and dispatches specific antibodies (also called immunoglobulins) that mount a substance-specific line of defense

addict a chronic user of drugs, either legal or illegal

Addison's disease (primary adrenal insufficiency) deterioration of the adrenal glands resulting in adrenal hypofunction

adduction movement toward the body center or midline

adenosine triphosphate (ATP) a chemical compound used for the storage of energy in cellular reactions

adhering sticking

adrenal cortex portion of the adrenal glands located on the superior kidney; they secrete hydrocortisone, which affects metabolism, and androgen hormone and aldosterone, which affect blood pressure and saline balance

adrenal glands glands located on the upper end of the kidneys; supply epinephrine, norepinephrine, and steroids to the body

adrenocorticotropin hormone (ACTH) governs the nutrition and growth of the adrenal cortex and stimulates its function

adult respiratory distress syndrome (ARDS) This term is obsolete. See Acute Respiratory Distress Syndrome

advance directive a document that makes patients' wishes regarding medical treatment known in the event they are unable to speak for themselves; as the name implies, advance directives are written in advance of need; also known as Do-Not-Resuscitate (DNR) Orders (DNRO)

Advanced Emergency Medical Technician (AEMT) trained EMS professional who possesses a limited number of advanced skills; this is the first level of the ALS level caregiver

advanced life support (ALS) the care that AEMTs and paramedics offer that includes advanced airway management, defibrillation, intravenous therapy, and medication administration

adventitious sounds abnormal breath sounds heard in addition to, or in place of, normal lung sounds

adverse drug reactions (ADR) a cause of accidental poisoning; occur when a patient has an adverse event while using a medication appropriately

advocacy active support; especially the act of pleading or arguing for patients who cannot speak for themselves

AEIOU-TIPS mnemonic used to determine possible causes of unconsciousness: alcohol, acid-base disorders, arrhythmias; encephalopathy, endocrine disorders, electrolyte disorders; insulin issues (hypo or hyper glycemia); opiates; uremia; trauma, tumor, thermal insult (hypothermia); infection, intracerebral vascular disorders; poisonings, psychogenic shock (fainting); seizures

aeroallergens airborne proteins and glycoproteins from a variety of sources that can cause an allergic reaction

aerobic reactions physiologic reactions that require an oxygen environment

aerobic respiration a two-part process to generate ATP (which is the energy-storing molecule in cells); this process is the most efficient form of human metabolism compared to anaerobic respiration

affective (mood) disorders a group of illnesses that is characterized by long-term sadness (unipolar) or a combination of sadness and mania (bipolar)

afferent nerves nerve fibers that transmit impulses from the peripheral to the central nervous system

afferent (or sensory) neurons the neurons that detect stimuli and changes in the environment and carry electrical signals into the central nervous system (CNS)

afferent pathways neurologic pathways where electrical and chemical messages are passed from peripheral receptors to control (integration centers)

affinity the degree to which the forces of attraction exist between a drug (or a chemical) and a receptor site

afterload the pressure against which the heart ventricle must pump; measured as systolic blood pressure. It pertains to both the left and right ventricle, but is often spoken of in terms of the pressures exerted against the left ventricle

Agenda for the Future a federally funded position paper completed in the 1990s by the National Association of EMS Physicians (NAEMSP) in conjunction with the National Association of State EMS Directors (NASEMSD) that set the vision for future EMS developments

agent of injury some form of energy, for example mechanical, thermal, electrical, radiation, etc., that is transmitted to the host (the patient) through a vehicle (an object such as a car, a metal fragment, or some other moving object) or a vector (some micro or macro organism)

agglutination the process by which cells adhere and form into clumps

aggregation gathering together and clumping of blood cells

agonists drug capable of binding with receptors to initiate a reaction

air hunger respiratory distress that is characterized as gasping labored breathing

air purifying respirator (APR) [**cartridge respirators, purified air powered respirators (PAPR)**] a device that filters ambient air through hazard-specific cartridges or canisters before inhalation; does not provide a presupplied source of air

airpack (positive pressure self-contained breathing apparatus) SCBA that supplies air to a facemask from a tank

alcoholic hepatitis an alcohol-related inflammatory liver disease

aldosterone the hormone that causes increased salt and water reabsorption in the kidney, which allows the body to retain fluids instead of excreting them; the result is to preserve or increase blood pressure

alimentary tract (gastrointestinal tract) the system responsible for ingesting, processing, absorbing, digesting, and eliminating food

alkalemia condition when excess bicarbonate levels of the blood overwhelms the pH buffering capacity and pH rises above 7.45

alkalosis an abnormal condition in which plasma pH rises above 7.45

allergen a substance that causes an allergic reaction

allergic reaction a hypersensitive or exaggerated immune response to the exposure of a foreign substance

allergy condition when a substance is identified as a potential threat by the body's immune system causing the release of histamine and other chemicals

alopecia hair loss

alveolar duct part of the respiratory passage; the terminal air passageway from which the alveolar sacs and alveoli arise

alveolar membrane a thin membrane one to two cell layers thick in the alveoli; this is the primary location where oxygen and carbon dioxide gasses exchange between the patient and the environment

alveolar plateau phase III on a normal capnogram waveform; it represents the concentration of CO_2 from the alveoli

alveolar sacs The individual terminal units of the lung where gas exchange takes place

alveolar ventilation (VA) the air that comes into contact with the alveolar-capillary membrane surfaces that participates in the exchange of gasses between the lung and blood

alveolar-capillary membrane walls of the alveoli and of the capillaries where gas exchange takes place

alveoli microscopic air sacs (see alveolar sacs)

Alzheimer's disease the most common form of dementia; characterized by the loss of memory and inability to learn, this slow, progressive disease robs an individual of the ability to reason, make judgments, communicate, or carry out day-to-day normal functions

American College of Emergency Physicians (ACEP) emergency medicine physician group, involved in the training of physicians about how to direct EMS services and the science that defines Paramedic practice

American College of Surgeons Committee on Trauma (ACS COT) surgeon physician group focusing on setting standards for the elements of paramedic practice pertinent to trauma topics

amniotic fluid embolism (AFE) extremely rare condition when amniotic fluid enters the maternal circulation usually during labor or birth; patient may experience a drop in blood pressure and decreased cardiac function, which leads to a maternal mortality rate of 60–80%

amniotic sac (bag of waters) sac that surrounds the developing fetus and contains amniotic fluid

amputation the cutting off of a limb or part of a limb, the breast, or other projecting part; may be accidental or surgical; surgical amputations typically include the removal of bone or cartilaginous tissues from the body

amyotrophic lateral sclerosis (ALS) a degenerative disease caused by the selective destruction of motor neurons in the peripheral nervous system, also known as "Lou Gehrig's disease"

anabolic reactions reactions that consume energy; used to synthesize large biomolecules by combining smaller ones into larger ones. The opposite of catabolic reactions

anaerobic metabolism type of metabolism that does not utilize oxygen in the metabolic process, is not very efficient in that it does not generate much ATP

anal fissures (varices) linear ulceration or laceration of the skin of the anus

anaphylactic reaction severe exaggerated allergic reaction that can be life-threatening due to either respiratory, circulatory compromise, or both

anaphylactic shock the most severe, systemic, and life-threatening reaction; different from allergic reaction. It results in massive vasodilation and a severe drop in blood pressure

anaphylactoid reaction term used at one time by physicians and other hospital clinicians to describe the reaction that was IgE mediated; used interchangeably with "anaphylactic"

anaphylaxis against or without protection; the most severe, systemic, and life-threatening reaction; more extreme than an allergic reaction

anatomic dead space, components of the airway such as the trachea, primary and secondary bronchi, etc. that are not sites of gas exchange but that are required to provide structure and passageways to the components (such as the alveoli) that are used to exchange gasses

anatomical position a body position with the subject standing erect (upright), with eyes facing forward, hands hanging down at sides, palms facing forward

anatomy branch of study that deals with the structure and organization of living things

anchoring heuristic problem-solving strategy that begins with the most likely cause as the anchor and then the signs and symptoms needed to confirm that cause are the ones assessed for first

anemia decrease in hemoglobin

aneurysm a focal dilation or expansion of an artery compared to an adjacent arterial segment; may lead to leakage or rupture

angina retrosternal chest pain, pressure, burning, heaviness; can radiate to jaw, neck, epigastrum, shoulders or arms; produced by blockage in the coronary circulation of the heart leading to myocardial ischemia. Angina occurs because of plaque build-up, thus some damage exists to the vessels supplying the heart, but actual cardiac tissue is not damaged unless a blockage (clot) results inside the damaged vessel

angina pectoris *see* angina

angioedema a rare and specific form of localized allergic reaction (usually involving swelling of the lips, tongue, oral cavity, and upper airway) that is usually of short duration, and frequently resolves itself

angiospastic (or variant) angina capable of producing symptoms identical to angina, but is related to a spasm of a coronary artery rather than an actual blockage

angiotensin converting enzyme (ACE) chemical located on the walls of blood vessels that converts angiotensin I to angiotensin II. The result is increased blood pressure

angiotensin converting enzyme (ACE) inhibitor medications class of medications used to mediate ACE reactions; the net result is a decrease in blood pressure

angiotensin I is formed by the action of renin on angiotensinogen; it appears to have no biological activity and exists solely as a precursor to angiotensin II

angiotensin II an oligopeptide in the blood that causes vasoconstriction, increased blood pressure, and release of aldosterone from the adrenal cortex; it is derived from the precursor molecule angiotensinogen, a serum globulin produced in the liver, and plays an important role in the renin-angiotensis system

angulation fractures a transverse fracture with a concave surface along the long axis of a bone

anhydrous ammonia chemical that can be used by a terrorist as a weapon of mass destruction, is very damaging to human tissue and is widely available; it is also a component in one of several methamphetamine manufacturing processes

anisocoria condition in which one eye is noticeably larger than the other

antagonism two chemicals working in opposition to each other

antagonists drugs that bind to receptors that then inhibit (or prevent) the binding of the agonist

antegrade amnesia when a patient has no recollection of the events occurring immediately after the incident causing a concussion

antepartum factors variables that are present before labor begins

anterior anatomic term meaning toward the front of the body

anterior cerebral artery (ACA) stroke stroke that produces deficits of one of the legs, which the patient usually describes as a feeling of heaviness, numbness, or weakness

anterior chamber forward chamber of the eye in front of the iris that contains the aqueous humor

anterior horns structures on the spinal cord that are primarily responsible for motor functions that control movement

anterior infarctions myocardial infarctions that represent problems with the left ventricle

anterior spinal cord injuries injuries that can occur from direct trauma to the anterior cord or injury to the anterior spinal artery resulting in ischemia to the cord

anthrax *Bacillus anthracis,* a spore-forming, rod-shaped organism; may be used as a weapon of mass destruction; see also cutaneous anthrax, gastrointestinal anthrax, and inhalation anthrax

antibiotics medications that treat bacterial infections

antibodies immunoglobulins

antibody substance produced by the body to attack antigens

anticoagulants medications that work to thin the blood

antidiuretic hormone (ADH) hormone from the pituitary gland that acts on the kidneys to increase water retention (also known as vasopressin)

antidotes treatments that specifically reverse the effects of a poison

antifungals medications that treat fungal infections

antigen a substance unknown or foreign to the body that may trigger an immune system response when detected

antihistamine medication that is especially helpful in counteracting the effect of histamine; used to treat allergic reactions

antiinflammatory medicines medications used to reduce inflammation, used for a variety of diseases including asthma

antimicrobials medications with actions against microorganisms

antiseptics cleansing agents capable of destroying or inhibiting the growth of most microorganisms; they are nontoxic to living tissue

antivirals medications used to treat viral infections

anxiety an uneasy feeling that is commonly experienced when a person is fearful or anticipating harm, even if the fear appears irrational

aorta the largest artery in the human body, originating from the left ventricle of the heart and bringing oxygenated blood to all parts of the body in the systemic circulation

aortic arch rupture a sudden deceleration force that causes the arch to tear just beyond its point of attachment; the result is almost universally fatal hemorrhage

aortic dissection separation of the luminal layers of the aorta that frequently results in death. The patient often reports "ripping" excruciating pain that typically starts suddenly, and anteriorly but radiates to the back

aortic valve one of the valves of the heart; it lies between the left ventricle and the aorta

aortic valve stenosis thickening or obstructing of the aortic valve; occurs in approximately 5 in 10,000 persons, usually males and may not present any symptoms until later in life

apathetic hyperthyroidism associated with older patients in which the signs and symptoms seen in younger patients are less obvious; symptoms of cardiovascular compromise may be noted in the latter case

APGAR score a tool for neonatal assessment that evaluates the appearance (skin color), pulse rate, grimace (responses to stimuli), activity level and muscle tone, and respiratory efforts

aphasia language disorder that result from damage to the language centers of the brain

aplastic anemia loss of blood cell creating function in bone marrow that causes a deficiency in circulating blood cells

apnea the absence of respirations

apneic not breathing at all

apneustic breathing abnormal breathing pattern (prolonged inspiration followed by a period of apnea) that indicates lesions in the respiratory center of the brain

apparent life threatening event (ATLE) a pediatric condition of a period of apnea accompanied by other respiratory symptoms (such as choking or gagging), skin color change, or change of muscle tone; also known as near miss SIDS

appendicitis inflammation of the vermiform appendix

appendicular skeleton refers to the paired long bones of the body of the upper and lower extremities (the appendages)

appendix hollow, muscular, close-ended tube that arises from the posterior medial surface of the cecum, just a few centimeters below the ileocecal valve

aquaporins channels that provide a mechanism for water that was filtered out in the kidneys to return to the bloodstream

arachnoid mater the middle covering of the brain under and around which run a network of small arteries and veins; the second layer of the meninges, it has a spiderweb-like appearance

arachnoid membrane one of the three layers of tissues insulating and protecting the brain and spinal cord that lies between the pia and dura mater

area command this type of command provides oversight to the management of one or more incidents when several ICS structures exist within close proximity to each other

areflexia (spinal shock) the temporary loss of spinal reflex activity that occurs below a near-total or total spinal cord injury

arm drift the inability to hold one or both arms straight out in front for longer than a few seconds or to hold them at the same height; testing for arm drift is a component of stroke evaluation

arrhythmia an ECG that is without a rhythm, often inaccurately used interchangeably with dysrhythmia

arterial gas embolism (AGE) pulmonary barotrauma that results when air bubbles are forced across the alveolar-capillary membrane into the pulmonary venous circulation and then through the left atrium and ventricle and into the arterial circulation, as a result of increased pressure; AGE can also result from a right-to-left shunt of venous bubbles

arterial oxygen content the amount of oxygen in blood

artertial blood gasses (ABGs) a laboratory test performed in the hospital that measures the pH and partial pressures of oxygen and carbon dioxide in an arterial blood sample

arthritis inflammation of a joint, characterized by pain, stiffness, swelling, and redness

articular cartilage cartilage that covers the ends of a bone

articulate to attach directly to or come together to form a joint

articulation disorders (dysarthria) disorders caused by the inability of an individual to produce sounds

arytenoids (arytenoid cartilages) a pair of tiny, pivoting cartilages located next to the vocal cords

ascending phase phase II on a normal capnogram waveform; represents the initiation of exhalation

ascites, the build up of fluid in the peritoneal cavity resulting in a distended abdomen with a fluid wave

asepsis maintaining the cleanliness of all supplies by preventing contamination

Asperger syndrome developmental disorder characterized by a lack of social communication skills, average to above-average intelligence and no language delays

aspirate process by which blood or fluid is pulled into a syringe by pulling back on the plunger creating negative pressure; it is used to confirm the patency of an IV line prior to injecting medication or, during IM injections, it is used to confirm placement of the needle into tissues other than an artery or vein

assault placing a patient in a position where he or she fears for his or her safety or perceives the paramedic means to do some sort of injury or harm

assist/control (A/C) A/C mode senses the patient's attempt to breathe as a negative pressure and triggers the ventilator to deliver a prescribed volume of air; initial mode of ventilation in patients who are breathing, but are tired from the work of breathing

assisted ventilation the use of a device to push air into a patient's lungs to improve the delivery of oxygen and the removal of CO_2

asthma a chronic reactive and inflammatory disorder of the lungs where the bronchioles spasm and constrict, causing a decrease in diameter and in increase in airflow restriction, mucus is excreted within the airway walls, and a fluid shift occurs within the cells of the airway, causing further restriction and increasing the potential of air trapping

asymptomatic inflammatory prostatitis the presence of white blood cells in the semen in the absence of symptoms or a causative agent

asystole the absence of electrical activity in the heart

atelectasis a condition within the lung involving collapse of the alveolar air spaces that permits blood to pass from the right side of the heart to the left side of the heart without meeting air for gas exchange

atherosclerosis fatty plaque buildup in arteries that causes an artery to become blocked so that it can no longer supply muscles or organs with the oxygen needed for metabolism (commonly referred to as "hardening of the arteries")

athetosis slow writhing movements of the extremities noted with some diseases such as cerebral palsy or motor disorders

atmosphere-supplying respirators self-contained breathing apparatus (SCBA) that contains its own air supply, and the supplied-air respirator (SAR)

atmospheric pressure the total pressure of the atmospheric air

atria plural of "atrium," the upper chambers of the heart

atrial fibrillation a disorganized rhythm of the atria that is the result of multiple ectopic sites within the atria, causing an atrial depolarization rate of 350–600; it is the number one cause of strokes. If the ventricular rate is affected, either too rapid or too slow, it will compromise cardiac output

atrial flutter a rapid, regular rhythm that is the result of a well-defined ectopic pacemaker within the atria, firing at a rate of 250–350 times a minutes. If the ventricular rate is affected, either too rapid or too slow, it will compromise cardiac output

atrial flutter with variable block atrial flutter is most commonly a very regular rhythm, but under certain circumstances displays varied conduction into the ventricles If the ventricular rate is disorganized, too rapid or too slow, it will compromise cardiac output

atrial kick the movement of blood into the ventricles associated with the very end of the atrial contraction; it is responsible for providing a little extra blood to the ventricles beyond what would flow passively once the valves open. The loss of atrial kick can impact cardiac output by as much as 25%

atrial natriuretic peptide (ANP) a peptide hormone produced by atrial myocardial cells that acts as an antagonist to aldosterone and ADH

atrial septal defect (ASD) a defect between the right and left atrial wall allowing oxygenated blood returning from the lungs to mix with the unoxygenated blood from the vena cava; present in 4 out of every 100,000 people; children with ASD may be asymptomatic and are susceptible to infective endocarditis, atrial fibrillation, and heart failure; symptoms include palpitations, shortness of breath, and difficulty breathing

atrial tachycardia a dysrhythmia originating from an ectopic site within the atria that exceeds 100 beats per minute

atrioventricular block an interruption or termination of cardiac conduction along normal pathways; occurs when the pathway is blocked within the AV node, bundle of His, or in the bundle branches

atrioventricular dissociation rare condition when ventricles begin to depolarize at a more rapid rate than the atria, creating a condition similar to complete heart block

atrioventricular node (AVN) the tissue between the atria and the ventricles of the heart, which conducts the normal electrical impulse from the atria to the ventricles; also known as the Aschoff-Tawara node

atrium low pressure, upper chamber of the heart

atropine an anticholinergic (parasympatholytic) agent sometimes administered as part of a rapid sequence intubation routine or to poisoned or cardiac patients; it blocks the effects of the vagus nerve

audible sounds noises that can be heard by the examiner without a stethoscope

auditory cortex the region of the brain that is responsible for processing of auditory (sound) information

aura a smell or visual disturbance or other sensation signaling a seizure is coming

auricle what we commonly think of as the ears on the outside of the head, also refers to a portion of the atrium

auscultation the technique of using a stethoscope

autism spectrum disorders (ASDs) disorders that affect the brain's normal development of social, communication, and sensory skills

autoclaving extreme heat from steam under pressure used to sterilize nonliving tissues

autoimmunity a malfunction of the immune system that causes it to overreact and turn against its own body's cells

automatic internal cardiac defibrillator (AICD) a small computer and cardiac monitor that is programmed to defibrillate a patient when it senses the onset of ventricular fibrillation or ventricular tachycardia, works in a similar fashion to an internal cardiac pacemaker

automaticity A unique property of cardiac muscle that allows the heart to depolarize and contract spontaneously without an external stimulus

autonomic branch the branch of the efferent division of the nervous system that controls cardiac muscle, smooth muscle, and glands

autonomic nervous system (ANS) "involuntary" nervous system; a subdivision of the peripheral nervous system (PNS) that controls involuntary functions like respiration, circulation, and digestion

autonomy self-dependent; having the right to choose a course of treatment based on personal beliefs independent of the influence of others

auto-PEEP a reduction in venous return and cardiac output resulting from increased intrathoracic pressure, often from too rapid positive pressure ventilation

availability heuristic making judgments based on the frequency of similar situations occurring

avian flu (H5N1) disease of poultry (primarily) that is caused by H5N1 virus that has been found in humans in Southeast Asia who handled infected poultry, epidemiologists are concerned that person to person transmission of H5N1 will result in a worldwide pandemic of flu with a high mortality rate

AVPU scale mnemonic used to determine the four basic levels of responsiveness: awake, verbal, painful, and unresponsive

avulsion total displacement of a tooth from its socket; the tearing away of soft tissues (muscle) and cartilage from the body

Awareness Color Coding System simple color coding system that describes a spectrum of awareness for personal safety; taught in many law enforcement academies designed to remind public safety workers to maintain vigilance for scene safety

axial load force that is applied to the top of the cranium that results in pushing together of the spinal cord and perhaps damage to the muscles, bones or nervous system tissues

axial skeleton the central (longitudinal) axis of the body and includes the skull, vertebral column, and bony thorax

axillary arteries continuation of the subclavian artery that passes through the axilla

axon part of the neuron that carries the electrical signal away from the cell body

azygos veins a vena cava that fails to form vein of the thorax (chest) that drains into the superior

B

B cells Specialized blood cells that comprise between 15-30% of all lymphocytes which are important in immunity because they produce immunoglobins (antibodies) in response to antigen

Babinski plantar response test an assessment made by stroking the foot; a positive finding is extension and spreading of the toes which can indicate a lesion (damage) to the pyramidal tract of the nervous system; positive finding in a newborn is acceptable

Bachmann's bundle part of the conduction system of the heart that facilitates conduction to the left atria; also called the interatrial pathway

bacteremia the presence of bacteria in the bloodstream

bacteria single-celled organisms that are found in all environments on Earth; capable of reproducing without the aid of host cells, and cause disease by direct infection of cells or by release of toxins that destroy cells

bacterial meningitis inflammation of the meninges caused by a bacterial infection

bag of waters (amniotic sac) sac that surrounds the developing fetus and contains amniotic fluid

bagging deliberate inhalation of hydrocarbons to produce intoxication; spraying volatile substance into a bag and placing the bag over one's head; slang term for mechanical bag-mask ventilation performed by health care providers

bag-mask ventilation manual technique for assisting ventilation

Bainbridge (right atrial) reflex response that allows the heart to eject a volume of blood that is equal to the volume it receives

balanitis chronic low-level infection of the glans of the penis

ballistics the study of the motion and trajectory caused by projectiles as energy is transferred to tissue

bandages materials used to hold dressings in place and to help provide pressure to a bleeding wound. Bandages typically do not come into direct contact with wounds, and therefore do not need to be sterile

baroreceptors pressure receptors found in the carotid arteries

barotitis condition that occurs in the ear during diving descent as gas-filled structures have a tendency to be "squeezed" into half their volume, also called aerotitis

barotrauma pressure-related trauma typically noted in the lungs, but it can occur in any air-filled space in the body

Bartholin's abscess infection (typically bacterial) of the Bartholin's gland; causes extreme localized pain, localized erythema, and sometimes walking difficulties from the swelling and pain, a fistula may develop from one or both of the glands and extend to the vagina, anus or perineum

basal ganglia masses of gray matter located deep within the cerebral hemispheres

base station two-way radios in a fixed location; may be small enough to fit on a desk top or so large they require banks of consoles to contain them; they have larger antennas than portable or mobile radios and more power enabling them to transmit over greater distances

bases locations where primary logistical and administrative functions are coordinated and administered under the Incident Command System

basilar artery stroke a stroke that can produce symptoms such as vertigo, facial weakness, diplopia, and difficulty swallowing or speaking depending on how much of the brain stem area is affected

basophils white blood cells that promote inflammation

battery touching of or contact with another person without that person's consent

Battle's sign a bluish hue to the bony prominence behind the auricle caused by bleeding from a basilar skull fracture into the mastoid air cells

Baux index or score a simple but highly predictive tool for mortality from burn injuries; add the age of the patient and the total body surface area burned (including relatively minor burns) to get a prediction of chance of dying

Beck's triad three classic clinical manifestations of cardiac tamponade: jugular vein distention, muffled heart tones, and hypotension. All patients with tamponade exhibit at least one of these signs but few manifest all three

Bell's palsy thought to be a viral immune-mediated disease that involves the segmental demyelination of the facial nerve (cranial nerve VII); acute inflammation can affect the patient from the eye to the mouth causing eyelid, mouth and facial droop on the affected side

beneficence kind, charitable, benefiting; acting in the best interest of the patient

benign prostatic hypertrophy a condition in which the prostate gland enlarges for unknown reasons; occurs as men age

benzodiazepines sedative medications; the first-line pharmacologic therapy used to terminate active seizures during status epilepticus, they can also be used to sedate patients prior to painful procedures such as cardioversion or to manage pain from illness or injuries

beta 2 agonist a medication that stimulates the beta 2 sympathetic receptor; one of the most common medications used to treat asthma in the prehospital setting, they dilate bronchioles improving ventilation in the lungs

beta blockers medications that block the effect of the beta adrenergic receptor site; used to depress myocardial contractility. They are also used to control hypertension

bias in regard to the critical thinking process, a tendency or prejudice

biased information prejudicial information, born of preconceived judgment or opinion by the provider; it is subjective based on past experience

bicuspid valve also called the mitral valve, this valve is between the left atrium and left ventricle

bifasicular block a left anterior heart block producing a classic right bundle branch block pattern with left axis deviation; a complete heart block is very possible

bi-level positive airway pressure (BiPAP) BiPAP allows the provider to set a separate level of inspiratory positive airway pressure (IPAP) and expiratory positive airway pressure (EPAP)

biliary tract the system consisting of the hepatic bile canaliculi (which produce bile), the bile ducts, and the gallbladder

bilirubin a product of hemoglobin breakdown or metabolism, which is then conjugated in the liver and excreted from the body

bioavailability the amount of drug that is available for the body to use following biotransformation and the first-pass events

bioethics the study of the ethical and moral implications of biological discoveries and biomedical advances, as in the fields of genetic engineering and drug research

biohazard container a container specifically designed for disposal of needles and anything capable of piercing the skin; also called a sharps container

biohazard exposure plan a plan required by law for all medical organizations; provides direction to the workforce should a body fluid exposure occur

biological clock the internal rhythm of the body's function; also referred to as circadian rhythm

Biot's (ataxic) breathing alternating pattern of increased respiratory rate and depth with apnea periods similar to Cheyne-Stokes, but unlike Cheyne-Stokes, the pattern is irregular

bioterrorism the intentional use of infectious agents in terrorist activities

biotransformation a specific type of metabolism that takes place in the liver where drugs are altered into metabolites of their original state; often the target tissue requires the altered metabolite instead of the original state

BiPAP A variation of CPAP that allows the provider to set a separate level of inspiratory positive airway pressure (IPAP) and expiratory positive airway pressure (EPAP)

biphasic anaphylaxis symptoms that re-occur after a previously resolved allergic reaction, they can occur as medications like epinephrine and benadryl wear off or because the offending allergen is still present in the body

bipolar disorder a condition characterized by erratic thinking and extreme changes in mood, energy and behavior (formerly known as manic-depression)

bladder a muscular organ that can distend to hold great volumes of urine

bladed stance body position in which the paramedic stands sideways at a slight angle with their weight on the back leg so as to be less imposing, a smaller target, and be able to turn and flee easily

blast cell a primitive cell capable of building tissue

blast injuries a combination of compression and shearing injuries from the pressure wave associated with the conversion of a solid or liquid explosive into a gas, as well as penetrating trauma from flying debris and shrapnel

bleb a "blister" on the surface of the lung that can rupture and leak air into the pleural space; also the name for misshapen, barely functional alveoli that develop following injury to the lung tissues from long term smoking

blind insertion airway devices devices that are placed into the airway without the direct visual aid of equipment such as a laryngoscope

blister agents (vesicants) chemicals that cause burn-like reactions in the body by disrupting cells, tissues, and organs; include sulfur mustard and Lewisite; may be used as weapons of mass destruction

blood gas analysis a blood test that is performed to determine the concentration of oxygen, carbon dioxide and bicarbonate, as well as the pH, in the blood

blood pressure (BP) the measurable pressure inside the arterial blood vessels which results from a combination of factors, including heart rate, stroke volume, blood volume, and the relative diameter of the peripheral arteries. BP = SV × HR × PVR

blood products the various components that make up blood and that can be administered intravenously, either alone or in combination for patients in hypovolemic shock (e.g., packed red blood cells)

blood substitutes intravenous fluids that have oxygen carrying capability (e.g., human polymerized hemoglobin) and which can be used for patients in hemorrhagic shock; can help to maintain blood pressure

blow-by a method of oxygen delivery that allows the FIO_2 level of the environment to be increased. This method is better tolerated in some patients, particularly infants and small children

blue bloater a slang term for a chronic bronchitis patient exhibiting the hypoxic drive to breathe

blunt thoracic aortic injury (BTAI) a life-threatening traumatic injury involving complete or partial tearing of one or more of the layers of the thoracic aorta after blunt trauma

blunt trauma trauma caused as the body absorbs energy; a direct blow that causes compression, shearing, deceleration, or crushing forces to the patient. It may not cause disruption of the skin which can result in "hidden" injuries

body the main or largest part of any structure or organ

body composition the ratio of fat weight to total body weight

body packers people who ingest a large amount of well-packaged illegal drugs in order to smuggle the drug into a secured area

body stuffers people who ingest illegal drugs or insert them in another body cavity such as the rectum or vagina in order to avoid arrest

body substance isolation (BSI) the practice of treating all bodily fluids as if they were infected; types of BSI equipment include gloves, goggles, a mask to cover the mouth, a combination face mask with eye shield, and a gown

Boerhaave's syndrome (esophageal rupture) spontaneous, life-threatening esophageal perforation from trauma, foreign bodies, or severe retching

bolus a single dose of medication that is given intravenously at one time to a patient

borderline personality disorder a condition in which a person's mood, interpersonal relationships, self-image, and identity are unstable

botulinum toxin a neurotoxin produced by *C. botulinum* causing the disease botulism; may be used as a biological warfare agent

botulism food poisoning caused by the bacterium *Clostridium botulinum;* symptoms include double vision, drooping eyelids, slurred speech, muscle weakness, difficulty swallowing, and respiratory paralysis

brachial arteries continuation of the axillary artery as it crosses the teres major muscle in the arm

bradycardia slowness of the heartbeat, usually defined as a rate under 60 beats per minute

bradypnea a slower than normal respiratory rate; breathing rate less than 12 respirations per minute in an adult

brainstem the part of the brain that extends from the base of the brain to the spinal cord and consists of the midbrain, pons, medulla oblongata and reticular formation

brand name drug name selected by the manufacturer to use when it sells the drug

Braxton Hick's contractions warm-up uterine contractions, occurring as early as second trimester, also called "false labor"

breach of duty the provider fails to meet their obligation to provide the standard of care for the need of a patient

breech presentation occurs when at birth the baby presents with their buttocks, foot, or knees first, rather than head first

bronchi plural of "bronchus"

bronchiectasis a dilation of one or more bronchi due to injury from infection

bronchioles series of small, branching tubules within the lung tissues

bronchiolitis inflammation of the bronchioles caused by respiratory syncytial virus (RSV) or other viruses; can mimic asthma because of the wheezing it produces

bronchitis an infection and/or inflammation of the main bronchi and some of the smaller branches

bronchophony a type of chest assessment where the patient is asked to speak while the health care professional auscultates the chest; used to detect lung consolidation as can occur with pneumonia

bronchospasm constriction of the smooth muscle in the bronchi and bronchioles

bronchovesicular sounds sounds heard over the mainstem bronchi, which are located below the manubrium and to the left and right of the center of the sternum which represent a combination of the airway (broncho) and lung tissues (vesicular)

Brown-Sequard syndrome a unique partial spinal cord syndrome that involves injury to a lateral half of the cord with a motor function deficit on the side of the injury and a sensory (pain and temperature) deficit on the opposite side

Brudzinski's sign involuntary flexion of the hips when the neck is flexed; symptom of meningitis

bruise closed soft tissue injury characterized by discoloration and swelling beneath the surface of the skin

bruit the sound of blood rushing through a damaged or constricted artery, organ or gland; a murmur-like sound present during auscultation

bubonic plague the most common form of plague, often spread by rodents, which is characterized by painful swollen lymph nodes (buboes) in the neck, groin, or axilla, treated by antibiotics

buckle (torus) fracture a fracture characterized by a buckling of one side of the cortex, usually in the metaphyseal region, and most often results from compressive forces

buffer system the chemical system that permits the precise control of pH, which is the acid concentration in the body fluids and within cells

buffers substances that act to prevent fluctuations in pH

bulk flow the movement of water and dissolved solutes because of osmotic and hydrostatic pressure

Bundle branch and fascicular blocks may appear in normal hearts, but they are usually associated with heart disease. They are caused by disruption in the flow of electricity through a component of the electrical conduction pathway

bundle of His a collection of heart muscle cells specialized for electrical conduction that transmits the electrical impulses from the AV node (located between the atria and the ventricles) to the point of the apex of the fascicular branches

burn a form of traumatic injury caused by heat, electricity, chemicals, scalds or radioactivity

burn depth thickness of a burn that is directly related to the temperature of the burning agent and the duration of contact with body tissue

BURP maneuver the larynx is manually displaced posteriorly (backward) against the cervical vertebrae, superiorly (upward), and laterally to the right (rightward pressure) that may be helpful during airway procedures like laryngoscopy

burst fracture occurs when forces that exceed the ability of the vertebrae to resist them cause the vertebral body to shatter outward from within

C

calcaneus heel (also referred to as "os calcis")

calcium channel blockers medications that depress myocardial contractility by interfering with the ability of calcium to enter the muscle cells, resulting in a weakened force of contraction

camps locations where resources are kept to support incident operations under the Incident Command System

cancellous bone the spongy type of bone tissue that makes up the inner portion of the bone

cancer condition that develops when cells in the body grow out of control

candidiasis (yeast) most common infection of the female reproductive tract; other infections include all nonsexually transmitted infections such as bacterial vaginosis, gardnerella and the sexually transmitted infections such as syphilis, gonorrhea, chlamydia, herpes, condyloma, human papilloma virus (HPV), molluscum contagiosum, and trichomonas vaginalis

capillary refilling refers to tissue perfusion (the amount of blood flow to tissue); tested by compressing the nailbed and determining how quickly the normal color returns; normal capillary refill time is less than 2 seconds

capillary sludging a stage during the late phase of shock which occurs following RBC agglutination and the formation of microemboli impairing the flow of blood through the capillaries

capillary stagnation phase the event in which little blood flow is occurring and little perfusion or circulation of nutrients and wastes is occurring at the level of the capillary bed

capacitance size change of the vascular system

capnograph device that calculates the partial pressure of CO_2 in exhaled air; it illustrates the findings as a continuous numerical printout or waveform

capnography a monitor that measures the amount of carbon dioxide in exhaled air and displayed as a waveform

capnos smoke; capnography in humans is determining the amount of exhaled carbon dioxide which represents the smoke from the fire of metabolism

carbohydrates chemical compounds that are usually ingested and metabolized to supply energy to the cells of the body

carbonic acid H_2CO_3

carbonic anhydrase enzyme that converts carbonic acid to its components of carbon dioxide and water; found in many tissues in the body

carboxyhemoglobin chemical compound formed when carbon monoxide binds to hemoglobin

carcinogenic a substance or chemical capable of causing cancer

cardiac cycle the time period extending from one heart beat to the next heart beat

cardiac dysrhythmia an abnormal cardiac rhythm; may be life threatening

cardiac enzymes cardiac troponin, creatine kinase (CK) and creatine kinase MB isoenzyme (CK-MB) are chemicals that are released by dying cardiac cells; they circulate in the blood and can be detected by blood studies; their presence generally indicates damage has occurred and they are a reliable indicator for AMI

cardiac muscle muscle of the heart that is involuntary and striated

cardiac myocyte an individual cardiac muscle cell

cardiac output the volume of blood ejected by one ventricle per minute; a measure of the heart's pumping effectiveness. It is represented by the equation: stroke volume times heart rate (SV × HR = CO)

cardiac reserve the difference between resting cardiac output and maximum cardiac output. The cardiac reserve is what is drawn upon by an individual in times of stress. Patients with a good cardiac reserve tolerate stressors better than those with a low reserve

cardiac tamponade a condition in which fluid, commonly blood, accumulates between the heart and the pericardium, compressing the heart and reducing blood flow through the heart

cardiogenic shock condition in which the output from the heart is inadequate to meet tissue needs; a severe and deadly complication of AMI is shock due to low cardiac output

cardiopulmonary resuscitation (CPR) an emergency first aid procedure for a victim of cardiac arrest that includes a combination of artificial ventilation (to provide oxygen and eliminate wastes) and chest compressions (to circulate the blood)

cardiovascular disease (CVD) a group of diseases that affect the heart and blood vessels, includes coronary artery disease (CAD), stroke, and peripheral vascular disease (PVD)

cardiovascular endurance the ability of the heart, lungs, and blood vessels to supply the muscles of the body with oxygen and fuel during prolonged exercise

cardioversion delivery of electrical energy synchronized with the cardiac cycle (with the QRS complex) to avoid delivery during the relative refractory period

carina the point of splitting of the trachea into the right and left mainstem bronchi

carotid pulses located in the neck, just to either side of the trachea

carpal bones the eight bones of the wrist

cartilage the connective tissue that covers the epiphysis of joints and allows bones to attach to other bones

cartilaginous joints joints that play a role early in life promoting growth and later become immobile

cartridge respirators [air purifying respirator (APR), purified air powered respirators (PAPR)] device that filters ambient air through hazard-specific cartridges or canisters before inhalation; does not provide a presupplied source of air

catabolic reaction a reaction that releases the energy contained in the chemical bonds of complex molecules by breaking them down; the opposite of anabolic reactions

cataract a film that clouds the lens of the eye causing double or blurred vision

catecholamine chemicals (e.g., dopamine, epinephrine, and norepinephrine) produced from the adrenal medulla and via synthetic means that are responsible for stimulating the sympathetic nervous system

cathartics medications that increased intestinal movement; used in the past to try to move poisons through the intestines before systemic absorption can occur; cathartics literally means "to bring to the surface"

cauda equina the terminal structure of the spinal cord that consists of nerve roots and rootlets from above; it fans out in a manner similar to a horses tail which is the literal translation of the term

caudad anatomic term meaning toward the tail

causation the action of a defendant likely caused or created the harm sustained by the plaintiff

cavitation wave during penetration of the body by a fast moving projectile, a wave of pressure pushes ahead of the object causing a temporary cavity to form as tissues are pressed out of the way; after the projectile passes through, a permanent cavity results when the tissues move back; all of the tissues affected by both the temporary and permanent cavity suffer some level of damage in the process

celiac trunk the branch of the abdominal aorta below the diaphragm that supplies the intestines

cell-mediated-immunity the response by various white blood cells (including T cells) that attack antigens one-on-one at the cellular level

cellular respiration the process used by cells to extract energy from nutrient molecules

Centers for Disease Control and Prevention (CDC) one of the 13 major operating components of the Department of Health and Human Services (HHS), which is the principal agency in the United States government for protecting the health and safety of all Americans and for providing essential human services, especially for those people who are least able to help themselves

central cyanosis the condition manifested by a bluish discoloration of the body, especially the mucous membranes, that reflects a whole body lack of adequate oxygenation

central integrative area the area in the CNS that interprets input from the thermosensors and regulates the thermoregulatory effectors to maintain a set point temperature

central nervous system (CNS) the brain and spinal cord

central neurogenic hyperventilation breathing that occurs as very deep, rapid respiratory rates of 40–60 breaths per minute; found in association with mid-brain lesions or dysfunction

central spinal cord syndrome injury to the central portion of the spinal cord that presents with variable sensory loss, but with abnormal motor findings that are more pronounced in the upper extremities than the lower extremities

central venous pressure (CVP) the blood pressure in the large veins of the body, particularly the vena cava; measured with catheters inserted in the large vessels; not currently a common prehospital skill

cephalad anatomic term meaning toward the head

cerebellum part of the brain located in the occipital region of the skull, composed of white matter with a thin layer of gray matter located inferior to the cerebrum; coordinates fine motor control, posture and balance; responsible for unconscious control of somatic motor activity

cerebral aqueduct connection between the third and fourth ventricles that contains cerebrospinal fluid

cerebral contusion bruise of the brain caused by a primary or secondary brain injury

cerebral cortex thin layer of gray matter (neuron cell bodies) that makes up the outer portion of the cerebrum

cerebral hemispheres part of the brain responsible for most of what are considered human abilities, including senses, memory and personality

cerebral ischemia brain cell hypoxia that if uncorrected will lead to cell death and neurologic damage

cerebral palsy a blanket term describing a group of chronic conditions affecting body movements and muscle coordination

cerebral perfusion pressure (CPP) the amount of blood flow to the brain; mean arterial pressure (MAP) minus the intracranial pressure (ICP) or (CPP = MAP − ICP)

cerebrospinal fluid (CSF) an electrolyte-rich fluid produced in the ventricular system of the brain that circulates throughout the subarachnoid space and constantly bathes the brain and spinal cord

cerebrum the upper part of the brain that includes the basal ganglia and the cortex; responsible for higher functioning and thought

certification a process that indicates proficiency has been attained, but it does not actually establish the permission to practice prehospital care as an EMS provider

certified nursing assistants also known as nursing aides, assist other healthcare professionals (especially nurses, physical therapists, and occupational therapists); their duties include taking vital signs and assisting patients with their activities of daily living (ADLs)

cerumen ear wax

cervical spine the upper seven vertebrae of the spinal column

cervix the lower portion of the uterus that opens into the vagina

cesarean section surgical removal of a baby from the uterus

chain of command an orderly line of authority

chancre painless ulceration of the genitals; symptom of primary syphilis

Charcot triad symptoms of right upper quadrant pain, fever, and jaundice; indicates possible diagnosis of cholangitis

Charcot's paralysis (keraunoparalysis) "lightning paraplegia" characterized by the victim's inability to move the extremities

(continued)

after being struck by lightning; accompanied by cool, pale skin, and diminished peripheral pulses

CHART Organizational framework of the patient care report: chief complaint, history, assessment, Rx (meaning prescriptions or drugs) and treatment

chemical buffering system the system that buffers the acid base balance by combining bicarbonate with hydrogen ions or water with carbon dioxide

chemical burn burn that occurs as acids or alkalis of varying pH levels (in liquid, solid or gaseous state) come into contact with external and internal body tissues

chemical name drug name that describes the exact chemical structure of the drug

chemoreceptors built-in sensors in the medulla and the carotid artery that monitor CO_2 and pH levels

chemotaxis the process of attracting responding white cells in response to the chemicals released while fighting an infection or antigens

Cheyne-Stokes pattern a regular cyclic pattern of increased respiratory rate and depth with periods of apnea

chickenpox disease caused by varicella zoster virus, transmitted through airborne droplets

chief complaint the reason care is being sought

chief the person in charge of each section under the Incident Command System

chilblains (pernio) a superficial injury that results from skin inflammation and tissue hypoxia from cold-induced vasoconstriction

child abuse any act or failure to act on the part of parents or caregivers that results in the death, serious physical injury, emotional harm, sexual abuse or exploitation of a child; or an act or failure to act that presents an imminent risk of serious harm

child neglect failure to provide for a child's basic needs; includes physical, emotional, medical, and educational neglect

children with special health care needs (CSHCN) children with medically complex needs

chiropractic treatments that focus on joint manipulation in order to treat a variety of problems

chitin an algae-derived polysaccharide biopolymer used to manufacture dressings designed to limit bleeding

chitosan an algae-derived polysaccharide biopolymer used to manufacture dressings designed to limit bleeding

chlamydia sexually transmitted disease caused by the bacterium *Chlamydia trachomatis;* transmitted through unprotected sexual intercourse, but can also be spread through clothing, towels, and hand-to-hand transfer

chlorine a greenish-yellow gas that has a characteristic pungent odor, when combined with water produces hydrochloric acid; may be used as a weapon of mass destruction

cholecystitis an acute inflammation of the gallbladder that usually occurs when the neck of the gallbladder or cystic duct is obstructed, often by a gallstone, and intraluminal pressure increases

chordae tendinae specialized fibers that attach the atrioventricular valve leaflets to the ventricular papillary muscles that aid in the opening and closing of the heart valves

chorea an abnormal movement characterized by irregular, unpredictable, involuntary muscle jerks that impair voluntary activity

chronic atrial fibrillation an irregularly irregular heart rhythm caused by uncoordinated contraction of the atria

chronic bacterial prostatitis an acute infection that persists, whether treated or not, due to a defect in the prostate that allows the continued existence of bacteria in the urinary tract

chronic lifestyle diseases diseases that take many years to develop and are directly related to lifestyle habits and choices such as poor diet, excess weight, lack of exercise, drinking, smoking, etc.

chronic obstructive pulmonary disease (COPD) a group of respiratory diseases other than asthma characterized by dyspnea, cough, sputum production, airflow limitation, and impaired gas exchange

chronic prostatitis a poorly understood syndrome of symptoms and signs of bacterial prostatitis, including at times the presence of white cells in the semen or urine, but with no evidence of a bacterial causative agent

chronic renal failure (CRF) a disease characterized by the gradual permanent and irreversible loss of kidney function due to destruction of the nephrons

chronic renal insufficiency (CRI) a condition in which the glomerular filtration rate in the kidneys is reduced on a chronic basis, but not to a degree sufficient to cause clinical symptoms

chronic venous insufficiency increased venous pressure caused by obstruction in venous outflow, deterioration of venous valves in the extremities and defects in the normal pumping physiology of the venous system

chronotropic effect describes influence on the heart rate; a positive chronotropic effect would speed up the heart rate

chyme a soft mixture of food with fluids and enzymes produced by the stomach

cilia hair-like cellular structures that move particulate matter out of the trachea and into the mouth where it can be removed by swallowing or coughing

Cincinnati Prehospital Stroke Scale (CPSS) a stroke screening tool that assesses arm drift and coordination, facial symmetry, and the ability to follow simple commands and speaking ability that is used to evaluate for the presence of stroke

circadian rhythm the internal rhythm of the body's function; also referred to as the biological clock

circumflex artery a coronary artery that circles and winds around the surface of the heart providing perfusion to the left atrium and ventricle

cirrhosis the end-stage of liver disease marked by the permanent destruction of hepatocytes

civil law the area of the law that concerns itself with issues such as professional malpractice and other types of tort actions

clammy cold and damp skin condition

classical heat stroke the form of heat stroke that usually strikes elderly or debilitated victims or those living in under-ventilated dwellings without air conditioning, manifested by elevated body temperature and altered mentation

clavicle a doubly curved long bone that forms part of the shoulder girdle, also known as the collar bone

clearance the measurement of the body's ability to eliminate the drug

closed fracture a break in a bone that is not associated with an over lying skin wound tissue

CO_2 narcosis high levels of CO_2 in the blood stream that cause disorientation and depression of consciousness similar to that seen with narcotic overdose

coagulation cascade a complex chemical and biological process designed to control bleeding (hemostasis)

coarse crackle the lower pitched, rumbling heard in the larger bronchi or trachea that is caused by air traveling through larger masses of debris

coccyx the vertebrae that together with the sacrum form the posterior, or back, of the pelvis

cochlea cone shaped structure of the inner ear

cold zone (support zone) area in a hazmat incident that is safe and isolated from contamination

colic a condition marked by recurrent episodes of prolonged and uncontrollable crying and irritability in an otherwise healthy infant that is of unknown cause and usually subsides after 3 to 4 months of age

collagen the most abundant protein in the body that helps to hold and connect tissues together

colloquialism terms or phrases that have meaning only within a certain culture

colon the large intestine between the cecum to the rectum; primary purpose is to extract water from feces

colorimetric capnometer a device for assessing for proper ETT placement that utilizes a pH sensitive paper that changes color in the presence of CO_2

colostomy surgical diversion procedure to create an opening into the large intestine to collect waste

Combitube™ a double-lumen tube with one blind end which functions as an esophageal obturator airway and the other as a standard cuffed ET tube; it is inserted blindly and "seals" the oral and nasal pharyngeal cavities

comfort care (palliative care) active total care of patients whose disease is not responsive to curative treatment; control of pain, of other symptoms, and of psychological, social, and spiritual problems

command staff the individuals that provide information, safety and liaison services, and section oversight; they report directly to the incident commander (IC) under the Incident Command System

comminuted fracture a fracture that involves several breaks in a bone

communicable disease a disease that can be transmitted from one person to another

communicable stage of infection period during which an infectious agent can be spread to another host

communication the exchange of information between two people; it can be in the form of verbal and nonverbal messages

compartment syndrome syndrome that is caused by increased pressure in an enclosed space that leads to compromise of circulation and function of tissues within the space

compassion a desire to alleviate someone's distress

compensated shock the condition that occurs as the body adjusts to fluid loss and organ perfusion is maintained

compensatory pause a pause that occurs in an ECG tracing following an ectopic beat

complement system collection of proteins in the blood that help to kill pathologic organisms. The complement system is part of the immune system

complete fracture a fracture that involves all of the layers of a bone

complete neurologic lesion the absence of sensory and motor function below the level of injury

complex partial seizure seizure that occurs in the frontal or temporal lobe and can produce bizarre behavior that may mimic a psychiatric disorder

compliant a patient who has adhered to the medication dosing regimen prescribed by the physician

compression a squeezing together; the exertion of pressure on a body in such a way as to tend to increase its density

compression injuries injuries that occur when a part of the body gets crushed

compressive cardiogenic shock mechanical impairment of cardiac output, as from pericardial tamponade

concealment anything that provides visual protection but does not provide an appropriate barrier to stop projectiles

concurrent medical direction or control the situation that occurs when a paramedic consults with a physician or other advanced health care professional via telephone, radio, or other electronic means, in real time, permitting the physician and paramedic to collaboratively decide on the best course of action in the delivery of patient care

concussion a temporary and brief interruption of neurological function after head trauma with no demonstrable evidence of injury on radiologic study such as CT scan of the brain

conduction a method of heat transfer from warmer to cooler objects by direct physical contact

conduction fibers specialized fibers in the heart that are capable of conducting impulses and a much faster rate than the average cardiac cell

conductive hearing loss hearing loss that results from damage to the middle or outer ear

conductivity the ability to spread impulses

condyloma lata large, wart-like lesions in the inguinal or perineal area that are highly contagious; symptom of secondary syphilis

confined space situation when a patient has been unconscious in a fire and will likely have respiratory distress

confirmation bias the tendency to search for and interpret information in a way that confirms your preconceptions

congenital anomaly a physical abnormality that is present at birth

congenital phimosis a condition that occurs when the foreskin of the penis in young, prepubescent males is too tight to retract or pull back over the head of the glans penis

congestive heart failure (CHF) common clinical name for many cardiac diseases that result from inadequate cardiac output

conjugate gaze eyes spontaneously open, face, and move in the same direction

conjunctiva a membrane that covers the sclera (white part of the eye) and lines the inside of the eyelids

consent informed permission given by a competent patient, or the patient's legally responsible decision-maker, for care or transportation by EMS providers

consolidation a form of blockage that occurs when areas of lung tissue become filled with fluid, pus or other material

constipation the delayed or infrequent passage of dry, hardened feces

contact and cover a scene management strategy whereby the contact member is responsible for patient care and the cover member is responsible for continued scene safety

contact burn burn that results from direct skin contact with very hot substances or chemicals such as metal, plastic, glass, gasoline or hot coals

contamination reduction zone (warm zone) the area in a hazmat incident that surrounds the hot zone; serves as a safety buffer area between the public in the cold zone and the hazardous material; area where decontamination occurs

continuing education an ongoing process to gain new knowledge

continuous ambulatory peritoneal dialysis (CAPD) a type of dialysis in which a silicone rubber catheter is inserted into the peritoneal cavity through a hole made in the abdominal wall and dialysate fluid is circulated through the catheter into the cavity

continuous positive airway pressure (CPAP) ventilator mode that applies pressure during the entire respiratory cycle; used for patients who are breathing on their own, but would benefit from positive pressure to expand atelectatic lungs, to ease the work of breathing, or as a weaning mode

contractility the ability of muscle cells to shorten; equivalent to the force each cardiac myocyte (muscle cell) generates during systolic contraction

contraindication identifies factors under which a drug should not be used; hypersensitivity is always a contraindication to medication use

contrecoup a second impact that occurs to the brain when it strikes the inside of the skull on the opposite side of the initial (coup) impact

control (integration) center a nervous system center that assesses information registered by a receptor, compares it to its normal set point and initiates a corrective change to regulate metabolism

controlled hypoventilation (permissive hypercapnia) proper technique for ventilation that includes slow ventilations. The benefit to this procedure is that intrathoracic pressures are allowed to remain near normal which enhances return of blood to the heart

controlled mandatory ventilation (CMV) the mode on a ventilator that is used when the patient is not breathing; the ventilator does all of the work of breathing for the patient

contusion bruise that is the result of blunt force trauma and can occur in any part of the body

convection heat transfer from a warm object into the surrounding atmosphere

cor pulmonale right heart failure resulting from hypertension of the pulmonary circulation

cord prolapse occurs when the umbilical cord presents through the open cervix during labor before the baby's presenting part and is observed in the vagina or outside of the vagina, if the cord becomes compressed during delivery it will stop providing oxygenated blood to the baby, resulting in high risk of brain damage to the infant

cornea the outermost convex transparent portion of the eye

corniculate cartilage tiny cartilages that tighten the vocal cords, changing the pitch of the voice

coronary artery artery that originates in the aorta and spreads over the heart and from which the heart receives its nutrients

coronary sinus a wide venous channel that drains the five coronary veins on the surface of the heart back to the right atrium

corpus callosum a structure in the brain that connects the left and right cerebral hemispheres and appears as a wide, flat region just ventral to (below) the cortex; most communication between regions in different halves of the brain are carried over the corpus callosum

cortex the outer portion of an organ

cortical bone the compact type of bone tissue that forms the hard outer layer of the bone

corticosteroid chemical (e.g., aldosterone and cortisol) from the adrenal cortex; steroid medications frequently prescribed by physicians to combat inflammation

cortisol hormone released by the adrenal cortex that primarily affects carbohydrate, protein, and fat metabolism with the objective of improving nutrient storage and supply to tissues

costal margin the lower border of the ribs and their cartilages

costochondral junction the junction between the ribs and their cartilages

costovertebral angle (CVA) the point in the back where the twelfth rib attaches to its corresponding vertebra

cough a modified form of respiration used to clear debris from the lower airways

coup commonly, an impact to the head (from the French term for *blow*)

course crackle auscultatory sound resulting from the presence of fluid in the alveoli. It is heard with a stethoscope as the alveoli "pops" open during inspiration

cover anything that protects someone from view as well as provides a barrier to stop projectiles like knives or bullets

crackle a respiratory sound generally heard on inspiration and presents as a discontinuous bubbling noise; reflects air passing through fluid

craniad anatomic term meaning toward the head

cranial nerves twelve pairs of nerves that originate in the brain and communicate with other parts of the body

crepitus air under the skin from an underlying injury to the trachea, esophagus, lung, or larynx or the crackling feeling when the two broken ends of a bone rub against one another

cricoid cartilage a small ring of cartilage located beneath the thyroid cartilage in the neck

cricoid pressure (Sellick's maneuver) applying pressure to the cricoid cartilage in such a way as to occlude the esophagus and prevent stomach contents from getting into the airway and aspirated into the lungs

cricothyroid membrane membrane between the cricoid and thyroid cartilages of the larynx

cricothyrotomy incision through the skin and cricothyroid membrane for relief of respiratory obstruction; used prior to or in place of tracheotomy in certain respiratory obstructions

criminal law law that describes actions that are forbidden and which is enforced by the government—including the local, state or federal government

critical incident stress (CIS) events that elicit strong emotional reactions in the paramedic

critical thinking the ability to think about the processes used to solve problems as well as the ability to solve problems

Crohn's disease a chronic, inflammatory bowel disease

croup (laryngotracheitis) an infection of the tissues within and below the larynx that results in a deep barking cough

crush fractures a comminuted or transverse fracture associated with extensive soft tissue injury that usually results in significant morbidity

crush injury a mechanism of injury in which skeletal muscle, as well as the overlying skin, subcutaneous tissue, and associated structures such as bones, nerves, and blood vessels, are locally compressed by high-pressure forces causing cellular disruption

crush syndrome a systemic disorder of severe metabolic disturbances resulting from the crush of skeletal muscle

crystalloid solutions intravenous fluids that can be used for patients in hypovolemic shock (e.g., saline, lactated ringers) that are composed of electrolytes, glucose, amino acids, lactate and other small particle molecules

Cullen's sign a bluish discoloration visible on the surface of the abdomen when a large amount of blood is present in the peritoneum

cultural bias beliefs and values based on a person's own cultural background as well as the experiences that have shaped a person's views over time

culture the customary beliefs, social forms, and material traits of a racial, religious, or social group

CUPS Assessment Scale assessment tool developed by the Critical Illness and Trauma Foundation to assist in determining the criticality of patients

Cushing's reflex the combination of bradycardia and hypertension; indicative of increased intracranial pressure and impending brain herniation

Cushing's triad Three common findings with increased intracranial pressure: hypertension, bradycardia, and respiratory patterns that change as various parts of the damaged brain attempt to compensate

Cushing's syndrome a metabolic disorder that results from excessive cortisol production, excessive use of steroids (topically, in pill form or in injections), or other similar steroid (glucocorticoid) hormones

cutaneous anthrax skin infections with *B. anthracis* caused through direct contact; symptoms include a raised bump at the site of inoculation that becomes necrotic

cyanide (hydrogen cyanide, cyanogen chloride) may be used as a weapon of mass destruction and are also common byproducts from the combustion of many materials; interferes with the ability of the cell to utilize oxygen for metabolism

cyanosis a bluish discoloration that can be observed in the nail beds or other tissues that results from hemoglobin that does not have oxygen bound to its binding sites; categorized as peripheral or central

cystic fibrosis an autosomal disorder of the exocrine glands resulting in physiological changes in the respiratory, GI, integumentary, and muscoskeletal systems; it is an inherited disorder found predominately in Caucasian children of both genders

cystitis bladder infection

cytokines proteins that are released into the blood by white blood cells

cytolytic cell cutting; any process or substance that damages cells

D

daily value (DV) the amount of a particular nutrient you should be getting each day

damages harm or other losses sustained by an injured party (the plaintiff) as a result of the action of a defendant

DCAP-BTLS mnemonic used to assess musculoskeletal injuries: deformity, contusions, abrasions, penetrations or punctures, burns, tenderness, lacerations, swelling

dead space gas (VD) the total amount of gas contained in the physiologic and anatomic deadspaces, those areas that do not exchange oxygen for carbon dioxide; the anatomic dead space in a normal respiratory system is approximately 150 ml; diseased lungs will have a greater dead space

death the state in which the brain ceases to function

deceleration slowing down

decerebrate posturing involuntary reflexive movements of abnormal extension, due to a lower brain injury

decibel (dB) a measurement of the loudness of a sound or strength of its vibration

decompensated shock stage of shock after compensated shock and before irreversible shock where the body's compensatory mechanisms are no longer effective, manifested by rapid pulse and diminished blood pressure

decompression illness (DCI) disease that results from the formation of small bubbles of nitrogen gas in the blood and tissues after ascent from scuba diving

decontamination the process of removing or reducing hazards that have accumulated on people or equipment to eliminate or reduce the toxic effect

decorticate posturing involuntary reflexive movements characterized by abnormal flexion inward, toward the core, due to a lesion higher in the brain

decubitus ulcers ulcers that result from the breakdown of skin and underlying tissue; also known as bed sores

deep anatomic term meaning toward the interior of the body

deep femoral artery extension of the inguinal artery, passing through the thigh

deep frostbite the degree of frostbite in which subdermal and deep tissues are affected

deep partial thickness second degree burn, involves blister formation

deep venous thrombosis (DVT) thrombosis of larger veins; serious condition due to risk of embolism to the pulmonary arteries

defamation saying or publicizing something untrue about a person that injures that person's character or reputation

defibrillation the administration of an unsynchronized electrical shock with the intent of depolarizing a critical mass of vulnerable cardiac cells to terminate ventricular fibrillation

deglutition reflex the act of swallowing

degradation occurs when the protective qualities of the material of protective clothing are altered through contact with chemical substances

delirium a disturbance in thought and reasoning that has a more rapid onset than dementia and is usually temporary

dementia the most severe form of cognitive impairment, resulting in a progressive impairment spanning memory deficits and the inability to carry out motor functions, aphasia, inability to identify objects, or higher-level thought processes, usually gradual onset and permanent

denatured unfolding of a protein

dendrites the projections of a nerve cell that contain receptors for specific substances and carry electrical signals toward the cell body of the neuron

dentoalveolar trauma mouth and dental injuries

denude remove; similar to degloving or avulsing

depolarization the change in ion balance as ions move into and out of the cell; the process allows a cell to pass an electrical current along to the next adjacent cell

depression a progressive mood disorder that involves a persistent sadness, dysphoria, or loss of interest in usual activities

dermatome the area of skin sensed by a single nerve root

dermis the middle layer of the skin; lies beneath the epidermis; contains hair and hair follicles, sweat glands, sebaceous (oil) glands, sensory nerves, muscles, and pressure receptors

descending phase phase IV on a normal capnogram waveform; represents the inspiratory limb

Destot's sign a superficial hematoma of the scrotum or perineum

detoxification a liver function that involves the breakdown of any drug not used by the target tissues until what remains is a harmless chemical

deviate move away from

dextrocardia when a person's heart is tipped to the right, instead of to the left

diabetes mellitus—type I disease caused by the inability of the pancreas to secrete insulin; patients require exogenous insulin; also called insulin dependent diabetes mellitus (IDDM) or juvenile onset diabetes mellitus (JODM)

diabetes mellitus—type II endogenous insulin is insufficient to allow for optimal glucose metabolism, but is sufficient to prevent ketoacidosis; also called adult onset diabetes mellitus (AODM) or noninsulin dependent diabetes mellitus (NIDDM)

diabetic ketoacidosis (DKA) results from a lack of insulin and an overabundance of glucose in the circulating blood. It involves a change in metabolism; normal glucose utilization does not occur, the7refore alternative energy sources, including muscles and lipids, are metabolized resulting in production of excessive waste products

diabetic retinopathy a complication of diabetes resulting from damage to the tiny blood vessels inside the retina which leads to visual changes and ultimately blindness

diagnosis of exclusion a diagnosis that is arrived at when all other reasonable causes are suspected and then carefully eliminated as more information from history, physical examination, or via testing results comes to light

dialysis the therapeutic process of filtering blood to maintain homeostasis; it reestablishes the proper electrolyte balance and rids the body of wastes normally filtered out by the kidneys

diaphoresis sweating

diaphysis the part of the bone between each epiphysis (growth plate); the shaft of the bone

diastole relaxation of the ventricles of the heart

diastolic arterial pressure the lowest pressure during the resting phase of the cardiac cycle

diencephalon the part of the brain that includes the thalamus and the hypothalamus

diffuse axonal injury (DAI) significant traumatic brain injury caused by deceleration that results in shearing forces on the connections within the brain

digital intubation intubation procedure performed by passing the ET tube over the curved fingers of the gloved hand into the trachea; the hand is placed into the mouth and the fingers locate the epiglottitis

dilation of the cervix when the cervix changes during the first stage of labor from being closed to stretched open at its widest, 10 centimeters

diplopia when the two eyes no longer move in tandem, causing the patient to complain of double vision

direct strike direct contact with a lightning bolt

disaster a mass casualty incident that overwhelms resources both on-scene and at the receiving facilities

Disaster Medical Assistance Teams (DMATs) specialized federal teams that are equipped to provide care to victims of a mass casualty incident

disaster mortuary operational response teams (DMORTs) specialized federal teams that are equipped to work with the dead patients

disease period The stage of the infection process when symptoms occur

disequilibrium syndrome cerebral edema due to osmolar differences between the newly filtered blood and brain tissue; it can occur following dialysis

disinfectants cleansing agents capable of destroying or inhibiting the growth of most microorganisms; they are toxic to living tissue

dislocated joint the condition that occurs when the articular surfaces (bone ends) that normally meet to form a joint are displaced completely out of contact with each other

dislocation the disruption of a joint where the bones are pulled out of their normal relationship and tendon or ligament damage occurs, manifested by abnormal, restricted and painful movement

displaced fracture a fracture where there is movement of the two bone fragments away from one another

disseminated intravascular coagulation (DIC) process in the body where the blood starts to coagulate throughout the whole body

disseminated intravascular coagulopathy (DIC) a systemic hemorrhagic state

distal anatomic term meaning farther from the trunk when compared to another point

distraction injuries the injuries that result when one part of the body is pulled away from the adjacent part, commonly occurs in the cervical spine

distress stress that results in negative consequences

distributive shock hypoperfusion caused by peripheral vasodilatation and maldistribution of blood

diuretics medications that cause volume depletion by causing body fluids to be lost through urination

diverticulitis inflammation of diverticulum (pouches of tissue within the colon that become filled with fecal matter)

diverticulosis the presence of diverticulum in the colon

diverticulum sacs or pouches protruding out from the bowel

Do not resuscitate order (DNR or DNRO) program an order that the paramedic shall withhold cardiac compressions, intubation, artificial ventilation, resuscitative drugs, defibrillation and other invasive resuscitative measures; also known as advance directive

documentation written factual evidence that reflects patient care during the patient encounter

domestic violence (DV) violence and abuse between intimate partners; in a broad sense may refer to intimate partner violence, spousal abuse, elder abuse, and child abuse

dopamine a catecholamine chemical naturally produced in the body; also a medication administered to support blood pressure

dorsal anatomic term meaning toward the back of the body

dorsalis pedis the pulse located on the top of the foot

dorsiflex lifting the toes upward and flexing (bending) the ankle and foot upwards

dose a single amount of medication administered via any route at a single point in time

dose response critical concept in toxicology; as the dose increases, the severity of the toxic response increases

Down syndrome (trisomy 21) a chromosome abnormality caused by an extra copy of the 21st chromosome, characterized by developmental delay, short stature and a characteristic facial appearance

dressings sterile absorbent materials applied directly on a wound to prevent contamination or to stop bleeding

dromotropic effect describes the excitability, or willingness, of the heart to conduct an impulse through the cardiac cells; a drug with a negative dromotropic effect on the heart would slow down the rate of electrical conduction

drowning death by suffocation after submersion

drug abuse taking a substance with nontherapeutic, nonself-harming intent

drug misuse taking a substance with therapeutic intent but knowingly using it in a nonstandard dose (usually excessive)

dual lumen airway device tube designed for difficult or emergency airway intubation and ventilation; dual lumen means it has two passages for air to move through and care must be taken to ensure the proper passage is used during ventilation

due process the legal process that involves, at a minimum, notice of the charges or proposed disciplinary action, and an opportunity to be heard regarding those charges, prior to any disciplinary action being taken

duodenum the first 10 inches of the small intestine

duration the length of time an event takes place

dura mater thick outer covering of the brain that is located against the skull, and under which lies a large system of bridging veins

duty the obligation that the paramedic must act with due regard for a patient, and provide the applicable standard of care with respect to that patient

dynamic ambulance deployment ambulances are deployed to various locations based on anticipated needs

dysarthria (articulation disorders) disorders that are caused by the inability of an individual to produce sounds

dysbarisms conditions that result from exposure to increased ambient pressure causing volume-pressure changes within the air-filled cavities in the body and from increased dissolution of gasses, particularly nitrogen, in body tissues

dysphagia difficulty swallowing

dysphasia difficulty speaking

dyspnea shortness of breath and difficulty breathing

dyspnea on exertion (DOE) shortness of breath when exercising or during exertion

dysrhythmia abnormal electrical cardiac pattern resulting in an abnormal heart beat that could lead to death if untreated

dysrhythmia on ECG, an abnormal rhythm

dystonia sustained abnormal postures

E

ear canal the structure leading from the outside into the middle ear

ear squeeze the condition that occurs during diving descent when gas-filled structures have a tendency to be "squeezed" into half their volume

early labor the early part of the first stage of labor when the cervix dilates from 0 cm to 4 cm

ecchymosis discoloration and bruising from subcutaneous bleeding

echolalia communication using repetitive words from someone else, often present in children with autism spectrum disorders

eclampsia condition in pregnant patients who have severe preeclampsia and are actively seizing or in coma

ectopic pregnancy a fertilized egg that has implanted somewhere outside its normal position in the uterus, 98% in the fallopian tube; most often results in rupture of the structure unless diagnosed early enough and has a maternal death of about 10%

edema swelling of body tissues; fluid that is third-spaced into the extra-vascular spaces

effacement the thinning and stretching of the cervix during the first stage of labor

effectors the structures of the body that accomplish the desired effect

efferent (or motor) neurons the neurons that carry electrical signals away from the brain and spinal cord to the effector cell such as a muscle or gland

efferent nerves conduct stimulatory signals from the central nervous system to the muscles and glands

efferent pathways pathways where electrical and chemical messages are passed from control centers to effectors

efficacy the process of change that occurs as the result of drugs binding to a receptor; when speaking of drugs it refers to the resultant degree of desired effects being present, high efficacy has more desired effects

egophony a type of chest assessment where the patient is asked to speak while auscultation is occurring

egress escape; movement away from an area

Einthoven's triangle relationship that can be expressed mathematically as the electrical sum of current in Lead I plus Lead III is equal to the current measured in Lead II

elder abuse abuse of the elderly by caregivers or self; may be physical abuse, sexual abuse, emotional abuse, financial exploitation, neglect, abandonment, or self-neglect

electrical alternans an alternating high and low amplitude QRS complex on the cardiac monitor

electrical axis the overall direction of the electrical depolarization wave in the heart, can be determined from the ECG

electrical burn burn caused as a result of electrical current flowing through the patient

electrocardiograph (ECG) the graphic tracing of the electrical patterns resulting from the flow of electricity throughout the heart

electron transport chain the metabolic process that takes $NADH_2^+$ $FADH_2$ molecules and converts them to NAD^+ and FAD; in doing so, a significant amount of ATP and hydrogen ions are produced

emancipated minor a minor legally capable of providing consent for medical care for self, typically a self-supporting

(continued)

minor; this status is often dependent upon the minor receiving an actual court order of emancipation

embolic stroke a stroke that arises from a clot that travels from another location in the body (usually the heart) to the brain where it lodges in one of the cerebral arteries causing obstruction of blood flow to the portion of the brain beyond the obstruction

embryo the developing human from the time of conception through the second month of gestation

emergency medical dispatcher (EMD) trained individuals who work in 9-1-1 centers, and other police, fire medical, and public safety agencies receiving telephone calls from persons needing emergency assistance and dispatching the appropriate aid with the help of computer aided dispatching systems and two-way radio

emergency medical responder (EMR) trained professional who has the skills necessary to be a bridge between the immediate event and the arrival of personnel with more training, equipment and supplies

emergency medical technician (EMT) trained professional who provides basic life support and may also transport patients

emergency operations center (EOC) a facility that coordinates support functions and provides resources support for larger or long duration incidents

emotional abuse a pattern of behavior that impairs a patient's emotional development or sense of self-worth

empathy a form of understanding, both intellectually and emotionally, that involves the ability to see other people as they see themselves

EMS Education Agenda for the Future: A Systems Approach the document that proposed an improved and structured education system to train the next generation of EMS professionals

EMS Systems Act under the Department of Health Education and Welfare, the act that provided for funding for planning, implementation and coordinating EMS systems

encephalitis inflammation or infection of the brain

end diastolic volume the volume of blood in the ventricle after it has finished filling (preload)

end systolic volume the volume of blood remaining in the ventricle after systole

endocardium the inner lining of the four chambers of the heart

endocrine organ an organ whose primary function is hormone secretion

endocrine system the system that provides the chemicals (hormones) needed to turn on and off the various systems of the body

endogenous agonists naturally occurring chemicals found within the body that bind to and activate receptors

endometritis postpartum infection of the internal layer of the uterus

endometrium the lining of the uterus; it develops and thickens during each menstrual cycle in order to be receptive to the implantation of an embryo

endothermic heat consuming chemical reaction

endotracheal intubation (ETI) the process of introducing a plastic tube into the trachea though the oropharynx for the purpose of providing ventilations

end-stage renal disease (ESRD) kidney function that is less than 10% of baseline; irreversible loss of renal function

end-tidal carbon dioxide (ETCO$_2$) detector device used to measure the amount of CO$_2$ that is exhaled; the information is displayed on a numeric readout as a waveform printed on a graph, or via pH sensitive paper that exhibits a color change in the presence of CO$_2$

enteral the medication route that brings a drug into the body via the gastrointestinal tract

enteric coating a special coating on a pill to ensure absorption from a specific location within the GI tract, typically somewhere beyond the stomach

Environmental Protection Agency (EPA) an agency of the federal government of the United States charged with protecting human health and with safeguarding the natural environment: air, water, and land

enzymes complex proteins, made by cells, that catalyze (promote) a chemical reaction

ependymal cells the cells that line the ventricles of the brain

epicardium outermost layer of the heart; serves as the "skin" of the heart and is a protective layer that contains most of the heart's blood vessels, lymph vessels and nerve fibers

epidemiology the branch of medical science that deals with the incidence, distribution, and control of disease in the population

epidermis the outermost layer of the skin mostly made of dead, flattened, and hardened (keratinized) cells called the stratum corneum

epididymitis inflammation or infection of the epididymis, a convoluted, worm-like structure that lies against the posterior surface of the testicle

epididymo-orchitis inflammation or infection of the epididymis and testicle

epidural hemorrhage bleeding into the space between the skull and dura mater covering the brain

epidural space a "potential" space located between the inside of the skull and the dura mater

epigastric region the section of the abdomen immediately above the periumbilical region and just inferior to the xiphoid

epigastrium the upper central region of the abdomen

epiglottis a somewhat stiff, cartilage-containing, flap of tissue that protects the airway (trachea) from food during swallowing

epiglottitis a bacterial infection of the epiglottis; can quickly lead to complete airway obstruction

epilepsy an umbrella term for a variety of disorders that cause electrical disturbances within the central nervous system that are characterized by convulsing motor activity

epinephrine a catecholamine hormone also known as adrenalin

epiphyseal plate fracture a fracture near, or through, the epiphyseal plate that can result in alternations to growth of the bone

epiphysis the portion of bone just beyond the growth plate

epistaxis hemorrhage from the nose

eponyms conditions that are named after those who first discovered or described something, or first diagnosed a disease, such as Beck's triad or Down syndrome

erector spinae the muscles that maintain erect posture and extend from the sacrum and iliac crest to the back of the head

erythema migrans red, painless rash at the site of bite from deer tick; first symptom of Lyme disease

erythema redness, used in describing a burn or coloration of the skin

erythematous reddened

erythrocytes red blood cells

erythropoiesis red blood cell production

erythropoietin EPO is a glycoprotein hormone released by the kidneys into the bloodstream. It increases the rate at which RBCs are produced above the normal rate of 3 million per second

escape in cardiology, escape refers to an ectopic beat or rhythm that results following the failure of a higher pacemaker site. Escape beats serve a temporary protective function but are often an indication of cardiovascular compromise

eschar the inelastic dead dermis (scar) tissue that over time separates from the underlying tissues; if it is circumferential (goes all the way around a part of the body) it may restrict blood flow or movement

escharotomy a surgical procedure involving an incision made with a scalpel through burned, devitalized, dead, eschar tissue to allow the muscles to move and blood to flow

esophageal detector device (EDD) consists of a bulb that is compressed and attached to the endotracheal tube; if the tube is in the esophagus (positive result for an EDD), the suction created by the EDD will collapse the lumen of the esophagus or pull the esophageal tissue against the tip of the tube, and the bulb will not re-expand

esophageal gastric airway a version of an EOA that includes a tube that allows air to be released from the stomach to prevent gastric distention

esophageal obturator airway (EOA) a tube inserted into the esophagus that obstructs the esophagus, attached to a mask so that air delivered into the mask enters the trachea. This device is fallen out of favor in the Prehospital setting but has served as the basis of the development of the more modern dual lumen airway devices

esophageal reflux the regurgitation of stomach acid or contents into the esophagus, causing burning pain, often epigastric but can be as high as into throat

esophageal rupture (Boerhaave's syndrome) esophageal perforation from trauma, foreign bodies, or severe retching

esophageal varices dilated veins in the esophagus resulting from increased venous pressure resulting from liver damage, that can lead to severe or life threatening bleeding

esophagitis inflammation of the esophagus

esophagus 10-inch muscular tube located posterior and lateral to the trachea in the mediastinum; transports food from the mouth to the stomach by way of voluntary and involuntary muscles during the process of swallowing

estrogen a hormone present in both men and women but usually at significantly higher levels in women of reproductive age

ethics personal or professional standards relating to character and what is right or wrong; the set of principles and standards that determine what is right and wrong conduct within the paramedic profession

eupnea easy normal breathing that has a regular pattern

eustachian tube the canal between the middle ear and the nasopharynx that balances pressures in the middle ear

eustress a stress that results in positive consequences, sometimes called "good stress"

evaporation an endothermic (heat-consuming) process; a manner of heat loss caused by sweat drying in moving air or hot temperatures

evidenced-based medicine (EBM) an approach that places emphasis on the scientific basis of medical practice; EBM is the preferred method for guiding the development of prehospital protocols and guidelines; however, limited research has been conducted on EMS to date; as more research come along, guidelines and protocols will change to reflect the best recommended practices

evisceration intraabdominal contents found to be protruding out of a wound

EVM-456 scale a method to remember the Glasgow Coma Scale (GCS) score; EVM = eyes, verbal and motor and 4-5-6 is the top score possible in each category

excitability the ability of cardiac and other cells to readily receive and respond to an electrical impulse

exclusion zone (hot zone) the area of contamination in a Hazmat situation into which no one who is unprotected by appropriate PPE should enter

excursion the ability of the chest wall to expand evenly and fully

exertional heat stroke form of heat stroke that usually strikes young and healthy victims and occurs secondary to predictable causes like working in a hot environment without adequate fluid replenishment, manifested by elevated body temperature and altered mentation

exothermic heat generating chemical reactions

expiratory reserve volume (ERV) the amount of additional air that can be forcibly expelled from the lungs following a normal exhalation

expressed consent consent that the patient desires treatment, given by a patient or his or her responsible decision-maker either verbally or through some physical action

expressive aphasia the inability to speak as a result of the inability to remember or express words or terms

exsanguination the loss of blood from the vascular system; also called "bleeding out"

extensibility the ability of muscle cells to lengthen, within limits, without damage

extension the act of straightening a limb; also when the head and spine move backward, or in a posterior direction, relative to the torso

external contamination when toxins, poisons, or radioactive gasses, liquids, or solids contaminate skin and clothing

external ear barotrauma (EEBT) when diving, if air becomes trapped in the external ear canal because of obstruction from cerumen, stenosis, earplugs, or a tight-fitting wet suit hood, a relative negative pressure will develop in the external canal

external irradiation when the victim is exposed to penetrating radiation from an external source

external laryngeal manipulation (ELM) intubation method where intubator moves trachea into visual position by manipulating the thyroid cartilage

external oblique muscle muscle that originates at the fifth through twelfth ribs and extends down over the lateral abdomen to the pelvis

extracellular fluid (ECF) the water found outside the cells; it is divided between plasma (5% of total body weight) and interstitial fluid (15% of total body weight)

extrapulmonary tuberculosis tuberculosis infections outside the lungs

F

facial barotrauma the condition that results from compression of the air within a dive mask over the eyes and nose

facilitated diffusion (active transport) a process whereby molecules diffuse across membranes, with the assistance of transport proteins

factitious disorder a disorder in which a patient is consciously, actively working to deceive the medical practitioner

fallacy something that is not true

fallopian tubes tubes leading from the ovaries to the uterus through which mature eggs travel

false imprisonment the confinement of a person without any good cause against his or her will, or without the person's consent

false ribs ribs 8, 9, and 10; their anterior connection is to the costal cartilage of the seventh rib rather than their own costal cartilage

fascia a connective tissue that encases each skeletal muscle; the sheath of tendon covering the muscle

fasciotomy a procedure in which a skin incision is made and the fascia (tissue sheath covering the muscle) overlying the affected compartment tissues is cut open to allow the compartment to decompress and allow for spontaneous return of perfusion

fat embolism syndrome fat globules that are released into the blood when a long bone is fractured

fats a form of energy storage and fuel used for metabolism

Federal Emergency Management Agency (FEMA) the lead federal agency responsible for emergency management activities after natural and terrorist disasters

Federal Interagency Committee on EMS (FICEMS) function is to coordinate various Federal agencies that are involved in EMS, including the Department of Health and Human Services, Homeland Security and the National Highway Traffic Safety Administration (NHTSA)

femoral artery extension of the inguinal artery, passing through the thigh

fertilization process of a sperm cell from the male combining with the female's ovum to become a conceptus, which is also called an embryo

fetal distress irregularities in the fetal heart rate pattern—tachycardia, bradycardia, deep variable decelerations or late decelerations—that generally indicate that there is some problem affecting the fetus; following birth, the presence of meconium indicates the newborn was in fetal distress

fetus an infant while it is still living inside the uterus in the mother

fiberoptic bronchoscope device that allows direct visualization of the trachea

fibrillation chaotic, disorganized electrical signals within the myocardium not originating from a pacemaker site that can lead to minimal or no mechanical response (contractions)

fibrillatory threshold the point at which fibrillation is likely to occur

fibrin a network of protein fibers, a component of the blood clotting process that is necessary for clot formation and hemostasis

fibrinogen a globulin of the blood plasma that is converted into fibrin by the action of thrombin in the presence of ionized calcium to produce coagulation of the blood

fibrinolysis the process where a fibrin clot, the product of coagulation, is broken down

fibroblasts a type of cell that synthesizes and maintains the extracellular matrix of many animal tissues, provides a structural framework (stroma) for many tissues, and plays a critical role in wound healing; the most common cells of connective tissue in animals

fibrocartilaginous composed of fibrous cartilage

fibrous joints joints that are made of dense connective tissue that provide stability and permit only very slight movement

fibula the smaller of the two bones in the calf; it is nonweight-bearing

fight-or-flight response the physiological reaction to a stressor; also called stress response

first stage of labor the initiation of the delivery process manifested by regular, increasingly forceful and frequent contractions of the uterus that ends with complete dilatation and effacement of the cervix

first-degree AV block a conduction delay occurring within the AV node manifested on ECG by a P-R segment that exceeds 0.2 seconds in duration with all impulses conducted through AV node

first-degree burn burn that involves only the outermost layer of skin tissue (the epidermis) manifested by redness of the skin associated with pain

first-pass effect passage of a drug through the liver and the renal (kidney) circulation that results in chemical changes to the drug and in elimination of some of the drug from the body

fixed tidal volume average volume of gas inhaled or exhaled in one respiratory cycle

flail chest a free-floating segment of the chest wall that occurs when three or more adjacent ribs are fractured in two or more places

flank common name for the postero lateral aspect of the abdomen

flash pulmonary edema (acute pulmonary edema) rapid fluid increase within the pulmonary interstitium and alveoli, resulting in shortness of breath, hypoxia, pulmonary rales, a "frothy" cough, and usually tachycardia with hypertension

flexion the act of bending a limb; when a force moves part of the spine forward relative to the rest of the spine

floating ribs ribs 11 and 12, which do not have any anterior attachment to the sternum

flow restricted oxygen-powered ventilation device (FROPVD) a device that is attached directly to the regulator on the oxygen cylinder to control the pressure of oxygen flow delivered, formerly called the demand valve

focalism the tendency to place too much importance on one aspect of an event that causes an error in accurately predicting a future outcome

Foley catheter plastic tube inserted into the urinary bladder for drainage

follicle stimulating hormone (FSH) hormone that targets the reproductive organs

Food and Drug Administration an agency of the United States Department of Health and Human Services that is responsible for regulating food (humans and animal), dietary supplements, drugs (human and animal), cosmetics, medical devices (human and animal) and radiation emitting devices (including nonmedical devices), biologics, and blood products in the United States

Food Guide Pyramid an outline of what to eat each day that is based on the principles of moderation, variety, and balance

foreign body airway obstruction (FBAO) foreign body lodged in the throat partially or fully occluding the airway

formulary a list of approved medications

Fournier's gangrene a polymicrobial necrotizing infection of the fascia of the perineal, perianal, or genital areas that can occur in males or females, though males are affected 10 times more frequently

fourth-degree burn outdated term for a burn that penetrates deep into the body (such as a burn into muscle and bone); now called a deep third-degree burn or full thickness burn

Fowler's position a position in which the patient is sitting (bent at the hip) from a supine position anywhere from a few degrees up to 90 degrees; "semi-Fowlers" position is a Fowler's position that is 45 degrees or less

fraction of inspired air (FIO$_2$) concentration of oxygen in inspired air; room air is 21% oxygen so the FIO$_2$ is 21

fracture a break in the continuity of a bone or cartilage; the term fracture also applies to torn tissue in a solid organ such as the liver

Frank-Starling mechanism of the heart the force of blood ejected by the heart is determined primarily by the length of the fibers of its muscular wall; the more a cardiac muscle is stretched, the harder it will contract

Frank-Starling relationship cardiac ventricular distention just prior to contraction (end-diastolic volume) is directly correlated to the volume of blood ejected with systole (stroke volume)

free radicals dangerous chemicals that are unstable and highly reactive and that quickly interact with other molecules in the cell, especially membrane phospholipids, cellular proteins and nucleic acids, in an effort to "steal" another electron to complete their pair

fremitus a palpable vibration on the human body when the patient is speaking, a respiratory assessment tool

frontal any structure that is toward the anterior surface of the body

frontal lobes an area in the brain located at the front of each cerebral hemisphere

frostbite a tissue injury that results from macrovascular, microvascular, and direct cellular disruption from freezing

frostnip the most superficial form of frostbite damage

full term newborns of 37 weeks of gestation and above; normal gestation length is 40 weeks

full-thickness burn also called third degree burn; involves burn damage to all layers of the skin and underlying tissue

functional residual capacity (FRC) the measurement of the total amount of air forcibly exhaled (ERV) plus the reserve volume (RV), which is the amount of air remaining in the lungs following this forcible exhalation

fundal massage massaging the uterus externally postpartum

fundamental attribution error the tendency for paramedics to overemphasize personality-based explanations for behaviors in others while underemphasizing the role of the situation on the same behavior in themselves

fundus the superior portion of the uterus that can stretch from 5 cm to the size of a newborn baby; at full term it is palpable just under the rib cage

fungi multicelled organisms with capsules that protect them from the host's immune response; fungal infections are rare in a host with a normally functioning immune system

futility having no practical result, all interventions are failing, or the interventions will not result in a positive outcome

G

gap junctions specialized plasma membrane channels inside the intercalated disks within cardiac cells; they allow ions and small molecules to pass between cells

gastric lavage ("stomach pumping") a technique for irrigating (washing) the interior of the stomach by insertion of a large-bore plastic tube; used to remove ingested poisons, has fallen from favor over the past 10 years, but it is occasionally still useful for high-risk poisonings

gastritis inflammation of the lining of the stomach

gastroenteritis an inflammation of the lining of the stomach or intestine; a collection of symptoms including nausea, vomiting, abdominal pain, and diarrhea that are caused by a variety of infectious agents

gastroenterology the study of the gastrointestinal tract

gastroesophageal reflux disease (GERD) reflux of gastric contents into the esophagus; also known as heartburn

gastroesophageal sphincter a ring-like band of fibers located between the esophagus and the stomach

gastrointestinal anthrax disease caused by ingesting *B. anthracis;* causes abdominal pain, vomiting blood, and diarrhea

gastrointestinal system the body system that breaks down complex nutrients into a form that the body can use for energy

gastrointestinal tract (alimentary tract) the system responsible for ingesting, processing, absorbing, digesting, and eliminating food

gastrostomy (G) tube surgically inserted tube that extends from the surface of the abdomen into the stomach; used for long-term nutritional support

general adaptation syndrome (GAS) a theory of stress and its relationship to disease that encompasses three stages: the initial stage, the alarm stage, and the resistance exhaustion stage

general staff the individuals in charge of each section under the Incident Command System

generalized convulsive status epilepticus (GCSE) the most dangerous type of seizure that results in continual tonic-clonic (severe muscle jerking) activity with no post ictal stage

generic name drug name created by a drug manufacturer to shorten the chemical name or create a variation of it

genetic immunity the immune system's inherited list of known "enemies" and its defense against them

genitourinary system consists of the kidneys, ureters, bladder and urethra; responsible for the elimination of waste products

genitourinary tract the tract made up of several organs including the kidneys, ureters, bladder, urethra, prostate, and testicles

German measles (rubella) disease caused by rubella virus; spread through respiratory droplets; causes low-grade fever, swollen lymph nodes, and generalized rash; now largely preventable by immunization

gerontology the scientific study of the process and problems of aging

gestational diabetes mellitus (GDM) any degree of glucose intolerance with an onset of or first recognition during pregnancy

glans the head of the penis

Glasgow Coma Score (GCS) a quantifiable tool that assesses level of consciousness based on how the patient responds to the environment and external stimuli by evaluating eye, verbal and motor response

glaucoma a group of eye diseases caused by increased intra-ocular pressure that results in gradual visual impairment; the two main types are open angle glaucoma and angle closure glaucoma

glial cell a type of cell that forms the blood-brain barrier

global positioning system (GPS) a satellite-based system that can pinpoint the position of a GPS unit within 100 feet anywhere on earth

globe rupture a rupture of the eye caused by blunt or penetrating trauma

glomerulus the filtering unit of the kidney

glottis the opening to the trachea just under the epiglottis, right above the vocal cords that marks the entrance into the lower airway

glucagon protein hormone that is produced and secreted by the alpha cells of the pancreas; acts on the same cells as insulin, but has opposite effects

glucometer a device that measures glucose blood levels using either capillary blood via a fingerstick or through venous blood obtained during venipuncture

glucometry a method of evaluating blood glucose levels

glycogen a glucose polymer that is used to store glucose in the cells of the body

glycolysis the process where a glucose molecule is broken down into two pyruvate molecules

goiter enlarged, palpable and often visible thyroid gland

Golden Hour the concept of rapid evacuation of critically injured patients from the scene of injury to the trauma center and the provision of definitive emergency and surgical care, now referred to as the "Golden Period"

Golden Period over the years the Golden Hour concept has been changed to refer to a Golden Period rather than one 60 minute hour; it is now recognized that while some patients may have "one hour," others have a shorter time in which to reach definitive care and some may have a longer period of time

gonads male and female reproductive glands (testes and ovaries) that produce and secrete a variety of hormones related to sexual maturation and function

gonorrhea sexually transmitted disease caused by the bacterium *Neisseria gonorrhoeae;* typically affects the genital tract, but can colonize the oropharynx or rectum, or can be disseminated; transmission is through direct contact with the purulent exudates that form on infected mucous membranes

good faith acting honestly and without deception

Good Samaritan Law law that protects anyone (including EMS providers who are not officially on duty) who provides medical assistance

Goodpasture's syndrome an autoimmune disease that creates inflammation of the alveolar-capillary membrane, reducing diffusion

grand mal (tonic-clonic) seizure seizure characterized by several distinct phases: unconsciousness, muscle tensing and spasms, jerking motions, relaxation, slow return to consciousness (post ictal state)

Grave's disease severe form of hyperthyroidism where the thyroid is swollen (it forms a goiter on the anterior surface of the neck), exophthalmos occurs (bulging eyes), and toxic signs of hyperthyroidism are present

gravid pregnant

greenstick fracture a fracture resulting from an angular force applied to a long bone that causes a break in the convex side of the cortex and a bowing of the concave side of the cortex; it may result in a bent deformity of the extremity

gum elastic bougie a device used during a difficult endotracheal intubation; it is placed into the trachea and the endotracheal tube is then inserted over it into the trachea and the bougie is then removed

gumma large painless ulcerations on the skin; can also occur on bone, causing deep, gnawing pain; symptom of tertiary syphilis

H

Haddon's Matrix the matrix that correlates the precrash, crash, and postcrash phases of injury with factors that are potentially changeable

half-life the amount of time it takes for half of the quantity of given drug to be metabolized and eliminated from the body. It serves as the basis of determining when additional doses are required

halo test a test for cerebrospinal fluid performed by placing bloody fluid on filter paper (a coffee filter or a fibrous paper towel) and a "halo" or double ring may be seen as the blood and CSF separate as they dry

Hamman's sign a crunching sound heard with each heart beat as a result of mediastinal emphysema

Hamstrings common name for muscles at the back of the thigh and the tendons on either side of the knees

Hangman's fracture bilateral fractures of the pedicles of the second cervical vertebra

Hantavirus pulmonary syndrome disease caused by virus found in mouse feces; spread when virus is dispersed into air by disturbing mouse droppings; presents with fever, chills, myalgias, cough, abdominal pain, nausea, and vomiting; patients rapidly develop pulmonary pneumonia and hypotension that resembles septic shock

hard palate the structure that runs from the back of the upper teeth posteriorly until it terminates just in front of the posterior pharynx

hazardous material any solid, liquid or gas that when released is capable of harming people, the environment, or property

hazmat hazardous material

Health Insurance Portability and Accountability Act (HIPAA) law that details strict guidelines for patient privacy for both personal and medical information

health the state of being free from illness, disease, and debilitating conditions

healthcare power of attorney a document created by a competent adult to appoint a legal representative to exercise the healthcare decision-making powers specified in the document in the event the patient becomes incapacitated

heart rate (HR) number of cardiac cycles (beats) per minute

heartburn a reflux of gastric contents into the esophagus; also known as gastroesophageal reflux disease (GERD)

heat cramps heat related intermittent muscle cramping, due to dehydration and sodium fluxes; it subsides with IV fluid replacement but it can cause severe pain

heat exhaustion (heat prostration) the condition that results from intravascular volume depletion brought on by heat stress; caused by the same mechanisms as heat cramps, but the electrolyte imbalances are more severe and systemic (vital organ systems are affected); failure to identify the seriousness of the situation and to provide aggressive supportive care may result in severe neurological, cardiopulmonary, or metabolic system collapse

heat stroke a severely elevated core body temperature (more than 40.5°C) and multisystem dysfunction that results when the body's compensatory mechanisms for handling environmental heat stress fail; most serious of all the hyperthermia related injuries; it is life threatening

HEENT abbreviation for **h**ead, **e**ars, **e**yes, **n**ose, and **t**hroat

Heimlich maneuver a first aid procedure for clearing an obstructed airway using abdominal thrusts

Heimlich® valve a commercially available device that is meant to allow for air to exit the chest and designed to then collapse when air tries to reenter into the chest at that site

helibases locations for helicopter operations under the Incident Command System

helispots temporary locations that function as helicopter landing zones under the Incident Command System

HELLP syndrome a complication of pre-eclampsia manifested by hemolysis, elevated liver enzymes, and low platelets that can lead to increased mortality

hemarthrosis blood that accumulates in a joint

hematemesis vomiting bright red blood

hematochezia stools containing frank, undigested blood

hematocrit the measurement of the ratio of red blood cells to plasma fluid

hematology the study of blood

hematoma a localized collection of blood, usually clotted, in an organ, space, or tissue, due to a break in the wall of a blood vessel

hematuria blood in the urine

hemiazygos a vein on the left side of the vertebral column which drains blood from the left ascending lumbar vein to the azygos vein

hemiblock a conduction block in either the anterior or posterior fascicles of the left bundle branch of the Purkinje system of the heart

hemithorax division of the thorax into two sides; each contains one lung

hemodialysis medical procedure that removes blood from a surgically constructed blood vessel, cleansing the blood (by removing metabolic wastes and excess water through a process of filtration, diffusion, osmosis and pressure gradients) with an artificial kidney (the dialysis machine) and returning it to the patient through another peripheral vein or the same surgically created blood vessel

hemodilution an increase in the volume of plasma, resulting in a reduced concentration of red blood cells in blood

hemodynamically unstable a patient with blood pressure less than 90 mmHg or exhibiting clinical signs from low blood pressure

hemolytic anemia a blood disorder in which blood cells are prematurely destroyed

hemophelia a hereditary blood disease in which there is a deficiency of one of the two factors that allow for coagulation or clotting of blood, can cause uncontrolled bleeding

hemopneumothorax the condition where blood and air accumulating inside the pleural space between the chest wall and the lung.

hemoptysis blood in the sputum

hemorrhage the loss of blood from the vascular system that results from a break in blood vessels

hemorrhagic (hypovolemic) shock condition in which there is inadequate blood volume to provide adequate tissue perfusion

hemorrhoids swollen, distended veins in the recto-anal area

hemostasis the process by which bleeding is controlled

hemothorax the accumulation of blood in the pleural space between the chest wall and the lung, usually as a result of injury

hemotypanum bleeding within the middle ear caused by penetrating or blunt trauma, often associated with fracture at the base of the skull, manifested by a bluish discoloration behind the eardrum

hepatic encephalopathy altered mental status from a build up of ammonia in the blood as a result of chronic liver disease

hepatitis A most common form of viral liver infection in the United States comprising almost half of all cases of hepatitis; virus is transmitted by the fecal-oral route and has an incubation period of approximately 28 days

hepatitis B comprises one-third of all cases of viral liver infection in the United States; transmitted through the parenteral route with an incubation period of 12 weeks

hepatitis B virus (HBV) one of several unrelated viral species which cause viral liver infection

hepatitis C accounts for 15% of cases of viral liver infection each year; transmission is through the parenteral route, but is far more virulent than Hepatitis B

hepatitis inflammation or infection of the liver

hepatocyte a liver cell

hepatorenal syndrome combined liver and renal failure of unclear cause

herbalism the study and use of plant-based and mineral-based remedies

hernia a protrusion of an abdominal organ through an opening in the abdominal wall; femoral, inguinal, and umbilical hernias are common types

herniation condition in which an organ is pushed or squeezed through an opening in its usual container, most commonly refers to the brain being squeezed through the tentorium or the base of the skull

herpes simplex virus type 1 (HSV1) causes painful blisters, also called cold sores, on the lips, face, and oropharynx

herpes simplex virus type 2 (HSV2) sexually transmitted disease that is genetically similar to HSV1; causes painful genital lesions; transmission is through close contact

heuristic any strategy or technique that helps direct attention and focus while thinking; see also representativeness heuristic, availability heuristic, and anchoring heuristic

hiatal hernia protrusion of the stomach up through the esophageal hiatus in the diaphragm

hiccough a spasm of the diaphragm that is a modified form of respiration

high-altitude cerebral edema (HACE) syndrome that includes ataxia, severe headache, nausea and vomiting, altered mentation, seizures, and, finally, coma in patients who have ascended to altitude (usually greater than 8000 feet elevation)

high-altitude pulmonary edema (HAPE) syndrome that includes dyspnea at rest, cough, fatigue, headache, anorexia, cyanosis, rales, tachypnea, and tachycardia in patients who have ascended to altitude (usually greater than 8000 feet elevation)

high-density lipoprotein (HDL) the "good cholesterol"

high-grade 2nd degree AV block occurs when two or more consecutive atrial beats fail to reach the ventricles due to an obstruction

high-risk pregnancy a pregnancy in which certain predisposing factors or complications increase the likelihood of jeopardizing the successful carrying of the pregnancy; factors include alcohol or substance abuse, chronic illness, gestational diabetes or hypertension, maternal age

hindsight the tendency to see past events as being predictable for future outcomes

histamine a substance that causes dilation of blood vessels, increased vascular permeability (which causes edema), bronchospasm, increased mucus production and contraction of the smooth muscle in the intestinal tract, often released as a result of allergic reaction

history of present illness (HPI) gathering of information from the patient concerning symptoms through an interview process to aid in developing a diagnosis

histrionics melodramatic or hysterical behavior

holistic therapies therapies that focus on the mind-body connection and recognize that disease is an imbalance that includes both psychoemotional and physiological components

hollow visceral organs the organs of the abdomen that comprise the intestinal tract

Holter monitors portable ECG machines used to record the heart rhythm of a patient over a period of time, usually 24 hours

home health aids (HHA) trained individuals who assist healthcare professionals such as nurses with the care of patients in the home care setting

home healthcare caring for chronically ill patients in their home by family, support network, and/or paid caregivers

homeopathy the study and use of substances designed to illicit and amplify the symptoms produced by the body's own immune response to help the body fight disease

homeostasis the process of constant regulation the body requires in order to remain in balance and stay alive

hormones chemicals produced by living cells that circulate in the blood to signal organs and tissues to release other chemicals or affect processes and systems

hospice a coordinated program providing palliative care to terminally ill patients and supportive services to patients, their families, and significant others 24 hours a day, 7 days a week

hot zone (exclusion zone) the area of contamination in a hazmat situation into which no one should enter unless wearing appropriate PPE

huffing deliberate inhalation of hydrocarbons to produce intoxication; holding a piece of clothing soaked in a volatile substance and breathing through it

human immunodeficiency virus (HIV) virus that infects and compromises the function of the T white blood cells that are responsible for mediating the immune response

human papilloma virus (HPV) over 100 types of viruses that cause genital warts; some types cause cervical cancer

humerus the long bone in the upper arm

humoral immunity an immune response that responds to antigens such as bacteria and foreign tissue; it is the result of the development and continued presence of circulating antibodies

hydrolysis the splitting of the bonds holding ATP together and adding a water molecule

hydrophobia fear of drinking water

hydrostatic pressure the pressure exerted by a liquid

hydroxycobalamine a cyanide antidote recently approved for use in the U.S

hymenoptera bees and wasps

hyoid bone bone in the anterior part of the neck, it is the only bone that does not articulate directly with another bone in the body

hypercalcemia increased calcium levels; can be caused by several disorders, including hyperparathyroidism, malignancy, and certain medications

hypercapnic (or ventilation) failure a type of respiratory failure that occurs as the result of increased carbon dioxide levels within the blood

hypercarbia condition of excess carbon dioxide in the blood

hypercarbic respiratory drive the dominant stimulus for breathing in a healthy person that comes from an increase in carbon dioxide triggering a respiratory cycle

hyperemesis gravidarum (morning sickness) nausea and vomiting in pregnancy that lasts excessively long, throughout the entire pregnancy or is severely pronounced and interferes with normal daily functioning

hyperglycemia elevation of the blood glucose level

hyperkalemia the accumulation of potassium in the body that can result in skeletal muscle weakness and cardiac arrest

hyperlipidemia an increased cholesterol level in the blood; a significant risk for CAD

hypermagnesemia excessive magnesium in the bloodstream; more common in patients with chronic renal disease or rhabdomyolysis

hypernatremia increased sodium level

hyperosmolar hyperglycemic nonketotic syndrome (HHNS) severe hyperglycemia in diabetic patients in which the blood sugar often exceeds 600 mg/dl and electrolyte imbalances occur; also called hyperosmolar hyperglycemic state (HHS) or hyperosmolar hyperglycemic nonketotic syndrome (HHNS)

hyperpnea a rapid respiratory rate

hyperpyrexia a core temperature greater than 41°C

hypersensitivity abnormal exaggerated response to an antigen

hypertension high blood pressure

hyperthyroidism occurs from an overactive thyroid gland; patients tend to be younger with multiorgan involvement; subset of thyrotoxicosis, which is caused by excess synthesis and secretion of thyroid hormone by the thyroid

hypertonic saline (HTS) a concentrated intravenous solution that pulls fluid into the vascular space via its osmotic effect, as opposed to normal saline where a great deal of it is lost out of the blood vessels by the same process

hyperventilating breathing too fast leading to an imbalance in the CO_2 level, resulting in dizziness

hyperventilation an increased rate of artificial ventilation; indicated for patients with evidence of brain herniation due to increased ICP

hyperventilation syndrome a rapid respiratory rate (hyperpnea) or a condition resulting in the lowering of $PaCO_2$ levels producing mild respiratory alkalosis and symptoms such

(continued)

as perioral tingling, numbness and tingling of the fingers and toes, and carpo-pedal spasm

hypervolemia an excessive amount of circulating blood volume resulting in pulmonary edema, hypertension, or other problems

hyphema an injury to the anterior chamber of the eye that disrupts the vessels resulting in bleeding; when the quantity is significant enough the blood tends to form a layer and gravity will cause it to pool and level when the patient is sitting upright

hypocalcemia low calcium levels; caused by the impaired ability to mobilize calcium from bone stores, abnormal binding of calcium, abnormal losses from kidneys, or the decreased absorption of calcium from the intestines

hypochondriac region the left and right lateral sections of the abdomen

hypodermis subcutaneous tissue that lies directly under the dermis

hypogastric region (suprapubic region) the section of the abdomen just below the periumbilical region and just superior to the symphysis pubis

hypoglycemia low blood sugar; involves a glucose level that is inadequate to effectively fuel the body's blood cells

hypokalemia low potassium, can result from a variety of causes, including renal or GI losses, inadequate diet, transcellular shift (movement of potassium from serum into cells), and the ingestion of certain medications

hypomagnesemia magnesium deficiency; caused by a variety of conditions that increase magnesium losses or shift the electrolyte balance, including renal disease and diuretic therapy, hyperthyroidism, pancreatitis, diabetes, parathyroid gland disorders, and diarrhea

hyponatremia low sodium level; can occur by itself or as a complication of other conditions; becomes clinically significant when it results in a reduction in serum osmolality

hypoperfusion inadequate perfusion; shock

hypopharynx the area at the back of the tongue where the opening of the gastrointestinal tract, called the esophagus, and the opening of the trachea meet

hypoproteinemia a decrease in blood protein levels

hypotension reduced arterial blood pressure

hypotensive condition in which individual has diminished perfusion to organs

hypothalamic-pituitary-adrenomedullary (HPA) axis refers to a complex set of direct influences and feedback interactions between the hypothalamus, a hollow, funnel-shaped part of the brain; the pituitary gland, a pea-shaped structure located below the hypothalamus; and the adrenal or suprarenal gland, a small, paired, pyramidal organ located at the top of each kidney

hypothalamus part of the brain; secretes hormones that stimulate or suppress the release of hormones in the pituitary gland; influences water balance, sleep, temperature, appetite, and blood pressure

hypothermia condition that occurs when the body's core temperature drops below 35°C; infants and children are especially prone to hypothermia; primary hypothermia is usually the result of an environmental exposure; secondary hypothermia occurs in patients with with a predisposing illness, frailty, or intoxication

hypothyroidism an endocrine-mediated disease process that involves diminished function of the thyroid gland

hypoventilation a decreased rate or depth of ventilation

hypovolemia low circulating blood volume

hypovolemic shock widespread hypoperfusion resulting from decreased intravascular (blood) volume

hypoxemia a low level of oxygen in the blood

hypoxia a low oxygen state; also used to describe the condition of insufficient oxygen delivery to body tissues

hypoxic drive a drop in oxygen levels that signals the patient's brain to take another breath; patients with chronic lung diseases such as emphysema switch respiratory control from CO_2 levels (hypercarbic) to O_2 levels (hypoxic)

I

iatrogenic caused by medical treatment

ictus (seizure) a temporary disruption in normal neuronal activity resulting in abnormal repetitive and synchronous firing (action potentials) of neurons in the brain

idiopathic unknown cause

ileostomy a surgical opening into the small intestine, also a surgical diversion procedure designed to collect waste products from the ileum

ileum the final section of the small intestine

iliac (inguinal) the left and right lower sections of the abdomen

iliac crest lateral bony ridge that is a landmark of the pelvis

immediately dangerous to life and health (IDLH) concentration of a toxin that causes immediate threat to life

immersion foot (trench foot) a nonfreezing injury from prolonged contact with cold water; can result in loss of soft tissues and infection

immersion syndrome sudden death upon submersion in very cold water (at least 5°C lower than body temperature)

immunity protection for the patient from foreign invaders to the immune system

immunity provisions laws that protect paramedics for acts of ordinary negligence, or for acts or omissions done in good faith (often called Good Samaritan laws)

immunocompetent persons with fully functional immune systems

immunoglobulin a purified solution of antibodies from a person or animal that has been infected with a specific disease

immunoglobulin E (IgE) an antibody

immunosupressed or immunodeficient people whose immune systems are not fully functional; they are less able to fight off infection

immunotolerance the process by which the body's immune system is coded to consider the molecules of "self" as friendly cells and to tolerate and not harm them

impact munitions weapons that are meant to strike and incapacitate a person without killing or causing serious bodily harm; rubber bullets and bean bags are examples

impaling injuries injuries generally caused by low-velocity penetrating force; damage is usually limited to the structures located along the object's pathway into and out of the body

impedance threshold device a device that will resist the flow of air from moving into the airway for a tiny instant, creating a few centimeters of water of negative pressure within the airway as the chest recoils which improves circulation of blood into the atria

impingement pinching

implied consent the concept that patients who are ill or injured and, for any reason unable to give consent (unconscious, incapacitated, minors, etc.), would consent to the delivery of emergency health care necessitated by their condition

In SAD CAGES mnemonic for remembering the classic elements of depression: interest, sleep, appetite, depressed mood, concentration, activity, guilt, energy, and suicide

incident action plan (IAP) an oral or written plan containing the general objectives that reflects the overall strategy of managing an incident under the Incident Command System

incident command post (ICP) the location where the IC oversees all incident operations under the Incident Command System

Incident Command System (ICS) an incident management system that utilizes common and consistent terminology, a chain of command, and flexible structure; formal incident management system approved by the approved by the National Incident Management System (NIMS)

incident commander (IC) the person with overall responsibility for managing an incident under the Incident Command System; the only position always staffed in every incident

incompetent patients who are not capable of making decisions that would represent their best interest

incomplete fracture fracture that involves only one side of the bone

incomplete neurologic lesion sensory, motor, or both functions that are partially present below the neurologic level of injury

incubation phase of infection period between initial infection and the onset of symptoms

indication the reason a drug is given

infant baby from the time of birth until the child has reached the first birthday

infection occurs when a pathogen invades a body and begins reproducing; not every infection causes disease; many infections are cleared by the immune system before they ever cause symptoms

infectious diseases diseases caused by various pathogens or disease-causing agents such as viruses, bacteria, and fungi

inferior term meaning toward the feet

inferior (lowest) concha a shelf of bone within the nares

inferior myocardial infarction myocardial infarction that is the result of blockage of the right coronary artery involving the right ventricle

inferior vena cava the large vein that carries deoxygenated blood from the lower half of the body into the heart

infestation presence of a parasite

inflammation pathologic process that develops when the body is injured; signs include swelling, redness, and heat; the process leads to healing

inflammatory bowel disease (IBD) disease that consists of two chronic intestinal disorders: ulcerative colitis and Crohn's disease

inflammatory response the phase in healing that creates an environment for the repair to begin

influenza disease caused by influenza virus; spread through respiratory droplets; symptoms include fever, runny nose, cough, body aches, and nausea

informed consent a legal condition whereby patients can give consent based upon an appreciation and understanding of the facts and implications of an action. Individuals needs to be in possession of all of his faculties, such as not being mentally retarded or mentally ill and without an impairment of judgment at the time of consenting. Such impairments might include illness, intoxication, drunkenness, using drugs, insufficient sleep, and other health problems

informed refusal a legal condition whereby a person can refuse case based upon an appreciation and understanding of the facts and implications of an action. The individual needs to be in possession of all of his faculties, such as not being mentally retarded or mentally ill and without an impairment of judgment at the time of consenting. Such impairments might include illness, intoxication, drunkenness, using drugs, insufficient sleep, and other health problems

ingestion introduction of drugs and other substances to the body by swallowing or eating so the drug enters the bloodstream by absorption from the gastrointestinal tract

inguinal (iliac) the left and right lower sections of the abdomen

inguinal hernia a hernia that occurs in the inguinal or groin region

inhalation anthrax disease caused by breathing in aerosolized *B. anthracis;* symptoms are flu-like, with fever, chills, myalgias, and cough followed by respiratory failure

inhalation the process by which air (as well as other chemicals and biologicals) enter the body through the respiratory system

inhibit to prevent something

initial assessment the primary survey to detect and treat any problems threatening the airway, breathing, and perfusion status

initial isolation distance the safe perimeter to which all persons should be evacuated

injection the process by which a chemical can enter the body via a needle or through a punctured place on the skin into an underlying structure such as the vascular system, muscle, bone, organ, joint or other tissue or structure

in-line manual stabilization manually maintaining the cervical spine in a neutral in-line position

inner ear internal structure of the ear containing the receptors for hearing

inner ear barotrauma (IEBT) the result of the development of negative pressure in the middle ear if a diver is unable to equalize pressure during descent; sudden equilibration of pressure in the middle ear or a vigorous Valsalva maneuver may rupture the round window and may cause hemorrhage into the inner ear or tearing of the labyrinthine (Reissner's) membrane

inotropic effect refers to the strength of the cardiac contraction; a cardiac property

insensitive a test that is not accurate as a predictor of illness or injury

inspection using sight to locate findings during a physical examination

inspiratory capacity (IC) a respiratory measurement determined by adding the inspiratory reserve volume and tidal volume together

inspiratory positive airway pressure (IPAP) pressure level that is maintained during the inspiratory phase

inspiratory reserve volume (IRV) the measure of additional air drawn into the lungs forcibly following a normal inhalation

institutional abuse abuse of the elderly who live in institutions, such as nursing homes or other healthcare facilities, by paid staff, caregivers, or other residents

insulin produced by the beta cells of the pancreas; is required by almost all of the body's cells; major targets include the liver, fat cells, and muscle cells; has several key functions: stimulates the liver and muscle cells to store glucose in glycogen and create proteins; a key element for glucose to enter the cell

integumentary system the skin, nails, sweat glands, and sebaceous glands

interatrial pathway part of the conduction system of the heart that facilitates conduction to the left atria; also called Bachmann's bundle

internal acoustic meatus a canal in the temporal bone of the skull that carries nerves from inside the cranium towards the middle and inner ear compartments

internal contamination when radioactive materials move through a "portal of entry" (e.g., mouth, nose, eyes, wounds or other skin breaks)

internal ear a series of cavities between the middle ear and the internal acoustic meatus

internal oblique muscle muscles that lie beneath the external oblique muscles of the abdominal wall

interneurons the cells that carry electrical signals from one neuron to another

internodal pathways part of the conduction system of the heart where impulses from the sinus node are moved quickly to the atrioventricular (AV) node and junction

interstitial space the space that surrounds all cells and is the location for transport of materials across cell walls

interventricular septum the wall separating the lower chambers (ventricles) of the heart from one another

intervertebral foramina spaces created by adjacent vertebrae through which pass the nerves that go to various parts of the body (nerve roots); also referred to as neuroforamina

intervertebral located between the vertebrae

intimate partner violence (IPV) violence and abuse between intimate partners; similar to domestic violence

intracellular fluid (ICF) the water found inside cells; it makes up approximately 40% of the total body weight with the greatest amount of water in the intracellular compartment found within the skeletal muscle mass

intracerebral bleeding (intraparenchymal hemorrhage) bleeding within the brain

intracranial hemorrhage any bleeding that occurs within the skull, may be epidural, subdural, subarachnoid, or intracerebral

intracranial pressure (ICP) the amount of pressure within the skull; normal ICP is 0-15 mmHg

intramuscular (IM) injection given directly into a muscle

intraocular pressure (IOP) the fluid pressure inside the eye

intraparenchymal hemorrhage (IPH) (intracerebral bleeding) bleeding within the brain

intrapartum factors variables that occur during labor or the birthing process

intraperitoneal structures the structures that are found inside the peritoneum, including the liver, spleen, stomach, small bowel (with the exception of the duodenum), colon, gallbladder, and female reproductive organs

intravenous (IV) within a vein; the route that allows direct placement of drugs into the blood stream for rapid circulation

intubation a common method for securing the airway that involves the introduction of a plastic tube into the trachea through the mouth or nose

intussusception when a length of intestine slips into an adjacent portion; usually produces an obstruction

ionic drugs with an electrical charge in their atomic structure

ionized the gain or loss of electrically charged particles (protons or electrons)

iris the colored part of the eye

irregular rhythm on ECG, when the difference between the shortest R-R and the longest R-R interval is greater than 0.16 sec (4 small boxes)

irregularly irregular rhythms cardiac rhythms that have no predictable pattern to their irregularity

irreversible shock final stage of shock; resuscitative efforts will be unsuccessful

irritability the abnormal ability or increased sensitivity to respond to external stimuli; increased irritability in cardiac cells results in dysrhythmias

ischemia hypoxia; lack of oxygen due to poor circulation or as failure of ventilation or diffusion

ischemic (pressure) ulcer an ulcer that develops in areas with a lack of blood flow usually due to pressure preventing adequate circulation

ischemic phase condition that occurs as tissue blood flow decreases due to peripheral vasoconstriction and hypovolemia and tissues do not receive adequate amounts of oxygen

ischemic strokes neurologic impairment as a result of obstruction of blood flow in vessels supplying the brain

islets of Langerhans the endocrine portion of the pancreas and the source of insulin and glucagon

isoelectric line the flatline, or baseline on the ECG

isolated septal infarctions rare infarction involving only the septum of the ventricles

isolette a specially sized bed that is heated and has full neonate access for monitoring and performing procedures

isthmus the narrow band of tissue that connects two lobes of tissue

J

J point on ECG, the point at which the S wave ends, a common landmark to use to determine ST elevation on depression

jargon a hybrid language of technical terminology characteristic of a special activity or group

jaundice a yellowing of the skin, sclera, and other tissues due to excess circulating bilirubin

Jefferson fracture injury where the ring of C1 verte-bra is pushed down on C2 resulting in a break in the ring of C1

Jejunum the central of the three divisions of the small intestine and lies between the duodenum and the ileum

job stress the harmful physical and emotional responses that occur when requirements of the job do not match the capabilities, resources, or needs of the worker

Joint Commission on Accreditation of Healthcare Organizations (JCAHO) a U.S. based nonprofit organization formed in 1951 with a mission to maintain and elevate the standards of healthcare delivery through evaluation and accreditation of healthcare organizations

joule the unit of energy in the meter-kilogram-second system

jugular vein distension (JVD) engorgement of the jugular vein visible as a rope-like appearance of the vein on the neck

jumpSTART triage a pediatric adaptation of the START triage method

junctional escape rhythm the AV junction serving as the secondary pacemaker in the event of failure of the SA node; typically the rate is between 40–60 (the inherent rate for the AV note) and cardiac output may be compromised

junctional tachycardia identifies any rhythm originating from the A-V junction at a rate greater than 100 beats per minute

justice the quality of being fair; especially regarding allocating proper healthcare resources to patients

K

keep the vein open (KVO) or TKO (to keep open) to administer fluids at low maintenance rate with the intent of maintain an unclotted line but minimize the volume of fluid given to the patient

Kehr's sign referred pain to the shoulder caused by injuries to organs that result in bleeding that irritates the diaphragm

keratinized hardened skin

keraunoparalysis (Charcot's paralysis) "lightning paraplegia" characterized by the victim's inability to move the extremities; accompanied by cool, pale skin, and diminished peripheral pulses after being struck by lightning

Kernig's sign an inability to extend the knee when the hip is flexed to 90 degrees due to irritation of the meninges; symptom of meningitis

ketoacidosis a metabolic condition that results from the deficiency or lack of insulin; fats and proteins are broken down resulting in acidosis and ketosis

kidney stones stones that form when crystals precipitate out from urine and build up on the inner surfaces of the kidney or its collecting system

kidneys organs that excrete urine

Kiesselbach's plexus site along the anterior and superior aspect of the nasal septum where numerous arteries that supply the nasal mucosa converge; a common site for many anterior nose bleeds to occur

kinematics the mechanism or science of trauma and what the forces of energy do to the body

kinetic energy a property of a moving object or particle that depends on its motion and also on its mass (size)

kissing disease (mononucleosis) disease caused by the Epstein-Barr virus (EBV); frequently transmitted by kissing; causes sore throat, swollen tonsils, fever, and swollen lymph nodes

Koplik's spots small white spots on the mucous membranes of the mouth; symptom of measles (rubeola)

Korotkoff sounds the arterial pressure sounds heard when a stethoscope is applied over the brachial artery during blood pressure measurement; used to determine the systolic and diastolic blood pressure readings

Korsakoff amnesic state (Korsakoff psychosis) a unique mental disorder in which retentive memory is impaired out of proportion to all other cognitive functions in an otherwise alert and responsive patient associated with cronic alcohol use

Krebs cycle the metabolic process where pyruvate is converted through a series of steps into a variety of different compounds resulting in the formation of ATP

Kussmaul's respiration fast and deep respiration without any periods of apnea, commonly associated with diabetic ketoacidosis

Kussmaul's signs elevated jugular venous pressure and pulsus paradoxus seen during inspiration

kyphosis a curvature of the spine that causes the patient to appear hunched or stooped forward

L

lacrimal duct the tear duct

lacrimal glands oval, almond structures located superior and lateral to the eye that secrete tears

lactic acidosis condition that occurs when the ability of the body to process lactate becomes overwhelmed, resulting in metabolic acidosis

lacunar infarcts small areas of brain destruction, usually related to microemboli

lancet a needle-like device that pricks the finger of the patient so a drop of blood can be obtained, usually for the glucometer

Laplace's Law the law that states that the pressure within a spherical structure with surface tension is inversely proportional to the radius of the sphere

laryngeal mask airway (LMA) a device inserted to assist ventilation of the patient whose level of conscious is such that a large device in the posterior hypopharynx and supraglottic area can be tolerated

laryngopharynx the lowest part of the upper airway

laryngospasm when the vocal cords go into spasm, becoming tight and closing off the airway

laryngotracheitis (croup) an infection of the tissues within and below the larynx

larynx the organ of voice production; the part of the respiratory tract between the pharynx and the trachea; also known as the voicebox

latent stage of infection occurs when the infectious agent is present, reproducing, but causes no signs or symptoms

lateral anatomic term meaning away from the midline

lateral horns projections on each side of the midline of the spinal cord

lateral recumbent anatomic term meaning lying on the side; record which side, left or right

lateral ventricles two curved shaped cavities located within the cerebrum, filled with cerebrospinal fluid

lateral wall ischemia or infarctions involve the circumflex coronary artery, and like the septal wall infarction, the isolated lateral wall infarction is rare

latex a natural rubber product derived from tree sap, a common cause of allergy

latissimus dorsi a triangular, flat muscle that covers the lumbar region and the lower half of the thoracic region

leachate hazardous material that carries soluble toxic materials through the soil and potentially into public water source

LEAPS mnemonic used to practice good communication skills: listen, empathize, ask, paraphrase, and summarize

LeFort fractures injury to bones on both sides of the face; classified as LeFort I, II, or III, depending on the location of the zygoma (cheekbones) and maxilla fractures

left anterior descending arteries (LAD) one of two branches of the left main coronary artery, the LAD provides oxygen to septum and left ventricular walls of the heart

left main coronary artery one of two major vessels arising from the aorta that divides into the left anterior descending (LAD) and circumflex arteries

legal blindness uncorrectable visual acuity of 20/200 or greater

legal capacity the legal age of majority for a given state or jurisdiction

legal guardian typically someone with court-appointed authority or other authority recognized under the law to make decisions for a minor or incapacitated patient

lens the eye structure that focuses images and light onto the retina

lesion a wound, injury, abnormality or pathologic change in body tissues

lethal dose (LD) concentration or dose of a toxin that results in death of a defined percentage of test subjects

leukotrienes substances that cause dilation of blood vessels, increased vascular permeability (which causes edema), bronchospasm, increased mucous production and contraction of the smooth muscle in the intestinal tract

levator scapulae a muscle situated at the back and side of the neck

level I trauma center regional trauma center located in large urban center; has 24/7 in-house capability for managing all aspects of trauma

level II trauma center area wide centers at large community hospitals equipped to handle the most common types of injuries 24/7; may refer complex injuries and specialty patients to level I centers

level III trauma center center at a local community hospital equipped to stabilize and treat common injuries; has limited surgical capabilities and limited specialists; transfers more complex injury to level II or I centers

level of consciousness (LOC) degree of a patient's ability to respond assessed through a series of questions and tests

Levine sign classic chest pain gesture of patients demonstrating a clenched fist over their chest when asked to describe what they are feeling

Lewisite a toxic vesicant (blister agent) that is rapidly absorbed by the eyes, skin, and lungs

liaison officer the person that serves as the primary contact for supporting agencies assisting in an incident under the Incident Command System

lice insects that infest human skin—head, body, and pubic area.; transmitted by close contact with infested person, clothing, or bedding; symptoms include intense itching caused by bites

licensed practical nurses (LPN) provide patient care to the sick and the injured, as well as the physically and mentally disabled; some of their responsibilities include obtaining vital signs, administering injections, administering certain medications, applying and changing dressings, and assisting the patient with their ADLs

licensed vocational nurse (LVN) an entry-level nurse who provides basic nursing care under the direction of a physician or a registered nurse

licensure a recognized authority grants permission to an individual to engage in a business or occupation that would be otherwise unlawful

ligament of Treitz the suspensory ligament of the duodenum

ligaments bands of connective tissue that support joints by attaching bone to bone

ligamentum arteriosum a piece of fibrous tissue that is a remnant of the embryological circulatory system; it tethers the aortic arch to the pulmonary artery outflow tract

ligand a group of cells, ions, or molecules that connects to a central atom in a complex of cells or tissues; an ion or molecule that is a component of a larger substance

lighted stylet a light wand inserted into an endotracheal tube used to assist in proper placement of the ET tube

limbic system the part of the brain that controls emotional responses

line of demarcation the line between areas of positive and negative findings

lipid an oily fat

liver the organ that secretes bile to digest fats; also detoxifies many substances

Locard's Principle the principle named for Dr. Edmond Locard (a historical authority of investigative science) that in the EMS realm means for every scene entered and for every patient cared for, paramedics will leave their mark (important for evidence preservation)

long backboard carrying device used for trauma patients who have sustained falls, were struck by motor vehicles, assaults to the head, neck, or spine by either blunt force trauma, or penetrating trauma

long term beta two agonist mediation that provides continuous protection against an asthma attack by stimulating the Beta-two receptor site

Longitudinal Emergency Medical Technician Attributes and Demographics Study (LEADS) conducted annually, this study seeks to define and describe the make up of the EMS profession; includes profiles of the people in EMS and examines their working conditions

loose leads common artifact on ECG related to leads that are not in good contact with the skin

Los Angeles Prehospital Stroke Screen (LAPSS) a stroke screening tool

low-density lipoprotein (LDL) "bad cholesterol"

lower airway that position of the airway from below the larynx to the alveoli; the respiratory exchange of oxygen and carbon dioxide occurs here

lower urinary tract infection (UTI) a bladder infection

Lown-Ganong-Levine syndrome condition that produces shortened PR intervals and is also capable of producing PSVT although the slurred QRS (delta wave) is usually not seen; less common cause of preexcitiation syndromes than WPW

LPN licensed practical nurse

LVN licensed vocational nurse

lucid interval period of time when a patient awakens from unconsciousness with little to no signs of obvious damage after which the patient becomes unconscious again, commonly associated with epidural hematoma

Ludwig's angina condition in which the area under the tongue can become infected with bacteria and possibly obstruct the airway

lumbar region the left and right middle sections of the abdomen

lumbar spine the five vertebra below the thoracic spine

lumen opening, or space, within a needle, ET tube, artery, vein, or other hollow vessel

Lund and Browder Chart the most accurate tool for estimating burn size and the standard tool utilized in burn centers in the U.S.

luteinizing hormone (LH) hormone that targets the sex organs

luxation the complete dislocation of a joint

Lyme disease caused by the bacteria *Borrelia burgdorferi;* spreads to humans through bites of the deer tick; earliest sign is erythema migrans at site of tick bite; later signs include nervous system involvement

lymphocytes type of white blood cells

lyse cut

lysis cell destruction

M

macrophage type of white blood cell that is essential to the healing process

macular degeneration causes blurred vision and loss of central vision

MADFOCS mnemonic for possible causes of altered behavior: memory deficits, activity, distortions, feelings, orientation, cognition, some other findings

Magill forceps a scissor-like device that has a flattened open circle at the tips, used to remove aspirated foreign bodies

mainstem bronchi the right and left air passages formed after the trachea divides

malaise a generalized feeling of discomfort

malicious poisonings uncommon, intentional poisoning of another individual

Mallampati classification classification that is helpful in determining if an airway may be difficult to intubate; it requires patients' cooperation as patients are asked to open their mouth, stick out their tongue and say "Ahhhh"

Mallory-Weiss syndrome a tear of the esophagus after vomiting that often results in hematemesis

malpractice professional negligence that causes injury

malpractice insurance insurance coverage where the insurer (provided it is given prompt notice of the claim) is obligated to provide a defense for the organization's paramedics in an allegation of negligence

mammalian dive reflex a reflex triggered by cold water stimulating receptors in the skin; vasoconstriction then shunts blood away from the skin, mesentery, and extremities toward the brain and heart; bradycardia results from vagal nerve stimulation in response to the increased central blood volume

mandible the jaw bone

manual suction a device that removes fluids romitus, or blood when mechanical suction devices are unavailable or nonfunctional

manubrium the smaller upper portion of the sternum

manufacturer's safety data sheets (MSDS) standard sheet that has ingredient information and may have some initial treatment suggestions for poisonings, and is produced by the manufacturer of common products; employers are required to maintain copies of the MSDS for products used in the workplace;

march (stress) fracture a break in a bone caused by repetitive, long-term, or abnormal stress such as seen with soldiers on long marches

mass casualty incident an emergency incident in which the number of patients and the severity of their injuries exceed the capacity of area medical systems and facilities

MAST (military antishock trousers) a pants-like, inflatable device to treat hemorrhagic shock

mast cells part of the immune system, cells containing granules with heparin, serotonin, bradykinin and histamine which are released in response to injury or infection

mastication breaking up of food by the teeth

maxilla bone of the upper jaw

mean arterial pressure (MAP) the average, over time, of the difference between the systolic blood pressure and the diastolic blood pressure; obtained by weighting the averages to account for normal pressure changes occurring on a continual basis; also the average pressure in elastic arteries, which drives blood flow

measles (rubeola) disease caused by measles virus; spread through respiratory droplets; causes fever, a red bumpy rash, and Koplik's spots in the mouth, no longer common in the U.S. as a result of immunization

mechanical suction a device that removes fluids, blood, romitus, and debris from the airway or other body cavity

mechanical ventilator a machine that allows for a specific concentration of oxygen to be warmed and humidified and delivered in a specific volume to patients who are not able to breathe on their own, or have an impaired ability to breathe in a manner that will sustain them

mechanism of injury (MOI) the nature of forces that injured a patient

meconium the material that makes up an infant's first stools; occasionally passed while in utero; meconium-stained amniotic fluids are indicative of a compromised baby (fetal distress)

medial anatomic term meaning toward the midline

medial malleolus the prominence at the medial aspect of the ankle bone

median effective dose (ED$_{50}$) a drug dose that is calculated through observing for the desired effects for 50% of the patients taking the drug

median lethal dose (LD$_{50}$) a drug dose that measures the point where half of the animals die with a given dose

mediastinal structures the structures in the center part of the chest, between the two lungs

mediastinum the space between the lungs that houses the heart, great vessels, esophagus, thoracic duct, and some major nerves including the phrenic and the vagus

medical asepsis technique used to help assure that the medical environment is kept free of pathogens to reduce contamination and infection

medical durable power of attorney a document created by a competent adult to appoint a legal representative to exercise the medical decision-making powers specified in the document once the patient is incapacitated

medically clean handling sterile equipment in such a way as to prevent contamination

medulla oblongata the part of the brain that is a continuation of the spinal cord; it extends from the foramen magnum of the skull up to the pons; it controls respiration and cardiac activity

megoblastic anemia blood disorder characterized by the production of large dysfunctional red blood cells

melanin the substance that gives skin its pigmentation

melena black or tarry stools resulting from the presence of digested blood

membrane threshold the point at which enough sodium gates have opened to start the massive influx of sodium into a cell

memory B cells the white blood cells that do not secrete antibodies, but remember the antigen and the defensive measures required for future attacks

menarche the first menstrual cycle; happens, on average, for girls between the ages of 12 and 13 years

meninges membranous protective layers that surround the brain and spinal cord

meningismus the physical findings of meningeal irritation, manifested by nuchal rigidity, Kernig's sign, and Brudzinski's sign; symptoms of meningitis

meningitis inflammation or infection of the meninges; a medical emergency seen in people of all ages and caused by bacterial, viral, and other organisms; the bacterial form can be life threatening and is a major cause of death and disability in children worldwide

meningococcus most virulent and dangerous agent that causes meningitis; bacterium *Neisseria meningitides*

menopause the cessation of menses; happens between the ages of 45–52 years on average

menorrhagia a large amount, >80 mL, or prolonged duration, >7 days, of menstrual bleeding

menstrual cycle occurs every month during a woman's reproductive years; the ovary prepares to release an egg and a system of hormonal preparations are undertaken to increase the potential for successful pregnancy; if fertilization does not occur, the cycle ends in menstruation

menstrual period the time interval during the menstrual cycle when the lining of the uterus sloughs off

mental capacity an assessment of the patients mental ability (or disability) for decision-making that takes into account any physiologic compromise from injury or illness; it is typically documented as level of consciousness along with orientation to the surroundings

mental illness the general term for any form of psychiatric disorder

mesencephalon (midbrain) a short section of the brainstem between the diencephalon and pons; controls eye movements and motor coordination

mesenteric ischemia a condition where the vascular supply to the bowel provided by the mesenteric artery or vein is compromised and the bowel is not receiving enough oxygen

metabolic acidosis results from production of acids; may be the result of vomiting, diarrhea, diabetes, and certain medication use; develops when there is a build up of acid

metabolic alkalosis results from acid loss or alkali gain; may be associated with the use of diuretics

metabolic shock hypoperfusion resulting from toxic disruption of cellular function

metabolic syndrome a condition resulting from the combination of abdominal obesity, hypertension, diabetes, and hyperlipidemia

metabolism a term that includes all of the chemical reactions that take place in an organism

metastasis the process of cancer cell migration

methylxanthine a class of medication to which aminophylline, theophylline, and caffeine belong, used for the treatment of asthma/COPD

microemboli microscopic blood clots

microporous polysaccharide hemosphere (MPH) a compound (sold as TraumaDEX™) that absorbs water and other inactive substances in blood, which then concentrates the clotting factors that are present in a wound to stop bleeding

microthrombosis small blood clots forming and blocking blood vessels

midbrain (mesencephalon) a short section of the brainstem between the diencephalon and pons; controls eye movements and motor coordination

middle cerebral artery (MCA) stroke a stroke of the brain that produces hemiparesis of the opposite side and face; may produce a syndrome known as "neglect"

middle concha a shelf of bone within the nares

middle ear a cavity in the temporal bone that contains the 3 bones that convert sound waves into electrical impulses for hearing

middle ear barotrauma (MEBT) condition that occurs during diving descent when gas-filled structures such as the ear have a tendency to be "squeezed" into half their volume

midsagittal plane the plane that passes through the midline of the body and divides it into equal left and right halves

military antishock trousers (MAST) an inflatable pants-like device used to treat hemorrhagic shock

mineral zeolite powder substance (sold as QuikClot™) that functions similarly to MPH; it adsorbs water and concentrates clotting factors at the wound to stop bleeding

minerals essential in many chemical reactions and body functions

minimum standard the absolute lowest level of acceptable performance

minute ventilation (MV) the volume of air exchanged between the environment and the alveoli in 60 seconds calculated as the number of breaths in a minute multiplied by the depth (tidal volume) of those breaths

miosis constriction of one or both pupils

mitochondria intracellular organelles that serve as the metabolic workhorse for all cells by converting oxygen, glucose, fatty acids, and some amino acids into adenosine triphosphate (ATP), which is the principal form of energy for all cells

mitosis cellular divisions

mitral valve heart valve located between the left atrium and ventricle

mixed nerves nerves that include both sensory and motor fibers

MMR shot measles, mumps and rubella vaccination

mobile radios two-way radios mounted in a vehicle; they have more power and a larger antenna than portable radios

mode of entry place in which disease enters into the body; unless the correct mode of entry is used, disease will not result

MONA mnemonic for medications used to treat acute coronary syndrome: morphine, oxygen, nitroglycerine, aspirin; although this is a helpful mnemonic, it is not the recommended order to administer the medication

monocytes large mononuclear white blood cells

mononucleosis (mono) disease caused by the Epstein-Barr virus (EBV); frequently transmitted by kissing; causes sore throat, swollen tonsils, fever, and swollen lymph nodes

mood (affective) disorders a grouping of illnesses that are characterized by a long-term sadness (unipolar) or a combination of sadness and mania (bipolar)

morals social standards; specifically how humans act (either good or bad), in a society

morbidity rates statistics that show how many people get sick from various diseases or are injured from accidents

morbidly obese anyone more than 100 pounds overweight

moro reflex primitive reflex that occurs when a newborn grasps anything placed into the palm of its hands; also having the appearance of being startled when the sense of falling is involved or a sudden loud noise is heard; also called the startle reflex

mortality the number of individuals who die from the illness or injury being studied; it is a component of morbidity

motility movement

motor function the ability for muscles to function when stimulated

motor (or efferent) neurons the neurons that carry electrical signals to the effector cell such as a muscle

motorsensory function the ability of the nervous system to detect a stimulus as well as use voluntary muscles

mucoviscidosis (cystic fibrosis [CF]) a genetic disease that most commonly affects breathing and digestion

multifocal atrial tachycardia (MAT) an irregular rapid rhythm on ECG

multiphasic anaphylaxis symptoms that re-occur after a previously resolved allergic reaction

multiple casualty incident an emergency incident that produces more patients than a jurisdiction is routinely capable of handling

multiple sclerosis (MS) a progressive disease of the central nervous system, whereby scattered patches of myelin in the brain and spinal cord are destroyed as a result of repeated inflammation of the myelin sheath

multisystem organ failure (MSOF) when more than one organ shows signs of failure

multisystem trauma trauma involving two or more body systems

mumps disease caused by mumps virus; spread through respiratory droplets; causes swelling of parotid glands in the cheeks, now easily prevented by immunization

murmurs sounds produced by turbulent blood flow within the heart

Murphy sign momentary inspiratory arrest during palpation of the right upper quadrant associated with gall bladder inflammation

muscarinic effects a drug that mimics the effects of acetylcholine (that are also selectively antagonized by atropine)

muscle tetany spasms brought on by mineral imbalance

muscular dystrophies (MD) group of genetic diseases characterized by slow but progressive weakness and degeneration of the skeletal muscles that control movement

muscular endurance the ability to contract muscles repeatedly under submaximal resistance

muscular flexibility the capacity to move joints through their full range of motion

muscular strength the amount of force produced by a muscle during a single maximal contraction

musculoskeletal injury any injury involving bones, cartilage, muscles, tendons, and ligaments

mutagenic causing abnormal changes in DNA that may result in genetic mutations

myalgias muscle aches

myasthenia gravis an autoimmune disease in which the immune system attacks the body's own tissues resulting in muscle weakness

myelin the sheath or covering around some nerve cells that allows for faster transmission of the nerve impulse down the length of the neuron

myocardial concussion a direct blow to the thorax and transfer of energy that stuns the heart

myocardial contusion bruising of heart muscle that typically occurs from blunt trauma

myocardial infarction (traumatic) an acute myocardial infarction sustained by a significant trauma to the chest wall and underlying heart

myocardial rupture the injury that occurs when the heart is compressed with such force that it ruptures; it can also occur when an area of previous injury (particularly an AMI) is weakened and the myocardium tears

myocardial septum the wall between the chambers of the heart

myocardial stunning postischemic contractile dysfunction where cardiac myocytes that are not technically dead are unable to contract normally

myocardium the bulk of cardiac muscle tissue

myoclonus a sudden involuntary jerking movement that is caused by a sudden contraction of a muscle or group of muscles followed by relaxation

myosin (myocin) a protein found in muscle fibers

myxedema coma a severe and potentially life-threatening condition that can occur during the progression of hypothyroidism

N

N95 mask a protective mask used for respiratory protection that filters extremely small particles

nares two openings into the external nose divided by the nasal septum

narrowing pulse pressure an increase in diastolic blood pressure along with a drop in systolic pressure with a decrease in the difference between the two

nasal cannula device that allows for delivery of oxygen by the placement of two prongs into or adjacent to the nares

nasal cartilage cartilage of the nose that provides and maintains the shape of the nose

nasal cavity a large air-filled space above and behind the nose in the middle of the face

nasal septum separates the left and right airways in the nose, dividing the two nostrils, made of cartilage

nasal vestibule small space just beyond the nares, lined by skin and filtering hair follicles

nasogastric (NG) tube device designed to empty the stomach contents (including air from gastric distension) or to occasionally deliver material into the stomach

nasopharyngeal airway (NPA) soft plastic or rubber device that is placed through the nose into the nasopharynx, and pharynx, lifting the tongue forward off of the posterior pharynx to maintain a patent airway

nasopharynx uppermost portion of the three regions of the throat, it is located behind the nose

nasotracheal intubation blind insertion of an endotracheal tube into the trachea via the nose without the use of the laryngoscope or stylet

National Association of EMS Educators (NAEMSE) professional organization made up of EMS educators, instructors, program directors, clinical coordinators, field training coaches,

(continued)

and any other person interested in educating any level of EMS provider

National Association of EMS Physicians (NAEMSP) physician group instrumental in the training of physicians on directing EMS services and the science that defines prehospital practice

National Association of EMTs (NAEMT) association that represents EMTs on a national level by participating in policy development and consensus building

National Association of State EMS Officials (NASEMSO) formed in 2006 when the National Association of State EMS Directors (NASEMSD) and the National Association of State EMS Training Coordinators (NASEMSTC) merged into a single organization

National Disaster Management System (NDMS) a federal program that works within the NIMS ICS structure during a national disaster to coordinate the care and movement of patients from a disaster area to a nonimpacted location

National Highway Traffic Safety Administration (NHTSA) an agency of the Executive Branch of the U.S. Government, part of the Department of Transportation; its mission is "save lives, prevent injuries, reduce vehicle-related crashes"

National Incident Management System (NIMS) the system responsible for developing a process that creates a clear chain of command and a consistent approach for federal, state, local, and tribal governments to work together

National Institute for Occupational Safety and Health (NIOSH) the United States federal agency responsible for conducting research and making recommendations for the prevention of work-related injury and illness; part of the Centers for Disease Control and Prevention (CDC) within the U.S. Department of Health and Human Services

National Registry of Emergency Medical Technicians (NREMT) often called "the Registry"; nonprofit group that credentials all levels of EMTs

National Response Plan (NRP) the plan created by the Department of Homeland Security that establishes a comprehensive all-hazards approach to enhance the ability of the United States to manage domestic incidents

National Special Security Events (NSSE) events of national significance that are potential terrorist targets and that fall under the jurisdiction of the United States Secret Service for overall management

natural killer (NK) cells special lymphocytes that provide protection against infection by secreting cytolytic (cell cutting) substances called perforans that lyse (cut) cell membranes

nature of the illness (NOI) a component of the patient assessment when the paramedic seeks information to determine what is wrong with the patient

necrose die

needle cricothyrotomy an emergency insertion of a hollow needle into the airway (larynx) at the cricothyroid membrane to treat life-threatening upper airway obstruction

needle decompression (needle thoracostomy) insertion of a needle into the pleural space in order to evacuate air trapped between the pleural layers that is causing a tension pneumothorax

negative feedback mechanisms mechanisms that work either by shutting down or reacting to a change in process and are designed to minimize deviation from the normal setpoint and to maintain homeostasis as much as possible

negative pressure breathing when air is sucked into the lungs by expanding the volume of the chest cavity (by the action of the diaphragm or costal muscles), creating negative pressure

negative-pressure pulmonary edema pulmonary edema that follows acute upper airway obstruction

neglect a syndrome in which patients are unaware of their own bodies and body space in one-half of their field of vision (usually the left) *or* the failure to provide for a patient's basic needs; includes physical, emotional, medical, and educational neglect

negligence the failure to act as a reasonably prudent and careful person with similar training would under similar circumstances

neonatal respiratory distress syndrome (RDS) often caused by hyaline membrane disease or meconium aspiration; newborns will present with decreased breath sounds, labored tachypnea rates of 70 to 120 breathes per minute, retractions, paradoxical respirations, grunting, cyanosis, and slow capillary refill

neonate term for infants during the hospitalization phase immediately following birth

neoplasm abnormal growth of cells

nephrology the study and treatment of disorders of the kidney, primarily from a medical rather than surgical point of view

nephron the unit within the kidneys made up of a glomerulus and the fluid-collecting tubule

nephrotic syndrome kidney disease characterized by high levels of protein in the urine (proteinuria), low levels of protein in the blood, and swelling that results in third spacing of fluid and decreased perfusion of the kidneys

nerve agents the most toxic of all the man-made chemical agents; may be used as weapons of mass destruction; include tabun (GA), sarin (GB), soman (GD), and VX; block the effect of acetylcholinesterase at the neural junction

nerve cells neurons

nerve roots branches that come off the spinal cord and leave the spinal column through each intervertebral space; in total, there are 31 nerve roots that originate from either side of the spinal cord

net filtration pressure the measure of how much pressure is acting on fluid to move it through the wall of a capillary

neurogenic shock condition where alterations in vascular tone due to sympathetic interruption after spinal cord injury result in poor tissue perfusion; presents as hypotension, dry, warm skin, normal capillary refill, and bradycardia

neuromuscular junction the junction between a nerve fiber and a muscle cell

neuron nerve cell; the functional unit of the nervous system

neuroses diseases related to personality

neurosyphilis disease characterized by high levels of *T. pallidum* in the cerebrospinal fluid; symptoms include dementia, blindness, numbness, decreased coordination, and paralysis

neurotransmitter chemicals that serve to move (or transmit) a nerve impulse across a synapse

neurovascular bundle refers to the association of nerves and blood vessels in close proximity to one another

neutrophils one type of white blood cell; responsible for phagocytosis (cell eating), which removes bacteria, cellular debris and solid particles from the body

newborn an infant who was just delivered from the mother's body

newly born an infant who was just delivered from the mother's body

Newton's First Law: Law of Inertia a body at a constant state remains at that constant state until some outside force acts upon it

Newton's Second Law: Law of Acceleration Force = Mass × Acceleration

Newton's Third Law: Law of Reciprocal Action for every action, there is an equal and opposite reaction

nightstick (tapping) fractures a linear fracture resulting in two segments, often as a result of being struck on the arm with a stick

nitrogen narcosis known as "rapture of the deep," the condition that results from the intoxicating effects of increased tissue nitrogen concentration at depth

nodal artery coronary artery that supplies oxygen to the sinus and atrioventricular nodes

nodes of Ranvier spaces along the myelin sheath that allow the nerve impulse to jump from node to node and thus speed up nerve impulse transmission

noncardiogenic pulmonary edema accumulation of fluid in the lungs that is not the result of impaired cardiac pumping ability as after an MI

nondisplaced fracture a fracture where a break through the bone results in the two fragments remaining in alignment with one another

nonmalfeasance without misconduct or wrongdoing

nonrebreather mask (NRBM) a device that allows for the administration of supplemental oxygen

nonsteroidal antiinflammatory (NSAID) medications a class of medications that are used to control inflammation, pain, or reduce fever. Includes drugs such as aspirin and ibuprofen

norepinephrine a catecholamine hormone that is released when a host of physiological changes are activated by a stressful event

normal intestinal flora bacteria that are normally present in the digestive tract that aid in normal digestive functions

normal sinus rhythm the most common rhythm on ECG; the electrical impulse originates within the sinus node and follows normal conduction pathways to the AV node and then the ventricles

normotensive condition in which blood pressure is adequate for perfusion to all organs and tissues of the body

not yet sick description of patients in between sick and not sick; those patients whose illness or injury provides significant likelihood for becoming "sick"

NPO allowing nothing to be taken by mouth (os is Latin for mouth)

nuchal cord umbilical cord that is wrapped around the infant's neck during birth

nuchal rigidity stiff muscles of the back of the neck; symptom of meningitis

O

obdundation dullness to pain or sensations, altered mental status

obesity adult female is considered obese when her weight is 25% more than the maximum desirable weight for her

height; a male is considered obese when his weight is more than 20% over the maximum

objective assessment the paramedic's report of signs found during the physical examination

objective findings findings that can be observed, evaluated, and recorded in a factual and impartial manner by the examiner; objective data are generally observable clinical signs and symptoms, physiologic data; technology-derived

oblique fractures fractures of bones that occur at a slanting angle

obsessive compulsive disorder (OCD) a condition in which intrusive ideas, strange images, or fears bother the patient, who cannot eliminate them

obstructive breathing a prolonged expiratory phase due to increased airway resistance

obstructive renal failure (postrenal failure) obstruction of the urinary tract at any level

obstructive shock widespread hypoperfusion that results from a condition that obstructs forward blood flow from the heart

obstructive sleep apnea a partial airway obstruction that commonly occurs during sleep and is manifested by snoring

obtund blunt or lessen

obtundation condition that occurs as a patient's mental state deteriorates to the point that the patient is virtually unresponsive to the environment

obturator device used to assist in the insertion of a tracheostomy tube

occipital cortex posterior part of the brain responsible for vision

occipital lobe the smallest of four lobes in the human brain; it is located in the rearmost portion of the skull, and is the visual processing center

occiput posterior part of the skull and head

occult cord prolapse when the umbilical cord is not visible, but is coming down the birth canal next to the baby

occult injuries injuries that are either missed or not appreciated on initial examination, despite a thorough evaluation, that can be life threatening

Occupational Safety and Health Administration (OSHA) an agency of the United States Department of Labor, its mission is to prevent work-related injuries, illnesses, and deaths by issuing and enforcing rules (called standards) for workplace safety and health

oculomotor nerve the third cranial nerve

odynophagia pain with swallowing

off-gassing when a chemical agent is trapped in a patient's clothing and converts to a gas

official name drug name listed in official government publications like the *United States Pharmacopeia* (USP) or *National Formulary* (NF); usually has the initials USP or NF following the drug name

olfactory fatigue when your senses become accustomed to a smell and you no longer perceive its presence

olfactory receptors provide the sense of smell

olfactory region the region of the nasal cavities that contains the olfactory receptors

oligodendrocyte the myelin-producing cells of the central nervous system

oliguria decreased urine output

oncotic pressure the pressure exerted by molecule concentration in blood

ongoing assessment an assessment of the patient's condition that is being continuously performed

onset start

open fracture any soft tissue wound adjacent to a suspected fracture; the term "compound" for describing an open fracture is dated and is no longer used

open pneumothorax a wound that allows air to pass unimpeded between the outside and the pleural space with each breath

open stance body position used to approach a patient in a nonthreatening manner; palms facing out, hands out of pockets so that the patient sees there is nothing to hide

open wounds any distinction in the integrity of the skin, such as abrasions, lacerations, incised wounds, punctures, avulsions, amputations, and human or animal bites

opportunistic infections infections that do not occur in immunocompetent patients but are related to immunodeficiency

OPQRST mnemonic used to evaluate the complaint of pain or discomfort: onset, provoke/palliate, quality, radiate, severity, time

optic nerve the structure that transmits visual impulses to the brain where they are interpreted as images, cranial nerve II

oral cavity the opening through which an individual takes in food and water; more commonly known as the mouth

orchitis an infection or inflammation of the testicle

organelle an internal cell structure

oropharyngeal airway (OPA) a curved plastic device which, when properly placed, holds the tongue off of the back of the pharynx and helps maintain a patent airway

oropharynx the inside of the mouth and throat

orotracheal intubation insertion of an endotracheal tube through the mouth into the trachea with the aid of a laryngoscope and stylet

orthopedic stretcher (Robinson stretcher) carrying device used as a backup to the Reeves stretcher if there are multiple patients that need to be carried lying flat; it should not be used for patients with head, neck or spine injuries or injuries of the arms and legs that require a splint, because the orthopedic stretcher does not protect or support the spinal column

orthopnea dyspnea (shortness of breath) when lying supine

orthostatic vital sign vital signs of a person that are assessed in a variety of positions, sitting, lying and standing; the purpose is to determine if the patient's normal regulatory mechanisms can respond adequately and readjust the blood pressure

osmosis water molecule movement in an effort to equalize the concentrations between two body compartments

osmotic pressure the pressure created by the presence of solutes (particles) in blood plasma and in interstitial fluid

osteoblast bone-forming cell

osteoclast cell that serves to reabsorb bone for the purpose of growth and repair

osteocyte cell that is imprisoned within the mineralized matrix of the bone, becoming a component of the bone

osteogenisis imperfecta a congenital birth defect causing abnormally fragile bones

osteopathy a traditional healing therapy that emphasizes the body's innate ability to heal itself; osteopaths focus their efforts accordingly

osteoporosis low bone mass and density combined with microarchitectural deterioration results in bone fragility and fractures

ostomy a surgically created opening between the surface of the body and an underlying structure such as the colon, ileum, or urinary bladder, often as an avenue by which fecal or urinary waste are emptied, typically into a collection pouch, and then discarded on a regular basis

otitis externa infection of the auricle or the external auditory canal

otitis media infection of the middle ear; typically occurs when inflammation narrows the eustachian tube, trapping fluid and infectious organisms

otoscope a medical device used to look into the ears

ovarian cyst a cyst that is formed if follicular development is stopped for some reason; a ruptured cyst can lead to severe sharp pain and is localized to one side; may become complicated by bleeding and lead to a life-threatening emergency

ovary female reproductive gland containing ovum (eggs)

overdrive suppression occurs when a cell is driven to depolarization by a higher or stronger pacemaker

overshoot hypothermia hypothermia caused by cooling measures used to treat heatstroke

over-the-counter (OTC) medications drug preparations that contain doses of medication that are available without a prescription

overtriage erring on the side of the patient during triage and transporting to the higher level of care

ovulation when an ovary releases an ovum (egg)

oxygenation the introduction of oxygen from the lungs to the circulation

oxyhemoglobin dissociation curve a graphic representation of the binding characteristics of oxygen with hemoglobin

oxytocin hormone that stimulates uterine contraction and lactation in women who have just delivered a baby

P

P wave the first deflection noted with the start of the cardiac cycle; it identifies atrial depolarization and shows the impulse originating in the sinus node

PACE mnemonic used to remember good communication techniques: problem, audience, constraints, and ethical presence

pacemaker cells cells that initiate depolarization waves at the appropriate time

package insert the accompanying literature from the medication package box

palate the roof of the mouth

palliated pain pain that is relieved

palliative care (comfort care) active total care of patients whose disease is not responsive to curative treatment; control of pain, of other symptoms, and of psychological, social, and spiritual problems is paramount

pallor paleness or blanching of the skin

palpation the technique of applying mild to moderate pressure to the body to detect abnormalities such as masses, tenderness, deformity, or swelling

palpitations fluttering or odd beating sensations that the patient feels in the chest when the heart is beating erratically or fast

pancreas organ located across the back of the abdomen, behind the stomach; plays a role in digestion as well as hormone production; secretes insulin and glucagon

pancreatitis an inflammation of the pancreas generally resulting in abdominal pain that is usually located in the midepigastric area or right upper quadrant

panic attack a sudden onset of acute anxiety

papillary muscles muscles attached to the valves of the ventricles of the heart, these muscles pull open the valve allowing for blood flow between the chambers and hold the valve closed to prevent backflow

paracrine regulation factors released by one cell that act on an adjacent cell in the same tissue

paradoxical respirations when inhaling, a patient's chest will rise, but the abdomen contracts as it works harder to create negative pressure to pull air into the lungs; when the patient exhales, the chest wall falls, but the abdomen rises as the patients increase their intraabdominal pressure to boost exhalation

paralysis the complete loss of muscle function that can affect a small area (localized) or be widespread (generalized)

paraphimosis condition that occurs when a tight foreskin is retracted over the glans penis and becomes entrapped

paraphrase to restate what has been heard

paraplegic a person paralyzed from the "waist" down as a result of injury to the spinal cord below the 7th cervical vertebrae

parasites animals that infest a host; most common are protozoa (amoeba), helminths (tapeworms), and insects (lice)

parasympathetic nervous system (PNS) a subdivision of the autonomic nervous system; controls vegetative functions; also called cholinergic. The vagus nerve is the primary nerve regulating the major organs for the PNS

parathyroid glands the four small endocrine glands located posterior to the thyroid gland; they regulate the level of calcium in the body

parenchyma the functional tissue of an organ

parenteral the medication route that introduces drugs into any part of the body other than the gastrointestinal tract

paresthesia odd or abnormal sensations such as numbness, prickling, tingling, etc.

parietal lobe a lobe in the brain positioned above the occipital lobe and behind the frontal lobe

parietal pain (somatic pain) pain that is caused by irritation of fibers that innervate the parietal peritoneum or abdominal wall

parietal pericardium tough outer layer of the pericardium

parietal pleura the membrane lining the interior of the chest wall

Parkinson's disease a brain disorder in which nerve cells are impaired or die rendering them unable to produce dopamine, an essential chemical messenger that transmits signals through the brain structures, manifested by extremity tremors, unsteady gait and a mask-like facial appearance

Parkland formula the formula used to estimate the amount of fluid to be given in the first 48 hours following burn trauma (4cc × patient weight in Kg × percent burn)

paroxysm something that starts or ends abruptly

paroxysmal atrial tachycardia (PAT) abrupt onset atrial tachycardia initiated by reentry of the stimulus into the conducting system

paroxysmal nocturnal dyspnea (PND) shortness of breath when trying to sleep

paroxysmal supraventricular tachycardia any tachycardic rhythm originating from somewhere above the ventricles

partial pressure a measurement of the percentage of gas dissolved in the plasma of the blood

partial seizure seizure that begins in a specific region or focus of the brain

PASTE mnemonic for determining symptoms associated with shortness of breath: provoke and progression, associated chest pain, sputum color and amount, time and trauma, and temperature, exertion and exercise tolerance

patella disc shaped bone that forms the anterior portion of the knee, also called the knee cap

patency of the airway the lack of obstruction encountered when air passes from the outside environment into the lower airway; also describes the ability of the patient to maintain the airway in an open and clear state

patent ductus arteriosus (PDA) a persistent congenital connection in the pulmonary artery and aortic arch allowing oxygenated blood from the aortic arch to mix with un-oxygenated blood from the right ventricle; there is a 10% prevalence of PDA in children with congenital heart disease

pathogen any organism (protein, bacteria, virus, etc.) that is capable of causing a disease

pathogenecity (virulence) the ease with which an agent causes disease

pathological fracture a fracture that occurs through diseased bone due to an inherent underlying weakness

patient assessment problem-orientated evaluation of patient and establishment of priorities based on existing and potential threats to human life

patient autonomy the right of the patient to be the primary decision maker with regard to the medical care received

patient care report (PCR) a permanent record of events that transpired on the ambulance call

patient self-determination the right of a competent patient to be the primary decision maker with regard to the medical care received

patient-controlled analgesia (PCA) pump pumps designed to allow patients to deliver their own IV pain medication according to their perceived level of discomfort with the touch of a button

peak expiratory flow rate (PEFR) a measurement of the flow rate of air during expiration that is an objective indicator of the severity of the asthma attack and the response to treatment administered

PEARL abbreviation for "pupils are equal and reactive to light"

Pediatric Assessment Triangle (PAT) assessment tool shaped like a triangle developed by the American Academy of Pediatrics; the three sides are appearance, work of breathing, and circulation

pediatric trauma score (PTS) assessment tool used to triage injured children

pelvic inflammatory disease (PID) a spectrum of infections in the female upper reproductive tract; causes pelvic pain and discomfort, abdominal tenderness and possibly signs and symptoms of fever

pelvis the large ring-shaped bone at the bottom of the trunk

penetrating cardiac injuries direct injury to one or more of the heart chambers, laceration of a coronary artery, or bleeding

(continued)

into the space between the pericardium and the myocardium causing a pericardial tamponade

penetrating fracture a fracture of bone that is the result of a penetrating injury such as a gunshot that results in fragmentation of the bone

penetrating trauma the direct injury to tissues as an offending object passes through, or as energy released from the penetrating object transmits through the tissues

penetration when the barrier of protective clothing is punctured or breached or when seams or openings allow a hazard to enter the suit

peptic ulcer disease (PUD) manifested by prolonged burning, epigastric pain; a common cause of gastrointestinal bleeding, felt to arise when there is an imbalance between the production of acid within the stomach and the ability of the gastric mucosa lining the stomach to prevent itself from being damaged by erosion of the protective lining

percent daily value (% DV) the amount of a particular nutrient found in a food

percussion tapping the surface of the chest or abdomen hard enough to send sound waves into the body

percutaneous coronary intervention (PCI) commonly known as coronary angioplasty; an invasive cardiologic therapeutic procedure to treat the stenotic (narrowed) or thrombosed coronary arteries of the heart, often performed as an emergency in a patient having an acute MI

percutaneous endoscopic gastrostomy (PEG) tube surgically inserted tube that extends from the surface of the abdomen into the stomach; used for long-term nutritional support

perfusion the delivery of oxygen and nutrient rich blood to each cell of the body and the removal of waste products from the cellular environment via this circulating blood

pericardial effusion excess fluid that accumulates between the two layers of the pericardium, can cause compression of the heart with obstruction of blood flow (tamponade)

pericardial friction rub a scratchy sound that can be heard at any point within the cardiac cycle that is produced by the pericardial layers rubbing against each other, occurs with infection or inflammation of the pericardium

pericardial space the potential space between the parietal and visceral layers of the pericardium

pericardial tamponade condition caused by illness or injury that results in the accumulation of fluid within the pericardial sac surrounding the heart. It can lead to compromise in pumping function and may result in death

pericardiocentesis the procedure whereby a needle is inserted into the pericardial sac and excess blood or fluid is drawn out with a syringe; this is typically not a paramedic skill although it is allowed in a few jurisdictions

pericarditis an infection or inflammation between the layers of the heart that causes sharp, pleuritic chest pain (worse with breathing); worse with position changes or swallowing, better with leaning forward, and the pain is of variable duration

pericardium a sac that surrounds the heart and is divided into two layers, the visceral pericardium adheres directly to the epicardium and the parietal pericardium is the outermost layer, contains a thin layer of fluid to allow for smooth heart contraction and movement

perimeter the area established by law enforcement to contain a situation within it and to establish a built-in buffer of safety so anyone outside the perimeter does not get hurt

perineum the area between the external genitalia and the anus

periorbital ecchymosis raccoon eyes; bruising and edema noted around the eyes that often accompanies a skull fracture

periosteum a double layer of connective tissue that covers bone

peripheral arterial disease (PAD) atherosclerosis obstructing the blood supply to the extremities

peripheral arteriosclerosis fatty buildup in peripheral arteries

peripheral cyanosis a newborn with a pink body and bluish-colored extremities; the condition that occurs as the body attempts to shunt the circulating volume of blood to the core of the body

peripheral nervous system (PNS) made up of the 12 pairs of cranial nerves (that arise directly from the brain) and the 31 pairs of spinal nerves. The PNS is divided into the somatic and autonomic systems

peripheral neuropathy peripheral nerve damage, commonly occurs with diabetes

peripheral vascular resistance (PVR) resistance to blood flow as produced by the blood vessels, primarily the arterioles, against which the heart must pump; also called afterload

peripherally inserted central catheter (PICC) a central venous access device inserted through veins in the antecubital area

peristalsis the rhythmic movement of the smooth muscles of the digestive system that propel the chyme through the body for processing

peritoneal dialysis (PD) a form of dialysis that allows the patient to receive their treatment in the home setting; a catheter is inserted through the wall of the abdomen and diasylate fluid is introduced into the abdomen and removed after a prescribed period of time

peritoneum a large, essentially closed membrane sac that contains most of the gastrointestinal tract distal to the esophagus

peritonitis inflammation or infection of the peritoneal lining of the abdomen

peritonsillar abscess collection of pus that forms beside the tonsils that can obstruct the airway

periumbilical region the center section of the abdomen over the belly button

permanent cavity the cavity that remains after a projectile has passed through the body

permeability the ease with which a chemical can pass through a barrier such as a cell or protective clothing

permissible exposure limit (PEL) the maximum amount or concentration of a chemical that a worker may be exposed to under OSHA regulations

permissive hypercapnea (controlled hypoventilation) proper technique for ventilation that includes slow ventilations to prevent a buildup of pressure within the chest that can decrease blood return to the heart and compromise blood pressure

pernio (chilblains) a superficial injury that results from skin inflammation and tissue hypoxia from cold-induced vasoconstriction

PERRL abbreviation for describing pupils that are equal, round, and reactive to light

PERRLA abbreviation for describing pupils that are equal, round, and reactive to light and accommodation

perseveration the repetition of comments or questions; it is common following a head injury like a concussion or during the post ictal phase of a seizure

persistent fetal circulation (PFC) the maintenance or resumption of fetal circulation caused by a persistent acidotic state that

(continued)

re-opens the fetal shunts that were closing and decreases the flow of blood to the lungs

persistent pulmonary hypertension–newborn (PPHN) the condition in which blood being shunted away from the lungs causes a hypoxemic (low blood oxygen level) state; caused by meconium-filled alveoli that prevent normal expansion causing increased pressure within the chest that keeps blood from flowing to the lungs

personal protective equipment (PPE) wide range of equipment—gloves, masks, N95 masks, eye protection, gowns, shoe covers, powered respirators, hoods, etc.—available to the healthcare provider to prevent the transmission of communicable diseases or to prevent chemical contamination

personality disorders a category of mental disorders characterized by long-lasting rigid patterns of thought and behavior that over time cause distress and impair social and occupational functioning

pertinent negatives critical findings (or more accurately non-findings) from the assessment or history provided by the patient that are important to include in the patient care report as they support the final assessment

pertussis (whooping cough) disease caused by bacterium *Bordetella pertussis;* spread by respiratory droplets; causes bursts of coughing followed by distinctive "whoop" sound

pervasive development disorders (PDDs) neurobiological disorders that are present from birth: autism, Asperger syndrome, PDD-NOS, etc.

pH the amount, or concentration, of hydrogen ions in the body measured on a standard scale (values < 7 are labeled acidic; 7 is neutral and values > 7 are labeled basic or alkaline); in the human body, normal pH is 7.35 to 7.45, less than 7.35 is considered acidosis and greater than 7.45 is considered alkalosis

phagocytes cells programmed to identify nonself cells, surround them, and consume them

phagocytize the process by which white blood cells consume bacteria and tissue debris

phagocytized broken down and engulfed

phalanges the bones of the fingers and toes

pharmacodynamics the study of how drugs interact with the living tissues in the body

pharmacokinetics the study of how drugs are delivered to, and removed from, affected organs

pharmacology the study of drugs

pharynx the open portion of the alimentary canal (GI tract) and respiratory tract between the inside of the lips and the top of the esophagus

phlebotomy the establishment of venous access; a phlebotomist is a health care provider who draws blood or starts IVs in the hospital setting

phobia a persistent and irrational fear due to an external factor

phonation speaking

phosgene a colorless gas that has a characteristic odor of freshly mown hay; may be used as a weapon of mass destruction causes pulmonary damage

photophobia light sensitivity that accompanies certain infections, toxicities, trauma or medical conditions

phrenic nerve the nerve that innervates the diaphragm and is involved with respiration

physical abuse physical injury of an individual at the hands of another

physical fitness the body's ability to meet the requirements and demands of work and leisure activities

physician extender nonphysicians educated to perform some procedures, such as chest decompression and surgical airway techniques, that previously only licensed physicians were allowed to perform; paramedics are often referred to as physician extenders

physiologic dead space the area in the lung that is not available for exchange of oxygen and carbon dioxide

physiology the branch of the biological sciences that studies the functions of a living organism and its component parts, including all chemical and physical processes

physis the distal ends of a bone

pia mater the innermost layer of the meninges that adheres closely to the brain and spinal cord

pill esophagitis irritation of the esophagus as a result of pills becoming lodged

piloerection "goose bumps"

pineal body located in the brain; produces melatonin

pin-index system a special configuration on oxygen cylinders and regulators that prevents the regulator from another type of gas from being used on an oxygen cylinder

pink puffer a descriptive term for an emphysema patient

pinna the part of the exterior ear that projects outward that directs sounds in to the inner ear.

pitch frequency of breath sound, described as high or low

pituitary gland located at the base of the brain; controls many functions of the other endocrine glands; secretes hormones to stimulate the adrenals, thyroid, pigment-producing skin cells and gonads (ovaries and testes); also secretes growth hormone, an antidiuretic hormone, prolactin, and oxytocin

placenta an organ that serves as the interface between the mother and the fetus to deliver oxygen and nutrients to and remove wastes from the fetus

placenta previa occurs when the placenta implants over the cervical os or internal opening of the cervix patients with complete placenta previa where the placenta has been perforated require rapid surgical intervention to prevent exsanguination and maternal and fetal death

plague *Yersinia pestis,* a gram-negative, rod-shaped organism that is nonmotile (cannot move around) and does not sporulate (reproduce by spores); may be used as a weapon of mass destruction

planes anatomical term meaning imaginary lines that slice through the body

plantar flexion bending the foot downward and extending the ankle

plaque a build-up of fatty deposits within the lining of the blood vessels; atherosclerosis or arteriosclerosis

plasma cells the cells produced from a single antigen activated B cell that can either be short- (a few days) or long-lived (months), producing and secreting 2,000 antibody molecules per second while they are alive

plateau phase Phase 2 of the action potential when calcium is accumulating inside the cell

platelets (thrombocytes) free-floating structures in the bloodstream that come together to form a plug when they encounter damaged or injured blood vessels

pleura connective tissues that cover the lungs; the visceral pleura covers the lungs and is insensate; the parietal pleura lines the thoracic cavity and contains nerve fibers

pleural fluid fluid that is secreted by the pleura, lubricates the two linings to allow for smooth movement of the lungs during breathing

pleural friction rub a condition where an infection or inflammation has caused the visceral and parietal pleura to rub against each other causing pain and a harsh grating sounds that can be heard on auscultation over the affected area

pleural space the space between the visceral and perietal pleura that normally contains a small amount of pleural fluid that lubricates the lung during the movement associated with breathing

pleuritic chest pain a sharp, stabbing pain worsened by breathing

Plummer disease (toxic multinodular goiter) occurs in 15–20% of patients with thyrotoxicosis; excess of thyroid hormone develops gradually over time

pneumatic antishock garment (PASG) a pants-like, inflatable device used to treat hemorrhagic shock

pneumomediastinum air collected within the mediastinal space

pneumonia a condition of infection and inflammation in distal sections of the lung including small airways and alveoli; symptoms include cough, abnormal breath sounds, abnormal respiratory patterns, tachypnea, and elevated fever

pneumothorax the collection of air within the pleural space causing collapse of the lung on the affected side

point of maximal impulse (PMI) the part of the heart closest to the chest wall; the apex is located just left of the sternum at the fifth rib and can be palpated on physical examination

point-of-care testing the provision of a test at the patient's bedside that can be used to make an immediate care decision

polarization the resting or ready state of a cell

polarized carrying a relative negative charge

poliomyelitis (polio) a highly contagious viral disease that can involve the nervous system and cause paralysis of the extremities or muscles of the trunk

polycythemia an abnormally high number of red blood cells; a condition often seen in patients with chronic lung diseases like emphysema

polydipsia excessive thirst often caused by diabetes

polyphagia excessive hunger caused by diabetes

polyps small, tumor-like growths

polyurea excess water lost from body from increased urination that accompanies diabetes

pons the part of the brain that separates the midbrain from the medulla oblongata; it relays messages between the cerebrum and medulla and between the cerebrum and cerebellum

pooling function of the venous system where it serves as a reservoir for blood not currently needed by the body

popliteal artery artery located behind the knee

popliteal pulse the pulse located behind the knee from the popliteal artery

portable radios lightweight, hand-held, two-way communication devices; they have shorter transmission ranges than mobiles and base stations, because they have less power and shorter antennas

portal hypertension increased venous pressure in the portal circulation

portal venous system a group of veins that receive blood from the gastrointestinal organs so that it can be taken directly to the liver for processing

positive chronotropic effect factors that elevate heart rate

positive end expiratory pressure (PEEP) a method of maintaining enough residual volume and pressure in the alveoli so that they do not completely empty and collapse during exhalation

positive feedback mechanisms mechanisms in which the effectors act to move the stimulus farther away from its setpoint

positive inotropic (contractile) effect factors that increase contractility

positive pressure self-contained breathing apparatus (SCBA) airpack that supplies air to a facemask from a tank

positive pressure ventilation (PPV) assisted ventilation

posterior anatomic term meaning toward the back of the body

posterior cerebral artery (PCA) stroke a stroke that results in a visual field deficit on the opposite side of the stroke (a right PCA stroke will result in a left visual field deficit)

posterior descending artery a branch of the right coronary artery which runs in the posterior interventricular sulcus to the apex of the heart, where it meets with the anterior interventricular artery

posterior horns structures on the spinal cord that receive the incoming sensory fibers that transmit pain, temperature, and vibration

posterior pharynx upper back part of the mouth or throat

posterior tibial arteries arteries located behind the medial malleolus

postictal phase of recovery that occurs following a seizure; the patient is exhausted and confused and often wants to sleep

postimmersion syndrome development of the respiratory distress syndrome hours or days after the initial resuscitation; occurs in up to 5% of submersion patients

postrenal failure (obstructive renal failure) obstruction of the urinary tract at any level

post-traumatic stress disorder (PTSD) a disorder in which a memory of a previous overwhelming or traumatic event is repeatedly reexperienced

posturing involuntary reflexive movements; an abnormal involuntary contraction of the limbs

potential spaces areas of the body where two tissues come together and may produce or contain fluid that serves to lubricate the layers, but could be separated if fluid, air, blood or pus were to accumulate,

Pott's disease active tuberculosis in the spine

power of attorney a document created by a competent adult to appoint a legal representative to exercise the powers granted in the document

pox any disease that causes vesicles

PR interval (PRI) calculated by determining the time from the beginning of the P wave to the end of the P-R segment

P-R segment straight line on ECG from the end of the P wave until the beginning of the QRS complex, approximately .08 sec long indicating ventricles are filling; may be shorter if the P wave comes from an ectopic site

precision the degree with which a measurement is clustered around a mean value (or average finding)

precordial thump a sharp blow to the chest; it is thought to produce an electrical depolarization of between 2 and

(continued)

5 Joules; this extremely small shock may disrupt a re-entrant pathway dysrhythmia if delivered at the right moment

preeclampsia (toxemia) pregnancy induced hypertension accompanied by edema or an increased excretion of proteins in the urine

pregnancy induced hypertension (PIH) blood pressure > 140/90 diagnosed on two or more occasions at least six hours apart in a pregnant female not previously diagnosed with hypertension

preload how tightly stretched the ventricular myocardium is just prior to contraction, measured by the ventricular pressure just before each heart contraction; end diastolic volume

premature atrial contraction (PAC) a beat originating from somewhere in the atria other than the sinus node

premature baby born before 37 weeks of gestation

premature junction contraction (PJC) a complex that originates from within the AV junction; it is an ectopic beat that occurs earlier than the next expected normal beat

premature labor labor that occurs after 20 weeks and before the mother completes 37 weeks of pregnancy

premature newborn a newborn less than 37 weeks gestational age

premature rupture of membranes (PROM) the spontaneous rupture of the amniotic sac, when there are no signs of labor

premature ventricular contractions (PVC) a premature heart beat that originates from an ectopic site in the ventricle

prerenal failure any condition that decreases perfusion before blood reaches the kidneys

presbycusis age-related hearing loss

presence the ability to project a sense of self confidence and show that you are at ease with the situation

pressure (ischemic) ulcer an ulcer that develops in areas of lack of blood flow usually due to pressure preventing adequate circulation

pressure dressings dressings that can be utilized to maintain pressure on a bleeding site

pressure points areas of the body where an artery is either lying close to the surface of the skin or is found directly over a bone; occlusion of a pressure point slows or stops the flow of blood into the distal tissues

preterm premature rupture of membranes (PPROM) when premature rupture of the amniotic sac occurs before 37 completed weeks of pregnancy

priapism a persistent erection of the penis, it may accompany spinal cord injuries, urinary calculi, or acute leukemia

prickly heat an acute inflammatory skin disorder that occurs in tropical environments

primary adrenal insufficiency (Addison's disease) inadequate function of the adrenal glands

primary apnea a period of rapid respirations followed by a period of apnea; the newborn's futile attempt to compensate while fatigued (tired)

primary brain injury injuries that occur during impact and result from bruising, bleeding, or shearing of the brain

primary hypothermia hypothermia that is usually the result of an environmental exposure

primary pacemaker (sinus node) initiates depolarization in the heart at a rate of 60–100 times per minute

primary prevention strategies deliberate life style choices designed to reduce the likelihood of developing diseases or sustaining injury

primary survey a quick determination by the paramedic to see if the patient requires life-saving interventions; the initial assessment designed to detect and treat any problems threatening the airway, breathing, and perfusion status

Primum non nocere Latin phrase meaning "first do no harm"

Prinzmetal's variant angina coronary artery spasm that occurs at rest but may also be triggered by exertion or periods of high stress

professional ethics the rules, regulations, and codes of conduct that distinguish paramedics in their profession

professional liability insurance insurance coverage where the insurer (provided it is given prompt notice of the claim) is obligated to provide a defense for the organization's paramedics in cases of alleged negligence

progesterone a hormone produced by the ovaries and sometimes referred to as the "hormone of pregnancy" because it is necessary for implantation of the fertilized egg and maintenance of the uterine lining throughout the pregnancy

projectile injuries penetrating injuries caused by any airborne high-velocity object (such as bullets) that enter the body

prolactin a hormone secreted by the pituitary gland in order to stimulate the mammary glands to produce milk

pronation the act of rotating the arm so that the palm of the hand is facing downward

prone anatomic term meaning lying horizontal with the face downward

prophylaxis to protect; immunizations are considered a form of prophylaxis

proprietary name drug name selected by the manufacturer to use when it sells the drug

proptosis bulging of the eyes from the orbit

prospective medical control the development of clinical practice standards such as training curricula, protocols, and other clinical standards that govern the care of patients in the prehospital setting; they may or may not require on-line medical direction to initiate or continue care

prostaglandin D substance that causes dilation of blood vessels, increased vascular permeability (which causes edema), bronchospasm, increased mucus production and contraction of the smooth muscle in the intestinal tract

prostatitis any of four different infectious or inflammatory entities involving the prostate: acute bacterial prostatitis, chronic bacterial prostatitis, chronic prostatitis, or asymptomatic inflammatory prostatitis

protected health information (PHI) individually identifiable health information that is protected from release by HIPPA regulations unless specific permission is granted by the patient

proteins chemical compounds that help build muscles, hormones, enzymes, antibodies, and cell membranes as well as supplying energy when needed

proteinuria high levels of protein in the urine

prothrombin a chemical that is part of the clotting cascade

prothrombin activator chemical triggered during stage I of blood clot formation following injury; PTA activates prothrombin to create thrombin

proximal anatomic term meaning nearer to the trunk of the body when compared to another point

pruritus itching

pseudomembranous colitis bloody diarrhea in patients who have been taking broad-spectrum antibiotics

psychosis disorder caused by complex biochemical disease of the brain; characterized by thought disorders and loss of contact with reality

public health emergencies incidents usually involving infectious diseases that broadly threaten the public health

public information officer (PIO) person who serves as a conduit for information to internal and external stakeholders during an emergency incident, including the media, under the Incident Command System

public safety answering point (PSAP) communications center that coordinates the deployment of emergency personnel and other resources

puerperal infection infection of the birth canal or associated structures that occurs in the post-partum period

pulmonary agents phosgene, chlorine, and ammonia when used as weapons of mass destruction that enter the body via the respiratory system and cause damage primarily in the lungs

pulmonary arteries arteries that carry deoxygenated blood from the heart to the lungs

pulmonary barotrauma any of five conditions (arterial gas embolism, pneumothorax, pneumomediastinum, subcutaneous emphysema, and alveolar hemorrhage) that can result from a rapid, uncontrolled ascent from diving

pulmonary contusion contusion (bruise) of the lung

pulmonary edema the accumulation of fluid in the alveoli of the lung, usually as a result of heart failure and the diminished ability of the left vertride to puag blood; may also occur from direct toxic injury to the alveoli from inhead toxins or chemicals

pulmonary emboli (PE) clots that lodge in blood vessels of the lungs; marefested by sudden onset of pain and shortness of breath; typically pleuritic pain; result in areas of the lung that are not receiving any blood to exchange oxygen with carbon dioxide

pulmonary hypertension condition that occurs when the small blood vessels of the lungs become damaged and it becomes harder for the right side of the heart to pump blood through the lungs; also called cor pulmonale

pulmonary laceration laceration of a lung

pulmonary tuberculosis active tuberculosis occurring in the lungs

pulmonary valve stenosis a defect causing a partial obstruction of the pulmonary valve and restricting blood flow to the lungs; there is a 10% prevalence of PVS in children with congenital heart disease; symptoms include fatigue, shortness of breath, cyanosis, poor weight gain or failure to thrive, and chest pain

pulmonary vascular resistance (PVR) the sum of all resistance in the pulmonary circulation

pulmonic valve one of two semilunar valves responsible for regulating the blood flow between the right ventricle and the pulmonary trunk (arteries)

pulmonic veins veins that carry oxygenated blood from the lungs to the heart; the only veins that carry oxygenated blood

pulse deficit a difference between the apical and peripheral pulse rates

pulse oximeter a reliable, portable, and noninvasive method to assess a patient's oxygenation in the prehospital environment

pulse points nine places on the human body where arteries are found and a pulse can be taken

pulse pressure the difference between the systolic arterial pressure and the diastolic arterial pressure

pulseless electrical activity (PEA) electrical activity seen on the cardiac monitor when the patient is without a pulse

pulseless ventricular tachycardia (VT) a condition in which there is rapid contraction of the cardiac muscle of the ventricles in the heart without any palpable pulse

pulsus alternans a pulse intensity that alternates between weak and strong

pulsus paradoxus a 10 mmHg or greater drop in the systolic blood pressure that occurs during inspiration

pupil the central opening of the eye through which light enters

purified air powered respirators (PAPR) [air purifying respirator (APR), cartridge respirators] device that filters ambient air through hazard-specific cartridges or canisters before inhalation; does not provide a presupplied source of air

purkinje network network of conduction fibers in the heart; location of third pacemaker

purulent drainage cloudy yellow drainage from an infected wound

push-to-talk (PTT) button button on two-way radio that you press when you want to transmit a message and release when you are through

pyelonephritis kidney infection

pyriform sinuses small recesses located to either side of the vallecula in the throat

Q

QRS complex on ECG, represents depolarization of the right and left ventricles

QT interval on ECG, the time represented from the start of the QRS complex to the end of the T wave

quadriceps the muscles in the thigh

quadriplegia paralysis of both arms and both legs, as well as the trunk, caused by injury to the cervical spinal cord

quick acting electrical signals electrochemical signals that cause the cells to change their resting membrane potential; also know as action potentials

R

R on T phenomenon a PVC that occurs within a T wave of the preceding complex, thought to increase the risk of developing ventricular fibrillation

rabies disease that is caused by rabies virus; transmitted through saliva/biting; symptoms include anxiety, headache, fever, altered mental status progressing to weakness, delirium, convulsion, and paralysis of pharynx, causing hydrophobia

radial pulse located on the thumb side of the wrist

Radiation Emergency Assistance Center/Training Site (REACTS) founded in 1944, the United States Department of Energy's group that monitors radiation incidents and collects data from around the world

radiation heat transfer by electromagnetic waves; a major source of heat loss or gain

radioactive agents substances that give off energy either in the form of electromagnetic energy or particles and that result in damage and destruction at a cellular level

radiographs x-rays

radius one of the bones in the forearm

rales fine, moist crackling sounds associated with fluid in the smaller airways

rapid sequence intubation intubation performed with the aid of sedative and paralytic drugs

reactionary gap the space that allows you to maintain a safe distance between yourself and the person you are interacting with until you can determine whether they represent a threat to you

reactive airway disorders (RAD) condition of mucus production, inflammation, edema, and bronchospasm that occurs when an irritant, bacteria, virus, irritant, or allergen invades the airway; asthma is classified as a reactive airway disease

re-bleeding when bleeding starts again following initial control

receptive aphasia difficulty understanding spoken language

receptor a molecule that is activated when a variable moves outside of its desirable range; also a specific site on or inside a cell, a whole cell, or a group of cells together that receive messages

recertification a process of verifying that the competencies required for each level of provider have been maintained over time

reciprocal changes on ECG, a reversal of ST changes seen in a lead or leads opposite from the actual location of infarction or ischemia

recommended exposure limit (REL) the highest allowable airborne concentration that is not expected to injure a worker; expressed as a celling limit or time-weighted average for an eight- or 10-hour day

rectus abdominus muscle of the abdominal wall

recurrent anaphylaxis symptoms that re-occur after a previously resolved allergic reaction; it may be triggered by the continued presence of the allergen or because the medication used to control the reaction has worn off

reduction the movement of misaligned bone ends or a displaced joint to restore proper alignment

Reeves stretcher carrying device used for unconscious, unresponsive patients, overdose, CVA, patients with a decreased level of consciousness such as diabetics, seizure patients, choking, unknown, bed bound elderly patients, respiratory and/or cardiac arrest, shooting, stabbing, and trauma not involving the head, neck, or spine

referred pain pain that is felt at a location distant from the site of the pathology causing the pain; often the pain follows dermatomal pathways

refusal of care when a competent patient (or legally responsible decision-maker) who is properly informed of the risks of nontreatment and the benefits of treatment chooses to refuse medical care and/or transportation, even if that care would save the person's life

registered nurse (RN) a healthcare professional who provides direct patient care under the direction of a physician, works in conjunction with other healthcare professionals and directs the care provided by HHAs, CNAs, LVN/LPNs, etc.

regularly irregular rhythm any time an irregular rhythm is encountered and there is a definite pattern to the rhythm; could occur as a result of grouped or paired beats, with cer-tain heart blocks occurring rhythmically, or with a beat being dropped consistently as you look across the ECG strip

relative contraindication caution must be used in a particular circumstance because there is not enough evidence to absolutely confirm the medication is safe to administer; the benefit of administration must be weighed against the potential risk

relative hypovolemia instead of an actual blood loss as seen in hemorrhage, movement of body fluids or a change in the vascular container size (dilation) causes the patient to exhibit shock symptoms; nitroglycerin may create a perceived loss of volume due to the vasodilation effects

relative refractory period small period of time during phase 3 of the cardiac action potential when enough of an electrical gradient has been achieved to theoretically cause tissue to respond to a new electrical impulse if it is of sufficient size; it ranges from the middle of the T wave to the end of the T wave on ECG

reliability a measure of how similar the results will be when the test, such as an interview, is performed by someone else

remodeling the phase in fracture healing when the bone tends to return to its normal shape and contours; the callus is reabsorbed and replaced by new bone laid down following the original lines of stress of the bone

renal arteries arteries that supply the kidneys

renin chemical released from the kidneys and functions as an enzyme that converts angiotensinogen (a protein circulating in the blood) to angiotensin I

renin-angiotensin mechanism the mechanism that releases renin from kidney cells into the blood; it is activated when renal pressure falls, or when the renal filtrate is dilute or slow moving

renin-angiotensin system the system that plays an important role in maintaining adequate blood volume, blood pressure, and cardiac and vascular function

reparative phase the phase in fracture healing when granulation tissue begins to infiltrate the area, forms callus, and stabilizes fractured bone ends

repolarization the process of moving (pumping) ions back to their original positions on either side of the membrane to return the membrane to the original ready state

representativeness heuristic the situation provides enough information for the paramedic to believe that the current signs and symptoms represent a particular disease

reproducible pain pain that can be caused following a stimulus such as pressing and releasing the involved body part

reservoir an animal, person, or environment in which an infectious agent reproduces without causing disease in the reservoir

residual volume (RV) the volume of air remaining at the end of the maximal, forced exhalation

resistance ability of the body to stave off infection

resonance the sound vibration quality that can be heard with percussion on the chest wall or during phonation

respiration the exchange of oxygen and carbon dioxide that occurs in the lung and tissues; enzymatic consumption of high-energy materials taking place inside of cells

respiratory acidosis results from the retention of CO_2; may be caused by the depression of the central respiratory center secondary to a variety of causes such as chest injuries, COPD, pneumonia, or pneumothorax

respiratory alkalosis results from increased respirations and excessive removal of CO_2; can result from a variety of

(continued)

causes including hyperventilation, anxiety, overventilation of patients on assisted ventilation, CNS disorders, liver failure, coma, and fever

respiratory arrest no, or few, spontaneous respirations

respiratory baseline phase I on a normal capnogram waveform; represents the end of inspiration

respiratory bronchioles a bronchiole at the beginning of the respiratory zone in the lung where oxygen and carbon dioxide gasses are exchanged in the blood

respiratory depression condition that occurs when the respiratory rate is slow for a prolonged period of time, or if chest wall expansion is inadequate to inflate the lungs, resulting in a lack of adequate perfusion; uncorrected respiratory depression leads to respiratory failure

respiratory droplets small particles of water, saliva, or mucus expelled from the respiratory system, particularly during a sneeze or cough, which can transmit infectious agents

respiratory failure decreasing respiratory effort, depth, or adequacy of breathing creating a life-threatening condition for the patient including hypoxia and hypercertia

respiratory insufficiency failure of the respiratory system to maintain adequate ventilation or perfusion of the lungs; it is very similar to respiratory depression

respiratory rate number of times a person breathes in one minute

respiratory syncytial virus (RSV) virus that causes bronchitis

responder a generic term used to describe a person with any level of credential in the EMS profession

resting membrane potential the difference in the electrical charge (voltage) when the inside of the cell is more negatively charged than the outside of the cell

reticular activating system (RAS) (reticular formation) a complex network of nerve fibers scattered throughout the medulla, pons, and midbrain responsible for maintaining an individual's level of consciousness

reticuloendothelial system (RES) the collection of white blood cells found outside the bloodstream, namely in the liver, spleen, lungs, lymph nodes, bone marrow, and intestines, that help to clear the blood of any debris that results from fighting an infection

retina light- and color-sensing tissue lining the posterior chamber of the eye

retraction the sinking of the suprasternal notch during inhalation or noted as the intercostals muscles pull inward during respiratory distress

retrobulbar hemorrhage bleeding behind the globe of the eye

retrograde amnesia when a patient has no recollection of the events immediately leading up to the incident causing a concussion

retroperitoneal cavity the posterior part of the abdominal cavity created by a fold of the peritoneum that separates the anterior component from the posterior portion

retroperitoneum the posterior abdominal cavity

retropharyngeal abscess collection of pus that develops in the posterior pharynx

retrospective medical direction or control medical oversight of the EMS service that is typically exercised through quality improvement mechanisms such as chart reviews, case reviews, and other methods after patient care has been completed

reverse Trendelenburg position where the patient is supine with the foot of the bed elevated up to 45 degrees

reverse triage occurs in a mass casualty incident when the threat of continued danger is minimial and patient care focuses on treating the patients in the worst conditions first, for example, in a lightning mass casualty incident, the first triage priority goes to those who are not moving and not breathing

revised trauma score (RTS) a physiological scoring system used to allow medical personnel to triage trauma patients

rhabdomyolysis a condition that results from necrosis of skeletal muscle; the dead cells release the protein myoglobin and other cellular components that circulate in the blood and "clog up" the kidneys resulting in bleeding and damage to the organs

rhinitis inflammation of the nasal passages causing a runny nose

rhinorrhea nasal secretions

rhomboideus major a muscle on the back that connects the scapula with the vertebrae of the spinal column

rhomboideus minor a muscle that arises from the lower part of the ligamentum nuchae and from the spinous processes of the seventh cervical and first thoracic vertebrae

rhonchi the sound produced by rattling vibrations as air flows through mucus or around an obstruction

ricin a lethal cytotoxin that is derived from castor beans and is a byproduct of castor oil production; may be used as a biological warfare agent

ricochet when a projectile deflects in an entirely different direction after striking something such as bone within the body; for example, a bullet may enter under the right axilla, strike the rib cage on the left side and slice back across the body and lodge in the liver

right atrial (Bainbridge) reflex the response that allows the heart to eject a volume of blood that is equal to the volume it receives

right coronary artery one of two main coronary arteries arising from the aorta that supplies the right atrium and right ventricle

RN registered nurse

Rocky Mountain spotted fever (RMSF) disease caused by a bacterium, *Rickettsia rickettsii,* spread through the bite of infected wood ticks; symptoms include fever, malaise, and rash of red spots all over the body, including on palms of hands and soles of feet

rotation injuries the injuries that occur when forces cause one side of a skeletal structure to act as a fulcrum against which the opposite side turns, commonly noted in knee and spinal injuries

rotator cuff muscles that work as a group to support the shoulder

RPM system mnemonic for evaluating patient: respiration, pulse, mental status; it is a component of the START triage system

rubella (German measles) disease caused by rubella virus; spread through respiratory droplets; causes low-grade fever, swollen lymph nodes, and generalized rash

rubeola (measles) disease caused by measles virus; spread through respiratory droplets; causes fever, a red bumpy rash, and Koplik's spots in the mouth

rule of nines method for estimating the size of a burn; the body of an adult is divided into nine parts and each portion of the body equals approximately 9% of the total body surface area; modified charts must be used for children and infants

rule of the palm the patient's palm (which is the entire hand surface, including the fingers) is estimated to equal approximately 1% of the patient's total body surface area (TBSA); used for estimating burn size

runsheet jargon for patient care report

S

Sacco Triage Methodology (STM) assessment tool created by Dr. William Sacco for assessing the criticality of pediatric and adult patients

sacrum the vertebrae that together with the coccyx form the posterior, or back, of the pelvis

safety officer (SO) person who monitors the safety conditions and develops measures to ensure the safety of the workers on the scene of a mass casualty under the Incident Command System

sagittal plane any dividing line that runs parallel to the midsagittal plane which divides the body into right and left halfs down the midline

salivary glands three glands (parotid, submandibular, and sublingual) that lubricate food and release digestive secretions into the oral cavity

SAMPLE mnemonic for gathering medical history: signs and symptoms, allergies to medications, medications, past medical history, last meal, events

sanguinous blood-tinged fluid

sarcomere muscle cell fiber

SARS acronym for severe acute respiratory syndrome, it is a highly infectious respiratory disease in humans caused by the SARS coronavirus

scabies parasitic infestation of the skin by *Sarcoptes scabei;* transmitted through close contact with infested persons; symptoms include intense itching with redness at site of insect burrows

scald traumatic injury that occurs as superheated liquids or gaseous steams come into contact with tissues

scapula also known as the shoulder blade; the bone that connects the humerus bone with the collar bone

scene size-up an assessment of the scene to ensure safety for crew, patients, and bystanders

schizophrenia a psychological disorder marked by a deterioration in thought and functioning

Schwann cells the cells that form the myelin sheath around neurons of the peripheral nervous system

sclera the white of the eye

scope of practice the foundation for the out-of-hospital competencies and expectations for the profession

scrofula lymph node infection in the neck caused by tuberculosis

scrotum pouch formed by the dartos muscle and skin in which the testes lie surrounded by the tunica vaginalis

seat belt sign ecchymosis over the inferior abdominal wall that is associated with intestinal injury; in motor vehicle crashes this injury is often seen from seat belts

sebaceous glands glands that secrete sebum (a wax-like substance) into the hair follicles

second degree AV block type I block resulting from a progressive delay in conduction through the AV node until an impulse is blocked entirely; also known as the Wenckebach rhythm

second degree AV block type II a block that is lower in the conducting system of the heart than type I; it is essentially regular with consistent P-P and PR intervals until a QRS complex is dropped

second stage of labor (expulsion stage) the time period from when the cervix is completely dilated and the baby moves down into the birth canal with pushing until birth of the infant; can last as short as one push or up to an average of 2.5 hours in a first-time labor

secondary (or lobar) bronchi arise from the primary bronchi, with each one serving as the airway to a specific lobe of the lung

secondary adrenal insufficiency caused by injury or illnoss to the pituitary gland resulting in inadequate function of the adrenal glands

secondary apnea when an infant ceases to breath and there is a considerable drop in both heart rate and blood pressure that occurs when primary apnea is unrecognized and untreated

secondary brain injury injuries that occur following the primary brain injury when the patient is allowed to become hypotensive or hypoxic

secondary diabetes diabetes caused by medication or the presence of another illness such as pancreatitis, cystic fibrosis, pheochromocytoma, acromegaly, or Cushing syndrome

secondary hypothermia hypothermia that occurs in patients with a predisposing illness, frailty, or intoxication

secondary survey detailed questions about the patient's condition and history

second-degree burn burn that involves the dermal layer and is subdivided into categories of thickness: partial or full, depending upon the final depth of the burn

secondhand smoke the smoke that nonsmokers are ekposed to that enters the air from the burning end of a cigarette, cigar, or pipe that has not been inhaled into the lungs; because it is unfiltered, it is believed to contain more carcinogens than the smoke inhaled by the smoker

seizure (ictus) a temporary disruption in normal neuronal activity resulting in abnormal repetitive and synchronous firing (action potentials) of neurons in the brain

self-neglect a concept unique to elder abuse; it describes behaviors of competent elderly persons that threaten their health or safety; examples include dehydration, malnutrition, untreated or improperly attended medical conditions, poor personal hygiene, and unsafe living conditions

self-serving bias the tendency to claim more responsibility for successes than failures; it also manifests itself as a tendency for people to evaluate information in a way that is beneficial to their interests

sella turcica a protective bone that surrounds the pituitary gland in the skull

Sellick's maneuver (cricoid pressure) applying pressure to the cricoid cartilage in such a way as to occlude the esophagus and prevent stomach contents from getting into the airway and being aspirated into the lungs

semipermeable membrane a membrane that will allow some, but not all, substances to pass through by diffusion

semispinalis capitis and **cervicis** back muscles that pull the back posteriorly

sensitivity of a test the proportion of people who truly have a particular disease identified by the test

sensorineural hearing loss hearing loss that is usually the result of damage to the cochlea or auditory nerve or due to brain damage itself

sensory (or afferent) neurons the neurons that detect stimuli and changes in the environment and carry electrical signals into the central nervous system

sensory function ability of the peripheral nervous system to receive external impulses and transmit them to the central nervous system

sensory function the brain function located in the postcentral gyrus of the parietal lobe; responsible for receiving, evaluating, and recognizing stimuli received from the environment

sepsis a syndrome caused by the presence of bacteria or bacterial toxins in the bloodstream

septic shock condition caused by infection resulting in organ dysfunction that leads to vascular bed changes so that blood is no longer adequately perfusing the body's tissues; usually accompanied by a blood pressure measurement below 90 mmHg

septicemia a generalized bacterial infection in the bloodstream

septum a structure that divides two sides of an organ or body part, i.e., the cartilaginous septum that divides the nose into right and left nares or the cardiac septum between the right and left ventricles

serous drainage yellowish, clear-colored fluid so called because of its resemblance to blood serum

serratus anterior a muscle that originates on the surface of the upper eight ribs at the side of the chest and inserts along the entire anterior length of the medial border of the scapula

setpoint the acceptable value for any variable

sexual abuse involves nonconsensual physical acts such as fondling, genital or oral stimulation, intercourse, or sodomy as well as nonphysical acts such as indecent exposure or obscene phone calls

sexual assault any genital, anal, oral, or manual penetration of the victim's body by way of force and without the victims consent

sexually transmitted diseases (STD) diseases transmitted through sexual contact

shaken baby syndrome a severe form of child abuse in which the child is usually held and violently shaken back and forth that frequently results in death or serious permanent neurological disability; the infant most commonly presents with seizures, coma, or respiratory distress from intracranial bleeding

shamanism a traditional healing therapy that relies on the innate ability of a shaman to transcend the visible world and manipulate invisible lines of force in order to diagnose disease and induce healing

sharps container a container specifically designed for disposal of needles and anything capable of piercing the skin; also called a biohazard container

shearing forces forces caused by rapid deceleration, usually occurs when one part of an organ is fixed in place and the adjacent part is mobile

shingles (zoster) disease caused by re-activated varicella zoster virus in patients who have had chickenpox, manifested by a vesicular rash that follows a dermatome distribution

shock a complex clinical entity in which there is inadequate oxygen and nutrient delivery to tissues leading to a cascade of events that, if left untreated, ultimately results in death

shock lung acute respiratory distress syndrome (ARDS) leading to hypoxia

shock position a position where the patient is placed supine or laterally recumbent, with the legs 12 inches or more above the level of the heart if possible

sickle cell anemia an inherited disorder in which the red blood cells become malformed and sickle-shaped in conditions of hypoxemia; causes vascular blockage and tissue damage

side flash (splash) injury an injury that occurs when an object is struck by lightning and the dissipating current, flowing along the path of least resistance, "jumps" to a person or group of people nearby

sigh a modified form of inhalation, occurs when the patient takes an excessively large volume breath; it is used to re-open alveoli in the lower distal parts of the airway that may have not been used in a while due to shallow breathing

simple diffusion when molecules of water move freely through a semipermeable membrane

simple partial seizure seizure that occurs in the motor area of the frontal lobe or the sensory area of the parietal lobe and produces focal motor or focal sensory seizures

simple pneumothorax the partial or complete collapse of a lung due to the entry of air into in the pleural space without the building up of pressure inside the chest

simultaneous intermittent mandatory ventilation (SIMV) ventilator mode that combines spontaneous breathing with A/C mode

sinoatrial node (SAN or SA node) heart tissue that normally generates the impulse that sets the heart rate and functions as a primary pacemaker

sinus arrest or pause occurs when the sinus node fails to initiate an impulse at the expected time

sinus arrhythmia a rhythm that slows down slightly with inhalation and speeds up slightly with exhalation

sinus bradycardia a regular rhythm originating from the sinus node, occurs when the sinus node fires at a rate less than 60 beats/min

sinus node specialized structure in the heart that is the dominate pacemaker

sinus tachycardia identifies a regular rhythm originating from the sinus node, beating at a rate greater than 100

sinuses plural of sinus, which is hollow cavity found in many of the bones of the face and skull

60-cycle interference common artifact on ECG caused by proximity to other electrical devices

skeletal muscle major muscles associated with the musculoskeletal system; they are made up of striated, cylinder-shaped cells, and can be controlled by choice (voluntary)

skilled nursing facility (SNF) a facility with the services and equipment needed to provide for the needs of patients with chronic illnesses

skin the outer covering of the body; it is made up of three layers; the largest organ in the body, the main part of the integumentary system; it is the first layer of defense against infection and protection from the environment

smallpox highly contagious disease caused by the variola virus; has a presentation similar to chickenpox; may be used as a biological warfare agent

smooth muscle the type of muscle that is found in organs and is involuntary

sneeze a modified form of respiration that is involuntary and used to clear debris from the nasopharynx

sniffing position a position in which the patient juts the jaw and lifts the chin slightly in an attempt to align the airway into a better position for breathing

snoring sound made during sleep or unconsciousness by the motion of the tongue and soft palate as a result of partial airway obstruction

SOAPIER organizational framework of the patient care report: subjective information (chief complaint and patient history using SAMPLE mnemonic); objective information; analysis of assessment; protocol to be used; implementation of protocol; evaluation of treatment and revised care plan

soft palate the flap of skin lying just below the inferior and posterior portions of the nasal structures and just beyond the posterior border of the hard palate

solid visceral organs solid organs that are highly vascularized; primary concern with injuries to these organs (mainly the liver and spleen) is the potential to cause substantial or even fatal blood loss

solubility how readily or easily a drug is able to combine with substances such as water or oil and enter into solution

soma the cell body of a neuron; also refers to the whole of the human body in general

somatic branch the branch of the efferent division of the nervous system that is used to activate skeletal muscles

somatic nervous system a subdivision of the peripheral nervous system that controls voluntary movement of skeletal muscle

somatic pain (parietal pain) a sharp, well-defined pain that originates in the skin, bones, tendons, or blood vessels

somatoform disorders disorders in which patients consciously believe their physical symptoms are being caused by a medical problem; however no obvious physical cause can be found, may be psychological in origin

span of control the number of people one supervisor can effectively manage; usually between three and seven under the Incident Command System

species resistance the body's innate, nonspecific defensive measures

specific immunity in response to an antigen entering the body, the immune system attempts to recognize the antigen from its list of known "hostiles" and dispatches specific antibodies that mount a substance-specific line of defense

specificity of a test the ability of a test to "rule out" or dismiss a problem

spectrophotometry the technique used by a pulse oximeter where red and infrared lights are emitted from a device to measure the percentage of oxygenated blood

sphygmomanometer device used to measure blood pressure

spike term used to describe the process of inserting the upper chamber of IV tubing into an IV bag

spina bifida (SB) a neural tube birth defect involving incomplete development of the brain, spinal cord, and/or their protective coverings; caused by the failure of the fetus' spine to close properly during the first month of pregnancy, may be associated with neurologic abnormalities

spinal cord structure that carries messages back and forth between the brain and the rest of the body

spinal cord injury without radiographic abnormality (SCIWORA) injury to the spinal cord demonstrable by magnetic resonance imaging, but shows as normal on imaging of the bony structures

spinal cord ischemia when the blood supply to the spinal cord is disrupted

spinal nerves the nerves that originate from the spinal cord and communicate with other parts of the body

spinal shock (areflexia) the temporary loss of spinal reflex activity that occurs below a near-total or total spinal cord injury

spiral fracture a break in a bone that is caused by a rotational force or twisting motion

splash (side flash) injury lightning injury that occurs when an object is struck and the dissipating current, following the path of least resistance, "jumps" to a person or group of people nearby

splenius capitis a rotator muscle in the neck

spontaneous abortion (SAB) (miscarriage) pregnancy loss occurring before 20 weeks gestation; about 80% of miscarriages happen in the first trimester of pregnancy, < 12 weeks gestation; patients will most often present with abdominal cramping, lower backache and vaginal bleeding

spontaneous bacterial peritonitis infection of ascites fluid in the peritoneum

spontaneous pneumothorax a sudden collection of air or gas in the chest that causes the lung to collapse in the absence of a traumatic injury to the chest or lung

sprains the damage that occurs as joints are stretched and ligaments are damaged

ST segment on ECG, the segment between the end of the S wave and the beginning of the T wave

stable angina ischemic cardiac chest pain, usually brought on with exertional activity, relieved by rest and is similar to previous episodes of cardiac-related chest pain; can become unstable angina, which can lead to acute myocardial infarction

staging areas temporary locations where personnel and equipment are kept until they are needed on the scene of a mass casualty under the Incident Command System

stair chair carrying device often used for patients with chest pain, respiratory distress, medical emergencies, anaphylaxis, and wheelchair bound patients

standard of care the actions expected of like-trained competent individuals within a profession when confronted with a medical or traumatic problem

Star of Life symbol that identifies EMS vehicles and personnel

Starling's Law of the Heart the force of contraction generated by a cardiac muscle fiber is directly related to its resting length

START (simple triage and rapid treatment) triage a triage method that evaluates respiratory rate, pulse, and mental status

startle reflex primitive reflex that occurs when a newborn grasps anything placed into the palm of its hands; also having the appearance of being startled when the sense of falling is involved or a sudden loud noise is heard; also called the Moro reflex

static ambulance deployment ambulances are based at fixed locations such as hospitals, fire stations, or other type of quarters; they are then dispatched to assignments that they are closest to

station position of fetus in relation to the ischial spine during the first stage of labor; the ischial spines are considered 0 station; if the top of the baby's head is above the spine it is noted in minus numbers (–2 means the baby is about 2 cm above the spine); when the top of the baby's head has moved past the spine, the station is then called "plus"

status epilepticus a continuous seizure that lasts longer than five minutes or two or more seizures that occur with no intervening period of consciousness

stem cells undifferentiated cells in the bone marrow that are capable of creating lymphocytes and many other types of cells

stenosis narrowing

step voltage (stride voltage) injuries received when the lightning current propagates outward from a ground strike under the earth

stereotype an incomplete or oversimplified attempt to draw conclusions about groups of people with a particular defining characteristic

sterilization the process by which the environment or equipment is made free of all forms of life, including bacterial spores, which are very difficult to kill

sternal angle of Louis (sternal angle) the junction between the manubrium and the body of the sternum

sternal notch hollow of the neck at the top of the sternum where the neck joins the rest of the body

sternocleidomastoid the muscle in the neck that helps to turn the head from side to side

sternum located in the middle of the front of the chest; the breastbone; it is a point of attachment of the ribs on the anterior chest

stoma openings; surgical opening

stomach the organ that continues digestion started by saliva by secreting hydrochloric acid which further breaks down the food

strains injury to the tendons of muscles

strategic documentation deliberate strategies employed to maximize the information contained within the patient care report

stratum corneum the dead, flattened, and hardened (keratinized) cells of the epidermis

stress (march) fracture break in a bone caused by repetitive, long-term, or abnormal stress, usually occurs in the foot, common in athletes and soldiers

stress response the physiological reaction to a stressor

stressor the circumstance that causes stress

striated striped

stride voltage (step voltage) injuries received when lightning current propagates outward from a ground strike under the earth

stridor a high-pitched whistling sound or harsh raspy sound that results from air passing through an abnormally narrowed portion of the upper respiratory tract during inspiration; often caused by the presence of a foreign body in the glottic opening, it can be heard without a stethoscope during inspiration

stroke a disruption in the blood supply to the brain that can be caused by either a hemorrhage or a clot (from embolus or thrombus) of one or more of the cerebral arteries resulting in neurologic impairment in the area of the brain affected

stroke volume (SV) the amount of blood pumped with each contraction of the left ventricle

subacute thyroiditis an inflammatory disease of the thyroid that causes increased release of thyroid hormones; accounts for approximately 20% of the cases of hyperthyroidism

subarachnoid hemorrhage (SAH) hemorrhage between the arachnoid membrane and the pia mater covering the brain

subarachnoid space the space between the arachnoid membrane and the pia mater that contains the cerebrospinal fluid

subclavian artery supplies the upper limb and thoracic structures

subcutaneous (SC) refers to the location under the skin and above the muscle; a common site for injection of medication

subcutaneous emphysema air under the skin from an underlying injury to the trachea, lung, or larynx

subdural hemorrhage bleeding into the space between the outer (dura mater) and inner covering (arachnoid mater) of the brain

subjective assessment the patient's report of symptoms

subjective findings findings that the patient (or someone else) tells you

subjective information information provided by patients or family members that they state or express, such as the chief complaint(s) and information regarding past medical history, medication history, allergies, etc

subluxation partial or incomplete dislocation of a joint; can result in damage and instability of the joint

submersion incident the adverse affects from being submerged in water; may or may not result in a fatal outcome

substance abuse a chronic pattern of chemical use that leads to clinically and socially significant impairment or distress

sucking chest wound a chest wound in which air can enter or exit; manifested by audible gurgling of air or visible bubbling of air through the wound; an open pneumothorax

sudden cardiac death (SCD) sudden cessation of cardiac function, whether or not resuscitation or spontaneous reversion of the dysrhythmia occurs

sudden infant death syndrome (SIDS) the sudden, unexplained death of children under the age of one year; also known as crib death

sudoriferous glands glands in the skin that secrete sweat

sulfur mustard a vesicant (blister agent) that poses both an inhalation and liquid contact hazard causing injury to the eyes, skin, airways, and some internal organs, chemical weapon that may be used as a weapon of mass destruction

superficial anatomic term meaning toward the surface

superficial burn first-degree burn involving only the outer layer of skin, manifested by erythema

superficial frostbite the degree of frostbite in which the dermis and portions of the subcutaneous tissues are damaged

superficial partial thickness burn second-degree burn that includes the upper portion of the dermis and the epidermis, it may present with blisters

superior anatomic term meaning toward the top

superior concha a shelf of bone within the nares

superior vena cava a large but short vein that carries deoxygenated blood from the upper half of the body to the heart's right atrium

supination body position or movement resulting in the body or palms of the hand facing upward

supine term meaning lying horizontal with the face upward

support zone (cold zone) area in a hazmat incident that is safe and isolated from contamination

suprapubic region (hypogastric region) the section of the abdomen just below the periumbilical region and just superior to the symphysis pubis

suprasternal notch the landmark or depression noted just above the top of the sternum

surface water water in the form of pools, ponds, lakes, quarry pits, or any other form of water that is not rapidly moving

surfactant a chemical that is slippery and soapy and it breaks up the surface tension inside of the alveoli, which allows them to remain open

surgical cricothyrotomy surgical incision through the skin and cricothyroid membrane for relief of upper airway obstruction

sustained ventricular tachycardia ventricular tachycardia that goes on for a long period of time

sutures stitches

swift water water in the form of rivers, streams, flood control systems, low head dams, and even flooded streets, water that is flowing

swimmer's ear otitis externa caused by maceration of the external tissue of the ear canal and changes in its surface pH through frequent exposure to water

sympathetic eye movement the movement that occurs when one eye moves and the other follows

sympathetic nervous system (SNS) a subdivision of the autonomic nervous system that prepares the body for stressful situations (fight or flight)

sympathomimetic effects drugs that mimic epinephrine-like effects on the sympathetic nervous system

sympathy feeling sad or sorry for someone

synapse the small space between the presynaptic membrane of a neuron and the postsynaptic membrane of another neuron or effector cell, such as muscles or glands

synaptic gap the small space between the presynaptic membrane of a neuron and the postsynaptic membrane of another neuron or effector cell, such as muscles or glands

syncope a temporary loss of consciousness and postural tone usually due to a brief, sudden drop in cerebral perfusion

synergistic effect an effect that occurs when the final effect seen with the administration of two drugs is greater than the sum of the effects of the administration of each drug individually

synovial joints joints that are fluid-filled to lubricate the articulations

syphilis sexually transmitted disease caused by the bacterium *Treponema pallidum*

system status management (SSM) unit deployment system that relies on historical data to deploy ambulances based on anticipated need

systemic a reaction affecting more than one organ; pertaining to the whole body

systemic inflammatory response syndrome (SIRS) early stage of septic shock; characterized by release of proteins into the blood by white blood cells; changes in the metabolic, cardiovascular, gastrointestinal, and coagulation systems that follow a deep burn; results in the release of inflammatory mediators like cytokines, arachidonic acid metabolites, free radicals, etc

systemic vascular resistance (SVR) pressure within the vasculature that the ventricle must overcome to eject blood into the arteries; also called afterload

systole contraction of the ventricles of the heart

systolic blood pressure (SBP) pressure reading determined when the heart is at the peak of its contraction pressure wave

T

T cells lymphocytes that reach maturity in the thymus gland

T helper cells cells that secrete substances called lymphokines that cause other white blood cells to migrate to the area

T killer cells cells that help kill pathogens

T lymphocytes a type of white blood cell that helps bridge the transition from the inflammatory phase to the proliferative phase of healing

T suppressor cells help to stop the immune response after the pathogen has been cleared

tachycardia a rapid heart rate; a heart rate greater than 100 beats per minute in an adult

tachypnea an increased respiratory rate; breathing rate greater than 20 respirations per minute in an adult; its presence can signify anxiety, pain, shock, or metabolic problems

tactical EMS a specialty team that provides medical support within the perimeter of high risk law enforcement operations

tactile fremitus a type of chest assessment whereby the patient's chest is palpated while phonating (speaking) and the provider feels for the transmission of sound through the vibrations

tapping (nightstick) fractures linear fracture resulting in two segments, often in the forearm after being stuck directly

tarsal foot bone

Taser a device that fires two metal probes with 4 mm barbs on their ends that are designed to attach to a subject's skin or clothing to deliver electrical pulses; considered a nonlethal method of subduing a patient, although some deaths associated with its use have been reported

tempered glass glass that is designed to shatter into many small beads of glass

temporal lobes part of the cerebrum; they lie at the sides of the brain, beneath the lateral or Sylvian fissure

temporary cavity the cavity that is created when the walls of a permanent cavity are temporarily pushed aside by the force as a bullet travels past them; can cause stretching and tearing of adjacent tissues thus increasing the amount of damage beyond the permanent cavity

temporomandibular joint (TMJ) hinges on both sides of the jaw just below the ear

tenderness pain upon palpation

tendons bands of connective tissue that bind muscles to bones

tension headache the most common type of headache, the pain can radiate from the neck, back, eyes, or other muscle groups in the body

tension pneumothorax (TP) condition when air is actively entering the pleural space and is not able to escape; if enough air is trapped, it begins to put pressure on the heart, great vessels, and opposite lung

teratogenic causing alteration in the development of a fetus or embryo, leading to birth defects

terminally ill a patient in an advanced stage of disease where the prognosis is grim or there is no known cure

terminus end

tertiary (or segmental) bronchi arise from the secondary bronchi; each of the tertiary bronchi serves a specific bronchpulmonary segment; there are 10 tertiary bronchi in the right lung, and 8 in the left

testes male reproductive organs that release sperm and also make and secrete testosterone, also referred to as testicles

testicular torsion occurs when the testicles become twisted around their attachment within the scrotum, the most common cause of testicular loss; if a proper diagnosis is made within 6 hours from onset, organ recovery is 80–100%

tetanus disease caused by the bacteria *Clostridium tetani;* spores enter the body through contaminated wounds and produce a toxin that releases into the bloodstream causing tetany; symptoms include trismus (spasm of the jaw muscles or lockjaw), tightening of neck muscles, and contraction of trunk muscles

tetany painful, prolonged contraction of the muscles; symptom of tetanus infection

tetralogy of Fallot a complex of abnormalities that includes a ventricular septal defect, pulmonary valve stenosis, overriding aorta and right ventricular hypertrophy; this congenital defect represents 10% of all congenital heart defects; symptoms include cyanosis (especially with exertion or crying), difficulty breathing that worsens with exertion or squatting, a low birth weight, and small for age growth

thalamus part of the brain that receives all incoming sensory messages

therapeutic abortion (TAB) the deliberate termination of a pregnancy before 24 weeks gestation

therapeutic error accidental delivery of an incorrect dose of medication or delivery via an incorrect route

therapeutic index (TI) a drug measurement that is determined by comparing the amount of drug needed to provide the desired effect to the toxicity and side effects

therapeutic massage a traditional healing therapy that uses healing touch to manipulate muscle and body parts to facilitate healing and relieve stress

therapeutic window difference between the dose of a medication that causes the desired effects and the dose that causes toxic effects

thermal burn burn caused by contact with flame or extremely hot surfaces on the exterior of the body

thermoregulatory effectors the body components that carry out heat loss or conservation primarily through skin blood flow (by vasoconstriction or vasodilation), sweating, and shivering

thermosensors temperature-sensitive neurons located in the skin, spinal cord, limb muscles, and the anterior hypothalamus

third degree AV block occurs with a complete blockage of the transmission of the electrical activity from the atria to the ventricles

third spacing the process that occurs as fluid leaves the blood stream and moves into extravascular tissues causing edema

third stage of labor final stage of labor, timed from the birth of the baby until the complete delivery of the placenta

third-degree burn burn that has penetrated through both layers of the skin (epidermis and dermis) and has extended into the subcutaneous layers; now called full-thickness burn

third-service EMS model an EMS service that is separate from police and fire (the first two public services) and may be operated by a private or public entity

thoracic aortic aneurysm aneurysm in the thoracic aorta; occurs in 6 per 100,000 patients; men are affected two to four times more commonly than women

thoracic spine the twelve vertebrae below the cervical spine; there is one vertebra for each pair of ribs in the thoracic cage

thoracostomy needle or surgical hole made in the chest in order to decompress a pneumothorax

thoracotomy a surgical incision to open the chest cavity

thorax the region of the body formed by the sternum, the thoracic vertebrae and the ribs. It extends from the neck to the diaphragm, not including the upper limbs

three Ps memory aid for the three "poly" symptoms and signs common to diabetic patients: polyuria, polyphagia, polydipsia.

threshold limit value/ceiling level (TLV/CL) maximum concentration of a toxin that should never be exceeded, not even for a moment

threshold limit value/short-term exposure limit (TLV/STEL) maximum concentration of toxin a person can be exposed to for 15 minutes without suffering adverse effects (not to be exceeded or repeated more than four times daily, with 60 minutes rests between each exposure)

thrill a humming vibration, described as a "cat purring" sensation, felt at the carotid artery; represents an area of turbulent blood flow, usually as a result of atherosclerosis

thrombi (plural of thrombus) blood clots

thrombin a coagulation protein that in the presence of calcium converts fibrinogen to stable fibrin, which then traps blood cells and more platelets to form a clot

thrombolysis the process of breaking up or dissolving blood clots, also refers to clot dissolving drugs

thrombosis formation of a clot

thrombotic stroke a stroke that occurs because of a thrombus (blood clot) that develops within a cerebral artery or one of the smaller branches

thrombus a blood clot

thymus gland located in the upper part of the chest that produces T lymphocytes, which are white blood cells that fight infections and destroy abnormal cells

thyroid cartilage (Adam's apple) a cartilaginous structure at the top of the trachea, visible on the neck as the Adam's apple

thyroid gland an endocrine organ that secretes thyroxine, triiodothyronine, and calcitonin, which affect metabolism, body heat, and bone growth

thyroid stimulating hormone (TSH) hormone that targets and regulates the endocrine function of the thyroid gland

thyroxine also known as T_4, it is a thyroid hormone that stimulates cell metabolism

tibia larger of the two bones in the lower leg, responsible for weight bearing

tidal volume (VT) the volume of air moved into and out of the lungs with each inhalation and exhalation of a respiratory cycle

tilt test obtaining vital signs of a patient in multiple positions for the purpose of determining if hypovolemia is present

time-weighted average (TWA) maximum concentration of a toxin a person can be exposed to eight hours/day, 40 hours/week without suffering adverse effects

tinnitus abnormal perception of sound when no external stimulus is present; often described as "ringing in the ears"

tissue plasminogen activator (t-PA) a fibrinolytic medication for used in acute ischemic stroke within 3 hours of the onset of symptoms in patients who meet a specific set of criteria or in cases of acute myocardial infarction in order to dissolve the obstructing blood clot causing the patient's symptoms

titrate to adjust the treatment regimen incrementally until the desired outcome is achieved; in fluid or medication therapy, "titrated to effect" means to give enough fluid or medication to achieve the desired effect, (i.e., reverseal of hypotension)

tonic-clonic (grand mal) seizure type of seizure characterized by several distinct phases including stiffening of muscles and violent shaking followed by a postictal phase

topical medication route that introduces drugs into the body through the skin

torque twisting force

torsade de pointes French for "twisting of the points"; malignant form of polymorphic ventricular tachycardia

torsion of the adnexa (fallopian tube, ovary) rotation of the ovary resulting in ischemia, often due to cyst formation; causes 3% of emergency surgeries in women

tort law the common area of civil law; torts can be either unintentional or intentional

torus (buckle) fracture a fracture characterized by a buckling of one side of the cortex, usually in the metaphyseal region, and most often result from compressive forces

total body surface area (TBSA) the amount of area involved in a burn

total body water (TBW) the total amount of water within the body; it is divided into two functional fluid compartments: the extracellular and intracellular (ICF) spaces

total lung capacity (TLC) the measurable volume of air in the lungs after a maximum inhalation has occurred

tourniquet a device used to stop blood loss by compressing the artery proximal to the bleeding wound

toxic epidermal necrolysis syndrome (TENS) an immune system reaction when the dermal layer of the skin reddens, necroses and sloughs off leaving the appearance of a scald and perhaps the formation of scars. The origin of the disease is unknown but it is believed to be caused by toxic or hypersensitivity reactions, particularly to certain drugs

toxic multinodular goiter (Plummer disease) occurs in 15–20% of patients with thyrotoxicosis; excess of thyroid hormone develops gradually over time

toxidromes poisons that produce a characteristic combination of symptoms

trachea the passageway that allows for the entry of air from the mouth and nose to the bronchi and lungs, made up of semicircular, ring-shaped cartilages that are like stiff plastic within the wall of the trachea to keep it open, the rings look like the letter C

tracheal sounds sounds that are heard over the trachea, primarily around the manubrium of the sternum

tracheal deviation movement of the trachea usually due to tension pneumothorax or a massive hemothorax; the trachea deviates away from the injured side toward the uninjured side

tracheal transection disruption of the integrity of the trachea, may be partial or complete; may occur secondary to trauma or during intubation

tracheobronchial injury a disruption of the tracheobronchial airways

tracheobronchitis infection or inflammation of the trachea and bronchi; a potentially very serious condition, most commonly occurring in children, produced by bacteria including staphylococcus

tracheostomy a surgical opening in the neck that extends into the trachea

tracheostomy tube a curved tube that is inserted into the surgical incision (stoma) in the trachea

traction (tension) fracture type of fracture that occurs where bone is pulled apart, resulting in a transverse fracture

traction headache (also referred to as inflammatory headache) a symptom of other disorders, ranging from stroke to sinus infection

trade name drug name selected by the manufacturer to use when it sells the drug; also known as brand name or proprietary name

trajectory the path a projectile follows

transection a right-angle, or lateral, shearing force; an injury that goes all the way through the involved organ, in effect severing it into two pieces

transfer of command process where an incident commander is replaced by another individual assuming command under the Incident Command System

transient ischemic attack (TIA) a syndrome that occurs when a patient exhibits the neurologic signs and symptoms of stroke; lasts less than 24 hours and resolves without any intervention

transition phase the end of the first stage of labor as the cervix approaches 8 cm dilation, contractions will last anywhere from 40–60 sec; the amount of discomfort will be peaking

translaryngeal jet insufflation a method for the emergency delivery of oxygen to a patient with an obstructed airway, involves an intravenous needle attached to a high flow oxygen source that is inserted across the cricothryoid membrane, removing the metal needle and leaving the plastic catheter inside of the tracheal lumen to administer high flow oxygen directly into the trachea

translation motion along a path from one place to another; also refers to the interpretation of a foreign language into English and vice versa

transverse fracture type of fracture that occurs in a bone at a right angle to its long part

transverse planes planes that section the body crosswise into top and bottom pieces and run at 90 degree angles to sagittal planes

transversus abdominus muscle of the abdominal wall

trapezius muscle that helps to turn the head from side to side

trauma a disease process that causes injury to the body as a result of the transfer of energy from one object to the patient's body tissues

trauma center designation the process by which the capability of hospitals to manage patients with traumatic injury is assessed and evaluated, based upon the hospital capability, a designation of the degree of preparedness is assigned: Level I: regional trauma center located in large urban area with 24/7capabilities to treat all types of injury; Level II: large community hospital equipped to handle most common injuries, refers complex cases to Level I facility; Level III: local community hospital equipped to stabilize and treat common injuries—has limited surgical and specialty capabilities, transfers complex injuries to Level II or I centers

traumatic asphyxia a rare entity caused by compression of the thorax forcing blood backward into the pulmonary system and into the veins of the neck and head

traumatic brain injury (TBI) a term that specifically refers to injury of the brain as opposed to that of the external structures of the head

traumatic injury injury that occurs when the body is exposed to more energy than its tissues and organs can tolerate

traumatic retinal detachment separation of the posterior elements of the globe resulting in immediate visual changes including possibly blindness. It may be treatable in the immediate aftermath with laser surgery or other techniques

tremors rhythmic oscillatory movements around a joint

trench foot (immersion foot) a nonfreezing injury from prolonged contact with cold water that results in the sloughing of water logged tissues

Trendelenburg position a position established for the operating room; patient lies supine with the head of the table angled downward at about a 45 degree angle and arms hanging loosely off the bed; EMS uses a modified version of this when they elevate the feet above the head to treat for shock

trending the evaluation of repetitive monitoring of vital signs to detect changes in patient condition

triage prioritization of patient care based on the severity of illness, prognosis, and availability of resources

tricuspid valve also known as the right atrioventricular valve, it has three leaflets, or cusps and is located on the right side of the heart, between the right atrium and the right ventricle

triiodothyronine also known as T_3, it is a thyroid hormone that stimulates cell metabolism

triple A (AAA) jargon for an abdominal aortic aneurysm

tripod position a position in which a patient with respiratory distress leans over and supports his or her weight on the hands and arms, juts the jaw, and lifts the chin slightly in an attempt to align the airway into a better position for breathing; this position allows the weight of the chest to be distributed off the diaphragm

trismus inability to open the mouth; symptom of tetanus and other infections

trisomy 21 (Down syndrome) a chromosome abnormality caused by an extra copy of the 21st chromosome manifested by developmental delay, short stature and characteristic facial appearance

trocar a rigid metal needle inserted inside a catheter to assist with insertion into the appropriate body site; for example, intraosseous needles have trocars inside the metal cannula to stiffen the device for insertion into the bone

true ribs defined as those ribs that connect directly to the sternum anteriorly through the costal cartilage; ribs 1 through 7

tuberculosis (TB) a disease caused by *Mycobacterium tuberculosis;* spread through droplet transmission; symptoms include a history of weight loss, fever, persistent cough, wheezing, potentially decreased breath sounds

tumor classically defined as swelling; commonly used to refer to a mass of tissue, either benign or malignant

tunica adventitia the outermost fibrous layer of a blood vessel; defines the maximum lumen size when the muscles relax

tunica intima the innermost layer of a blood vessel; it is smooth and allows the free flow of blood

tunica media the middle muscular level of a blood vessel; it controls the size of the lumen

tunnel vision to focus on one aspect of the patient's history and ignore important information

turbinates three shelf-like structures (inferior, middle and superior) inside the nose that cause turbulent flow of the air as it enters the nose; they precipitate particulate matter

T-Wave component of the ECG that represents the electrical repolarization of the ventricles

two-point discrimination a test used to determine sensation, it assesses the smallest distance between the two points that the patient can correctly detect in two out of three trials

tympanic membrane lateral wall of the tympanic cavity in the ear, also called the ear drum, responsible for transmitting sound waves to the auditory nerve of the ear

U

U wave the final stage of ventricular repolarization; not commonly seen; may be noted in patients with hypokalemia

ulcerative colitis an inflammatory condition of the large intestine

ulna inner bone of the forearm

umbilical cord the structure that connects the placenta to the fetus

uncal the most common type of herniation in the brain

unified command (UC) system a shared command structure that allows each agency to retain autonomy and also allows the agencies to work together to solve problems under the Incident Command System

unintentional tort a tort that the defendant did not mean to commit; it is simply a case where a bad outcome may occur due to the failure to exercise reasonable care

United States Pharmacopeia (USP) the official standards-setting authority for all prescription and over-the-counter medicines, dietary supplements, and other healthcare products manufactured and sold in the U.S.

unity of command under the Incident Command System, throughout the management of an incident, every individual has one supervisor at any given time

universal precautions set of procedures used by healthcare providers to prevent transmission of infectious disease

unstable angina (UA) ischemic cardiac chest pain that has changed from previous patterns, meaning angina that is either new, occurring at rest, changing from its previous state (pain lasts longer, is more severe, comes on with less exertion, new location, etc.), or is more frequent; also referred to as accelerated angina

upper respiratory infections (URI) infections that occur in the upper respiratory tract; caused predominantly by viruses, typically manifested by nasal congestion, rhinorrhea, low grade fever, cough and sometimes sputum production

uremia the clinical syndrome associated with elevated levels of urea in the blood as a result of chronic renal failure

ureterolithiasis the presence of a kidney stone in the ureter

urethra canal leading from the bladder through which urine is voided

urethritis inflammation of the urethra due either to trauma or infection

urinary outlet obstruction blockage of urine flow out of the kidney or bladder

urinary tract infection (UTI) an infection of the urinary tract

urology the study and treatment of diseases that affect the entire urinary tract from the kidneys to the genitalia, primarily focusing on surgical problems

urostomy surgical diversion procedure designed to collect waste products from the urinary bladder or urethra

uterine prolapse physical condition when the cervix and neck of the uterus is seen in the vaginal canal or extending beyond the vaginal opening; can be caused by over-stretching or damage to the ligaments, muscles and organs in the pelvis; patients report pelvic or vaginal pressure, heaviness in the lower abdomen, backache, and changes in urination or bowel habits; if it occurs during childbirth it is a life threatening condition

uterine rupture occurs when the scar from a previous uterine surgery, such as a cesarean section, opens up and the contents of the uterus, amniotic sac, and baby spill into the peritoneal space with extensive bleeding

uterus hollow muscular organ in female in which the fetus develops during pregnancy

V

V/Q defect one of many terms used to describe an abnormality between ventilation (V) and perfusion (Q)

vagina a structure connecting the cervix to the perineum

vagus nerve cranial nerve X, helps to control the heart rate

vallecula a small pouch located in front of the epiglottis

vascular compromise impairment of the flow of blood within a blood vessel either secondary to trauma or obstruction due to atherosclerosis or external compression of the blood vessel

vascular headache headache where blood vessel swelling or disturbance causes the pain, such as cluster headache, migraine headache or toxic headache

vascular permeability the degree to which the fluid within the blood stream stays there

vascular pooling process that results in the redistribution of the circulating blood volume into the venous side. The therapeutic benefit is to help decrease workload on the heart and lower blood pressure.

vascular resistance also called afterload, is the pressure that the heart must overcome as it pumps blood out into the arterial circulation

vascular shock failure of the vasomotor center to maintain vasomotor tone

vascular tone the relative degree to which the size of the vascular system is appropriate to maintain blood pressure within the normal range

vasoconstriction when arteries, arterioles, and some veins constrict in response to injury, sympathetic stimulation or medication administration

vasomotor tone the degree of vascular constriction

vasopressin a hormone from the pituitary gland that acts on the kidneys to increase water retention; also known as antidiuretic hormone

vas deferens the excretory duct of the testes

vectored moved

vectors the linear pathway a depolarization wave takes as it travels through the heart. A summation of all the vectors produces the characteristics waves and segments that make up the ECG

vehicle a substance added to a drug preparation to provide for or enhance delivery of the drug to the body tissues

velocity speed

venous return the amount of blood returning to the heart from the peripheral circulation of the body

venous thrombosis formation of a blood clot within a vein

ventilation (or hypercapnic) failure a type of respiratory failure that occurs as the result of increased carbon dioxide levels within the blood

ventilation rate the number of breaths given when performing bag-mask ventilation or when the patient is connected to a ventilator or other device delivering air into the patient

ventilation the mechanical process of air flowing into and out of the structures of the respiratory system; removal of carbon dioxide from the circulation to the lungs and out of the body

ventral anatomic term meaning toward the front of the body

ventricles a cavity, as in the brain or heart

ventricular activation time (VAT) the time it takes for an impulse to depolarize the septum, right ventricle, and most of the left ventricle; normally is less than 0.05 sec

ventricular assist devices (LVADs, RVADs and BiVADs) artificial devices that are implanted internally or externally in the heart, which take the functional place of the diseased ventricle and assist in the circulation of blood

ventricular dysrhythmias abnormal heart beats or rhythms that originate from a focus in the ventricles; the most significant of all dysrhythmias; they often degrade into life-threatening conditions leading to cardiopulmonary arrest

ventricular escape rhythm (idioventricular rhythm) the result of failure of the sinus and AV nodes; rhythm resulting from the third and final pacemaker site within the purkinje network doing its job; purkinje fibers have an inherent pacemaker rate of 20–40 beats/min; this rhythm can appear within about 1.5–2.0 sec after a higher impulse fails to arrive within the ventricles; this is often the final rhythm before ventricular standstill occurs, and is also a rhythm seen after successful defibrillation

ventricular fibrillation (VF) a disordered electrical activity resulting in unsynchronized depolarization within the

(continued)

ventricles and no circulation of blood; the leading cause of sudden cardiac death in the U.S.

ventricular septal defect (VSD) a defect in the septal wall between the ventricles; the size and location of the defect will dictate the significance of the clinical presentations; approximately 1% of all newborns have VSD

ventricular tachycardia an ectopic rhythm originating from one of the ventricles resulting in a heart rate of 100 to 250 beats per min or in a run of three or more beats during another rhythm

Venturi mask device that allows for a precise delivery of a specific FiO_2; often used for patient with chronic lung diseases like COPD or emphysema

veracity telling the truth and being honest

vertebra basic skeletal element of the spinal column that consists of a body, lamina, pedicle, transverse process, and spinous process

vertebral bones the bones that surround and protect the spinal cord

vertex position the head first, face down position of a baby that promotes drainage of secretions from the mouth and nose during birth when the mother is supine or sitting

vertical compression a force applied to either the top or bottom of the spine that is directed along the length of the spine

vertigo sudden disruption of balance; abnormal perception by individuals that either they or the surrounding environment is in motion

vesicants (blister agents) chemical agents that cause the appearance of a burn-like injury, include sulfur mustard and Lewisite; may be used as weapons of mass destruction

vesicles a rash characterized by small collections of fluid or pus

vesicular sounds sounds heard over the lung fields that represent movement of air in and out of the distal airways

vestibular labyrinth middle part of the inner ear

viral hemorrhagic fevers (Ebola, Marburg) a diverse group of illnesses caused by a variety of RNA viruses with a wide range of morbidity and mortality; may be used as a biological warfare agent

viral meningitis inflammation and infection of the meninges caused by a viral infection

virtue moral excellence and righteousness; goodness

virulence (pathogenicity) the ease with which an agent causes disease

viruses an organism comprised of genetic material wrapped in a protein coat; when a virus infects a cell, it uses that cell's reproductive mechanisms to create new copies of itself; viruses are unable to reproduce without the help of the host cell; a virus has only one function—to replicate itself

visceral abdominal pain a vague, aching, difficult-to-localize pain that originates in the organs of the abdomen and pelvis; caused by the stretching of pain fibers which are located in the walls of the affected hollow organs (such as intestines or the gallbladder) and the capsules of solid organs (such as the liver, spleen, and kidneys)

visceral pericardium the inner layer of the pericardium that covers the heart

visceral pertaining to the internal organs in the trunk of the body

visceral pleura thin serous membrane that covers each lung

vital capacity (VC) the measurement of complete expiration following the deepest inspiration

vital signs the measurements that assess the heart (rate, rhythm and character), respirations (rate, rhythm and character), and the blood pressure; as more devices and equipment come into the prehospital setting the vital signs are expanding to include skin assessment, pupil assessment, lung sounds, blood sugar, pulse oximetry and capnometry

vitamins essential in many chemical reactions and body functions

vitreous humor the gelatinous substance through which the images focused through the lens travel to the retina at the posterior aspect of the vitreous chamber

vocal cords the structures responsible for generating sound and speech, the dividing point between the upper and lower airway; usually appear as white bands seen on either side of the airway, when viewed through a laryngoscope

volume of dead space gas (VD) the total amount of gas contained in the physiologic and anatomic deadspace; the anatomic dead space in a normal respiratory system is approximately 150 ml; diseased lungs will have a greater dead space

voluntary muscle the type of muscle that can be controlled by choice

vortices the whirling pathway or flow pattern the air takes as it travels through the lungs

W

wandering atrial pacemaker (WAP) a sinus dysrhythmia that results from multiple different ectopic atrial or junctional beats occurring in fairly regular timing intervals replacing sinus generated beats

warm zone (contamination reduction zone) the area in a hazmat incident that surrounds the hot zone that serves as a safety buffer area between the public and the hazardous material and is the site for decontamination activities

washout phase the period during which accumulated toxins, gasses or medications are removed from the site of accumulation

weapons of mass destruction (WMD) weapons designed to kill large numbers of people; includes biological, nuclear (including radiological weapons), chemical, and explosive weapons

wedge fracture a fracture to the anterior aspect of the vertebral body

wellness a multidimensional state of being of positive health; it encompasses the physical, intellectual, and emotional dimensions of the individual as well as social, environmental, and spiritual dimensions

Wenckebach rhythm block resulting from a progressive delay in conduction through the AV node until an impulse is blocked entirely; also known as second degree AV block type I

Wernicke disease (Wernicke encephalopathy) neurologic disorder characterized by nystagmus (rapid side-to-side eye movements), abducens nerve abnormalities (the 7th cranial nerve is damaged and the eyes cross), conjugate gaze palsies (conjugate means moving together), ataxia (halting movements) of gait, and mental confusion

Wernicke-Korsakoff syndrome arises when Wernicke disease is combined with a learning or memory deficit

wheeze a high-pitched musical sound that is caused by high velocity air flow through a very narrowed or constricted

(continued)

airway, usually heard during expiration, most commonly heard in asthma

whiplash term used by the lay public to describe sprains and strains to the spinal cord

whispered pectoriloquy a type of chest assessment whereby the patient is asked to whisper a phrase over and over while the provider auscultates the chest looking for areas of consolidation

white blood cell leukocytes, the blood component that fights infection by attacking foreign organisms in the bloodstream.

white paper any formal document that provides a vision for change that has a national or international scope

whole bowel irrigation (WBI) oral administration of a polyethylene glycol bowel preparation; used to try to expedite the movement of poisons through the intestines before systemic absorption can occur

whooping cough (pertussis) disease caused by bacterium *Bordetella pertussis;* spread by respiratory droplets; causes bursts of coughing followed by distinctive "whoop" sound

Wolf-Parkinson-White syndrome characterized by a flaw in the development of the annular fibrous rings that make up the cardiac skeleton, leaving a short circuit present in the skeleton, manifested on ECG by a short (< 0.12 secs) P-R interval and a delta wave (slurring of the initial deflection of the QRS complex)

work of breathing (WOB) physical effort and energy used in respiration

X

xiphoid process the structure at the distal tip of the sternum

Y

yeast (candidiasis) most common infection of the female reproductive tract; other infections include all nonsexually transmitted diseases such as bacterial vaginosis, gardnerella and the sexually transmitted infections such as syphilis, gonorrhea, chlamydia, herpes, condyloma, human papilloma virus (HPV), molluscum contagiosum, and trichomonas vaginalis

Z

zone of coagulation the deepest part of the full-thickness burn

zone of safety the cold zone of a hazardous materials incident, or location where bystanders, patients and rescuers, may be safely staged

zone of stasis a combination of living and dead tissue in an area of burned tissue

zoster (shingles) (herpes zoster) disease caused by re-activated varicella zoster virus in patients who have had chickenpox; causes painful, itchy vesicles in the distribution of a dermatome

zygoma cheekbone

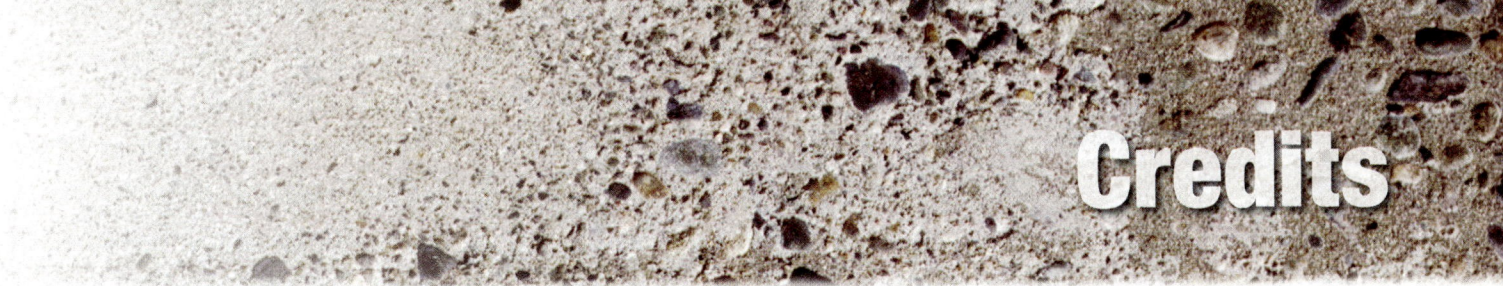

Credits

Chapter 1

Opener: Courtesy David Page; **1.1**: ©The McGraw-Hill Companies, Inc./Carin Marter, photographer; **1.2**: National Library of Medicine; **1.3**: National Library of Medicine; **1.4a–d**: Provided by David Rogers/Hennepin County Medical Center—Emergency Medical Services; **1.6**: Safar Center for Resuscitation Research University of Pittsburgh; **1.7**: Courtesy Federal Highway Administration; **1.8**: Courtesy Angel Clark Burba, MS, EMT-P.; **1.9**: The NENA logo is a registered trademark of the National Emergency Number Association and is used with permission; **1.10**: Courtesy Angel Clark Burba, MS, EMT-P.; **1.11**: NBC/Photofest; **1.12**: Courtesy David Page; **1.13**: ©McGraw-Hill: Aehlert: Emergency Medical Responder; **1.14, 1.15**: ©McGraw-Hill Higher Education, Inc./Rick Brady, photographer.

Chapter 2

Opener: ©McGraw-Hill Higher Education, Inc./Rick Brady, photographer; **Table 2.1**: National Center for Disease Control and Prevention; **Table 2.2**: From the Nebraska Rural Health and Safety Coalition. Funded by a grant from the W. K. Kellogg Foundation. Nebraska Rural Health and Safety Coalition, University of Nebraska.

Chapter 3

Opener: Courtesy David Page; **3.1**: Texas Department of State Health Services; **3.2, 3.3, 3.4**: ©McGraw-Hill Higher Education, Inc./Rick Brady, photographer; **Box 3.2**: Written by Charles Gillespies, M.D. Reprinted with permission from The National Association of Emergency Medical Technicians; **Box 3.3**: Written by Charles Gillespies, M.D. Reprinted with permission from The National Association of Emergency Medical Technicians.

Chapter 4

Opener: ©McGraw-Hill Higher Education, Inc./Rick Brady, photographer; **4.1**: Courtesy David Page; **4.2**: ©McGraw-Hill: Aehlert: Emergency Medical Responder; **4.3**: Courtesy David Page; **4.4**: ©McGraw-Hill Higher Education, Inc./Rick Brady, photographer; **4.5**: Courtesy David Page; **4.6**: ©McGraw-Hill: Aehlert: Emergency Medical Responder; **4.7**: 911 Pictures.

Chapter 5

Opener, **5.1** Courtesy Allina Hospitals & Clinics; **5.2, 5.3**: ©McGraw-Hill Higher Education, Inc./Rick Brady, photographer; **5.4, 5.5**: Courtesy David Page. **7.5, 7.6, 7.7, 7.8, 7.16** (right):

©McGraw-Hill: Companies, Inc./Timoty L Vacula, photographer; **7.25c**: © Phototake; **7.33a**: ©The McGraw-Hill companies, Inc.

Chapter 6

Opener: ©McGraw-Hill: Aehlert: Emergency Medical Responder

Chapter 7

7.1, 7.3: ©The McGraw-Hill Companies, Inc./Joe DeGrandis, photographer; **7-2**: Courtesy of Hennepin County Medical Center, Minneapolis, MN; **7.5, 7.6, 7.7, 7.8, 7.16** (right): ©The McGraw-Hill Companies, Inc./Timoty L Vacula, photographer; **7.25c**: © Phototake; **7.33a**: ©The McGraw-Hill companies, Inc.

Chapter 8

Opener: ©P. Motta/SPL/Photo Researchers, Inc.; **7.1, 7.3**: © The McGraw-Hill Companies, Inc./Joe DeGrandis, photographer; **7.5, 7.6, 7.7, 7.8, 7.16** (right): © The McGraw-Hill Companies, Inc./Timoty L Vacula, photographer; **7.25c**: © Phototake; **7.33a**: © The McGraw-Hill Companies, Inc.

Chapter 9

Opener: Courtesy Arthur Hsieh, NREMT-P.; **9.1** ©AP Wide World Photo; **9.2**: Courtesy David Page; **9.3**: ©McGraw-Hill Higher Education, Inc./Rick Brady, photographer; **9.4**: 911 Pictures; **9.5, 9.6, 9.7, 9.9, 9.10**: Courtesy David Page; **Box 9.2**: Reprinted from *Accident Analysis and Prevention*, vol. 35, L. R. Becker, E. Zaloshnja, N. Levick, L. Guohua, and T. R. Miller, "Relative Risk of Injury and Death in Ambulances and Other Emergency Vehicles," pages 941–948. Copyright © 2003, with permission of Elsevier.

Chapter 10

Opener: ©McGraw-Hill Higher Education, Inc./Rick Brady, photographer; **10.1a, b, 10.2a, b**: ©McGraw-Hill Higher Education, Inc./Rick Brady, photographer; **10.3**: Courtesy David Page; **10.4**: ©McGraw-Hill Higher Education, Inc./Rick Brady, photographer.

Chapter 11

Opener: Courtesy Arthur Hsieh, NREMT-P.; **11.1**: Courtesy David Page; **11.2**: Courtesy Arthur Hsieh, NREMT-P.; **11.3, 11.4, 11.6, 11.7**: ©McGraw-Hill Higher Education, Inc./Rick Brady, photographer; **11.8, 11.9**: Courtesy

David Page; **11.10**: ©McGraw-Hill: Aehlert: Emergency Medical Responder; **11.11, 11.12, 11.13a, b, 11.14a, b, c, 11.15a, b, c, d, 11.16, 11.17, 11.18a, b**: ©McGraw-Hill Higher Education, Inc./Rick Brady, photographer; **11.19**: ©McGraw-Hill: Aehlert: Emergency Medical Responder; **11.20, 11.21**: ©McGraw-Hill Higher Education, Inc./Rick Brady, photographer.

Chapter 12

Opener: ©Eddie Sperling; **12.3b, 12.4**: ©McGraw-Hill Higher Education, Inc./Rick Brady, photographer; **12.6**: ©CNRI/PhotoTake; **12.7**: Reprinted with permission of the American Academy of Otolaryngology—Head and Neck Surgery Foundation, copyright © 2006. All rights reserved; **12.8a, b**: ©McGraw-Hill Higher Education, Inc./Rick Brady, photographer; **12.14**: Courtesy David Page; **12.21**: EMSC Slide Set (CD-ROM). 1996. Courtesy of the Emergency Medical Services for Children Program, administered by the U.S. Department of Health and Human Service's Health Resources and Services Administration, Maternal and Child Health Bureau; **12.22d, 12.23, 12.24, 12.25, 12.27, 12.29a, b, 12.30, 12.31**: ©McGraw-Hill Higher Education, Inc./Rick Brady, photographer; **12.28a, b**: ©McGraw-Hill Higher Education, Inc./Rick Brady, photographer.

Chapter 13

Opener: ©McGraw-Hill Higher Education, Inc./Rick Brady, photographer; **13.3, 13.4**: EMSC Slide Set (CD-ROM). 1996. Courtesy of the Emergency Medical Services for Children Program, administered by the U.S. Department of Health and Human Service's Health Resources and Services Administration, Maternal and Child Health Bureau; **13.5, 13.6, 13.7**: ©McGraw-Hill Higher Education, Inc./Rick Brady, photographer.

Chapter 14

Opener: Courtesy David Page; **14.3**: ©McGraw-Hill Higher Education, Inc./Rick Brady, photographer; **14.4**: Courtesy David Page; **14.5, 14.6, 14.7, 14.8, 14.9**: ©McGraw-Hill Higher Education, Inc./Rick Brady, photographer; **14.11**: Courtesy David Page.

Chapter 15

Opener: Courtesy David Page; **15.1, 15.2**: ©McGraw-Hill Higher Education, Inc./Rick Brady, photographer; **Table 15.7**: Adapted from the American Heart Association Guidelines for Cardiopulmonary Resuscitation and Emergency Cardiovascular Care, *Circulation*, 2005.

Chapter 16

Opener: ©McGraw-Hill Higher Education, Inc./Rick Brady, photographer; **16.1, 16.2, 16.3:** Courtesy David Page; **16.4:** ©The McGraw-Hill Companies, Inc./Jill Braaten, photographer; **16.5:** Courtesy David Page; **16.6, 16.7:** © McGraw-Hill Higher Education, Inc./Rick Brady, photographer; **Table 16-1:** ©McGraw-Hill Higher Education, Inc./Rick Brady, photographer.

Chapter 17

Opener: Courtesy David Page; **17.1:** ©McGraw-Hill: Aehlert: Emergency Medical Responder; **17.2, 17.3:** Courtesy Will Chapleau; **17.4:** Courtesy David Page; **17.5:** ©McGraw-Hill Higher Education, Inc./Rick Brady, photographer; **17.6:** Courtesy David Page; **17.7:** ©McGraw-Hill Higher Education, Inc./Rick Brady, photographer; **17.8:** Courtesy David Page.

Chapter 18

Opener: Courtesy Col John P. Gritz, USA-Ret.; **18.1a, b:** Courtesy Col John P. Gritz, USA-Ret.; **18.2:** Courtesy of City of Tempe Fire Department, Tempe, Arizona; **18.3b, 18.4b, 18.5a, b, 18.6 (2):** Courtesy David Page; **18.7a:** Courtesy Col John P. Gritz, USA-Ret.; **18.7b:** Courtesy David Page; **18.9:** Courtesy Deputy Chief Michael Camilli, Chicago Heights Police Department; **18.10:** Courtesy Peter T. Pons, MD; **18.11:** Trauma.org Image; **18.12:** Courtesy University of Iowa Hospitals & Clinics; **18.13:** ©McGraw-Hill Higher Education, Inc./Rick Brady, photographer; **Table 18.3:** National Center for Disease Control and Prevention; **Tables 18.4, 18.6, 18.7:** Copyright © The McGraw-Hill Companies, Inc. All rights reserved.

Chapter 19

Opener: Courtesy Kevin Boone; **19.2b, 19.3:** ©McGraw-Hill Higher Education, Inc./ Rick Brady, photographer; **19.4a** both photos: Tactical Medical Solutions, Inc.; **19.4b:** American Forces Information Service/DVIC; **19.5, 19.6:** ©McGraw-Hill Higher Education, Inc./Rick Brady, photographer.

Chapter 20

Opener: ©Eddie Sperling; **20.3a, b:** ©McGraw-Hill Higher Education, Inc./Rick Brady, photographer; **20.4:** Courtesy Mark Lindquist; **20.5:** Copyright © 2006 McGraw-Hill Companies, Inc, Schwartz Principles of Surgery; **20.6:** Courtesy Peter T. Pons, MD.; **20.7a:** ©McGraw-Hill Higher Education, Inc./Rick Brady, photographer; **20.7b:** Courtesy David Page: **20.8** photo: ©The McGraw-Hill Companies, Inc./ Photo by Christine Eckel; **20.12:** Courtesy Mark Lindquist; **20.13:** ©Photo Researchers, Inc.

Chapter 21

Opener: ©Eddie Sperling; **21.1** photo: ©Victor Eichler, Ph.D.; **21.6, 21.7:** Courtesy Peter T. Pons, MD.; **21.9a, b, 21.10:** ©McGraw-Hill Higher Education, Inc./Rick Brady, photographer; **21.11:** Courtesy Arthur Hsieh, NREMT-P.

Chapter 22

Opener: Courtesy North Memorial Ambulance; **22.4:** Courtesy Peter T. Pons, MD.; **22.5, 22.6, 22.7:** Courtesy David Page; **Table 22.1:** Reprinted from "Emergency Medicine Secrets," 2nd edition, by V. Markovchik and P. Pons, page 426, Copyright 2000, with permission from Elsevier.

Chapter 23

Opener: ©McGraw-Hill Higher Education, Inc./Rick Brady, photographer; **23.11, 23.12, 23.13:** Courtesy John L. Kendall; **23.17a:** ©Yoav Levy/Phototake; **23.17b:** ©The McGraw-Hill Companies, Inc./Rick Brady, photographer; **23.18:** ©McGraw-Hill: Aehlert: Emergency Medical Responder; **23.19:** ©McGraw-Hill Higher Education, Inc./Rick Brady, photographer.

Chapter 24

Opener: Courtesy David Page; **24.4:** 1966 C. R. Wheeless/Wheeless' Textbook of Orthopaedics; **24.7:** Courtesy David Page; **24.8:** Courtesy David Page; **24.9:** Courtesy Peter T. Pons, MD.; **24.11:** Trauma.org Image; **24.12** both photos, **24.13:** ©The McGraw-Hill Companies, Inc./Rick Brady, photographer; **24.13** ©McGraw-Hill Higher Education, Inc./Rick Brady, photographer; **24.14, 24.15:** ©McGraw-Hill: Aehlert: Emergency Medical Responder; **24.16:** ©McGraw-Hill Higher Education, Inc./Rick Brady, photographer; **24.17, 24.18, 24.19:** ©McGraw-Hill: Aehlert: Emergency Medical Responder.

Chapter 25

Opener: Courtesy Stephen Kotch, MD.; **25.5:** Courtesy Mark Lindquist; **25.6:** Courtesy Peter T. Pons, MD.; **Box 25.2 photos a, c:** Trauma. org Image, **photos b, d:** Courtesy David Page, **photo e:** The McGraw-Hill Companies, Inc./ Carin Marter, photographer, **photo f:** Courtesy Stephen Kotch, MD., **photo g:** Courtesy Peter T. Pons, MD.; **25.7:** Courtesy David Page; **Box 25.3 a-d:** ©The McGraw-Hill Companies, Inc./Rick Brady, photographer.

Chapter 26

Opener: Courtesy David Page; **26.1a, b, c:** Courtesy Regions Hospital; **26.1d:** Courtesy David Page; **26.2:** EMSC Slide Set (CD-ROM). 1996. Courtesy of the Emergency Medical Services for Children Program, administered by the U.S. Department of Health and Human Service's Health Resources and Services Administration, Maternal and Child Health Bureau; **26.3:** The McGraw-Hill Companies, Inc./Electronic Publishing Services Inc.

Illustration Team/Kellie Marsh Holoski; **26.7:** ©McGraw-Hill: Aehlert: Emergency Medical Responder; **26.8:** EMSC Slide Set (CD-ROM). 1996. Courtesy of the Emergency Medical Services for Children Program, administered by the U.S. Department of Health and Human Service's Health Resources and Services Administration, Maternal and Child Health Bureau; **26.9, 26.10, 26.11:** Courtesy Lana Parsons; **Box 26.4 photo:** ©Royalty-Free/ CORBIS; **26.14:** Courtesy Mark Lindquist; **26.15:** EMSC Slide Set (CD-ROM). 1996. Courtesy of the Emergency Medical Services for Children Program, administered by the U.S. Department of Health and Human Service's Health Resources and Services Administration, Maternal and Child Health Bureau; **26.16:** ©AP Wide World; **26.17:** Trauma.org Image; **26.18:** Courtesy Lana Parsons; **26.19:** ©McGraw-Hill: Aehlert: Emergency Medical Responder; **Box 26.5 photo:** ©Getty Images; **Box 26.6:** Excerpted from Guidelines for the Operations of Burn Units (pp. 55–62), Resources for Optimal Care of the Injured Patient: 1999: Committee on Trauma, American College of Surgeons.

Chapter 27

Opener: ©McGraw-Hill Higher Education, Inc./Rick Brady, photographer; **27.1, 27.2:** ©McGraw-Hill Higher Education, Inc./Rick Brady, photographer; **27.3:** Courtesy David Page; **27.4:** ©AP Wide World; **p. 558:** ©Jeremy Hoare/Life File/Getty Images.

Chapter 28

Opener: ©McGraw-Hill Higher Education, Inc./Rick Brady, photographer; **28.5, 28.6:** ©McGraw-Hill Higher Education, Inc./Rick Brady, photographer; **28.11:** ©Photodisc Collection/Getty Images; **28.12:** Courtesy David Page; **28.13a, b, 28.14a, b:** ©McGraw-Hill Higher Education, Inc./Rick Brady, photographer.

Chapter 29, I

Opener Section I: Courtesy David Page; **29.2:** Science Museum/Science & Society Picture Library; **29.36:** ©McGraw-Hill Higher Education, Inc./Rick Brady, photographer; **29.39:** Courtesy David Page; **Box 29.7 photo:** Courtesy Angel Burba; **29.95:** Courtesy Medtronic, Inc; **29.96:** ©Jim Wehtje/Getty Images; **29.97:** ©Getty Images.

Chapter 29, II

Opener Section II: ©McGraw-Hill Higher Education, Inc./Rick Brady, photographer; **29.114:** American Heart Association Guidelines for Cardiopulmonary Resuscitation and Emergency Cardiovascular Care, *Circulation*, 2005; **29.117a, b, c:** Courtesy David Page; **29.118a, b:** ©McGraw-Hill Higher Education, Inc./Rick Brady, photographer; **29.119, 29.120, 29.121:** American Heart Association Guidelines for Cardiopulmonary Resuscitation and Emergency Cardiovascular Care, *Circulation*,

2005 **29.122a:** ©McGraw-Hill Higher Education, Inc./Rick Brady, photographer; **29.122b:** Courtesy David Page; **29.123:** ©McGraw-Hill Higher Education, Inc./Rick Brady, photographer; **29.124:** Courtesy David Page; **29.125:** Courtesy Jolife; **29.126:** Revivant Corp.; **29.127:** ©L. Bassett/Visuals Unlimited; **29.128:** ©McGraw-Hill Higher Education, Inc./ Rick Brady, photographer; **29.136:** Courtesy Peter T. Pons, MD.; **29.137:** ©Vital Images, Inc.; **29.139:** Harrison's Online, Chapter 232.

Chapter 30

Opener: Courtesy David Page; **Table 30.3:** Reprinted from the *Annals of Emergency Medicine*, **33(4)**, R. Kothari, A. Pancioli, T. Liu, and J. Broderick, Cincinnati Prehospital Stroke Scale, **pp.** 373-378. Copyright © 1999, with permission from The American College of Emergency Physicians. **Box 30.5 photo:** Courtesy Laura Horowitz; **30.14:** From J. Dankmeiger, H.G. Lambers & J.M.F. Landsmeer.

Chapter 31

Opener: ©McGraw-Hill Higher Education, Inc./ Rick Brady, photographer; **31.3:** Courtesy Will Chapleau; **31.4:** ©Imagingbody.com.; **31.5:** ©L.V. Bergman/The Bergman Collection; **31.6a, b:** From "Atlas of Pediatric Physical Diagnosis," 3/e, by Zitelli & Davis; **31.10:** Courtesy Will Chapleau.

Chapter 32

Opener: Courtesy David Page; **32.3, 32.5:** Courtesy Paul Satterlee, MD.

Chapter 33

Opener: ©The McGraw-Hill Companies, Inc./Christopher Kerrigan, photographer; **33.3:** Phototake; **33.4:** ©Photo Researchers, Inc.; **33.5:** CDC/Dr. K.L. Hermann; **33.6:** CDC; **33.7:** ©Photo Researchers, Inc.; **33.8:** CDC/Dr. Hermann; **33.9, 33.10:** ©Photo Researchers, Inc.; **33.11:** ©Dr. Ken Greer/Visuals Unlimited; **33.12:** National Geographic/Getty Images; **33.13:** Courtesy Bernard Cohen, MD, Dermatlas, http://www.dermatlas.org; **33.14:** ©Dr. Ken Greer/Visuals Unlimited; **33.15:** ©CDC/Corbis; **33.16:** ©Mediscan/Visuals Unlimited.

Chapter 34

Opener: Courtesy David Page; **34.4, 34.5, 34.7:** Courtesy Will Chapleau; **34.8:** ©Susan Leavines/Photo Researchers; **34.9:** Courtesy Peter T. Pons, MD.

Chapter 35

Opener: ©McGraw-Hill Higher Education, Inc./Rick Brady, photographer; **35.1, 35.2:** Courtesy Will Chapleau; **35.3:** Courtesy Fire Preventer; **35.4:** ©Patrick Johns/Corbis; **35.5:** Courtesy Jeffrey S. Guy, MD, FACS; **35.6:** ©Jason Cohn/Reuters/Corbis; **35.7:** ©Jacques M. Chenet/Corbis.

Chapter 36

Opener: Courtesy David Page; **36.6:** Hank Morgan/Photo Researchers, Inc.; **36.7:** Courtesy Peter T. Pons, MD.

Chapter 37

Opener: ©McGraw-Hill Higher Education, Inc./ Rick Brady, photographer; **37.1:** ©J&L Weber/ Peter Arnold, Inc.; **37.3:** ©Bill Longcore/photo Researchers, Inc.; **37.11:** ©Meckes/Ottawa/Photo Researchers, Inc.

Chapter 38

Opener: ©McGraw-Hill Higher Education, Inc./Rick Brady, photographer; **38.2:** London Ambulance Service; **38.3:** ©Getty Images; **38.4:** ©AP Wide World Photo; **38.5:** ©McGraw-Hill Higher Education, Inc./Rick Brady, photographer; **38.6:** ©Johan Copes Van Hasselt/Sygma/Corbis; **38.7:** ©Bart's Medical Library/Phototake; **38.8:** ©Getty Images; **38.9:** ©Patti Sapone/Star Ledger/ Corbis; **38.10:** ©Photo Researchers, Inc.; **38.11a:** ©Dr. Gary D. Gaugler/Phototake; **38.11b:** Courtesy CDC Public Health Image Library; **38.12:** ©Photo Researchers, Inc.; **38.13a:** ©E.R. DEGGINGER/ Animals Animals-Earth Scenes; **38.13b:** ©Scott Camazine/Phototake; **Table 38.1:** Reprinted from *Rosen's Emergency Medicine: Concepts and Clinical Practice*, 5e, by J. Marz, R. Kockberber, and R. Walls, "Accidental Hypothermis," page 1984, Copyright © 2002, with permission from Elsevier; **Box 38.5:** Reprinted from *Rosen's Emergency Medicine: Concepts and Clinical Practice*, 5e, by J. Marx, R. Hockberber, and R. Walls, "Heat Illness," page 2004, Copyright ©2002, with permission from Elsevier; **Box 38.14:** Reprinted from *Wilderness Medicine*, 4e, P. S. Auerbach, "Submersion Incidents," page 1341, Copyright ©2001, with permission from Elsevier; **Box 38.15:** CDC: Nonfatal and fatal drownings in recreational water settings—United States, 2001–2002. MMWR Morb Mortal Wkly Rep. June 4, 2004; 53(21): 447–452.

Chapter 39

Opener: Courtesy David Page; **39.2** both photos: © McGraw-Hill Higher Education, Inc./Rick Brady, photographer; **39.5:** Courtesy Will Chapleau; **39.7:** Courtesy David Page; **39.8a, b, 39.9a, b:** ©McGraw-Hill Higher Education, Inc./Rick Brady, photographer; **39.10:** Photo Researchers, Inc.

Chapter 40

Opener: ©McGraw-Hill Higher Education, Inc./ Rick Brady, photographer; **40.1:** Courtesy David Page; **40.2:** ©McGraw-Hill Higher Education, Inc./Rick Brady, photographer; **40.3, 40.4, 40.5:** Courtesy David Page; **40.6, 40.7:** ©McGraw-Hill Higher Education, Inc./Rick Brady, photographer.

Chapter 41

Opener: Courtesy David Page; **41.8:** ©McGraw-Hill Higher Education, Inc./Rick Brady, photographer; **41.10a-d:** ©Scott Camazine/Phototake; **41.11a-d:** Dr. Kurt Benirschke; **41.17:** Courtesy Kerry Dixon; **41.18:** ©AP Wide World.

Chapter 42

Opener: Courtesy David Page; **42.2(1):** Photonica/Getty Images; **42.2(2):** RF Corbis; **42.6:** Adapted from 2005 *American Heart Association Guidelines for CPR and ECC*; **42.8, 42.9, 42.10, 42.11, 42.12, 42.15:** ©McGraw-Hill Higher Education, Inc./Rick Brady, photographer; **42.16:** ©CNRI/Phototake; **42.17:** Courtesy David Page; **42.18:** ©Photo Researchers, Inc.; **42.19a, b, c:** ©McGraw-Hill Higher Education, Inc./Rick Brady, photographer.

Chapter 43

Opener: ©McGraw-Hill Higher Education, Inc./Rick Brady, photographer; **43.1, 43.2a, b, c:** Courtesy Laura Horowitz; **43.3, 43.4, 43.5:** ©McGraw-Hill Higher Education, Inc./Rick Brady, photographer; **43.6:** Courtesy David Page; **43.9, 43.10:** ©McGraw-Hill Higher Education, Inc./Rick Brady, photographer; **43.12b:** ©James Shaffer; **43.15, 43.16a, b, 43.17, 43.18, 43.19, 43.20, 43.21, 43.22a, b, c, 43.23, 43.24, 43.25:** ©McGraw-Hill Higher Education, Inc./Rick Brady, photographer; **43.26:** Reprinted with permission of the American Academy of Otolaryngology— Head and Neck Surgery Foundation, copyright ©2006. All rights reserved; **43.27:** ©McGraw-Hill: Aehlert: Emergency Medical Responder; **43.28:** EMSC Slide Set (CD-ROM). 1996. Courtesy of the Emergency Medical Services for Children Program, administered by the U.S. Department of Health and Human Service's Health Resources and Services Administration, Maternal and Child Health Bureau; **Box 43.5:** Copyright ©American College of Emergency Physicians and American Academy of Pediatrics; **Table 43.1:** Adapted from TRIPP Paramedic; **Table 43.2:** Health Survey for England 1998: Children's Reference Table, Normal Weight Ranges for Boys and Girls, Department of Health, 1998. Reproduced under the terms of the Click-Use License; **Table 43.6:** Medical Algorithms Project, www. medal.org.; **Box 43.6:** Reprinted with permission from ThinkSharp, Inc. All rights reserved.

Chapter 44

Opener: ©McGraw-Hill Higher Education, Inc./ Rick Brady, photographer; **44.1:** ©Digital Vision/ PunchStock; **44.2:** ©Royalty-Free/CORBIS; **44.3:** ©Photodisc; **44.4:** McGraw-Hill Higher Education, Inc./Digital Asset Library; **44.5:** ©McGraw-Hill: Aehlert: Emergency Medical Responder; **44.6:** ©Yoav Levy, Phototake; **44.7, 44.8, 44.9:** ©McGraw-Hill Higher Education, Inc./Rick Brady, photographer; **44.10:** ©Garry Watson/Photo Researchers, Inc.; **44.11, 44.12:** Courtesy David Page.

Chapter 45

Opener: ©McGraw-Hill Higher Education, Inc./Rick Brady, photographer; **45.1:** ©Getty Images; **45.2, 45.3:** EMSC slide set (CD-ROM).

1996. Courtesy of the Emergency Medical Services for Children Program, administered by the U.S. Department of Health and Human Services' Health Resources and Services Administration, Maternal and Child Health Bureau; **45.4:** ©McGraw-Hill Higher Education, Inc./Rick Brady, photographer; **45.6:** ©Eddie Sperling; **45.7:** Courtesy David Page.

Chapter 46

Opener: Courtesy Charles Kauffman; **46.2: Box 46.6:** Courtesy Laura Horowitz; **Box 46.7 photo:** Courtesy Charles Kauffman; **46.4:** ©Getty Images; **46.5:** ©Biophoto Associates/Photo Researchers, Inc.

Chapter 47

Opener: ©LEXINGTON HERALD/Corbis Sygma; **Box 47.1 photo:** ©Getty Images; **47.1a, b, c, 47.2:** Courtesy Will Chapleau; **47.4, 47.5a** (both photos): ©McGraw-Hill Higher Education, Inc./Rick Brady, photographer; **47.7:** ©McGraw-Hill Higher Education, Inc./Digital Asset Library; **47.8:** ©David M. Grossman/Phototake; **47.9:** Courtesy Will Chapleau.

Chapter 48

Opener: ©McGraw-Hill Higher Education, Inc./Rick Brady, photographer; **48.1:** ©McGraw-Hill Higher Education, Inc./Rick Brady, photographer; **48.4:** ©Mark De Fraeye/ Photo Researchers, Inc.; **48.5:** Dermatology of Pigmented Skin, www.ethnomed.org. Harborview Medical Center, University of Washington; **48.6:** ©McGraw-Hill Higher Education, Inc./Rick Brady, photographer; **Table 48.1:** U.S. Census Bureau, 1999; **Table 48.2:** The Annie E. Casey Foundation/ KIDS Count. http://www.aecf.org/kidscount/ sld/auxiliary/race-child.jsp; **Table 48.3:** U.S. Census Bureau, 2004.

Chapter 49

Opener: ©McGraw-Hill Higher Education, Inc./Rick Brady, photographer; **49.1a, b, c:** Courtesy David Page; **49.2a, b, c:** Courtesy Will Chapleau; **49.3a, b, c:** Courtesy David Page; **49.4, 49.5:** Courtesy Will Chapleau; **49.7:** ©McGraw-Hill Higher Education, Inc./Rick Brady, photographer.

Chapter 50

Opener: Courtesy David Page; **50.1:** ©Acadian Ambulance Service/Ray Bias, photographer; **50.2:** ©McGraw-Hill Higher Education, Inc./ Rick Brady, photographer; **50.3:** Courtesy of AirEvac Services, Phoenix, Arizona; **50.15:**

Developed by Deputy Chief Richard Freas, Howard County Department of Fire & Rescue; **50.16:** ©Getty Images; **50.18:** Reprinted with permission from the Critical Illnesses & Trauma Foundation; **50.19:** Courtesy David Page; **50.20:** Reprinted with permission from the Critical Illnesses & Trauma Foundation; **50.21:** JumpStart developed by Dr. Lou Romings, MD, Miami Children's Hospital, Miami, FL. www.jumpstarttriage.com/ TheJumpSTARTAlgorithm.html ©Lou Romig MD, 2002; **50.22:** Courtesy David Page; **50.23:** Howard County Department of Fire & Rescue; **50.24:** ©Acadian Ambulance Service/Dr. Chuck Burnell, photographer.

Chapter 51

Opener: Courtesy David Page; **51.1:** ©McGraw-Hill Higher Education, Inc./Rick Brady, photographer; **51.2:** Courtesy David Page; **Box 51.1 photo:** Rescue pack photo courtesy of www.conterra-inc.com; **51.3:** ©McGraw-Hill Higher Education, Inc./Rick Brady, photographer; **51.4:** Courtesy David Page; **51.5:** ©McGraw-Hill: Aehlert: Emergency Medical Responder; **51.6:** Courtesy David Page; **51.7:** ©McGraw-Hill Higher Education, Inc./Rick Brady, photographer; **51.8, 51.9:** Courtesy David Page; **51.10:** ©Salem Krieger/ZUMA/ Corbis; **51.11:** Courtesy David Long; **51.12:** ©David Woods/Corbis; **51.13, 51.14, 51.15:** ©McGraw-Hill Higher Education, Inc./Rick Brady, photographer; **51.16:** Courtesy David Page; **51.17:** US Army Corps of Engineers; **51.18a, b, 51.19:** ©McGraw-Hill Higher Education, Inc./Rick Brady, photographer; **51.20:** Courtesy of City of Mesa Fire Department, Mesa, Arizona.

Chapter 52

Opener: ©McGraw-Hill Higher Education, Inc./ Rick Brady, photographer; **52.1:** EMS Supervisors Representing: Allina Medical Transportation, Hennepin County Medical Center—Emergency Medical Services, North Memorial Ambulance Service; **52.2:** The McGraw-Hill Companies, Inc./Carin Marter/photographer; **52.3:** ©McGraw-Hill Higher Education, Inc./Rick Brady, photographer; **52.4:** Courtesy Mark Lindquist; **52.5:** ©AP Wide World; **52.6:** Courtesy David Page; **52.7:** ©Acadian Ambulance Service/ Ray Bias, photographer; **52.8:** Reprinted with permission from Minnesota Emergency Medical Services Regulatory Board (EMSRB).

Chapter 53

Opener: ©McGraw-Hill Higher Education, Inc./Rick Brady, photographer; **53.1:** ©McGraw-Hill: Aehlert: Emergency Medical Responder;

53.2: Agency for Toxic Substances and Disease Registry, "Managing Hazardous Material Incidents, Vol. I, Section 3." 2001. June 12, 2005, http://www.atsdr.cdc.gov/mhmi.html, page 48; **53.4:** Agency for Toxic Substances and Disease Registry, "Managing Hazardous Material Incidents, Vol. II, Appendix A." 2001. June 12, 2005, http://www.atsdr.cdc. gov/mhmi.html, page A10; **53.5:** Reprinted with permission from NFPA 704, System for the Identification of the Hazards of Materials for Emergency Response, Copyright © 2007, National Fire Protection Association, Quincy, MA 02269. This warning system is intended to be interpreted and applied only by properly trained individuals to identify fire, health, and reactivity hazards of chemicals. The user is referred to certain limited number of chemicals with recommended classifications in the Fire Protection Guide to Hazardous Materials, which would not be used as a guideline only. Whether the chemicals are classified by NFPA or not, anyone using the 704 system to classify chemicals does so at their own risk. **53.6:** U.S. Department of Transportation; **53.8:** Courtesy David Page; **Box 53.2 photo:** ©McGraw-Hill: Aehlert: Emergency Medical Responder; **53.9:** ©McGraw-Hill Higher Education, Inc./Rick Brady, photographer.

Chapter 54

Opener: London Ambulance Service Alistair Drummond Communcations Department; **54.1:** ©Acadian Ambulance Service/W. Keith Simon, photographer; **54.2:** ©AFP/Getty Images; **54.3:** ©McGraw-Hill: Aehlert: Emergency Medical Responder; **54.4, 54.5:** London Ambulance Service Alistair Drummond Communcations Department; **54.6:** Courtesy David Page.

Chapter 55

Opener: ©Neville Elder/CORBIS; **55.1:** ©Getty Images; **55.2:** ©TOKYO SHIMBUN/Corbis Sygma; **55.3:** ©Bettmann/Corbis; **55.4:** ©Getty Images; **55.5:** ©AP Wide World; **55.6:** ©Dr. Arshad Kahan, Dermatlas; **55.7:** ©Mary Evans/ Photo Researchers, Inc.; **55.8:** ©CDC/PHIL/ Corbis; **55.9:** ©Fayyaz Ahmed/epa/Corbis; **55.10:** ©Getty Images; **55.11:** ©AP Wide World; **55.12:** ©McGraw-Hill: Aehlert: Emergency Medical Responder.

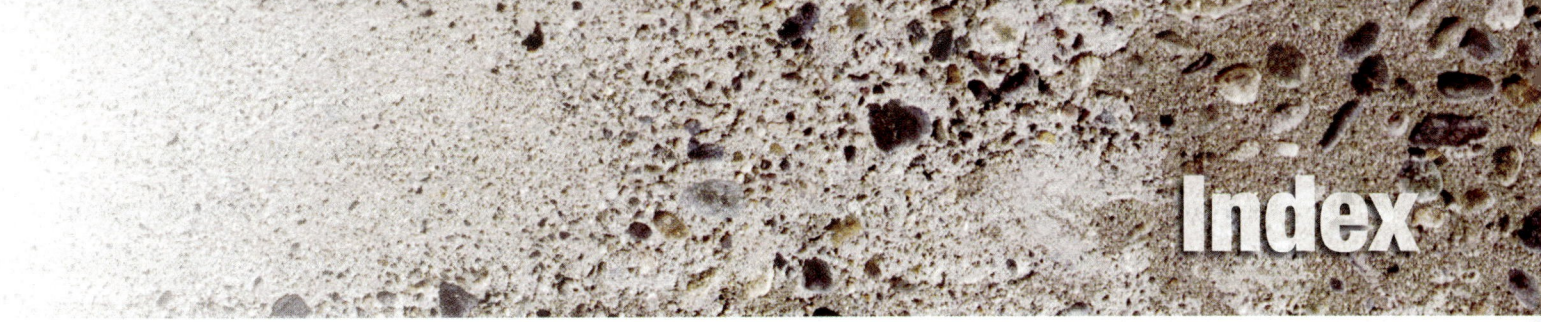

Note: Page numbers followed by f indicate figures; t, tables; and b, boxes.

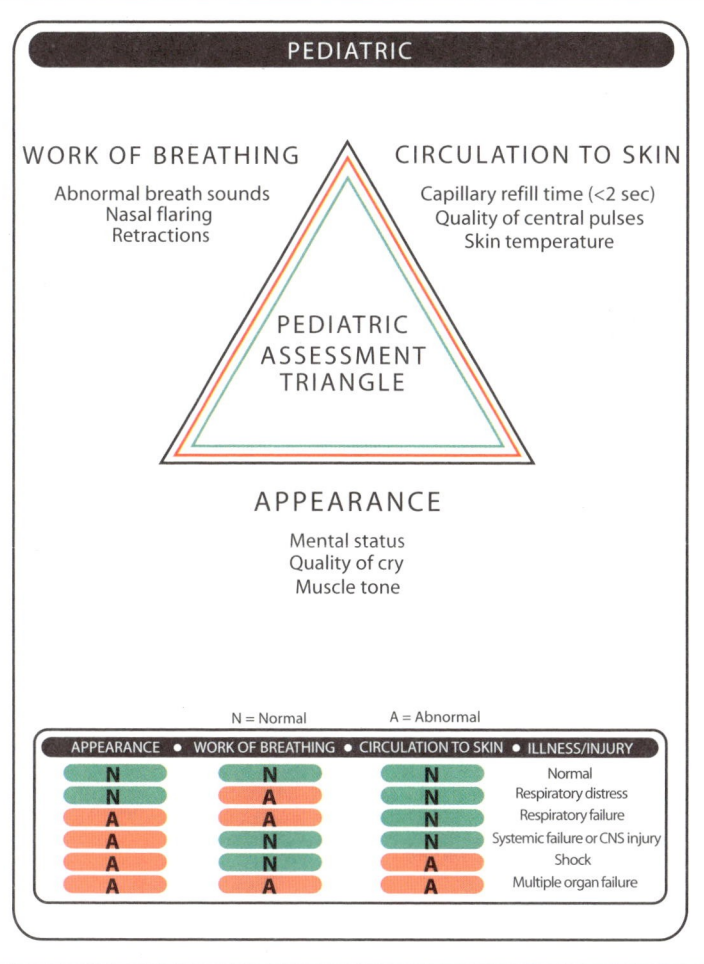

PEDIATRIC

WORK OF BREATHING
Abnormal breath sounds
Nasal flaring
Retractions

CIRCULATION TO SKIN
Capillary refill time (<2 sec)
Quality of central pulses
Skin temperature

PEDIATRIC ASSESSMENT TRIANGLE

APPEARANCE
Mental status
Quality of cry
Muscle tone

N = Normal   A = Abnormal

APPEARANCE	WORK OF BREATHING	CIRCULATION TO SKIN	ILLNESS/INJURY
N	N	N	Normal
N	A	N	Respiratory distress
A	A	N	Respiratory failure
A	N	N	Systemic failure or CNS injury
A	N	A	Shock
A	A	A	Multiple organ failure

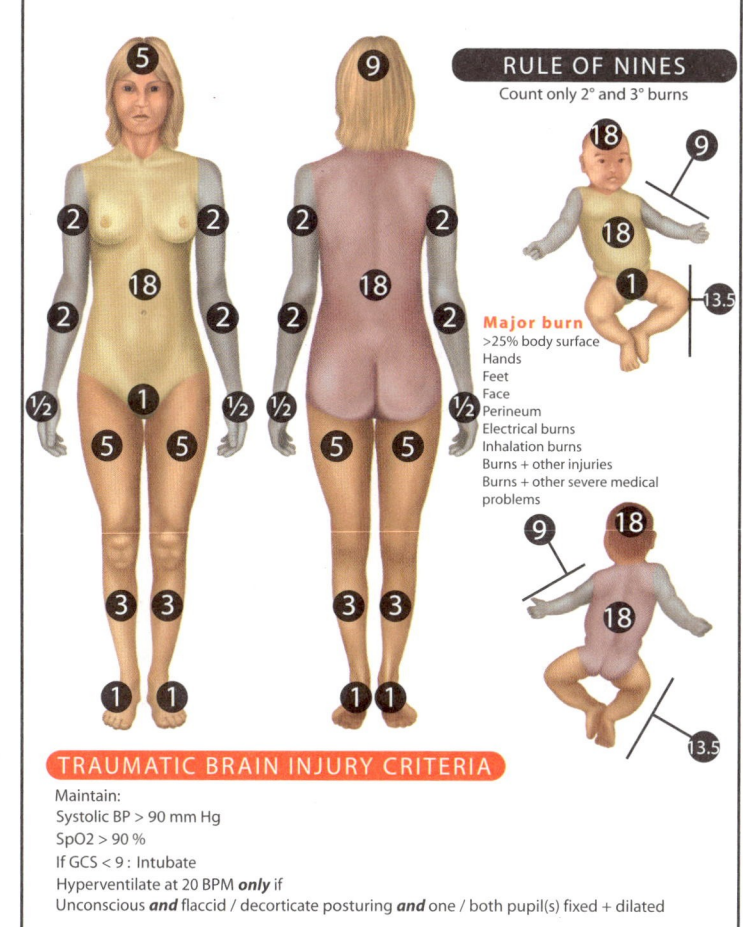

RULE OF NINES
Count only 2° and 3° burns

Major burn
>25% body surface
Hands
Feet
Face
Perineum
Electrical burns
Inhalation burns
Burns + other injuries
Burns + other severe medical problems

TRAUMATIC BRAIN INJURY CRITERIA
Maintain:
Systolic BP > 90 mm Hg
SpO2 > 90 %
If GCS < 9 : Intubate
Hyperventilate at 20 BPM *only* if
Unconscious **and** flaccid / decorticate posturing **and** one / both pupil(s) fixed + dilated

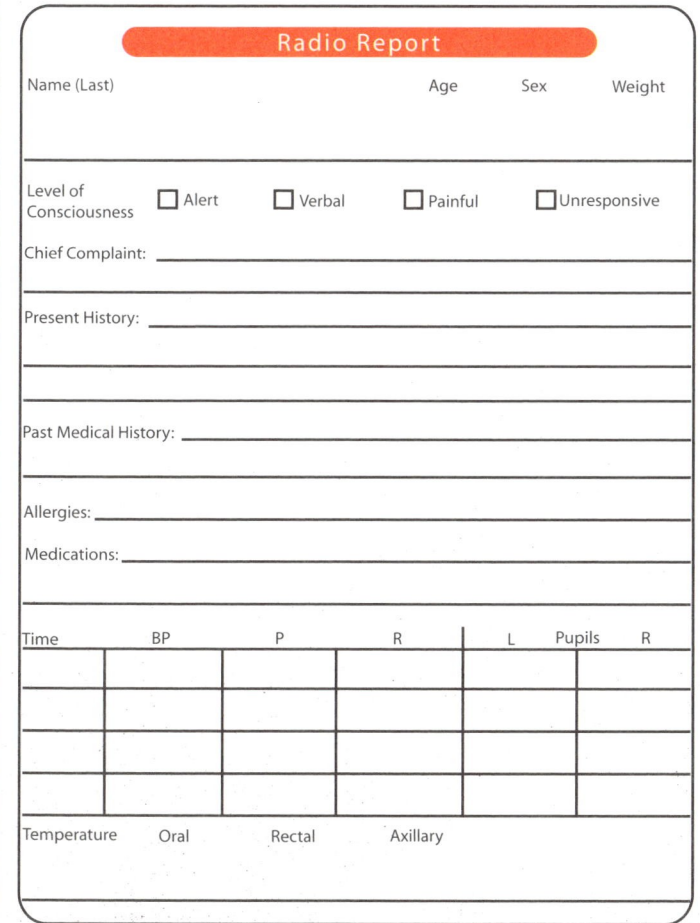

Radio Report

Name (Last)   Age   Sex   Weight

Level of Consciousness   ☐ Alert   ☐ Verbal   ☐ Painful   ☐ Unresponsive

Chief Complaint: _____

Present History: _____

Past Medical History: _____

Allergies: _____

Medications: _____

Time	BP	P	R	L	Pupils	R

Temperature   Oral   Rectal   Axillary

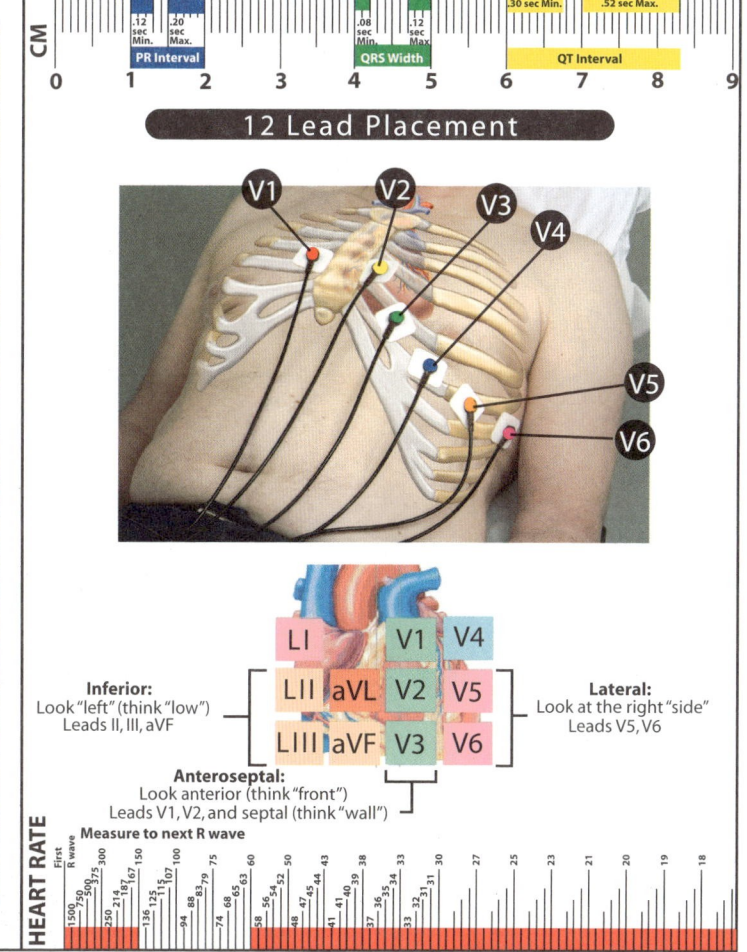

12 Lead Placement

Inferior:
Look "left" (think "low")
Leads II, III, aVF

Lateral:
Look at the right "side"
Leads V5, V6

Anteroseptal:
Look anterior (think "front")
Leads V1, V2, and septal (think "wall")

LI		V1	V4
LII	aVL	V2	V5
LIII	aVF	V3	V6

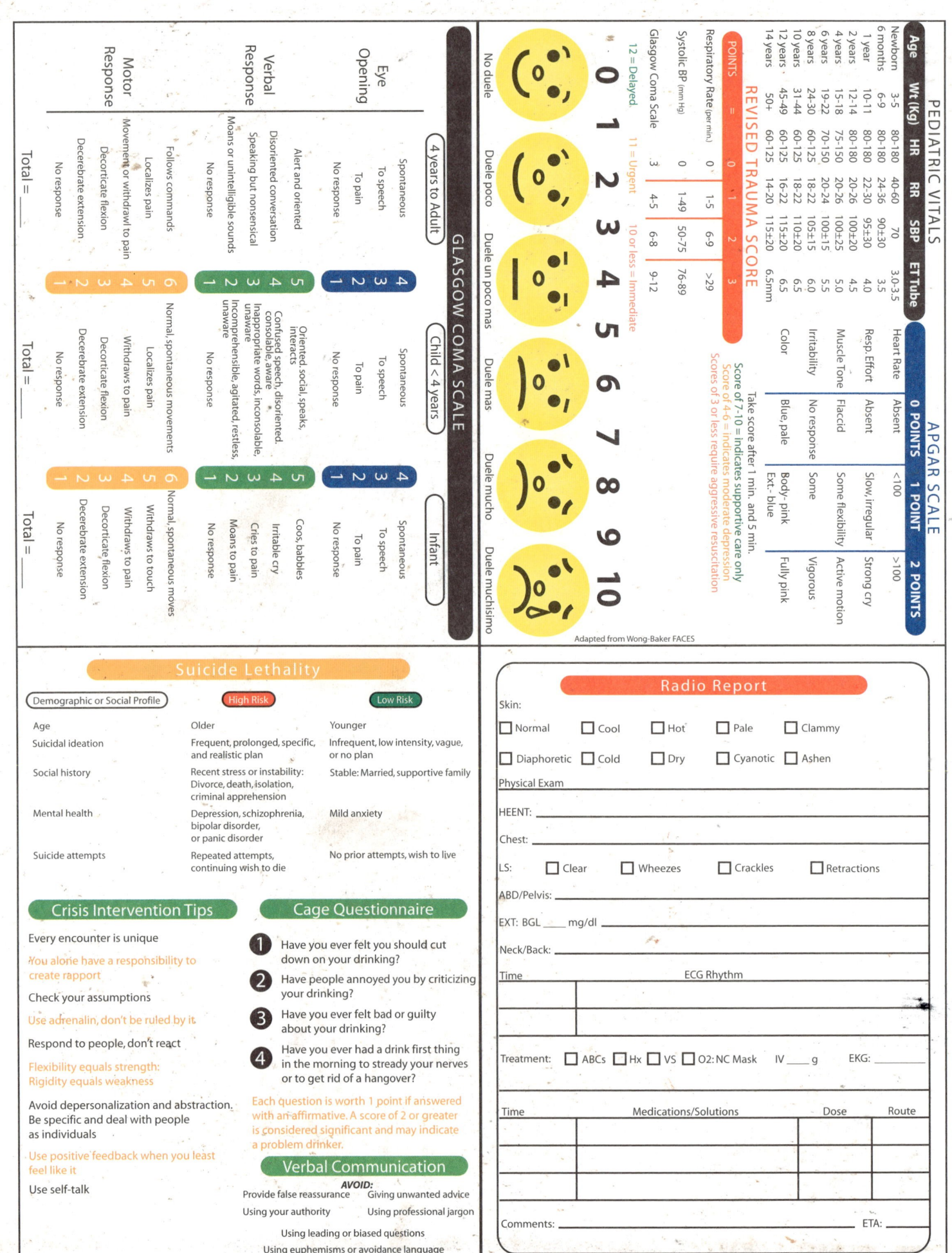

PEDIATRIC VITALS

Age	Wt (Kg)	HR	RR	SBP	ET Tube
Newborn	3-5	80-180	40-60	70	3.0-3.5
6 months	6-9	80-180	24-36	90±30	3.5
1 year	10-11	80-180	22-30	95±30	4.0
2 years	12-14	80-180	20-26	100±20	4.5
4 years	15-18	75-150	20-26	100±20	5.0
6 years	19-22	70-150	20-24	100±15	5.5
8 years	24-30	70-150	18-22	105±15	6.0
10 years	31-44	60-125	18-22	110±20	6.5
12 years	45-49	60-125	16-22	115±20	6.5
14 years	50+	60-125	14-20	115±20	6.5mm

REVISED TRAUMA SCORE

POINTS	Respiratory Rate (per min)	Systolic BP (mm Hg)	Glasgow Coma Scale
0	0	0	3
1	1-5	1-49	4-5
2	6-9	50-75	6-8
3	>29	76-89	9-12

12 = Delayed 11 = Urgent 10 or less = Immediate

APGAR SCALE

Take score after 1 min. and 5 min.

	0 POINTS	1 POINT	2 POINTS
Heart Rate	Absent	<100	>100
Resp. Effort	Absent	Slow, irregular	Strong cry
Muscle Tone	Flaccid	Some flexibility	Active motion
Irritability	No response	Some	Vigorous
Color	Blue, pale	Body-pink Ext.-blue	Fully pink

Score of 7-10 = indicates supportive care only
Score of 4-6 = indicates moderate depression
Scores of 3 or less require aggressive resuscitation

Wong-Baker FACES: 0 No duele 2 Duele poco 4 Duele un poco mas 6 Duele mas 8 Duele mucho 10 Duele muchisimo

0 1 2 3 4 5 6 7 8 9 10

Adapted from Wong-Baker FACES

GLASGOW COMA SCALE

	4 years to Adult	Child < 4 years	Infant
Eye Opening	4 Spontaneous / 3 To speech / 2 To pain / 1 No response	4 Spontaneous / 3 To speech / 2 To pain / 1 No response	4 Spontaneous / 3 To speech / 2 To pain / 1 No response

Verbal Response

4 years to Adult:
- 5 Alert and oriented
- 4 Disoriented conversation
- 3 Speaking but nonsensical
- 2 Moans or unintelligible sounds
- 1 No response

Child < 4 years:
- 5 Oriented, social, speaks, interacts
- 4 Confused speech, disoriented, consolable, aware
- 3 Inappropriate words, inconsolable, unaware
- 2 Incomprehensible, agitated, restless, unaware
- 1 No response

Infant:
- 5 Coos, babbles
- 4 Irritable cry
- 3 Cries to pain
- 2 Moans to pain
- 1 No response

Motor Response

4 years to Adult:
- 6 Follows commands
- 5 Localizes pain
- 4 Movement or withdrawl to pain
- 3 Decorticate flexion
- 2 Decerebrate extension
- 1 No response

Child < 4 years:
- 6 Normal, spontaneous movements
- 5 Localizes pain
- 4 Withdraws to pain
- 3 Decorticate flexion
- 2 Decerebrate extension
- 1 No response

Infant:
- 6 Normal, spontaneous moves
- 5 Withdraws to touch
- 4 Withdraws to pain
- 3 Decorticate flexion
- 2 Decerebrate extension
- 1 No response

Total = ____   Total = ____   Total = ____

Suicide Lethality

Demographic or Social Profile	High Risk	Low Risk
Age	Older	Younger
Suicidal ideation	Frequent, prolonged, specific, and realistic plan	Infrequent, low intensity, vague, or no plan
Social history	Recent stress or instability: Divorce, death, isolation, criminal apprehension	Stable: Married, supportive family
Mental health	Depression, schizophrenia, bipolar disorder, or panic disorder	Mild anxiety
Suicide attempts	Repeated attempts, continuing wish to die	No prior attempts, wish to live

Crisis Intervention Tips

Every encounter is unique

You alone have a responsibility to create rapport

Check your assumptions

Use adrenalin, don't be ruled by it

Respond to people, don't react

Flexibility equals strength: Rigidity equals weakness

Avoid depersonalization and abstraction. Be specific and deal with people as individuals

Use positive feedback when you least feel like it

Use self-talk

Cage Questionnaire

1. Have you ever felt you should cut down on your drinking?
2. Have people annoyed you by criticizing your drinking?
3. Have you ever felt bad or guilty about your drinking?
4. Have you ever had a drink first thing in the morning to stready your nerves or to get rid of a hangover?

Each question is worth 1 point if answered with an affirmative. A score of 2 or greater is considered significant and may indicate a problem drinker.

Verbal Communication

AVOID:
- Provide false reassurance
- Giving unwanted advice
- Using your authority
- Using professional jargon
- Using leading or biased questions
- Using euphemisms or avoidance language

Radio Report

Skin:
☐ Normal ☐ Cool ☐ Hot ☐ Pale ☐ Clammy
☐ Diaphoretic ☐ Cold ☐ Dry ☐ Cyanotic ☐ Ashen

Physical Exam

HEENT: _____

Chest: _____

LS: ☐ Clear ☐ Wheezes ☐ Crackles ☐ Retractions

ABD/Pelvis: _____

EXT: BGL ____ mg/dl _____

Neck/Back: _____

Time	ECG Rhythm

Treatment: ☐ ABCs ☐ Hx ☐ VS ☐ O2: NC Mask   IV ____ g   EKG: ____

Time	Medications/Solutions	Dose	Route

Comments: _____   ETA: ____